Physiologic and Pharmacologic Bases of Anesthesia

Physiologic and Pharmacologic Bases of Anesthesia

Vincent J. Collins, M.D., SC.D.

Professor Emeritus
Department of Anesthesiology
University of Illinois College
  of Medicine at Chicago
Chicago, Illinois
  and
Professor Emeritus
Department of Anesthesiology
Northwestern University Medical School
Chicago, Illinois

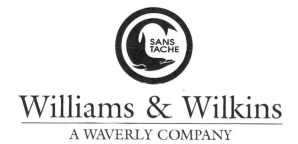

Williams & Wilkins

A WAVERLY COMPANY

BALTIMORE • PHILADELPHIA • LONDON • PARIS • BANGKOK
BUENOS AIRES • HONG KONG • MUNICH • SYDNEY • TOKYO • WROCLAW

1996

Editor: Carroll Cann
Managing Editor: Tanya Lazar
Production Coordinator: Pete Carley
Book Project Editor: Susan Sfarra
Designer: Tom Scheuerman
Typesetter: University Graphics, Inc.
Printer: Maple Press
Binder: Maple Press

Rose Tree Corporate Center
1400 North Providence Road
Building II, Suite 5025
Media, Pennsylvania 19063-2043 USA

Accurate indications, adverse reactions, and dosage schedules for drugs are provided in this book, but it is possible that they may change. The reader is urged to review the package information data of the manufacturers of the medications mentioned.

Printed in the United States of America

Library of Congress Cataloging in Publication Data

Physiologic and pharmacologic bases of anesthesia/edited by Vincent J. Collins.
     p.   cm.
    Includes index.
    ISBN 0-683-02011-0
    International ISBN 0-683-18022-3
    1. Anesthesiology.   I. Collins, Vincent J. (Vincent Joseph)
1914–
    [DNLM: 1. Anesthetics.   WO 200 P577 1995]
    RD81.P48   1995
    617.9'6—dc20
    DNLM/DLC
    for Library of Congress   95-14786
                               CIP

96 97 98 99
1 2 3 4 5 6 7 8 9 10

Reprints of chapters may be purchased from Williams & Wilkins in quantities of 100 or more. Call Isabella Wise in the Special Sales Department, (800) 358-3583.

This work is dedicated to my wise and patient wife, Florence, and to my loving and understanding children, Katherine, Patricia, Michael, Gregory, Peter, Delia, Mary-Claire, and Vincent Jr.

PREFACE

In preparing this text on the basic elements of physiology and pharmacology applicable to the practice of anesthesia, it was considered that the subject matter should be brought together in a separate volume. The chapter titles noted in the Contents represent the subjects chosen. To a large extent, this objective contrasts with our textbook, *Principles of Anesthesiology*, 3rd Edition, wherein emphasis is placed on fundamental procedural and technical aspects.

To do justice to the subjects, I have assembled a team of contributors from various clinical specialties, internal medicine, and from outstanding practicing anesthesiologists who have sub-specialty interests in different organ systems. Five contributors have assisted me in the selection process. They are as follows:

Dr. Mark Boswell, M.D., Ph.D., Assistant Professor of Anesthesiology at Case-Western University in Cleveland, Ohio, has been instrumental in having members of the Department of Anesthesiology at the University of Arizona Health Science Center author specific chapters: Dr. James DiNardo wrote Neurohumoral Control of Circulation; Blood Pressure Pulse and Blood Flow Physiology; The Pharmacology of Vasoactive Agents and Nitric Oxide. Dr. Stuart Hameroff of Arizona and Dr. Mark Boswell authored a "cutting edge" chapter on Mechanisms of Pleural Anesthesia. Mark also assumed the responsibility for the chapters on Volatile Anesthetics and on Inorganic Gas Anesthetics.

Dr. Ramez Salem, Professor of Anesthesiology, Rush-Presbyterian Medical Center and Chairman of Department of Anesthesiology at Illinois Masonic Hospital for providing unstinting assistance. Members of his staff have made many valuable contributions in both Physiology and Pharmacology: George Crystal, Ph.D., Associate Professor and Director of Research wrote an excellent chapter on Blood Transport of Oxygen and Carbon Dioxide, while Edward Czinn, M.D. contributed a comprehensive work on Abnormalities of Hemoglobin Synthesis and the Management of Bleeding Disorders. Harold Heyman, Chief of Obstetrical Anesthesia prepared a basic chapter on the Physiology of Pregnancy and drugs affecting uterine motility. Another Associate of Dr. Salem, Dr. Nimmagadda, has updated the pharmacology of anticholinergic agents for their role in anesthesia practice.

Members of the Medical and Anesthesia Faculty at *Northwestern University Medical School* have been prolific in contributing chapters. Dr. Rahim Behnia of the Department of Anesthesiology has been outstanding in his reports, first on Renal Physiology and then on Anesthesia for Genitourinary Surgery including renal transplantation. He also enlisted Dr. Tabatabai, of the University of Pittsburgh, for the splendid chapter on Neurochemical Regulation of Respiration.

Dr. Colin Shanks, Professor of Anesthesiology, has prepared a lucid chapter on the Principles of Pharmacokinetics and Pharmacodynamics. Dr. Hak K. Wong has completed a new chapter on the use of non-opioid analgesics in the perioperative period.

From the Department of Medicine at Northwestern, recognition is given to Gerald Soff, M.D., Professor of Medicine, for his contribution on Coagulation Mechanisms; while Dr. James Perkins and Dr. Jeffrey Vender of Evanston Hospital have prepared a practical and informative report on Transfusion Therapy.

Loyola University Medical Center Faculty have been prolific in their contributions. Dr. Brian Olshansky, Associate Professor of Medicine, has written a comprehensive chapter on Cardiac Physiology. In addition, he has collaborated with Dr. Bruce Kleinman in the Department of Anesthesiology for the preparation of the practical chapter on Perioperative Arrhythmias and their management. An outstanding contributor is Dr. Theodore C. Smith, Clinical Professor of Anesthesiology. He has been in the forefront of investigations on the pharmacological role of carbon dioxide. With Dr. Mark Chaney, he has prepared the basic chapter on Anesthetic Drug Effects on Respiratory Control.

Dr. Michael Roizen, Chairman of the Department of Anesthesia and Critical Care at the University of Chicago, has stimulated members of his staff to write several chapters. He, together with Jonathan Moss, M.D., Ph.D., developed the chapter on Immune Responses and Hypersensitivity Responses during Anesthesia. Dr. Roizen recommended Dr. Dennis Carlson to write the chapter on Hepatobiliary Disease. Besides a concise overview of hepatic physiology, there is an intensive review of the effects of anesthetic drugs on hepatic function. This is followed by medical and surgical management of portal hypertension and liver transplantation.

The subject of gastrointestinal physiology has been extensively presented by Dr. Paula Craigo. Aspiration of gastric contents and prevention and management, is clearly described. Included is the subject of postoperative nausea and vomiting, and an impressive review of antiemetic drugs.

In addition, Dr. J. Lance Lichtor of the University of Chicago has written a comprehensive review of the pharmacology and use of benzodiazepines.

Special mention is directed to Dr. Raghubar Badola for assisting me in writing the chapter on Selected Acute and Chronic Diseases—Anesthetic Implication. He is also to be credited for the outstanding presentation of carcinoid tumors and the carcinoid syndrome, in addition to a current review of neurofibromatosis.

To complete the team of major contributors is Dr. Kenneth Candido, a friend and colleague and former resident of Dr. Alon Winnie. As a resident, he completed an exhaustive report on shock. This has become the basis for two chapters: The Pathophysiology of Shock and the Management of Shock States. At present, Dr. Candido is in private practice with a staff appointment in anesthesia at Lenox Hill Hospital in New York City. He also conducts a Pain Management Service. Dr. Candido has been a prolific writer for me in completing other chapters. These include Antagonists to Opioids and Dysfunctional States of the Autonomic Nervous System.

Other contributors must be mentioned. Dr. Verna Baughman, Associate Professor of the Department of Anesthesiology at the University of Illinois Medical Center in Chicago, completed an updated chapter on tranquilizers and hallucinogens. Dr. Marc J. Shapiro, Professor of Surgery at St. Louis University School of Medicine in St. Louis, Missouri, completed for me a simplified and practical chapter on Acid Base Balance. Dr. Terry Yemen, Associate Professor of Anesthesiology at the University of Virginia Medical Center at Charlottesville, Virginia, prepared an excellent chapter on the normal physiology of the pediatric patient and the pharmacodynamic and pharmacokinetic patterns in pediatric subjects.

For chapters which I have written, I have been greatly helped by eminent experts, and wish to acknowledge and thank them for their suggestions and corrections. Dr. Barry Shapiro, Professor of Anesthesia at Northwestern University Medical Center and Director of Respiratory Care, was kind enough to review my chapter on Dynamic Aspects of Ventilation and found the information to be current and well documented.

The chapter on Temperature Regulation was reviewed by Dr. Daniel Sessler, University of California Medical School, San Francisco. He provided many suggestions and additions which I have included and appreciate.

Thanks are extended to David Visintine, Research Assistant at the University of Illinois College of Medicine Department of Anesthesiology for his excellent photography work and his preparation of glossy prints as illustrations for many of the chapters.

Invaluable secretarial assistance has been received from Karen Senger for organizing references and writing letters requesting permission.

Special thanks are due to the executive family of Williams & Wilkins. Carroll Cann, Executive Editor, is particularly noted for his overall suggestions and Tanya Lazar, Development Editor, implemented the suggestions. The artistic work of Grant Lashbrook in improving the illustrations and graphs is greatly appreciated. The patience of Peter Carley in production is extraordinary.

Finally, I take responsibility for my efforts in editing all chapters written by my contributors. I hope that not too many errors have been allowed, and, for any omissions, I apologize. I found the reading and editing of the chapters informative and edifying; and I wish to congratulate and thank all of the contributors for their splendid cooperation and excellent writing.

Vincent J. Collins
Chicago, Illinois

CONTRIBUTORS

RAGHUBAR P. BADOLA, M.D.
Assistant Professor of Anesthesiology
Albert Einstein College of Medicine
Montefiore Medical Center
Bronx, New York

VERNA L. BAUGHMAN, M.D.
Associate Professor of Anesthesiology
Department of Anesthesiology
University of Illinois at Chicago
Chicago, Illinois

MARK V. BOSWELL, Ph.D., M.D.
Assistant Professor
Case Western Reserve University and
  University Hospitals
Cleveland, Ohio

RAHIM BEHNIA, M.D., Ph.D.
Associate Professor of Clinical Anesthesia
Northwestern University Medical School
Chicago, Illinois

KENNETH D. CANDIDO, M.D.
Associate Attending
Department of Anesthesiology
Lenox Hill Hospital
New York, New York

MARK A. CHANEY, M.D.
Assistant Professor of Anesthesiology
Loyola University
Stritch School of Medicine
Maywood, Illinois

DENNIS W. COALSON, M.D.
Assistant Professor
Department of Anesthesia and Critical Care
University of Chicago Pritzker School of Medicine
Chicago, Illinois

VINCENT J. COLLINS, M.D., Sc.D.
Professor Emeritus
Department of Anesthesiology
University of Illinois College of Medicine at Chicago
Chicago, Illinois

PAULA A. CRAIGO, M.D.
Assistant Professor
Department of Anesthesiology and Critical Care
Medical Director, Post Anesthesia Care Unit
University of Chicago Pritzker School of Medicine
Chicago, Illinois

GEORGE J. CRYSTAL, Ph.D.
Associate Professor of Anesthesia, Physiology and
  Biophysics
Department of Anesthesiology
University of Illinois College of Medicine
Director of Research
Illinois Masonic Medical Center
Chicago, Illinois

EDWARD A. CZINN, M.D.
Clinical Assistant Professor of Anesthesiology
University of Illinois College of Medicine
Attending Anesthesiologist
Illinois Masonic Medical Center
Chicago, Illinois

JAMES A. DiNARDO, M.D.
Clinical Associate Professor of Anesthesiology
Director of Cardiothoracic Anesthesia
Department of Anesthesiology
University of Arizona Health Sciences Center
Tucson, Arizona

STUART R. HAMEROFF, M.D.
Associate Professor of Anesthesiology
Department of Anesthesiology
University of Arizona Health Sciences Center
Tucson, Arizona

HAROLD J. HEYMAN, M.D.
Associate Professor of Anesthesiology
Director of Obstetrical Anesthesia
Illinois Masonic Medical Center
Chicago, Illinois

DUNCAN A. HOLADAY, M.D.
Professor of Anesthesiology
University of Miami
Miami, Florida

WADE C. JONES, Jr., R.R.T.
Administrative Director
Respiratory Care Services
University of Illinois Hospital
Chicago, Illinois

BRUCE S. KLEINMAN, M.D.
Associate Professor of Anesthesiology
Department of Anesthesiology
Foster G. McGraw Medical Center
Loyola University of Chicago
Maywood, Illinois

JERROLD H. LEVY, M.D.
Associate Professor of Anesthesiology
Emory University College of Medicine
University Hospital
Atlanta, Georgia

J. LANCE LICHTOR, M.D.
Associate Professor
Department of Anesthesiology and Critical Care
University of Chicago Medical School
Chicago, Illinois

RICHARD L. McCAMMON, M.D.
Associate Professor of Anesthesiology
Department of Anesthesiology
Indiana University Medical Center
Indianapolis, Indiana

JONATHAN MOSS, M.D., Ph.D.
Professor of Anesthesiology
Department of Anesthesia and Critical Care
University of Chicago Pritzer School of Medicine
Chicago, Illinois

CRAIG NELSON, D.O.
Department of Anesthesiology
Foster G. McGaw Medical Center
Loyola University of Chicago
Maywood, Illinois

USHARANI NIMMAGADDA, M.D.
Attending Anesthesiologist
Illinois Masonic Medical Center
Chicago, Illinois

BRIAN OLSHANSKY, M.D.
Associate Professor of Medicine
Division of Cardiology
Foster G. McGaw Medical Center
Loyola University of Chicago
Maywood, Illinois

JAMES T. PERKINS, M.D.
Assistant Professor of Clinical Pathology
Northwestern University College of Medicine
Director of Blood Bank
Evanston Hospital
Evanston, Illinois

ERNESTO PRETTO, M.D., M.P.H.
Associate Professor
Department of Anesthesiology
 and Critical Care Medicine
School of Medicine
University of Pittsburgh
Pittsburgh, Pennsylvania

MICHAEL F. ROIZEN, M.D.
Professor and Chairman
Department of Anesthesia and Critical Care
University of Chicago Pritzker School of Medicine
Chicago, Illinois

M. RAMEZ SALEM, M.D.
Professor of Anesthesiology
Rush Medical College
Chairman, Department of Anesthesiology
Illinois Masonic Medical Center
Chicago, Illinois

COLIN A. SHANKS, M.D., Ch.B.
Professor of Anesthesiology
Northwestern University Medical School
Chicago, Illinois

MARC JEROME SHAPIRO, M.D.
Professor of Surgery
Department of Surgery
St. Louis University School of Medicine
St. Louis, Missouri

THEODORE C. SMITH, M.D.
Clinical Professor of Anesthesiology
Loyola University Medical Center
Stritch School of Medicine
Maywood, Illinois

GERALD A. SOFF, M.D.
Assistant Professor of Medicine
Division of Hematology
Northwestern University Medical School
Chicago, Illinois

MAHMOOD TABATABAI, M.D., Ph.D.
Associate Professor
Department of Anesthesiology
University of Pittsburgh School of Medicine
Presbyterian University Hospital
Pittsburgh, Pennsylvania

JEFFREY S. VENDER, M.D.
Associate Professor of Clinical Anesthesia
Northwestern University Medical School
Director, Medical-Surgical Intensive Care Unit
Evanston Hospital
Evanston, Illinois

HAK YUI WONG, M.D.
Clinical Associate Professor
Department of Anesthesiology
Northwestern University Medical School
Chicago, Illinois

TERRY YEMAN, M.D.
Associate Professor of Anesthesiology
Department of Anesthesiology
University of Virginia Medical Center
Charlottesville, Virginia

CONTENTS

Chapter 1

ANATOMICAL ASPECTS OF RESPIRATION

VINCENT J. COLLINS

Respiration is the exchange of gases between a living organism and its environment. Some organisms, such as insects, have such an efficient system of ramifying tracheal tubes that oxygen is brought directly to cells and the need for a circulatory system is eliminated. The frog on the other hand depends on a combination of systems; approximately 50% of its respiration occurs through the skin, whereas the other 50% occurs through a pulmonocirculatory system.[1]

Gas exchange in humans is affected entirely by a complex pulmonocirculatory system, whereby oxygen is supplied to all the body cells and carbon dioxide is eliminated from them.

RESPIRATION

Respiration in humans may be divided into external and internal respiration.

External respiration is the exchange of gases between the blood and the air in the surrounding environment. It involves four sequential processes:[2]

1. Ventilation: The mass displacement of air from outside to the alveoli and the even distribution of this air in the alveoli.
2. Mixing: Intrapulmonary distribution of gas molecules (alveolar).
3. Diffusion: The passage of gases across the alveolar-capillary membrane.
4. Alveolar perfusion–capillary circulation: The uptake of gases by an adequate pulmonary blood flow.

Internal respiration is the exchange of gases between the blood and tissues. It involves the following processes:

1. Cardiocirculatory efficiency in moving oxygenated blood;
2. Capillary distribution;
3. Diffusion, the passage of gases into interstitial spaces and thence across cellular membranes; and
4. Cellular metabolism involving the respiratory enzymes.

In this discussion, consideration is given to external respiration, the mechanics of which have both static and dynamic features. Fundamentally, ventilation varies with the metabolic rate of the individual and with the chemical reaction of the blood. These parameters set the activity level. A minimum amount of effort should be ex-

pended to accomplish the given goal, and the value of this effort determines the efficiency.

The four requisites for efficient ventilation are as follows:[3]

1. Normal structures
2. Coordinate muscular action
3. Gradient of gas pressures
4. Neuromuscular integration

ANATOMY

The pulmonary system consists essentially of two anatomic parts with two distinct functions:[4] (1) a system of conduits or connecting tubes, the nasal and oral passages, the pharynx, larynx, trachea, bronchi and bronchioles, and (2) a respiratory part, consisting of the respiratory bronchioles, the alveolar ducts, atrium, alveolar sacs, and alveoli.

Basically, the lung is the sum total of the branching of the embryologic tracheal bud into undifferentiated mesoderm. The trachea undergoes 18 divisions (Table 1–1). The primary buds form the main stem bronchi. Each of these in turn has three branches forming secondary bronchi. Finally, tertiary bronchi are formed by each secondary bronchus dividing into three branches that, together with the extension of the main stem, result in 10 independent bronchopulmonary segments (Fig. 1–1).[5]

These segmental bronchi are third-order branches and a companion division represents the fourth-order branch or subsegmental bronchus. The segmental bronchi further subdivide five times up to the tenth order; these branches unnamed are known only as small bronchi.

Further branches are known as bronchioles and represent six further divisions or branching order 11 through 18.

The mesoderm into which the stem bronchi extend develops into the respiratory portion of the lung. The ensemble of alveolar ducts, alveolar sacs, and alveoli with their accompanying vessels and nerves constitutes a primary lobule (Fig. 1–2).

The alveoli present a surface area of approximately 55 m^2 in the adult,[3] an amount some 25 times greater than the surface area of the skin. The alveoli have a dense ramification and network of capillaries that allow red cells to pass through almost single file. Practically 100% oxygen saturation occurs. Certain measurements of pulmonary anatomy are important to the anesthesiologist, such as distances from: lips to larynx, 12 cm; top of thyroid carti-

Table 1–1. Classification of Airways by Order of Branching and by Structural Characteristics (after Weibel and Nunn 1963)

Common Name	Generation (mean)	Number	Mean Diameter (mm)	Area Supplied	Cartilage	Muscle	Nutrition	Emplacement	Epithelium
Trachea	0	1	18	Both lungs	U-shaped	Links open end of cartilage			
Main bronchi	1	2	13	Individual lungs					
Lobar bronchi	2 → 3	4 → 8	7 → 5	Lobes	Irregular shaped and helical plates	Helical bands	From the bronchial circulation	Within connective tissue sheath alongside arterial vessels	Columnar ciliated
Segmental bronchi	4 → 5	16 → 32	4 → 3	Segments Secondary lobules					
Small bronchi	11	2,000	1			Strong helical muscle bands			Cuboidal
Bronchioles	12	4,000	1						
Terminal bronchioles	16 → 17	65,000 → 130,000	0.5			Muscle bands between alveoli		Embedded directly in the lung parenchyma	
Respiratory bronchioles	19	500,000	0.5	Primary lobules	Absent		From the pulmonary circulation		Cuboidal to flat between the alveoli
Alveolar ducts	20	1,000,000	0.3	Alveoli		Thin bands in alveolar septa		Forms the lung parenchyma	Alveolar epithelium
Alveolar sacs	22 → 23	4,000,000 → 8,000,000	0.3						

(After Weibel, E. R.: *Morphometry of the Human Lung.* Berlin, Springer, 1963.)

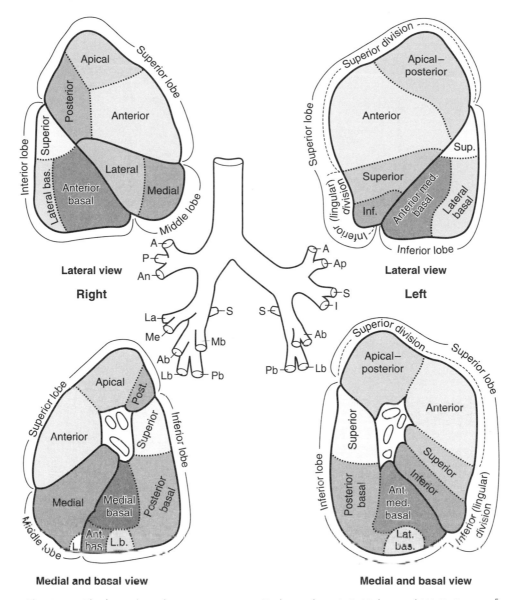

Fig. 1–1. The bronchopulmonary segments. Redrawn from J. F. Huber and W. B. Stewart.[5]

lage to bottom of cricoid, 4–5 cm; larynx to carina, 12–13 cm; diameter of average adult trachea, 2.5 cm.

The position of the carina with reference to the midline of the trachea and the take-off angles of the stem bronchi are presented in Chapter 22 of Volume I, *Endobronchial Technique*.

PEDIATRIC STRUCTURAL DIFFERENCES

These differences are detailed in Table 1-2.

SUBDIVISIONS OF LUNG AIR[6,7]

The total air capacity of the lung is approximately 5000 ml (5 l). This value can be estimated by the rule of 70 ml/kg of body weight. By means of simple volume recorders and a spirometer, various subdivisions (Fig. 1-3) can be determined. Because confusion existed over definitions, a group of physiologists met in 1950 under the chairmanship of Pappenheimer and standardized the

various terms. They recognized volumes as the primary subdivisions and defined four such volumes without overlap. They also recognized the term capacity and defined four such capacities, each of which includes two or more primary subdivisions or volumes (Table 1-3).

Lung Volumes

TIDAL VOLUME (TV)

This is the quantity of air breathed in and out with each ordinary respiratory effort, amounting to approximately 500 ml in the adult at rest: The tidal volume can be calculated approximately on the basis of 6.0 to 7.5 ml/kg body weight. In the newborn full-term baby and through the neonatal period, the value of 6.0 ml/kg is used. After the first month and through infancy, the base value used is 7.0 ml/kg, and in the adult, the value is set at 7.5 ml/kg.

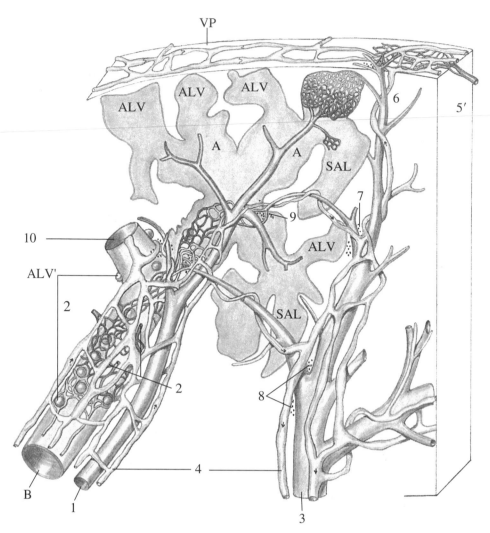

Fig. 1–2. General scheme of a primary lobule, showing the subdivisions of (B) a respiratory bronchiole into two alveolar ducts; and the atria (A), alveolar sacs (S.AL.) of one of these ducts. ALV, alveoli scattered along the bronchioles; P, pleura; 1, pulmonary artery, dividing into smaller radicles for each atrium, one of which terminates in a capillary plexus on the wall of an alveolus; 2, it branches to the respiratory bronchiole and alveolar duct; 3, pulmonary vein with its tributaries from the pleura 6, capillary plexus of alveolus, and wall of the atrium 9 and alveolar duct 10; 4, lymphatics; dotted areas at 7, 8, 9 and 10, indicating areas of lymphoid tissue; 5, bronchial artery terminating in a plexus on the wall of the bronchiole; 5′, bronchial artery terminating in pleura. Redrawn from Miller, The Lung, Charles C Thomas.

Inspiratory Reserve Volume (IRV)

This is the maximal amount of gas that can be inspired beyond the end-inspiratory position. It is the additional volume of air that can be drawn into the lungs if after an ordinary tidal volume inspiration a further maximal inspiratory effort is made. It is approximately 40 to 50% of total lung capacity (TLC) and amounts to approximately 2000 to 3000 ml in 70-kg adults. In young subjects, the IRV amounts to 3000 to 3500 ml. In individuals 50 years of age or older, the IRV approaches 2500 ml.

Expiratory Reserve Volume (ERV)

This is the maximal volume of gas that can be expired from the end-expiratory (normal) position. It is the additional quantity of air that can be expelled from the lungs if further maximal expiratory effort is made after normal expi-

ration. This volume is approximately 20% of TLC, is constant with age, and amounts to approximately 1000 to 1200 ml.

Residual Volume (RV)

This is the volume of air remaining in the lungs at the end of a maximal expiration. It amounts to 20% of TLC, or 1200 ml. It varies with age, averaging approximately 1300 ml at ages 20 to 30 years, 1500 ml at ages 30 to 40 years, and approximately 2000 ml at ages 40 to 60 years. In the elderly, it increases to 2400 ml.[2] It cannot be measured directly on a spirogram, but it can be determined by indirect means. Two methods are available that depend on the use of insoluble gases. In the open circuit method, all the nitrogen in the lungs (80% of the volume) is washed out by the subject inspiring oxygen and expiring into a spirometer acting as a collecting reservoir. The volume of expired gas is then measured and the nitrogen content is calculated.[8]

Table 1–2. Structural Differences in Respiratory System of Pediatric Patients

	Anatomic Characteristic	Importance
All pediatric patients	Narrow larynx and trachea	Increased susceptibility to upper airway obstruction from mucosal edema, granulation tissue, and so on
	Short tracheal length	Position of endotracheal tube critical to prevent accidental dislodgement or endobronchial intubation
	Smaller terminal airways and alveoli	Increased tendency to small airway obstruction and alveolar collapse
Infants	Greater dependence on diaphragm for respiratory work	Significant respiratory impairment from interference with movement of diaphragm (phrenic nerve palsy, abdominal distention)
Newborn	Greater elasticity of chest wall	Tendency to retraction of thoracic cage with inspiration; inefficient ventilatory effort
	Increased thickness of muscular layer of wall of pulmonary arterioles; smaller lumina	Increased pulmonary vascular resistance
Premature	Immature central control of respiration	Periodic breathing; apneic episodes
	Surfactant deficiency	Increased surface tension and tendency to atelectasis; respiratory distress syndrome

(Compiled from Motoyama, E. K. and Cook C. D.: Respiratory physiology. In *Anesthesia for Infants and Children*, 4th Ed. Edited by R. M. Smith. St. Louis, C. V. Mosby, 1980, pp. 38–86; Doershuk, C. F., et al.: Pulmonary physiology of the young child. In *Pulmonary Physiology of the Fetus, Newborn and Child*. Edited by E. Scarpelli and P. Auld. Philadelphia, Lea & Febiger, 1975; Polgar, G. and Weng, T. R.: Functional development of the respiratory system. Am. Rev. Respir. Dis., *120*:625, 1979.)

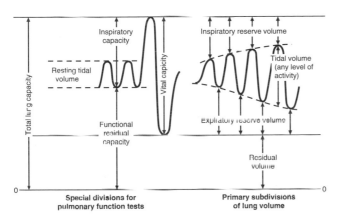

Fig. 1–3. Subdivisions of total lung air capacity. Redrawn from Pappenheimer, Fed Proc 1950.

In the closed circuit method, helium is used in a known volume and concentration (10%) and is breathed from a reservoir until mixing with the alveolar gas is complete. The change in percent in the reservoir permits calculation of lung volume.[9]

The *end-inspiratory position* is the position of the thorax at the end of a normal inspiration. The *end-expiratory position* is the position to which the thorax returns at the end of a quiet expiration. The end-expiratory position is the point of reference from which all measurements of capacity are made.

Lung Capacities

As previously mentioned, various combinations of the primary lung volumes are termed capacities, of which four are defined.

Inspiratory Capacity

This is the maximal volume of air that can be inspired from the resting end-expiratory position. It combines TV and the IRV.

Vital Capacity (VC)

This is the total amount of air that can be inspired from a point of maximal expiration. It thus combines the expiratory reserve volume, the tidal volume, and the inspiratory reserve volume (ERV + TV + IRV = VC). Normal ranges for vc values depend on age and habitus (Table 1–4).[10,11]

Functional Residual Capacity (FRC)

This is the volume of gas remaining in the lungs in the resting end-expiratory position. It amounts to approximately 2500 ml and represents the combined RV and ERV.

The FRC decreases on assumption of the supine position as compared to the sitting position because of upward displacement of the diaphragm. Substantial increases in the FRC occur, however, in awake subjects who turn from the supine to the prone position.[12]

The FRC usually decreases during general anesthesia, to the extent of 0.5 liters in the average adult.[13] This change is related to greater cephalad displacement of the position of the diaphragm at end expiration. The FRC is reduced in obese patients and increases with age.[14]

Total Lung Capacity (TLC)

This is the maximal amount of air that can be contained in the lungs when they are fully expanded.

Table 1–3. Nomenclature for Lung Volumes and Capacities with Normal Values in Adults*

Terminology	Explanation	Normal Values M.	F.
Tidal volume	Volume of air inspired or expired at each breath.	660 (230)	550 (160)
Inspiratory reserve volume	Maximum volume of air that can be inspired after a normal inspiration.	2240	1480
Expiratory reserve volume	Maximum volume of air that can be expired after a normal expiration.	1240 (410)	730 (300)
Residual volume	Volume of air remaining in the lungs after a maximum expiration.	2100 (520)	1570 (380)
Vital capacity	Maximum volume of air that can be expired after a maximum inspiration.	4130 (750)	2760 (540)
Total lung capacity	The total volume of air contained in the lungs at maximum inspiration.	6230 (830)	4330 (620)
Inspiratory capacity	The maximum volume of air that can be inspired after a normal expiration.	2900	2030
Functional residual capacity	The volume of gas remaining in the lungs after a normal expiration.	3330 (680)	2300 (490)

*Normal values taken from Needham et al. Figures are mean values, with the standard deviation in brackets; 98% of the population lie within ± 2 S.D. of the mean.
(From Needham, C. D., Rogan, M. C., and McDonald, I.: Normal standards for lung volumes, intrapulmonary gas mixing and maximum breathing capacity. Thorax, 9:313, 1954.)

Table 1–4. Measurements of Principal Lung Volumes and Formulas for Their Prediction in Normal Subjects

	Age 16–34 yrs		Age 35–49 yrs		Age 50–69 yrs	
	Range ♀	Range ♂	Range ♀	Range ♂	Range ♀	Range ♂
Vital capacity, supine (ml)	2300–4200	2800–4900	2200–3400	3300–5200	1600–3500	2200–5400
Maximum breathing capacity, standing (L/min)	64–118	80–170	50–110	85–140	50–100	60–140
Ventilation L/min/m² body surface, resting	2.5–4.3	3.0–4.5	2.5–3.7	2.6–4.0	2.5–4.0	3–5
O₂ consumption, ml/min/m² body surface, resting	110–150	130–190	110–140	120–160	100–150	100–170
Predicted (calculated) total capacity, (supine)	$\dfrac{\text{Vital capacity}}{80} \times 100$		$\dfrac{\text{Vital capacity}}{76.6} \times 100$		$\dfrac{\text{Vital capacity}}{69.2} \times 100$	
Ratio $\dfrac{\text{Residual air}}{\text{Total cap. (supine)}} \times 100$	♀ and ♂ 20		♀ and ♂ 23.4		♀ and ♂ 30.8	

Predicted (calculated) vital capacity, supine (ml)

$$\dfrac{♂/27.63 - (0.112 \times \text{age in yrs})/ \times \text{height in cm}}{♀/21.78 - (0.101 \times \text{age in yrs})/ \times \text{height in cm}}$$

Predicted (calculated) maximum breathing capacity, standing (L/min)

$$\dfrac{♂/86.5 - (0.522 \times \text{age in yrs})/ \times \text{m}^2 \ \text{body surface}}{♀/71.3 - (0.474 \times \text{age in yrs})/ \times \text{m}^2 \ \text{body surface}}$$

(From Matheson, H. W.: Ventilatory function tests. II. Factors affecting the voluntary ventilation capacity. J. Clin. Invest., 29:682, 1950; Baldwin, E. de F., Cournand, A., and Richards, Jr., D. W.: Pulmonary insufficiency: Methods of analysis, physiologic classification, and standard values in normal subjects. Medicine, 27:243, 1948.)

RESPIRATORY CHANGES IN THE NEWBORN[15]

Measurements of respiratory function at birth (after 2 hours) and during the first 24 hours of life have been made and show important adaptive changes. No signifi-cant increases in minute volume, TV, and respiratory rate occur. The FRC increases significantly, however, from a mean of 65 to 85 ml, i.e., from approximately 22 to 28 ml/kg. At the same time, a 33% increase occurs in alveolar ventilation, from 383 to 511 ml/min. The increase in alveolar ventilation parallels the increase in oxygen consumption. Hill determined the oxygen consumption 3 hours after birth in term infants to be 4.5 ml/kg, with an increase to 6.5 ml/kg noted by 26 hours.[16]

Surfactant Effect on Pulmonary Mechanics[17]

The administration of 90 mg of exogenous surfactant to infants with respiratory distress syndrome produced a large decrease in the ratio of alveolar oxygen to arterial oxygen. This change correlates with improved gas exchange. During spontaneous breathing with continuous positive airway pressure, large and consistent improvement in pulmonary mechanics occurs: TV increases by over 30%; dynamic compliance by 30%; and minute ventilation by 38%. Inspiratory flow rates increase by 54% or more.

SPIROGRAMS

Simple tracings of the volume changes resulting from breathing into a bellows or reservoir can be recorded. The graph is called a spirogram and its examination provides useful information regarding the lung volumes and breathing patterns.

Respiratory Cycle

The cycle begins with the onset of one inspiration and ends with the onset of the next inspiration. It includes the inspiratory phase, the expiratory phase, and the respiratory pause. The pattern of the normal cycle is noted in the Fleisch Curve (Fig. 2-2). The cycle lasts approximately 3 seconds and the expiratory pause approximately 1 second.[18]

Times for Normal Inspiration and Expiration

In normal breathing, expiration lasts approximately 1.2 times as long as inspiration. Thus, one may state that normal inspiration is a little less than ½ seconds and expiration a little more than 1½ seconds.

In certain diseases wherein the elastic recoil of the lung is lost (emphysema), expiration is prolonged. Expiration is also prolonged when lower airway obstruction exists.

Subdivisions of Lung Volume

Certain measurements of lung volumes and capacities may be made and are of value in estimating pulmonary re-

serve and function.[19] Three commonly used determinations vc, timed vc or forced expiratory volume, and maximum breathing capacity. The normal range of values, depending on age and sex, are presented in Table 1-5. Values for vc and maximum breathing capacity may be calculated on the basis of age, height, and body surface area by the prediction formula of Baldwin.[11]

Dead Space

Space in the bronchial tree through which no significant gas exchange occurs is termed *dead space.*[2,3] It represents the proximal portion of the pulmonary system concerned with the conduction of air from outside to the lung periphery or the respiratory portion. Of the 500 ml of tidal air, approximately 150 ml are used to fill this conduit part of the bronchial tree. Modifications of this space alter efficiency of respiration.

Anatomic Dead Space

This extends from the nostrils to the respiratory bronchioles. During ordinary inspiration, air is drawn into the respiratory tree and into the alveoli. Air in the dead space is displaced into the lung periphery, while some of the fresh air fills the dead space. The air not filling this space mixes with the residual and supplemental air. Thus, anatomic dead space air is air that does not enter the alveolar structure.[9]

Normal Values

Normal values for anatomic dead space are illustrated in Figure 1-4. In ordinary circumstances, *the anatomic dead space in milliliters is approximately equal to the weight of the subject in pounds.*[20] This correlation can be applied in practice. The anatomic respiratory dead space may be subdivided into the intra- and extrathoracic parts. The boundary between these two components has been taken to be the upper border of the manubrium sterni, which is approximately 6 cm above the carina and 8 cm below the vocal cords. (This is the point usually reached in an adult male by the tip of an endotracheal tube or a tracheostomy). The volume of intrathoracic dead space in living subjects has a mean value of 66 ml or 0.43 times the body weight in pounds.[21] Measurements of extrathoracic dead space in cadavers and in living subjects provide a mean value of 70 ml, which is roughly

Table 1–5. Age-Related Respiratory Variables

Age	Respiratory Rate (per min)	Tidal Volume (ml)	Minute Ventilation (L/min)	Estimated Alveolar Ventilation (ml/min)	Closing Volume (% of vital capacity)
Term newborn	50 ± 10	21.0	1.05	385	28
6 months	30 ± 5	45	1.35	—	24
12 months	24 ± 6	78	1.78	1245	22
3 years	24 ± 6	112	2.46	1760	20
5 years	23.5 ± 5	270 ± 80	5.5	1800	16
12 years	18.5 ± 5	476 ± 90	6.15	2790	10
Adults	12.5 ± 3.5	575 ± 10	6.38	3070	8

(Adapted from Polgar, G., Weng, T. R.: Functional development of the respiratory system. Am. Rev. Respir. Dis., *120*:625, 1979; Scarpelli, E. and Auld, P. (eds.): *Pulmonary Physiology of the Fetus, Newborn and Child.* Phildelphia, Lea & Febiger, 1975.

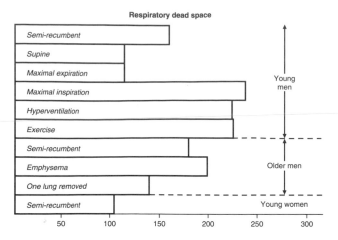

Fig. 1–4. Anatomical respiratory dead space. Redrawn from Comroe, Am J Med.

0.55 times the body weight in pounds. The sum of these two ratios is nearly unity and is the value for the ratio of total anatomic dead space to body weight in pounds suggested by Radford.[20]

Variations

Values for females are usually smaller than those for males; values for older men are usually larger. Tracheotomy reduces dead space by approximately one half. An endotracheal tube similarly reduces dead space. Protrusion of the jaw to the sniffing position (no endotracheal tube) increases anatomic dead space by 25 ml,[22] whereas jaw depression causes a mean decrease of 46 ml. Separation of the teeth increases the dead space by 50 to 100 ml simply by enlarging the mouth. Increased dead space during anesthesia was first observed by Nunn. The increase, approximately 70 ml, was subcarinal and in the alveolar component. This increase correlated with the increased geometric dimensions of the lower respiratory tract.

Recent studies indicate that minute amounts of oxygen and carbon dioxide are exchanged in the supraglottic portion of the respiratory tract. It is insignificant, however, as regards physiologic needs.

Physiologic Dead Space

Physiologic dead space is the total lung space occupied by fresh air just before expiration and represents air that does not come in contact with respiratory epithelium. It includes anatomic dead space plus the space in the alveoli occupied by air not participating in gas exchange. The latter has been termed *alveolar dead space*.[23] The physiologic dead space is a function of tidal volume.

Normal Values

The mean volume of physiologic dead space for healthy patients is 0.3 times the tidal volume. Higher tidal volumes increase the alveolar dead space because a larger tidal volume will increase the expansion of the alveoli. The increase as related to the end-inspiratory lung volume is of the order of 40 ml/L of tidal volume.[24] Thus, physiologic dead space varies with depth of respiration. Ordinarily, it is larger than the anatomic dead space in that fresh air goes beyond respiratory bronchioles, but it may not contact alveolar epithelium, except by diffusion.

Infants and Children[25]

Measurement of dead space based on sampling arterial PCO_2 is the best measure of true physiologic dead space ($VD_{physiol}$). This amount can be estimated closely from accurate measurements of end-tidal PCO_2 (DET). Lindahl conducted a study of infants and children to age 9 years. In healthy children or in children with acyanotic heart disease, end-tidal CO_2 tensions correlate closely with arterial CO_2 tension. The dead space volume was calculated as 3.0 ml/kg, and the VD/VT ratio was approximately 3.5.

In children with cyanotic congenital heart disease, the end-tidal CO_2 underestimates arterial CO_2 with underestimation of physiologic dead space, and overestimates alveolar ventilation. The VDET in the cyanotic group was 25% lower than VDa. Thus, a noninvasive technique is available to provide practical information on dead space.

In the cyanotic group, large differences exist in the $PaCO_2$ and the end-tidal CO_2 (P(a-ET)CO2). A tension gradient of 27% results, and the alveolar ventilation is 27% greater. The DD/VT ratio was calculated as 25% lower calculated from end-tidal rather than arterial CO_2 tension (Fig. 1–5).

Mechanical Dead Space

This is additional space imposed on a subject by devices and anesthetic appliances in which there is no gas exchange. Thus, in closed system anesthesia, it is that space containing respiratory gases that are not brought into contact with the absorbent.

Investigations by Guedel and Waters reveal that proper use of endotracheal equipment can reduce anatomic dead space.[26] They measured the cubic content of the mouth, nose, and pharynx of adults and found it to be 60 to 75 ml. Because an endotracheal tube of approximate size (ID 11 and ID 12) has a volume of approximately 20 ml, its use reduces the dead space of the upper respiratory tract. This advantage is offset, however, by the unscientific use of long tubes extending beyond the lips as well as the use of extensions and tubular connections. Besides creating dead space, resistance is introduced, and the practice should be condemned. Other practices imposing mechanical dead space include large, poorly fitting masks and partially exhausted absorbents. The burden of external dead space may reach a critical point where rises in PCO_2 and marked physiologic adjustments occur. Hamilton[27] determined that a volume of 125 ml represents critical external (mechanical) dead space.

Some pathophysiologic conditions may also increase physiologic dead space (Fig. 1–6). Alveoli with diminished or absent blood flow increase dead space. This situation can occur in shock and interstitial edema. Physiologic dead space is also increased during hyperpnea. At such times, the alveolar ventilation may be in excess of the blood flow.

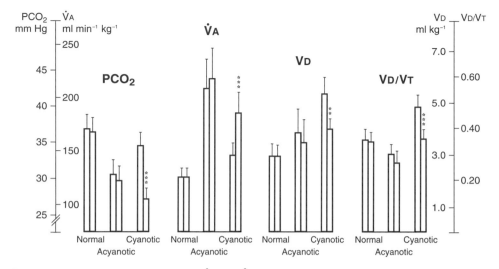

Fig. 1–5. Mean values (±SEM) of PaCO2 − PETCO2, $\dot{V}$Aa − $\dot{V}$AET, VDa − VDET, and VDa/VT − VDET/VT in normal (n = 18), acvanotic (n = 7), and cyanotic (n = 11) children. Open columns represent PaCO2 or values calculated from PaCO2 tensions, while hatched columns represent PETCO2 or values calculated from PETCO2 tensions. ☆☆ = P < 0.01 and ☆= P < 0.001 for differences between arterial and end-tidal values. Redrawn from Lindahl S. G. E., Yates A. P., Hatch D. J.: Anesthesiology 66:168, 1987.

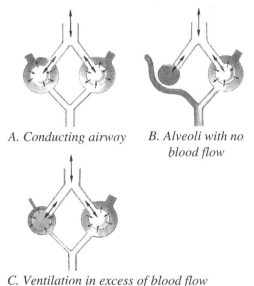

A. Conducting airway   *B. Alveoli with no blood flow*

C. Ventilation in excess of blood flow

Fig. 1–6. Types of respiratory dead space. A. Basic anatomical dead space of the conducting air passage. (VD anat) i.e. The portion of tidal volume not in alveoli. B. Extreme of alveolar dead space in which the air volume in the entire alveolus does not participate in gas exchange (VD alv) i.e. The portion of tidal volume in non-perfused alveoli. C. Hyperpnea in which the ventilation of alveoli is out of proportion to the ability of the capillary blood flow to pick up oxygen—much of the air thus merely flows in and out without exchange occurring. TOTAL DEAD SPACE (VV PHYSIOL.) = ANATOMICAI D.S. (VD anat) + ALVEOLAR D.S. (VD alv). Redrawn from Comroe, The Lung, Mosby Year Book.

RESPIRATORY THORACIC SYSTEM GEOMETRY

Supine-Awake Position

In the awake state, the average functional residual capacity (FRC) in the supine position is approximately 2.5 to 3 liters, and represents a reference value (Grimby) for healthy adults with an average weight of 70 kg. The cross-sectional areas of the lung and rib cage, as well as the abdomen, have been carefully measured by Hedenstierna and coworkers.[28] The average rib cage area in the upper portion of the thorax is approximately 220 cm². In the midchest region, the cross-sectional area averages 300 cm², and in the lower thoracic region, the cross-sectional area is 350 cm². For healthy subjects weighing 70 kg and in the age range of 35 to 75 years, while supine, the abdomen shows an overall cross-sectional area between 40 and 80 cm² throughout the upper middle and lower portions, with minimal variations (Table 1–6).

Thoracic volume in the supine position is approximately 5 l (4.87 ± 0.39 l) and the abdominal volume at approximately 10 l (compared with values in the upright or sitting positions of a thoracic volume of 6.0 l and an abdominal volume of 8.0 l). Total thoracic lung water volume is 2.3 l, of which 1.7 l (75%) is represented by the central blood volume (lung blood volume and blood in the cardiac chambers and thoracic blood vessels[29]) and 0.6 l or 600 ml represents the extravascular lung water (essentially 8 ml/kg of body weight).

Supine Position in Anesthetized Subjects

In 1963, Bergman reported decreases in the FRC on induction of general anesthesia in the supine patient. The average reduction is approximately 18%, or approximately 500 ml in a 70-kg subject.[31] Of the changes in geometry, the following are established.[28] The diaphragm moves cranially, and the dome is elevated by approximately 2 cm, resulting in a reduced rib cage dimension, although the abdominal cross-sectional area is not changed significant. Consequently, the abdominal volume increases by approximately 400 ml. The thoracic volume is reduced by 750 ml, which is somewhat greater than the reduction in FRC of 450 ml. The reduction in the total

Table 1–6. Functional Residual Capacity (FRC) and Chest and Abdominal Dimensions ($\bar{x} \pm$ SE)

| | | Cross-Sectional Area (cm²) | | | | | | Cranial Shift of Diaphragm (cm) | Thorax Volume (liters) | Abdomen Volume (liters) |
| | | Lungs (rib cage) | | | Abdomen | | | | | |
	FRC (liters)	Upper	Middle	Lower	Upper	Middle	Lower			
Awake	3.08 ± 0.37	222 ± 18	308 ± 22	348 ± 25	473 ± 37	441 ± 45	443 ± 43	0	4.87 ± 0.39	9.87 ± 0.99
Anesthetized	2.57* ± 0.43	206 ± 19	288* ± 21	335† ± 26	467 ± 40	435 ± 44	435 ± 40	1.9* ± 0.5	4.12* ± 0.41	10.21† ± 1.06

*Significantly different from the awake value: $p < 0.01$.
†Significantly different from the awake value: $p < 0.05$.

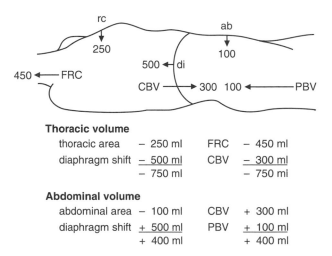

Thoracic volume

thoracic area	– 250 ml	FRC	– 450 ml
diaphragm shift	– 500 ml	CBV	– 300 ml
	– 750 ml		– 750 ml

Abdominal volume

abdominal area	– 100 ml	CBV	+ 300 ml
diaphragm shift	+ 500 ml	PBV	+ 100 ml
	+ 400 ml		+ 400 ml

Fig. 1–7. Mean changes in thoracic and abdominal dimensions and in gas and blood volumes after induction of general anesthesia and mechanical ventilation. Data from the present study and a previous one on peripheral blood volume have been "smoothed" to fit each other. Volumes in milligrams, rc = rib cage; di = diaphragm; ab = abdomen; CBV = central blood volume; PBV = peripheral blood volume. Redrawn from Hedenstierna G., Strandberg A., Brismar B., et al.: Anesthesiology 62:247, 1985.

thoracic volume is attributable to a combined cephalad diaphragmatic shift of 500 ml plus the change in thoracic dimensions of approximately 250 ml. At the same time, these changes are accompanied by a reduction in air volume; approximately a 400- to 500-ml gas volume reduction occurs, along with the 300-ml reduction of central blood volume. By actual measurement, the total lung water is reduced by an average of 340 ml, mostly related to the diminished central blood volume of 0.3 liter or 300 ml. No decrease in extravascular lung water is noted (Fig. 1–7).

The abdominal volume actually increases by approximately 500 ml because of the shift of the diaphragm. Thus, a relative balancing of volume changes apparently exists between the abdominal volume and the intrathoracic total volume. Rehder et al. pointed out that in the supine position, the reduction in FRC in the anesthetized patient occurs soon after induction, that it is not progressive, quickly attains a value of 18%, and is not affected by muscle paralysis. They also noted that if induction of anesthesia is carried out while the patient is sitting, the FRC shows no reduction.

Mechanisms for Functional Reserve Capacity Change in Anesthetized Subjects

The increase in abdominal volume is associated with a combined shift of blood from the thorax (300 ml) and from the periphery (100 to 200 ml) into the abdomen. The diaphragm appears to be the major muscle maintaining FRC in the supine position.[32] An interaction between the tension of the diaphragm and the changes in rib cage and thoracic dimensions is evident. A tense diaphragm expands the rib cage whereas a relaxed diaphragm causes a narrowing of the rib cage. This effect is a readily recognized from ordinary observations of respiration.[37] Thus, changes in the elastic recoil of the chest wall may then become a major factor in changes in FRC. At resting FRC, the inward recoil of the lung is balanced by the outward recoil of the chest wall. An imbalance between these two recoils then alters the FRC. Anesthesia apparently reduces muscle tone of the respiratory muscles, as demonstrated by the loss of tonic electromyographic activity of the diaphragm, which occurs on induction of anesthesia (in the supine position), associated with the cephalad displacement of the diaphragm. Thus, the reduction of the outward recoil of the chest supplements the inward recoil of the lungs and thereby reduces the overall FRC.

ENLARGEMENT OF THE BONY CAGE[34]

The chest may be considered a truncated cone attached to a fixed axis, the spinal column. The lower end of the cone is covered by the diaphragm, which consists of a central tendon with two sets of muscles, the sternocostal and the lumbocostal.[35] In addition, an upper group of muscles covers the rib cage and consists of internal and external intercostals and to some extent the strap muscles of the neck, the serratus anterior, and the latissimus dorsi. The respiratory muscles serve as an "air pump" and the work of breathing is carried out primarily by the inspiratory muscles.[36] On inspiration, all dimensions of the thorax increase (Fig. 1–8).[34] Each group of muscles participates in the ventilatory effort and the volume change resulting from each group effort can be quantitatively partitioned.[37] The diaphragm is the most important muscle but is complemented by the inspiratory intercostal muscles. In stress, these muscles are supported by the scaleni, the stenocleidomastoid, and the strap muscles of the neck.

Tonic postural activity predominates in the intercostal muscles and phasic ventilatory activity in the diaphragm.[38]

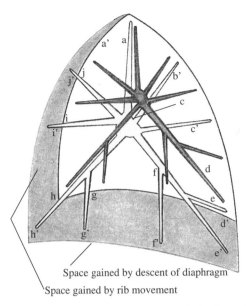

Space gained by descent of diaphragm

Space gained by rib movement

Fig. 1–8. Diagrammatic representation of the bronchial tree with freely movable lung root. Root shown from the side. All bronchi are free to elongate in inspiration (open lines), and shorten in expiration (solid black), thus permitting the lung to expand equally in all directions. Redrawn from Macklin, Am Rev Tubercul.

The diaphragm is richly supplied by α-motoneurons; the intercostals have τ-neurons and a fusimotor system.

Up and Down

The roof of the diaphragm on full expiration is at the level of the fifth costal cartilage. During normal breathing, it is usually at the level of the sixth, or seventh costal cartilage. The diaphragm moves up and down like a piston. The range of movement is approximately 1.5 cm during quiet respiration; in deep breathing, the distance moved may be 6 to 10 cm. In the supine position, it accounts for 60% of the air ventilated during ordinary respiration, and in the erect position, 70% of the air. These figures refer to males; the diaphragmatic component is some 10 to 20% less in females. Movement of 1.0 cm downward the diaphragm causes approximately 250 ml of air to enter the lungs. In resting tidal ventilation of approximately 500 ml, the movement of the diaphragm is approximately 1.5 cm down.

Dorsoventral

Thoracic lid consists of the first ribs, the manubrium, and the articulations, which are fixed by the scalene muscles. When the scaleni contract, the upper chest moves upward and forward.

Upper costal series or ribs, 2 through 6, act rather similarly. They slope outward and downward and each succeeding rib is longer than its higher neighbor. The axis of rotation of these ribs is parallel to the neck of the rib. Hence, during inspiration, these ribs become more horizontal, that is, the body moves up and the anterior part of the upper chest moves upward and forward.

Lateral

Lower costal series or ribs 7 through 10 slope outward and downward at first and then upward. Their anteroposterior axis of rotation passes between the point of articulation in the midline anteriorly and the neck of the ribs posteriorly. During inspiration, these ribs swing outward and upward in the so-called bucket-handle movement. The subcostal arch is widened and the transverse diameter is thereby increased.

DIAPHRAGMATIC LOADING[39]

In the adult, the contractility of each hemidiaphragm is proportional to the length of the resting muscle fibers. Maximal contractile force is generated at low lung volumes when the length of the diaphragmatic muscle fibers is the longest.[40] The muscle fiber length itself is determined by the preload on the diaphragm and, in part, this is the weight of the abdominal contents and intra-abdominal pressure against the undersurface of the hemidiaphragm. The preload or pressure against the undersurface of the diaphragm is similar for both hemidiaphragms. In the prone posture, the overall preload is symmetrically increased as the anterior abdominal wall is compressed.[41] In contrast, in the lateral decubitus postures, the weight of the abdominal contents preferentially loads the dependent hemidiaphragm, lengthens these fibers, and thus improves contractility. Consequently, the fractional ventilation to the dependent lung in a spontaneously breathing individual adult is greater, as demonstrated by bronchospirometric studies[42] and by scanning radiographs in subjects breathing radioactive krypton 81.

Anesthetics and Muscle Paralysis

The functional advantage of diaphragmatic loading disappears in patients who are paralyzed or who are apneic and undergoing intermittent positive pressure ventilation. Pressure on the diaphragm is decreased when the abdominal wall is relaxed. The usual increased ventilation to the dependent lung is reversed in anesthetized subjects.[43]

Induction of Anesthesia

In the awake, supine, healthy adult subject, the mean excursion of the dome of the diaphragm (which shows the greatest tidal movment) from the high end-expiratory position to completion of a normal tidal volume inspiration has been measured as 1.56 ± 0.52 cm. After induction, the position of the dome of the diaphragm was displaced in a caudad direction by 0.35 ± 0.52 cm.[44]

INFLUENCE OF SEX[2]

The mechanism of quiet breathing is influenced by sex. This fact was first demonstrated by Hutchinson in 1846.[45] The difference lies in the fact that breathing in males is chiefly abdominal, i.e., diaphragmatic; in females, breathing is predominantly thoracic. In males, 70% of the respiration is accomplished by diaphragmatic action, in females, 50% of the respiration is accomplished by the diaphragm. A possible explanation is that thoracic breathing in women is a preparation for the time when the abdomen contains a gravid uterus and the diaphragm is restricted.

ZONES OF EXPANSIBILITY

Accompanying the increased size of the thoracic cage during inspiration is an increase in pulmonary expansion. Different areas of the lung vary as to degree of expansion. Keith[46] outlined three distinct zones:

1. *Root Zone.* The hilar area of the lungs moves down forward and laterally on inspiration. Pulmonary parenchyma in this area has little room for expansion because of the rather rigid structures.
2. *Intermediate Zone.* Located approximately midway between the hilus and the periphery of the lung, this zone exhibits a moderate amount of expansion.
3. *Outer Zone.* In the periphery of the lung parenchyma, i.e., the outer 2 to 4 cm, there is no cartilage and the vessels are fine branches so that no rigidity is apparent and the greatest amount of pulmonary expansion is allowable.

REFERENCES

1. Walter, H. E.: Biology of the Vertebrates. New York, MacMillan, 1939.
2. Comroe J. G., et al.: The Lung, 2nd Ed. Chicago, Year Book, 1962.
3. West, J. B. (ed.): Best and Taylor's Physiological Basis of Medical Practice, 12th Ed. Baltimore, Williams & Wilkins, 1990.
4. Miller, W. S.: The Lung. Springfield, Charles C Thomas, 1947.
5. Jackson, C. L., Huber, J. F.: Correlated applied anatomy of the bronchial tree and lungs with a system of nomenclature. Dis Chest 9:319, 1944.
6. Weibel, E. R.: Morphometry of the Human Lung. Berlin, Springer, 1963.
7. Staub, N. C.: Airways: Order of branching. Anesthesiology 24:831, 1963.
8. Darling, R. C., Cournand, A., Richards, Jr., D. W.: Functional residual lung volume open circuit technique. J Clin Invest 19:609, 1940.
9. Comroe, J.: Interpretation of commonly used pulmonary function tests. Am J Med 10:363, 1951.
10. Matheson, H. W.: Ventilatory function tests. II. Factors affecting the voluntary ventilation capacity. J Clin Invest 29:682, 1950.
11. Baldwin, E. de F., Cournand, A., and Richards, Jr., D. W.: Pulmonary insufficiency: Methods of analysis, physiologic classification, and standard values in normal subjects. Medicine 27:243, 1948.
12. Craig, A. B.: Effects of position on expiratory reserve volume of the lungs. J Appl Physiol 15:59, 1960.
13. Westbrook, P. R., Stubbs, S. E., Sessler, A. D.: Effect of anesthesia and muscle paralysis on the respiratory mechanics in man. J Appl Physiol 34:81, 1973.
14. Don HF, Wahba, W. M.: The effects of anesthesia and 100% oxygen on the functional residual capacity of the lungs. Anesthesiology 32:521, 1970.
15. Sandberg, K., et al.: Analysis of alveolar ventilation in the newborn. Arch Dis Child 59:542, 1984.
16. Hill, J. R., Rahimtulla, K. A.: Heat balance and the metabolic rate of newborn babies. J Physiol (Lond.) 180:239, 1965.
17. Davis, J. M., et al.: Changes in pulmonary mechanics after administration of surfactant to infants with respiratory distress syndrome. N Engl J Med 319:476, 1988.
18. Fleisch, A.: Der Pneumotachograph: ein Apparat zur Geschwindigkeits registrierung atemluft. Pflugers Arch 209:719, 1925.
19. Meier, H. C.: The value of respiratory function studies in pulmonary surgery. Surg Gynecol Obstet 88:537, 1949.
20. Radford, E. P.: Ventilation standards for use in artificial respiration. J Appl Physiol 7:451, 1955.
21. Nunn, J. F., Hill, D. W.: Respiratory dead space and arterial to end-tidal CO_2 tension difference in anesthetized man. J Appl Physiol 15:383, 1960.
22. Nunn, J. F., Campbell, E.J.M., Peckett, B. W.: Anatomical subdivisions of the volume of respiratory dead space and effect of position of jaw. J Appl Physiol 14:174, 1959.
23. Severinghaus, J. W., Stupfel, M.: Alveolar dead space as an index of distribution of blood in pulmonary capillaries. J Appl Physiol 10:335, 1957.
24. Shepard, R. H., et al.: Factors affecting the pulmonary dead space as determined by single breath analysis. J Appl Physiol 11:241, 1957.
25. Lindahl, S.G.E., Yates, A. P., Hatch, D. J.: Relationship between invasive and non-invasive measurements of gas exchange in anesthetized infants and children. Anesthesiology 66:168, 1987.
26. Guedel, A. E. and Waters, R. M.: A new intratracheal catheter. Anesth Analg 7:238, 1928.
27. Clappison, G. B. and Hamilton, W. K.: Respiratory adjustments to increases in external dead space. Anesthesiology, 17:643, 1956.
28. Hedenstierna, G., et al.: Functional residual capacity, thoraco-abdominal dimensions and central blood volume during general anesthesia with muscle paralysis and mechanical ventilation. Anesthesiology 62:247, 1985.
29. Dolovich, M. B., et al.: Regional distribution of ventilation and perfusion as a function of body position. J Appl Physiol 21:767, 1966.
30. Bergman, N. A.: Distribution of inspired gas during anesthesia and artificial ventilation. J Appl Physiol 18:1085, 1963.
31. Rehder, K., Camerson, P. D., Krayer, S.: New dimensions of the respiratory system (editorial). Anesthesiology 62:230, 1985.
32. Froese, A. B., Bryan, A. C.: Effects of anesthesia and paralysis on diaphragmatic mechanics in man. Anesthesiology 41:242, 1974.
33. Saunders, N. A., et al.: Effect of curare on maximum static PV relationships of the respiratory system. J Appl Physiol 44:589, 1978.
34. Macklin, C. C.: The dynamic bronchial tree. Am Rev Respir Dis 25:393, 1932.
35. Koepke, G. H., et al.: Sequence of action of diaphragm and intercostal muscles during respiration. Part I. Arch Phys Med 39:426, 1958.
36. Campbell, E.J.M.: An electromyographic examination of the role of the intercostal muscles in breathing in man. J Physiol (Lond.) 129:12, 1955.
37. Konno, K., Mead, J.: Measurements of separate colume changes of rib cage during breathing. J Appl Physiol 22:407, 1967.
38. Campbell, E.J.M.: The Respiratory Muscles and the Mechanics of Breathing. Chicago, Year Book, 1958.
39. Svanberg, L.: Influence of posture on the lung volumes, ventilation and circulation in normals; a spirometric-broncho-spirometric investigation. Scand J Clin Lab Invest (Suppl) 25:1, 1957.

40. West, J. B., Dollery, C. T.: Distribution of blood flow ventilation-perfusion ratio in the lung measured with radioactive CO_2. J Appl Physiol *15*:405, 1960.

41. Remolina, C., et al.: Positional hypoxemia in unilateral lung disease. N Engl J Med *304*:523, 1981.

42. Svanberg, L.: Bronchospirometry in the study of regional lung function. Scand J Respir Dis (Suppl.) *62*:91, 1966.

43. Rehder, K., et al.: The function of each lung of anesthetized and paralyzed man during mechanical ventilation. Anesthesiology *37*:16, 1972.

44. Drummond, G. B., Allan, P. L., Logan, M. R.: Changes in diaphragmatic position in association with induction of anesthesia. Br J Anaesth *58*:1246, 1986.

45. Hutchinson, J.: Respiration. Med Chir Trans *29*:137, 1846.

46. Keith, A.: The Mechanism of Respiration in Man. London, Edward Arnold & Co., 1909.

Chapter 2

DYNAMIC ASPECTS OF VENTILATION

VINCENT J. COLLINS

The anatomic features of the pulmonary system have been reviewed, and this chapter reviews the mechanical changes that occur during breathing. To bring about the movement of air and gases into the lungs and circulation, a gradient of pressure must be established between the mouth and the alveoli. Three principles of ventilation are involved: (1) pressure-volume relations; (2) alveolar gas law (mixing); and (3) capillary-alveolar equilibrium (diffusion).

PRESSURE-VOLUME RELATIONS[1]

This is a simple problem of mechanics dealing with the relation of *Stress* to *Strain*. It is a fundamental physical law of elasticity that an applied force produces a proportionate change or strain in the medium affected and that stress divided by strain is constant:

K Modulus = Stress / Strain

When dealing with pulmonary ventilation, stress is numerically equal to pressure and strain is the fractional change in volume.

When effort is exerted by the respiratory muscles to enlarge the chest, work is performed. This work must overcome three opposing forces: (1) elasticity of lungs-thorax system; (2) nonelastic opposition due to weight and friction of movement of all tissues; and (3) resistance to air flow.

It is estimated[3] that of the energy expended, 60% is directed at overcoming elastic opposition, 10% to moving tissues, and 30% to move air against resistance.

For passive inspiration and passive expiration, the values of developed pressures and the corresponding volumes are related in a curve called "the relaxation pressure curve," which has an "S" shape (Fig. 2–1). Such a curve can be obtained by (1) measuring volume changes resulting from different pressures (Bernoulli 1911), or (2) measuring pressure changes occurring at different volumes (Rahn 1946).

Fundamental data have been obtained by Rahn and coworkers[4] using the second method. The steps in this method are as follows:

1. Subject voluntarily inflates the chest to a known volume.
2. Lungs are connected to manometer by a tube inserted through nares.
3. Inflated chest is allowed to relax and pressure is measured.

From the fact that pressures are measured at time of beginning of relaxation, the resultant curve derives its name as a relaxation pressure curve.

Certain requirements necessary for accurate measurement have been enumerated by Gaensler[6] as: (1) intact thoracic cage, (2) muscular paralysis, and (3) no movement or flow of gas at time of measurement.

Compliance

Over the physiologic range, the expansion of the lungs is a linear function of the pressure. The slope of the line represents the degree to which the respiratory structures are able to respond or comply, hence, the term compliance (a mechanical property). A lung that does not distend or expand to an adequate applied pressure is stiff and has poor elasticity. Compliance is a measure of the distensibility of the lungs and of the restriction to expansion imposed by the surrounding structures.

In specific terms, compliance is the change in volume (ΔV) in the respiratory system per unit increase in intrapulmonary pressure. It is expressed as the milliliters gas per centimeter or $\Delta V/\Delta P$ water pressure change. In the physiologic range, it is 100 ml/cm H_2O (120 ml/mm Hg) for the normal lung-thorax system.

In healthy males over the physiologic range of tidal volumes, compliance values are as follows:

For the lung-thorax system:
100 ml/cm H_2O
For lung compliance alone:
200 ml/cm H_2O
For thoracic cage compliance only:
200 ml/cm H_2O

These various values may be related by the following equation:

$$\frac{1}{C\ total} = \frac{1}{C\ lungs} + \frac{1}{C\ thoracic\ cage}$$

Compliance of the lungs varies with the initial volume of the alveoli. Specifically, the volume change as a fraction of the original lung volume should be related to pressure; i.e., compliance varies direction with functional reserve capacity (FRC). This is specific compliance.

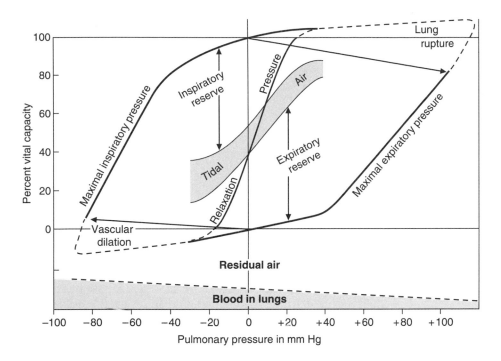

Fig. 2–1. The pressure-volume diagram. Ordinates are the difference between intrapulmonary and extrathoracic pressure in mm. Hg. Abscissas are lung volume as a percentage of vital capacity. Redrawn from Fenn, Am J Med.

Elasticity

Normally, the lungs are in a stretched condition. The lungs tend to pull away from the chest wall. At the end of normal expiration, the lungs are still capable of further contraction to the extent of about 5 mm Hg pressure; at the height of full expansion, the tendency to contract is measured in terms of 30 mm Hg intrapulmonary pressure. These are relaxation curve pressures.

On the other hand, the chest that is elastic is normally in a slightly compressed state and has a tendency to expand to its resting position. It is similar to a coiled spring ready to extend itself.

Elasticity of the respiratory system has two components, namely, lung elasticity and thorax elasticity. Each component structure has its resting position. For example, the resting state of the lungs outside the thorax and exposed only to the atmosphere has a measurable air capacity of about 20% of the vital capacity. The resting position of the thorax alone without the lungs is estimated at 53 to 72% of the vital capacity (i.e., a full expression of the tendency of the thorax to expand). The figure of 72% is predicted on the basis of the fact that, in emphysema, the chest is expanded to accommodate this lung volume, there being no elastic recoil of the lungs. The intact thorax (with lungs) at the position of end-expiration or rest allows a lung volume of 40% of vital capacity.

Inspection of Figure 2-1 shows the solid line relaxation pressure curve of the intact chest. This is essentially the consequence of the probable pressure volume relations of the lungs and thorax separately. At the point Vr, called the relaxation volume, the pressures exerted by the lungs and the thorax are equal and opposite. The chest tends to expand by a pressure equal to the collapsing pressure of the lungs. Where the curve crosses the vertical axis is the point at which the thorax alone attains its resting state. As previously noted, this value in normal subjects is about 53% of vital capacity.

The elasticity of the isolated lung has been investigated, and the pressure volume relations have been determined. The lung behaves as a rubber bag and the extensibility follows the "S" shape curve similar to rubber. One, therefore, recognizes compliance of the lungs alone. Thus, a volume change occurs in response to each change in pressure. The value of this compliance for lungs alone is approximately 220 ml/cm of water pressure.

Surface Tension Forces in Lungs

Recoil of the lung is related to elastic tissue fibers, but it also depends on a special surface film lining the alveoli. In 1929, von Neergaard[7] concluded from studies of pulmonary pressure-volume relationships that each alveolus has a liquid-air interface that tends to retract or shrink to the smallest possible area. This action is a manifestation of attracting forces between molecules; at an interface, the intermolecular forces cause the surface to retract and diminish the size of an alveolus.

The surface tension for fully inflated lungs has been calculated at 50 dynes/cm; the surface tension recoil of the lung is 20,000 dynes/cm and exerts a pressure of 20 cm H_2O. At normal lung volumes, the actual measured surface tension is 5 to 10 dynes/cm. Clements[9] considered that some substance with surface active properties must be present in the liquid surface to account for this difference. This substance has been termed pulmonary surfactant. In the presence of surfactants, the alveoli are maintained open, even at low transpulmonary pressures.

Lung Surfactants

The principal pulmonary surface active agent is the lipid dipalmitoyl phosphotidyl choline (dipalmitoyl-lecithin)—a desaturated lecithin—made from long-chain fatty acids. This material forms an alveolar surface layer. The sites of origin, synthesis, and storage appear to be within alveolar type II cells (pneumatocyte).

Synthesis of long-chain fatty acids from acetate has been reported to be a function of the microsomal fraction of subcellular particles derived from alveolar cells. The mitochondrial activity in such synthesis is 50% of the microsomal activity. Both particles incorporate palmitic acid into lecithin and glycerides.

Two major paths for biosynthesis are recognized. The cytidine diphosphocholine (CDP-choline) pathway is quantitatively most important for production of total lecithin. This synthesis of saturated lecithin is depressed by decreased pulmonary blood flow (bronchial), atelectasis, and hypoxia. This is an "in situ" action.

Synthesis and storage of surfactant, as with secretory capacity, is augmented by thyroxine. Thyroxine also accelerates maturation of the fetal lung.[14] Surfactant[13] capacity is reduced, however, by intrauterine asphyxia. The storage site appears to be the subcellular lamellar bodies.

Synthesis of lecithin by N-methyltransferase is less important. This process involves the methylation of phosphatidyl-ethanolamine to lecithin. The turnover rate for the choline and palmitate is 45 hours and 16 hours, respectively. It is depressed by high concentrations of oxygen. The methyltransferase path is less depressed by pulmonary artery ligation and is increased by hypoxia in the fetus.

Factors Affecting Compliance

Certain physiologic, pharmacologic, and mechanical factors affect compliance (Table 2-1). Belonging to the first grouping are such features as position; the lateral and supine positions diminish compliance by an average of 10%. The physical condition of a patient influences compliance greatly. Thus, obesity and compliance are inversely related. The heavier the patient, the less the compliance. In obese patients or those with large pendulous breasts, the lateral position actually improves the respiratory physiology by increasing compliance. The weight and restriction to chest movements are removed.

In the following pulmonary and cardiac diseases, decreased compliance is of practical significance: pulmonary fibrosis, pneumonitis, pulmonary hypertension, pleural effusion, pleural fibrosis, and thoracic wall rigidity. Conditions of edema, generalized or pulmonary, and especially in the presence of cardiac failure, diminish compliance extensively.

General anesthesia and depressant drugs decrease compliance and the extent of the decrease is proportional to the depth of anesthesia. Relaxant drugs have a variable influence on compliance. Blocking agents such as *d*-tubocurarine greatly reduce compliance. Safar[15] reported reductions in dogs of 50 to 86% of control values, presumably related to the release of histamine. The administration of diphenhydramine hydrochloride intravenously (Benadryl) prevents this change in compliance. Gallamine also reduces compliance. Other explanations include possible changes in the chest wall itself, changes in the stiffness of the lung, and bronchoconstriction. On the other hand, succinylcholine and decamethonium do not significantly alter compliance.

Operative factors are most influential. For example, opening the chest results in a 45% increase in compliance.[16] This change is expected. Packs and retractors reduce compliance however, and the net effect in thoracic surgery is usually a reduction. Similarly, retractors and packs in the upper abdomen and especially any that impinge on the diaphragm reduce compliance. The rapid intravenous administration of crystalloid solutions causes a reduction in lung-thorax compliance.

Thoracic Pressures

That the lungs are in a stretched condition normally and tend to pull away from the chest wall while the latter is in a slightly compressed state has been described. The pressure-volume relationship of the relaxation pressure curves were determined under conditions of relaxation and with no air flow, hence, they are static quantities. It is, therefore, of practical importance to know the intrapulmonary and intrapleural pressure changes during breathing.

The intrapulmonary space is exposed to atmospheric pressure and has a mean pressure equal to the atmospheric pressure. The intrapleural pressure is subatmospheric or "negative." These pressures vary with the phase of respiration.[17]

Table 2–1. Factors Affecting Compliance

1. Anesthesia:	44% decrease; more with depth
2. Obesity:	Decrease proportional to weight
3. Hypoxia:	Decreases
4. Position:	Lateral—decrease
5. Postoperative factors:	Progressive decrease to fifth day
6. Operative factors:	Retraction lung—17% decrease

7. Physical status:
  a. Edema, generalized
  b. Pulmonary edema
  c. Cardiac failure
  d. Pulmonary fibrosis
  e. Splinting
	Decreased

8. Open chest:	Increase, 45%

INTRAPLEURAL PRESSURE
Inspiration 4.5 to 8.0 mm Hg below atmospheric
Expiration 2.5 to 4.0 mm Hg below atmospheric
INTRAPULMONARY PRESSURE
Inspiration 2.0 to 4.0 mm Hg below atmospheric
Expiration 1.0 to 4.0 mm Hg above atmospheric

NonElastic Resistance[1]

Opposition to ventilation is imposed by the nonelastic properties of the respiratory system and surrounding tissues. This opposition is simply due to the inherent weight of tissues and the frictional resistance offered during movement. It is related to the speed of motion in that rapid movements result in more friction.

PHYSIOLOGY OF AIR FLOW

The pressure required to move a fluid through a system of tubes depends on three factors:

1. The volume rate of air flow.
2. The nature of the flow.
3. The dimensions of the airway.

These factors are interrelated in Poiseuille's Law of flow of fluids through tubes of varying diameter.

Mass of Air

Air has weight and approximates 1.3 g/L at standard conditions. Although some work is done to move the mass of air, it is negligible in most calculations.

Normal Volume Flow Rates[18]

In normal breathing, gases do not flow in a continuous stream. On the contrary, the volume of flow is variable. At the beginning of inspiration, it is zero. As inspiration progresses, the volume flowing per unit time accelerates until a peak is reached about one third of the interval through the inspiratory phase. In the remaining interval of inspiration, the instantaneous volume flow rate of gas decreases until no gas is flowing at the completion of inspiration. The converse of this pattern occurs during expiration.

Plotting the rate of flow of gases in liters per minute against time during a respiratory cycle produces a curve referred to as the Fleisch curve (Fig. 2-2).[19] In an adult

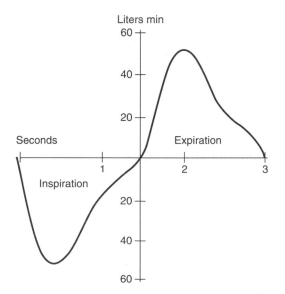

Fig. 2–2. Fleisch curve. Volume rate of flow of gases during respiratory cycle.

breathing quietly a volume of 8 L/min, the maximum flow rate reaches 25 L/min. If a subject breathes deeply, the flow rate may reach a peak of 60 L/min. These facts are of importance in determining resistance of equipment. It is necessary to analyze any apparatus with respect to the highest flow rates to which it will be subjected in patients.

The upper limit of the velocity of air flow in the human trachea is about 10 m/sec. The velocity of air flow in the different parts of the airway (relative to tracheal velocity of 1.0) is 3.39 for glottis, 1.70 at nasal openings, and 1.6 in the bronchioles.

Nature of Air Flow

For large volumes of flow, a greater pressure is required to advance the fluid through a tubular system than for a small volume.

The nature of flow is contributory. Turbulent air flow prevails in the upper airway passages and laminar flow predominates in the trachea, bronchi, and straight conduits. Increasing the rate of ventilation increases the percentage of the total resistance because of turbulence.

Airway Size and Resistance

The dimensions of the airway represent the third important factor affecting the pressure required to advance a fluid in a tubular system. Small tubes require a greater pressure to advance a given volume of fluid than large tubes. Long tubes and narrow tubes offer more resistance. The pressure is determined by the length and cross-sectional area. Again, Poiseuilles law is applicable and it is seen that the pressure required for flow is directly proportional to length of tube and indirectly proportional to cross-sectional area.

Reflex Effects of Airway Resistance

Increased airway resistance has a reflex effect on respiration: slowing of respiratory frequency[20] and an increase in tidal volume.)[73]

The larynx also exerts an important regulatory function on respiration by acting as a valve. When resistance to expiration increases, the valvular resistance of the larynx decreases and vice versa. The time course of inspiration/expiration is also attended by changes in resistance. The time of inspiration is determined by respiratory effort as related to compliance and nonelastic resistance; the time course of expiration (passive) is determined by elastic recoil and airway resistance.[21]

Physical Effects on Airways

Pulmonary airways can be enlarged or partially collapsed by internally or externally applied pressures. The physical effect of the act of breathing is to change the size of all airways but especially the bronchioles, which have no cartilages. On inspiration, the overall enlargement of the lung pulls on and widens the conducting tubes. As the lung volume increases, airway resistance becomes less. During quiet inspiration, the changes are not remarkable because the airways on inspiration also elongate, but during maximal inspiration, resistance is measurably reduced. A maximal or forced expiration increases resistance significantly in normal subjects, but especially in patients with emphysema. Conversely, forced expiration raises intrapleural pressure enough to compress or collapse flaccid alveolar ducts or respiratory bronchioles.

Coughing causes a decrease in the cross-sectional area of the trachea up to one sixth of normal; because of the high intrathoracic pressure, the noncartilaginous portion of the intrathoracic trachea is inverted.

Airway Patency

Patency is determined by airway compliance (determined by intrinsic airway wall compliance and elastic forces in adjacent lung) and transmural pressure. This is not merely a passive affair but a dynamic airway compression and expansion. When the pressure outside peripheral airways exceeds that inside, airway closure occurs. The airways may be critically narrowed (so-called closing volume, CV) at some percentage of vital capacity between 15 and 50%.

Airway Closure[22]

During slow inspiration, starting from residual volumes, the upper zones of the lungs in all lobes begin to fill before the lower zones. At total lung capacity (TLC), all alveoli in normal subjects are evenly inflated. On subsequent slow exhalation, emptying persists from the upper zones after lower zones have ceased to empty. Leblanc and colleagues[23] explained this "first-in-last-out pattern" of filling and emptying that occurs with closure of small airways, especially bronchioles, at low lung volumes and in dependent portions of the lung. Critical narrowing of the airways may also account for the phenomenon. The closure or critical narrowing of the small airways occurs when tissue and airway distending pressure forces are minimal and prevent air flow and alveolar emptying, especially from the dependent parts of the lung.

The term closing capacity (CC) is defined as the fraction of the TLC below which rapid airway closure occurs and peripheral dependent zones cease to ventilate.[24] The determination of volume can be made on a single breath nitrogen washout test of Comroe and Fowler[25]: A vital capacity inhalation of pure oxygen is followed by determination of nitrogen concentration in the exhaled air.[26] This volume occurs below FRC and between it and residual volume (RV).[27] In childhood, however, airways close above FRC. During growth, the CC decreases to an optimum in early adult life below FRC. The CC then increases with age, until at 40 years, the CC begins to exceed FRC (Fig. 2–3). Corresponding changes occur in alveolar-arterial oxygen differences, which are large in childhood, least in young adulthood, and increase with age.

Any effect of airway closure on gas exchange depends on whether it occurs below, in, or above the tidal volume range. Gas exchange is impaired when CC is high and closure is at or above FRC.

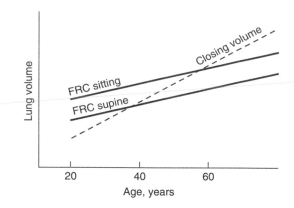

Fig. 2–3.   Relationship of 'closing volume' to age and posture. In the seated subject the closing volume exceeds the FRC at the age of 60 years. In the supine position, closing volume exceeds the FRC at an earlier age. Redrawn from Gray and Nunn, Butterworth & Co., Ltd.

Both CC and FRC are reduced in the supine position and during anesthesia.[28] When CC exceeds FRC, ventilation of lower zones is reduced, even during tidal breathing, which may produce hypoxemia. A concomitant increase in pulmonary shunting then occurs. This situation occurs in middle-aged and elderly populations, in the supine position, and in obese subjects. The rapid administration of intravenous fluids also causes closure at or above FRC.

The percentage of TLC at which airway closure occurs correlates with gas trapping. Gas trapping occurs in normal subjects breathing at low lung volumes and is a result of closure of airways with diameters of 1 mm or less (respiratory bronchioles).

During anesthesia, a reduction in FRC occurs while CC remains unchanged so that airways close during tidal ventilation. Simultaneously, an increase in volume of trapped gas occurs. In general, as lung volume decreases, three events are likely: airway narrowing; airway closure with gas trapping; and alveolar collapse.

Premature closure of the small airways in lower zones may occur after acute myocardial infarction. This occurrence may explain the persistent arterial hypoxemia and increase in alveolar-arterial oxygen gradient in these patients.[29]

Increased Resistance

As lung volume decreases, airway caliber decreases and airway resistance increases. It has been demonstrated that breathing in the supine position in the region of the FRC results in decreased airway caliber and increased airway resistance. Inhalational volatile agents offset much of the decreased lung volume by their bronchodilatory action (Fig. 2–4).[30]

Neural Effect on Airways

Smooth muscle extends from the trachea to the alveolar ducts and is arranged in a geodesic network. In the trachea, transverse smooth muscle fibers narrow the lumen, and longitudinal fibers can shorten it. In the bronchi, con-

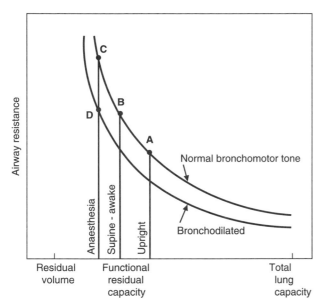

Fig. 2–4. Airway resistance as a function of lung volume with normal bronchomotor tone and when bronchodilated. A = upright and awake; B = supine and awake; C = supine and anaesthetized without bronchodilatation; D = supine, anaesthetized and with the degree of bronchodilatation which normally occurs during anaesthesia. Note that the airway resistance is similar at B and D with bronchodilatation approximately compensating for the decrease in FRC. Redrawn from Nunn, J. F., Utting, J. E., and Brown Jr., B. R. General Anaesthesia, Fifth Edition, Butterworth's, London, 1989.

traction of both the circular and longitudinal smooth muscle produces narrowing of lumen and some shortening of the conduit. Bronchioles and alveolar ducts are rich in circular smooth muscle fibers, and constriction may produce almost complete obstruction. Alveolar ducts are ringed by smooth muscle to form a sphincter-like mechanism and can produce complete obstruction.

The autonomic nervous system exerts a profound effect on the size of pulmonary airways by regulating the tone of the smooth muscle fibers in the walls of all airways.

Parasympathetic System

Efferent fibers arising in the dorsal motor nucleus of the vagus run in the vagus to the chest and form plexuses on the main pulmonary artery and its branches. These plexuses communicate with hilar parasympathetic ganglia and intermingle with the sympathetic pulmonary artery and hilar plexuses. The preganglionic vagal fibers to the plexuses and the postganglionic sympathetic fibers from the stellate and middle cervical ganglia are separate in their course in man.

The intrapulmonary distribution of parasympathetic fibers is to bronchi, blood vessels, and mucus glands.

Sympathetic System

The distribution of sympathetic fibers is mainly to pulmonary and bronchial blood vessels. Good physiologic

evidence shows, however, the existence of sympathetic nerves to lower airways and to bronchi.

From trachea to alveoli, sympathetic efferent impulses cause relaxation of smooth muscle, while parasympathetic impulses cause constriction. Vagal stimulation reduces the caliber of airways and atropine prevents this reduction. In unanesthetized man, atropine decreases airway resistance and increases anatomic dead space. On the other hand, electrical stimulation of the stellate ganglion dilates the trachea and bronchi and decreases airway resistance.

Distribution of Bronchodilatation Versus Bronchoconstriction

Studies of density dependence of maximal expiratory flow to assess the relative contributions of large versus small airways to air flow indicate a greater cholinergic influence manifest on the upper airways, whereas sympathetic influence predominates on the lower airways.

A comparison of a parasympatholytic agent (atropine) and a β-adrenergic agonist (isoetharine) by inhalation shows a similar increase in specific airway conductance of about 80% (atropine, 78%; isoetharine, 88%), but anatomic dead space is increased significantly (by 17%) after atropine administration.[31]

Constriction at any level increases airway resistance. Constriction at terminal bronchioles, however, is the most determinative mechanism for increasing resistance. Simultaneously, anatomic dead space is reduced while lung volume is increased because of obstruction to outflow of air from alveoli during expiration.

Reflex initiation of airway constriction may be caused by any inhaled irritant, such as smoke, dust, chemicals, or foreign bodies.[32] Other constricting influences include arterial anoxemia, elevated $PaCO_2$, cold air, single deep inspiration,[33] and pulmonary emboli. These stimuli excite subepithelial sensory receptors, which send impulses over afferent fibers via the sympathetic-parasympathetic nerves. Impulses in the efferent arc over the same paths excite the contraction of the muscle.[34]

Bronchoconstriction

Such reflex bronchoconstriction to nonantigenic stimuli can be prevented by atropine, vagal cooling, or vagotomy. Forced inspiratory and expiratory efforts also stimulate irritant receptors.[35]

Antigen-induced bronchoconstriction, as in human asthma, also involves a parasympatholytic reflex as well as mediator release of histamine. Inhalation of antigen aerosols will increase airway resistance up to 80% in susceptible subjects. Intravenous administration of atropine after such inhalation decreases resistance to only 12% above control levels. When atropine is administered before the challenge, the increase in airway resistance is prevented. Parasympatholytic activity is of critical importance in both antigen and nonantigen induction of bronchoconstriction.[36]

Bronchodilatation

Relaxation of bronchiolar muscle also occurs reflexly during normal inspiration and when systemic arterial pressure is increased.

Chemical Effects on Bronchial Muscle

Many drugs and agents affect bronchiolar muscle directly or indirectly via intermediary chemicals or reflexes. Isoproterenol epinephrine and norepinephrine, in that order of activity, inhibit bronchial smooth muscle tone at receptor sites (beta 2) to produce bronchodilatation. Acetylcholine and anticholinesterases stimulate the same receptors and produce constriction. Histamine also produces constriction.

Carbon dioxide exerts both a central neural effect and a peripheral direct effect on bronchiolar muscle and on airway resistance. The magnitude of response to changes in arterial carbon dioxide depends on levels of alveolar carbon dioxide tension and vice versa. Arresting pulmonary blood flow to one lung or to a segment of one lung and allowing alveolar ventilation to continue induces bronchoconstriction in this lung.[37] Ventilation then shifts to the other lung or to segments that are perfused. If the lung or segment without blood flow is ventilated with a 3 to 5% carbon dioxide breathing mixture, no constriction occurs, indeed, bronchodilatation results. In the isolated or denervated lung, this effect also occurs and is thus a local response that results from direct action of alveolar carbon dioxide on the bronchiolar muscle.

Effect of Alveolar CO₂ on Ventilatory Compliance

The interrelationship between levels of alveolar and arterial carbon dioxide have been studied by Patterson and Sullivan (Table 2–2).[38]

When arterial PCO_2 is maintained constant in human subjects (30 mm Hg), a stepwise increase in alveolar carbon dioxide tension by ventilating with mixtures at 6 to

40 mm Hg produces an increase in compliance of 35% accompanied by a decrease of 40% in resistance to work of breathing (25% decrease in resistive [air flow breathing] and 15% in elastic resistance).

Pulmonary Resistance =

$$\frac{\text{Mouth Pressure} - \text{Intrapleural Pressure}}{\text{Flow (L/min.)}}$$

At a normal arterial oxygen tension, hypocapnia induces bronchoconstriction and, in general, the greater the arterial carbon dioxide tension, the greater the bronchoconstriction or resistance to breathing. Thus, hypocapnia and hypercarbia have an additive effect on increasing airway resistance.

When alveolar carbon dioxide tension is held constant at 6 mm Hg, a stepwise increase in arterial PCO_2 of 20 mm Hg produces a 25% increase in resistance and a decrease in compliance. If alveolar carbon dioxide is maintained at normal or higher than normal levels, minimal alteration of mechanics occurs in response to changes in arterial PCO_2.

Normal Values for Resistance

Resistance is a calculated value and not a measured quantity. One must measure the pressure difference between two points and know the volume flow of air. An equation similar to Ohm's electrical law of resistance is applied: part of pulmonary resistance is related to frictional resistance of the tissues themselves estimated at 20% of the whole, whereas 80% is related to flow resistance.

The overall resistance is expressed in centimeters of water pressure per liter of air flow. A normal value for airway flow resistance in the adult, when measured by body plethysmography at an arterial PCO_2 of 30 to 40 mm Hg, is 1.5 to 2.0 cm H_2O/L. About one half of airway resistance during quiet breathing occurs in the nasal passages; less resistance occurs through the mouth. Some resistance occurs at the glottis and the remainder is in the bronchioles principally.

WORK OF BREATHING[1,3,39]

Measurement

The work of breathing represents all the energy needed to ventilate the lungs; it is the work required to move air. The three opposing forces to this effort are the elastic resistance, the force needed to move nonelastic tissues, and the force needed to overcome resistance to air flow.

Three approaches have been used to measure work of breathing:

1. Measurement of difference in oxygen consumption between that at rest and during vigorous ventilation. This value is the amount needed for the increased work done in breathing.
2. Use of a tank respirator after abolition of respiration. The work of breathing performed by the machine is

Table 2–2. Dependency of Resistance on the Alveolar and Arterial Carbon Dioxide Tensions

		$F_{ET_{CO_2}}$	
		(6 mm Hg) <1%	(40 mm Hg) 6%
$PaCO_2$ (mm Hg)	25 (18–30)	9.5	3.9
	38 (30–45)	11.0	3.7

Average values obtained from 10 cases for lung-tissue resistance in cm H_2O/L/sec. The columns give resistance values when the end tidal carbon dioxide ($F_{ET_{CO_2}}$) was about 6 mm Hg tension and when it was about 40 mm Hg. Reading across the rows gives the resistance values that were obtained when the arterial carbon dioxide tension was 25 mm Hg (with a range of 18 to 30) or 38 mm Hg (with a range of 30 to 45). (From Patterson, R. W. and Sullivan, S. F.: Inter-relation between $PaCO_2$ and $PaCO_2$ in the control of the mechanisms of breathing in man. Bull. N.Y. Acad. Med., *44*:1265, 1968.)

considered equivalent to the work performed by the subject.

3. Measurement of pressure difference between intrapleural space and the mouth.

Work is defined as exerting a force through a distance, i.e., Work = Force × Distance. In ventilation, this is equivalent to Pressure × Volume and is expressed as kilogram meters per minute. The total work required to breathe in an adult subject at rest amounts to 0.3 kg m/min. On exercise, the value goes up to 80.0 kg m/min.

The work required to move the lungs alone is parallel to the elastic resistance of the lungs.

Oxygen Cost of Breathing[40]

Oxygen consumed by the respiratory muscles in breathing at rest is a small fraction of the total metabolism. It amounts to about 1 to 2% for normal resting ventilation, but increases to 10% of the oxygen consumed during activity and 15% for strenuous work or exercise.

A more accurate method for describing the oxygen cost of breathing is on the basis of milliliters of oxygen consumed per liter of air ventilated. In the resting normal subject, this amount ranges from 0.3 to 1.8 ml of oxygen per liter for minute volumes of respiration ranging from 5 to 50 L/min. The actual consumption by the respiratory pump is between 3.0 to 15.0 ml of oxygen per minute for 70-kg man. The oxygen cost of breathing during voluntary hyperventilation is approximately 3.2 ml/L of ventilation or up to 10% of oxygen consumed; if ventilation is 50 l or more per minute, the requirement may be 25 to 30% of total oxygen consumption. In patients with emphysema, the oxygen cost of breathing at rest varies between 4 to 10 times that of normal.[41] At low levels of ventilation, this amount may be 25% of total oxygen consumption. For patients in congestive heart failure, it is about twice the normal cost. For obese subjects, the oxygen cost of breathing is four times normal.[42] The amount of oxygen needed by those 20% overweight is of the order of 4.0 ml/L of air moved (normal average at rest is 1.0 ml/L), which represents 12 to 16% of the total oxygen consumed. For patients in congestive heart failure, the oxygen cost of breathing is doubled.

Efficiency of Breathing

For the mechanical work performed, the amount of oxygen required for ventilation is 10 to 20 times greater than that needed for a similar amount of work performed by other systems. The mechanical efficiency of the respiratory muscles is thus low and of the order of 5 to 10% at rest. Nevertheless, the respiratory system attempts to use a pattern that provides optimal alveolar ventilation with minimal expenditure of energy. The tidal volume in fact determines the work required to overcome elastic recoil on each breath. The flow rate determines the work to overcome airway resistance on each breath. As tidal volume increases, elastic work becomes greater, and as the rate becomes faster, the "resistive work" increases. Normal humans chose a combination of rate and volume that

performs the least work, namely, tidal volume of 400 ml at a rate of approximately 15 times per minute.[43]

Ventilatory Muscle[44]

The two types of muscle fibers found in the human ventilatory muscles are as follows:

Type I—Slow-twitch, high-oxidative, low-glycolytic capacity fibers with great endurance and resistance to fatigue. About one half of the fibers in the human diaphragm are of this type.

Type II—Fast-twitch fibers represent the other half and are of two subtypes.

A—high-oxidative, low-glycolytic capacity fibers that are resistant to fatigue and compose 20% of the fibers in the diaphragm.

B—Low-oxidative, high-glycolytic capacity fibers that fatigue easily and account for 30% of the fibers in the diaphragm.

The resistance of skeletal muscle to fatigue correlates with the type of muscle fiber and the proportion of high-oxidative fiber types.[44]

Development

The respiratory muscle fibers resisting fatigue develop gradually during gestation and this development continues post partum. Thus, the premature and newborn baby is easily subject to fatigue and tolerates respiratory loads poorly. Up to 30 weeks gestation, the fetus has few type I fibers.[45] Type I fiber development progressively increases until birth and during the 8 months to 1 year postpartum.[46]

In the diaphragm, before 37 weeks gestation, only approximately 10% of fibers are type I; in the full-term newborn, 25% of the fibers are of this type. A gradual increase in the proportion of type I fibers occurs during infancy, and by 8 months of age, it reaches 55%.[47] The intercostal muscles show a similar pattern of development. Premature infants have approximately 20% type I fibers and the full-term baby has approximately 45%; by 2 years of age, approximately 65% of the fibers are type I, and this proportion continues into adulthood. Premature and newborn infants are susceptible to fatigue until both diaphragm and intercostal muscles mature.

During sleep, an inhibition of intercostal muscle tone decreases the stability of the rib cage.[48] As a consequence, most of the work of the diaphragm is used to overcome rib cage distortion, and this muscle must work harder to maintain adequate tidal volumes.

Ventilatory support is necessary in the premature infant, and in early infancy, during general anesthesia of even short duration, decreases the extra effort usually needed to stabilize the chest during sleep.

Efficiency[49]

The work of the inspiratory muscles represents the primary "air pump" mechanism. The endurance of the respiratory muscles is determined by the type of fibers, the blood supply, and the force of contraction.[50] The diaphragm is the most important inspiratory muscle. As stated previously, the human diaphragm consists of approximately 50% slow-twitch (type I) fibers and approximately 20% fast-twitch (type IIa) fibers. Both have high-oxidative and low-glycolytic capacities and great endurance. The other type of fast-twitch fiber (IIB) is easily fatigued.

Diaphragmatic force is greatest near the normal breathing position. At high lung volumes, force decreases. The rate of contraction also plays a role in the development of the contractile force.[51] Experimentally, force is maximal when the phrenic nerve is stimulated at 100 Hz; at 50 Hz, the force of contraction is 94% maximal; at 20 Hz, 70%; and at 10 Hz, 25%. Normal phrenic nerve activity is approximately 15 Hz; doubling to 30 Hz produces a 50% increase in force. A neural drive of 50 Hz augments contractility to the most efficient level.[52]

The diaphragm as a whole becomes fatigued when the force of contraction demanded exceeds 40% of the maximal force that it can generate. Hypoxia, rapid respiratory rates, and breathing at high lung volumes (diaphragm fiber length shortened) diminish the force of contraction, decrease diaphragmatic endurance, and increase oxygen demand. In obstructive lung disease, lung volume is increased and diaphragmatic muscle fiber length decreases, which impose a mechanical disadvantage and decrease respiratory force. Fatigue from contracting against increased respiratory resistance may be at the muscle itself or at the neuromuscular junction. Hypoxia and hypercapnia hasten fatigue.[53]

Studies by Aubier and coworkers show that aminophylline in therapeutic doses enhances the contractile force of the human diaphragm by 15%.[54] This drug also antagonizes the fatigue of the diaphragm induced by inspiratory resistance loading, resulting in an increase in efficiency. The plasma level of theophylline (aminophylline is converted to theophylline) for therapeutic purposes is approximately 20 mg/ml, but most is protein bound and the free form is 50 μmol/L. The mechanism of the antifatigue action may be blockade of adenosine receptors with release of catecholamines, which enhance neuromuscular transmission.

Diaphragmatic Blood Supply

During normotensive states and spontaneous breathing, the blood flow to the respiratory muscle mass (5 kg in a 70-kg man) varies from 3 ml/100 g for intercostal muscle to 6 ml/100 g for the diaphragm (total 285 ml/min in a 70-kg man). This amount may represent 3 to 5% of the cardiac output.[55] During respiratory resistance loading and spontaneous breathing, the blood supply to the diaphragm may increase to 200 ml/100 g/min.

In hypotensive states and shock from any cause—oligemic, septic, or cardiac temporal[56]—the proportion of blood flow to the diaphragm increases, which reduces blood flow to other organs. In this distribution, the respiratory muscles may receive up to 20% of the cardiac output. The increased demand by the diaphragm and respiratory muscles is compensated to some extent by maintained blood flow at the expense of other organs. Thus, anaerobic metabolism with lactate production and metabolic acidosis ensues.

If the energy demands of the respiratory muscles exceed the actual blood supply, diaphragmatic fatigue ensues, with hypoventilation and hypoxia. Experimentally, such shock states may cause death from respiratory failure. Shock patients should be managed by paralysis, endotracheal tube placement, and mechanical ventilation. In experimental studies, these efforts lowered the fatality rate and improved outcome and prognosis.[57]

Energetics[53]

The respiratory muscles represent a vital pump function to supply the body with oxygen and to remove carbon dioxide. The mass of the respiratory skeletal muscles—the diaphragm and intercostals—is estimated at 5.0 kg in a 70-kg man. At resting breathing in a healthy man, the blood flow to these muscles is approximately one third of the blood flow of the total skeletal muscle mass of 30 kg, which is 850 ml/min. Thus, the blood flow to respiratory muscle is 285 ml/min. Flow to the diaphragm and inspiratory muscles occurs largely during relaxation (as with the heart, where blood flow occurs during diastole). Thus, each kilogram of respiratory muscle receives 57 ml of flow or 5.7 ml/100 g/min. The remainder of the skeletal muscles receive 2.26 ml/100 g/min. In terms of oxygen consumption at rest, the respiratory muscle mass requires 3.3 ml O_2/kg/min (16.5 ml O_2/min/5 kg). Other skeletal muscle requires less—approximately 1.3 ml/kg.

As part of its pump action, respiratory muscle contributes to its own oxygen requirements.[58] Pump failure may occur from any one of three major causes: (1) inadequate neurologic drive; (2) mechanical defects of chest wall or intrinsic passageway obstruction; or (3) reduction in energy capacity of respiratory muscles to meet the body's demands, causing fatigue.

Carbon Dioxide Effects

In the presence of hypercapnia, contractility of the diaphragm is reduced. The ability of the diaphragm to generate pressure, as shown by the time-tension index and electromyographic changes, is curtailed during hypercapnia (breathing 7.5% CO_2). Signs of fatigue appear and a decrease in endurance time of the diaphragmatic contractility occurs with acute respiratory acidosis.[59]

Hypophosphatemia[60]

Among the electrolytes affecting skeletal muscle activity is the phosphate ion. The lack of the phosphate ion produces significant respiratory muscle weakness in both the intercostal muscles and the diaphragm. The diaphragm is particularly susceptible to fatigue and weaning from mechanical ventilation may be difficult.[59]

Clinical Information

Conditions associated with hypophosphatemia and respiratory insufficiency include the following:[61] pre-existing wasting illness, cancer, anorexia nervosa, intestinal dysfunction, malnutrition, chronic obstructive lung disease, emphysema, respiratory failure, and induction by hyperalimentation.

The normal serum value of phosphate is set at 1.2 ± 0.10 mmol/L. When phosphate levels decrease below 1.0 mmol to the range of 0.5 to 0.8 (< 1.5 mg/dl) or less, transdiaphragmatic pressure is significantly reduced.[60]

Treatment[60,61]

Treatment of hypophosphatemia is carried out with the use of monopotassium (or sodium) phosphate, as KH_2PO_4, which is administered intravenously in a continuous infusion covering 2 to 4 hours. The dose is set at 10 mmol phosphorus, which, at the conclusion of administration, usually restores diaphragmatic contractility.

In difficult conditions of mechanical ventilation, it is particularly important to obtain phosphate levels of the plasma to be assured that the phosphate level is sufficient to maintain muscle strength. In the absence of adequate phosphorus, weaning is both difficult and prolonged.

Hyperphosphatemia also has an impact on respiratory gas exchange. The mechanism is in regard to oxygen saturation of hemoglobin. Excess PO_4 ions decrease the affinity of oxygen for hemoglobin in the lungs.[62]

Role of Plasma Lidocaine[63]

When lidocaine is administered intravenously for the purpose of controlling cardiac arrhythmias, a significant plasma level (between 2.0 and 5.0 μg/ml) is usually desired. Large doses of lidocaine solution administered in epidural anesthesia likewise provide a significant plasma lidocaine level, such that within 15 minutes, the plasma level is 1.8 μg and by 25 minutes, the plasma level is 2.25 μg/ml.

Studies by Labaille and colleagues are consistent with most of the studies on absorption of lidocaine from the epidural space. These authors demonstrated ventilatory stimulation in response to carbon dioxide at these levels of lidocaine. In their careful study of patients, they determined that the carbon dioxide ventilatory response curve is shifted to the left. In fact, the slope of the ventilatory response is increased by 20 to 40%; i.e., the response to carbon dioxide causes a significant increase in resting minute ventilation.

ALVEOLAR AIR MIXING

Alveolar Gas Law[1,64]

Consideration of the volume of gas that reaches the alveoli during normal inspiration reveals that it is only part of the total amount inspired. The other part is allocated to filling the tracheobronchial tree and is the dead space air. The air that actually reaches the alveoli may be determined by subtracting the dead space volume from the tidal volume. During the course of 1 minute, the amount of air that ventilates the alveoli and participates in gas exchange is the effective alveolar ventilation, which is equal to (Tidal volume [TV] − Dead space) × rate. For example, if dead space is 150 ml and the tidal volume is 350 ml with a respiratory rate of 15/min, effective alveolar ventilation = (350 − 150) × 15 = 3000 ml/min.

Additional factors may be involved in a precise mathematic calculation, but the essence of effective alveolar flushing is the above relationship and is basically the alveolar gas equation.

Alveolar Air Equation[1]

This equation has been used extensively to solve complex problems in gas exchange. The underlying principle is simple and the following is extracted from Comroe.

The equation states that, at sea level, the the total pressure of gases (O_2, CO_2, N_2, and H_2O) in the alveoli equals 760 mm Hg and that if the partial pressures of any three of these four are known, that of the fourth can be obtained by subtraction. Suppose, for example, it is desired to calculate the partial pressure of oxygen in alveolar gas at ambient conditions:

$$760 \text{ mm Hg} = P_{O_2} + P_{CO_2} + P_{N_2} + P_{H_2O}$$
$$-47 \text{ mm Hg } P_{H_2O}$$
$$\overline{713 \text{ mm Hg} = P_{O_2} + P_{CO_2} + P_{N_2}}$$
$$-563 \text{ mm Hg } P_{N_2} \text{ (assumed)}$$
$$\overline{150 \text{ mm Hg} = P_{O_2} + P_{CO_2}}$$
$$-40 \text{ mm Hg } P_{CO_2} \text{ (measured as arterial } P_{CO_2})$$
$$\overline{110 \text{ mm Hg} = P_{O_2}}$$

Inherent in the process of determining P_{O_2} by subtracting the P_{H_2O}, P_{CO_2}, and P_{N_2} are certain value measurements and assumptions.

First, the water vapor pressure at 37° C is approximately 47 mm Hg.

Second, values for arterial P_{CO_2}, which can be measured with reasonable accuracy (±2 to 3 mm Hg), are used as representative of mean alveolar P_{CO_2}. This is done because the arterial blood coming from all the alveoli approaches an integrated value of alveolar P_{CO_2} with respect to the different regions of the lung and to different times during the respiratory cycle. Further, carbon dioxide diffuses through body membranes so readily that its partial pressure in blood leaving any alveolus is always equal to its partial pressure in the gas of that alveolus. Although it is true that nonuniformity of alveolar ventilation with respect to alveolar capillary blood flow throughout the lung can produce a difference between the P_{CO_2} of mixed capillary blood and mixed alveolar gas in spite of diffusion equilibrium across any single individual alveolus, this difference is relatively small, except in the presence of extreme nonuniformity of alveolar ventilation/alveolar blood flow or large venous-to-arterial shunts.

Third, it is also assumed in the foregoing calculation that $P_{N_2} = 563$ mm Hg and is not metabolized or particularly diluted. This statement would be true if the respiratory quotient were 1.0, i.e., if the amount of carbon dioxide added to the alveoli were exactly equal to the amount of oxygen removed from the alveoli each minute; in this case, the inspired nitrogen would be neither diluted nor concentrated as it entered the alveoli, and alveolar P_{N_2} would equal moist inspired P_{N_2} (79.03% × 713 = 563 mm Hg). Actually, in most cases, more oxygen is removed per minute than carbon dioxide is added. The usual respiratory exchange ratio is

$$(R) = \frac{200 \text{ ml } CO_2/min}{250 \text{ ml } O_2/min} = 0.8 \; \frac{\dot{V}_{CO_2}}{\dot{V}_{O_2}},$$

which results in the nitrogen molecules being slightly more concentrated, because the same number of nitrogen molecules is now present in a smaller gas volume. If the alveolar nitrogen level rises to 81%, the alveolar P_{N_2} would rise to 577 and the alveolar P_{O_2} would fall to 96 mm Hg. It is therefore essential to calculate alveolar P_{N_2} accurately by determining the respiratory exchange ratio.

Finally, inspired carbon dioxide is zero and the only source of carbon dioxide in the alveoli is from the capillary blood.

Calculation of Composition of Alveolar Air (Alveolar Air Equation)

The determination of alveolar P_{O_2} and P_{CO_2} from analyses of a spot sample of expired alveolar gas is subject to considerable error. The mean alveolar P_{O_2}, however, can be calculated with reasonable accuracy. The basis for the calculation was outlined previously. The precise formula (assuming that inspired P_{CO_2} is zero) is:

$$\underset{\text{(unknown)}}{P_{A_{CO_2}}} = \underset{\text{(known)}}{P_{I_{O_2}}} - \underset{\text{(measured)}}{P_{A_{CO_2}}}$$

$$\underbrace{\left[FI_{O_2} + \frac{1 - FI_{O_2}}{R} \right]}_{\text{(correcting factor)}}$$

in which P_{IO_2} is inspired oxygen tension (moist); at sea level, this value is 20.93% of $(760 - 47) = 149$ mm Hg. The alveolar carbon dioxide (P_{AO_2}) tension assumed to be equal to arterial P_{CO_2}, and the latter is measured. The "correcting factor" introduces no correction when R, the respiratory exchange ratio $\dot{V}_2/\dot{V}_{O_2}$, 1.0.

If $R = 1$, the correcting factor is

$$\left[FI_{O_2} + \frac{1 - FI_{O_2}}{R} \right] = 0.2093 + \frac{1 - 0.2093}{1} = 1$$

Usually, R is less than 1.0 (the volume of oxygen absorbed exceeds the amount of carbon dioxide excreted), so that the volume of expired gas is slightly less than the volume of inspired air. This slight difference cannot be ignored if great accuracy is desired.

Thus, if $R = 0.8$, the usual respiratory quotient, the correcting factor is 1.2. The latter is calculated as follows:

$$\left[FI_{O_2} + \frac{1 - FI_{O_2}}{R} \right] = 0.2093 + \frac{1 - 0.2093}{0.8} = 1.2$$

When $R = 1.0$ and $P_{A_{CO_2}} = 40$ mm Hg, the correcting factor is 1.0, then, $P_{AO_2} = 109$ mmHg.
When $R = 0.8$ and $P_{A_{CO_2}} = 40 \times 1.2$ or 4g, the correcting factor is 1.2, then, $P_{AO_2} = 100$ mmHg.

Derivation of Alveolar Air Equation[1]

The actual derivation of the alveolar air equation follows. It is based on the knowledge that nitrogen is not metabolized in the body and that, under steady state conditions, the quantity of nitrogen entering the alveoli per minute in the inspired gas must equal the quantity leaving the alveoli each minute in expired gas.

$$\dot{V}_{AI} (1 - FI_{O_2} - FI_{CO_2}) = \dot{V}_{A_E} (1 - FA_{O_2} - FA_{CO_2}) \quad (1)$$

This equation is based on the fact that when oxygen, nitrogen, and carbon dioxide are the only gases present in the lungs (the gases here are measured as dry gases), the sum of their fractional concentrations must add up to 1.0. Therefore, $1 - F_{O_2} - F_{CO_2}$ must equal FN_2. Note that the volumes of alveolar ventilation on inspiration and on expiration are given different symbols ($\dot{V}_{A_I}$ and $\dot{V}_{A_E}$, respectively) because these volumes differ when R is less than or greater than 1.0. Because the number of nitrogen molecules must be the same in inspired and expired gas but the total volume of gas in which they are contained may change on expiration, it is obvious that FN_2 may be different in inspired and expired gas.

If we rearrange this equation,[1] considering FI_{CO_2} negligible when the patient breathes air,

$$\frac{\dot{V}_{A_I}}{\dot{V}_{A_E}} = \frac{1 - FA_{O_2} - FA_{CO_2}}{1 - FI_{O_2}} \quad (2)$$

The correction factor requires knowledge of $\dot{V}_{O_2}$ and $\dot{V}_{CO_2}$. Oxygen consumption ($\dot{V}_{O_2}$) equals the quantity of oxygen entering the alveoli in inspired gas less the quantity leaving the alveoli in expired gas.

$$\dot{V}_{O_2} = \dot{V}_{A_I} FI_{O_2} - \dot{V}_{A_E} FA_{O_2} \quad (3)$$

Carbon dioxide production ($\dot{V}_{CO_2}$) equals the quantity expired because no appreciable amount of carbon dioxide is inspired while the patient breathes air.

$$\dot{V}_{CO_2} = \dot{V}_{A_{E_F}} A_{CO_2} \quad (4)$$

Respiratory exchange ratio is

$$R = \frac{\dot{V}_{CO_2}}{\dot{V}_{O_2}} \quad (5)$$

Substituting equations 3 and 4 in equation 5 yields

$$R = \frac{\dot{V}_{A_E} FA_{CO_2}}{\dot{V}_{A_I} FI_{O_2} - \dot{V}_{A_E} FA_{O_2}} = \frac{FA_{CO_2}}{\left[\dfrac{\dot{V}_{A_I} FI_{O_2}}{\dot{V}_{A_E}} \right] - FA_{O_2}} \quad (6)$$

Substituting equation 2 in equation 6 yields

$$R = \frac{FA_{CO_2}}{\left[\dfrac{1 - FA_{O_2} - FA_{CO_2}}{1 - FI_{O_2}} \right] FI_{O_2} - FA_{O_2}} \quad (7)$$

Clearing and solving for FAO_2

$$FAO_2 = FIO_2 - FACO_2\left[FIO_2 + \frac{1 - FIO_2}{R}\right] \quad (8)$$

If PAO_2 is desired, the equation becomes

$$PAO_2 = FIO_2(713) - PACO_2\left[FIO_2 + \frac{1 - FIO_2}{R}\right] \quad (9)$$

Alveolar—Arterial Oxygen Difference [(A-a)O₂]

Ordinarily, in a subject breathing room air, the alveolar oxygen PAO_2 is higher than the arterial PaO_2, reflecting the normal anatomic shunt. The (A-a)O₂ difference is 5 to 6 mm Hg. If the FIO_2 is increased to 0.4 (40% oxygen), the difference is increased to 12 mm Hg, and with 100% oxygen, the difference is increased to 35 mm Hg. Indeed, the A-a DO₂ stabilizes at approximately 35 mm Hg when alveolar oxygen reaches 150 mm Hg.[4] When breathing high concentrations of oxygen, however, the A-a DO₂ may be higher than 35 mm Hg.

The A-a DO₂ is often used as an index of gas exchange and in shunt calculations, despite great variability and, in healthy young subjects breathing 100% oxygen, the A-a DO₂ may be as high as 190 mm Hg. Because A-a MD4DO₂ changes as FIO_2 changes, its usefulness to calculate and predict PaO_2 at any given FIO_2 is limited. It has been recommended that the arterial-to-alveolar oxygen partial pressure ratio is more stable and more useful in predicting and comparing gas exchange, especially when FIO_2 is greater than 0.3 and when PaO_2 levels are less than 100 mm Hg.[65]

Calculation of Arterial Oxygen Tension

Arterial oxygen tension PaO_2 can be closely predicted by the following calculation: the alveolar oxygen tension PAO_2 is calculated from alveolar air equations; the alveolar-arterial oxygen tension gradient, (A-a)O₂ Diff, is subtracted. The usual (A-a)O₂ gradients are as follows:

Breathing room air (A − a) difference	= 6 mm Hg
40% Oxygen	= 12 mm Hg
60% Oxygen	= 20 mm Hg
100% Oxygen	= 35 mm Hg

Relation of Alveolar PO₂ to PCO₂

The alveolar air equation has numerous applications. It essentially describes the relationships between the tensions of carbon dioxide and oxygen in the alveoli (and arterial blood). If other variables are constant, the alveolar carbon dioxide and oxygen tensions vary in opposite directions. A hyperbolic relation exists between ventilation and PAO_2 (Fig. 2–5).

When alveolar hyperventilation occurs, more oxygen is supplied than the metabolic rate may require. The alveolar and arterial oxygen pressure rises while the carbon dioxide level falls. If fresh air is continuously supplied and metabolic rate remains low, the alveolar PO₂ and PCO₂ approaches that of moist tracheal air, i.e., 149 mm

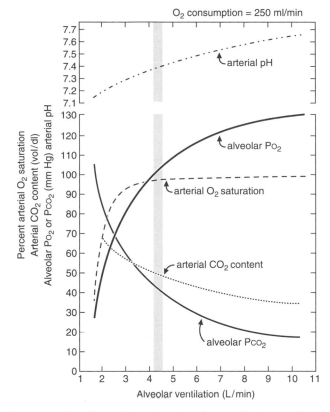

Fig. 2–5. The effect of changing alveolar ventilation on alveolar gas and arterial blood O₂, CO₂ and pH. Vertical hatched line represents values in a "normal" man with alveolar ventilation of 4.27 l/min, O₂ consumption of 250 ml/min and R (gas exchange ratio) of 0.8. NOTE: (1) When alveolar ventilation exceeds this value, alveolar and arterial PO₂ rise, but there is little increase in arterial O₂ saturation because Hb is almost maximally saturated at the PO₂ achieved by "normal" alveolar ventilation. (2) When alveolar ventilation decreases to less than 3 L/min, arterial O₂ saturation falls sharply because of the steep slope of the O₂ dissociation curve at this PO₂. (3) The line for blood CO₂ content, unlike that for arterial O₂ saturation, shows no abrupt inflection and is not flat until very high ventilations are achieved. Thus an increase in ventilation which is ineffective in increasing the O₂ saturation is effective in decreasing the CO₂ content. This chart applies approximately in a great variety of conditions. The lines apply exactly when (1) barometric pressure is 760 mm Hg, (2) O₂ consumption is 250 ml/min, (3) R is 0.8 and (4) gas tensions are the same in all alveoli and in the arterial blood. Redrawn from Comroe et al., The Lung, Mosby Year Book.

Hg for oxygen and 0.3 mm Hg for carbon dioxide (Table 2–3).

Bohr's Equation for Respiratory Dead Space[1]

Bohr's equation as it applies to a particular gas (g) is developed as follows:

Total volume of expired gas (VE) equals the volume of alveolar gas portion (VA) + volume of dead space portion (VD), or

$$VE = VA + VD \quad (1)$$

Expired gas is defined as the total volume of gas that leaves the nose and mouth between the onset and end of

Table 2–3. Effect of Normal, Increased and Decreased Alveolar Ventilation on Arterial Blood (Comroe et al.: The Lung, courtesy of Year Book Medical Publishers)

| Type of Ventilation | Alveolar Ventilation (L/min) | Alveolar and Arterial Gas Tensions* | | Arterial Blood Gas Contents | | Arterial pH Units |
		O_2 (mm Hg)	CO_2 (mm Hg)	O_2 (% sat.)	CO_2 (mM/L)	
Hypoventilation	2.50	67	69	88.5	27.2	7.24
Normal	4.27	104	40	97.4	21.9	7.40
Hyperventilation	7.50	122	23	98.8	17.5	7.56

*In each case, respiratory exchange ratio of 0.8 and O_2 consumption of 250 ml/min are assumed, and the values are calculated from the CO_2—O_2 diagram of Rahn and Fenn. It is also assumed that arterial and alveolar O_2 tensions are the same, although this would not be true in example 2 in which the alveolar PO_2 is low.
Conversely, hypoventilation results in anoxemia and CO_2 tension when the patient is breathing air. The administration of oxygen may improve the oxygenation of arterial blood but will not help to eliminate carbon dioxide, which may indeed be elevated. (From Comroe, J. H., et al.: *The Lung*. Chicago, Year Book, 1962.)

a single expiration. VA is used here to denote the volume of alveolar gas contributed to the expired gas and does not refer to the total volume of gas in the alveoli.

The amount of gas (g) in VE, VA, or VD is its fractional concentration, F_x, time the total gas volume in which gas x is contained. Therefore, as in (1)

$$FE_x \cdot VE = FA_x \cdot VA + FD_x \cdot VD \qquad (2)$$

The gas in the dead space at the beginning of expiration is inspired gas; therefore, $FD_x = FI_x$ and

$$FE_x \cdot VE = FA_x \cdot VA + FI_x \cdot VD \qquad (3)$$

Because the volume of the alveolar gas portion (VA) = volume of expired gas (VE) minus the volume of dead space gas (VD), equation 3 becomes:

$$FE_x \cdot VE = FA_x \cdot (VE - VD) + FI_x \cdot VD \qquad (4)$$

Algebraic rearrangement results in the following equation:

$$VD = \frac{[FA_x - FE_x] \cdot VE}{[FA_x - FI_x]} \qquad (5)$$

When the gas in question is carbon dioxide, equation 5 is simplified because inspired air contains practically no carbon dioxide and $FICO_2 = O$. Therefore:

$$VD = \frac{VE [FACO_2 - FECO_2]}{FACO_2} \qquad (6)$$
$$\text{BOHR EQUATION}$$

If alveolar and arterial carbon dioxide concentrations are equal ($FACO_2 = FaCO_2$) and we replace the concentrations by partial pressures, we have Enghoff modification:

$$VD = \frac{VE [PACO_2 - PECO_2]}{PaCO_2} \qquad (7)$$
$$\text{ENGHOFF EQUATION}$$

Diffusion[1,17]

The process of movement of gases across the alveolar-capillary membrane is that of diffusion. Several factors influence this transfer.

Surface Area of Diffusion

The surface area for pulmonary gas exchange has been estimated as 75 to 90 mm^2, approximately 50 times the total surface area of the body. It is important to realize the critical pulmonary surface area is actually the number of functioning alveoli in contact with functioning capillaries.

Distance of Diffusion

Gas molecules must pass through the following (Fig. 2-6):

1. Alveolar membrane
2. Interstitial fluid
3. Capillary endothelium
4. Plasma layer
5. Red cell membrane
6. Intracellular fluid

Passage through these layers is governed by physical laws of partial pressure of a gas, and the solubility of the gas in plasma membranes and in body fluids.

Tissue Characteristics

Changes in thickness of tissues (fibrosis) or presence of excess fluid alter rate of diffusion.

Diffusing Capacity[1]

The diffusing capacity of the lung is a measurement of the quantity of a gas that can be transferred across all structures from the alveolus to the hemoglobin molecule *per* unit time *per* unit area of alveolar surface. This capacity is designated as DL or total diffusing capacity of lung. Most tests of diffusion measure all the processes together. Carbon monoxide or oxygen are the usual test gases used. The units of expression are milliliters of oxygen or carbon monoxide transferred per minute for each millimeter of mercury of pressure difference for each gas across the lung. It is expressed in the following formula:

$$\frac{1}{D_L} = \frac{1}{D_M} + \frac{1}{\theta V_c}$$

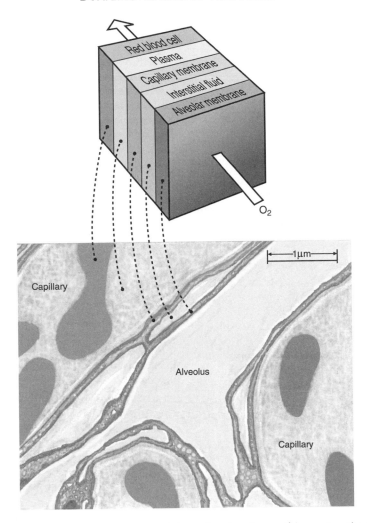

Fig. 2–6. Photograph of tissues through which oxygen passes from the alveolus until it reaches the red cell hemoglobin. Electron-microscopy of rat lung (×20,000). Redrawn after Low, Anatomical Record and Comroe et al., The Lung, Mosby-Year Book.

The rate of diffusion depends on four primary factors:

1. Character of gas—the difference in partial pressure between gas in the alveolus and in the plasma.
2. Distance of diffusion through several tissues—membrane variables (DM) of alveolar wall and capillary wall.
   a. Thickness of tissue.
   b. Surface area available.
   c. Membrane properties and diffusion coefficients of gas; solubility of gas; physiochemical properties.
3. The concentration of red cells in the pulmonary capillary bed and the average volume of blood in a capillary (V$_c$).
4. Rate of gas uptake by normal blood capillaries (θ) per average red cell per capillary volume per millimeters of mercury pressure.

In addition other variables are considered:
   a. Dco increases with body surface area.
   b. Maximal Do$_2$ diffusion capacity for o$_2$ decreases with advancing age.
   c. Dco is increased when lung volume is increased.
   d. Exercise increases Dco or Do$_2$.
   c. Dco is greater in the supine position.
   f. Differences in gas partial pressure and influence of other gases are important.
   g. Increased alveolar oxygen tension diminishes the carbon monoxide uptake and therefore gives low measurements. This is a test factor variable.
   h. Alveolar carbon dioxide tension when elevated usually increases Dco.
   i. Nonuniform blood distribution.

Values of Pulmonary Diffusing Capacity[1,66]

In experimental testing using a carbon monoxide technique and controlling most of the variables (supine breath method), the range of values for DLCO in healthy men is from 28 to 30 ml/min/mm Hg at rest and 34 to 36 ml/min/mm Hg with exercise.

A reduction in DM may be brought about by several conditions:

1. Alveolar-capillary block, early pulmonary fibrosis, interstitial edema.
2. Chronic obstructive emphysema decreases area for exchange.

3. Loss of pulmonary tissue (pneumonectomy; space-occupying lesions).
4. Vascular disorders with occlusion or obstruction of capillary bed.
5. Anemia—diminished number of red cells per cubic millimeter; decreased mean corpuscular hemoglobin volume (MCHV); decreased blood volume in capillary bed.

VENTILATION-PERFUSION RELATIONS

Concept

The major function of the respiratory system through the process of ventilation is to maintain the partial pressure of oxygen and carbon dioxide in the pulmonary alveoli and therefore in the pulmonary arterial blood at physiologic levels.

The major function of the cardiocirculatory system is to supply an adequate volume of blood to all tissues of the body to meet their total metabolic needs, and especially to supply oxygen and remove carbon dioxide. This gas-exchange function depends on the pulmonary-capillary circulation or pulmonary perfusion.

To effect a balanced relationship and permit pulmonary alveolar-capillary membrane equilibration, the two processes of the circulation and the ventilation should match each other appropriately (Fig. 2-7). Regional variations exist, however, and the differences are due largely to significant increasing perfusion as one progresses from top to bottom, whereas only slight increases in ventilation occur in the same direction. Thus, the distribution of ventilation and distribution of perfusion appear to be gravity dependent, and each process is considered separately.

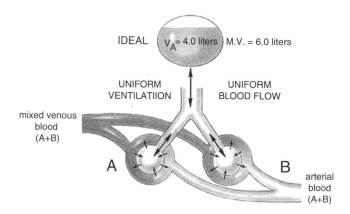

Fig. 2–7. Ideal Ventilation Blood Flow Relationship. Ideal case with uniform ventilation and uniform blood flow to all parts of the lungs. Total area of the rectangle signifies minute volume of ventilation, and shaded area, alveolar ventilation/min. Mixed alveolar gas (A + B) has the same P_{O_2} as gas in alveoli A and B. Mixed capillary blood (A + B) has the same P_{O_2} as blood in capillaries A and B. There is no alveolar-arterial P_{O_2} difference. (For the sake of simplicity, mixed blood from pulmonary capillaries A and B is called arterial blood; this is true only when there is no anatomical shunt from right to left.) Redrawn from Comroe, et al., The Lung, Mosby-Year Book.

Distribution of Ventilation

As early as 1934, Björkman,[67] using bronchospirometry, showed changes in both the partition of ventilation and difference in oxygen uptake between the lungs. The right lung accounts for 54% of the minute ventilation and the left lung for 46% (S. J. Ostrand) of the ventilation.[68] The ventilation is not uniform, however, and greater ventilation occurs in dependent compared with superior regions.[69]

A descriptive model of the differences of the changes in ventilation and gas composition of the alveolar gas and postcapillary pulmonary blood is that of West.[65] By using radioactive carbon dioxide and noting its disappearance and by xenon 133 distribution (the latter technique is particularly suitable for study of effects of changes in position of activity), absolute ventilation and perfusion values can be assigned to nine levels of the lung topographically (Fig. 2–8). The data demonstrate regional inhomogeneity as well as the influence of gravity on regional lung air volumes and alveolar size.

Alveoli in dependent lung regions are considerably smaller than superior alveoli, which is explained by the gradient in pleural pressure relative to a uniform alveolar pressure. Normally, the average intrapleural pressure is 7.5 cm H_2O. But the weight of blood in the lungs causes the intrapleural pressure to be more negative in the upper than in the lower pleural space. The pleural pressure shows a vertical gradient of 0.3 cm of water per centimeter. As a result of this pressure gradient, the apical lung (in the upright posture) is pulled out with more force than the basilar regions, so the upper lobe alveoli are held at a larger volume than the basilar alveoli. This situation can be viewed another way, because of a constant alveolar pressure associated with the changing intrapleural pressure, the transpulmonary pressure shows a decreasing vertical gradient of distending pressure. The highest net distending pressure is in upper alveoli and the lowest distending pressure is in the basal segments. A fourfold difference in volume may be noted (in dogs) between highest and lowest alveoli.

A second factor in air distribution is that of pulmonary compliance, which is greater at low lung volumes. Therefore, during inspiration, the additional negative intrapleural pressure will have a greater effect at the bases; i.e., the volume change per unit pressure change will be greatest at the base. During inspiration, the dependent smaller alveoli expand more per unit pressure than superior larger and already distended alveoli. In normal breathing, inspired gas is preferentially distributed to alveoli in dependent regions. In summary, a progressive, but slight increase in ventilation occurs from the superior to the lower portions of the lung.

Postural Effect on Ventilation[72]

When a subject is moved from the supine or erect posture to a lateral decubitus position, readjustments of ventilation and perfusion occur.[67]

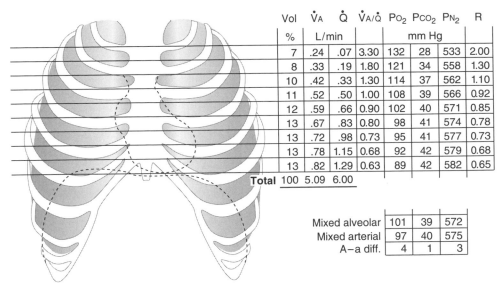

Vol	V̇A	Q̇	V̇A/Q̇	PO₂	PCO₂	PN₂	R
%	L/min				mm Hg		
7	.24	.07	3.30	132	28	533	2.00
8	.33	.19	1.80	121	34	558	1.30
10	.42	.33	1.30	114	37	562	1.10
11	.52	.50	1.00	108	39	566	0.92
12	.59	.66	0.90	102	40	571	0.85
13	.67	.83	0.80	98	41	574	0.78
13	.72	.98	0.73	95	41	577	0.73
13	.78	1.15	0.68	92	42	579	0.68
13	.82	1.29	0.63	89	42	582	0.65
Total 100	5.09	6.00					

Mixed alveolar	101	39	572
Mixed arterial	97	40	575
A–a diff.	4	1	3

Fig. 2–8. Effects of observed distribution of ventilation and perfusion on regional gas tension. The lung is divided into nine horizontal slices, and the position of each slice is shown by its anterior rib marking. Table shows relative lung volume (Vol.), ventilation (V̇A), perfusion (Q̇), ventilation-perfusion ratio (V̇A/Q̇), gas tensions (PO₂, PCO₂, PN₂) and respiratory exchange ratio (R) of each slice. Redrawn from West, J. B., J Appl Physiol.[70]

Adjustments in Adults

In the right lateral position (right lung dependent), changes are noted as follows:

1. The FRC of the right lung decreases from 55% of the total to 45%.
2. But the right lung takes a larger percentage of the tidal volume, with an increase from 53 to 57% to 62 to 68% of total.
3. Dead space of the right lung is reduced from 60 to 53% of the total.
4. The oxygen uptake (V̇O₂) by the right lung increases from a supine value of 52% of the total to 59 to 81% of the total. In the left lateral position (right lung uppermost), the oxygen uptake by the right lung decreases from the supine value of 52% to a range of 14 to 47% of the total.

Postural Adjustments in Infants

In contrast to the effect of position on pulmonary gas distribution in the adult, the infant shows better pulmonary gas exchange in the upper lung when placed in the lateral position. In the presence of unilateral pulmonary disease, oxygenation is better when the good lung is uppermost and the diseased lung is dependent. The proportion of ventilation to the good lung is greater when the good lung is uppermost. No significant changes with position are noted in the FRC, the tidal volume, or dynamic lung compliance in infants.[72]

Fractional Ventilation in Infants

Confirming the preceding information is the study of fractional ventilation using krypton 81m ventilation scanning in both infants and very young children up to the age of 1 to 2 years.[73] When the patients were supine, the mean fractional ventilation to the right lung was 56.6% ± 12.3. When the right lung was dependent, the fractional ventilation fell to 40.6% ± 16.8, and when the right lung was uppermost, the fractional ventilation rose to 69.9% ± 14.2.

Children with radiographic evidence of unilateral or bilateral parenchymal changes behaved identically, whether the affected lung was uppermost or dependent.[74] In either instance, the fractional ventilation of the affected lung increased from a dependent value of 29.0% to 45.0% when it was uppermost. Similarly, the fractional ventilation to the unaffected lung was 53.0% when it was dependent and rose to 70.0% when it was uppermost. Thus, in either the normal or the abnormal state, if the affected lung is placed in the upper position and is not dependent, overall ventilation is improved significantly.

Mechanism of Adjustment

In adults and older children, there is a resting negative pleural pressure attributable to the opposing elastic recoil of the lungs on the chest wall. This negative pleural pressure has a distending effect on the intrapulmonary tissues and helps to maintain the patency of peripheral intrapulmonary airways, but it is not uniformly distributed throughout the thorax. Thus, in the erect posture, the weight of the lungs distends the uppermost regions of the pulmonary system more than the dependent regions, creating a vertical intrathoracic pleural pressure gradient, with the most negative values in the uppermost portion of the pleura.[75]

In explanation of the differences between the adult and the infant and very young child, two factors are pertinent.[73] First, the chest of the infant is unstable when compared to that of the adult, and the resting pleural pressure in an infant is closer to atmospheric; hence, early closure of peripheral airways is more likely to occur in dependent lung regions. In the lateral decubitus posture, the pleural pressure in the dependent thorax approaches atmospheric pressure and airway closure is likely to occur. In turn, ventilation is distributed toward the uppermost portions of the lung.

A second feature is that of diaphragmatic function in the lateral decubitus postures, which differs in infants relative to the adult.[73] In the infant, little difference exists between the preload on the uppermost and that on the dependent hemidiaphragm because of the narrow abdominal cavity. Therefore, effects on the lungs and their fractional ventilation are minimal. The uppermost portions of the lung are well ventilated.

Distribution of Circulation[71]

Perfusion changes considerably more than ventilation as one progresses from apex to base. Gravity causes the largest portion of the right ventricular output to go to the lower lobes, a lesser amount to the middle zones, and the least amount to the apices.

The lung can be arbitrarily divided into three functional zones, designated as upper, middle and lower. This division is largely determined by the distribution of blood flow and to the effective pulmonary circulatory pressures.[77] There is a steady increase in blood flow from top to bottom of the lung in an erect human. The relative magnitudes of the pulmonary arterial and venous pressures to alveolar pressure is explained schematically (Fig. 2-9).

In zone 1, the arterial capillary (prealveolar) pressure is less than the alveolar pressure so that vessels are subject to collapse, resulting in minimal or no flow.

In zone 2, arterial pressure exceeds the alveolar pressure, but the alveolar pressure exceeds the venous pressure and produces some impedance at the outflow side of the alveolus. Blood flow is thus determined by arterial pressure minus the alveolar pressure to which the vessels are exposed. Because arterial capillary pressure increases linearly as one progresses from upper lung levels to lower levels owing to hydrostatic gradient, a linear increase in flow occurs from above downward. A steady increase in blood flow occurs in regional levels from top to bottom of lung in an erect human.

In zone 3, venous pressure exceeds alveolar pressure and flow is determined by the alveolar-venous difference. Because the transmural pressure is increasing from above downward in this zone, the more dependent vessels have a larger caliber, and flow increases linearly.

Ventilation-Perfusion Ratios

The interaction of these two factors produce a series of ventilation/perfusion ($\dot{V}/\dot{Q}$) ratios throughout the lung. In normal resting man, the alveolar ventilation is approximately 4.0 L/min, (MV—6.0 L/min), and the pulmonary blood flow is approximately 5.0 L/min. Therefore, the overall $\dot{V}/\dot{Q}$ ratio is 0.8 for ventilation perfusion (Fig. 2-10).

At the apices, a small amount of air is distributed, but it is greatly in excess of the blood flow so that the $\dot{V}/\dot{Q}$ ratio is high. In the middle lung zones, the quantity of air inspired and the blood flow are nearly equal, so that the $\dot{V}/\dot{Q}$ ratio is nearly 1.0. In the lower lung zones, blood flow is large compared with air distribution and the ratio is less than 1.0. The $\dot{V}/\dot{Q}$ ratios range from 3.3 at the top of the lung to approximately 0.6 at lowest lung zones.

Matching of V and Q-Positional[43]

Gravity affects pulmonary blood flow and ventilation. With respect to blood flow, gravity causes a vertical gradient of pressure downward so that the bases or the dependent parts of the lung are favored with flow.[76] With respect to ventilation in the normal lung, a vertical gradient of pleural pressure also exists so that ventilation is favored in the dependent parts. This ventilation effect is related to the design and structure of the lungs. In the upper portions of the lung, the alveoli are relatively distended so that at their level of inflation, compliance is decreased.[70] Conversely, the lower alveoli are smaller and not greatly distended; therefore, their compliance is greater and when inspiratory forces are imposed, they are distended more easily. Also, neurochemical and reflex factors enhance ventilation of lung bases because of the stimulus of the increased blood flow.

Lung disease alters the normal anatomic relationship. In left ventricular failure with interstitial edema, blood flow is diverted from the lung base and redistributed to upper areas. Mismatching occurs in interstitial fibrosis

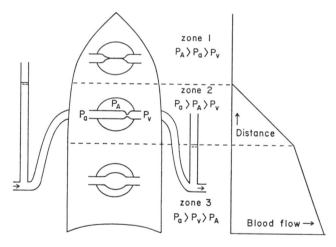

Fig. 2–9. Diagram to explain the topographical distribution of blood flow in the lung. The lung is divided into 3 zones by the relative magnitudes of the pulmonary arterial, venous, and alveolar pressures. In zone 1, arterial pressure is less than alveolar, and there is no flow presumably because collapsible vessels are directly exposed to alveolar pressure. In zone 2, arterial pressure exceeds alveolar, but alveolar exceeds venous. Here the vessels behave like Starling resistors and flow is proportional to the difference between arterial pressure (which is increasing down the lung) and alveolar pressure (which is constant). In zone 3, venous pressure exceeds alveolar and flow is determined by the arterial-venous difference. Flow increases down this zone because the transmural pressure of the vessels increases so that the vessels have a larger caliber. However, it is not surprising that the slopes of zones 2 and 3 are dissimilar, since they are caused by different mechanisms. Reprinted with permission from West, J. B., J Appl Physiol.

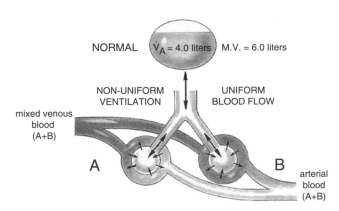

Fig. 2–10. Ventilation/Blood Flow Relationship in Normal Man—This differs from the "ideal" in that there is some uneven ventilation. Blood flow may also be uneven in normal individuals. The degree of uneven ventilation present is responsible for an alveolar-arterial PO_2 difference of approximately 4.0 mm Hg; the remainder of the normal PO_2 difference is due to anatomical shunts, which are ignored in this illustration (arterial blood assumed to be the identical to mixed blood from the pulmonary capillaries). Redrawn from Comroe, J. Jr., et al. The Lung. Mosby-Year Book.

and in obstructive lung disease. When parenchymal disease is diffusely and equally distributed to each side, arterial oxygen tension is higher when the right lung is dependent (lateral position). This situation is observed in patients with atelectasis or pneumonia.[78]

In patients with unilateral lung disease, improvement in oxygenation occurs when the diseased lung is uppermost. Remolina and colleagues found an average increase of 29 mm Hg of arterial oxygen tension when the "good" lung is dependent.[74] Hence, the rule "down with the good lung."[79]

Clinical Abnormalities (Fig. 2–11)

Actual abnormal ratios may be classed as increased or decreased. Conditions in which an increased ratio exists (inadequate perfusion or uneven blood flow) include the following:

1. Pulmonary embolism
2. Ligation of pulmonary artery or branches
3. Reduction of capillary vascular bed shunts; emphysema (extensive fibrosis)
4. Hyperventilation (inhalation of 5% carbon dioxide)

On the other hand, a decreased ratio (inadequate ventilation or uneven ventilation) can exist in the following:

1. Regional obstruction to ventilation, as in cysts, asthma, peribronchial and intrabronchial pathology; obstructive emphysema
2. Regional changes in elasticity
3. Reduction in alveolar bed (restricted expansion), atelectasis, pneumothorax, compression by tumors, congestion, fluid exudate in alveoli
4. Hyperventilation

In some situations, diffusion between the mixed alveolar gas and the mixed venous capillary blood are also important. Besides hypoxia resulting from inadequate perfusion and that from inadequate ventilation, one also recognizes hypoxia related to disorders of diffusion. The latter can usually be corrected by breathing oxygen.

Thus, abnormal variation in the ratio may be brought about by uneven ventilation, uneven blood flow, or diffusion derangements.

In clinical situations, respiratory insufficiency (RI) and respiratory failure (RF) are brought about by increased shunting, increased dead space, increased work of breathing, and decreased oxygen transport.

In a cancer-containing lung or lobe, there is a disproportionate reduction in pulmonary function.

Pulmonary Shunt[43]

A shunt is defined as that part of cardiac output that does not participate in pulmonary blood-gas exchange.

As blood traverses the pulmonary circuit, some bypasses the gas exchange surfaces. This pulmonary physiologic shunt, or venous admixture effect, is attributable to certain constant anatomic pathways, and also to a variable amount of ventilation-perfusion inequality (Fig. 2–12). Subdivisions of the physiologic shunt, as indicated by Bendixen,[81] are as follows:

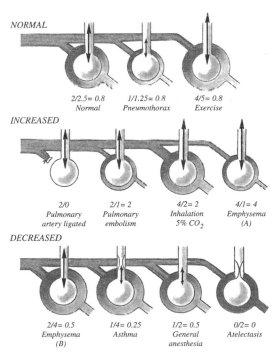

Fig. 2–11. Clinical abnormalities in ventilation/blood flow ratios. Each circle represents one lung with its pulmonary capillary blood flow. Redrawn from Comroe, J. Jr., et al.: The Lung. Mosby-Year Book.

Constant shunt
Anatomic shunt ($\dot{Q}s_{anat}$)
   Bronchial veins
   Pleural veins
   Thebesian veins
Total shunt ($\dot{Q}s_{phys}$) Abnormal arteriovenous communications
Variable shunt
Capillary shunt ($\dot{Q}s_{cap}$)
   Atelectasis
   Uneven distribution of $\dot{V}_A$ and $\dot{Q}$
   Diffusion gradient

The anatomic shunt does not exceed 2% of the cardiac output in normal subjects. When pathologic pathways exist (intrapulmonary anastomoses or intracardiac right-to-left shunts), the anatomic shunt may cause arterial hypoxemia when breathing air.

Atelectasis (miliary, alveoli, plate-like) is used to define gas exchange units that are not ventilated. This situation is in contrast to the classic clinical picture of atelectasis (lobular or segmental) in which there is a superimposed infiltration. The mechanism of physiologic atelectasis may be a bronchial occlusion with absorption of trapped gases; primary air space collapse as in small alveoli that are completely emptied at the end of expiration. If these units are perfused, increased physiologic shunting results.

Mismatching of alveolar ventilation and of perfusion can produce a shunt effect. Mixing of inspired gas in the lung is at best neither uniform nor complete. Uneven ventilation or underventilation may produce a shunt when air or a gas mixture with a "third inert gas" is present. Breathing 100% oxygen in patients who are hypoventilating or in patients with emphysema, fibrosis, obesity, and mitral disease clear up a shunt seen when air is breathed. In atelectasis, however, breathing 100% oxygen will not have a significant effect on the shunt.

Diffusion block, in which pulmonary gases are impeded in their passage from alveoli to red cell or vice versa, is rare. Most clinical situations are related to a severe maldistribution of ventilation to perfusion. Diffusion capacity, which includes the area factor, is more often related to atelectasis or decreased perfusion.

Shunt Equation[43,81]

In the presence of a shunt, a negative gradient in oxygen content exists between end-pulmonary blood and systemic arterial blood: the systemic arterial blood has a lower oxygen content than the pulmonary end-capillary blood, or the systemic arterial oxygen tension is lower than either the pulmonary end-capillary tension or the alveolar oxygen tension, i.e. an (A-a) O_2 tension difference exists (Fig. 2–13).

From the Fick principle, it follows that the ratio of the pulmonary physiologic shunt to cardiac output may be represented by the classic shunt equation:

$$\frac{\dot{Q}s}{\dot{Q}t} = \frac{C\acute{c}o_2 - Cao_2}{C\acute{c}o_2 - C\bar{v}o_2}$$

Arterial and mixed venous blood can be obtained so that Cao_2 and $C\bar{v}o_2$ may be measured. They are often derived indirectly from electrode measurements of oxygen tension, pH, base excess, and the hemoglobin content after reference to a standard oxyhemoglobin dissociation curve to obtain oxygen saturation.

Pulmonary end-capillary samples are unobtainable. But the assumption is made that nonshunted blood ($\dot{Q}t-\dot{Q}s$) is

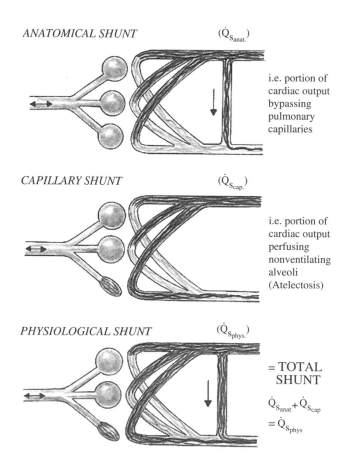

ANATOMICAL SHUNT   ($\dot{Q}_{S_{anat.}}$)

i.e. portion of cardiac output bypassing pulmonary capillaries

CAPILLARY SHUNT   ($\dot{Q}_{S_{cap.}}$)

i.e. portion of cardiac output perfusing nonventilating alveoli (Atelectosis)

PHYSIOLOGICAL SHUNT   ($\dot{Q}_{S_{phys.}}$)

= TOTAL SHUNT

$\dot{Q}_{S_{anat}} + \dot{Q}_{S_{cap}}$
= $\dot{Q}_{S_{phys}}$

Fig. 2–12. Subdivisions of the physiological shunt. Redrawn from Bendixen, Respiratory Care, C. V. Mosby Co.

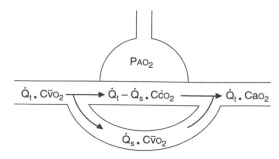

Fig. 2–13. Schematic shunt. Permits visualization of factors for calculation of amount of shunt on Fick principle. Redrawn from Leigh, Anesthesiology.

in ideal equilibrium with alveolar gas so that the ideal alveolar oxygen tension is equal to pulmonary end-capillary tension. A healthy subject has practically no alveolar to end-capillary P_{O_2} gradient when breathing room air. The alveolar oxygen tension is then used to calculate the pulmonary end-capillary content indirectly. The "end-capillary" $\dot{P}_{O_2}$ is really a contrived P_{O_2}.

The final value of $\dot{Q}_s/\dot{Q}_t$ is that of the "physiologic shunt," which includes not only anatomic shunts, but also the capillary shunt or a quantity of blood coming from regions with a low ventilation/blood flow ratio as well as nonventilated but perfused alveoli (pulmonary shunt) (Table 2-4).

The quantity of blood flowing through the anatomic shunt can be revealed by allowing a patient to breathe 100% oxygen for a period long enough (10 minutes) to wash out all the nitrogen from alveoli. Alveolar P_{O_2} is then 760—PA_{H_2O} − PA_{CO_2} or approximately 673 mm Hg, and is the same in all ventilated alveoli. With such there is no alveolar to end-capillary gradient and the influence of ventilation-perfusion inequalities is eliminated, i.e. poorly ventilated but perfused alveoli.

Therefore, the $P(A\text{-}a\ D_{O_2})$ reflects "true" physiologic shunt. The "true" physiologic shunt now includes perfused but nonventilated alveoli plus anatomic shunt.

When PA_{O_2} is high enough to ensure full saturation ($FI_{O_2} = 100\%$), and is uniformly distributed throughout patent alveoli, the shunt equation can be expressed in tensions and simplified as follows (see Leigh for simplified equations):[83]

$$\dot{Q}_s/\dot{Q}_t = \frac{P(A-a\ D_{O_2}) \times 0.0031}{P(A-a\ D_{O_2} \times 0.0031 + C(a-\bar{V}\ D_{O_2})} \times 100$$

in which .0031 is the factor converting tension to content; only two measurements are needed, i.e., the tensions of arterial blood and the oxygen content of mixed venous blood of a pulmonary artery sample.

Table 2–4. Common Causes of the Components of Total Physiologic Shunt

---

Anatomic shunt
  Bronchial veins
  Pleural veins
  Thebesian veins
Capillary shunt
  Atelectasis
  Consolidating pneumonia
  Pneumothorax
  Complete airway obstruction
Ventilation/perfusion inequalities
  Partial airway obstruction
  Regional increases in fibrotic tissue
  Decreased tidal volumes
  Bronchiolar mucosal edema

(After Dimas, S. and Kaemarek, R. M., in Shapiro, B. A., Harrison, R. A., and Walton, I. R.: *Clinical Applications of Blood Gases.* Chicago, Year Book.)

CLEARING OF THE RESPIRATORY TRACT

The prevention and resolution of material accumulating in the tracheobronchial tree is based upon the natural capacity to remove foreign material and accumulated natural secretions, which is accomplished by mucus production and transport, ciliary action, peristaltic movement of the bronchi and trachea, and the cough reflex.

Respiratory Tract Mucus

One of the chief defenses of the respiratory tract against inhaled particulate matter and other pollutants is respiratory tract mucus. It is secreted throughout the respiratory tract, from the nose through the peripheral airways as far as the cartilaginous bronchi. Several types of cells are responsible for mucus secretion, but goblet cells located in the submucosal glands contribute most to this production. The volume of mucus-producing cells, aggregated in the submucosal glands, is normally approximately one third of the volume of the epithelial wall. Other cells may be stimulated to secrete mucus under abnormal conditions of irritation. In bronchitis, the volume of mucus-secreting cells increases to one half or more of the epithelial wall.[84]

Neural mechanisms and a direct chemical effect control mucus secretion.[85] Vagal stimulation causes the submucosal glands to empty mucus into the respiratory tract. Irritation of the mucosa by chemicals or pollutants also stimulates secretion of mucus by goblet cells and recruits other cells to secrete mucus.

Composition and Production

The composition of mucus is mostly water (95%) with approximately 1% glycoprotein, which confers the fundamental property to the mucus.[86] These long peptide chains with short-branched side chains tend to become intrinsically entangled. Ordinarily, mucus exists in solid state, but when compressed or agitated, adjacent molecules may join by disulphide bridging. The mucus then enters into a gel state and takes on elastic properties. Ciliary action appears to be essential to form the gel state by moving the mucus blanket on the epithelial surface and entangling foreign particles. The pH of mucus varies between 7.4 and 8.2 and is in equilibrium with carbon dioxide. It possesses, thereby, a buffering capacity.

The daily production of mucus is approximately 100 ml from the nose and another 100 ml from the remainder of the tracheobronchial tree, under normal circumstances. Ordinarily, a total of approximately 2.0 ml of mucus is distributed at any moment over the epithelium in a thin (0.5 μm) sheet.[87]

Continuous production of mucus into the blanket on the epithelial surface maintains movement and the blanket is moved steadily toward the larynx by the steady beat of the cilia. The beat frequency of cilia is approximately 20 per second and thus maintains the mucus in an agitated and compressed or gel state, which traps particles.

Some pathologic changes in mucus composition are especially noted in asthmatics, smokers, and individuals with chronic bronchitis. In asthmatics, the mucus contains more glycoprotein than normal; the pH is low and varies between 7.0 and 5.3. This acidic mucus increases the viscosity as well as the buffering capacity.[88]

Rate of Transport[89]

Animal studies show that the rate of mucus transport increases progressively from distal to proximal airways.[90,91] Transport can be diminished by increasing viscosity of the serous fluid layer over the cilia or by diminishing the depth of this layer. Aspirin in modest single doses (16 mg/kg) significantly decreases lung mucociliary clearance and the tracheal mucociliary transport rate. The removal of inhaled particles, bacteria, and cellular debris by the mucociliary system is an important clearance function.[89]

Cilia

Structure (Fig. 2–14)

Electron microscopy of normal cilia in cross section reveals a highly organized configuration of microtubules.[92] Nine peripheral pairs of microtubules surround a central doublet, which are interconnected by elements designed as dynein arms and radial spokes. Motility is accomplished by a bending motion of the ciliary shaft accomplished by sliding of the peripheral microtubules.[93] The ciliary shafts are related to one another by an alignment of these central microtubules, which provides a synchronized action.[94] The structure of respiratory epithelial cilia is the same in the cilium of a spermatozoa.[93]

Various defects of the cilia may be acquired. These defects are especially evident in the nasal epithelium of children consequent to acute viral upper respiratory tract infections.[95]

Action[89]

Cilia are minute hairs found on the cells of membranes lining the nasal and respiratory passages. Examination of the motion of cilia reveals a similarity to a wind-blown field of hay. The individual cilium bends suddenly in one direction like a whip. The point of bending appears like a lever or joint. The cilium straightens gradually. Thus, the major force of ciliary motion is in one direction. The rate of ciliary beating is approximately 1200 to 1500 per minute.[89] The concerted action of moving cilia results in a significant force capable of carrying appreciable weights of material. For good function, the viscosity or stickiness of the material in contact with cilia must not be too great. Thus, dehydration impairs their motion. Action is depressed by cold and by most anesthesia.

The work performed by ciliated frog membrane (pharynx) for example is astonishing. If a flat piece of cork is placed on the membrane and various weight is applied, it is carried a distance of 1½ cm in rapid order as follows:[90]

Weight Moved	Time	Work
20 mg	6.0 sec	30 ergs
50 mg	7.0 sec	75 ergs
100 mg	13.0 sec	150 ergs

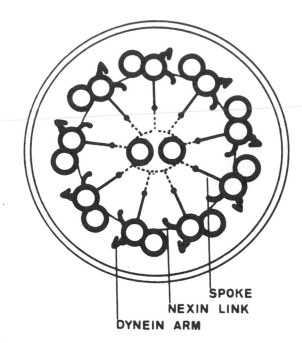

Fig. 2–14. Diagram of the cross-section of a cilium or of the central portion of a sperm tail. The assembly of the nine outer microtubular doublets and the two central microtubules is held together by three kinds of connections: the dynein arms, the nexin links and the spokes. The dynein arms are believed to be responsible for the motility. Redrawn from Eliasson, N Engl J Med 297:1, 1977.

Effects of Drugs on Ciliary Action

The effect of various drugs on ciliary activity is of importance in the clearing of the respiratory tract.

Hibnia and Curreri showed that a therapeutic dose of morphine reduces ciliary motion by 60%. Thus, the number of beats of cilia are reduced from 1500 per minute to 500 per minute.[96]

Explants of human respiratory ciliated epithelium have been cultured in a plasma clot and effects of added chemicals were studied. Such explants tend to round up and form a rotating globe in the culture chamber. Perfusion of the chamber with various solutions reveals the following:[97,98]

Acetylcholine 0.1 to 1.0%
   Increases rotary motion
   Smaller concentrations have no effect
Acetylcholine 2.5 to 5.0%
   Causes progressive depression and arrest at higher concentration
Physostigmine concentrations .001 to 0.5%
   Cause an initial slight stimulation followed by depression for 30 minutes and then stimulation
Atropine sulfate concentrations 0.01%
   Show stimulatory action followed by a return to a normal level of activity. Higher concentrations first stimulate, then cause reversible arrest.
Local anesthetic depressant effect

The degree of depression varies with the drug and its concentration. Procaine and lidocaine produce the least depression, which is reversible at all concentrations up to 20%. Pontocaine and dibucaine produce the greatest depression when in small concentrations of 0.1%; higher concentrations may cause irreversible depression.

Functional Activity [98]

Observations of functional activity can be carried out using a frog preparation. By dividing the lower jaw of a pithed frog and carrying the incision to the esophagus, an area containing ciliated epithelium is obtained. The flaps formed are set aside and the mucous membrane is kept moistened by Ringer's solution. A thin piece of cork can be used as a shuttle for carrying weights from one point on the membrane to another. Charcoal sprinkled at one point can be observed microscopically and grossly to move in the proper direction.

Movements of the Tracheobronchial Tree[99]

In large measure, the zones of expansibility are allied to the movements of the tracheobronchial tree.

As the chest expands on inspiration, the root of the lung descends and moves forward and laterally. The bronchial arborization at this time elongates and increases in diameter. The trachea also lengthens and dilates while the apex of the lung tends to descend. This occurrence allows segments of pulmonary tissues located between various bronchi to expand.

Although the trachea stretches and widens during quiet inspiration, the glottis tends to narrow slightly. Thus, the watchdog mechanism is altered. During passive expiration, the arborizations shorten and narrow.

Bronchial Peristalsis

The anatomic structure of the bronchiolar system has been described by Miller in Chapter 1. The segmental bronchi and small bronchi in man are built in spirals, with a rich but ever-decreasing cartilaginous framework. These spirals are unrolled during respiration. Bands of smooth muscle and of elastic fibers are richly distributed to provide contraction and relaxation and to withstand pressure maximally.[99]

Luminal changes are of fundamental importance. The bronchiolar and tertiary bronchial muscles relax and lengthen during inspiration; they contract and foreshorten during expiration. These changes are passive but depend on two factors: (1) volume changes of the whole lung (static factor) and (2) pressure difference inside and outside bronchi (dynamic factor). With enlargement of the thoracic cage, the pleural pressure decreases and causing particularly the large and intermediate size bronchi to widen. Also with the volume enlargement of the lung is radial traction on the small bronchi and bronchioles so as to enlarge their lumina.[100]

Peristalsis of the bronchiolar tree has been clearly described by Fleischer.[101] Using bronchographic techniques, wavelike bands of contraction can be seen to pass from the periphery toward the trachea. The action mimics that of the intestinal tract. The movements apparently assist in the removal of foreign material.

Respiratory Tract Reflexes[102]

A variety of reflexes originate in the respiratory tract. They are typical reflexes with an afferent path, central nervous system coordination, and an efferent path producing motor effects (Fig. 2-15).

These reflexes are designed to protect the lungs from environmental interference and to maintain the normal pattern of breathing. Any disturbance modifies respiratory activity and evokes adjustments (Table 2-5).

Cough Mechanism[100]

Definition of Cough Act

Coughing is a reflex with a stimulus and response resulting in the explosive removal of material from the tracheobronchial tree.

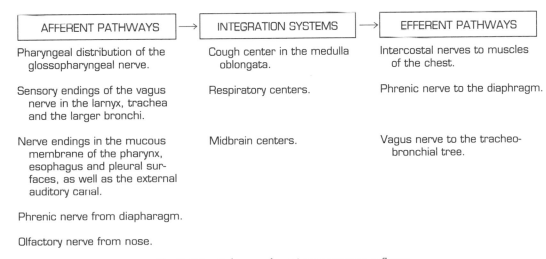

Fig. 2–15. Scheme of respiratory system reflexes.

Table 2–5. Summary of Effects of Reflexes from the Respiratory System (Widdicombe, J. G., courtesy Anesthesiology.)

Reflex	Responses			
	Respiratory	Blood Pressure	Heart Rate	Bronchomotor
Hering-Breuer inflation	Inspiratory inhibition	? Hypertension	? Tachycardia	? Dilation
Hering-Breuer deflation	Inspiratory stimulation	? Hypotension	? Bradycardia	? Constriction
Head's paradoxical inflation	Inspiratory stimulation	Unknown	Unknown	Unknown
Nasal irritation	Apnea	Hypertension	? Bradycardia	Constriction
Tracheal mechanical irritation	Cough	Unknown	Unknown	Constriction
Pulmonary chemical irritation	Hyperpnea	? Hypotension	? Bradycardia	Constriction
Multiple pulmonary embolism	Apnea and rapid shallow	Hypotension	Bradycardia	Constriction

(From Widdicombe, J. G.: Clinical significance of reflexes from the respiratory system. Anesthesiology, *23*:434, 1962.)

The cough reflex is initiated chiefly by stimuli applied to the mucosa of the tracheobronchial tree. Mechanical irritation of the pharynx, tracheobronchial tree, pleura, pericardium, and diaphragm is the most common cause. Postnasal drip, cigarette smoking, chronic obstructive lung disease, and hyperventilation from exercise are also effective stimuli. In anesthesia practice, common causes of both bronchoconstriction and coughing is the inhalation of dry air, especially cold, dry air.

Neurologic Paths[103]

The afferent impulses travel over the superior laryngeal nerve and the vagus to the medulla oblongata. Here integration occurs and efferent impulses pass to various respiratory muscles. Hypoxia sensitizes this reflex.

Description of Cough Act

The act itself consists of three phases:[104] (1) inspiratory, (2) compressive (tussic), and (3) expulsive (bechic).

A strong, deep inspiratory act creates a large negative intrapleural pressure and a large lung volume change up to four times the volume at expiration. The diaphragm contracts strongly to form a rigid floor and simultaneously the glottis closes tightly. The inspired air is thus entrapped.[100]

The thoracic and accessory respiratory muscles contract and squeeze the lung tissue for approximately one-fourth of a second to compress the contained air. This action is called the tussic squeeze. The interpleural pressure is raised to a high level of 100 to 150 mg Hg and the intrapulmonary pressure is similarly raised. Because the lung is an elastic organ, pressure adjustments occur toward a uniform distribution. Such adjustment occurs also in the bronchioles and bronchi. As soon as it reaches a maximum, the glottis opens the respiratory and abdominal muscles continue to contract, and the compressed air is expelled with a semiexplosive force. The expulsion is aided by a strong lung elastic record as the glottis opens.

In the initial phase, the "pressure" in the large bronchi is lower than in the bronchiolar system. The surrounding tissue pressure also compresses the bronchi and narrows them. The trachea is also narrowed (Fig. 2-16). Thus, a greater speed of air flow is achieved. A volume air flow of 12 L/sec is usual and is called the bechic blast. This blast of air passes through the glottis at a velocity of approximately 150 to 360 ft/sec and carries any loose or foreign material with it (Fig. 2-16).

The effectiveness of a cough depends, therefore, on the velocity of air flow. A greater speed of air flow creates a shearing force, which aids in the expulsion of mucus and foreign matter.[105] In a normal subject, the maximal expiratory flow rate in a vigorous cough approaches 9.8 L/sec. During various disease states, this rate is naturally decreased. In pulmonary emphysema, maximal expiratory flow rates approximate 3000 ml/sec; in poliomyelitis, a similar rate is obtained even with most vigorous effort.

Mechanical Cough[105,106]

Expiratory flow rates surpassing the capacity of human coughing may be mechanically produced. The principle involved is that of explosive decompression. The first step is to inflate the patient's lungs; when inflation is maximal, sudden termination of this step is followed by active deflation. A patient's lungs are inflated by application of positive tracheobronchial pressure up to 40 mm Hg using, a face mask. To achieve full inflation and dilatation of the bronchial tree, pressure is applied over a period of 1.5 to 2.5 seconds. Termination of the pressure then uses the relaxation pressure of the elastic lung and surrounding structures to empty the lungs of a

TRACHEA DURING NORMAL BREATHING

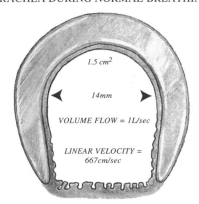

TRACHEA DURING COUGH

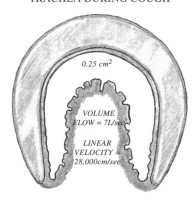

Fig. 2–16. Tracheal air velocity during cough. A, Contours and dimensions of trachea during normal breathing. B, During cough, the positive intrathoracic pressure inverts the noncartilaginous part of the intrathoracic trachea and decreases its cross-sectional area to ⅙ of normal. This, added to a 7-fold increase in flow rate, increases the linear velocity 42-fold. Redrawn from Olsen, J Appl Physiol.

large volume of air. If the termination of the positive pressure is abrupt, i.e., in approximately 0.04 second and accompanied by a decreasing negative pressure + 040 mm Hg below atmosphere, the expiratory air flow velocity will be high. This process is called exsufflation with negative pressure. The velocity of the current of air at the peak of expiration is as high as those currents produced by a normal subject during a maximal normal cough, which may reach between 8 and 10 L/sec. This type of mechanical cough enables a patient to eliminate secretions with minimal effort.

Barach and coworkers evaluated the effect of mechanical cough on intragastric pressure.[105] They determined the peak pressure is not as high as with natural cough and therefore is safe postoperatively (Fig. 2–17).

Hiccoughs (Singultus)107

The treatment of hiccoughs during general anesthesia includes inhalation of carbon dioxide, deepening anesthesia, increases in the dosage of morphine or meperidine (Demerol), and administration of muscle relaxants to paralyze the diaphragm. Methylamphetamine and amyl-nitrite, and recently metoclopramide, have been used but have not been effective. In the postoperative period, phrenic nerve block has been used. Kumar and Mehta found that droperidol in doses of 5 mg has been successful in stopping hiccoughing during anesthesia.[107]

Sighing

Normal breathing has an irregular pattern whereby both depth and rate are influenced by position and activity. The sigh has been defined by Bendixen[108] as "a breath having a volume three or more times larger than the mean tidal volume." It is a slow-deep inspiration followed by a slow exhalation.

Sighing occurs irregularly in normal healthy subjects. The frequency of sighing is inversely related to body size. Thus, it occurs an average of 10 times per hour in women and 9 times per hour in men. Infants sigh more frequently than children or adults. The rate of sighing increases in the supine position. Physiologically, the role of such deep breaths is apparently that of providing periodic hyperinflation of the lungs to re-inflate atelectatic air spaces, and thus, keeping pulmonary compliance, work of breathing,

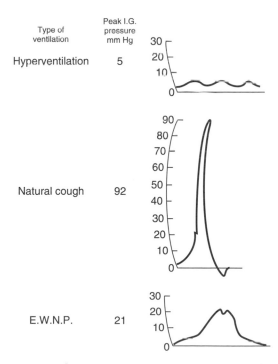

Fig. 2–17. Intragastric pressure curves in a normal subject show a markedly higher peak during a spontaneous cough than during E. W. N. P. and hyperventilation.

and venous admixture within normal limits. Sighing is more frequent in acute circulatory hypotension and in anxious subjects.

Such a role seems to be confirmed by the work of Bendixen and others[109] who have shown that when sighing is absent, as in the anesthetized patient, a significant decrease in compliance, functional residual capacity, and arterial oxygen tension results from closure of underinflated alveoli with venous admixture. Simultaneously, there is decreased venous return to the heart and a transient lowering of stroke output. Egbert and colleagues[109] subsequently showed that all of these changes that occur under anesthesia could be reversed by a passive deep breath or artificial sigh by the anesthesiologist. A pharmacologic sigh can be induced by a small dose of doxapram (0.2 mg/kg).[110] This drug is effective in the postanesthetic period and has been shown to diminish atelectasis and transpulmonary shunting and to raise arterial oxygen tension.[111]

In the postoperative patient, the sigh mechanism may be inhibited by pain, as is tidal volume. Whereas narcotics improve tidal volume by reducing the pain of breathing, they also abolish the sigh completely, even in doses that do not affect respiration. Thus, most hypoxemic episodes occur in the postoperative period, and some means of providing a sigh artificially is essential to prevent the development of postoperative pulmonary complications.

Yawning [43]

A yawn is a sustained maximal inspiration (SMI) with the mouth and glottis wide open. A negative intrathoracic pressure of (-40 mm Hg) is developed with a good steady inspiratory flow of air (200 ml/sec) and an increase in lung volume to total lung capacity. Right atrial pressure decreases, mean pulmonary artery pressure decreases (up to 5 to 10 mm Hg), and venous return increases. Yawning occurs in babies, and under conditions of weariness, boredom, or when there is decreased awareness of the environment.

A mechanical yawn has been recommended by Bartlett. The technique involves an incentive spirometer in which the patient is encouraged to prolong inspiratory effort by maintaining a red light.

TESTS OF VENTILATORY FUNCTION

An analysis of pulmonary function reveals that determinations made through testing can be divided into three basic aspects:

1. Overall ventilation, i.e., all those mechanisms responsible for the pumping into the lungs of air and the distribution of air to different parts of the lung;
2. Overall pulmonary circulation, i.e., all those mechanisms responsible for the pumping of blood into the lungs and the distribution of the blood to different parts of the lungs; and

3. The alveolar-diffusion mechanisms, designed to permit the gas phase to interchange with the blood phase.

These processes are interdependent. It is especially important to emphasize the parallelism between ventilation and circulation. Each may be considered a continuous process. Each possesses a pump. The bellows action of the chest-diaphragm pumps blood into the lungs and it is distributed to the alveolar capillaries. Distribution depends on pressure relationships in lung segments and on patency of either airway or vessels. These mechanisms are then beautifully united in the diffusion process.

The present objective is to outline tests that permit evaluation of overall ventilation. In considering the process of moving air into and out of the lungs, interest is directed at both the qualitative features of the mechanism and the quantitative effectiveness in terms of specific volumes of air moved.

Physical Examination

Qualitative features of ventilation are revealed by physical examination. By inspection of the chest while a patient is breathing normally, one can observe the overall shape and size of the thorax, the pattern of motion of chest and diaphragm, and the amplitude of movements. Deformities are apparent. Costal breathing can be distinguished from diaphragmatic breathing. Auscultation can furnish further information regarding the aeration of the lung alveoli and indeed the patency of the bronchioles. It provides some indication of volumetric exchange.

Fluoroscopy

Fluoroscopy can give supplementary information also of a qualitative nature for estimation of pulmonary function. In the examination of the various respiratory structures during fluoroscopy, the recommendations of the section on Diseases of the Chest of the American Medical Association are most valuable. One can visibly note the following:

1. The speed with which air can be drawn in and forced out.
2. The mechanics of breathing: (*a*) diaphragmatic; (*b*) abdominal; (*c*) intercostal; (*d*) accessory.
3. The extent of aeration and relative lucency during inspiration and expiration in: (*a*) apex; (*b*) base.
4. Abnormal motility or fixation: (*a*) hila; (*b*) mediastinum; (*c*) other midline structures; (*d*) peripheral lung markings.
5. Differences between the lungs and segments of a lung with respect to the above.
6. Evidence of the nature of cysts and other pathologic processes.

The diaphragm can be evaluated as to position, contour, and motion. Any delayed or prolonged ascent may indicate expiratory air trapping.

Midline structures are readily observed. Any shift in structures in normal breathing is attributable to inequality or intrathoracic pressures. In deep inspiration, the mediastinum and heart ordinarily shift to the right approximately 2 cm.

The hila ordinarily moves up and down some 2.0 cm. Reduced motion may be caused by restricted diaphragmatic motion, pulmonary fibrosis, or inflammatory or neoplastic fixation. Hilar compression may be seen in emphysema. Rotational movement of the hilum may be related to relative fixation.

Intercostal activity can be evaluated. Intercostal motion is seen best during deep breathing. Normally, any motion is less over the upper lung fields. Inequalities of costal movement should be noted.

Spirometry

Some quantitative features of ventilation are determined by spirometry. The equipment is basically simple. It is necessary to have a mask and tubing assembly, a one-way, no-resistance, high-velocity valve and either a direct measuring gas meter or a direct recording respirometer. Of practical utility in anesthesia practice is the simple gas meter. For more detailed evaluation, a Collins Recording Ventilograph is recommended. Terminology for tests of ventilatory capacity are listed and defined (Table 2–6). This table lists the primary sources for standard terminology. All relevant later literature refers back to these sources.

By these means, both static and dynamic aspects of ventilation are assessed. One can determine the various subdivisions of lung air and relate the capacities and volumes to time (Table 2–7).

It is important to appreciate that ventilatory function tests can provide objective information regarding impairment or disability of respiration. They cannot provide a diagnosis or distinguish between processes producing the impairment.

Vital Capacity

This screening procedure provides information about the potential of the lung to respond to a single effort. It is essentially a "single stroke volume" of ventilation and measures the total volume of gas displaced by a single muscular action.

> "A vital capacity measurement in any single healthy individual may deviate from the group mean by as much as 20%. Thus, there is difficulty in evaluating a single border-line (low) vital capacity measurement. However, vital capacity measurements are useful when measuring changes in the same individual over a period of time. Variations in excess of 200 ml have real significance."[38]

Vital capacity is most consistently related to body surface area, but a fairly close relationship is found between height and vital capacity:

	Men	Women
Vital capacity (in ml/mV of body surface)	2500	2000
Vital capacity (in ml/cm height)	25.0	20.0

The capacity is reduced in association with many abnormal or diseased conditions. A loss of vital capacity occurs when the lesion is of a restrictive nature. Encroachment on the pulmonary space, loss of lung substance, mechanical interference with enlargement of thoracic cavity, and engorgement of pulmonary vessels in heart diseases all reduce vital capacity.

By considering the values of three successive vital capacity measurements, the observer can determine the presence of air trapping. When trapping occurs, successive values are each smaller than the preceding determinations. This pattern most often reflects obstruction. If this sequence is consequent to increased bronchomotor tone, improvement occurs after epinephrine administration.

Forced Expiratory Volume[116]

The shortcoming of the vital capacity measurement is that it is a static value. It is solely a volume measurement and lacks relationship with time or effort, both of which are important in respiratory efficiency. By relating the single stroke volume against time, one is furnished with additional information concerning the speed of air exchange and the ease of movement of this air. Such a test is thus a measure of the speed of performance. A spirographic recording with a known rapid drum speed permits measurement of the time element as well as the breathing pattern and respiratory level.[43]

In normal subjects, the time of exhalation of tidal air is approximately 1.2 times as long as inspiration and the total time for a respiratory cycle is approximately 3 seconds. In these same subjects, the time of exhalation of vital capacity volume is itself approximately 3 seconds. Analysis of this period of time reveals the following percentages of vital capacity for the units of time noted.

Fraction of Air Expelled as Percent of Vital Capacity

Vital Capacity (%)	Time Required for Exhalation (sec)
65	0.5
84	1.0
94	2.0
97	3.0

A timed vital capacity on measurement of forced expiratory volume is the simplest method of differentiating obstructive from restrictive respiratory abnormalities. A diminished 0.5-sec vital capacity indicates obstruction and/or loss of elasticity. A diminished 1.0-sec vital capacity indicates even greater impairment.

The results of a total vital capacity measurement calcu-

Table 2–6. Terminology for Measurements of Ventilatory Capacity

Measurement Expressed in Terms of:	Name of Test (Synonyms)	Abbreviation	Remarks
A. Single breath 1. Volume	Forced vital capacity* (Fast vital capacity)	FVC*	Always refers to expiratory effort unless qualified by "inspiratory."
2. Volume in a unit time	Forced expiratory volume* (Timed vital capacity)	FEV_t*	Must be qualified by a time interval. $FEV_{1.0''}$ = vol. expired in 1 sec.; $FEV_{0.25-0.75''}$ = vol. expired between 0.25 and 0.75 sec.
	Percentage expired* (Percent timed vital capacity)	% FEV_t/VC*	Refers to volume of forced expiration (in time specified) related to vital capacity.
		% FEV_t/FVC*	Refers to volume of forced expiration (in time specified) related to forced vital capacity.
3. Volume time	Maximal expiratory flow rate	MEFR	Refers to L./min. for specified portion of a forced expiration; MEFR 200–1200 is flow rate for the liter of expired gas after 200 ml. has been expired.
	Maximal inspiratory flow rate	MIFR	Refers to L./min. for specified portion of a forced inspiration.
	Maximal mid-expiratory flow	MMF	Refers to L./min. measured for the middle half of FVC.
B Repeated breaths 1. Volume/time	Maximal breathing capacity	MBC	Usually attained by voluntary effort; occasionally exercise produces greater values.
	Maximal voluntary ventilation	MVV*	Maximal volume obtained by voluntary effort.

*Data from Comroe, J. H., et al.: *The Lung.* Chicago, Year Book, 1962; Pappenheimer, J. R.: Standardization of definitions and symbols in respiratory physiology. Fed. Proc., *9*:602, 1950; Ganderia, L. and Hugh-Jones, R.: New terminology for measurements of ventilatory capacity. Thorax, *12*:290, 1957.

lated as percent of the ideal or normal vital capacity may be related to the half-second expiratory capacity evaluated as percent of normal. When such is plotted quadrimetrically, the ventilatory pattern of a given subject is readily determined. Differentiation between obstructive and restrictive lesion is thereby possible (Fig. 2–18).

Maximal Breathing Capacity[117]

Also termed the maximal minute ventilation, it is the maximal volume of air a subject can move in and out of the lungs per unit of time. To some extent, this test is a measure of muscular efficiency and of airway resistance. This parameter can be measured and recorded on a spirometer or ventilometer. It is most accurately determined by using low-resistance valves in a large gasometer or by collecting expired air in a Douglas bag through a nonresistance valve, after which it is measured in a gas meter. By using the simple gas meter with inhaler assembly and one-way, low-resistance valve, slightly lower values are obtained.

In this test, the patient is instructed to breathe as deeply and as rapidly as possible for 15 seconds. The patient should determine his or her own rate. It is usually between 40 and 70 per minute. These values reflect both volume defects and resistance and demonstrate the mechanical effectiveness of the chest bellows.

Nominal ranges of maximal capacity are as follows:

	Males	Females
Gas meter	70–80	50–90
Respirometer	80–120	70–100
Open circuit (Douglas)	100–150	100–120

Calculated Values of Function

Breathing Reserve

The maximal breathing capacity minus the resting minute ventilation of a subject represents his ventilatory

Table 2–7. Selected Pulmonary Function Tests and Normal Values

Test	Symbol	Normal Value (Adults)
Lung Volumes (BTPS)		
Slow vital capacity	SVC	4.8 L*
Residual volume	RV	1.2 L*
Total lung capacity	TLC	6.0 L*
Residual volume/total lung capacity	RV/TLC	<30%
Ventilatory Performance and Air Flow Parameters		
Forced vital capacity	FVC	4.8 L*
Forced expiratory volume in 1 second		
as % predicted	$FEV_{1.0}$	>80%*
as % observed FVC	$FEV_{1.0}\%$	
		>75—80%
Forced expiratory volume in 3 seconds		
as % observed FVC	$FEV_{3.0}\%$	>95%
Maximum breathing capacity	MBC	>150 L/min*
(maximum voluntary ventilation)	(MVV)	
Maximal expiratory flow rate	MEFR	>300 L/min*
Peak expiratory flow rate	PEFR	>350 L/min*
Alveolar Gas		
Alveolar oxygen tension	P_{AO_2}	95–105 mm Hg
Alveolar carbon dioxide tension	P_{ACO_2}	38–42 mm Hg
Alveolar-arterial oxygen gradient	A-a O_2	5–15
Gas Distribution		
Single breath N_2 test	SBN_2	<2.5% N_2 (between 750–1,250 ml expired)
Arterial Blood		
Arterial oxygen tension	Pa_{O_2}	85–95 mm Hg
Arterial carbon dioxide tension	Pa_{CO_2}	38–42 mm Hg
Oxygen saturation, rest	Sa_{O_2}	95–98%
Arterial pH	pH_a	7.38–7.42
Hydrogen ion concentration (activity)	(H^+)	40.0 ± 2.0 nM/L.
Bicarbonate concentration	(HCO_3)	22–27 mM/L.
Oxygen content	Ca_{O_2}	19.5 vol %
Oxygen capacity	Cap	20.0 vol %
Ventilation/Ventilation-Perfusion† Gas Exchange		
Alveolar ventilation	V_A	4.0–7.5 L/min
Physiologic dead space	V_D	100–200 ml
Minute ventilation	V_E	6.0–10.0 L/min
Tidal volume	V_t	0.5–0.8 L/breath
Physiologic dead space tidal volume ratio	V_D/V_t	<0.33
Venous admixture/cardiac output × 100	Q_s/Q_T	<2–4%
CO_2 evolution	V_{CO_2}	200–240 ml/min
O_2 consumption	V_{O_2}	250–300 ml/min
Respiratory quotient V_{CO_2}/V_{O_2}	R.Q.	0.8
Diffusion capacity of lung (STPD)		
for carbon monoxide	DL_{CO} (steady state)	15–20 ml/min/mm Hg
for oxygen	DL_{O_2}	>15 ml/min/mm Hg
Mechanics of Breathing		
Compliance of lungs	C_L	0.2 L/cm H_2O
Total (lungs + thorax)	C_T	0.1 L/cm H_2O
Airway resistance	R_a	1.5–2.5 cm H_2O/L/sec (Lung volume specified)
Work of breathing (rest)		0.5 kg M/min

*Illustrative value only for a normal young male at rest. Observed normal values should be at least 80% of predicted.
†Approximate values for a normal male at rest.
(From Weiss, E. B., *Acute Respiratory Failure in Chronic Obstructive Lung Disease*. Chicago: Year Book; Shapiro, B., Peruzzi, W., and Templin, S.: *Respiratory Blood Gases*, 5th Ed. St. Louis, C. V. Mosby, 1994.)

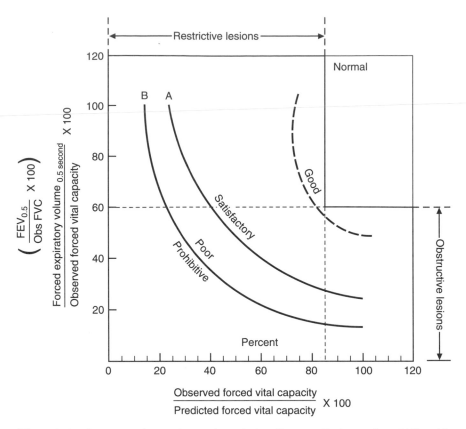

Fig. 2–18. Shows the differentiation between obstruction and restrictive diseases. Redrawn from Miller, Nu and Johnson, Anesthesiology.[119]

reserve (VR). It indicates capabilities under demand and hence is a measure of pulmonary fitness.

Air Velocity Index

This determination was introduced by Gaensler to aid in differentiation of obstruction from restrictive lesions of the pulmonary system. It is calculated as follows:[6]

$$\text{Air velocity index (AVI)} = \frac{\% \text{ of Predicted MBC}}{\% \text{ of Predicted VC}}$$

The AVI is normally 1.0. In obstruction, the reduction of the observed maximal breathing capacity (MBC) in percent of the predicted MBC is greater than any reduction in percent of the vital capacity (VC). The index is thus less than 1. In restrictive lesions involving loss of effective aerated pulmonary tissue, the reduction in the VC in percent of the normal VC is greater than any reduction in MBC. Hence, the AVI will be greater than 1.0.

Ventilatory Insufficiency

Capacity Ratio

Failure to meet normal requirements for ordinary activity is termed insufficiency. Such subjects are often referred to as respiratory cripples. It has been indicated that two types of insufficiency may exist. One is restrictive, in which there is primary loss of effective pulmonary tissue, and the other is obstructive, in which there is resistance to air movement. A summary of the characteristic findings in each follows:

Restrictive ventilatory insufficiency
  Decreased vital capacity
  No significant slowing in expiratory VC; i.e., no significant changes in timed VC
  Normal MBC. If decreased, the reduction is disproportionately less than the decrease in VC.
Obstructive ventilatory insufficiency
  Total vital capacity is normal or decreased
  Prolonged expiratory vital capacity time
  Maximal breathing capacity is decreased

Bronchospirometry

This technique allows the measurement of function in each lung separately. A double-lumen tube is introduced under topical anesthesia into the left bronchus, at least 2 cm but no more than 4 cm. By inflating an appropriate cuff, this lung is sealed from the right side. Respiration through the tube represents function of the left lung. Respiration of the right lung is accomplished via a side opening higher on the tube. Oxygen consumption can be measured on each side and the volume ventilation of each lung can be determined by separate spirometers. Also, oxygen uptake is slightly greater in the right lung.

In normal subjects, the right lung ventilates 55% of the air and the left lung 45% of the minute volume.

Distribution of Inspired Air to Different Parts of Lungs

The proper distribution of air through the lungs is essential for efficient gas exchange. Uneven distribution of inspired air leads to poor oxygenation and carbon-dioxide removal. Techniques for measuring the efficiency of intrapulmonary mixing are available. Inert gases such as helium, hydrogen, or nitrogen are used under controlled circumstances and the extent of dilution or residual concentrations determined.

In the helium dilution technique,[118] a measured volume of the gas is introduced into the system and then into the patient's respiratory system. By application of the Fick Principle of Proportionality, the capacity of lung air and the residual volumes may be determined.

Analysis of the course of nitrogen elimination when a patient breathes pure oxygen follows a normal pattern. Departures from this predicted curve reflect ineffective washing out of certain pulmonary areas.

Pulmonary Diffusing Capacity

A rapid single-breath test of pulmonary diffusing capacity is useful in detecting various pulmonary diseases. It is particularly useful in dyspneic patients who have a normal vital capacity and a normal maximal expiratory flow rate. Among the diseases to be detected are infiltrative lung diseases, pulmonary-vascular disease, and disease associated with the loss of alveolar-capillary surface area.

The test is performed by requiring the patient to inhale a low, nontoxic concentration of carbon monoxide (0.3%). The patient holds his or her breath for 10 seconds and then exhales. The equipment needed is that for delivering the gas and for measuring the concentration of the expired gases. The entire test, including calculations, requires approximately 10 minutes. It is safe, easy to perform, and may be repeated several times.

This test measures the rapidity of the transfer of molecules of carbon monoxide across the capillary alveolar membrane, and their combination with hemoglobin in the red cells in the pulmonary capillaries. The procedure depends on the area, thickness, and characteristics of the alveolar membranes, and on the total functioning area of contact between ventilated alveoli and alveolar capillaries.

Determination of Gas-Blood Distribution

Several screening tests are available to show one or another of three conditions: (1) distribution of inspired air to the airways and pulmonary alveoli; (2) distribution of blood flow to the pulmonary capillaries; and (3) matching of blood and gas in the pulmonary alveoli.

Single-Breath Oxygen Test[119]

This test requires the continuous measurement of nitrogen concentration of expired gas following the single inhalation of 100% oxygen. The nitrogen is measured by an electrical analyzer. Abnormal values indicate that the filling and emptying of the lungs are uneven and may be related either to an abnormality of the airway or of lung structure. If the abnormal value returns to normal after inhalation of isoproterenol, the abnormality is probably related to constriction of smooth muscle and is reversible. The test indicates maldistribution of air but not the region.

Single-Breath Xenon

After a single inhalation of gas containing radioactive xenon, the continuous recording of the radioactivity from both lungs is required. Determinations are made at the end of inspiration, during breath-holding, and during subsequent exhalation and clearance of radioactive xenon from the lungs. This measurement gives information about the distribution of gas to different parts of the lungs. Good geographic location of large lesions can be realized. The test is safe and the exposure to radiation is no greater than that during an ordinary radiographic evaluation of the chest. It is painless and requires no injections or blood samples.

Screening Bronchographic Test

Radiographic outlines of the airways can detect abnormalities of the trachea, bronchi, and bronchioles. Radiopaque material is introduced into the trachea through a bronchoscope or catheter or by a needle through the cricothyroid membrane. These materials are irritating locally, somewhat toxic systemically, and occasionally block airways.

A newer technique involving insufflation of powdered tantalum and inhalation of the particulate cloud provides excellent bronchograms without the disadvantages just cited.

Intravenous Injection of Tagged Albumin

Macroaggregates of radioactive iodinated serum albumin are injected intravenously and, because of their size, lodge in the pulmonary arterioles or capillaries. The radiation detector maps out the perfused areas of the lung. If a branch of the pulmonary artery is obstructed, the material does not reach the arterioles and therefore reveals nonperfused areas. With technetium, the procedure can be done in 10 minutes. Of these macroaggregates, only a small percentage of pulmonary capillaries are blocked, and the injected particles are rapidly removed. The test may be repeated every 24 hours. It is useful in detecting pulmonary embolism.

REFERENCES

1. Comroe, J. H.: Physiology of Respiration, 2nd Ed., Chicago, Year Book, 1974.
2. Altman, P. L., Dittmer, D. S.: Biological Handbook: Respiration Circulation, Chap. IV. Fed Am Soc Exp Biol 1970.
3. Fenn, W. O.: Mechanics of Respiration. Am J Med 10:77, 1951.
4. Rahn, H.: The pressure-volume diagram of the lungs and thorax. Am J Physiol 146:161, 1946.
5. Fenn, W. O.: Mechanics of respiration. Am J Med 10:77, 1951.
6. Gaensler, E. A.: Analysis of the ventilatory speed by timed capacity measurements. Am Rev Tuberc 64:256, 1951.
7. von Neergaard, K.: Neue Auffassungen uber einen Grund-

begriff der Atemmechanik. Die Retraktionskraft der Lunge, abhangig von der Oberflachenspannung in den Alveolen. Z Ges Exp Med 66:373, 1929.

8. Scarpelli, E. M.: The Surfactant System of the Lung. Philadelphia, Lea & Febiger, 1968.

9. Clements, J. A.: Pulmonary surfactant. Am Rev Respir Dis 101:984, 1970.

10. Gluck, L., et al.: Biochemical Development of Surface Activity in Mammalian Lung. IV. Pulmonary Lecithin Synthesis in the Human Fetus and Newborn and Etiology of the Respiratory Distress Syndrome. Pediatr Res 6:81, 1972.

11. Morgan, T. E.: Pulmonary Surfactant. N Engl J Med 284:1185, 1971.

12. Niden, A. H.: Bronchiolar and Large Alveolar Cell in Pulmonary Phospholipid Metabolism. Science 158:1323, 1967.

13. Brumley, G. W., Hodson, W. A., Avery, M.D.: Lung phospholipids and surface tension correlations in infants with and without hyaline membrane disease and in adults. Pediatrics 40:13, 1967.

14. Redding, R. A., Douglas, W. H., Stein, M.: Thyroid hormone influence upon lung surfactant metabolism. Science 175:994, 1972.

15. Safar, P., Bachman, L.: Compliance of the lungs and thorax in dogs under the influence of muscle relaxants. Anesthesiology 17:334, 1956.

16. Brownles, W. E. and Allbritten, Jr. F. F.: The significance of the lung-thorax compliance during thoracic surgery. J Thorac Surg 32:454, 1956.

17. Brobeck, J. R.: Best and Taylor's *Physiological Basis of Medical Practice,* 9th Ed. Baltimore, Williams & Wilkins, 1973.

18. Fleisch, A.: Pneumotachygraph. Helv Physiol Pharm Acta 14:363, 1956.

19. Fleisch, A.: Der Pneumotachograph: ein Apparat zur Geschwindigkeits registrierung der atem luft. Pfugers Arch 209:719, 1925.

20. McIlroy, M., et al.: The effect of added elastic and non-elastic resistances on the patterns of breathing in normal subjects. Clin Sci 15:337, 1956.

21. Rattenborg C: Laryngeal regulation of respiration. Acta Anaesthesiol Scand 58:129, 1961.

22. Fairley, H. B.: Airway closure. Anesthesiology 36:529, 1972.

23. Leblanc, P., Ruff, F., Milic-Emili, J.: Effect of age and body position on airway closure in man. J Appl Physiol 24:448, 1970.

24. Don, H. F., Wahba, W., Craig, D. R.: Airway closure, gaws trapping and functional residual capacity during anesthesia. Anesthesiology 36:533, 1972.

25. Comroe, Jr., J. H., Fowler, W. S.: Nitrogen washout by inhalation of a single breath of oxygen. Anes J Med 10:408, 1951.

26. Miller, W. F., Wu, N., Johnson, R. L.: Convenient method of evaluating pulmonary function with a single breath test. Anesthesiology 17:480, 1956.

27. Sutherland, J. V.: Airway closure during lung deflation. J Appl Physiol 25:566, 1968.

28. Bergman, N. A., Tien, Y. K.: Contribution of the closure of pulmonary units to impaired oxygenation during anesthesia. Anesthesiology 59:395, 1983.

29. Hales, C. A., Kaxemi, H.: Small airways function in myocardial infarction. N Engl J Med 290:761, 1974.

30. Heneghan, C. P. H., et al.: Effect of isoflurane on bronchomotor tone in man. Br J Anesth 58:24, 1986.

31. Hensley, M. J., et al.: Distribution of bronchodilatation in normal subjects: Beta agonist versus altropine. J Appl Physiol 45:616, 1962.

32. Widdicombe, J. G., Kent, D. C., and Nadel, J. A.: Mechanism of bronchoconstriction during inhalation of dust. J Appl Physiol 17:613, 1962.

33. Lloyd, Jr., T. C.: Bronchoconstriction in man following single deep inspirations. J Appl Physiol 18:114, 1963.

34. Nadel, J. A. and Widdicombe, J. G.: Reflex effects of upper airway irritation on total lung resistance and blood pressure. J Appl Physiol 17:861, 1962.

35. Simonson, B. G., Jacobs, F. M., Nadel, J. A.: Role of eutonic nervous system and the cough reflex in the increased responsiveness of airways in patients with obstructive lung disease. J Clin Invest 46:1812, 1967.

36. Yu, D., Y. C., Galant, S. P., and Gold, W. M.: Inhibition of antigen-induced bronchoconstriction by atropine in asthmatic patients. J Appl Physiol 32:823, 1972.

37. Severinghaus, J. W., et al.: Unilateral hypoventilation produced in dogs by occluding one pulmonary artery. J Appl Physiol 16:53, 1961.

38. Patterson, R. W. and Sullivan, S. F.: Inter-relation between $PaCO_2$ and $Paco_2$ in the control of the mechanics of breathing in man. Bull NY Acad Med 44:1265, 1968.

39. Campbell, E. J. M.: The Respiratory Muscles and the Mechanics of Breathing. Chicago, Year Book, 1958.

40. Cherniack, R., Cherniack, L., Naimark, A.: Respiration in Health and Disease, 2nd Ed. Philadelphia, W.B. Saunders, 1972.

41. Murray, J.F.: Oxygen cost of ventilation. J Appl Physiol 14:187, 1959.

42. Bedell, G.N.: Pulmonary function in obese person. J Clin Invest 37:1049, 1958.

43. Comroe, Jr., J. H., et al.: The Lung. Chicago, Year Book, 1962.

44. Burke, R. E., et al.: Physiological types and histochemical profiles in motor units of the cat gastrochemius. J Physiol (Lond.) 234:723, 1973.

45. Dubowitz, V.: Enzyme histochemistry of skeletal muscle. J Neurol Neurosurg Psychiatry 28:516, 1965.

46. Fenichel, G. M.: A histochemical study of developing human skeletal muscle. Neurology 16:741, 1966.

47. Keens, T. B., et al.: Developmental pattern of muscle fiber types in human ventilatory muscles. J Appl Physiol 44:909, 1978.

48. Hagan, R., et al.: The effect of sleep state on intercostal muscle activity and RC motion (abstract). Physiologist 19:214, 1976.

49. Rochester, D. F. and Briscoe, A. M.: Metabolism of the working diaphragm. Am Rev Respir Dis 119 (Suppl) 110:1, 1979.

50. Roussos, C. S., Macklem, P. T.: Diaphragmatic fatigue in man. J Appl Physiol 43:198, 1977.

51. Moxham, J., et al.: Contractile properties and fatigue of the diaphragm in man. Thorax 36:164, 1981.

52. Rochester, D. F.: Is diaphragmatic contractility important? N Engl J Med 305:178, 1981.

53. Roussos, C., Macklem, P. T.: The respiratory muscles. N Engl J Med 307:786, 1982.

54. Aubier, M., et al.: Aminophylline improves diaphragmatic contractility. N Engl J Med 305:249, 1981.

55. Viires, N., et al.: Regional blood flow distribution in the dog during induced hypotension and low cardiac output. Spontaneous breathing versus artificial ventilation. J Clin Invest 72:935, 1983.

56. Hussain, S., Roussos, C.: Distribution of respiratory muscles and organ blood flow during endotoxin shock in dogs. J Appl Physiol 59:1802, 1985.

57. Roussos, C.: Diaphragmatic fatigue and blood flow distribution in shock. Can J Anaesth 33:S361, 1986.

58. Fitts, R. H., Holloszy, J. O.: Lactate and contractile force in

frog muscle during development of fatigue and recovery. Am J Physiol *231*:430, 1976.

59. Juan, G., et al.: Effect of carbon dioxide on diaphragmatic contractility in patients with acute respiratory failure. N Engl J Med *313*:447, 1985.

60. Aubier, M., et al.: Effect of hypophosphatemia on diaphragmatic contractility in patients with acute respiratory failure. N Engl J Med *313*: 420, 1985.

61. Knochel, J. P.: The clinical status of hypophosphatemia: An update (editorial). N Engl J Med *313*:447, 1985.

62. Card, R. T., Braun, M. C.: The anemia of childhood: Evidence for a response to hyperphosphatemia. N Engl J Med *288*:388, 1973.

63. Labaille T., et. al.: Ventilatory response to CO_2 following intravenous and epidural lidocaine. Anesthesiology *63*:179, 1985.

64. Riley, R. L., et al.: On the determination of the physiologically effective pressures of oxygen and carbon dioxide in alveolar air. Am J Physiol 191, 1946.

65. Gilbert, R., et al.: Stability of the arterial/alveolar oxygen partial pressure ratio. Effects of low ventilation/perfusion regions. Crit Care Med 7:267, 1979.

66. Bedell, G. N., Adams, R. W.: Pulmonary diffusing capacity during rest and exercise. J Clin Invest *41*:1908, 1962.

67. Bjorkman, S.: Bronchiospiroetrie: eine kliniache Methode, die Funktion der menschlichen Lungren getrennt und gleichzeitig zu untersuchen. Acta Med Scand Suppl 56:1, 1934.

68. Etsten, B: Anesthesia for thoracic surg. NY State J Med *43*:1980.

69. Svanberg, L.: Bronchospirometry in the study of regional lung function. Scand J Resp Dis Suppl *62*:91, 1966.

70. West, J. B.: Regional differences in gas exchange in the lung of erect man. J Appl Physiol *17*:893, 1962.

71. Svanberg, L.: Influence of posture on lung volumes, ventilation and circulation in normals: A spirometric-broncho spirometric investigation. Scand J Clin Lab Invest (Suppl), 25:1, 1957.

72. Heaf, D. P., et al.: Postural effects of gas exchange in infants. N Engl J Med *308*:1505, 1983.

73. Davies, H., et al.: Regional ventilation in infancy: Reversal of adult pattern. N Engl J Med *313*:1626, 1985.

74. Remolina, C., et al.: Positional hypoxemia in unilateral lung disease. N Engl J Med *304*:523, 1981.

75. Milic-Emili, J., Mead, J., Turner, J. M.: Topography of esophageal pressure as a function posture in man. J Appl Physiol *19*:212, 1965.

76. West, J. B., Dollery, C. T.: Distribution of blood flow ventilation-perfusion ratio in the lung, measured with radioactive CO_2. J Appl Physiol *15*:405, 1960.

77. West, J. B., Collery, C. T., Naimark, A.: Distribution of blood flow in isolated lung: Relation to vascular and alveolar pressures. J Appl Physiol *19*:713, 1964.

78. Zack, M. B., Pontoppidan, H., Kazemi, H.: The effect of lateral positions on gas exchange in pulmonary disease: A prospective evaluation. Am Rev Respir Dis *110*:49, 1974.

79. Fishman, A. P.: Down with the good lung (editorial). N Engl J Med *304*:537, 1981.

80. Rehder, K., Hatch, D. J., Sessler, A. D., Fowler, W. S.: The function of each lung of anesthetized and paralyzed man during mechanical ventilation. Anesthesiology *37*:16, 1972.

81. Bendixen, H., et al.: Respiratory Care. St. Louis, C. V. Mosby, 1965.

82. Shapiro, B. A., Harrison, R. A., Walton, I. R.: Clinical Application of Blood Gases. Chicago, Year Book.

83. Leigh, J. M., Tyrell, M. F., Strickland, D. A. P.: Simplified versions of shunt and oxygen consumption equations. Anesthesiology *30*:468, 1969.

84. Raid, L.: Measurement of the bronchial mucous gland layer: A diagnostic yardstick in chronic bronchitis. Thorax, *15*:132, 1960.

85. Widdicombe, J. G.: Control of secretion of tracheobronchial mucus. Br Med Bull *34*:57, 1978.

86. Clamp, J. R., et al.: Chemical aspects of mucus. Br Med Bull *34*:25, 1978.

87. Lopez-Vidriero, M. T., Reid, L.: Bronchial mucus in health and disease. Br Med Bull *34*:63, 1978.

88. Respiratory mucus. (editorial). Lancet 1978;1473.

89. Dahlman T: A method for determination in vivo of the role of ciliary beat and mucous flow in the trachea. Acta Physiol Scand *33*:1, 1955.

90. Collins, V. J.: Experiments in Physiology. Providence, Brown University, 1937.

91. Asmundsson. (see Lopez-Vidriero, Ref. 77)

92. Satir, P.: Further studies on the cilium tip and "sliding filament" model of ciliary motility. J Cell Biol *39*:77, 1968.

93. Eliasson, R., et al.: The immotile-cilia syndrome: A congenital ciliary abnormality as an etiologic factor in chronic airway infections and male sterility. N Engl J Med *297*:1, 1977.

94. Busuttil, A., More, I. A., McSeveney, D.: A reappraisal of the ultrastructure of the human respiratory nasal mucosa. J Anat *124*:445, 1977.

95. Carson, J. L., Collier, A. M., Hu, S. S.: Acquired ciliary defects in nasal epithelium of children with acute viral upper respiratory infections. N Engl J Med *312*:463, 1985.

96. Hibnia, Jr., D. V. and Curreri, A. B.: A study of the effect of morphine, atropine, and scopolamine on the bronchi. Surg Gynecol Obstet 74:851, 1942.

97. Corssen, G., Allen, C. R.: Acetylcholine: Its significance in controlling activity of human respiratory epithelium in vitro. J Appl Physiol *14*:901, 1959.

98. Corssen, G., Allen, C. R.: Cultured human respiratory epithelium: Its use in the comparison of the cytotoxic properties of local anesthetics. Anesthesiology *21*:237, 1960.

99. Macklin, C. C.: The Musculature of the bronchi and lungs. Physiol Rev 9.1, 1929.

100. Coryllos, P. N.: Action of diaphragm in cough. Am J Med Sci *194*:523, 1937.

101. Fleischer, F. G.: Bronchial peristalsis. Am J Roentgenol *62*:65, 1949.

102. Widdicombe, J. G.: Clinical significance of reflexes from the respiratory system. Anesthesiology *23*:434, 1962.

103. Merendine, K. A., et al.: The intradiaphragmatic distribution of the phrenic nerve. Surgery *38*:180, 1954.

104. Huizinga, E.: The tussic squeeze and the bechic blast. Ann Otol Rhinol Laryngol 76:923, 1967.

105. Barach, A. L., Beck, G. J., Smith, W.: Mechanical production of expiratory flow rates surpassing the capacity of human coughing. Am J Med Sci *226*:241, 1953.

106. Beck, G. J., Scarrone, L. A.: Physiological effects of exsufficiation with negative pressure. Chest 29:1, 1956.

107. Kumar, C., Mehta, M.: Hiccoughs during general anesthesia. Anesthesia, *39*:1035, 1984.

108. Bendixen, H. H., Smith, G. M., Mead, J.: Pattern of ventilation in young adults. J Appl Physiol *19*:195, 1964.

109. Egbert, L. D., Loves, M. B., Bendixen, H. H.: Compliance in anesthetized patients. Anesthesiology *24*:57, 1963.

110. Winnie, A. P., Collins, V. J.: The doxapram test: A new test for differential diagnosis of apnea. Anesthesiology *26*:27, 1965.

111. Winnie, A. P.: Search for a pharmacologic ventilator. Acta Anaesthesiol Scand [Suppl.] 10P: 19, 1966.

112. Meneely, G. R.: Pulmonary Function Testing. Dis Chest *31*:125, 1957.

113. Comroe J. H., Foster, R. E., Dubois, A. R., et al: The Lung, 2nd Ed. Chicago, Yearbook Publishers, 1962.

114. Gandevia, L., Hugh-Jones, R.: New terminology for measurements of ventilatory capacity. Thorax *12*:290–296, 1957.

115. Weiss, E. B. Acute Respiratory Failure in Chronic Obstructive Lung Disease. Year Book Medical Publishers, Inc.

116. Segal, M. S., Herschfus, J. A., Dulfano, M. J.: A sample method for determination of vital capacity-time relationship. Chest *22*:123, 1952.

117. Worten, E. W., Bedell, G. N.: Determination of vital capacity and maximal breathing capacity. JAMA *165*:1652, 1957.

118. Snyder, J. C.: Determination of the residual air volume by helium dilution technic. U.S. Armed Forces Med J 1597, 1954.

119. Miller, W. F., Wu, N., Johnson, R. Convenient method of evaluating pulmonary ventilatory function with a single breath test. Anesthesiology *17*:480–484, 1956.

120. Shapiro, B., Peruzzi, W., Templin, S.: Respiratory Blood Gases. 5th Edition. St. Louis. 1994.

Chapter 3

NEUROCHEMICAL REGULATION OF RESPIRATION

MAHMOOD TABATABAI, RAHIM BEHNIA, AND ERNESTO PRETTO

The neurochemical regulation of respiration deals with the mechanisms that maintain homeostasis of arterial oxygen and carbon dioxide partial pressures (PaO_2 and $PaCO_2$, respectively) and arterial pH by adjusting the level of ventilation. Oxygen (O_2) uptake and carbon dioxide (CO_2) elimination vary considerably in accordance with the metabolic demands of the body. For example, the resting O_2 uptake of 250 ml/min and CO_2 elimination of 200 ml/min may increase more than tenfold during strenuous exercise, yet the controlled variables, namely, PaO_2, $PaCO_2$, and pH, are kept within close limits. This remarkable constancy of the variables in the face of ever-changing metabolic needs is made possible by the respiratory control system (Fig. 3–1), which consists of the following:

1. The sensors (receptors), both peripheral and central, which sense the information and deliver it via their afferent nerve fibers to:
2. The central controller, i.e., the brain stem respiratory neurons, located in the medulla and pons, which process and integrate the information and send motor impulses via:
3. Efferent respiratory nerves, consisting of spinal (phrenic and intercostal) and cranial (vagus, accessory, and hypoglossal) nerves, to:
4. Effectors (respiratory muscles), the contraction of which brings about ventilation.

SENSORS (RECEPTORS)

Peripheral Chemoreceptors

An immediate increase in ventilation occurs when the inspired O_2 concentration is decreased to less than 10% (Table 3–1).[1,2] This response is common in all mammalian species, and depends on specialized chemoreceptors that sense PaO_2. These receptors are located in the carotid arteries, at the bifurcation of the common carotid arteries, and in aortic bodies scattered around the aortic arch.

The neurovascular nature and probable chemoreceptor function of the carotid bodies were first reported by DeCastro in 1926,[3] but it was Heymans and coworkers who demonstrated the role of the carotid bodies in response to hypoxemia and hypercarbia in 1930.[4] In 1938, Heymans was awarded the Nobel prize in medicine and physiology for his discovery. In 1939, Comroe established the chemosensitivity of the aortic bodies.[5]

The afferent impulses from the carotid chemoreceptors travel in a branch of the carotid sinus nerve (Her-

ing's nerve) and reach the brain stem respiratory neurons in the glossopharyngeal (ninth cranial) nerve; those from the aortic chemoreceptors travel along the vagus (tenth cranial) nerve. The afferent impulses carried by the glossopharyngeal and vagus nerves reach the nucleus tractus solitarius (NTS) in the medulla oblongata, where they exert their stimulatory effects on the medullary respiratory neurons to increase ventilation by increasing the depth and rate of breathing.

The carotid chemoreceptors are stimulated by decreased PaO_2, decreased pH, and increased $PaCO_2$.[6-11] The aortic body chemoreceptors are also stimulated by decreased PaO_2 and increased $PaCO_2$, but not by decreased arterial pH.[12] Interaction between various stimuli occurs such that an increase in chemoreceptor activity in response to low PaO_2 is potentiated by high $PaCO_2$ and, in the carotid body, also by low pH.[9-11]

Studies in humans have revealed that the carotid bodies are entirely responsible for hypoxic ventilatory drive, account for about 30% of the response to hypercarbia, and provoke all the ventilatory compensation for the acute metabolic acidosis of exercise.[13] In fact, in the absence of the carotid bodies, severe hypoxemia depresses respiration, presumably through a direct inhibitory effect on the brain stem respiratory centers. Complete loss of hypoxic

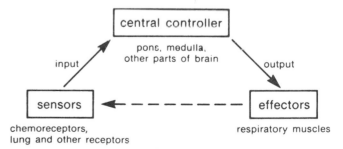

Fig. 3–1. Basic elements of the respiratory control system. The central controller in the brain stem has its own inherent rhythmicity, but is modulated by incoming information (input) from various sensors (receptors) such as chemoreceptors, mechanoreceptors, thermoreceptors, and nociceptors. The output (i.e., the processed integrated information) from the central controller gets to the effectors (respiratory muscles) via respiratory efferent nerves. By changing ventilation, the respiratory muscles reduce perturbations of the sensors (negative feedback, dashed arrow). From West, J. B. (ed.): Best and Taylor's Physiological Basis of Medical Practice, 12th Ed. Baltimore, Williams & Wilkins, 1992, p. 580.

Table 3–1.   Effect of Decreased Inspired O_2 Concentration on Pulmonary Ventilation in Healthy Men*

Concentration of O_2 in Inspired Air (%)	Tidal Volume (ml)	Frequency (Breaths/min)	Respiratory Minute Volume (L/min)	Alveolar Ventilation (L/min)
20.93	500	14	7.0	4.9
18.0	500	14	7.0	4.9
16.0	536	14	7.5	5.4
12.0	536	14	7.5	5.4
10.0	593	14	8.3	6.2
8.0	812	16	13.0	10.4
6.0			18.0	
5.2			22.0	
4.2	933	30	28.0	23.2

*All data are mean values. Predicted anatomic dead space was used to calculate alveolar ventilation. (From Dripps, R. D. and Comroe, Jr., J. H.: The effect of the inhalation of high and low oxygen concentrations on respiration, pulse rate, ballistocardiogram and arterial oxygen saturation (oximeter) of normal individuals. Am. J. Physiol.,*149*:277, 1947.)

ventilatory drive has been shown in patients with bilateral carotid body resection.[14]

Plots of single-fiber or whole-nerve chemoreceptor activity versus PaO_2 show a nonlinear relationship. An arterial PO_2 of 500 mm Hg or higher is associated with no nerve activity. A progressive increase in the nerve firing rate develops as the PaO_2 falls from 500 mm Hg, with a rapid rise in activity occurring below 100 mm Hg.[8,11,15] Maximum response occurs when the arterial PO_2 is lower than 50 mm Hg (Fig. 3–2). When the PaO_2 is lower than 30 mm Hg, the chemoreceptor activity is not sustained and gradually decreases with time.[11] In contrast, the response of the carotid chemoreceptors to $PaCO_2$ and pH, and that of the aortic chemoreceptors to $PaCO_2$, are almost linear over a range of $PaCO_2$ from 20 to 60 mm Hg, and with an arterial hydrogen ion concentration from 20 to 60 nanoequivalent per liter (pH from 7.2 to 7.6).[11,15]

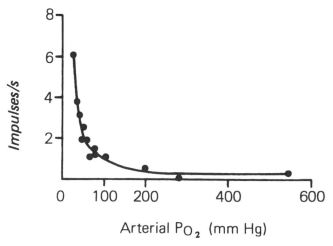

Fig. 3–2.   Rate of discharge of a single chemoreceptor afferent fiber from the carotid body plotted against arterial blood oxygen tension. Little increase in rate occurs as arterial PO_2 decreases from 550 to 100 mm Hg, more between 100 and 50 mm Hg, and a sharp increase below 50 mm Hg. Courtesy of S. Sampson; from Ganong, W. F.: Review of Medical Physiology, 16th Ed. Norwalk, CT, Appleton and Lange, 1993, p. 614.

Good correlation exists between the preceding observations and the ventilatory response to low PaO_2 or high $PaCO_2$. For example, the increase in ventilation in response to decreased inspired O_2 concentration is nonlinear; little increase in ventilation occurs until the inspired O_2 concentration is less than 10% (O_2 concentration in room air is approximately 21%).[16] In contrast is the linear correlation between the increase in $PaCO_2$ and the increase in ventilation—an increase of 1.5 to 2.5 l/min per 1 mm Hg increase in $PaCO_2$[17] (Fig. 3–3; Table 3–2). Interaction between various stimuli occurs (Figs. 3–4 and 3–5).

Carotid bodies are highly vascular with rich blood flow: 2000 ml/100 g/min compared with brain blood flow of 50 ml/100 g/min or renal blood flow of 400 ml/100 g/min. Decreased blood flow to the carotid bodies, because of either hypotension or sympathetic stimulation resulting in vasoconstriction of vessels supplying the carotid bodies, provokes increased chemoreceptor activity. Powerful stimulation is also produced by drugs that interfere with the tissue consumption of O_2 by their inhibiting action on cytochrome oxidase, such as sodium cyanide[18] (Table 3–3).

Chemosensitive Elements Within the Carotid Bodies

The carotid bodies contain two main cell types; type I cells (also called glomus cells), and type II cells (also called supporting cells). Nerve fibers in contact with glomus cells are free unmyelinated nerve endings, which join each other to form the chemoreceptor branch of the carotid sinus nerve (Hering's nerve). Fluorescent microscopy has shown that glomus cells are intensely fluorescent because of the presence of catecholamines, primarily dopamine.

Originally, it was thought that the glomus cells themselves are the chemoreceptors. The prevailing theory at present, however, is that the afferent nerve terminals (free nerve endings) of the carotid sinus nerve within the carotid body are the chemoreceptors, a notion based in part on the observation that neuromas that form on the

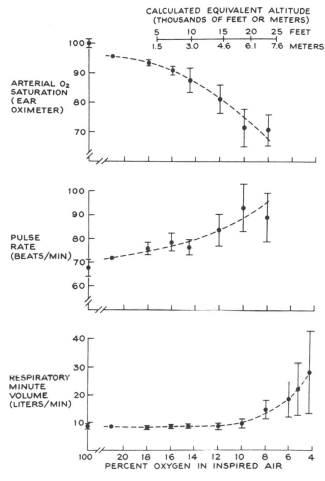

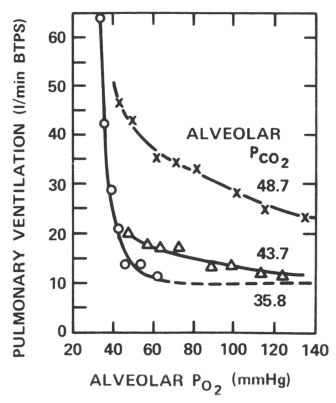

Fig. 3–3. Effect of changes in inspired oxygen concentration in humans. Healthy men breathed gas mixtures high or low in O_2 for 8 minutes. Measurements are mean values ±1 SD of arterial O_2 saturation, pulse rate, and respiratory minute volume for the last 3 minutes. From Dripps, R. D. and Comroe, Jr., J. H.: The effect of the inhalation of high and low oxygen concentrations on respiration, pulse rate, ballistocardiogram and arterial oxygen saturation (oximeter) of normal individuals. Am J Physiol 149:277, 1947.

Fig. 3–4. Increase in ventilation related to hypoxia associated with low and high levels of CO_2. Alveolar PCO_2 ($PACO_2$) was maintained at about 35.8 mm Hg, (bottom curve), 43.7 mm Hg (middle curve), and 48.7 mm Hg (top curve) in a subject breathing low O_2 gas mixtures. Each curve starts at a higher level because of the effect of higher CO_2 tensions. Between 80 and 120 mm Hg, the slope of the upper curve is steeper than that of the lower ones because of interaction between the low O_2 and high CO_2 stimuli. Volume of ventilation corrected to BTPS (body temperature and pressure, saturated with water vapor). Data of Loeschke, H. H. and Gertz, K. H., reproduced from West, J. B. (ed.): Best and Taylor's Physiological Basis of Medical Practice, 12th Ed. Baltimore, Williams & Wilkins, 1992, p. 585.

Table 3–2. Pulmonary Ventilation in Response to CO_2 Excess*

Concentration of CO_2 in Inspired Air (%)	Tidal Volume (ml)	Frequency (Breaths/min)	Minute Volume (L/min)	Alveolar Ventilation (L/min)
0.03	440	16	7	4.6
1.0	500	16	8	5.6
2.0	560	16	9	6.6
4.0	823	17	14	11.3
5.0	1,300	20	26	22.5
7.6	2,100	28	52	47.9
10.4	2,500	35	76	69.0

*More than 20 normal subjects were studied at each concentration of CO_2.
All data are mean values; alveolar ventilation was calculated using predicted anatomic dead space, taking into account increases in tidal volume.
From Forster, R. E., et al.: The Lung: Physiological Basis of Pulmonary Function Tests, 3rd Ed. Chicago, Year Book, 1986, p. 118.)

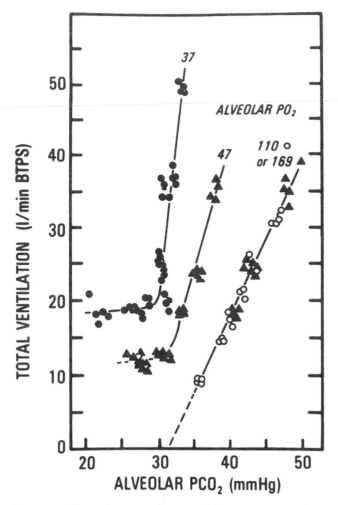

Fig. 3–5. Effect of varying degrees of hypoxia on ventilatory response to CO_2. The alveolar PO_2 (in mm Hg) is indicated at the top of each curve. Note the increase in slope of the curves as the alveolar PO_2 decreases. In this study, no difference was observed in the ventilatory response between an alveolar PO_2 of 110 and one of 169 mm Hg, although some investigators have found that the slope of the line is slightly less at the higher alveolar PO_2. Volume of ventilation is corrected to BTPS (body temperature, pressure, saturated with water vapor). Data of Nielsen and Smith, reproduced from West, J. B. (ed.): Best and Taylor's Physiological Basis of Medical Practice, 12th Ed. Baltimore, Williams & Wilkins, 1992, p. 584.

Table 3–3. Factors Stimulating Peripheral Chemoreceptors

Low PaO_2
High $PaCO_2$
Low pH (only effective on carotid chemoreceptors)
Decreased blood flow to the chemoreceptors as in hypotension, or sympathetic stimulation resulting in vasoconstriction of blood vessels supplying the chemoreceptors
Cytochrome oxidase inhibitors that interfere with O_2 utilization, such as sodium cyanide.

cut end of the carotid sinus nerve are chemosensitive in the absence of carotid body tissue.[19] It has been suggested that the glomus cell is a dopaminergic inhibitory interneuron that modulates the generation of impulses in the afferent nerve terminals. According to this theory, chemical stimulation of the sensory nerve endings in the carotid bodies generates impulses directed toward the medulla, and also causes secretion of an excitatory neurotransmitter that evokes release of dopamine from glomus cells.[20] Dopamine, in turn, acts on the free nerve endings to inhibit impulse generation.

Central Chemoreceptors

After denervation of the peripheral chemoreceptors, the ventilatory response to increased $PaCO_2$ does not disappear, but is slightly diminished. Further, under such conditions, the response is delayed by about 60 to 90 seconds,[21,22] which suggests that in contrast to the peripheral chemoreceptors, the central chemoreceptors do not equilibrate with the arterial blood instantly.

The central chemosensitivity does not arise from the brain stem respiratory neurons, but from chemosensitive areas (CSA) of the medulla, situated near its ventrolateral surface[23,24] (Fig. 3–6). The CSA is believed to lie 200 to 400 μm below the surface of the medulla,[25] lateral to the pyramids and medial to the roots of the seventh through tenth cranial nerves,[23] and that the afferent fibers from the CSA project to the medullary respiratory neurons, which process and integrate the incoming information and adjust ventilation by their efferent impulses to the respiratory muscles.

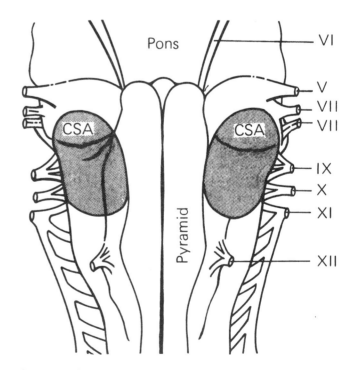

Fig. 3–6. Chemosensitive areas (CSA) on the ventrolateral surface of the medulla. From Ganong, W. F.: Review of Medical Physiology, 16th Ed. Norwalk, CT, Appleton and Lange, 1993, p. 615.

The central chemoreceptors respond to the hydrogen ion (H^+) concentration in their surrounding environment, i.e., the local interstitial fluid. As the local H^+ concentration increases, ventilation increases, and as local H^+ concentration decreases, ventilation decreases. The composition of the interstitial fluid surrounding the receptors is governed by the cerebrospinal fluid (CSF), local blood flow, and local metabolism. Of these, the CSF is apparently the most important.

The normal pH of the CSF is 7.33 and its PCO_2 is 50 mm Hg, in contrast to pH of 7.4 and PCO_2 of 40 mm Hg for arterial blood. The CSF has little protein (15 to 45 mg/100 ml) and therefore less buffering capacity in contrast to blood, which has hemoglobin and plasma proteins, that can act as buffers to maintain a constant blood pH. Consequently, the change in CSF pH for a given change in PCO_2 or H^+ concentration is greater than that in blood.

The CSF is separated from the blood by the blood-brain barrier. This barrier accommodates CO_2, which diffuses rapidly from the blood to the CSF, but is impermeable to H^+ and bicarbonate ion (HCO_3) (Fig. 3–7). When the $PaCO_2$ increases, CO_2 diffuses into the CSF from the cerebral blood vessels, increasing it H^+ concentration. The increased H^+ concentration of the CSF stimulates the chemoreceptors, which in turn, increase ventilation. Thus, the CO_2 level in blood regulates ventilation chiefly by its effect on the pH of the CSF. The resulting hyperventilation lowers the PCO_2 in the blood and, therefore, in the CSF, resulting in adjustment of the CSF pH.

The location of the central chemoreceptors near the surface of the medulla and their response to changes in the H^+ concentration of CSF suggest that their function is to guard the pH or H^+ concentration of the CSF, which bathes the central nervous system, whereas the carotid and aortic bodies regulate the PO_2 and, under extreme

conditions, the PCO_2 and pH of the arterial blood. If cerebral blood flow stops, the environment of the H^+ receptors is influenced largely by the composition of the local interstitial fluid, but more importantly by the CSF, because these receptors are fairly close to the surface of the medulla. On the other hand, if cerebral blood flow becomes unusually rapid, the environment of the receptors is influenced largely by the plasma composition.

A prolonged change in the pH of the CSF results in a compensatory change in CSF HCO_3 because of slow HCO_3 transport across the blood-brain barrier in an effort to adjust the CSF pH, (although it may not return to 7.33). The importance of CSF pH in the control of ventilation is demonstrated in patients with chronic lung disease and longstanding CO_2 retention. Such patients may have near normal CSF pH, and therefore, abnormally low ventilation for their arterial PCO_2. A similar situation is seen in normal subjects who are exposed to an atmosphere containing 3% CO_2 for some days.

Pulmonary Receptors

The three types of lung receptors[26] can all respond to mechanical changes, hence they may be regarded as mechanoreceptors. They are the pulmonary stretch receptors (PSR), irritant receptors, and J receptors (juxtapulmonary capillary receptors). The afferent fibers of these receptors travel in the vagus nerves and end in the nucleus tractus solitarius (NTS) of the medulla. They modulate the medullary respiratory neuronal output in order to change the rate and depth of breathing or to bring about changes in airway muscle tone.

Pulmonary Stretch Receptors (PSR)

These receptors for the Hering-Breuer reflex are believed to lie in the smooth muscle of airways from the trachea to bronchioles. They are activated by stretch of the airways (not by stretch of the alveoli), and their activity is sustained with maintained lung inflation; that is, they show little adaptation. The afferent impulses from the PSR travel to the medulla via large myelinated fibers in the vagus nerves. The primary reflex effect of activation of these receptors is termination of inspiration, which is the classic Hering-Breuer inhibito-inspiratory reflex or inflation reflex. Therefore, as the lung is inflated, inspiration is inhibited and expiration is promoted. Lung deflation, on the other hand, inhibits expiration and promotes inspiration, which is known as the Hering-Breuer excito-inspiratory reflex, or deflation reflex.

These reflexes can provide a regulatory mechanism to maintain rhythmic breathing through negative feedback. Of the two, the inflation reflex is more potent, and carries more weight in determining the rate and depth of respiration. Bilateral cervical vagotomy, which interrupts the reflex arc, results in slow deep breathing in most animals.

As early as 1868, Hering and Breuer observed the inflation and deflation reflexes in anesthetized animals.[27] Although the Hering-Breuer inflation reflex is active in animals during tidal volume breathing,[28] it does not operate

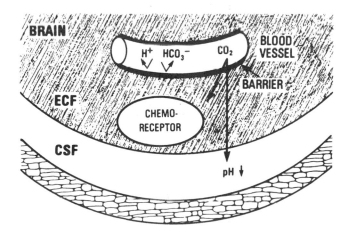

Fig. 3–7. The central chemoreceptors of the medulla are bathed in the brain interstitial fluid through which CO_2 easily diffuses from the brain blood vessels to the cerebrospinal fluid (CSF). H^+ and HCO_3^- ions cannot readily cross the blood-brain barrier. ECF, extracellular fluid. From West, J. B. (ed.): Best and Taylor's Physiological Basis of Medical Practice, 12th Ed. Baltimore, Williams & Wilkins, 1992, p. 581.)

in man breathing at normal tidal volume, unless the tidal volume is about 1 liter or more.[29] The reflex does operate in newborn babies at tidal volume breathing, but decreases in effectiveness during the first 5 days of life as higher centers become more active.[16]

Because inflation and deflation reflexes terminate inspiration and expiration, respectively, they may play a role in the off-switch, on-switch mechanisms of the medullary inspiratory center, respectively. Evidence also shows that the inflation reflex regulates the rate and depth of breathing in such a way that optimal alveolar ventilation occurs with the least amount of muscular effort.[16]

Inhalational anesthetics such as halothane tend to increase the frequency of breathing, probably by sensitizing the inflation receptors, and thus earlier termination of inspiration.[16]

Irritant Receptors

These receptors respond to chemical as well as mechanical stimulation, and are located among airway epithelial cells in the trachea, bronchi, and bronchioles. They include intrapulmonary epithelial irritant receptors and extrapulmonary tracheal and bronchial cough receptors.[16] They are excited by irritant gases and vapors (ammonia, sulfur dioxide), chemical mediators released in the lung during allergic reactions (histamine, leukotriene C4, bradykinin), inert particles (dust, smoke), and inhaled antigents (pollens). Unlike PSR, they adapt quickly to stimulation. Their afferent impulses travel in small myelinated fibers of the vagus to reach the medulla.

When stimulated, the receptors produce cough, bronchoconstriction, and tachypnea. These responses may limit penetration of potentially harmful substances into the lungs, thereby preventing reaction of these substances with the gas-exchanging surfaces. The irritant receptors may also help to maximize lung compliance by initiating periodic sighs or large breaths that occur during normal breathing. These sighs expand the alveolar surface area and replenish the surface active molecules.[30]

J Receptors

The term J or juxtapulmonary-capillary receptor is used because of the belief that these receptors are in the intersitial tissue between pulmonary capillaries and alveoli.[26] The afferent impulses, carried by unmyelinated vagal C fibers, are stimulated by distortion of the lung's interstitium, such as by intersititial lung edema, pulmonary capillary congestion, capillary hypertension, and some chemicals, such as histamine and capsaicin (the active irritant in pepper). Their activation causes laryngeal closure and apnea followed by rapid shallow breathing. They may play a role in the tachypnea experienced by patients with pulmonary edema, pulmonary emboli, and pneumonia.

Other Receptors

Upper Airway Receptors

The nose, nasopharynx, larynx, and trachea have receptors that respond to chemical and mechanical stimulation. The afferent pathways for nasal receptors lie in the trigeminal and olfactory nerves. The primary reflex effects of activation of these receptors in anesthetized animals are apnea, bradycardia, and sneezing.

Receptors in the larynx, probably irritant receptors, also respond to chemical and mechanical stimulation.[31] The afferent fibers from these receptors are located in the internal branch of the superior laryngeal nerve and inferior laryngeal nerve (recurrent laryngeal nerve). The responses to stimulation of these receptors are variable and include coughing, slow deep breathing, apnea, laryngeal spasm, bronchoconstriction, and hypertension.[32,33]

Joint Receptors

Active and passive movements of joints produce afferent impulses that reflexly increase the rate and depth of respiration. This response probably plays a role in exercise-induced hyperpnea.

Muscle Receptors

The two types of muscle receptors are the muscle spindles and the Golgi tendon organs. The former is responsible for stretch reflex and the latter are involved in the inverse stretch reflex. These receptors are abundant in intercostal and abdominal wall muscles, but scarce in the diaphragm. Afferent impulses from these receptors are mainly integrated at the spinal segmental level; their contribution to tidal volume regulation is negligible.[34] Muscle spindles appear to help coordinate breathing during changes in posture and speech, whereas Golgi tendon organs monitor the force of muscle contraction and tend to inhibit inspiration.[30] Spindle afferent fibers also seem to project to the cerebral cortex to provide conscious information about respiratory movements.[30]

The motor nerve supply to the muscle spindles (consisting of intrafusal muscle fibers) is through the gamma efferent system, whereas that to the regular contractile units (the extrafusal fibers) is through the alpha efferent system, both orginating from the anterior horn cells of the spinal cord.

Pain Receptors

Pain receptors are free nerve endings. Pain may cause either respiratory stimulation or inhibition, depending on the character, origin (visceral or somatic), and intensity.[17]

Temperature Receptors

An increase in body temperature increases pulmonary ventilation, sometimes to such an extent that severe alkalosis and tetany may follow. This effect results in part from stimulation of the hypothalamic thermoreceptors. Heating of skin may also prompt hyperventilation, resulting from stimulation of the peripheral thermoreceptors. The increase in ventilation after stimulation of the peripheral and hypothalamic heat-sensitive receptors is one of the thermoregulatory responses that occurs as the surface or deep body temperature goes up and the need to increase heat loss through the respiratory system is recognized.

CONTROLLER

Although breathing is an involuntary automatic process, it can be controlled, to some extent, by motor impulses from the cerebral cortex during wakefulness. Examples are voluntary hyperventilation, voluntary hypoventilation, and breath holding, all under voluntary control. Thus, the respiratory controller within the central nervous system consists of two anatomically and functionally distinct parts: the brain stem, which regulates automatic respiration, and the cerebral cortex, which regulates voluntary respiration.

The descending voluntary respiratory tract travels separately from the descending involuntary respiratory tract. The former travels from the cortex to the spinal cord respiratory motoneurons through corticospinal tracts, bypassing the medullary respiratory neurons. The latter travels from the medulla to the spinal cord respiratory motoneurons in the white matter between the lateral and ventral corticospinal tracts. Therefore, both systems project to the spinal cord respiratory neurons in the cervical and thoracic segments, where motor impulses in the two descending systems integrate. Spinal respiratory motoneurons in the anterior horn serve as the final common pathway to the respiratory muscles. In the following discussion, the principal focus is on the automatic regulation of respiration.

EFFERENT RESPIRATORY SYSTEMS

Anatomic Organization of the Brain Stem Respiratory Neurons and Spinal Projection

Historical Perspective

Ever since Legallois[35] and Flourens[36] showed that rhythmic breathing depends on the anatomic and functional integrity of some structures in the pons and medulla, a great deal of work has been done to localize the brain stem respiratory neurons and to determine their role in the normal pattern of breathing.

The pioneering studies of Legallois,[35] Flourens,[36] and others,[37] which included the use of such techniques as brain transection at various levels and ablation of different parts of the brain showed that the structures responsible for breathing rhythmicity were within the pontomedullary region. These early investigative techniques were rather crude, and the results fell short of precise localization of the respiratory neurons.

Another technique involved electrical stimulation of pinpoint areas of the brain.[38-41] The region of the medulla where electrical stimulation produced sustained deep inspiration was named the "inspiratory center," and that region where electrical stimulation produced sustained deep expiration was named the "expiratory center" by Pitts et al.[38] Still another technique involved the production of macro-[42] and microlesions[43] in the brain stem to determine the location, or to assess the function, of respiration-related structures.

Currently, the technique of microelectrode recording (extracellularly or intracellularly) is used for localization of the respiratory neurons.[44-49] Cells whose firing activity is synchronous with phrenic nerve activity or with the tracheal inspiratory air flow are considered inspiratory neurons (Figs. 3-8 and 3-9). Cells whose firing activity is synchronous with the silent phase of the phrenic nerve or with the tracheal expiratory air flow are considered expiratory neurons (Fig. 3-10).

In the cat, data from microelectrode recording coupled with information from histochemical studies and ortho- and antidromic stimulation of nerve fibers has led to more clarity concerning the organization of the brain stem respiratory neurons (Fig. 3-11) and their axonal projections.[50-53]

Medullary Respiratory Neurons

Within the medulla oblongata are two anatomically distinct groups of respiratory neurons located bilaterally and symmetrically. The dorsal respiratory group (DRG), composed primarily of inspiratory cells, is in the dorsomedial part of the medulla.[50,54] The ventral respiratory group (VRG), composed of both inspiratory and expiratory cells, is located in the ventrolateral part of the medulla.[50,52]

Dorsal Respiratory Group

The DRG is associated with the nucleus tractus solitarius (NTS), which is the projection site for visceral afferents in the ninth and tenth (glossopharyngeal and vagus) nerves. On the basis of response to lung inflation, three types of neurons have been recognized in the DRG. One type, called I alpha[55] or R alpha[56] (I and R stand for inspiratory and respiratory, respectively), is inhibited by lung inflation. The axons of these cells project to both the phrenic and external intercostal motoneurons of the spinal cord. Another type, called I beta[55] or R beta,[56] is excited by lung inflation. Whether the I beta axons project into the spinal cord respiratory motoneurons is controversial. The rhythmic firing activity of the I alpha and I

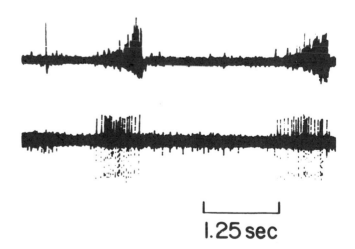

Fig. 3–8. Simultaneous recording of the phrenic neurogram (upper tracing) and a medullary inspiratory neuronal discharge (lower tracing). The neuronal discharge is synchronous with that of the phrenic nerve; hence, the neuron is an inspiratory neuron. From Tabatabai, M., et al.: Effects of halothane on medullary inspiratory neurons of the cat. Anesthesiology 66:176, 1987.

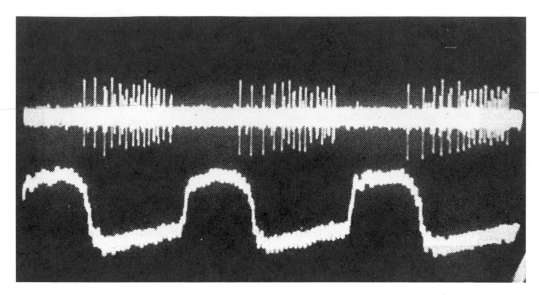

Fig. 3–9. Simultaneous recording of the discharge activity of a few medullary neurons in the rat (upper tracing) and tracheal air flow (pneumotachogram) (lower tracing). Inspiration is indicated by upwards movement on the pneumotachogram. The discharge activity of the neurons is synchronous with inspiration; therefore, they are inspiratory neurons.

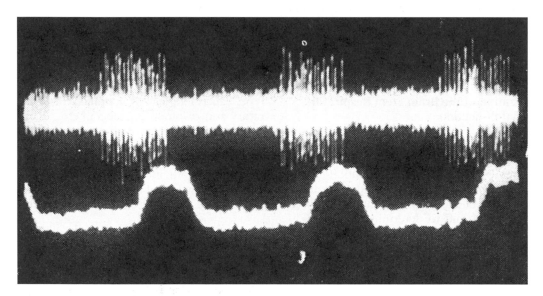

Fig. 3–10. Simultaneous recording of the discharge activity of two or three medullary neurons in the rat (upper tracing) and tracheal air flow (pneumotachogram) (lower tracing). Inspiration is indicated by upward movement on the pneumotachogram. The discharge activity of the neurons is synchronous with expiration; therefore, they are expiratory neurons.

beta cells continues even when lung inflation is stopped or the vagus nerves in the neck are severed, suggesting that these cells receive excitatory input from the central pattern generator (CPG) for breathing.[55,57]

The DRG also includes a number of cells without input from the CPG for breathing. The firing activity of these cells closely follows lung inflation during either spontaneous or controlled ventilation; these are called pump or "P" cells, and are assumed to be interneurons.

Because excitation of the I beta neuron discharge by lung inflation is associated with shortening of inspiration, it has been suggested that the I beta neurons function to promote the inspiration-to-expiration phase switching by inhibitory actions on I alpha neurons,[51,55] and that this network is thus responsible for the Hering-Breuer reflex

inhibition of inspiration by lung inflation, i.e., the Hering-Breuer inflation reflex or Hering-Breuer inhibito-inspiratory reflex.[56]

Ventral Respiratory Group

The VRG extends from the rostral to the caudal end of the medulla and has three subdivisions. The Botzinger complex,[58] located in the most rostral part of the medulla, contains mainly expiratory neurons that send inhibitory connections to DRG inspiratory neurons[58] to ensure inspiratory neuronal silence during expiration (reciprocal inhibition) and to take part in inspiratory off-switch mechanisms.

The nucleus ambiguus (NA) and nucleus para-am-

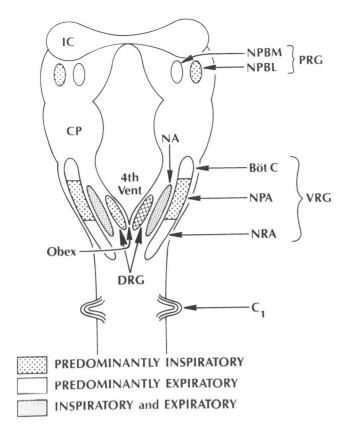

Fig. 3–11. Respiratory neurons on the dorsal surface of the brain stem. Cross-hatched areas, contain mainly inspiratory neurons; blank areas, contain mainly expiratory neurons; dotted areas contain both inspiratory and expiratory neurons. Böt C, Bötzinger complex; C_1, first cervical spinal nerve; CP, cerebellar peduncle; DRG, dorsal respiratory group; 4th Vent, fourth ventricle; IC, inferior colliculus; NA, nucleus ambiguus; NPA, nucleus para-ambigualis; NPBL, nucleus parabrachialis lateralis; NPBM, nucleus parabrachialis medialis; NRA, nucleus retroambigualis; PRG, pontine respiratory group; VRG, ventral respiratory group.

bigualis (NPA) lie side by side in the intermediate portion of the VRG. The NA contains respiratory motoneurons the axons of which exit the brain along with other vagal efferent fibers and innervate the laryngeal abductor (inspiratory) and adductor (expiratory) muscles via the recurrent laryngeal nerve.[59] The NPA[60] contains mainly inspiratory neurons, referred to as I gamma neurons to distinguish them from I alpha and I beta neurons of the DRG.[55] The I gamma neurons respond to lung inflation in a manner similar to I alpha neurons. The axons of these neurons project to both the phrenic and the external (inspiratory) intercostal motoneuron pools in the spinal cord.

The nucleus retroambigualis (NRA),[61] occupying the caudal part of VRG, contains expiratory neurons with axons that project into the spinal motoneuron pool for the internal (expiratory) intercostal and abdominal muscles.[61,62]

Pontine Respiratory Neurons

The dorsolateral portion of the rostral pons contains both inspiratory and expiratory neurons (Fig. 3-11), the latter in the region of the nucleus parabrachialis medialis (NPBM) and the former in the nucleus parabrachialis lateralis (NPBL).[63] The respiratory neurons of these nuclei are referred to as the pontine respiratory group (PRG),[52] which is also called the pneumotaxic center, a term coined by Lumsden in 1923.[64] Electrical stimulation of the PRG produces rapid breathing with premature switching of the respiratory phases.[65] Conversely, transection of the brain at a level caudal to the PRG, or lesions that impact the PRG prolong inspiration, resulting in slow deep breathing.[66,67] Bilateral cervical vagotomy produces a similar pattern, i.e., slow deep breathing. Bilateral cervical vagotomy in combination with transection caudal to PRG or lesions of the PRG results in apneusis (sustained inspiration or cessation of respiration in inspiration) (Table 3-4) or apneustic breathing (slow rhythmic respiration with increased inspiratory time) (Fig. 3-12).[66,68]

In summary, there are three groups of brain stem respiratory neurons; one in the pons and two in the medulla. Of the latter two, one group occupies the dorsomedial part of the medulla, and is called the dorsal respiratory group (DRG), and the other lies in the ventrolateral part of the medulla, and is called the ventral respiratory group (VRG). The pontine respiratory neurons are located in the rostral pons, and referred to as the pontine respiratory group (PRG) or pneumotaxic center.

Breathing Rhythmogenesis

In all species studied, rhythmic breathing can occur in the absence of feedback from peripheral receptors, indicating that respiratory rhythm is produced by a CPG and not peripheral input. Because transection of the brain at a level rostral to the pons has little effect on the respiratory pattern, and transection below the level of the medulla eliminates rhythmic breathing, the CPG must reside in the lower brain stem, i.e., pons and medulla. Most authorities agree that the CPG for basic breathing rhythmicity is in the medulla,[51] but its precise location within the medulla remains unclear. The DRG, VRG, and PRG have been considered as possible sites, but the neural elements constituting the CPG appear to be separate from the identified respiratory neurons studied so far.[69]

The mechanism of breathing rhythm generation is also unclear and has been a subject of much debate and extensive research. In short, rhythmic breathing may result from the activity of pacemaker cells or neural networks or both. Pacemaker cells do not require interaction with other neural elements to produce rhythmic output; rather they are capable of self-depolarization and hyperpolarization alternately. Although an attractive hypothesis, to date, no evidence exists to either confirm or deny the existence of pacemaker cells and their role in breathing rhythmogenesis. Because of technical difficulty in showing pacemaker cells, most investigations regarding the mechanisms of breathing rhythm generation have focused on neural network interactions such as reciprocal inhibition (i.e., inhibition of expiratory neurons by inspiratory neurons during inspiration and inhibition of inspiratory neurons by expiratory neurons during expiration), although reciprocal inhibition alone cannot explain the

Table 3–4. Normal and Abnormal Patterns of Breathing*

Eupnea: normal breathing—repeated rhythmic inspiratory-expiratory cycles without inspiratory or expiratory pause; inspiration is active and expiration passive.

Hyperpnea: increased breathing; usually refers to increased tidal volume with or without increased frequency.

Polypnea, tachypnea: increased frequency of breathing.

Hyperventilation: increased alveolar ventilation in relation to metabolic rate (i.e., alveolar alveolar P_{CO_2} <40 mm. Hg).

Hypoventilation: decreased alveolar ventilation in relation to metabolic rate (i.e., alveolar P_{CO_2} >40 mm. Hg).

Apnea: cessation of respiration in the resting expiratory position.

Apneusis: cessation of respiration in the inspiratory position.

Apneustic breathing: apneusis interrupted periodically by expiration; may be rhythmic.

Gasping: spasmodic inspiratory effort, usually maximal, brief, and terminating abruptly; may be rhythmic or irregular.

Cheyne-Stokes respiration: cycles of gradually increasing tidal volume followed by gradually decreasing tidal volume.

Biot's respiration: originally described in patients with meningitis by Biot (Lyon med., 23, 517, 561, 1876) as irregular respiration with pauses; today, it refers to sequences of uniformly deep gasps, apnea, then deep gasps.

Comroc, Physiology of Respiration, 2nd Ed., Year Book, 1977.

alteration of respiratory phases, i.e., switching of inspiration to expiration and vice versa.

As has been stated, the CPG for breathing is located in the medulla. The activity of CPG is influenced by input from chemoreceptors (peripheral and central), mechanoreceptors (pulmonary stretch, irritant, J, and muscle and joint), thermoreceptors (peripheral and central), nociceptors, and higher central structures, such as the PRG. The function of this input is to adapt the breathing pattern to ever-changing metabolic and behavioral needs.

In summary, basic breathing rhythmicity is generated by a central pattern generator (CPG) located somewhere in the medulla, whose activity is modulated by a host of afferent inputs such that its output may meet the ever-changing metabolic and behavioral demands.

Tests of Respiratory Control

Respiratory control is tested by providing a stimulus to perturb the respiratory control system and measuring the resulting ventilatory response.[17] Because there are various components in the respiratory control system, no single test can measure the efficiency and integrity of all the components. Thus, the ventilatory response to hypercarbia mainly tests the central chemoreceptors, the ventilatory response to hypoxia mainly tests the peripheral

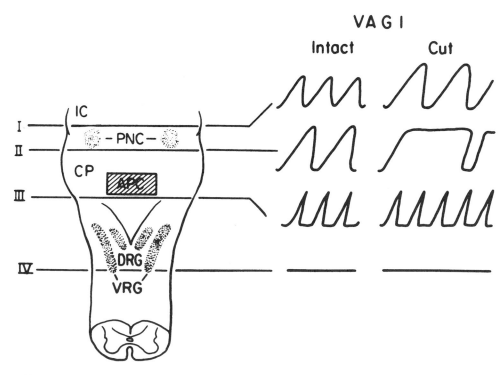

Fig. 3–12. Effects of brain stem transections at four different levels (left side) on patterns of respiration (right side) with the vagus nerves intact or cut. Section below the medulla results in cessation of breathing. APC, apneustic center; CP, cerebellar peduncle; DRG, dorsal respiratory group; IC, inferior colliculus; PNC, pneumotaxic center; VRG, ventral respiratory group. (From Berger, A. J., et al.: Regulation of respiration. N Engl J Med *297*:92–97, 138–143, 194–201, 1977.

chemoreceptors, and voluntary hyperventilation can assess the efficiency of the neuromuscular system.

Measurement of respiratory-center output, the so-called respiratory drive, is more difficult to quantitate. Direct measurement of the inspiratory neuronal activity would be ideal, but this approach is not yet possible. Indirect methods used to evaluate the output of the respiratory center are (1) integrated electrical activity of the phrenic nerve, (2) integrated electrical activity of the diaphragm (electromyography), (3) mouth occlusion pressure as a measure of inspiratory force generated by inspiratory muscles, and (4) lung ventilation.

Response to Carbon Dioxide

Two types of CO_2 response tests are available: the steady-state and rebreathing methods. In the steady-state method, the subject breathes a gas mixture containing increased concentrations of CO_2 and the change in ventilation (or one of the other parameters of respiratory center output) at steady state is measured. Normally, it takes 10 to 15 minutes to reach a steady state of ventilation. Five percent CO_2 in O_2 is commonly used as a test gas, although greater reliability is achieved by using several CO_2 concentrations, such as 0, 3%, 5%, and 7%. Normal subjects show about a fourfold increase in ventilation while breathing 5% CO_2, or an increase in ventilation of 1.5 to 2.5 L/min/mm Hg rise in arterial PCO_2.[17] Figure 3–13 illustrates the results of the steady-state CO_2 response test performed in a person with normal respiratory function, one with emphysema, and one with a depressed respiratory center.

In the rebreathing methods, the subject breathes from a bag prefilled with 7% CO_2 and 93% O_2. The minute ventilation and the end-tidal CO_2 concentration or partial pressure are recorded continuously.

The ventilatory response to CO_2 decreases with age and during sleep, and it can be severely depressed by a variety of sedatives, narcotics, and anesthetics. The response is also decreased in patients with obstructive pulmonary disease. This depression can be reproduced in normal subjects when they are breathing with added mechanical loads.[70]

Response to Hypoxia

By gradually decreasing the concentration of O_2 in the inspired gas mixture and measuring the corresponding changes in ventilation, it is possible to evaluate a subject's response to hypoxia. The relationship between arterial PO_2 and ventilation is hyperbolic (Fig. 3–14A) and differs depending on whether arterial PCO_2 is allowed to fall, as it normally does when ventilation increases, or is held constant by adding CO_2 to the inspired mixture, as is the case during an isocapnic hypoxia-response test. Because hyperbolic curves are cumbersome to analyze, the response to hypoxia is now often expressed as the relationship between minute ventilation and arterial O_2 saturation, monitored with a pulse oximeter (Fig. 3–14B).

To avoid systemic effects of hypoxia and to minimize

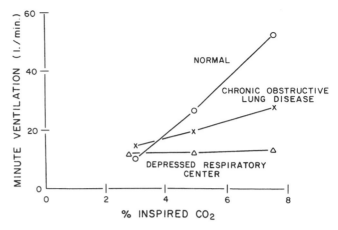

Fig. 3–13. Steady-state CO_2 response test. Subjects breathed gas mixtures containing 3%, 5%, and 7.5% CO_2 in air until a steady level of minute ventilation was attained. Subjects breathed room air for about 10 minutes between each test gas. The normal subject (○) shows an approximately linear increase in minute ventilation over this range of inspired CO_2. The subject with chronic obstructive lung disease related to moderately severe emphysema (X) shows a blunted ventilatory response to CO_2. The subject with depressed respiratory center (△), in this case from previous inflammatory disease of the brain, shows essentially no ventilatory response to exogenous CO_2. From Forster, R. E., et al.: The Lung: Physiologic Basis of Pulmonary Function Tests, 3rd Ed. Chicago, Year Book, 1986, p. 125.

fluctuations in alveolar CO_2, the test can also be accomplished by taking one to three breaths of 100% nitrogen, which in healthy individuals results in prompt stimulation of ventilation by stimulation of carotid chemoreceptors.

Hypoxic sensitivity decreases with increasing age and the administration of sedatives, narcotics, and anesthet-

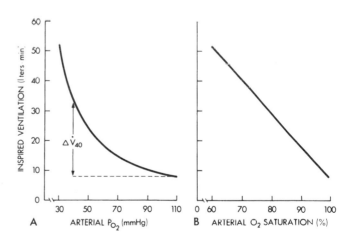

Fig. 3–14. Mean hypoxic response of four normal men at standard constant arterial PCO_2 (isocapnic hypoxia response test). A. Hyperbolic relationship between arterial PO_2 and ventilation. Also shown is the hypoxic sensitivity index ($\Delta \dot{V}_{40}$), defined as the increment in ventilation when PaO_2 is reduced from above 150 to 40 mm Hg. B. Linear response between arterial O_2 saturation and ventilation. From Berger, A. J., et al.: Regulation of respiration. N Engl J Med *297*:92–97, 138–143, 194–201, 1977.

ics, and is characteristically depressed or even absent in long-term residents of high altitudes.[71,71] In the absence of the carotid bodies, hypoxia (PaO_2 of 45 to 55 mm Hg) reduces ventilation through a direct depressive effect on the respiratory center.[73]

The CO_2 response and the hypoxia response tests provide useful information about chemosensitivity, but interpretation is limited because both tests are influenced by mechanical abnormalities anywhere in the respiratory system.

Mouth Occlusion Pressure

This test is used as an indirect method of measuring the respiratory-center output, the so-called respiratory drive.[74,75] The force generated by the inspiratory muscles in response to the inspiratory center output is estimated by measuring the negative pressure at the mouth with the onset of inspiration against a closed shutter, hence the name occlusion pressure. The subject breathes through a mouthpiece with separate inspiratory and expiratory valves. During expiration at a time unknown to the subject, the operator closes the inspiratory valve so that the subject begins the next breath in the usual way. Because there is no air flow, the mouth pressure reflects the static mechanical forces in the respiratory system generated by the inspiratory muscles in response to the respiratory center output. The pressure change is measured 0.1 second (Po.1) after closure of the shutter to minimize conscious or reflex changes in muscle tone that occur during longer occlusions. Therefore the Po.1 reflects both the neuronal drive to the muscles of inspiration and the contractile capabilities of these muscles. This test can be used to study the respiratory sensitivity to CO_2, hypoxia, and other factors as well.

Breathing Cycle Timing

Duty cycle of respiration, calculated as the inspiratory time (t_i) divided by the total time of the respiratory cycle (t_{tot}), i.e., t_i/t_{tot}, is a reflection of "respiratory timing."[76] Mean inspiratory flow rate, calculated as the tidal volume (V_t) divided by the inspiratory time (t_i), i.e., V_t/V_i, is a measure of "inspiratory drive."[76]

Causes of Abnormal Tests

Abnormal CO_2 Response

When the CO_2 response test is abnormal, it implies that an abnormality exists with one or more components of the respiratory control system: sensors (receptors), controllers, or effectors. Clinically, three general conditions account for most of the abnormalities in CO_2 response. The first is failure (decreased sensitivity) of the central chemoreceptors or inadequate response of brain stem respiratory neurons to impulses from the central chemoreceptors (Fig. 3–13). In this category, the neural output from the respiratory center in response to CO_2 is decreased. These conditions could involve congenital defects or may be acquired after inflammatory or traumatic lesions of the brain. Sedatives, narcotics, and anesthetics

also work on the central chemoreceptors-controller system to decrease CO_2 response. Chronic CO_2 retention, as it occurs in patients with chronic pulmonary disease, results in the decreased response of the central chemoreceptors. The ventilatory response to CO_2 is also reduced during sleep and old age.

The second condition that accounts for an abnormal CO_2 response test is disease of the neuromuscular system, so that although the respiratory center output in response to CO_2 administration is normal, the neuromuscular apparatus fails to respond to the increased respiratory center output. Examples include poliomyelitis, with damage to anterior horn cells innervating the respiratory muscles, and myasthenia gravis. These conditions are also associated with decreased force of the inspiratory muscles, such that the mouth occlusion pressure (Po.1) will be low.

The third condition with which the CO_2 response is abnormal involves mechanical limitations to chest expansion, such as occurs in patients with obstructive or restrictive lung disease or thoracic wall deformity (Fig. 3–13). In this situation, the respiratory-center output and the neuromuscular response to CO_2 challenge are normal, but because of altered lung or chest wall mechanisms, respiratory muscle activity is not effective in producing an expected increase in ventilation. Measurement of the diaphragmatic electromyogram or the force of contraction of the inspiratory muscles (mouth occlusion pressure) are normal, however, indicating adequate response of central chemoreceptors to exogenous CO_2.

Patients with chronic obstructive pulmonary disease who have CO_2 retention have decreased ventilatory response to exogenous CO_2, in part because of decreased sensitivity of central chemoreceptors to the H^+ concentration of the CSF and in part because of mechanical lung dysfunction, i.e., increased airway resistance.

Abnormal Hypoxia Response

This test has limited clinical applications. Subjects with longstanding hypoxemia, such as those born and raised at high altitude, patients with cyanotic congenital heart disease, and patients with surgical removal of carotid bodies, may lose much or all of their oxygen chemosensitivity. The degree of depression of O_2 chemosensitivity in these individuals can be evaluated by a hypoxia response test.

Patients with chronic obstructive pulmonary disease and CO_2 retention have decreased ventilatory response to CO_2, as explained previously. These patients may depend on hypoxic drive for their ventilation. It is possible to determine the extent to which hypoxemia is responsible for maintaining a patient's ventilation by measuring ventilation when the patient is breathing air and again when O_2 is substituted for air. In healthy individuals with normal arterial PO_2, inhalation of 100% O_2 decreases minute ventilation only slightly and only for a few breaths.[17] In patients with decreased central chemosensitivity to CO_2 who depend on hypoxic ventilatory drive, inhalation of 100% O_2 may decrease ventilation substantially by removal of the hypoxic stimulus.[17]

EFFECTOR RESPIRATORY MUSCLES

The respiratory muscles consist of inspiratory and expiratory muscles.

Inspiratory Muscles

This muscle group includes the diaphragm, external intercostal, scalene (anterior, middle, and posterior), and sternocleidomastoid muscles. In severe muscular exercise or during maximal voluntary ventilation, accessory inspiratory muscles are active, including the trapezius and back muscles. Strap, laryngeal, and tongue muscles aid inspiration not by enlarging the thorax but by reducing the resistance to airflow.[16]

The Diaphragm

This large, dome-shaped sheet is the principal muscle of inspiration. During quiet breathing at rest, movement of the diaphragm accounts for at least 75% of the increase in intrathoracic volume. During contraction, it moves downward and pushes on the abdominal contents and displaces the abdominal wall outward. During maximal inspiration, its downward stroke may be as much as 10 cm.[16] The main action of the diaphragm is to enlarge the thoracic cavity downward. Although primarily an inspiratory muscle, it remains active (contracted) during the early part of expiration, presumably to let the thorax decrease in volume less abruptly in order to smooth out expiration. The motor nerve supply to the diaphragm is through the phrenic nerve, which arises from the third to the fifth cervical spinal cord segments, but mainly from the fourth.

External Intercostal Muscles

Contraction of these muscles lifts the anterior end of each rib and pulls it upward and outward, thus increasing the anteroposterior diameter of the thorax. They are innervated by the intercostal nerves, which arise from the first to the twelfth thoracic spinal cord segments.

Other Muscles of Inspiration

The scalene muscles (anterior, middle, and posterior) have rhythmic activity during quiet breathing at rest.[77] They elevate the upper two ribs, thus increasing the intrathoracic volume, and are innervated by way of the cervical spinal nerves.

Sternocleidomastoid muscles elevate the sternum by their contraction, thereby increasing the intrathoracic volume. They become active as an inspiratory muscle during strenuous breathing[77] and are supplied by the accessory nerves (eleventh cranial nerves).

In severe muscular exercise or during maximal voluntary ventilation, all of the accessory muscles of inspiration, including the trapezius and back muscles, are active.

Other accessory muscles aid inspiration by reducing the resistance to air flow. These consist of glossal, laryngeal, and strap muscles.[16] One of the external glossal muscles, the genioglossus, has earned recognition for its possible role in sleep apnea and upper airway obstruction. This muscle contracts rhythmically in phase with inspira-

tion and pulls the tongue forward.[78,79] In cats, interference with its activity was noted during anesthesia.[80,81] It is reasonable to assume that induction and maintenance of anesthesia may interfere with activity of the genioglossus in humans, causing the tongue to fall back against the posterior pharyngeal wall and explaining the airway obstruction that occurs commonly when anesthesia is induced. One cause of the obstructive type of sleep apnea appears to be failure of the genioglossus muscle to contract during inspiration in sleep, causing the tongue to fall back and then obstruct the airway.[82]

Maximal contraction of the inspiratory muscles can lower intrapleural pressure to as much as 60 to 100 mm Hg below atmospheric pressure, i.e., to -60 to -100 mm Hg.[16]

Expiratory Muscles

Expiration is passive and occurs by recoil of the stretched elastic tissues and release of energy stored in the elastic tissues during inspiration. At high rates of ventilation or with moderate to severe airway obstruction, the expiratory muscles, which are supplied by intercostal nerves, contract. The internal intercostal and the abdominal muscles belong to this group. Contraction of the internal intercostal muscles moves the ribs downward and inward, thus reducing the intrathoracic volume. Contraction of the abdominal wall muscles (rectus abdominis, external oblique, internal oblique, and transversus abdominis) depresses the lower ribs and flexes the trunk, but above all, it increases intra-abdominal pressure, which pushes the diaphragm upward.

Vigorous contraction of the expiratory muscles can generate a sustained intrapulmonary pressure of 120 mm Hg. Maximal contraction of the abdominal muscles during straining can generate intra-abdominal pressure of 150 to 200 mm Hg, enough to stop blood flow through the abdominal aorta.[17]

REGULATION OF VENTILATION DURING SLEEP

Sleep is not a homogeneous state, but a cyclic phenomenon, which, on the basis of electroencephalographic (EEG) and electro-oculographic (EOG) characteristics, has two distinct phases: rapid eye movement (REM), or active, sleep, and nonrapid eye movement (nonREM), or quiet, sleep. NonREM sleep has four stages of progressively deepening levels, of which the deepest two (stages 3 and 4) are called slow-wave sleep because of the characteristic EEG pattern. In adults, each cycle lasts about 90 minutes, and, on average, four to five episodes of REM sleep occur per night.

Stage 1 is dozing; the EEG is characterized by fast waves of low amplitude. Stage 1 progresses into stage 2, in which the background EEG is similar to stage 1, but with periodic sleep spindles (frequency, 12 to 14 Hz). Stage 3 is characterized by slow, large-amplitude (delta) waves and fewer sleep spindles. Stage 4 has mainly delta waves (2 to 7 cycles/sec, greater than 75 µV in amplitude). In REM sleep, the EEG is the same as in stage 1, but the EOG shows frequent rapid eye movements. REM sleep is associated with dreaming.

During slow-wave sleep (stages 3 and 4 of nonREM sleep) in normal healthy subjects, the neural drive from the brain stem respiratory center is diminished and minute ventilation is decreased. Consequently, arterial PCO_2 increases 4 to 6 mm Hg, arterial PO_2 decreases 4 to 9 mm Hg, and arterial pH decreases 0.03 to 0.05 units.[83] Similar changes in arterial blood gas and pH are present during REM sleep.[84] The ventilatory response to CO_2 is decreased and the CO_2 response curve is shifted to the right in slow-wave sleep and in REM sleep,[85] indicating reduced sensitivity of the central chemoreceptors. In contrast, the ventilatory response to low arterial PO_2 is spared during sleep, although this is a point of controversy.[86,87]

The most common abnormality of regulation of respiration during sleep is the occurrence of apneic episodes, i.e., sleep apnea, whether of central or obstructive type. The apneic episode lasts more than 10 seconds, recurs at least 11 times per hour during sleep,[88] and may be associated with reductions in arterial O_2 saturations to 75% or less.[30]

Central apnea is characterized by a cessation of all breathing efforts, i.e., complete cessation of central respiratory drive. In obstructive apnea, despite persistent breathing efforts, air flow ceases because of obstruction of the upper airway. The role of the external glossal muscle genioglossus in obstructive sleep apnea was discussed previously.

In central sleep apnea, the automatic respiratory controller in the brain stem does not generate respiratory impulses during sleep. This situation may result from impairment of ascending spinal pathways that normally carry afferent impulses from peripheral receptors to brain stem respiratory neurons.[89,90] This condition is reversible with arousal. In Ondine's curse, the automatic brain stem respiratory center fails even while awake.[91] Patients with Ondine's curse breathe on command, or they breathe if they can remember to breathe. These patients depend totally on their voluntary system of breathing for survival. Patients with this intriguing condition generally have bulbar poliomyelitis or disease processes that compress the medulla. The condition has also been inadvertently produced in patients who have been subjected to bilateral anterolateral cervical cordotomy for pain. This procedure cuts the pathways that bring about automatic respiration while leaving intact the voluntary efferent pathways in the corticospinal tracts.[82]

Snoring is a manifestation of partial upper airway obstruction.

REGULATION OF VENTILATION DURING EXERCISE

The mechanisms underlying tight coupling of increased ventilation to increased metabolic demands of exercise remain elusive. Several good reviews are available on this topic.[92-94]

In adults at rest, O_2 uptake is 250 ml/min. During severe vigorous exercise, it may increase to as much as 5500 ml/min, an 22-fold increase.[17] The body meets this enormous increase in O_2 demand by a great increase in cardiac output and a tremendous increase in alveolar ventilation

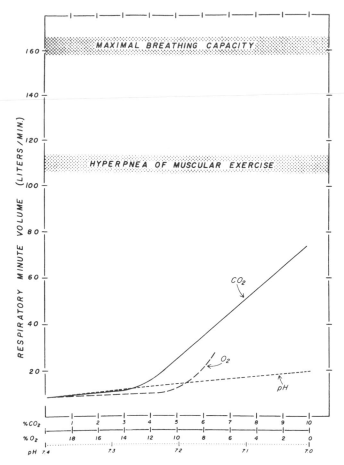

Fig. 3–15. Hyperpnea of severe muscular exercise is contrasted with hyperpnea produced by breathing low O_2 or high CO_2 mixtures in normal man and in patients with acidosis and with hyperpnea of maximal breathing capacity. From Forster, R. E., et al.: The Lung: Physiologic Basis of Pulmonary Function Tests, 3rd Ed. Chicago, Year Book, 1986, p. 120.

(Fig. 3–15). The highest level of work that can be performed without inducing a sustained metabolic acidosis is called the anaerobic threshold. Acid-base balance is normal during steady-state exercise (up to about a sixfold increase in O_2 consumption), when O_2 delivery to the mitochondria is adequate to meet all energy requirements.[30] Further increases in the level of exercise, however, cross the anaerobic threshold, after which energy requirements can be satisfied only by a combination of aerobic metabolism and anaerobic glycolysis. The lactic acid formed during glycolysis diffuses into the blood and increases the H^+ concentration. Below the anaerobic threshold, the arterial PO_2, PCO_2, and pH are virtually unchanged, although venous values are altered.[30]

Because no significant change in arterial PO_2, PCO_2, or pH occurs during moderate exercise in a normal subject, an increased "chemical drive," acting on central or peripheral chemoreceptors, does not exist to explain the increase in ventilation. Different theories proposed to explain the hyperpnea of exercise in the face of normal arterial PO_2, PCO_2, and pH[17] include the following: (1) increased sensitivity of the central chemoreceptors to normal levels of arterial PCO$_2$ caused in part by release of adrenergic mediators; (2) bombardment of the brain stem respiratory centers by impulses from the motor cortex en route to the exercising muscles, thus increasing the output of the brain stem respiratory neurons; (3) an increase in body temperature stimulating respiration by acting on the respiratory center either directly or indirectly via central or peripheral thermoreceptors; (4) increased stimulatory input to the brain stem respiratory center from mechanoreceptors in the joints, tendons, and muscles; and (5) an unidentified X-substance formed during muscular exercise and acting on the brain stem respiratory centers. No single theory proposed so far is adequate, and it is likely that multiple factors are responsible for the hyperpnea of exercise.

REFERENCES

1. Heymans, J. F., Heymans, C.: Sur les modifications directes et sur la régulation reflexe de l'activité du centre respiratorie de la tête isolée du chien. Arch Int Pharmacodyn Ther 33:273, 1927.
2. Dripps, R. D., Comroe, Jr., J. H.: The effect of the inhalation of high and low oxygen concentrations on respiration, pulse rate, ballistocardiogram and arterial oxygen saturation (oximeter) of normal individuals. Am J Physiol 149:277, 1947.
3. De Castro, F.: Sur la structure et l'innervation de la glande intercarotidienne (glomus caroticum) de l'homme et des mammifères, et sur un nouveau système d'innervation autonome du nerf glosspharyngien. Études anatomiques et experimentales. Trab Lab Invest Biol Univ Madrid, 24:365, 1926.
4. Heymans, C., Buckaert, J. J., and Dautrebande, L.: Sinus carotidien et réflexes respiratoires. II. Influences respiratoires réflexes de l'acidose, de l'alcalose, de l'anhydride carbonique, de l'ion hydrogène et de l'anoxémie. Sinus carotidien et échanges respiratoires dans les poumons et du-delà des poumons. Arch Int Pharmacodyn Ther 39:400, 1930.
5. Comroe, Jr., J. H.: The location and function of the chemoreceptors of the aorta. Am J Physiol 127:176, 1939.
6. Eyzaguirre, C., Lewin, J.: Chemoreceptor activity of the carotid body of the cat. J Physiol (Lond) 159:222, 1961.
7. Neil, E., Joels, N.: The carotid glomus sensory mechanism. In The Regulation of Human Respiration. Edited by D.J.C. Cunningham, and B.B. Lloyd. Oxford, Blackwell, 1963, pp. 163–172.
8. Hornbein, T. F., Roos, A.: Specificity of H ion concentration as a carotid chemoreceptor stimulus. J Appl Physiol 18:580, 1963.
9. Fitzgerald, R. S., Parks, D. C.: Effect of hypoxia on carotid chemoreceptor response to carbon dioxide in cats. Respir Physiol 12:218, 1971.
10. Lahiri, S., DeLaney, R. G.: Relationship between carotid chemoreceptor activity and ventilation in the cat. Respir Physiol 24:267, 1975.
11. Lahiri, S. and DeLaney, R. G.: Stimulus interaction in responses of carotid body chemoreceptor single afferent fibers. Respir Physiol 24:249, 1975.
12. Sampson, S. R., Hainsworth, R.: Responses of aortic body chemoreceptors of the cat to physiological stimuli. Am J Physiol 222:953, 1972.
13. Whipp, B. J., Wasserman, K.: Carotid bodies and ventilatory control dynamics in man. Fed Proc 39:2668, 1980.
14. Lugiani, R., et al.: Effect of bilateral carotid-body resection on ventilatory control at rest and during exercise in man. N Engl J Med 285:1105, 1971.
15. Biscoe, T. J., Purves, M. J., Sampson, S. R.: The frequency of nerve impulses in single carotid body chemoreceptor afferent fibers recorded in vivo with intact circulation. J Physiol (Lond.) 208:121, 1970.
16. Comroe, J. H.: Physiology of Respiration, 2nd Ed. Chicago, Year Book, 1977.
17. Forster, R. E., et al.: The Lung: Physiologic Basis of Pulmonary Function Tests, 3rd Ed. Chicago, Year Book, 1986, pp. 115–135.
18. Comroe, Jr., J. H., Mortimer, L.: The respiratory and cardiovascular responses of temporally separated aortic and carotid bodies to cyanide, nicotine, phenyldiguanide and serotonin. J Pharmacol Exp Ther 146:33, 1964.
19. Mitchell, R. A., Sinha, A. K., McDonald, D. M.: Chemoreceptive properties of regenerated endings of the carotid sinus nerve. Brain Res 43:681, 1972.
20. McDonald, D. M.: Regulation of chemoreceptor sensitivity in the carotid body: The role of presynaptic sensory nerves. Fed Proc 39:2627, 1980.
21. Berger, A. J., Krasney, J. A., Durron, R. E.: Respiratory recovery from CO$_2$ breathing in intact and chemodenervated awake dogs. J Appl Physiol 35:35, 1973.
22. Gelfond, R., Lambertson, C. J.: Dynamic respiratory response to abrupt change of inspired CO$_2$ and normal and high PO$_2$. J Appl Physiol 35:903, 1973.
23. Mitchell, R. A., et al.: Respiratory responses mediated through superficial chemosensitive areas on the medulla. J Appl Physiol 18:523, 1963.
24. Fukuda, Y., Honda, Y.: pH-sensitive cells at ventrolateral surface of rat medulla oblongata. Nature 256:317, 1975.
25. Berndt, J., et al.: Untersuchungen gum zentralen chemosensiblen mechanismus der atmung. II. Die steuerung der atmung durch das extracelluläre pH in gewebe der medulla oblongata. Pflugers Arch 332:146, 1972.
26. Paintal, A. S.: Vagal sensory receptors and their reflex effects. Physiol Rev 53:159, 1973.
27. Breuer, J., Hering, E.: Self-steering of respiration through the nervus vagus (translated by Ullmann, E.) In Breathing: Hering-Breuer Centenary Symposium. Edited by R. Porter. London, J.A. Churchill, 1970, p. 358.
28. von Euler, C., Herrero, F., Wexler, I.: Control mechanisms determining rate and depth of respiratory movements. Respir Physiol 10:93, 108, 1970.
29. Guz, A., et al.: The role of vagal inflation reflexes in man and other animals. In Breathing: Hering-Breuer Centenary Symposium. Edited by R. Porter. London, J.A. Churchill, 1970, pp. 17–40.
30. Staub, N. C.: The respiratory system. In Physiology, 3rd Ed. Edited by R.M. Berne and M.N. Levy. St. Louis, Mosby-Year Book, 1993, pp. 547–611.
31. Boushey, H. A., et al.: The response of laryngeal afferent fibers to mechanical and chemical stimuli. J Physiol (Lond.) 240:153, 1974.
32. Boushey, H. A., Richardson, P. S., Widdicombe, J. G.: Reflex effects of laryngeal irritation on the pattern of breathing and total lung resistance. J Physiol (Lond.) 224:501, 1972.
33. Tomori, Z., Widdicombe, J. G.: Muscular, bronchomotor and cardiovascular reflexes elicited by mechanical stimulation of the respiratory tract. J Physiol (Lond.) 200:25, 1969.
34. Duron, B.: Intercostal and diaphragmatic muscle endings and afferents. In Regulation of Breathing, Part I. Edited by T. F. Hornbein. New York, Marcel Dekker, 1981, pp. 473–540.
35. Legallois, C. J. J.: Experiences sur le principe de la vie. Paris, D'Hautel, 1812.
36. Flourens, M. J. P.: Note sur le point vital de la moelle allongée. CR Acad Sci 33:437, 1851.

37. Brown-Sequard, C. E.: Recherches sur les causes de mort aprés l'ablation de la partie de la moelle allongée qui a ete nommée point vital. J Physiol (Paris), *1*:217, 1858.

38. Pitts, R. E., Magoun, H. W., Ranson, S. W.: Localization of the medullary respiratory centers in the cat. Am J Physiol *126*:673, 1939.

39. Magoun, W. H., Beaton, L. E.: Respiratory responses from stimulation of the medulla of the cat. Am J Physiol *134*:186, 1941.

40. Tabatabai, M.: Respiratory and cardiovascular responses resulting from heating of the medulla oblongata in cats. Am J Physiol *222*:1558, 1972.

41. Tabatabai, M.: Respiratory and cardiovascular responses resulting from cooling of the medulla oblongata in cats. Am J Physiol *223*:8, 1972.

42. Tabatabai, M., et al.: Respiratory arrest induced by unilateral lesion(s) of the medullary inspiratory center in cats. Proc Soc Exp Biol Med *145*:1333, 1974.

43. Speck, D. F., Feldman, J. L.: The effects of microstimulation and microlesions in the ventral and dorsal respiratory groups in medulla of cat. J Neurosci *2*:744, 1982.

44. von Baumgarten, R., von Baumgarten, A., Schaefer, K. P.: Beitrag zur lokalisationsfrage bulboreticularer respiratorischer Neuron der Katze. Pflugers Arch *264*:217, 1957.

45. Haber, E., et al.: Localization of spontaneous respiratory neuronal activities in the medulla oblongata of the cat: A new location of the expiratory center. Am J Physiol *190*:350, 1957.

46. Howard, B. R., Tabatabai, M.: Localization of the medullary respiratory neurons in rats by microelectrode recording. J Appl Physiol *39*:812, 1975.

47. Tabatabai, M., Howard, B. R., Vazir, H.: Localization of the medullary respiratory neurons in rats by microelectrode sounding. IRCS Med Sci *3*:495, 1975.

48. Tabatabai, M., Kitahata, L. M., Collins, J. G.: Disruption of the rhythmic activity of the medullary respiratory neurons and phrenic nerve by fentanyl and reversal with nalbuphine. Anesthesiology *70*:489, 1989.

49. Tabatabai, M., et al.: Enflurane depresses activity of the medullary inspiratory neurons in the cat. Proc Soc Exp Biol Med *195*:79, 1990.

50. Berger, A. J., Mitchell, R. A., Severinghaus, J. W.: Regulation of respiration. N Engl J Med *297*:92–97, 138–143, 192–201, 1977.

51. von Euler, C.: Brain stem mechanisms for generation and control of breathing pattern. In Handbook of Physiology, Section 3: The Respiratory System, Vol. II, Part I. Edited by N. S. Chermack and J. G. Widdicombe. Bethesda, American Physiology Society, 1986, pp. 1–67.

52. Feldman, J. L.: Neurophysiology of breathing in mammals. In Handbook of Physiology, Section 1: Nervous System, Vol. IV. Edited by F. E. Bloom Bethesda, American Physiology Society, 1986, pp. 463–524.

53. von Euler, C.: Neural organization and rhythm generation. In The Lung: Scientific Foundations. Edited by R. G. Crystal and J. B. West. New York, Raven Press, 1991, pp. 1307–1318.

54. Berger, A. J.: Dorsal respiratory neurons in the medulla of cat: Spinal projections, responses to lung inflation and superior laryngeal nerve stimulation. Brain Res *135*:231, 1977.

55. Cohen, M. I.: How is respiratory rhythm generated? Fed Proc *40*:2372, 1981.

56. von Baumgarten, R., Kanzow, E.: The interaction of two types of inspiratory neurons in the region of the tractus solitarius of the cat. Arch Ital Biol *96*:361, 1958.

57. Feldman, J. L., Speck, D. F.: Interactions among inspiratory neurons in dorsal and ventral respiratory groups in cat medulla. J Neurophysiol *49*:472, 1983.

58. Merrill, E. G., Lipski, J., Kukin, L.: Origin of the expiratory inhibition of nucleus tractus solitarius inspiratory neurons. Brain Res *263*:43, 1983.

59. Barillot, J. C., Bianchi, A. L.: Activité des motoneurons larynés pendant reflexes de Hering-Breuer. J Physiol (Paris) *63*:783, 1971.

60. Kalia, M. P.: Anatomical organization of central respiratory neurons. Annu Rev Physiol *43*:105, 1981.

61. Merrill, E. G.: The lateral respiratory neurons of the medulla: Their association with nucleus ambiguus, nucleus retroambigualis, the spinal accessory nucleus and the spinal cord. Brain Res *24*:11, 1970.

62. Miller, A. D., Ezure, K., Suzuki, I.: Control of abdominal muscles by brain stem respiratory neurons in the cat. J Neurophysiol *54*:155, 1985.

63. Cohen, M. I., Wang S. C.: Respiratory neuronal activity in pons of cat. J Neurophysiol *22*:33, 1959.

64. Lumsden, T. L.: Observations on the respiratory centers in the cat. J Physiol (Lond.) *57*:153, 1923.

65. Cohen, M. I.: Switching of the respiratory phases and evoked phrenic responses produced by rostral pontine electrical stimulation. J Physiol (Lond.) *217*:133, 1971.

66. Feldman, J. L., Gautier, H.: Interaction of pulmonary afferents and pneumotaxic center in control of respiratory pattern in cats. J Neurophysiol *33*:31, 1976.

67. Knox, C. K., King, G. W.: Changes in the Breuer-Hering reflexes following rostral pontine lesion. Respir Physiol *28*:189, 1976.

68. Stella, G.: On the mechanism of production, and the physiological significance of "apneusis." J Physiol (Lond.) *93*:10, 1983.

69. Mitchell, R. A., Berger, A. J.: Neural regulation of breathing. In Regulation of Breathing. Edited by T. F. Hornbein. New York, Marcel Dekker, 1981, pp. 541–601.

70. Eldridge, F., Davis, J. W.: Effect of mechanical factors on respiratory work and ventilatory responses to CO_2. J Appl Physiol *14*:721, 1959.

71. Severinghaus, J. N.: Hypoxic respiratory drive and its loss during chronic hypoxia. Clin Physiol *2*:57, 1972.

72. Weil, J. V., et al.: Acquired attenuation of chemoreceptor function in chronically hypoxic man at high altitude. J Clin Invest *50*:186, 1971.

73. Wade, J. G., et al.: Effect of carotid endarterectomy on carotid chemoreceptor and baroreceptor function in man. N Engl J Med *282*:823, 1970.

74. Milic-Emili, J., Whitelaw, W. A., Derenne, J. P.: Occlusion pressure—a simple measure of respiratory center's output. N Engl J Med *293*:1029, 1975.

75. Whitelaw, W. A., Derenne, J. P., Milic-Emili, J.: Occlusion pressure as a measure of respiratory center output in conscious man. Respir Physiol *23*:181, 1975.

76. Milic-Emili, J., Grunstein, M. M.: Drive and timing components of ventilation. Chest *70* (Suppl):131, 1976.

77. Raper, A. J., et al.: Scalene and sternomastoid muscle function. J Appl Physiol *21*:497, 1966.

78. Önal, E., Lopata, M., O'Conner, T. D.: Diaphragmatic and genioglossal electromyogram responses to CO_2 rebreathing in humans. J Appl Physiol *50*:1052, 1981.

79. Drummond, G. B.: Influence of thiopentone on upper airway muscles. Br J Anaesth *63*:12, 1989.

80. Ochiai, R., Guthrie, R. D., Motoyama, E. K.: Effects of varying concentrations of halothane on the activity of the genioglossus, intercostals, and diaphragm in cats:

An electromyographic study. Anesthesiology 70:812, 1989.

81. Nishino, T., et al.: Comparison of changes in the hypoglossal and phrenic nerve activity in response to increasing depth of anesthesia in cats. Anesthesiology 60:19, 1984.

82. Ganong, W. F.: Review of Medical Physiology, 15th Ed. Norwalk, CT, Appleton and Lange, 1991, pp. 623–632.

83. Philipson, E. A.: Control of breathing during sleep. Am Rev Respir Dis 118:909, 1978.

84. Cherniack, N. S.: Sleep apnea and its causes. J Clin Invest 78:1501, 1984.

85. Philipson, E. A.: Respiratory adaptations in sleep. Am Rev Physiol 40:133, 1978.

86. Hedemark, L. L., Kronenberg, R. S.: Ventilatory and heart rate response to hypoxia and hypercapnia during sleep in adults. J Appl Physiol 53:307, 1982.

87. Douglas, N. J., et al.: Hypoxia ventilatory response decreases during sleep in man. Am Rev Respir Dis 125:286, 1982.

88. Guilleminault, C., Tilkian, A., Dement, W. C.: The sleep apnea syndromes. Annu Rev Med 27:465, 1976.

89. Krieger, A. J., Rosemoff, H. L.: Sleep-induced apnea. I. A respiratory and autonomic syndrome following bilateral and percutaneous cervical cordotomy. J Neurosurg 40:168, 1974.

90. Krieger, A. J., Rosomoff, H. L.: Sleep-induced apnea. II. Respiratory failure after anterior spinal surgery. J Neurosurg 40:181, 1974.

91. Severinghaus, J. W., Mitchell, R. A.: "Ondine's curse"; failure of respiratory center automaticity while awake. Clin Res 10:122, 1962.

92. Wasserman, K.: Breathing during exercise. N Engl J Med 298:780, 1978.

93. Whipp, B. J.: The control of exercise hyperpnea. In Regulation of Breathing. Edited by T. F. Hornbein. New York, Marcel Dekker, 1981, pp. 1069–1139.

94. Forrster, H. V., Pan, L. G.: Exercise hyperpnea. In The Lung: Scientific Foundations. Edited by R. G. Crystal and J. B. West. New York, Raven Press, 1991, pp. 1553–1564.

Chapter 4

ANESTHETIC DRUG EFFECTS ON RESPIRATORY CONTROL

MARK A. CHANEY AND THEODORE C. SMITH

NORMAL PHYSIOLOGY OF RESPIRATORY CONTROL

Respiration is a recurring diphasic cycle. Muscles contract (exerting force on bones, cartilage, ligaments, and organs) and enlarge the thorax. This action creates a lower than atmospheric pressure in alveoli, and air moves into the alveoli (inspiration). Muscles relax. Elastic recoil causes positive alveolar pressure and outflow of air (expiration). Neurons clumped in several centers in the central nervous system control the cycle timing (Fig. 4–1). These neurons stimulate motor neurons in the cervical and thoracic spinal cord and thus modulate tidal volume. The respiratory centers also receive afferent impulses from neurons in the medulla, pons, cerebellum, and cerebral cortex, and receptors in lung, aorta, carotid artery, muscles, and ligaments. The most important afferent input arrives from chemoreceptors. These chemoreceptors, largely sensitive to oxygen partial pressure in blood and hydrogen ion concentration in cerebrospinal fluid, play important roles in minute-to-minute involuntary control of respiration.[1]

The major function of this complex control system is to regulate hydrogen ion concentration in body fluids and to provide sufficient oxygenation of pulmonary capillary blood. The sum of these actions, therefore, maintains a level of overall alveolar ventilation that provides homeostasis, compensation for pulmonary, circulatory, and metabolic diseases, and facilitation of the voluntary efforts of alimentation, elimination, communication, and transportation.

Respiratory Center

The principle neurons controlling respiration are located in the medulla as part of the nucleus tractus solitarius and nucleus ambiguous. These medullary neurons have extensive neural connections with the pons. Neural input to the respiratory center also comes from pulmonary lung receptors (stretch, irritant, and juxtacapillary) via the vagus nerve, other cranial nerves (trigeminal, facial, and glossopharyngeal), somatic afferents from muscles and ligaments, as well as the cerebral cortex (voluntary control). There is still no universal agreement as to how the intrinsic rhythmicity of respiration is generated in the neural network that is the respiratory center. For a fuller discussion of the neural physiology of respiration, see Chapter 3.

Effectors of Respiration

These effectors are essentially the muscles of respiration, which include the diaphragm, intercostals, abdominals, and accessories. Coordination of contraction and relaxation in these muscles is important in achieving efficient respiration, a task performed by neurons in the respiratory center.

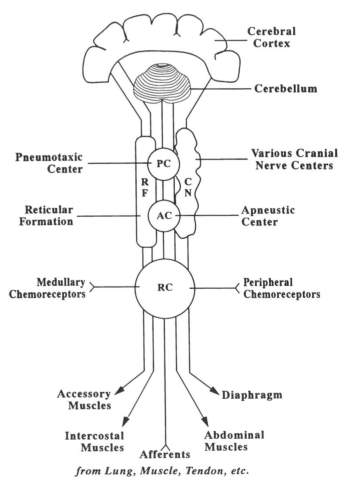

Fig. 4–1. Diagram of the central nervous system elements of respiratory control. All structures are bilaterally symmetrical. The respiratory center (RC) consists of both dorsal and ventral groups of neurons.

Chemoreceptors

The most important afferent input to the neurons of the respiratory center arrives from the central chemoreceptors and the peripheral chemoreceptors. The central chemoreceptors are located on the ventral surface of the medulla in an area that is separate from the neurons of the respiratory center. These chemoreceptors are responsive to cerebrospinal fluid hydrogen ion concentration and provide the most important afferent activity during normal control of respiration. Hypoxia depresses the central chemoreceptors.

The peripheral chemoreceptors are located in the carotid and aortic bodies and are responsive to hypoxia, acidosis, hypercarbia, and certain drugs in the blood that bathes them. The peripheral chemoreceptors are not as vital as the central chemoreceptors during normal control of respiration, but they may provide important afferent input to the respiratory center under certain environmental conditions or disease states. Atherosclerotic vascular disease or surgical dissection may ablate these receptors with little effect on quiet respiration.

Ventilatory Response To Carbon Dioxide (VERCO$_2$)

A straight line describes the increasing ventilation that results from inspiratory CO$_2$, either exogenous CO$_2$ or rebreathing expired CO$_2$ (Fig. 4–2). Afferent input from the central chemoreceptors to the respiratory center provides the major modulation. The slope of the response is normally 2 to 3 l/min/mm Hg. The abcissal intercept where ventilation is zero is called the apneic threshold. It is found by extrapolating the ventilatory response to zero ventilation and is normally approximately 36 mm Hg. The apneic threshold is a name for a point, and not a fact. Healthy humans do not usually become apneic after hyperventilation lowers arterial carbon dioxide tension.

Characteristically, the VERCO$_2$ increases or decreases in slope as level of consciousness changes. It may also shift left or right with or without a change in slope. If the slope is altered, no conclusion regarding displacement of the curve can be made, unless the point about which the curve rotates when the slope changes is known.

As a useful generalization, pharmacologic effects that do not cause loss of consciousness shift the position of the response left or up (stimulation) and right or down (depression) with no change in slope. Pharmacologic effects that do alter consciousness change the slope. Sleep, anesthesia, and coma all depress the response; fear, arousal, and hypoxia steepen the response.

Ventilatory Response to Hypoxia (VER ↓ O$_2$)

Approximately 10 percent of resting ventilation can be attributed to peripheral chemoreceptors, as evidenced by the small decrement in ventilation noted with breathing air with an oxygen concentration of 50% or more. Lowering oxygen concentrations below normal ambient levels increases ventilation mainly by afferent activity input from the peripheral chemoreceptors. Two different dis-

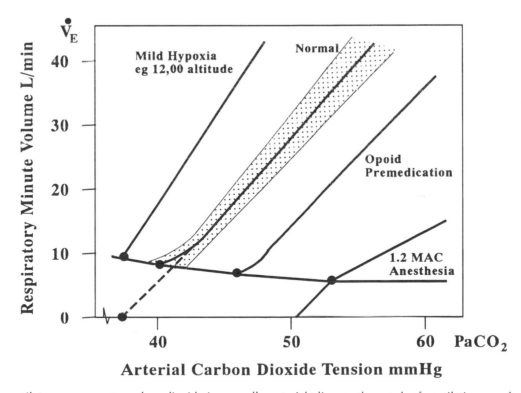

Fig. 4–2. The ventilatory response to carbon dioxide is normally a straight line on the graph of ventilation as a function of arterial CO$_2$ tension. It has a slight dog-leg or hockey stick shape near the resting point. Extrapolation of the straight line to zero ventilation defines the apneic threshold, although normal man does not usually become apneic with the slight reduction of CO$_2$ tension. Hypoxia increases the slope of the response while sleep and anesthesia decreases it. Some depressants, typically opioids, slight the response right or down with little or no change in slope.

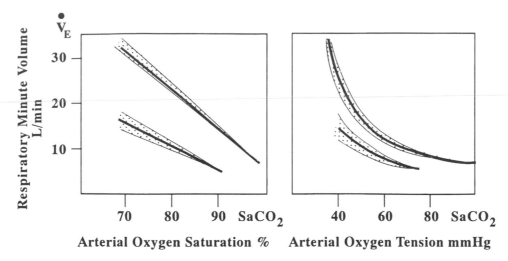

Fig. 4–3. The ventilatory response to hypoxia may be shown in two different ways, depending on whether the hypoxia is quantitated by arterial oxyhemoglobin saturation (left panel) or by arterial oxygen tension (right panel). In the former a straight line results. In the latter a hyperbolic response is fitted, assuming asymptotes for infinite ventilation and 100% oxygen breathing. The choice is made as a matter of taste.

plays of the results follow from two different choices to represent the stimulus (hypoxia): arterial oxyhemoglobin tension or arterial oxygen saturation (Fig. 4–3). The latter representation, an older technique, provides more of the data, although it makes certain assumptions that have not been examined regarding their implications in pharmacologic analysis. Two variables (asymptotes) are guessed and the response is "quantified" by fitting a hyperbola to the data and calculating its curvature, a parameter known as A. In the alternate method, arterial oxyhemoglobin saturation is used to estimate the stimulus. The data are characterized by a straight line with a negative slope, normally about 1 l/min/percent desaturation, with increasing depression. The choice between the two different displays is largely a matter of taste.

ASSESSMENT OF ANESTHETIC DRUG EFFECTS ON RESPIRATORY CONTROL

Assessment of anesthetic drug effects on respiratory control is difficult, because the complex mechanism underlying normal respiratory control is still incompletely understood as is the mechanism of action of many anesthetic drugs. Several tests, however, have been developed to examine respiratory control that may be used to assess anesthetic drug effects.[2] Simple tests include examination of respiratory rate, tidal volume, arterial blood gas tensions, minute ventilation, and spirometry. More involved tests include tidal volume partitioning, airway occlusion pressure, electrical measurements, work of breathing, and oxygen cost of breathing. The tests used most often, however, are the VERCO$_2$ and VER $\downarrow$ O$_2$, because they are relatively easy to perform and are clinically applicable.

Many factors, other than the drug being studied, have significant effects on respiratory control mechanisms and must be considered when interpreting results of investigations. In addition to primary stimuli of hydrogen ion concentration and hypoxia, respiration is affected by age, sex, blood pressure, metabolic rate, temperature, time of

day, genetic factors, exercise, mechanical loads, instrumentation apparatus, interindividual variability, posture, psychologic profile, and concomitant use of other central nervous system or muscle-affecting drugs. The mere awareness by a patient that an investigator is studying their breathing significantly affects respiratory rate and tidal volume. The level of consciousness, in and of itself, exerts profound influence on respiratory control mechanisms. Anesthetic drugs, therefore, may alter respiratory control via specific receptor mechanisms or by simply decreasing the level of consciousness in a nonspecific manner.

Significant differences exist between species. A 70-kg human may need 0.2 mg/kg of morphine for premedication. A 7-kg dog requires 2.0 mg/kg for the same clinical effect, whereas a cat given 2 mg/kg exhibits gross hyperactivity and sham rage. For this reason, the following discussion regarding anesthetic drug effects on respiratory control concerns data obtained only in humans.

Most importantly, even if an investigation proves beyond doubt that an anesthetic drug causes "respiratory depression," this information does not necessarily translate into problems when the drug is used in the clinical setting. "Respiratory depression" may be defined in many ways. Furthermore, statistically significant respiratory depression may be not only clinically acceptable, but even desirable.

INHALATION AGENTS

All inhalation agents cause dose-dependent depression of the slope of the VERCO$_2$. Interestingly, the least depressing (fluroxene, cyclopropane, ether, and methoxyflurane) are no longer used, whereas the most potent respiratory depressants (halothane, enflurane, and isoflurane) are in common clinical use. Agents in the former group activate the sympathetic nervous system and those in the latter do not; nitrous oxide is intermediate in both slope and catecholamine effects.

Common Halogenated Agents

Halothane, enflurane, isoflurane, and (to the extent that the present studies are available) the newest agents sevoflurane and desflurane share many similarities in respiratory effects.[3]

Effects on Resting Ventilation

All of the halogenated agents decrease tidal volume and increase respiratory rate in proportion to the administered dose. Minimal differences exist between the agents at equipotent concentrations. At subanesthetic concentration, little change is observed in alveolar ventilation. With increasing inspired levels, however, consciousness is altered and alveolar ventilation begins to decrease. The increase in rate is not enough to compensate for the decrease in tidal volume. The decrease in alveolar ventilation causes an increase in arterial carbon dioxide tension (Fig. 4-4).

Effects on Ventilatory Response to Carbon Dioxide

Much like their effects on resting ventilation, halogenated agents cause a dose-dependent depression of the slope of the VERCO_2, with little differences noted between the agents at equipotent concentrations (Fig. 4-5). At high levels of the halogenated agents (2.5 MAC), essentially no increase in ventilation is observed after a carbon dioxide challenge.[3]

Effects on Ventilatory Response to Hypoxia

Contrary to older opinions, anesthetics depress the ventilatory response to hypoxia (VER $\downarrow$ O_2) as much or even more than they depress VERCO_2. Although low levels of halothane (0.1 MAC) cause little depression of the VERCO_2, this same level causes significant depression of the VER $\downarrow$ O_2 (Fig. 4-6)[3] by reducing activity of chemoreflexes from the carotid and aortic bodies. Higher levels (1.1 MAC) totally abolish the hypoxic response. The effects of newer agents may be as great or greater. This impairment in a normal patient with a normal and intact hypercarbic response does not necessarily pose a problem. In patients who depend on their hypoxic drive to breathe, however, such as those with chronic obstructive pulmonary disease, surgical or disease-induced ablation of the carotid reflex, or acute metabolic acidemia, and those who have taken other drugs known to depress the VERCO_2 (opioids, benzodiazepines, etc.), this impairment places them in danger. Sedating or subanesthetic levels of

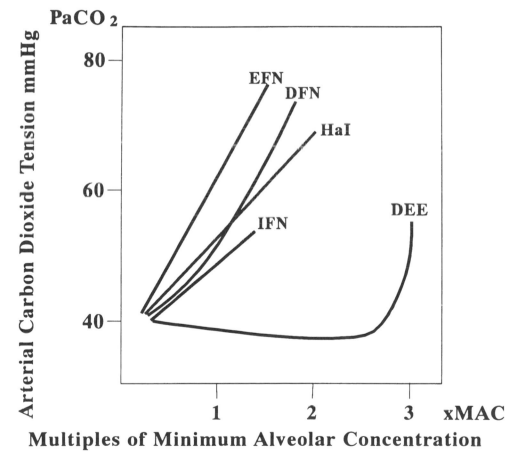

Fig. 4-4. Typical effects of selected anesthetic agents at increasing depth of anesthesia, represented by multiple of minimum alveolar concentration, on the arterial tension of carbon dioxide. Most halogenated agents give a progressive rise in resting carbon dioxide tension. Diethyl ether is exceptional, stimulating breathing at lighter planes of surgical anesthesia, probably due to sympathetic nervous system arousal. EFN = enflurane; DFN = desflurane; HaL = halothane; IFN = isoflurane; SFN = sevoflurane; C_3H_6 = cyclopropane; DEE = di-exthyl ether; FXE = fluorexene; NI = nitrous oxide.

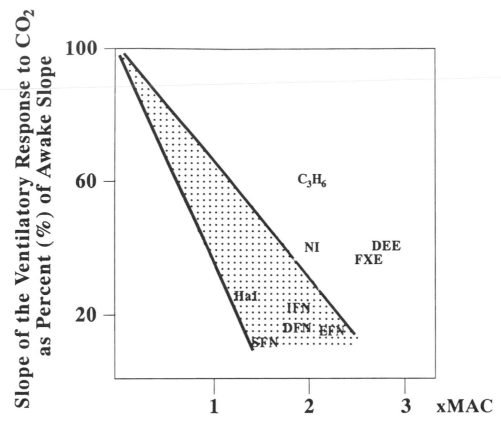

Fig. 4–5. Typical effects of selected anesthetic agents at increasing depth of anesthesia, on the slope of the ventilatory response to carbon dioxide. Most halogenated agents cause a proportional flattening of the response as anesthetic concentration increases, all within the shaded area on the diagram. But those older agents which were capable of sympathetic stimulation, such as di-ethyl ether (Dee), cyclopropane (C_3H_6), fluroxene (FXE) and even to a lesser extent nitrous oxide (NI) with Innovar, were less depressing, especially in concentration in the one to two MAC ranges. EFN = enflurane; DFN = desflurane; HaL = halothane; IFN = isoflurane; SFN = sevoflurane; C_3H_6 = cyclopropane; DEE = di-ethyl ether; FXE = fluroxene; NI = nitrous oxide.

the halogenated agents often persist into the recovery period after general anesthesia. Patients may also receive other drugs that depress the $VERCO_2$. Therefore, on arrival in a postanesthesia care unit, patients initially are at risk of hypoxemia. Appropriate monitoring and delivery of supplemental oxygen are warranted.

Effects on Apneic Threshold

Healthy humans may but do not usually become apneic after hyperventilation-lowered arterial carbon dioxide. By contrast, nearly uniform apnea occurs in anesthetized man when the arterial carbon dioxide tension is lowered even slightly below their current resting level.[4]

Surgical Stimulation

In patients anesthetized with halogenated agents, minute ventilation increases and arterial carbon dioxide tension decreases with onset of surgical stimulation.[5] Although surgical stimulation increases minute ventilation, it does not appear to affect chemoresponsiveness, in that the slope of the $VERCO_2$ remains unchanged. Effects of surgical stimulation on VER $\downarrow O_2$ are comparable. No mechanism for these effects is known, but the rapidity of

the ventilatory changes suggests a neurogenic mechanism involving peripheral nerve fibers.

Time Adaptation

The magnitude of ventilatory depression induced by the halogenated agents is affected by time.[6] A small but distinct tendency toward reversal of ventilatory depression over time has been demonstrated for halothane, enflurane, and isoflurane. It is unclear as to why time adaption occurs, the clinical impact, if any, is minor.

Chronic Obstructive Pulmonary Disease

Ventilatory depression induced by anesthesia is significantly greater in patients with emphysema than in normal patients. Controlled or assisted ventilation is strongly recommended when using halogenated agents in these patients because of their greater susceptibility.

Sevoflurane And Desflurane

Sevoflurane and desflurane are the most recently introduced halogenated agents. Few studies exist regarding their ventilatory depressant effects, but investigations performed indicate they behave much like the other halo-

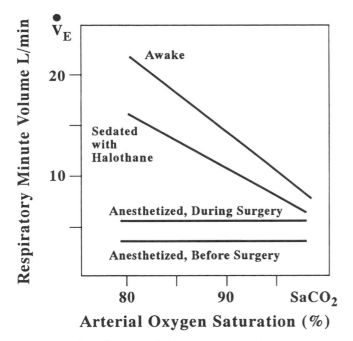

Fig. 4–6. The effect of halothane in subanesthetic and anesthetic concentrations, on the ventilatory response to hypoxia. Low concentration (0.1 × MAC) significantly depress the response, and anesthetic concentration (1.1. × MAC) nearly abolish it. Newer halogenated agents such as sevoflurane may not be as quantitatively depressant, according to abstracts published in 1993.

genated agents. Both cause a dose-dependent decrease in tidal volume and in alveolar ventilation despite an increase in respiratory rate. Arterial carbon dioxide tension increases. Both agents cause dose-dependent depression of the slope of the $VERCO_2$. The effects on $VERCO \downarrow O_2$, as reported in 1993, are not certain because reported results are contradictory.

Nitrous Oxide

Nitrous oxide has low potency. Therefore, its effects can be investigated only in subanesthetic doses or under hyperbaric conditions. Winter et al. exposed nine normal volunteers in a hyperbaric chamber to 1.55 atm nitrous oxide and 0.32 atm oxygen.[7] The volunteers displayed a dramatic increase in respiratory rate (15 breaths/minute baseline to 47 breaths/minute) and a dramatic decrease in tidal volume (0.72 L baseline to 0.33 L). Minute ventilation increased significantly (9.95 L/min baseline to 15.4 l/min) yet arterial carbon dioxide tension remained unchanged from baseline (38 to 40 mm Hg). The slope of the $VERCO_2$ was significantly decreased when compared to baseline (from 3.2 L/min/mm Hg to 0.75 L/min/mm Hg).

Nitrous oxide, when substituted for a portion of a halogenated agent, results in less ventilatory depression and a lower arterial carbon dioxide tension than is caused by equipotent concentrations of the halogenated agents alone. Simply stated, a mixture of 0.5 MAC halogenated agent and 0.5 MAC nitrous oxide causes less ventilatory depression than 1.0 MAC halogenated agent. This "venti-

latory sparing" effect of nitrous oxide has been well documented with halothane, enflurane, and isoflurane. The underlying mechanism may involve sympathetic nervous system stimulation.

Nitrous oxide also affects the $VER \downarrow O_2$. Even at low concentrations (0.1 MAC), nitrous oxide decreases the hypoxic response to approximately 60% of awake control values.

SYSTEMATICALLY ADMINISTERED OPIOIDS

Opioids are perhaps the oldest and best studied drugs known to humans. Opium use, for its euphoric effects, can be traced back over 4000 years. Respiratory effects were first noted approximately 600 years ago.

Mechanism of Respiratory Effects

Opioid receptors of several types have been found in high concentrations in areas of the human brain and play significant roles in control of respiration. Minute amounts of opioids, when injected into the cerebrospinal fluid bathing the medulla, result in profound respiratory depression. Analgesic and respiratory depressant effects of opioids are mediated via different receptor mechanisms. The mu-1 receptor subtype mediates analgesia, whereas the μ2-receptor subtype mediates respiratory depression. Kappa receptors appear to mediate analgesia with little effects on respiration, whereas contributions from δ, ε, and σ-receptors are unclear. Endogenous peptides possessing μ-receptor agonist properties are found in the central nervous system. Their role in normal respiratory control is uncertain. They may, however, be important in states characterized by abnormal respiratory control, such as infant apnea syndromes or chronic obstructive pulmonary disease.

The many drugs possessing μ-receptor agonist properties induce qualitatively similar dose-dependent depression in respiration. Quantitative differences do exist, however, and are dictated by the dose, route of administration, pharmacokinetic profile, and pharmacodynamic profile of the drug given. Not all opioids are capable of producing maximal μ-effect. These drugs are called partial agonists or agonist-antagonists. A few drugs bind to receptors with no effect; these are called antagonists. Often, a characteristic decrease in respiratory rate occurs after the administration of opioids, with normal to slightly increased tidal volume. A decrease in alveolar ventilation and corresponding increase in arterial carbon dioxide tension results.

When used clinically, opioids may produce only subtle changes in alveolar ventilation by reduction of the respiratory rate, tidal volume, or both. Doses that retain consciousness displace the $VERCO_2$ down or to the right. In some patients, high doses of opioids (>3 mg/kg morphine or >25 μg/kg fentanyl) halt breathing without producing complete unresponsiveness. These narcotized patients will breathe if directed to do so, although their attention span is measured in seconds. When unconsciousness does occur, a decreased slope of the $VERCO_2$ is appreciated. The differing effects of opioids on the $VERCO_2$ at increasing doses is likely related to changing levels of consciousness.[8]

Influence of Level of Consciousness

Augmentation of opioid-induced ventilatory depression by a decreased level of consciousness has important clinical implications. Opioids may be confidently administered without much concern for ventilatory depression so long as the dose is titrated to partial relief of pain. If pain that stimulates consciousness persists, it prevents augmented ventilatory depression. Patients who exhibit significant opioid-induced ventilatory depression can be partially "reversed" by arousal (physical stimulation) to increase the level of consciousness. Any concomitant decrease in consciousness from other factors (fatigue, benzodiazepines, anesthesia, coma, etc.) augments opioid-induced ventilatory depression.

Opioids also decrease the $VER \downarrow O_2$. As after the administration of inhalation agents, the hypoxic response is more sensitive to depression than the response to carbon dioxide.

Specific Opioid Agonists

Morphine

This classic natural opioid produces dose-dependent depression of ventilation characteristic of μ-receptor agonists. With increasing doses, morphine decreases alveolar ventilation and increases arterial carbon dioxide tension, but changes in respiratory rate and tidal volume are variable. Slow breathing is not a reliable clinical indicator of the magnitude of ventilatory depression. Bradypnea may be absent even when arterial carbon dioxide tension exceeds 90 mm Hg. Morphine decreases hypercarbic and hypoxic responses when administered subcutaneous in doses as low as 7.5 mg.[9] Peak ventilatory depressant effects of morphine occur within 10 minutes of intravenous injection and nearly 1 hour after subcutaneous injection. Intramuscular effect is intermediate, depending on muscle blood flow. The slight delay after intravenous usage is attributed to morphine's relative lipophobic nature, compared with the newer opioids. Morphine (10 mg intravenously) may measurably reduce the $VERCO_2$ for up to 10 hours.

Fentanyl

This synthetic opioid causes ventilatory depression that is qualitatively similar to but quicker in onset and shorter in duration than equianalgesic doses of morphine. Fentanyl is approximately 580 times more lipophilic than morphine. Therefore, its quick onset is likely the result of rapid entry of the drug into the cerebrospinal fluid. Maximum ventilatory depression from an intravenous dose of fentanyl occurs within 5 minutes of delivery. Duration is shorter than that of morphine because of more rapid detoxification in the liver. Fentanyl, in small doses, may cause significant depression of the $VERCO_2$ lasting 4 hours. Even though fentanyl is a relatively short-acting drug, delayed ventilatory depression after its use has been reported. Secondary increases in plasma fentanyl concen-

trations may occur 30 to 90 minutes after injection and initiate delayed, clinically significant, ventilatory depression.[10] Possible mechanisms underlying the secondary increase in plasma fentanyl concentration include enterosystemic recirculation or drug sequestration in lung or muscle. Whatever the cause, delayed ventilatory depression is possible with the use of fentanyl.

Sufentanil and Alfentanil

Newer congeners of fentanyl both cause ventilatory depression similar to equianalgesic doses of fentanyl. Sufentanil and alfentanil are highly lipophilic drugs, and are approximately 1270 and 104 times more lipophilic than morphine, respectively. Ventilatory depression after intravenous use is quick in onset. Pharmacokinetic data predict, and studies have demonstrated, that alfentanil produces ventilatory depression that is shorter in duration than equianalgesic doses of fentanyl, a fact attributed to quicker metabolism as well as faster redistribution. Sufentanil is intermediate between the two. Several cases have been described in which severe delayed postoperative ventilatory depression, responsive to naloxone, occurred after continuous intravenous infusion of alfentanil. This depression occurred as late as 70 minutes after termination of the infusion. Secondary increases in plasma alfentanil concentrations do occur, but they have not been linked to episodes of delayed ventilatory depression. Alfentanil, much like fentanyl, may delay ventilatory depression, especially when used as a continuous intravenous infusion.

Meperidine

Ventilatory depression similar to morphine occurs with meperidine in equianalgesic doses. Meperidine is approximately 28 times more lipophilic than morphine, and its ventilatory effects are somewhat quicker in onset. Maximum ventilatory depression from an intramuscular injection of meperidine varies widely, from 15 to 110 minutes.

Methadone

This potent μ-receptor agonist is given to prevent withdrawal symptoms in opioid addicts. The drug has a long elimination half-life (15 to 25 hr). A single dose of methadone (30 mg intravenously) can cause measurable ventilatory depression for up to 8 days. Patients receiving methadone provide a unique model to examine whether tolerance develops to the ventilatory depressant effects of μ-receptor agonists.[11] Patients that receive methadone for more than 5 months do develop full tolerance to depression of the $VERCO_2$ and partial tolerance to depression of the $VER \downarrow O_2$.

Partial Opioid Agonists

The goal of opioid analgesia without respiratory depression has led to a search for drugs with μ- or κ-receptor-mediated analgesia without μ-receptor-mediated ventilatory depression. There is no doubt that the opioid agonist-antagonists demonstrate a "ceiling effect" on ventilatory depression, i.e., administering more of the drug does not necessarily initiate additional ventilatory depression. A disadvantage of this class of drugs, however, is that they also demonstrate a ceiling effect on analgesia, which may limit clinical applicability. The opioid agonist-antagonists may be useful in reversing ventilatory depression initiated by μ-receptor agonists without fully reversing analgesia. Clinically, the opioid agonist-antagonists used most often are butorphanol, buprenorphine, and nalbuphine.

Butorphanol

This weak μ-receptor partial agonist and κ-receptor agonist is five to eight times as potent as morphine in producing analgesia and ventilatory depression effects. A ceiling effect exists at doses of 0.03 to 0.06 mg/kg. Increasing the dose above this level does not increase arterial carbon dioxide tension above about 500 mm Hg, but it does increase the duration of ventilatory depression. Butorphanol may be useful in decreasing fentanyl-induced ventilatory depression without reversing analgesia.

Buprenorphine

This drug is a μ-receptor partial agonist with very high affinity as well as a weak κ-receptor partial agonist. Despite very high μ receptor affinity, receptor association and dissociation is slow. Peak effects, therefore, may not occur until 3 hours after a dose is administered and effects may persist up to 10 hours. Buprenorphine is 30 times as potent as morphine in producing analgesia. A ceiling effect on ventilatory depression, with arterial carbon dioxide tension attaining a level of approximately 50 mm Hg, occurs at intravenous doses of 0.15 to 1.2 mg in adults. Buprenorphine may also be useful in decreasing fentanyl-induced ventilatory depression without reversing analgesia.

Nalbuphine

A μ-receptor agonist and κ-receptor partial agonist, nalbuphine is equipotent to morphine in small doses. Maximum analgesia and ventilatory depression is obtained with 20 to 30 mg, intravenously, equivalent to that induced by 15 mg of morphine, intravenously, in adults. Arterial carbon dioxide tension attains a level of approximately 50 mm Hg in adults, but is not equivalent to that achieved with the same amount of morphine.

INTRATHECAL* AND EPIDURAL OPIOIDS

The intrathecal and epidural use of opioids in humans, first reported in 1979, has enjoyed widespread popularity because of the possibility of obtaining excellent analgesia without motor, sensory, or autonomic deficits typically induced by intrathecal and epidural local anesthesia. The major disadvantage of the technique, however, is development of respiratory depression. Early respiratory depression occurs 30 to 120 minutes after administration of the opioid and is likely caused by vascular uptake of the drug. Early respiratory depression is typically associated with epidural use of opioids, but it has been reported in at least one case of intrathecal use. Delayed respiratory

depression occurs 4 to 18 hours after opioid administration and is thought to be caused by cephalad spread of the drug in cerebrospinal fluid. Delayed respiratory depression can occur with intrathecal or epidural use of opioids.

When administered epidurally, highly lipophilic fentanyl and sufentanil traverse the dura rapidly when compared to the less lipophilic morphine. Once the opioid is present in cerebrospinal fluid, whether by intrathecal or epidural administration, physiochemical properties of the drug again dictate the amount of opioid allowed to spread cephalad. Fentanyl and sufentanil, being highly lipophilic, dissolve readily into neural tissue, limiting the amount of drug available for cephalad spread. Conversely, morphine, being less lipophilic, is allowed to travel cephalad to a greater extent in the cerebrospinal fluid and is associated with a higher incidence of delayed respiratory depression.

Intrathecal Morphine

Numerous case reports describe delayed respiratory depression after intrathecal use of morphine. Most of such instances involve a relative overdose (3 to 20 mg) that occurs by design, drug error, or intrathecal migration of an epidural catheter. Respiratory depression typically occurs 4 to 12 hours after injection and is responsive to naloxone. Intrathecal doses of morphine in the range of 0.1 to 1.0 mg may be used to obtain excellent analgesia with minimal respiratory depression. The most important factor influencing the development of delayed respiratory depression after intrathecal morphine use is the dose of drug administered. Larger doses are clearly associated with a higher incidence of delayed respiratory depression.

Epidural Morphine

Early or delayed respiratory depression may result from epidural morphine. After lumbar epidural injection of 10 mg of morphine, peak serum concentrations of the drug from vascular uptake are noted at 8 minutes and peak cervical cerebrospinal fluid concentrations of the drug occur at 120 minutes.[12] Therefore, initial vascular uptake of the drug may cause early respiratory depression and late cephalad spread of the drug in cerebrospinal fluid may cause delayed respiratory depression. Findings of large studies suggest the incidence of clinically significant respiratory depression that follows conventional doses of epidural morphine is less than 1% and is extremely rare in healthy patients when the use of additional parenteral opioids is avoided. These studies also stress the insensitivity of relying on respiratory rate alone to diagnose respiratory depression. A global assessment, focusing on level of consciousness, is more useful. Life-threatening, delayed respiratory depression after epidural morphine administration has been reported with doses as low as 2.5 mg and as much as 22 hours after injection.

Intrathecal Fentanyl

As stated previously, fentanyl, being highly lipophilic, does not travel cephalad in cerebrospinal fluid to the same extent as morphine. Clinical experience documents

---

*Refers to subdural or subarachnoid placement.

an extremely low incidence of delayed respiratory depression when fentanyl is delivered intrathecally. Prudence dictates, however, that patients receiving intrathecal fentanyl warrant close monitoring for the appearance of early as well as delayed respiratory depression.

Epidural Fentanyl

Clinically significant respiratory depression after epidural fentanyl use is rare. After lumbar epidural injection of fentanyl (1.0 μg/kg), serum concentrations of the drug from vascular uptake are negligible and lumbar cerebrospinal fluid concentrations of the drug peak 5 to 30 minutes after injection.[13] Cervical cerebrospinal fluid concentrations of fentanyl from cephalad spread peak 10 to 45 minutes after injection, but peak cervical concentrations are only 10% of peak lumbar concentrations.[13] Data indicate that respiratory depression after epidural fentanyl delivery may be, but is not likely related cephalad spread of the drug in cerebrospinal fluid.

Recommendations

The incidence of clinically significant respiratory depression from intrathecal and epidural opioids administered in conventional doses is probably less than 1%. Certain techniques, however, do increase the risk, including the use of hydrophilic opioids (morphine), large doses, repeated doses, intrathecal as opposed to epidural administration, concomitant use of intravenous opioids or other central nervous system depressants, and the use of a thoracic catheter as opposed to a lumbar catheter. Certain patients are also at increased risk of developing respiratory depression. These persons include the elderly, the debilitated, the opioid "virgin," those with coexisting pulmonary disease, and possibly those with increased intrathoracic pressure from coughing, vomiting, or mechanical ventilation. Even in the absence of any identifiable risk factors, however, some patients develop life-threatening respiratory depression after intrathecal or epidural administration of opioids.[14]

SEDATIVE/HYPNOTICS

Many drugs are administered to patients with the goal of decreasing anxiety (sedation) and the level of consciousness (hypnosis). All possess the ability to initiate significant, life-threatening respiratory depression, especially in patients concomitantly receiving other drugs that induce respiratory depression.

Barbiturates

Barbiturates are similar to all sedative/hypnotics in that respiratory depression tends to parallel the decrease in level of consciousness. In the small doses used for premedication, oxybarbiturates have a negligible stimulating effect on breathing. Given for induction of anesthesia, however, major effects occur. The thiobarbiturates thiopental and thiamylal, along with the oxybarbiturate methohexital, may be considered together when discussing their respiratory effects, for all three exert clinical effects via the same specific receptor mechanism that modulates central nervous system chloride ion channels. In larger doses, unconsciousness comes with decreased

alveolar ventilation, increased arterial carbon dioxide tension, and a decrease in the slope of the VERCO$_2$. Larger doses also cause apnea. The VER $\downarrow$ O$_2$ is significantly decreased by barbiturates, much more so than the VERCO$_2$.

Thiopental (4.0 mg/kg intravenously) decreases the VERCO$_2$ maximally within one vein-to-brain circulation time. Redistribution, however, terminates the action of a single dose of thiopental quickly, and the response is nearly restored in 6 minutes after the same dose. Methohexital, 1.5 mg/kg intravenously, acts similarly. Apnea is common after administering induction doses of barbiturates, but episodes rarely last longer than 30 seconds. The elimination half-lives of thiopental and methohexital are 6 to 18 hours and 2 to 6 hours, respectively. If large or multiple doses are administered, prolonged respiratory depression may occur.

Benzodiazepines

The benzodiazepines, like the barbiturates, may be considered together when discussing their respiratory effects, for they also exert clinical effects via the same specific receptor mechanism that modulates central nervous system chloride ion channels.

Benzodiazepines likely exert respiratory depressant effects simply by decreasing the level of consciousness. The many available benzodiazepines do not differ in magnitude of respiratory depression induced when administered in clinically equivalent amounts. Along with dose-dependent depression of alveolar ventilation is a corresponding increase in arterial carbon dioxide tension. Their effects on respiratory rate and tidal volume are variable. In sedative doses, benzodiazepines have little effect on the slope of the VERCO$_2$ in normal humans, yet larger hypnotic doses decrease the slope progressively. Benzodiazepines also decrease the VER $\downarrow$ O$_2$.

Diazepam. The respiratory effects have been studied often with conflicting results. The majority of investigations document a decrease in the slope of the VERCO$_2$ that parallels the decrease in level of consciousness. Some patients, however, demonstrate an increase in the slope of the VERCO$_2$.[15] Failure to account for this small subgroup of patients who demonstrate respiratory stimulation when given diazepam may explain the conflicting results of investigations detailing the respiratory effects of this drug.

Diazepam, in small doses that do not affect the VERCO$_2$, significantly decreases the VER $\downarrow$ O$_2$. Respiratory effects associated with diazepam begin within 1 minute of intravenous injection, peak at 3 minutes, and are minimal at 30 minutes. Life-threatening apnea and Cheyne-Stokes breathing have resulted from as little as 2.5 mg intravenously. The elimination half-life 20 to 90 hours, and an active metabolite (desmethyldiazepam) has been identified. Therefore, larger doses or multiple doses of diazepam may cause significantly prolonged respiratory effects.

Lorazepam. This drug exhibits respiratory effects that are similar to those of diazepam when administered in clinically equivalent amounts. Few cases of life-threatening respiratory depression following use of lorazepam have been reported. In normal subjects, doses as high as 7.5 mg orally, 6.0 mg intramuscularly, and 5.0 mg intravenously, have produced minimal clinical respiratory effects. With these high doses, however, it is difficult for the patient to remain awake and prolonged sedation and distressing amnesia are likely. The elimination half-life of lorazepam is 11 to 22 hours, which suggests that prolonged respiratory effects may occur if large or multiple doses are administered.

Midazolam, the first clinically useful water-soluble benzodiazepine, exhibits respiratory effects that are similar to those of diazepam: a decrease in the slope of the VERCO$_2$ with doses that decrease the level of consciousness and a decrease in the VERCO$_2$ with smaller doses that do not affect consciousness. Clinically important respiratory depression is usually minimal in healthy subjects receiving doses up to 0.1 mg/kg intravenously. Effects of 0.2 mg/kg intravenously begin within 1 minute of injection, peak at 3 minutes, and are minimal at 15 minutes. The elimination half-life is 1.7 to 2.6 hours, making it the most attractive benzodiazepine for use as a continuous intravenous infusion.

Propofol

The respiratory effects of propofol appear similar to those of other sedative/hypnotics. Interestingly, the VERCO$_2$ decreases maximally within 90 seconds of an intravenous injection, yet may remain significantly decreased 20 minutes later despite recovery of consciousness. The incidence of prolonged apnea associated with propofol also appears to be greater than after other intravenous induction agents. Induction doses of propofol may initiate apneic episodes lasting more than 3 minutes.

Etomidate

The respiratory effects of etomidate are similar to those of all sedative/hypnotics: respiratory depression tends to parallel the decrease in level of consciousness. Quantitatively less respiratory depression than is noted with other agents used for intravenous induction may result. Even brief periods of hyperventilation may occur. The increase in minute ventilation may be desired during induction of anesthesia, but apnea may still occur. Its incidence is influenced significantly by concomitant use of other drugs that induce respiratory depression.

OTHER SEDATIVE-LIKE DRUGS

Ketamine

Ketamine has unique respiratory effects that separate it from other anesthetics, intravenous or inhalational. Characteristic effects of ketamine include an increased tidal volume with a variable effect on respiratory rate. Most investigators report minute ventilation is unchanged, whereas others document increased minute ventilation for up to 20 minutes after a single injection. Ketamine appears to be the only anesthetic, intravenous or inhalational, to preserve, or actually increase, the functional residual capacity by increasing the inspiratory time:expiratory time ratio and preserving intercostal muscle function. Ketamine causes dose-dependent displacement to the right of the VERCO$_2$, yet even in doses large enough to reliably produce unconsciousness, the slope remains

unchanged.[16] This ability to maintain a normal slope of the VERCO$_2$, despite producing unresponsiveness, is unique to ketamine. Paradoxically, the incidence of apnea associated with ketamine is high, 60% in some studies, and may be prolonged.

Droperidol

The respiratory effects of droperidol are minor. Doses as high as 0.44 mg/kg intravenously produce no clinical respiratory effects. Although droperidol produces little change in the VERCO$_2$, it measurably increases the VER$\downarrow$O$_2$. A single 2.5-mg, dose intravenously almost doubles the VER$\downarrow$O$_2$, probably an effect mediated by dopaminergic blockage in the carotid bodies.[17] The respiratory effects of Innovar (a mixture of droperidol and fentanyl) are caused solely by the fentanyl it contains. Droperidol does not augment fentanyl-induced respiratory depression.

REVERSAL AGENTS

Many agents have been used to reverse drug-induced respiratory depression. Some act via a specific receptor mechanism, and others attempt to reverse respiratory depression by nonspecific central nervous system arousal.

Opioid Antagonists

The ability of naloxone to antagonize μ-receptors has led to its widespread clinical application in reversing the respiratory depression caused by opioids.[18] Intravenous naloxone promptly reverses morphine-induced respiratory depression.[19] The slope of the VERCO$_2$ normalizes with return of consciousness, and with further doses, the VERCO$_2$ shifts to the left (Fig. 4–7). Minute ventilation in-

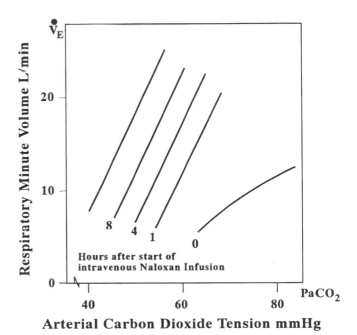

Fig. 4–7. The VERCO$_2$ before and after administration of morphine and reversal with naloxone. The slope of curve normalizes with return of consciousness. Further doses shift the curve left.

creases and arterial carbon dioxide tension decreases. Naloxone is also an antagonist for Kappa Sigma and Delta receptors, but its affinity for each opioid receptor population is not equal. Therefore, the dose of naloxone may be manipulated to reverse respiratory depression yet maintain some analgesia.

Peak clinical effects after intravenous, intramuscular, and subcutaneous administration of naloxone occur 3, 15, and 30 minutes, respectively. Clinical effects of a single injection last only 30 to 90 minutes, depending on the dose administered. Repeated intravenous injections or a continuous intravenous infusion of naloxone, therefore, is often required to maintain reversal of opioid-induced respiratory depression. Multiple case reports describe reappearance of opioid-induced respiratory depression after single intravenous injections of naloxone.

Administration of large doses of naloxone to normal conscious humans does not appear to affect respiratory control. No discernible physiologic changes are observed with daily doses of naloxone, 90 mg subcutaneously, for 2 weeks or upon its abrupt withdrawal from this regimen. Naloxone does, however, appear to influence respiratory control in patients with chronic obstructive pulmonary disease, suggesting that endogenous opioids may play a significant role in respiratory control in these patients.

Benzodiazepine Antagonists

Flumazenil (Romazicon) is the only clinically available benzodiazepine receptor antagonist. It has high affinity and great specificity for benzodiazepine receptors. Flumazenil is not a pure antagonist and does possess very weak agonist and possible inverse agonistic properties. Flumzenil reliably reverses benzodiazepine-induced hypnosis, yet its ability to reverse benzodiazepine-induced respiratory depression is inconsistent. Flumazenil may improve the slope of the VERCO$_2$ or may have no effect. Some investigators have actually demonstrated augmentation of benzodiazepine-induced decrease in the slope of the VERCO$_2$. Large doses of flumazenil, 0.1 mg/kg intravenously, cause no discernible clinical effects in patients not receiving benzodiazepines.

Clinical effects of a single dose of flumazenil, intravenously, peak within five minutes of administration and persist 45 to 60 minutes. Sedation and respiratory depression may reappear following initial reversal by a single dose because flumazenil's clearance is higher, and its half-life shorter, than all of the clinically utilized benzodiazepines. Repeated intravenous injections or a continuous intravenous infusion of flumazenil, therefore, may be required to maintain reversal of benzodiazepine-induced clinical effects, including respiratory depression.

Anticholinesterases

Physostigmine may arouse the central nervous system after a variety of diverse compounds including opioids, benzodiazepines, butyrophenones, tricyclic antidepressants, and antihistamines. The highly unpredictable improvement in sedation and respiratory depression relate to the drugs nonspecific mechanism of action. Physostigmine rapidly crosses the blood brain barrier and inhibits acetylcholinesterase, increasing acetylcholine levels, thus causing generalized central nervous system arousal. Clinical effects of a single dose of physostigmine, 1–2 mg intravenously, peak within ten minutes of administration and last approximately 60 minutes.

With the development of more specific receptor antagonists such as naloxone and flumazenil, clinical use of physostigmine in drug-induced respiratory depression is waning. However, when significant respiratory depression occurs following administration of a drug with no clinically available specific receptor antagonist, physostigmine remains an option in treatment.

RESPIRATORY STIMULANTS

Doxapram

Doxapram produces selective respiratory stimulation of carotid chemoreceptors. The inducing displacement up or to the left of the VERCO$_2$, increasing respiratory rate, tidal volume, and increases minute ventilation. Significant side effects include tachycardia, hypertension, restlessness, agitation, frank psychosis, and convulsions. Utilization of doxapram to stimulate respiration in the immediate postoperative period following general anesthesia with the halogenated inhalation agents may be unproductive. Doxapram's respiratory stimulant properties are profoundly depressed by very low levels of halogenated inhalational agents, much in the same way that they depress the VER $\downarrow$ O$_2$.

Doxapram, therefore, is a drug with very limited clinical applications. Its primary use appears to be in situations where short-term respiratory stimulation is desired. This time period of respiratory stimulation is beneficial in that other modes of therapy (oxygen, bronchodilators, pulmonary toilet, etc.) can be utilized that may prevent the need for endotracheal intubation and mechanical ventilatory support.

Catecholamines

Norepinephrine, epinephrine, and dopamine effect respiration.[20] The latter to exerting the most significant respiratory effects. Endogenous dopamine is present in human carotid bodies and likely plays a central role in peripheral chemoreceptor neurotransmission. Dopaminergic receptor stimulation decreases the VER $\downarrow$ O$_2$ and VERCO$_2$, Beta adrenergic receptor stimulation increases resting ventilation and the slope of the VERCO$_2$, while alpha receptor stimulation decreases resting ventilation. Dopaminergic and beta receptor effects appear to be mediated via peripheral chemoreceptors located in the carotid bodies, whereas alpha receptor effects do not.

Progesterone

Progesterone is a respiratory stimulant, increasing both the VERCO$_2$ and VER $\downarrow$ O$_2$. Increased levels of progesterone in pregnancy and during the luteal phase of the menstrual cycle are accompanied by increases in minute ventilation and decreases in arterial carbon dioxide tension. In normal patients, male or female, exogenous progesterone increases tidal volume and minute ventilation and decreases arterial carbon dioxide tension. Little or no effect on respiratory rate is seen. Progesterone, for its respiratory stimulant properties, has been utilized clinically in the treatment of Pickwickian syndrome and in sleep apnea syndromes without an obstructive component. The mechanism underlying progesterone's ability to stimulate respiration is uncertain but likely involves the central nervous system.

Hormones other than progesterone may also influence respiration by poorly understood mechanisms.[21] These include other gonadal hormones, thyroid hormones, adrenocortical hormones, and adrenocorticotrophic hormones.

MUSCLE RELAXANTS

There are no consistent central nervous system effects of muscle relaxants. Their respiratory effects originate solely from their ability to paralyze muscles. Partial paralysis causes no consistent change in the $VERCO_2$.[22] Some investigations document an increased respiratory drive in patients partially paralyzed without sedation, but this likely reflects patient anxiety.

Characteristic respiratory changes in patients with partial paralysis include a decreased tidal volume and increased respiratory rate. Eventually the increase in respiratory rate is unable to compensate for the decrease in tidal volume and a decrease in alveolar ventilation occurs along with an increase in arterial carbon dioxide tension. The magnitude of the decrease in alveolar ventilation is dependent on the degree of respiratory muscle paralysis.

Respiratory muscles exhibit significant differences in sensitivity to muscle relaxants. The pharyngeal muscles of the upper airway and the accessory muscles of respiration appear to be the most sensitive to neuromuscular blockade. Abdominal muscles and expiratory intercostals are more sensitive than are inspiratory intercostals. The diaphragm is the least sensitive. Clinically adequate ventilation can be maintained with significant amounts of partial paralysis (hand-grip strength 6% of control) if a patent airway is maintained.[22] At these levels of partial paralysis, however, significant impairment of vital respiratory functions such as coughing, swallowing, and deep breathing are severely impaired.

Normal breathing matches gas exchange with metabolic rate without voluntary effort such that breathing is proportional to demands. The major drive to breathe originates from the central chemoreceptors in the medulla that are responsive to cerebrospinal fluid hydrogen ion concentration. Additional input arrives from the peripheral chemoreceptors in the carotid bodies that are responsive mainly to hypoxia. Assessment of anesthetic drug effects on respiratory control is difficult, for the complex mechanism underlying normal respiratory control is still incompletely understood, as is the mechanism of action of many anesthetic drugs. All anesthetic drugs may alter respiratory control via specific receptor mechanisms or by a decreased level of consciousness in a nonspecific manner.

REFERENCES

1. Berger, A. J., Mitchell, R. A., Severinghaus, J. W.: Regulation of respiration. N Engl J Med 297:92-97, (Part One) 138-143 (Part Two) 194-201 (Part Three), 1977.

2. Lourenco, R. V. (editor): Clinical methods for the study of regulation of ventilation (Report of Symposium). Chest 70:Supplement 109-105, 1976.

3. Knill, R. L., Gelb, A. W.: Ventilatory responses to hypoxia and hypercapnia during halothane sedation and anesthesia in man. Anesthesiology 49:244-251, 1978.

4. Hickey, R. F., Fourcade, H. E., Eger, E. I., et al: The effects of ether, halothane, and forane on apneic thresholds in man. Anesthesiology 35:32-37, 1971.

5. Lam, A. M., Clement, J. L., Knill, R. L.: Surgical stimulation does not enhance ventilatory chemoreflexes during enflurane anaesthesia in man. Can J Anaesthes 27:22-28, 1980.

6. Fourcade, H. E., Larson, C. P., Hickey, R. F., et al. Effects of time on ventilation during halothane and cyclopropane anesthesia. Anesthesiology 36:83-88, 1972.

7. Winter, P. M., Hornebein, T. F., Smith, G., et al: Hyperbaric nitrous oxide anesthesia in man: determination of anesthetic potency (MAC) and cardiorespiratory effects. Abstracts of Scientific Papers-American Society of Anesthesiologists Annual Meeting 103-104, 1972.

8. Forrest, W. H., Bellville, J. W.: The effect of sleep plus morphine on the respiratory response to carbon dioxide. Anesthesiology 25:137-141, 1964.

9. Weil, J. V., McCullough, R. E., Kline, J. S., et al.: Diminished ventilatory response to hypoxia and hypercapnia after morphine in normal man. N Engl J Med 292:1103-1106, 1975.

10. Stoeckel, H., Schuttler, J., Magnussen, H., et al.: Plasma fentanyl concentrations and the occurrence of respiratory depression in volunteers. Br J Anaesthes 54:1087-1095, 1982.

11. Santiago, T. V., Pugliese, A. C., Edelman, N. H.: Control of breathing during methadone addiction. Am J Med 62:347-354, 1977.

12. Gourlay, G. K., Cherry, D. A., Plummer, J. L., et al.: Armstrong PJ, Cousins MJ. The influence of drug polarity on the absorption of opioid drugs into CSF and subsequent cephalad migration following lumbar epidural administration: application to morphine and pethidine. Pain 31:297-305, 1987.

13. Gourlay, G. K., Murphy, T. M., Plummer, J. L.: Pharmacokinetics of fentanyl in lumbar and cervical CSF following lumbar epidural and intravenous administration. Pain 38:253-259, 1989.

14. Etches, R. C., Sandler, A. N., Daley, M. D.: Respiratory depression and spinal opioids. Can J Anaesthes 36:165-185, 1989.

15. Bailey, P. L., Andriano, K. P., Goldman, M., et al: Variability of the respiratory response to diazepam. Anesthesiology 64:460-465, 1986.

16. Bourke, D. L., Malit, L.A., Smith, T. C.: Respiratory interactions of ketamine and morphine. Anesthesiology 66:153-156, 1987.

17. Ward DS: Stimulation of hypoxic ventilatory drive by droperidol. Anesth Analg 63:106-110, 1984.

18. Sawynok, J., Pinsky, C., LaBella, F. S.: Minireview on the specificity of naloxone as an opiate antagonist. Life Sci 25:1621-1631, 1979.

19. Johnstone, R. E., Jobes, D. R., Kennell, E. M., et al: Reversal of morphine anesthesia with naloxone. Anesthesiology 41:361-366, 1974.

20. Heistad, D. D., Wheeler, R. C., Mark, A. L.: Effects of adrenergic stimulation on ventilation in man. J Clin Invest 51:1469-1475, 1972.

21. Lyons, H. A.: Centrally acting hormones and respiration. Pharmacol Therapeut Bull 2:743-751, 1976.

22. Gal, T.J., Smith, T.C.: Partial paralysis with d-tubocurarine and the ventilatory response to CO_2: an example of respiratory sparing? Anesthesiology 45:22-28, 1976.

Chapter 5

TRANSPORT OF OXYGEN AND CARBON DIOXIDE

GEORGE J. CRYSTAL AND M. RAMEZ SALEM

The volume of oxygen consumed per minute by the average adult is approximately 225 ml. Carbon dioxide production is slightly less, and it varies with the foodstuffs in the diet. A person on a high carbohydrate diet will consume a volume of oxygen and produce a volume of carbon dioxide which are about equal, whereas a person on a high fat diet will consume a relatively greater volume of oxygen. The ratio of expired carbon dioxide to inspired oxygen is called the respiratory exchange ratio.

OXYGEN TRANSPORT

The cardiovascular system acts in concert with the respiratory system in transporting oxygen to cellular mitochondria from its store in environmental air. The oxygen serves as an electron acceptor in oxidative phosphorylation, permitting production of adenosine triphosphate (ATP) along efficient aerobic pathways. The high-energy phosphate bonds of ATP provide energy for functional and biochemical processes within the cell, such as the contraction of muscle proteins and the metabolic activity of enzymes.

Figure 5–1 presents the influence of partial pressure of oxygen (PO_2) on oxygen consumption ($\dot{V}O_2$) of isolated mitochondria.[1] It shows that above approximately 0.1 mm Hg, $\dot{V}O_2$ is independent of PO_2. Accordingly, the objective of the integrated oxygen delivery system *in vivo* is

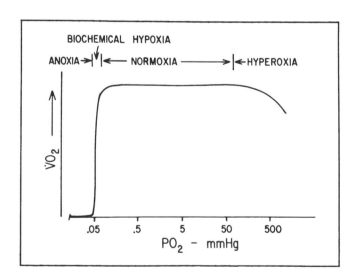

Fig. 5–1. Oxygen consumption of isolated mitochondria as a function of PO_2. From Honig C. R.: Modern cardiovascular physiology, Boston, 1981, Little, Brown and Company.

to ensure that a PO_2 is maintained above 0.1 mm Hg in the vicinity of all mitochondria. The only function of a PO_2 above 0.1 mm Hg is to provide sufficient driving force for diffusion of oxygen to mitochondria remote from capillaries.

Determinants of Convective Oxygen Delivery

The amount of oxygen carried from the lungs to tissues by circulating blood, i.e., the convective systemic oxygen delivery (DO_2), is given by the equation:

$$DO_2 = CaO_2 \times CO \qquad (1)$$

where CaO_2 is the arterial oxygen content in vol %, and CO is systemic blood flow or cardiac output in L/min.

Arterial Oxygen Content

Arterial oxygen content is composed of oxygen bound to hemoglobin (Hb) and oxygen dissolved in plasma:

$$CaO_2 = O_2 \text{ bound} + O_2 \text{ dissolved} \qquad (2)$$

Oxygen Bound to Hemoglobin

The structure of a human Hb molecule, which is characteristic for all Hb molecules in vertebrates, is presented (Fig. 5–2). The Hb molecule is composed of two basic portions.[2] The protein or globin portion is made up of identical polypeptide chains: two α and two β chains. The polypeptide chains are folded and assembled as a tetramer. Each of these chains contains one heme group, which serves as an iron-containing, reversible carrier of one molecule of oxygen. Thus, each molecule of Hb can bind four molecules of oxygen. Oxygen bound is a function of Hb concentration, oxygen-carrying capacity for Hb (1.39 mL O_2/gram Hb), and oxygen saturation of Hb (SaO_2), according to the equation:

$$O_2 \text{ bound} = (Hb \times SaO_2 \times 1.39) \qquad (3)$$

Dissociation Curve

SaO_2 is a function of PO_2 and the oxyhemoglobin dissociation curve, which is a plot of oxyhemoglobin saturation as a function of PO_2 (Fig. 5–3). The sigmoid shape of the curve reflects the fact that the four binding sites on a given Hb molecule interact with each other.[3] When the

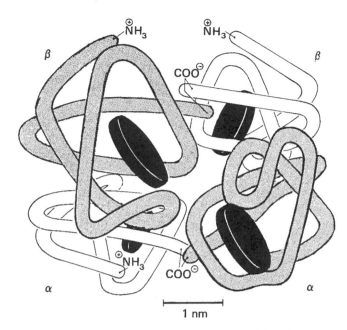

Fig. 5–2. Molecular model of human hemoglobin showing its four polypeptides- two α and two β chains, each having one heme (indicated by disk) to which oxygen can bind. Reproduced with permission from Harper H. A. et al., Physiologische Chemie. Springer-Verlag, 1975.

first site has bound a molecule of oxygen, the binding of the next site is facilitated, and so forth. The result is a curve that is steep up to PO_2 of 60 mm Hg and then becomes more shallow thereafter, approaching 100% saturation asymptotically. At a PO_2 of 100 mm Hg, the PO_2 to which human arterial blood is normally equilibrated, 97 percent of the hemes have bound oxygen; at 40 mm Hg, a

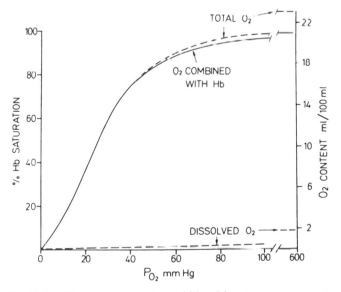

Fig. 5–3. The oxygen content of blood has two components: oxygen binding to hemoglobin follows an S-shaped curve up to full saturation; the amount of oxygen in solution increases linearly with PO_2 without limit. From West J. B.: Best and Taylor's Physiological Basis of Medical Practice, 12th ed., 1990, Baltimore, Williams & Wilkins.

typical value for the mixed venous oxygen tension ($P\bar{v}O_2$) in a resting person, the saturation declines to about 75%.

The shape of the oxyhemoglobin dissociation curve has important physiological implications. The flatness of the curve above a PO_2 of 80 mm Hg ensures a constant oxyhemoglobin saturation for arterial blood despite wide variations in alveolar oxygen pressure. The steep portion of the curve between 20 and 60 mm Hg permits unloading of oxygen from Hb at relatively high PO_2 values, which permits the delivery of large amounts oxygen into the tissue by diffusion.

The oxygen binding properties of Hb are influenced by a number of factors, including pH, PCO_2, and temperature (Fig. 5–4). These factors cause shifts of the oxyhemoglobin dissociation curve to the right or left without changing the slope of the curve. For example, an increase in temperature or a decrease in pH, such as may occur in active tissues, decreases the affinity of Hb for oxygen, and shifts the oxyhemoglobin dissociation curve to the right. Thus, a higher PO_2 is required to achieve a given saturation, which facilitates unloading of oxygen at the tissue. To quantify the extent of a shift in the oxyhemoglobin dissociation curve, the so-called P_{50} is used, i.e., the PO_2 required for 50% saturation. The P_{50} of normal adult Hb at 37°C and normal pH and PCO_2 is 26 to 27 mm Hg.

Fetal Hemoglobin

Fetal Hb differs structurally from adult Hb in that two of its polypeptide chains are of the ν rather than β type.[1] The oxyhemoglobin dissociation curve of the fetus is similar to that of the adult except that the curve is shifted to the left, resulting in a P_{50} of 20 mm Hg.

Methemoglobin

Methemoglobin is the ferric form of heme. The ferrous and ferric concentrations of iron are in equilibrium but only about 0.1% of the iron is normally ferric. This ferric form does not bind reversibly with oxygen and thus cannot deliver oxygen to tissues. When the concentration of methemoglobin exceeds 8–10% of the total (to reach 1.5 to 2 grams) cyanosis may appear. Symptoms of hypoxia appear if 30% of the hemoglobin is in the ferric form.

Certain drugs cause the production of methemoglobin: the divalent iron is oxidized to the trivalent form. Methylene blue and benzocaine form the met compound; other agents that oxidize the ferrous iron include nitrates, chlorates and some sulfa compounds.

Oxygen Releasing Factor

The compound 2,3-diphosphoglycerate (2,3-DPG) is an intermediate in anaerobic glycolysis (the biochemical pathway by which red blood cells produce ATP) which binds to Hb. Increases in intraerythrocytic 2,3-DPG concentration reduce the affinity of Hb for oxygen, i.e., they shift the oxyhemoglobin dissociation curve to the right, whereas decreases have opposite effects. Several factors influence red cell 2,3-DPG concentrations. For example, after storage in a blood bank of only one week, 2,3-DPG concentrations are one-third normal, resulting in a shift to the left of the oxyhemoglobin dissociation curve. On the other hand, conditions associated with chronic hypoxia, e.g., living at high altitude or chronic anemia, stimulate production of 2,3-DPG which causes a rightward shift of the oxyhemoglobin dissociation curve. P_{50} shifts from 26 to 29 mm Hg when a 15% increase in 2,3-DPG occurs.

Oxygen Capacity of Hemoglobin

The amount of oxygen that can be carried per one gram of Hb is controversial.[4] Originally 1.34 was used, but with the determination of the molecular weight of Hb, the theoretical value of 1.39 became popular. On the basis of extensive human studies, Gregory observed that the appropriate value was 1.306 in human adults.[5] Nevertheless, 1.39 remains in use in most studies.

Dissolved Oxygen in Plasma Water

Oxygen is also transported by the blood in simple physical solution with plasma water. Dissolved oxygen is linearly related to PO_2 and obeys Henry's Law (Figure 5-3). At 37°C it is defined by the equation:

$$O_2 \text{ dissolved} = 0.003 \text{ vol\% / mm Hg } PO_2 \quad (4)$$

Dissolved oxygen normally accounts for only 1.5 percent of total oxygen but this contribution increases when the bound component is reduced during hemodilution. Because Hb is completely saturated at PO_2 of 100 mm Hg, increases in arterial PO_2 (PaO_2) to levels above 100 mm Hg increase CaO_2 by raising the dissolved component.

Characteristics Values for Parameters of Oxygen Delivery

For an individual with a Hb concentration of 15 g/100 mL, PaO_2 of 100 mm Hg, $P\bar{v}O_2$ of 40 mm Hg, and cardiac output of 5000 mL/min:

$$CaO_2 = (15 \times 0.97 \times 1.39) + (0.003 \times 100)$$
$$= 20.5 \text{ vol\%;}$$
$$DO_2 = (5000 \times 20.5/100) = 1025 \text{ mL/min;}$$

$$C\bar{v}O_2 = (15 \times 0.75 \times 1.39) + (0.003 \times 40)$$
$$= 15.8 \text{ vol\%;}$$

and the arteriovenous oxygen content difference ($CaO_2 - C\bar{v}O_2$) is:

$$(CaO_2 - C\bar{v}O_2) = 20.5 - 15.8 = 4.7 \text{ vol\%.}$$

Carbon Monoxide

Carbon monoxide interferes with the oxygen transport function of blood by combining with Hb to form carboxyhemoglobin (COHb). The dissociation curves of oxy- and carboxyhemoglobin have similar shapes. However, CO has approximately 250 times the affinity of oxygen for Hb; this means that CO will combine with the same amount of Hb as oxygen when the CO partial pressure is 250 times lower. For example, at a PCO of only 0.16 mm Hg, 75% of the Hb is combined with CO as COHb. Therefore, when plotted on the same scale (Fig. 5-5), the CO dissociation curve has almost a right-angled bend near a PCO of zero.

The higher affinity of CO for Hb implies that people inadvertently exposed to small concentrations of CO in the air (for example, during a building fire) may have a large proportion of their Hb combined with CO, and thus unavailable for oxygen transport. Under this condition, the Hb concentration and PO_2 of the blood may be normal, but the oxygen content may be grossly reduced. Small amounts of COHb also shift the oxygen dissociation curve to the left thus making it difficult for the blood to unload the oxygen that it does carry. Figure 5-5 also presents the oxygen dissociation curve of blood containing 60% COHb as contrasted to the curve for anemic blood.

A patient with CO poisoning is treated by giving him pure oxygen or 95% with 5% CO_2 to breath. The addition of 5% CO_2 to the inspired gas accelerates washout of CO from the blood. In specialized medical centers, hyperbaric oxygen therapy is often given by increasing the inspired PO_2 to 2,000 mm Hg, the oxygen demands of the body tissues can be satisfied by the amount of oxygen dissolved in the plasma.

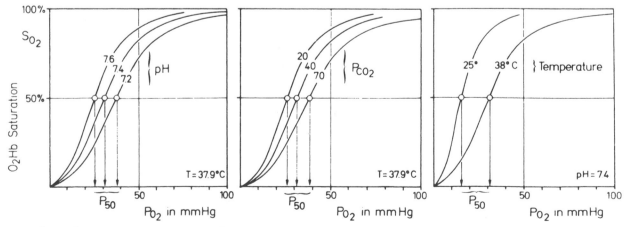

Fig. 5-4. Effects of variations in pH, PCO_2, and temperature on oxyhemoglobin dissociation curve. Reprinted with permission from Weibel E. R.: The pathway for oxygen, Cambridge, 1984, Harvard University Press.

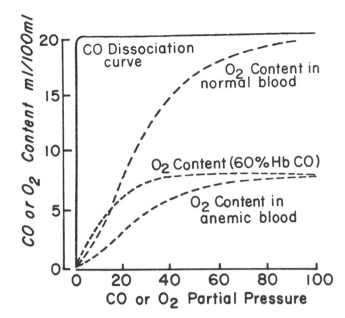

Fig. 5–5. Comparison of dissociation curves for CO and oxygen. Hemoglobin is almost completely saturated with CO at a very low partial pressure. The CO dissociation curve for 60% HbCO is displaced to the left compared with the oxygen dissociation curve for anemic blood. From West J. B.: Best and Taylor's Physiological Basis of Medical Practice, 12th ed., 1990, Baltimore, Williams & Wilkins.

Blood Flow to Peripheral Tissues—Principles of Blood Rheology

In addition to arterial oxygen content, blood flow is a primary determinant of tissue oxygen delivery (Eq. 1). Tissue blood flow is a function of the arteriovenous pressure gradient (Pa − Pv) and local vascular resistance (R), according to the equation:

$$F \text{ (flow)} = (Pa - Pv)/R \qquad (5)$$

This is analogous to Ohm's law in an electrical circuit. Because arterial and venous blood pressures are normally well maintained within narrow limits, tissue blood flow usually varies inversely as a function of vascular resistance.

Poiseuille's Law

Poiseuille performed studies that yielded an equation describing the resistance to flow in a straight, rigid tube of length (l) and radius (r):

$$R \text{ (resistance)} = \eta 8l/\pi r^4 \qquad (6)$$

where η is the viscosity. Blood flow resistance varies inversely with tube radius raised to the fourth power. Thus, small changes in tube radius cause large changes in resistance.

Geometric Factors

Because the length of blood vessels *in situ* is fixed, geometric changes in blood flow resistance occur by variations in vessel radius. These adjustments are the result of contraction or relaxation of the smooth muscle investing the arterioles, which are the principal site of vascular resistance. Chemical factors, which are linked to the metabolic activity of the tissue, e.g., adenosine, modulate vascular resistance so that blood flow (and oxygen delivery) is commensurate with the prevailing local oxygen demands.

Viscosity

Viscosity is the internal friction resulting from the intermolecular forces operating within a flowing liquid. The term internal friction emphasizes that as a fluid moves within a tube, laminae in the fluid slip on one another and move at different speeds. This produces a velocity gradient in a direction perpendicular to the wall of the tube. This velocity gradient is termed the shear rate. In the circulation, shear rate shows a direct correlation to rate of blood flow. An intuitive understanding of the term viscosity can be gained from the experiment shown in Figure 5-6. In this experiment, a homogeneous fluid is confined between two closed spaced, parallel plates (analogous to playing cards). Assume the area of each plate is A, the distance between the plates is Y, and the bottom plate is stationary. If a tangential force (a shear stress) is applied to the upper plate, this plate will move with velocity v in the direction of the applied force and a velocity gradient (or shear rate) is developed in the fluid. Viscosity is defined as the factor of proportionality relating shear stress and shear rate for the fluid.

$$\text{Viscosity} = \text{shear stress/shear rate} \qquad (7)$$

Newton assumed that viscosity was a constant property of a particular fluid and independent of shear rate. Fluids that demonstrate this behavior are termed Newtonian. The units of viscosity are dynes per second per square centimeter or poise.

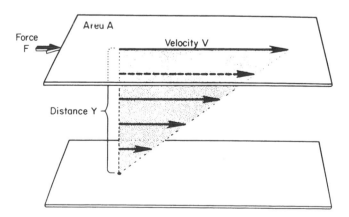

Fig. 5–6. Relationship between shear stress and shear rate when a fluid is sheared between two parallel plates. Details included in text. From Fahmy N. R.: Techniques for deliberate hypotension: haemodilution and hypotension. In: Enderby GEH, ed, Hypotensive anaesthesia, London, 1985, Churchill-Livingstone, p. 164, with permission.

Factors Affecting Blood Viscosity

Factors that affect blood viscosity are presented on Table 5-1. The viscosity of blood varies as direct function of hematocrit (Hct) (Fig. 5-7), i.e., the greater the Hct, the more friction there is between successive layers. Plasma is a Newtonian fluid, even at high protein concentrations (Fig. 5-7). However, because blood consists of red cells suspended in plasma, it does not behave like a homogeneous Newtonian fluid; the viscosity of blood increases sharply with reductions in shear rate (Fig. 5-7). This non-Newtonian behavior of blood has been attributed to changes in the behavior of red cells at low flow rates: 1) red cells lose their axial position in the stream of blood (Fig. 5-8); 2) red cells lose their ellipsoidal shape; 3) red cells form aggregates; this tendency toward aggregation appears dependent upon the plasma concentration of large protein molecules, such as fibrinogen, which form cell to cell bridges; 4) red cells adhere to the endothelial walls of microvessels. Figure 5-9 demonstrates that non-Newtonian behavior is localized *in vivo* on the venous side of circulation because of its lower shear rates, but that this behavior can be attenuated or abolished by hemodilution.

Table 5–1. Factors Affecting Viscosity of Whole Blood

HCT
Plasma proteins
RBC deformability
RBC aggregation
Temperature

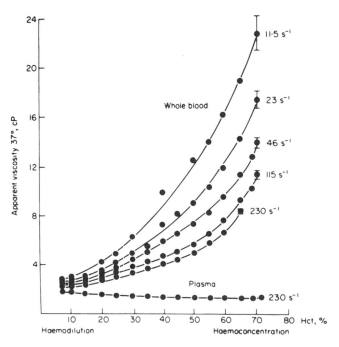

Fig. 5–7. Viscosity of whole blood at various hematocrits as a function of shear rate. Hematocrit was varied by addition of dextran and packed red blood cells. Whole blood viscosity increases with hematocrit and that these increases in viscosity are greatest at the lower shear rates. Reprinted with permission from Messmer K: Hemodilution, Surg Clin North Am 55:662, 1975.

Effect of Vessel Size

The tendency for increased Hct to increase blood viscosity is attenuated when blood flows through tubes of capillary diameter (Fig. 5-10). This is because red cells are deformable, and with a diameter similar to that of the capillary, they can squeeze through the vessel lumen in single file with minimal extra force required. Thus, the rate at which red cells pass through the capillary has little influence on blood viscosity there; viscosity remains close to that of plasma.

Effect of Temperature

Blood viscosity varies inversely with temperature (Fig. 5-11). A decrease in Hct is required to maintain a constant viscosity during hypothermia. It indicates that at 20°C a reduction in Hct from 45 to 25% is required to restore viscosity to the same value evident at 37°C. This is an important consideration during hypothermic cardiopulmonary bypass. After circulatory arrest, the shear stress required to reinitiate flow and to break up red cell aggregates is likely to be high. Additional rheologic benefit may be gained by a further decrease in Hct.

Turbulent Flow

The Poiseuille equation assumes that energy dissipation is entirely viscous in nature. However, inertial or kinetic energy dissipation may occur at high Reynold's numbers. The Reynold's number (Re) is equal to:

$$Re = (\rho \, v \, r)/\eta \qquad (8)$$

where ρ is the fluid density and v is the linear velocity of flow. With a high Reynold's number, the inertial dissipation associated with turbulent flow increases the pressure drop from that predicted from the Poiseuille equation (Fig. 5-12). Tissues with extremely pulsatile flow patterns and highly complicated vascular geometry, e.g., myocardium, are most vulnerable to inertial dissipation of pressure.

Diffusion of Oxygen to Tissues

Capillary to Cell Oxygen Delivery

The final step in the delivery of oxygen to cellular mitochondria is diffusion from the capillary blood. According to the law of diffusion, this process is determined by the capillary-to-cell PO_2 gradient and the diffusion parameters, capillary surface area and blood-cell diffusion distance. In 1919 Krogh[9] formulated the capillary recruitment model to describe the processes underlying oxygen transport at the tissue level. This basic model was later expanded and refined by Honig. Although Krogh's model is limited by multiple simplifying assumptions, it has value as a tool for appreciating the role of vascular control mechanisms in the transport of oxygen to tissue.

General Features of Krogh Model

The Krogh model consists of a single capillary and the surrounding cylinder of tissue that it supplies (Fig. 5-13). Two interrelated oxygen gradients are involved: a longitu-

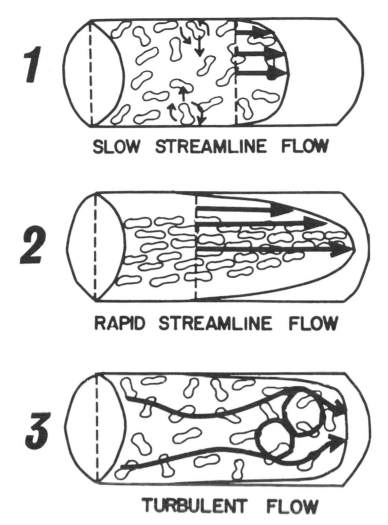

1 SLOW STREAMLINE FLOW

2 RAPID STREAMLINE FLOW

3 TURBULENT FLOW

Fig. 5–8. Diagram representing different features of streamline and turbulent flow. Reprinted with permission from Keele C. A. and Neil F: Sampson Wright's applied physiology, London, 1971, Oxford University Press.

dinal gradient within the capillary (upper panel), and a radial oxygen gradient extending into the tissue (lower panel). Most oxygen in capillary blood is bound to Hb and cannot leave the capillary. This bound oxygen is in equilibrium with the small amount of oxygen dissolved in the plasma. The consumption of oxygen by the tissue creates a transcapillary gradient for oxygen. Diffusion of oxygen into the surrounding tissue shifts the equilibrium between bound and dissolved oxygen, so that more oxygen is released from Hb. By this mechanism, oxygen dissociation from Hb is controlled by tissue oxygen consumption.

Longitudinal Oxygen Gradient

The longitudinal oxygen gradient within the capillary is created by the extraction of oxygen by tissue as blood passes from the arterial to venous ends of the capillary. In accordance with the Fick equation (Eq. 10), the arteriovenous oxygen difference is equivalent to the ratio of oxygen consumption to blood flow. An increase in oxygen consumption, a decrease in blood flow, or both, will steepen the longitudinal oxygen gradient (Fig. 5–13). Proportional changes in VO_2 and blood flow are required for the longitudinal oxygen gradient to remain constant.

A corresponding value for capillary PO_2 (PcO_2) can be estimated from the value for CcO_2 taking into account Hb concentration and the oxyhemoglobin dissociation curve. The shape of the longitudinal gradient in PO_2 within the capillary is approximately exponential because of the influence of the oxyhemoglobin dissociation curve. The PcO_2 is the driving force for diffusion of oxygen into the tissue. Since PcO_2 is minimum at the venous end of the capillary, the mitochondria in this region are most vulnerable to oxygen deficits.

Radial Oxygen Gradient (Capillary Recruitment)

The radial PO_2 gradient can be described by a value for mean tissue PO_2 (PtO_2), as calculated according to equation:

$$\text{Mean } PtO_2 = PcO_2 - A(\dot{V}O_2 \cdot r^2/4D) \qquad (9)$$

where PcO_2 is blood oxygen tension at a midway point in the capillary, A is a constant related to the relationship between capillary radius and tissue cylinder radius, $\dot{V}O_2$ is oxygen consumption of the tissue cylinder, r is the radius of the tissue cylinder (½ intercapillary distance), and D is

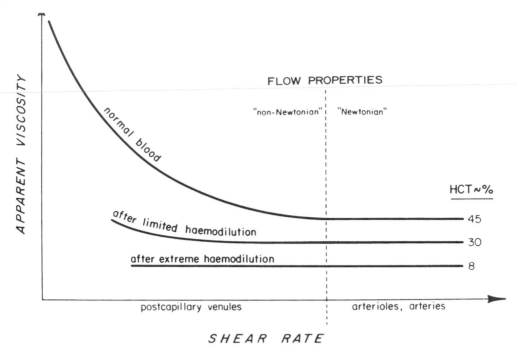

Fig. 5–9. Graphic representation of the effect of hemodilution on blood viscosity as related to shear rate in the different vascular compartments. The most pronounced decrease in blood viscosity, and thus resistance to flow, occurs within the postcapillary venules when hematocrit (HCT) is decreased from control level (45%) to 30%, i.e., during limited hemodilution. Further decreases in hematocrit (extreme hemodilution) reduced viscosity remarkably less. Reprinted with permission from Messmer K, Sunder-Plassman L: Hemodilution. Prog Surg *12*:208, 1974.

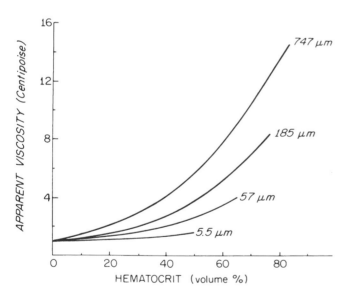

Fig. 5–10. Hematocrit on viscosity of blood in tubes of varying radii. In wide tubes, increasing hematocrit raises viscosity, whereas in narrow tubes it has no effect. Reprinted with permission from Feigl E. O.: Physiology and biophysics II: circulation, respiration and fluid balance. Philadelphia, W. B. Saunders, 1974.

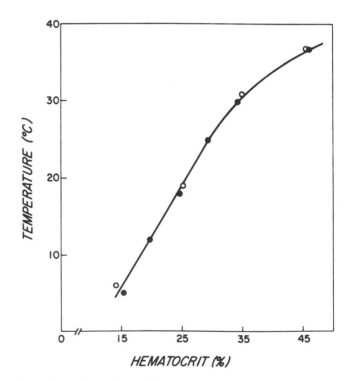

Fig. 5–11. Illustration of decrease in hematocrit that must accompany a reduction in temperature to hold viscosity constant. The measurements were made at low shear rate with an initial hematocrit of 45% at 37°C. Data were obtained with whole blood from two normal adults. From Larson L: Changes in flow properties in human blood (Master's thesis), Bozeman, Montana, 1973, Montana State University.

the oxygen diffusion coefficient. r is determined by the number of capillaries perfused with red cells per volume of tissue and is controlled by the precapillary sphincters. The favorable influence of capillary recruitment on tissue PO_2 is evident (Fig. 5-13, lower panel). If only capillaries "1" and "3" are open, diffusion distance is so large that

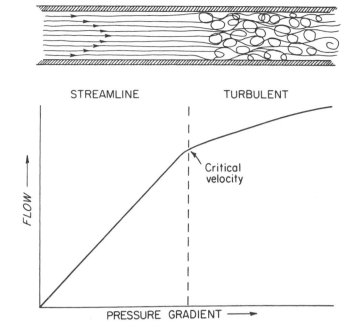

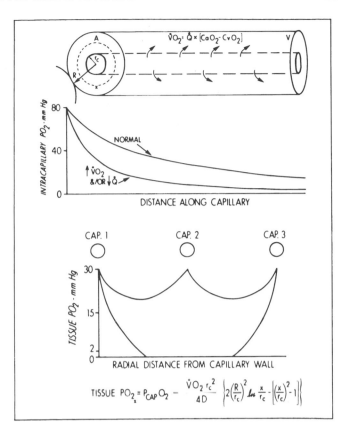

Fig. 5–12. The linear relationship between pressure gradient and flow is shown. Beyond a critical velocity, turbulence begins and relationship between pressure and flow is no longer linear. Reprinted with permission from Feigl E. O.: Physiology and biophysics II: circulation, respiration and fluid balance, Philadelphia, W. B. Saunders, 1974.

Fig. 5–13. Longitudinal and radial oxygen gradients within tissue in accordance with Krogh cylinder model. Details provided in text. VO_2, oxygen consumption; Q, blood flow; $[CaO_2-CvO_2]$, arteriovenous oxygen content difference; r_c, capillary radius; R, tissue cylinder radius; A, arterial end of capillary; V, venous end of capillary; x, point within tissue cylinder; $P_{cap}O_2$, oxygen tension of capillary blood; D, diffusion coefficient for oxygen. Reprinted with permission from Honig C. R.: Modern cardiovascular physiology, Boston, Little, Brown and Company, 1981.

PO_2 falls to zero toward the center of the tissue cylinder. The low PtO_2 causes relaxation of the precapillary sphincter controlling capillary "2." Perfusion of capillary "2" decreases diffusion distance, and increases PtO_2 to an adequate level throughout the tissue.

Mean PtO_2 is a reflection of the overall balance between oxygen supply and demand within a particular tissue.[10,11] For example, an increase in blood flow without a change in oxygen demand, i.e., luxuriant perfusion, raises mean PtO_2 whereas a reduction in blood flow without a change in oxygen demand lowers mean PtO_2. If mean PtO_2 falls below a critical level, tissue oxygen consumption will become impaired (Fig. 5–1). Measurements of mean PtO_2 have been obtained in laboratory animals in various tissues, including the myocardium and skeletal muscle, by use of a polarographic technique involving bare-tipped platinum electrodes.[10,11] The invasiveness of the technique has curtailed the use of mean PtO_2 measurements in patients. Measurements of local venous PvO_2 provide an approximation for average end-capillary PO_2, and although they neglect the radial PO_2 gradient, they generally show a reasonable correlation to mean PtO_2.[12]

Oxygen Consumption and Other Measurable Variables In Vivo

Oxygen Consumption

In a clinical setting, there are several methods to measure VO_2 of the body tissues:[13,14] 1) oxygen loss or replacement into a closed breathing system, 2) subtraction of expired from inspired volume of oxygen, and 3) use of the Fick principle.

The first method, oxygen loss or replacement into a closed breathing system, is the most fundamental, is well validated, and has an accuracy well in excess of clinical requirements. However, it is cumbersome and requires meticulous attention to detail if used safely during intensive care. The second method, subtraction of expired from inspired volume of oxygen, is a difficult and potentially inaccurate method to determine VO_2. The major source of problem is that VO_2 is a small number calculated as the difference between two large numbers. Recent technical advancements have reduced the impact of this limitation.[14]

Under steady-state conditions, the Fick equation can be used to calculate $\dot{V}O_2$:

$$\dot{V}O_2 = CO \times (CaO_2 - C\bar{v}O_2) \qquad (10)$$

where $C\bar{v}O_2$ is expressed in vol%, and $(CaO_2 - C\bar{v}O_2)$ is the systemic arteriovenous oxygen content difference. This approach is commonly referred to as the reversed Fick technique. In this technique, CO is usually measured by thermodilution using a Swan-Ganz catheter situated in the pulmonary artery. Samples of blood are collected from an artery and from the pulmonary artery (mixed venous sample) and analyzed for oxygen content. The values for blood oxygen content are used to calculate the systemic arteriovenous oxygen content difference. Using values for CO and $(CaO_2-C\bar{v}O_2)$ at rest, the Fick equation can be used to calculate a value for whole body oxygen consumption.

Indices of Mixed Venous Oxygenation

Oxygen Extraction Ratio

Oxygen extraction ratio (ER in %) is defined by the equation:

$$ER = (CaO_2 - C\bar{v}O_2)/CaO_2 \qquad (11)$$

Combining equations and rearranging terms, it can be demonstrated that ER is also equal to the ratio of $\dot{V}O_2$ to DO_2, and, thus that it reflects the balance between systemic oxygen demand and delivery. Measurements of ER, as well as of $P\bar{v}O_2$, are frequently used clinically to assess the overall adequacy of DO_2 (and CO) in critically ill patients.[17-19]

"Critical Oxygen Delivery"

At rest DO_2 greatly exceeds VO_2 (in our example above 1025 vs. 228 mL/min) and thus ER is modest (approximately 25%), resulting in a substantial reserve for oxygen extraction.[20] At normal or high levels of DO_2, VO_2 is constant and independent of DO_2 (Fig. 5-14A). As DO_2 is gradually reduced, an increased ER maintains VO_2 (Figure 5-14B). Eventually a critical point is reached where oxygen extraction cannot increase adequately, and VO_2 begins to fall. Below this threshold, the so-called "critical DO_2",[21] the level of VO_2 is limited by the supply of oxygen. In anesthetized dogs, the critical DO_2 was found to be approximately 10 mL/min/kg (Fig. 5-14A).[21] In some studies, oxygen increases further as DO_2 is reduced below critical DO_2,[22] whereas in others oxygen extraction was maximum at critical DO_2 (Fig. 5-14B).[23] The normal biphasic DO_2-VO_2 relationship has been demonstrated in patients without respiratory failure undergoing coronary artery surgery,[24] whereas a direct linear relationship between DO_2 and VO_2 has been demonstrated in patients with acute adult respiratory distress syndrome,[25,26] implying a pathologic impairment to tissue extraction of oxygen in these patients.[20]

Factors Decreasing Oxygen Delivery

A decrease in DO_2 can be produced by a reduction in Hct, PaO_2, or cardiac output. Old terminology referred to these conditions as anemic, hypoxic, or stagnant hypoxia. If the reduction in DO_2 is severe, it can produce tissue hypoxia, i.e., cause a decrease in PtO_2, that is sufficient to limit VO_2 and to stimulate lactate production. Although the value for critical DO_2 appears to be similar regardless of the etiology, the corresponding value for critical $P\bar{v}O_2$ differs.

The critical $P\bar{v}O_2$ during acute anemia (hemodilution) was 40 mm Hg compared to 17 mm Hg and 31 to 36 mm

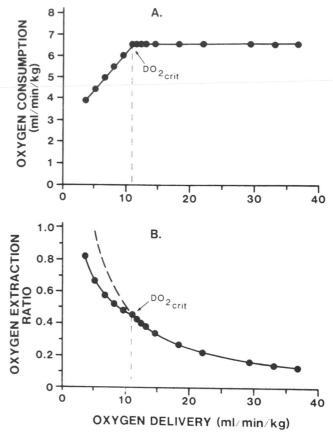

Fig. 5–14. Changes in systemic oxygen consumption (A) and oxygen extraction ratio (B) during progressive reduction in oxygen delivery. An increased oxygen extraction ratio maintains oxygen consumption constant until oxygen delivery is lowered to a critical value (DO_{2crit}). The dashed line demonstrates the theoretical increase in oxygen extraction required to maintain oxygen consumption for levels of oxygen delivery below DO_{2crit}. Modified from Schumaker P. T., Cain S. M.: The concept of critical oxygen delivery. Intensive Care Med *13*:223, 1987.

Hg during hypoxemia and reduced cardiac output, respectively.[21,27,28] A high value for critical $P\bar{v}O_2$ suggests that hemodilution may impair tissue oxygen extraction. This may be attributable to decreased transit time for red cells through the capillary circulation, thus limiting the available time for unloading of oxygen at the tissue, i.e., capillaries within tissues became functional shunts for oxygen.[29] In terms of the Krogh model (Eq. 11), this means that the effective open capillary density was reduced resulting in a steeper PO_2 gradient between the capillary blood and tissue cells. Another potential explanation for the higher values for critical $P\bar{v}O_2$ during hemodilution relates to the possibility that certain regions of the body with high flow rates, e.g., the kidneys, were overperfused with respect to oxygen demands, which increased values for $P\bar{v}O_2$, while other underperfused regions were producing lactate.

Equations 1, 12, and 13 can be applied to individual tissues by substituting local blood flow for cardiac output

Table 5–2. Interorgan Variation in Baseline Values Blood Flow, Oxygen Consumption, and Oxygen Extraction

	Blood Flow (ml/min/100g)	Oxygen Consumption (ml/min/100g)	(a-v) O_2 Difference (vol%)	Oxygen Extraction (%)
Left ventricle	80	8	14	70
Brain	55	3	6	30
Liver	85			
		2	6	30
GI tract	40			
Kidneys	400	5	1.3	6.5
Muscles	3	0.15	5	25
Skin	10	0.2	2.5	12.5
Rest of body	3	0.15	4.4	22

From Folkow, B., Neil, E. Circulation. New York, Oxford University Press, 1971, with permission.

and local venous oxygen measurements for $P\bar{v}O_2$ measurements. The individual body tissues vary widely with respect to the relationship between baseline DO_2 and VO_2, and in their baseline ER (Table 5–2). For example, in the left ventricle baseline ER is 70 to 75%, whereas in the kidney it is 5 to 10%. The high baseline ER of the left ventricle renders it dependent on changes in blood flow to maintain adequate oxygen transport.

CARBON DIOXIDE TRANSPORT

Combustion of foodstuffs, by cellular metabolism, is the source of body carbon dioxide. At the cell level the partial pressure of carbon dioxide is greatest and a gradient exists from cell → interstitium > blood → lungs. Diffusion occurs in this direction. Upon entering the blood, carbon dioxide is hydrated to carbonic acid which is quickly buffered and contributes to the formation of bicarbonate or enters into chemical reaction with amino groups. Carbon dioxide is found in blood in three principal forms and is so transported. It is physically dissolved, as bicarbonate, and combined with hemoglobin as a carbamino compound (Fig. 5–15).

Dissolved Carbon Dioxide

Physically dissolved carbon dioxide obeys Henry's Law. Accordingly, it is chiefly in plasma; only small portion is contain in the erthyrocyte cytoplasm. Carbon dioxide is about 20 times more soluble than oxygen in plasma.

Carbon Dioxide as Bicarbonate

Bicarbonate is formed in the blood by the following sequence of reactions:

$$CO_2 + H_2O \rightleftarrows H_2CO_3 \rightleftarrows H^+ + HCO_3^- \qquad (12)$$

The formation of carbonic acid (H_2CO_3) is very slow in plasma but rapid within the red blood cell because of the presence there of the enzyme carbonic anhydrase. This is a zinc-containing protein which is present in high concentration in the red cell but not in the plasma. Ionization of the carbonic acid within the red cell occurs rapidly

and does not require an enzyme. When the concentration of H^+ and HCO_3^- ions in the cell rises, HCO_3^- ions diffuse out, but H^+ ions cannot move out easily because the cell membrane is relatively impermeable to cations. Therefore, in order to maintain electical neutrality, Cl^- ions diffuse into the cell from the plasma, the so-called chloride shift.

Most H^+ ions that are liberated become bound to hemoglobin, which is the prominent buffer in the blood:

$$H^+ + HbO_2 \rightleftarrows H \cdot Hb + O_2 \qquad (13)$$

This reaction occurs because reduced Hb is a better proton acceptor than the oxygenated form. Therefore, the presence of reduced Hb in the peripheral blood facilitates loading of carbon dioxide, while the reoxygenation of the blood in the lung facilitates unloading of carbon dioxide. The ability for deoxygenation of the blood to enhance the carriage of carbon dioxide is often referred to as the "Haldane effect."

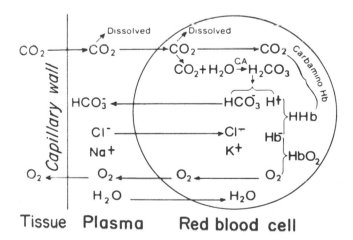

Fig. 5–15. Scheme of delivery of oxygen and removal of carbon dioxide from tissue in systemic capillaries. Exactly opposite events occur in the pulmonary capillaries. Reprinted with permission from West J. B.: Best and Taylor's Physiological Basis of Medical Practice, 12th ed., Baltimore, Williams & Wilkins, 1990.

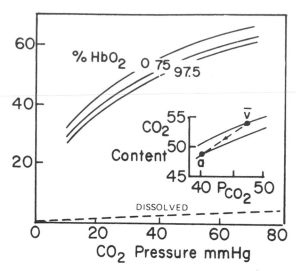

Fig. 5–16. CO_2 dissociation curves for blood of different oxygen saturations. Oxygenated blood carries less CO_2 for the same P_{CO_2}. The "physiological" curve between arterial and mixed venous blood is also shown in the inset. Reprinted with permission from West J. B.: Best and Taylor's Physiological Basis of Medical Practice, 12th ed., Baltimore, Williams and Wilkins, 1990.

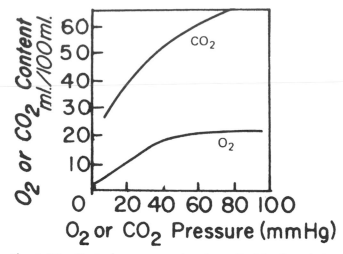

Fig. 5–17. Typical oxygen and carbon dioxide dissociation curves plotted with the same scales. The carbon dioxide curve is much steeper. Reprinted with permission from West J. B.: Best and Taylor's Physiological Basis of Medical Practice, 12th ed., Baltimore, Williams & Wilkins, 1990.

Carbamino Compounds

The carbamino compounds are formed by the combination of carbon dioxide with the terminal amine groups of blood proteins. The most important protein is the globin of hemoglobin, and the reaction can be represented:

$$CO_2 + Hb \cdot NH_2 \rightleftarrows Hb \cdot NH \cdot COOH \rightleftarrows Hb \cdot NH \cdot COO + H^+ \quad (14)$$

This reaction occurs rapidly without an enzyme, and most of the carbamic acid is in the ionized form. Reduced Hb can bind more carbon dioxide than can HbO_2. Deoxygenation of blood in the peripheral capillaries facilitates the loading of carbon dioxide while oxygenation in the pulmonary capillaries facilitates unloading of carbon dioxide (Haldane effect).

The contributions of the various forms of carbon dioxide in arterial blood can be approximated as follows:

1. Physically dissolved 5%
2. Bicarbonate 90%
3. Carbamino 5%

Dissociation Curve

The relationship between P_{CO_2} and the total carbon dioxide content of the blood is presented in Figure 5–16. The carbon dioxide dissociation curve is much more linear than the oxygen dissociation curve (Fig. 5–3). The lower the saturation of Hb with oxygen, the larger the carbon dioxide content for a given P_{CO_2}. As cited, this Haldane effect can be explained by the better ability of reduced Hb to mop up the H^+ ions produced when carbonic acid dissociates and the greater facility of reduced Hb to form carbaminohemoglobin.

Figure 5–17 shows that the dissociation curve for carbon dioxide is much steeper than that for oxygen. For example, in the range 40–50 mmHg, the carbon dioxide content changes about 4.7 ml/100 ml compared with the oxygen content of about 1.7 ml/100 ml.

REFERENCES

1. Honig, C. R.: Modern Cardiovascular Physiology. Boston, 1981, Little, Brown and Company.
2. Weibel, E. R.: The pathway for oxygen. Cambridge, 1984, Harvard Univ Press.
3. Mines, A. H.: Respiratory Physiology. New York, 1981, Raven Press, p 62.
4. Benumof, J. L.: Respiratory physiology and respiratory function during anesthesia. In: Miller R. D., editor, Anesthesia, 2ed, New York, 1986, Churchill Livingstone, pp. 1115-1163.
5. Gregory, I. C.: The oxygen and carbon monoxide capacities of foetal and adult blood. J Physiol 236:625, 1974.
6. Fahmy, N. R.: Techniques for deliberate hypotension: haemodilution and hypotension. In: Enderby GEH, ed, Hypotensive anaesthesia, London, 1985, Churchill-Livingstone, p. 164.
7. Laver, M. B., Buckley, M. J., and Austen, W. G.: Extreme hemodilution with profound hypothermia and circulatory arrest. Bibliotheca Haematol 41:225, 1975.
8. Hofling, B., von Restorff, W., Holtz, J., et al: Viscous and inertial fractions of total perfusion energy dissipation in the coronary circulation of the *in situ* perfused dog heart. Pflugers Arch 358:1, 1975.
9. Krogh, A.: The number and distribution of capillaries in muscles with calculations of the oxygen pressure head necessary for supplying the tissue. J Physiol (London) 52:409, 1919.
10. Crystal, G. J., and Weiss H. R.: VO_2 of resting muscle during arterial hypoxia: role of reflex vasoconstriction. Microvasc Res 20:30, 1980.
11. Crystal, G. J., Downey H. F., and Bashour, F. A.: Small vessel and total coronary blood volume during intracoronary adenosine infusion. Am J Physiol 241:H194, 1981.
12. Tenny, S. M.: Theoretical analysis of the relationship be-

tween venous blood and mean tissue oxygen pressure. Respir Physiol *20*:283, 1975.

13. Nunn, J. F., Makita, K., and Royston, B: Validation of oxygen consumption measurements during artificial ventilation. J Appl Physiol *67*:2129, 1989.

14. Makita, K., Nunn, J. F., and Royston, B.: Evaluation of metabolic measuring instruments for use in critically ill patients. Crit Care Med *10*:638, 1990.

15. Smithies, M. N., Royston, B., Makita, K., et al: A comparison of the measurement of oxygen consumption by indirect calimetry and the reversed Fick method. Crit Care Med *19*:1401, 1991.

16. Webster, N. R., and Nunn J. F.: Molecular structure of free radicals and their importance in biological reactions. Br J Anaesth *60*:98, 1988.

17. Astiz, M. E., Rackow, E. C., Kaufman, B., et al: Relationship of oxygen delivery and mixed venous oxygenation and to lactate acidosis in patients with sepsis and acute myocardial infarction. Crit Care Med *16*:655, 1988.

18. Pinsky, M. R.: Assessment of adequacy of oxygen transport in the critically ill. Appl Cardio Pathophysiol *3*:271, 1990.

19. Levy, P. S., Chavez, R. P., Crystal, G. J., et al: Oxygen extraction ratio: A valid indicator of transfusion need in limited coronary vascular reserve? J Trauma *32*:769, 1992.

20. Schumacker, P. T., and Cain, S. M.: The concept of critical oxygen oxygen delivery. Intensive Care Med *13*:223, 1987.

21. Cain, S. M.: Oxygen delivery and uptake in dogs during anemic and hypoxic hypoxia: J Appl Physiol *42*:228, 1977.

22. Cain, S. M.: Peripheral oxygen uptake and delivery in health and disease. Clin Chest Med *4*:39, 1983.

23. Cain, S. M., and Bradley, W. E.: Critical O_2 transport values at lowered body temperatures in rats. J Appl Physiol *55*:1713, 1983.

24. Shibutani, K., Komatsu, T., Kubal, K., et al: Critical level of oxygen delivery in anesthetized man. Crit Care Med *11*:640, 1983.

25. Danek, S. J., Lynch, J. P., Weg, J. G., et al: The dependence of oxygen uptake on oxygen delivery in the adult respiratory syndrome, Ann Rev Resp Dis *122*:387, 1980.

26. Mohsenifar, Z., Goldbach, P., Tachkin, D. P., et al: Relationship between O_2 delivery and O_2 consumption in the adult respiratory distress syndrome. Chest *84*:267, 1983.

27. Cain, S. M.: Appearance of excess lactate in anesthetized dogs during anemic and hypoxic hypoxia. Am J Physiol *209*:604, 1965.

28. Heusser, F., Fahey, J. T., and Lister, G.: Effect of hemoglobin concentration on critical cardiac output and oxygen transport. Am J Physiol *256*:H527, 1989.

29. Gutierrez, G.: The rate of oxygen release and its effect on capillary O_2 tension. A mathematical analysis. Respir Physiol *63*:79, 1986.

Chapter 6

CARDIAC PHYSIOLOGY

BRIAN OLSHANSKY AND CRAIG NELSON

The heart delivers oxygenated blood and other nutrients to the tissues (including the heart) and delivers deoxygenated blood to the lungs.[1-8] After blood returns to the right atrium from the vena cavae, it flows through the tricuspid valve to the right ventricle where it is pumped through the pulmonic valve into the pulmonary arteries and the pulmonary capillary bed. The blood, now oxygenated, flows into the left atrium through the mitral valve into the left ventricle where it is then pumped into the aorta (Fig. 6-1). When functioning normally, the heart delivers enough blood to the organs to meet metabolic demands. For this to occur effectively, the heart is endowed with specific physiologic properties (Table 6-1) discussed in this chapter.

CARDIAC ULTRASTRUCTURE[2-5,9-13]

The chambers of the heart are composed of atrial and ventricular myocytes oriented and arranged on a *cardiac cytoskeleton,* a supporting structure, composed of fibrous and elastic connective tissue. These cells are surrounded by the *sarcolemma,* the *sarcoplasmic reticulum* and are connected by *intercalated discs,* a portion of which, the *gap junctions,* provides electrical communication between cells (Fig. 6-2). The *T-tubular system* helps transport electrical signals from the sarcolemma to the cell interior. The cells are composed of multiple contractile proteins that include *troponin, actin* and *myosin* arranged longitudinally in structures called *sarcomeres.* There is an intracellular cytoskeleton composed of *vinculin* which runs under the sarcolemma and helps bind it to the Z-line.

The muscle bundles wind spirally around the pumping chambers. Their insertion ends in the fibrous portion of the heart surrounding the heart valves (Fig. 6-3). In the left ventricle, the endocardium courses in a counterclockwise direction, the mid-myocardium in a horizontal direction and the epicardium in a clockwise direction. The fibers in the mid-myocardium run perpendicular to the long axis; the endocardial and epicardial fibers run parallel to the long axis (Fig. 6-4).

There are specialized conduction and pacemaker fibers (Fig. 6-5), parasympathetic and sympathetic nerve fibers, nerve terminals and valve structures. Epicardial coronary arteries supply an extensive vascular network that drains into the coronary sinus. Each structure is important for the heart to function properly.

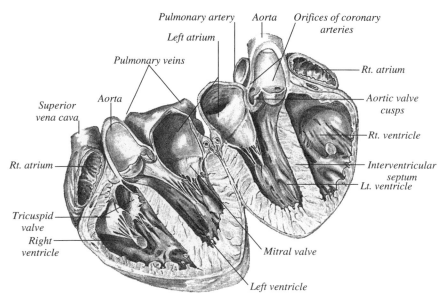

Pulmonary artery — Aorta — Orifices of coronary arteries
Left atrium
Pulmonary veins
Superior vena cava
Aorta
Rt. atrium
Rt. atrium
Aortic valve cusps
Rt. ventricle
Interventricular septum
Lt. ventricle
Tricuspid valve
Right ventricle
Mitral valve
Left ventricle

Fig. 6–1. The heart transected slightly anterior to its midline. Note the more elongated left ventricle, which has thicker walls than the right ventricle. Modified from Berne and Levy: Cardiovascular Physiology. Mosby, St. Louis, 1967. Redrawn and modified from Katz[4] with permission.

GENERAL PROPERTIES OF HEART MUSCLE[1-8,14-18]

Electrical activation of myocytes is essential for the heart to contract. Electrical activation is linked to subsequent mechanical contraction (Fig. 6–6). Cardiac contraction, caused by a series of biochemical processes, ultimately leads to expulsion of blood from the heart. Relaxation follows.

Table 6–1. Five Principal Properties of Heart Muscle

1. Excitability (*Bathmotropic*)
2. Conductivity (*Dromotropic*)
3. Rhythmicity and Rate (*Chronotropic*)
4. Contractility (*Inotropic*)
5. Relaxation (*Lusitropic*)

The events of the normal cardiac cycle can be divided into: electrical activation ("excitation"), excitation-contraction coupling, and mechanical contraction and relaxation (Fig. 6–7). These processes are regulated by the nervous system, mechanical, electrical, and chemical factors. These aspects of the cardiac cycle will be discussed later in the chapter.

THE CARDIAC CYCLE[19-21]

The cardiac cycle consists of systole and diastole. Events in systole occur during cardiac contraction. Diastole includes the events that occur for the remainder of the cardiac cycle. Systolic and diastolic events are energy dependant although eighty-five percent of energy use occurs in systole. The sequence of events in the cardiac

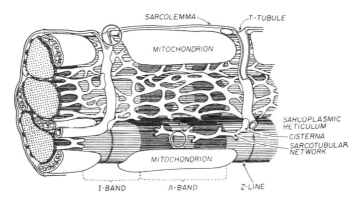

Fig. 6–2. Ultrastructure of the working myocardial cell. Contractile proteins are arranged in a regular array of thick and thin filaments (seen in cross section, left). The A-band represents the region of the sarcomere occupied by the thick filaments into which thin filaments extend from either side. The I-band is the region of the sarcomere occupied only by thin filaments: these extend toward the center of the sarcomere from the Z lines, which bisect each I-band. The sarcomere, the functional unit of the contractile apparatus, is defined as the region between a pair of Z-lines, and contains two half I-bands and one A-band. The sarcoplasmic reticulum, a membrane network that surrounds the contractile proteins, consists of the sarcotubular network at the center of the sarcomere, and the cisternae, which abut the t-tubules and the sarcolemma. The transverse tubular system (t-tubule) is lined by a membrane that is continuous with the sarcolemma, so that the lumen of the t-tubules carries the extracellular space toward the center of the mycardial cell. Mitochondria are shown in the central sarcomere and in cross section at the left. Redrawn from Katz A. M.: Congestive heart failure: Role of altered myocardial cellular control. N Engl J Med *293*:1184–1191, 1975.

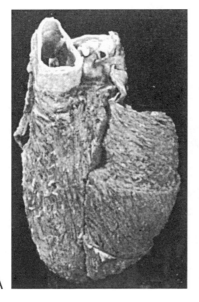
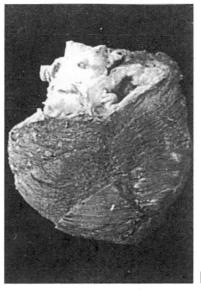

Fig. 6–3. Spiral musculature of the ventricular walls. A. Human heart viewed from the left and anteriorly. The right ventricle (*left*) and left ventricle (*right*) have been dissected to show differing fiber orientations at two depths. B. Posterior surface of the same specimen. C and D. Schematic drawing of heart viewed from the apex (C) and anteriorly (D). Redrawn and modified from Opie, L. H.: The Heart: Physiology and Metabolism, 2nd ed. New York, Raven Press, 1992.

A
B

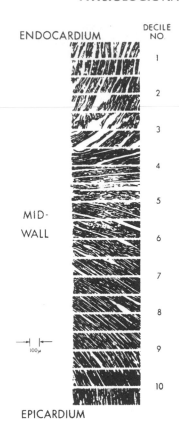

Fig. 6–4. Reconstruction of the left ventricular wall, prepared from a series of microphotographs, showing changing fiber angles at different depths. Reprinted with permission from Streeter et al., American Heart Association, 1969.

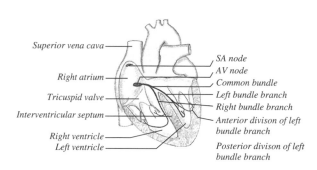

Fig. 6–5. Conducting system of the human heart, showing anatomical features of the heart (labels at *left*) and the conducting structures (labels at *right*). Redrawn from Benninghoff: Lehrbuch der Anatomie des Menschen, J. F. Lehmanns Verlag, Munich, 1944.

cycle (volume, pressure and electrical), graphically represented, characterized initially by Wiggers (Fig. 6–8), represent the features crucial to effective cardiac performance.

Ventricular Systole

This is the period of active contraction of the ventricles. The average duration is 0.25 to 0.3 seconds. It is sub-

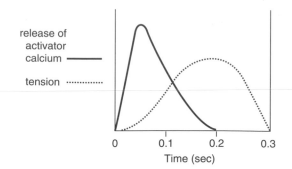

Fig. 6–6. The release of activator calcium (*solid-line*) precedes the development of tension in cardiac muscle. Redrawn from Katz[4] with permission.

divided according to blood flow patterns out of the ventricle.

Isovolumetric (Isometric) Contraction

This phase of the cardiac cycle occurs with the cardiac valves closed. No blood is ejected during this initial phase. Contraction of the ventricular muscle causes the ventricular pressure to rise. The increase in ventricular pressure is isometric. The ventricular pressure rises until it exceeds arterial (pulmonary artery and aortic) pressure, this is known as the *pre-ejection period (PEP)*.

Rapid Ejection Phase

Once the ventricular pressure exceeds the pressure in the aorta and pulmonary artery, the aortic and pulmonic valves open and blood is ejected rapidly out of the ventricles. This is the initiation of isotonic contraction but, despite the decrease in the blood volume within the ventricle, the continued ventricular contraction causes a continued increase in ventricular pressure. The arterial pressures beyond the valves have a parallel increase in pressure. During this phase, peak systolic ventricular and arterial pressure is achieved.

Reduced Ejection Phase

Ventricular contraction continues but it starts to lose its strength. This loss of contractile strength coupled with the decrease in ventricular volume, causes the pressure within the ventricle to decrease. Ejection continues during this phase, but decreases in volume. The period for the total left ventricular ejection of blood is called the *left ventricular ejection time (LVET)*.

Ventricular Diastole

This aspect of the cardiac cycle, when the ventricles relax and dilate, has gained much recent attention. It is no longer viewed as a time of rest, during which the ventricle is refilled with blood. It is recognized as an active complex process. Ventricular compliance, a diastolic property, has an important influence on ventricular func-

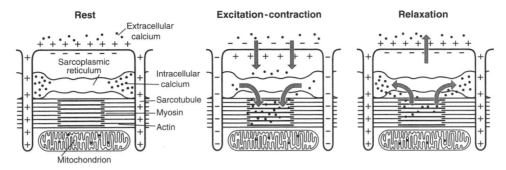

Fig. 6–7. Redrawn from Braunwald[2] with permission.

tion. The average duration of 0.5 seconds is quite variable; the duration of diastole parallels the heart rate closely. As with systole, diastole is subdivided into component parts.

Protodiastole

Immediately after the end of the ventricular contraction, ejection from the ventricle stops. The pressure within the ventricles drop below the aortic and pulmonary artery pressures causing closure of the aortic and pulmonic valves.

Isovolumetric (Isometric) Relaxation

During this phase, the ventricular volume does not change but most relaxation occurs. The pressure drops

rapidly until the atrial pressure exceeds the ventricular pressure which then cause the mitral and tricuspid valves to open.

Rapid Filling (Inflow) Phase

After the AV valves open, approximately 80% of ventricular filling occurs. Isotonic ventricular relaxation occurs in this phase. This phase encompasses the first third of diastole.

Diastasis

Blood flow into the ventricles slows. There is little change in the diastolic pressure during this phase. Relaxation is complete. The time for this portion of diastole is most influenced by changes in heart rate.

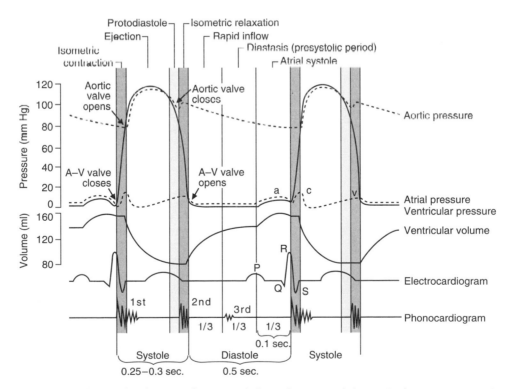

Fig. 6–8. The events of the cardiac cycle, showing changes in left atrial pressure, left ventricular pressure, aortic pressure, ventricular volume, the electrocardiogram, and the phonocardiogram. Redrawn from Guyton, Textbook of Medical Physiology, W.B. Saunders Co.

Atrial Systole

The atria contract increasing the blood flow into the ventricles. Atrial systole has a duration of approximately 0.1 second. Although the ventricular pressure increases only slightly as it fills, this portion of diastole contributes more than 20% of the end-diastolic volume.

Atrial Diastole

The atria relax. Their contraction stops as does the flow of blood into the ventricle. The duration is approximately 0.7 seconds and lasts throughout ventricular systole. Ventricular pressure decreases just before the ventricles contract initiating the cardiac cycle again with the ventricular systolic phase.

Figure 6-8 summarizes graphically the pressure changes that occur during the cardiac cycle. Also represented is electrical activation of the heart and its relation to mechanical events. The QRS complex (electrical activation of both ventricles) is inscribed during the isovolumetric phase of the ventricular systole.

Pressure–Volume Relationships[22–34]

The pressure, volume, and electrical changes during phases of the cardiac cycle can be represented graphically. Ventricular chamber size can be related to instantaneous ventricular pressures measured throughout the cardiac cycle. The relationship may be plotted, producing an external work diagram or pressure-volume loop, demonstrating four phases of the cardiac cycle (Fig. 6–9).

Phase I is that of diastolic filling (point D to A). A slight decrease in ventricular pressure occurs due to ventricular relaxation (lusitropy) and distensibility. Closer to A, an increase in ventricular pressure occurs as ventricular filling continues. This gives the final ventricular end-diastolic volume and pressure. The mitral valve closes at point A.

Phase II describes isovolumetric contraction (point A to B). A significant pressure increase occurs without an accompanying volume increase. A point B, the aortic valve opens.

Phase III represents systolic ejection (point B to C) with both rapid and reduced ejection components. The aortic valve closes at the end of this phase.

Phase IV represents isovolumetric relaxation (point C to D) during which a pressure drop occurs, unaccompanied by a change in volume. Isovolumetric relaxation may be impaired by conditions such as myocardial ischemia or ventricular hypertrophy. Small changes in loading conditions do not influence isovolumetric relaxation in a normal ventricle. It is, however, influenced by the inotropic state. At the end of this phase, the mitral valve opens.

The pressure-volume loops may be used to assess ventricular performance. Using these loops obtained under different loading conditions, the contractile state of the ventricle can be described. By connecting end-systolic points of several loops made at different preloads and afterloads, an isovolumic pressure line is obtained. An approximation of this, the end-systolic pressure-volume relation (ESPVR), represent the end-systolic state of the ventricle. The end systolic volume varies inversely with contractility while the end-systolic pressure varies directly with it. The end-diastolic pressure-volume relation represents the end-diastolic state of the ventricle. End-diastolic volume varies directly whereas end diastolic pressure varies indirectly with it (Fig. 6–10).

ELECTRICAL PROPERTIES OF THE HEART[16–18,35–46]

Mechanical systole is preceded by electrical activation (depolarization) of cardiac myocytes. Several properties of the heart are responsible for adequate cardiac activa-

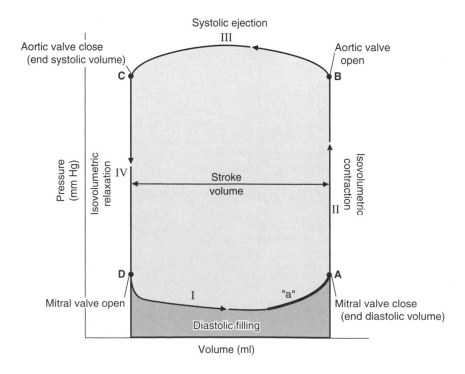

Fig. 6–9. Pressure-volume loop of the left ventricle for one cardiac cycle (D A B C). Note the slight decrease in ventricular pressure occurring in phase I owing to ventricular relaxation and distensibility. Stroke volume is the difference between ventricular volume at end-diastole and end-systole. Redrawn with permission from Barash P. G., Kopriva C. J.: Cardiac pump function and how to monitor it. In Thomas S. J. (ed): Manual of Cardiac Anesthesia. New York, Churchill Livingstone, 1984, pp 1–34.

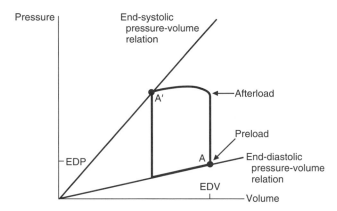

Fig. 6–10. Schematic pressure-volume loop showing its constraint between the end-diastolic pressure-volume relation (**lower line**) and the end-systolic pressure-volume relation (**upper line**). Systole begins at the end-diastolic point (A) and ends at the end-systolic point (A′). The ventricle encounters its afterload when the aortic valve opens, so that the end-systolic point reflects both contractility and afterload. After isovolumic relaxation the ventricle begins to fill, and the preload is initially encountered when the mitral valve opens; the preload of the ventricle is defined by the pressure and volume at end-diastole. For simplicity, the ventricle is shown to fill along the end-diastolic pressure-volume curve; however, complete relaxation often does not occur until well after the onset of filling, especially in diseased hearts. EDP = end-diastolic pressure; EDV = end-diastolic volume. Redrawn from Katz, A. M.: Influence of Altered Inotropy and Lusitropy on Ventricular Pressure-Volume Loops. J Am Coll Cardiol 11:438, 1988.

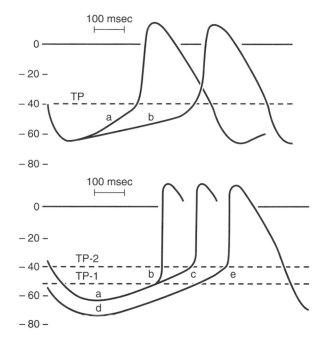

Fig. 6–11. Drawings of transmembrane action potentials from fiber located in mammalian sino-atrial node to show ways in which frequency of pacemaker discharge can be altered. Upper diagram illustrates decrease in frequency of discharge caused by slowing of rate of diastolic depolarization from rate shown in *a* to that in *b*, resulting in increase in length of time required to reach threshold potential, *TP*, for generation of action potential. Lower diagram shows effects of reduction in level of threshold potential from 50 mv., *TP-1*, to 40 mv., *TP-2*, which results in slowing of rate. Also evident in this diagram is effect of change in level of "resting" potential from *a* to *d*, resulting in slowing of rate of discharge (see *a-b, a-c, d-e*). Redrawn from Hoffman and Cranefield, Electrophysiology of the Heart. Courtesy of McGraw-Hill Book Co.

tion. These properties include excitability, automaticity and conduction.

Excitability (bathmotropic property)[21,46] is the ability of the heart to activate electrically and contract in response to electrical, mechanical or chemical stimulation. An excitable stimulus may be influenced by pH, temperature, mechanical stress, ionic balance, nutrition or ischemia.

Automaticity (chronotropic property)[16–18,35,38,41,42,44] is the ability of the heart to initiate impulses spontaneously to cause self-excitation. Spontaneous depolarization that occurs during electrical diastole is responsible for normal automaticity (Fig. 6-11). Most of the conducting system is capable of automaticity at varying rates. The SA node usually has the fastest rate while the Purkinje fibers have the slowest rate (Table 6-2).

Conduction (dromotropic property)[38,39,43,47] is the ability of the heart to propagate electrical impulses from one cell to another. The conduction of electrical impulses through the heart may be due to active depolarization (*propagated action potentials*) or passive electrical activation (*electrotonic influences*). The speed of conduction may be slow or fast; it is related in part to the tissue involved. The speed of conduction is caused by the force and speed of electrical depolarization of the impulse, the electrical communication between cells (*gap junctions*), and the direction of the electrical activation (*anisotropic properties*).

Table 6–2. Automaticity of the Heart—Normal Rates (beats/minute)

SA Node	60–100
AV Node	40–60
His-Purkinje System	20
Ventricular muscle	20–40

Action Potential of Single Cardiac Cells[36,37,41–43]

Single Cell Activation

The transmembrane potential difference of a quiescent atrial or ventricular myocyte is normally 80–90 mV. It is less negative, 50–70 mV, for AV nodal and SA nodal cells (Fig. 6-12). The cell interior is negative relative to the outside and is denoted the *resting membrane potential*. On excitation, an action potential is produced with a rapid change in voltage over time (Fig. 6-13).

Four phases of the action potential are recognized (Fig. 6-13): *Phase 0,* the initial, rapid depolarization (also called dV/dT_{max}), is the upstroke toward and overshoot

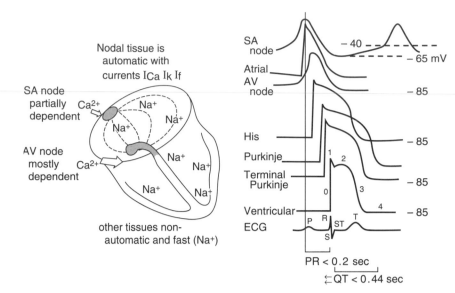

Fig. 6–12. Patterns of conduction from sinoatrial (SA) node to ventricles. The SA node has three depolarizing currents, of which the slow upstroke is largely calcium-dependent. In other tissues, such as atrial muscle, Purkinje fibers, and ventricular muscle, the impulse travels very rapidly because the initial phase of depolarization is much faster and sodium-dependent. Conduction between atria and ventricles is slowed by the calcium-dependent AV node. The patterns of the cardiac action potential in different sites are modified from Singer et al. Prog Cardiovasc Dis *24*:97, 1981. Redrawn from Opie with permission.

above the zero potential. It is due to opening of the sodium channels with rapid movement of and increased permeability to Na^{+1} into atrial and ventricular myocytes or slower movement of Ca^{+2} (without Na^{+1} movement) into SA and AV nodal cells. This phase, as it occurs throughout the ventricular myocardium results in a QRS complex and, as it occurs in the atria, results in a P wave on the electrocardiogram. A rapid repolarization period, designated *phase 1,* follows in select atrial and epicardial ventricular myocytes. A plateau phase, unique to cardiac myocytes (not present in skeletal muscle or nerves), is designated *phase 2.* This continued depolarization is caused by a slower inward movement of Ca^{+2}. *Phase 3* of the action potential then occurs. During this phase, repolarization occurs, with return to the resting membrane potential. Phase 3 is caused by opening of potassium channels with inward movement of K^+. Many types of potassium channels responsible for repolarization are present on myocardial membranes. This phase is responsible for the T-wave in the electrocardiogram (Fig. 6–13). Atrial repolarization is not visible on the electrocardiogram. *Phase 4* is the period that occurs during electrical diastole. During this phase, the equilibration phase of the action potential, there is an active sodium and potassium exchange across the cell membrane.

Normal myocardial cells differ with respect to their action potential configuration, characteristics, and magnitude of depolarization (Fig. 6–12). Phase 0 of the action potential is approximately 10 times slower in the AV node and the SA node compared to the atrial and ventricular myocardium. In automatic cells, such as those present in the SA and the AV nodes, there is slow diastolic depolarization during phase 4 (Fig. 6–11).

Maintenance of the normal resting potential during phase 4 depends primarily on the concentration gradient of potassium ions across the membrane. This relationship is defined by the Nernst equation which at normal body temperature yields the expression:

$$E_m = 62 \text{ mV } \log[K_i^+]/[K_o^+]$$

E_m is the resting membrane potential. In mammalian nerve, skeletal and cardiac muscles, the ratio of K_i^+ to K_o^+ is approximately 30:1. The ionic changes occurring during the action potential are reestablished by active metabolic processes. Excitability of cardiac fibers is related to the transmembrane action potential. Excitation depends upon raising the transmembrane action potential to a certain critical value, the threshold potential or lowering the threshold of excitability.

The Refractory Period[18,41–43]

The *absolute refractory period* is the interval in which the cell cannot be activated. The absolute refractory period lasts nearly throughout the action potential duration. When the transmembrane potential is less than -45 to -55 mV (in atrial and ventricular tissue), the tissue remains unexcitable.

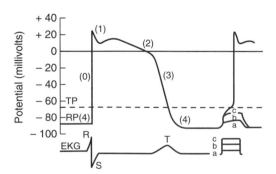

Fig. 6–13. Diagrammatic representation of the transmembrane action potential and unipolar electrogram recorded from an isolated preparation of cardiac muscle. Depolarization and the various phases of repolarization are designated by the symbols *(0), (1), (2), (3), (4).* Shown on the right are the changes in transmembrane potential produced by subthreshold stimuli. Stimulus *(c)* is sufficient to produce a local response which reaches threshold (TP) and merges with the upstroke of the action potential. Redrawn from Hoffman and Cranefield, Electrophysiology of the Heart, McGraw-Hill.)

The refractory period of cardiac muscle differs from skeletal muscle. Whereas skeletal muscle responds to a stimulus any time after it begins to contract, cardiac muscle, in contrast, will not respond to a stimulus since the cell remains depolarized. The absolute refractory period eliminates the occurrence of summation or tetanic contracture seen in skeletal muscle. It can be shortened by an increase in temperature and by vagal stimulation (most prominently in atrial myocardium) and can be lengthened by class Ia and class III antiarrhythmic drugs such as quinidine or sotalol. The refractory period of atrial muscle is shorter than ventricular muscle. The specialized conduction tissue (His-Purkinje system) has a longer refractory period than ventricular muscle.

Excitability follows repolarization. When repolarization restores the negative resting membrane potential, the tissue again becomes excitable in atrial and ventricular myocytes but not immediately in AV nodal and SA nodal cells. In AV nodal and SA nodal cells, the refractory period outlasts the repolarization phase. This phenomena, unique to these cardiac cells, is known as *post-repolarization refractoriness.*

Automaticity (Rhythmicity)[9–11,18,38,41]

Normal Pulse Formation

There are two predominant sources of normal impulse formation: the SA node and the AV node. However, all cardiac tissue can exhibit spontaneous impulse formation. The SA node appears as a group of elongated, pale cells with single nuclei (Fig. 6–14) and the human node is approximately 25–30 mm long and 2–5 mm thick. It was first identified histologically by Keith and Flack in 1912. It is located in the posterior right atrial wall, at the junction of the right atrium and the superior vena cava. The SA node is less than 1.0 mm below the epicardial surface and is surrounded by an abundance of sympathetic and parasympathetic nerve endings.

The SA node consists of three types of cells: P (pacemaker), T (transitional), and Purkinje cells (Fig. 6–14). The P cells, located in a collagen matrix in the central region of the sinus node, usually have the highest degree of automaticity of all cardiac cells. Therefore, the SA node is the dominant cardiac pacemaker. Transitional cells surround the dominant P cells and are responsible for trans-

mitting the generated impulses. Purkinje cells located beyond the transitional cells at the junction of the SA node transmit impulses from the transitional cells to the atrial myocardium and to the internodal pathways (James fibers).

The primary point of automaticity in the SA node is the P cells. When the central area of the SA node is stimulated, a normal P wave on the electrocardiogram results, while stimulation of other areas of the atria and ventricles results in abnormal activation patterns evident on the electrocardiogram.

The principal blood supply of the sinus node is the SA nodal artery which courses to the center of the node. This originates from the first few centimeters of the right coronary artery in 55% and from the first few millimeters of the left circumflex artery in 45% of individuals.

The AV node is located on the posterior aspect of the right side of the interatrial septum near the coronary artery ostium. It is located in the triangle of Koch which represents structures bounded by the tendon of Todaro, the coronary sinus ostium, the tricuspid valve ring and the atrial septum. The chief blood supply of the AV node in 90% of individuals is a septal branch of the right coronary artery originating from the portion on the diaphragmatic surface. When the blood supply to the AV node arrives from the right coronary artery, the circulation is considered *right-dominant.* In 10% of individuals, the arterial supply is from the left circumflex. When this occurs, the coronary circulation is considered *left-dominant.* As opposed to the SA node, the AV node is deep and not affected by epi- or pericardial disease. However, acute block in the AV node readily follows posterior-inferior wall infarctions. The mechanism of this form of AV nodal block may be at least in part autonomically mediated (see below). Like to SA node, the AV node is richly innervated by the autonomic nervous system and is affected by changes in sympathetic and parasympathetic stimulation. The area of delay at the AV node is larger than the morphological node. Three functional zones with distinct electrophysiologic properties have been identified in the region of the AV node (James): 1. **AN region**—a transitional zone between the atrium and the remainder of the AV node; 2. **N region**—the middle portion of the AV node; 3. **N-H region**—the zone in which nodal fibers gradually merge with the bundle of His.

Mechanism of Automaticity[10,11,35–38,40–42]

Pacemaker Electrophysiology

Slow diastolic depolarization ("pacemaker activity") is the process underlying intrinsic rhythmicity of cardiac pacemaker cells. Pacemaker activity has been studied by micro-electrodes inserted into SA node and AV node cells (Fig. 6–15). Transmembrane action potentials from SA and AV nodal fibers show the following characteristics: lower resting potential, an unsteady resting potential with slow depolarization, a slowly rising action potential and a minimal electric potential overshoot. The resting potential normally depends on potassium concentrations and these fibers have an altered permeability to this ion. There is likely either a lowered intracellular content of

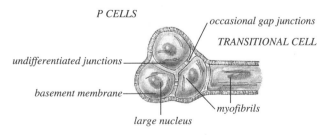

Fig. 6–14. The heart beat originates in the P (pacemaker) cells of the sinoatrial node. Note very low content of myofibrils. Transitional T cells, closer to normal myocardial cells in histology, help to conduct the impulse away from the P cells. Redrawn and modified from James, 1974 and from Opie.[5]

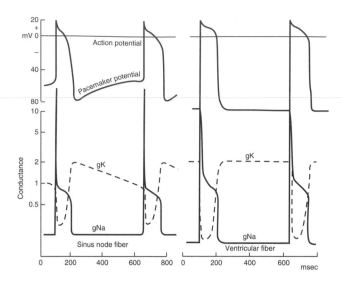

Fig. 6–15. Schematic diagram of estimated sodium and potassium conductances (gNa and gK, lower traces) underlying pacemaker potential and action potential (upper traces). A, Sinus node fiber; B, ventricular fiber from isolated rabbit heart. Note that "resting," diastolic, sodium conductance is higher in sinus node than in ventricular muscle fiber. Also in nodal fiber, potassium conductance declines throughout diastole but remains at constant level in ventricular fiber. Redrawn from Trautwein, Pharmacol Rev *15*:277, 1963.

K^+ or a greater inward Na^+ current. Compared to ventricular muscle fibers, SA nodal fibers do not show a steady level of resting potential during pacemaker diastole. Upon reaching a maximum negative electrical value at the end of repolarization, the transmembrane potential slowly increases until a threshold potential is reached. Then, there is a merging with and triggering of a developing action potential.

Other cardiac tissue can exhibit slow depolarization but the rate or rise of phase 4 is much slower and may not occur at all unless the rate of tissue activation is slow. Fibers of the His-Purkinje system and ventricular and atrial myocardium show very little slow depolarization under normal conditions.

Ionic Mechanism

Slow diastolic depolarization (phase 4) characteristic of pacemaker cell electrical activity results from alterations in sodium and potassium conductance (g_{Na+} g_{K+}) across the cell membrane (Fig. 6-15). Depolarization results from a change in the membrane potential away from the potassium equilibrium potential to the sodium equilibrium potential. When sodium permeability increases relative to potassium or if potassium permeability decreases, depolarization occurs.

In the SA node, a greater resting diastolic sodium permeability exists compared to atrial or ventricular muscular fibers and to other portions of the conduction system (Fig. 6-15). During diastole, potassium permeability (g_{K+}) decreases slowly allowing sodium permeability (g_{Na+}) to be more effective in determining the membrane potential.

As the membrane potential decreases slowly, the po-

tential reaches a threshold and sodium permeability increases suddenly reducing membrane potential to zero or above and produces an action potential.

With the sudden increase in sodium permeability at threshold potential, there is a precipitous decrease in potassium permeability accompanying the action potential. The combination of these changes result in the membrane potential approaching the sodium equilibrium potential with a reversal of polarity.

An equally rapid and sudden decrease in sodium permeability occurs (sodium conductance is "shut off"). This is accompanied by a rapid rise in potassium permeability as the sodium permeability returns to its resting diastolic potential. These changes bring the membrane potential toward the potassium equilibrium potential and produce the repolarization phase of the action potential.

Autonomic mediators alter the slope of slow depolarization. Vagal stimulation, or acetylcholine, decreases the rate at which the membrane potential approaches threshold levels. Sympathetic stimulation increases the rate at which the membrane potential approaches the threshold level.

Cardiac Conduction System (Dromotropic Property) (Fig. 6–5)

The cardiac conduction system[4,10,11,38,39,47] is myogenic in origin. The human heart beats at 3 weeks' gestation, although nerve elements are not present until 2 weeks later. Tissue in the great veins without neural elements exhibits rhythmical contraction.

Impulses originating in the SA node pass in the subendothelial layer of the atrium at a concentric speed of approximately 1.0 m/sec. There is spread by muscle fasciculi over three internodal paths to the AV node. A special branch (Bachman's bundle) passes to the left atrium.

The anterior intranodal pathway is the shortest path and is the most direct route of electrical spread to the upper AV node. The middle intranodal tract, described by Wenckebach, is a posterior tract, which passes behind the superior vena cava to the intraatrial septum and then to the top of the AV node. The third tract (Thorel's) passes from the posterior end of the SA node, along the crista terminalis to the intraatrial septum and then reaches the AV node at its upper margin. These pathways are a continuum of myocardial cells, with the SA node and, subsequently, with the Purkinje cells. The importance of these pathways in myocardial conduction to the AV node are disputed. The AV node has a long refractory period. Slowing of conduction of electrical impulses occurs here. The velocity of impulses in the Bundle of His and its branches is 3 to 5 m/sec. In contrast, conduction through the AV node is one tenth this speed.

Electrical impulses pass from the AV node through the His-bundle to two main bundle branches. Septal activation occurs first followed by left and then right ventricular activation. The right bundle continues as a single pathway. The left is more complex, is longer and is thinner and divides into two parts, namely the smaller anterior and larger posterior division. In addition, a small branch of the left bundle enters the septum between the two ventricles. Normally, there is nearly simultaneous arrival of electrical impulses through the bundles to the ventricular myocardium and nearly simultaneous contraction of both ventricles. Electrical activation however proceeds from the septum to the mid-endocardium then to the epicardium, base and apex of the ventricles. The endocardial surfaces, particularly of the septum and papillary muscles, are excited first and within 0.4 second.

Excitation-Contraction Coupling (Figs. 6–6, 6–7)[14,15,48–51]

Excitation-contraction coupling represents the ability of the heart to respond with a mechanical contraction when the muscle is activated electrically. Following electrical activation (depolarization) of atrial and ventricular myocytes, there is release of Ca^{+2} for the terminal cisternae of the sarcoplasmic reticulum. This process has been called *calcium-induced calcium release.* In effect, depolarization of the myocardium causes release of calcium in the sarcoplasmic reticulum that then, through an amplification mechanism, releases additional calcium. This additional calcium release, whose concentration is approximately 1000 times that present during the initial release, triggers the contractile response by repressing troponin. By doing so, the cross bridges between actin and myosin can form causing the myocardial fibers to shorten and therefore contact.

The interaction between the two contractile proteins and the two regulatory proteins is controlled by the intercellular calcium ion concentration. The process by which the intercellular calcium ion concentration changes in the muscle cell is called *excitation contraction coupling.* A generalized idea of the process has become understood: When a wave of depolarization crosses over the cell membrane, calcium is allowed to pass through the cell membrane and into the cell. This small increase in calcium concentration triggers the sarcoplasmic reticulum to release larger quantities of calcium. This sudden large rise in calcium concentration starts the contraction process described previously.

MECHANICAL PROPERTIES OF THE HEART

The ultimate action of the heart is to *pump* blood. Some of the important mechanical properties responsible for generating cardiac output are described[1-8,52-58] and depend on factors intrinsic and extrinsic to the myocardium (Table 6-3).

Stroke Volume

The quantity of blood expelled with each beat is the *stroke volume.* approximately 74 ml of blood are ejected with each beat during rest and approximately 120 ml during maximal effort. Cardiac reserve is the difference between output at maximum effort and output at rest. If the stroke volume is divided by the body surface area, the average stroke index is 43 ml at the age of 40 years. At 20 years, the stroke volume index averages 50 ml and decreases to 37 ml by age 80. There is a decrease in stroke index of 26% between the ages of 20 and 80 years and there is a 19% decrease in rate over the same interval. Al-

Table 6–3. Determinants of Mechanical Performance of the Heart (from Katz)

Factors intrinsic to the myocardium
    Number of active cross bridges (P_O)
    Rate of cross-bridge cycling (V_{max})
    Time courses of activation and inactivation
    Initial sarcomere length
External factors, most important of which is load

though each ventricle has a potential capacity of approximately 200 ml, it is not filled completely under normal conditions. A typical end diastolic volume is 160 to 180 ml. At end-systole, a there is a residual volume of 100 ml.

Ejection Fraction

Ejection phase indices can be used to assess contractile properties of the ventricles. The ejection fraction is the best and most reproducible parameter to measure in this regard. The ratio of the stroke volume (SV) to the end diastolic volume (EDV) is defined as the ejection fraction (EF).

$$EF = SV/EDV$$

This measurement provides an index of intrinsic myocardial function; it is less susceptible to loading conditions compared with the other measurements such as fractional shortening the ventricular myocardium, velocity of circumferential fiber shortening (V_{cf}).

When considering pumping function of the ventricle, it is important to assess segmental wall motion abnormalities. All walls of the ventricles contract uniformly. Segmental wall motion abnormalities suggest impairment of myocardial contractility.

Cardiac Output

The quantity of blood ejected over time by the heart is the *cardiac output.* The minute cardiac output is described as the liters of blood ejected from each ventricle every minute. Cardiac output is dependant on the heart rate and the stroke volume and is calculated to be the product of the heart rate (HR) and the stroke volume (SV).

$$Cardiac\ Output = SV \times HR$$

While the formula appears straightforward, measurements can be complicated and fraught with error. The major factor in increasing cardiac output is heart rate. The stroke volume and heart rate are influenced by many physiologic variables, especially loading conditions and the inotropic state of the heart. The effect of different heart rates on cardiac output is well illustrated by Rushmer (Fig. 6-16).

Cardiac Index

The cardiac output for a normal adult male of 160 lbs with a body surface area of 1.7 m^2 is 5.2 L/min. *Cardiac*

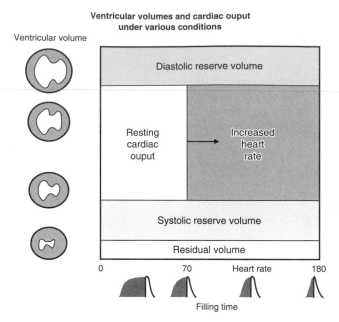

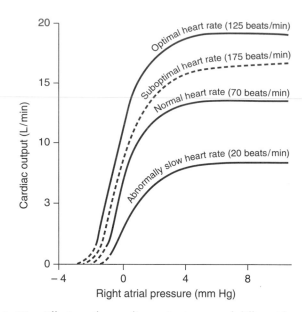

Fig. 6–16. The normal resting cardiac output, approximately 5 liters per minute (dark stippled area) is the product of stroke volume (approximately 70 cc.) and heart rate (approximately 70 beats per minute). The cardiac output can increase maximally to approximately six times the resting value (total crosshatched area) if heart rate and stroke volume increase simultaneously. Heart rate can increase to approximately 180 beats per minute, which would increase cardiac output two and a half times if the reduced filling time did not diminish stroke volume. Stroke volume can also increase through utilization of the systolic reserve and diastolic reserve volumes. The residual volume is the quantity of blood remaining in the ventricle after a maximal systolic ejection. Redrawn from Rushmer, R. F.: Cardiovascular Dynamics. Philadelphia, W.B. Saunders, 1970.

Fig. 6–17. Effect on the cardiac output curve of different heart rates, showing that when the heart is driven electrically, the output becomes optimal at approximately 125 beats per minute. Redrawn from Guyton, Circulatory Physiology, W.B. Saunders Co.

index is a way to normalize cardiac output to body surface area:

Cardiac Index $(L/min/m^2)$

$$= \text{Cardiac output } (L/min)/\text{Body Surface area } (m^2)$$

A formula to calculate body surface area (BSA) is:

BSA (m^2)

$$= 0.007184 \times \text{weight}^{0.425}(kg) \times \text{height}^{0.725}(cm)$$

When cardiac output is expressed in relation to the body surface area, cardiac index values range from 3.0 to 3.6 $L/min/m^2$. In proportion to weight, cardiac output averages 62 ml/kg/min. These are resting values as cardiac output can rise as much as 600% with exercise, is critically dependant on loading conditions on heart rate and on autonomic tone (Figs. 6–16 to 6–18).

Ventricular End-Diastolic Pressure

The diastolic pressure prior to the onset of ventricular contraction is related closely to the end diastolic myocardial fiber length and end-diastolic ventricular volume.

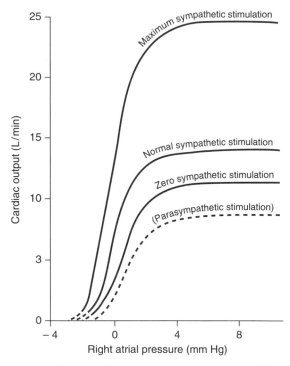

Fig. 6–18. Effect on the cardiac output curve of different degrees of sympathetic and parasympathetic stimulation. Redrawn from Guyton, Circulatory Physiology, W.B. Saunders Co.

This property, known as preload, is related to the compliance of the ventricle (Fig. 6–19).

Ventricular Stroke Work

External useful work performed by the ventricle per stroke is expressed in gram-meters, and is related to the potential energy imparted to the blood leaving the ventri-

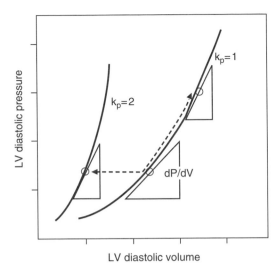

Fig. 6–19. The compliance reflects the relation between the increase in heart volume for a given increase in pressure (dP/dV). On the right, the heart has become stiffer because it operates at a high end-diastolic pressure. On the left, the compliance is decreased because the modulus of chamber stiffness (k_p) is increased. Such a true increase of stiffness can occur in acute myocardial infarction. Redrawn from Gaasch et al. Am J Cardiol 38:645, 1976.

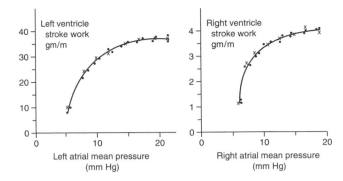

Fig. 6–20. Right and left ventricular function curves in a dog, depicting ventricular stroke work output as a function of the respective right and left mean atrial pressures. Curves reconstructed from data in Sarnoff, 1955. Redrawn from Guyton, Circulatory Physiology, W. B. Saunders Co.

cle during ejection. Stroke work increases with end-diastolic and therefore atrial pressures (Fig. 6–20). The values are obtained by multiplying the ventricular stroke volume and mean arterial pressure.

Duration of Systole

The interval between the onset and the cessation of ventricular ejection is determined from the arterial pressure-time curve. It is the time interval between the abrupt rise in arterial pressure and the dicrotic notch. It is often called the left ventricular ejection time.

Ventricular Stroke Power

Ventricular stroke power is the rate of doing work and is usually expressed in watts. The average rate of performing external useful stroke work by a ventricle is calculated by dividing stroke work in gram-centimeters by duration of systole in seconds.

Mean Ejection Rate

The average velocity of blood flow during systole, the ratio of stroke volume (ml per beat) to the duration of systole (seconds), is defined as mean ejection rate. When the size of the heart remains relatively constant, the mean ejection rate is indicative of the rate of change in ventricular volume, or mean shortening velocity of a ventricle.

Ventricular Contractile Force

A strain gauge sutured to the ventricle can be used to record contractile force. The maximal force of contraction is measured when the myocardial fiber is prevented from shortening by an external constraint.

Ventricular Function Curve (Fig. 6–20)

The ventricular function curve is the relationship between the ventricular end-diastolic pressure (fiber length, "preload", usually equivalent to mean atrial pressure) and external useful work performed by a ventricle (stroke work). The slope of the ventricular function curve indicates the rate of performing ventricular stroke work at a given preload level.

Contraction and Contractility

Inotropic Properties[31,59–66]

Contraction is the ability of heart muscle to shorten over time. The heart has been modelled as a series of elastic, viscous and contractile elements arranges in series and parallel (Fig. 6–21).

Contractility is the rate of the potential strength of myocardial contraction. It is independent of loading conditions. Contractility is increased when the potential rate of force development increases. This is a *positive inotropic* response. Contractility is decreased if the potential rate of increase in force development is impaired. This is a *negative inotropic* response.

Muscle fibers exhibit an "all or none" phenomenon (Bowditch), that is, when a threshold stimulus is applied, a complete response occurs. Otherwise, the muscle does not contract. Contractility depends on the end-diastolic ventricular pressure (preload), the arterial pressure (afterload), and the inotropic state of myocardium (force-velocity relationships).

Mechanism of Contraction[67–74]

Myocardial muscle cells contract secondary to the interaction of two proteins, that have a fixed position within the myocardial cell (Figs. 6–2, 6–7). During contraction, these contractile proteins, named actin and myosin, slide over one another, causing the cell to shorten. Also involved, are two regulatory proteins, troponin and tropomyosin, that interact with the actin and myosin. Regulation of the sliding process is complex, but the major factor controlling contraction is the intercellular concentration of calcium ions.

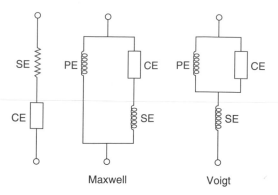

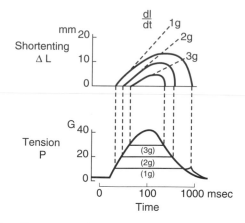

Fig. 6–21. Hill's original two-element model for skeletal muscle (left) consists of a contractile element (CE) and a series elastic element (SE). Cardiac muscle has significant resting tension (Table 3.2). Since the CE is assumed to be freely extensible at rest, the parallel elastic element (PE) has been added to account for this resting tension. The PE may be in series with the SE (Voigt model) or in parallel with the SE (Maxwell model). Redrawn from Smith, N. T.: Myocardial Function and Anaesthesia. In Prys-Roberts, C. (ed.): The Circulation in Anaesthesia, Oxford, Blackwell Scientific Publications, 1980, pp 69.

Fig. 6–22. Shortening of the muscle (Δ L) and developed tension (P) are shown as functions of time after electrical stimulation with three different afterload levels. The initial slope (dl/dt) of the time-shortening curve is velocity of shortening. Redrawn from Etsten after Sonnenblick.

Raising the intercellular calcium ion concentration, will cause the calcium ions to bind on sites of the troponin protein. The troponin protein undergoes a change in its configuration secondary to the binding of the calcium. This configuration change exposes active sites on the contractile protein actin. Cross bridges alternately will form and then break between the actin and myosin proteins at these active sites, with the end result being the sliding movement of the proteins over one another. The result is that the interaction between the two contractile proteins and the two regulatory proteins is controlled by the intercellular calcium ion concentration.

The Force-Velocity Relationship[67–75]

This is the relationship between the initial maximum velocity of muscle shortening and developed force. The unique characteristic is that the force developed by the contractile components of the heart, depends upon its own state of motion. This was first demonstrated in skeletal muscle but later, a similar force-velocity relationship in cat papillary muscle.

With different total loads against which a muscle contracts, shortening of the muscle as related to time, and tension of the muscle as related to time, produces different curves of performance (Fig. 6–22).

The slope (the change in length (1) over time, dl/dt) of the time-shortening curve is the velocity of shortening. The peak height of the time-shortening curve is the net shortening of the muscle. When afterload is increased, there is a decrease in the shortening of the fibers, in the shortening velocity, and an increase in the maximum tension or amplitude of contraction. When the load (force) is related to velocity of shortening, a graph of force-velocity relationship may be obtained and results in a rectangular hyperbolic curve (Fig. 6–23). The velocity of shortening becomes the maximum value (V_{max}) when the muscle is carrying no load. When the load is so great that the mus-

cle cannot shorten at all, the velocity of shortening becomes zero and isometric tension (P_o) is obtained.

Power and work may be calculated from data obtained by the force-velocity curve. *Power* is a function of velocity of shortening and force (shaded and crosshatched areas in Figure 6–23 show the difference in power as related to two different force-velocity curves). *Work* performed by the heart muscle may be obtained by either integrating the power with respect to the time or multiplying stroke volume by mean arterial pressure (force). When the curve shifts from M to M as shown in Figure 6–23, a new force-velocity curve is identified as a negative inotropic effect. Conversely, when the curve shifts from M' to M, this indicates a positive inotropic effect.

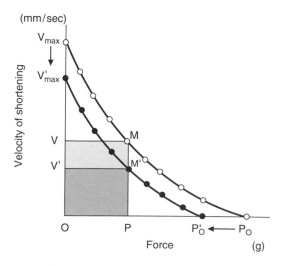

Fig. 6–23. Alteration of force-velocity relationship. Ordinate: Velocity of shortening; Abscissa: Total load or force (preload plus afterload); V max: Maximal velocity of shortening; Po: Isometric tension. Power performed by the muscle is demonstrated by the shaded rectangular area (MPOV). The crosshatched area (M'POV') represents decreased power resulting from the shift of the curve to the left (negative inotropism). Redrawn from Etsten.[2]

Both work and power are zero at either end of the curve (V_{max} and P_o).

Cardiac muscle, therefore, may alter the power and work from any given initial fiber length (preload) and any given loading condition (afterload) simply by shifting the force-velocity curve.

DETERMINANTS OF WORK (TABLE 6–4)[76–81]

Preload

The force applied to ventricular muscle in diastole just before contraction is called *preload*. It is determined by venous return and end-diastolic compliance. The ventricular end-diastolic and atrial pressures correlate closely with the end-diastolic fiber length. The *pulmonary capillary wedge pressure* measurement made by the Swan-Ganz catheter usually correlates with left atrial mean pressure and also the left ventricular filling pressure. These represent left ventricular preload. End-diastolic ventricular blood volume also correlates with preload.

Fiber length prior to systolic contraction will influence stroke volume. Generally the greater the fiber length, the greater the strength of contraction and the greater the developed pressure. This phenomena is the Frank-Starling law of the heart. This relationship is illustrated in Figure 6-24.

With excessive myocardial stretch (from preload), the strength of contraction and stroke volume decrease (or not change). This "descending limb of the Starling curve" may be related to sarcomere stretch and loss of effective cross bridge linkages, however, there is evidence against this. The point at which this occurs varies with the disease state and myocardial contractility.

Venous Return[7,54,82]

Guyton and others have emphasized the importance of the venous return to the heart on the cardiac output. As systemic venous return increases, the cardiac output increases until a maximal value is achieved based on the Frank-Starling relationship. Generally, the greater is the filling of the ventricle the greater is the stroke volume.

Venous return is determined by: 1. Ventricular force. A residual pressure from the arterial side exists in the veins. This "force from behind", or impelling force, pushes blood back to the heart. It represents a pressure gradient from the systemic circulation to the right atrium. 2. Suction. This "force from the front" represents the forward pull from atrial and ventricular diastole (a back pressure also exists at time of atrial and ventricular systole, but is of shorter duration than diastole). 3. Extramural factors: (a) skeletal muscle tone, support of veins, and venous massage, (b) containing effect of all tissues, (c) gravity. 4. Venous tone. 5. Unidirectional venous valves. 6. Thoracic respiratory pump.

Afterload

Afterload is the pressure that the ventricles must exceed to eject blood. The added force required to overcome aortic and pulmonary artery pressure during ventricular contraction in systole (during fiber shortening) is *afterload*. The ventricles encounter this dynamic increase

Table 6–4. Determinants of the Work of the Heart

Diastolic
  Preload: systemic and pulmonary venous return
  Lusitropic State: relaxation
  Compliance: diastolic pressure-volume relation

Systolic
  Afterload: systemic and pulmonary vascular impedance
  Inotropic State: end-systolic pressure-volume relation

Heart Rate
  A major factor in the work of the heart
  All diastolic and systolic determinants are affected

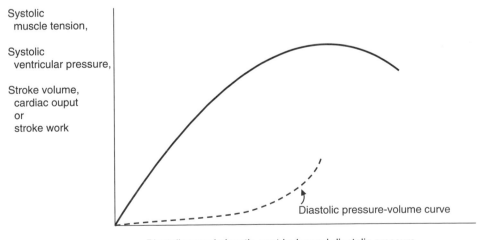

Fig. 6–24. Diagrammatic representation of the Frank-Starling type curves of cardiac function. The dashed curve represents a diastolic pressure-volume curve relating end-diastolic pressure on the ordinate to end-diastolic volume or muscle length on the abscissa. Redrawn and modified from Spann and Mason, Concepts of Cardiovascular Disease *39*:79, 1970.

Table 6–5. Normal Physiologic Values

Systemic artery pressure	90–140/60–90 mm Hg
Pulmonary artery pressure	15–30/4–12 mm Hg
Cardiac (output) index	2.6–4.2 liters/minute/m²
Pulmonary vascular resistance	20–130 dynes-sec-cm⁻⁵
Systemic vascular resistance	700–1600 dynes-sec-cm⁻⁵
Pulmonary capillary wedge (left atrial) pressure (mean)	2–12 mm Hg
Right atrial pressure	2–8 mm Hg
Left ventricular pressure	90–140/3–12 mm Hg
Right ventricular pressure	15–30/2–8 mm Hg
Stroke (volume) index	30–65 ml/beat/m²
MVO₂	110–150 L/min/m²
Left ventricular stroke work index	30–90 gram-meters/m²
Left ventricular minute work index	1.8–6.6 Kg-meters/m²/min

in aortic or pulmonary artery resistance ("impedance") at the onset of and throughout ventricular contraction. The higher the afterload, the more energy the heart must use to raise the intraventricular pressure. Hence, less energy is available to eject ventricular blood.

Systemic arterial systolic pressure reflects left ventricular systolic pressures and therefore left ventricular afterload. The pulmonary arterial pressure reflects right ventricular systolic pressure and therefore right ventricular afterload (Table 6-5).

Vascular Resistance (Impedance)

Vascular impedance is the continuously changing resistance present in the two circulatory beds: the pulmonary and the systemic circulation. *Resistance* is the mean of the impedance values throughout systole. The resistance to blood flow on the arterial (systemic) side of the circulation is called *the systemic vascular resistance (SVR)*. Calculation of this measurement is important since it provides an indicator for the systemic afterload. SVR can be derived from Ohm's law. This law states that flow is proportional to the change in pressure within the system divided by the resistance. If the equation is solved for the resistance, the resistance becomes proportional to the change in pressure divided by flow.

$$Resistance = (Change\ in\ Pressure/Flow) \times Constant$$

In the cardiovascular system, flow is cardiac output (CO). The change in pressure depends on which resistance is being determined. For systemic vascular resistance (SVR), the change in pressure is the mean arterial pressure (MAP, the pressure going into the circuit) minus the central venous pressure (CVP, the pressure coming out of the circuit). The constant for the equation is 80.

$$SVR = \{(MAP - CVP)/CO\} \times 80$$

Resistance in the pulmonary arterial circuit, the *pulmonary artery resistance (PVR)*, the right ventricular afterload can be calculated similarly. The same cardiac out-

put and constant pertains to this calculation, but the calculation requires different pressure measurements. The pressure entering the circuit is the mean pulmonary artery pressure (PAP) and the pressure leaving the circuit is the pulmonary venous pressure. The pulmonary venous pressure is difficult to measure, so use an estimate of the pulmonary venous pressure, the pulmonary artery wedge pressure (PCWP) is used. The equation becomes:

$$PVR = \{(PAP - PCWP)/CO\} \times 80$$

Cardiac Function Curves

Pressure-Volume Relationships-The Frank-Starling Law

The Frank-Starling law[25,26,31,33,59,83-91] states that the strength of ventricular contraction depends on the initial fiber length (Fig. 6–24). Fiber length is dependent on the end-diastolic volume. Ventricular diastolic volume can be determined but there can be difficulty in measuring individual ventricular volumes accurately. As a practical substitute for ventricular volumes, based on previously described pressure-volume relationships, filling pressures may be used. Starling's law may then be restated: The strength with which ventricles contract is a function of the "filling" (end-diastolic) pressure. In this way, systolic function is related to is a function of diastolic function.

Modified Cardiac Function Curves

There is a consistent relationship between atrial pressure and ventricular stroke work. Mean right atrial pressure can be plotted against right ventricular stroke work; and left atrial pressure can be plotted against left ventricular stroke work. Such ventricular function curves are modified Starling curves. Ventricular stroke work and output are functions of mean right and left atrial pressure (Fig. 6–20).

Coronary artery blood flow influences ventricular function. When mean coronary artery blood flow is plot against left ventricular function or work, a direct quantitative relationship is apparent. When impaired coronary artery blood flow is present, ventricular function is depressed and myocardial failure can develop. Failure can be reversed by increasing coronary flow.

Guyton has also shown that the ventricular function curves can be correlated to a cardiac output curve provided the systemic resistance is known. The ability of a heart to pump blood can be expressed by such cardiac output curves. In these curves cardiac output is depicted as a function of mean atrial pressure.

Relaxation (Lusitropic Property)

Relaxation[92-97] occurs when the contractile proteins slide back over one another so that the original cellular length is restored. Following contraction, there is re-uptake of Ca^{+2} by the sarcoplasmic reticulum through a protein embedded in the membrane. This protein, phospholamban, has a high affinity for calcium and causes active transport of Ca^{+2} from the cell to the sarcoplasmic reticulum. *Lusitropy* is the diastolic property describing the ability of the heart to relax.

Compliance-Diastolic Pressure–Volume Relationships

Diastolic *compliance*[32-34,95,96,98-104] is defined as the distensibility of the heart throughout diastole (Fig. 6–19). A highly compliant ventricle con accept blood more readily in diastole whereas an incompliant ventricle will only fill at higher pressures. Compliance is now known to be an important contributor to overall cardiac function. For any given diastolic ventricular volume, there is a ventricular pressure. The pressure-volume relationship (i.e., compliance) varies throughout diastole. By the end-diastole, the ventricles are maximally filled with blood and the pressure rises. Compliance is partially due to the passive and active visco-elastic priorities of the heart muscle and partially due to the degree of active relaxation. There is a relationship of relaxation to diastolic compliance but compliance is also influenced by factors which do not necessarily change the ability of the heart to relax. Diastolic compliance is decreased by ventricular hypertrophy, ischemia, restrictive disease and heart failure as is relaxation; constriction may decrease ventricular compliance without influencing relaxation. Catecholamines generally increase compliance and facilitate relaxation.

MEDIATORS OF MECHANICAL AND ELECTRICAL CARDIAC PERFORMANCE[105-112]

Chemical Mediators

Various substances exert a direct effect on cardiac excitability. Alterations in excitability are the direct result of changes in the critical level of transmembrane (threshold) potential. Ringer, as early as 1882, observed the effects of various ions on excitability. Cardiac muscle, in physiological sodium chloride solution, is excitable initially but contractions eventually become weak and stop. Adding calcium chloride to the solution will cause heart muscle to contract strongly, while potassium chloride and magnesium sulfate solutions will result in prompt muscle relaxation. When all sodium, potassium and calcium salts are present, the muscle contracts normally and vigorously for prolonged periods.

Hydrogen Ion

pH Effect

Changing the pH can alter excitability and contractility. Ringer observed that an isolated, perfused heart lost its contractility while beating in Ringer's solution. Contractility could be restored by sodium bicarbonate. A high pH (alkalosis) causes more rapid initiation of excitation, accelerated cardiac conduction and increased excitability. Alkalies (high pH) increase contractility and excitability, similar to Ca^{+2}.

A low pH (acidosis) causes cardiac muscle to stop beating (to become asystolic), similar to the effect of high K^+. Excitability and contractility are depressed. Small increases in lactic acid may impair contractility; skeletal muscle requires a concentration a lactic acid concentration 32 times greater to impair contractility.

Carbon Dioxide Effect

Carbon dioxide initially enhances excitability but ultimately causes acidosis and impairs cardiac excitability. Small increases in carbon dioxide slow the heart rate and increase vagal tone. Large increases in carbon dioxide depress cardiac conduction and contractility largely by producing an uncompensated acidosis. At a pH of 7.0, AV block can occur. Often associated with hypercarbia and acidosis, hypoxemia tends to accelerate heart rate.

Calcium Ion

The extracellular calcium ion changes the threshold potential and has a pronounced limiting effect on inward sodium flux during depolarization. It has a marked positive inotropic effect. Calcium can limit the occurrence and magnitude of depolarization; a high calcium level lowers excitability, causes an action potential of lower magnitude and permits easier repolarization. At very high levels there is decreased excitability and cardiac arrest may occur. Unrestricted contracture can result. A low concentration of calcium enhances excitability and may result in appearance of multiple pacemakers, especially in Purkinje fibers.

That all cardiac tissue is influenced by calcium in a similar qualitative manner is evident. However, there are quantitative dissimilarities. Atrial muscle is more sensitive to changes in calcium than the Purkinje fibers and the ventricular (papillary) muscle in that order. Ventricular muscle and Purkinje fibers maintain normal excitability in the presence of moderately elevated calcium levels whereas atrial muscle may show marked limitation of depolarization and require an intense stimulus to respond. As concentrations of calcium increase, Purkinje fibers become unexcitable.

Studies on anesthetized subjects (halothane-oxygen) reveal that a calcium infusion ($CaCl_2$ solution) improves cardiac performance, even in the presence of a negative inotropic anesthetic drug (halothane). The cardiac index, left ventricular work index, and stroke index can increase; the heart rate, peripheral vascular resistance decrease. Calcium administration exerts this effect by increasing the intracellular calcium availability for actinomycin interaction.

Potassium Ion

Increasing extracellular potassium ion concentrations cause progressive decrease in transmembrane potential. Moderate lowering of extracellular K^+ mildly increases resting membrane potential but marked lowering produces depolarization of ventricular muscle and Purkinje fibers.

The relationship between calcium and potassium ions on transmembrane potentials is important. Calcium and potassium ions are antagonistic: A low calcium ion concentration prevents the depolarizing effect of low potassium while high calcium ion concentration decreases the loss of resting potential produced by potassium excess.

Magnesium Ion

Magnesium ions counteract the actions of calcium. An excess of magnesium will block and a deficiency will potentiate the action of calcium. It moderates the movement of calcium across and within the cell membrane of cardiac and vascular tissues. It is a cofactor of the enzyme systems involved in the phosphate transfer reaction.

Magnesium can block directly calcium influx during slow current activity in neural axons and at motor nerve endings. Within the myocardium, magnesium: 1) inhibits the release of calcium from the sarcoplasmic reticulum; 2) drives extracellular calcium into the sarcoplasmic reticulum; 3) competes with calcium at some binding sites; 4) inhibits calcium ion increase in muscle tension and 5) reduces the development of muscle tension directly. Magnesium depresses myocardial contractility through its interaction with calcium at the sarcolemma. The normal plasma levels of magnesium range from 2.0–2.5 mEq/L. Even when the levels are not low, magnesium administration may help control ventricular tachycardias and prevent death following myocardial infarction.

Severe magnesium deficiency (1.10 mEq/L or less), however, is associated with both supraventricular and ventricular tachycardias. In magnesium deficiency, there is a loss of cellular potassium with no change in sodium and an increase in calcium. Several disease entities are associated with magnesium deficiency: toxemic cardiomyopathy, endomyocardial fibrosis of malnutrition. Vasospasm of many organs including the placenta can occur. When present, magnesium deficiency can be treated with 1–8 grams of magnesium sulfate given slowly intravenously.

Adenosine

Adenosine, a metabolite of ATP, can have a potent effect on AV conduction and on AV nodal and SA nodal automaticity. When administered intravenously, adenosine can interrupt conduction in the AV node and prevent SA node activation.

Indirect Mediators

In contrast to direct chemical effects, indirect and reflex effects can have an opposite effect. Anoxia that causes hypoxemia is frequently accompanied by acidosis and accelerates the heart rate. This reflex is not initiated through the chemoreceptors; it is initiated through peripheral vasodilatation and baroreceptors. High oxygen tension reduces cardiac rate and cardiac output.

Asphyxia (combined elevated carbon dioxide tension and lowered oxygen values), causes initially impairs excitability but this is followed by tachycardia.

Thyroxine and adrenaline can increase the heart rate while acetylcholine decreases the rate.

NEURAL INFLUENCES[113–125]

Cardiac muscle can maintain rhythmic contractions automatically; nevertheless, such actions are responsive to extrinsic neural influences.

Central Mechanisms

Stimulation of the anterior temporal lobe, the cingulate gyrus, and orbital surface of the frontal lobe will produce changes in rhythm mediated through the hypothalamus. A cardio-inhibitory center is located in the dorsal nucleus of the tenth (X) cranial nerve in the medulla.

Autonomic Mechanisms

Cardiac rate and rhythm are modulated by the mutually antagonistic influences of the sympathetic and parasympathetic nervous systems. Classical studies hold that the atrium and the nodal system are innervated by both the sympathetic and parasympathetic systems while the ventricles are innervated chiefly by the sympathetic nerves. However more recent data demonstrates that the parasympathetic nervous system also supplies the ventricles and may influence contractility. When both sympathetic and parasympathetic nervous systems are activated simultaneously, the vagal influences predominate. This effect is known as *accentuated antagonism.*

Parasympathetic Nervous System

The vagus nerve can have a profound and continuous influence on the heart. This influence, called vagal tone, acts as a "brake" mechanism. Stimulation of the vagus nerve suppresses contractility in all cardiac chambers, lengthens diastole and stops the heart in a state of relaxation. All properties and actions of the heart are depressed. The heart rate (the SA node) slows. The force of contraction decreases, especially in the atria. Electrical conduction is slowed, especially in the AV node. Excitability decreases.

Right vagal stimulation causes the greatest slowing of the heart particularly by impairing SA nodal automaticity. Less prominent slowing of the SA node will also occur on stimulation of the left vagus. The right vagus terminates mainly in ganglion cells near the SA node while the left vagus terminates mainly in the AV node. AV nodal conduction block can also occur with vagal stimulation.

Stimulation of the vagus shortens the refractory period of the atria, but there is no pronounced direct effect on the ventricular refractory period. Continuous stimulation also results in an escape phenomena. This is often manifested by sudden increase in amplitude of contraction. Vagal effects are abolished by anticholinergic agents such as atropine. Vagal nerve block to prevent cardio-circulatory depression from surgery has been advocated and used with good results during pulmonary hilar dissection.

Sympathetic Nervous System

The sympathetic nervous system exerts an excitatory influence on heart activity. The sympathetic fibers influence the atria and the ventricles. All properties and actions of the heart are augmented: 1. The heart rate is increased; 2. Systole is shortened (more than diastole); 3. Myocardial contraction is stronger; 4. The coronary arteries dilate; 5. Conduction is enhanced; 6. Excitability and automaticity are increased; 7. The refractory periods are shortened.

There is apparently a sympathetic cardioaccelerator center located in the posterior hypothalamus. Impulses from this region influence cells in the antero-lateral column of the spinal cord from where sympathetic fibers arise. These fibers are preganglionic in type and emerge at thoracic levels one through five. These synapse at thoracic sympathetic ganglia and at superior, middle and inferior cervical ganglia. From these ganglia, postganglionic fibers pass to the heart.

Specific Peripheral Neural Reflexes That Affect the Heart (Table 6–6)

Various cardiac reflexes are influenced by the nervous elements described. The afferents involved influence the cardiac centers where integration occurs causing alteration in efferent vagal output. Among specific reflexes modifying cardiac function are:

---

the oculo-cardiac reflex, the nasal branch reflex of the (V) fifth cranial nerve, the pressorceptor reflex (aortic and carotid depressor reflexes). These reflexes work through the vagal efferents slow the heart rate and cause peripheral vasodilatation. They act as a homeostatic mechanism to maintain the blood pressure. The pulse rate varies inversely with blood pressure during these reflexes. This inverse relationship is known as Marey's law.

With carotid sinus stimulation alone, the usual response is to increase cardiac output by 10–15%. If the aortic pressoreceptors are also stimulated, a 25% increase in cardiac output may be expected. The Bainbridge Reflex is an increase in heart rate due to an increase in venous return. This is brought about by the stimulation of vagal afferent receptors beneath the endothelium in the walls of the great veins which subsequently initiates a response over the cardio-accelerator nerve. Distention of the right atrium is the effective stimulus.

Another specific important neural reflex is the somatic nerve reflex. Pain causes heart rate acceleration and elevated blood pressure by augmenting sympathetic stimulation. Pulmonary afferent stimulation slows the heart rate.

The central nervous system ischemic reflex (the Cushing Reflex) causes a powerful sympathetic and vagal discharge due to central nervous system ischemia caused by increasing intracranial pressure. The blood pressure can increase and sinus bradycardia then occurs.

The abdominal compression reflex occurs when pressure in the thoracic vessels falls to low levels. A reflex is elicited which causes the abdominal muscles to tighten. Abdominal contracture can increase the mean systemic pressure by 100% by aiding venous return.

Specific Local Reflexes from the Heart and Lungs (Table 6-7)

Reflexes specific to heart and lung tissue receptors are as follows.

Right Atrial Reflex

Receptors have been found in the walls of the right atrium that respond to pressure. Afferent nerve fibers carry impulses from these points over the vagus and produce an efferent vagal response. The receptors are stimulated by increased pressure at the right atrium and produce bradycardia and hypotension. Atropine abolishes the bradycardia but not the hypotension.

This reflex contrasts to the Bainbridge reflex which was shown originally in the anesthetized dog to be the opposite response, i.e., a tachycardiac response to the intravenous administration of fluids increased venous return.

Pulmonary Depressor Reflex

Elevation of the pressure in the pulmonary artery can produce a decrease in systemic blood pressure and can cause bradycardia. Chemoreceptors may exist in pulmonary veins which causes this depressor response. The vagus nerve carries the impulses.

Left Ventricular Pressoreceptor Reflex

Elevation of left ventricular pressure causes bradycardia and marked peripheral vasodilatation manifest as systemic hypotension. The effect is abolished by vagal section by anticholinergic drugs or by inhibition of the initial elevation of left ventricular pressure by beta adrenergic blockade.

The aortic pressoreceptors are known to extend into the left side of the heart. Since the receptors are similar in each situation these may be the same reflex.

The Bezold-Jarisch Reflex (Coronary Chemoreflex)

Strong vagal efferent responses occur when vagal afferents located at the posterior portion of the left ventricle

---

Table 6–6. Specific Neural Reflexes Affecting the Heart

Oculo-cardiac reflex
Nasal branch reflex of the (V) fifth nerve
Pressoreceptor reflex (Aortic and Carotid Depressor Reflexes)
Bainbridge reflex
Somatic nerve reflex
Pulmonary afferent reflex
Central nervous system ischemic reflex (the Cushing Reflex)
Abdominal compression reflex

Table 6–7. Specific Reflexes from the Heart (and Lungs)

Right atrial reflex
Pulmonary depressor reflex
Left ventricular pressoreceptor reflex
Bezold-Jarisch reflex (coronary chemoreflex)
Left atrial (and pulmonary vein) vagal receptors

near termination of the left circumflex and right coronary arteries become stimulated. This reflex induces sinus bradycardia and peripheral vasodilation causing systemic hypotension.

Left Atrial (and Pulmonary Vein) Vagal Receptors

These sensory endings respond to pulmonary congestion. The resultant effect is a marked diuresis that follows. This was shown first during negative pressure breathing. This effect is felt to be mediated by a peptide, atrial natriuretic peptide, which possess natriuretic, vasorelaxant and aldosterone-inhibiting properties.[126-128] Its release is regulated by both right and left atrial pressure elevation.

MYOCARDIAL METABOLISM[80,81,129-137]

Excitation, contraction, and relaxation are dependent on proper metabolic processes. The human heart is an obligate aerobic organ that uses adenosine triphosphate (ATP) most efficiently for fuel to maintain cellular integrity and to contract effectively. The ATP generated for aerobic metabolism comes from substances taken from the blood. As anaerobic metabolism (using glycolytic pathways) in the heart is limited, the heart becomes reliant on the coronary artery blood supply for oxygen and fuel.

All the energy for cardiac function must come from oxidation of various substrates (glucose, lactate, pyruvate, esterified and non-esterified fatty acids, and, to some extent, acetate, ketone bodies and amino acids). Without glucose, free fatty acids can be used if ample oxygen is available. Increased nutritional and energy demands are met by increasing coronary blood flow that occurs with increasing coronary vasodilatation. A large coronary artery flow reserve can increase blood flow by over 5 times resting values. The mechanisms for this are complex but are, in part, related to ischemic metabolites, such as adenosine and changes in adrenergic tone. A highly simplified mechanism for such increased coronary artery blood flow is: Increased myocardial work that causes more metabolic breakdown products leading to vasodilation that evokes greater blood flow.

Oxygen Consumption

The human heart is considered to be an aerobic organ with little or no anaerobic capability; no oxygen debt can be incurred. All energy for cardiac function must come from oxidation of various substances available immediately to the heart. The utilization of these substances (glucose, lactate, pyruvate, esterified and non-esterified fatty acids, and to some extent, acetate, ketone bodies and amino acids) is influenced by the concentration of the substances in arterial blood and by the state of nutrition. In the absence of glucose, free fatty acids are used preferentially.

The total amount of oxygen that the heart consumes, *myocardial oxygen consumption* ($M\dot{V}O_2$), varies with several physiological factors (Table 6-8). $M\dot{V}O_2$ is a measure of the myocardial energy requirements of the heart but it is also related to the efficiency of energy utiliza-

Table 6–8. Determinants of Oxygen Consumption

Major determinants
  Myocardial wall stress (tension)
    Preload and isometric contraction: 40% (internal work).
    Afterload and isotonic contraction: 20% (external work).
  Contractile state and velocity of contraction
    Maximum velocity of contraction: 20%.
    Shortening against a load (Fenn effect): 5%.
  Heart Rate
    Influences the above.
    Most critical determinate of MVO_2.

Minor determinants
  Depolarization—0.5% of total energy consumed by heart.
  Activation-deactivation energy: 1%.
  Basal (non-contracting) metabolism: 20%.
  Direct metabolic effect of catecholamines: variable

tion. While normal values for oxygen consumption by left ventricular muscle are approximately 8.0 ml to 15 ml/min/100 g of tissue during active beating, mechanical efficiency of the heart is only approximately 20%. This includes the amount needed for basal cellular metabolism and cell integrity.

Basal Oxygen Consumption

The total metabolism of the arrested non-contracting heart (basal oxygen consumption) requires an average of 2.3 ml oxygen/min/100 g tissue; the range is 1-4 ml/min/100 g tissue. This basal oxygen consumption (non-contracting) is small and covers the needs for maintenance of cell integrity (10%) and of the electrophysiologic processes at the cell membrane (8-10%). The resting oxygen consumption of cardiac tissue is thus roughly 10-20% of that of the contracting organ on an equal time basis.

Total oxygen consumption can be calculated from the product of the (arterial oxygen content—coronary sinus oxygen content difference) multiplied by (the coronary blood flow) and expressed in milliliters of oxygen consumed per 100 g tissue per minute during active beating at rest (flow 8-15 ml/100 g tissue/min). The MVO_2 is expressed as milliliters of oxygen consumed per gram of cardiac tissue per minute.

Because the normal cardiac A-V O_2 difference is high (approximately 11.5 volumes%) and maximal (oxygen availability is determined by coronary flow), all of the increased oxygen demands from increased work must be met by an increase in coronary blood flow. The heart cannot incur and sustain an oxygen debt.

There must be a continuous source of oxygen. Cardiac muscle can accumulate only an extremely small oxygen debt. The oxygen requirement is 3.24 ml/g/hr and this high oxygen need is further seen by the observation that coronary venous blood contains far less oxygen than systemic venous blood. It is characteristically very dark and contains only 4 to 6 volumes % oxygen. There is almost complete oxygen extraction from blood flowing through cardiac muscle.

When coronary artery blood flow stops, myocardial

contraction stops almost immediately. However, recent data indicates that myocardium does not die immediately; myocardium can remain *stunned* for hours or days with subsequent return of normal function. This can occur despite several hours of impaired metabolism. *Hibernation* is a related phenomenon that occurs when there is compromised delivery of nutrients and oxygen to myocardium chronically. After return of impaired myocardial blood flow, metabolic properties can return to the muscle with subsequent resumption in muscle contraction.

Major Determinants[129–137]

Myocardial Work

Oxygen consumption of the contracting heart is related directly to the total amount of work performed. Left ventricular stroke work (LVSW) is the product of the developed pressure (the difference of the mean of the LV systolic and diastolic pressures) and stroke volume (SV).

$$LVSW \propto LV \text{ developed pressure} \times SV$$

Although this formula represents one of the major determinants of $M\dot{V}O_2$, it does not represent total $M\dot{V}O_2$ accurately. Also, minute LVSW has a large normal ranges (from 1.5–7.0 kg/meter) and varies with the cardiac output.

When venous input to the heart is enhanced or peripheral resistance is increased, the heart must do more work but there is also increased cardiac output. Such work is accomplished by greater stretching of the muscle fibers with development of increased tension during contraction. Oxygen consumption increases. These observations have been incorporated in Starling's law of the heart. This law states that the energy for contraction is a function of fiber length: greater filling increases fiber length and the force of contraction.

Heart rate, wall stress, and the contractile state all influence the extent the heart must work; these are the major determinants of MVO_2.

Heart Rate

Myocardial contractile proteins use energy each time they contract. The faster the heart contracts, the more energy and, therefore, the more oxygen is required.

Wall Stress[81]

The forces applied against the myocardium is known as *wall stress* (or tension, in a one dimensional model). As wall stress increases, energy need is increased and oxygen consumption rises. The two forces responsible for wall stress on heart muscle are called *preload* and *afterload*. The stretch on the ventricle before contraction is the preload (the ventricular end-diastolic volume) and the pressure against which the ventricle must contract is the afterload (generated left ventricular systolic pressure). The wall stress developed during isometric contraction demands a great amount of energy. The largest portion of the oxygen consumed is in this aspect of the cardiac cycle.

Two indirect indices of $M\dot{V}O_2$ reflecting wall stress can be calculated easily. These are the *Rate-Pressure Product (RPP)* and *the Tension-Time Index (TTI)*. Rhode showed that MVO_2 varies directly with the product of developed systolic pressure (SP) and heart rate (HR):

$$MVO_2 \propto RPP = SP \times HR$$

This calculation is still useful as it is easily calculated. The TTI may be more accurate an indicator of MVO_2. A relation exists between "tension set-up on contraction and the metabolism of contracting tissue". Developed wall tension (or more precisely, stress) is a fundamental determinant of MVO_2 and is related linearly. Maintenance of wall stress (in contrast to development of wall stress) is a minor determinant of oxygen utilization. A simple relationship expresses MVO_2 conveniently and accurately in an empiric formula called the Tension-Time Index:

$$MVO_2 \propto TTI = HR \times SP \times LVET$$

(left ventricular ejection time)

A more definitive and accurate determination of myocardial energy use (The Law of LaPlace) indicates that developed myocardial stress is related directly to the radius of the ventricular cavity and to the intraventricular pressure and is related indirectly to the ventricular wall thickness.

LAW OF LAPLACE

WALL STRESS = VENTRICULAR PRESSURE

$\times$ RADIUS/2 $\times$ WALL THICKNESS

Contractility

Raising the speed and force of contraction (i.e., increasing myocardial contractility) for any given degree of wall stress will increase the amount of energy needed for contraction and consequently will increase the MVO_2.

Velocity of Contraction (V_{max})

The maximum velocity of contraction of left ventricular myocardial muscle (V_{max}) is the peak rate of left ventricular ejection. Change in the velocity of contraction reflects the contractile state of the heart. Shortening the duration of ventricular ejection increases MVO_2 when it occurs with an increased velocity of ejection.

Muscle Shortening Against a Load (the Fenn Effect)[81]

Fenn showed that shortening of skeletal muscle against a load results in a proportional increase in work performed. There is an additional need for oxygen and an excess release of heat; MVO_2 increases. This represents systolic wall stress developed during the ventricular ejection period and represents most of the oxygen required. This is the external contractile component of work in contrast to the internal tension development component of work. Comparing MVO_2 requirements for isometric myocardial contraction, MVO_2 for isotonic contraction at equal levels of stress indicates that there is excess oxygen consumption when there is shortening and external work performed.

The total oxygen needs for isometric tension development and for isotonic contraction account for 75–80% of the myocardial oxygen consumption.

Minor Determinants of Oxygen Consumption

Depolarization

Electrophysiologic processes (depolarization, repolarization and propagation of the action potential) at the myocardial cell membrane require some energy. However, only a small amount of oxygen is used by the normal working heart for depolarization amounting to approximately 0.5% of the total amount consumed by the heart (or 0.04 ml/100 gram muscle). Increase in the frequency of depolarization is accompanied by only trivial increases in oxygen use.

Activation–Deactivation of Contraction

The contractile machinery is activated by calcium. On activation, the calcium is released from the sarcoplasmic reticulum and diffuses into myofibrils. Sliding of actin along myosin filaments follows. This and removal of calcium to produce relaxation is an active process and requires energy. The amount of chemical energy associated with myocardial muscle deactivation is small and approximates 1.0% of the total MVO_2 of the normal beating heart.

Other Contributors to Myocardial Oxygen Consumption

Catecholamines

Beta$_1$ adrenergic stimulants and sympathetic stimulation produce large increases in MVO_2 in the contracting heart. In contrast, in the non-contracting or arrested heart, catecholamines produce only a small increase (5–10%) in MVO_2. Catecholamines induce significant increase in energy demand in the beating heart by augmenting contractility.

Temperature

During hypothermia, there is a marked increase in total body oxygen requirements. A decrease of 0.8°C (2°F) in core body temperature induces an increase of 40% in total body oxygen demand. Hyperthermia also augments MVO_2.

MEASUREMENTS OF CARDIAC OUTPUT AND CARDIAC INDEX[138–150]

Several techniques are available to measure of cardiac output. Commonly used methods are invasive and require access to the patients central blood system. Some newer methods are non-invasive. All methods have specific weaknesses and each can incur its own specific source of error.

Fick Cardiac Output

The Fick principle is based on the observation that cardiac output is related directly to the rate oxygen consumption in body tissues and related indirectly to the difference between the amount of oxygen entering the tissues (arterial oxygen content) and amount of oxygen leaving the tissues and reentering the heart (central venous oxygen content). If there variables are know, it is possible to calculate the speed that blood is being pumped throughout the body. Therefore:

Cardiac Output

$$= \text{Oxygen consumption} / \text{Arterial } O_2 \text{ Content}$$
$$- \text{Venous } O_2 \text{ Content}$$

Oxygen content is calculated from three factors: The amount of oxygen 1 gram of fully saturated hemoglobin can carry, the grams of hemoglobin present and the saturation of hemoglobin.

O_2 carrying capacity (ml O_2/L blood)

$$= 1.36 \times \{\text{Hemoglobin (gm/d)}\}$$
$$\times \{\text{Hemoglobin saturation (\%)}\} \times 10$$

Arterial and venous samples taken from the patient at approximately the same time are required for this calculation. More cumbersome (and inaccurate) in the clinical setting is the calculation of the oxygen consumption. This measurement requires detailed analysis of the patients exhaled volume of expired gas.

Dilution Cardiac Output

Dilutional techniques which can also measure cardiac output require injection of an indicator and measurement of the indicator concentration distal in the circulation. The cardiac output is related directly to the speed at which a known volume of indicator is diluted in the body. The higher the cardiac output the faster the dilution will occur. There are two dilution methods used: indicator (dye) dilution and thermodilution.

Indicator (Dye) Dilution Method

A dye, usually indocyanine green, is injected into the central venous system. Its concentration is measured in the arterial system using a spectrophotometer. The calculation is completed and is performed by a computer, which allows a rapid reading of the cardiac output. This technique is now rarely used.

Thermodilution Method

A fluid of known temperature, colder than body temperature, and of known volume is injected through a pulmonary arterial catheter at the proximal port (central vein or right atrium). A thermistor, present at the distal tip of the catheter in the pulmonary artery, measures the temperature change brought about by the cold injection. From the changes in temperature observed at the recording tip over time with the injection an approximation of right sided cardiac output can be measured.

Transesophageal Echocardiographic Cardiac Output

Using the change in the volume of the ventricular chamber between end-diastole and end-systole in the echocardiographic view of the heart, computer derived cardiac output can be obtained. The diameter of the ventricle in each view is traced and labeled. Once the computer has the information it will present a variety of cardiac values, including end-diastole and end-systole volumes, stroke volume, ejection fraction, and cardiac output.

Aortic Pulse-Wave Contour Analysis

This technique uses another computer-based analysis method that is directed at the change in the diameter of the thoracic aorta. This measurement is dependent on a properly placed catheter, which allows a perpendicular view of the aorta. Any change in the orientation of the catheter from perpendicular will invalidate the values obtained.

REFERENCES

1. West J. B.: Best and Taylor's: The Physiologic Basis of Medical Practice. 12th Ed., Baltimore, The Williams & Wilkins Co. 1990.
2. Braunwald E.: Heart Disease: A Textbook of Cardiovascular Medicine, 4th edition, W.B. Saunders, Philadelphia, 1992.
3. Berne R. M., Levy M. N.: Cardiovascular Physiology. St. Louis, CV Mosby Co. 1986.
4. Katz A. M.: Physiology of the Heart, second edition, Raven Press, New York, 1992.
5. Opie L. H. The Heart: Physiology and Metabolism, second edition, Raven Press, New York, 1991.
6. Streeter D. D., Jr: Gross morphology and fiber geometry of the heart. In Handbook of Physiology, Section 2. Edited by R. M. Berne, et al. Washington D.C., American Physiologic Society, 1979.
7. Guyton A. C.: Textbook of Medical Physiology, seventh edition, Philadelphia, W B Saunders Co. 1986.
8. Hurst J. W., Schlant R. C.: The Heart, seventh edition McGraw-Hill, Inc New York, 1990.
9. Lev M.: Normal anatomy of the conduction system in man. Ann NY Acad Sci 1964; 111:817.
10. James T. N.: Ultrastructure of the human atrioventricular node. Circulation 37:1049, 1968.
11. James T. N.: Anatomy of the cardiac conduction system in the rabbit. Circ Res 20:638, 1967.
12. Greenbaum R. A., Ho S. Y., Gibson D. G., et al: Left ventricular fibre architecture in man. Br Heart J 28:1323-1367, 1981.
13. James T. N., Scherf L: Ultrastructure of Myocardial Cells. Am J Cardiol 22:289, 1968.
14. Noble M. I. M.: Excitation-contraction coupling. In: Drake-Holland A. J., Noble M. I. M., eds. Cardiac Metabolism. Chichester: John Wiley. 1983:49-71.
15. Brady A. J.: Active state in cardiac muscle. Physiol Rev 48:570, 1968.
16. Fozzard H. A., Gibbons W. R.: Action potential and contraction of heart muscle. Am J Cardiol 31:182, 1973.
17. Noble D.: The Initiation of the Heartbeat. New York. Oxford University Press, 1979.
18. Hoffmann B: Origin of the heart beat, in Luisada A. A. (ed.): Cardiology: An Encyclopedia of the Cardiovascular System. New York, McGraw-Hill Brook Company. 1959.
19. Wiggers C. J.: Studies on the consecutive phases of the cardiac cycle. I. The duration of the consecutive phases of the cardiac cycle and the criteria for their precise determination. Am J Physiol 56:415-432, 1921.
20. Wiggers C. J.: Dynamics of ventricular contraction under abnormal conditions (the Henry Jackson Memorial Lecture). Circulation 5:321, 1952.
21. Szent-Gyorgi A.: Contraction in the heart muscle fibre. Bull NY Acad Med 28:3, 1952.
22. Gilbert J. C., Glantz S. A.: Determinates of left ventricle filling and of the diastolic pressure-volume relation. Circ Res 64:827-852, 1989.
23. Suga H., Hayashi T., Shirahata M.: Ventricular systolic pressure-volume area as predictor of cardiac consumption. Am J Physiol 240:H39, 1981.
24. Suga H., Yamakoshi K.: Effects of stroke volume and velocity of ejection on end-systolic pressure on canine left ventricle. Circ Res 40:455, 1977.
25. Sagawa K., Maughan L., Suga H., et al: Cardiac contraction and the pressure-volume relationship. Oxford University Press, New York, 1988.
26. Kass D. A., Maughan W. L.: From "Emax" to pressure-volume relations: A broader view. Circulation 77:1203, 1988.
27. Kass D. A., Yamazaki T., Burkhoff D., et al: Determination of left ventricular end-systolic pressure-volume relationships by conductance (volume) catheter technique. Circulation 73:586, 1986.
28. Lee J., Tajimi T., Widmann T. F., et al: Application of end-systolic pressure-volume and pressure-wall thickness relations in conscious dogs. J Am Coll Cardiol 9:136, 1987.
29. Kaseda S., Tomoike H., Ogaa I., et al: End-systolic pressure-volume, pressure-length, and stress-strain relations in canine hearts. Am J Physiol 18:H648, 1985.
30. Mehmel H. C., Stocking B., Ruffmann K., et al: The linearity of the end-systolic pressure-volume relationship in man and its sensitivity for assessment of left ventricular function. Circulation 63:1216, 1981.
31. Grossman W., Braunwald E., Mann T., et al: Contractile state of the left ventricle in man as evaluated from end-systolic pressure-volume relations. Circulation 56:845, 1977.
32. Maughan W., Sunagawa K.: Factors affecting the end-systolic pressure-volume relationship. Fed Proc 43:2408, 1984.
33. Sagawa K.: The end-systolic pressure-volume relation of the ventricle: Definition, modifications and clinical use. Circulation 63:1223, 1981.
34. Glantz S. A., Parmley W. W.: Factors which affect the diastolic pressure volume curve. Circ Res 42:171, 1978.
35. Hoffman B. F. and Cranefield P. F.: Electrophysiology of the Heart. New York, McGraw-Hill Book Co., 1960.
36. Hoffman B. F.: Electrophysiology of single cardiac cells. Bull NY Acad Med 35:689, 1959.
37. Hoffman B. F., Suckling E. E.: Effect of several cations on transmembrane potentials of cardiac muscle. Am J Physiol 186:317, 1956.
38. Trautwein W.: Generation and conduction of impulses in the heart as affected by drugs. Pharmacol Rev 15:277, 1963.
39. Speralakis N.: The slow action potential and properties of the myocardial slow channels. J Gen Physiol 85:159, 1985.
40. Reuter H.: Ion channels in cardiac cell membrane. Ann Rev Physiol 46:473, 1984.
41. Sperelakis N.: Origin of the cardiac resting potential. In: Berne R. C., et al (eds): Handbook of Physiology, Section 2, The Cardiovascular System. Baltimore, Williams & Wilkins Co., 1979.
42. Trautwein W.: Membrane currents in cardiac muscle fibers. Physiol Rev 53:793, 1973.
43. Vanhoutte P. M.: Symposium. Calcium entry blockers and the cardiovascular system. Fed Proc 40:2851, 1981.
44. Cranefield P. F., Wit A. L., Hoffman B. F.: Genesis of cardiac arrhythmias. Circulation 47:190, 1973.
45. Wantabe Y., Dreifus L. S.: Factors controlling impulse

transmission with special reference to A-V conduction. Am Heart J 89:79, 1975.

46. Fozzard H. A.: Cardiac muscle: Excitability and passive electrical properties. Prog Cardiovasc Dis 19:343, 1977.

47. Hurst J. W., Myerberg R. J.: Cardiac arrhythmias-evolving concepts. Mod Concepts Cardiovasc Dis 37:73, 1968.

48. McDonald T. F.: Excitation-contraction coupling: Relationship of the slow inward current to contraction. In: Sperelakis N, (ed.): The Physiology and Pathophysiology of the Heart. Boston, Martinus Nijhoff. 1984; 187.

49. Blinks J. R.: Intracellular Ca^{2+} measurements. In: Fozzard H. A., Haber E, Jennings R. B., et al (eds.): The Heart and Cardiovascular System. New York, Raven Press. 1986; 671.

50. McDonald T.: Excitation-contraction coupling: Relation of the slow inward current to contraction. J Gen Physiol 85:187, 1985.

51. Tada M., Katz A.: Phosphorylation of the sarcoplasmic reticulum and sarcolemma. Ann Rev 44:401, 1982.

52. Sonnenblick E. H.: Implications of muscle mechanics in the heart. Fed Proc 21:975, 1962.

53. Braunwald E.: Determinants and assessment of cardiac function. N Engl J Med 296:86, 1977.

54. Guyton A. C.: Regulation of cardiac output. N Engl J Med 227:805, 1967.

55. Vatner S. F., Boettcher D. H.: Regulation of cardiac output by stroke volume and heart rate in conscious dogs. Circ Res 42:557, 1978.

56. Fifer M. A., Grossman W.: Measurement of ventricular volumes, ejection fraction, mass and wall stress. In Grossman W., (ed.): Cardiac Catheterization and Angiography. 3rd Ed. Philadelphia, Lea and Febiger. 1986; 282–300.

57. Grossman W.: Evaluation of systolic and diastolic function of the myocardium. In: Grossman W. (ed.): Cardiac Catheterization and Angiography, 3rd ed. Philadelphia, Lea and Febiger. 1986; 301–319.

58. Rushmer R. F.: Cardiovascular Dynamics. Philadelphia: W.B. Saunders, 1970.

59. Katz A. M.: Influence of altered inotropy and lusitropy on ventricular pressure-volume loops. J Am Coll Cardiol 11:438–455, 1988.

60. Karliner J. S., et al: Mean velocity of fiber shortening. A simplified measure of left ventricular myocardial contractility. Circulation 44:323, 1971.

61. Van Den Box G. C., Elzinga G., Westerhof N., et al: Problems in the use of indices of myocardial contractility. Cardiovasc Res 7:834, 1973.

62. Mason D. T., Braunwald E., Covell J. W., et al: Assessment of cardiac contractility: The relation between the rate of pressure rise and ventricular pressure during isovolumic systole. Circulation 44:47, 1971.

63. Ross J.: Cardiac function and myocardial contractility: A perspective. J Am Coll Cardiol 1:52, 1983.

64. Etsten B. E., Shimosato S: Myocardial contractility: Performance of the heart during anesthesia. Clin Anesth 3:56–78, 1964.

65. Quinones M. A., Gaasch W. H., Alexander J. K.: Influence of acute changes in preload, afterload, contractile state and heart rate on ejection and isovolumic indices of myocardial contractility in man. Circulation 53:293, 1976.

66. Braunwald E: On the difference between the heart's output and its contractile state. Circulation 43:171, 1971.

67. Sonnenblick, E. H., Skelton C. E.: Reconsideration of the ultrastructural basis of cardiac length-tension relations. Circ Res 35:517, 1974.

68. Allen D. G., Kentish J. C.: The cellular basis of length-tension relation in cardiac muscle. J Mol Cell Cardiol 17:821, 1985.

69. Brutsaert D. L.: The force-velocity-length-time interrelation of cardiac muscle. In the Physiological Basis of Starling's Law of the Heart. Ciba Foundation Symposium 24. Elsevier, North-Holland, Amsterdam. 1974.

70. Ross J., Sobel B. E.: Regulation of cardiac contraction. Annu Rev Physiol 34:47, 1974.

71. Weber K. T., Janicki J. S., Hunter W. C., et al: The contractile behavior of the heart and its functional coupling to the circulation. Prog Cardiovasc Dis 24:375, 1982.

72. Weber K. T., Janicki K. T.: The dynamics of ventricular contraction: Force, lengthening, and shortening. Fed Proc 39:188, 1980.

73. Winegrad S.: Regulation of cardiac contractile proteins. Circ Res 55:565, 1984.

74. Sunagawa K., Maughan W. L., Burkhof F. D., et al: Left ventricular interaction with arterial load studied in isolated canine ventricle. Am J Physiol 245:H773, 1983.

75. Brutsaert D. L., Sonnenblick E. H.: Force-velocity-length relationship in the contractile elements in heart muscle of the cat. Circ Res 24:137, 1969.

76. Sonnenblick E. H., Downing S. E.: Afterload as a primary determinate of ventricular performance. Am J Physiol 204:604.

77. Ross J.: Afterload mismatch and preload reserve: A conceptual framework for the analysis of ventricular function. Prog Cardiovasc Dis 18:255, 1976.

78. Lang R. M., Borow K. M., Neumann A., et al: Systemic vascular resistance: An unreliable index of left ventricular afterload. Circulation 74:1114, 1986.

79. Milnor W. R.: Arterial impedance as ventricular afterload. Circ Res 36:565, 1975.

80. Fenn W. O.: A quantative comparison between the energy liberated and the work performed by the isolated sartorious muscle of the frog. J Physiol 58:175–203, 1923.

81. Yin F. C. P.: Ventricular wall stress. Circ Res 49:829, 1981.

82. Rothe C. F.: Physiology of venous return: An unappreciated boost to the heart. Arch Intern Med 146:977, 1986.

83. Sarnoff S. J., Berglund E.: Ventricular function. I. Starling's law of the heart studied by means of simultaneous right and left ventricular function curves in the dog. Circulation 9:706, 1954.

84. Kentish J. C.: The length-tension relation in the myocardium and its cellular basis. Heart Failure 4:125, 1988.

85. Paterson S., Starling E. H.: On the mechanical factors which determine the output of ventricles. J Physiol 48:357, 1914.

86. Frank O.: Zur dynamik des herzmuskels. Z Biol 32:370, 1895.

87. Jewell B. R.: A reexamination of the influence of muscle length on myocardial performance. Circ Res 40:221, 1977.

88. MacGregor D. C., Covell J. W., Mahler F., et al: Relations between afterload, stroke volume, and the descending limb of Starling's curve. Am J Physiol 227:884, 1974.

89. Linderer T., Chatterjee K., Parmly W. W., et al: Influence of atrial systole on the Frank-Starling relation and the end-diastolic pressure-diameter relation of the left ventricle. Circulation 67:1045, 1983.

90. Guyton A. C., Coleman T. G., Granger H. J.: Circulation: Overall regulation. Annu Rev Physiol 34:13, 1972.

91. Lakatta E. G.: Starling's law of the heart is explained by an intimate interaction of muscle length and myofilament calcium activation. J Am Coll Cardiol 10:1157–1164, 1987.

92. Brutsaert D. L., et al: Diastolic Failure Pathophysiology and therapeutic implications J Am Coll Cardiol 22:318–325, 1993.

93. Blaustein A. S., Gaasch W. H.: Myocardial relaxation. VI. Effects of adrenergic tone and asynchrony on left ventricular relaxation rate. Am J Physiol 244:H417, 1983.

94. Starling M. R., et al: Load independence of the rate of iso-volumic relaxation in man. Circulation 56:1274, 1987.

95. Grossman W., McLaurin L. P.: Diastolic properties of the left ventricle. Ann Intern Med 84:316, 1976.

96. Gaasch W. H., Ariel Y., McMahon T. A.: Dynamics of left ventricular diastolic filling. J Am Coll Cardiol 7:243A, 1986.

97. Brutsaert D. L., Rademakers F. E., Sys S. U.: Analysis of relaxation in the evaluation of ventricular function of the heart. Prog Cardiovasc Dis 28:143, 1985.

98. Plotnick A. D.: Changes in diastolic function-difficult to measure, harder to interpret. Am Heart J 118:637–641, 1989.

99. Bonow R. O., et al.: Impaired left ventricular diastolic filling in patients with coronary artery disease: Assessment with radionuclide angiography. Circulation 64:315, 1981.

100. Shapiro L. M., Gibson D. G.: Patterns of diastolic dysfunction in left ventricular hypertrophy. Br Heart J 59:438, 1988.

101. Rankin J. S., Arentzen C. E., McHale P. A., et al: Viscoelastic properties of the diastolic left ventricle in the conscious dog. Circ Res 41:37, 1977.

102. Mirsky I.: Assessment of diastolic function: Suggested methods and future considerations. Circulation 69:836, 1984.

103. Gaasch W. H., Levine H. J., Quinones M. A., et al: Left ventricular compliance: Mechanisms and clinical implications. Am J Cardiol 38:645, 1976.

104. Carabello B. A., Spann J. F.: The uses and limitations of end-systolic indexes of left ventricular function. Circulation 69:1058, 1984.

105. Bellett S., Wasserman F.: Effect of molar sodium lactate in increasing cardiac rhythmicity. JAMA 160:1293, 1956.

106. Denlinger J. K., Kaplan J. A., Lecky J. H., et al: Cardiovascular responses to calcium administered intravenously to man during halothane anesthesia. Anesthesiology 42:390, 1975.

107. Lang R. M., et al: Left ventricular contractility varies directly with blood ionized calcium. Ann Intern Med 108:524, 1988.

108. Moore M. J.: Magnesium sulfate and digitalis-toxic arrhythmias. (Letter to Editor). JAMA 253:513, 1985

109. Iseri L. T., French J. H.: Magnesium: nature's physiologic calcium blocker. Am Heart J 108:188, 1984.

110. Katz B., Miledi R.: Spontaneous evoked activity of motor nerve endings in calcium Ringer. J Physiol 203:689, 1969.

111. Seeling M. S.: Magnesium Deficiency in the Pathogenesis of Disease. New York/London: Plenum Medical Book Co. 1980:185.

112. Sheehan J. P.: Magnesium sulfate and digitalis-toxic arrhythmias. (Letter to editor) JAMA 253:513, 1985.

113. Katz A. M.: Role of the contractile proteins and sarcoplasmic reticulum in the response of the heart to catecholamines: a historical review. Adv Cycl Nucl Res 2:303–343, 1979.

114. Randall W. C., (ed.): Neural Regulation of the Heart. New York, Oxford University Press. 1977, 440 pp.

115. Higgins C. B., Vatner S. F., Braunwald E.: Parasympathetic control of the heart. Pharmacol Rev 25:119, 1973.

116. Randall W. C.: Nervous Control of the Heart. Baltimore, The Williams & Wilkins Co. 1965.

117. Levy M. N., Martin P. J.: Neural control of the heart. In Sperelakis N, (ed.): Physiology and Pathophysiology of the Heart. Boston, Martinus Nijhoff. 337–354, 1984.

118. Pace J. B., Randall W. C., Wechsler J. S., et al: Alterations in ventricular dynamics induced by stimulation of cervical vagosympathetic trunk. Am J Physiol 214:1213, 1968.

119. Levy M. N.: Cardiac sympathetic-parasympathetic interactions. Fed Proc 43:2598, 1984.

120. Schaefer S., et al: Effect of increasing heart rate on left ventricular performance in patients with normal cardiac function. Am J Cardiol 61:617, 1988.

121. Hutter O. F., Trautwein W.: Vagal and sympathetic effects on the pacemaker fibers in the sinus venosus of the heart. J Gen Physiol 39:715, 1956.

122. Heymans C., Bouckaret J. J.: Role of the cardioaortic and carotid sinus nerves in the reflex control of the respiratory center. N Engl J Med 219:157, 1938.

123. Schmidt C. F.: Carotid sinus reflexes to the respiratory center. Am J Physiol 102:94, 1932.

124. Gilfoil T. M., Youmans W. B., Turner J. K.: Abdominal compression reaction. Am J Physiol 196:1160, 1959.

125. Vatner S. F., Rutherford J. D.: Control of the myocardial contractile state by carotid chemo- and baroreceptor and pulmonary inflation reflexes in conscious dogs. J Clin Invest 61:1593, 1978.

126. Laragh J.: Atrial natriuretic hormone, the renin-aldosterone axis and blood pressure-electrolyte homostasis. N Engl J Med 313:1329, 1985.

127. Lang R. E., Tholken H., Ganten D., et al: Atrial natriuretic factor—a circulating hormone stimulated by volume loading. Nature 314:264–266, 1985.

128. Raine A. E. G., et al: Atrial natriuretic peptide and atrial pressure in patients with congestive heart failure. N Engl J Med 315:533, 1986.

129. McKeever W. P., Gregg D. E., Canney P. C.: Oxygen uptake of the non-working left ventricle. Circ Res 6:612, 1958.

130. Braunwald E.: Control of myocardial oxygen consumption physiologic and clinical considerations. Am J Cardiol 27:416, 1971.

131. Sonnenblick E. H., Ross J., Braunwald E.: Oxygen consumption of the heart. Am J Cardiol 22:328, 1968.

132. Sarnoff S. J., Braunwald E., Case R. B., et al: Hemodynamic determinants of oxygen consumption of the heart with special reference to the tension-time index. Am J Physiol 192:148, 1958.

133. DuBois E. F.: Basal metabolism in health and disease. Philadelphia, Lea & Febiger. 1936.

134. Graham T. P., Covell J. W., Sonnenblick E. H., et al: Control of myocardial oxygen consumption: Contractile state and tension development. J Clin Invest 47:375, 1968.

135. McKeever W. P., Gregg D. E., Canney P. C.: Oxygen uptake of the non-working left ventricle. Circ Res 6:612–623, 1958.

136. Hoffman J. I. E., Buckberg G. D.: Pathophysiology of subendocardial ischemia. Br Med J 1:76, 1975.

137. Braunwald E., Sarnoff S. J., Case R. B., et al: Hemodynamic determinants of cardiac output on the relationship between myocardial oxygen consumption and coronary flow. Am J Physiol 192:157–163, 1958.

138. Fick A.: Mechanische Arbeit u. Warmeentwicklung bei derMuskeltatigkeit. Leipzig: F.A. Brockhaus. 1982.

139. Brandfonbrener M., Landowne M., Shock N. W.: Changes in cardiac output with age. Circulation 12:557, 1955.

140. Ganz W., Swan J. H. C.: Measurement of blood flow by thermodilution. Am J Cardiol 29:241, 1972.

141. Ganz W., Donoso R., Marcus A. S., et al: A new technique for measurement of cardiac output by thermodilution in man. Am J Cardiol 27:392, 1971.

142. Heneghan C. P. H., Brantwaithe M. A.: Non-invasive measurement of cardiac output during anaesthesia. Br J Anaesth 53:351, 1981.

143. Davies G, Jebson P. J. R., Glasgow B. M., Hess D. R.: Continuous Fick cardiac output compared to thermodilution cardiac output. Crit Care Med 14:881, 1986.

144. Carpenter J. P., Nair S., Staw I.: Cardiac output determination: Thermodilution versus a new computerized Fick method. Crit Care Med 13:576, 1985.

145. Matsumoto M., Oka Y., Strom J., et al: Application of transesophageal echocardiography to continuous intraoperative monitoring of left ventricular performance. Am J Cardiol *46*:95, 1980.

146. Terai C., Vensihi M., Sugimoto H., et al: Transesophageal echocardiographic dimensional analysis of four cardiac chambers during positive end-expiratory pressure. Anesthesiology *63*:640, 1985.

147. Kronik G., Slany J., Moslacher H.: Comparative value of 8 M-mode echocardiographic formulas for determining left ventricular stroke volume. A correlative study with thermo-dilution and left ventricular single-plane cineangiography. Circulation *60*:1308, 1979.

148. Mark J. B., Steinbrook R. A., Gugino L. D., et al: Continuous non-invasive monitoring of cardiac output with esophageal Doppler ultrasound during cardiac surgery. Anesth Analg *65*:1013, 1986.

149. Freund P. R.: Modification in the transesophageal Doppler: Comparison with thermodilution measurement during cardiac output in anesthetized man (abstract). Anesthesiology *65A*:144, 1986.

150. Roewer N., Bednarz F., Dridha A., et al: Intraoperative cardiac output determination from transmitral and pulmonary blood flow measurements using transesophageal pulsed Doppler echocardiography. Anesthesiology *65A*:639, 1987.

Chapter 7

PERIOPERATIVE ARRHYTHMIAS

BRUCE S. KLEINMAN, BRIAN OLSHANSKY, AND VINCENT J. COLLINS

In this chapter, we assume that the anesthesiologist has a passing familiarity with the differential diagnosis of simple rhythm disturbances. We will not go into great detail on how to differentiate a premature ventricular beat from a premature atrial beat or ventricular tachycardia from a supraventricular tachycardia.

Many causes exist for the occurrence of arrhythmias during the administration of anesthesia care. These can be broken up into two broad categories: rhythm disturbances caused by anesthetic drugs per se and those to surgical manipulation or other ancillary factors. These other factors include hypoxemia, hyper- or hypocarbia, electrolyte disturbance, "light" anesthesia, and malignant hyperthermia.

This chapter presents an overview of rhythm disturbances, particularly those common in the perioperative period. Mechanisms, incidence, and treatment are discussed.

PATHOPHYSIOLOGY OF THE GENESIS OF ARRHYTHMIAS

Cardiac arrhythmias may be classified descriptively into two major groups.[1,2] One group consists of abnormalities of impulse generation (automaticity). The other consists of abnormalities of impulse conduction (propagation). Abnormalities of impulse generation or impulse conduction may be seen in patients during the perioperative period. In addition, changes in autonomic tone can cause some ventricular arrhythmias.[3] A thorough understanding of arrhythmogenic mechanisms is helpful for diagnosis and subsequent rational treatment (Table 7-1).

Abnormalities in Automaticity

Normally, impulse formation occurs from the spontaneous slow depolarization during electrical diastole (phase 4) of specialized automatic cells. These cells are located in the sinoatrial node (SAN) and other specialized tissue such as the atrioventricular (AV) junction[4] (Fig. 7-1). The upstroke of SAN and AV junctional cell action potentials are produced by a slow inward calcium current. This is in direct contrast to normal Purkinje fiber automaticity which is mediated by a fast inward sodium current. Myocardial muscle cells, under normal conditions, do not undergo diastolic depolarization (Fig. 7-2).

Cells with the fastest rates of diastolic depolarization serve as the primary pacemaker. Under normal conditions the cells in the sinoatrial (SA) node serve as the pri-

mary pacemaker; the cells in other areas of the heart—such as specialized atrial tissue, AV junction, and His-Purkinje system—serve as latent pacemakers. These pacemakers will exhibit spontaneous depolarization in response to sinus slowing or failure of the sinus impulse to reach the ventricle because of AV block. This phenomena typically will lead to AV dissociation. For instance, a very slow sinus bradycardia will lead to the spontaneous depolarization of junctional pacemakers. Since the junctional pacemaker will be the faster, the ventricle will usually be under control of junctional pacemakers, whereas the atrium will be under control of sinus pacemakers; hence, AV dissociation secondary to sinus bradycardia.

The discharge rate of an automatic or potentially automatic cell can be altered in one of three ways:

1. changing the slope of phase 4
2. changing the threshold potential
3. changing the resting membrane potential

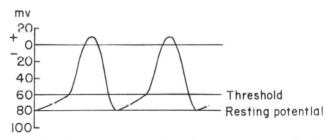

Fig. 7-1. The action potential of an automatic cell. The threshold potential is reached spontaneously (phase 4 diastolic depolarization) in specialized conductive tissue.

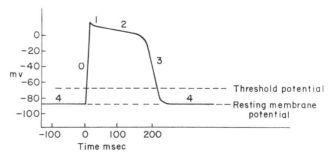

Fig. 7-2. The action potential of a single myocardial cell. Rapid depolarization is represented by phase 0. Repolarization represented by phases 1 to 3 restores the cell to its resting transmembrane potential (phase 4).

The implications of the above are that any factor that decreases the intrinsic rate of the normal SA node pacemaker or increases the automaticity of more distal latent pacemakers can lead to an automatic escape rhythm. For example, ischemic areas in a patient with coronary disease can cause an increase rate of phase 4 depolarization in Purkinje tissue leading to premature ventricular beats (PVBs).[4] Hypokalemia, hypocalcemia and acidosis all increase the rate of spontaneous depolarization in automatic tissue below the SA node.[5] This too, can lead to ectopic foci.

Rhythms typically caused by disturbances in automaticity are slow atrial, junctional and ventricular escape rhythms. Some atrial tachycardias secondary to digoxin, non-paroxysmal junctional tachycardia and idioventricular and parasystolic rhythms are also felt to be secondary to disturbances in automaticity.[4]

Triggered activity refers to oscillatory changes in transmembrane potential which follow or are triggered by a preceding impulse.[4,5] These oscillatory after-depolarizations (which may be early [EAD] or delayed [DAD]) may arise during or after repolarization of a previous action potential. Triggered activity is unrelated to any demonstrable re-entry and never arises spontaneously; an action potential is always required to initiate or trigger it.[6] Therefore, triggered activity while clearly being an abnormality in impulse generation, is in the strictest sense not an example of abnormal automaticity. Triggered activity is felt to be the primary mechanism in tachyarrhythmias induced by cardiac glycosides. None the less its overall importance to the genesis of tachyarrhythmias in the clinical setting is still quite speculative.

Abnormalities of Impulse Propagation

Abnormalities of the pattern of normal atrio-ventricular activation may lead to slow conduction and eventually block. The slow conduction is also critical for the manifestation of reentrant arrhythmias.

Reentry

Reentry (Fig. 7–3) is a term used to describe an impulse which excites a region of myocardium, conducts slowly around an area of inexcitable tissue and finally reexcites the original region. Reentrant circuits depend upon three conditions for their existence[4] (Fig. 7–3):.

1. Initial unidirectional block in one limb of the circuit
2. Relatively short refractory period in the previously excited region
3. Prolonged conduction time in one limb of the circuit

Reentry circuits have been described involving circular pathways and also involving transmission of impulses back and forth along the same myocardial fiber—so called reflection.[1,4] More recently a figure of eight reentry circuit has been described.[7] This figure of eight circuit is felt to be the mechanism for most ventricular tachycardias.

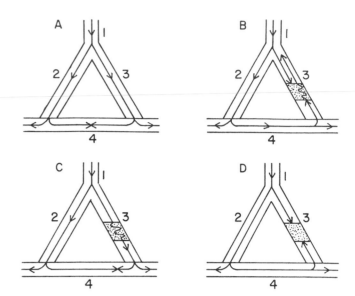

Fig. 7–3. Schematic representation of Purkinje fiber 1 with terminal branches 2 and 3 into the ventricular muscle 4. *A,* Normal conduction. Conduction occurs at the same speed through both limbs of a terminal Purkinje fiber bundle to activate the myocardium. *B, Shaded area,* area of unidirectional antegrade block due to disease or drug effect. Slow retrograde conduction is established in limb 3. An impulse from 1 passes down branches 2 and 3 but is blocked proximally at the area of unidirectional block in 3. It passes normally through 2 and enters the ventricular tissue (4). From 4 it may enter limb 3 distally and conduct slowly through 3 to the bifurcation. If limb 2 has recovered its excitability, the impulse may re-enter limb 2 and excite the ventricular muscle, resulting in a premature ventricular beat. *C and D,* two methods of suppression of re-entrant arrhythmias. In *C,* the area of unidirectional block is abolished and antegrade conduction is restored. In *D,* a bidirectional block is established in antegrade and retrograde directions. (From Pratila M. G., Pratilas V.; Anesthetic agents and cardiac electromechanical activity. Anesthesiology 1978; 49:344.

Reentry is felt to be the cause of many clinically important tachyarrhythmias. Among these are atrial flutter and fibrillation, paroxysmal junctional tachycardias and ventricular tachycardia.

BASIC DIAGNOSTIC PROBLEMS

Ventricular Rhythms vs Supraventricular Rhythms

Most of the rhythm disturbances that anesthesiologists will be confronted with are rather straightforward. One common problem is being able to distinguish a premature ventricular beat from a premature atrial beat with aberrant conduction. A variation on this theme is being able to distinguish ventricular tachycardia from a supraventricular tachycardia with aberration. This is the classic problem of the correct diagnosis of wide QRS complex tachycardia.

Premature Ventricular Beats vs Premature Atrial Beats

Generally speaking, premature ventricular beats are not conducted retrogradely to the atria and hence do not reset the sinus node. One reason for this is that the premature beat is usually early enough such that the AV junction is still in its effective refractory period. Hence, the sinus rate will remain undisturbed. This leads to the so called 'compensatory pause.' A premature atrial beat, on the other hand does reset the sinus node (Fig. 7–4). As far as morphology goes a premature ventricular beat is likely to show a monophasic R or biphasic qR complex in lead V_1. With aberrancy, a triphasic RSR complex is likely to be seen in V_1.[8]

Ventricular Tachycardia vs Supraventricular Tachycardia

Being able to distinguish ventricular tachycardia from a wide QRS complex supraventricular tachycardia can be difficult.[9] Stability of vital signs is not helpful.[10] Ventricular tachycardia should be considered the likely cause of a regular wide QRS complex tachycardia in the conscious adult patient especially if a history of remote myocardial infarction is elicited.[11] In addition, there are many electrocardiographic criteria which help distinguish supraventricular tachycardia with a wide QRS complex from ventricular tachycardia.[12] One of these criterion is the demonstration of atrio-ventricular dissociation.[9,11,12] The hall marks of atrio-ventricular dissociation are (1) demonstrating that the atria and ventricles are under control of different pacemakers (2) presence of capture beats (3) presence of fusion beats. (Figs. 7–5, 7–6). Demonstrating atrio-ventricular dissociation, strongly favors the diagnosis of ventricular tachycardia. Unfortunately lack of atrio-ventricular dissociation does not rule out the diagnosis of ventricular tachycardia, since upwards of 40–60% of documented ventricular tachycardias do not exhibit atrio ventricular dissociation.

Hence, in the middle aged or elderly patients, a wide QRS complex tachycardia is in our opinion most likely to be ventricular tachycardia until proven otherwise. We take this approach because ventricular tachycardia is often seen in the presence of organic heart disease. In the aforementioned population of hospitalized patients the prevalence of organic heart disease is moderately high. Therefore, when in doubt, we recommend treating wide QRS complex tachycardia in this age group as ventricular tachycardia—with intravenous lidocaine or cardioversion. Do not use calcium channel blockers when in doubt

about whether the wide QRS complex tachycardia is truly ventricular tachycardia or supraventricular with aberrancy. This can lead to cardiovascular collapse if ventricular tachycardia is the problem. Fortunately, the use of adenosine has safely decreased our diagnostic uncertainty. The use of this drug will be discussed later.

Torsades de Pointes: A Special Case of Ventricular Tachycardia

This type of ventricular tachycardia is morphologically distinct. It is characterized by oscillation around the baseline of the peaks of successive QRS complexes. In addition there is an association between torsade and marked QTU prolongation. It may be congenital or acquired (quinidine toxicity, hypokalemia, subarachnoid hemorrhage). Torsade has been divided into two major groups or settings.[13] The ventricular tachycardia may occur in the setting where it is preceded by a long pause, so called pause dependant long QT interval syndrome. This is characteristic of torsade occurring in patients receiving antiarrhythmic medications such as quinidine.

The other setting in which this rhythm abnormality may occur is with prolonged QT intervals during excessive adrenergic stimulation—so called adrenergic-dependent long QT interval syndrome. Patients who develop torsade in this setting typically experience heightened sympathetic tone as would occur during sudden exertion, fright, pain or disease pathology such as a subarachnoid hemorrhage.

Obviously, appropriate immediate therapy would depend upon the setting the tachycardia occurs in. Whereas, isoproterenol might be appropriate for torsade of the "long pause type" this would not be appropriate for the "adrenergic-dependent type." In the latter case beta blockers might prove helpful.

ARRHYTHMIAS DURING ANESTHESIA

Sinus bradycardia, wandering atrial pacemaker (changing p wave morphology with bradycardia or normal heart rate), and junctional rhythms are common during general anesthesia. These rhythms are mediated by the vagal nerve through surgical stimulation or by the administration of drugs having potent parasympathomimetic activ-

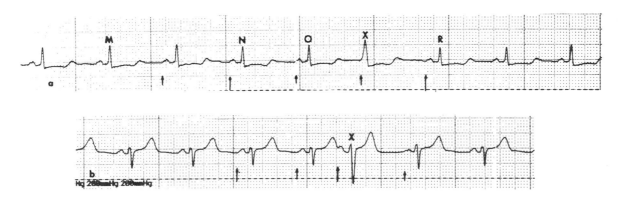

Fig. 7–4. Premature ventricular beat versus premature atrial beat. 'x' signifies a PVB. The arrows show that the sinus rate is constant—not interrupted by the PVB. Therefore a 'compensatory' pause is noted. (Interval OR equals interval MN) b) The third arrow shows a PAB with its subsequent ventricular conduction signified by 'x'. The sinus rate is reset by the PAB and therefore there is no compensatory pause.

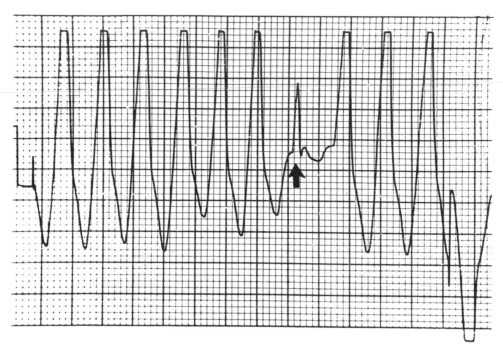

Fig. 7–5. A wide QRS tachycardia. The arrow shows a fusion beat strongly suggesting AV dissociation and therefore the diagnosis of ventricular tachycardia. (Courtesy of David Wilber, M.D.)

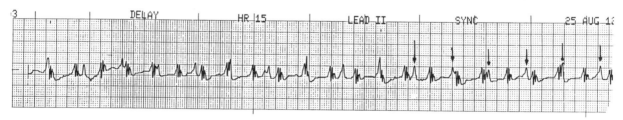

Fig. 7–6. Ventricular tachycardia. The atria are under control of the sinus mode. The ventricles under control of an ectopic foci; hence AV dissociation. (Arrows signify P waves.)

ity. In and of themselves these rhythm disturbances are not life threatening. The potential hemodynamic consequences of junctional bradycardia or wandering atrial pacemaker relate to the decrease in cardiac output that occurs. This may be due to the absence of the "atrial kick". Generally speaking, the change in cardiac output in patients with normal hearts is not clinically important. However, this may not be the case in patients with impaired diastolic or systolic function.

Bradyarrhythmias

The causes of bradyarrhythmias during the administration of anesthesia are multifactorial. Drug related factors such as the combination of sufentanil and vecuronium or the administration of beta-blockers are predisposing factors. Intrinsic disease of the sinus node may also predispose to bradyarrhythmias. The aforementioned vagal responses—reflex excitement of the peritoneum, nasopharynx or nares,[14] or drugs related to acetylcholine, also play a part.

Halogenated agents such as halothane, enflurane, and isoflurane directly depress the automaticity of the sinus node.[15,16] In addition the above drugs depress conduction through the AV junction.[15,16,17,18,19] These effects often lead

to a sinus bradycardia. When administering halothane or enflurane, blood pressure frequently decreases as a result of their vasodilating properties. However, because both drugs markedly depress the baroreflex[20,21] a compensatory tachycardia will not be observed. On the other hand isoflurane (also a vasodilator) has less depressant effects on the baroreflex than halothane or enflurane,[22] hence sinus tachycardias may sometimes be observed with this anesthetic.

Many intravenous drugs also can produce bradyarrhythmia. Generally speaking, barbiturates prolong AV junctional conduction time.[17] The bradycardia associated with morphine and even more so with fentanyl is due to central stimulation of the vagal cardioinhibitory center, in the medulla, leading to an increased release of acetylcholine at the cholinergic fiber endings in the heart.[17] In addition, fentanyl is found to have a direct effect on cardiac conduction. It increases AV junctional conduction time.[23]

Incidence

Early Studies

The incidence of arrhythmias due to anesthetic drugs per se is difficult to determine. Many factors other than anesthetic drugs could be arrhythmogenic. Intubation, surgical manipulation, hypoventilation, and hypoxemia, all can be contributory factors.[24] This issue was addressed in a large study by Vanik in 1968.[25] He looked at over 5,000 patients, most of whom underwent a halothane anesthetic. He found a 16.9% incidence (defined as any rhythm other than normal sinus) of arrhythmia with halothane. Vanik's study however had two major drawbacks: (1) some patients were not monitored during induction and intubation, and more importantly, (2) hard copy data were not obtained. This last point undoubtedly would cause underestimation of arrhythmic events.

Many studies that tried to quantify the problem of rhythm disturbances during the administration of anesthesia suffer from the same drawback:[24] continuous hard copy data was not obtained. A frequently quoted figure is that there is a 62% incidence of perioperative arrhythmias. This figure is based on Kuner's classic study of 154 surgical patients, of which 108 had a general anesthetic.[26] This study has much more credibility than Vanik's and others because hard copy data (Holter monitor) was obtained. Sinus tachycardia was not considered an arrhythmia.

Most of the rhythm disturbances were supraventricular. They consisted of wandering atrial pacemaker, isorhythmic A-V dissociation, (atria and ventricles under control of different pacemakers, but both at nearly the same rate—such that the P waves moves in and out and around the QRS complex) and junctional rhythm. Premature ventricular beats were also noted. Only five patients had ventricular tachycardia. By far the most frequent disturbance were rhythms of a vagotonic nature: wandering atrial pacemakers, isorhythmic A-V dissociation and junctional rhythms. This study, although frequently quoted is hard to generalize to today's patient population. Classic "arrhythmogenic" agents were used. For instance, 61% of Kuner's general anesthesia patients received halothane, 11% received ether and 12% received cyclopropane. Therefore, Kuner's study may not be very relevant to contemporary anesthetic practices in the United States.

Studies Since 1980

More recent literature on perioperative arrhythmias in patients, aged 0–72 years of ASA PS 1 to 3 who received general anesthesia has been reviewed.[27-33] The anesthetic drugs were halothane, enflurane, and fentanyl. All patients were supplemented with N_2O-O_2. Induction was mostly accomplished with thiopental. If sinus tachycardia is excluded, 242 patients or 42% had some type of arrhythmia. Some patients had more than one type of rhythm disturbance. Premature ventricular beats were by far the most common; occurring in 190 or 33% of the patients. Ventricular tachycardia on the other hand was by far the most uncommon arrhythmia, occurring in only 2 patients or 0.8%. There were no fatalities due to arrhythmias. As with some earlier studies, not all studies (most, but not all) obtained hard copy. Also in some study groups (patients receiving halothane and patients receiving enflurane) beta-blocking drugs were given preoperatively.

Enflurane Arrhythmias

If we divide the group of patients into those who received enflurane versus those who received halothane major differences are obvious. There were 302 patients age 16–72 years in ASA physical status class 1–3 who received enflurane-nitrous oxide-oxygen.[28-31] Only 67 (22%) of those patients developed arrhythmias. None developed ventricular tachycardia. Premature ventricular beats were noted in 30 patients or 10%.

In one study, Pratila,[31] found only an 8% incidence of rhythm disturbances (excluding sinus bradycardia) in 40 PS 1 and PS 2 patients receiving enflurane anesthesia. This study avoided beta-blockade and collected hard copy data prior to the beginning of surgery. No observations were made during actual surgery.

Halothane Arrhythmias

A review of reports of patients, who received halothane-nitrous oxide-oxygen,[30,32,33] who ranged in age between 12–60 years, and who were all ASA physical status class 1, showed that 62% developed some sort of arrhythmia—a figure similar to Kuner's study. Two patients (1%) developed ventricular tachycardia. Almost 37% or 72 patients exhibited premature ventricular beats. The incidence of slow rhythm disturbances was quite similar between those receiving halothane versus enflurane (8% vs 5%). In some of these studies, beta-blocking drugs were given for sinus tachycardia. This occurred in both halothane and enflurane groups. The trend however implies that the incidence of reentrant rhythm disturbances, such as premature ventricular beats and ventricular tachycardia, is less with enflurane. This would seem to make sense and not be surprising since enflurane has a reputation to maintain stable cardiac rhythm during surgery for pheochromocytoma, despite very high circulating catecholamine levels.[34]

This finding was confirmed in a study involving one of the largest number of patients receiving general anesthesia. In analyzing the results in over 17,000 general anesthetics, Forrest[35] found that halothane was associated with a higher incidence of ventricular excitability (PVBs, ventricular tachycardia) than other anesthetics. He further found that general anesthesia involving a narcotic was associated with a higher incidence of bradycardias and not surprisingly severe tachycardia (presumed sinus) was associated with isoflurane rather than other anesthetic regimens.

One factor that should be approached is that almost all studies on the incidence of arrhythmias have involved the concomitant use of nitrous-oxide. Arrhythmias have not been attributed to this anesthetic. This may be inappropriate. Nitrous-oxide may be a cause of intraoperative junctional rhythms.[36]

GENERAL APPROACH TO PERIOPERATIVE RHYTHM DISTURBANCES

The key to the management of an arrhythmia prior to, during, or immediately after an anesthetic is to treat the underlying cause. An arrhythmia should be thought of as a symptom: treat its cause and only treat the symptom if it is in itself dangerous. The importance of a rhythm disturbance, preoperatively, largely relates to the setting in which it occurs. For instance, premature ventricular beats may be more ominous in someone who has coronary artery disease as opposed to someone who is otherwise healthy. Rhythm disturbances intraoperatively, as discussed below may be caused by anesthetic drugs, surgical manipulation or unrecognized preoperative conditions (valvular disease or coronary artery disease).

When confronted with an arrhythmia postoperatively the anesthesiologist should do the following: he or she should review the patients history to ensure that important medical conditions were not missed preoperatively. Some important conditions might be 1) valvular heart disease; 2) coronary artery disease; 3) obstructive lung disease, and; 4) thyroid disease. The anesthesiologist should also determine the patient's functional class. For instance, a (New York Heart Association) class IV heart patient may not tolerate a rhythm disturbance. Whereas a class I patient may tolerate easily the same disturbance. In addition the anesthetic record should also be reviewed. The anesthesiologist should quickly examine the patient, paying particular attention to the patient's level of consciousness, temperature, hemodynamic status and adequacy of ventilation. A twelve lead electrocardiogram should be obtained. This will help to clarify a rhythm easier by looking at 12 different views (leads) rather than just one i.e. a rhythm strip. Whether treatment is indicated depends upon many considerations to be discussed.

Slow Rhythms

Many of the slow rhythm disturbances in and of themselves are benign and need no treatment. Possible exceptions could be seen in patients who have very stiff hearts and therefore have a significant portion of their cardiac output dependent on the booster pump function of the atrium.[37,38] When this mechanism is lost as in junctional rhythm disturbances or isorhythmic dissociation, blood pressure may precipitously decrease.[28,39] If this occurs intraoperatively, a change in anesthetic drug may be indicated.

Rapid Rhythms

The most common "fast" rhythm disturbances seen during anestheses are sinus tachycardia, and premature ventricular beats. Sinus tachycardia in general needs no treatment. A search for its cause is mandatory. Some common causes include "light" anesthesia, hypoxemia and hypercarbia from any cause. Depending upon the choice of anesthetic agent hypovolemia may or may not cause a sinus tachycardia. Rarely, after these entities are ruled out the sinus tachycardia may persist. Occasionally what one thought was sinus tachycardia is really atrial flutter or paroxysmal atrial tachycardia masquerading as such.

More commonly it may be a patient taking beta-blocker medication whose plasma drug level is decreasing. If the patient has coronary artery disease then treatment with beta-blockade is indicated. Generally speaking, cardiac glycosides are not good drugs to treat sinus tachycardia. Clearly if the sinus tachycardia is secondary to congestive heart failure, the administration of digoxin for instance

will result in slowing of the heart rate. But in this section, the poor pump function with subsequent low cardiac output leads to increased sympathetic tone causing the sinus tachycardia. With improvement in pump function, as would occur with the administration of a cardiac glycoside, and hence a decrease in sympathetic tone, the tachycardia will abate.

In other cases where the sinus tachycardia is not due to congestive heart failure, for instance fever of any cause or pain and anxiety (or rarely a sinus node reentrant tachycardia) cardiac glycosides will not slow the sinus rate. In these examples the sympathetic tone overwhelms any effect that the cardiac glycoside may have in slowing the heart rate. These drugs have been used to slow ventricular rate in patients with atrial fibrillation but not to slow ventricular rate (unless in heart failure) in patients in sinus rhythm who are tachycardic.[40,41] The reason is twofold: One, cardiac glycosides have little if any direct effect on the sinus node.[42] Also their vagal effect on the sinus node is *not very pronounced.*[43] Two, their effect in slowing ventricular rates in atrial fibrillation is largely due to superimposing their vagal effects on the AV junction *on top of* the effect that concealed conduction has on the effective refractory period of the AV junction.[42]

Concealed Conduction

Concealed conduction classically refers to the effects of incomplete penetration of the action potential into a part of the AV conduction system. The term was applied, and to some extent still is, to unexpected electrophysiologic phenomena observed on the surface electrogram, that were compatible with the effects of incompletely penetrating impulses. Now with the extensive use of intracardiac electrophysiologic recording, the presence of these impulses can be directly observed and recorded—hence they are in the strictest sense not truly concealed.

One of the classic manifestations of concealed conduction—the electrophysiologic effects of incomplete penetration of an impulse—is unexpected prolongation of conduction i.e. 1° AV block. In atrial fibrillation there is varying depth of penetration of the many wavefronts bombarding the AV junction. And in fact the AV junction may be bombarded by 400–600 stimuli per minute. However because of concealed conduction only 1 in 3 may be propagated to the ventricle. The slight increase in AV junction refractoriness caused by a cardiac glycosides vagal effects may be sufficient to result in 1 to 4 conduction. However, in 1 to 1 conduction, in the absence of concealed conduction, as occurs in sinus tachycardia, a slight increase in AV junction refractoriness is easily overridden by the increased sympathetic tone causing the sinus tachycardia. This really is not surprising. A patient who is in atrial fibrillation whose ventricular rate is well controlled with digoxin for instance will become quite tachycardic with minimal exercise (i.e., walking). The increased sympathetic tone easily overwhelms any slowing effect of digoxin.

One may ask why not give a lot of digoxin? The reason is that digoxin as is characteristic of all cardiac glycoside has a narrow therapeutic window. You certainly can give large amounts of the drug; but this will also increase the likelihood of rhythm disturbances secondary to the drug itself.

If one must treat a sinus tachycardia primarily the drugs of choice are the beta blockers. Unfortunately they are negative inotropic agents. Fortunately, esmolol, is a beta blocker with such a short serum half life that this drug probably can be safely used when in doubt about the patients hemodynamic status and how that patient would tolerate beta blockade.

Premature Ventricular Beats

Other than sinus tachycardia, (and sinus bradycardia), premature ventricular beats are probably the most common rhythm disturbance in the perioperative setting. What has been said for sinus tachycardia can also be said for premature ventricular beats: look for the cause. Patients who have premature ventricular beats preoperatively in the absence of demonstrable organic heart disease are not at increased risk from sudden cardiac death.[43] Obviously if these patients undergo anesthesia and surgery they very likely will have premature ventricular beats during surgery. There may be no need to treat these. It cannot be over emphasized that premature ventricular beats which are not present preoperatively but appear intraoperatively at a sufficiently "deep" level of anesthesia may signify hypoxemia, inadequate ventilation, or perhaps malignant hyperthermia. The occurrence of ventricular tachycardia is rare. This is a potentially serious disturbance that must be treated first and then seek its cause.

Atrioventricular Dissociation

Atrioventricular dissociation is not synonymous with AV block. It is not a primary rhythm disturbance per se. Normally, the ventricle will be under the control of the most rapidly firing pacemaker. Most often that is the sinus node. Atrioventricular dissociation is a physiologic response to either slowing of the sinus node or acceleration of other pacemakers. For instance, disease of the sinus node may cause marked sinus node slowing. The physiologic response to this would be for a normal junctional pacemaker to discharge at a rate of 60 and thereby control the ventricular rate. The atrium would probably be under control of the slow sinus rate. Therefore there would be atrioventricular dissociation secondary to marked sinus bradycardia. The primary pathology is not the atrioventricular dissociation but rather the **sinus bradycardia.** During ventricular tachycardia, the ventricles are frequently under control of a reentrant focus in the ventricle. The atria are under sinus control. This is by definition atrioventricular dissociation. But this is not the physio-pathology—**the ventricular tachycardia** is.

If the ventricles are beating slowly, much slower than the sinus node, we will again have atrioventricular dissociation. But in this case the atrioventricular dissociation is probably due to atrioventricular block—a pathological situation. An interesting variant of the above is isorhythmic atrioventricular dissociation. This phenomenon is rele-

vant to the anesthetic state because of the possible wide swings in arterial blood pressure—as the P wave appears to dance around the QRS complex.[28] The mechanism here is complex and is related to the interaction of vagal tone and arterial baroreceptors.[44]

Reentry and the "Sensitized" Myocardium

Kuner's data and the more recent data presented earlier seem to imply that anesthetics such as ether, cyclopropane and halothane are associated with a higher incidence of premature ventricular beats than other anesthetics. This has led to the frequently heard statement that halothane sensitizes the myocardium to endogenous and exogenous catecholamines. What are the proposed mechanisms?

The exact mechanisms are still largely unknown. Halothane depresses intraventricular conduction.[15,16,17] Hence, one condition for possible reentry is established. In the canine model at least, halothane has a marked slowing effect on the sinus node.[45] This would allow for the emergence of a ventricular pacemaker in response to epinephrine. Therefore, this mechanism is one of increased automaticity. However, the evidence for automaticity was found weak in another study.[46] Hence, by exclusion reentry was felt to be the mechanism of arrhythmogenesis, even though it could not be proved. However, the mechanism for arrhythmogenesis may be multifactorial. Depression of primary pacemakers and depression of conduction creates conditions that are conducive both to automatic rhythms and reentrant rhythms.[47] In addition triggered activity may also be involved.[15,47]

Elevations in blood pressure with subsequent stretch of latent pacemakers fibers is probably also a cause of ectopic foci induction during halothane anesthesia.[47,48] In many ways halothane can be thought of as an antiarrhythmic drug.[49] And like antiarrhythmics in general, it has proarrhythmic potential. A proarrhythmic drug is one that will induce arrhythmias that otherwise would not occur in the absence of the drug. Halothane will promote reentry as previously discussed. Hence, a condition for arrhythmogenesis exists. However, in infarcted hearts (in the dog) halothane tends to depress automaticity,[50] thereby acting as an antiarrhythmic. Hence, the halothane story, like so many other proarrhythmic and antiarrhythmic drugs, is indeed a complex one.

Halothane may have important interactive effects with nonanesthetic drugs. Halothane can depress digitalis induced ectopic pacemakers.[51] In addition, quinidine and halothane have synergistic actions on Purkinje fibers resulting in both prolongation of conduction time.[52] The clinical significance of this is not known.

Although the exact electrophysiologic mechanism of arrhythmogenesis with halothane remains unknown, myocardial α_1 adrenergic, and β_1 adrenergic receptors mediate the sensitization by halothane to the arrhythmogenic effects of catecholamines.[53] Halothane concentration does not alter the threshold for the development of catecholamine (epinephrine) induced ventricular arrhythmias.[54]

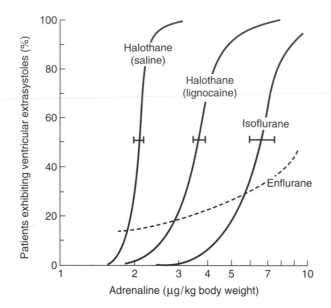

Fig. 7–7. Effect of different inhalation anesthetics in sensitizing the heart to adrenaline. Statistical analysis suggest that the two halothane and the isoflurane curves are parallel, and that the ED_{50}s for the production of arrhythmias are significantly different from each other (p. 01), but not the enflurane curve. The bars indicate the standard deviation from ED_{50}. (From Johnson et al.[56])

Other Inhalational Anesthetics55

Sensitization of the myocardium is seen to some extent with isoflurane and less so with enflurane.[56] In addition, lidocaine protects against the development of epinephrine induced ventricular arrhythmias, in the presence of halothane. This is probably true in the presence of isoflurane and also enflurane.[56]

Epinephrine: Interaction With Volatile Anesthetics—Arrhythmias[55]

During halothane anesthesia, ventricular arrhythmias frequently occur in adults. The incidence varies from 3–7% and is increased when exogenous adrenaline is administered.[57] The incidence also increases with increased $PaCO_2$.

The interaction of adrenaline during anesthesia with the commonly used volatile agents shows significant differences in the arrhythmic potential. The threshold concentration, that is, the lowest concentration at which *any* patient may develop an arrhythmia, shows halothane to sensitize the heart significantly more than either enflurane or isoflurane[55] (Fig. 7-7).[56] The ED_{50} for production of arrhythmias has been defined as the concentration of adrenaline administered submucosally, which produces three or more ventricular extrasystoles in 50% of patients. Low doses of adrenaline are effective in the presence of halothane, while enflurane is the least provocative of ventricular arrhythmia, and requires a dose five times[58] the ED_{50} of halothane and twice the ED_{50} of isoflurane (Table 7-2).

Lidocaine will increase the arrhythmia threshold and the provocative dose of epinephrine by two- to threefold.[59]

Table 7–1. Brief Classification of Rhythm Disturbances

Disturbances in impulse generation
  Disturbances in Automaticity
    Supraventricular arrhythmias
      Changes in vagal tone
      (1) Sinus arrhythmia
      (2) Sinus bradycardia
      Sinus tachycardia
      Nonparoxysmal junctional tachycardia
    Ventricular arrhythmias
      Idioventricular rhythms
      Parasystole
  Triggered Activity
    Toxic rhythms due to cardiac glycosides
    Multifocal atrial tachycardia
Distrubances in propagation or conduction
  Reentry
    Supraventricular arrhythmias
      Premature atrial beats
      Atrial flutter
      Atrial fibrillation
      Atrioventricular nodal reentry: paroxysmal junctional tachycardias
      Wolf—Parkinson—White syndrome
    Ventricular arrhythmias
      Premature ventricular beats
      Ventricular tachycardias
  Block
    Sinus
      SA block
      Sick Sinus Syndrome
    Atrioventricular block
      First degree
      Second degree
      (1) Mobitz type I
      (2) Mobitz type II
      Third degree
    Bundle branch block

Table 7–2. Adrenaline Doses Associated with Arrhythmias

Agent	Arrhythmic Threshold Dose ($\mu g\ kg^{-1}$)	ED_{se} Dose ($\mu g\ kg^{-1}$)
Halothane	1.8	2.1
Isoflurane	5.4	6.7
Enflurane	3.6	10.9

Johnston, R., Eger, E. I., Wilson, C.: *Anesth. Analg. 55*: 709, 1976. (Data from Johnston, Eger and Wilson (1976) and Horrigan, Eger and Wilson (1978)).

ANESTHETICS THAT AFFECT AV JUNCTIONAL CONDUCTION

Intravenous Drugs

As noted before, barbiturates prolong AV junctional conduction time.[17] Other than increasing the PR interval on surface electrocardiogram, heart rates very well could remain unchanged. However, sinus bradycardia and junctional rhythms are occasionally seen. Most often however due to perhaps some venodilation and the fact that many patients have mild volume deficits upon induction, sinus tachycardia will be seen. Barbiturates, in addition, may potentiate ventricular arrhythmias. Specifically thiopental has been found (in the dog) to potentiate epinephrine induced ventricular arrhythmias with enflurane and isoflurane.[60] Similar findings are seen with thiopental and halothane.[61] Ketamine increase sinus rate by its sympathetic stimulation and parasympathetic inhibition.[17]

Narcotics are generally associated with bradycardias. For instance, fentanyl which regularly causes a slowing of the sinus node, is felt to do this through its central stimulation of vagal cardioinhibitory centers.[17] In dogs fentanyl prolonged AV junction conduction.[62] However, when pancuronium is given after fentanyl, AV junction conduction increases as does heart rate.[62] Sufentanil is also associated with bradycardias.[63,64] Experience with alfentanil has shown little effect on heart rate.[65,66] Etomidate has little direct effect on cardiac rhythm in isolated hearts[67] but is frequently associated with sinus tachycardia shortly after tracheal intubation in the clinical setting.[68] Although propofol is not usually associated with disturbances in cardiac rhythm, propofol will depress cardiac excitability[67] and occasionally propofol will promote bradycardias partly by inhibiting the baroreceptor reflex.[69] Interestingly enough, this agent has also been implicated as one that can "sensitize" the (canine) myocardium.[70]

Muscle Relaxants

Succinylcholine can cause bradycardias. It is believed that succinylcholine acts as does acetylcholine, stimulating the pressor receptors in great vessel walls with secondary intense vagal stimulation.[17] Succinylcholine is also believed to have a direct action on the myocardium. It directly stimulates cholinergic receptors in the heart.[17] Most of the slow rhythm disturbances with succinylcholine usually include sinus bradycardia, junctional rhythms, and sinus arrest. An accelerated ventricular rhythm has been described after administration of a second dose of succinylcholine.[71] Succinylcholine has also been associated with ventricular arrhythmias. The genesis of this may be related to the presence of hypoxemia, hypercarbia, acidosis or inhalational anesthetic drugs which sensitize the myocardium.[72] This point is further emphasized by the fact that in the presence of hypoxemia and halothane, succinylcholine can induce premature ventricular beats and ventricular tachycardia. The mechanism for these ventricular rhythm disturbances is sympathetic stimulation.[73] These arrhythmias do not occur with enflurane anesthesia.

Pancuronium is frequently associated with increased sinus rates. This effect is largely due to its vagolytic activity because of its ability to block cardiac muscarinic receptors.[17] In addition, AV conduction can also be enhanced by pancuronium. This effect may be important clinically—especially in patients with coronary artery disease. The increased heart rate with pancuronium may cause ischemic events.[74] In the setting of fentanyl anesthesia vecuronium is associated with sinus bradycardias.[75,76] Atracurium has little effect on sinus rates;[76] although bradycardias after its use have been reported.[77]

Spinal Anesthesia

Subarachnoid block to the T_5 level in normovolemic patients will produce a sinus bradycardia.[78] The mechanisms of sinus bradycardia and other bradyarrhythmias is multifactorial. The decreased venous return and subsequent low right atrial pressure may produce a vagal discharge.[79] In addition, spinal block at this level could conceivably block the efferent cardiac sympathetic nerves (T_1–T_5). This may be particularly true when one considers the fact that sympathetic blockade occurs several segments above the level of the sensory blockade. The bradyarrhythmias that normally occur are most often benign.

However, unexpected catastrophic cardiac events have been reported during subarachnoid block in healthy volunteers[79] and otherwise healthy patients.[80] In these events, often there was a preceding bradyarrhythmia. Some patients exhibited true asystole; implying total failure of escape of subsidiary pacemakers. How many of these patients were really in fine ventricular fibrillation cannot be determined. The cause of these events is not clear. Certainly the likelihood of unrecognized hypoxemia must strongly be considered. And in fact there seemed to be a relationship between verbal nonresponsiveness due to sedation and the detection of cyanosis. Therefore it would seem prudent to frequently evaluate the patient's state of consciousness in those patients undergoing spinal anesthesia. Also evaluation of the level of the block should occur throughout the case. We would like to believe that the universal use of pulse oximetry will make these uncommon events even more uncommon.

RHYTHM DISTURBANCES NOT ASSOCIATED WITH ANESTHETICS

Arrhythmias in the perioperative period can be caused by factors other than the anesthetic drugs per se.

Sinus bradycardias can frequently be seen in the presence of intrinsic disease of the sinus node, or increased intracranial pressure or secondary to other drugs (betablockers, cardiac glycosides). Reflex responses may be elicited during the surgery itself, for instance, stimulation of the oral pharynx during intubation; or tugging of the peritoneum during surgery. Fast rhythm disturbance can be seen with electrolyte disturbance, hypoxemia, hypercarbia, pain or hyperthermia. Causes of the rhythm disturbance from surgical manipulation can interact with the causes of rhythm disturbances due to the anesthetic drugs per se. For instance, tugging on the peritoneum may cause a more profound bradycardia in the presence of narcotic anesthesia with vecuronium for muscle relaxation, than inhalation anesthesia with pancuronium for muscle relaxation.

Ventricular ectopic beats may be seen preoperatively in the setting of hypokalemia. In addition, it is believed that preoperative hypokalemia predisposes to potentially life threatening arrhythmias during general anesthesia, although this has never been documented. It has been found however that in patients with moderate levels of hypokalemia (2.6–3.4 mEq/L) who are not taking cardiac glycosides, and in the absence of serious heart disease, hypokalemia per se is not a risk factor for the occurrence of intraoperative arrhythmia.[81] In addition the same conclusion can be applied to patients who are chronically hypokalemic but in addition have serious heart disease and are taking cardiac glycosides.[82] Hence, the general practice of ensuring normal potassium values in all hypokalemic patients scheduled for elective surgery is certainly now open to question. It seems reasonable at this point in time to proceed with elective surgery in patients who are otherwise well and have mild to moderate levels of hypokalemia. Whether hypokalemia per se is a risk factor for sudden death in the perioperative setting (for instance ventricular fibrillation could occur without any premonitory signs of other rhythm disturbances) would require enormous numbers of patients to answer this question.

Supraventricular Rhythm Disturbances

Any rhythm disturbance is of concern because it frequently is a sign of underlying systemic disease. Common rhythm disturbances of the supraventricular type that are encountered in the perioperative period are 1) atrial fibrillation, and 2) premature atrial beats.

Atrial Fibrillation

Atrial Fibrillation (atrial flutter) (Figs. 7–8, 7–9, 7–10) is usually seen in the presence of organic heart disease or other systemic disease. Frequently encountered "causes" are a) mitral valve disease, b) coronary artery disease, c) "sick sinus syndrome," d) obstructive pulmonary disease, e) hyperthyroidism. This list is by no means all inclusive but points to the fact that the anesthesiologist must ask the question "in what setting does this patient have atrial fibrillation?" Rarely patients may have atrial fibrillation in the absence of demonstrable organic heart disease or systemic disease, so-called lone atrial fibrillation.

Atrial fibrillation is the most common supraventricular tachyarrhythmia in hospitalized adults after surgery.[83] The occurrence of this rhythm as well as other supraventricular tachycardias, postoperatively, does not correlate with a preoperative history of heart disease, obstructive lung disease or preoperative atrial beats.[83] The key to the management of this disturbance once the underlying cause has been defined is, whether the underlying cause is controlled? If the answer is yes, the next question to ask is "should the patient be restored to sinus rhythm?" The reason for this question is that atrial fibrillation in and of itself is associated with decreased long term survival.[84] This is probably due to the occurrence of thromboembolism. Often times restoration to sinus rhythm is impossible. Then the key is, to control the ventricular rate appropriately before undergoing elective surgery. Beta blockers and or cardiac glycosides may be used to control the ventricular rate. We now know that cardiac glycosides by themselves will not convert patients with atrial fibrillation to sinus rhythm.[85] We also now know that cardiac glycosides are not effective for suppressing recurrences of atrial fibrillation.[86]

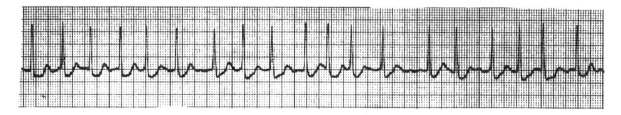

Fig. 7–8. Atrial fibrillation. The key to diagnosis is to note that the ventricular rate is 'irregularly irregular.'

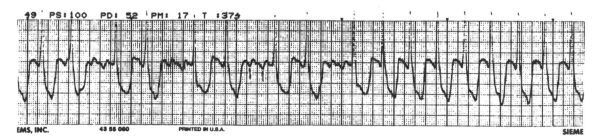

Fig. 7–9. Atrial flutter with variable block. Arrows show flutter waves. Generally speaking the treatment of choice for this rhythm disturbance is electrical cardioversion.

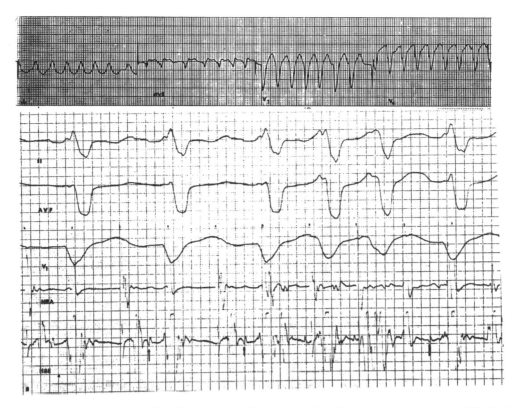

Fig. 7-10. A. Wide QRS complex tachycardia. The rhythm is slightly irregularly irregular suggesting atrial fibrillation with a bundle branch block. However, given the wide QRS complex it may well be ventricular tachycardia. B. His bundle recording (HBE) shows a His spike (arrow) prior to QRS complex. Therefore this is a supraventricular tachycardia—specifically atrial fibrillation and not ventricular tachycardia.

Preoperative Prophylaxis of Atrial Fibrillation

Another issue that the anesthesiologist will often face is whether a patient who is scheduled for a thoracotomy should be given cardiac glycosides (digitoxin or digoxin) for prophylaxis against atrial fibrillation and other postoperative supraventricular rhythm disturbances. These rhythm disturbances are fairly common after this type of surgery.[87,88] Several authors have suggested that the incidence of supraventricular rhythm disturbances could be reduced by preoperative digitalization.[87-89] And certainly if not reduced, the ventricular rate in patients who were prophylactically 'digitalized' would be slower in the face of a postoperative supraventricular rhythm disturbances than if they were not prophylactically 'digitalized'. However, one study[90] actually showed an increase in post operative rhythm disturbances in those patients receiving 'prophylactic digitalization'.

One must appreciate the following pharmacologic character of all cardiac glycosides: (1) They are drugs with a narrow therapeutic window. (2) They are mild inotropes. (3) Large doses of these drugs may be necessary to slow the ventricular response in the setting of atrial flutter or fibrillation. (4) They can be proarrhythmic. Therefore prophylactic 'digitalization' is of questionable benefit and should not be used routinely in patients undergoing thoracotomy unless there are other indications for their use.

Premature Atrial Beats

Premature atrial beats may also be seen in the presence of organic heart disease, but they are also frequently seen in normal people. In and of themselves they are benign. Frequent premature atrial beats may be premonitory to the onset of a supraventricular tachycardia—although this was not borne out in one study.[83]

Preexcitation Syndromes

In 1970 Durrer at al gave the following definition.[91] "Preexcitation exists, if in relation to atrial events, the whole or some part of the ventricular muscle is activated earlier by the impulse originating from the atrium than would be expected if the impulse reached the ventricles by way of the normal specific conduction system only." Characteristic of these syndromes is premature activation of the ventricular musculature.

Anatomical Basis

Studies have identified five principle accessory pathways to the normal conduction system. By these paths, impulses can pass from the atrium to the ventricle and activate a part of or the whole ventricle before the normal impulse arrives (Table 7-3).[92]

Table 7–3. Old and New Nomenclature of Accessory Connections*

Nomenclature			
Old	Symbol in Fig 1	New	Connections
Kent's bundle	K	Accessory atrioventricular pathway	Atrium to ventricle
Mahaim fiber	M_1	Nodoventricular pathway*	Atrioventricular node to ventricle
Mahaim fiber	M_2	Fasciculoventricular pathway	His bundle or bundle branch to ventricle
Atrio-Hissian fiber	A	Atriofascicular bypass tract	Atrium to His bundle
James fiber	J	Intranodal bypass tract	Atrium to atrioventricular node

*The fiber may insert into the bundle branch and is then called a *nodofascicular fiber.*
From Wellens, H. J. J., Brugada, P., Penn, O. C.: *JAMA,257*:2325, 1987.

Mechanism

A normal impulse spreads from the sinus node through the atrium to the A-V node, undergoes delay and then passes via the His bundle to the Purkinje system. But in pre-excitation syndromes, an impulse is carried simultaneously via anomalous conduction pathways originating in the atrium, which enter low in the A-V node or which bypass the A-V node and, without A-V delay, reach the ventricular musculature before the normal impulse. The most common dysrhythmia in these syndromes is paroxysmal supraventricular tachycardia.

Any event that increases the rate of conduction over the anamlous pathway will produce ventricular tachycardia. Events which decrease the effective refractory period will permit retrograde conduction and atrial dysrhythmias. The most common developing dysrhythmia is a paroxysmal supraventricular tachycardia.

Incidence[92]

By far, the most common type of extra connection between the atrium and the ventricle is the accessory atrioventricular pathway or bundle of Kent. It also leads to the most common disorder, the WPW Syndrome. The true incidence is unknown; reports vary from 0.1–3.0% per 1,000 ECG's (Chung).

Recognized Syndromes[92]

Three types of pre-excitation syndrome are clinically recognized (Fig. 7–11). The classic form is the Wolff-Parkinson-White syndrome. A sinus impulse is conducted simultaneously down the normal path and the anomalous bundle of Kent pathway. Ventricular excitation is usually a composite of the two impulses, which produce a fusion beat. In the electrocardiogram, the PR interval is short (0.12 sec), but the QRS is prolonged with an elevation in the PQ segment, called a delta wave, replacing the normal Q. In all precordial leads, the vector of the delta wave is upright and the QRS resembles right bundle branch block (RBBB) (K in Fig. 7–11). This is the common ECG pattern of WPW, in which the path of impulses crosses the A-V sulcus on the left. In Type B traces, the Kent fibers preexcite the lateral margin of the right ventricle and produce a negative delta wave.

A frequent variant is LGL (Lown-Ganong-Levine) syndrome, in which the anomalous path is the James-Lev fibers, which may enter the low part of the AV node or bypass the A-V node to enter high in the His-bundle (J in Fig. 7–11). There is a short PR interval, but a normal QRS complex. The time gap between the arrival of normal and premature impulse is shorter than in WPW. The arrhythmia most commonly seen in this syndrome is atrial flutter-fibrillation with rapid conduction over accessory path.

A less common variant is due to the presence of Mahaim fibers, which arise at a lower part of the A-V node (M_1 fibers) or which arise in the H-s bundle (M_2) but pass directly to the ventricular muscle (M in Fig. 7–11). There is usually a normal PR interval, but a delta wave appears in the QRS complex.

These conditions are significant in causing serious tachycardias and in being associated with cardiac anomalies (Ebstein's anomaly, balloon mitral valve, coronary artery disease). Because of the anomalous pathways, patients are subject to episodes of arrhythmias.

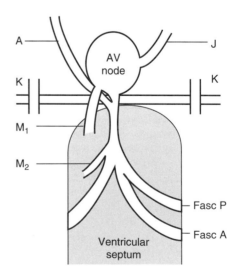

Fig. 7–11. Scheme of atrioventricular conduction system and possible accessory connection(s) partially or totally bypassing that system. A indicates atrioventricular bypass tract; J, Intranodal bypass tract; K, accessory atrioventricular pathway; M_1, nodoventricular pathway; M_2, fasciculoventricular pathway; Fasc P, fasciculus posticus of left bundle branch; and Fasc A, fasciculus anticus of left bundle branch. Redrawn from Wellens H. J. J., Brugada P., Penn O. C.: JAMA *257*:2325, 1987.

Associated Tachyarrhythmias

The most frequent arrhythmia in the WPW syndrome is a reciprocal supraventricular tachycardia.[92] This is the classic orthodromic circus movement tachycardia using the AV-Node-His pathway for antegrade conduction and the accessory pathway for retrograde conduction.

An antidromic circus movement tachycardia may also occur. In this situation, the A-V conduction is primary over the accessory pathway, while retrograde conduction from ventricle to atrium over His-AV node path occurs over the normal path i.e., in the reverse direction.

A regular ventricular tachycardia of 120–130 beats/min may be seen. This is often accompanied by chest pain, congestive heart failure or syncope.

The origin of the ventricular tachycardia may also be due to atrial fibrillation which ensues from the retrograde conduction up the accessory pathway and this, in turn, may induce rapid antegrade conduction with development of ventricular tachycardia.

In the LGL syndrome, atrial flutter/fibrillation is most frequently seen. It is of the re-entrant type with retrograde conduction over the James fibers to the atrium.

General Management

Quinidine and procainamide are the principle drugs used to increase block in the anomalous pathway. Propanolol and digitalis increase the refractory period of the normal path and block re-entry. Digitalis, however, may shorten the refractory period of the anomalous paths and should not be used if atrial fibrillation is present.

Anesthetic Management[93]

Stimulation of the sympathetic system must be avoided. Physiologic, pharmacologic and psychologic stresses must be minimized.

- All preoperative medication for cardiac control must be continued.
- Preanesthetic medication should include a sedative (barbiturate) or tranquilizer (Diazepam) and morphine or a morphinone derivative. Meperidine and its derivatives are not recommended because of their negative inotropic effect.
- As part of preanesthetic medication and prior to induction of anesthesia, droperidol may be administered in doses of 250 ug/kg.[94] This drug has been found to prevent the typical tachyarrhythmias of WPW. Both the antegrade and retrograde effective refractory period of the accessory pathways are increased. Neither fentanyl nor diazepam modify the conduction system nor refractory period in this condition (Gomez-Arnau).
- An anticholinergic is recommended, such as scopolamine or glycopyrrolate. Atropine has been used safely in very small doses. These drugs have some therapeutic advantages, since they usually produce normal A-V conduction with disappearance of delta wave and prevent tachycardias (rates over 120 beats/min).
- Induction to a stage of sleep with thiopental is safe at doses up to 3 mg/kg. Midazolam is equally recommended and has other advantage.

- Anesthetization and maintenance with an inhalation anesthetic is recommended. Enflurane is the recommended anesthetic, administered in a nitrous oxide-oxygen mixture.[95] Enflurane blocks chromaffin cell membranes and reduces sympathetic out-flow, and is preferred. It prolongs A-V nodal conduction without prolonging His-Purkinje conduction. Halothane may sensitize the myocardium to adrenergic stimulation, but prolongs His-Purkinje conduction in contrast to enflurane, thereby favoring ventricular arrhythmias and is not recommended.[96]
- For muscle relaxation, vecuronium or atracurium are preferred. D-tubocurarine can be used. Pancuronium is prone to cause tachyarrhythmias and is not recommended. Succinylcholine is associated with K^+ release and disturbances of cardiac rhythm and should be avoided.
- For a paroxysmal supraventricular tachycardia, phenylephrine will abolish the dysrhythmia; the mechanism involves stimulation of arterial baroreceptors with enhanced vagal output.[97]
- Other technics of conversion of tachyarrhythmias may be used. These include carotid sinus massage, calcium channel block (verapamil 5.0 mg doses repeated), edrophonium and procainamide synchronized cardioversion up to 200 watt/sec.

The Wolff-Parkinson-White Syndrome (Fig. 7–12)

As noted earlier, this syndrome can be associated with rapid supraventricular arrhythmias. Atrial fibrillation in this syndrome can be particularly devastating due to the exceedingly rapid ventricular rates. The successful anesthetic management of these patients depends on avoiding tachyarrhythmias by avoiding sympathetic stimulation.[91] An understanding of this syndrome requires that one know the effects of various anesthetics on the refractory periods of the accessory pathways. Thiopental and Vecuronium do not affect the refractory period of the accessory pathways. Neither does diazepam or fentanyl. Droperidol does increase the antegrade and retrograde refractory periods of the accessory pathways, and hence may be a useful drug in preventing tachyarrhythmias.[93] If tachyarrhythmias do occur, generally speaking, a beta-blocker is a useful drug for treatment.[91] All cardiac glycosides by shortening the refractory period of the accessory pathways, are contraindicated in the presence of atrial fibrillation, or in patients with a history of atrial fibrillation. One should know however, that asymptomatic patients with this syndrome have a good prognosis. It seems a considerable number of these patients lose their capacity for antegrade conduction over the accessory pathway thereby making it less likely that they develop life threatening rapid ventricular rates.[98]

Ventricular Rhythm Disturbances

Premature Ventricular Beats

Of more serious concern is the evaluation of patients with premature ventricular beats. This is a complex issue in cardiomyopathies, and valvular heart disease. It is im-

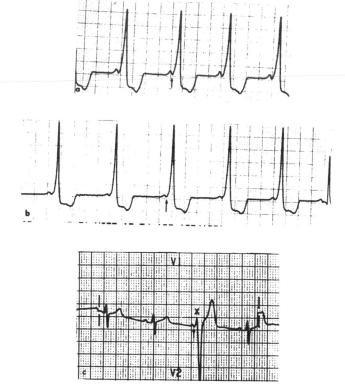

Fig. 7–12. Wolf-Parkinson-White Syndrome. a) Electrocardiographic tracing from lead I. b) Tracing from lead V_5. c) Intermittent WPW. Complex 'x' was originally misinterpreted to be a PVB. In all three panels the arrow depicts the characteristic delta wave—the electrocardiographic manifestation of early depolarization leading to the short PR interval.

portant to realize that premature ventricular beats may be seen in patients who otherwise have no clinical evidence of organic heart disease.[99] Cardiac catheterization of these people will reveal slight abnormalities in myocardial function,[100,101] but most will have normal coronary anatomy.[101] Should they be treated with antiarrhythmic drugs just because they are about to undergo an anesthetic-surgical experience? There are no studies that address this issue, but the answer is no. Treatment of these patients with potentially toxic antiarrhythmic drugs such as quinidine just to suppress ectopic activity may do more harm than good.[102] What about acute suppression with lidocaine intraoperatively? Again, there are no hard and fast answers.

The patient who has ventricular ectopy in the presence of organic heart disease presents a different set of problems. Clearly, the goal here is to try as best one can to treat the underlying cause. That underlying cause can range from uncontrolled hypertension to severe coronary artery disease. The dilemma here is that suppression of premature ventricular beats in and of themselves is not necessarily correlated with prevention of ventricular tachycardia.[103] Complex ventricular ectopic activity is associated with a high risk of sudden cardiac death.[104] But the absence of such activity does not rule out the possibility of sudden cardiac death.[104,105]

Preventing Sudden Cardiac Death

Antiarrhythmic drugs used to prevent sudden cardiac death by preventing ventricular fibrillation or ventricular tachycardia may be helpful despite the lack of suppression of chronic premature ventricular beats.[106] The issues are quite complex. Overall, the benefits of antiarrhythmic drug treatment in preventing sudden death have not been proved.[107] In fact only one class of drugs has been found to improve long term survival after myocardial infarction. That is the beta-blockers.[107] This efficacious effect does not appear to be related to any antiarrhythmic effect of beta-blockers per se.[108]

One must also realize that the commonly used antiarrhythmic drugs (except for lidocaine) are all potentially arrhythmogenic[109-111] (Table 7-4). This feature is emphasized by the sudden partial discontinuation of the Cardiac Arrhythmia Suppression Trial (CAST).[112] This study was designed to determine whether antiarrhythmic drugs could reduce cardiac death in post-myocardial infarction patients with ventricular arrhythmias. Three antiarrhythmic drugs were evaluated. Two of them were encainide and flecainide. The part of the study using these drugs was stopped when it was found that those patients receiving encainide and flecainide had a much higher death rate than the placebo group. Some of these patients died of arrhythmia thereby implying a proarrhythmic effect of these drugs.

In addition to any proarrhythmic effects, drugs such as quinidine, procainamide, mexiletine, and amiodarone exhibit many clinically significant side effects. These include

Table 7–4. Common Classification of Drugs Used to Treat Arrhythmias

Principle Mechanism	Example
Depresses Phase O Depolarization	
Membrane Stabilizers	
(Sodium Channel Block)	
A (Moderate)	Quinidine
	Procainamide
	Disopyramide
B (Weak)	Aprindine
	Tocainide
	Mixiletine
	Lidocaine
C (Strong)	Encainide*
	Flecanide*
	Propanfenone
Beta-Blockers	Propranolol
Beta-adrenergic Antagonists	Esmolol
	Sotalol†
Prolonged Repolarization	Amiodarone
Antiadrenergic	Bretylium
Calcium Channel Blockers	Verapamil

*No longer on the market.
†Also has Class III properties.
Modified from Nestico, P. F., DePace, N. L., and Morganroth, J.: Therapy with conventional antiarrhythmic drugs for ventricular arrhythmias. Medical Clinics of North America, 1984; 68:1297.

nausea, fever, lupus like syndrome, hypotension, pulmonary infiltrates, ataxia, and hypothyroidism.[113] Therefore the key for the anesthesiologist is to determine what is the setting that the premature ventricular beats are in. If the patient is known to be otherwise healthy, then premature ventricular beats are probably of little consequence in the perioperative period. If however, this is not the case, the problem is as stated, a complex one. Cardiology consultation may be helpful in sorting this problem out.

Atrio-Ventricular Blocks

Atrio-ventricular dissociation, as stated before, implies that the atrium and ventricle are dissociated i.e. each under the control of different pacemakers. It can be physiologic—namely the ventricle under junctional control in the face of a marked sinus bradycardia or pathologic or due to block. We will focus now on the rhythm disturbance due to AV block. In passing it should be pointed out that many of the things said about AV block may also be said about SA block.

Type I Second—Degree AV-Block

This type of block is characterized by progressive prolongation of the P-R interval until a P wave is no longer conducted to the ventricle (Fig. 7-13). This is the classic Wenckebach pattern of progressive prolongation of the P-R interval so that the R-R intervals become progressively shorter. Generally the conduction delay is in the AV junction. Subsidiary pace makers are stable; so generally speaking pacemakers are not indicated unless the ventricular rate is very slow and no response to atropine is seen. Occasionally a type I phenomenon may occur within the His-Purkinje system.[114] This may progress to complete heart block and therefore a pacemaker is indicated. However, this phenomenon is uncommon and His bundle studies are needed for diagnosis.

Type II Second—Degree AV—Block

This type of block is distinguished by an unexpected blocked P wave on the surface electrocardiogram. The PR intervals remain constant as well as the RR intervals. The block here is typically below the His bundle.[114] Type II AV block usually progresses to complete heart block. Therefore permanent pacemaking is recommended even if the patient is asymptomatic.

High Degree AV Block

By high degree AV block we mean 2:1, 3:1 AV conduction ratio. The block may be in the AV junction, bundle of His or even the bundle branch-Purkinje system. Often times it is impossible to tell from the surface electrogram whether the block is type I (localized to the AV junctional region) or type II (block below the His bundle). Narrow QRS complexes in conducted beats imply type I. Bundle branch block in conducted beats suggest type II.[114]

Atrio-Ventricular Dissociation Secondary to Complete Heart Block

If complete heart block is due to block in the AV junction, the ventricles will be driven by a junctional pacemaker. These pacemakers are relatively stable. When complete heart block is due to block within or below the His bundle, the ventricle will be under the control of pacemaker tissue localized to the His bundle or distal Purkinje system (Fig. 7-14). These pacemakers are unstable. A permanent pacemaker is indicated.

It is now felt that ischemia induced AV block may be mediated by adenosine which has been released from hypoxic myocardial cells.[115] Therefore, in this setting the known adenosine antagonist aminophylline—may have a therapeutic role.[116,117]

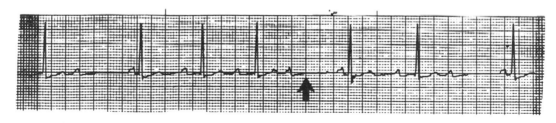

Fig. 7–13. Type I AV block with characteristic prolongation of PR intervals and subsequently dropped ventricular beat (arrow).

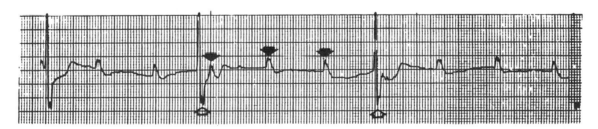

Fig. 7–14. A-V dissociation secondary to complete heart block. The atria are under control of a sinus pacemaker. The ventricles are under control of a ventricular pacemaker. Even though the atrial rate is much faster than the ventricular rate, there is no ventricular capture, i.e. there is complete block. (Solid arrows depict atrial activity; clear arrows denote QRS complex.)

Bundle Branch Block, Bifascicular and Trifascicular Block

In patients presenting for surgery with either chronic right or left bundle branch block, there is little chance that the block will acutely progress to complete heart block. In one situation this may not (at least theoretically) be so. That is in patients who have a left bundle branch block who also need the insertion of a pulmonary artery catheter. In these patients causing right bundle branch block will lead to acute complete heart block. However, the incidence of the phenomenon appears to be quite low. In fact, in one very large series[109] the incidence of inducing complete heart block with a pulmonary artery catheter in patients with preexisting left bundle branch block was less than 1% (1 out of 113).

In asymptomatic patients with chronic bifascicular block undergoing elective surgery temporary pacemaking is not indicated.[119] This is probably also true for chronic trifascicular block.[120] However, if a patient has transient symptoms such as syncopal episodes or vertigo then pacemaking may be indicated. This depends on many things including the results of electrophysiologic studies.

The occurrence of type I block preoperatively or intraoperatively may often be due to medications such as cardiac glycosides or beta-blockers. In and of itself this is normally quite benign and usually can be ignored. Type II block on the other hand has a much more ominous significance; implying the need for artificial pacemaking.

Pacemaker-Mediated Rhythm Disturbances

A three letter code for describing pacemaker function was initiated in 1974 by the Pacemaker Study Group of the Intersociety Commission for Heart Disease Resources.[121] The first letter represents the chamber paced: that is V (ventricular), A (atrium), or D (both). The second letter refers to the chamber sensed, for instance V, A, D, or O (absent sensing). The third letter describes the mode of response: T (triggered), I (inhibited), D (both), or O (asynchronous). Currently two additional letters have been added to describe programmable functions and anti-tachycardiac functions,[122] but as of yet are not widely used.

The classic concern of rhythm disturbances occurring with pacemakers had to do with radio frequency inhibition of normally functioning VVI pacemakers. The result would be to inhibit the pacemaker causing failure to discharge. If the patient's underlying rhythm was a serious bradycardia or complete heart block, the results could be catastrophic. Therefore it is useful to know the reasons the pacemaker was inserted. Fortunately, in our experience, most patients with cardiac pacemakers, are not pacemaker dependent. The options presented to the anesthesiologist consist of the following: 1) Use a magnet to convert the VVI pacemaker to the VOO mode. 2) Make sure that the surgical unit's return electrode is as far away from the pulse generator as possible. 3) Use low energy settings. Other options include limiting the frequency and duration of use of the electrosurgical unit.

Practically speaking with the latest generation of VVI pacemakers these problems were not as serious as first thought since sophisticated filter circuits are employed to screen out extraneous signals such as radiofrequency. Also if the radiofrequency signals do interfere with later generation pacemakers, they convert to the VOO mode. Problems with these pacemakers can occasionally get quite complex. For instance, one case report describes a particular pacemaker where the magnet did not convert the pacemaker to the VOO mode.[123] With multiprogrammable pacemakers things are even more complicated. The use of a magnet in some models activates a receiver that receives rate programming instructions. Hence, in the presence of extraneous radiofrequency signals, the use of a magnet could reprogram some of the pacemakers in an unpredictable manner.[124] The only way really to know the effect of magnet activation for program reception and radiofrequency signals is to check the manual of that particular pacemaker. Hence, it may become important to know the brand and model number of the patient's particular pacemaker.

However, pacemaker technology is getting so complex that if the anesthesiologist is confused, then by all means consult your cardiology colleague. Prior to checking with your cardiology colleague there are some things an anesthesiologist should know about pacemaker patients: One, most of these patients carry a card in their wallet describing the type of pacemaker, and when it was inserted. Two, chest x-ray pacemaker profiles are distributed by pacemaker manufacturers. Cardiology departments usually have a few. Three, most pacemaker manufacturers keep a registry of all patients who have received their products.

Dual Chamber Pacemakers

These can actually mediate rhythm disturbances. A commonly described rhythm disturbance in the DDD mode is artificial circus movement tachycardia (Pacemaker Mediated Tachycardia, PMT). In this mode it is possible that a premature ventricular beat may be conducted retrogradely to the atrium generating a retrograde P wave which will be sensed as an atrial event leading to ventricular discharge at the programmed AV interval. The resulting QRS complex again will be conducted retrogradely and the cycle will repeat itself, leading to a rapid repetitive rhythm disturbance, often at the programmed upper rate limit of the pacemaker[125] (Fig. 7-15). This problem can be handled in two ways: 1) increase the atrial refractory period of the pacemaker beyond the retrograde VA conduction time (post ventricular atrial refractory period—PVARP), 2) reprogram the DDD pacemaker to a mode where atrial events are not sensed i.e., DOO, DVI or VVI. Some late generation models automatically extend the atrial refractory period of the pacemaker following a premature ventricular beat. In addition, some actually terminate the reentry circuit by failing to pace for one beat in the ventricle.

Pacemaker mediated tachycardia, can also occur by mechanisms other than a reentry loop as described above. It is possible for the pacemaker sensing circuits to interpret various extraneous signals as its own atrial events thereby leading to ventricular discharge at the rate

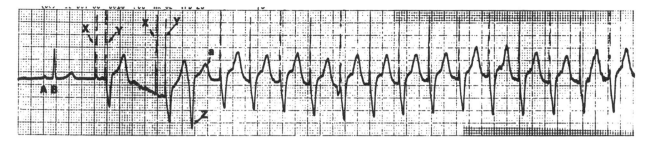

Fig. 7–15. DDD Pacemaker with PMT. A, sinus p wave. B, normal QRS complex. X, atrial spike. Y, ventricular spike. Z, PVB; 'a' denotes retrograde p wave. The retrograde p wave is sensed as a atrial event which subsequently activates the ventricular circuit leading to a ventricular spike and ventricular activation with retrograde conduction. The cycle repeats generating a PMT.

of those signals. This has been reported with the use of somatosensory evoked potentials.[126] Namely the pacemaker discharge rate tracked the somatosensory stimulus—although not in a 1:1 relation.

In our experience, patients with pacemakers scheduled for surgery do not present a major problem. However, one possible adverse consequence of surgery should be kept in mind. A significant percentage of patients will, unbeknownst to themselves or their physicians, have their pacemakers unintentionally reprogrammed due to the electrocautery used during the surgery.[127]

Automated Internal Cardioverter Defibrillators

Automated internal cardioverter defibrillators (AICD) are being used more frequently in patients with life threatening rhythm disturbances not responsive to other measures.[128,129] Some patients with AICDs will come for surgery for reasons other than their heart problem. Here in lies a potential problem. Radiofrequency waves, generated by the electrosurgical unit can be sensed by the AICD as a rapid ventricular rate. This will cause the device to discharge even though the patient may be in sinus rhythm. For this reason we deem it appropriate that the device be deactivated during the surgery. Application of adhesive defibrillator pads directly to the patient's chest and attached to an external defibrillator, will allow for external defibrillation if necessary. The internal defibrillator patches could theoretically shield the heart from shocks from an external defibrillator. Therefore we recommend that the external pads be placed in an anterior—posterior fashion. Now it is important to keep in mind, that when the AICD is deactivated, that the patient is attached to a working defibrillator and monitor. And, that in fact qualified medical personnel are watching the monitor at all times.

Athlete's Heart ("Vagotonia of Atheletes")

Intensive and prolonged isotonic "aerobic" physical training programs frequently result in the "athlete's heart". During training, the following body adjustments occur: increase in skeletal muscle mass, increase in blood volume, increase in myocardial mass and continuous adaptation of the autonomic nervous system to produce adjustments of cardiovascular and pulmonary function.

Cardiomegaly is evident on X ray. Both right and left ventricles are enlarged. The left ventricular wall thickens and cavity size is increased up to 20%.

Clinically, a slow heart rate due to high resting vagal tone is evident in athletes.[130] At rest, a rate of 30–60 beats is common. The stroke volume is increased. During exercise, the heart rate does increase, but not to the same extent as in an untrained individual. The ejection fraction is high and on exercising there is further increase in stroke volume and cardiac output.

The ECG at rest is frequently abnormal. There are large QRS complexes. In precordial leads, the depolarization R and S waves are of a high amplitude. The repolarization ST segment is elevated and the T wave may be low or inverted. U-waves are often seen.[131] At rest, the rhythm is usually sinus, but it may be irregular. A marked sinus arrhythmia, often present, is indicated of high vagal tone. The rate regularized with exercise. There may be an exaggerated sinus bradycardia or a wandering atrial pacemaker. First degree heart block (impaired conduction usually in the AV node with a PR interval greater than 0.2 second); or second-degree Mobitz I (Wenckebach) due to progressive delay in AV node conduction until a beat is blocked before resuming conduction (the PR interval becomes progressively longer and then a P-wave is not conducted to the ventricle). This is generally benign in marathoners.[132] Some have symptomatic bradycardia at rest.

Bradycardias seen at rest are attributed to increased vagal tone. Also, local changes in myocardium may make the neurogenic mechanisms less sensitive to sympathetic influences and normal vagal tone dominant. It should be appreciated that other systems, such as the gastrointestinal and respiratory systems, do not show enhanced vagal activity. Exercise often reverts these abnormal rhythms to normal rhythms. In the differential diagnosis, the sick sinus syndrome should be considered. Atropine does not distinguish between the two, but exercise results in complete improvement in the sinus node function of the athlete's vagotonia and regularization of the sinus rate. The sinus node often continues to malfunction in those with sick sinus syndrome ("chronotropic incompetence") malfunctioning.

When symptoms occur, such as syncope at rest or minor cerebral symptoms, fatigue, or dizziness, theophylline may be considered or an anticholingeric drug such as transdermal scopolamine or oral disopyramide. Rarely, a pacemaker is needed.

Sinus Node Dysfunction (Sick Sinus Syndrome)

This syndrome, first so termed by Ferrer in 1968,[133] consists of three features: (1) symptoms of dizziness, feelings of light headedness, occasional symptoms of syncope and diaphoresis, and complaints of palpitations; (2) an abnormally slow pulse on examination (at least below 60 BPM); (3) electrocardiographic confirmation of sinus bradycardia, sinoatrial block (first, second and third degree), alternating brady- and tachyarrhythmias, and/or carotid hypersensitivity. More than 100,000 Americans are affected, approximately one-third having serious symptoms.

Causes of Dysfunction

Dysfunction of the sinus node may occur during the course of reversible illnesses or from chronic irreversible sinus node disease (Table 7–5). Pathophysiologic mechanisms are either intrinsic disturbances in electrophysiologic properties of sinus pacemaker cells or disturbances in extrinsic regulation. The latter includes autonomic nervous system dysfunction with blockade in the perinodal buffer zone, disturbed coronary blood flow (sinus node artery originates from proximal 2–3 cm of right coronary artery in 55% of subjects and from proximal 1.0 cm of left circumflex artery in 45% of subjects), and endocrine dis-

turbances. Many pharmacologic causes are recognized but are self-limited (Table 7–6).

Pathogenesis and Clinical Course[134]

In the early stages of the sick sinus syndrome, there is progressive decreased sinus node (P cell) automaticity to sinus bradycardia at rates of 30–60 BPM. Progressively, there ensues dysfunction of the transitional cells, as well as the atrial Purkinje's cells, with sinoatrial block.

Later stages are characterized by prolonged periods of sinus arrest and profound bradycardia at rates under 36 BPM. Such may be replaced by "rescue rhythms" due to pacing by atrial, AV junctional, ventricular or supraventricular tachyarrhythmias.

Clinical Manifestations[135]

Dysfunction may occur in young individuals (athletes) but is more common in elderly adults. Symptoms show up during the seventh and eighth decade of life. Dizziness, syncope and seizures are seen. If atrial flutter or fibrillation occurs, it may lead to low cardiac output and pulmonary congestion.

Tests of Appropriate Responsiveness of the Sinus Node[134]

Normally the sinus node output increases with graded exercise. Tests are of two types: (1) challenge of the SA node by sympathetic stimulation, using a beta stimulant

Table 7–5. Pathological Causes of Sinus Node Dysfunction

Reversible or self-limited causes
  Excessive vagal tone
  Ischemia involving sinus node
  Surgical injury to stress node
  Myocarditis (including diphtheric and rheumatic)
  Acute pericarditis
  Thyrotoxicosis
  Hyperkalemia
  Hypothermia

Chronic causes
  Nonspecific aclerodegenerative disease of sinus node
  Ischemic heart disease
  Amyloidosis
  Hemochromatosis
  Systemic lupus erythematosus
  Duchenne and myotonic muscular dystrophy
  Friedreich's ataxia
  Surgical injury to sinus node
  Familial disease of sinus node
  Metastatic cancer
  Systemic embolism
  Mitral valve prolapse
  Hypothyroidism
  Carotid sinus hypersensitivity*

*May produce sinus arrest or other bradyarrhythmias in patients with normal intrinsic sinus node function, or may uncover occult sinus node dysfunction.
Alpert, M. A., Flaker, G. C.: Arrhythmias associated with sinus node dysfunction. JAMA *250*:2160, 1983.

Table 7–6. Pharmacologic Causes of Sinus Node Dysfunction

Drugs that may cause sinus node dysfunction in patients with normal intrinsic sinus node function
  Digitalis*
  Quinidine sulfate or gluconate*
  Lidocaine hydrochloride*
  Atropine sulfate*
  Lithium carbonate
  Cimetidine†
  β-blocking agents‡
  Reserpine‡
  Guanethidine sulfate‡
  Clonidine hydrochloride‡

Drugs that may further impair sinus node function in patients with intrinsic sinus node disease
  β-blocking agents
  Digitalis
  Quinidine sulfate or gluconate
  Procainamide hydrochloride
  Disopyramide phosphate
  Verapamil
  Methyldopa
  Reserpine
  Clonidine hydrochloride

*At toxic serum levels.
†After intravenous administration; controversial.
‡Decreased sinus node automaticity is an expected pharmacologic response.
Alpert, M. A., Flaker, G. C.: Arrhythmias associated with sinus node dysfunction. JAMA *250*:2160, 1983.

such as isoproterenol in a slow low dose intravenous infusion of 1-2 ug/min; an increase in rate of 25% or more is normal; failure of sinus rate to exceed 90 BPM is evidence of dysfunction; (2) parasympathetic stimulation using a small dose of edrophonium; this normally produces some cardiac slowing, and in these patients a hypersensitivity response with profound slowing may occur. This test is dangerous and not used; (3) parasympathetic block—an alternative or concomitant test is the IV administration of a bolus of 1-2 mg of atropine. A normal increase of 25% of beats is expected. However, with a sinus node dysfunction, little or no change will occur.

Aside from documenting symptomatic sinus bradycardia on a monitor, sinoatrial node function can be assessed by the electrophysiology test. Atrial pacing can be used to measure the ability of the SA node to generate an impulse and respond to overdrive suppression. This is called the sinoatrial node recovery time (SNRT).[134] The test is performed by placement of an electrode in the upper part of the right atrium under fluoroscopic control and stimulating the atria at rates greater than the sinus rate. When pacing is stopped the response of the sinus node is observed and measured.

Once measured, the response is "corrected" for sinus rate (CSNRT). A noninvasive pacing technique to measure CSNRT employs transesophageal electrical stimulation of the heart. Another pacing method to assess sinus node function is the SA conduction time (SACT). This is a way to determine if there is block between the SA impulse generated and the atria. The sinoatrial conduction time (SACT) can be measured by direct or indirect means. These two methods do not necessarily correlate with each other nor do they correlate with the clinical condition of the patient, however.

Management[135]

Acute management begins with the use of pharmacologic agents. Atropine is rarely effective; isoproterenol has been helpful. Temporary pacing may be needed in highly symptomatic patients. Patients who demonstrate the capacity of the SA node to generate an impulse and who show normal sinus node recovery time (SNRT) and normal conductivity (SACT) may undergo pharmacologic treatment. Theophylline and anticholinergic drugs may be effective.

Arrhythmias associated with SA node dysfunction rarely cause sudden death. If the patient is asymptomatic, pacing may be deferred. Of those with severe cardiac neurological symptoms from bradycardia, permanent pacing is warranted. If symptoms become frequent or alarming or if there is progressive sinus node dysfunction with no treatable cause, a permanent pacemaker is necessary and should be implanted before major complications occur.

The traditional pacemaker has been a ventricular demand pacer (VVI), but with this modality there is loss of AV synchrony often with symptoms. Technical advances and electrophysiologic knowledge has resulted in the use of atrial (AAI) and "universal" (DDD) pacing. Atrial function is preserved and thereby reduces the risk of low cardiac output or heart failure. Multiprogrammable pacemakers are now available. The rate and output of these can be tailored to provide a stimulation rate low enough to maintain an effective endogenous rhythm, but high enough to prevent symptoms.

Also, since many of these patients have "chronotropic incompetence" (the inability of the SA node to accelerate appropriately with exercise), newer pacemakers have circuitry and provides an increase in pacing rate with exercise. Dual chamber pacemakers (DDD) have the capability to sense and pace in both chambers, and to "track" the atrial impulse and trigger ventricular pacing. If the dual chamber pacer is rate responsive it is called "DDDR". Single chamber demand atrial or ventricular pacers with rate response are called AAIR or VVIR respectively.

The prognosis with pacing in sinus node dysfunction is good. Present survival rates are 88% at one year or more and 75% at 10 years. Death is usually due to coronary artery disease or stroke.

DRUG TREATMENT OF ARRHYTHMIAS

When the cause of a rhythm disturbance is not immediately known or known but cannot be eliminated; and if the disturbance is or potentially is physiologically disturbing to the patient, then drug therapy is indicated. Some common drugs that the anesthesiologist might determine that a patient is using are listed in Table 7-2. Most anesthesiologists have 'hands on' experience with lidocaine, propranolol, esmolol and verapamil. The electrophysiologic effects of some of these drugs are listed in Table 7-7. The efficacy of antidysrhythmic drugs in the treatment of some specific dysrhythmias is presented in Table 7-8.

Quinidine

Quinidine (Fig. 7-16) depresses myocardial excitability, conduction velocity and contractility. Large doses of the drug can cause hypotension by causing peripheral vasodilation (α_1 sympathetic blockade). Gastrointestinal symptoms are common and may require discontinuation of the drug. There is an interaction with digoxin such that digoxin levels may rise when a patient is initially started on quinidine.[136] The anesthesiologist should understand that this drug is usually given for maintenance therapy and rarely if ever given for control of acute rhythm disturbances. Virtually any antiarrhythmic drug is arrhythmogenic. Quinidine is the prototype of this. "Quinidine syncope" is a clinical syndrome associated with this drug that has been described for generations.[137] It is now felt that the cause of this is ventricular tachycardia in the setting of an increased QT interval (torsades de pointes). As pointed out earlier, halothane and quinidine act in a synergistic manner to depress conduction.[51]

Quinidine interferes with normal neuromuscular transmission and can enhance the action of neuromuscular blocking agents.

Procainamide

Procainamide (Fig. 7-17) reduces conduction velocity in the atria, ventricles and Purkinje fibers.[138] It is metabo-

Table 7-7. Comparative Electrophysiological Effects and Pharmacokinetics of Cardiac Antidysrhythmic Drugs

	Automaticity (phase 4)	Excitability (phase 0)	Duration of Action Potential	Effective Refractory Period	P–R Interval	QRS Duration	Principal Clearance Mechanism	Protein Binding (%)	Elimination Half-Time (hours)	Therapeutic Plasma Concentration
Membrane Stabilizers										
Group 1A										
Quinidine	D	D	I	I	I	I	Hepatic	70–80	6	2–8 μg ml^{-1}
Procainamide	D	D	I	I	NC,I	I	Renal and hepatic	20	2.5–5	4–12 μg ml^{-1}
Disopyramide	D	D	I	I	NC	NC	Renal	68	7–8	2–4 μg ml
Group 1B										
Lidocaine	D	NC,D	D	D	NC	NC	Hepatic	55	1.5	1–5 μg ml^{-1}
Tocainide	D	NC,D	D	D	NC	NC				1–5 μg ml^{-1}
Phenytoin	D	NC,D	D	D	NC,D	NC	Hepatic	>90	24	8–16 μg ml^{-1}
Beta-adrenergic Antagonists										
Propranolol β_1–β_2	D	D	I	I	NC,I	NC	Hepatic	90–95	2–4	10–30 ng ml^{-1}
Esmolol β_1	D	D	I	I	NC	NC	Esterases in RBC	55	0.15	
Repolariation Prolongation										
Antiadrenergic Drugs										
Bretylium	NC	NC	I	I	NC,I	NC	Renal	0–8	13.5	75–100 ng ml^{-1}
Amiodarone	NC	NC	I	I	I	I	Hepatic	>90	29 days	0.5–2.5 μg ml^{-1}
Calcium Entry Blockers										
Verapamil	D	NC	D	D	NC,I	NC	Renal	90	3–7 days	100–300 ng ml^{-1}

I—Increase; D—decrease; NC—no change.
Data from: Nestico, P. F., DePace, N. L., and Morganroth, J.: Therapy with conventional antiarrhythmic drugs for ventricular arrhythmias. Medical Clinics of North America, 1984; 68:1297; Bigger, J. T., and Hoffman, F. F. Antiarrhythmic Drugs. In Goodman and Gilman's Pharmacological Basis of Therapeutics. Ed 8, 1990. McGraw-Hill, Inc.; Stoelting, R. K.: Cardiac Antidysrhythmic Drugs: In Pharmacology and Physiology in Anesthetic Practice, Philadelphia, 1987, pp 323, J. B. Lippincott Co.

Table 7–8. Efficacy of Antidysrhythmic Drugs for Treatment of Specific Cardiac Dysrhythmias

Class	Drug	Conversion of Atrial Fibrillation	Atrial Premature Depolarizations	Paroxysmal Supraventricular Tachycardia	Premature Ventricular Contractions	Ventricular Tachycardia	Digitalis-induced Arrhythmias
IA	Quindine	2	2	2–3	3	3	1
	Procainamide	2	2	2–3	3	3	1
	Disopyramide	2	2	2	2	2	1
IB	Lidocaine	0	1	1	2	2	3
	Phenytoin	0	1	1	2	2	3
	Tocainide	0	1	1	2	2	3
II	Propranolol	2	1	3	2	1	2
III	Bretylium	0	0	0	0	1–2	0
	Amiodarone	+	0	0	0	2	0
IV	Verapamil	1	+	3	0	0	0

The utility score is based on an estimate of efficacy, convenience and toxicity. The scale is as follows: O. none; 1. fair; 2. good; 4. excellent. Modified from Antiarrhythmic Drugs, J. T. Bigger, Jr., and Brian F. Hoffman in Goodman and Gilman's The Pharmacological Basis of Therapeutics, Eighth Edition 1990, McGraw-Hill, Inc.

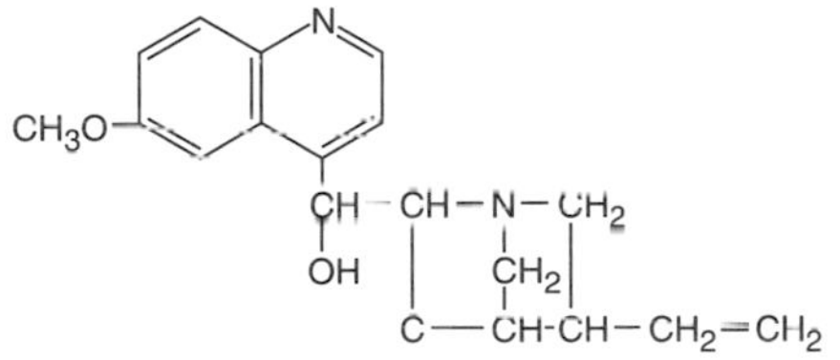

Fig. 7–16. Quinidine. Quinidine is one of the alkaloids derived from the bark of the cinchona tree found in certain regions of South America. It has a structure similar to quinine and differs only with respect to the configuration of the secondary alcohol. The drug is metabolized in the liver principally by hydroxylation at the quinoline and quinlucidine rings.

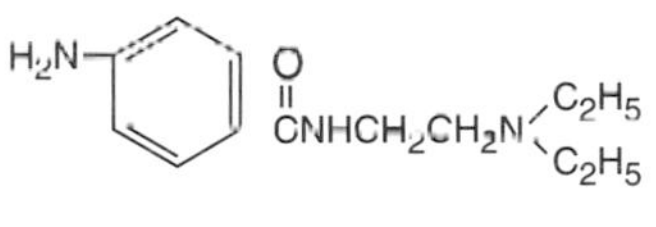

Procainamide.

Fig. 7–17. Procainamide. Replacement of the ester—linkage of procaine with an amide linkage results in procainamide with a significant prolongation of action over procaine. Unlike procaine it is not bitransformed by esterases in the blood plasma but is metabolized by acetylation in the liver by N-acetyltransferase. Up to 70% of the drug is excreted unchanged in the urine.

lized by the liver (to an active compound-N-acetyl-procainamide [NAPA]) and excreted by the kidney.[139] This drug is used to treat or prevent paroxysmal supraventricular tachycardia (PSVT), atrial fibrillation and flutter. Like quinidine, it is useful for treating ventricular arrhythmias such as ventricular tachycardia. It is a useful drug for the emergency treatment of ventricular tachycardias unresponsive to lidocaine. This drug can also be used for the treatment of supraventricular arrhythmia associated with

the Wolf-Parkinson-White (WPW) syndrome. Procainamide will increase the refractoriness of the accessory AV pathway in the WPW syndrome, thereby terminating some of the reentrant arrhythmias in these patients. Unfortunately there is a very high incidence of adverse side effects which thereby limits chronic therapy with procainamide (lupus-like syndrome in 15%).[140] Like most other antiarrhythmic agents, procainamide is proarrhythmic and can cause torsade de pointes.[141]

The oral dose is about 500–750 mg every 4-6 hours. The IV dose is a bolus 500–600 mg infused over 30 minutes followed by 2-4 mg/kg/hr.

Disopyramide (Phosphate)

Disopyramide is a Class IA antidysrhythmia. Chemically, it is a carbamoylester (Fig. 7-18). It is available as a ra mixture approved for oral use.[141a]

For the pharmacology of the drug, see Tables 7-6 and 7-7 for references. The electron effects resemble those of quinidine: disopyramide slows the rate of cardiac depolarization, rate of rise of the O-phase, increases action potential duration (AP), and extends the refractoriness into the diastolic period. Hence, conduction velocity and automaticity are reduced. The effective refractory period (ERP) is increased. A direct depressant action on the myacardium is present, so that cardiac output is reduced.[141b]

Electrocardiographic effects include an increased QT interval as a result of increased duration of both the QRS complex and the ST interval.[141c]

Autonomic effects are due to disopyramide's strong capacity to block muscarinic receptors. It is about 10% as potent as atropine, and is associated with dry mouth, urinary retention, and some blurring of vision. Gastrointestinal adverse effects are less than with quinidine or procainamide. There is no adrenergic blockade of either the alpha or beta receptors.

Molecular mechanism of action is due to the blockage of the sodium channels. There is also some ability to block calcium (Ca^{2+}) channels.[141d]

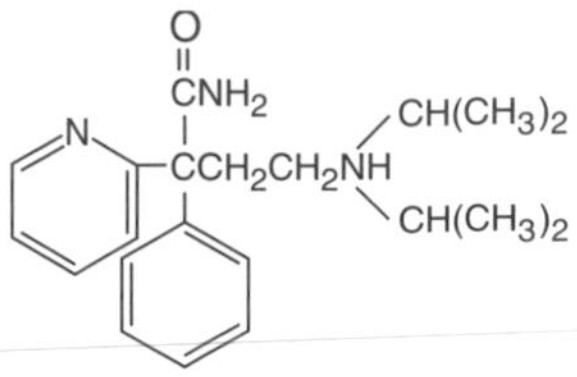

Disopyramide.

Fig. 7–18. Disopyramide. Disopyramide is a derivative of phenyl-2 pyridine acetamide phosphate. Less than 50% of the drug is metabolized in the liver. About 20% appears as the mono-N-dealkylated metabolite and 10 to 20% appears as unidentified metabolites in the urine. About 50% of the drug is excreted unchanged by the kidney. Gastrointestinal adverse effects are less common than after quinidine; however, strong anticholinergic effects are to be noted, with dry mouth and blurred vision.

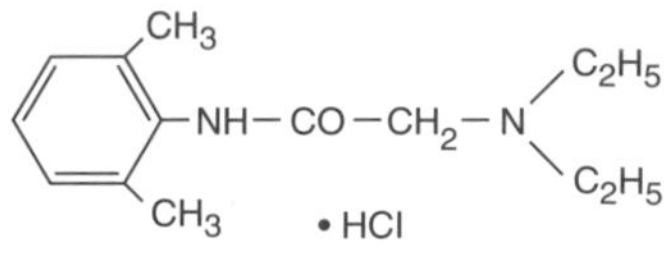

Therapeutic use is primarily to prevent or suppress chronic ventricular arrhythmias, including premature ventricular contractions (PVCs) and ventricular tachycardia. The usual dose is 100–150 mg four times a day (400–600 mg daily). About 90% of an oral dose is absorbed (Table 7-7).

Disopyramide is also effective against paroxysmal supraventricular tachycardia and is an alternative to quinidine. For atrial fibrillation, direct current cardio version is the usual method for producing a sinus rhythm; however, this drug is also useful for maintenance of the sinus rhythm post-defibrillation as is procainamide.

Pharmacokinetic studies reveal that about 70% is bound to plasma protein. The half life is 4 to 6 hours, and the effective plasma concentration is greater than 1.5 mg/ml. About 50% of the drug is excreted in the urine unchanged, while an additional .10% is excreted in the bile. The remainder of the drug, about 40%, is metabolized in the liver.

Besides the atropine side effects, disopyramide may have significant hemodynamic adverse effects with hypotension due to the myocardial depression. Arteriolar vasoconstriction occurs, and heart failure may be observed.[141e]

Lidocaine

Lidocaine (Fig. 7–19) is undoubtedly the most common drug used by anesthesiologists to suppress perioperative ventricular ectopy. Lidocaine is thought to abolish unidirectional block but also increase block in ischemic myocardium[142] thereby eliminating conditions for reentry. In addition, lidocaine also depresses automaticity. Lidocaine is metabolized by the liver and hence serum lidocaine levels are greatly affected by drugs or pathological processes that affect the liver. This is particularly true with patients in congestive heart failure. Lidocaine clearance is affected greatly by alterations in hepatic blood flow. Common side effects are related to the central nervous system: dizziness, paresthesia, and tinnitus. A large bolus of the drug injected quickly can cause convulsions. One of the major

Fig. 7–19. Lidocaine. Lidocaine belongs to the amide series of local anesthetic agents but has been found to be quite effective in the treatment of ventricular ectopic arrhythmias especially in the ischemic myocardium. Specifically it is the acetic derivative of xylidide. It is about twice as potent as procainamide for the treatment of arrhythmias. About 90% of a dose is metabolized in the liver and 10% is excreted unchanged by the kidney.

benefits of this drug is that in therapeutic concentration, lidocaine has minimal effects on myocardial contractility. Also it has little effect on sinus node function. However, lidocaine can decrease conduction (in atrial tissue) and thereby accelerate the ventricular rate in atrial flutter or fibrillation.[143] Few if any reports of lidocaine induced ventricular tachycardia or fibrillation have been published. It is probably the least proarrhythmic of the classic antiarrhythmic drugs.

Bupivacaine, also an amide local anesthetic, is notorious for its ability to induce life threatening cardiac arrhythmias.[144,145] Why is one amide local anesthetic an efficacious and safe antiarrhythmic and the other amide local anesthetic a devastating proarrhythmic drug? One of the reasons for the marked proarrhythmic affect of bupivacaine include its prolonged duration of binding to sodium channels (as compared to lidocaine).[144] This prolonged binding to sodium channels and subsequent slow recovery provides a reason why conduction can be seriously depressed in the face of bupivacaine overdose.[146] In addition, lidocaine is much less potent than bupivacaine in depressing purkinje fiber-ventricular muscle conduction as well as other factors that contribute to the genesis of reentry arrhythmias.[147]

Another major difference is that bupivacaine is much more potent.[148] Though both drugs are amides bupivacaine is definitely much more proarrhythmic.[149] The exact reason for this is not clear. It is not related to the piperidine moiety of bupivacaine since mepivacaine, which contains this moiety, is not proarrhythmic per se.[150] Suffice it to say, the previously described intense conduction block by bupivacaine (as opposed to lidocaine) does establish a necessary condition for reentry arrhythmias.

While there are to date no reports of lidocaine being proarrhythmic in man, it has been demonstrated to be proarrhythmic in the cat—with the induction of ventricular tachyarrhythmias.[151]

The role of lidocaine in resuscitation in the setting of acute ischemia is being reevaluated. There is some concern that its indiscriminate use can lead to diminished countershock efficacy and lidocaine-induced asystole.[152-154]

A bolus dose of 200–400 mg is administered intravenously followed by an infusion of 1–2 mg/kg/hour.

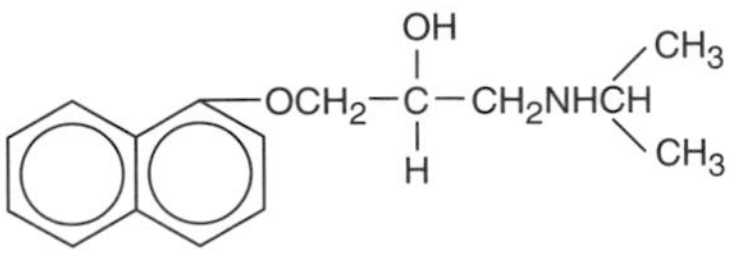

Nonselective Antagonists   Propranolol.

Fig. 7–20. Propranolol. This drug belongs to the class of phenyl-oxy propanol amines. Specifically it is 1-(isopropyl amino)-3-(naphthyl-oxy)-2 propanol. In one sense it can be considered a derivative of the alcohol of propane. Pharmacologically, it is a non-selective β-adrenergic receptor antagonist and has equal affinity for both B_1 and B_2 receptors. It has no agonist activity. After oral administration, the bioavailability during passage through the portal circulation only 25% reaches the systemic circulation. The drug enters the central nervous system to some extent and can control panic reactions. Propanolol binds to plasma protein to 90%. It is extensively metabolized in the liver and the metabolites are excreted by the kidney. The plasma half-life is short at about 4 hours; however the antihypertensive and antidysrhythmic effect may last up to 24 hours. A quinidine-like effect is to be noted on the heart. Exercise-induced tachycardia is suppressed.

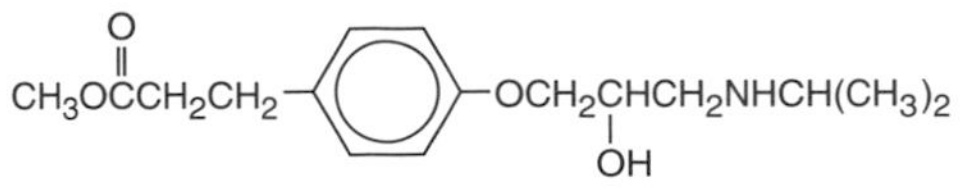

Esmolol.

Fig. 7–21. Esmolol. This is a selective Beta$_1$ adrenergic antagonist and has neither Beta$_2$ activity or any sympathomimetic action. In its interaction with the adrenergic receptor it combines within the plane of the receptor membrane and not on extracellular surfaces. Furthermore this drug differs from most of the other beta adrenergic antagonists structurally in having an ester linkage, and is thus rapidly metabolized by the esterases in the erythrocyes. The plasma half-life is about 8 minutes. Dosage consists of a loading dose of 500 μg/kg administered over a period of one minute follwed by a maintenance dose of 50 μg/kg administered over a period of 4 minutes. This procedure may be repeated 3 or 4 times if a therapeutic response is not seen in five minutes; the endpoint is a lowering of the heart rate or blood pressure. A peak effect may last for 8 to 10 minutes after discontinuing the infusion. The rapid degredation in the blood produces a carbolic acid metabolite which has a half lifelonger than 4 hours but has little or no potency and is excreted in thermofurine.

Beta-Blockers

Propranolol

The prototype of this classification of drugs is propranolol (Fig. 7-20). This drug is usually used to slow ventricular response in supraventricular arrhythmias. Side effects include 1) myocardial depression 2) excessive slowing of the heart rate 3) AV block 4) bronchospasm.

Esmolol

Esmolol (Fig. 7-21) works in a similar manner, with similar side effects. Its major advantage lies in the fact that it has a rapid onset of action and its action may be terminated within minutes of discontinuing the infusion. Because this drug can be used efficaciously as an infusion, it is becoming more and more important in anesthesis practice. Major advantages over other beta-blockers are as follows: It has a very short half life (elimination half-life of 9 minutes) and the effect of esmolol on heart rate is absent within 5 minutes after discontinuing an infusion.[152] Plasma levels are generally undetectable 15 minutes after discontinuation.[152] Hence, it is a drug whose effects can be quickly initiated or terminated. Esmolol can attenuate increases in blood pressure and heart rate resulting from surgical stimuli.[155] Esmolol has been used successfully to treat intraoperative sinus tachycardias (when other serious causes of sinus tachycardia have been ruled out).[156] This drug would seem to be an ideal drug to control ventricular rates in atrial fibrillation (or other supraventricular rhythm) when the anesthesiologist is unsure about the patient's ventricular function. It is no longer necessary to use extremely large doses of cardiac glycosides to control heart rates in atrial fibrillation or other supraventricular rhythm disturbances.

Bretylium

Bretylium (Fig. 7-22) has two main antiarrhythmic actions: adrenergic and direct myocardial effects. Bretylium (depending upon dose) can release norepinephrine from the adrenergic nerve endings. It also can potentiate the action of norepinephrine and epinephrine. The direct effects of bretylium on the myocardium are related to its ability to increase the duration of the action potential and prolong the effective refractory period of Purkinje fiber and ventricular muscle fiber.

Common side effects include hypotension, nausea, and vomiting. Its main clinical use has been in the treatment of ventricular rhythms not responsive to lidocaine. Of particular interest, is the fact that this drug may be the drug of choice for treating bupivacaine induced ventricular tachycardia.[157,158]

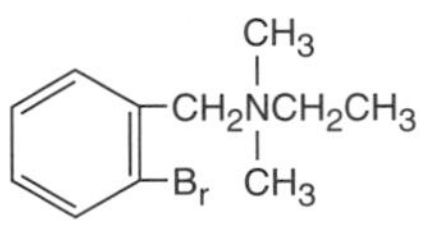

Bretylium.

Fig. 7–22. Bretylium. Bretylium is a brombenzyl quaternary amine. Metabolism if any is minimal. Over 70% is excreted intact in the urine within the first 24 hours after administration and 98% or more is excreted by 48 hours. The drug selectively accumulates in sympathetic ganglia and their postganglionic adrenergic neurones. The release of norepinephrine is inhibited by depression of the exitability of the adrenergic nerve terminal. The plasma half-life is 9.0 hours. The mechanism of action is to delay repolarization.

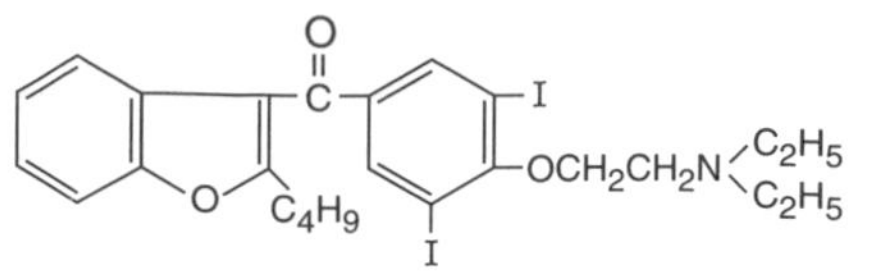

Amiodarone.

Fig. 7–23. Amiodarone. Amiodarone is a benzofurane deriva-tive and its structure is similar to thyroxine. The drug was ap-proved for treating recurrent ventricular fibrillation and ventric-ular tachycardia in 1986 when these disorders were resistent to other drugs. The mechanism of action is to delay repolariza-tion. The drug is long lasting with a therapeutic effect of over 45 days; the half-life for elimination is between 25 and 60 days.

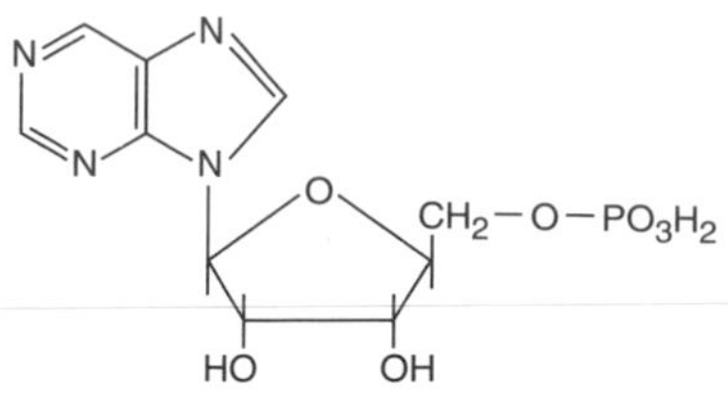

Amiodarone

Amiodarone (Fig. 7–23) is another class III antidys-rhythmic drug with similar actions to bretylium except the very long elimination time.

Verapamil

Verapamil is a calcium channel blocker which prolongs the effective refractory period and increases action poten-tial duration in the AV junction. Its main use is in slowing the ventricular response to supraventricular rhythms. Some rhythms (paroxysmal supra ventricular tachycardia) will convert to a sinus mechanism when verapamil is given. This drug can marked slowing of heart rate particu-larly in the presence of beta-blockade. Being a strongly negative inotropic drug, it reduces myocardial oxygen consumption. These effects are additive to the effects of halothane.[159] In addition, at least in the dog, verapamil can induce heart block in the presence of the potent in-halation anesthetics (enflurane, isoflurane, halothane).[160]

Besides its usefulness in supraventricular rhythm distur-bances it may have a use for ventricular arrhythmias par-ticularly in the operative setting. For instance, verapamil has been found to raise the dose of epinephrine required to induce a ventricular rhythm disturbance during halothane anesthesia in the dog.[161] There is some reason to believe that some ventricular rhythm disturbances, oc-curring in the setting of myocardial ischemia, may be de-pendent on calcium ionic currents. Verapamil has been used successfully in the treatment of intractable ventricu-lar arrhythmias (ventricular tachycardia and ventricular fibrillation) after cardiopulmonary bypass.[162]

Adenosine

Adenosine (Fig. 7–24) is an endogenous nucloside that can cause marked AV conduction block. It has proven very useful to safely aid in the distinction between a wide QRS complex tachycardia secondary to supraventricular tachycardia with aberrancy versus ventricular tachycar-dia.[163] The serum half life of the drug is 0.6 to 1.5 sec.[163]

If the rhythm disturbances is a supraventricular tachy-cardia, adenosine will induce AV block and noncon-ducted atrial activity will become apparent. If on the

Fig. 7–24. Adenosine. Adenosine is a purine derivative and present in all cells of the body. As such it is known as an auta-coid and the effects are mediated by specific receptors in the plasma membrane of nearly all cells. Its function is to assist in the maintenance of a balance between available oxygen and its utilization. Thus it participates in many local regulatory mecha-nisms at brain synapses and at peripheral neuroeffector junc-tions. Its specific structure is adenine-D-ribose 6-amino purine, a cyclin nucleoside.

other hand the disturbance is ventricular tachycardia, the ventricular rate will remain unaffected. In the past vera-pamil was used. Unfortunately this resulted in some in-stances of cardiopulmonary collapse when given to pa-tients who in fact had ventricular tachycardia.[163] Adeno-sine has also been used for the successful cardioversion of supraventricular tachycardia during open heart surgery.[164]

REFERENCES

1. Cranefield P. F., Witt Al, Hoffman, B. F.: Genesis of cardiac arrhythmias. Circ 1973; 47:190–202.
2. Bigger T. J.: Antiarrhythmic treatment: An overview. Am J Cardiol 1984; 53:8B–16B.
3. Olshansky B., Martins J. B.: Usefulness of isoproteronol fa-cilitation of ventricular tachycardia induction during ex-trastimulus testing in predicting effective chronic therapy with beta-adrenergic blockade. Am J Cardio 1987; 59:573–577.
4. Gilmour R. F., Zipes D. P.: Basic electrophysiologic mecha-nisms for the development of arrhythmias. Medical Clinics of North America 1984; 68:795–814.
5. Singer D. H., Baumgarten C. M., Ten Eick R. E.: Cellular electrophysiology of ventricular and other dysrhythmias: Studies on diseased and ischemic heart. Progress in Cardio-vascular Diseases 1981; 24:97–111.
6. Rosen M. R., Reder R. F.: Does triggered activity have a role in the genesis of cardiac arrhythmias? Ann Int Med 1981; 94:794–801.
7. El-Sherif N., Gough W. B., Restuo M.: Reentrant ventricular arrhythmias in the late myocardial infarction period: 14. Mechanisms of resetting, entgrainment, acceleration, or termination of reentrant tachycardia by programmed elec-trical stimulation. PACE 1987; 10:341–371.
8. Marriott H. J. C., Lacamera F.: Diagnosis of arrhythmia. JAMA 1968; 203:527–528.
9. Stewart R. B., Bardy G. H., Greene L. H.: Wide complex tachycardia: Misdiagnosis and outcome after emergent therapy. Ann Int Med 1986; 104:766–771.
10. Morady F., Baerman J. M., DiCarlo L., DeBustleir M., Krol R., Wahr D. W.: A prevalent misconception regarding wide-complex tachycardia. JAMA 1985; 254:2790–2792.
11. Steinman R. T., Herrera C., Schinger C. D., Lehman M. A.: Wide QRS tachycardia in the conscious adult. JAMA 1989; 261:1013–1016.

12. Akhtar M., Shenasa M., Jazayeri M., et al.: Wide QRS complex tachycardia. Ann Intern Med 1988; 109:905-912.
13. Jackman W. M., Clark M., Friday K. J., Aliot E. M., Anderson J., Lazzara R.: Ventricular tachyarrhythmias in the long QT syndromes. Med Clin of North America 1984; 68:1079-110.
14. Baxandall M. L., Thorn V. L.: The nasocardiac reflex. Anaesthesia 1988; 43:480-481.
15. Atlee J. L., Bosnjak Z.: Mechanisms for cardiac dysrhythmias during anesthesia. Anesthesiology 1990; 72:347-374.
16. Atlee J. L.: Anesthesia and cardiac electrophysiology. European Journal of Anesthesiology 1985; 2:215-256.
17. Pratila M. G., Pratilas V.: Anesthetic agents and cardiac electromechanical activity. Anesthesiology 1978; 49:338-360.
18. Atlee J. L., Brownlee S. W., Burstrom, R. E.: Conscious-state comparisons of the effects of inhalation anesthetics on specialized atrioventricular conduction times in dogs. Anesthesiology 1986; 64:703-710.
19. Wilton N. C. T., Landau S. N., Knight P. R. Electrophysiological effects of the volatile anesthetic agents: An alternative approach. Anesthesiology 1986; 64:A57.
20. Duke P. C., Fownes O., Wade J. G.: Halothane depresses baroreflex control of heart rate in man. Anesthesiology 1977; 46:184-187.
21. Morton M., Duke P. C., Ong B.: Baroreflex control of heart rate in man awake and during enflurane and enflurane-nitrous-oxide anesthesia. Anesthesiology 1980; 52:221-223.
22. Kotrly K., Ebert T. J., Vucins E., Ogler F., Barney I. A., Kampine V. P.: Baroreceptor reflex control of heart rate during isoflurane anesthesia in humans. Anesthesiology 1984; 60:173-179.
23. Royster R. L., Keeler D. K., Haisty W. K., Johnston W. E., Prough O. S.: Cardiac electrophysiologic effects of fentanyl and combinations of fentanyl and neuromuscular relaxants in pentobarbital-anesthetized dogs. Anesth Analg 1988; 67:15-20.
24. Katz P. L., Bigger T. J.: Cardiac arrhythmias during anesthesia and operation. Anesthesiology 1970; 33:193-213.
25. Vanik P. E., Davis H. S.: Cardiac arrhythmias during halothane anesthesia. Anesth Analg 1968; 47:299-307.
26. Kuner J., Enescu V., Utsu F., Boszormeny E., Bernstein H., Corday E.: Cardiac arrhythmias during anesthesia. Dis Chest 1967; 52:580-587.
27. Ostroft L. H., Goldstein B. H., Pennock R. S., Weiss W. W.: Cardiac dysrhythmias during outpatient general anesthesia: A comparison study. J Oral Surgery 1977; 35:793-797.
28. Chander S.: Isorhythmic atrioventricular dissociation during enflurane anesthesia. Southern Medical Journal 1982; 75:945-950.
29. Rollason W. N., Bennetts F. E., Clarke I.: Cardiac dysrhythmias during outpatient dental anaesthesia with enflurane. The role of beta-blockade. Acta Anaesthesiol Scand 1984; 28:497-502.
30. Willatts D. G., Harrison A. R., Groom J. F., Crowthe A.: Cardiac arrhythmias during outpatient dental anaesthesia: Comparison of halothane with enflurane. Br J Anaesth 1983; 53:399-402.
31. Pratila M. G., Pratilas V., Smith H.: Dysrhythmias and enflurane anesthesia. Mount Sinai Journal of Medicine 1979; 46:500-503.
32. Fisch C., Oehler R. C., Miller J. R., Redish C. H.: Cardiac arrhythmias during oral surgery with halothane—nitrous oxide—oxygen anesthesia. JAMA 1969; 208:1839-1842.
33. Hanna M. H., Heap D. G., Kimberley A. P. S.: Cardiac dysrhythmia associated with general anaesthesia for oral surgery. Anaesthesia 1983; 38:1192-1194.
34. Kreul J. F., Dauchot P. J., Anton, A. H.: Hemodynamic and catecholamine studies during pheochromocytoma resection under enflurane anesthesia. Anesthesiology 1976; 44:265-268.
35. Forrest J. B., Cahalan M. K., Rehder K., Goldsmith C. H., Levy W. J., Strunin L., et al.: Multicenter study of general anesthesia. II. Results. Anesthesiology 1990; 72:262-268.
36. Roizen M. R., Plummer G. O., Lichtor L.: Nitrous oxide and dysrhythmias. Anesthesiology 1987; 66:427-431.
37. Mitchell J. H., Gilmore V. P., Sarnoff S. J.: The transport function of the atrium. Am J Cardiol 1962; 9:237-247.
38. Braunwald E.: Comments on the hemodynamic significance of atrial systole. Am J Med 1964; 37:665-669.
39. Boba A.: Significant effects on the blood pressure of an apparently trivial atrial dysrhythmia. Anesthesiology 1978; 48:282-283.
40. Russell R. O., Reeves T. J.: The effect of digoxin in normal man on the cardiorespiratory response to severe effort. Am Heart J 1963; 66:381-388.
41. Beiser G. D., Epstein S. E., Stampfer M., et al.: Studies on digitalis. N Engl J Med 1968; 278:131-137.
42. Smith T. W., Braunwald E.: The management of heart failure, in Braunwald E (ed): Heart Disease: A Textbook of Cardiovascular Medicine. Philadelphia, WB Saunders, 1984 pp 524.
43. Kennedy H. L., Whitlock J. A., Sprague M. K., Kennedy I. J., Buckinghan T. A., Goldberg R. J.: Long-term follow-up of asymptomatic healthy subjects with frequent and complex ventricular ectopy. N Engl J Med 1985; 312:193-7.
44. Levy M. N., Edelstein J.: The mechanism of synchronization in isorhythmic A-V dissociation. II. Clinical Studies. Circulation 1970; 42:689-699.
45. Hashimoto K., Hashimoto K.: The mechanism of sensitization of the ventricle to epinephrine by halothane. Am Heart J 1972; 83.652-658.
46. Hashimoto K., Endoh M., Kimura T., Hashimoto K.: Effects of halothane on automaticity and contractile force of isolated blood-perfused canine ventricular tissue. Anesthesiology 1975; 42:15-25.
47. Reynolds A. K.: On the mechanism of myocardial sensitization to catecholamine by hydrocarbon anesthetics. Can J Physiol Pharmacol 1984; 62:183-198.
48. Zink J., Sasyniuk B. I., Dresel P. E.: Halothane—epinephrine—induced cardiac arrhythmias and the role of heart rate. Anesthesiology 1975; 43:548-555.
49. Atlee J. L.: Halothane: Cause or cure for arrhythmia. Anesthesiology 1987; 67:617-618.
50. Turner L. A., Bosnjak Z. J., Kampine J. P.: Actions of halothane on the electrical activity of purkinje fibers derived from normal and infarcted canine hearts. Anesthesiology 1987; 67:619-628.
51. Morrow D. H., Townley N. T.: Anesthesia and digitalis toxicity: An experimental study. Anesth Analg (Cleve) 1964; 43:510-519.
52. Gallagher J. D., Gessman L. J., Moura P., Kerns D.: Electrophysiologic effects of halothane and quinidine on canine purkinje fibers. Evidence for a synergistic interaction. Anesthesiology 1986; 65:278-285.
53. Maye M., Smith C. M.: Identification of receptor mechanism mediating epinephrine—induced arrhythmias during halothane anesthesia in the dog. Anesthesiology 1983; 59:322-326.
54. Metz S., Maye M.: Halothane concentration does not alter the threshold for epinephrine—induced arrhythmias in dogs. Anesthesiology 1985; 62:470-474.

55. Halsey M.: Drug Interactions in Anaesthesia. Br. J. Anaesth. 1987; 59:112-123.
56. Johnston R. R., Eger E. L., Wilson C.: Comparative interaction of epinephrine with enflurane, isoflurane, and halothane in man. Anesth Analg 1976; 55:709-712.
57. Katz R. L., Matteo R. S., Papper E. M.: The Injection of Epinephrine During General Anesthesia With Halogenated Hydrocarbons and Cyclopropane in Man. Anesthesiology, 1962; 23:597.
58. Konchigeri H. N., Shaker M. H., Winnie A. P.: Effect of Epinephrine During Enflurane Anesthesia. Anesth. Analg., 1974; 53:894.
59. Horrigan R. W., Eger E. I., Wilson C.: Epinephrine-Induced Arrhythmias During Enflurane Anaesthesia in Man: A Non-Linear Dose-Response Relationship and Dose-Dependent Protection from Lidocaine. Anesth. Analg., 1978; 57:547.
60. Atlee J. L., Roberts F. L.: Thiopental and epinephrine-induced dysrhythmias in dogs anesthetized with enflurane or isoflurane. Anesth Analg 1986; 65:437-443.
61. Atlee J. L., Malkinson C. E.: Potentiation by thiopental of halothane-epinephrine induced arrhythmias in dogs. Anesthesiology 1982; 57:285-288.
62. Royster R. L., Keeler K., Haisty W. K., Jonston W. E., Prough D. S.: Cardiac electrophysiologic effects of fentanyl and combinations of fentanyl of neuromuscular relaxants in pentobarbital—anesthetized dogs. Anesth Analg 1988; 67:15-20.
63. Sherman E. P., Lebowitz P. W., Street W. C.: Bradycardia following sufentanil—succinylcholine. Letter. Anesthesiology 1987; 66:106.
64. Starr N. J., Sethna D. H., Estafanous F. G.: Bradycardia and asystole following the rapid administration of sufentanil with vecuronium. Anesthesiology 1986; 64:521-523.
65. Bovill J. G., Sehel P. S., Stanley T. H.: Opioid analgesics in anesthesia: With special reference to their use in cardiovascular anesthesia. Anesthesiology 1984; 61:731-755.
66. Nanta J., Koopman D., Spierdijk J., Van Kleif J., de Lange S., Stanley T. H.: Alfentanil, a new narcotic anesthetic induction agent. Anesth Analg 1982; 61:267-271.
67. Stowe D. F., Bosnjak Z. J., Kampine J. P.: Comparison of etomidate, ketamine, midazolam, propofol, and thiopental on function and metabolism of isolated hearts. Anesth Analg 1992; 74:547-558.
68. Giese J. L., Stockham R. J., Stanley T. H., Pace N. L., Nelissen R. H.: Etomidate versus thiopental for induction of anesthesia. Anesth Analg 1985; 64:871-876.
69. Ebert T. J., Muzi M., Berens R., Goff D., Kampine J. P.: Sympathetic responses to induction of anesthesia with propofol or etomidate. Anesthesiology 1992; 76:725-733.
70. Kamibayashi T., Hayashi Y., Sumikawa K., Yamatodani A., Kawabata K., Yoshiya I.: Enhancement by propofol of epinephrine-induced arrhythmias in dogs. Anesthesiology 1991; 75:1035-1040.
71. Elia S. T., Lebowitz P.: Succinylcholine induced idioventricular rhythm. Anesth Analg 1988; 67:588-589.
72. Nigrovic V., McCullough L. S., Wajskol A., Levin J. A., Martin J. T.: Succinylcholine-induced increases in plasma catecholamine levels in humans. Anesth Anagl 1983; 62:627-632.
73. Leiman B. C., Katz J., Butler B. D.: Mechanisms of succinylcholine-induced arrhythmias in hypoxic or hypoxic: hypercarbic dogs. Anesth Analg 1987; 66:1292-1297.
74. Thomson I. R., Putnins C. L.: Adverse effects of pancuronium during high-dose fentanyl anesthesia for coronary artery bypass grafting. Anesthesiology 1985; 62:708-713.
75. Salmenpera M., Peltola K., Takkunen O., Heinonen J.: Cardiovascular effects of pancuronium and vecuronium during high-dose fentanyl anesthesia. Anesth Analg 1983; 62:1059-1064.
76. Heinonen J., Salmenpera M., Suomivuiori M.: Contribution of muscle relaxant to the hemodynamic course of high-dose fentanyl anaesthesia: A comparison of pancuronium, vecuronium and atracurium. Can Anaesth Soc J 1986; 33:597-605.
77. Carter M. L.: Bradycardia after the use of atracurium. British Medical Journal 1983; 287:247-248.
78. Kennedy W. F., Bonica J. J., Akamats T. J., Ward R. J., Martin W. E., Grinstein A.: Cardiovascular and respiratory effects of subarachnoid block in the presence of acute blood loss. Anesthesiology 1968; 29:29-35.
79. Wetstone D. L., Wong K. L.: Sinus bradycardia and asystole during spinal anesthesia. Anesthesiology 1974; 41:87-89.
80. Caplan R. A., Ward R. J., Posner K., Cheney F. W.: Unexpected cardiac arrest during spinal anesthesia: A closed claims analysis of predisposing factors. Anesthesiology 1988; 68:5-11.
81. Vitez T. S., Soper L. E., Wong K. C., Soper P.: Chronic hypokalemia and intraoperative dysrhythmias. Anesthesiology 1985; 63:130-133.
82. Hirsh I. A., Tomlinson D. L., Slogoff S., Keats A. S.: The overstated risk of preoperative hypokalemia. Anesth Analg 1988; 67:131-136.
83. Goldman L.: Supraventricular tachyarrhythmias in hospitalized adults after surgery. Chest 1978; 73:450-454.
84. Gajewski J., Singer R. B.: Mortality in an insured population with atrial fibrillation. JAMA 1981; 245:1540-1544.
85. Falk R. H., Knowlton A. A., Bernard S. A.: Digoxin for converting recent-onset atrial fibrillation to sinus rhythm. Ann Intern Med 1987; 106:503-506.
86. Marcus F. I., Huang S. K.: Digitalis. In: The Heart. Hurst, J. W. (ed.). McGraw-Hill, New York 1990; 1748-1761.
87. Shields T. W., Vjiki G. T.: Digitalization for prevention of arrhythmia following pulmonary surgery. Surg Gynecol Obstet 1968; 126:743-746.
88. Burman S. O.: The prophylactic use of digitalis before thoracotomy. Ann Thorac Surg 1972; 14:359-368.
89. Deutsch S., Salem J.: Indication for prophylactic digitalization. Anesthesiology 1969; 30:648-656.
90. Juler G. L., Stemmer E. A., Connolly J. E.: Complications of prophylactic digitalization in thoracic surgical patients. J Thorac Cardiovasc Surg 1969; 58:352-360.
91. Durrer D., Schuelenberg R. M., Wellens H. J. J.: Preexcitation revisited. Am J Cardiology 1970; 25:690.
92. Wellens H. J. J., Brugada P., Penn O. C.: The management of preexcitation syndromes. JAMA 1987; 257:2325.
93. Sadowski A. R., Moyers J. R.: Anesthetic management of the Wolff-Parkinson-White syndrome. Anesthesiology 1979; 51:553.
94. Gomez-Arnau J., Marquez-Montes J., Avello F.: Fentanyl and droperidol effects on the refractoriness of the accessory pathway in the Wolff-Parkinson-White syndrome. Anesthesiology 1983; 58:307.
95. Gothert M., Wendt J.: Inhibition of adrenal medullary catecholamine secretion by enflurane. Anesthesiology 1977; 46:400.
96. Jones R. M., Broadbent M. P., Adams A. P.: Anesthetic considerations in patients with paroxysmal supraventricular tachycardia. Anaesthesia 1984; 39:307.
97. Jacobson L., Turnquist K., Masley S.: Wolff-Parkinson-White syndrome. Anaesthesia 1985; 40:657.
98. Klein G. J., Yee R., Sharma A. D.: Longitudinal electrophysiologic assessment of asymptomatic patients with the Wolf-Parkinson-White electrocardiographic pattern. N Engl J Med 1989; 320:1229-1233.

99. Ruskin J.: Ventricular extrasystoles in healthy subjects. N Engl J Med 1985; 312:238-239.
100. Kennedy H. L., Pescarmona J. E., Bouchard R. J., Goldberg R. J., Caralis D. G.: Objective evidence of occult myocardial dysfunction in patients with frequent ventricular ectopy without clinically apparent heart disease. Am Heart J 1982; 104:57-65.
101. Kennedy H. L., Pescarmona J. E., Bouchard R. J., Goldberg R. J.: Coronary artery status of apparently healthy subjects with frequent and complex ventricular ectopy. Ann Int Med 1980; 92 (Part 1):179-185.
102. Stanton M. S., Prystowsky E. N., Fineberg N. S., Miles W. M., Zipes D. P., Heger J. J.: Arrhythmogenic effects of antiarrhythmic drugs: A study of 506 patients treated for ventricular tachycardia or fibrillation. J Am Coll Cardio 1989; 14:209-215.
103. Myerburg R. J., Kessler K. M., Kiem I., Petkaros K. C., Conde C. A., Cooper D., Castellanos A.: Relationship between plasma levels of procainamide, suppression of premature ventricular complexes and prevention of recurrent ventricular tachycardia. Circulation 1981; 64:280-289.
104. Ruberman W., Weinblatt E., Goldberg J. D., Frank C. W., Chandhary B. S., Shapiro S.: Ventricular premature complexes and sudden death after myocardial infarction. Circulation 1981; 64:297-304.
105. Fletcher A. F., Cantwell J. D.: Ventricular fibrillation in a medically supervised cardiac exercise program. JAMA 1977; 238:2627-2629.
106. Myerburg R. J., Conde C., Sheps D. S., Appel R. A., Kiem F., Sung R. J., Castellanos A.: Antiarrhythmic drug therapy in survivors of prehospital cardiac arrest: Comparison of effects on chronic ventricular arrhythmias and recurrent cardiac arrest. Circulation 1979; 59:855-863.
107. May G. S.: A review of long-term beta-blocker trials in survivors of myocardial infarction. Circulation 1983; 67(suppl I):46-49.
108. Friedman L., Byington R. P., Capone R. J., Furberg C. O., Goldstein S., Lichstein E.: Effect of propranolol in patients with myocardial infarction and ventricular arrhythmia. J Am Coll Cardiol 1986; 7:1-8.
109. Velebit V., Podrid P., Lown B., Cohen B., Graboys T. B.: Aggravation and provocation of ventricular arrhythmias by antiarrhythmic drugs. Circulation 1982; 65:886-894.
110. Rinkenberger R. L., Prystowsky E. N., Jackman W. M., Naccarelli G. V., Heger J. J., Zipes D. P.: Drug conversion of nonsustained ventricular tachycardia to sustained ventricular tachycardia during serial electrophysiologic studies: Identification of drugs that exacerbate tachycardia and potential mechanisms. Am Heart J 1982; 103:177-184.
111. Ruskin J. N., McGovern G., Garan H., DiMarco J. P., Kelly E.: Antiarrhythmic drugs: A possible cause of out-of-hospital cardiac arrest. N Engl J Med 1983; 309:1302-1305.
112. The Cardiac Arrhythmia Suppression Trial (CAST) Investigators: Preliminary report: Effect of encainide and flecainide on mortality in a randomized trial of arrhythmic suppression after myocardial infarction. N Engl J Med 1989; 321:406-412.
113. Nygaad T. W., Sellers D. T., Cook T. S., DiMarco J. P.: Adverse reactions to antiarrhythmic drugs during therapy for ventricular arrhythmias. JAMA 1986; 256:55-57.
114. Gomes J. A. C., El-Sherif N.: Atrioventricular block. Medical Clinics of North America 1984; 68:955-967.
115. Wesley R. C., Lerman B. B., D'Marco J. P., Berne R. M., Belardinelli L.: Mechanism of atropine-resistant atrioventricular block during inferior myocardial infarction: Possible role of adenosine. J Am Coll Cardiol 1986; 8:1232-1234.
116. Shah P. K., Nalos P., Peter T.: Atropine resistant post infarction complete AV block: Possible role of adenosine and improvement with aminophylline. Am Heart J 1987; 113:194-195.
117. Stemp L. I.: Treatment of complete heart block in a patient with coronary artery disease. Anesthesiology (Letter) 1992; 77:612.
118. Shah K. B., Rao T. L. K., Laughlin S., El-Etr A.: A review of pulmonary artery catheterization in 6,245 patients. Anesthesiology 1984; 61:271-275.
119. Wertz H. H., Goldman L.: Non cardiac surgery in the patient with heart disease. Medical Clinics of North America 1984; 68:413-432.
120. Goldman L., Caldera D., Southwick F., et al.: Cardiac risk factors and complication in non-cardiac surgery. Medicine 1978; 57:357-367.
121. Parsonnet V., Furman S., Smyth N., Bilitch M.: Implantable cardiac pacemakers: Status report and resource guideline. Circulation 1974; 50:A21-35.
122. Parsonnet V., Furman S., Smyth N. P. D., Bilitch M.: Implantable cardiac pacemakers: Status report and resource guideline, 1982. Pacemaker Study Group, Intersociety Commission for Heart Disease Resources (ICHD). Circulation 1982; 68:227A.
123. Shapiro W. A., Roizen M. F., Singleton M. A., Morady F., Bainton C. R., Gaynor R. L.: Intraoperative pacemaker complications. Anesthesiology 1985; 63:319-322.
124. Domino K. B., Smith T. C.: Electrocautery-induced reprogramming of a pacemaker using a precordial magnet. Anesth Analg 1983; 62:609-612.
125. Luceri R. M., Castellanos A., Zaman L., Myerburg R. J.: The arrhythmias of dual-chamber cardiac pacemakers and their management. Ann Int Med 1983; 99:354-359.
126. Merritt W. T., Brinker J. A., Beattie C.: Pacemaker-mediated tachycardia induced by intraoperative somatosensory evoked potential stimuli. Anesthesiology 1988; 69:766-768.
127. Hayes D. L., Trusty J., Christiansen J.: A prospective study of electrocautery's effect on pacemaker function. PACE 1987; 10:442.
128. Thomas A. C., Moser S. A., Smutka M. C., Wilson P. A.: Implantable defibrillation. Eight years clinical experience. PACE 1988; 11:2053-2058.
129. Marchlinski F., Flores B. T., Buxton A. E., Hargrove W. C., Addonizio V. P., Stephenson L. W., Harken A. H., Doherty J. U., Grogan E. W., Josphyson M. E.: The automatic implantable cardioverter defibrillator: Efficacy complications and device failure. Ann Int Med 1986; 104:481-488.
130. Beckner G. L., Winsor T.: Cardiovascular adaptations to prolonged physical effort. Circulation 1954; 9:835.
131. Bullock R. E., Hall R. J. C.: Athletic dysrhythmias: A case report and review of the phenomenon of the 'athlete's heart'. Anaesthesia 1985; 40:647.
132. Zeppilli P., et al: Wenkebach second-degree A-V block in top-ranking athletes: An old problem revisited. Am Heart J 1980; 100:281.
133. Ferrer M. I.: The sick sinus syndrome in atrial disease. JAMA 1968; 206:645.
134. Jordan J. L., Yamguchi I., Mandel W. J.: The sick sinus syndrome. JAMA 1977; 237:682.
135. Alpert M. A., Flaker G. C.: Arrhythmias associated with sinus node dysfunction. JAMA 1983; 250:2160.
136. Doering W.: Quinidine-digoxin interaction. Pharmokinetics underlying mechanism and clinical implications. N Engl J Med 1979; 301:400-404.
137. Selzer A., Wrag H. W.: Quinidine syncope. Circulation 1964; 30:17-26.
138. Josephson M., Caracta A., Riccuitti M.: Electrophysiologic

properties of procainamide in man. Am J Cardiol 1974; 33:596–603.

139. Roden D. M., Reele J. B., Higgins J. B.: Antiarrhythmic efficacy, pharmokinetics and safety of N-acetyl procainamide in human subjects: comparison with procainamide. Am J Cardiol 1980; 46:463–468.

140. Anderson R. J., Gentsin E.: Procainamide—induced pericardial effusion. Am Heart J 1972; 83:798–800.

141. Strasberg B., Schlarasky S., Erdberg A.: Procainamide—induced polymorphous ventricular tachycardia. Am J Cardiol 1981; 47:1309–1313.

141a.LeCorré P., Gibassier D., Sado P., and LeVerge R.: Stereoselective metabolism and pharmacobinetics of disopyramide enantiomers in humans, Drug Metab. Dispos 1988; 16:858–64.

141b.Mirro M. J., Watanabe A. M., and Barley J. C.: Elect physiological effects of disopyramide and quinidine on guinea pig and canine Purkinje fibers. Dependence on underlying cholmergic tone, Circ. Res. 1980; 46:660–669.

141c.Birkhead J. S., and Vaughan Williams E. M.: Dual effect of disopyramide on atrial and atrioventricular conduction and refractory periods, Br. Heart J. 1977; 39:657–660.

141d.Gilman A. G.: Goodman and Gilman's The Pharmacologic Basis of Therapeutics, 8th Ed. New York, McGraw-Hill, 1990.

141e.Purdy R. E., and Boucek R. J.: Handbook of Cardiac Drugs, Little, Brown and Co., Boston Third Printing 1988.

142. Kupersmith J.: Electrophysiological and antiarrhythmic effects of lidocaine in canine acute myocardial ischemia. Am Heart J 1979; 97:360–365.

143. Danahy D. T., Aronow W. S.: Lidocaine-induced cardiac rate changes in atrial fibrillation and atrial flutter. Am Heart J 1978; 95:474–481.

144. Nath S., Haggmark S., Johansson G., Reiz S.: Differential depressant and electrophysiologic cardiotoxicity of local anesthetics: An experimental study with special reference to lidocaine and bupivacaine. Anesth Analg 1986; 65:1263–1270.

145. Albright G. A.: Cardiac arrest following regional anesthesia with etidocaine or bupivacaine. Anesthesiology 1979; 51:285–286.

146. Clarkson D. W., Hondeghem L. M.: Mechanism for bupivacaine depression of cardiac conduction: Fast block of sodium channels during the action potential with slow recovery from block during diastole. Anesthesiology 1985; 62:396–405.

147. Moller R. A., Covino B. G.: Cardiac electrophysiologic effects of lidocaine and bupivacaine. Anesth Analg 1988; 67:107–114.

148. Wheeler D. M., Bradley E. L., Woods W. T.: The electrophysiologic action of lidocaine and bupivacaine in the isolated, perfused canine heart. Anesthesiology 1988; 68:210–212.

149. Kotelko D. M., Shnider S. M., Dailey P. A., Brizgys R. V., Levinson G., Shapiro W. A., Koike M., Rosen M. A.: Bupiva-

caine-induced cardiac arrhythmias in sheep. Anesthesiology 1984; 60:10–18.

150. Covino B. G.: Toxicity of local anesthetics. Advances in Anesthesia 1986; 3:37–59.

151. Heavner J. E.: Cardiac dysrhythmias induced by infusion of local anesthetics into the lateral cerebral ventricle of cats. Anesth Analg 1986; 65:133–138.

152. Wesley R., Resh W., Zimmerman D.: Reconsideration of the routine preferential use of lidocaine in the emergent treatment of ventricular arrhythmias. Crit Care Med 1991; 19:1439–1444.

153. Zeisler J., Camp J., Gaardner T., Misuraca L., Saketkhoo K., Shah M., O'Brien A., Imparato B., Sadowinski W.: Reconstruction of the routine and preferential use of lidocaine in the emergent treatment of ventricular arrhythmias. (Letter). Crit Care Med 1993; 21:305.

154. Calvin J. E., Parrillo J. E.: Lidocaine and acute coronary care. Crit Care Med 1993; 21:179–181.

155. Menkhaus P. G., Reves J. G., Kissin I., Alvis J. M., Govier A. V., Samuelson P. N., Lell W. A., Henling C. E., Bradley E.: Cardiovascular effects of esmolol in anesthetized humans. Anesth Analg 1985; 64:327–334.

156. Gold M. I., Sacks D., Grosnoff D. B., Herrington C., Skillman C. A.: Use of esmolol during anesthesia to treat tachycardia and hypertension. Anesth Analg 1989; 68:101–104.

157. Kasten G. W., Martin S. T.: Successful cardiovascular resuscitation after massive intravenous bupivacaine overdosage in anesthetized dogs. Anesth Analg 1985; 64:491–497.

158. Kasten G. W., Martin S. T.: Bupivacaine cardiovascular toxicity: Comparison of treatment with bretylium and lidocaine. Anesth Analg 1985; 64:911–916.

159. Schulte-Sasse U., Hess W., Markschies-Hornung A., Tarnow J.: Combined effects of halothane anesthesia and verapamil on systemic hemodynamics and left ventricular myocardial contractility in patients with ischemic heart disease. Anesth Analg 1984; 63:791–798.

160. Atlee J. L., Hamann S. R., Brownlee S., Kreigh C.: Conscious state comparisons of the effects of the inhalation anesthetics and diltiazem, nifedipine, or verapamil on specialized atrioventricular conduction times in spontaneously beating dog hearts. Anesthesiology 1988; 68:519–528.

161. Kapur P. A., Flacke W.: Epinephrine-induced arrhythmias and cardiovascular function after verapamil during halothane anesthesia in the dog. Anesthesiology 1981; 55:218–225.

162. Kapur P. A., Norel E., Dajee H., Cimochowski G.: Verapamil treatment of intractable ventricular arrhythmias after cardiopulmonary bypass. Anesth Analg 1984; 63:460–463.

163. Camm A. J., Garratt C. J.: Adenosine and supraventricular tachycardia. N Engl J Med 1991; 325:1621–1629.

164. Stemp L. I., Roy W. L.: Adenosine for the conversion of supraventricular tachycardia during general anesthesia and open heart surgery. Anesthesiology 1992; 76:849–852.

Chapter 8

NEUROHUMORAL CONTROL OF CIRCULATION

JAMES A. DI NARDO

This chapter is intended to be an overview of the factors controlling circulation in the major vascular beds of the body. In addition, the effect of anesthetic agents on these vascular beds will be addressed.

SYSTEMIC CIRCULATION

Discussion of the systemic circulation will be divided into sections on the peripheral arterial, venous, and capillary circulations (Fig. 8–1).[1]

Peripheral Arterial Circulation Controls

The peripheral arterial circulation is under the control of both intrinsic and extrinsic factors, which are summarized.

Nervous System Control (Fig. 8–2)

The sympathetic nervous system innervation of the peripheral circulation is reviewed in Vasoactive and Inotropic Agents. Some remarks are appropriate at the point.

Central Nervous System Control

Suprasegmental regulation of blood vessels consists of a large number of intracranial regions that exert significant effects.[2] Many levels of the central nervous system have independent long-fiber pathways directly (and without intermediate relay at medulla) to spinal centers, as well as the classical pathways interconnecting, the various areas in the brain which are known to contribute to the control of blood vessels.

Final Pathway

Ultimate control of sympathetic outflow to the blood vessels is determined by the discharge rate of sympathetic cell bodies in the spinal cord. These are in the lateral cell column. Within the physiologic discharge rate, postganglionic discharge frequency has a 1:1 relation to the discharge frequency in the preganglionic fiber. The preganglionic cell bodies, therefore, serve as the final common pathway for central autonomic discharge to the blood vessels.

Humoral Factors

Atrial natriuretic peptide (ANP)

Atrial natriuretic peptide is a peptide released by myocytes in the right atrium in response to increases in atrial volume and pressure, increase of salt intake, and infusions of phenylephrine, angiotensin II, and vasopressin.[3] ANP induces peripheral vasodilation, suppression of ADH and aldosterone release and direct renal effects.

Renin-angiotensin System

Renin is a proteolytic enzyme produced by the juxaglomerular cells of the kidney. Renin is released in response to epinephrine, stimulation of the sympathetic nervous system, stimulation of intrarenal baroreceptors, and reduced sodium delivery to the macula densa. Renin in turn cleaves angiotensinogen to angiotensin I. Angiotensin I is converted to angiotensin II by angiotensin-converting enzyme in the lungs. Angiotensin II stimulates release of aldosterone and is the most potent vasopressor produced by the body.

Endothelium-derived Relaxing Factor (EDRF)

Endothelium-derived relaxing factor, which appears to be NO is described in the chapter Vasoactive and Inotropic Agents. Basal release of EDRF/NO by vascular endothelium is responsible for modulation of peripheral vascular tone.

Baroreceptor Reflexes

Baroreceptors are located in the aortic arch and the carotid sinuses. These receptors communicate with the medullary vasomotor center via the vagus and glossopharyngeal nerves respectively. Increased stretch of these receptors due to increased blood pressure results in decreased sympathetic nervous system output and vasodilation. Other reflexes are of lesser importance for normal control but include somatic reflexes for pain and cold.

Chemical Effects

Elevated PCO_2 stimulates output from the medullary vasomotor center resulting in peripheral vasoconstriction. This effect is attenuated by the local vasodilating effect of PCO_2 on vascular smooth muscle. PCO_2 and a reduction in oxygen tension or of pH cause vasodilatation locally.

Peripheral Venous Circulation

The peripheral venous circulation serves both a conduit and a reservoir function. The unstressed volume of the venous capacitance system is 50 ml/kg or approximately 3.5 liters. This is the volume of blood that can be

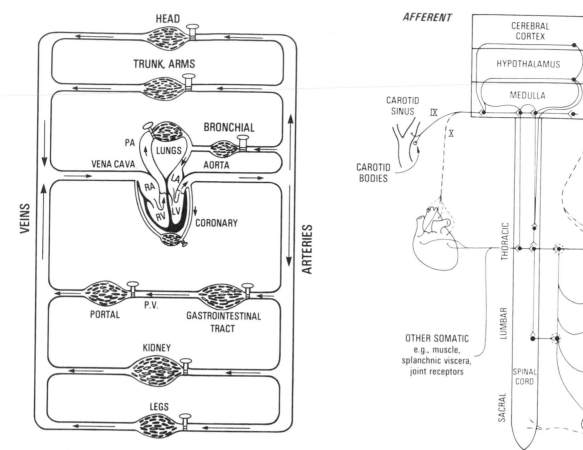

Fig. 8–1. The pulmonary and systemic circulations. The pulmonary circulation is connected in series to the remainder of the circulation (blood flows first through the chambers of the right heart and lungs, and then through chambers of the left heart). The organ systems operate in parallel from the systemic circulation. The small bronchial arteries supply oxygenated blood to the tissue of the lungs. *PA*, pulmonary artery; *RA*, right atrium; *LA*, left atrium; *LV*, left ventricle; *RV*, right ventricle; *PV*, portal vein. From Ross, J. Jr.: Introduction to the Cardiovascular System. In Best and Taylor's Physiological Basis of Medical Practice, 12th ed. Edited by J. B. West. Baltimore, Williams & Wilkins, 1990.

Fig. 8–2. Schematic diagram of the neural connections important in circulation control. Although the system is bilaterally symmetrical, in this schematic drawing inputs (afferent fibers to the *left*) and outputs (sympathetic and parasympathetic efferent fibers, to the *right*) are shown only on one side. From Covell J. W.: Neurohumoral Control of the Circulation. In Best & Taylor's Physiological Basis of Medical Practice, 12th ed. Edited by J. B. West. Baltimore, Williams & Wilkins, 1990; Adapted from Korner, 1979.

contained in the venous system at a mean pressure of 0 mm Hg,[4,5] and represent a normal nervous capacity of about 65% of the active circulating volume. The stressed volume is the additional smaller volume increment (1.5 L) necessary to create the pressure gradient from peripheral veins to the right atrium. The unstressed volume will be reduced by venoconstriction and increased by venodilation. All the intrinsic and extrinsic factors described under control of the peripheral arterial system influence the venous system as well.

Capillary Circulation

The arterioles have several metarterioles that give rise to innumerable precapillaries, which in turn are divided into capillaries. The precapillary sphincters are under sympathetic control but local factors such as pressure and metabolites may be more important in determining tone.

Net fluid capillary filtration is described by Starling's law of capillary filtration:

$$Q = kA[(P_c - P_i) + \sigma(\pi_i - \pi_c)]$$

Q = fluid filtration
k = capillary filtration coefficient, this is a measure of water conductivity
A = capillary membrane area
P_c = capillary hydrostatic pressure
P_i = interstitial hydrostatic pressure
σ = albumin reflection coefficient, 0 is free permeability and 1.0 is no permeability. Most capillaries have a reflection coefficient of 0.6 to 0.9
π_i = interstitial colloid oncotic pressure
π_c = capillary colloid oncotic pressure

Anatomy (Fig. 8–3)

For study of the microcirculation the anatomy of the arteriolar system is basic. Arterioles may be defined as branches of the small arteries with diameters less than

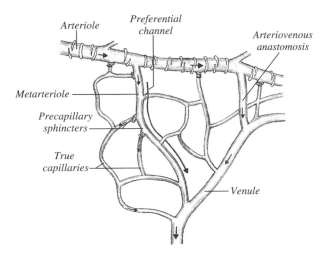

Fig. 8–3. Basic scheme of capillary unit. Sketch according to Chambers and Zweifach. The capillary network is an organized system. Redrawn from Sketch by Thomas E. Nelson, Jr., from Fulton, Medical Physiology. W.B. Saunders Co.

Table 8–1. Listing of the Average Size of All Vessels Analyzed in this Study

Order	Type	Average Size (μm)
First	Arteriole	99.6
	Venule	160.3
Second	Arteriole	71.5
	Venule	90.8
Third	Arteriole	38.5
	Venule	53.9
Fourth	Arteriole	17.4
	Venule	25.0

Hutchins, P., Goldstone, J., and Wells, R. Microvascular Research 5:131, 1973.

150 μm. There are four orders of arterioles in descending size to the capillary bed. The size of the first order arteriole averages 100 μm with a range from 75 to 125 μm. The second order arteriole has an average internal diameter of 75 μm and a range of 50 to 100 μm. The third order has an average diameter of 40 μm, and the fourth order averages 15 μm.[6,7] The metarteriole is considered the terminal part of the fourth order of arteriole and immediately precedes the precapillary sphincter and the capillary bed. Each arteriole is accompanied by a venule of appropriate size (Table 8–1).

The capillary channel is approximately 5–7 μm in diameter and can accommodate a red blood cell. The volume of the capillary is small being about 4% of the total blood volume. The precapillary resistance vessels represent the largest pressure drop in the circulation from a mean pressure of about 85 mm Hg in the aorta to 38 mm Hg across the metarterioles while across the capillary vessels the pressure decreases to 25 mm Hg. The remainder of the pressure fall occurs in the postcapillary venules to reach the venous pressure of 5 mm Hg. Plasma volume tends to be preserved because capillary oncotic pressure is greater than interstitial oncotic pressure.

CORONARY CIRCULATION

Anatomy

The majority of patients (85%) have a right dominant system of coronary circulation. The right coronary artery extends to the crux cordis in the atrioventricular groove and gives rise to the posterior descending branch, the left atrial branch, the AV nodal branch, and one or more posterior left ventricular branches. In a left-dominant system (8%), these branches are supplied by the left circumflex artery and the right coronary artery supplies only the right atria and ventricle. In 7% of patients the system is balanced with the right coronary artery supplying the posterior descending, left atria and AV nodal branches

while the left circumflex artery supplies the posterior left ventricular branches.

Coronary perfusion pressure (CPP)

Coronary perfusion can only occur in the time intervals when aortic root pressure exceeds subepicardial and subendocardial pressure. Myocardial back pressure, which is the sum of factors that collapse microvessels, is important in determining coronary perfusion pressure.[8] For practical, clinical purposes myocardial back pressure can be assumed to be equal to myocardial tissue pressure. The best estimate of myocardial tissue pressure is the ventricular intracavitary pressure. In diastole this will be the ventricular end diastolic pressure. The best clinical estimate of left ventricular end diastolic pressure is the pulmonary capillary wedge pressure (PCWP) while the best estimate of right ventricular end diastolic pressure is the central venous or right atrial pressure (RAP).

Coronary perfusion pressure will differ during systole and diastole. In the left ventricle intracavity pressure during systole is equal to or in the case of aortic stenosis greater than aortic root pressure. For this reason the vast majority of coronary blood flow to the left ventricle occurs during ventricular diastole. Aortic blood pressure gradually falls during diastole because of peripheral runoff and thus reference to mean aortic diastolic blood pressure (MADBP) is often made. In the absence of obstruction to flow within the coronary arterial system left ventricular CPP = MADBP-PCWP (Figure 8–4). In the right ventricle where intracavitary systolic and diastolic pressures are both considerably less than aortic root pressure coronary blood flow is more evenly distributed between systole and diastole.

Autoregulation

Changes in coronary vascular resistance are necessary if the myocardium is to be able to regulate coronary blood flow in response to changes in myocardial oxygen consumption. When myocardial oxygen consumption is constant it is desirable for the myocardium to maintain coronary blood flow constant. The intrinsic ability of the myocardium to maintain coronary blood flow constant

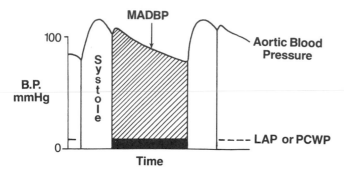

Fig. 8–4. Left ventricular coronary perfusion pressure (CPP) is the difference between aortic diastolic blood pressure and left ventricular diastolic pressure (LVEDP). Clinically LVEDP is estimated by left atrial pressure (LAP) or pulmonary capillary wedge pressure (PCWP). The diastolic CPP is represented by the cross-hatched area and can be seen to decrease as diastole progresses. The average diastolic CPP can be obtained by taking the difference between the mean aortic diastolic blood pressure (MADBP) and the LAP or PCWP.

over a variety of perfusion pressures when myocardial oxygen consumption is constant is referred to as coronary autoregulation.[9] As Figure 8-5 illustrates, coronary autoregulation maintains coronary blood flow constant between perfusion pressures of 60 to 140 mm Hg. Below and above these pressures myocardial blood flow is pressure dependent; that is, myocardial blood flow will vary linearly with pressure and with the time available for perfusion (diastole for the left ventricle, systole and diastole for the right ventricle).

Autoregulation is dependent on changes in coronary vascular resistance. The primary source of resistance in the coronary arterial system is the intramyocardial arterioles. Currently the stimulus for changes in resistance is poorly understood. Autoregulation may be tied to myocardial oxygen metabolism and coronary venous PO_2 although the exact mediators at the vascular level are unknown.[5] During exercise reductions in coronary vascular resistance increase coronary blood flow. Likewise as CPP decreases coronary vascular resistance decreases so that coronary blood flow is maintained. At the lower pressure limits of autoregulated coronary blood flow coronary vascular resistance is minimal. This is referred to as exhaustion of autoregulatory coronary vasodilator reserve. Because further reductions in coronary vascular resistance are impossible through the autoregulatory process, coronary blood flow decreases linearly with coronary perfusion pressure once the lower pressure limits of autoregulation are reached. The autoregulatory vasodilator reserve of the subendocardium appears to be exhausted before that of the subepicardium.[5]

Collateral Blood Flow

The development of collateral blood flow in humans is dependent on enlargement of pre-existing anastomoses between coronary arteries. These anastomoses may be either serial (prestenosis to post stenosis from the same artery) or parallel (one artery to another). These existing collateral pathways enlarge in response to pressure gradients. Once the collateral pathways have enlarged the direction and magnitude of collateral blood flow remains pressure dependent. For this reason, collateral blood flow to a poststenotic segment can be drastically reduced if perfusion pressure at the origin of the collateral is reduced.

INCREASED MYOCARDIAL OXYGEN DEMAND

Three factors are primarily responsible for determining myocardial oxygen consumption (MVO_2): wall tension, contractility, and heart rate.

Wall tension

Myocardial wall tension (T) is determined by the relationship between intraventricular radius (r), intraventricular pressure (P) and ventricular wall thickness (h) according to Laplace's law: $T = Pr/h$. Ventricular wall tension is constantly changing during the cardiac cycle. For example during isovolumic contraction intraventricular pressure and wall thickness will be increasing while ventricular radius remains unchanged. During ventricular ejection ventricular pressure will remain constant while radius decreases and wall thickness increases. Inherent in the analysis of wall tension are the concepts of preload, afterload, and hypertrophy. Increases in end diastolic volume (preload) will increase ventricular radius and will reduce wall thickness if dilation is severe. These changes will increase wall tension. Increases in the impedance to ventricular ejection (afterload) will necessarily increase intraventricular pressure and will also increase wall tension. Concentric ventricular hypertrophy will increase wall thickness and reduce wall tension.

Important differences exist between the increase in MVO_2 induced by increases in preload and by those in-

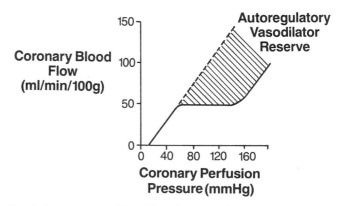

Fig. 8–5. Coronary blood flow is seen to be constant (autoregulated) over coronary perfusion pressures from 60 to 140 mm Hg in this illustration. When coronary perfusion pressure reaches 60 mm Hg there will be maximal autoregulatory vasodilation to maintain coronary blood flow. Further decreases in coronary perfusion pressure will result in decreases in coronary blood flow. At pressures above 60 mm Hg maximal autoregulatory vasodilation will provide autoregulatory vasodilator reserve. This reserve provides the increased coronary blood flow necessary to meet increases in myocardial oxygen consumption such as those induced by exercise.

duced by increases in afterload. Work done in the isovolemic phase of ventricular contraction is energy consumptive. Increases in the impedance to ventricular ejection increase the pressure required to begin ventricular ejection and thus increase the work done in the isovolemic contraction phase. The ejection phase of ventricular contraction on the other hand is a more energy efficient process. Increases in preload induce ejection of a larger stroke volume and an increase in the work done in the ejection phase. For these reasons when equal quantities of work are compared, the increase in MVO_2 induced by an increase in preload (volume work) is much less than that induced by an increase in afterload (pressure work).[10]

Contractility

Contractility is defined as the state of myocardial performance independant of preload and afterload. Increasing the contractile state of the heart increases MVO_2. However, an increase in contractility may actually result in a MVO_2, which is reduced or unchanged under certain conditions. If ventricular dilation (increased ventricular radius) exists as the result of exhaustion of preload reserve to maintain cardiac output wall tension and MVO_2 will be high. Improving contractility through use of an inotropic agent will reduce ventricular radius by reducing reliance on a large preload to maintain cardiac output. The reduction in MVO_2 that accompanies an reduction in wall tension may more than offset the increase in MVO_2 which accompanies an increase in contractility.

Heart rate

It is important to review the manner in which increases in heart rate affect myocardial oxygen balance. Myocardial oxygen balance must be examined on a beat to beat basis. Myocardial ischemia is not induced with tachcardia simply because there are more beats per minute but because supply per beat is inadequate to meet demand per beat. Increases in heart rate increase MVO_2 per beat by increasing contractility via the Bowditch effect. Normally an increase in heart rate is accompanied by a decrease in end diastolic volume. This reduction in preload reduces wall tension and MVO_2 per beat. Thus the increase in MVO_2 per beat caused by tachycardia enhanced contractility is in large part offset by the reduction in MVO_2 per beat that accompanies reduced wall tension. Oxygen delivery on the other may be compromised by tachycardia-induced reductions in the length of diastole per beat.

REDUCED MYOCARDIAL OXYGEN DELIVERY

Adequate myocardial oxygen supply is dependent on delivery of the appropriate volume of oxygenated coronary blood flow. The following factors may compromise myocardial oxygen delivery.

Reduction in CPP

Left ventricular CPP can be reduced either by a reduction in mean aortic diastolic blood pressure or by an increase in left ventricular end diastolic pressure. A commonly overlooked cause of reduced CPP is bradycardia. Bradycardia encourages diastolic runoff from the proximal aorta and may result in a wide pulse pressure and a reduced mean aortic diastolic blood pressure. Furthermore, maintenance of cardiac output with bradycardia requires an increased stroke volume. The increased stroke volume will be maintained primarily by an increase in left ventricular end diastolic volume and pressure. This further reduces CPP.

Reduction in the Time Available for Coronary Perfusion

Because the left ventricle receives the majority of its perfusion during diastole reductions in the time per beat spent in diastole are potentially detrimental. Figure 8–6 illustrates that as heart rate increases the length of time per beat spent in diastole is diminished while the length of systole remains more constant. Because MVO2 per beat is minimally affected by tachycardia the primary disadvantage of tachycardia is a reduction in diastolic perfusion time per beat.

Coronary Artery Obstruction

Any obstruction to flow in a coronary artery results in a pressure drop across the obstruction. The high velocity of blood flow in the area of a stenosis or spasmotic segment necessarily results in the conversion of pressure energy to kinetic energy. On the distal side of the obstruction turbulent eddies form and dissipate. The transfer of kinetic energy to this turbulent energy and the subsequent dissipation of the turbulence reduces the quanity of kinetic energy available for reconversion to pressure energy.[11] This results in a pressure decrease across the obstruction. The pressure decrease across the obstruction will increase in direct proportion to any increase in flow across the obstruction as a greater proportion of kinetic energy is dissipated as turbulence. For this reason requirements for increased coronary blood flow such as those which accompany exercise will increase the hemodynamic significance of any obstructive lesion.

Arteriolar dilatation distal to the obstruction will help compensate for this pressure loss until the stenosis becomes critical. A stenosis is said to be critical when the autoregulatory vasodilator reserve distal to it is nearly exhausted to maintain coronary blood flow at rest. Some vasodilatory reserve is needed to maintain basal coronary blood flow with stenoses as small as 30–45% and this reserve is nearly exhausted with stenoses greater than 90%.[12] When reserve is exhausted and the pressure distal to the stenosis falls below 55–60 mm Hg coronary blood flow will decrease linearly with further decreases in perfusion pressure and the subendocardium will be at risk for developing ischemia. Therefore, in the presence of an obstructive coronary lesion proximal coronary artery pressure (mean aortic diastolic pressure) will have to be greater than 60 mm Hg to ensure a distal pressure above 60 mm Hg.

The main coronary artery epicardial branches have lumens 2–4 mm in diameter. Exertional angina occurs when lumen area is reduced to 1.0 mm^2 (a 60% diameter reduction).[8,13] The threshold for the onset of ischemia at

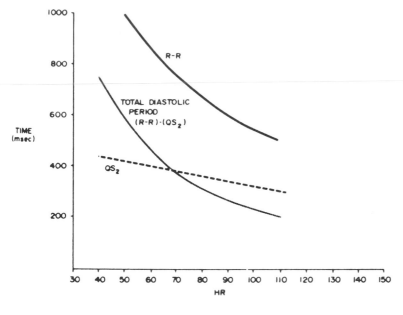

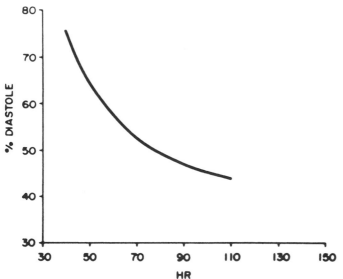

Fig. 8–6. Top, Increases in heart rate cause a decrease in the lenght of each cardiac cycle (R-R interval). The decreases in the lenght of systole (QS2) with increases in heart rate are far less dramatic than the decreases in the lenght of diastole (R-R minus QS2). Bottom, Percent of each cardiac cycle (R-R interval) spent in diastole at various heart rates. Small changes in heart rate are seen to cause large decreases in the percent of time spent in diastole.

rest appears to be a lumen area of 0.63 mm² or approximately a 72% reduction in lumen diameter.[8] Subendocardial infarction has been associated with a lumen area of 0.35 mm² (76% diameter reduction) while transmural infarctions involve lumens with areas of 0.26 mm² (81% diameter reduction).[8]

Several factors are responsible for reducing or obstructing flow within the coronary arterial system. Not all the factors are active in a given patient manifesting myocardial ischemia. However various combinations of these factors are necessary to explain the wide clinical variation in the ischemic, preinfarction, and infarction patterns of patients. The following factors deserve attention.[14]

Atherosclerotic Disease

Atheromatous lesions may be localized to one area of the arterial wall. As these eccentrically located lesions enlarge they enchroach upon the arterial lumen. Because the remainder of the arterial wall is free of plaque it remains responsive to vasoactive stimuli and is capable of contraction. Such contraction will cause the fixed atheromatous lesion to occupy a greater portion of the arterial lumen and will result in a larger pressure decrease across the lesion. Therefore the severity of the stenosis is not static but is dynamic and dependent on the vasomotor activity of the free arterial wall. This phenomena is known as dynamic coronary stenosis.[16] A normal change in coronary vasomotor tone resulting in a 10% circumferential shortening of the outer arterial wall can convert a nonsignificant 49% eccentric stenosis to a 76% stenosis. This will result in rest ischemia (Fig. 8-7). Likewise, a normal increase in arterial tone can convert an eccentric stenosis, which causes ischemia on exertion (60% stenosis) to one which also causes ischemia at rest (76% stenosis) (Fig. 8-7).

Atheromatous lesions may be static if the atheromatous changes involve the entire circumference of the arterial wall. In this instance the lumen area is fixed and is unaltered by changes in arterial vasomotor activity (Fig. 8-7). A lesion that occupies the entire circumference of the ar-

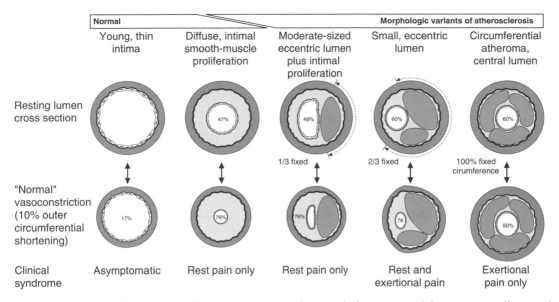

Fig. 8–7. Cross-sections of normal and diseased coronary arteries. The morphologic state of the arteries is illustrated. The percent reduction in lumen diameter for each morphologic state at rest and following a normal degree of vasoconstriction is also illustrated. The clinical syndromes associated with both the resting and vasoconstricted state of the normal and diseased arteries are summarized at the bottom of the diagram. See text for discussion.

terial wall and causes exertional ischemia (60% stenosis) will be unaffected by changes in arterial vasoconstriction.

Variations in Coronary Vasomotor Tone

The extent of coronary vasomotor activity manifested by patients varies. At one end of the spectrum is the normal 10% reduction in outer arterial wall circumference which occurs with α-adrenergic stimulation such as that induced by isometric hand grip, hand emersion in ice water, or emotional upset.[8,15] At the other end of the spectrum is the intense vasoconstriction or spasm that occurs with variant or Prinzmetal's angina. Spasm is defined as inappropriate active vasoconstriction of a segment of coronary artery resulting in total or subtotal occlusion in response to stimuli which cause only minimal constriction in individuals who do not have variant angina.[16] In patients with physiologic coronary vasoconstriction myocardial ischemia will occur only if coronary stenoses also exist. In patients with coronary spasm myocardial ischemia may develop in the absence of coronary stenoses.

Intermediate to these two extremes is the coronary vasoconstriction induced in the region of coronary stenoses by a variety of vasoactive substances. Platelet activation occurs at the site of coronary narrowing and endothelial disruption. The release of the potent coronary vasocontrictors thromboxane A2 and serotonin by platelets may enhance normal coronary vasomotor tone and may enhance coronary vascular response to vasoconstrictors.[7] Such responsiveness can convert a nonsignificant eccentric atherosclerotic lesion to a significant one.[10] Likewise leukotrienes can enhance coronary arterial tone. These arachidonic acid derivatives seem to be released in greater amounts by atherosclerotic vessels.[11]

Platelet Activation in Narrowed Arteries

In addition to enhancing coronary vasomotor tone through release of vasoactive substances platelet activation in narrowed arteries may result in further narrowing of the vessel lumen and eventually even complete occlusion of the lumen through thrombus formation.[9]

Coronary Steal

Recently the phenomena of coronary steal has received a great deal of attention. It must be emphasized that for patients with coronary artery disease to develop coronary steal their coronary anatomy must meet certain criteria and they must be exposed to a potent arteriolar dilator. Two types of coronary steal exist[17]:

1) **Collateral dependent to collateral independent** (pressure dependent to pressure independent): or this type of steal to exist the following anatomic criteria must be met (Figure 8-8)[14,18]:

- An occluded coronary artery
- Collateral blood flow to the area distal to the occlusion
- A hemodynamically significant stenosis of the vessel supplying the collaterals

Approximately 23% of the 16,249 patient angiograms contained in the CASS registry met these anatomical criteria.[19]

Once these anatomical criteria are met the administration of an agent which is an arteriolar dilator such as dipyridamole or adenosine is necessary to produce a steal. Autoregulation induced arteriolar dilation in the collateral dependent region will be maximal at rest in order to maintain blood flow to this compromised region. In other words, coronary autoregulatory vasodilator reserve will be exhausted in this region and perfusion will be

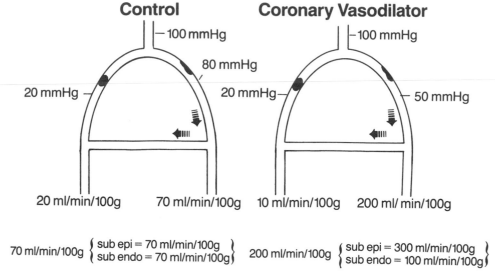

Fig. 8–8. Schematic representation of the coronary anatomy present in patients at risk for coronary vasodilator induced coronary steal. Control In the control state the myocardium distal to the completely obstructed vessel is supplied via collaterals from the partially stenosed vessel. In this collateral dependent myocardium autoregulatory vasodilation is maximal and perfusion to this zone is pressure dependent. The pressure gradient for perfusion of this area is 60 mmHg (80-20 mmHg) and flow is 20 ml/min/100g in the direction of the arrows. The myocardium distal to the partially stenosed vessel retains coronary vasodilator reserve. Flow to this area is 70 ml/min/100 g and this flow is evenly distributed between the subepicardium and the subendocardium.

pressure dependent. Exposure to an arteriolar dilator will have little additional effect on collateral dependent arteriolar tone but will dilate arterioles in the collateral independent region. This will cause a increase in flow across the stenosis and a reduction in the perfusion pressure distal to the stenosis. The result will be a reduction in flow to the pressure dependent collateralized region. Blood will be shunted from this collaterized region to the region supplied by the stenosed vessel which provides the collaterals (Fig. 8-8) Ischemia in the collateral dependent region may then develop.

2) **Subendocardial to subepicardial (transmural):** for this type of steal to exist, only a severe stenosis in a coronary artery and exposure to an arteriolar dilator such as dipyridamole or adenosine is required.[14] Autoregulation induced arteriolar dilatation in the subendocardium distal to a stenosis will be maximal at rest to maintain subendocardial blood flow. When this occurs subendocardial perfusion will be pressure dependent. Exposure to an arteriolar dilator will have little additional effect on subendocardial arteriolar tone but will dilate arterioles in the subepicardium. This will cause a increase in flow across the stenosis and a reduction in the perfusion pressure distal to the stenosis. The result will be a shunting of blood away from the subendocardium toward the subepicardium with resultant subendocardial ischemia (Fig. 8-8).

PULMONARY CIRCULATION

Anatomy

Branches of the pulmonary artery ramify extensively through the lung substance and the ramifications accompany the respiratory tract. Each bronchiole is accompanied by an arteriole and within the lung parenchema a dense plexus of capillaries is formed around the alveoli.

The bronchial circulation arises from the thoracic aorta and intercostal arteries and receives about 1-2% of the total cardiac output. This circulation provides nutrients to the lung. A portion of the bronchial vessels anastomose with pulmonary alveolar capillaries with subsequent drainage to the left atrium. There may be impressive enlargement of these connections in the presence of chronic low pulmonary blood flow as seen with cyanotic congenital heart disease. Another smaller portion of the bronchial circulation joins the bronchial venous system at the bronchial and bronchiolar level; drainage is into the right atrium via the ayzgos and hemiayzgos veins. Finally, a small (1-2%) anatomic shunt is created by blood from bronchial arteries which reach the pulmonary parenchema and deliver deoxygenated blood to the left atrium via the pulmonary veins.

Blood Flow

The pulmonary circulation is a high-flow low-pressure system. The pulmonary bed performs several important functions:

Transport Through the Lungs

The distribution of pulmonary blood flow is illustrated (Fig. 8-9). In zone 1, alveolar pressure exceeds pulmonary capillary pressure creating physiologic dead space. In zone 2, pulmonary capillary pressure exceeds alveolar pressure which exceeds pulmonary venous pressure. In this situation reductions in pulmonary venous pressure will not increase pulmonary blood flow. This is the hydraulic equivalent of the Starling resistor. In zone 3, both pulmonary capillary and pulmonary venous pressure exceed alveolar pressure. Zone 1 regions normally occur at the apices while zone 3 regions are

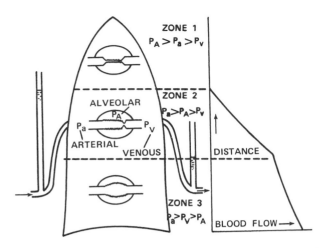

Fig. 8–9. Model to explain the uneven distribution of blood flow in the lung based on the pressures affecting the capillaries. Zones of pulmonary blood flow. P_A = alveolar pressure, P_a = pulmonary arterial pressure, P_v = pulmonary venous pressure. In Zone 1 there is alveolar dead space as there is ventilation but no perfusion. In Zone 2 pulmonary venous pressure is not a determinant of pulmonary blood. Pulmonary blood flow is determined by the difference between pulmonary artery and alveolar pressure. In Zone 3 pulmonary blood flow is determined by the difference between pulmonary artery and venous pressure. From West, J. B., et al. J Appl Physiol 19:713–724, 1964. In Best and Taylor's Physiological Basis of Medical Practice. Williams & Wilkins, Baltimore, 1990.

present at the bases. An acute reduction in pulmonary capillary pressure or an increase in alveolar pressure can convert a zone 2 region to a zone 1 and a zone 3 to a zone 2.

Pulmonary Vascular Resistance

This is influenced by a number of factors.

Oxygen Tension (PO₂)

Both alveolar hypoxia and arterial hypoxia induce pulmonary vasoconstriction.[20,21] Hypoxic pulmonary vasoconstriction is the homeostatic mechanism which diverts blood away from hypoxic regions of the lung. This mechanism helps to maintain a more balanced ventilation/perfusion relationship by reducing shunt.

Hypercarbia (PCO₂)

Hypercarbia increases PVR independent of arterial pH.[22] Hypocarbia on the other hand only reduces PVR through production of an alkalosis.[23] Maximal reduction in PVR occurs at an arterial PCO_2 of 20 mm Hg and a pH of near 7.60.[24]

Acid-Base Balance (pH)

Both respiratory and metabolic alkalosis reduce PVR,[17,20,21] whereas both respiratory and metabolic acidosis increase PVR.[17,18]

Variation in Lung Volumes

At small lung volumes atelectasis results in compression of extra-alveolar vessels, while at high lung volumes hyperinflation of alveoli results in compression of intra-alveolar vessels. Therefore, pulmonary vascular resistance is normally lowest at lung volumes at or near the functional residual capacity.

Vasodilator Agents

At present no oral or intravenously delivered drug is available which acts as a selective pulmonary vasodilator. Drugs such as PGE_1, nitroglycerin, sodium nitroprusside, and tolazoline all induce some degree of systemic vasodilation as well. There is increasing enthusiasm for nitric oxide (NO) which delivered as an inhalant (10–40 ppm) is proving to be a potent selective pulmonary vasodilator in patients with pulmonary hypertension.[25-28]

Inhalation Anesthetics

Inhalation anesthetics do not selectively reduce pulmonary vascular resistance. Clinically relevant concentrations (1–1.5 MAC) of enflurane, halothane, and isoflurane inhibit hypoxia pulmonary vasoconstriction while intravenous agents have no effect.[29] In clinical practice the attenuation of hypoxic pulmonary vasoconstriction by inhalation agents is mitigated by anesthetic induced reductions in cardiac output, mixed venous oxygen saturation, and pulmonary artery pressure.[30] As a result the use of these agents during one lung ventilation usually has little effect on shunt and PaO_2.[31-33]

Compliance

The compliance of the pulmonary venous system attenuates acute changes in left atrial and ventricular compliance. This helps prevent pulmonary vascular congestion and pulmonary edema.

Capillary Filtration

This role is described in detail in the section on capillary circulation. Cardiogenic pulmonary edema results from an increase in P_C (capillary hydrostatic pressure) while noncardiogenic pulmonary edema results from an increase in k (capillary permeability)

Vascular Endothelial Functions

The pulmonary vascular endothelium is responsible for biosynthesis and removal of a wide variety of vasoactive substances including catecholamines, prostaglandins, leukotrienes, and peptides.

CEREBRAL CIRCULATION (TABLE 8–2)

Anatomy

The cerebral circulation is provided by two paired arteries, the internal carotids and the verterbrals. These arteries together with the anterior and posterior communicating arteries form the circle of Willis in the cranial cavity at the base of the brain. This system allows collateral blood flow in the presence of an arterial occlusion.

Table 8–2. Normal Values, Units and Abbreviations

Full Name	Abbreviations	Normal Values and Units
Cerebral blood flow	CBF	44 ml/100 g/min
Regional cerebral blood flow	rCBF	20–80 ml/100 g/min
Cerebral perfusion pressure*	CPP	80 torr
Cerebrovascular resistance†	CVR	1.8 torr/ml/100 g/min
Arteriovenous oxygen content difference	$(A-V)O_2$	6.8 ml/100 ml
Cerebral metabolic rate for oxygen	$CMRO_2$	3.0 ml/100 g/min
Cerebral metabolic rate for glucose	CRMglucose	4.5 mg/100 g/min
Cerebral metabolic rate for lactate	CMRlactate	2.3 mm/100 g/min
Cerebral venous oxygen tension	PvO_2	35–40 torr
Oxygen-glucose index	OGI	90–100%
Lactate-glucose index	LGI	0–10%
Cerebral blood flow equivalent	$CBF/CMRO_2$	14–15 ml/blood/ml O_2

*Definded as mean arterial minus mean cerebral venous pressure or mean arterial pressure minus intracranial pressure.
†Defined as CPP/CBF.

Cerebral Perfusion Pressure (CPP) and Intracranial Pressure (ICP)

Cerebral perfusion pressure is defined as the difference between the mean arterial pressure and the ICP. Normally ICP is less than 10 mm Hg and varies directly with central or jugular venous pressure. Three major components comprise the contents of the skull; the brain, the cerebrospinal and extracellular fluids, and blood. An increase in the volume of one or more of these components in the closed cranium will eventually increase ICP. As illustrated in Figure 8-10, initial increases in intracranial volume will not increase ICP owing to the compressibility of the intracranial structures. In addition the ability of CSF and blood to be translocated extracranially provides a buffer for acute changes in volime. As volume increases, ICP increases precipitously as the compressibility of structures in the closed compartment is exhausted. Increases in ICP reduce CPP and can also cause herniation of brain tissue.

Blood Flow

Cerebral blood flow (CBF) is influenced by a variety of factors which are discussed below and some of which are summarized in Figure 8-11. Under normal conscious conditions, CBF in the adult human averages 40 to 60 ml/100 g of brain tissue per minute. As regional CBF (rCBF) falls, neuronal function and metabolism change. When rCBF decreases to approximately 20 mls · 100 gm^{-1} · min^{-1} neuronal electrical function ceases, as manifested by flattening of the electroencephalogram (EEG) and loss of evoked potentials. A rCBF approaching 15 mls/100 gm/min can be tolerated for about 2 hours without ill effect if perfusion is subsequently restored. If perfusion is restored after this time, significant cerebral edema results.

Flows less than 15 to 20 mls/100 gm/min, if lasting longer than 2 to 3 hours, lead to cerebral infarction. A CBF of 10 mls/100 gm/min, for even a brief period of time (3-6 minutes), results in intracellular ATP depletion and consequent failure of membrane ion pumps. The re-

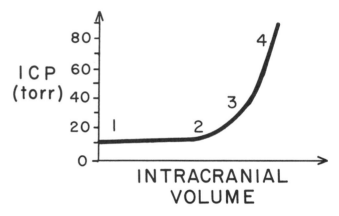

Fig. 8–10. Intracranial pressure volume curve. At low volumes (1-2) compliance is high and changes in volume have little or no influence on ICP. As volume increases compliance diminishes and volume changes result in gradual (2–3) and then precipitous (3–4) increases in ICP.

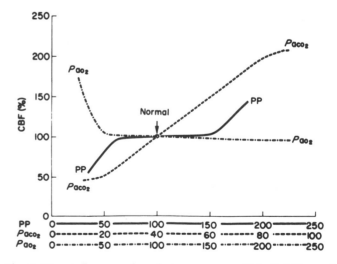

Fig. 8–11. Influence of perfusion pressure (PP), PaCO$_2$, and PaO$_2$ on CBF in the autoregulated brain. One parameter is varied while the other two are held constant.

sult of this failure is a massive efflux of potassium from the ischemic neuron. Potassium efflux heralds a series of irreversible chain reactions and subsequent subcellular events which inexorably lead to neuronal necrosis, irrespective of subsequent perfusion.

PCO₂

Between 20 and 80 mm Hg, there is a linear relationship between PCO_2 and cerebral blood flow due to changes in cerebral vascular resistance (CVR). For each 1 mm Hg increase in PCO_2, there is a 1 ml/100 g/min increase in CBF and approximately a 30 ml change in cerebral blood volume. Hypercarbia (PCO_2 greater than 40 mm Hg) induces cerebral vasodilatation and increases CBF while hypocarbia (PCO_2 less than 40 mm Hg) induces cerebral vasoconstriction and reduces CBF. These changes are believed to be secondary to changes in the hydrogen ion concentration of the extracellular fluid of vascular smooth muscle.[34]

With maintenance of hypo or hypercarbia PCO_2 induced changes in CBF are relatively short lived. Cerebral spinal fluid bicarbonate adjustments begin to return CBF to normal in 4-6 hours with complete return to normal in 24-36 hours.

In areas of focal cerebral ischemic there can be near maximum cerebral vasodilation and loss of cerebral autoregulation. Intentional hypocarbia will reduce CBF to regions of the brain with retained autoregulation and will increase flow to the vasodilated ischemic areas. This is known as inverse steal or the Robin Hood effect. Conversely hypercapnia will result in over perfusion of normal regions and underperfusion of ischemic regions a phemonena known as luxury perfusion.

PaO₂

At arterial oxygen tensions below 50 mm Hg there is a reduction in CVR and an increase in CBF.

Cerebral Perfusion Pressure

CBF is constant when arterial blood pressure is between 50 and 150 mm Hg in normal patients. This intrinsic ability of the brain to maintain CBF constant over a variety of perfusion pressures when cerebral metabolic rate for oxygen ($CMRO_2$) is constant is refered to as cerebral autoregulation. Autoregulation is dependent on changes in cerebral vascular resistance. These resistance changes are myogenic in origin with the cerebral arterioles constricting or dilating in response to distending pressure. The response time is not immediate and takes 2-3 minutes. Thus acute changes in CPP will result in transcient changes in CBF. Chronically hypertensive patients have a shift of the upper and lower limits of the autoregulatory curve to the right.

When vasodilatory mechanisms are unable to provide adequate oxygen delivery, cerebral tissues extract a greater fraction of arterial oxygen content. Normally, cerebral tissues extract 35-40% of the available arterial oxygen content, but under conditions of ischemia may extract up to 80-90%.

CMRO₂

CBF is intimately coupled to $CMRO_2$ both regionally and globally with increases and decreases in $CMRO_2$ leading to increases and decreases in CBF. The mechanism is unclear but may be related to changes in potassium or hydrogen ions in the extracellular fluid surrounding resistance vessels.

Normal, conscious $CMRO_2$ is 3.5 ml/100gm/min. Approximately 50% of metabolic activity, and consequent ATP generation, is directed toward neuronal electrical (synaptic) function, while the remainder is devoted to membrane ion pumps and cellular homeostasis. Since the brain has little reserve of oxygen or glucose, it is dependent on a constant supply of these substrates.

Hypothermia

With hypothermia cerebral requirements for oxygen and glucose decrease. The relative decrease in metabolism over a range of 10 degrees is quantitated by the term O_{10}. For the brain this value equals about 2.2.[35] Hence, from 37°C to 27°C $CMRO_2$ would be expected to decrease from 3.5 ml/100gm/min to 1.6 ml/100gm/min. With further cooling the EEG slows, and at <18-20°C becomes flat.

Inhalation Anesthetics

The effects of inhalation anesthetic agents on CBF and $CMRO_2$ are summarized in Table 8-3. Halothane, enflurane and isoflurane all decrease $CMRO_2$. Preliminary evidence suggests that sevoflurane and desflurane do as well. Isoflurane depresses $CMRO_2$ more than enflurane and halothane.[32] With appropriate coupling of $CMRO_2$ and CBF this should produce a reduction in CBF. However, all these agents are cerebral vasodilators, which tend to increase CBF. Halothane is a more potent vasodilator than enflurane or isoflurane. As a result halothane uniformly increases CBF while isoflurane at inspired concentrations less than 1 MAC is the most favorable to the CBF/$CMRO_2$ relationship. At this concentration there is a reduction in $CMRO_2$ with little or no increase in CBF.

The same appears to be true for sevoflurane.[36] To date

Table 8-3. Relative Effects of Anesthetic Drugs on CBF and $CMRO_2$

	CBF	$CMRO_2$	CBF/$CMRO_2$ Coupling
Halothane	↑ ↑ ↑	↓	No
Enflurane	↑ ↑	↓	No
Isoflurane	↑	↓ ↓	Yes
Sevoflurane	↑	↓ ↓	Yes
N₂O	↑	↑	?
Barbiturates	↓ ↓ ↓	↓ ↓ ↓	Yes
Narcotics	↓ ↓	↓	?
Ketamine	↑ ↑	↑	Yes
Midazolam	↓ ↓	↓ ↓	Yes
Etomidate	↓ ↓ ↓	↓ ↓	Yes
Propofol	↓ ↓	↓ ↓	Yes

no human studies looking at $CMRO_2$ and CBF have been done with desflurane. Desflurane and isoflurane produce similar increases in CBF and show similar preservation of CO_2 reactivity.[37] Isoflurane is commonly used as an adjuvant agent during neuroanesthesia; at inspired concentrations exceeding 1 MAC, the increasing cerebral vasodilation caused by isoflurane progressively uncouples cerebral metabolism and blood flow.

Cerebral vascular responsiveness to PCO_2 is maintained with inhalation agents. This means that inhalation agent induced cerebral vasodilation can be attentuated by hyocarbia. Unfortunately, enflurane can induce seizure activity which is potentiated by hypocarbia. Seizures dramatically increase $CMRO_2$ and CBF.

Intravenous Anesthetics

The effects of some commonly used intravenous anesthetic agents on CBF and $CMRO_2$ are summarized in Table 8-3. Barbiturates dramatically decrease $CMRO_2$ and as a result decrease CBF in parallel. The reduction in metabolic rate produces cerebral vasoconstriction. When an isoelectric EEG is produced with thiopental $CMRO_2$ and CBF are reduced by 50%. Etomidate also reduces $CMRO_2$ and CBF in parallel. However, some cerebral vasoconstriction occurs prior to the reduction in $CMRO_2$.[38] Propofol in combination with N_2O maintains coupling of CBF with PCO_2[39] and propofol alone appears to reduce $CMRO_2$ and CBF in parallel.[40] Ketamine can increase regional $CMRO_2$ and CBF.[41]

Opioids have traditionally been believed to reduce $CMRO_2$ and CBF. Some recent investigations have demonstrated fentanyl and sufentanil to increase CBF[42] and sufentanil to increase ICP[43,44] while others have demonstrated no change in CBF[45] or ICP[46] with sufentanil. It should be noted that that the ICP elevations noted were transient. The benzodiazepine midazolam reduces $CMRO_2$ and CBF in parallel.[47]

Muscle Relaxants

Succinylcholine administration produces increases in muscle afferent activity, $CMRO_2$ and CBF. This can result in an increase in ICP in patients with reduced intracranial compliance. Both a paralyzing dose of vecuronium[48] and a defasculating dose of metacurine[49] prevent this ICP increase. Atracurium, vecuronium, and pancuronium have no effect on ICP in neurosurgical patients.[50-52]

UTERINE AND PLACENTAL CIRCULATION

Anatomy

The uterine placenta is composed of three important units: 1) the fetal component composed of chorionic villi, 2) the maternal component composed of the decidua basalis and its blood vessels, and 3) the intervillous space between the fetal and maternal components.

The villus is a core of connective tissue with capillaries at its tip. These capillaries are supplied by branches of the umbilical arteries and are drained by branches of the umbilical vein. The maternal decidua basalis contains spiralling arteries which pass through into the intervillous space. These are branches of the uterine arteries. Extensive endometrial venules are also located in the decidua basalis. These drain into the uterine veins.

Blood Flow

Approximately 80% of the 500 ml/min of total uterine blood flow enters the intervillous space per minute. At any given time there is approximately 175 ml in the intervillous space. The spiral uterine arteries spurt blood into the low pressure intervillous space where exchange with villous blood occurs across the syntrophoblastic layer of the villi and the villous capillary endothelium. Following each sput blood drains form the intervillous space into the endometrial venous system.

Several factors can reduce uteroplacenta blood flow. Reductions in uteroplacenta blood flow are deleterious because they predispose to fetal distress. These factors are summarized.

Aortocaval Compression

Fifty percent of pregnant patients have narrowing of the lower aorta and its branches in the supine position as the result of uterine compression in the second and third trimesters.[53] This can lead to uteroplacenta insufficiency and fetal distress. 90% of pregnant women have complete obstruction of the inferior vena cava by the uterus in the supine position beginning in the second trimester.[54] Brachial artery blood pressure is maintained in this circumstance by an increase in peripheral resistance and near normal venous return by shunting of blood from the distal vena cava to the proximal vena cava and superior vena cava via collateral return from the ovarian, iliolumbar, paraverterbral, and azygos veins. In 10% of women, this compensation is incomplete and supine hypotensive syndrome characterized by tachycardia, hypotension, pallor, and faintness occurs.[55] Left lateral uterine displacement will prevent aortocaval compression in the pregnant patient.

Uterine Contractions

Uterine contractions reduce perfusion to the intravillous spaces by increasing intramyometrial pressure. Labor contractions reduce placental perfusion by one fifth with complete cessation of flow at peak contraction.

Hypotension

Apart from aotocaval compression hypotension is most likely to result from hemorrhage and induction of regional anesthesia. Obviously maternal hypotension can seriously compromise the fetus by reducing placenta blood flow. Maternal hypotension should be promptly treated with left lateral uterine displacement, infusion of a balanced salt solution and supplemental oxygen to the mother. If vasoactive agents are deemed necessary ephedrine is the drug of choice because uterine blood flow improves linearly with blood pressure.

Pre-eclampsia/Eclampsia

Pre-eclampsia is diagnosed on the basis of hypertension, proteinura, or edema, or both. Eclampsia is diagnosed when convulsions or coma occur as well. Although the precise mechanism of these disorders is unknown, uteroplacental ischemia and uteroplacental insufficiency is a hallmark. An inbalance between uteroplacental thromboxane and prostacyclin with an overproduction of thromboxane is probably involved.[56] This thromboxane overproduction leads to vasoconstriction, endothelial damage, platelet aggregation, and enhanced uterine activity. Pre-eclampsia/eclampsia produces dysfunction in multiple end organs as a result of these changes.

Placental Transfer of Drugs

Transfer of drugs across the placenta occurs by simple diffusion as defined by the Fick principle:

$$Q/t = \frac{KA\,(C_m - C_f)}{D}$$

Q/t = rate of diffusion
K = diffusion constant
A = diffusion surface area
C_m = concentration of free drug in maternal blood
C_f = concentration of free drug in fetal blood
D = thickness of diffusion barrier

The diffusion constant of a drug is determined by drug molecular size, ionization status, and lipid solubility. Drugs with a molecular weight less than 500 daltons easily cross the placenta while those with weights of 500–1000 are more restricted. Most commonly used anesthetic drugs are of low molecular weight. Lipophilic drugs cross the placenta easily and drugs that are unionized are more lipophilic. The pK_a is the pH at which the concentrations of free base and cation are equal. When the pK_a of a drug is close to physiologic pH (such as amide local anesthetics) potential for ion trapping in the fetus exists. If the fetus is acidotic drug which crosses the placenta to the fetus will have a greater tendency to be converted to the ionized form which has a lesser tendency to cross back to the maternal side of the placenta. This will result in accumulation of drug in the fetus.

REFERENCES

1. Ross, J. The Cardiovascular System. In Best and Taylor's The Physiological Basis of Medical Practice, 12th Ed. John B. West, Ed. Baltimore, Williams & Wilkins, 1990.
2. Korner P. I. Central nervous control of autonomic cardiovascular function. In Handbook of Physiology. Section 1, Vol 1. The Cardiovascular System. Washington, DC: The American Physiologic Society, p 691–739, 1979.
3. Needleman P., Greenwald J. E. Atriopeptin: A cardiac hormone intimately involved in fluid, electrolyte, and blood pressure homeostasis. N Eng J Med 314:829, 1986.
4. Rothe C. F. Physiology of venous return. An unappreciated boost to the heart. Arch Int Med 146:977, 1986.
5. Shoukas A. A. Overall systems analysis of the carotid sinus baroreceptor reflex control of the circulation. Anesthesiology 79:1402, 1993.
6. Zweifach B. W., Lowenstein B., and Chamber R. Responses of blood capillaries to acute hemorrhage in the rat. Am J Physiol 142:80–93, 1944.
7. Hutchins P. M., Goldstone J., and Wells R. Effects of hemorrhagic shock on the microvasculature of skeletal muscle. Microvasc Res 5:131–140, 1973.
8. Klocke F. J., Weinstein I. R., Klocke J. F., et al. Zero-flow pressures and pressure-flow relationships during single long diastoles in the canine coronary bed before and during maximal vasodilation. J Clin Invest 68:970, 1981.
9. Dole W. P. Autoregulation of the coronary circulation. Prog Cardiovasc Dis 29:293, 1987.
10. Suga H., Hayashi T., Suehiro S., Hisano R., Shirahata M., Ninomiya I. Equal oxygen consumption rates of isovolumic and ejecting contractions with equal systolic pressure-volume areas in canine left ventricle. Circ Res 49:1082, 1981.
11. Brown B. G., Bolson E. L., Dodge H. T. Dynamic mechanisms in human coronary stenosis. Circulation 70:917, 1984.
12. Gould K. L., Lipscomb K. Effects of coronary stenoses on coronary blood flow reserve and resistance. Am J Cardiol 34:48, 1974.
13. Brown B. G. Coronary vasospasm. Observations linking the clinical spectrum of ischemic heart disease to the dynamic pathology of coronary atherosclerosis. Arch Intern Med 141:716, 1981.
14. Conti C. R., Mehta J. L. Acute myocardial ischemia: role of atherosclerosis, thrombosis, platelet activation, coronary vasospasm, and altered arachidonic acid metabolism. Circulation 75(suppl 5):84, 1987.
15. Brown B. G., Lee A. B., Bolson E. L., Dodge H. T. Reflex constriction of significant coronary stenosis as a mechanism contributing to ischemic left ventricular dysfunction during isometric exercise. Circulation 70:18, 1984.
16. Maseri A. Role of coronary artery spasm in symptomatic and silent myocardial ischemia. J Am Coll Cardiol 9.249, 1987.
17. Gross G. J., Warltier D. C. Coronary steal in four models of single or multiple vessel obstruction in dogs. Am J Cardiol 48:84, 1981.
18. Becker L. C. Conditions for vasodilator-induced coronary steal in experimental myocardial ischemia. Circulation 57:1103, 1978.
19. Buffington C. W, Davis K. B., Gillispie S., Pettinger M. The prevalance of steal-prone coronary anatomy in patients with coronary artery disease: An analysis of the Coronary Artery Surgery Study registry. Anesthesiology 69.721, 1988.
20. Fishman A. Hypoxia on the pulmonary circulation: How and where it acts. Circ Res 38:221–231, 1976.
21. Abman S. H., Wolfe R. R., Accurso F. J. Pulmonary vascular response to oxygen in infants with severe bronchopulmonary dysplasia. Pediatrics 75:80–84, 1985.
22. Malik A. B., Kidd B. S. L. Independent effects of changes in H^+ and CO_2 concentration on hypoxic pulmonary vasoconstriction. J Appl Physiol 34:318–323, 1973.
23. Schreiber M. D., Heyman M. A., Soifer S. J. Increased arterial pH, not decreased PCO_2, attenuates hypoxia-induced pulmonary vasoconstriction in newborn lambs. Pediatr Res 20:113–117, 1986.
24. Drummond W. H., Gregory G. A., Heyman M. A. The independent effects of hyperventilation, tolazoline and dopamine on infants with persistent pulmonary hypertension. J Pediatr 98:603–611, 1981.
25. Frostell C., Fratacci M. D., Wain J. C., et al. Inhaled nitric oxide: A selective pulmonary vasodilator reversing hypoxic pulmonary vasoconstriction. Circulation 83:2038–2047, 1991.
26. Girard C., Lehot J. J., Pannetier J. C., et al. Inhaled nitric oxide after mitral valve replacement in patients with chronic pulmonary hypertension. Anesthesiology 77:880–883, 1992.
27. Rich G. F., Murphy G. D., Roos C. M., et al. Inhaled nitric oxide. Selective pulmonary vasodilation in cardiac surgical patients. Anesthesiology 78:1028, 1993.
28. Sellden H., Winberg P., Gustafsson L. E., et al. Inhalation of

nitric oxide reduced pulmonary hypertension after cardiac surgery in a 3.2 kg infant. Anesthesiology 78:413, 1993.

29. Eisenkraft J. B. Effects of anaesthetics on the pulmonary circulation. Br J Anesth 65:63, 1990.

30. Benumof J. L. Isoflurane anesthesia and arterial oxygenation during one-lung ventilation. Anesthesiology 64:419, 1986.

31. Rees D. I., Gaines G. Y. One-lung anesthesia—a comparison of pulmonary gas exchange during anesthesia with ketamine or enflurane. Anesth Analg 63:521, 1984.

32. Rogers S. M., Benumof J. L. Halothane and isoflurane do not decrease PaO$_2$ during one-lung ventilation in intravenously anesthetized patients. Anesth Analg 64:946, 1985.

33. Benumof J. L., Augustine S. D., Gibbons J. A. Halothane and isoflurane only slightly impair arterial oxygenation during one-lung ventilation in patients undergoing thoracotomy. Anesthesiology 67:910, 1987.

34. Messick M. M., Newberg L. A., Nugent M., et al. Principles of neuroanesthesia for the neurosurgical patient with CNS pathophysiology. Anesth Analg 64:143, 1985.

35. Michenfelder J. D., Theye R. A. Hypothermia: Effect on canine brain and whole-body metabolism. Anesthesiology 29:1107, 1968.

36. Kitaguchi K., Ohsumi H., Kuro M., et al. Effects of sevoflurane on cerebral circulation and metabolism in patients with ischemic cerebrovascular disease. Anesthesiology 79:704, 1993.

37. Ornstein E., Young W. L., Fleischer L. H., Ostapkovich N. Desflurane and isoflurane have similar effects on cerebral blood flow in patients with intracranial mass lesions. Anesthesiology 79:498, 1993.

38. Milde L. N., Milde J. H., Michenfelder J. D. Cerebral functional, metabolic and hemodynamic effects of etomidate in dogs. Anesthesiology 63:371, 1985.

39. Fox J., Gelb A. W., Enns J., et al. The responsiveness of cerebral blood flow to changes in arterial carbon dioxide is maintained during propofol-nitrous oxide anesthesia in humans. Anesthesiology 77:453, 1992.

40. Van Hemelrijck J., Fitch W., Mattheussen M., et al. Effect of propofol on cerebral circulation and autoregulation in the baboon. Anesth Analg 71:49, 1990.

41. Takeshita H., Okuda Y., Sari A. The effects of ketamine on cerebral circulation and metabolism in man. Anesthesiology 36:69, 1972.

42. Trindle M. R., Dodson B. A., Rampil I. J. Effects of fentanyl versus sufentanil in equipotent doses on middle cerebral artery blood flow velocity. Anesthesiology 78:454, 1993.

43. Sperry R. J., Bailey P. L., Reichman M. V., et al. Fentanyl and sufentanil increase intracranial pressure in head trauma patients. Anesthesiology 77:416, 1992.

44. Albanese J., Durbec O., Viviand X., et al. Sufentanil increases intracranial pressure in patients with head trauma. Anesthesiology 79:493, 1993.

45. Mayer N., Weinstabi C., Podreka I., Spiss C. K. Sufentanil does not increase cerebral blood flow in healthy human volunteers. Anesthesiology 73:240, 1990.

46. Weinstabl C., Mayer N., Richling B., et al. Effects of sufentanil on intracranial pressure in neurosurgical patients. Anaesthesia 46:837, 1991.

47. Forster A., Juge O., Morel D. Effects of midazolam on cerebral blood flow in human volunteers. Anesthesiology 56:453, 1982.

48. Minton M. D., Grosslight K. R., Stirt J. A., et al. Increases in intracranial pressure from succinylcholine: Prevention by prior non-depolarizing block. Anesthesiology 65:165, 1986.

49. Stirt J. A., Grosslight K. R., Bedford R. F., et al. "Defasiculation" with metacurine prevents succininylcholine-induced increases in intracranial pressure. Anesthesiology 67:50, 1987.

50. Minton M. D., Stirt J. A., Bedford R. F., et al. Intracranial pressure after atracurium in neurosurgical patients. Anesth Analg 64:1113, 1985.

51. Stirt J. A., Maggio W., Haworth C., et al. Vecuronium: Effect on intracranial pressure and hemodynamics in neurosurgical patients. Anesthesiology 67:570, 1987.

52. McLeskey C. H., Cullen B. F., Kennedy R. D., et al. Control of cerebral perfusion pressure during induction of anesthesia in high-risk neurosurgical patients. Anesth Analg 53:985, 1974.

53. Bieniarz J., Crottogini J. J., Curuchet E., et al. Aortocaval compression by the uterus in late human pregnancy. II. An angiographic study. Obstet Gynecol 100:203, 1968.

54. Kerr M. G., Scott D. B., Samuel E. Studies of the inferior vena cava in pregnancy. Br Med J 1:532, 1964.

55. Howard B. K., Goodson J. H., Mengert W. F. Supine hypotensive syndrome in late pregnancy. Obstet Gynecol 1:371, 1953.

56. Walsh S. W. Preeclampsia: An imbalance in placenta prostacyclin and thromboxane production. Am J Obstet Gynecol 152:335, 1985.

Chapter 9

BLOOD PRESSURE, PULSE, AND FLOW

JAMES A. DI NARDO AND VINCENT J. COLLINS

Blood pressure is the pressure exerted by the blood on the walls of the vessels in which it is flowing.[1,2] To study blood pressure, a cannula can be inserted into a large artery of the body, such as the carotid, and connected to a transducer; the pressures are recorded electronically. Such a record of blood pressure reveals four types of waves representing normal variations in pressure over a period of 1 or more minutes.[3]

1. *Cardiac Contraction.*
2. *Mechanical Effects of Respiration.* Changes in pressure within the thorax are reflected in the vessels and in cardiac output. During inspiration, cardiac rate increases and overall arterial pressure increases slightly.
3. *Vasomotor Tone Changes.* In the central nervous system, fluctuations in vagal efferent activity synchronous with respiration also account for some of the changes in the heart rate and blood pressure[2] During inspiration, vagal tone decreases and increases during expiration. Similarly cyclic variations in activity of areas of the brainstem influence efferent autonomic activity to the cardiovascular system. Interactions between the respiratory "pacemakers" and cardiovascular centers alter autonomic output and affect heart rate and blood pressure. The blood pressure variations induced have the same periodicity as that of respiration. The waves of increased blood pressure are called Traube-Hering and occur at a rate of 5-10 per minute.
4. *Alteration of Splenic Volume.* The spleen contracts and relaxes rhythmically. The contractions occur approximately every 50 seconds, which increases blood volume and this in turn increases the pressure.

Analysis and magnification of each blood pressure pulse due to cardiac action reveals a maximum or systolic pressure occurring at the height of cardiac contraction and representing total heart energy and a minimum or diastolic pressure occurring during cardiac relaxation and reflecting the integrity of the vessels—it is the sum of the forces acting contrary to cardiac force.

Pulse pressure is the difference between systolic and diastolic pressures. It represents the efficient work of the heart and indicates the extent to which cardiac action overcomes peripheral resistance. It is the excess of pressure over and above that required to equalize the diastolic pressure, to open the aortic valves, to develop potential energy in arterial walls, and to force blood into capillaries.

SCHEMA OF BLOOD PRESSURE

Blood pressure shows a gradient of fall from the heart and aorta through the arteries and arterioles.[4] At the arterioles there is a sharp decrease in pressure followed by a more gradual decrease in the capillary bed. Pressure continues to decrease in the venules so that in the large veins of the chest and at the entrance of the great veins into the right auricle, a negative or subatmospheric pressure occurs (Fig. 9-1).

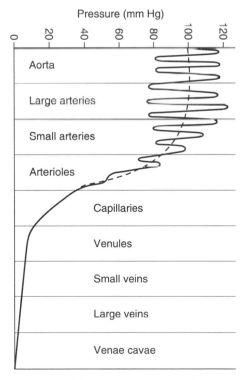

Fig. 9-1. Schema of blood pressures in the functionally differentiated segments of the vascular bed. Redrawn from Mellander and Johansson, 1968.

155

DYNAMICS OF PULSATILE-PRESSURE FLOW

With pulsatile flow caused by intermittent pressure pulses in a stiff system (a visceroelastic arterial tree),[5] the flow velocity wave lags behind the driving pressure wave. The pressure wave precedes the flow velocity wave in the peripheral arteries and can be palpated as a pulse. Initially[6] the ventricular contraction imparts a driving force on the column of blood in the ascending aorta, which is accelerated to move the blood ahead of the pressure wave into the arterial tree; at this point the pressure wave however advances at a greater velocity than the flow of blood. Blood continues to move as long as there is a dynamic pressure difference but ceases when the difference is zero, that is when ventricular ejection ceases.

With increased frequency of the ventricular contractions, the driving pulse pressures become continuous and the flow approaches a steady state. The musculature of the arterial and arteriolar tree also contribute to the steady flow.[5]

PHYSIOLOGY OF PULSATILE PRESSURE FLOW

The left ventricle and the arterial tree are coupled. The generation of blood pressure and the arterial pulse is the direct consequence of the interaction between the contractile left ventricle and the viscoelastic arterial tree. The arterial tree influences ventricular performance through alterations in aortic input impedance. Similarly arterial blood pressure is directly related to the volume ejected by the left ventricle into the arterial tree.

Aortic Input Impedance

Aortic input impedance is defined as the ratio of pulsatile pressure and flow wave forms obtained throughout the cardiac cycle and expressed as frequency moduli.[7] Fourier analysis allows a pressure or flow wave form to be defined by a unique set of sine waves or harmonics. Each harmonic has a modulus (amplitude), a phase angle (relative timing of pressure and flow waves) and a frequency. The ratio of the pressure harmonic to the flow harmonic at a given frequency is defined as impedance. An aortic input impedance spectra is a graphic display of this ratio over an appropriate frequency range (Figure 9-2). From this type of analysis, for a given impedance spectra, the aortic pressure wave form will be uniquely determined by the aortic flow wave form. Likewise for a given impedance spectra and aortic pressure wave form, there can only be one pattern of flow ejected from the left ventricle into the aorta.

Aortic input impedance can also be defined as the sum of external factors that oppose ventricular ejection. Thus it can serve as a ready measure of afterload. Aortic input impedance is determined by both pulsatile (the density of blood, the diameter and compliance of the aorta, and the reflected pressure and flow waves generated in the peripheral arterial tree) and non-pulsatile (the peripheral resistance) components. Normally, frequency-dependent impedance is 5-10% of total input impedance.[8]

A example of an aortic input impedance spectra is illustrated in Figure 9-2. The characteristic impedance Z_0 describes the elastic properties of the arterial tree. Wave reflections exert most influence at low frequencies (<2 Hz), and thus, at higher frequencies the input impedance approaches the characteristic impedance. The input impedance at frequency 0 is the non-pulsatile component, which is commonly called the peripheral resistance and is comprised of arteriolar tone and the viscosity of the blood.[9,10]

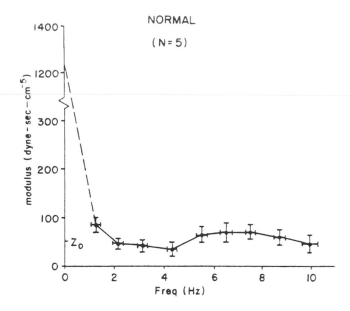

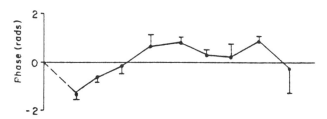

Fig. 9-2. Input impedance in normal human subjects (top). Z_0 is characteristic impedance. Impedance at frequency 0 is peripheral resistance. Impedance phase is shown below. The phase is initially negative (flow leads pressure) and subsequently positive (pressure leads flow).

Mean Arterial Blood Pressure

Mean arterial blood pressure is the average pressure that exists in the arterial tree during a cardiac cycle. It is the non-pulsatile component of blood pressure on which the pulsatile components (systolic and diastolic) are superimposed. As such mean arterial blood pressure is determined by the volume of blood ejected by the left ventricle (stroke volume) and the peripheral resistance (impedance at frequency 0). Thus for a given stroke volume mean arterial pressure will increase as peripheral resistance increases. After an increase in stroke volume, the magnitude of the mean arterial pressure increase depends only on peripheral resistance while the rate at which the increase develops depends on aortic compliance (Z_0).

Pulse Pressure

Pulse pressure is the difference between systolic and diastolic pressure. It is largely determined by the stroke volume and the characteristic impedance. When aortic compliance is low (high Z_0) the delivery of pulsatile flow will create a wide pulse pressure. This is analogous to delivery of pulsatile flow into a rigid pipe. Conversely, delivery of pulsatile flow to a very compliant system (infinite Z_0) will result in the generation of a constant pressure, that is no pulse pressure.

Normally the difference between the systolic pressure and the mean pressure will be greater than the difference between the mean and the diastolic pressure. Typically 80% of the stroke volume ejected is involved in distension of the aorta during systole while only 20% runs off to the periphery during this same phase.

Systolic Blood Pressure

Systolic blood pressure is the culmination of the ejection phase of aortic contraction. Ejection commences when left ventricular pressure exceeds aortic diastolic pressure. Ejection terminates when the stroke volume is ejected and left ventricular end-systolic volume is reached. The aortic valve closes when left ventricular pressure falls below aortic pressure.

Systolic pressure is the peak pressure during the ejection phase. It is largely determined by the stroke volume and the viscoelastic properties of the aorta (Z_0). However, other factors also contribute the increases in systolic pressure. Increased peripheral resistance increases mean arterial blood pressure. This in turn alters factors which influence pulsative aortic blood flow. Increased mean arterial pressure causes an increase in arterial wall tension. This in turn increases Z_0 which increases arterial pulse wave velocity.[11]

For a given amount of flow the peak of the arterial trace (systole) will be greater in a person with reduced aortic compliance (increased Z_0) from primary causes or from increased peripheral resistance. An increased Z_0 causes the timing of reflected wave from the periphery to change. In normal young people the timing of reflected waves from the periphery is such that pressure is augmented during diastole. With increasing age, Z_0 increases and the reflected wave velocity increases such that it augments pressure during systole. These concepts are illustrated in Figure 9-3.

Acutely an increase in ventricular contractility is necessary to maintain flow in the face of such increased impedance to ejection. Chronic elevations in impedance will stimulate the development of concentric ventricular hypertrophy and an increase in ventricular mass.

Diastolic Blood Pressure

Diastolic blood pressure is the nadir of aortic blood pressure, which occurs after aortic valve closure but before commencement of the next ejection phase. Diastolic blood pressure will be determined by the end-diastolic aortic volume and Z_0. Diastolic pressure can be expected to be reduced in situations where peripheral runoff is high. Clinically this situation exists in the presence of low

Effects of Hypertension

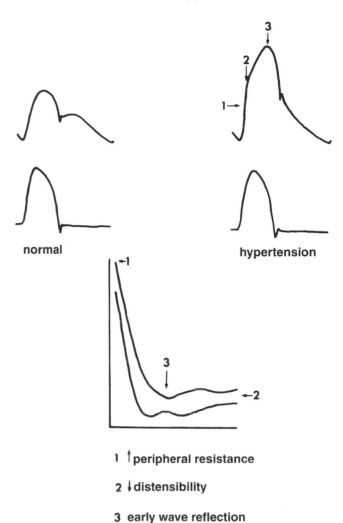

normal   **hypertension**

1 ↑**peripheral resistance**

2 ↓**distensibility**

3 early wave reflection

Fig. 9–3. Effects of hypertension on an aortic input impedance and the shape of aortic pressure wave. 1 is increased peripheral resistance which increases impedance at frequency 0 and increases mean arterial pressure. 2 is a decrease in aortic distensibility which increases Z_0 and increases systolic pressure at the anacrotic shoulder when early peak aortic flow is high. 3 is early wave reflection which increases peak systolic pressure.

peripheral resistance, with systemic to venous shunts and with aortic insufficiency.

Diastolic pressure will be reduced in situations in which there is isolated elevation of Z_0 and hence reduced aortic compliance. In this setting peripheral runoff will be enhanced by the high driving pressure in the aorta during diastole.[12] Diastolic pressure will also be reduced with bradycardia as more time is available for equilibration prior to the next systole.

Blood Velocity and Flow

Blood velocity is the speed of the average drop of blood while flow wave velocity is the speed with which motion in blood is transmitted. At least two heartbeats are required to move a drop of blood from the aortic

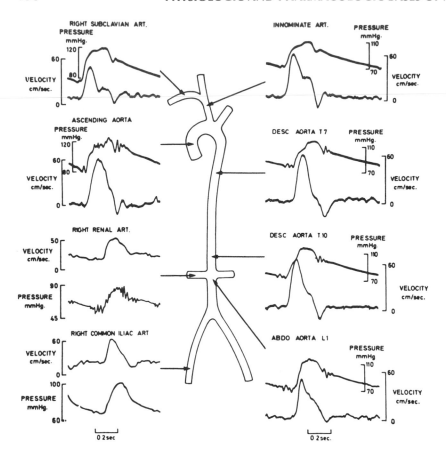

Fig. 9-4. Simultaneously recorded pressure and flow waves in the central and peripheral arterial tree. Peripheral augmentation of arterial pressure is accompanied by a diminution in arterial flow.

valve to the distal aorta yet only 0.1 seconds are required for the flow wave to travel this distance. Average blood velocity is 0.5 m/sec while flow wave velocity is 5 m/sec.

As the pulse wave travels the arterial system reflected waves from the periphery affect the shape of the arterial wave form. The effects of wave reflection on flow and velocity are the opposite of the effects on pressure. The peak arterial pressure and the pulse pressure increases as arterial pressure is sampled more distally in the arterial tree (Figure 9-4). Conversely, the amplitude of the flow and velocity profiles diminish as they are sampled more distally.

Three general types of reflected wave patterns in the ascending aorta have been described[13] (Figure 9-5). The type A pattern is seen in older individuals. In this pattern the reflected wave from the lower portion of the body occurs prior to aorta valve closure. As discussed previously this results in augmentation of systolic pressure. The type C pattern is seen in children. Here the reflected wave occurs after aortic valve closure (during diastole). The type B pattern is intermediate in character with the reflected wave occurring during aortic valve closure.

Ventriculoarterial Coupling

In an ideal circulatory system ventricular stroke work is maximized because ventricular and arterial elastances are matched.[14] Not surprisingly, when arterial and ventricular elastance are equal the effective ejection fraction is

50%.[14] When impedance and flow are considered, conditions are ideal when maximal values for flow harmonics occur at minimal values of impedance. Unfortunately, in man such matching of flow and impedance exists only during childhood. As aging occurs Z_0 increases and maximal flow occurs when aortic impedance is high. As previously discussed this results in augmented afterload and the requirement for ventricular concentric hypertrophy to keep the ventricular and arterial systems matched.

NORMAL VARIATIONS IN BLOOD PRESSURE[15]

There are no ironclad rules regarding such a variable factor as the systolic blood pressure. In all probability, it is not the same in any two consecutive movements. The usual systolic pressure in adults ranges from 105 to 145 mm Hg. The normal diastolic pressure ranges 25 to 50 mm lower than systolic. A systolic pressure below 100 mm Hg or above 150 mm Hg and a pulse pressure below

AORTIC PRESSURE

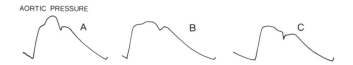

Fig. 9-5. The three types of aortic pressure waves are illustrated.

25 mm Hg or above 50 mm Hg may be regarded as abnormal. A diastolic pressure of 110 mm Hg or over is almost always pathological.

1. *Age.* Pressure in children depends largely on height and weight. There is a rapid elevation of systolic pressure at the age of puberty. Systolic pressures for some life spans are as follows: Ages 20 to 35-123 mm Hg; 36 to 50-128 mm Hg; 51 to 65-133 mm Hg. Old age is usually accompanied by higher pressures; this is due to loss of fats, general tissue shrinkage and increased rigidity of vascular system.

2. *Sex.* In females, the pressure is approximately 10 mm Hg less than in males. Pressure in children is seemingly uninfluenced by sex.

3. *Habitus.* Obese individuals have a higher systolic pressure as compared with normal individuals.

4. *Humidity.* High temperatures and high atmospheric humidity materially lower both systolic and diastolic pressures. Excessive increases in temperature raise systolic and lower diastolic pressure.

5. *Altitude.* This temporarily increases both systolic and diastolic pressures. A given amount of exercise at a high altitude raises pressure more than the same amount at a lower altitude.

6. *Posture.* Posture affects chiefly diastolic pressure. It is highest standing and lowest in recumbency. Systolic pressure changes similarly but to a lesser extent. Hence, the pulse pressure in standing position is lower than in recumbency.

7. *Psychic Influence.* Emotional outbursts may cause marked increases or profound decreases in pressure; the contemplation of exercise will cause a significant increase in systolic pressure.

8. *Regional Variations.* Different parts of the body show variations; readings in legs are usually higher than in arms. Pressures in the two arms vary a little, the left being higher.

9. *Physical Stress.* Transitory influences that increase pressure include digestion and exercise.

10. *Nutrition.* High caloric and saturated fat intake and hypercholesterolemia all increase blood pressure.

NEONATAL BLOOD PRESSURES[16]

Arterial blood pressures have been taken by the Doppler ultrasound method in unselected mature neonates (birth weights 2.6-3.9 kilograms). The ultrasound method is in close agreement with values obtained by direct intra-aortic measurement in small infants and newborns when measures at the brachial artery. Blood pressures were measured at 3-5 minutes, 10, and 30 minutes of life and intermittently during the following 24-48 hours. (Table 9-1). The following findings are of importance: Left and right arm pressures were identical or varied by less than 2 mm Hg. Lower than normal blood pressures were found in infants born by cesarean section; those recovering from intrauterine asphyxia, those exposed to maternal antihypertensive therapy and those whose mothers received thiopenta within four minutes of delivery.

Table 9-1. Systolic and Mean Pressures at Birth of 101 Nondepressed Neonates According to Mode of Delivery

Mode of Delivery	No.	Birth Weight (grams)	Systolic Pressure (mm Hg)	Mean Pressure (mm Hg)
Spontaneous	62	3.238 ± 56	65.7 ± 0.9	46.3 ± 0.8
Operative	39	3.216 ± 70	64.9 ± 1.4	46.2 ± 1.0

From Marx, G. F., Cabe, C. M., Kim, Y.I. and Eldelman, A. I. Neonatal blood pressures. Anaesthetist 25:318–322. 1976. With permission.

MAINTENANCE OF PRESSURE

The following factors are involved: (1) pumping action of heart, (2) peripheral resistance, (3) volume of blood, (4) viscosity of blood, and (5) elasticity of arteries.

PULSE

The pulse is the pressure change produced by ventricular ejection and propagated as a wave through the arterial tree to the periphery. The blood actually ejected does not move this distance but merely transmits its energy of motion to adjacent quantities of blood. Particles of blood change their position with respect to the vessel walls, but in regard to each other the relative positional changes are small. Blood velocity in the aorta, for instance, is approximately 0.5 m./sec., while the pulse pressure wave travels at a rapid rate of 5 m./sec.

Study of the form of a pulse wave is accomplished by sphygmography (Fig. 9-6). Such a wave shows an ascending limb called the anacrotic wave and a descending limb or catacrotic wave. On the descending limb is the dicrotic notch followed by the dicrotic wave. This is caused by closure of aortic valves, and the dicrotic wave is a reflected move. The peak of the wave corresponds to the systolic pressure, and the lowest point corresponds to the diastolic pressure.[17]

Variations

Certain pulse changes occasionally noted should be described. Thus, with exaggerated thoracic breathing the pulse may become imperceptible during inspiration. This is the *paradoxic pulse* since usually during ordinary inspiration the pulse is fuller because of pressure increase. *Pulsus alternans* is the alteration of a strong with a weak pulse wave irrespective of respiratory activity.

Peripheral Pulse Waves

Tracings of finger pulse waves can be obtained by use of an inflatable cuff 2.5cm in width applied about the middle finger and inflated to a desired pressure. The maximum tracing are observed just below the diastolic blood pressure level. Pressure changes in the cuff are then transduced and recorded. The important aspect of the pulse wave is the dicrotic notch (Figs. 9-5, 9-6). On the basis of the appearance of the dicrotic notch vasculograms (pulse wave contours) can be divided into four classes[18]:

Arterial pressure pulse

A Distortion of the arterial pulse wave along the aorta

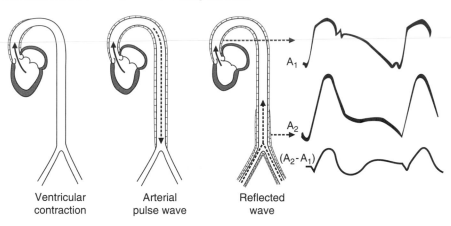

Ventricular contraction　　Arterial pulse wave　　Reflected wave

B The velocity of blood flow and arterial pulse in the aorta

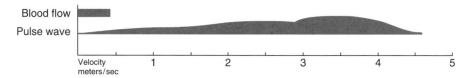

Blood flow
Pulse wave

Velocity meters/sec　　1　　2　　3　　4　　5

Fig. 9–6. A, The arterial pressure pulse is a wave of pressure which passes rapidly along the arterial system. Blood suddenly ejected into the ascending aorta at the beginning of systole has insufficient energy to overcome all the inertia of the long columns of blood in the arteries. Therefore, blood tends to pile up and distend the ascending aorta, causing a sudden local increase in pressure. Blood is then forced into the next portion of the aorta, extending the region of distention and inititating a pulse of pressure which travels rapidly along the arteries toward the periphery. These waves of pressure, reflected by peripheral structures, travel back toward the heart and become superimposed on the advancing pulse wave. This produces a higher peak of systolic pressure, a slurring of the incisura and a lower diastolic pressure in the femoral artery. If the peripheral arterial pulse wave is subtracted from the pulse recorded at the arch of the aorta, the resulting wave form ($A_2 + A_1$) suggests a natural frequency of the peripheral arterial system. B, The pulse wave velocity (4 to 5 m. per second) is much faster than the velocity of blood flow (less than 0.5 m. per second). The pulse wave velocity is determined by the elasticity of the arterial walls which, in turn, depends upon their distensibility in relation to the blood pressure. Redrawn from Rushmer, Cardiovascular Dynamics, W. B. Saunders Co.

Class I—A distinct incisura is inscribed on the downward slope of the pulse wave

Class II—No incisura develops but the line of descent becomes horizontal

Class III—No notch is present but a well-defined change in the angle of of descent is observed

Class IV—No evidence of a notch is seen

The normal wave shows a dicrotic notch (Class I). Variations include age and sex with increasing age in males. The number of "normals" decrease to less than 50% by age 50 years and to less than 10% at 65–75 years.

Women have fewer normal waves (only 5%) than men. Normal waves are seen in 28% of a population of men below 40 years. This may indicate a greater degree of vasospasm in the female. More females have class III vasculograms.

In the presence of coronary artery disease there is a progressive loss of the dicrotic incisura. High blood pressure is associated with a loss of the incisura but a well defined change in the slope of the dicrotic wave.

The pulse-wave contour represents an interaction of three principal variables: 1) the distensibility of the vessel walls, 2) the pulse velocity and 3) cardiac function, inclu-

sive of the vis a tergo force, the ejection fraction and ejection volume for cardiac output. The height of the dicrotic notch is principally determined by the systemic vascular resistance and the diastolic run-off of the pulse force, as well as the cardiac output.

CIRCULATION TIMES

The time for a particle within the vascular tree to travel from one point to another is the circulation time. Total circulation time is the time required by a particle to travel through both systemic and pulmonary circulation and return to its starting point. Various methods have been used to measure circulation time. Using fluorescein the total circulation time, i.e., from arm to arm, is approximately 21 seconds and with histamine, whose endpoint is flushing of face, the total circulation time is approximately 24 seconds. By use of radioactive salts, the arm-to-heart circulation time averages 6.6 seconds.

Pulmonary circulation time has been measured by Radium$-C^{14}$. Over the distance from the right atrium to the brachial artery, the time averages 11.0 seconds. Measurement by thorotrast over the distance from right ventricle to left ventricle gives values of approximately 1.7 to 2.0

seconds. This is considered to be the true pulmonary circulation time.

BLOOD FLOW

Velocity

The mean linear velocity of blood flow in the aorta of humans is 0.5 m/sec and in the capillaries 0.5 mm/sec. As the vascular bed widens, the velocity decreases; velocity increases in the venous side and is rapid in the great veins (Figs. 9–7, 9–8).

Distribution of Blood Volume (Table 9–2)

Blood volumes that exist in different parts of the vascular system have been approximated. In the arterial or high pressure system the total content is quite small and amounts to approximately 800 ml or 15%. The aorta contains 100 ml or 2% of the blood volume; the arteries approximately 8% and the arterioles approximately 1%.

The capillaries contain approximately 250 ml in the systemic area and 60 ml in the pulmonary area or a total of approximately 5% of the blood volume.

The systemic venous system contains a major portion of the blood volume, holding 75% or more. The heart cavities together contain 400 ml of blood or approximately 8% of the volume.

Volume Blood Flow (Fig. 9–8)

The volume of blood that flows through an organ or region has been determined by several methods including the thermostromuhr, the plethysmograph and the calorimeter. The plethysmograph is particularly useful in recording volume changes of the extremities. The hand or other part is placed in an air-tight chamber which communicates with a sensitive pressure transducer. Any increase or decrease in volume will be recorded through a selected channel of an electronic instrument.

The volume of a part is affected by the individual heart beat, respiration, vasomotor changes, the cross-sectional area of the vascular bed and the arteriolar resistance. The volume flow of blood per minute for representative tissues is noted (Table 9–3).

Most of the cardiac output supplies a relatively minor mass of tissue which can be collectively called the "vis-

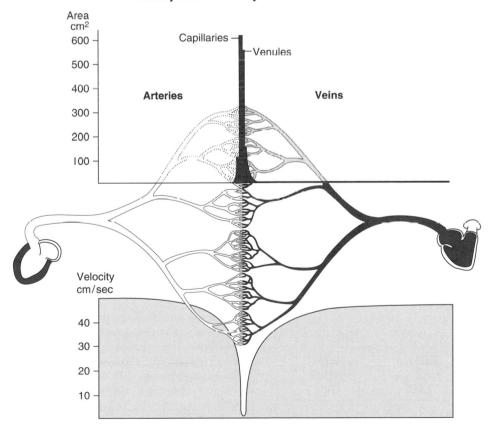

The relation between cross-sectional area and the velocity of flow in the systemic circulation

Fig. 9–7. Cross-sectional areas of various segments of the systemic circulation computed for a 13 kg. dog. Note the tremendous area in the arterioles, capillaries and venules. The velocity of blood flow is inversely proportional to the cross-sectional area so that blood flows through the capillaries at approximately 0.07 cm. per second. It should be emphasized that volume of fluid flowing in a unit time past any vertical line drawn through the vascular bed must be equal to the quantity entering and leaving the system.

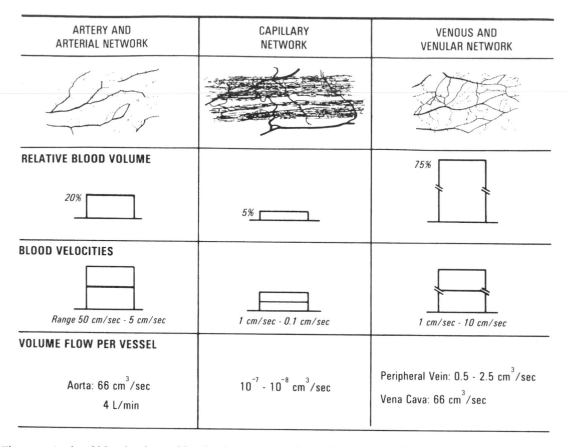

Fig. 9–8. The magnitude of blood volume, blood velocity, and volume flow per vessel. The volume flow changes over many orders of magnitude in the circulation due, in part, to vessel diameter variations. From Ross, J., Jr.: Structure–Function Relations in Peripheral Circulation. In Best and Taylor's Physiological Basis of Medical Practice, 12th Ed. Edited by B. West. Baltimore, Williams & Wilkins, 1990.

Table 9–2.   Estimated Distribution of Blood in Vascular System of Hypothetical Adult Man

Region	Volume	
	ml	%
Heart (diastole)	360	7.2
Pulmonary		
Arteries	130 ⎫	2.6 ⎫
Capillaries	110 ⎬ 440	2.2 ⎬ 8.8
Veins	200 ⎭	4.0 ⎭
Systemic		
Aorta and large arteries	300 ⎫	6.0 ⎫
Small arteries	400	8.0
Capillaries	300 ⎬ 4,200	6.0 ⎬ 84.0
Small veins	2,300	46.0
Large veins	900 ⎭	18.00 ⎭
	5,000	100

From Ross, J., Jr. Chapter 6 Structure-Function Relations in periphral Circulation. In Best and Taylor's Physiological Basis of Medical Practice. Ed John B. West Twelfth Edition, Baltimore 1990 Williams & Wilkins. Data from Milnor, W. R. Pulmonary Circulation in Medical Physiology Ed. V. B. Mountcastle. St. Louis Vol. 1:24–34, C. V. Mosby. 1968.

ceral mass" namely the renal, hepatoportal, central nervous system and cardiac tissues. These represent 70% of the cardiac output. Renal blood flow is extraordinarily high and this probably reflects the clearing and excretory function of the kidney. The myocardium has a small total blood flow but in relation to its mass shows a high flow rate. This flow might be higher if it were not limited by the fact that myocardial perfusion occurs chiefly during diastole and is difficult during systole. The small flow in relation to its needs is reflected in the high extraction rate.

Normal Oxygen Extraction

The quantity of oxygen presented to all the tissues of the body is approximately 1000 ml/min or 19 ml/100 ml of blood. The average A-V oxygen difference at rest or average extraction value of oxygen is approximately 4 to 6 ml of oxygen per 100 ml/min.; so that the venous blood oxygen content is approximately 14 ml/100 ml of blood (Fig. 9–9).

Each organ of the body has an extraction value. In terms of A-V oxygen difference the myocardium shows the highest extraction level. Approximately 14 ml of oxygen is removed by the cardiac muscle for each 100 ml of

Table 9–3. Distribution of Cardiac Output and Oxygen Usage in Resting Humans (Compare with Exercise)

Region	Weight kg	Weight % Total	Blood Flow 1/min	Blood Flow % Total	Blood Flow ml/100 g/min	Oxygen Usage ml/min	Oxygen Usage % Total	Oxygen Usage ml/100 g/min	O$_2$ Extraction Venous O$_2$ ml/100 ml blood	O$_2$ Extraction AVO$_2$
Total	70	100	5.4	100		250	100		14.5	4.5
Brain	1.54	2.2	0.83	15	54	63	23	3.7	12.5	6.5
Heart	0.33	0.5	0.22	4	70	23	9	7.0	7	12
Liver, intestines	2.86	4.0	1.54	29	54	55	20	1.95	15	4.0
Kidney	0.33	0.5	1.43	27	430	20	7	6.0	17	2.0
Skeletal muscle	34.0	50.0	0.92	17	2.7	55	20	0.16	12.5	6.5
Skin	3.6	5.1	0.45	8	14	12	5	0.33	18	1.4
Residue	27.2	38.0	0.35	5	1.4	40	2	0.21	20	1.0
Exercise			35.0	80	100	2700	90	7.9	3	16.0

Modified from Ross, J., Jr. Chapter 13. Intracardiac and Arterial Pressures and the Cardiac Output. In Best and Taylor's Physiological Basis of Medical Practice. Ed. John B. West, Twelfth Edition, Baltimore, Williams & Wilkins, 1990. Includes data on skin and residue from P. Bard, **Medical Physiology**.[3]

The arteriovenous oxygen differences in various tissues

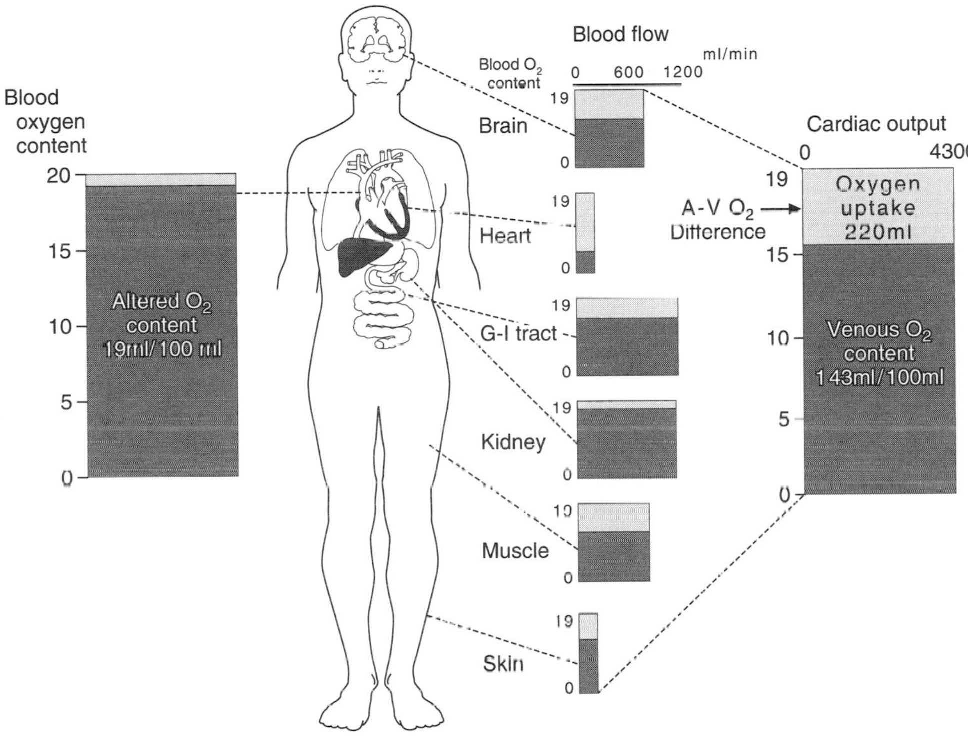

Fig. 9–9. The blood flow through some tissues is voluminous in relation to the oxygen requirements (kidney and skin). In contrast, the myocardium extracts most of the oxygen from the blood. The arteriovenous oxygen differences represent the relationship between blood flow and oxygen utilization in various tissues. Redrawn from Rushmer, Cardiovascular Dynamics, W.B. Saunders.

Table 9–4. Age Related Circulatory Variables

Age	Heart Rate per min	Stroke Vol ml/beat	Cardiac Index L/min/m^2	O$_2$ Consumption ml/kg/min	Hgb Concentration g/dl
Term newborn	133 ± 18	4.5 ± 5.0	2.5 ± 0.6	6.0 ± 1.0	16.5 ± 1.5
6 months	120 ± 20	7.4 ± 2.0	2.0 ± 0.5	5.0 ± 0.9	11.5 ± 1.0
12 months	120 ± 20	11.5 ± 3.0	2.5 ± 0.6	5.2 ± 0.9	12.0 ± .75
2 years	105 ± 25	16.9 ± 4.5	3.1 ± 0.7	6.4 ± 1.2	12.5 ± 0.5
5 years	90 ± 10	27.8 ± 7.5	3.7 ± 0.9	6.0 ± 1.1	12.5 ± 0.5
12 years	70 ± 17	53.5 ± 14.5	4.3 ± 1.1	3.3 ± 0.6	13.5 ± 1.0
Adult	75 ± 5	85.5 ± 6.0	3.7 ± 0.3	3.4 ± 0.6	14.0 ± 10.

Konvetz, L. J. and Goldbloom, S.: Normal standards for cardiovascular data. Johns Hopkins Med J *130*:174–186, 1972.[21]

blood passing through. This represents a 70% extraction. With such a high value, increased demands by the heart can be met only by increasing flows. On the other hand, the kidney has one of the smallest extraction values of only 2.0 ml/100 ml of blood passing. The liver A-V oxygen difference is 10 ml and that of the brain is approximately 6.0 ml/100 ml of blood circulating (Table 9-4).

Resting skeletal muscle is the predominant body mass, approximately 50%. However, it receives only 16% of the cardiac output and extracts approximately 30% of the oxygen presented to it, that is, approximately 6.6 ml/100 ml of blood flowing. It consumes 20% of the total body oxygen.

REFERENCES

1. Ross, J., Jr.: Introduction to Cardiovascular System In *Best & Taylors' Physiologic Basis of Medical Practice.* Ed. John B. West Twelfth edition, Williams & Wilkins, Baltimore, 1990.
2. Hales, Stephen.: Statical Essays: Containing Haemostaticks. London 1733. Published under the auspices of the New York Academy of Medicine. Reprinted by Hafner Publishing Company, New York, 1964.
3. Bard, P.: Medical Physiology. Eleventh Ed. St. Louis, The C.V. Mosby Company. 1961.
4. Mellander, S. and Johansson, B.: Control of resistance, exchanges and capacitance functions of the peripheral circulation. Pharmacol. Rev. 20:117-196, 1969.
5. Fung, Y. C.: *Biodynamics: Circulation.* New York, Springer, 1984.
6. Milnor, W. R.: Arterial Impedence as ventricular afterload. Circul. Res. 36:565-576, 1975.
7. Pepine, C. J. and Nichols, W. W.: Aortic input impedance in cardiovascular disease. Prog Cardiovasc Dis 24:307, 1982.
8. O'Rourke, M. F. and Taylor M. G.: Input impedance of the systemic circulation in man. Circ Res 20:365, 1967.
9. Nichols, W. W. and Pepine, C. J.: Left ventricular afterload and aortic input impedance: Implications of pulsatile blood flow. Prog Cardiovasc Dis 24:293, 1982.
10. Cohn, J. N.: Blood pressure and cardiac performance. Am J Med 55:351, 1973.
11. Merillon, J. P., et al: Aortic input impedance in normal man and arterial hypertension; its modification during changes in arterial pressure. Cardiovas Res 16:646, 1982.
12. Elzinga, G. and Westerhof, N.: Pressure and flow generated by the left ventricle against different impedances. Circ Res 32:178, 1973.
13. Murgo, J. P., et al: Aortic input impedance in normal man: Relationship to pressure wave forms. Circ 62:105, 1980.
14. Sunagawa, K., Maughan, W. L. and Sagawa, K.: Optimal arterial resistance for the maximal stroke work studied in the isolated canine ventricle. Circ Res 56:586, 1985.
15. Master, A. H., Goldstein, I. and Walters, M. B.: New and old definitions of normal blood pressure. Bull. N.Y. Acad. Med., 27:442-446. 1951.
16. Marx, G. F., Cabe, C. M., Kim, Y. I. and Eidelman, A. I. Neonatal Blood Pressures. Anaesthetist 25:318-322, 1976.
17. Rushmer, R. F.: *Cardiovascular Dynamics* 3rd, Philadelphia, W. B. Saunders Co., 1970.
18. Dauber, T. R., Thomas, H. E. and McNamara, P. M. Characteristics of the dicrotic notch of the arterial pulse wave in coronary heart disease. Angiology 24:244-248, 1973.
19. Milnor, W. R.: Pulmonary Circulation. In *Medical Physiology.* Ed. V.B. Mountcastle. Vol 1: 24-34; 209-220. St. Louis, C.V. Mosby, 1968.
20. Ross, J. Jr., Gault, J. H., Mason, D. T., et al. Left ventricular performance during muscular exercise in patients with and without cardiac dysfunction. Circulation 34:597-608, 1966b.
21. Konvetz, L. J. and Goldbloom, S.: Normal standard for cardiovascular data. Johns Hopkins Med. J. 130:174-186, 1972.

Chapter 10

FLUIDS AND ELECTROLYTES

VINCENT J. COLLINS

The environment in which we live is neither air nor water but body fluids of constant composition. It has been aptly said that we are a "bag of salt water" encased in a semipermeable membrane.[1] Life could not be maintained without an accurate means of defending this internal environment against permanent change. This biological fact was the basis for Claude Bernard's statement—"The stability of the internal environment is an absolute requirement for free life."[2] Yet transient changes occur which allow exchanges with external environment. To accomplish this goal and maintain a dynamic equilibrium *systems of fluids have* been provided.

The transport of nutrient material to all the cells of the body and removal of waste products to organs of excretion are accomplished by these systems. The present objective is to review the physiology of the systems of fluids the components of which are water and electrolytes.

EXCHANGES WITH EXTERNAL ENVIRONMENT

Normally water enters the body by ingestion. This is usually in form of liquids but some water is obtained by the body as a result of oxidative processes of food stuffs within cells. The average adult in temperate climate receives about 2,500 ml. of water each day: 1200 ml. from liquids; 1000 ml. from water in solid food and 300 ml. as water of oxidation.[3]

Water leaves the body by four routes: (1) the kidney—1200 ml.; (2) The skin: insensible—800 ml., sensible sweat varies; (3) The lungs: insensible—400 ml.; (4) intestinal discharge—100 ml. The values given are for an adult male at rest in a temperate climate. The quantity of fluid eliminated through the skin, lungs and intestine is relatively constant. Darrow[4] has shown that a more accurate estimation of water needs can be made based on the number of calories metabolized (Table 10-1).

Water balance may be further analyzed by summarizing the various losses into a single value of daily water requirement.[5] This is also based for the sake of accuracy on the number of ml. per 100 calories metabolized (Table 10-2).

The kidneys are responsible for the major losses of body fluids and therefore for the major control of the volume of body fluids and their concentration. Renal function is a complex process and is determined by the integration of cardiovascular mechanism, the neurohypophysis; the capillary system and hormonal influences.

It has been stated that our internal environment is thrown out of the body in the form of a glomerular filtrate 16 times a day. However, most of this water is recaptured by the tubules.[7] Actually of the water excreted by the glomeruli about 85% is reabsorbed by the tubules without changing the osmotic pressure of the urine in the proximal tubules. The rate and variation in volume of tubular reabsorption is in large measure determined by the amount of sodium and chloride excreted. In the distal tubules, water, sodium, and bicarbonate are reabsorbed by independent processes. The rate of water reabsorption is under the control of the antidiuretic hormone of

Table 10-1. Water Loss for Normal Activity

1. Loss
   Adult = 42 ml/100 calories metabolized skin — 800 ml
               lungs = 400 ml
   Child = 300–600 ml/each day
   Infant = 75–300 ml/each day

2. Sweat
   Adult = 10–20 ml/100 cal minimal activity
           50 ml/100 cal—(light clothing; temp. 85° 98°F; humidity = 50%)
   Infant = Insignificant

3. Urine water volume (varies inversely with specific gravity)
   Adult = 84 ml/100 cal (sp. gr. = 1.012) = 1500 ml
   Child = 90 ml/100 cal (sp. gr. = 1.010) = 500–800 ml
   Infant = 100 ml/100 cal (sp. gr. = 1.008) = 200–500 ml

4. Stool water
   All = 4 ml/100 calories

Table 10-2. Fluid Balance—Daily Water Requirements (Based on Caloric Consumption—After Darrow)

	Caloric Needs		Water Needs	
	Cal/kg	Cal/Total	ml/100 cal	ml/kg
Infants	125	1000–1200	120	125
Children	100	1500–2000	100–150	150
Adolescents	80	2200–3000	125	100
Adults				
Bed rest	20–25	1,600	90	25
Not sweating	30	2,100	90–125	30
Sweating	35	3,500	144	40–45
Work	45	3000–5000	125–150	60

165

the hypophysis; the rate of sodium reabsorption is under the control of the adrenal cortical hormone aldosterone.[8,9] The rate of potassium reabsorption may be both influenced directly by adrenal corticoids and indirectly via a relationship with sodium. The rate of bicarbonate absorption appears to be an inherent function of tubular cells. The tubular cells appear to have the ability to exchange hydrogen ions for other cations. Lastly these cells are able to form ammonium which can be substituted for other cations. Thus, it is apparent that the kidney controls not only water volume of the body fluids, but also the electrolyte content and the acidity—basicity of the fluids.

DIVISIONS OF BODY FLUIDS[10]

The importance of total body water cannot be over-emphasized.[3] It comprises about 60% of the composition of the living body and is anatomically distributed into three main compartments (Table 10-3) with approximate values as follows:

  I. Plasma Compartment: 7.5% of body weight.
 II. Interstitial Fluid: 20%.
III. Intracellular Compartment: 55% (includes Erythrocyte Compartment [3%]).

The movements of substances within the organism and the exchange of these substances with the external environment are effected by water as the medium of transportation (Fig. 10-1).[11]

The membranes which separate these compartments are semipermeable and permit water as well as selected constituents to move freely from one compartment to another. Darrow has noted that water like other body constituents is in a dynamic state. A change in one compartment is followed by an alteration in the constituents of the other.[4]

Values for Adults

Total body water (TBW) actually varies[10] with the habitus of the healthy subject[3] and is primarily a function of

Table 10–3. Body Fluid Compartments

Compartment	Percent of Total Body Water[a]	Percent of Total Body Weight Normal Adult Man	Percent of Total Body Weight Normal Adult Woman
Intracellular fluid	55	33	27.5
Extracellular fluid	45	27	22.5
Interstitial	20	12	10
Plasma	7.5	4.5	3.75
Bone	7.5	4.5	3.75
Dense connective tissue	7.5	4.5	3.75
Transcellular	2.5	1.5	1.25
Total body water	100	60	50

(From Edelman, I. S., and Leibman J.: Anatomy of body water and electrolytes. Am. J. Med., *27*:256, 1959.)

the amount of adipose tissue. Skeletal muscle is over 75% water, skin is over 70% while organs such as heart, lungs and kidneys are about 80% water. In contrast adipose tissues has less than 10% water (Table 10-4). The percent decreases with age.[12] Asthenic individuals have a high per cent of water and obese individuals, a lower per cent than the normal person. Females in each category have a lower body water content than males (Table 10-4). Of the extracellular water the sum of the plasma and interstitial water is known as the ciscellular fluid. There is an additional volume of water amounting to 5.5% known as transcellular water. Such fluid consists of fluids in serous and synovial cavities, in gastrointestinal tract, in lower urinary tract in bile and in cerebrospinal fluid.[11,13]

Values for Infant and Children

In the newborn, the ECF[6,14] volume is approximately 50% (45% ISF + 5% plasma); at 2 months of age, the ECF is approximately 35%, whereas at 4-6 years of age the total ECF is approximately 25%. This is compared to the adult volumes of 20% or 15% ISF + plasma values of 5%. Muscle cell mass of an infant is 20-25% of body water (BW) compared with muscle cell mass of 40-50% in the adult.[14]

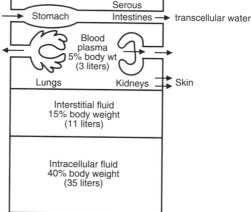

Body fluid compartments

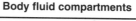

Fig. 10–1. Body fluid compartments diagrammatically represented in normal %-kilogram weight. Transcellular fluid consists of water in serous and synovial cavities, in gastrointestinal tract, in bile and in cerebrospinal fluid (F. Moore). Extracellular water of the plasma and interstices of red cells and the interstitium is known as cis-cellular water.

Table 10–4. Body Water Percent Body Weight

Males	Lean	Normal	Obese
Water	70	60	50
Fat	4	18	32
Females			
Water	50	50	42
Fat	18	32	42

Rule: More Fat—Less Water (Talbott)

EXCHANGES WITH CELLS

The volume of fluid in the vascular compartment is adjusted to the function of maintaining an exchange of metabolites with cells. Movement of materials is accomplished through the capillaries and the interstitial space.[15]

The relative distribution of extracellular fluid between the intravascular and interstitial compartment is determined by a capillary balance.[16] This scheme was first advanced by Starling in 1896,[17] and confirmed experimentally by Pappenheimer.[18]

A balanced exchange is maintained by the operation of the following basic factors:

Capillary hydrostatic pressure
Colloid osmotic pressure
Semipermeability of capillary wall and cell membrane
Lymph drainage
Tissue turgor
Physiochemical equilibrium of electrolytes

The intracapillary hydrostatic pressure and the colloid osmotic pressure of the perivascular fluids favor the outward movement of water and diffusible substances from the vascular compartment.[18] This situation prevails at the arterial side of the capillary where the capillary hydrostatic pressure is high. The return of substances into the vascular compartment is favored at the venous side by the lowered hydrostatic intracapillary pressure and the higher interstitial fluid pressure plus the colloid osmotic pressure of the protein in the plasma. Filtration thus occurs at the arterial side of a capillary and absorption at the venous side (Fig. 10–2).[19]

Besides the passage of materials through capillaries as a result of changes in capillary blood pressure, there is also a gradient of capillary membrane permeability depending on actual differences in the permeability property of the endothelium, at the venous vs. arterial end. Rous has demonstrated that water and crystalloids can pass more readily through the walls of veins than arterial walls.[20]

Osmosis[21]

Whenever a membrane between two fluid compartments is freely permeable to water but not to some solutes, it is called a *semipermeable membrane.* Most biological membranes are partially or completely impermeable to large molecules such as dextrose and proteins but do allow small molecules and water to pass freely. The relation that exists between ions of a solution of elec-

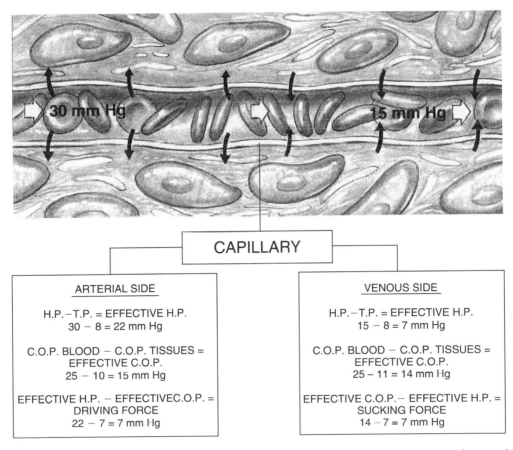

Fig. 10–2. Starling's Equilibrium of Capillaries. Diagrammatic representation of the forces governing exchange of fluids between capillaries and tissues. Arrows indicate direction of fluid movement. H.P. = capillary hydrostatic pressure, which is approximately 30 mm. Hg on the arterial side and approximately 15 mm. on the venous side. T.P. = tissue tension, which is approximately 8 mm Hg. C.O.P. = colloid osmotic pressure, which is approximately 25 mm Hg in the blood plasma and approximately 10 mm Hg in the interstitial fluid. Redrawn from Wakim, K. G. and Gatch, W. D., Q Bull Indiana Univ Med Center, 6:51, 1994.

trolytes and molecular particles separated by such semipermeable membranes is defined by the Gibbs-Donnan theory of membrane equilibrium. For example, if a solution containing a large number of dissolved particles, including a non-diffusible ion or molecule, is placed on one side of a membrane, and a solution containing a smaller number of particles is on the other, water will pass across the membrane from the less concentrated to the more concentrated solution. This phenomenon is called *osmosis*.

Osmotic Pressure[21]

Osmotic flow will continue until an equilibrium is established. This equilibrium is governed by the First and Second Laws of Thermodynamics, and at equilibrium the *products of the concentrations of the diffusible ions on each side of the membrane are equal.* Because there are more particles on one side, a larger volume will result on that side. The particles exert a force of attraction for water. Osmotic pressure is the force required to oppose the transfer of water. It is a function solely of the number of particles independent of their nature and is actually governed by the general formula of the ideal-gas law. (PV = n RT − Nernst Equation.) This law states that the *osmotic pressure exerted by any substance in solution is the same as it would exert if it were a gas in the same volume as that occupied by the solution.*

The unit of measurement of osmotic activity of a solution is the *osmol. One osmol is equal to 1 gram-molecular weight of a solute.* In biological systems, it is the milliosmol or 1/1000 of an osmol. This measures the amount of work *that all* dissolved particles, both ions and non-ionized molecules, can perform in drawing water through a membrane. For univalent ions, the milliosmol value is identical to the milliequivalent value, whereas for multivalent ions the milliosmolar value is the milliequivalent divided by the valence.

Osmotic pressure in cellular fluid is determined mainly by potassium ions. In the extracellular fluid, OP is determined mainly by sodium ions. Measurement of the *number of particles,* both cations and anions, will provide the milliosmolarity. That of plasma will reflect osmolarity in other compartments.

Osmolarity of Body Fluids

The total osmolarity of each of the three fluid compartments is almost 300 milliosmols per liter (Fig. 10–3). Plasma has a value of 1.3 milliosmols greater than interstitial or intracellular fluid. This provides an excess osmotic pressure of 24 mm Hg (often referred to as the blood oncotic pressure). Almost four-fifths of the osmolarity of the plasma and interstitial fluid is caused by sodium and chloride ions, whereas half of the intracellular osmolarity is

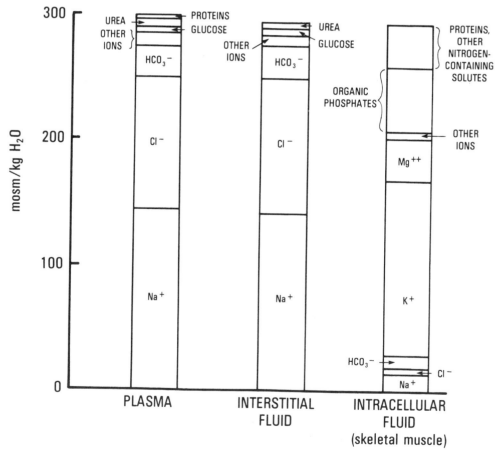

Fig. 10–3. Osmotic composition of the major body fluids. From Best and Taylor's Physiological Basis of Medical Practice, 12th Ed. Edited by J. B. West Baltimore, Williams & Wilkins, 1990.

due to potassium ions. Intermolecular attraction forces reduce the osmotic activity so that the corrected activity is only approximately 93% of that calculated from the milliosmols present. This is approximately 280 milliosmols per liter.

VOLUME CONTROL OF BODY FLUID[21,22]

Total body water fluctuates between rather narrow limits in health. Conceptually, regulation is determined by simple physiochemical forces and laws modulated by reflex and hormonal factors. Fundamentally, there are two general regulatory systems:

1. Osmolar control
2. Non-osmolar control

The osmotic forces in the body fluid compartments predominantly determined by electrolytes, provide the basic control of the fluid volume. Osmotic equilibrium is considered to exist between the fluids in the cellular space and extracellular space. Calculations of cation concentrations results in a figure for intracellular osmolarity that is almost identical with extracellular fluid. Further, the two compartments behave as if in equilibrium by the following observations:

1. Potassium deficiency is accompanied by shrinking of extracellular space.
2. Hypertonic sodium chloride intravenously administered causes a shift of water from intracellular space to extracellular space.
3. A large water load is evenly distributed between the two spaces.

As the extracellular fluid volume and composition is altered, the intracellular fluid is appropriately modified.

Osmolar Regulation of ECF Volume[22]

The *osmolar control* is the dominant and the most effective regulation of extracellular volume and extracellular osmotic pressure and involves two mechanisms:

I. Osmoreceptors (Hypothalamic)-Antidiuretic Hormone ADH (Neurohypophyses) System.[23]
II. Renal Receptors (Juxtaglomerular Apparatus)-Angiotensin-Aldosterone System.

Osmoreceptor—ADH System

Special neurons exist in the anterior hypothalamus close to or part of the supra-optic nuclei known as osmoreceptors. These cells contain large fluid vesicles which swell or shrink in accordance with extracellular fluid osmolarity. They exibit continuous activity but at varying rates—when extracellular fluid becomes concentrated (increased osmolarity) the cells shrink and the impulse rate increases, whereas low osmolarity of the extracellular fluid decreases the receptor discharge. Impulses

from the osmoreceptors pass through the pituitary stalk to the supra-optic nuclei and regulate the release of antidiuretic hormone (vasopressin). Thus, ADH is secreted in accordance with the degree of stimulation by the hypothalamus consequent to changes in the osmolarity of extracellular fluids: *The greater the osmolarity, the greater the ADH secretion; the less the osmolarity, the less the ADH secretion.*

Vasopressor levels (and thirst) increase sharply at *osmolar pressures* above 280 mOsM/kg of body water.[24] Volume depletion is also a separate and distrust stimulus with absence of any changes in toxicity.[25]

Antidiuretic hormone acts on both the distal tubules and the collecting ducts of the kidney. Its function is to conserve water by promoting reabsorption. An increased reabsorption of water corrects excess concentration of extracellular fluids, and the urine volume is decreased but more concentrated. In the absence of ADH, the amount of water passing into the urine is 5 to 20 times the usual daily volume; in the presence of large amounts of ADH, enormous amounts of water are reabsorbed so that the urine volume may be only one third of normal. At the same time solutes continue to be lost in the urine; eventually a feedback to the osmoreceptor turns off the release of ADH.

Thirst Mechanism[26]

The osmoreceptor-ADH system is activated when there are changes in tonicity of ECF. Thus, water ingestion decreases tonicity; this abolishes thirst and inhibits the secretion of antidiuretic hormone. Lack of water and increased ECF tonicity has two effects: produces thirst which stimulates the "drinking center" of McCann located in the hypothalamus and stimulates the posterior pituitary to release ADH.

Renal Receptor-Aldosterone System[27]

Concentration of solute is not the only factor affecting body water. If changes in ECF volume are isotonic, then adjustments must be made in the *total amount* of extracellular solute. Regulation of total extracellular solute is brought about by control of sodium and especially the urinary Na^+ excretion. This in turn is determined by the interaction of (*a*) renal mechanisms and (*b*) adrenal cortical hormones. Sodium is regulated by a process of glomerular filtration and tubular reabsorption. Approximately 600 grams of sodium are filtered every day but over 95% is reabsorbed in renal tubules.

In humans, the filtration is fairly constant and is not increased during sodium diuresis which follows isotonic saline infusions. Reduction in tubular reabsorption explains the diuresis. A low salt diet increases tubular reabsorption after 48 hours. These responses are not under nervous control and most evidence indicates that the adrenal cortex profoundly affects tubular function.

The adrenal cortex is a major factor in maintaining ECF volume through its hormonal effects on sodium. Aldosterone is one of the important mineral-corticoids since it accounts for ⅔ (two-thirds) of the sodium-retaining activity of adrenal hormones. This hormone has a duration of action of approximately 8 hours. After intravenous saline solution, slow sodium diuresis occurs. This is in contrast to the rapid diuresis after water-only intake, which depends upon the inactivation of antidiuretic hormone (1 hr).

Renin-Angiotensin System[27]

Renin is a proteolytic enzyme synthesized, stored and secreted mainly by the kidney. Renin-like enzymes are also obtained from many other organs but do not have a significant physiologic role.

The sites of renin formation and storage in the kidney are special cells at the vascular pole of the glomerulus which appear to be derived from modified smooth muscle cells of the afferent arteriole. These are associated with a special group of cells at the origin of the distal tubule that form the macula densa. The combined structures form the *juxtaglomerular apparatus.*

The release of renin is considered to be brought about by renal baroreceptors. Two mechanisms operate. The first is an osmolar mechanism, the maculadensa concept—depending on changes in sodium load in the distal tubule. A high sodium content inhibits the maculadensa activity. A low sodium load is accompanied by a reduced tubular volume and a decreased content at the macula with arteriolar cells causing release of renin.

The second is a nonosmolar mechanism, the stretch-receptor complex, depending on changes in pressure and distention of the afferent arteriole. The JCA at the afferent arteriole responds to changes in pressure. In this sense, it is a volume receptor or baroreceptor mechanism: lowered pressures increase renin secretion and elevated pressures decrease renin secretion.

According to the first concept, a small sodium load is accompanied by a reduced tubular volume and decreased contact of the macula with arteriolar cells causing the release of renin. The second concept states that a decreased arteriolar volume or decreased perfusion (from hypovolemia or hyponatremia) is accompanied by decreased contact of arteriole with the macula densa which increases the release of renin. To some extent there is autonomic regulation of the receptors in juxtaglomerular apparatus and the degree of release of renin is partially dependent on β-adrenergic activity. Propranolol will attenuate the amount of renin released.

After the release of renin, a sequence of enzymatic reactions occurs. Cleavage of the renin substrate α_2-globulin from the liver forms angiotensin I, a decapeptide. A converting enzyme from the lung removes two other amino acids from angiotensin I to form the octapeptide angiotensin II. This substance is a powerful vasoconstrictor with a transient life of one to two circulations. It is simultaneously a powerful stimulator of aldosterone production. The role of angiotensin II in vascular homeostasis is for maintenance of blood pressure when there is volume reduction or salt depletion. An *indirect* pressor response also occurs due to action on the central nervous system. This effect may be due to inhibition of vagal centers.

The increased aldosterone production enhances sodium reabsorption and increased water retention. The physiologic consequences are an increased circulatory volume, raised blood pressure and improved tissue perfusion.

Nonosmolar Regulation of Fluid Volume[28]

In addition to osmotic control mechanisms several neural mechanisms, and others less specific regulate body fluid volume (Table 10–5). all hemodynamic responses are influenced by cardiovascular reflexes and these provide some regulation of fluid volume and of urinary output. When blood pressure falls or hypovolemia occurs, intrathoracic reflexes, extrathoracic pressor-receptor reflexes and a central ischemic response are evoked causing activation of hypothalamic mechanisms and of the sympathetic nervous system.

Vascular "Volume Receptors" and Reflex

Fullness of vascular compartment influences ADH secretion and presence or absence of urine formation.[29] In the low pressure intrathoracic circulatory system, a mechanism exists which senses changes in the relative size of the compartment, either distended or contracted, and provides a stimulus to change vasopressin secretion. Total volume may not alter but distribution may change, *i.e.* increases or decreases in intrathoracic volume may immensely affect vasopressin secretion. A *decrease* in central volume by such maneuvers as standing, exposure of lower part of body to negative pressure and positive pressure breathing increases vasopressin release and causes an antidiuresis. An *increase* in central volume from negative pressure breathing, from immersion of

Table 10–5. Nonosmolar Factors Affecting Renal Water Excretion

Changes in Plasma Volume—"Volume Receptors"

Changes in Systemic Arterial Pressure—"Baroreceptors"

Hormonal Factors
    Catecholamines
    Prostaglandins
    Adrenocortical hormones
    Renin-angiotensin
    Thyroid hormone

Physical and Emotional Stress

Chronic Renal Failure

Metabolic Disturbances
    Sodium balance
    Water balance
    Protein intake
    Hypercalcemia
    Hypokalemia

Sickle-Cell Disease

Pharmacologic Agents:
    Barbiturates
    Cholinergic agents

(From Schrier, R. W., and Berl, T.: Nonosmolar factors affecting renal water extraction. N. Engl. J. Med., *292*:81, 1975.)

lower part of body or other similar maneuvers, decreases vasopressin secretion and causes diuresis.

An atrial volume reflex has been established.[30] Stretch receptors in the left atrium are responsible. The degree of distention of the left atrium (or level of left atrial pressure) is the principal stimulus. Increased distention increases rate of firing of receptor; afferent impulses accordingly pass over parasympathetic vagal pathways to reach the hypothalamus and sequentially the pituitary is inhibited and vasopressin release is suppressed. Conversely, a low rate of receptor firing from low atrial pressures decreases afferent input to the hypothalamus, diminishes inhibition of the neurohypophysis and permits greater secretion of vasopressin. Cervical vagotomy abolishes the reflex, permits continuous vasopressin release and causes antidiuresis.

Under most circumstances the atrial volume receptor reflex works synergistically with osmotic regulatory mechanisms. The relative influence of each has been elucidated: The osmoreceptor mechanism is the more sensitive. A 1 to 2% change (average 3.5 mOsm/L.) in plasma osmolarity changes vasopressin levels. To activate the atrial volume reflex a depletion of 7 to 10% of blood volume is needed for significant vasopressin release.

Baroreceptor Regulation of Fluid Volume

In the high pressure systemic circulation a mechanism exists which also regulates the fluid volume. When volume changes occur, concomitant pressure changes affect presso-receptors and evoke the hypothalamic-pituitary mechanism; renal responses follow related to the level of vasopressin. Two principal reciprocal reflexes appear to exist.

- Carotid baroreceptors exist at the thyrocarotid junction and they respond to decreased arterial pressure and become inactive. The afferent path is over parasympathetic fibers of the glossopharyngeal nerve, whose rate of firing is decreased. Inhibition of activity of hypothalamus ensues which permits the pituitary to increase release of vasopressin. An antidiuresis follows.
- Aortic arch baroreceptors are stimulated by increases in pressures. Afferent impulses pass over vagal parasympathetic paths to the hypothalamus and sequentially suppress vasopressin release from the pituitary.

Catecholamines

Many non-osmolar stimuli, including stress of emotion, physical stresses (exercise) and chemical stresses (hypovolemia) increase the release of vasopressin and decrease urine formation. This appears to be related to beta-adrenergic stimulation of the hypothalamus and can be induced by low doses of isoproterenol and prevented by beta-blockers. Evidence also indicates that alpha-adrenergic stimulation by non-pressor doses of epinephrine and/or norepinephrine can inhibit the release of vasopressin and causes a diuresis of solute-free water. This oc-

curs in normal hydrated man and in the absence of changes in filtration rate, renal plasma or in osmolar changes. Experimental studies show that either alpha-adrenergic stimulation (NE infusion) causing diuresis or beta-adrenergic stimulation (isoproterenol) causing antidiuresis do not occur when baroreceptors are denervated. In summary enhanced renal water clearance by sympathetic agents is mediated primarily by changes in baroreceptor tone which then alters vasopressin secretion.

Miscellaneous Controls

Prostaglandins have a role in regulating renal function, including water and solute excretion. An antidiuresis occurs similar to that following stress. The hemodynamic effects of PGE_1, are similar to beta-adrenergic stimulation which causes decreased baroreceptor activity and permits release of vasopressin.

In contrast the infusion of angiotensin II results in the following specific sequence: Increased systemic arterial pressure and baroreceptor activity, followed by increased impulses over parasympathetic afferent vagal fibers which suppress vasopressin release. The net result is diuresis.

Hypothyroid subjects are not able to adequately excrete a water load, and often have impaired volume-regulating mechanisms. The exact role of thyroid hormone on water excretion needs to be clarified.

Summary of Volume Regulation

Two fundamental mechanisms are considered in the regulation of body water. One mechanism is that of osmoregulation, the other is non-osmolar volume regulation. Generally, in osmo-regulation the sodium balance of input and output is the key.

Sodium excretion is increased by any process which increases central circulatory volume such as infusion of isotonic saline or hypertonic salt solutions, lying down, compression of limbs, or closure of A-V shunts. On the other hand, sodium excretion is decreased by procedures which diminish blood volume or cause pooling; shock, hemorrhage, passive standing, obstruction to venous return.[20]

Simultaneously, a change in vascular volume evokes the stretch-receptor reflex originating in the left atrial wall. If a decrease in volume occurs, the reflex activates processes conserving water, increasing renal absorption and translocating fluid into the vascular compartment.

An interaction between volume receptors, baroreceptors and osmoreceptors is involved in the maintenance of vascular volume and body fluid tonicity. The maintenance of volume appears to have priority over maintenance of tonicity in most clinical circumstances. It is further considered that volume-receptor mechanisms in the low pressure intrathoracic system may predominate over the baroreceptor mechanisms in the systemic circulation. This is based on the observation that during volume contraction a release of vasopressin occurs before changes in arterial pressure.

ELECTROLYTE BALANCE

Chemical Terminology[21]

The most important constituents of the fluid compartments of the body are the electrolytes. Electrolytes are chemical compounds, chiefly salts, which dissociate into their component ions when placed in water.

Ions are electrically charged atoms. The *cations* are those groups that possess a positive charge and are represented in the body fluids by sodium, potassium, calcium and magnesium. The *anions* are the negatively charged particles and are represented by chloride, bicarbonate, phosphate, sulfate, organic acids and proteinate (Table 10-6).[7]

The term "base" has been used erroneously to refer to cations and the "acid" to refer to anions. Actually, the base value depends on the number of (OH^-) hydroxyl ions and the acid value depends on the number of hydrogen ions (H^+). (To remember which cation and which the anion, the following aid is recommended: the word cation has a crossed "t" in it, and this represents the positive charged particles).

Electroneutrality of Body Fluids

This requires a constant balance between the sum of the electropositive ions and the electronegative ions. The utilization of a unit of measurement of concentration which expresses chemical equivalence or values which have the same power of chemical and physiological activity is logical. Such a unit is the *equivalent. An equivalent is a unit of measure of the comparative weights of different compounds, elements, or groups which possess the same value of reaction.* It is the atomic weight of an element which in neutralization reactions is equivalent to one gram-atom of hydrogen.

Solutions are usually analyzed and prepared on the basis of weights.

A mol of a substance is equal to the molecular weight of that substance expressed in grams. When 1 mol of a substance is dissolved in a liter of solution, it is known as a 1.0 molar solution. Thus, if the weight in grams of NaOH, KOH, and HCl corresponding to the molecular weight of these substances is dissolved in enough water to make 1 liter, each solution will contain, respectively, 40 gm. of NaOH, 56 gm. of KOH, and 37 gm. of HCl. Since these salts are composed of univalent ions each contains the same number of electroactive particles per unit volume; but the weights of the substances per unit volume are not the same. For example, 1 mol of NaOH exhibits the same combining power as 1 mol of KOH, they are univalent, mol for mol, but the weights per liter are 40 gm. of NaOH and 56 gm. of KOH. Hence, one equivalent of any substance is 1 mol of the substance. It is evident that the comparison of electrolyte substances in terms of their equivalents provides more useful biochemical information in living systems than does the comparison in terms of weight. (If a mol of a substance is dissolved in 1000 grams of solvent [1 liter at 4°C.], the solution is designated as a molal solution).

Table 10-6. Approximate Concentrations of Solutes in Body Fluids*

	Plasma (mEq/L)	Plasma Water (mEq/L H_2O)	Interstitial Fluid (mEq/L H_2O)	Intracellular Fluid (Skeletal Muscle) (mEq/L H_2O)
Cations				
Na^+	142	153	145	10
K^+	4	4.3	4.1	159
Ca^{2+b}	2.5	2.7	2.4	<1
Mg^{2+b}	1	1.1	1	40
Total	149.5	161.1	152.5	209
Anions				
Cl	104	112	117	3
HCO_3	24	25.8	27.1	7
Proteins	14	15.1	<0.1	45
Other	7.5	8.2	8.4	154
Total	149.5	161.1	152.5	209

	mmol/L	mmol/L H_2O	mmol/L H_2O	mmol/L H_2O
Nonelectrolytes				
Glucose	4.7	5.0	5.0	
Urea	5.6	6.0	6.0	6.0

*The plasma water, interstitial fluid, and intracellular fluid concentrations are expressed as meq/liter of H_2O. While proteins and protein-bound ions are strictly not part of the aqueous phase of these fluids, their charges have an important role in understanding body fluid composition (see text). Thus, the table presents the compositions of these fluids as if proteins and protein bound ions were in fact part of the aqueous phase. *Total* concentrations are given; free ionized concentrations are lower. From Best and Taylor's Physiological Basis of Medical Practice. John B. West Editor 12th Edition, Williams & Wilkins, Publishers Baltimore, 1990. With permission.

Substances react also on the basis of their valence. The chemicals mentioned thus far are all univalent. But calcium (atomic weight = 40) is bivalent; that is, 1 mole of Ca^{++}, which is 40 gm., possesses twice the combining power of 1 mole of Na^+. Hence, 1 mole or 40 gm. of Ca provides two equivalents of Ca; and one equivalent of Ca^{++} is provided by 20 gm.

Equivalents

The same weight of different substances will not have the same power of reaction. Also, the custom of expressing concentrations of substances in terms of milligrams is illogical when applied to living systems. In living systems the chemical constituents of the body fluids react on the basis of their equivalents.

Because the concentrations of electrolytes in biological systems are low, the values are expressed in *milliequivalents* or 1/1000 of an equivalent.

Under ordinary conditions the extracellular fluid as well as the interstitial fluid contains approximately 155 mEq. per liter of cations and an equal number of anions (conjugate bases-ions which bear a negative charge). The average concentration of each electrolyte is represented in Table 10-6. All of the components except protein are readily diffusible in the interstitial fluid, so that, with the exception of protein, the concentration of these ions in the fluid surrounding the cells is essentially the same as that in the plasma. This table also illustrates the advantages of expressing the concentration of all components in the same unit, so that the total concentration of cations and anions can be obtained. The total concentration of cations must equal that of the anions.

Since reports are often in terms of milligrams per 100 ml. of body fluid it is desirable to convert such values to milliequivalents (Table 10-7). To do so, the following formula is applied:

$$\text{mEq./L.} = \frac{\text{mg per 100 ml} \times 10}{\text{atomic weight}} \times \text{valence}$$

Example: 360 mg/100 ml and chloride is converted to mEq/L

$$\frac{360 \times 10}{35} \times 1 = 103 \text{ mEq/L}$$

In the case of substances which under ambient conditions exist as gases (e.g. carbon dioxide) or are nonionized, advantage is taken of the fact that a molecular weight of gas occupies a volume of 22.4 liters under standard conditions. The formula used is as follows:

$$\text{mmol} = \frac{\text{Volume }\% \times 10}{22.4}$$

Example: CO_2 of 60.5 volume %

$$\frac{60.5 \times 10}{22.4} = 27 \text{ M/L}$$

Since this value represents carbon dioxide in the form of carbonic acid and bicarbonate a further correction must be introduced depending on the plasma ratio of bi-carbonate to carbonic acid $(HCO_3^-)/(H_2CO_3)$ or 20:1.0 $^{20}/_1$. When this is considered, a final formula for approximation of bicarbonate is as follows:

MilliMols of bicarbonate/L =

$$\frac{\text{Volume }\% \text{ of carbon dioxide}}{2.3}$$

Chemical Anatomy[31,32]

Changes in body water and changes in acid-base balance are governed by the exchanges in sodium, potassium, chloride and bicarbonate. The source of water and electrolytes is dietary, whereas the source of bicarbonate is chiefly metabolic. The distribution of these constituents in various body fluids is essential.

Analysis of the fluids within each compartment reveals distinctive chemical characteristics. A pronounced difference is noted between the extracellular and intracellular compartments (Fig. 10-4).

The extracellular fluid is denoted by a predominance of sodium as the cation; the chief anions are chloride and bicarbonate. In turn, the major distinction between plasma fluid and interstitial fluid is higher concentration of protein in the plasma (a difference of approximately 16 mEq). The composition of extracellular fluid in milliequivalents of electrolytes is illustrated in the classical diagram modified from Gamble. It is seen that there are a total of 155 mEq. of cations and an equal value of anions.

Intracellular fluid is more complex. The cation pattern is denoted by a predominance of potassium; this together with magnesium accounts for most of the intracellular cations. The chief anions are phosphate and proteinate. The total milliequivalent value for intracellular electrolyte cations amounts to 195 mEq., and there is an equivalent amount of anions. The composition is illustrated in a Gambelogram based on tissue analysis of Darrow.

Table 10–7. Data for Conversion of Serum (or Plasma) Electrolytes to mEq/L

Electrolyte	Calculated as	Atomic Weight	Valence	Equiv. Weight	Normal Ranges Serum or Plasma	
					mg/100 ml	mEq/L
Sodium	Sodium	23	1	23	310–340	135–147
Potassium	Potassium	35.5	1	39	16–22	4.1–5.7
Calcium	Total Ca	40	2	20	9.0–11.5	4.5–6.0
	Ionized Ca	40	2	20	4.25–5.25	2.1–2.6
Magnesium	Magnesium	24	2	12	1.8–3.6	1.5–3.0
				22.4	55–70	25–31
Bicarbonate	CO_2 capacity	—	—	Infants	45–60 (vol. %)	20–26 (mM/L)
Chloride	Chloride	35.5	1	35.5	350–375	98–106
	NaCl	58.5	1	58.5	570–620	98–106
Phosphate, inorganic	Phosphorus	31	1.8	17.2	2–4.5	1.2–3.0
				Children	4–7	2.5–4.5
Sulfate, inorganic	Sulfur	32	2	16	0.5–2.5	0.3–1.5
Protein	Protein	—	—	—	6.8 g	14.6–19.4
Glucose		180	1		60–100	3.3–5.5 (4.7)

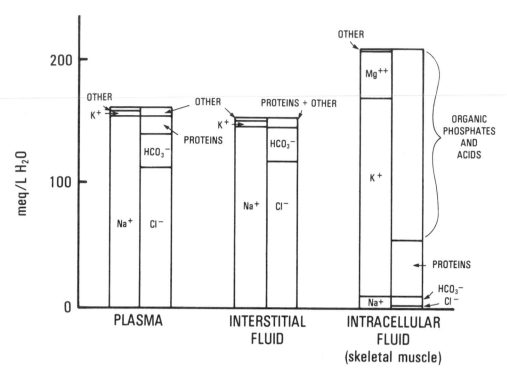

Fig. 10–4. Electrolyte composition of the major body fluids. From Best and Taylor's Physiological Basis of Medical Practice, 12th Ed. Edited by J. B. West, Baltimore, Williams & Wilkins 1990.

Each compartment is separated by some form of semi-permeable membrane and there is relatively easy transfer of all electrolytes (except proteinate). Despite the ease of transfer a selective distribution in concentration of certain ions in the different compartments exists and this is based on a Gibbs-Donnan type equilibrium.[32] In abnormal conditions much of the intracellular potassium may be replaced by sodium.

In general, changes in body water, electrolyte equilibrium and acid-base balance are explained chiefly by variations in sodium, potassium, chloride and bicarbonate. In ordinary states of health there is a daily obligatory loss of water and of electrolytes (Table 10-8). These electrolyte losses must be replaced (Table 10-9). Discussion will be limited to these.

Sodium Balance[7,32]

The great importance of sodium in body economy is on the osmotic stability of body fluid. Total body sodium amounts to 2700 to 3000 mEq. Most of the sodium is in the extracellular fluid compartment. It is "available" sodium and amounts to approximately 2000 mEq. (approximately 1000 mEq. in bone). Plasma sodium is maintained in normal states between 135 to 150 mEq. per liter (for calculations, 140 mEq. is taken as average). A like value is found in the interstitial fluid compartment whereas intracellular sodium amounts to 4 to 7 mEq. Many complex mechanisms are involved in maintaining this range. The kidneys are extremely effective in maintaining this range. The kidneys are extremely effective in handling sodium so that wide variations in plasma levels do not occur. A straight line relationship exists between

sodium load and the urinary excretion. When sodium load is heavy, tubular reabsorption is greatly reduced; when diet is low in sodium, tubular reabsorption is great.

In turn, tubular function is greatly dependent on adrenal cortex. Low sodium intake acts as a stress causing increased production of cortical hormones. Although in cardiac failure and in the immediate postoperative period restriction of sodium is valuable, it may lead to the complications of "low sodium syndrome." The sodium restriction may cause serum sodium levels to fall, diminish osmotic equilibrium, interfere with urinary excretion and cause reaccumulation of tissue fluid. The signs and symptoms are those of **water intoxication:** Anorexia, vomiting, weakness, fibrillary muscular twitchings and occasionally convulsions.

Hyponatremia

This electrolyte imbalance can occur in the perioperative period. Hyponatremia is unlikely to be encountered during anesthesia and surgery under current practices of fluid replacement, because of the liberal use of salt solutions. One exception is in urological cystoscopic procedures, when large volumes of salt-free solutions are used for irrigation purposes and a significant proportion enters into the circulation through the open venous sinuses of the prostatic beds. Hyponatremia may then be a result of intraoperative dilutional hypervolemia. This circumstance is commonly called the "TURP Syndrome."

Hyponatremia most often occurs in the postoperative period, whenever fluid intake is principally 5% dextrose in water.[33] approximately 4% of postoperative patients

Table 10–8. Daily Water and Electrolyte Loss—Adults, Based on Number of Calories Metabolized

	Sodium	Chloride	Potassium	Water
Urine	0.2–0.4 mEq/100 cal or 8.0 mEq	0.2–0.4 mEq/100 cal or 8.0 mEq	0.4–0.8 mEq/100 cal or 16 mEq	90–144 ml/100 cal or 2000–3500 ml
Sweat	0.5 mEq/100 cal or 15 mEq	0.5 mEq/100 cal or 15 mEq	0.2 mEq/100 cal or 6.0 mEq	10–20 ml/100 cal or 300 ml
Insensible	None	None	None	42 ml/100 cal or 1200 ml
Stool	0.1 mEq/100 cal	0.1 mEq/100 cal	0.4 mEq	4 ml/100 cal

develop some hyponatremia, but the serum sodium rarely falls below 120 mmol/liter and neurological sequelae are rare.[34] This postoperative mild to moderate hyponatremia results from the secretion of ADH, triggered by the surgical stress and postoperative decreases in extracellular fluid volume.[35]

Hazardous hyponatremia occurs when the serum sodium decreases to levels below 120 mmol/L. Conditions leading to this state include the following:

1. Maintenance of patients on hypotonic fluids or salt-free 5% dextrose in water
2. Medications that interfere with free water excretion and concomitant water retention, such as the thiazide diuretics, narcotics, phenothiazines, vasopressin, ACTH and oxytocin in obstetric practice
3. Pain and blood loss that stimulates ADH secretion
4. Female gender
5. Urologic procedures using large volumes of salt-free irrigating solutions

Symptoms and Signs

The development of neurologic complications from *acute* hyponatremia and concomitant water retention was clearly described in the postoperative period by Zimmerman and Wangesteen in 1952,[33] and entitled "water intoxication." Initial symptoms included progressive nausea, headache, vomiting, depression, hallucinations and disorientation. The critical serum sodium level for more serious CNS signs is below 120 mEq/L. At levels of 116 mEq/L, seizures, coma, respiratory arrest and death may occur. Patients may fully recover from the anesthesia, but will lapse into the above progression of complications approximately 48 hours post-surgery.

In the study of fatalities by Arieff,[36] the average plasma

Table 10–9. Daily Electrolyte Requirements

Adults		Infants
Sodium	40 mEq = 3.0 g	8 mEq = 0.5 g
Chloride	40 mEq NaCl	8 mEq NaCl
Potassium	40 mEq = 1.5 g KCl	8 mEq = 0.3g

(From Darrow, D. C. and Pratt, E. L.: Fluid Therapy, JAMA, *143*:365, 1950.)

sodium level was 108 mEq/L, the urinary sodium level was 68 mmol/liter, and the osmolality 501 mOsm/kg. These patients had received an average fluid load of 8.0 liters IV dextrose in water and a net water retention of 7.5 liters during the 2 postoperative days. This appears to produce cerebral edema and brain damage.

Deficit Correction

Rapid correction of plasma sodium may reverse the coma, but a relapse may occur 2–6 days later with coma, a persistent vegetative state or death. Sterns has described this outcome of rapid correction of chronic hyponatremia as the phenomenon of osmotic demyelination, which occurs when hypertonic (3%) sodium is administered at rates producing an increase in serum sodium concentration greater than 12 mmol/l over 24 hours.[37-39] It appears to be similar to the syndrome of central pontine myelinosis. This neurological disorder is related to rapid correction of hyponatremia, is fulminating in course and usually fatal.

The management of the acute hyponatremia syndrome, as it occurs in the immediate postoperative period, has been nicely outlined by Narins.[40] It is recommended that sodium be administered at a rate of 2.0 mmol/l/hr until the plasma sodium concentration reaches a level of 120–125 mmol/l. This can be accomplished with 3.0% saline and a diuretic. Thereafter, water intake should be restricted. When a hypertensive patient on a diuretic develops a hyponatremic state, it is recommended that the diuretic be discontinued. In patients with mild symptoms of hyponatremia and hypotension, the administration of physiologic saline to achieve intravascular expansion will suppress vasopressin release, normalize renal perfusion and aid in free water loss.

Intoxication

Guidelines to prevent and manage hyponatremia intoxication are as follows:[41]

1. During anesthesia, surgery, and in the immediate recovery period, sodium containing fluids should be administered to prevent postoperative hyponatremia.
2. Correct the sodium serum deficit at rates of 2.0 mmol/l/hour. Fluid/water restriction may be sufficient to correct mild states of hyponatremia between 135 to 120 mmol/liter.

3. Ventilatory care must be early and prompt when respiratory insufficiency or failure is evident to prevent hypoxic encephalopathy.
4. Monitor serum electrolytes postoperatively.

Potassium Balance[42]

Rapid changes in composition of intracellular fluid composition can occur. Such changes are particularly concerned with intracellular potassium and seriously affect acid-base balance of extracellular fluid. It is estimated that the total potassium content of the body is approximately 4,000 mEq (175 grams as KCl), approximately 55 mEq/kg for males and 50 mEq/kg for females. The total exchangeable potassium is approximately 3200 mEq. in males and 2300 mEq. in females. Only approximately 7 mEq. is in the extracellular compartment. The concentration in the plasma amounts to 3.5 to 5.0 mEq. per liter (4.5 mEq. value is used in the calculation).[43] Thus, potassium is predominantly an intracellular cation. It can freely pass the cell membrane in either direction and the interchange is affected by many pathophysiologic phenomena.

Serum potassium levels may not reflect the intracellular levels.[43] It requires between 200–400 mM body deficit before the serum level decreases. The serum K level is also influenced by the blood pH: for each 0.1 unit change in pH there is approximately and 0.6 mM reciprocal change in potassium. In diabetic acidosis, there is an increase in serum K whereas in alkalosis serum K may be depressed.

A metabolic deficit of approximately 600–800 mEq of total body potassium is required to reduce serum K by one mEq/L to a serum level below 3 mEq/L. However one can lower serum K rapidly by elevating pH as by hyperventilation without any change in total body potassium.

As a principle the body defends sodium balance at the expense of potassium:

1. K^+ ions exchange freely with H^+ ions. High serum H^+ ions enter cells in exchange for K^+ ions.
2. Hyponatremia for example increases K^+ excretion. In the distal tubules, serum potassium is exchanged for tubular sodium.

The escape of potassium from cells occurs under many circumstances. Of importance are the following:

1. Daily obligatory loss from body
2. Cellular anoxia
3. Agonal states and general hypoxia
4. During exercise
5. Deficient potassium intake in the intraoperative periods
6. Tissue trauma

In some of these conditions there may be an increase in the serum potassium, i.e. cellular anoxia and general hypoxia; during exercise; agonal states; convulsions. In some conditions the cellular and serum potassium levels may both be low, i.e. chronic nephritis; familial periodic paralysis.

Potassium Homeostasis[42]

The primary source of body potassium is that of dietary intake. The primary disposition of body potassium is by renal excretion, which dominates in adjusting the daily external potassium intake. The average intake is between 60–90 mEq/day, but may be as high as 200–300 mEq. Output is largely by renal excretion averaging 60–90 mEq/day. Some potassium is also excreted by the gastrointestinal tract (GITract) and skin approximately 5–10 mEq/day. However, it is clear that the function of most cells in the body, particularly muscle, nerve and secretory cells, depend critically on the electrical potential across the plasma membrane, which is determined by the ratio of intracellular to extracellular potassium.

Though renal excretion dominates the overall control, extra-renal devices are utilized when there are sudden changes in potassium levels. Two systems are involved principally in the regulation of extracellular and intracellular potassium. These systems are especially utilized at the time of meals. They are 1) insulin[44] and 2) the adrenergic nervous system.[45]

Insulin is an extra-renal mechanism for the disposal of acute potassium loads, and this is accomplished by accelerating skeletal muscle uptake. This mechanism is entirely independent of glucose metabolism.[44]

In addition, the adrenergic system is activated by eating. For example, the injection of epinephrine intravenously may produce a very transient rise in serum potassium related to an hepatic release of potassium, but this is quickly followed by prolonged hypokalemia which is brought about by the epinephrine's effect on increasing skeletal muscle uptake of potassium.

The adrenergic mechanism of potassium control is independent of other hormones including insulin, aldosterone or renal mechanisms themselves. It is mediated by beta$_2$ adrenergic receptors[46] A number of manifestations of this control are evident: a) after chemical sympathectomy with 6-hydroxydopamine, there is a reduction in potassium tolerance; b) beta adrenergic blockade impairs extra-renal disposal of intravenous potassium loads, whereas epinephrine increases the disposal of potassium by the aforementioned muscular uptake; c) beta adrenergic blockade also exaggerates the hyperkalemia of exercise; d) exercise is known to increase serum potassium; e) studies of a continuous infusion of epinephrine to levels that are seen in myocardial infarction bring about a fall in serum potassium by approximately 0.8 mM/L. The danger of hypokalemia in myocardial infarction is well recognized and, thus, selective beta$_2$ blockade has an additional salutary effect by maintaining normal or slightly elevated potassium levels and, thereby, reduces the frequency of ventricular arrhythmias.

Conditions that may be clinically encountered, producing hypokalemia, include the following: a) the administration of epinephrine; b) the increase of epinephrine related to myocardial infarctions; c) the hypokalemia related to delerium tremens; d) asthmatic patients who are treated with beta$_2$ agonists; e) patients given terbutaline in the treatment of asthma or for control of premature labor[47] (Table 10-10).

Hyperkalemic episodes may be encountered in the use of large doses of beta$_2$ blockers, following exercise, and in the presence of uncontrolled diabetes mellitus or renal failure. Elevations are also seen in the muscular disorder known as hyperkalemic periodic paralysis. The hyperkalemia of exercise, which is exaggerated by beta blockade, may be somewhat diminished in the presence of alpha adrenergic blockade.

Hypokalemia

Common Causes

Hypokalemia can result from mechanisms related to either decreased intake or increased elimination of potassium (Table 10-11).

Excessive losses of K^+ may be gastrointestinal (e.g., vomiting, nasogastric suctioning, bowel obstruction) or renal (diuretics, hyperaldosteronism). Hypokalemia may also occur without loss of total body potassium, as by a shift in K^+ from plasma into cells through maximal adrenal stimulation (shock), administration of epinephrine,[50,51] or administration of beta$_2$ agonists.[52]

Epinephrine is a non-selective adrenergic stimulant of both alpha and beta receptors. D'Silva first showed in 1934 its effect in producing hypokalemia. Epstein elaborated on this effect and demonstrated a two-phase response: An initial action results in a transient hyperkalemia due to alpha-adrenergic mediated hepatic release of potassium. The second action is a prolonged hypokalemia caused by beta$_2$-adrenergic mediated uptake of potassium in skeletal muscles.[53]

Beta$_2$-selective adrenergic agonists, such as terbutaline, are active in producing hypokalemia. A subcutaneous injection of 0.5 mg terbutaline induces a decline in plasma potassium, and this is related to and dependent upon the plasma concentration of the terbutaline. This effect can be antagonized by non-selective beta-antagonists, such as oxyprenolol.[52]

Clinical Signs and Symptoms[42,51]

The principle clinical findings are the skeletal muscular effects, manifested by skeletal muscular weakness and the electocardiographic changes. These two effects constitute the "low potassium syndrome". The muscular effects may progress to skeletal muscle paralysis, shallow respiration and respiratory failure.

Hypokalemia increases cardiac automaticity, conductivity and excitability particularly when acute.. The ECG findings are classic: ST segment depression; U-waves; tachycardia and ectopic beats. Chronic hypokalemia may not be predisposing to dysrhythmias (Fig. 10-5).[51,61]

Other pathophysiologic features of hypokalemia include: ileus, predisposing to vomiting and aspiration; accompanying the decreased skeletal muscle strength there is a potentiation of neuromuscular NMJ blockers.

Renal impairment is denoted by a conentrating defect with polyuria, sodium retention and edema; there is increased bicarbonate reabsorption and reduced GFR. Metabolic impairment is evidenced by glucose intolerance and hepatic encephalopathy. Neurologic features include confusion and depression.

Adverse Effects

Cardiac Arrhythmias

Normokalemia is usually defined as serum levels between 3.5 to 5.5 mEq/L. It has been generally regarded that patients with serum potassium levels below 3.0 mEq, and below 3.5 mEq/liter for those on digitalis, are candidates for various types of arrhythmias.[62] Postponement of elective surgery has even been suggested. This should not necessarily be decided unless a repeat serum potassium

Table 10-10. Clinical Conditions of Hypokalemia According to Loss or No Loss from the Body

Induced Without Loss of Body Potassium

    Pathophysiologic Causes

        Hypocarbia—normoxia by hyperventilation[48]
        Hypercarbia—airway obstruction with hypoxia and/or hypoxemia[49]
        Hypoxemia—epinephrine related

    Epinephrine Drug Induction

        Epinephrine[50,51]
            Initial hyperkalemia—due to α-adrenergic hepatic release of potassium
            β$_2$-Adrenergic action[52] uptake of potassium in skeletal muscles and other tissues[53]

    Other Drug Induction

        Nonselective and β$_2$-selective agonists—terbutaline (0.5 mg)
        β$_2$-blockers prevent hypokalemia

Induced With Loss of Body Potassium

    Gastrointestinal disturbances
    Renal: diuretics that inhibit Na^+ reabsorpt (at prox tubule /asc loop) produces hypokalemia and alkalosis.
    Diseases—hyperaldosteronism (principle mineral corticoid) Increases delivery of Na^+ to distal tubules
    Drugs—miscellaneous

Table 10–11. Mechanisms of Hypokalemia

1. Deficient oral intake.
2. Gastrointestinal loss: suction or vomitus diarrhea. The gastric juices contain 5 times the concentration of potassium present in serum. Villous adenoma.
3. Starvation.
4. Renal loss
   Osmotic-tubular diuretics
   Hyperglycemia
   Excess aldosterone secretion
   Excess endogenous or exogenous cortisol
5. *Altered Distribution of Potassium Between Intracellular and Extracellular Sites*
   Respiratory or metabolic alkalosis
   Glucose-insulin
   Familial periodic paralysis
6. *Trauma.* For every gram of nitrogen released from cellular breakdown about 2.5 gm. of potassium are released, which is excreted in the urine. This is accompanied by varying degrees of water and sodium retention and of potassium and magnesium excretion. The increase in body water is in the extracellular compartment so that the ratio of the extracellular water to the total body water (TBW) is increased.[54]
   Surgical stress (trauma) is also associated with the retention of sodium, chloride and water.[55] There is apositive sodium and water balance and a negative potassium-magnesium balance.[56] This response occurs early in the surgical period with the accumulation largely in skeletal muscle cells in both the injured and non injured portions of the body.[57] A major factor contributing to the retention is the increased release of antidiuretic pituitary hormone and the stimulation of aldosterone secretion.[58]
7. Routine operative parenteral therapy with saline and dextrose and lacking potassium. This possible *excess of sodium;* aggravates the effect of the low potassium; excesses of sodium enhance potassium excretion.
8. Administration of glucose rapidly.
9. Rapid alkalinization as with bicarbonate administration.
10. *Diuretic Therapy (except K-sparing agents) spirohalactone; amilorde.*
11. Drug Induced Hypokalemia
   Administration of Beta, agonist drug: The β_2-agonist drugs and epinephrine are capable of reducing serum potassium.[59] Terbutaline commonly used in obstetrics to inhibit contractions in premature labor is associated with lowered serum potassium.[60]

confirms the original values. An association between preoperative potassium levels below 3.5 mEq/L (and above 3.0 mEq/L) and arrhythmias has not been demonstrated.[61,63] Probably patients with serum levels above 3.5 mEq/L are not at unusual risk.[64] However, this does not answer the question with regard to potassium levels that are usually considered to be critical, namely those below 3.0 mEq/L.

Induced hypokalemia of an acute type, as with diuretic therapy, is always of concern. In these patients, normalization of the serum potassium may be brought about within 6–12 hours by minimal potassium therapy between 40–80 mEq. This observation is not necessarily similar to the hypokalemia in the debilitated or the patient with wasting disease. Furthermore, hypokalemia in the presence of ischemic heart disease may represent a greater hazard. In those patients with ischemic heart disease and not receiving digitalis, an increased susceptibility to ventricular arrhythmias has been shown.[64] Mild hypokalemia of values less than 3.3 mEq/L produced electrical instability in these patients. This minor reduction is associated with a greater risk in patients with ischemic heart disease.

Other Effects

The following adverse effects of hypokalemia are listed: 1) arrhythmias; 2) stress catecholamine release ex-

aggerated; 3) glucose intolerance; 4) increase in serum cholesterol; 5) decrease of blood pressure, especially in hypertensive patients; 6) decrease in renin serum plasma levels, and no increase in aldosterone.[65]

In several clinical situations, caution should be exercised in attempting potassium replacement in patients with hypokalemia.[66] This is especially so in patients with renal insufficiency; but the risks are also increased in patients who are hypertensive, in the elderly, those on drugs, including beta adrenergic blockers, the nonsteroid anti-inflammatory drugs and captopril. Diabetics are also quite susceptible to the development of hyperkalemia when deficiencies are being treated with intravenous potassium.[66,67]

Treatment[68]

Potassium salts may be administered orally or parenterally. In the intraoperative period the parenteral route is usual. The deficit should be calculated and this amount administered (observe clinical signs). It is usually safe to give 3 mEq./kg. per day. The solution used should be made of potassium chloride which is easiest to use since it does not alter pH. The concentration should not exceed 40 mEq./L. of potassium; that is a solution of 0.28;pc KCl is satisfactory.

Blood reaching heart, should not exceed 7 mEq/L, (except for cardioplegia) whereas total single dose

ECG changes in hypopotassemia (idealized)

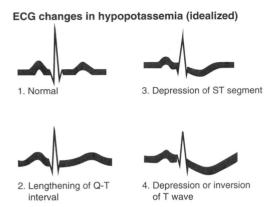

1. Normal

3. Depression of ST segment

2. Lengthening of Q-T interval

4. Depression or inversion of T wave

ECG changes in hyperpotassemia (idealized)

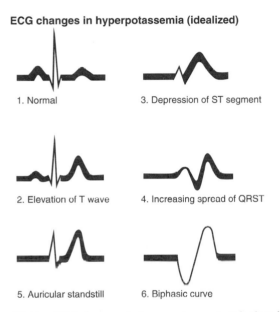

1. Normal

3. Depression of ST segment

2. Elevation of T wave

4. Increasing spread of QRST

5. Auricular standstill

6. Biphasic curve

Fig. 10–5. ECG changes in hyperpotassemia (idealized).

should not exceed 0.1 mEq./kg. or 7 to 8 mg./kg. (KCl) or rates greater than 20 mEq. per hour (500 ml. of 0.28% solution). Generally, it takes 5 to 6 days to replace a large deficit safely.

Potassium Replacement Therapy

Treatment should be based on the entire clinical situation, not on the serum potassium level alone.[68] Acute losses probably warrant aggressive replacement. This is likely if there are already serious dysrhythmias, a patient on digitalis therapy, drug therapy with aminophylline or beta$_2$ agonists (Table 10–12).

Potassium therapy is itself associated with hazard and is relatively contraindicated in oligemia or low cardiac output states.

Guidelines for safe potassium therapy include the following:

1. Concentration of solutions for infusion should not exceed 40 mEq/L.

Table 10–12. Indications for Rapid K Replacement

Severe hypokalemia (<2.5 mEq/L)
Diabetic ketoacidosis (even with normal serum K)
Ventricular arrhythmias secondary to K deficit
Digitalis intoxication
Severe metabolic Alkalosis: pH >7.55

2. Infusion rates should not exceed 10–20 mEq/hr.
3. Large total body K$^+$ losses or deficits usually require 36–48 hours of therapy.

For most conditions of hypokalemia the recommended rate is 10 mEq per hour of a potassium solution. For deficits in which the serum potassium is less than 2.5 mEq but more than 2.0 mEq/L faster rates of 20 mEq per hour may be safely administered. In rare instances a single bolus dose of 0.1 mEq/kg may be given over a 5 minute period. In digitalis intoxication 0.5 to 1.0 mEq can be administered as a bolus slowly over a 5 minute period and every 2–3 minutes until the electrocardiogram returns to normal.

If serum potassium is below 2.0 mEq/L potassium may be given at a rate of 40 mEq/hour at a concentration up to 60 mEq/L. A total dose of 400 mEq may be needed or 6 mEq/kg/day. Other indications for rapid replacement include:

- Diabetic Ketoacidosis (even with normal serum K),
- Ventricular Arrhythmias secondary to K deficit,
- Digitalis Intoxication,
- Severe Metabolic Alkalosis pH greater than 7.55.

Hyperkalemia

Causes

Failure to adequately excrete potassium from the body is the fundamental process leading to hyperkalemia. Renal failure is a common cause and may be aggravated by angiotension inhibitors (captopril) or by verapamil.

Elevated potassium levels have been observed in severe *renal disease,* in diabetic acidosis, Addison's disease, prolonged stress with adrenal failure and adrenal insufficiency. Of great practical importance to the anesthesiologists is the increased serum potassium which results from the following intraoperative situations: cellular hypoxia, general hypoxia, shock, dehydration, retained potassium in stress, agonal states, convulsions, and hypothermia.

Shock is particularly upsetting. Significant quantities of potassium are lost from the cells to the serum, whereas there is a gain in sodium. Both acidosis and alkalosis will increase potassium urinary excretion. As a preliminary to this is an elevated serum potassium.

During potassium therapy overdosage is not uncommon. If there is inordinate restriction of saline solution or any situation of reduced serum sodium, the effects of potassium are enhanced. Thus, it is advisable to administer at least the obligatory sodium losses and maintain a *normal* serum sodium.

In surgical-anesthesia practice, hyperkalemia is most often due to the following[68]:

Rapid infusion of blood
Rapid injection of penicillin
Prolonged heparin therapy
Too agressive treatment of hypokalemia
Administration of succinylcholine to patients with neuromuscular disorders, including:
   Muscular dystrophies
   CV accidents
   Cord injuries
   Burns
   Tetanus
Administration of high dose mannitol (2.0 mg/kg)[69]

Signs and Symptoms

Darrow has listed the following signs and symptoms of increased serum potassium.[4,42] (*a*) Listlessness and mental confusion; (*b*) Numbness and tingling of the extremities with a sense of weakness; (*c*) Bradycardia and irregular rhythms; (*d*) Peripheral vascular collapse and hypotension; (*e*) Ascending flaccid muscular paralysis; (*f*) Cardiac arrest.

Cardiac Clinical Effects

The cardiotoxic effects of excess potassium are by far the most important. Impaired excitability, automaticity, conductivity and contractility occurs. There are specific electrocardiographic changes with elevated levels of potassium. Thus, as the plasma levels exceed 7.5 mEq./L. (30 mg./100 ml.) the following changes appear: Elevation of T wave; depression and disappearance of P waves; depression of ST segment; widened QRS complex with spread of QRST which becomes biphasic.

Management

When evidence of hyperpotassemia develops, steps must be taken to control the condition. If parenteral potassium is being given, it should be stopped. Administration of glucose and insulin are most effective in reducing serum potassium. In the presence of normal renal function a saline infusion should be given.

Treatment

Acute hyperkalemia should be aggressively treated, especially when the P-R interval or QRS complex are abnormal in the ECG tracing. The following is recommended:[68,70]

- Calcium chloride administration is key.
  Concentration of solution 10% $CaCl_2$
- Dose is 10–20 ml of the solution with restored excitability and contractility in 2–3 minutes with duration of 15–20 minutes.
  Repeat as needed.
- Infusion of bicarbonate shifts serum potassium into cells.
  A bolus of 50 mEq of sodium bicarbonate (50 ml with 1.0 mEq/ml) will shift serum K^+ within 5 minutes. Duration of shift is variable and K^+ levels should be maintained and doses repeated.

- Hypocarbia by hyperventilation[48]: a rapid decrease in potassium occurs in parallel with a decrease in arterial carbon dioxide. A $Pa_{CO}2$ of 30 from 40 decreases K^+ by 0.5 mEq; from 40 to 20 $Pa_{CO}2$, a decrease in 1 mEq. This is a rapid response.[49]
- Infusion of glucose-insulin solution
  Solution of 50% dextrose with 10 units regular insulin in each 50 ml
  Initial bolus injection 50 ml of the above solution
  Maintenance 10% dextrose with 1 unit insulin over 30–60 minutes, with a decrease of 1.5–2.5 mEq in 30 minutes
- Beta$_2$ agonists: non-selective beta$_2$ epinephrine selective beta$_2$ terbutaline; ritodrine (uterine beta$_2$ receptors)
  Epinephrine is quite effective in lowering serum potassium.[50] An epinephrine infusion is administered to provide 20ug/min[70]
- Other Beta-$_2$ adrenergic agonists are successfully used to lower serum potassium. They are particularly effective when potassium levels are above 7.0 mEq/L[51,53] and are used to reduced potassium levels in renal failure patients requiring hemodialysis.

Exchange resins are useful in lowering serum potassium, especially in the presence of oliguria. Lastly, peritoneal dialysis should be used when derangement is severe or other measures are not quickly effective. Monitoring by the EKG is the best tool for determining effectiveness of therapy.

DEHYDRATION SYNDROME

One of the common surgical and anesthesia problems encountered is that of the "Dehydration Syndrome."[71] In this there is water and salt depletion, and in the early phases this is often unrecognized. It is due to a large extent to the obligatory losses that are incompletely replenished.[72]

The syndrome can be considered to represent progressive phases and severity.

In the early phase, the patient who is awake complains of thirst, and there is usually a slight pulse rise. This type of simple water depletion will occur when there is approximately a 2% loss of body weight or a deficit of 1,500 ml. of water. In this phase the electrolytes are not seriously out of balance.

In the moderate phase, thirst is significant and observation of the mucous membranes does reveal serious dryness, and the patient does indeed complain of some degree of skeletal muscle weakness. This represents approximately a 6% loss of body weight. It will occur in healthy subjects after 3 days of water deprivation.

Continued water deprivation will precipitate the advanced or severe state of dehydration and this is represented largely by a cardiocirculatory shock state. This occurs when there is a 7 to 15% deficit in body weight, or a loss of 5 to 10 liters of fluids. Failure to adequately replace, and above all to also replenish, the concomitant electrolyte disturbance deficits will usually bring about death. This will occur whenever there is a 15% or greater loss in body water.[73,74]

CALORIC REQUIREMENTS[75]

To provide the basic facts for complete parenteral therapy reference is given to caloric needs (Talbott). At bed rest the requirement is approximately *25 cal/kg/day*. Thus, a 70-kg man requires at least 1750 calories or 450 grams of carbohydrate. For protein sparing action at least 100 grams of carbohydrate per day are essential and at least 200 grams of carbohydrate per day are essential for antiketosis.[76]

PARENTERAL FLUID THERAPY

A number of solutions containing various constituents are available for water and electrolyte replacement (Table 10-13). Many of the constituents can be combined in one solution. However, they are available in separate solutions for specific balance needs.

Water Replacement

Glucose in 5 or 10% concentration is most effective in furnishing water.[74,77] The 5% solution is approximately isosmotic. The volume of water is based on the metabolic needs as previously reviewed, *i.e.*, for every 100 calories metabolized, 100 ml of water is needed. A one liter 5% glucose solution will (1000 ml.) spare protein. It will not prevent ketosis; it is inadequate in calories and should not be continued for long periods. A 10 or 15% glucose solution not only accomplishes the above goals, but provides more adequate calories.[76]

The *rate of administration* of glucose solutions is determined by assimilatory power.[78] If the rate is rapid, most of the glucose will be excreted in the urine. Glucose tolerance has been determined for preoperative and late postoperative periods as well as the anesthetic and intraoperative period. The overall tolerance is between 0.5 to 0.85 gm. per kg. per hour. To accomplish this rate of assimilation requires a quantitative infusion procedure. This is divided into an initial slow rate and an accelerated maintenance rate as follows:

Preoperative and Postoperative:

1. Initial rate: 25 gm. per hour for $^1/_2$ hour, *i.e.*, 250 ml. of 10% solution in $^1/_2$ hour or 5 to 10 ml. per minute.
2. Maintenance: 50 gm. per hour.

During Anesthesia and Surgery:

1. Initial rate: 10 gm. per hour for $^1/_2$ hour, *i.e.*, 100 ml. of 5% solution in $^1/_2$ hour or 2 to 4 ml. per minute.
2. Maintenance: 25 gm. per hour.

Electrolyte Replacement[73,74]

A number of solutions are available for replenishing body electrolytes.

Whenever a deficit is anticipated, the serum concentrations of sodium, potassium, chloride and bicarbonate should be determined. These values should then be used in calculating the actual deficit of the extracellular fluid compartment. Since the extracellular fluids represent 20% or one-fifth of the body weight the following formula is applicable:

$$\text{Amount in mEq.} = \frac{\text{Wgt. of pt.}}{5} \text{Kg} \times \left(\begin{array}{c} \text{Normal value of} \\ \text{ion in mEq./liter} \end{array} \right) - \left(\begin{array}{c} \text{Actual patient's} \\ \text{mEq./liter} \end{array} \right)$$

Replacement — ECF Vol in liters 40 mEq/L — X

Table 10-13. Electrolyte Fluid Balance Solutions for Parenteral Therapy

Solution	Composition	g/L	mEq/L Cations	mEq/l Anions	Indications
Isotonic saline 0.9% NaCl	Sodium chloride	9.0 g	Na-154	Cl-154	Limited use Not physiologic low salt syndrome
Ringers's Isotonic solution of three chlorides	Sodium chloride Potassium chloride Calcium chloride	8.6 g 0.3 g 0.3 g	Na-147 K-4.0 Ca-6.0	Cl-156	Acidosis Dehydration Vomiting
Darrow's (K-Lactate)	Sodium chloride Sodium lactate Potassium chloride	4.0 g 5.9 g 2.6 g	Na-121 K-35	Cl-103 Lactate-53	K⁺ deficiency Infant diarrhea
Hartman's Lactated-Ringer's Solution Resembles Interstitial Fluid Isotonic Solution of three chloride with lactate	Isotonic Sodium chloride Potassium chloride Calcium chloride Sodium lactate	6.0 g 0.3 g 0.2 g 3.1 g	Na-130 K-4.0 Ca-3.0 Na-28	Cl-109 Lactate-28	For routine parenteral therapy
Lactate Solution One sixth molar (mw sodium lactate-112)	Sodium lactate	18.6 mg	Na-166	Lactate-166 mM	For metabolic acidosis
Sodium bicarbonate 1.5%	Sodium bicarbonate	15.0 g	Na-178	Bicarb-178 mM	For metabolic acidosis

Physiologic saline solution 0.9% sodium chloride is isotonic with body fluids. It is limited in use to emergency circumstances and for sodium replacement. The basic solution for electrolyte therapy is Ringer's solution; it contains the principal extracellular ions but there is an excess of chloride. A mixture of 3 parts isotonic mixed salt solution and 1 part isotonic sodium lactate resembles interstitial fluid. This is available as lactated Ringer's or Hartman's solution and it provides the sodium and potassium needs without an excess of chloride. Sodium lactate may be given alone to correct a sodium deficit that is greater than the chloride deficit.

The potassium needs may be met by the addition of the daily requirement to 500 ml of 5% dextrose solution (i.e., 40 mEq or 1.5 g KCl to 500 ml). It is also provided in Ringer's lactate solution. If a patient must be continued on parenteral fluids (no resumption of oral intake in 2 days) for long periods, the potassium supplement can be based on a dose of 1.0 to 1.5 mEq/kg/day (2.5 to 3.0 mEq/lb).

Practical Summary

In planning parenteral fluid therapy, it is usually appropriate to determine the water needs. This is then supplied as 5 or 10% glucose solution. Part of the glucose solution should be combined with isotonic saline solution. Other electrolytes should be added for the deficits and for the daily expenditure. Isotonic saline solution in the amount required alone will not supply all of the water needs since this solution requires up to $1/2$ water to excrete the salt.

Out of every 100 ml. of water required approximately 20 ml. should be isotonic saline solution or other appropriate electrolyte solution and the remainder should be 5 to 10% of glucose.

In the presence of metabolic acidosis a mixture of 2 parts saline and 1 part isotonic sodium lactate is preferable. In alkalosis, saline alone or with the addition of calcium chloride is recommended.

During anesthesia and surgery, other factors than the normal requirements must be considered. Particular losses should be identified and measured (Table 10-14).

Acidity of Parenteral Solutions[79]

All common parenteral solutions are acidic in nature (Table 10-15). Saline solution 0.9% has a pH approximately of 5.6 and titrable acidity of 0.13 to 0.15 mEq/L. Ringer's lactated solution heat sterilized has a pH of 6.4 with a titrable acidity of 0.14, whereas the same solution prepared by ultrafiltration has a pH of 7.0 and acidity of 0.1 mEq/L. Dextrose solutions are the most acid. Dextrose 5% in water and heat sterilized has a pH of 4.9 and titrable acidity of 0.24 mEq/L. The accentuation of acidity of dextrose solutions by heating is due to formation of methylfurfural and mutarotation. Thus pH may vary as much as 1000 × between different commercial solutions, and the titrable acidity may vary 5-fold. Acid solutions may have a corrosive effect on blood vessels and can also contribute to body acidity. This should be appreciated in the fluid therapy of patients. Newer methods or preparations are needed and solutions buffered to pH 7.4 are desirable.[79]

Hazards with Intravenous Solutions[80]

A variety of complications and hazards directly related to establishing and maintaining a quality solution have been recognized. These hazards are summarized in Table 10-16.

Certain recommendations have been made to reduce these hazards by the Committee on Education of Therapeutics of the American Society for Clinical Pharmacology and Therapeutics. Among these recommendations are the following:[80,81]

1. Discontinue addition of drugs to intravenous fluids except in emergencies.
2. When addition of drugs is indicated, only one drug should be added to intravenous fluid. The fluids should preferably be a simple saline or other electrolyte solution or 5% dextrose in water.
3. Clear labeling of intravenous container with an added drug must be emphasized.
4. Administration equipment should be carefully reviewed by the Drug and Formulary Committee.

Table 10–14. Fluid Balance During Surgery and Anesthesia

Blood loss
1. Clinical conditions
2. Gravimetric determinations
3. Hematrocrit
4. Blood volume determinations
5. Estimates for children

Fluids and electrolytes
In shock, blood loss or anoxia cells lose K and gain sodium (Fox)
Insensible loss water nonsweating (80°F)
skin—30–50 m/hr = 800 q day
during op. air conditioned = 200 ml/hr
during op. nonconditioned = 600 ml/hr
lungs = 400 ml qd

Effects of agents
Morphine—antidiuresis
General anesthesia—decreased urine
decreased electrolytes

Table 10–15. Acidity of Parenteral Solutions

Solution	pH	Titrable Acidity (mEq/L)
Dextrose 10% (DW)	4.4	0.31
Dextrose 5% (DW) (Heat sterilized)	4.9	0.24
Saline 0.9%	5.6	0.15
Ringers Lactate (Heat sterilized)	6.4	0.14
Ringers Lactate (Ultrafiltration)	7.0	0.10

a. Volume control units should be more widely used.
b. Micropore filters should be included. It appears that commercially available filters with micropore size of 40×40 micra are effective. More complete protection is available by filters of 40×25 micra dimensions.
5. Visual inspection of container of solution in a clear light; note extent of particulate "floats"

INTRAVENOUS NUTRITIONAL CALORIC SUPPORT

Glucose Solutions

Glucose solutions are customarily administered as part of parenteral fluid therapy and in the presence of fasting

Table 10–16. Hazards Encountered with IV Solution Therapy

Microbiologic hazards

Solution nutrients for microorganisms
Supplies of carbon, nitrogen, phosphate and trace elements are sufficient to sustain microscopic organisms. Gram-negative organisms are easily sustained.
Solutions with dextrose—can support a 10-fold colony increase.

Contamination
By airborne microbes during opening of container
By an open system without filter during administration
By touch contamination
By addition of drugs
By pyrogens

Drug addition hazards
Contamination—8% rate
Drug incompatibility (related to difference in solvents, preservation, pH, ionic strength and redox potentials) many precipitates not visible
Drug bioavailability
adsorption of insulin to bottles and tubes
antibiotics—lose potency (Weisenfied, 1968)

Particulate Matter

Types—rubber, cellulose, glass crystals, fibers, fungus.
Size and number per ml: 0.5–2.0μm (2000–1000)
2.0–5.0μm (250–100) over 10–20μm (25–50)

Administration Sets

Disposable units—Cost disadvantage
Volume control devices—lack or misuse

Interactions (incompatibilities and instability of equipment)

Polyvinyl chloride—containers:
absorption of warfarin by plastic leaching of plasticizers into solution

Total parenteral nutrition (hyperalimentation)

The following adverse effects may occur:
Osmotic dehydration
Electrolyte depletion
Sensitization to peptides

(Vidt, D. G.: Use and abuse of intravenous solutions. JAMA,*232*:533, 1975.)

or limited oral intake. Perioperatively, glucose solutions are given for the following reasons:

- To provide a readily available fuel for metabolism
- To provide part of the free water requirements
- To prevent hypoglycemia
- To conserve protein by its sparing action. At least 100 grams of carbohydrate are essential.
- To lower blood levels of free fatty acids and ketone levels
- To prevent ketosis, at least 200 grams of carbohydrate are essential.[78]

Normal Caloric Requirements[75,77]

The caloric requirement at bed rest is approximately 25 calories/kg/day. For an adult man of 70 kg, this represents 1750 calories or 450 grams of carbohydrate.* In terms of carbohydrates, 5% or 10% glucose may be administered for caloric needs over a short period.[81] A rate of infusion of glucose of 12.5 g/hour will provide a blood glucose level of up to 200 mg/dl.

Caloric Requirements in Critically Ill Patients

Recent studies of hospitalized patients show that even the critically ill require no more than 2,000 calories/day.[82] The current practice of total parenteral nutrition, especially hyperalimentation, of the hospitalized patient is generally excessive.[83] The result is that there is an excessive CO_2 production, and the production of hypercapnea as a consequence of such nutritional support. This is not of great importance when patients are on mechanical respirators, but otherwise in the spontaneously breathing (room air) patient, this overproduction of CO_2 represents a burden and there is significant difficulty in weaning patients from ventilators because of the increased $PaCO_2$. Even at a caloric infusion of 1500–2000 kcal/day, the CO_2 production is still above normal, but can be handled by most patients.

Daily Water Requirement

This is related in ordinary circumstances to the rule that for every 100 calories of CHO metabolized, 100 ml of water is required.[77]

Hypoglycemia

Hypoglycemia is defined for the adult as a blood glucose concentration less than 50 mg/dl. This may occur after a 24 hour fast, as may be seen in some patients preoperatively. However, the anxiety and overall stress of the operative experience will increase the blood sugar levels to some extent. A normal or above level is assured by the administration of approximately 6–12 g/hr of glucose. An infusion of 250 ml of 5% dextrose in 1–3 hours will maintain blood sugar levels at 150 to 200 mg/dl.

The amount of glucose administered to satisfy fuel requirements, and for a protein-sparing effect, varies with the status of the patient. During starvation, the administration of 100–150 g/day of glucose reduces protein ca-

*Caloric value of glucose: 1.0 g glucose = 3.7 kcal or Cal is expressed in kilocalories.

tabolism by 50%.[83] However, in the intraoperative period, this amount and more does not cause a protein-sparing action.[84] In the postoperative period, the administration of 100 g of glucose during the first day produces little reduction in urinary nitrogen (20%)[85] or not at all.[86]

A decrease in blood free fatty acids can be accomplished to some extent by an infusion rate of approximately 12.5 g/hour in an adult man. This may reduce blood ketone levels, but not prevent ketosis. Free fatty acids have been shown to increase myocardial oxygen consumption,[87] hence reducing their level will benefit the myocardium. High levels of free fatty acids have been reported to increase cardiac arrhythmias.[88]

Hyperglycemia (Table 10–17)[89]

In the surgical situation, the stress reaction will increase blood sugar and the parenteral administration of glucose during surgery should be monitored. Blood levels greater than 200 mg/dl should be avoided. In otherwise healthy adult patients, administration of 5 g glucose (200 ml 5% glucose) will provide blood glucose levels between 100–150 mg/dl. A rate of 10 g glucose/hour will raise levels above 200 mg/dl and is not recommended.

Hypoglycemia is unlikely in procedures of short duration; i.e., less than 4 hours.[90] Hence, the administration of glucose may result in hyperglycemia and should be limited.

For surgery of 4 hours or more duration, glucose should be administered at rates up to 10 g/hr. If administered slowly, the glucose will be assimilated and blood vessels maintained at approximately 150 mg/dl.

Effect of Glucose Loads on Metabolism

Carbon dioxide is increased by the administration of glucose. Following ingestion of a single load of up to 100 g, no significant change in end-respiratory CO_2 tension (and hence in alveolar Pa_{CO_2}) has been noted, nor does blood lactic acid or CO_2 content increase.[91] Oral glucose loads over 200 g increase tidal volume minute ventilation, minute oxygen consumption and an increase in V_{CO_2}.[92] This may place a ventilatory load on patients with COPD.[93]

Table 10–17. Perioperative Complications of Hyperglycemia

Hyperosmolality
Nonketotic acidosis
Hyperosmolar-coma
Increase FF Acids increases Mvo_2
Delayed wound healing: Decreased tensile strength
Diminished phagocytosis by leukocytes (poor migration)
Diminished immunosuppression by lymphocytes
Increased infection
Maternal hyperglycemia induces fetal hypoglycemia

(Woodruff, R.: Perioperative complications of hyperglycemia. JAMA, 244:166, 1980.[89])

Parenteral glucose administration intraoperatively, however, does increase CO_2 production and metabolism. Patients receiving 100 g glucose intravenously over a period of 1–2 hours show an increased RQ (CO_2 production/O_2 consumption) and a 20% increase in CO_2 excretion (V_{CO_2}).[94] This places an additional load on ventilatory work, especially in recovery. However, the nutritional needs of patients on mechanical ventilatory support is decreased.[95]

Intracellular Lactic Acidosis

This occurs in the presence of hyperglycemia.

Experimental studies show that hyperglycemia will exacerbate the effects of brain ischemia and increased cerebral injury.[96,97]

In neurosurgical procedures, blood levels do not fall below 85 mg/dl when glucose is withheld. Withholding glucose initially and then administering glucose at one-half the usual rate after 3–4 hours will allow blood levels to remain close to 100–120 mg/dl.[98]

The main recommendation is to monitor blood sugar levels and provide glucose if needed.

The rate of gastric emptying is slowed. Hyperglycemia with blood glucose levels higher than 160 mg/dl delays emptying, especially of fat and protein.[99,100]

Hypoglycemia in Pregnancy

The clinical signs of hypoglycemia usually consist of developing hypotension of both systolic and diastolic pressures accompanied by nausea, sweating and often headache. The principal cause is fasting and/or starvation with high insulin levels from excessive secretion or inadvertent relative overdose of insulin. The normal blood sugar is set at 5.55 mMol/L or 100 mg/dl. In the non-pregnant subject, symptoms are likely to occur at levels of 50 mg/dl (2.78 mMol/L). However, the gravid subject is less tolerant of lowered levels and develops low levels more readily than other surgical patients.[101] The critical level of blood glucose in the pregnant subject is 60 mg/dl (3.33 mMol/L), at which clinical signs of hypoglycemia are likely.

The pregnant woman lives in a state of "accelerated starvation," a term applied by Marx.[102] She is likely to develop hypoglycemia from short periods of fasting. Furthermore, the administration of spinal or epidural anesthesia may permit the development of hypotension more readily and block adrenocortical or hypoglycemic response to surgical stress.[103]

When significant hypotension (more than 20% decrease) develops in the pregnant patient, a blood sugar level should be determined. Hypoglycemia should be carefully treated by the administration of glucose. Marx[102] recommends the following regimen:

- If blood glucose is 40 mg/dl or less, administer 25 g of glucose in intravenous bolus doses; raise the glucose level by repeated doses to a level of 100 mg/dl.
- If blood sugar is 60 mg/dl, administer 12–15 g of glucose in intravenous bolus doses to a blood glucose level of approximately 100 mg/dl.

Fetal Hypoglycemia Induced by Maternal Hyperglycemia

Caution should be exercised in administering glucose so that maternal hyperglycemia does not develop.[102] Glucose readily traverses the placenta and raises the fetal glucose levels. Since maternal insulin does not cross the placental boundary, the elevated blood glucose in the term infant stimulates fetal insulin secretion. After delivery, the neonate deprived of maternal glucose may develop reactive hypoglycemia with vomiting.[104]

Testing with Dextrostix is recommended when hypotension is resistant to fluids and/or ephedrine, as well as positron.

Indications for Glucose Administration

- After fasting for more than 12 hours,[105] administer glucose at a rate of 5.0 g/hour, whenever hypoglycemia may occur.
- In diabetics, on either oral hypoglucagon drugs or an insulin regimen
- In patients on total parenteral hyperalimentation, whenever the infusion is stopped. Hypoglycemia otherwise ensues.
- In prolonged operative procedures and duration of anesthesia of more than 4 hours. Note that in short duration or minor surgical procedures, normoglycemia is usual. No increases in blood sugar are likely.[106]
- Infants and children (in-hospital) are prone to develop hypoglycemia.[104] After a fast of 8–10 hours, approximately 15% of children have blood glucose levels below 40 mg/dl. After an 8 hour fast 28% of infants under 15.5 kg, or younger than 4 months, have hypoglycemia.

Note: Fasting outpatients, infants and children, frequently develop hypoglycemia.[107,108] They are presumably less sick and follow a more mandated intake regimen.

- Postoperative hypoglycemia may occur after removal of pheochromocytoma. Catecholamines have an inhibitory effect on pancreatic islet cells; when the levels of catecholamines decrease, a reactive increase in insulin secretion occurs.[109]
- Miscellaneous causes of hypoglycemia should be recognized and the patient provided intravenous glucose.[110] Such conditions include:
  Pancreatic islet cell tumors
  Hepatomas
  Alcoholism
  Hypopituitarism
  Adrenal insufficiency

REFERENCES

1. Smith H. W.: The kidney: Structure and function in health and disease. New York, Oxford University Press, 1951.
2. Bernard C.: Lecons sur les proprietes physiologiques et let alterations pathologiques des liquides de porganisme. Paris, Vol. 1, J. B. Bailliere et Fils, 1959.
3. N. B. Talbot, R. H. Richie, Crawford J. D.: Metabolic Homeostasis. Cambridge, Harvard University Press, 1959.
4. Darrow D. C., Pratt E. L.: Fluid therapy. JAMA 143:365, 1956.
5. Peters J. P., Van Slyke D. D.: Quantitative clinical chemistry, 2nd Ed. Vol. 1. Baltimore, The Williams and Wilkins Co., 1946.
6. Widdow E. M.: Changes in body proportions and composition during growth. In Scientific Foundation of Paediatrics. E. Davis (Ed.) W. B. Saunders Co., Philadelphia, PA, 1974.
7. Weisberg H. F.: Water, electrolyte, and acid base balance, 2nd Ed. Springfield, Charles C. Thomas, 1960.
8. Goldberger E.: A primer of waters, electrolyte and acid-base syndromes, 5th ed. Philadelphia, Lea & Febiger, 1975.
9. Ehrlich, E. N.: Electrolyte metabolism: Adrenal regulation of electrolyte and water metabolism. In: Endocrinology Ed. L. J. Degrout. W. B. Saunders, Philadelphia, p. 1582–1597, 1989.
10. Edelman I. S., Leibman J.: Anatomy of body water and electrolytes. Am J Med 27:256–277, 1959.
11. Moore F. D., Oleson K. M., McMurray J. D., Parker H. V., et al.: The body cell mass and its supporting environment. Philadelphia, W.B. Saunders Co., 1963.
12. Hays R. M.: Dynamics of body water and electrolytes. In: Clinical disorders of fluid and electrolyte metabolism. H. M. Maxwell, H. R. Keenan (Eds.), p. 1–36, New York, McGraw Hill, 1980.
13. Moore F. D.: Metabolic care of the surgical patient. Philadelphia, W.B. Saunders Co., 1959.
14. Friis-Hansen B.: Changes in body water composition during growth. Acta Paediatr 46(Sup 110):1–68, 1957.
15. Landis E. M.: The passage of fluid through capillary wall. Am J Med Sci 193:297, 1937.
16. Krogh A.: The anatomy and physiology of capillaries. New Haven, Yale University Press, 1929.
17. Starling E. W.: Physiological factors involved and the causation of dropsy. Lancet 1:1405, 1896.
18. Landis E. M., Pappenheimer J. R.: Exchange of substances through the capillary walls In Handbook of Physiology Section 2: Circulation. Washington, D.C. Amer Physiological Society Vol. 2 p. 961–1034, 1963.
19. Wakin K. G., Gatch M. D.: Q. Bull., Indiana University Medical Center, 6:51–54, 1944.
20. Rous P., Gilding H. P., Smith F.: The gradient of vascular permeability. J Exper Med 51:807, 1930.
21. White A., Handler P., Smith E.: Principles of biochemistry, 5th Ed. New York, McGraw-Hill Book Co., 1973.
22. Wrong O.: Volume control of body-fluids. Br Med Bull 13:10, 1957.
23. Verney E. B.: Absorption and excretion of water. Lancet 2:739, 1946.
24. Robertson G. L., Mahn E. A., Arthur S., Sinha T.: Development and clinical application of a new method for immunoassay of arginine vasopressin in human plasma. J Clin Investig 52:2340–2352, 1973.
25. Hays B.: Antidiuretic hormone. New Engl J Med 295:659–665, 1976.
26. Fitzsimmons J. T.: The physiological basis of thirst. Kidney Int 10:3–18, 1976.
27. Laragh J. H., Sealey J. F.: The renin-angiotensin aldosterone hormonal system and regulation of sodium, potassium, and blood pressure homeostasis. In: Handbook of Physiology: Renal Physiology. Am Physiol Soc, Washington, D.C., p. 831–908, 1973.
28. Schrier R. W., Berl T.: Nonosmolar factors affecting renal water excretion. N Engl J Med 292:81, 141, 1975.
29. Zerbe R. L., Robertson G. L.: Osmotic and non-osmotic

regulation of thirst and vasopressin secretion. In: Clinical Disorders of Fluid and Electrolyte Metabolism. Eds. M. H. Maxwell, C. R. Kleenan, and B. G. Marins. 4th Ed. p. 61–78, New York, McGraw-Hill, 1987.

30. deBold A. J.: Atrial natriuretic factor: Overview. Fed Proc 45:2081–2085, 1986.

31. Gamble G. L.: Chemical anatomy, physiology and pathology of extracellular fluids. Cambridge, Harvard University Press, 1953.

32. Best and Taylor's Physiological Basis of Medical Practice, 12th ed. John B. West. Ed. Williams & Wilkins, Baltimore, 1990.

33. Zimmermann B., Wangensteen O. H.: Observation on water intoxication in surgical patients. Surgery 31:654–69, 1952.

34. Chung H.-M., Kluge R., Schrier R. W., Anderson R. J.: Postoperative hyponatremia: A prospective study. Arch Intern Med 146:333–336, 1986.

35. Philbin D. M., Coggins C. H.: Plasma antidiuretic hormone levels in cardiac surgical patients during morphine and halothane anesthesia. Anesthesiology 49:95–98, 1978.

36. Arieff A. L.: Hyponatremia, convulsion, respiratory arrest, and permanent brain damage after elective surgery in healthy women. N Engl J Med 314:1529–1535, 1986.

37. Sterns R. H., Riggs J. E., Schochet S. S., Jr.: Osmotic demyelination syndrome following correction of hyponatremia. N Engl J Med 314:1535–1542, 1986.

38. Arieff A. L.: Rapid correction of hyponatremia: Cause of pontine myelinolysis? Am J Med 71:846–847, 1981.

39. Laurenco R.: Central pontine myelinolysis following rapid correction of hyponatremia. Ann Neurol 13:232–242, 1983.

40. Narins R. G.: Therapy of hyponatremia. N Engl J Med 314:1573–1575, 1986.

41. Carr D: Commentary. Hyponatremia leads to brain damage. Intelligence Report in Anesthesia 4:8 (Sept.–Oct.), No. 2., 1986.

42. Hoffman W. S.: Clinical physiology of potassium. JAMA 144:1157, 1950.

43. Finch C. A., Sawyer C. G., Flynn J. M.: Clinical syndrome of potassium intoxication. Am J Med 1:337, 1947.

44. Andres R., Baltzan M. A., Cader G., Zieler K. L.: Effect of insulin and carbohydrate metabolism and on potassium in the forearm of man. J Clin Invest 41:108–114, 1962.

45. Rosa R. M., Silva P., Young J. B., Landsberg L., Brown R. S., Rowe J. W., Epstein F. H.: Adrenergic modulation of extrarenal potassium disposal. N Engl J Med 302:431–434, 1980.

46. Epstein F. H., Rosa R. M.: Adrenergic control of serum potassium. Editorial. New Engl J Med 309:1450–1451, 1983.

47. Moravec M. A., Hurlbert B. J.: Hypokalemia associated with terbutaline administration in obstetrical patients. Anesth Analg 59:917–920, 1980.

48. Edwards R., Winnie A. P., Ramamurthy S.: Acute hypocapnic hypokalemia and iatrogenic anesthetic complication. Anesth Analg 56:786, 1977.

49. Kane P. B., Torretti J.: Hypokalemia and respiratory acidosis following partial obstruction of the airway. Can J Anaesth 34:380, 1987.

50. D'Silva J. H.: The action of epinephrine on serum potassium. J Physiol (Lond) 91:393, 1934.

51. Epstein F. H., Rosa R. M.: Adrenergic Control of serum potassium. New Engl J Med 309:1450, 1983.

52. Jonkers R., Van Boxtel C. J., Oosterhuis B.: Beta-2-adrenoceptor-mediated hypokalemia and its abolishment by oxprenolol. Clin Pharmacol Ther 42:627, 1987.

53. Brown M. J., Brown D. C., Murphy M. B.: Hypokalemia from beta-2-receptor stimulation by circulating epinephrine. New Engl J Med 309:1414, 1983.

54. Moore F. D.: Metabolic care of the surgical patient. Philadelphia/London, W. B. Saunders, Co., 1959.

55. Stillstrom A., Person E., Vinnars E.: Postoperative water and electrolyte changes in skeletal muscle: A clinical study with three different intravenous solutions. Acta Anaesthesiologica Scand. 31:284–288, 1987.

56. Vinnars E., Furst P., Gump F. E., Kinney J. M.: Influence of trauma and sepsis on water and electrolytes of human muscle tissue. Surg Forum 26:16, 1975.

57. Bergstrom J., Furst P., Holtrom B., et al.: Influence of injury and nutrition on muscle water and electrolytes. Ann Surg 193:810–816, 1981.

58. Cochrane J. P. S.: The aldosterone response to surgery and the relationship of this response to the postoperative sodium retention. Br J Surg 65:744–747, 1978.

59. Moravec M. A., Hurlbert B. J.: Hypokalemia associated with terbutaline administration in obstetrical patients. Anesth Analg 59:917–920, 1980.

60. Hurlbert B. J., Edelman J. D., David K.: Serum potassium levels during and after terbutaline. Anesth Analg 60:723–725, 1981.

61. Vietz T. S., Soper L. E., Wong K. C., Soper P.: Chronic hypokalemic and intraoperative arrhythmias. Anesthesiology 63:130, 1985.

62. Harrington J. F., Kassirer J. P.: Am J Med 73:155, 1982.

63. McGovern B.: Hypokalemia and cardiac arrhythmias. (Editorial) Anesthesiology 63:127, 1985.

64. Stewart D. E., Ikram H., Espiner E. A., Nicholls M. G.: Arrhythmogenic potential of diuretic-induced hypokalemia in patients with mild hypertension and ischemic heart disease. Br Heart J 54:290, 1985.

65. Struthers A. D., Whitesmith R., Reid J. L.: Prior thiazide diuretic treatment increases adrenaline-induced hypokaliemia. Lancet 1:1358, 1983.

66. Kassirer J. P., Harrington J. T.: Fending off the potassium pushers. (Editorial) New Engl J Med 312:785, 1985.

67. Kaplan N. M., Carnegie A., Raskin P., et al.: Potassium supplementation in hypertensive patients with diuretic-induced hypokalemia. N Engl J Med 312:746, 1985.

68. Vietz T.: Potassium and the anaesthetic (refresher course). Can J Anaesth 34:530, 1987.

69. Manninen P. H., Lam A. M., Gelb A. W., Brown S. C.: The effect of high-dose mannitol on serum and urine electrolytes and osmolality in neurosurgical patients. Can J Anaesth 34:442, 1987.

70. Vietz T. S.: Treatment of hyperkalemia with epinephrine. Anesthesiology 65:350–351, 1986.

71. Marriott C.: Water depletion. Springfield, Charles C. Thomas, 1950.

72. Elkington J. R.: Hemodynamic changes in dehydration. J Clin Invest 25:120, 1946.

73. Peters J. P.: Treatment of salt depletion. Surg 24:568, 1948.

74. Wakim J. G.: Basic considerations in the rectification of clinical disturbance of electrolyte and fluid balance. World Med J 2:237, 1956; 3:27, 1957.

75. Butler A. M., Talbot N. B.: Parenteral fluid therapy. I J Med 231:585–621, 1944.

76. Pareira M. D., Probstein J. G.: Glucose assimilation during anesthesia and surgery. Am J Surg 129:463, 1949.

77. Talbot N. B., Richie R. H., Crawford J. D.: Metabolic homeostasis. Cambridge, Harvard University Press, 1959.

78. Pereira M. D., Somiogyi M.: Rationale of parenteral glucose feeding in the postoperative state. Am J Surg 127:417, 1948.

79. Lebowitz M. H., Masuda J. Y., Beckerman J.: The pH and acidity of intravenous infusion solutions. JAMA *215*:1937, 1971.

80. Duma R. J., Latta T.: What have we done? The hazards of intravenous therapy. New Engl J Med *294*:1178, 1976.

81. Quebbeman E. J., Ausman R. K.: Estimating energy requirements in patients receiving parenteral nutrition. Arch Surg 117:1281, 1982.

82. Koretz R. L.: Nutritional support: Whether or not some is good, more is not better. (Editorial) Chest *88*:2, 1985.

83. Gamble J. L.: Physiological information gained from studies on the life raft ration. Harvey Lect *42*:247, 1947.

84. Sieber F. E., Smith D. S., Kupferberg J., Crosby L., et al.: The effects of intraoperative glucose on protein catabolism and plasma glucose levels in patients with supratentorial tumors. Anesthesiology *64*:453, 1986.

85. Askanazi J., Carpentier Y. A., Jeevanandam M., et al.: Energy expenditure, nitrogen balance and norepinephrine excretion after injury. Surgery *89*:478, 1981.

86. Giddings A. E. B.: The control of plasma glucose in the surgical patient. Br J Surg *61*:787, 1974.

87. Challoner D. R., Steinberg D.: Effect of free fatty acid on the oxygen consumption of perfused rat heart. Am J Physiol *210*:280, 1966.

88. Tansey M. J., Opie L. H.: Relation between plasma free fatty acids and arrhythmias within the first twelve hours of acute myocardial infarction. Lancet *2*:419, 1983.

89. Woodruff R.: Perioperative complications of hyperglycemia. JAMA *244*:166-68, 1980.

90. Sieber F. E., Smith D. S., Traystman R. J., Wollman H.: Glucose: A reevaluation of its intraoperative use. Anesthesiology *67*:72-76, 1987.

91. Edwards H. T., Bensley E. H., Dill D. B., Carpenter T.: Human respiratory quotients in relation to alveolar carbon dioxide and blood lactic acid after ingestion of glucose, fructose, or galactose. J Nutr *27*:241, 1944.

92. Saltzman H. A., Salzano J. V.: Effects of carbohydrate metabolism upon respiratory gas exchange in normal men. J Appl Physiol *30*.228, 1971.

93. Giescke T., Gurushanthaiah G., Glauser F. L.: Effects of carbohydrates on carbon dioxide excretion in patients with airway disease. Chest *71*:55, 1977.

94. Hagerdal M., Caldwell C. B., Gross J. B.: Intraoperative fluid management influences on carbon dioxide production and respiratory quotient. Anesthesiology *59*:48, 1983.

95. Hunger F. D., Bruton C. W., Hunker E. M., Durham R. M., Krumdieck C. L.: Metabolic and nutritional evaluation of patients supported with mechanical ventilation. Crit Care Med *8*:628, 1980.

96. Pusinelli W. A., Waldman S., Rawlinson D., Plum F.: Moderate hyperglycemia augments ischemic brain damage. Neurology *32*:1239-1246, 1982.

97. MacGregor G. A., de Wardner E.: Idiopathic brain oedema. Lancet *2*:355, 1979, *1*:397, 1979.

98. Pusinelli W. A., Levy D. E., Sigsbee L., Scherer P., Plum F.: Increased damage after ischemic stroke in patients with hyperglycemia with or without established diabetes. Am J Med *74*:540-544, 1983.

99. MacGregor I. L., Wiley Z. D., LaVigne M. E., Way L. W.: Slowed rate of gastric emptying of solid food in man by high caloric parenteral nutrition. Am J Surg *138*:652-654, 1979.

100. MacGregor I. L., Deveny C., Way L. W., Meyer J. H.: The effect of acute hyperglycemia on gastric emptying in man. Gastroenterology *70*:190-196, 1976.

101. Spellacy W. N., Goetz F. C., Greenberg B. Z., Ellis J.: The human placental gradient for plasma insulin and blood glucose. Am J Obstet Gynecol *90*:753, 1964.

102. Marx G. F., Domurat M. F., Costin M.: Potential hazards of hypoglycemia in the parturient. Can J Anaesth *34*:4, 1987.

103. Engquist A., Brandt M. R., Fernandez A., et al.: The blocking effect of epidural analgesia on the adrenocortical and hyperglycemic responses to surgery. Acta Anaesthesiol Scand *21*:330, 1977.

104. Thomas K., de Gasparo M., Hoett J. J.: Insulin levels in the umbilical vein and in the umbilical artery of newborns or normal and gestational diabetic mothers. Diabetologia *3*:299, 1967.

105. Doze Van A., White P. F.: Effects of fluid therapy on serum glucose levels in fasted outpatients. Anesthesiology *66*:223, 1987.

106. Clarke R. S. J.: The hyperglycemic response to different types of surgery and anaesthesia. Br J Anaesth *42*:45-53, 1970.

107. Stafford M., Jeon A., Pascucci R.: Pre and post induction blood glucose concentrations in healthy fasting children Anesthesiology *63*:A350, 1985.

108. Welborn L., Hannullah R. S., McGill W. A., et al.: What is the appropriate glucose concentration for routine infusions in pediatric outpatient surgery. Anesthesiology *65*:A434, 1986.

109. Meeke R. I., O'Keefe J. D., Gaffney J. D.: Pheochromocytoma removal and postoperative hypoglycemia. Anaesthesia *40*:1093-96, 1985.

110. Roizen M. F.: Anesthetic implications of concurrent diseases. In Anesthesia edited by Miller, R. New York p. 259-260, Churchill Livingstone, 1986.

Chapter 11

ACID-BASE BALANCE

MARC J. SHAPIRO

Homeostasis results in part from electrical neutrality due to hydrogen ion modification. Derangement of this balance leads to profound physiologic abnormalities that result in intracellular and organ death. This chapter explores the relationship of acids and bases in maintaining electrical neutrality for homeostasis.[1,2]

An acid is a compound that is a proton donor, such as the hydrogen ion [H+]. A base is a proton acceptor such as the hydroxide ion and may accept hydrogen ions. Simplistically:[3]

$$Acid \leftrightarrows base + hydrogen\ ion \qquad (1)$$

The hydrogen ion concentration in vivo can vary over the wide range of $-<20$ to >20 nmol/l; the normal concentration of hydrogen ion in the extra cellular fluid is 40 ± 4 nmol/l (0.00004 nmol/l). The concentration of hydrogen ions within a solution determines in part its ability to donate protons. Sorensen developed the commonly used nomenclature:[4]

$$pH = \log [H^+] = \log \frac{1}{[H^+]} \qquad (2)$$

The equation allows a relationship to exist between pH and hydrogen ion concentration.

Physiologic neutrality is 7.4, corresponding to a hydrogen ion concentration of 40 nmol/l (Fig. 11-1). In contrast a pH of 7.0 corresponds to 100 nmol/l. The logarithmic scale allows a large range of hydrogen ion concentration to be related to the simplistic logarithmic scale. For example, for every 0.1 decrease in pH, hydrogen ion concentration will increase by approximately 1.25 and for every 0.1 increase in pH, the hydrogen ion concentration will decrease by approximately 0.8. Because of its logarithmic relationship, a doubling or halving a hydrogen ion concentration will correspond to a pH change of .3. Figure 11-1 demonstrates the inverse relationship between the two measurements [H$^+$] and pH. Acidosis occurs as the [H$^+$] increases and the pH decreases below 7.4. Alkalosis occurs when the [H$^+$] decreases and the pH increases above 7.4.

ACID-BASE METABOLISM

An equilibrium exists between acids and bases in biologic systems. This equilibrium is expressed by the equation:

$$HA \leftrightarrows H+ + A \qquad (3)$$

The weak acid dissociates according to constant (K). The acid-base reaction always involves a conjugate acid-base pair made up of a proton donor and corresponding proton acceptor as shown in equation 1. For the acid or proton donor HA, the dissociation constant for a given temperature is:

$$k = [H^+] \frac{[A^-]}{HA} \qquad (4)$$

where the brackets indicate concentrations in mol/l. Equation 4 expressed for the hydrogen ion yields the Henderson equation:[5]

$$[H^+] = \frac{k\ (HA)}{[A^-]} \qquad (5)$$

Logarithmic transformation of equation 5 yields the Henderson Hasselbalch equation:[6]

$$-\log H^+ = -\log K - \log \frac{HA}{[A^-]} \qquad (6)$$

Substituting pH for $^-$log [H$^+$] with a $^-$log of a hydrogen ion concentration and pK for $^-$log k log.

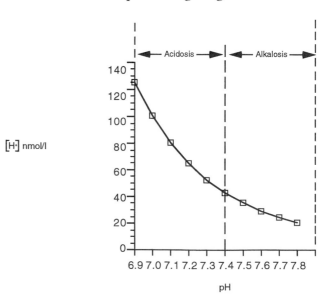

Fig. 11–1. Relationship between pH and hydrogen ion concentration [H$^+$].

188

$$pH = pK + \log \frac{[A^-]}{HA} \qquad (7)$$

In more general terms is pH = pK + concentration of the proton acceptor divided by the log concentration of the proton donor. This allows not only calculation of the pH but also with a known pH, calculation of the pK when the acid and the base concentrations are also known.[7]

BUFFERS AND pH REGULATION[8–10]

A buffer is a substance that is capable of receiving or donating hydrogen ions to maintain electrical neutrality in pH demonstrated how a buffer system works. When hydrogen is added to the mileu and combines with the weak base, the reaction in equation 3 is driven to the left forming the weak acid, HAC. When the reaction is driven to the right by adding the weak acid HA, hydrogen ions are released. Strong acids such as hydrochloric acid or hydrogen sulfate are not very effective buffers because they do not bind hydrogen ions. Weak acids such as ammonia are not good blood buffers because they tightly bind hydrogen ions even during systemic alkalosis. The ionization constant (K_{eq}) measures this dissociation ability. The pK_{eq} the negative logarithm of the ionization constant, is utilized to prioritize potency. The pK_{eq} is inversely proportional to the strength of the acid in that hydrogen chloride has a low pK and ammonium has a high pK. The most effective buffers have pK_{eq}s close to the physiologic pH 7.4; these are used to stabilize human blood pH.

Carbonic Acid/Bicarbonate Buffer System[8,14]

The carbonic acid/bicarbonate buffer system plays a central role in maintaining systemic acid-base balance. The following equation describes this role:

$$[H^+] + [HCO_3^-] \leftrightharpoons H_2CO_3 \leftrightharpoons H_2O + CO_2 \qquad (8)$$

Using the Henderson-Hasselbalch equation:

$$pH = pK + \log \text{ of } \frac{[HO_3^-]}{H_2CO_3} \qquad (9)$$

pK is equal to approximately 6.1.

When compensated by substituting dissolved CO_2 for true H_2CO_3 the following exists:

$$pH = pK + \log \frac{[HCO_3^-]}{P_{CO_2}} \qquad (10)$$

$$[H^+] = 24 \times \frac{P_{CO_2}}{[HCO_3^-]}$$

By combining the dissociation constant and solubility constant into the single value of 24. Kassirer and Bleich derived the following equation: From equation 10, the term ratio

$$\frac{P_{CO_2}}{[HCO_3^-]} \qquad (11)$$

reflects the $[H^+]$. The importance of this buffering system is evident in that concomitant changes in P_{CO_2} and

[HCO_3] will not change the hydrogen ion concentration or the pH of the individual, this allows the carbonic acid—bicarbonate system to act as a compensatory buffer mechanism. In many clinical laboratories, pH and P_{CO_2} are measured and $[HCO_3^-]$ is obtained from a nomogram. All modern blood gas analyzers report bicarbonate $[HCO_3^-]$ concentration not by direct measurement but by calculating its value from equation 10. Carbonate concentration is not equivalent to total CO_2 content, a value normally obtained from the serum electrolyte profile and a measurement of the total molar concentration of all CO_2 in serum. This measurement includes not only bicarbonate, but CO_2 gas in physical solution and serum, and CO_2 in the forms of carbonic acid and protein carbmates.

Hemoglobin as a Buffer System[11,12]

Hemoglobin functions as a primary noncarbonic buffer in extracellular fluid since it contains a large number of acidic or basic groups, such as carboxyl, amino, ammonium, or guanidino complexes. Because it exists as an isoionic protein in which the number of anionic groups equals the number of cationic groups, the net charge on the protein is 0. Hemoglobin exists within red cells as a potassium salt and its weak base existing in equilibrium with carbonic buffers. Both buffer systems are used when exogenous acid or alkali loads are administered. Due to it being a weak acid, hemoglobin is capable of buffering additional CO_2, resulting in a diffusion of $[HCO_3^-]$ into plasma in exchange for chloride to maintain electrical neutrality. This is known as the chloride shift.

The Phosphate Buffer System[2]

Phosphate ions exists in monohydrogen and dihydrogen phosphate forms five pH of 7.4 the monohydrogen form is five times more prevalent. The addition of a strong acid, such as HCl causes the following reaction:

$$HCL + Na_2HPO_4 \rightarrow NaCL + NaH_2PO_4 \qquad (12)$$

in which the strong acid (HCl) is converted to the neutral salt (sodium chloride, NaCl) and the weak acid (Na H_2 PO_4).

Similarly, if a strong base such as sodium hydroxide (NaOH) is administered, the following reaction would occur:

$$NaOH + NaH_2PO_4 \rightarrow Na_2HPO_4 + H_2O \qquad (13)$$

in which the strong base is converted into water and the phosphate buffer salt undergoes a change from a mild acid form to a mildly basic form (Na_2HPO_4).

Protein Buffer System

This buffer system exists primarily in tissue cells with proteins acting as anions.

pH Regulation System[1,8,10]

Respiration is regulated by sensors located in the central nervous system (CNS) and in the systemic circulatory system. CNS chemoreceptors located in the medulla are in contact with cerebrospinal fluid (CSF) and sensitive to small changes in pH and PCO_2 resulting in dramatic changes in ventilation. The CSF is more permeable to CO_2 than HCO_3^-, being responsive to changes in minutes rather than hours.

Peripheral chemoreceptors located in the aortic arch and carotid sinus are stimulated by change in PCO_2 or pH. Hypoxemia also stimulates the carotid sinus receptor. Stimulation of these chemoreceptors may result in an increase in ventilation such that an acid load hypercarbia or hypoxemia is counteracted with a rapid respiratory response. An alkaline load or decline in PCO_2 results in hypoventilation mediated through central and peripheral chemoreceptors. High PCO_2 is a stimulant of the central respiratory center. However, PCO_2 above 65 mm/Hg may act as a depressant, leading to carbon dioxide narcosis.

The pH also affects ventilation with acidosis stimulating respiration by compensatory Kussmaul hyperventilation. However a pH below 7 may abolish this response.

Regulation of pH by Kidneys[9]

Bicarbonate filtered by the glomerulus is reabsorbed by exchanging with hydrogen ion, which renal tubular cells secrete for sodium ions in the tubular urine. In a 24-hour period, more than 4,000 mEq of bicarbonate must be reabsorbed to maintain electrical neutrality. In addition, the body produces approximately 1 mEq/kg body weight per day of nonvolatile acids such as phosphoric and sulfuric acid in order to maintain pH. This also must be excreted by the kidney through acidification of buffer salts and by the excretion of $NH4^+$.

Hydrogen ions exist in tubular cells because of the enzyme, carbonic anhydrase, which catalyzes:

$$CO_2 + H_2O \rightarrow H^+ + HCO_3^- \qquad (14)$$

In the tubular urine, hydrogen ions combine with bicarbonate ions to form carbonic acid, which then forms water and carbon dioxide from equation 1. Water is secreted and the carbon dioxide absorbed. Sodium ions pass from the tubular urine into the tubular cells, uniting with the bicarbonate ions to form sodium bicarbonate, which passes into the plasma and extracellular water.

Hydrogen ions and sodium salts are similarly exchanged. As previously discussed in the phosphate buffer system, monohydrogen phosphate (Na_2HPO_4) dissociates into sodium and HPO_4 ions (equation 11). As the sodium gets reabsorbed, hydrogen ions move into the tubular urine to unite with $NaHPO_4$ to form the dihydrogen phosphate salt (NaH_2PO_4) which is secreted, removing hydrogen ions from the body.

Ammonia (NH_3) is found in the renal tubular cells due to the oxidation of the amino acid glutamine by glutaminase. This free ammonia is converted to ammonium ion ($NH4^+$) by uniting with hydrogen ion and is excreted as ammonium chloride (NH_4Cl). Thus hydrogen ions are removed from the body with the ammonia being converted to urea by the liver and excreted by the kidneys.

OSMOLALITY[15]

The osmolality of a solution is a measure of the total number of particles in that solution by weight. The higher the osmolality, the lower its specific activity. Although in clinical practice solute concentrations are measured per liter of solution (molal), the solute concentration of body fluids (mOsm) corresponds so closely to molal that the terms are used interchangeably. The principle electrolyte in extracellular fluid, NaCl, completely dissociates only in extremely dilute solutions and in vivo is approximately 93% intact.

The standard technique for the measurement of osmolality is based on the freezing temperature of vapor pressure of water. However, in all practicality, serum osmolality can be approximated from the molal concentrations of the three major solutes, sodium, glucose, and urea (Table 11-1). Because the solutes of glucose and urea are not polar, the calculation involves conversion of mg/dl into nmol/l. For glucose it is mg/dl $\times$ 10 $\div$ 180 = nmol/1cg and for BUN mg/dl $\times$ 10/28.

Discrepancy between the measured and calculated osmolality is caused by the fact that either the water content of the serum deviates widely from normal or an unaccounted solute is present in the plasma in significant amounts. Two major groups leading to >10 mOsm/kg H_2O discrepancy are categorized (Fig. 11-2). One reason is a decreased serum water content from hyperlipidemia or hyperproteinemia. Lipemic serum may be a tip-off or

Table 11-1. Serum Osmolality and Abnormalities

Osmolality (mOsm/kg H_2O) = 2 x sodium + glucose/18 + BUN/2.8

Measured − Calculated osmolality >10 mOsm/kg H_2O

    Decrease serum water:
        Hyperlipidemia
        Hyperproteinemia

    Additional low molecular weight solutes:
        Mannitol
        Ethanol
        Methanol
        Ethylene glycol
        Other

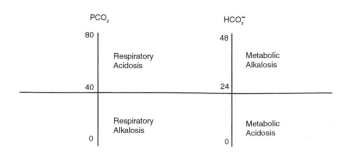

Fig. 11-2. Metabolic and respiratory physiologic derangement. The final pH determines if a primary or mixed acidosis or alkalosis exists.

the total protein concentration may be greater than 10 g/dl. Additional low molecular weight solutes being measured may be responsible for the measured and calculated discrepancy. A final reason for a discrepancy may be related to a laboratory error.

CLINICAL ACID-BASE BALANCE[2,7]

In the course of normal metabolism carbohydrates and fat are oxidized almost completely to carbon dioxide and water. Oxidation of these substances serves as a major energy source being responsible for oxygen consumption. The normal respiratory quotient:

$$\frac{CO_2 \text{ production}}{O_2 \text{ delivery}} \qquad (15)$$

is approximately .80 or 220 ml CO_2 produced per minute for every 260 ml of O_2 consumed. In addition with anaerobic metabolism incomplete carbohydrate and lipid metabolism may produce ketone bodies and lactic acid leading to a metabolic acidosis with a pH <7.4 and an elevated $PaCO_2$ (Fig. 11-2). Protein catabolism of amino acids containing sulfates and phosphates produce acidic compounds such as phosphoric acid and sulfuric acid also leading to a metabolic acidosis. With the average diet, about 60 mEq of strong acid (hydrogen ions) are produced per day under resting circumstances and this is why the buffering system is crucial to maintain a neutral pH for effective cellular respiration and function.

To counteract any metabolic component to acid-base equilibrium, carbon dioxide production is modified per the respiratory component of this equilibrium. The rates of CO_2 production and elimination vary on the basis alveolar ventilation. When changes occur in the metabolic component with an intact respiratory system, respiratory compensation may be triggered by the central and peripheral chemoreceptors (Fig. 11-2). In summary, four acid-base abnormalities are described in Figure 11-2 as follows:[7,17,18]

A. **Metabolic acidosis.** An abnormal physiologic process characterized by:
   1. a primary gain of strong acid by extracellular fluid; or
   2. a loss of bicarbonate from extracellular fluid.
B. **Metabolic alkalosis.** An abnormal physiologic process characterized by:
   1. a primary gain in bicarbonate; or
   2. a primary loss of strong acid by the extracellular fluid.
C. **Respiratory acidosis.** An abnormal physiologic process characterized by an elevation of $PaCO_2$ and a primary decrease in ventilatory rate relative to the rate of CO_2 production. The differential diagnosis is listed in Table 11-2.
D. **Respiratory alkalosis.** An abnormal process characterized by a decrease in $PaCO_2$ and increase in ventilatory rate relative to the rate of CO_2 production. The differential diagnosis is listed in Table 11-3.

Table 11-2. Differential Diagnosis of Respiratory Acidosis

Pulmonary Disorders
  Restrictive airway disease (fibrosis, flail chest)
  Chronic obstructive pulmonary disease
  Acute airway obstruction (tumor, foreign body, bronchospasm)
  Pulmonary edema
  Acute parenchymal pulmonary disease (pneumonia, aspiration, smoke inhalation)
  Impaired diaphragmatic excursion (paralyzed phrenic nerve, post CABG, obesity, ascites, pleural effusion)
  Increased CO_2 production (carbohydrates, $NaHCO_3$)
  Pickwickian syndrome (narcolepsy, sleep apnea)
Central Nervous System (CNS)
  Drug induced (sedative-hypnotic narcotics, anesthesia)
  CNS injury disease (trauma, tumor, ischemia, hemorrhage)
Neuromuscular System
  Primary (muscular dystrophy, myasthenia gravis, Guillain-Barre syndrome)
  Drugs/toxins (paralytics, botulism)
  Other (hypokalemia, periodic paralysis)
Mechanical Ventilation (malfunction, low rate, deadspace)

Table 11-3. Differential Diagnosis of Respiratory Alkalosis

Pulmonary disorder (pulmonary edema, pulmonary embolism, pneumonia, asthma)
CNS (hyperventilation syndrome, anxiety, hysteria, tumor, trauma, infection)
Hypoxia (high altitude, shunt, V/Q mismatch)
Endocrine system (pregnancy, progesterone excess)
Drugs (salicylates, progesterone, analeptics, catecholamines)
Other (mechanical ventilation)

The Anion Gap[11,16]

The serum anion gap may be useful in defining the cause of metabolic derangement. The anion gap is derived from simultaneously obtained values of serum sodium chloride and total bicarbmate according to the equation:

$$\text{Serum anion gap} = [Na^+] - [Cl^-] - [HCO_3^-] \quad (16)$$

The normal anion gap range is 8 to 16 nmol/l. Elevated levels in the presence of excessive concentrations of unmeasured organic anions such as lactate or acetoacetic acid or inorganic ions such as sulfates and phosphates might be due to any of the reasons listed in Table 11-4. If the anion gas is within normal limits, other causes listed in Table 11-4 must be considered. Increased plasma concentration of unmeasured cations other than sodium, such as hypercalcemia in multiple myeloma may lead to a positively charged protein acting as strong unmeasured cations and a normal gap.

Table 11–4. Differential Diagnosis of Metabolic Acidosis

Normal anion gap
  Hypokalemia
    Gastrointestinal bicarbonate loss (diarrhea, enterocutaneous fistula)
    Ureteral diversion
    Renal tubular acidosis (proximal, distal)
    Carbonic anhydrase inhibitors (acetazolamide, mafenamide)
    Posthypocapnia
    Diarrhea (villous adenoma)
  Normohyperkalemia
    Early renal failure
    Tubulo-interstitial renal disease
    Adrenal insufficiency
    Chloride containing acids (HCl, $NH_4 Cl$, Arginine)
  Other
    TPN
    Burns
    Dilutional (hypertonic saline)
Elevated anion gap
  Ketoacidosis (diabetic, alcoholic, starvation)
  Renal failure
  Lactic acidosis
  Toxins (methanol, ethylene glycol, salicylates, paraldehyde)
  Inborn errors of metabolism

Table 11–5. Differential Diagnosis of Metabolic Alkalosis

Chloride-responsive
  Gastrointestinal causes (vomiting, nasogastric suction, villous adenoma)
  Diuretic therapy
  Post-Hypercapnia
  Cystic fibrosis
  Drugs (carbenicillin, penicillin)
Chloride-resistant
  Adrenal disorder
    Hyperaldosteronism
    Cushing syndrome
      Pituitary
      Adrenal
      Ectopic ACTH
    Exogenous steroids (licorice, carbenoxalone)
  Profound potassium depletion
  Magnesium depletion
Unclassified
  Alkali ingestion
  Refeeding alkalosis

metabolic alkalosis may be chloride resistant (Table 11-5).

SUMMARY

Metabolic and respiratory acid-base disorders may be single or mixed. Various perturbations in PCO_2 bicarbonate, pH and serum electrolytes lead to simple or mixed disorders. Pathophysiology underlining the simple framework has been discussed and the differentials presented to interpret the abnormalities. Only when these disease states are considered can a diagnosis be obtained.

Some factors may decrease the anion gap. Albumen, a negatively charged protein, comprises largest fraction of normal unmeasured anion concentration and if presenting excessive amounts will lead to a normal or low anion gap.

The anion gap may also increase in severe metabolic acidosis as a result of polyanionic albumen releasing loosely bound hydrogen ions. Although, the serum albumen level may not change, the serum anion concentration increases yielding an increased anion gap.

Urine anion gap can be helpful in delineating the cause of metabolic acidosis associated with a normal serum anion gap. It is calculated as follows:

$$\text{Urine anion gap} = [Na^+] + [K^+] - [Cl^-] \quad (17)$$

Normally, the urine anion gap is positive in the face of metabolic acidosis due to ammonium chloride loading or gastrointestinal bicarbonate loss. The gap may decrease and become negative from increased renal ammonium production as the major unmeasured cation in urine. In distal renal tubular acidosis, the urine anion remains positive since renal ammonium impairs excretion. Thus, urine anion gap calculation is useful in differentiating hyperchloremic metabolic acidosis due to distal renal tubular acidosis from that of diarrhea.

As with the serum anion gap, any increase in the concentration of unmeasured anions will tend to increase the gap. This may be seen with increased renal excretion of organic anions such as ketoacid anions or anionic drugs such as penicillin and salicylates in the urine. This

REFERENCES

1. Astrup, P., Severinghaus, J. W.: The History of Blood Gases, Acids, and Bases, 1st Ed., Denmark, Munksgaard International Publishers, 1986.
2. Goldberger, E., and Brensilver, J. M.: A Primer of Water, Electrolyte and Acid-Base Syndromes, 7th Ed., Philadelphia, Lea & Febiger, 1986.
3. Kokko, J. P., Tannen, R. L.: Fluids and Electrolytes, 2nd Ed. Philadelphia, W. B. Saunders, 1990.
4. Sorensen, S. P. L.: Uber die Messung und die Bedeutung der Wasserstoff-zahle-koncentration bei enzymatischen Prozesses. Biochem. Zeitschr., *21*, 131, 1909.
5. Henderson, L. J.: Equilibrium Between Bases and Acids in the Animal Organism. Eregebn. Physiol. *8*, 254, 1909.
6. Hasselbalch, K. A.: Elektrometrische Reactions bestimmung Kohleusuarehaltiger Flussigkeiters. Biochem. Zeitschr. *30*, 317, 1911.
7. Shapiro, B. A., Harrison, R. A., Cane, R. D., et al: Clinical Application of Blood Gases, 4th Ed. Chicago, Year Book Medical Publishers, Inc., 1989.
8. Hill, L. L.: Body composition, normal electrolyte concentrations, and the maintenance of normal volume, tonicity, and acid-base metabolism. Pediatr Clin North Am *37*:241, 1990.
9. Cohen, R. D.: Roles of the liver and kidney in acid-base regulation and its disorders. Br J Anaesthes *67*:154, 1991.

10. Fencl, V., Leith, D. E.: Frontiers in respiratory physiology. Res Physiol *91*:1, 1993.
11. Haussinger: pH haemostasis: The conceptual. Contrib Nephrol *100*:58, 1992.
12. Carroll, H. J., Oh, M. S.: Whole body acid-base balance. Contrib Nephrol *100*:89, 1992.
13. Lehninger, A. L.: Biochemistry: The Molecular Basis of Cell Structure and Function. New York, Worth Publishers, Inc., 1970.
14. Editorial Review: The concept of bicarbonate distribution space: The crucial role of body buffers. Kidney Int *36*:747, 1989.
15. Gennari, F. J.: Medical intelligence concepts serum osmolality uses and limitations. N Engl J Med *310*:102, 1984.
16. Salem, M. M., Mujais, S. K.: Gaps in the anion gap. Arch Intern Med *152*:1625, 1992.
17. Winters, R. W.: Terminology of acid-base disorders. Ann. NY. Acad. Sci. *133,* 211, 1966.
18. Valtin, H., Gennari, F. J.: Acid-Base Disorders. Little, Brown and Company: Boston/Toronto.
19. Adrogue, H. J.: Acid-Base and Electrolyte Disorders. Churchill Livingstone Publication, New York, 1991.
20. Davenport, H. W.: The ABC of Acid-Base Chemistry. The University of Chicago Press, Chicago, Sixth Edition, 1984.

Chapter 12

TRANSFUSION THERAPY

JAMES T. PERKINS AND JEFFREY S. VENDER

Two thirds of all red blood cell transfusions occur in the perioperative period, and a majority of these are given in the operating room. In addition, maintenance of hemostasis in the operative setting may require transfusion of platelets and plasma components. Thus transfusion is an essential part of the armamentarium of the anesthesiologist.

The premise of transfusion medicine education is that each physician who prescribes blood must have a working knowledge of pretransfusion tests and their interpretation, the nature of the blood components to be transfused, the potential adverse consequences of such transfusion, and its demonstrated benefits. It is the general experience that blood components are often transfused unnecessarily, in situations in which the risks outweigh the potential benefits. In addition, unnecessary delays in patient care often result from a lack of understanding of pretransfusion tests; immunohematologic consultation should be available but is not a substitute for a basic knowledge of blood compatibility. Transfusion medicine is an area which should be, and is, receiving increasing attention, largely as a result of increased awareness of transfusion-transmitted disease.

IMMUNOHEMATOLOGY

Immune-mediated Destruction of Red Blood Cells[1]

Table 12–1 shows the spectrum of disorders that entail immune-mediated red blood cell (RBC) destruction. Immune hemolysis is generally considered to occur by one of two mechanisms, termed *intravascular* and *extravascular hemolysis*. Intravascular hemolysis refers to an entirely humoral mechanism that begins with the binding of a potentially complement-fixing antibody to a RBC antigen. Activation of the complete complement sequence yields a membrane attack complex that creates a channel for salt and water through the membrane and results in lysis of the cell. This form of RBC destruction is characteristic of antibodies directed against ABO groups. Because lysis is within the circulation, it is characterized by hemoglobinemia and, once the renal threshold of hemoglobin is exceeded, hemoglobinuria. Activation of the complete complement sequence leads to the release of several anaphylatoxins, which, directly and indirectly, cause vasodilatation and an increase in vascular permeability, activation of the coagulation cascade and release of a variety of cytokines, and other systemic effects. These in turn produce the much-feared clinical consequences of intravascular RBC destruction: shock, disseminated intravascular coagulation (DIC), and renal failure.

Extravascular hemolysis is also initiated by antibody, but in this case the effector mechanisms are cellular. The best-documented of such cellular mechanisms is complete or partial phagocytosis by macrophages, but extracellular lysis by monocytes or lymphocytes may also play a role. The destruction of RBCs by cellular mechanisms is enhanced by the fixation of early complement components to the RBCs, as monocytes have receptors both for the Fc portion of IgG and for C3b. The extravascular destruction of RBCs is characteristic of antibodies directed against antigens of the Rh blood group system-antibodies that, as a rule, do not fix complement. Such hemolysis has relatively mild clinical consequences. If complete phagocytosis were the only cell-mediated mechanism of hemolysis, one would not expect hemoglobinuria to accompany extravascular destruction. In fact, hemoglobinuria may accompany such hemolysis, even that caused by Rh antibodies.[1]

The concepts of intravascular and extravascular destruction are useful ways to think about hemolysis, but in actual practice many different, incompletely characterized factors determine the outcome when a given blood group antibody is combined in vivo with RBCs carrying the corresponding antigen. Because of the multiplicity of such factors, the clinical consequences of hemolysis form a continuum.

Table 12–1. Disorders of Immune-Mediated RBC Destruction

RBC destruction by alloantibody
  Hemolytic transfusion reactions
    Immediate hemolytic reactions
    Delayed hemolytic reactions
  Hemolytic disease of the newborn
RBC destruction by autoantibody
  Warm autoimmune hemolytic anemia
    Primary
    Secondary (i.e., in SLE, rheumatoid arthritis, etc.)
  Cold autoimmune hemolytic anemia
    Paroxysmal cold hemoglobinuria
    Cold agglutinin disease
      Primary
      Secondary (i.e. in CLL, infectious mononucleosis, etc.)
RBC destruction by drug-related antibodies

Blood Groups and Blood Group Antibodies

The term blood group refers to a RBC membrane antigen, and, like all antigens, a blood group is defined by its corresponding antibody. Blood groups are organized into systems by virtue of their allelic relationships, genetic linkage, and biochemical relationships. The antigenic activity of blood groups is carried either by oligosaccharides that form part of complex membrane lipids (as in the ABO, Lewis, P, and Ii systems) or by peptides or oligosaccharides of membrane proteins (as in the Rh, Kell, MNSs, Duffy, and Kidd systems).

Blood groups may stimulate formation of antibodies directed against self antigen or *autoantibodies,* antibodies directed against RBC antigens of individuals of the same species or *alloantibodies,* or antibodies directed against members of different species or *heterologous antibodies.* Blood group alloantibodies may be present in individuals who have never been exposed to foreign RBCs by transfusion or pregnancy. Such *naturally occurring* antibodies are made in response to the presentation of the same or similar antigens in the form of bacteria or other exogenous agents. ABO antibodies are of this type and, because such exposure appears to be universal, anti-A and -B are found in all normal individuals who lack the corresponding antigen. Alloantibodies of other specificities, including most Rh system antibodies, are usually found only in individuals who have been exposed to foreign RBCs; such antibodies are termed *immune.* The term *unexpected antibody* is reserved for all non-ABO antibodies, whether naturally occurring or immune.

Different blood groups are not equally immunogenic. The Rh antigen (more specifically, the Rho or D antigen) is the most immunogenic of such blood groups, with the Kell antigen, which is just one-tenth as immunogenic, being next.

Blood groups are clinically significant if they stimulate formation of antibodies that: (1) destroy RBCs in vivo; (2) are relatively common; or (3) cause hemolytic disease of the newborn (HDN). Although over 600 blood group antibody specificities have been defined, only 5% of these specificities are significant in ordinary clinical practice. A number of factors, such as the class (IgG vs. IgM) or subclass (IgG1, IgG2, IgG3, IgG4) of blood group antibodies, their thermal optima and complement-fixing abilities, the quantity and equilibrium constant of the antibodies, and the characteristics of the antigen (e.g., its density or mobility), have been demonstrated to determine the clinical significance of blood group antibodies. However, even with a knowledge of these factors, clinical significance is difficult to predict based on *in vitro* testing in a given case. Demonstration of the specificity of an antiserum and the comparison of that specificity with past clinical outcomes remains the most important predictor of significance for a specific individual.

In fact, the transfusion of ABO-compatible RBCs provides adequate safety in the vast majority of first transfusions, and additionally ensuring Rh specificity for Rh-negative individuals ensures the safety of most subsequent transfusions.

The ABO Blood Group System

ABO antigenicity is determined by terminal sugars of oligosaccharides, which are part of the complex lipids of the RBC membrane as well as of plasma and membrane proteins. As such, they are present in relatively large numbers. The presence of these antigens is determined by structural genes coding for formation of glycoseal transferases that add sugar moieties to a precursor substance. For this reason, the A and B genes are codominant alleles, the oligosaccharide product being detectable whenever the corresponding transferase is present. Group O individuals do not make an active transferase. A and B antigens are present on all cells and therefore are significant not only in transfusion, but also in the transplantation of solid organs. Although ABO antigens are present on platelets, when ABO-incompatible platelets are transfused, only a minor fraction is usually destroyed. (Exceptions to this rule occur among group O patients who have been repeatedly stimulated by transfusion of group A or B platelets).

ABO alloantibodies appear within the first 6 to 8 months of life in all individuals with normal immune systems who lack the corresponding antigen. Because of this fact, individuals can be ABO typed by tests of their RBCs for antigen (so-called *forward typing*) or their serum for antibody (*reverse typing*). Anti-A or -B antisera invariably contain IgM antibodies, but IgG with ABO specificity also occurs, particularly in group O individuals, and can cross the placenta to cause relatively mild HDN (High Dilution normovolemic). Group O individuals also make an antibody that reacts with both group A and group B RBCs, termed anti-A, B. These relationships are summarized (Table 12-2).

ABO antibodies typically cause intravascular hemolysis with severe clinical consequences. For this reason, and because of their common presence as expected antibodies, the ABO group is highly significant by the criteria cited above.

Table 12–2. ABO Blood Group System

Phenotype	Antigens	Antibodies	Gene product	Genotypes
O	Precursor H	Anti-A, -B, -AB	Inactive Transferase	*OO*
A	A(H)	Anti-B	A-transferase	*AO, AA*
B	B(H)	Anti-A	B-transferase	*BO, BB*
AB	A&B (H)	None	A- and B-transferase	*AB*

Rh Blood Group System

The terms Rh positive and Rh negative refer to the presence or absence of an antigen, "Rho" or "D" (the designation "Rh" is here used interchangeably with "D"). Eighty-five percent of individuals are Rh positive. No antibody has ever been found to define a blood group that is antithetical to D. The D antigen is highly immunogenic: 80% of Rh-negative recipients of a single unit of Rh-positive RBCs will form anti-D. Two other pairs of alleles—designated C and c, and E and e—are closely linked genetically to D. The clinical significance of these alleles is proportionate to their lesser immunogenicity.

Occasional Rh-positive individuals express a weakened form of the antigen, termed *weak D*. Such individuals may be misclassified as Rh negative if less sensitive tests are used. This is of significance for blood donors, as the RBCs of a weak D phenotype donor, misclassified as Rh negative, could immunize a truly Rh negative recipient. Conversely, such misclassification of a weak D phenotype recipient is of no significance. Because Rh typing tests of different sensitivity may be used in different situations apparent discrepancies may arise over time, to the consternation of some patients.

Rh system antibodies are virtually always formed in response to foreign RBC's and cause RBC destruction in vivo. As mentioned above, because such destruction does not involve complement, its clinical manifestations are relatively mild. However, anti-Rh causes the most severe form of HDN, and its clinical significance derives, in large part, from this fact as well as from the high immunogenicity of the D antigen.

Discussion of other blood group systems is beyond the scope of this chapter. The reader is referred to standard transfusion medicine texts.[2]

PRETRANSFUSION TESTING

Pretransfusion testing asks two questions: (1) Does this recipient have an antibody against this donor's RBCs? and (2) Could this recipient make an antibody against this donor's RBCs? The former question is embodied in the antibody screening test, the major crossmatch, and ABO typing of donor and recipient. The latter question underlies the logic of Rh typing the recipient and donor. Both questions focus on the incompatibility of recipient antibody with donor RBCs, so-called *major-side incompatibility.* The *minor-side* reactions of donor antibodies

against recipient antigens are of lesser importance and are largely ignored except for selection of whole blood or plasma blood types for transfusion (Table 12–5).

Routine pretransfusion tests are based on the ability of antibody in a given serum to agglutinate RBCs having the corresponding antigen. In the case of ABO typing, agglutination will occur after the simple admixture of serum containing anti-A or -B with dilute suspensions of RBCs having the corresponding antigens, and such tests can be performed very rapidly.

Use of Coombs' Serum

Some blood group antibodies are able to bind to or sensitize RBCs, but not to agglutinate them. In such cases, the addition of Coombs' serum or *anti-human globulin* (AHG), a heterologous antiserum directed against human immunoglobulin and/or complement, may cross-link the RBC-bound blood group antibody and achieve agglutination, thus demonstrating the presence of blood group antibody in the test serum. In immunohematology, the latter sequence is termed an indirect antiglobulin test (IAT). One of a variety of *enhancing agents* may also be used to speed the reaction or enhance its sensitivity.

AHG is also used to detect the *in vivo* sensitization of RBCs by antibody or complement in the disorders listed in Table 12–1. In such cases, patient RBCs are simply washed to remove unbound antibody, mixed with AHG, and examined for agglutination; this is a so-called direct Coombs' or direct antiglobulin test (DAT).

Hemagglutination tests can be used for several purposes, depending on the RBCs and antisera selected in the first step, as shown in Table 12–3. In each case, the IAT methodology has the greatest sensitivity, although important information, particularly about ABO incompatibility in a crossmatch, can be gained without the addition of AHG. In the antibody screening test, two or three RBC samples (provided as commercial reagents) are selected which express a set of blood group antigens that are clinically significant according to the criteria discussed above; these are reacted with patient or donor serum in an IAT. If the test indicates the presence of a blood group antibody, the unknown serum is reacted with additional reagent RBCs in the form of an *antibody identification panel,* and the specificity of the serum is determined by the pattern of reactivity. If a clinically significant antibody is detected and identified, compatible units of RBCs can be selected using reagent antisera of known specificity, a

Table 12–3. Applications of the Indirect Antiglobulin Test

Test Name	Serum	Cells
Antibody screen	Unknown antibodies (Recipient or donor)	Known antigen phenotypes (Reagent)
Antigen typing	Known antibody (Reagent)	Unknown antigen phenotype (Patient or donor)
Crossmatch (major)	Recipient	Donor
Antibody Identification	Antibody of unknown specificity	Known antigen phenotypes (Reagent panel)
Crossmatch (minor)	Donor	Recipient

so-called *antigen typing* procedure. The major-side crossmatch provides similar information in a single test, in which recipient antiserum is reacted with donor RBCs. The crossmatch has the limitation however that incompatibility due to clinically insignificant antibodies cannot be distinguished from incompatibilities that may indeed cause hemolysis. In addition, the antibody screen is often more sensitive since the antibody screening cells can be selected for strong expression of relevant antigens. Immunohematologic testing may be somewhat slow, with incubation steps as long as one half hour depending on the institution's IAT protocol, and complete antibody identification can take many hours depending on the complexity of the serologic abnormality.

Testing Protocol

The hemagglutination tests discussed above are combined into a pretransfusion testing protocol as shown in Table 12-4. ABO forward and reverse typing is typically performed multiple times on both donor and recipient blood samples. Note that the D^u test is only required for the donor, but many institutions will perform it on the recipient as well. Although the major crossmatch is often

Table 12–4. Standard Pretransfusion Testing Protocol

Donor	Recipient
ABO type	ABO type
Forward	Forward
Reverse	Reverse
Rh type	Rh type
including D^u	
Antibody screen	Antibody screen
Crossmatch (major side)—	

referred to as the *compatibility test,* it should be emphasized that no one test ensures compatibility: compatibility is determined by a battery of tests, of which correct ABO typing is the most important. In fact, it has been shown that if no serologic problems are detected in blood typing and the antibody screen, the antiglobulin phase of the major crossmatch can be omitted. This is the basis for the *type-and-screen* protocol used at many hospitals; if the recipient's antibody screen is negative, the crossmatch is abbreviated to a quick test that checks for ABO typing errors before issuing RBCs. This form of abbreviated pretransfusion testing offers many logistic advantages, since blood can be made rapidly available without reserving it for a specific patient in advance. A complete AHG-crossmatch will occasionally detect incompatibility in sera with a negative antibody screen, but mild, clinically evident hemolysis occurs very rarely—one in 250,000 crossmatches in the study of Shulman.[3] Table 12-5 specifies the selection of compatible ABO types for RBCs and plasma when *group specific* components are not available.

Type-and-Screen Application

The type-and-screen, followed by an abbreviated crossmatch if blood is needed, is particularly applicable to surgeries which rarely require blood transfusion. A recent, negative type-and-screen assures relatively safe transfusion in an emergency; "recent" is taken to refer to the FDA regulation that the sample must be less than 2 days old if the patient has been pregnant or transfused in the past 3 months. A positive type-and-screen prompts the laboratory immediately to begin antibody identification should transfusion be needed, and most hospital transfusion services automatically begin the search for compatible units if abnormalities that might otherwise delay transfusion are detected. If transfusion is not

Table 12–5. Properties of Blood Components

| Component | Contents | Storage | Blood Group Selection | |
			Recipient	Donor
RBCs	170–220 ml RBCs* 50–100 ml plasma (15 ml anticoagulant)	35 days 1–6°C	O A B AB	O A or O B or O AB or A, B, or O
FFP	200–250 ml plasma 1 U/ml of all factors (40 ml anticoagulant)	1 year <18°C	O A B AB	O or A, B, or AB A or AB B or AB AB
Platelet Concentrate	5.5–8.0×10^{10} platelets 50–60 ml plasma (10 ml anticoagulant)	5 days Room temp.	All	Type specific preferred; otherwise as available
Platelets, Apheresis	>3.0×10^{11} platelets 210–300 ml plasma (25 ml anticoagulant)	5 days Room temp.	All	Type specific preferred; otherwise as available
Cryoprecipitate	80–120U FVIII:c 40–70% original FVIII:vwf 200–300 mg fibrinogen 10–15 ml plasma	1 year <18°C	All	Type specific preferred; otherwise as available

*Volume ranges are approximate and do not represent the extremes.

needed, the patient who received only a type-and-screen is saved the cost of unnecessary crossmatches, and no units are taken out of the stock blood inventory where they might benefit other patients.

Compatibility testing for neonatal patients can be abbreviated because the formation of new RBC alloantibodies is rare in the first 4 months of life and because the relevant RBC alloantibodies are maternally derived, in a process that ceases at parturition. Therefore, the mother's serum is preferable for compatibility testing, and if her antibody screen is negative and all components transfused during the neonatal period are ABO compatible, no crossmatches or other compatibility tests need be done. Any RBCs transfused must be ABO compatible with the mother's and infant's sera, and transfused plasma must be compatible with the infant's ABO group. Cellular blood components transfused to neonates should be Rh specific.

Provision of Compatible RBCs in Emergencies

Immunohematologic testing is relatively time consuming, so it may have to be severely abbreviated in trauma cases or other hemorrhagic emergencies. Since ABO compatible components are entirely compatible in the vast majority of cases, particularly if the patient has never been transfused before, group O RBCs, which are ABO compatible with all recipients, are often used for emergency transfusion prior to completion of *any* compatibility tests. In this situation, Rh-negative RBCs should be used for girls and women of childbearing age because of the concern for immunizing such individuals and possibly causing a case of HDN. For men or women beyond their childbearing years, only the current presence of anti-D is a concern, and since this antibody is no more common than certain other blood group alloantibodies, Rh-positive RBCs can be used with similar safety.

Universal Donors

The use of so called *universal donor* RBCs, as discussed above, has several drawbacks. Group O RBCs are typically in short supply because of demographic differences between the donor and recipient populations in the United States, and universal donor practices accentuate this problem. ABO typing can be performed very quickly, and in most emergencies there is time for ABO typing of the recipient and provision of ABO specific components. Secondly, transfusion of large quantities of group O RBCs prior to obtaining a recipient blood sample may obscure subsequent immunohematologic testing. Therefore, even if universal donor RBCs are to be used, a blood sample should be obtained *prior* to transfusion; this is possible in all but the most dire cases of exsanguinating hemorrhage. Finally, unexpected blood group antibodies *can* cause fatal transfusion reactions. This can occur in multiply transfused patients such as those with sickle cell disease, presenting to an emergency room with severe anemia. Individuals caring for such patients must understand that correction of volume deficits is much more important than correction of deficits in oxygen carrying capacity, and that patients without severe coronary artery disease can tolerate very low hematocrits as long as perfusion is maintained, (vida infra).

Emergency situations should not be construed as justification for exceptions to strict identification of recipient blood samples. On the contrary, increased attention to patient identification is warranted, and one indication for use of universal donor RBCs is in multiple trauma in which recipient mixups are particularly common.

Many institutions require that physicians ordering transfusion prior to completion of standard compatibility tests document the need by signing some type of *emergency release form*. This documentation should only need to be completed after the emergency is dealt with, typically within 24 hours, and such forms should not be construed as a release of responsibility by the blood bank. The blood bank must insist on strict identification of samples, documentation of unit disposition, and documentation of the emergency status of the transfusion, but it also has the responsibility to avoid unnecessarily restrictive practices.

Safe Transfusion of "Incompatible" Blood

It is important for all physicians, particularly those who take care of surgical emergencies, to understand that, at times, transfusion must be performed in spite of certain blood group incompatibilities. For example, in platelet transfusion, ABO incompatibility of donor plasma (platelet units contain 50 to 60 ml of plasma) and recipient RBCs is frequently ignored. Hemolysis due to such *minor-side* incompatibility is very rare, and the risk is often overridden by the need to transfuse whatever platelets are available. Similarly, it may be necessary to transfuse Rh-positive platelets to an Rh negative individual. The small amount of RBCs contaminating the platelets carries a low risk of immunizing the recipient, and such immunization can be prevented by subsequent administration of RhIG if the recipient is a girl or woman of childbearing age at risk for having a future pregnancy complicated by HDN.

Another circumstance in which in vitro incompatibility between donor and recipient is ignored is that of patients with RBC autoantibodies. Warm-reacting *auto*antibodies may cause positive crossmatches with all donor RBCs. In such a circumstance, it is important to rule out concomitant blood group *allo*antibodies, the presence of which may be masked by autoantibody and which can cause significant transfusion reactions. However, once this is done, donor RBCs that react with the recipient's autoantibody are expected to survive no differently than the recipient's own RBCs. Similarly, as discussed above many blood group antibodies do not mediate hemolysis and can be ignored as long as significant alloantibodies can be ruled out. Unfortunately, this may be a time-consuming process and require the efforts of an experienced laboratory with access to rare RBC samples and sera. As long as ABO-compatible RBCs are available, no patient should be allowed to exsanguinate for lack of completely compatible blood components. Needless to say, in such a situation, consultation with an experienced immunohematologist should be sought.

The potential for hemolysis due to cold autoantibodies has been a concern in patients undergoing cold cardioplegia or other hypothermic procedures. We are unaware of any such case in which otherwise clinically insignificant cold autoantibodies have caused hemolysis. In general, cold autoantibodies are only significant if they react at 30°C or above.

BLOOD COMPONENTS AND PLASMA DERIVATIVES

The adoption in the early 1960s of plastic bags for blood collection and subsequent transfusion made it possible to easily separate whole blood into its components by differential centrifugation in a closed system. This technologically simple procedure accomplishes two powerful and related ends: first, it allows the physician to treat the individual patient's deficiency of a blood element, such as platelets, RBCs, or coagulation factors, with that specific element, rather than "shotgunning" all deficiencies with whole blood; second, it allows the storage of the separated components to be optimized, rather than sacrificing platelets and factor VIII for the optimization of RBC survival, as is the case when blood is stored whole.

Component Preparation

Blood component preparation begins with a donor who, in this country, is typically a volunteer. Voluntarism is the first step in providing safe transfusion since the volunteer donor has no financial incentive to donate in spite of personal knowledge of potentially transmissible disease. The donor is questioned regarding conditions that might compromise his or her own safety or that of the recipient, with a major focus on risk factors for HIV and hepatitis virus infection. Blood, generally 450 ml (±10%), is then drawn into a **primary bag** containing citrate for anticoagulation, dextrose as a glycolytic energy source, and phosphate and adenine to supplement adenosine triphosphate (ATP) generation. If components are to be made, the unit of whole blood is centrifuged at a relatively low speed to separate the RBCs from platelet-rich plasma, and the latter is expressed into an integrally connected **secondary** bag. The connecting tubing is heat-sealed and cut, yielding a unit of RBCs. The platelet-rich plasma is centrifuged at a higher rate that results in a platelet pellet and plasma supernatant. Most of the plasma is expressed into another secondary bag and immediately frozen, yielding fresh-frozen plasma (FFP); 50 to 60 ml of the plasma is used to resuspend the platelet pellet. The resulting unit of RBCs is stored at 4°C in order to slow glycolytic metabolism. FFP is stored at 18°C or lower to prevent activation of coagulation factors. Platelet concentrate is stored at room temperature in plastics which allow transpiration of oxygen and carbon dioxide, and with continuous agitation to prevent aggregation. The properties of the blood components resulting from these manipulations are summarized in Table 12–6.

Four variations on the above sequence are frequently used. In the first, an additive solution is combined with the separated RBCs, which extends their shelf life from 35 to 42 days. Second, the FFP may be thawed slowly, a procedure that precipitates coagulation factors VIII and

Table 12–6. Available Plasma Derivatives

Oncotic agents
  Albumin
  Plasma protein fraction
Coagulation factor concentrates
  Factor VIII concentrate
  Factor IX concentrate
  Anti-inhibitor concentrate
Immune globulins
  Rh immune globulin
  Intravenous immune globulin
  Gamma globulin (intramuscular)

XIII and fibrinogen; this cryoprecipitate is then pelleted, resuspended in a reduced volume of plasma, and refrozen. Third, the RBCs may be frozen after addition of glycerol as a cryoprotectant. Finally, platelets may be prepared by *apheresis* using a blood cell separator which performs the required centrifugation steps in on-line fashion, returning the donor's plasma and RBCs throughout the procedure. This yields a unit of platelets from a single donor that is equivalent in platelet content to 6 to 8 units of Platelet Concentrate.

Testing for Transmissible Diseases

Blood samples drawn at the time of donation are tested for markers for transfusion transmissible diseases including a serologic test for syphilis, hepatitis B surface antigen (HBsAg), alanine aminotransferase (ALT, synonym SGPT), and antibodies against HIV, hepatitis B core antigen (HBcAb), hepatitis C virus (anti-HCV), and human T-lymphotropic virus I (a human retrovirus causing T-cell leukemia and myelopathy). Disease and immunohematologic test results are carefully matched to the corresponding blood components, a procedure termed *component processing*, and then labelled as acceptable for transfusion.

Donors Selection

Blood donor selection, component preparation, disease testing, processing, and labelling procedures are all heavily regulated by the FDA, state laws, and the voluntary accreditation programs of the American Association of Blood Banks (AABB). The FDA regards blood component preparation as a manufacturing process subject to the same *good manufacturing practices* as pharmaceuticals. For these reasons there is little room for individual variation or discretion in the process. These processes and the strict quality controls they are subject to are also time consuming, a source of frustration to patients or families requesting *directed donations*. Because the FDA considers the item to be tested the donated unit, rather than the blood donor him or herself, programs for "fresh, warm whole blood" are essentially precluded.

Other manipulations are performed on blood components at the time of issue. RBCs can be washed in saline to remove plasma, anticoagulant, and some of the leukocytes. More efficient leukocyte removal can be achieved by filtration, either in the blood bank or at the bedside, and this procedure is more readily applicable to units of platelets than is washing. Multiple units of platelets or cryoprecipitate are frequently pooled into one bag for transfusion. FFP and cryoprecipitate must, of course, be thawed before issue. Pooling confers a short expiration time on the blood component, so terminal preparation steps should only be ordered immediately before the intended transfusion. Wastage often results when such blood components are ordered before the clinician has made a definite determination to transfuse.

Fractionation of Plasma

The component preparation sequences discussed are used by blood centers and hospital-based donor services. Further fractionation of plasma is performed on an industrial scale to yield the colloid agents albumin or plasma protein fraction (PPF), factor VIII (antihemophilic factor) concentrate, factor IX concentrate, anti-inhibitor complex (a concentrate containing variable levels of activated and precursor factors II, VII, IX, and X), antithrombin III concentrate, and the various preparations of immune globulins such as RhIG or intravenous immune globulin (IVIG). In the past, the coagulation factor concentrates listed above carried high risks of transmission of the hepatitis and AIDS viruses, but new methods of isolation or heat treatment have reduced or eliminated these risks.

For a more complete discussion of the specifics of each of these blood components and plasma derivatives, the reader is referred to the convenient handbook on blood transfusion therapy[4] published by the AABB, or to the *Circular of Information* for blood components available in every transfusion service.

AUTOLOGOUS TRANSFUSION

Blood for *autologous transfusion* is obtained by three different procedures: the deposit of blood before anticipated losses, such as those at surgery or delivery; hemodilution immediately before surgery; and intraoperative or postoperative salvage of shed blood, with or without washing of the RBCs.

Advance Deposit of Blood

Advance deposit is the source of autologous blood most often utilized, and its safety for patient/donors with a variety of medical problems has been demonstrated.[5] Absolute contraindications to this procedure include bacteremia and unstable angina. Aortic stenosis is often cited as a contraindication, but patients being operated for moderate disease may do well. Severe cerebral vascular disease is a major concern. In one study,[5] careful hemodynamic monitoring during phlebotomy of patients with cardiac disease demonstrated systolic hypotension (>20 mg Hg drop) in 20% of donors but most responded to fluids.

To be eligible for autologous blood collection patients must be able to replace the removed RBCs, so those with refractory anemias (e.g., a patient with rheumatoid arthritis having joint replacement surgery) may not be candidates. A hematocrit of 33 is used as a cutoff for eligibility

according to AABB standards, which generally ensures that phlebotomy will not result in preoperative hematocrits below 30. However, patients with a demonstrated ability to respond to phlebotomy and adequate time before surgery (2 weeks or more), may be drawn at slightly lower hematocrits at the discretion of the blood bank physician. AABB standards also require that there be 72 hours between donations and between the last donation and surgery, in order that volume losses can be replaced by plasma refill.

One large study[6] conducted at multiple academic institutions estimated that 10% of all RBC-containing units could come from autologous sources, but most hospitals do not achieve this goal.[7] This discrepancy may be due in part to lack of knowledge regarding autologous donation and local resources for obtaining such donations.[8] Advance deposit requires planning and attention to logistic details, and may delay surgery. In order to draw autologous donors, blood centers used to healthy volunteer donors must learn to be comfortable dealing with patients having significant medical conditions. Finally, physicians aware of exclusion criteria for volunteer donors may inappropriately apply these to the autologous donor/patient, for whom the benefits of donation are much higher than the usual juice and cookies provided to volunteer donors, justifying acceptance of a higher level of risk. The question "Which is safer, to give blood or to receive it?" helps to clarify many decisions regarding autologous donor eligibility.

The 35-day limitation for liquid storage of whole blood restricts the number of units that can be drawn before surgery. Women may be limited to donation of 2 or 3 units within this period, while men can often donate 4 units. Use of exogenous erythropoietin can increase the number of RBCs that can be drawn within this period,[9] but it is prohibitively expensive at this time. Units can be drawn over a longer period and frozen, but this is also a very expensive practice and the use of such units is difficult logistically, since many hospitals do not have the facilities for thawing and deglycerolization, thawing takes 1½ hours at best, and once thawed the units must be used within 24 hours. Autologous donations are often scheduled at weekly intervals, but it may help to draw 2 or 3 units at 3 day intervals in order to maximize endogenous erythropoietin release, and then allow the patient a longer time prior to surgery to restore his or her hematocrit.[10]

Because arrangements for autologous blood must be made well in advance of surgery, the anesthetist may be completely unaware that such units are available. The transfusion service is responsible for tracking the unit status, and when the anaesthetist requests more units than are available for a patient who has made autologous donation, homologous units should not be issued to the operating room until all of the autologous units are exhausted.

As public concern for transfusion safety has increased, so has the demand for autologous donation. Many patients request autologous donation before surgical procedures that are unlikely to require transfusion, and different transfusion services experience a 20 to 60% (mode 40 to 50%) discard rate for autologous donations.[7] Some institutions attempt to use such units for other patients, a procedure termed *crossover* of autologous units. In order for an autologous unit to be eligible for crossover, the donor/patient must meet all of the same criteria as homologous donors, and this is the case for only a small proportion. Autologous units need not be tested for disease markers as long as they are drawn and transfused within the same institution, which helps to keep the cost down and partially ameliorates the inefficiency posed by high discard rates. Nonetheless, the cost-effectiveness of autologous donation has been challenged based on recent improvements in the safety of homologous transfusion.[11] Collection of autologous units in situations with a low risk for transfusion may also be questioned on purely medical grounds; that is, if the rate of transfusion of patients scheduled for cesarian section (excluding placenta previa) is only 1 to 2%, is it appropriate to cause 98 to 99 women to lose 200 mg of iron with each donation, so that 1 or 2 women can have a safer transfusion? The obvious response is to attempt to restrict donation to patients having certain procedures, but arbitrary thresholds may have to be selected and individual patients will have difficulty accepting such limitations.

A second controversy regards the appropriate indications for transfusion of autologous units. Many would hold that risk/benefit analysis dictates a lower threshold for transfusion when autologous units are available. Others feel that, since the risks of misidentification of units and of bacterial contamination remain for autologous blood, criteria for appropriateness of autologous transfusion should be just as restrictive as those for homologous transfusion. Autologous units should not be returned to the patient simply because "it's the patient's blood."

Preoperative Hemodilution (ANH)

Preoperative *acute normovolemic hemodilution* (ANH) refers to the withdrawal of whole blood from the patient at the start of surgery with volume replacement. The units withdrawn are then reserved for transfusion later in the procedure. Net patient RBC conservation is achieved because a given volume of surgical blood loss contains a smaller volume RBCs when the patient has been previously hemodiluted. In contrast to advance deposit of autologous blood, this practice is almost entirely the purview of the anesthesiologist. A number of studies of ANH[12] suggest that it can reduce homologous transfusion, but these have typically used historical controls, and are thus subject to the concern that changes in the "transfusion trigger" may actually be responsible for the observed benefit. A recent calculation[13] suggests that the actual savings of patient RBCs is small, typically less than one unit, but this number will increase if more extreme hemodilution is performed. Hemodilution may actually improve regional perfusion because of its effect on whole blood viscosity, a fact of some interest to those performing neurosurgical anesthesia.[12]

Acute normovolemic hemodilution seems technically simple and correspondingly inexpensive, requiring only blood bags and replacement solutions. However, the time and labor required may be significant, particularly if the procedure is carried out in the operating room proper, so the cost may not be negligible. If units are to be available for transfusion in the postoperative period, the transfusion service must be involved in setting up the systems for closed system phlebotomy, unit identification, and control. ANH may be accepted by Jehovah's Witnesses, particularly if a continuous extracorporeal blood circuit can be maintained.

Intraoperative and Postoperative Blood Salvage

Blood salvage is the conceptually simple process of collecting shed blood and reinfusing it. This is typically done intraoperatively from open body cavities or large wounds using a suction wand connected via a reservoir to a vacuum system, or postoperatively from chest tubes or other drains left in body cavities such as joint spaces. Early experience with reinfusion of blood that was collected intraoperatively and simply filtered revealed an unacceptable rate of complications including frequent coagulopathies.[14] This led to the development of equipment to wash the collected RBCs, and there are now many devices on the market that can rapidly collect and wash shed RBCs using disposable collection sets. In cardiac surgery the same device that is used to collect and wash RBCs shed into the pericardial cavity can be used at the end of the case to concentrate RBCs from the blood that remains within the bypass pump. Procedures and devices have also been developed for the preparation of platelet-rich plasma before cardiac surgery for use after the patient is taken off bypass,[15] and this can be performed with the same device and disposable collection set. Manufacturers of devices for postoperative collection advocate reinfusion of the collected blood without washing, but many remain concerned about this practice.

Intraoperative blood salvage (IBS) is an appropriate form of transfusion only if the collected blood is free of, or can be washed free of, elements that might harm the patient when infused. These are typically said to include malignant cells, bacteria, exogenous and endogenous thrombin, squamous cells from amniotic fluid, betadine, avitene, and RBC-bound toxic agents. For these reasons, many institutions restrict use of IBS to clean surgical cases such as cardiac and vascular surgery, major joint replacement, spinal fusion, or bleeding from a ruptured liver, spleen or ectopic pregnancy. However, these restrictions are controversial.[16]

Some Jehovah's Witnesses patients will accept intraoperative RBC salvage if the salvaged blood can be returned through a continuous circuit, making operative procedures that otherwise could not be performed available to such individuals.

IBS with washing is relatively expensive since blood cell separator is required, someone must be paid to run it, and a disposable tubing and bowl set is used for each case. The breakeven point compared to banked blood is generally between 2 and 3 units. For cardiac surgery the perfusionist can run the blood salvage device. Otherwise, salvage should generally be restricted to cases in which the loss of at least 1000 ml of blood is anticipated, with the intent of salvaging 2 or more units of RBCs; patients can generally tolerate lesser degrees of blood loss without homologous RBC replacement. In a large operating suite where one or more staff trained in the procedure are always available, it may be reasonable to collect blood into a cardiotomy reservoir primed with anticoagulant, and only process the blood if a sufficient amount is collected.

ADVERSE CONSEQUENCES OF TRANSFUSION

Incidence and Recognition

Adverse reactions to transfusion are common, and they may have long-term negative consequences for the recipient. The transfusing physician must be able to recognize such transfusion reactions so that they are treated promptly, if necessary. Prompt reporting to the transfusion service is a key step in this process, enabling appropriate diagnostic testing, prevention of future reactions, and activation of quality assurance measures. In addition, the physician must understand the magnitude of transfusion risks so that they may be appropriately balanced against the potential benefits of transfusion. A high index of suspicion is required in order that transfusion reactions be identified as such. Although certain symptoms such as fever are well recognized as associated with transfusion reactions, any adverse reaction occurring at the time of transfusion is considered to be due to transfusion until proven otherwise, and the safest course is to stop the transfusion until the cause is identified. In cases of uncertainty, consultation should be sought.

Classification

Adverse reactions to transfusion can be classified in different ways. Although they are often listed as immediate versus delayed reactions, a pathogenetic classification is preferable that begins by distinguishing immune-mediated and nonimmune reactions. Because of their importance, infectious complications are treated separately.

Immune-mediated Reactions

All of the basic elements of blood can act as immunogens, and each element has a corresponding transfusion reaction, as shown in Table 12-7. With the exception of graft-versus-host disease (GVHD), the well-characterized reactions are all antibody mediated. Transfusion may also cause immune suppression but since this is still controversial, it is discussed separately.

Immunization itself is listed as a transfusion reaction, because it frequently results from transfusion and may eventually lead to such adverse consequences as high dilution normovolemia (HDN) transfusion reactions, or platelet refractoriness. For example, because immunization to platelets may cause later platelet refractoriness, prophylactic platelet transfusion is generally not indicated in patients with congenital thrombocytopathy or long-term thrombocytopenic states such as aplastic anemia; in such patients platelets are reserved for treatment of significant hemorrhage.

Hemolytic Transfusion Reactions

Hemolytic reactions may occur immediately upon the transfusion of donor RBCs, or they may be delayed. He-

Table 12–7. Immune-Mediated Transfusion Reactions

Type of Reaction	Site of Antigen
Immunization	
Hemolytic	Donor RBCs
Immediate	
Delayed	
Febrile	Donor WBCs
Allergic	Donor plasma proteins
Anaphylactic	
Anaphylactoid	
Urticarial	
Transfusion-related	Recipient WBCs
acute lung injury	
Post transfusion purpura	Donor platelets
Graft-versus-host disease	All recipient tissues

molysis in immediate hemolytic transfusion reactions (IHTRs) may be intravascular or extravascular, or it may occur by a combination of these mechanisms. The clinical consequences of the reaction are largely determined by the degree and rapidity of complement fixation and its resulting generation of anaphylotoxins. The most common manifestation of an IHTR is fever, which is often preceded by a rigor. The rapid lysis of RBCs is manifested by hemoglobinemia and hemoglobinuria and, within 5 to 7 hours, by icterus. The other manifestations classically associated with IHTR are usually limited to reactions due to ABO antibodies. Such reactions may be heralded by phlebitis, which is followed by flank pain and a general sense of discomfort. There may also be pain in the chest or abdomen, as well as nausea and vomiting. The release of anaphylatoxins is the presumed cause of urticaria, flushing, bronchospasm, and hypotension. DIC may occur, both because the membranes (stroma) of lysed RBCs are thromboplastic and because immune events such as complement fixation may activate the coagulation cascade. Renal failure occurs because of DIC, hypotension, other effects of the immune cascade, and direct effects of hemoglobin, the latter possibly related to nitric oxide binding, but it typically resolves if the patient can be supported by fluid and electrolyte management or dialysis. Because the anesthetized patient cannot complain of the early, subjective symptoms of an IHTR, the initial manifestation during operations may be DIC-related oozing or other severe complications.

Incidence

Several studies suggested an IHTR rate of 1 per 10,000 to 20,000 RBC transfusions and a mortality of approximately 10%,[17] in general agreement with the estimate by an NIH consensus statement[18] of 1 fatal IHTR per 100,000 RBC transfusions. Most fatal IHTRs are due to ABO mismatches between donor and recipient, and the vast majority of these are due to clerical error, in either specimen labeling, transcription of results, or identification of the recipient.[19] For this reason, hospital blood banks tend to be very exacting about specimen labeling, and emergency situations should not be considered an exception to required identification practices.

Delayed Hemolytic Transfusion Reactions (DHTRs)

Delayed hemolytic transfusion reactions occur in previously immunized recipients in whom the strength of the resulting blood group antibody has declined to a point at which it cannot be detected by the antibody screening test or crossmatches. Memory lymphocytes are present, however, and are able to generate an anamnestic antibody response with subsequent lysis of the donor RBCs carrying the corresponding antigen. RBC destruction is extravascular with mild clinical consequences. DHTRs are typically detected when a patient is found to have a declining hematocrit (Hct) about a week after transfusion and RBCs are ordered; pretransfusion testing then reveals a new blood group antibody. Review of the patient's record often will show that the patient had a fever spike in the time since transfusion, and the patient occasionally develops icterus, but the DHTR is seldom suspected on clinical grounds alone. Renal failure is uncommon in the absence of other causes. DHTRs are not uncommon, occurring after 1 in 1600 RBC transfusions, according to various studies,[17] and they cannot be prevented.

Reactions Due to Antibodies Directed Against Leukocytes (Febrile Reactions)

Febrile nonhemolytic transfusion reactions (FNHTRs) usually begin with a rigor soon after a transfusion of RBCs or platelets is started, followed by fever that develops over an hour or more. There may be mild dyspnea as well. Febrile reactions are classically thought to be due to recipient antibody directed against donor leukocyte antigens, including HLA antigens. These *leukoagglutinins* lyse donor leukocytes in units of RBCs or platelets, releasing endogenous pyrogen and causing fever. Because leukocyte antigens are highly immunogenic, such reactions are common in the parous or previously transfused patient, occurring in one case per 100 to 200 transfusions of cellular blood components.

If this pathogenic sequence were the sole cause of FNHTRs, use of high efficiency leukocyte depletion filters would be expected to prevent all such reactions, but this is not the case for many febrile reactions to platelet transfusion.[20] More recent data suggest that in addition to the above sequence, febrile reactions may be caused by release of lymphokines during storage.[21] Leukocyte filtration at the time of preparation might prevent reactions due to the postulated lymphokine mechanism.

Although febrile reactions can be very uncomfortable, their major importance is in their differential diagnosis: that is, fever at the time of transfusion may represent a hemolytic reaction or bacterial contamination of the unit, both of which can be devastating. For this reason, transfusion should always be stopped when fever occurs, and the reaction should be reported and investigated. The fever typically resolves soon after the transfusion is stopped. Preventative measures, particularly leukocyte filtration, are typically initiated after the patient has had 2 clear-cut reactions, a circumstance suggesting that the patient indeed is having leukoagglutinin-mediated reactions; in selecting patients to receive filtered units, it is useful to attempt to distinguish those patients who are having fever due to their underlying disease, simply coinciding

with transfusion. Acetaminophen prophylaxis is often tried; demerol is quite effective both in preventing FNHTRs and in treating them.

Transfusion-related Acute Lung Injury (TRALI)

This is thought to represent the minor-side equivalent of the febrile/leukoagglutinin reaction; that is, donors have been found to have potent antibodies against leukocytes of recipients developing respiratory failure during or soon after the transfusion of plasma-containing blood components.[22] In this syndrome, severe hypoxemia is associated with fever, hypotension, and the bilateral infiltrates characteristic of ARDS. The last is thought to be due to a capillary leak syndrome, which perhaps is initiated by pulmonary leukocyte sequestration and degranulation. Most cases require mechanical ventilation, but, if the patient can be supported successfully, the problem can resolve rapidly without sequelae.

Allergic Transfusion Reactions

Allergic reactions to transfusion are manifest by a spectrum of findings from urticaria to anaphylactic shock. It is generally thought that allergic reactions represent recipient allergy to antigens in donor plasma, but this has been documented only at the severe end of the spectrum in patients with IgA deficiency who react to donor IgA as a foreign antigen and make anti-IgA. At the mild end of the spectrum, the responsible antigen specificities are unknown. Hypotension and anaphylactoid symptoms are also associated with the infusion of solutions containing immunoglobulin aggregates and would occur if immunoglobulin preparations, such as RhIG, intended for intramuscular use were given intravenously.

Urticaria

The prevalence of urticaria is given as 1 to 3% or more, and its frequency is attested by the regularity with which antihistamines are prescribed before transfusion. Urticarial reactions constitute the only transfusion reaction after which infusion of the same unit can safely be restarted; this is acceptable if the patient has a history of urticaria and if the symptoms have resolved after antihistamine administration (25 to 50 mg of intravenous diphenhydramine). Urticaria generally is easily prevented with pretransfusion antihistamines.

Anaphylactic Reactions

Anaphylactic reactions are rare, occurring in one recipient per 20,000 or more transfusions, and are characterized by flushing, hypotension, dyspnea, and gastrointestinal symptoms that begin soon after initiation of transfusion. A chill may occur, but fever is characteristically absent. The differential diagnosis of hypotension associated with transfusion includes an IHTR and the transfusion of a unit contaminated with bacteria. Treatment is with epinephrine and supportive measures. Severe reactions can generally be prevented by repeatedly "washing" RBCs before transfusion. Platelets can be washed, but large numbers are lost in the process. If plasma-containing components must be given, they can be obtained from IgA-deficient blood donors.

Posttransfusion Purpura

Posttransfusion purpura (PTP) is a rare reaction in which the recipient, usually a multiparous woman, develops thrombocytopenic purpura 5 to 10 days after the transfusion of RBCs or whole blood. Serologic investigation reveals the presence of an alloantibody in the patient's serum directed against platelet antigens, but the reason that this leads to the destruction of both donor (allogeneic) and recipient (autologous) platelets is controversial. Without treatment, severe thrombocytopenia may last for 1 to 4 weeks, but most cases will respond to plasma exchange or IVIG.

Graft-Versus-Host Disease

Graft-versus-host disease (GVHD) can occur after the transfusion of blood components containing viable donor lymphocytes into recipients who are severely immunodeficient or individuals tolerant of the donor lymphocyte antigens.[23] The former group of patients includes children with congenital cellular immunodeficiencies, patients with a variety of malignancies, particularly Hodgkin's disease and neuroblastoma, and bone marrow transplant recipients; the latter group includes fetuses who receive intrauterine transfusion (IUT), or exchange transfusion subsequent to IUT and to recipients who share HLA haplotypes with the donor in the form of a *one-way HLA match* (donor homozygous for a complete HLA haplotype that is identical to one recipient haplotype). A one way match occurs more commonly when donor and recipient are related or within certain countries or ethnic groups,[24] and transfusion-associated GVHD (TA-GVHD) is thought to be the mechanism of a large number of postsurgical deaths in Japan.[25] The latter patients were originally said to have a syndrome of *postoperative erythroderma*, which was most often seen after cardiac surgery with fresh whole blood replacement, the form of blood transfusion which carries the highest number of viable lymphocytes.

TA-GVHD differs from GVHD occurring after bone marrow transplantation in that the transfusion recipient's marrow is histo*in*compatible with the engrafted lymphocytes, and death almost invariably results from bone marrow failure. Lymphocyte engraftment can be prevented by irradiation of cellular blood components intended for at-risk patients, a process that does not interfere with the function of the transfused cells. Leukocyte reduction by filtration does not appear sufficient for prevention of TA-GVHD.

Transfusion-Related Immunomodulation

Transfusion prior to renal transplantation improves graft survival, and this effect may be due to some form of immunosuppression. A large number of studies have also suggested that transfusion promotes postoperative wound infection and increases the risk of tumor recurrence after cancer surgery.[26] These effects are postulated to be caused by donor leukocytes or plasma factors such as donor anti-idiotypic antibodies. Although many students would regard these observations as controversial, we are unaware of any studies that have *not* shown a relationship between transfusion and postoperative wound infection, and magnitude of the effect seen in many studies is substantial. The effect of transfusion on postoperative infection is not seen when only autologous units are used,[27] and may be abrogated by leukocyte filtration.[28] The existence of a *transfusion effect* for cancer recurrence remains controversial; skeptics generally hold that transfusion is correlated with a poorer outcome simply because it is a marker for more advanced cancer rather being a causal factor. However, there is strong support for the effect in animal models,[29] and, if the effect is mediated by donor leukocytes, prospective studies using leukocyte filtered transfusions may provide confirmatory evidence. Many immune function tests change after transfusion, but the direction of such changes reported by various studies differs,[30] and the relevance of these changes is unknown. This is an area of active investigation; transfusion mediated immunomodulation may prove numerically to be one of the most important adverse consequences of transfusion.

Nonimmune-mediated Transfusion Reactions

Although blood bankers in the past tended to identify themselves most closely with immunohematologic investigation, no less effort is expended in preventing adverse reactions to transfusion that are not mediated by immune mechanisms. The recent focus on AIDS and other forms of virus transmission has, of course, greatly increased the latter role. Table 12–8 lists the important categories of such reactions.

Storage Lesions

The term *storage lesion* refers to those changes in a unit of blood, particularly whole blood, that are consequences of storage conditions optimized for the preservation of RBCs. These changes may have clinical consequences for the recipient:

1. **The citrate-calcium interaction.** The citrate used as an anticoagulant chelates ionized calcium when infused. Lower concentrations of ionized calcium may produce a tingling sensation (typically, in the face), muscle tremors, and, if very severe, myocardial depression and arrhythmias. In practice, however, the liver metabolism of citrate is fast enough that significant depression of the ionized calcium level occurs only when whole blood or plasma is being transfused at a rate above 1 unit every 4 to 5 minutes, and life-threatening cardiac events are not expected unless even higher rates are obtained. Citrate toxicity typically is a problem only in patients with very severe liver disease, during liver transplant surgery, or in rapid exchange transfusions of infants.

2. **Acid-base balance/potassium changes.** Other potential toxins accumulating in liquid-stored whole

blood and RBCs include organic acids and potassium, both of which have potential cardiac toxicity. In actual massive transfusion cases, however, metabolic alkalosis and hypokalemia are more commonly observed, probably as consequences of citrate metabolism, since for each milliequivalent of citrate metabolized, there is consumption of 1 mEq of hydrogen ion and 1 mEq of potassium is shifted from the extracellular to the intracellular space. Moreover, the total load of potassium in a unit of RBCs is only about 5 mEq after 35 days of storage. If there is a significant concern regarding potassium load, relatively fresh units can be selected; this is preferable to washing the units since the latter causes a loss of RBCs, is expensive, and is unnecessary.

Concern has also focused on the adenine used to extend storage and the plasticizers that accumulate in stored blood, but problems involving these elements have not materialized. Microaggregates that form unavoidably after a few days of storage were once thought to promote the pulmonary toxicity sometimes seen after massive transfusion, but the current concept is that this is caused by the patient's underlying problem, typically trauma and shock.

3. **Viability of RBCs with storage.** With storage, RBCs become progressively less viable and their level of diphosphoglycerate (2,3-DPG) declines, which increases their oxygen affinity. This increased oxygen affinity might be expected to affect the ability of transfused RBCs to deliver oxygen in massively transfused patients, but, here again, real problems have not been well documented, perhaps because 2,3-DPG is repleted in the transfused cells within 24 hours after infusion. In spite of this, RBCs less than 5 days old, which maintain their 2,3-DPG levels, are commonly used for exchange transfusion in neonatal patients and for intrauterine transfusion.

Massive Transfusion—The Role of Platelets

Of more concern is the dilutional coagulopathy that has been attributed to massive transfusion with stored whole blood that is deficient in platelets and, to a variable degree, clotting factors VIII and V. This coagulopathy was studied in Vietnam battle casualties by Miller and co-workers,[31] who demonstrated a progressive increase in the incidence of microvascular bleeding characteristic of a coagulopathy. Such bleeding began in some patients after approximately two blood volumes had been replaced, and affected all patients after replacement of a third blood volume. This clinical finding was paralleled by a decline in platelet counts and an increase in clotting times, both of which trends tended to progress with larger transfusion volumes in a fashion that suggested that the patients' own hemostatically effective blood was being diluted by the platelet- and coagulation-factor-deficient whole blood. When Miller et al. examined the coagulation variables, they discerned a clear relationship between the onset of bleeding and fall in the platelet count below 60,000. On the other hand, no such relationship

Table 12–8. Adverse Consequences of Transfusion Not Immune-Mediated

Clinical consequences of the "storage lesion"
  Accumulation of toxins
  Decline in function
  Cold
Intravascular volume overload
Iron overload
Nonalloimmune hemolysis
Transfusion of infected blood
  Transmission of infection
    Viruses (hepatitis, HIV, CMV, others)
    Bacteria (gram-negative bacilli, Treponemes, others)
    Parasites (Malaria, *T. cruzi*, others)
  Reaction to preformed endotoxin

could be determined between a patient's clotting times and the onset of bleeding. In addition, when patients with pathologic bleeding were treated with fresh whole blood—the only available source of active platelets—all stopped bleeding; when similar patients were treated with FFP, none stopped bleeding.

Subsequent studies have refined these observations. Significant platelet dysfunction has been demonstrated in massively transfused trauma patients.[32,33] Counts and co-workers[34,35] demonstrated the dilution of platelets and clotting factors V and VII but emphasized the variability of coagulation parameters in different patients. In their studies, the prothrombin time (PT) and partial thromboplastin time (PTT) were predictive of pathologic bleeding only when they were 1.5 to 1.8 times control. Better predictors of hemostatic failure were a fibrinogen level below 50 mg/dl and a platelet count below 50,000; consumption (DIC) was thought to be the major cause of these abnormalities. In a group of patients receiving similar numbers of transfusions, Harke and Rahman[36] correlated the degree of platelet and clotting abnormalities with the length of time the patient was hypotensive. Taking these data together, Collins[37] concluded that "... coagulopathy in heavily transfused patients was due to hypoperfusion, not transfusion."

Hypothermia—Cold Blood Transfusion

A final effect of storage is that RBCs or whole blood will be cold (4°C) when transfused, and hypothermia and even cold cardioplegia can result from their rapid transfusion. Again, cardiac arrest is likely to occur only when cold blood components are being transfused very rapidly, on the order of 50 ml or more per minute. However, hypothermia may impair platelet function and increase oxygen demand, so that a blood warmer should be used in massive transfusion.

Intravascular Volume Overload

This is a common complication of transfusion. Patients with chronic anemia are particularly at risk, as they may be compensating for their anemia with a hyperdynamic, hypervolemic circulation and may have myocardial damage as well. Volume overload can be prevented to some degree by prior treatment with diuretics. RBCs can be administered over 4 hours, or RBC units can be split in two, with one-half left in the blood bank refrigerator and transfused 12 hours later.

Iron overload is a major problem in thalassemia major patients or any other patients who are completely dependent on transfused RBCs. Each milliliter of RBCs contains 1 mg of iron, approximately the amount absorbed or lost by a normal adult in 1 day. Because the excretion of iron cannot be increased, a positive iron balance is inevitable in the chronically transfused. The manifestations of chronic iron overload include cirrhosis, heart failure, and diabetes. Transfusion hemochromatosis can be prevented by chelation therapy with desferoxamine.

Units of RBCs can be hemolyzed by nonimmune mechanisms, in particular by improper heating or cooling. RBCs are also hemolyzed by contact with dextrose or hypotonic solutions, and by many drugs. For this reason, blood components should come in contact with normal saline only in IV lines, and no drugs should be added to the unit. RBCs and whole blood should only be stored in temperature monitored refrigerators or in coolers that are specifically designated for this purpose. Likewise, blood warming should only be performed in quality controlled blood warmers. We have seen hemolysis of units issued to the operating room that were warmed in beakers of tap water and blanket warming ovens, and that were hung next to hot lights.

Transfusion-transmitted Viral Infections

It would be difficult to imagine a vector more efficient than transfusion for the transmission of an infectious agent with a hematogenous phase. In 1937, Ottenberg, the first individual to apply blood typing and crossmatching to actual transfusions, stated: "Today transfusion has become so safe . . . the chief problem it presents is the finding of large sums of money needed for the professional donors who now provide most of the blood."[38] The irony of this statement is obvious to us, in this era of transfusion-associated AIDS (TA-AIDS), but it highlights an important principle. Many agents that are transmitted by transfusion cause morbidity and mortality only years after the infection is acquired. This is particularly true for human immunodeficiency virus (HIV) and hepatitis C virus (HCV, an agent causing parenterally transmitted non-A, non-B hepatitis [NANBH]), and the prolonged incubation periods of diseases caused by these agents resulted in a corresponding delay in the recognition that such infections were occurring at all. Much of the overuse of blood components derives from this fact. For example, the vast majority of transfusion-associated hepatitis cases are occult, in spite of which there is a high rate of chronic infection, with progression to cirrhosis over 10 to 20 years course.[39] Because this manifestation is delayed, the transfusing physician is seldom reinforced negatively for having ordered the transfusion and is not prompted to reexamine whether the transfusion was truly needed. Recently developed tests have largely eliminated the transmission of HIV by transfusion and have re-

duced the rate of HCV transmission by several orders of magnitude. Thus, we are at a point at which we may become complacent about the infectious risks of transfusion. The examples of HIV and HCV should warn us that such complacency is dangerous. Other agents are undoubtedly being transmitted by transfusion; we cannot surmise what diseases they may cause.

Post Transfusion Hepatitis

Essentially all of the viral agents known to cause hepatitis have been found to be transmitted by transfusion. Although hepatitis A virus has the highest incidence of all hepatitis viruses in North America, because it does not have a chronic carrier state, it causes only occasional cases of posttransfusion hepatitis (PTH). When the test for hepatitis B surface antigen (HBsAg) was introduced in the early 1970s, it was discovered that most PTH cases were so-called NANBH caused by another agent(s) that until recently defied serologic detection. Nonetheless, the introduction of routine testing of donated blood for HBsAg, coupled with a concomitant shift in the nation's blood supply from commercial to volunteer donors, led to a drop in PTH incidence from as high as one-third of all blood recipients to approximately one-tenth by the end of the 1970s. A number of changes in blood donor recruiting and testing, initiated during the 1980s, undoubtedly led to very significant further reductions in PTH incidence, although the magnitude of their net effect is not precisely known; these changes included progressively intensified donor screening for AIDS risk factors, HIV antibody testing, and alanine aminotransferase (ALT, syn. SGPT) and hepatitis B core antibody (HBcAb) testing of donated units (the latter two are surrogate tests for NANBH).

Hepatitis C-Virus

Introduction of the first generation test for HCV in May, 1990, decreased the risk of HCV to 3 cases per 10,000 units transfused,[40] and more recent versions of the HCV antibody test have lowered this risk further.[41] At the present time PTH incidence may be indistinguishable from the background rate of infection.

Hepatitis Associated with Blood Components

The PTH risk posed by different blood components (RBCs, FFP, platelets, cryoprecipitate) is generally assumed to be the same. Hepatitis transmission by plasma derivatives, which are prepared in large batches, has in the past been almost inevitable. However, methods developed to inactivate HIV may considerably reduce this risk.

The high rates of infection cited above conflict with the common experience of physicians, because most patients with PTH are anicteric and asymptomatic; such high rates were found only in prospective studies in which NANBH is defined by elevations of the ALT level on two occasions within 6 months after exposure.[42] Such studies also demonstrated a 50% rate of chronicity in NANBH with 20% or more of the chronic cases progressing to cirrhosis.[39]

HIV and AIDS

TA-AIDS has focused the public's attention on the risks of transfusion as never before and has led to an increased scrutiny of the indications for transfusion, an increased use of autologous transfusion, public demand for directed-donor transfusions, the use of consent forms specifically for transfusion, and a heightened sensitivity within the blood banking community to the prevention of transfusion-transmitted disease. These changes have occurred in spite of the fact that HIV antibody testing has reduced the risk of TA-AIDS to very low levels. The risk is not zero, however; the transmission of HIV from seronegative individuals can occur early in the course of their infection. Studies have suggested that HIV is transmitted by 1 of 40,000[43] to 225,000[44] seronegative units of blood components, or approximately 80 to 450 components per year. In a layman's comparison, this roughly corresponds to the number of individuals per year who are struck by lightning in the United States. The rate of such HIV transmission does not appear to be reduced by tests for circulating HIV p24 antigen.[45,46]

Cytomegalovirus

Cytomegalovirus (CMV) commonly establishes latent infections in leukocytes, making transmission by transfusion likely; in recent studies,[47] approximately 1% of CMV-seronegative blood recipients became infected. Although most primary CMV infections are mild, intrauterine infections can have devastating sequelae, as can the infection of low-birth-weight (<1250 g) infants of seronegative mothers and other immunosuppressed individuals. The reactivation of latent recipient infection can occur after transfusion from either seropositive or seronegative donors, and therefore, it cannot be prevented. Transmission of CMV can be prevented by providing blood components from CMV-seronegative donors, or by leukocyte reduction procedures such as the freezing and deglycerolization of RBCs or leukocyte filtration; leukocyte filtration has been shown to be equivalent to use of CMV-seronegative units in several studies.[48,49,50] FFP and cryoprecipitate do not transmit CMV. CMV-safe (filtered of seronegative) blood components are indicated for seronegative pregnant women, seronegative newborn infants weighing less than 1250 gm, and seronegative bone marrow or organ transplant recipients whose transplant donor is seronegative.

Bacterial Blood Contamination

Bacterial contamination is uncommon, but units may be contaminated by skin flora (e.g., Staph epidermidis) or bacteria present in the donor's bloodstream at the time of draw (e.g., Yersinia enterocolitica). Bacteria may multiply in the unit causing accumulation of endotoxin. When such a unit is transfused the patient may rapidly develop a high fever, but the reaction may be distinguished from a febrile or leukoagglutinin reaction by the presence of hypotension. In any case the transfusion should be stopped and the reaction be reported to the blood bank.

Concept of Directed Donations

Concern for the risks of disease transmission have led many patients to request that they recruit their own blood donors to make so-called *directed donations.* Many blood bankers have condemned directed donations, citing philosophic concerns regarding the volunteer nature of such donations and confidentiality problems for directed donors with positive disease test results. Blood banks are continually frustrated in dealing with the logistic issues posed by directed donations, which are exacerbated by unrealistic expectations of patients and patient families, and this wastes energy that might be spent on more productive activities. There are important recipient safety issues involving directed donation. Transfusion from blood relatives poses an increased risk of TA-GVHD, necessitating irradiation of the units. We have often seen a demand for directed donation delay the delivery of a needed transfusion. A recent large national study[51] demonstrated that donor disease marker rates were higher in directed donors, although this was entirely explained by differences in donor demographic variables.

INDICATIONS FOR TRANSFUSION

Risk-Benefit Ratios

The decision to transfuse, like any other therapeutic decision, must be based on a comparison of the relevant risks and benefits. Although this is a simple truism, it often is neglected. Studies of the use of blood components invariably demonstrate overutilization. Decision-making in transfusion therapy has been studied. Avorn and co-workers[52] determined that the transfusing physicians could estimate accurately the risk of transfusion, but there was wide variation in their experimental subjects' estimation of the benefit of receiving blood components, or, as it was phrased in the study, the "risk of not transfusing." This deficit of knowledge appears not to reflect a specific blind spot on the part of physicians. Instead, there has been a dearth of hard data in this area, and many important efficacy questions have only recently begun to receive attention. This impression is bolstered by inspection of the National Institutes of Health (NIH) Consensus Conference statements on the use of FFP,[53] platelets,[54] and RBCs,[18] in which repeated reference is made to the need for further study of the purported indications for transfusion. The issue is further complicated by the fact that new technology is being introduced continuously to improve the efficacy and safety of all forms of hemotherapy; examples that are anticipated at the time of this writing include crosslinked hemoglobin solutions, solvent-detergent treated plasma, improved hemopoietic hormones, and improved methods of screening for transfusion-transmitted diseases.

Prophylaxis Versus Therapy

In most instances, the uncertainty or controversy regarding the use of blood components centers on prophylactic rather than therapeutic indications. Therapeutic indications include transfusion for clearcut clinical problems, such as hemorrhagic shock or pathologic bleeding, and the success of the transfusion often is readily seen in the reversal of the problem. Prophylactic indications generally relate to specific laboratory findings, such as thrombocytopenia in the absence of bleeding or anemia in the absence of symptoms. The rationale for transfusion to normalize such findings is based on the assumption that the abnormal laboratory result is predictive of an adverse consequence for the patient. However, this is not the case for many laboratory results, since the limits of normality are established from population statistics, not on the test's predictive value for specific clinical outcomes. Thus, the rationale for prophylactic modes of transfusion should not be simply to correct an abnormal laboratory value that *might* predict a given adverse outcome. Instead, prophylactic transfusion should be based either on a demonstrated efficacy in decreasing the rate of the relevant occurrence or, at the very least, on a demonstration that the laboratory value to be corrected is truly predictive of the occurrence to be prevented.

Red Blood Cells

RBCs are indicated for the treatment of oxygen-carrying deficits. Although RBCs and whole blood are excellent volume expanders, their use should be restricted to patients needing augmented oxygen carriage, with volume expansion being relegated to the status of a positive side effect. Occasionally transfusion is also used to replace abnormal RBCs, such as antibody-sensitized RBCs in HDN or RBCs affected by sickling hemoglobinopathies.

For years anesthesiologists have believed a minimum hemoglobin (Hgb) of 10 g/dl was necessary for the safe conduct of anesthesia. This dictum has been passed on for decades despite the absence of sound clinical or experimental evidence. Numerous articles have been published in the past decade addressing the elusive "transfusion trigger", the physiologic end point for initiating RBC therapy. However, no such number can be applied to all circumstances since Hgb level is not the sole criterion for transfusion. The indication for RBC's must be predicated on the maintenance of oxygen delivery to the tissues. Oxygen delivery is determined by the product of oxygen content and cardiac output, and must meet the oxygen demand of the various organ systems. Anemia will reduce O_2 carrying capacity since the majority of O_2 is transported by Hgb. Oxygen delivery is maintained in the face of *normovolemic* anemia by various compensatory mechanisms. These mechanisms include an increase and redistribution of cardiac output, capillary recruitment, alteration in capillary transit time, increased oxygen extraction, and alteration in Hgb affinity for O_2. In the situation of acute intra-operative bleeding with volume replacement (i.e., acute normovolemic hemodilution), the primary mechanism for increasing O_2 delivery is an increase in cardiac output due to the effects of decreased blood viscosity and increased sympathetic nervous activity. The importance of fluid resuscitation for the maintenance of normovolemia in the face of acute blood loss cannot be overemphasized.

Recent articles have addressed the newer physiologic concepts of critical oxygen delivery, oxygen supply-dependency, and oxygen debt.[55] Animal[56] and human[57] studies demonstrate an ability of the organism to compensate, in the absence of coronary artery disease, down to hematocrit levels of 10% or below. Even in the presence of severe experimental[58] and human[59] coronary artery disease, myocardial oxygenation may be maintained in the presence of hematocrits as low as 20%.

Factors Determining Need for RBCs

A better understanding of, and better means of monitoring, the relationship between O_2 delivery and oxygen consumption will eventually lead to a more precise delineation of the appropriate transfusion trigger. The true "transfusion trigger" must take into account the underlying disease process, the patient's age, cardiac reserves, and oxygen demands all contribute to the decision when to transfuse. No single index can be the basis for perioperative transfusion. Clinical judgment in conjunction with the monitoring of tissue oxygen delivery will determine the individual patient's "transfusion trigger", not the use of a categorical "magic number".

On the basis of such experiences, an NIH consensus panel on perioperative RBC transfusion[18] recommended that the "hematocrit 30 rule" be dropped and be replaced by clinical judgment based on multiple patient factors. The NIH panel concluded that there is no evidence that postoperative anemia impairs wound healing. Because of the magnitude of the risk of transfusions, the panel emphasized that they be kept to a minimum and that alternatives be explored in the form of autologous transfusion, aggressive use of volume expanders to support perfusion, and pharmacologic approaches, such as desmopressin to enhance hemostasis and erythropoietin to enhance hematopoiesis.

Outside of operative circumstances, the patient with chronic anemia has additional compensatory resources in the form of increased RBC levels of 2,3-DPG, which promote increased oxygen unloading by hemoglobin; this change occurs over the course of several days. The power of this mechanism was demonstrated in the elegant studies of Elwood and co-workers,[60] who showed that when the Hct was as low as 24%, the symptoms one classically associates with anemia, such as fatigue, decreased exercise tolerance, and palpitations, do not correlate with the degree of anemia; instead, the best predictors of the presence of such nonspecific symptoms were personality factors. Moreover, correction of the anemia by iron administration did not improve these symptoms to any greater degree than did placebo. Elwood's data were corroborated by physiologic studies showing that if arterial oxygenation is normal, this mechanism can normalize oxygen delivery in the presence of Hct as low as 24 to 25%.[61] Cardiac output at rest begins to increase at a Hct of approximately 21% in chronically anemic patients, but many individuals with the anemia of chronic renal failure or sickle cell anemia tolerate lower levels. These data behoove the physician electing to transfuse an anemic patient to consider whether the reported symptoms are severe enough to limit the patient's lifestyle and, if so, to follow the course of the symptoms after transfusion to ensure that they are reversed.

Surgical Blood Ordering Schedule

The JCAHO requires that a hospital have a *maximum surgical blood ordering schedule* (MSBOS) to aid in the appropriate ordering of RBCs for use in the operating room. A MSBOS specifies the number of units which should be crossmatched for a given surgical procedure; amounts in excess of these levels must be justified by specific clinical conditions. The intent of this process is to decrease the number of units of RBCs that are crossmatched and held ready for a patient, but not transfused. When the latter occurs, unnecessary charges are generated for the patient, unnecessary costs are generated for the hospital, and increased amounts of blood outdate. If most cases of the listed procedure do not require blood, but occasional cases do, the suggested preoperative order is for a type-and-screen. In some minor cases, not even a type-and-screen is justified. Although it may seem prudent to always order a large number of units crossmatched, because the blood bank can rapidly supply RBCs for patients with a negative type-and-screen, it is not necessary to routinely prepare for worst-case scenarios. If the type-and-screen is positive, crossmatches will take additional time and the laboratory should compensate by automatically crossmatching additional units. The MSBOS may also be useful as a guide for autologous donation planning and auditing.

Fresh Frozen Plasma

Fresh frozen plasma (FFP) is the blood component that probably is overused most frequently and the use of which most often generates controversy in blood utilization review committees. Again, a focus on whether a presumed indication for use of this component is therapeutic or prophylactic will often help resolve the issue: evidence for the prophylactic use of FFP is almost entirely lacking. The appropriate use of FFP has been considered by an NIH consensus development conference.[53] The panel's conclusions are summarized in Table 12–9, and several of them deserve comment.

Primary Indication

For the most part the use of FFP involves the treatment of deficiencies of multiple coagulation factors, as found in patients with liver disease, DIC, or dilutional coagulopathy or in patients receiving warfarin therapy. In such cases, if the patient is bleeding from multiple sites (such as needle punctures), if sites where hemostasis was previously established bleed again, or if the surgeon finds that there is poor clot formation by shed blood, it is reasonable to conclude that the patient would benefit from the replacement of clotting factors. The grounds for such replacement are less strong when there is bleeding from a specific lesion in the presence of coagulopathy. If surgical hemostasis has been attempted and coagulation times are elevated to more than 1.5 to 1.8 times the PT or PTT control value, it may be efficacious to attempt to correct the coagulopathy. When dilution is the presumed cause of the coagulopathy, thrombocytopenia or platelet dysfunction must first be ruled out, because, as discussed above, platelet problems more commonly limit hemostasis in this circumstance, and the correction of clotting times often does not lead to a cessation of bleeding.[31] Consumption coagulopathy must also be ruled out, as FFP replacement will not adequately replete fibrinogen, and cryoprecipitate is generally required in DIC.

Studies of massive transfusion generally have concluded that prophylactic formulas for FFP supplementation are not appropriate.[31,35,37,62] The major controversy focuses on the need for prophylactic coagulation factor replacement in patients with abnormal clotting times who are to have invasive procedures. There is little evidence that mildly to moderately elevated coagulation times predict bleeding complications of invasive procedures. In a particularly well-executed study, Ewe[63] was unable to show any relationship between PT or platelet count and the extent of bleeding from liver biopsy sites under direct laparoscopic visualization. Similarly, a study[64] of patients undergoing paracentesis or thoracentesis failed to show any relation of excess bleeding to coagulation times that were as much as twice the control level. In the face of such data, the generally low rate of bleeding complications after biopsy, and the known risks of transfusion, the principle of primum non nocere would seem to preclude FFP prophylaxis in most cases. Nonetheless, many texts advocate advance FFP treatment of patients with mild coagulopathies who are scheduled for biopsies. Certainly for some levels of coagulopathy, ei-

Table 12–9. NIH Consensus Conference Recommendations* for Use of FFP

FFP is not recommended for
    Volume expansion
    Nutritional source
    Routine management of massive hemorrhage (prophylaxis against dilutional coagulopathy)
Indications for FFP
    Isolated deficiencies of factor II, V, VII, IX, X, and XI when more specific components are unavailable or inappropriate
    TTP
    Reversal of coumarin effect in *bleeding* patients or before *emergency* surgery
    Massive transfusion (>1 blood vol) *and pathologic hemorrhage* if factor deficiencies are presumed to be the sole or principal
      derangement.
    Bleeding patients with multiple coagulation factor deficiencies (such as those with liver disease)

*Adapted from the NIH consensus statement on the use of FFP. [Consensus Development Panel, National Institutes of Health. Fresh frozen plasma. Indications and risks. JAMA *253*:551–3, 1985.]
Indications that have become obsolete since the original publication of this statement have been omitted.

ther FFP prophylaxis or avoidance of the procedure certainly appears rational. But the question is: At what level of coagulopathy is prophylactic coagulation factor replacement appropriate for this procedure? In the absence of better data, coagulation times 1.5-fold those of the control are a frequently cited indication for FFP transfusion.[65] However, such publications rarely make a distinction between different invasive procedures, and it seems self evident that the risk of bleeding complications from thoracentesis or paracentesis is less than that of lumbar puncture, liver biopsy, bronchoscopic biopsy, or subclavian catheter placement, which in turn is less than that of pancreatectomy.

Dose of FFP

When factor replacement is elected, the next issue is the appropriate dose. Coagulation abnormalities in patients with liver disease are notoriously resistant to correction, particularly if the patient has not responded to vitamin K supplementation. In one study,[66] only 20% of patients' PT values decreased after the infusion of 600 ml of FFP; 8 of 11 patients treated in another study[67] achieved partial correction with volumes from 600 to 1800 ml of FFP, but the PT returned toward baseline 2 to 4 hours after cessation of infusion. The infusion of volumes of plasma large enough to correct coagulopathies in such patients often leads to volume overload and pulmonary edema. For these reasons, the ability to correct and then demonstrate the correction of a coagulopathy in patients with liver disease prior to a procedure often proves to be impossible. Instead, if prophylaxis is to be attempted, we have suggested that rapid infusion of 2 to 4 units of FFP immediately before the procedure and additional supplementation during the procedure, particularly if excessive bleeding occurs.

DIC often accompanies trauma or other circumstances leading to hemorrhagic shock, such as abruptio placenta. It is important that an appropriate work-up for this problem be performed, since the treatment for simple dilutional coagulopathy will not be sufficient. Bleeding due to DIC reflects the consumption of platelets and labile clotting factors, particularly fibrinogen and FVIII, so that initial therapy should be a platelet transfusion—6 to 8 units of platelet concentrate for an adult—and a cryoprecipitate transfusion—generally 10 units. As factors V and II may also be consumed, additional supplementation with 2 units of FFP can be employed. Subsequently therapy should be guided by laboratory values, with the goal being to maintain a fibrinogen level greater than 100 units per deciliter and a platelet count greater than 50,000 μl.

Use of Cryoprecipitate

Cryoprecipitate is used for the treatment of von Willebrand's disease, hemophilia A (deficiency of FVIIIc), and fibrinogen deficiencies or abnormalities. Discussion of the treatment of congenital deficiencies of individual coagulation factors is beyond the scope of this chapter (see Chapter 13).

Platelets

The therapeutic and prophylactic indications for platelet transfusion are better understood than are those for FFP, and this form of treatment has undoubtedly had a major impact on the survival of many patient groups, particularly those with hematologic malignancies. Severely thrombocytopenic patients typically develop skin or mucosal bleeding that is manifest as petechiae, epistaxis, oral bleeding, hematuria, gastrointestinal blood loss, and delayed hemostasis after instrumentation. Intracerebral bleeding is the most feared complication of thrombocytopenia and in the past was a common cause of death in leukemia patients. In thrombocytopenic patients, once bleeding stops it rarely starts again unless there is associated coagulopathy. The frequency and gravity of such bleeding is directly related to the platelet count:[68] major visible hemorrhage occurs in some patients at platelet counts of 20,000/μl and becomes frequent at counts below 5,000. The bleeding time is also directly related to platelet count at levels below 100,000. The appropriate indications for platelet transfusion as outlined by an NIH consensus conference panel[64] are shown in Table 12-10.

Therapeutic Indications

These indications for platelet transfusions are relatively clearcut. When the platelet count is less than 50,000 and active bleeding is present in the absence of a lesion requiring surgical correction; elevation of the platelet count by 40,000 or more is expected to resolve bleeding.[69] If the platelet count cannot be increased because of immunologic or other factors, a response is not expected. A response is also expected in bleeding patients with normal numbers of platelets but with congenital or acquired platelet function abnormalities sufficient to elevate the bleeding time to more than twice normal. Finally, if pathologic bleeding develops in the setting of massive

Table 12–10. NIH Consensus Conference Recommendations* for the Use of Platelets

Platelets are not generally indicated for
  Aplastic anemia patients
  ITP patients in the absence of severe bleeding
  Prophylactic treatment before or following cardiopulmonary
    bypass
Indications for the use of platelets
  Actively bleeding patients with
    Platelet count less than 50,000
    Platelet function abnormality and bleeding time greater
      than twice normal
    Massive transfusion and documented thrombocytopenia
  Prophylaxis
    Temporary thrombocytopenia with platelet count less than
      20,000
    Before invasive procedure to correct bleeding time (esp. *if
      hemostasis cannot be observed*)

*Adapted from the NIH consensus statement on the use of platelets. [Consensus Development Panel. Platelet Transfusion Therapy. Transfus Med Rev *1*:195–200, 1987.]

transfusion and thrombocytopenia, platelet replacement is expected to stop the bleeding.[31]

Prophylactic Indications

These indications for platelet transfusion have a rationale based on the data cited above, and in prospective controlled trials prophylactic platelet transfusion has been effective in preventing hemorrhage but not in prolonging survival, probably because the trials have not been large enough.[70] In the study by Murphy and co-workers,[71] a disturbing finding was that, during the last month of life, there was an increase in the duration of hemorrhage experienced by patients who had been transfused prophylactically, presumably because these patients had a greater exposure to donor units and had become alloimmunized—and therefore refractory—to further platelet transfusion. This observation raises the caveat that prophylactic platelet transfusion is relevant only to patients in whom thrombocytopenia is expected to be a temporary condition; if thrombocytopenia or platelet dysfunction will be prolonged, the development of refractoriness can eventually be expected to limit the response to platelets, particularly if immune function is normal as it is in patients with aplastic anemia or congenital thrombocytopathies.

Preoperative Thrombocytopenia Prophylaxis

Patients with severe preoperative thrombocytopenia are generally assumed to benefit from prophylactic platelet transfusion, but this has not been demonstrated in experimental studies. In the utilization criteria of various hospitals, the threshold for such prophylaxis is typically set at platelet counts between 50,000 and 70,000. Prophylactic transfusion of platelets has been investigated in circumstances in which thrombocytopenia is expected to develop intraoperatively, either because of dilution[72] or cardiopulmonary bypass,[73] in both cases, prophylaxis was ineffective. Although it endorsed the logic of prophylactic platelet transfusion for thrombocytopenic patients undergoing surgery, the NIH consensus panel[54] suggested that such transfusions made the most sense for patients in whom hemorrhage could not be observed or in whom it occurred at a site where it could be critical in small amounts, (e.g., in the central nervous system); in this regard, it may be more important to infuse platelets prior to closing wounds, rather than prior to incision.

Patients with idiopathic thrombocytopenic purpura are generally not considered to be candidates for platelet transfusion for two reasons. The first is that, in spite of very low platelet counts, their bleeding times are often relatively normal, and life-threatening hemorrhage is rare. The second is that, as rapid destruction of transfused platelets is the rule, transfusion, particularly for prophylaxis, exposes the patient to a risk with little potential benefit. The same logic applies to patients with TTP. In addition to the usual transfusion reactions, the TTP patient may have an increased risk of complications of microvascular thrombosis when transfused with platelets, and this should particularly be avoided if there are CNS signs.

Poor Response to Platelet Transfusion

Poor responses to platelet transfusion are relatively common, either because of immune-mediated platelet destruction, or because of nonimmune-mediate destruction/consumption. The former may be due to HLA antibodies, platelet antigen-specific antibodies, or drug-related antibodies. Clinical factors leading to destruction/consumption include fever, infection, DIC, splenomegaly, and concomitant administration of amphotericin.[74] The approaches to these two groups of problems are quite different. In the former case, compatible platelets must be sought; in the latter, the dose must be increased if platelets are truly required. A poor response to platelets as measured at 10 minutes to 1 hour after transfusion, was previously held to favor immune-mediated causes of refractoriness, while nonimmune-mediated refractoriness was said to manifest as an adequate response at 1 hour, with a return to baseline by 18 to 24 hours.[75] This generalization has recently been challenged,[76] and a screen for HLA antibodies, is generally needed in order to make a decision as to the need for HLA-matched platelets.

REFERENCES

1. Mollison P. L., Engelfriet C. P., Contreras, M.: Blood transfusions in clinical medicine. 8th ed. Oxford: Blackwell Scientific Publications, 1987.
2. Rippee C., Myers J., Gindy L.: Blood groups. In, Petz LD, Swisher SN: *Clinical Practice of Blood Transfusion,* 2nd Ed. New York: Churchill Livingstone (1989).
3. Shulman I.: The risk of overt hemolytic transfusion reaction following the use of an immediate spin crossmatch. Arch Pathol Lab Med *114*:112–4, 1990.
4. Pisciotto P. T.: ed. Blood transfusion therapy; A physicians handbook 3rd Ed. Arlington, VA: American Association of Blood Banks, 1989.
5. Speiss B. D.: et al. Autologous blood donation: hemodynamics in a high-risk patient population. Transfusion *32*:17–22, 1992.
6. Toy P., Strauss R. G., Stehling L. C., et al.: Predeposited autologous blood for elective surgery; a national multicenter study. N Engl J Med *316*:517–20, 1987.
7. Renner S. W., Howanitz, P. J., Bachner, P.: Preoperative autologous blood donation in 612 hospitals; a College of American pathologists' Q-probes study of quality issues in transfusion practice. Arch Pathol Lab Med *116*:613–19, 1992.
8. Strauss R. G., Ferguson K. J., Stone G. G., et al.: Surgeons' knowledge, attitude, and use of preoperative autologous blood donation. Transfusion *30*:418–22, 1990.
9. Goodnough L. T., et al.: Increased preoperative collection of autologous blood with recombinant human erythropoietin therapy. N Engl J Med *321*:1163–8, 1989.
10. Lorentz A., et al.: Serial immunoreactive erythropoietin levels in autologous blood donors. Transfusion *31*:650–4, 1991.
11. AuBuchon J. P., Birkmeyer J. D.: Controversies in transfusion medicine; Is autologous transfusion worth the cost? Con Transfusion *34*:79–83, 1994.
12. Stehling L., Zauder H. L.: Acute normovolemic hemodilution. Transfusion *31*:857–868, 1991.
13. Brecher M. E., Rosenfield M.: Mathematical and computer

modeling of acute normovolemic hemodilution. Transfusion 34:176-9, 1994.

14. Williamson K. R. and Taswell H. F.: Intraoperative blood salvage: a review. Transfusion 31:662-75, 1991.

15. Giordano G. F., et al.: Autologous platelet-rich plasma in cardiac surgery: Effect on intraoperative and postoperative transfusion requirements. Ann Thorac Surg 46:416-9, 1988.

16. Dzik W. H., Sherburne B.: Intraoperative blood salvage: Medical controversies. Transfusion Med Rev 4:208-35, 1990.

17. Popovsky M. A.: Immune-mediated transfusion reactions. In: Nance S. J., ed. Immune destruction of red blood cells. Arlington, VA: American Association of Blood Banks, 1989:201-25.

18. NIH Consensus Conference. Perioperative red cell transfusion. JAMA 260:2700-3, 1988.

19. Honig C. L., Bove J. R.: Transfusion-associated fatalities: Review of Bureau of Biologics reports 1976-1978. Transfusion 20:653-60, 1980.

20. Mangano M. M., Chambers L. A., Kruskall M. S.: Limited efficacy of leukopoor platelets for prevention of febrile transfusion reactions. Am J Clin Pathol 95:733-8, 1991.

21. Muylle L., Joos M., Wouters E., De Bock, R., Peetermans M. E.: Increased tumor necrosis factor α (TNFα), interleukin 1, and interleukin 6 (IL-6) levels in the plasma of stored platelet concentrates: relationship between TNFα and IL-6 levels and febrile transfusion reactions. Transfusion 33:195-9, 1993.

22. Popovsky M. A., Moore S. B.: Diagnostic and pathogenetic considerations in transfusion-related acute lung injury. Transfusion 25:573-7, 1985.

23. Anderson K. C., Weinstein H. J.: Transfusion-associated graft-versus-host disease. N Engl J Med 323:315-21, 1990.

24. Ohto H., Yasuda H., Noguchi M., Abe R.: Risk of transfusion-associated graft-versus-host disease as a result of directed donations from relatives. Transfusion 37:691-3, 1992.

25. Juji T., Takahashi K., Shibata Y., et al.: Post-transfusion graft-versus-host disease in immunocompetent patients after cardiac surgery in Japan. N Engl J Med 321:56, 1989.

26. Triulzi D. J., Heal J. M., Blumberg, N.: Transfusion-induced immunomodulation and its clinical consequences. In Nance SJ. ed. Transfusion Medicine in the 1990's Arlington VA: American Association of Blood Banks, 1990.

27. Mezrow C. K., Bergstein I., Tartter P. I.: Postoperative infections following autologous and homologous blood transfusions. Transfusion 32:27-30, 1992.

28. Jensen L. S., et al.: Postoperative infection and natural killer cell function following blood transfusion in patients undergoing elective colorectal surgery. Br J Surg 79:513-6, 1992.

29. Blajchman M. A., Bardossy L., Carmen R., Sastry A., Singal D. P.: Allogeneic blood transfusion-induced enhancement of tumor growth: two animal models showing amelioration by leukodepletion and passive transfer using spleen cells. Blood 81:1880-2, 1993.

30. Blumberg N., Heal J. M.: Transfusion and recipient immune function. Arch Pathol Lab Med 113:246-53, 1989.

31. Miller R. D., Robbins T. O., Tong M. J., Barton S. L.: Coagulation defects associated with massive blood transfusions. Ann Surg 174:794-801, 1971.

32. Lim R. C., Olcott C., Robinson A. J., Blaisdell F. W.: Platelet response and coagulation changes following massive blood replacement. J Trauma 13:577-82, 1973.

33. Harrigan C., Lucas C. E., Ledgerwood A. M., et al.: Serial changes in primary hemostasis after massive transfusion. Surgery 98:836-43, 1985.

34. Counts R. B., Haisch C., Simon T. L., et al.: Hemostasis in massively transfused trauma patients. Ann Surg 190:91-9, 1979.

35. Ciavarella D., Reed R. L., Counts R. B., et al.: Clotting factor levels and the risk of microvascular bleeding in the massively transfused patient. Br J Haematol 67:365-8, 1987.

36. Harke H., Rahman S.: Haemostatic disorders in massive transfusion. Bibl Haematol 46:179-88, 1980.

37. Collins J. A.: Recent developments in the area of massive transfusion. World J Surg 11:75-81, 1987.

38. Ottenberg R.: Reminiscences of the history of blood transfusion. J Mt Sinai Hosp NY 4:264-71, 1937.

39. Alter H. J.: You'll wonder where the yellow went: a 15-year retrospective of posttransfusion hepatitis. In: Moore SB, ed. Transfusion-transmitted viral diseases. Arlington, VA. American Association of Blood Banks, 1987:53-86.

40. Donahue J. G., et al.: The declining risk of post-transfusion hepatitis C virus infection. N Engl J Med 327:369-73, 1992.

41. Watanabe M., et al.: Hepatitis C viral markers in patients who received blood that was positive for hepatitis C virus core antibody, with genetic evidence of hepatitis C virus transmission. Transfusion 34:125-9, 1994.

42. Aach R. D., et al.: Serum alanine aminotransferase of donors in relation to the risk of non-A, non-B hepatitis in recipients; The transfusion-transmitted viruses study. N Engl J Med 304:989-94, 1981.

43. Donahue J. G., et al.: Transmission of HIV by transfusion of screened blood. (letter) N Engl J Med 323:1709, 1990.

44. Dodd R. Y.: The risk of transfusion-transmitted infection. N Engl J Med 327:419-21, 1992.

45. Alter H. J., Epstein J. S., Swenson S. G., et al.: Collaborative study to evaluate HIV-antigen (HIV-ag) screening of blood donors (abstract). Transfusion 29 (suppl):56S, 1989.

46. Transfusion Safety Study Group. HIV-1 P-24 antigen screening of male blood donors from high anti-HIV prevalence areas (abstract). Transfusion 29 (suppl):56S, 1989.

47. Tegtmeier G. E.: Posttransfusion cytomegalovirus infections. Arch Pathol Lab Med 113:236-45, 1989.

48. de Graan-Hentzen Y. C. E., et al.: Prevention of primary cytomegalovirus infection in patients with hematologic malignancies by intensive white cell depletion of blood products. Transfusion 29:757-60, 1989.

49. Gilbert G. L., Hayes K., Hudson I. L., James J., and the Neonatal Cytomegalovirus Infection Study Group.: Prevention of transfusion-acquired cytomegalovirus infection in infants by blood filtration to remove leukocytes. Lancet 1:1228-31, 1989.

50. Bowden R. A., et al.: Use of leukocyte-depleted platelets and cytomegalovirus-seronegative red blood cells for prevention of primary cytomegalovirus infection after marrow transplant. Blood 78:246-50, 1991.

51. Conference addresses safe expansion of the donor pool. Blood Bank Week. Vol 10, #35:2-4, 1993.

52. Avorn J., Soumerai S. B., Salem S. R., Popovsky M.: Documenting and correcting inappropriate use of blood components. In: Kurtz SR, Summers S, eds. Improving transfusion practice: the role of quality assurance. Arlington, VA: American Association of Blood Banks, 1989:21-30.

53. Consensus Development Panel, National Institutes of Health. Fresh frozen plasma. Indications and risks. JAMA 253:551-3, 1985.

54. Consensus Development Panel. Platelet Transfusion Therapy. Transfus Med Rev 1:195-200, 1987.

55. Tuman K. J.: Tissue oxygen delivery. Anesth Clinics of North America 8:451-69, 1990.

56. Wilkerson D. K., et al.: Limits of cardiac compensation in anemic baboons. Surgery 103:665-70, 1988.

57. Leone B. J., Spahn D. R.: Anemia, hemodilution, and oxygen delivery. (editorial) Anesth Analg 75:651-3, 1992.

58. Levy P. S., et al.: Limit to cardiac compensation during acute isovolemic hemodilution: influence of coronary stenosis. Am J Physiol 265:H340-9, 1993.

59. Geha A. S., Baue A. E.: Graded coronary stenosis and coronary flow during acute normovolemic anemia. World J Surg 2:645-51, 1978.

60. Elwood P. C., Waters W. E., Creene W. J. W., Sweetnam P., Wood M. M.: Symptoms and circulating haemoglobin level. J Chronic Dis 21:615-28, 1969.

61. Hogman C. F.: Oxygen affinity of stored blood. Acta Anaesthesiol Scand 45 (suppl):53-61, 1971.

62. Mannucci P. M., Federici A. B., Sirchia G.: Hemostasis testing during massive blood replacement. Vox Sang 42:113-23, 1982.

63. Ewe K.: Bleeding after liver biopsy does not correlate with indices of peripheral coagulation. Dig Dis Sci 26:388-93, 1981.

64. McVay P. A., Toy P.: Lack of increased bleeding after paracentesis and thoracentesis in patients with mild coagulation abnormalities. Transfusion 31:164-71, 1991.

65. Willis J. L., ed.: Use of blood components. FDA Drug Bull, July 1989.

66. Gazzard B. G., Henderson I. M., Williams R.: The use of fresh frozen plasma or a concentrate of factor IX as a replacement therapy before liver biopsy. Gut 16:621-5, 1975.

67. Spector I., Corn M., Ticktin H. E.: Effect of plasma transfusion on the prothrombin time and clotting factors in liver disease. N Engl J Med 275:1032-7, 1966.

68. Gaydos L. A., Freireich E. J., Mantel N.: The quantitative relationship between platelet count and hemorrhage in patients with acute leukemia. N Engl J Med 266:905-9, 1962.

69. Djerassi I., Farber S., Evans A. E.: Transfusions of fresh platelet concentrates to patients with secondary thrombocytopenia. N Engl J Med 268:221-6, 1963.

70. Kelton J. G., Ali A. M.: Platelet transfusions—a critical appraisal. Clin Oncol 2:549-85, 1983.

71. Murphy S., Litwin S., Herring L. M., et al.: Indications for platelet transfusion in children with acute leukemia. Am J Hematol 12:347-56, 1982.

72. Reed R. L., Ciavarella D., Heimbach D. M., et al.: Prophylactic platelet administration during massive transfusion; a prospective, randomized, double-blind clinical study. Ann Surg 203:40-8, 1986.

73. Simon T. L., Akl B. F., Murphy W.: Controlled trial of routine administration of platelet concentrates in cardiopulmonary bypass surgery. Ann Thorac Surg 37:359-64, 1984.

74. Slichter S. J.: Mechanisms and management of platelet refractoriness. In: Nance SJ, ed. Transfusion Medicine in the 1990's. American Association of Blood Banks, Arlington, VA:1990.

75. Daly P. A., Schiffer C. A., Aisner J., Wiernik P. H.: Platelet transfusion therapy; One-hour posttransfusion increments are valuable in predicting the need for HLA-matched preparations. JAMA 243:435-8, 1980.

76. McFarland J. G., Anderson A. J., Slichter S. J.: Factors influencing the transfusion response to HLA-selected apheresis donor platelets in patients refractory to random platelet concentrates. Br J Haematol 73:380-6, 1989.

Chapter 13

COAGULATION MECHANISMS: HEMOSTASIS AND THROMBOSIS

GERALD A. SOFF

The need to control surgically associated bleeding remains a primary concern of the surgical and anesthesia services. Nature has provided a complex and elegant system to provide for hemostasis following trauma and surgery, which serves to limit blood loss. The term "the coagulation cascade" conveys the concept of amplification of the sequential coagulation reactions following a procoagulant stimulus, resulting in formation of a clot.[1] However, the coagulation system is better viewed as a balance between the procoagulant pathways and an equally complex system of physiologic anticoagulants that serve to limit the coagulation process to appropriate sites of vascular injury. Failure of the procoagulant or anticoagulant processes result in hemorrhage or thrombosis respectively, and thus coagulation is better viewed as a tightrope walk rather than a cascade. Balance is essential to insure normal blood flow throughout the vascular system.

PHYSIOLOGY OF COAGULATION

Procoagulant Mechanisms

Under normal circumstances following trauma to a blood vessel, three types of responses contribute to hemostasis: (1) vasoconstriction, (2) platelet adhesion and aggregation, and (3) formation of a fibrin clot. These are interrelated processes.

Vasoconstriction

Endothelial cells (EC) produce renin, an activator of angiotensin, and endothelin, a peptide hormone that induces contraction of the smooth muscle cells of the vascular media (2). A loss of, or reduction in, EC production of endothelium-derived relaxing factor (nitric oxide) and prostacyclin (PGI$_2$) also results in vasoconstriction as these agents are known to exert potent vasodilatory effects.[3,4] Vasoconstriction serves as an early response to trauma, stemming the flow of blood through a traumatized vessel.

Platelet Adhesion

Platelet adhesion to the vessel wall follows, mediated largely by the von Willebrand factor (vWF) and the platelet membrane vWF receptor, a complex of glycoproteins 1b, V and IX.[5,6] Other proteins may contribute to platelet adhesion, including fibronectin, laminin, thrombospondin, and vitronectin.[6] High shear stress may also contribute to platelet adhesion. Adhesion is followed by platelet activation, granule release, and aggregation.[7] Release of ADP from dense granules activates additional platelets,[8] while the proteins of the alpha granules, including vWF, fibrinogen, and factor V, contribute to platelet activation and aggregation, and the formation of a fibrin clot.[9] The activated platelet provides the surface for several reactions of the soluble coagulation factors (Fig. 13-1).[10]

Although numerous stimuli, including adhesion, shear stress, and exposure to thrombin, ADP, collagen, epinephrine, or thromboxane A2 may cause platelet activation, platelet aggregation is mediated via a single pathway. This is activation-dependent conversion of the membrane glycoprotein IIb/IIIa (GP IIb/IIIa) complex to a high affinity receptor. The cross-linking of platelets occurs via ligand bridging of GP IIb/IIIa complexes by one of a number of potential ligands, but predominantly fibrinogen.[6,11]

Fibrin Clot Formation

In conjunction with platelet activation and aggregation, interactions with the soluble coagulation factors facilitates formation of cross-linked fibrin clots. The coagulation cascade, as we currently know it, is illustrated in Figure 13-1. The primary mechanism of coagulation in vivo is via the "extrinsic pathway," also referred to as the tissue factor pathway. Tissue factor (TF) is released by vascular tissues upon injury and serves as a cofactor for the activation of factor VII.[12,13] Activated factor VII activates factors X and IX.[14] Exposure of circulating factor XII to negatively charged constituents of the damaged vessel wall results in activation of the "intrinsic pathway".[15] Factor XII, prekallikrein, and high molecular weight kininogen, together referred to as the contact system, are part of a positive feed-back loop which further activates the intrinsic system. The intrinsic system "proximal" to factor XI is believed to play a minor role in hemostasis, as defects in the contact factors are not associated with a hemorrhagic tendency.

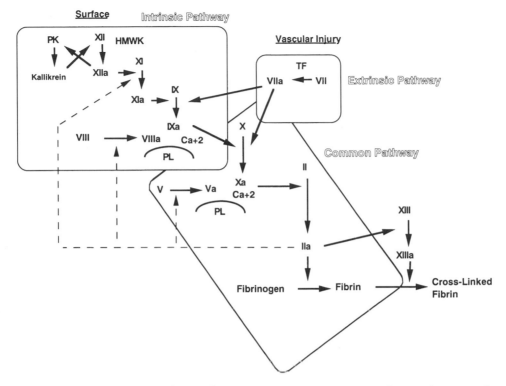

Fig. 13–1. Coagulation cascade. The current understanding of the coagulation cascade is illustrated. In vivo, the primary activation of the coagulation cascade is via the extrinsic (tissue factor) pathway. A calcium-dependent complex of factors VIIIa and IXa on platelet membrane activates factor X. A second complex of calcium, factors Xa and Va on platelet membranes activates prothrombin (Factor II) to thrombin. The cross-linking of fibrin by factor XIII is illustrated outside of the common pathway as the standard in vitro coagulation assays will not detect deficiencies of this process. Factors are represented by the respective Roman numerals. Factor II is more commonly referred to as prothrombin. PK = prekallikrein, HK = high molecular weight kininogen, PL = phospholipid membrane, TF = tissue factor.

Principal Coagulation Factors

Before 1950, the designation of clotting factors was in a chaotic state and an International Commission was formed under the chairmanship of Irving Wright.[16] This Commission assigned Roman numerals to the then recognized clotting factors (Table 13-1). It is noted that although a Roman numeral was assigned to fibrinogen, prothrombin and thromboplastin (also to calcium), these factors are rarely so designated. For factors in their activated state, the lower case letter "a" is added to the Roman numeral.

A number of the coagulation factors circulate as zymogens of serine protease enzymes, including factors II (prothrombin), (VII, IX, X, XI, XII).[17,18] Once activated, these enzymes may activate numerous molecules of their respective substrate factors, thus providing amplification of the coagulation system. Factors V and VIII are cofactors, but also require enzymatic cleavage to become active.[18] Factor VIII circulates as a complex with von Willebrand factor (vWF), which together are referred to as the factor VIII:vWF complex. Factors II, VII, IX, and X possess gammacarboxyl glutamic acid (Gla) residues, which mediate calcium binding, necessary for normal activity.[19] The physiologic anticoagulants, protein C and protein S, discussed below, also possess Gla residues. The post-translational synthesis of the Gla residues is dependent on vita-

Table 13–1. Coagulation Factors and Their Source of Production

Factor	Name	Produced
I	Fibrinogen	Liver
II	Prothrombin	Liver
III	Thromboplastin, tissue factor	—
IV	Calcium	—
V	Accelerator globulin, labile factor	Liver
VI	Now known to be activated, factor V	—
VII	Serum prothrombin conversion accelerator (SPCA), stable factor, proconvertin	Liver
VIII	Antihemophilic globulin platelet cofactor I, antihemophilic factor A	Endothelial cells + RES
IX	Plasma thromboplastin component (Christmas factor) platelet cofactor I, antihemophilic factor B	Liver
X	Stuart-Prower factor	Liver
XI	Plasma thromboplastin antecedent (PTA), antihemophilic factor C	Liver
XII	Hageman factor, glass factor	Unknown
XIII	Fibrin stabilizing factor	Liver

Wright, I.: *International Commission on Nomenclature of Clotting Factors.* New York, International Society of Hemostasis, 1954.

min K, and therefore factors II, VII, IX, and X and proteins C and S are referred to as the vitamin K-dependent factors (Table 13-2).

Anticoagulant Mechanisms

Under circumstances in which the vessel wall is intact, several physiologic anticoagulant mechanisms act to prevent, or limit, the coagulation process. Heparan sulfate, synthesized by vascular EC, is a cofactor for the circulating glycoprotein antithrombin III (AT III). AT III, when bound to heparan (or heparin) binds to activated serine proteases in a 1:1 stoichiometric ratio.[20] The AT III:enzyme complex then dissociates from the heparan sulfate molecule, and is cleared from the circulation. Thrombomodulin (TM) is an EC membrane receptor for thrombin. When thrombin binds to TM it undergoes a conformational change with reduced ability to cleave fibrinogen and a markedly increased ability to activate the anticoagulant, protein C.[21] Protein C, with its cofactor protein S, inactivates the activated forms of the procoagulant cofactors, factors Va and VIIIa. Activated protein C may also augment fibrinolysis. Heparin cofactor II is also activated by heparan or heparin and neutralizes thrombin. Tissue factor pathway inhibitor (TFPI) inactivates the complex of factors VIIa, Xa, and tissue factor, limiting the initiation of the coagulation cascade. TFPI may play a role in determining whether the primary in vivo substrate of activated factor VII is factor IX or factor X.[22]

The fibrinolytic system acts to degrade both physiologic and pathologic thrombi. The central component of the fibrinolytic system is plasminogen, which is converted to the fibrinolytic enzyme plasmin.[23,24] Two plasminogen activators are expressed by endothelial cells and other tissues, which convert plasminogen to plasmin; these are tissue plasminogen activator (tPA) and urokinase (urokinase-type plasminogen activator; u-PA). "Kringle" domains of the plasminogen activators and plasminogen facilitate binding of these factors to fibrin, which serve to localize plasmin generation to the surface of a fibrin clot. Plasminogen activator inhibitor-1, (PAI-1), rapidly neutralizes tPA, u-PA, and plasmin limiting the scope of fibrinolysis. $\alpha2$-Antiplasmin and $\alpha2$-macroglobulin neutralize plasmin as well.

ANALYSIS OF COAGULATION

A number of assays have been developed to guide the physician in evaluating the coagulation system. It is essential to remember that a thorough history and physical examination remain the most sensitive and valuable tools in predicting which patients are at increased risk of intraoperative, and postoperative hemorrhage.

History

Complaints of excessive bruising, particularly if not related to known injury, suggest defects of primary hemostasis (platelet and microvascular function). Mucosal bleeding (i.e., menorrhagia, epistaxis, gingival bleeding) also are common from defects of primary hemostasis. Complaints of post-traumatic hemorrhage, particularly delayed bleeding after trauma and deep muscle bleeding, suggest defects of the soluble coagulation factors. Symptoms beginning in infancy or childhood suggest a congenital hemostatic defect, while symptoms beginning in later life usually indicate an acquired disorder. It is equally important to document whether the patient has experienced hemostatic challenge without complication, such as circumcision, dental extraction, tonsillectomy/adenoidectomy, or fractures. A family history of excessive bleeding, whether characterized or not, is valuable in assessing potential for increased operative hemorrhage. Evidence by history, physical exam, or routine laboratory evaluation of diseases which are associated with defects in hemostasis may be very helpful. As discussed below, renal and hepatic disease, and other acquired disease processes are associated with hemostatic compromise and an increased risk of hemorrhage. A detailed drug history, including over-the-counter and recently discontinued drugs, is essential, as numerous drugs may effect hemostasis.

It is equally important to obtain a detailed history of thromboembolic events in the patient's past, as well as family history of these events. More surgical patients suffer fatal complications of a thrombotic nature than a hemorrhagic nature. Standard measures are readily available for reduction of this risk.

Physical Examination

A variety of skin abnormalities may provide evidence for vascular or hemostatic disorders. Petechiae and purpura result from thrombocytopenia, platelet dysfunction, or some vascular disorders. Obviously, evidence of recent blood loss in the mouth, GI tract, or in other parts of the exam indicates a possible hemorrhagic tendency. Deep hematomas or evidence of acute or chronic joint hemorrhage (hemarthrosis, ankylosis) may be observed from coagulation factor deficiencies.

Laboratory Tests

Although a great variety of coagulation assays are available, the literature indicates that performance of "routine coagulation tests" is of limited utility in predicting excessive surgical bleeding, if a thorough history and physical examination are obtained and indicate no risk for hemorrhage.[25] In general three tests are reasonable for an initial evaluation of hemostasis; the platelet count, the prothrombin time (PT), and the activated partial thromboplastin time (aPTT). The bleeding time, discussed below, has been shown to be a particularly poor screening test and should only be performed to characterize an evident hemorrhagic tendency.[26]

Complete Blood Count with Peripheral Smear

The platelet count is included in most standard "Complete Blood Counts" (CBC), performed on automated counters, and reduction in platelet number is readily detected by current automated cell counters. However, confirmation by examination of the peripheral smear is essential to confirm a reportedly deficient platelet count, to characterize the platelet morphology, and to detect abnormalities of the red and/or white cells which may aid in characterizing the process leading to thrombocytopenia. Alterations in platelet size or morphology may be observed in the peripheral smear as well. Circulation of large platelet forms suggests an increased rate of platelet production, as observed in immune thrombocytopenia.[27] Several hereditary disorders of platelet functional, discussed below, are associated with abnormal platelet morphology. Thrombocytosis (thrombocythemia) may result from myeloproliferative diseases, and the platelets may be dysfunctional. The dysfunctional platelets may be hypofunctional or hyperfunctional, leading to a hemorrhagic diathesis and/or thrombotic disorder.[28]

Activated Partial Thromboplastin Time

The activated partial thromboplastin time (aPTT) is a modified recalcification clotting time employing citrated platelet poor plasma, a source of phospholipid, and an activating agent.[29] The aPTT is particularly sensitive to deficiencies of (or inhibitors to) factors of the intrinsic pathway (Figs. 13-1 and 13-2), including factors XII, XI, IX, and VIII, prekallikrein, and high molecular weight kininogen. Deficiencies of the common pathway factors (factors II, V, X, and fibrinogen) may also prolong the aPTT. Mild factor deficiencies may be missed, as in general, reductions of levels to <50% must be achieved before the aPTT is prolonged. Inhibitors, which include heparin, antibodies to one or more of the factors, the lupus anticoagulant, and fibrin-degradation products, may also prolong the results.

Prothrombin Time

The prothrombin time (PT) is performed by addition of brain thromboplastin and calcium to citrated plasma.[29] The PT is prolonged by defects of the extrinsic and common pathways (Figs. 13-1 and 13-2), i.e., deficiencies of factors II, V, VII, and X, and fibrinogen. As noted for the aPTT, mild deficiencies may not result in a prolonged PT. Inhibitors may prolong the PT, but the PT is less sensitive to the effects of heparin than the aPTT.

Thrombin Time

The thrombin time (TT) is the clotting time when exogenous thrombin is added to citrated plasma, and reflects the conversion of fibrinogen to fibrin.[29] A prolonged TT may result from hypofibrinogenemia or dysfibrinogenemia. The most common settings in which a TT is prolonged is in the presence of heparin or fibrinogen-fibrin degradation products.[29,30]

Inhibitor Assays

The PT and aPTT may be modified to detect the presence of an inhibitor in a sample with a prolonged PT, aPTT. A 1:1 mixture of sample plasma and normal pooled plasma is prepared, and the assay repeated.[29] As 50% levels of each of the factors is sufficient for a normal PT or aPTT, the 1:1 mixture should yield a normal value if fac-

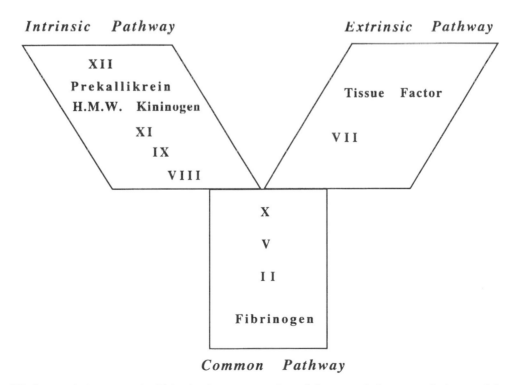

Fig. 13-2. Simplified coagulation cascade. This classic representation of the coagulation cascade is a useful tool for analysis of bleeding disorders. The prothrombin time (PT) measures the factors represented in the extrinsic and common pathways. The activated partial thromboplastin time (aPTT) measures the factors represented in the intrinsic and common pathways. In actuality, the in vivo coagulation process is more complex (Fig. 13-1), with feedback amplification at several points. Also, factor VIIa can activate factor IX directly. H. M. W. Kininogen = high molecular-weight kininogen.

tor deficiency caused the elevated PT or aPTT in the patient sample. In contrast, if the 1:1 mix is prolonged, then an inhibitor is suspected. Some inhibitors, such as antibodies to one or more of the factors, may only be detectable following incubation of the mixture at 37°C prior to the assay, while other inhibitors, such as fibrin split products or heparin, do not require prior incubation. The inhibitor assay may be modified to titer the antibody against a specific factor.

Fibrinogen

The PT and aPTT may be prolonged by deficiencies of fibrinogen, but this effect is variable and typically observed only if fibrinogen is reduced below about 100 mg/dl.[31] Therefore, fibrinogen functional levels are measured by a specific assay. Fibrinogen may also be measured as total clottable material or by an immunoassay, which measures fibrinogen antigen, independent of activity.[29,31]

Fibrinogen-Fibrin Degradation Products (FDP)/D-Dimer Test

These assays assist in detecting and quantitating the products of degradation of fibrin. The D-dimer assay, which has largely replaced the FDP assay, measures levels of cross-linked fibrin degradation products, the D-dimer.[29,32] D-dimer levels are elevated in various settings of intravascular coagulation. The FDP assay measures degradation products of fibrinogen, as well as fibrin, and therefore is less specific.

Bleeding Time

The bleeding time (BT) is a measure of the time required for clotting of a standardized cutaneous laceration. The BT reflects the primary mechanisms of hemostasis, i.e. platelet and microvasculature. The Ivy bleeding time (BT) is performed by making a cut in the skin with a standardized template, while a blood pressure cuff is applied.[29,33] Under normal circumstances, bleeding from the laceration ceases within 9 minutes, but due to variability of the assay between technicians, each institution must standardize its BT. Prolongation of the BT suggests a defect of the platelet-vessel interaction, due to (1) vascular abnormalities, (2) moderate-to-severe thrombocytopenia, or (3) platelet dysfunction. Mild thrombocytopenia will not prolong the BT if the platelet function and the vasculature are intact. Platelet levels below 100,000/ul will typically prolong the BT.[34] Hereditary or acquired platelet dysfunction will prolong the BT and vWD, in which platelet adhesion is defective, is associated with a prolonged BT. The BT is an imprecise test, with significant false positive and false negative rates. Therefore, it is not appropriate as a screening test, but is useful in characterizing the underlying cause of a clinically evident hemorrhagic diathesis.[26]

Platelet Aggregation/Agglutination Assays

In vitro platelet activation and aggregation in response to a number of agonists may be measured in an aggregometer. Addition of aggregating agents to samples of platelet-rich plasma normally results in an increase in light transmission, reflecting platelet activation and aggregation.[29] Commonly used aggregating agents include epinephrine, collagen, and ADP. Arachidonic acid and thrombin are also tested under some circumstances. Platelet aggregation to agonists such as ADP, is normally a biphasic process. The first phase is in response to the exogenous agonist, and the second phase follows the additional stimulation by the platelet components secreted in the release reaction. Ristocetin induces platelet agglutination in the presence of adequate levels of von Willebrand factor (vWF) and the platelet vWF receptor.[29,35] This process is referred to as agglutination since it is a passive process, independent of platelet metabolic activity. In contrast, true aggregation requires viable platelets. As Ristocetin-induced agglutination is a passive process, a single phase response is observed. Ristocetin-induced agglutination is routinely included in the panel of platelet "aggregation" studies.

Specific Factor Assays

Specific factor assays are based on mixing test plasma with an excess volume of a standardized plasma deficient in a single factor and performing a PT or aPTT. The resultant PT or aPTT will therefore be a function of the level of the specific factor in the test plasma. Immunoassays are also available to measure the amount of the specific factor proteins, independent of functional activity.

Other Tests

Numerous other assays are available to characterize the coagulation system in an individual. The activated coagulation time (ACT) is infrequently used, but is a valuable tool during some operative procedures, particularly during cardiopulmonary bypass, because of the rapidity of the results, and the ability of the test to be performed in the operative room. The ACT may be used in lieu of the aPTT to monitor heparin anticoagulation.[36]

The thromboelastogram (TEG) is an assay that measures several phases of the blood coagulation system, including the levels and activity of the soluble coagulation factors and platelets, and the fibrinolytic system. The TEG is infrequently used, but it has been used in intraoperative settings, where deficiencies of coagulation factors and platelets develop rapidly, and the rapidity of the TEG has been valuable to guide replacement therapy.[37]

Protein C, protein S, antithrombin III, heparin cofactor II, and plasminogen may currently be assayed by functional and/or immunoassay techniques. Immunoassays are also generally available for the procoagulant factors, and assist in characterizing the nature of the functional defects which may be found.

HEREDITARY HEMORRHAGIC DIATHESES

Hemophilia

Recorded descriptions of hemophilia date to ancient times, when Talmudic rabbis recognized the sex-linked inheritance of this hemorrhagic disease.[38] Hemophilia A and B are X-linked deficiencies of factor VIII and IX, re-

Table 13–2. Properties of Moeities Involved in Blood Coagulation

Type	Name*	Molecular Weight, daltons	Plasma Concentration		Intravascular Half-time, days
			μg/ml	nM	
Contact system	F XII	80,000	29	360	2
proenzymes	Prekallikrein	88,000	45	510	—
	F XI	160,000	4†	25^b	2.5
Vitamin K-dependent	F VII	50,000	0.5	10	0.2
coagulant	F IX	57,000	4	70	1
proenzymes	F X	57,000	8	140	1.5
	Prothrombin	70,000	150	2.1×10^3	3
Cofactors	Tissue factor	—	0	0	
	Platelet lipid	—	0	0	
	HMW kininogen	120,000	70	583	—
	Factor V	300,000	7	21	1.5
	Factor VIII	300,000	0.2	0.3	0.5
	Protein S	69,000	25	348	—
Factors of fibrin	Fibrinogen	340,000	2500	7.0×10^3	4.5
deposition	F XIII	320,000	8	25	7
Inhibitors	Protein C	62,000	4	66	0.3
	Antithrombin III	58,000	150	2.6×10^3	2.5
	EPI	~40,000	0.1	~3	—

*Abbreviations are as follows: F, factor; HMW, high molecular weight; EPI, extrinsic pathway inhibitor. EPI is also referred to as LACI (lipoprotein-associated coagulation inhibitor).
†A dimer with two active enzymatic sites per molecule; therefore, the functional concentration is double the value given.
From Rappaport, S. I.: Hemostasis. In *Best & Taylor's Physiological Basis of Medical Practice*, 12th Ed. Edited by J. B. West, Baltimore, Williams & Wilkins, 1990.

spectively. Approximately 1 in 5,000 males are born with hemophilia, 85% of them with factor VIII deficiency, 15% with factor IX deficiency.[39] These individuals experience a range of hemorrhagic complications, including hemarthroses (joint bleeding), and deep muscle and subcutaneous hematomas, posttraumatic and postoperative bleeding, and intracranial hemorrhage. The severity of the hemorrhagic tendency is a function of the factor levels. Hemophilia results in elevated aPTT with normal PT, fibrinogen, and platelet counts. Hemophilia A and B can not be distinguished by clinical criteria, but by measurement of the specific factor VIII and IX levels (Table 13–3).

Management

A number of measures are available to improve hemostasis in individuals with hemophilia A and B. Desmopressin (DDAVP) at 0.3 μg/kg administered intravenously acts to promote accelerated release of the preformed factor VIII complex, and leads to an increase in factor VIII levels of two to three fold within 30 to 60 minutes.[40] In mild and moderately affected individuals with hemophilia A (or von Willebrand's disease) this may provide adequate hemostasis for elective surgical procedures. Because of depletion of the factor VIII complex from the pre-released pool, repeat doses of DDAVP are less effective if administered within 24 hours.

The mainstay of therapy is factor replacement. While fresh frozen plasma (FFP) contains factors VIII and IX, and may be used in emergency settings, factor concentrates are the material of choice. Current factor concentrates include a variety of measures, including heat and detergent treatment, and/or monoclonal antibody purifi-

Table 13–3. Clinical Classification of Hemophilia

Classification	Factor Level (% of normal)	Clinical Features
Severe	≤1% (≤0.01 U/ml)	Spontaneous hemorrhage from multiple sites. At risk for development of inhibitor.
Moderate	1–5%	Postsurgical and posttraumatic hemorrhage. Occasional spontaneous hemorrhage.
Mild	6–50%	Variable postsurgical and posttraumatic hemorrhage. Spontaneous hemorrhage rare.

cation to eliminate the risk of viral pathogen transmission. The following are useful guidelines to predict the factor levels achieved with infusion of factor VIII and factor IX concentrates:[41]

Increase in factors VIII level = 2 X (Units of factor VIII) / Weight (kg)
Increase in factor IX level = 1 X (Units of factor IX) / Weight (kg)

The responses are approximations, in the absence of inhibitors. The differences in the dose calculation for factor VIII and IX reflect differences in the volume of distribution. Factor VIII should be administered every 12 hours and factor IX may be administered every 24 hours, reflecting the differences in half-life of the proteins in vivo. The factor level required is a function on the severity of the hemorrhagic challenge, and the risk of bleeding. For major risks; such as for head trauma, and major surgery, levels of 50% to 100% must be maintained. For intermediate risk situations, such as hemarthroses, and superficial hematomas, 30% to 50% levels are sufficient. Similarly the duration of therapy reflects the challenge. Following major surgery, maintenance of the factor level in the 30 to 50% range for up to 10 to 14 days may be necessary, while a single infusion may be adequate for individuals experiencing a hemarthrosis.[41]

Some factor IX concentrates are complexes of the vitamin K dependent factors, and therefore contain prothrombin (factor II), factors VII, IX, and X, as well as protein C and protein S. They are also referred to as prothrombin complex concentrate (PCC). Newer factor IX concentrates are more purified and have negligible levels of the other factors. All current products have been virally inactivated to reduce or eliminate the risk and hepatitis and eliminate the risk of HIV. While earlier generations of concentrate conferred a thrombotic risk due to the presence of activated factors, this too has been rectified in current products.

Antifibrinolytic agents include ε-aminocaproic acid (EACA) and tranexamic acid. These agents help to stabilize clots and are used as an adjuvant in settings of dental procedures.[42,43] They are also used to block severe systemic fibrinolysis (Table 13–4).

Inhibitors in Hemophilia

One of the most problematic complications which may occur in a patient with hemophilia is the development of antibodies to the deficient factor. Typically, inhibitors occur in patients who have the most severe variants of hemophilia (factor levels of <1%).[45] The antibodies are usually of the IgG class. Management of patients with inhibitors is problematic. Replacement therapy with large amounts of factor concentrates may provide temporary control of hemorrhage, but will also stimulate an increase in the antibody titer. An alternative approach is the infusion of agents that "bypass" the inhibitor. These agents include activated prothrombin complex concentrates (APCC) which contain partially activated vitamin K-dependent enzymes, and recombinant factor VIIa. APCC

(Autoplex, FEIBA) is infused at 75 U/kg, and may be repeated every 12–24 hours. Recombinant factor VIIa is not yet available in the U.S.A. except on a compassionate basis. These preparations "bypass" the inhibitor, due to activated forms of one or more of the vitamin K-dependent enzymes.[46] They are indicated for control of hemorrhage, but are inappropriate as prophylactic agents. Other agents include porcine factor VIII, which may be sufficiently distinct antigenically, yet functionally related, to allow for hemostasis despite the presence of an anti-human factor VII antibody. A number of protocols have been tested to reduce the titer of the antibodies, with varying results.[47-49]

von Willebrand's Disease

von Willebrand's disease (vWD) is the most common hereditary hemorrhagic diathesis. Incidence estimates are as high as 1 to 2%.[50] Affected individuals experience a mucocutaneous pattern of bleeding, demonstrating epistaxis, gastrointestinal bleeding, menorrhagia, petechiae, and purpura. The majority of individuals have one of the dominant types of vWD (types I and II), but rare individuals are homozygous (type III). The vWD types reflect the electrophoretic patterns of the multimers of the von Willebrand factor protein complex.[51,52] The larger molecular weight species possess markedly greater ability to facilitate platelet adhesion in vitro and in vivo. In type I vWD all of the multimers are symmetrically reduced, in type II the large multimers are disproportionately reduced, and in type III all multimers are absent. More subtle variations have led to subtyping of vWD.[52]

Clinical and laboratory manifestations of vWD are variable between individuals, and within an affected patient with time. Typical laboratory abnormalities include prolonged BT, elevated aPTT, and defective Ristocetin-induced platelet agglutination. Levels of von Willebrand factor (Ristocetin cofactor activity), factor VIII coagulant activity, and vWF antigen (factor VIII associated antigen) are also typically reduced.[52] The degree of deficiencies of these factors varies with time, and the absence of one or more factor VIII or vWF-related parameter does not rule out the presence of vWD.

DDAVP and replacement therapy are the primary mode of management.[40] As noted, DDAVP induces accelerated release of the factor VIII:vWF complex, particularly the large molecular weight forms. Dosage is 0.2 to 0.4 μg/kg administered intravenously in 50 ml of saline over 15 to 30 minutes. The response is typically within 30 minutes and lasts 6 or more hours. The response to DDAVP is related to the subtype of vWD. In the majority of patients with types I and some with IIA vWD, the factor VIII:vWF complex levels will rise and the clinical picture will improve temporarily with DDAVP therapy. Type III vWD does not improve with DDAVP. DDAVP is contraindicated in patients with Type IIB vWD, as altered interactions between their vWF and platelets may induce platelet activation and thrombocytopenia.[40,52] Because of the variable response to DDAVP, it is recommended to give a test dose of DDAVP to determine the potential efficacy in any newly diagnosed case of vWD. Individuals who are within a pedigree of type IIB, or known to have

Table 13–4. Recommended Doses of Antifibrinolytic Agents

Agent	Route of Administration	Recommended Dose
ε-Aminocaproic Acid	Intravenous or Oral	4g/4 hr
Tranexamic Acid	Intravenous	0.5g/8 hr
	Oral	1.5g/8 hr
	Mouthwashes	1.0g/6 hr

Modified from Mannucci, P. M.: Nontransfusional modalities. In *Thrombosis and Hemorrhage.* Edited by J. Loscalzo and A. Schafer. Boston, Blackwell Scientific, 1994, pp. 1117–1135.

type IIB based on aggregation and multimer studies, should not be given a DDAVP trial. Because of tachyphylaxis, DDAVP is less effective if administered within 24 to 48 hours of the previous dose.

Cryoprecipitate, derived from normal donor plasma, is enriched for vWF, and has been the replacement fluid of choice.[41,52] One unit of cryoprecipitate is derived from the plasma from a single unit of whole blood. The dosing is less precise than for hemophilia, but a useful guideline for significant hemorrhage or surgical hemostasis, is infusion of 1 unit of cryoprecipitate per 10 kg, which may be repeated every 8 to 24 hours. Dose adjustment and duration depend upon the hemostatic challenge. Volume overload may limit the dose of cryoprecipitate, and cryoprecipitate is associated with a risk of transfusion-associated viral infection. While most factor VIII concentrates contain vWF antigen, the multimers present are the smaller forms with limited platelet cofactor activity. Therefore they are not appropriate for treatment of vWD.[41,52] A new concentrate, Humate-P (Armour), possesses a richer complement of the larger multimers and is now available for treatment of vWD. Because Humate-P is virally inactivated, and provides less of a volume load than cryoprecipitate, it offers distinct advantages for the management of patients with vWD in whom DDAVP does not provide sufficient correction.

Factor XI Deficiency

Factor XI deficiency is an autosomal disorder which is extremely rare except among Ashkenazi (Eastern European) Jews. Some heterozygous individuals and most homozygous individuals exhibit a bleeding tendency following trauma and/or surgery. There is only limited correlation between factor XI activity levels and the hemorrhagic tendency in a given patient.[53] The aPTT will be prolonged by the factor XI deficiency, and factor XI deficiency should be included in the differential diagnosis of an individual with a prolonged aPTT and a normal PT, particularly if the patient is an Ashkenazi Jew. The management of factor XI deficiency is with FFP infusion 6 to 8 hours prior to scheduled surgery, or as soon as possible for trauma or urgent surgery. A dose of 15–20 ml/kg of FFP as a loading dose, followed by 3 to 6 ml/kg every 12 to 24 hours will provide hemostasis.[54] The required duration of therapy is dependent upon the severity of the hemostatic challenge. As with hemophilia A and B, inhibitors to the deficient factor (factor XI) may develop.

Other Hereditary Hemorrhagic Disorders

A number of other hereditary hemorrhagic disorders have been identified, but these are uncommon. Hereditary deficiencies of factors II (prothrombin), V, VII, X have each been described, and are associated with varying degrees of a hemorrhagic tendency.[54] These are autosomal diatheses. Management of these deficiencies may be with infusion of FFP, or PCC for deficiencies of prothrombin, factor VII, or factor X. Hereditary deficiencies of the contact system (factor XII, prekallikrein, and high molecular weight kininogen) are associated with a markedly prolonged aPTT, a normal PT and BT, but no hemorrhagic tendency. Factor XII deficiency is paradoxically associated with a thrombotic tendency. If deficiency of factor XII, prekallikrein, and high molecular weight kininogen has been identified as the only cause of prolonged aPTT, surgery may be carried out with only routine measures.[54]

Factor XIII deficiency is a rare autosomal recessive diathesis characterized by slow wound healing, and often delayed bleeding from an operative site.[54,55] Often a history of umbilical bleeding as a neonate is present. It is important to note that the routine screening tests including the PT, aPTT, and BT are normal, and therefore only the history will provide warning of the presence of this disorder. In vitro tests of clot solubility or specific assays of factor XIII will confirm the diagnosis.[54,56]

A variety of hereditary fibrinogen disorders have been described, including relative and absolute deficiencies of the protein (hypofibrinogenemia, afibrinogenemia), or structural abnormalities of the protein (dysfibrinogenemia).[31,54] In some instances the disorder is characterized by both hypo- and dysfibrinogenemia. Hypofibrinogenemia is very rare and may be autosomal recessive or dominant. It is usually associated with a hemorrhagic tendency. Dysfibrinogenemias are autosomal dominant, and cause a more varied clinical picture. Different mutations may be associated with clinical syndromes of a hemorrhagic tendency, a thrombotic tendency, a mixed picture of both hemorrhage and thrombosis, or may be asymptomatic. Abnormalities or deficiencies of fibrinogen may prolong the aPTT and PT, but these tests are relatively insensitive to mild or moderate abnormalities, and the degree of prolongation is variable. The thrombin Time (TT) is a more sensitive test for the adequacy of fibrinogen and a modified TT is the standard functional measurement for fibrinogen. The presence of heparin or fibrin degradation products will prolong the TT and may result in spuriously reduced fibrinogen functional measurements. Therefore, these must be considered in the differential diagnosis of a laboratory report of fibrinogen deficiency, as they are more common than a true fibrinogen deficiency. If a dysfibrinogen is suspected, immunologic measurements may indicate if the patient has a dysfibrinogen or hypofibrinogenemia. Therapy for hypofibrinogenemia or dysfibrinogenemia is by replacement with cryoprecipitate.

Hereditary Platelet Function Abnormalities

Hereditary disorders of platelet function are rare and are associated with mild to moderate spontaneous and posttraumatic bleeding. The bleeding pattern is usually of a mucocutaneous nature. The BT is variably prolonged and there is a poor correlation between the degree of hemorrhagic tendency and the BT. Bernard Soulier syndrome (BSS) is an autosomal recessive deficiency of the vWF receptor, and is characterized by defects in Ristocetin-induced agglutination of platelet rich plasma.[57,58] The vWF levels, by immunologic and functional measurements, are normal. The platelets may be abnormally large, and often mild thrombocytopenia is present.

Glanzmann's thrombasthenia, also autosomal recessive, is characterized by absent aggregation to all agents, except Ristocetin, due to deficiency of the GP IIB/IIIA receptor complex.[59] Storage pool diseases (SPD) represent deficiencies of the dense granules (δ-SPD), the alpha granules (α-SPD or Gray platelet syndrome), or both ($\alpha\delta$-SPD).[58,60] Aggregation studies in SPD reveal a loss of the second wave of platelet aggregation due to deficient release of granule content. Bernard Soulier syndrome, Glanzmann's thrombasthenia, and storage pool disease are characterized by a mucocutaneous pattern of bleeding, discussed above. Therapeutic approaches for patients with hereditary disorders of platelet function is largely supportive. When essential for hemostatic control, platelet infusions may be administered. However, platelet transfusions in patients with BSS or GT often results in alloimmunization, with subsequent refractoriness to platelet transfusion. Therefore platelet transfusions should be employed only if the necessity is clear.[58]

A number of rare hereditary syndromes are associated with thrombocytopenia, including Thrombocytopenia-Absent Radii (TAR) syndrome, Chediak Higashi syndrome (oculocutaneous albinism, and recurrent infection with thrombocytopenia), and Wiskott-Aldrich syndrome (X-linked syndrome of eczema, recurrent infections, and failure of lymphoid maturation).

Vascular Disorders Associated with a Bleeding Tendency

A number of congenital syndromes are associated with localized abnormalities of the vasculature. Hemangiomas of infancy or childhood represent a localized malformation of capillaries, and may be associated with a marked tendency to bleed. Kasabach-Merritt syndrome is characterized by a consumptive coagulopathy with microangiopathic hemolytic anemia resulting from a giant cavernous hemangioma.[61]

Hereditary hemorrhagic telangiectasia is an autosomal dominant diathesis, also referred to as Osler-Weber-Rendu syndrome.[62] Telangiectasias are observed on oral, nasal, and gastrointestinal mucosa, and less frequently, cutaneous surfaces and internal organs. For unknown reasons, the lesions may not become apparent until adulthood. The fragile vessels of the telangiectasias are prone to hemorrhage, and epistaxis and gastrointestinal hemorrhage are common. Local measures, such as cautery, may contribute to hemostasis. This syndrome may complicate tracheal intubation, as the intubation may result in marked hemorrhage.

Osteogenesis imperfecta, Marfan's syndrome, and Ehlers-Danlos syndrome are disorders of connective tissue and may be associated with friability of the vasculature, with an increased risk of bleeding.[63]

ACQUIRED HEMOSTATIC DEFECTS

A great number of acquired diseases are associated with an increased risk of hemorrhage. The more common, or more significant of these is discussed below, but this list is not all inclusive.

Thrombocytopenia

Thrombocytopenia is one of the most common acquired hemostatic defects. Thrombocytopenia may result from decreased production of platelets, increased destruction, or splenic sequestration. The approach to the patient with thrombocytopenia requires an evaluation of the complete blood count with peripheral smear, measurement of the PT, aPTT, and fibrinogen level, and often a bone marrow aspirate and biopsy. Platelet clumping in the peripheral smear may suggest the presence of EDTA-dependent antiplatelet antibodies, which results in a spurious reduction in the platelet count in individuals who actually have normal counts.[64] Anisocytosis and/or poikylocytosis of red cells suggests a more disseminated process. Presence of immature white cells, or nucleated red cells in the peripheral circulation, may result from marrow infiltration with metastatic cancer, a myeloproliferative disorder, leukemia, or some infectious processes. If the PT and aPTT are prolonged, with a reduction in fibrinogen, disseminated intravascular coagulation (DIC) is suggested. DIC is discussed below.

Although normal platelet counts are from 150,000 to 450,000/μl, if platelet function is intact, increased post-traumatic or operative bleeding is observed only when the platelet count drops below 50,000. Post-traumatic bleeding and purpura will be observed if the count decreases to less than 30,000 to 50,000/μl. Spontaneous bleeding is observed with counts less than 20,000 to 30,000/μl.[65]

Immune Thrombocytopenic Purpura

Immune thrombocytopenic purpura (ITP) had previously stood for idiopathic thrombocytopenic purpura, but is now known to be due to the presence of antiplatelet antibodies. In general, ITP is characterized by preservation of the red and white cell numbers, and an increase in megakaryocytes in the bone marrow.[66-68] ITP may be drug induced, AIDS associated, post-viral infection, or idiopathic. An acute form, more common in children and young adults, may manifest as a single episode of thrombocytopenia with petechiae, purpura, and a mucocutaneous pattern of bleeding. The majority of adults will experience a chronic relapsing form of ITP. The diagnosis of ITP is supported by the presence of moderate to severe thrombocytopenia, with normal PT, aPTT, and fibrinogen. Certain drugs, or metabolites of the drugs, can form circulating complexes with plasma proteins, and induce an antibody to this complex. The antibody:antigen complex may then bind to circulating platelets, followed by premature clearance via the Fc receptors of macrophages of the reticuloendothelial system in the spleen and other organs. Platelets may also be lysed intravascularly by complement activation. Numerous drugs may cause immune-mediated thrombocytopenia. Quinine, quinidine, chlorothiazides, procainamide, valproic acid, sulfonamides, penicillin and other β-lactam-containing antibiotics are well known to cause immune-mediated thrombocytopenia, but numerous other drugs may cause this syndrome as well.[68] Heparin-dependent antiplatelet antibody may be associated with activation of platelets, and a microangiopathic syndrome, as well as thrombocytopenic purpura. As the antibody binding requires the presence of the drug or its metabolite, discontinuation of the offending agent leads to prompt normalization of thrombocytopenia, within days or weeks.

The clinical manifestations of ITP are a function of the degree of thrombocytopenia, as the remaining platelets are usually normal in function. In a minority of patients, the antiplatelet antibody may inhibit function, thus compounding the hemorrhagic risk. Several approaches are available for the management of ITP. If an inciting drug is suspected, of course discontinuation of the agent is essential. For chronic ITP, in a non-emergent setting, glucocorticoid therapy (prednisone at 1 mg/kg/day) is the first choice. Improvement in platelet counts may follow within several days to several weeks. The effect is due to inhibition of macrophage clearance of the platelets, and/or reduction in antibody titers. A majority of patients with idiopathic ITP will respond to glucocorticoids, but treatment failure results in approximately a third of patients treated with glucocorticoids.

For a more prompt response, as would be indicated for a patient with an active hemorrhage or impending need for surgery, high dose intravenous gammaglobulin (IVIG) may be helpful. This is given as 2 g/kg intravenously, in divided doses over 2 or 5 days.[69] Because a rare patient may experience anaphylaxis due to IgA deficiency, a small test dose is essential before administering the full dose. The beneficial effect is believed due to blockade of the macrophage Fc receptors. Improvement in platelet counts may be as soon as two or three days after therapy. The improvement is only temporary, often only weeks or less, and the cost is significantly greater that glucocorticoids. However, in the setting of a patient in urgent need for surgery, IVIG may be clearly indicated.

Patients with chronic relapsing ITP, who fail to experience durable remissions with glucocorticoids, may undergo splenectomy.[70] Splenectomy will often reduce the frequency and severity of thrombocytopenic relapses. If this is to be performed nonemergently, normalization of the platelet count by glucocorticoids or IVIG may reduce the operative bleeding. However, splenectomies have been performed for chronic ITP, during acute thrombocytopenic episodes, without undo hemorrhagic complications.

Platelet transfusions have been of some benefit as well, and should be considered in life-threatening situations. Although the magnitude and the duration of the increment to platelet transfusion will be blunted in ITP, platelet transfusions may provide a clinical benefit if IVIG or glucocorticoid therapy have not been implemented. If drug-induced ITP is present, and the drug has been discontinued for sufficient time for the offending drug and/or its metabolites to be cleared, the patient should experience a normal increment to platelet infusion.

Other Immune-Mediated Thrombocytopenia Syndromes

Post-transfusion purpura is a rare syndrome in which patients develop profound thrombocytopenia approximately 6 to 10 days after receiving a red cell transfusion. Many of the cases occur in multiparous women, or individuals who have been previously transfused. The mechanism is believed to be related to the recipient having a rare platelet antigen type, such as PLA1 negative, and developing antibodies to the PLA1 positive platelets in the donor blood product. Why the patients' platelets, which lack the PLA1 antigen, are also affected is not known.

Nonimmune Thrombocytopenia

Thrombotic thrombocytopenic purpura (TTP), and hemolytic-uremic syndrome (HUS) are two related syndromes. TTP is characterized by the clinical pentad of (1) thrombocytopenia, (2) microangiopathic hemolytic anemia, (3) fever, (4) fluctuating neurologic signs, and (5) renal abnormalities.[71] In HUS there are similar findings, except neurologic signs and fever are rare. The etiology of these syndromes remains unknown, although some evidence suggests endothelial cell dysfunction may contribute. Patients experience tissue ischemia due to microangiopathic hemolytic anemia, which contributes to the neurologic and renal abnormalities. The thrombocytopenia is due to platelet consumption, but normal PT and aPTT, and fibrinogen levels are the rule, indicating the consumption is distinct from disseminated intravascular coagulation (DIC). Laboratory findings will include thrombocytopenia, anemia, elevated LDH, schistocytes in the peripheral blood smear, and often hematuria, and/or azotemia.

Up until the 1980s, the mortality from TTP and HUS exceeded 75%. Fortunately, management has improved markedly and the survival rate is currently over 75% if patients are appropriately managed.[72,73] Firstly, platelet transfusion, regardless of the level of thrombocytopenia, is strictly contraindicated, as activation of the platelets contributes to the MAHA, tissue ischemia, and morbidity and mortality. Secondly, immediate transfusion of fresh frozen plasma (FFP), followed by plasmapheresis with FFP replacement, has been shown to dramatically reduce the pathologic process. The mechanism for the improvement with plasmapheresis and FFP transfusion is still unknown. Because of the marked contraindication to platelet transfusion, it is incumbent on all practitioners to consider TTP or HUS in any patient with thrombocytopenia before platelet transfusions are given.

Sequestration

Normally, approximately one third of the platelet mass is in the splenic circulation, but a variety of disorders are associated with hypersplenism, and increased sequestration of platelets. Cirrhosis and secondary portal hypertension, splenic lymphoma, sarcoidosis, or metabolic disorders such as Gaucher's disease, also may result in hypersplenism, and thrombocytopenia. The thrombocytopenia from hypersplenism/sequestration is typically mild. However, splenic sequestration may contribute an additive effect in the setting of other causes of thrombocytopenia.

Other Causes of Thrombocytopenia

Two situations related to surgery may contribute to thrombocytopenia. Dilutional thrombocytopenia is observed in the patient who requires massive transfusion due to trauma or complications of surgery, typically with replacement of the patient's blood volume with red cells and fresh frozen plasma.[74] The resultant thrombocytopenia is typically mild to moderate (50,000 to 100,000/μl), and unless a systemic coagulopathy is present, platelet transfusions are not indicated. Extracorporeal circulation, as occurs in cardiopulmonary bypass, is associated with a low level of platelet activation, and degranulation. Thrombocytopenia may ensue, and the degranulated platelets may exhibit an acquired storage pool deficiency phenotype, deficient in their ability to sustain and propagate a clot in vivo.

Decreased Platelet Production

The bone marrow, the site of platelet production by megakaryocytes as well as production of other blood cell components, is prone to injury by a variety of agents. Chemotherapy and/or radiation therapy for cancer treatment, will often acutely suppress the bone marrow. Usually within several weeks of therapy the blood counts return to normal. High cumulative doses of these therapies may irreversibly reduce hematologic precursors, resulting in permanent pancytopenia. Some drugs, and chemical toxins such as alcohol, are also known to cause marrow toxicity, with resultant thrombocytopenia, and possibly, pancytopenia. Other drugs which induce thrombocytopenia do so via an immune-mediated mechanism.[75]

Infiltration of the bone marrow by a variety of disease processes may also cause pancytopenia. Leukemia, lymphoma, and metastatic carcinoma are neoplastic processes which often reduce platelet (and other blood cell) production. Disseminated tuberculosis, and some fungal infections may also invade and suppress normal marrow function.

Myelodysplastic syndromes are associated with a primary refractory anemia, typically with suppression of the white cells and platelets as well. Agnogenic myelofibrosis with myeloid metaplasia is a myeloproliferative disorder, associated with reticulin deposition in the marrow, presumably due to fibroblast stimulation by an abnormal population of megakaryocytes. The reticulin prevents the hematopoietic precursors from normally proliferating and maturation. Other myeloproliferative disorders, such as polycythemia vera, may result in a "spent phase" in which normal hematopoietic precursors are depleted, often with associated toxic changes in the marrow.

Megaloblastic anemia results from folate or vitamin B12 deficiency. Defective DNA synthesis leads to pancytopenia, with hypersegmented granulocytes in the peripheral circulation, and a distinct pattern of abnormal nuclear chromatin in the erythroid precursors in the bone marrow. Aplastic anemia may be idiopathic or in response to various toxic injuries to the bone marrow. Aplastic anemia is associated with pancytopenia, although the severity of involvement of the different hematologic lines may vary.

Acquired Platelet Defects

A number of disease processes, as well as drugs, may result in acquired platelet dysfunction. Uremia and nonsteroidal anti-inflammatory drugs are two of the more common ones.

Uremia

The association of acquired platelet dysfunction with uremia has been well recognized although the mechanism for this dysfunction is not known.[76] Uremic individuals experience an increased tendency for mucocuta-

neous-type bleeding. Administration of 0.3 to 0.4 $\mu g/kg$ IV of DDAVP (desmopressin)[40] and cryoprecipitate transfusion[77] have been associated with improvement in the BT and the hemorrhagic tendency. These two therapies increase the large molecular weight multimers of vWF, suggesting a possible pathophysiologic role of vWF in the uremic bleeding tendency. Normalization of the anemia typically associated with chronic renal failure, by erythropoietin or transfusion will also improve the hemorrhagic tendency.[78,79]

Nonsteroidal Anti-Inflammatory Drugs

Aspirin acetylates and permanently inactivates platelet cyclooxygenase. The resultant defect in platelet thromboxane A2 synthesis from arachidonic acid is associated with reduced platelet activity. Other nonsteroidal anti-inflammatory drugs, such as ibuprofen and indomethecin, also inhibit platelet cyclooxygenase, therefore inhibiting platelet function. Therefore, patients who have ingested nonsteroidal anti-inflammatory drugs may experience a mild defect in the primary phase of hemostasis.

OTHER COAGULATION DISORDERS

Disseminated Intravascular Coagulation

Disseminated intravascular coagulation (DIC) results from a wide spectrum of clinical disorders, and is characterized by an inappropriate activation of the coagulation system. (Further details are provided in Chapter 14). DIC may range from clinically mild, and only detectable by abnormal laboratory results, to a severe life-threatening hemorrhagic diathesis.[80] Sepsis, particularly with gram-negative bacteria, and obstetrical complications, such as retained products of conception, are well recognized to cause fulminant DIC. Endotoxin from bacteria is a major stimulus for DIC, but other microorganism and leukocyte constituents may also cause intravascular coagulation. Tissue factor and possibly other factors released from necrotic tissue may result in DIC, as in obstetrical complications as well as from malignancies, tissue injuries from trauma and ischemia.[81]

Management of DIC requires correction of the underlying pathologic process. Replacement of depleted coagulation factors with fresh frozen plasma and cryoprecipitate, and platelet transfusions for thrombocytopenia, may reduce the hemorrhagic complications (see Chapter 14). Concerns that transfusions could worsen the DIC by adding "fuel to the fire" have not been borne out,[82] but prudence is always warranted in administering transfusions. Administration of antithrombin III concentrate has shown promise in managing acute DIC.[83]

Liver Failure

As the liver is the site of synthesis of most of the coagulation factors, many diseases associated with reduced hepatic function result in a hemorrhagic tendency. Empirically, in most individuals with hepatic dysfunction, the PT will be prolonged in greater proportion to the aPTT from decreased factor production.[84,85] Liver failure is also often associated with acquired dysfibrinogenemia and platelet dysfunction. Portal hypertension leading to hypersplenism, may contribute to thrombocytopenia. If surgery or other invasive intervention is necessary, transfusion of FFP and possibly cryoprecipitate, will improve the factor deficiencies. Vitamin K deficiency is at times superimposed upon hepatic dysfunction, and an empiric trial of vitamin K may further contribute to hemostasis.

Acquired Inhibitors

Acquired immune inhibitors to one or more of the coagulation factors may arise in the adult patient. Although acquired inhibitors often occur spontaneously, they occur more often in elderly patients, postpartum women, and patients with autoimmune diseases, lymphoproliferative diseases, or cancer. These inhibitors bind to the involved factor and lead to factor deficiency and a significant hemorrhagic diathesis.[86] Management of these patients may be as difficult as the severe hemophiliac who develops an inhibitor, except factor infusion is not associated with an increase in the antibody titer. For emergent hemostatic control, administration of high doses of factor concentrate or fresh frozen plasma may be of benefit.

The Lupus Anticoagulant

The lupus anticoagulant (LA) is an antiphospholipid antibody that characteristically prolongs the aPTT.[87] Although patients with systemic lupus or other connective tissue diseases may manifest the LA, many patients with the LA do not have a connective tissue disorder. A syndrome of arterial or venous thrombosis, recurrent spontaneous abortion, and thrombocytopenia is associated with the LA.[87,88] Patients with the LA syndrome may also experience cardiac valvular lesions.[87] Although the LA prolongs the aPTT, typically there is no hemorrhagic tendency, unless the PT is also prolonged. In this subset of patients, an anti-prothrombin antibody has been described,[89] which may cause a hemorrhagic diathesis.

Vascular Lesions

Henoch-Schonlein purpura (HSP) may follow viral or bacterial infection, or exposure to chemical (or pharmaceutical) toxins. Usually occurring in children, HSP is a result of immune complex deposition in the vascular tissue, with secondary complement activation and neutrophil recruitment, and vascular injury.[90] The disorder is characterized by purpura, arthralgias, glomerulonephritis, and abdominal pain. The purpuric lesions are raised, and referred to as "palpable purpura." Patients with Cushing's syndrome, or patients receiving long-term glucocorticoids will experience altered collagen and connective tissue synthesis, and prone to purpura. Elderly individuals also manifest vascular fragility. A variety of syndromes may include a component of vascular fragility and a tendency to purpura.

THROMBOEMBOLIC DISEASE

Pathogenesis

Although operative hemorrhage has appropriately been a great concern of physicians and surgeons, a greater number of patients suffer operative-related mortality from venous thrombosis and associated pulmonary embolism. Virchow's triad, dating from the nineteenth century, remains the fundamental understanding of the pathophysiology of thrombosis. Thrombosis results from three factors, (1) an alteration in the blood vessel, (2) an alteration in the blood flow, and (3) an increase in the inherent coagulability of the blood.[91] In the surgical patient, decreased activity and ambulation is associated with venous stasis (alteration in flow). Tissue damage, from surgery or trauma, is associated with release of tissue factor, and possibly other factors which leads to an increase in activation of the clotting system (alteration in the coagulability of the blood). Alteration of specific portions of the vasculature may result from trauma or surgery. Prior venous thrombosis (post-phlebitic syndrome) will predispose to recurrent thrombosis due to a loss of the venous valves as well as other sequellae of the previous luminal thrombus. Hereditary deficiency of antithrombin III, protein C, protein S, or plasminogen, as well as some variants of hereditary dysfibrinogenemia, are known to predispose to thromboembolism.[92,93] Other hereditary defects may also be associated with a thrombotic risk, such as heparin cofactor II deficiency, homocystinemia, and excess plasminogen activator inhibitor levels (Table 13-5).

Incidence

In general surgical patients who do not receive prophylaxis for thrombosis, there is a 25% incidence of thrombosis,[94] and 40 to 70% incidence in high risk orthopedic patients.[94,95] The general medical inpatient, particularly those at bed rest such as following myocardial infarction or stroke, are also at risk for development of thrombosis. Routine use of minidose heparin prophylaxis reduces mortality during hospitalization in the medical as well as surgical patient.[94,96]

Prophylaxis

The most important consideration is prevention of thromboembolic disease with appropriate prophylactic measures. While intermittent compression boots are useful in reducing the incidence of thrombosis in immobilized and postoperative patients, they are not as effective as anticoagulant therapy (Table 13-6)[94,97] summarizes current guidelines for prophylaxis of thromboembolism in the hospitalized patients. The general medical and sur-

Table 13–5. Acquired Hypercoagulable States

Disease State	Mechanism of Hypercoagulability
Cancer	Release of tissue factor
Lupus anticoagulant	Possible endothelial cell toxicity
Myeloproliferative diseases	Alteration in platelet activity
	Hyperviscosity in setting of polycythemia
Nephrotic syndrome	Deficiency of antithrombin III, and altered levels of other factors
Heparin-induced thrombocytopenia (immune based)	Antibody: antigen complex activates platelets

Table 13–6.   Recommendations for Prophylaxis of Deep Vein Thrombosis

Risk	Patients	Recommendation
Low	Surgical patients under 40 years old, surgery under 30 minutes with no additional risk factors	Early ambulation, leg exercises
	Medical patients without risk factors	
Moderate	Surgical patients over 40 years old having abdominal or thoracic surgery	Heparin 5000 units S.C., every 12 hours (beginning 2 hours postoperatively)
	Hospitalized medical patients with risk factor (myocardial infarction, congestive heart failure, prolonged bed rest)	
	Neurosurgery or other patients with high risk for bleeding	Pneumatic compression boots
High	Hip fracture	Warfarin, LMWH
	Hip replacement	Warfarin, heparin, LMWH
	Knee replacement	Warfarin, pneumatic compression, LMWH
	Open prostatectomy	Pneumatic compression boots
	Gynecologic malignancy	Pneumatic compression boots

LMWH, low molecular weight heparin.
Modified from Francis, C. W.: Prevention and treatment of venous thromboembolic disease. In *Thrombosis and Hemorrhage*. Edited by J. Loscalzo and A. Schafer. Boston, Blackwell Scientific. 1994, pp. 1287–1311.

gical patient should receive 5000 units of heparin S.C. every 12 hours. Patients who have had a history of thromboembolic disease should receive 10,000 units of heparin S.C. every 12 hours.[94] These doses of heparin will not prolong the aPTT. Orthopedic patients, who are at particular risk of thrombosis, benefit from dose adjusted warfarin.[94] Low molecular weight heparins have recently become available and have shown promise in the prevention of thromboembolic disease.

Diagnosis

Venous thrombosis and pulmonary embolism remain a major cause of morbidity and mortality in the hospitalized patient, and a high index of suspicion is necessary to identify their occurrence promptly. Edema, pain and tenderness, and erythematosus discoloration are signs of venous thrombosis, but minimal physical signs may be all that is evident. Similarly, pleuritic chest pain, hemoptysis, tachycardia, and tachypnea may result from a pulmonary embolism, but more often definitive signs are lacking. Doppler ultrasonography and ultrasound imaging studies are the more commonly performed first-line studies to detect a deep vein thrombosis in the leg.[98] Impedance plethysmography (IPG) is another noninvasive test which may detect a deep vein thrombosis, but the definitive study for diagnosis of venous thrombosis is the venogram. Similarly, the ventilation/perfusion scan is a valuable tool in the diagnosis of a pulmonary embolism, but if the scan is of intermediate probability, a pulmonary arteriogram may be necessary for the definitive diagnosis of a pulmonary embolism.

Therapy

Heparin

Treatment of a deep vein thrombosis or pulmonary embolism has remained largely unchanged for several decades. While new agents are being developed, evaluated, and now entering clinical practice, the mainstay of anticoagulation therapy remains heparin and warfarin. Heparin is a naturally occurring mucopolysaccharide, which functions similarly to endothelial cell heparan sulfate, described above, and acts to neutralize activated enzymes of the coagulation system.[99] Intravenous heparin is initiated with a bolus followed by an intravenous drip. For uncomplicated adults, a bolus of 5,000 units of heparin is followed by an infusion of 1300 units per hour. If a patient is already anticoagulated, the heparin dose may need to be reduced. The aPTT is checked in 4 to 6 hours, with a target of 1.5 to 2.5 times control value.[100] A therapeutic aPTT must be achieved within the initial 24 hours to reduce the morbidity and mortality of the thrombosis or embolism. Current guidelines are for 5 days of heparin therapy.[100]

As discussed, heparin therapy may cause thrombocytopenia. A mild idiosyncratic form is more common, and self-limited, but a more severe immunologically based form of heparin-associated thrombocytopenia is associated with platelet activation, thrombosis and microangiopathic hemolytic anemia.[99] Prompt discontinuation of heparin is required if thrombocytopenia develops. A number of alternative agents are available or are under clinical trial. Low molecular weight heparin compounds have reduced, but not absent, cross-reactivity with the heparin-dependent antibody.[68] ORG10172 (Organon), a heparinoid that functions similarly to heparin but lacks antigenic cross-reactivity, is in clinical trial. Dextran has been used as an anticoagulant, although its utility as an alternative to heparin for acute thrombosis has yet to be demonstrated conclusively. Ancrod, derived from a snake venom, induces hypofibrinogenemia which inhibits platelet aggregation and clot formation, and is another alternative anticoagulant in the patient with heparin-induced thrombocytopenia.[68] It is not yet available, except on a compassionate basis.

Warfarin

On the first or second day of heparin therapy, warfarin is initiated at an oral dose of 10 mg daily for 2 days, and then the dosage is adjusted by the prothrombin time. Warfarin (coumadin) is the standard oral anticoagulant agent. It is a competitive inhibitor of vitamin K, and therefore results in reduction in the gamma-carboxylation of factors II, VII, IX, and X, as well as protein C and protein S. Warfarin administration prolongs both the PT and the aPTT, but empirically, the PT is more sensitive to warfarin effects. In an attempt to normalize the PT to the various commercial agents available, most hemostasis labs now report the PT as an INR (International Normalized Ratio). The INR corrects for the variability of the reagents used in different hospital laboratories. For thromboembolic disease the INR target is 2.0 to 3.0.[100] Warfarin therapy reduces the functional levels of all of the vitamin K-dependent factors, but as the factors have different half-lives, a stable prolonged PT is the desired end-point.[100] Therefore only when the INR is therapeutic for two consecutive days on a constant dose of warfarin, may the patient be considered adequately anticoagulated. It often may require three of four days to achieve adequate warfarin-mediated anticoagulation, hence the recommendation to begin warfarin on the first one to two days of heparin.

Warfarin-induced skin necrosis is a severe complication observed during the first several days of warfarin therapy. Capillary and venule thrombosis is observed in the subcutaneous tissues. It is more likely to occur in patients who are protein C deficient.[101] The physiological anticoagulant, protein C, has a short half-life of seven hours, and is one of the first factors to decline following warfarin therapy. Therefore, warfarin may induce a severe protein C deficiency in heterozygous protein C deficient individuals. If warfarin is initiated at an excessive dose, skin necrosis is also more likely to develop as severe protein C deficiency may be induced before the patient is therapeutically anticoagulated. Anticoagulation with heparin, when warfarin therapy is initiated, will reduce the risk of skin necrosis.

Numerous drugs alter warfarin metabolism, and warfarin doses may need to be adjusted if there is a change in one or more medicine which the patient is taking. As a major source of vitamin K is through the diet and bacterial flora of the bowel, antibiotic therapy or poor nutrition may lead to an acquired vitamin K deficiency, and an excessive anticoagulant effect of warfarin. If a patient exhibits evidence of warfarin toxicity, this may be reversed by fresh frozen plasma or vitamin K administration.

Fibrinolytic Agents

Fibrinolytic agents (also referred to as thrombolytic agents) may be administered for treatment of thromboembolic disease. In the setting of a massive pulmonary embolism, or hemodynamic compromise, fibrinolytic agents may lyse a thrombus and restore pulmonary blood flow more promptly than by heparin alone. Several fibrinolytic agents are currently available for management of thrombosis. Streptokinase, urokinase, tissue plasminogen activator (tPA), and an isolated plasminogen:streptokinase activator complex (APSAC) are currently available and are administered intravenously. These drugs act by activating plasminogen to plasmin, which in turn lyses fibrin clots. All of these agents will lyse fibrinogen as well as fibrin, and result in hypofibrinogenemia when administered in therapeutic doses. The advantage of these agents is they may reestablish vascular patency more rapidly than heparin alone, but there is an increased risk of hemorrhagic complication. Thrombolytic agents have been extensively studied in the setting of myocardial infarction, with few clinical questions receiving as much interest from the medical community and public. The data on the use of these agents in the setting of deep vein thrombosis and pulmonary embolism are much more limited and the appropriate indications are still incompletely defined.[102,103]

Reversal of Anticoagulation

If a patient is on heparin, and this needs to be reversed for anticipated surgery, discontinuation of heparin for at least three hours prior to surgery is usually sufficient as the in vivo half-life is approximately 90 minutes.[99] If more emergent reversal of heparin therapy is required, protamine sulfate may be administered.

Warfarin has a long in vivo half-life and, therefore, reversal requires specific intervention if surgery or other invasive intervention is required. Vitamin K, administered at 10 mg subcutaneously, will reverse the warfarin effect, unless an overdose of warfarin has been ingested. In this case higher doses of vitamin K may be required. Vitamin K may be associated with greater side effects when administered intravenously, with no therapeutic advantage over the subcutaneous route. Transfusion of fresh frozen plasma will help to restore hemostasis in an emergency setting and should be considered if there is inadequate time for vitamin K repletion to normalize the synthesis of the vitamin K-dependent factors.

EHLERS-DANLOS SYNDROME

Classification

This is an inherited connective tissue disorder denoted by lax joints and skin, easy bruising, and bleeding.[104] In most patients the condition is inherited as an autosomal dominant and at least four varieties may be recognized. More recently, the condition has been genetically broadened to include several rarer recessive conditions. McKusick classified the condition into nine variations. Other subtypes have been proposed based on the tissue pathology.[104]

Pathology

The abnormality appears to be related to a defect in fibronectin of the connective tissue. The bleeding tendency is thus due to a connective tissue defect of the vascular walls. It has been reported that a similar fibronectin defect is present in certain platelet abnormalities of aggregation.[105]

Clinical Characteristics

This generalized systemic disorder affects many organs. Hypermobility of joints and hyperextensibility of the skin are prominent features; joint dislocations are frequent and deformities occur. The skin can be easily stretched but returns to normal. Scars occur over bony prominences.

Presenting Signs and Symptoms

These are listed but vary widely depending on the gene mutation and the phenotype.

1. Bruising is common and bleeding is present but not always troublesome. Ecchymotic sites are seen. Minor trauma may cause wide gaping wounds but little bleeding.
2. Wound healing is poor and related to deep tissue fragility.
3. Synovial effusions and hemoarthroses are frequent.
4. Skeletal deformites are seen: spinal kyphoscoliosis is present in 75% of patients, thoracic deformity in 20% and talipes equinovarus in 5%. Pes planus is present in 90% of adults.
5. Gastrointestinal hernias and diverticula are common. The gastrointestinal tract is often dilated but visceral rupture is rare.
6. Spontaneous rupture of large arteries and dissecting aneurysm of the aorta rarely occur.
7. Tissue fragility of women may complicate pregnancy.
8. An increased incidence of dilatation of the esophagus and trachea is seen.
9. The incidence of of pneumothorax is high.
10. The incidence of varicose veins and inguinal hernias is abnormally high.

Anesthetic Considerations

Technical problems are challenging especially in the performance of venipuncture and other invasive procedures. Positional problems are related to the ease of injury of the extremities. Blood requirements are often high.

Pre-anesthetic Preoperative Requirements

1. Genetic consultation
2. Hematology consultation; coagulation disorders to be ruled out.
3. Cardiologic evaluation. Mitral valve prolapse should be considered.
4. Antibiotics should be administered for possible endocarditis.

Summary of Anesthetic Recommendations[106]

1. Avoid subcutaneous and intramuscular injections.
2. Establish an intravenous line peripherally prior to operation.
3. Avoid arterial lines and central venous catheters if possible.
4. Choice of anesthesia is general. Regional anesthesia is avoided.

5. Airway Management
Mask with cotton padding and spontaneous breathing if possible.
Endotracheal Intubation requires utmost care.
No nasal intubation.
Provide excellant relaxation for endotracheal intubation and avoid bucking.
6. Maintenance
Spontaneous respiration is desirable.
If assisted respiration is needed low pressures are desired.
Hypertension and arrhythmias must be prevented or controlled.

Correction of Fibronectin Deficiency

Some evidence has indicated that the fibronectin deficiency of at least one type of the ED syndrome (type X) can be corrected by the administration of cryprecipitate since this product contains considerable amounts of fibronectin. It also appears to correct the platelet dysfunction seen in this EDS subtype.

MARFAN SYNDROME

In 1895, Marfan described the clinical features of a 5-year-old patient with long thin extremities initially with some contractures and subsequently developed severe scoliosis; arachnoidactly was included in the description. McKusick extensively investigated and described this syndrome.[107]

The Marfan syndrome is a relatively rare familial disorder of unknown etiology. It is transmitted as an autosomal dominant trait with variable phenotypes. The prevalence of the classic syndrome is placed at 4-6 per 100,000 people.[108]

Pathogenesis

It is a generalized connective tissue disorder specifically of elastic tissue. An abnormality of the protein microfibrillan appears to be the principal microscopic defect and shows cystic degeneration and fragmentation of the elastic strands. This is prominant in the media of the walls of the aorta and great vessels. This degenerative condition also occurs in other tissues.[109]

Clinical Characteristics

Widespread abnormalities of three systems are encountered, skeletal, cardiovascular, and ocular, but show great variability in severity. These three systems represent the classic triad of McKusick along with the familial history.[108]

Skeletal Deformities

Extremities are disproportionally long, especially the fingers and toes, which are long and thin with contractures and/or webbing (arachnoidactyly). Arm span often exceeds height while the height is more than 95 percentile for age in over 30% of the patients. Deformities of the sternum are frequent with forward or inward pectus displacement (60%). Scoliosis is common with a variable incidence of over 49%; it is often severe and painful and may interfere with pulmonary function; it is associated with cystic disease of the lung and spontaneous pneumothorax occurs. Surgical correction is necessary for the severe conditions to prevent mortality.[110]

Hyperextensibility of joints with backward curvature of knees (Genu recurvatum) and flat feet may be found alone and is referred to as the Marfanoid syndrome.

Other characteristics of a less serious nature are to be observed including sparse subcutaneous fat; a lack of skeletal muscle tone is common. A high arched palate is frequent but has not been a factor in making intubation difficult.[111]

Cardiovascular Changes

These are of a serious nature and are related to weakness of the media in the walls of the aorta and great vessels. The ascending aorta undergoes progressive dilation. Dissection of the aorta beginning in the coronary sinus develops early and continues throughout life in many patients. An acute episode with formation of an aneurysm imposes a disastrous burden on the heart and may be lethal. Aortic regurgitation is an early sign and often related to mitral valve prolapse and redundant cusps or chordae tendeni. Mild systolic clicks may be heard in over 30% of patients.

Ocular Abnormalities

Dislocation of the lens is often associated with tremulousness of the iris, a peculiar sign. Severe myopia is frequent. Spontaneous detachment of the retina may occur.

Diagnosis

A positive family history along with the clinical triad of McKusick is essential. There are many patients with only a partial "set" of clinical abnormalities. Homocystinuria is one condition that has many similar features and should be differentiated from Marfan syndromes by urine testing.

Prognosis and Management

Complications relate to the severity of the skeletal or cardiovascular abnormalities. To prevent girls from attaining unusual heights precocious puberty may be induced before age 10–12 years by administration of an estrogen/progesterone course. Propanolol reduces the abruptness of ventricular ejection and may prevent aortic dissection. Scoliosis can be corrected and replacement of the aorta has been successful in selected cases.[112]

Surgical-Anesthesia Morbidity-Mortality

For the correction of scoliosis morbidity has not been different than for the surgery of idiopathic scoliosis.[112] For the correction of cardiovascular lesions the mortality has been reported to be between 5 and 12%.[110]

HEREDITARY ANGIONEUROTIC EDEMA

In 1887, William Osler described a pediatric patient with chronic intermittent "attacks of transient swelling in various fleshy parts of the body". He further identified a genetic basis by his review of the family history in whom similar episodes occurred in five generations. Many basic and clinical investigations in later years have defined the molecular basis of the disorder.[113]

Pathogenesis

Deficiency of the serum inhibitor of the activated first component of complement was identified as $C'1$ esterase inhibitor ($C'1$ INH).[114] In 85% of patients the deficiency is due to a lack of the inhibitor.[115] The result is imcontrolled activation of the classical pathway of the complement cascade.

Genetic Basis

The biochemical abnormality is inherited as an autosomal dominant trait.[116] Two types of the condition have been defined and both are rare:

Type 1—The common form shows decreased serum levels of the $C'1$ inhibitor protein, an α_2-globulin that blocks the esterolytic activity of the first component. This form is due to impaired biosynthetic production.

Type 2—The variant form is less common but shows elevated concentrations of the inhibitor protein which is functionally deficient due to abnormal biosynthesis.[117]

Both types are associated with low titers or absence of complements C_2, C_4 and total hemolytic complement (CH 50)

A third type of HAE is an acquired form that appears in middle age. It is rare, not associated with heredity but associated with lymphoproliferative diseases. The synthesis of $C'1$ inhibitor is normal but there is accelerated catabolism. In some instances abnormal antibodies against the $C'1$ inhibitor have been found.[118]

Clinical Characteristics

The edema is unifocal, indurated, and painful, not pruritic. Cutaneous and mucosal attacks may be precipitated by trauma or viral illness and aggravated by emotional stress. The face, lips, tongue and larynx are often involved and fatal airway obstruction may occur, episodes may occur as often as every 2 to 3 weeks or once a month.

Attacks of abdominal pain indicate involvement of the mucosa of the gastrointestinal tract; this is accompanied by nausea, vomiting, colic, and signs of intestinal obstruction.

Treatment

An acute attack may be managed by ε amino caproic acid, which may terminate an attack. An airway must be provided if there is respiratory obstruction. Epinephrine and glucocorticosteroids are ineffective.

For short-term prophylaxis and prior to elective surgery 2 units of fresh frozen or a purified C'1-INH fraction of plasma can be given with some advantage. For long-term prophylaxis, however, androgens are effective in preventing attacks and ameliorating an acute attack. Danazol (200 mg tid) and oral stanazolol (2.0 mg tid) (less expensive) are effective, and are the drugs of choice.[119] These agents reduce the severity and frequency of symptoms and attacks. The androgens increase the level of C'1 INH as well as C4 in the plasma toward normal of patients with the disorder.

REFERENCES

1. Davie E. W., Fujikawa K., Kisiel W.: The coagulation cascade: Inititation, maintenance, and regulation. Biochemistry 30:10363–70, 1991.
2. Lilly L. S., Pratt R. E., Alexander R. W., et al.: Renin expression by vascular endothelial cells in culture. Circ Res 57:312–318:1985.
3. Furchgott R. F., Vanhoutte P. M.: Endothelium-derived relaxing factors. FASEB J 2:2007–2018, 1989.
4. Moncada S., Vane J. R.: Arachidonic acid metabolites and the interactions between platelets and blood-vessel walls. N Engl J Med 300:1142–1147, 1979.
5. Ruggeri Z. M., De Marco L., Gatti L., Bader R., Montgomery R. R.: Platelets have more than one binding site for von Willebrand factor. J Clin Invest 72:1–12, 1983.
6. De Groot P. G., Sixma J. J.: Platelet adhesion. Br J Haematol 75:308–312, 1990.
7. Hawiger J.: Platelet secretory pathways: An overview. Methods Enzymol 169:191–195, 1989.
8. Fukami M. H., Dangelmaier C. A., Bauer J., Holmsen H.: secretion, subcellular localization, and metabolic status of inorganic pyrophosphate in human platelets, a major constituent of the amine-storing granules. Biochem J 192:99, 1980.
9. Wencel-Drake J. D., Painter R. G., Zimmerman T. S., et al.: Ultrastructural localization of human platelet thrombospondin, fibrinogen, fibronectin, and von Willebrand factor in frozen thin sections. Blood 65:929–938, 1985.
10. Mann K. G., Nesheim M. E., Church W. R., et al.: Surface-dependent reactions of the vitamin K-dependent enzyme complexes. Blood 76:1–16, 1990.
11. Peerschke E. I. B.: The platelet fibrinogen receptor. Semin Hematol 22:241–259, 1985.
12. Spicer E. K., Horton R., Bloom L., et al.: Isolation of cDNA clones coding for human tissue factor: primary structure of the protein and cDNA. Proc Natl Acad Sci USA 84:5148–5152, 1987.
13. Bach R., Gentry R., Nemerson Y.: Factor VII binding to tissue factor in reconstituted phospholipid vesicles: induction of cooperativity by phosphatidylserine. Biochemistry 25:4007–4020, 1986.
14. Rao L. V. M., Robinson T., Hoang A. D.: Factor VIIa/tissue factor-catalyzed activation of factors IX and X on a cell surface and in suspension: a kinetic study. Thromb Haemost 67:654–659, 1992.
15. Griffin J. H.: The role of surface in the surface-dependent activation of Hageman factor (blood coagulation factor XII). Proc Natl Acad Sci USA 75:1998–2002, 1978.
16. Wright I.: International Commission on Nomenclature of Clotting Factors. New York, Society of Hemostasis, 1954.
17. Rappaport S. I.: Hemostasis. In Best and Taylor's Physiological Basis of Medical Practice, 12th Ed. Edited by J.B. West. Baltimore, Williams & Wilkins, 1990.
18. Furie B., Furie B. C.: Molecular and cellular biology of blood coagulation. N Engl J Med 326:800–806, 1992.
19. Park B. K.: Warfarin: metabolism and mode of action. Biochem Pharmacol 37:19–27, 1988.
20. Bauer K. A., Rosenberg R. D.: Role of antithrombin III as a regulator of in vitro coagulation. Semin Hematol 28:10, 1991.
21. Esmon C. T.: The roles of protein C and thrombomodulin in the regulation of blood coagulation. J Biol Chem 164:4743, 1989.
22. Rapaport S. I.: The extrinsic pathway inhibitor: A regulator of tissue factor dependent blood coagulation. Thromb Haemost 66:6, 1991.
23. Henkin J. et al.: The plasminogen-plasmin system. Prog Cardiovasc Dis 34:135, 1991.
24. Wiman B.: Hamsten A. The fibrinolytic enzyme system and its role in the etiology of thromboembolic disease. Semin Thromb Hemost 16:207–16, 1990.
25. Rapaport S. I.: Preoperative hemostatic evaluation: Which test if any? Blood 61:229–231, 1983.
26. Rodgers R. P., Levin J.: A critical reappraisal of the bleeding time. Semin Thromb Hemost 16:1, 1990.
27. Dumoulin-Lagrange M., Capelle C.: Evaluation of automated platelet counters for the enumeration and sizing of platelets in the diagnosis and management of hemostatic problems. Semin Thromb Hemost 9:235–244, 1983.
28. Schafer A. I.: Bleeding and thrombosis in the myeloproliferative disorders. Blood 64:1–12, 1984.
29. Bockenstedt P. L.: Laboratory methods in hemostasis. In Thrombosis and Hemorrhage. J. Loscalzo, A.I. Schafer (Eds.), Blackwell Scientific Publications, Boston, 1994, pp. 455–513.
30. Penner J. A.: Experience with a thrombin clotting time assay for measuring heparin activity. Am J Clin Pathol 61:645–653, 1974.
31. Mammen E.: Fibrinogen abnormalities. Semin Thromb Hemost 9:1–9, 1983.
32. Grau E., Linares M., Estany A., et al.: Utility of D dimer in the diagnosis of deep vein thrombosis in outpatients. Thromb Haemost 66:510, 1991.
33. Mielke C. H.: Measurement of the bleeding time. Thromb Haemost 52:210–211, 1984.
34. Harker L. A., Slichter S.: The bleeding time as a screening test for evaluation of platelet function. N Engl J Med 187:155–159, 1972.
35. Coller B. S.: Biochemical and electrostatic considerations in primary platelet aggregation. Ann NY Acad Sci 416:693, 1983.
36. Palkuti H. S.: Laboratory monitoring of anticoagulant therapy. J Med Tech 2:81–86, 1985.
37. Martin P., Horkay F., Rajah S. M., et al.: Monitoring of coagulation status using thrombelastography during paediatric open heart surgery. Int J Clin Monitor Comput 8:183–7, 1991.
38. Rosner F.: Hemophilia in the Talmud and rabbinic writings. Ann Intern Med 70:833, 1969.
39. Gitschier J., Kogan S., Diamond C., Levinson B.: Genetic basis of hemophilia A. Thromb Haemost 66:37–39, 1991.
40. Mannucci P. M.: Desmopressin: a nontransfusional form of treatment for congenital and acquired bleeding disorders. Blood 72:1449–1455, 1988.
41. Brugnara C., Churchill W. H.: Plasma component therapy. In Thrombosis and Hemorrhage. J. Loscalzo, A.I. Schafer (Eds.), Blackwell Scientific Publications, Boston, 1994, pp. 1091–1116.
42. Walsh P. N., Rizza C. R., Matthews J. M., et al.: Epsilon-aminocaproic acid therapy for dental extractions in

haemophilia and Christmas disease: A double blind controlled trial. Br J Haemat 20:463–75, 1971.

43. Sindet-Pedersen S., Ingerslev J., Ramstrom G., Blomback M.: Management of oral bleeding in haemophiliac patients. Lancet 2:566, 1988.

44. Mannucci P. M.: Nontransfusional modalities. In Thrombosis and Hemorrhage. J. Loscalzo, A.I. Schafer (Eds.), Blackwell Scientific Publications, Boston, 1994, pp. 1117–1135.

45. Schwarzinger I., Pabinger I., Korniger C., et al.: Incidence of inhbitors in patients with severe and moderate hemophilia A treated with factor VIII concentrates. Am J Hemat 24:241–245, 1987.

46. Sultan Y., Loyer F.: In Vitro evaluation of factor VIII-bypassing activity of activated prothrombin complex concentrate, and factor VIIa in the plasma of patients with factor VIII inhibitors: thrombin generation test in the presence of collagen-activated platelets. J Lab Clin Med 121:444–452, 1993.

47. Brackmann H. H., Gormsen J.: Massive factor VIII infusion in hemophiliac with factor VIII inhibitor, high responder. Lancet 2:933, 1977.

48. Sultan Y., White C. G., Aronstam A., et al.: Hemophiliac patients with an inhibitor to factor VIII treated with a high dose factor VIII concentrate: results of a collaborative study for the evaluation of factor VIII inhibitor titer, recovery and half life of infused factor VIII. Nouv Rev Fr Hematol 28:85–89, 1986.

49. Green D.: Suppression of an antibody to factor VIII by a combination of factor VIII and cyclophosphamide. Blood 37:381–387, 1971.

50. Miller C. H., Lenzi R., Breen C.: Prevalence of von Willebrand's disease among U.S. adults. Blood 70:377, 1987.

51. Hoyer L. W., Rizza C. R., Tuddenham E. G., Carta C. A., Armitage H., Rotblatt F. von Willebrand factor multimer patterns in von Willebrand's disease. Br J Haemat 55:493–507, 1983.

52. Cooney K. A., Ginsburg D., Ruggeri Z. M.: von Willebrand disease. In Thrombosis and Hemorrhage. J. Loscalzo, A.I. Schafer (Eds.), Blackwell Scientific Publications, Boston, 1994, pp. 657–682.

53. Seligsohn U.: High gene frequency of factor XI (PTA) deficiency in Ashkenazi Jews. Blood 51:1223–1228, 1978.

54. Roberts H. R., Eberst M. E.: Other coagulation factor deficiencies. In Thrombosis and Hemorrhage. J. Loscalzo, A. I. Schafer (Eds.), Blackwell Scientific Publications, Boston, 1994, pp. 701–728.

55. Duckert F.: Documentation of the plasma factor XIII deficiency in man. Ann NY Acad Sci 202:190–198, 1972.

56. Francis J. L.: The detection and measurement of factor XIII activity: a review. Med Lab Sci 37:137–147, 1980.

57. Berndt M. C., Fournier D. J., Castaldi P. A.: Bernard-Soulier syndrome. Baillière's Clin Haemat 2:585–607, 1989.

58. Dunlop L. C., Andrews R. K., Berndt M. C.: Congenital disorders of platelet function. In Thrombosis and Hemorrhage. J. Loscalzo, Al Schafer (Eds.), Blackwell Scientific Publications, Boston, 1994, pp. 615–633.

59. George J. N., Caen J. P., Nurden A. T.: Glanzmann's thrombasthenia: the spectrum of clinical disease. Blood 75:1383–1395, 1990.

60. Rao A. K.: Congenital disorders of platelet function. Haemat Oncol Clin North Am 4:65–86, 1990.

61. Larsen E., Zinkham W., Eggleston J., et al.: Kasabach-Merritt syndrome: Therapeutic considerations. Pediatrics 79:971–980, 1987.

62. Peery W. H.: Clinical spectrum of hereditary hemorrhagic telangiectasia (Osler-Weber-Rendu disease). Am J Med 82:989–997, 1987.

63. Byers P. H.: Inherited disorders of collagen gene structure and expression. Am J Med Genet 34:72–80, 1989.

64. Payne B. A., Pierre R. V.: Pseudothrombocytopenia: a laboratory artifact with potential serious consequences. Mayo Clin Proc 59:123–125, 1984.

65. McMillan R., Imbach P. A.: Immune thrombocytopenic purpura. In Thrombosis and Hemorrhage. J. Loscalzo, A.I. Schafer (Eds.), Blackwell Scientific Publications, Boston, 1994, pp. 575–595.

66. Garg S. K., Amorosi E. L., Karpatkin S.: Use of the megakathrombocyte as an index of megakaryocyte number. N Engl J Med 284:11–17, 1971.

67. Mueler-Eckhardt C.: Idiopathic thrombocytopenic purpura (ITP): Clinical and immunologic considerations. Semin Thromb Haemost 3:125–159, 1977.

68. McCrae K. R., Cines D. B.: Drug-induced thrombocytopenia. In Thrombosis and Hemorrhage. J. Loscalzo, A.I. Schafer (Eds.), Blackwell Scientific Publications, Boston, 1994, pp. 545–573.

69. Blanchette V., Adams M., MacMillan J., et al.: Initial therapy of childhood acute ITP: results of a randomized study comparing IVIgG, oral prednisone, and IV anti-D. Blood 78:345a, 1991.

70. Berchtold P., Harris J. P., Tani P., et al.: Autoantibodies to platelet glycoproteins in patients with disease-related immune thrombocytopenia. Br J Haematol 73:365–368, 1989.

71. Bukowski R. M.: Thrombotic thrombocytopenic pupura: a review. Prog Hemost Thromb 6:287–337, 1982.

72. Rock G. A., Shumack K. H., Buscard N. A., et al.: Comparison of plasma exchange with plasma infusion in the treatment of thrombotic thrombocytopenic purpura. N Engl J Med 325:393–397, 1991.

73. Bell W. R., Braine H. G., Ness P. M., Kickler T. S.: Improved survival in thrombotic thrombocytopenic purpura-hemolytic uremic syndrome. Clinical experience in 108 patients. N Engl J Med 325:398–403, 1991.

74. Krevans J. R., Jackson D. P.: Hemorrhagic disorder following massive whole blood transfusions. JAMA 159:171–177, 1955.

75. Kelton J. G., Meltzer D., Moore J., et al.: Drug-induced thrombocytopenia is associated with increased binding of IgG to platelets both in vivo and in vitro. Blood 58:525–529, 1981.

76. Remuzzi G.: Bleeding in renal failure. Lancet 1:1205–1208, 1988.

77. Janson P. A., Jubelier S. J., Weinstein M. J., et al.: Treatment of the bleeding tendency in uremia with cryoprecipitate. N Engl J Med 303:1318–1322, 1980.

78. Livo M., Gotti E., Marchesi D., et al.: Uraemic bleeding: role of anaemia and beneficial effect of red cell transfusion. Lancet 2:1013–1015, 1982.

79. Vigano G., Benigni A., Mendogni D., et al.: Recombinant human erythropoietin to correct uremic bleeding. Am J Kid Dis 18:44–49, 1991.

80. Bell W. R.: Disseminated intravascular coagulopathy. Johns Hopkins Med J 146:289–299, 1980.

81. Carr J. M., McKinney M., McDonagh J.: Diagnosis of disseminated intravascular coagulation. Role of D-dimer. Am J Clin Pathol 91:280–287, 1989.

82. Goldberg M., Ginsburg D., Mayer R., et al.: Is heparin necessary during induction chemotherapy for patients with acute promyelocytic leukemia? Blood 69:187–191, 1987.

83. Fourrier F., Iestavel P., Chopin C., et al.: Meningococcemia and purpura fulminans in adults: acute deficiencies of proteins C and S and early treatment with antithrombin III concentrates. Intens Care Med 16:121–124, 1990.

84. Martinez J., Barsigian C.: Coagulopathy of liver failure and vitsamin K deficiency. In Thrombosis and Hemorrhage. J. Loscalzo, A.I. Schafer (Eds.), Blackwell Scientific Publications, Boston, 1994, pp. 945-963.
85. Kelly D. A., Tuddenham E. G. D.: Haemostatic problems in liver disease. Gut 27:339-349, 1986.
86. Green D., Lechner K.: A survey of 215 non-hemophilic patients with inhibitors to factor VIII. Thromb Haemost 45:200-203, 1981.
87. Alving B. M.: Lupus anticoagulants, anticardiolipin antibodies, and the antiphospholipid syndrome. In Thrombosis and Hemorrhage. J. Loscalzo, A.I. Schafer (Eds.), Blackwell Scientific Publications, Boston, 1994, pp. 749-766.
88. Harris E. N., Gharavi E. A., Boey M. I., et al.: Anticardiolipin antibodies: detection by radioimmunoassay and association with thrombosis in systemic lupus erythematosus. Lancet 2:1211-1214, 1983.
89. Bajaj S. P., Rapaport S. I., Fierer D. S., et al.: A mechanism for the hypofibrinogenemia-lupus anticoagulant syndrome. Blood 61:684-692, 1983.
90. Lanzkowsky S., Lanzkowsky L., Lanzkowsky P.: Henoch-Schoenlein purpura. Pediatr Rev 13:130-137, 1992.
91. Luzzatto G., Schafer A. I.: The prethrombotic state in cancer. Semin Oncol 17:147-159, 1990.
92. Comp P. C.: Hereditary disorders predisposing to thrombosis. Prog Hemost Thromb 8:71-102, 1987.
93. Schafer A. I.: The hypercoagulable state. Ann Intern Med 102:814-828, 1985.
94. Clagett G. R., Anderson F. A. Jr., Levine M. N., et al: Prevention of venous thromboembolism. Chest 102: 391S-407S, 1992.
95. Hull R. D., Raskob G. E., Hirsh J.: Prophylaxis of venous thromboembolism: an overview. Chest 89:374S-383S, 1986.
96. Halkin H., Goldberg J., Modan M., et al: reduction of mortality in general medical in-patients by low-dose heparin prophylaxis. Ann Intern Med 96:561-565, 1982.
97. Francis C. W.: Prevention and treatment of venous thromboembolic disease. In Thrombosis and Hemorrhage. J. Loscalzo, A.I. Schafer (eds.), Blackwell Scientific Publications, Boston, 1994, pp. 1287-1311.
98. Creager M. A., O'Leary D. H., Doubilet P. M.: Noninvasive vascular testing. In Vascular Medicine, Loscalzo J, Creager MA, Dzau VJ, eds., Little Brown, Boston, 1992, pp. 419-451.
99. Hirsh J.: Heparin. N Engl J Med 324:1565-1574, 1991.
100. Hyers T. M., Hull R. D., Weg J. G.: Antithrombotic therapy for venous thromboembolic disease. Chest 102:408S-425S, 1992.
101. Broekmans A. W., Bertina R. M., Loeliger E. A., Hofmann V., Klingemann H. G.: Protein C and development of skin necrosis during anticoagulant therapy. Thromb Haemost 49:251-258, 1983.
102. Goldhaber S. Z., Burning J. E., Lipnick R. J., et al.: Pooled analyses of randomized trials of streptokinase and heparin in phlebographically documented acute deep vein thrombosis. Am J Med 76:393-397, 1984.
103. Levine M. N., Goldhaber S. Z., Califf R. M., et al: Hemorrhagic complications of thrombolytic therapy in the treatment of myocardial infarction and venous thromboembolism. Chest 102:364S-373S, 1992.
104. McKusick V. A.: Mendelian Inheritance in Man. 5th Ed. Johns Hopkins University Press, 1978.
105. Hammerschmidt D. E., Arenson M. A., Larson S. L. et al.: Maternal Ehlers-Danlos syndrome Type X. Successful Management of pregnancy and parturition. JAMA 248: 2487-2488, 1982.
106. Dolan P., Sisko F., and Riley E.: Anesthetic consideration for Ehlers-Danlos Syndrome. Anesthesiology 52:266-269, 1980.
107. McKusick V. A.. Heritable Disorders of the connective tissue. The Marfan syndrome. J Chronic Dis 2:609-44, 1955.
108. McKusick V. A.: Heritable disorders of the connective tissue. 3rd Ed. Chapter 3. St Louis, Mosby 1972.
109. Pyeritz R. E., McKusick V. A.: The Marfan Syndrome. Diagnosis and management. N Engl J Med 300:772-7, 1979.
110. Gallotti R., Ross N.: The Marfan Syndrome: surgical technique and follow up in 50 patients Ann Thorac Surg 29:428-33, 1980.
111. Verghese C.: Anaesthesia in Marfan's syndrome. Anaesthesia 39:917-922, 1984.
112. Gott V. L., Pyeritz R. E., McGovern G. J. Jr., et al.: Surgical treatment of the ascending aorta in the Marfan Syndrome. Results of composite-graft repair in 50 patients. N Engl J Med 314:1070-1074, 1986.
113. Colten H. P.: Hereditary angioneurotic edema 1887-1987. N Engl J Med 317:43-44, 1987.
114. Pensky J., Levy L. R., Lepow I. H.: Partial purification of a serum inhibitor of C′1-esterase. J Biol Chem 236:1674-9, 1961.
115. Donaldson V. H., Evans R. R.: A biochemical abnormality in angioneurotic edema: absence of serum inhibitor of C′1 esterase. Am J Med 35:37-44, 1963.
116. Rosen F. S., Charche P., Pensky J., Donaldson V.: Hereditary angioneurotic edema: two genetic variants. Science 148:957-8, 1965.
117. Stoppa-Lyonnet D., Tosi M., Laurent J. et al.: Altered C′1 inhibitor gene in Type 1 hereditary angioedema. N Engl J Med 317:1-7, 1987.
118. Alsenz J., Bork K., Loos M.: Autoantibody mediated acquired deficiency of C′1 inhibitor. N Engl J Med 316:1360-6, 1987.
119. Gelfand J. A., Sherins R. J., Alling D. W., et al.: Treatment of hereditary angioedema with danazol. N Engl J Med 295:1444-8, 1976.

Chapter 14

ABNORMALITIES OF HEMOGLOBIN SYNTHESIS AND PERIOPERATIVE MANAGEMENT OF ACQUIRED BLEEDING DISORDERS

EDWARD A. CZINN

Anemia is defined as a reduction in red blood cell mass or total body hemoglobin. States of anemia impose tremendous physiologic burdens on the human organism because oxygen is primarily transported throughout the body via hemoglobin. The decreased oxygen carrying capacity associated with anemia results in multiple physiologic derangements including chronic tissue hypoxia, increased cardiac output, and redistribution of blood flow. The etiology of anemia is traditionally considered under the general pathophysiologic categories of decreased red blood cell production, increased red blood cell destruction, and blood loss (Table 14–1).

Anemias are often classified according to the size of the red cell. *Macrocytic or megaloblastic* anemias are typical of folic acid, vitamin A, and vitamin B_{12} deficiencies in which DNA synthesis is impeded during the maturation of red blood cells. *Normocytic* anemias are associated with gross hemorrhage, hemolytic anemias, sickle cell anemia and thalassemias, chronic infections, and splenic anemias. *Microcytic, hypochromic* anemias are the result of chronic blood loss and nutritional deficiencies.

The first part of this chapter focuses on disorders associated with abnormal hemoglobin production and synthesis, which may lead to a state of anemia. In addition, common diseases associated with hemolysis and decreased red cell survival are addressed. The second part of this chapter focuses on acquired disorders that contribute to abnormal bleeding and anemia during surgery and the perioperative period. Special emphasis is given to diagnosis, treatment, and anesthetic management.

HEMOGLOBINOPATHIES AND DISEASES OF RED BLOOD CELLS

Hemolytic anemias are characterized by premature destruction of red blood cells or hemolysis. The normal life span of red blood cells is approximately 90 to 120 days; however, *intravascular* hemolysis associated with mechanical and complement-mediated injury, and *extravascular* hemolysis in the spleen, reduce this life span. Many hemolytic anemias are hereditary and involve alterations in hemoglobin structure (hemoglobinopathies), abnormalities in red cell membranes, and enzyme defects.

Sickle Cell Disease[1]

First described by Herrick in 1910, sickle cell disease is manifested by the presence of large quantities of mutant hemoglobin in the blood. The disease is a genetically determined hemoglobinopathy, and inheritance of the disease essentially follows the Mendelian principles of autosomal recessive genes. Heterozygous individuals are considered to have sickle cell trait and have both normal and abnormal hemoglobin. The concentration of abnormal hemoglobin S in individuals with sickle cell trait varies between 20 and 40%. Homozygous individuals have sickle cell anemia with a concentration of hemoglobin S ranging from 80 to 100 percent.

The sickle cell gene has worldwide distribution and is not confined to one race or skin color. Although the gene

Table 14–1. Pathophysiologic Classification of Anemia

Decreased production of red cells
  Congenital
    Red cell aplasia
    Infections (rubella)
    Leukemia
  Acquired
    Nutritional deficiencies: iron, B_{12}/folic acid
    Drugs and toxic agents
    Infections and sepsis
    Marrow infiltrates
    Chronic renal failure
Increased destruction of red cells
  "Immune" hemolytic anemia
    Incompatibility
    Autoimmune
    Drug-induced
  Infections
  Vitamin deficiency
  Red cell membrane disorders
    Spherocytosis
    Elliptocytosis
  Red cell enzyme deficiencies
    Glucose-6—phosphodiesterase deficiency
    Pyruvate kinase deficiency
  Hemoglobinopathies
  Thalassemias
Blood loss
  Acute
  Chronic

---

[1]This section was contributed by V. J. Collins.

is most concentrated in West Central Africa, it has been found in such diverse areas as Saudi Arabia, India, southern Italy, northern Greece, southern Turkey and has also been reported in Caucasian and other populations. The incidence of sickle cell anemia (SS) in African-Americans in the United States is 1 in 625 births (0.16%), whereas that of sickle cell trait (AS) is 8 to 9%.[1]

Pathophysiology

Hemoglobin is made up of four polypeptide chains that are held together by noncovalent interactions. Hemoglobin A (Hb A), the principal hemoglobin in adults, consists of two chains of one kind, called α chains, and two chains of another kind called β-chains. The subunit of hemoglobin A is $\alpha_2\beta_2$. Sickle-cell hemoglobin or hemoglobin S (Hb S) differs from Hb A in that the amino acid valine is substituted for glutamate at position 6 of the β-chain. The side chain of valine is distinctly nonpolar, whereas the side chain of glutamate is highly polar. This substitution of valine for glutamate places a nonpolar residue on the outer surface of hemoglobin S. When hemoglobin S is deoxygenated, a complementary site that is able to bind to this nonpolar residue is exposed. Binding of the complementary site to the nonpolar residue results in the formation of long double stranded aggregates. As oxygen tension decreases, the concentration of deoxygenated hemoglobin S increases producing complex, multistranded fibers that deform the red blood cell into the characteristic sickle shape. Dehydration increases the concentration of Hb S and enhances the tendency for aggregate formation. When hemoglobin S is oxygenated, the complementary site is masked and unable to bind to the nonpolar residue, preventing aggregate formation.

These distorted red cells with their less elastic membranes have difficulty moving through the microcirculation and are associated with an increased blood viscosity.[1,2,3] When oxygenated, there is no difference in viscosities of blood containing normal hemoglobin (AA), heterozygous hemoglobin (AS), or homozygous sickle cell hemoglobin (SS), even at a hematocrit of as high as 60%. However, deoxygenation of SS or AS hemoglobin results in disproportionate rise in viscosity as a function of hematocrit when compared to normal hemoglobin. This increased viscosity leads to stasis, sludging, vascular occlusion, tissue ischemia, anoxia, and acidosis. This initiates a vicious cycle where ischemia, anoxia, and acidosis precipitate further sickling.[2] Vaso-occlusion can occur at both the arterial and venous ends of the capillary bed, and may result in chronic end-organ damage. The presence of dehydration, diuresis, and infection further increase viscosity and sickling.

In SS blood, some irreversibly sickled and fragile red cells may be observed at even 100 percent oxygen saturation. Sickling in SS blood, however, usually begins when O_2 saturation is 85 percent; at an O_2 saturation of 65 percent, three-fourths of the red cells are sickled; and at 50 percent, all red cells are sickled.[2,3] The low shear rates and low PO_2 associated with the venous circulation tend to promote sickling. Sickling is further enhanced in the presence of low cardiac output and increased O_2 consumption. In patients with sickle cell trait, sickling begins

at or below an O_2 saturation of 40%. The speed of the sickling process is increased by hypoxemia, acidosis, hypothermia, and increased 2,3 DPG levels. The sickling process is lessened in the presence of other hemoglobins such as hemoglobin F (Hb F), hemoglobin A, and to a certain extent hemoglobin C (Hb C).[2,3,4] The presence of these hemoglobins, as well as thalassemia and malaria, offer some protection against sickling and may modify the clinical severity of the disease. Newborns who have SS and a high concentration of Hb F are usually asymptomatic, although extreme conditions may still promote sickling. However, when Hb F concentrations fall after the neonatal period, the clinical disease is manifested.

The anemia of sickle cell disease is related primarily to accelerated destruction of red blood cells. The life span of sickled red cells is 10 to 12 days as opposed to 120 days in normal red cells.[1,4] Other factors contributing to anemia and hemolysis include decreased deformability of sickled cells, adherence of the sickled cells to vessel walls, and polymerization.[3]

Clinical Syndrome

The severity of the clinical syndrome is related to the proportion of Hb S, with homozygous individuals (SS) being at particular risk. Sickle cell trait is a benign and asymptomatic condition, frequently discovered incidentally by laboratory testing.[5,6] These individuals usually live a normal life and there is no evidence of increased morbidity or mortality. However vaso-occlusive crises may occur under extreme nonphysiologic conditions. Sequestration of blood with splenic infarctions has been reported during nonpressurized, high altitude flying.[7] Sickling can also occur in these individuals during extremes of low-flow states and hypoxemia.[3] Conditions reported to predispose to such sickling crises include respiratory depression from drug overdose,[8] severe alcohol intoxication[9] and high spinal anesthesia resulting in hypotension and splenic pooling.[10]

Sickle cell anemia is a chronic disorder associated with acute crises which are described in four forms: 1) hemolytic crisis, which depletes the circulatory red cell mass, is not common unless associated with glucose-6-phosphate dehydrogenase deficiency; 2) aplastic crisis, which is characterized by bone marrow depression accompanying an infectious process; 3) sequestration crisis, common in children and occurs when red blood cells are trapped in the spleen and reticuloendothelial cells; and 4) vaso-occlusive crisis, which is usually characterized by ischemic pain. Patients with sickle cell anemia are also more prone to develop infections as compared to the rest of the population.

Diagnosis

A reliable history and physical examination are essential to making a diagnosis and improving long-term survival. Hemoglobin electrophoresis is recommended for those newborns of African or Caribbean descent because the history and physical exam may be inconclusive during this period. In older children and adults of African or Caribbean ancestry, a sickle preparation test may be performed as a screening test. In this test, a sample of blood is added to a solution of sodium metabisulfite, a reducing agent. A positive indicates sickling of the red blood cells. The test is positive in the presence of both SS and AS hemoglobin and does not differentiate sickle cell anemia from sickle cell trait. The differentiation can only be made by hemoglobin electrophoresis.

Early screening in newborns permits early vaccination and prophylactic antibiotics, which reduce the incidence of infections. Folic acid is commonly prescribed to prevent megaloblastic anemia associated with impaired folate turnover.[3] Preventive therapy of vaso-occlusive crises consists of hydration, avoiding conditions that promote sickling, and prompt and aggressive treatment of infections.

Homologous red blood cell transfusions containing hemoglobin A blood is a mainstay in the treatment of this disease. This not only corrects the decreased oxygen-carrying capacity of anemia, but also decreases erythropoiesis, which would produce more Hb S red cells. Transfusion is recommended for situations associated with increased morbidity, such as severe cerebral ischemic events, acute lung disease with hypoxia, overwhelming infections, high-risk pregnancy, and preoperatively before major surgery.[3] The need for repeated transfusions runs the increased risk of transfusion reactions, iron overload, increased blood viscosity, and compromised immunocompetency in these patients. Alloimmunizations from these transfusions may result in crossmatching difficulties and increase the risk for severe delayed hemolytic reactions.[11] Hydroxyurea therapy has been shown to be effective for treating adult patients with sickle cell disease. The principal therapeutic effect is believed to be the increase in the fraction of "F cells." These cells contain approximately 20% fetal hemoglobin and 80% hemoglobin S. The dilution of the S-hemoglobin delays the polymerization of the S hemoglobin as it becomes deoxygenated in the capillary bed, and permits the cells to pass through without occluding the vessels.[11a]

Perioperative Management

Patients with sickle cell trait (AS) require no special perioperative treatment, although a rare sickle cell crisis can occur in the presence of severe hypoxemia, acidosis, and hypotension. Although patients with sickle cell anemia are at increased risk for perioperative morbidity and mortality, improved preoperative screening, transfusion therapy, and improved anesthetic and monitoring techniques have contributed to improved outcomes.[3] Major considerations prior to elective surgery include the extent of the operation, the concentration of Hb S in the patient's blood, the anticipated blood loss, and preoperative physical condition. Preoperative medical preparation focuses on maintenance of adequate oxygenation, prevention of dehydration, control of infections including prophylactic antibiotics, treatment of pre-existing diseases, and having an adequate hemoglobin level. Preoperative blood transfusion therapy may be necessary to increase the levels of hemoglobin A and reduce the amount of hemoglobin S. The preoperative hemoglobin level should be greater than 10 g/dl with Hb S levels less than 40 to 50%. In certain situations, lower Hb S levels may be recommended.[3]

Both general and regional anesthetic techniques are acceptable for patients with sickle cell disease.[12-14] Intraoperatively, attention is directed toward maintaining adequate tissue oxygenation, perfusion, and hydration, while preventing vasoconstriction, acidosis, and hypothermia. When cardiac output is decreased, oxygen extraction is increased and PvO_2 may decrease to dangerously low levels, resulting in sickled red cells underscoring the need to maintain hydration and normal cardiac output in these patients. Acidemia should be prevented and treated promptly; a mild degree of alkalemia maintained by sodium bicarbonate (50 mEq added to each liter of fluids administered) may render hemoglobin S resistant to sickling. Hypothermia not only causes stasis, but may also increase the blood viscosity and tendency to sickling. Aseptic techniques must be practiced and antibiotics may be administered as indicated. Proper patient positioning and avoiding venous stasis is of prime concern. The use of tourniquets has been discouraged because it may lead to circulatory stasis, acidosis, and hypoxemia leading to sickling; however, recent studies suggest that it is safe to use a tourniquet in patients with sickle cell disease provided optimum acid-base status and oxygenation are maintained throughout the surgical procedure.[15,16] Vasoconstrictors, particularly α-agonists, should be used with extreme caution as they may produce undesirable peripheral vasoconstriction.

Appropriate monitoring is essential during anesthesia and surgery. For major procedures, monitors should include those for cardiac function (pulse, blood pressure, ECG), hydration (urine output), oxygenation (pulse oximetry, blood gases, pH), capnography, and temperature. It may be helpful to monitor SvO_2 or PvO_2 in these patients. The critical levels for the PvO_2 are 30 mm Hg for patients with sickle cell disease and 20 mm Hg for those with sickle cell trait. A sickle cell crisis can occur intraoperatively and the presence of excessive hemolysis or rapid deterioration in the patient's condition should arouse suspicion. A crisis may be manifested as cardiac, pulmonary or central nervous system dysfunction. Management includes maintenance of oxygenation, hydration and blood transfusion. The need for urgency in these circumstances may be sufficient to warrant the transfusion of fresh uncross-matched O-negative blood.

Postoperative care is particularly important in these patients. Complications including sickle cell crises are most common during the postoperative period, when the potential for hypoxemia is greatest.[3] Attempts to prevent shivering must be considered during recovery from anesthesia since it may cause a marked increase in O_2 production to 300 percent above normal. Close monitoring, adequate hydration, early ambulation, and prevention of infection are imperative. Administration of oxygen and the use of respiratory therapeutic maneuvers may be necessary.

Pregnancy

Pregnant patients with sickle cell disease are at an increased risk for spontaneous abortion, intrauterine growth retardation, and possible neonatal death; however, improved perinatal care has decreased maternal and perinatal morbidity and mortality.[17] All pregnant patients with sickle cell anemia should receive the usual prenatal iron and extra folic acid. Prophylactic transfusions are not recommended. Transfusion should be reserved for complications such as preeclampsia, septicemia, acute renal failure, severe anemia, hypoxemia, or anticipated surgery.[17] Exchange transfusion should be aimed at decreasing the Hb S level below 50% if general anesthesia is to be employed for cesarean section. The pregnant patient with sickle cell trait requires no special treatment other than counseling regarding possibility of having offsprings with sickle cell anemia.

Cardiopulmonary Bypass

Patients with sickle cell anemia who undergo hypothermic cardiopulmonary bypass (CPB) require special consideration because both hypothermia and stasis may lead to sickling. Exchange transfusion, either preoperatively or intraoperatively to reduce the quantity of Hb S to no greater than 50 percent before the initiation of hypothermic CPB has been recommended;[18,19] however, other investigators have found that prebypass exchange transfusion is not necessary as long as care is given to maintaining adequate oxygenation, and avoiding acidosis and dehydration.[20] Additional prophylactic measures include avoidance of profound hypothermia, use of vasodilators to improve peripheral perfusion, maintenance of low viscosity, and monitoring SvO_2. Patients with sickle cell trait have successfully undergone CPB procedures without the need for special therapeutic maneuvers.

Thalassemia

The thalassemias are a group of hereditary anemias in which the rate of synthesis of one of the chains of hemoglobin is reduced or impaired. The word thalassemia is derived from the Greek word for the sea and refers to the many patients of Mediterranean ancestry who have the disease. Thalassemia major and minor refer to the homozygous and heterozygous states, respectively, whereas the prefix α and β designate which chain is synthesized at a reduced rate.

Beta-Thalassemia

Pathophysiology

Beta-thalassemia is often classified into two categories: (1) β°-thalassemia, a syndrome associated with a total absence of β-chains in the homozygous state; and (2) β^+-thalassemia, characterized by reduced but detectable synthesis of the β-chain in the homozygous state. Two factors are responsible for the anemic state of β-thalassemia. First, the reduced or lack of synthesis of β-chain leads to inadequate Hb A formation and results in a hypochromic red cell secondary to an overall reduction of hemoglobin in the cells. Second and more importantly, the synthesis of α chains continues unimpaired and forms highly unstable aggregates that precipitate in the red cell precursors in the form of insoluble inclusions.[21] These inclusions contribute to cell membrane damage and destruction of the red cell precursors within the bone marrow, a process known as *ineffective erythropoiesis*. As many as 75% of marrow normoblasts are destroyed in severely affected patients and those that survive are at increased risk for destruction in the spleen. In severe cases, erythropoietin secretion is stimulated and leads to massive erythropoiesis within bones resulting in skeletal abnormalities and impairment of bone growth. Extramedullary hematopoiesis in the liver and spleen is also common. The marked anemia associated with ineffective erythropoiesis, hemolysis, combined with the need for repeated blood transfusions, leads to a state of iron overload and accumulation of iron within parenchymal organs.

Clinical Syndrome

Patients with *β-thalassemia minor* or trait are heterozygous with one normal gene and usually have enough β-chain synthesis so that they are asymptomatic with only a mild hypochromic and microcytic anemia. β-thalassemia minor must be differentiated from the hypochromic, microcytic anemia of iron deficiency because iron supplementation in these patients may enhance iron absorption and worsen the complications of iron overload. Patients with *β-thalassemia intermedia* have a disorder characterized by several variants of homozygous and heterozygous β-thalassemia. β-thalassemia intermedia is a heterogeneous disorder that is associated with a severe anemia but afflicted individuals do not usually require regular blood transfusions. Patients with homozygous β-thalassemia (β° or β^+) have the most severe form of anemia called *β-thalassemia major*.

β-thalassemia major is first manifest in infancy, as hemoglobin synthesis switches from Hb F to Hb A. Hemoglobin levels range from 3 to 5 g/dl in untransfused patients and is associated with growth retardation and early death. With blood transfusions, patients may live into the second and third decades of life. Transfusions not only improve the anemia but also minimize the effects of extramedullary hematopoiesis. The increased production of red blood cells results in characteristic skeletal changes including thinning of cortical bone and cephalofacial abnormalities. Hepatosplenomegaly is common and cardiac disease results from progressive iron overload and secondary hemochromatosis.[22]

Perioperative Management

This is geared toward maintaining hemoglobin concentrations greater than 9 g/dl with blood transfusions. Maxillofacial abnormalities associated with severe forms of the disease may make visualization of the glottis difficult during direct laryngoscopy. A pulmonary artery catheter and/or transesophageal echocardiography may be useful in managing left ventricular dysfunction associated with secondary hemochromatosis.

Alpha Thalassemia

Alpha-thalassemias are characterized by reduced synthesis of α-chains in hemoglobin. Normally, there are four genes for the α chain and the severity of the disease reflects the number of defective genes. The clinical syndrome can range from a silent carrier state (one abnormal gene), to α-*thalassemia trait* (two abnormal genes) in which a mild hypochromic and microcytic anemia exists, to *hemoglobin H disease* (three abnormal genes) which clinically resembles β-thalassemia intermedia. The most severe form of α-thalassemia is the homozygous genotype in which no α-chains are synthesized. This homozygous state, often called hydrops fetalis, is incompatible with life and associated with early neonatal death.

Porphyria

The porphyric diseases of humans are rare metabolic disorders with a genetic basis in which the biochemical lesion involves the pathway for the production of heme. Porphyrins are tetrapyrrole pigments that are stepping stones in the biochemical pathway for the production of heme proteins including hemoglobin, myoglobin, various cytochromes and enzymes. Heme compounds serve two purposes: 1) for transport of oxygen, e.g., heme is the base for hemoglobin formation and respiratory activity; and 2) for interactions with toxic substances, e.g. hepatic heme protein cytochrome P-450 is essential for binding of molecular oxygen in hydroxylation reactions of chemical substrates brought to liver for detoxification. The porphyric diseases involve a partial deficiency of enzymes involved in heme synthesis which lead to an accumulation of one or more porphyrin intermediates.[23,24]

The synthetic (Fig. 14-1) pathway of heme begins with two simple molecules, the amino acid glycine and succinyl-CoA. These two molecules are combined by enzymatic action of aminolevulinic acid (ALA) synthetase to form an aminoketone aminolevulinic acid (ALA). The formation of ALA is the rate limiting step for heme formation. The enzyme ALA dehydrase combines two ALA molecules to form the ring-shaped monopyrolle, porphobilinogen (PBG). ALA and PBG are the essential building blocks for heme production. Four monopyrolles PBG molecules are combined by uroporphyrinogen (UPG) synthetase to form the tetrapyrrole uroporphyrinogen and other *porphyrinogen* compounds. Porphyrinogens differ from porphyrins only in the nature of their side-chains and serve as intermediate chemical precursors

for the synthesis of heme. Porphyrinogens are colorless, but when oxidized, become porphyrins that appear wine red under visible light. They are also capable of absorbing UV radiation and render patients photosensitive.

Hepatic Porphyrias

There are four principal subtypes: acute intermittent porphyria, variegate porphyria, hereditary coproporphyria, and cutanea tarda (cutaneous porphyria). Each is related to a specific enzyme deficiency in porphyrin synthesis. During attacks large quantities of colorless PBG are excreted in the urine. If allowed to stand, the PBG is oxidized to pigmented porphyrins and the urine darkens to a "port wine" color. Laboratory measurement of the actual porphyrin produced is available. Acute symptoms associated with the hepatic porphyrias may be precipitated by exposure to a variety of drugs, including anesthetic agents (Table 14-2).

Acute Intermittent Porphyria

The most common and best studied of all porphyrias is the acute intermittent porphyria (AIP) or Swedish type. The incidence of AIP is approximately 1 in 70,000. It is the most common type of hepatic porphyria and represents 75% of all cases. It is inherited in an autosomal dominant manner, appears in adults in the 2nd and 3rd decade of life, and affects more females than males in a ratio of 3 to 2. The enzymatic defect in this form of porphyria is a deficiency of uroporphyrinogen (UPG) synthetase and there may be a relative or actual excess of ALA synthetase. Hence, there is accumulation of ALA and PBG. Most of the symptoms and signs are relative to accumulation of the intermediate metabolites ALA, PBG, and the porphyrinogens.

Clinical Characteristics

A porphyric attack is often precipitated by drugs, infections, and endocrinologic variations. In women, the premenstrual period and pregnancy exacerbate the disease. Tension and emotional stress are common precipitants while fasting and dehydration are initiating factors. Clini-

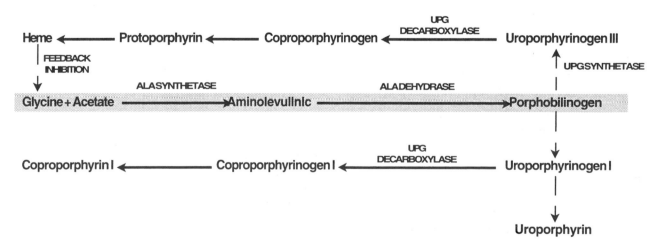

Fig. 14–1. Porphyrin and hemesynthesis.

Table 14–2. Porphyrogenic Drugs: Inducers of Porphyria

Hypnotics	Steroids
Barbiturates	Birth control pills; estrogen
Benzodiazepines	Sulfonylureas
Local anesthetics	Tolbutamide
Lidocaine	Analgesics
Muscle relaxant reversal agents	Acetaminophen
Neostigmine	Miscellaneous
Anticonvulsants	Ethyl alcohol
Phenytoin	Ergot preparations
Antibiotics/Antifungals	Methyldopa
Sulfa drugs; griseofulvin	

cal characteristics include gastrointestinal, neurologic, cardiovascular, and psychiatric abnormalities.

Patients often present with gastrointestinal symptoms that may mimic virtually any surgical abdominal emergency. Colic, generalized abdominal pain, vomiting, ileitis, constipation, or diarrhea are common. Fever, leucocytosis, proteinuria and tachycardia accompany an attack. The abdominal pain may be related to neurological involvement particularly of the autonomic nervous system. Neurologic involvement of the peripheral, central, and autonomic nervous systems are common. Porphyria precursors ALA and PBG produce partial axonal degeneration that results in denervation of some muscle fibers combined with normal nerve conduction in other muscle fibers. Weakness of muscles is frequent and the precursors inhibit neuromuscular transmission by inhibiting the release of acetylcholine.[25] Central neurological manifestations include convulsions and paralysis. These may be related to the hypo-osmolality and hyponatremia. Cardiovascular lability is often present. Tachycardia and hypertension are common. Hypotension is easily precipitated by stress. Such pulse and blood pressure changes are probably secondary to autonomic neuropathy. Psychiatric disturbances range from the behavioral disorders to frank psychosis. Depression is prominent during attacks and even manifested during remission. The incidence of porphyria in mental institutions appears to be higher than in the general population.

The signs and symptoms of a porphyric crisis are severe and are exacerbated by porphyrogenic drugs. A rapidly fatal course may occur in 25% of the patients. The cause of death is usually secondary to extensive axonal degeneration by the porphyrin precursors of peripheral nerves including motor, sensory, and autonomic fibers; cranial nerves are also involved and similar lesions occur in the parenchyma of the brain. Paralysis of visceral and skeletal muscle is evident and respiratory paralysis occurs.

Treatment

Treatment is focused on preventing attacks, supporting care particularly neurologic dysfunction, and reversing the fundamental disease process. In the event of an acute attack, care should be given to avoiding porphyrogenic drugs that may exacerbate symptoms. Somatic pain can be safely obtunded by morphine; codeine is especially effective for bone pain; meperidine is more satisfactory for abdominal and visceral pain. Infection needs to be treated with appropriate antibiotic therapy; penicillins and tetracyclines are safe and beneficial. Tachycardia may be safely treated with β-blockers. Psychiatric symptoms may be safely treated with chlorpromazine, but other phenothiazines may not be tolerated. Fluid and electrolyte balance must be normalized as dehydration may precipitate or further exacerbate an attack. However, inappropriate anti-diuretic hormone (ADH) secretion is usually present and overhydration may occur. Finally, respiratory function must be evaluated: hypoxemia must be corrected and mechanical ventilation should be considered in the face of muscular weakness.

Glucose, β-blockade, and hematin have a role in the management of an acute attack. A high carbohydrate diet has been shown to limit the frequency of attacks and their severity.[26] The induction of porphyrinogenic enzymes is repressed by glucose. Generous amounts of intravenous glucose with an elevation of blood glucose level specifically suppress *ALA synthetase*. The porphyrin precursors and their excretion are usually decreased, i.e., overproduction of ALA and PBG is curtailed. Also, the response to drugs that accelerate hepatic porphyria is blocked. Glucose, in amounts of 10 to 15 g per hour for 24 hours (200 g/day supplemental to a high carbohydrate diet) ameliorates attacks. Complete symptomatic relief has been reported following β-blockade in AIP and other forms of hepatic porphyria.[27,28] Propanolol, in particular, reduces the formation and excretion of urinary porphyrins.

The rate-limiting enzyme ALA synthetase is normally stimulated by a heme deficiency while ordinary levels provide a negative feedback to modulate its presence (Fig. 14-1). On this basis, exogenous intravenous hematin has been recommended to repress ALA synthetase activity.[29,30] The administration of 200 to 400 mg (2 to 3 mg/kg) of hematin ameliorates attacks of AIP and other hepatic porphyria.[31]

Anesthetic Management

During the preanesthetic period, special attention should be given to hydration and electrolyte status. A thorough neurologic evaluation is warranted and cardiovascular abnormalities should be addressed. Preanesthetic medications should be limited to those that have no porphyrogenic potential.[32] Benzodiazepines may precipitate an acute attack. Fentanyl and meperidine are well tolerated, as are anticholinergic agents.

Regional anesthesia is best avoided because of the frequent and sometimes masked neurological symptoms, although epidural anesthesia has been performed safely in patients undergoing obstetric procedures.[33] General anesthesia is preferred utilizing a glucose intravenous infusion for reasons described previously. Safe anesthetic induction agents include ketamine, etomidate, and propofol.[34,35,36] The influence of barbiturates in precipitating an attack of porphyria is long established including the adverse effect of intravenous thiopental in anesthesia practice.[37] It appears porphyrogenic drugs, including thiopental, induce the mitochondrial enzyme ALA synthetase and probably the ALA dehydrase. Other drugs that have been alleged to induce acute attacks of porphyria include lidocaine,[33] intravenous steroid agents, and phonytoin. Nitrous oxide and all narcotics are well tolerated. Volatile agents which are probably safe, although enzyme inducing agents such as halothane are best avoided. Muscle relaxants are safe. Anticholinesterase drugs appear to be safe; however, neostigmine has been porphyrogenic[38,39] and should probably be avoided. Postoperative attention to ventilation as the development of respiratory insufficiency and failure is often insidious and sudden.

Variegate Porphyria

Variegate porphyria is an hereditary autosomal dominant hepatic disorder of porphyrin synthesis with presenting manifestations of both skin lesions and neuropsychiatric symptoms. The large majority of individuals with variegate porphyria are photosensitive and develop eczematous lesions and vesicle formation. About 20% of hepatic porphyrias are represented by this variety. It is also known as South African porphyria with an incidence in 1 to 100 whites of Dutch extraction. Onset is later than AIP occurring in the fourth to fifth decade. Acute episodes are accompanied by a mortality of about 25%. Neurologic disturbances are usually present and abdominal pain frequent. Both sexes are equally affected. However, more men have skin lesions while women are prone to show neurologic signs. In the quiescent stage, urine findings are normal, but high levels of porphyrin are present in stools. The disorder is due to an enzymatic defect in the terminal portion of heme biosynthesis. A decrease in protoporphyrin permits the precursor protoporphyrinogen to accumulate; the excess is excreted in bile and is auto-oxidized to protoporphyrin.[40] A variant of the disorder involves a deficiency of heme synthetase needed for conversion of protoporphyrin to heme. Treatment and anesthetic management of variegate porphyria is similar to that of acute intermittent porphyria.

Hereditary Coproporphyria

Coproporphyria resembles variegate porphyria, but is distinguished by little or no photosensitivity and the absence of skin lesion, and only mild neurologic symptoms. It comprises approximately 5% of patients with hepatic porphyria. It is inherited as a dominant trait and both sexes are equally affected. Between attacks, the unique features are the marked increase in fecal coproporphyrin with low fecal protoporphyrin and normal urinary coproporphyrin. During an acute attack, urinary coproporphyrin is also elevated. Porphyrogenic drugs are able to precipitate acute attacks.

Cutanea Tarda

Cutanea tarda (cutaneous porphyria) is a familial and hereditary variant transmitted as an autosomal dominant trait. The defect is a deficiency of UPG decarboxylase

leading to an accumulation of uroporphyrinogen III. The disease is characterized by photosensitivity, lesions of the skin, liver disease, and increased uroporphyrin in the urine. It affects males in the fifth and subsequent decades of life. Skin lesions of the face may be followed by disfiguration and scarring. Neurologic signs are not seen. Alcohol, iron compounds, phenols, and estrogens are precipitating agents. Certain diseases such as lupus, hemolytic anemias, and hepatomas have been associated with this disorder. Urine levels of ALA and PBG are normal, but the urine is pink or brown due to the increased uroporphyrinogen III. Treatment is largely symptomatic, but patients should not ingest alcohol or expose themselves to sunlight or benzene type chemicals.

Erythropoietic Porphyrias

Of the porphyrias, the erythropoietic types represent less than 20%. Two subtypes are recognized and both are inherited. *Congenital erythropoietic porphyria* is a very rare autosomal recessive disorder. It is seen between birth and five years of age and associated with extreme photosensitivity. Chemically, there is a marked over-production of uroporphyrin I and coproporphyrin I in circulating erythrocytes and bone marrow cells. Clinically, patients have a dramatic appearance of red urine soon after birth. They show pronounced vesicle and bullae formation, ulceration of skin, and secondary infection. A brownish red discoloration of the teeth and nails is seen due to deposition of porphyrins. Hemolytic anemia with splenomegaly occurs; splenectomy ameliorates the anemia. There is a marked increase in urinary and fecal uroporphyrins. Mortality is appreciable and death frequently occurs in childhood.

Congenital erythropoietic protoporphyria is a genetic disease transmitted in an autosomal dominant manner. Excessive amounts of protoporphyria are produced in circulating erythrocytes and bone marrow. In contrast to the previous type, there is *no* increase in fecal or urinary porphyrins. Some increase in hepatic production of porphyrins may occur; therefore, this disease may have biochemical defects in both erythropoietic and hepatic cells. The prognosis is good without disability, but cholelithiasis appears to be a common complication. Clinically, there is mild photosensitivity. Eczema is frequent and inflammatory reactions of skin occur on exposure to sun. Hypersplenism is occasionally seen with a hemolytic anemia. Onset is in the first years of life, but may not be expressed until after adolescence. This subtype may be more common than formerly believed and could explain many light-sensitive skin reactions. Porphyrogenic drugs do not induce reactions in this form of porphyria.

Hereditary Spherocytosis

Hereditary spherocytosis is an autosomal dominant disorder that is characterized by an intrinsic defect in the red cell membrane that causes the red cell to be spheroidal in shape, less deformable, and vulnerable to sequestration and destruction in the spleen. These spherocytes are particularly vulnerable to osmotic lysis induced by intravascular hypotonic salt solutions. The disease is most prevalent in people of North European descent and characteristic clinical features include anemia, splenomegaly and jaundice.[41] The severity of the disease varies from patient to patient. It may manifest at birth with marked jaundice requiring exchange transfusion, while in others, the mild anemia is well compensated by increased erythropoiesis. This compensatory mechanism may be overwhelmed in the presence of infection leading to a *hemolytic crisis* characterized by massive hemolysis accompanied by abdominal pain, nausea, vomiting, fever, and hypotension. During active hemolysis, the patient is typically markedly jaundiced. Transfusion may be necessary to support the patient. Cholelithiasis secondary to chronic hemolysis and elevated plasma bilirubin is common in these patients.

Diagnosis is made primarily by family history, hematologic findings, and laboratory evidence of spherocytosis and osmotic fragility. These patients benefit from elective splenectomy if anemia is severe. Although splenectomy does not affect the spheroidal shape of the cell, it greatly reduces hemolysis and increases the life span of the cell to 80 percent of normal.

Glucose-6-phosphate Dehydrogenase Deficiency

Glucose-6-phosphate dehydrogenase (G-6-PD) deficiency is a common inherited x-linked disorder that enables endogenous and exogenous oxidants to damage red blood cells and their membranes. Normally these oxidants are inactivated by intracellular reduced glutathione, which is usually produced via metabolic processes dependent on the activity of the enzyme G-6-PD. The deficiency of this enzyme and resulting lack of glutathione, reduces the ability of the red cell to protect itself from oxidative injuries leading to hemolysis.[42] Although many variants of G-6-PD deficiency exist worldwide, two variants designated as G-6-PD A^- and G-6-PD Mediterranean, lead to clinically significant hemolysis. G-6-PD A^- is found in approximately 10 percent of African American males, whereas G-6-PD Mediterranean is found largely in middle eastern populations. In the G-6-PD A^- variant, the amount of enzyme synthesized in red cell precursors are normal, but it is rapidly inactivated during the life span of the red cell making older cells prone to oxidative injury. In G-6-PD Mediterranean, enzyme activity is markedly reduced throughout the life span of the red cell suggesting impaired synthesis of the enzyme.

The pathophysiology of hemolysis appears to involve infection or exposure to oxidant drugs that cause oxidation of the reduced glutathione via the production of hydrogen peroxide. Because regeneration of reduced glutathione is impaired in G-6-PD deficient cell, peroxides accumulate and damage both hemoglobin and red cell membranes. These defective red cells are ultimately sequestered and phagocytized in the spleen. Drugs that interact with oxyhemoglobin to form peroxides include antimalarials (primaquine and quinacrine), sulfonamides, acetaminophen, and various antibiotics (nitrofurans, penicillin, streptomycin, and isoniazid). The clinical course is generally mild in those patients with the G-6-PD A^- variant, while those with the G-6-PD Mediterranean variant have more severe and prolonged hemolysis when exposed to oxidant injuries. Although anesthetic agents have not been associated with oxidant injuries, patients with G-6-PD deficiency may develop hemolysis and jaundice in the early postoperative period.[43]

Paroxysmal Nocturnal Hemoglobinuria

Paroxysmal nocturnal hemoglobinuria (PNH) is a rare disorder of unknown etiology that is characterized by chronic intravascular hemolysis with acute exacerbations. The basic defect involves an unusual sensitivity of red blood cells to complement-mediated lysis. The disease is most common in young adults and is variable in clinical manifestation. Patients classically have intravascular hemolysis that tends to get worse at night. Some patients present with hemoglobinuria upon awakening. Anemia is often severe enough to require blood transfusion. Chronic loss of blood and iron eventually leads to iron deficiency. Many patients develop venous thromboses in the hepatic, portal, or cerebral veins which or often fatal. Perioperative anticoagulation may be warranted in these patients.

PERIOPERATIVE MANAGEMENT OF ACQUIRED BLEEDING DISORDERS

Normal hemostasis is dependent on precisely regulated interactions between (1) subendothelium and endothelial cells of the blood vessel wall, (2) platelets, and (3) the plasma coagulation system. Excessive bleeding may occur during the perioperative period if the hemostatic system is overwhelmed by large wounds to major blood vessels, or if the hemostatic machinery is impaired by congenital or acquired bleeding disorders. Occasionally, excessive bleeding is the result of dilution and/or consumption of coagulation factors and platelets. Essential information necessary to evaluate and manage abnormal perioperative bleeding is discussed in this following section.

Vitamin K Deficiency

Vitamin K is a fat-soluble vitamin which is necessary for the carboxylation of glutamic residues on factors II, VII, IX, and X. This enzymatic action is required for the biologic function of these coagulation factors. In the process of doing this, vitamin K is converted into an epoxide by liver microsomes, making vitamin K nonfunctional. Vitamin K epoxide is subsequently converted back to its functional state by a liver membrane reductase. Warfarin, a coumarin derivative, inhibits the action of the reductase enzyme and competitively inhibits the coagulation effects of vitamin K.

Dietary vitamin K is absorbed in the small intestine in the presence of bile salts and is stored in the liver. Vitamin K is also synthesized in varying quantities by endogenous bacterial flora resident in the small intestine and colon. The major causes of vitamin K deficiency are (1) inadequate dietary intake, (2) intestinal malabsorption, and/or (3) antibiotic-induced elimination of intestinal bacterial flora. Although a normal liver can store vitamin K for 30 days, acutely ill patients can become deficient within 7 to 10 days. Patients recovering from biliary tract surgery without dietary intake of vitamin K and on broad spectrum antibiotics are particularly prone to deficiencies. Neonatal vitamin K deficiency causes hemorrhagic disease of the newborn; however, routine supplemental administration of vitamin K has virtually eliminated this disease.

Vitamin K deficiency results in a reduction in all vitamin K-dependent coagulation factors. Because factor VII has the shortest half-life, a mild vitamin K deficiency will be readily reflected in the PT, while the APTT is normal. As the deficiency persists, the other factors fall and the APTT will also become prolonged. The treatment for vitamin K deficiency depends on the urgency of the situation. Parenteral administration of vitamin K restores vitamin K levels in the liver and permits production of affected coagulation factors within 6 to 8 hours. In the face of active hemorrhage, FFP immediately corrects the hemostatic defect.[44] Patients with malabsorption problems and receiving total parenteral nutrition require regular supplementation of vitamin K. Patients receiving long-term antibiotic therapy should be considered for supplementation as well.

Drug-induced Platelet Abnormalities

Antiplatelet Medication

Antiplatelet medications are often used in the management of patients with arterial vascular and thromboembolic diseases.[45] These medications are associated with mild bleeding disorders, the most common of which result from the ingestion of aspirin and nonsteroidal anti-inflammatory agents (NSAIDs). These drugs inhibit platelet cyclo-oxygenase, which, in turn, inhibits the platelet production of thromboxane A_2, an important mediator of platelet aggregation.

Aspirin is the most potent of these agents and the most widely studied. Aspirin irreversibly acetylates cyclo-oxygenase[46] and inhibits thromboxane production with a single dose that is lower than 160 mg. This inhibition lasts for the normal lifespan of the platelets, which is 8 to 11 days. The other NSAIDs are competitive and reversible inhibitors of cyclo-oxygenase and have more transient effects. Patients with drug-induced cyclo-oxygenase inhibition usually have prolonged bleeding times. At higher chronic doses, aspirin also decreases the production of prothrombin, leading to an increased PT. Patients taking oral warfarin may have increased plasma concentrations of free warfarin secondary to reduced protein binding in the presence of aspirin.

Patients have minimal symptoms but will occasionally have prolonged oozing after surgery, particularly with procedures involving mucous membranes, such as periodontal and oral surgery. The antiplatelet effect of these drugs may be particularly dramatic in patients with underlying defects like von Willebrand's disease and hemophilia. Evidence is also accumulating that aspirin is particularly hazardous to patients undergoing CPB surgery, in that perioperative bleeding may be severe[47] (See Cardiopulmonary Bypass). Therefore, it is reasonable to defer elective surgical procedures associated with significant blood loss until the effects of antiplatelet medications have worn off. Epidural and spinal anesthesia is often avoided because of the associated prolongation of the bleeding time and potential risk for hematoma formation; however, recent studies suggest that patients receiving preoperative antiplatelet medication can safely undergo these anesthetic procedures.[48] Nonetheless, caution should be used when performing major regional blocks on patients receiving higher doses of antiplatelet medications.

Antibiotics

The administration of high doses of antibiotics, particularly the penicillins, has been associated with platelet dysfunction by apparently interfering with ADP receptors on the platelet membrane, leaving them unavailable for agonists to induce aggregation.[49] An increased bleeding time in patients undergoing antibiotic therapy is associated with an increased risk of clinical bleeding.[50]

Nitrates

The preservation of platelet function needs to be considered when using nitrates to control arterial blood pressure and vascular resistance. Traditionally, sodium nitroprusside and nitroglycerine have been used for this purpose during cardiac surgery and procedures requiring induced hypotension (i.e., scoliosis, head and neck procedures); however, these two agents significantly alter hemostatic mechanisms and inhibit platelet function resulting in increased bleeding times at clinically relevant doses.[51,52] Studies suggest that this platelet inhibition is related to the generation of nitric oxide (NO) or endothelium-derived relaxing factor.[53,54] Trimethaphan, a ganglionic blocker, is also used to control arterial blood pressure and vascular resistance. Unlike the nitrates, platelet function is preserved in the presence of trimethaphan and is not associated with increased bleeding times.[55] Trimethaphan may be a more appropriate vasodilator during surgical procedures that are associated with abnormalities in hemostasis (i.e., cardiopulmonary bypass).

There are many other drugs that affect platelet function (Table 14-3) and bleeding times, including bronchodilators, β-adrenergic blockers,[56] calcium-channel blockers,[57] dipyridamole,[58] and inhaled anesthetic agents including nitrous oxide.[59,60] In addition to affecting platelet function, many drugs including antibiotics, diuretics, and certain cardiovascular drugs can cause thrombocytopenia resulting in increased bleeding times (Table 14-4).

Anticoagulant Medications

Heparin

Heparin is a water soluble, organic acid that is present in high concentrations in the liver and in the granules of mast cells and basophils. The anticoagulant effect of heparin stems from its ability to bind with antithrombin III (ATIII), inducing a conformational change that greatly enhances the ability of ATIII to inhibit factors XIIa, XIa, IXa, Xa, and IIa (thrombin).[61] Commercially, heparin is prepared from bovine lung and bovine or porcine gastrointestinal mucosa. It is a heterogeneous biochemical substance, and its anticoagulant activity may vary per unit weight. Therefore, the anticoagulant potency of heparin is measured in standardized units and should always be prescribed in units.

Table 14–3. Drugs Inhibiting Platelet Function

Anti-inflammatory agents (inhibitors of thromboxane synthesis)	Anesthetic agents
Aspirin	Halothane, isoflurane
Nonsteroidal anti-inflammatory agents	Nitrous oxide
Corticosteroids	Local anesthetics (procaine, lidocaine)
Furosemide	Cardiovascular drugs
Antibiotics	Adenosine
Penicillin derivatives	β-adrenergic blockers (propanolol)
Nitrofurantoin	Calcium channel blockers (verapamil, diltiazem)
Bronchodilators	Dipyridamole
Methylxanthines (aminophylline, theophylline)	Hydralazine
β-sympathomimetic agents (isoproterenol)	Nitroglycerine
Psychoactive drugs	Nitroprusside
Diazepam	Protamine
Phenothiazines	Miscellaneous drugs
Tricyclic antidepressants (amitriptyline)	Ethanol
	Antihistamines (chlorpromazine)
	Caffeine

Table 14–4. Drugs Causing Thrombocytopenia

Antibiotics	Cardiovascular drugs
Cephalothin	Heparin
Gentamicin	Protamine
Sulfonamides	Quinidine
Diuretics	Miscellaneous drugs
Acetazolamide	Acetaminophen
Chlorothiazide	
Ethacrynic acid	
Furosemide	

Clinically, heparin is primarily used to produce anticoagulation, although it also induces a release in lipid-hydrolyzing enzymes that reduce plasma triglyceride concentrations. The clinical uses of heparin are multifold, including anticoagulation for cardiopulmonary bypass, prophylaxis to reduce the risk of deep vein thrombosis and pulmonary embolism, and as a continuous intravenous infusion to maintain the patency of intravascular catheters.

The anticoagulant effect of heparin is instantaneous when given intravenously and occurs within 20 to 30 minutes after subcutaneous injection. It is not effective when given orally. Intramuscular injection is avoided, as there is risk of hematoma formation.

Heparin is metabolized to inactive metabolites in the liver and is excreted by the kidney. It has an elimination half-life of approximately 150 minutes and a duration of action that is less than 6 hours. Larger doses are eliminated more slowly and hypothermia prolongs the anticoagulant effect as well. The duration of action is also prolonged in patients with hepatic and renal disease.

The heparin effect is monitored by the APTT and/or the ACT. A therapeutic APTT that inhibits thrombus formation is considered to be 1.5 to 2.5 times the patient's predrug baseline value. Very prolonged APTT values are readily managed by either omitting a single dose of heparin or reducing the dose because the half-life is very short. The ACT is widely used to monitor the effectiveness of heparin therapy during CPB and extracorporeal circulation.

Adverse Effects of Heparin

Hemorrhage

Hemorrhage is the most serious complication associated with the use of heparin; however, close monitoring of laboratory measurements should minimize the risk of bleeding complications. Heparin should not be administered to patients with a history of a bleeding disorder and should be used cautiously in patients taking antiplatelet medication. Patients at risk for subclinical vitamin K deficiency (i.e., antibiotic therapy, malnutrition) may develop severe hemorrhage with even small amounts of heparin[62] and should receive parenteral vitamin K prior to heparin administration. Heparin is best avoided in patients undergoing intraocular or intracranial surgery.

The use of major regional anesthetic techniques is controversial in patients who are receiving or will subsequently receive heparin. With spinal or epidural anesthesia, the concern is related to the potential for an epidural hematoma to develop if a blood vessel were punctured and subsequent compression of the spinal cord.[63] Performing a peripheral nerve block might also result in hematoma formation and compression of peripheral nerves in a heparinized patient. There are studies that demonstrate that major regional techniques can be done safely in anticoagulated patients.[64] However, the potential severe complications associated with these techniques make it prudent to avoid them in patients with prolonged PT and APTT (more than 20 percent above control). This issue is even less clear in patients who receive heparin anticoagulation after receiving spinal or epidural anesthesia. Many institutions use regional anesthetic techniques for major vascular surgery. Again, studies using a large number of patients have shown no increased incidence of hematoma formation with subsequent heparin administration.[65,66] Despite this, it would seem prudent to delay surgery if the regional technique is associated with bleeding at the time of administration. The use of regional techniques is probably safe in patients receiving subcutaneous heparin injections as prophylaxis for deep vein thrombosis; however, APTT should be done and confirmed to be normal before performing the regional block.

Allergic Reactions

Such responses are rare but do occur and are associated with fever and urticaria. Heparin should be given cautiously to patients with a history of allergy to beef or pork products.

Decreased Antithrombin III (ATIII) Activity

Patients receiving intermittent or continuous heparin therapy develop a reduction in ATIII activity to approximately 10 to 20% of normal.[67] This heparin-induced reduction may cause a paradoxical tendency for thrombotic complications in patients with a mild ATIII deficiency. These patients may require increased dose requirements for adequate anticoagulation from heparin.[68] The administration of FFP or ATIII concentrate restores adequate levels of ATIII and will promote adequate anticoagulation in these patients showing resistance to heparin secondary to acquired or congenital decreases in ATIII.

Heparin-induced Thrombocytopenia

Heparin-induced thrombocytopenia (HIT) is an uncommon but well documented complication of heparin therapy. Most studies show a higher incidence of HIT when bovine-lung heparin is used.[69] Two types of HIT exist: one that occurs early and another that is delayed.[70,71] Type I HIT has an early onset, appearing 1 to 5 days after onset of heparin therapy and occurs in about 15 percent of patients. In type I HITP, platelet counts fall significantly but are usually greater than 50,000/mm^3. The platelet count improves during continued therapy and often returns to normal. Type I has few clinical sequelae and is probably due to a direct heparin-induced platelet aggregation.

Type II is more severe and referred to as *heparin-associated thrombosis* (HAT). It occurs in approximately 6 percent of patients between 4 and 15 days after initiation of heparin therapy. Type II is characterized by a severe reduction in platelets, often to 10,000/mm^3, and is commonly associated with thromboembolic complications. In general, the lower the platelet count, the higher the incidence of thromboembolic complications. Thrombocytopenia is the result of an immune mediated platelet aggregation caused by IgG and IgM bound to platelets. Treatment consists of discontinuing heparin, following antibody titers, and switching to oral anticoagulant therapy. In most instances, platelet counts improve and thromboembolic events resolve 5 to 6 days after discontinuing heparin; however, antibody titers can persist from several weeks to months. Intravenous immunoglobulin has been used to correct particularly severe HAT.[72] Early re-exposure to heparin can result in a catastrophic secondary immune response. If patients require re-exposure to heparin (e.g., cardiopulmonary bypass), pretreatment

with platelet-inhibiting drugs, such as aspirin and dipyridamole, and strict abstinence from heparin after surgery can minimize the severity of HIT and associated thromboembolic complications.[71,73] Iloprost, a stable PGI$_2$ analogue with a short half-life of 15 to 30 minutes, is a potent anti-platelet drug that has been successful in preventing HITP in patients requiring re-exposure to heparin.[74,75]

Effect on Protein-binding Sites

After the acute administration of heparin, the circulatory plasma concentrations of drugs like diazepam and propanolol increase. This is probably due to displacement of these alkaline drugs from their protein binding sites by heparin. These drugs may have increased pharmacologic effects in the presence of acute heparin administration.

Neutralization of Heparin: Protamine

Protamine is commercially prepared from fish sperm and is the only drug currently available in the United States to neutralize heparin.. The high arginine content of protamine makes it strongly cationic, enabling it to form a stable complex with the strongly anionic heparin. The heparin-protamine interaction is based on weight, and, in general, 1.0 mg of protamine is necessary to neutralize 100 units of circulating heparin. However, as much as 3.0 mg of protamine for every 100 units of heparin may be necessary to effectively neutralize heparin.

Hypotension

Hypotension is the most common side effect and is usually associated with rapid administration. The hypotension appears to be associated with histamine release[76] and is generally minimized by administering protamine slowly over 5 minutes.[77] Administering protamine slowly through a peripheral vein may also dilute the protamine, minimizing the release of histamine in the lungs.

Allergic Reactions

A high incidence of anaphylactic and anaphylactoid reactions to protamine have been reported in patients with true fish allergies, diabetic patients receiving NPH (neutral-protamine-Hagedorn) insulin, and prior exposure to protamine.[78] True protamine allergies with antiprotamine IgE and IgM exist,[79] but anaphylactoid reactions are more common. These allergic reactions can be life threatening, and treatment includes intravascular fluid administration, supplemental oxygen, epinephrine, antihistamines, and steroids.

Patients who require heparin anticoagulation and are known to be hypersensitive to protamine are a clinical dilemma. Clinical options include (1) avoidance of protamine, allowing heparin to be eliminated by the liver and kidney, (2) pretreatment with H$_1$ and H$_2$ antagonists followed by slow infusion of protamine, (3) neutralizing heparin with hexadimethrine bromide, an agent not currently available in the United States.[80] Allowing heparin to be metabolized without protamine neutralization may be associated with excessive bleeding requiring blood and

FFP. Hexadimethrine bromide may be associated with a greater degree of hypotension than protamine and may have its own inherent anticoagulant effect.[81] At the pres-ent time, pretreatment with antihistamines and slow administration of protamine with a test dose prior to initiation of the full neutralizing dose is probably the best option.

Pulmonary Hypertension

Occasionally the administration of protamine is associated with complement activation and release of platelet thromboxane A_2, which presents as severe pulmonary vasoconstriction and bronchoconstriction.[82,83] Pretreatment with cyclo-oxygenase inhibitors such as aspirin or NSAIDs diminish these effects,[84] however, these drugs may cause bleeding secondary to platelet dysfunction.

Coumarin Derivatives

The anticoagulant effect of coumarin is related to its ability to interfere with the hepatic synthesis of vitamin K-dependent clotting factors resulting in a reduction of their plasma concentrations. Among the coumarin derivatives, warfarin is the most commonly used and can be administered both orally and intravenously. The anticoagulant effect of warfarin is delayed for 8 to 12 hours with either oral or intravenous administration. It takes 3 to 5 days of therapy before vitamin K-dependent factors reach their lowest levels. Warfarin has a long half-life (24 to 36 hours) and is metabolized in the liver to inactive metabolites that are conjugated and excreted in the bile and urine.

Clinically, warfarin is primarily used to reduce the incidence of thromboembolism associated with prosthetic heart valves and atrial fibrillation. Warfarin therapy is generally initiated slowly with 5 to 10 mg daily for the first few days, after which the dose is adjusted according to the PT. The PT is very sensitive to reductions in factors VII and X. Since factor VII has a short half-life of 7 hours, its concentration is reduced the earliest and reflected in the PT. A therapeutic PT, one that inhibits thrombus formation, generally corresponds to about 17 to 18 seconds. The World Health Organization, along with the International Committee on Thrombosis and Haemostasis have recommended that the reporting of PT results for patients on oral anticoagulant therapy include the use of INR (International Normalized Ratio) values.[85,86] INR results are independent of reagents and methods used, and are specifically intended for assessing patients on long term warfarin therapy. An INR of 3 to 4 is considered to be therapeutic. Unlike heparin, an excessively prolonged PT is not readily reduced by omitting a dose of warfarin because of the long elimination half-life. Likewise, an inadequate PT is not increased quickly with one additional dose of warfarin.

To avoid risks of excessive hemorrhage, warfarin should be discontinued 2 to 3 days before elective surgery to reduce the PT to less than 14 seconds.[87] This approach is reasonable in patients with aortic prosthetic valves because of a low incidence of thromboemboli (1 to 3%). Patients with mitral prosthetic valves have a higher risk for thromboemboli (5%) and may be better managed by reversal of warfarin therapy with vitamin K the day before surgery. In high-risk patients, intravenous heparin should be given while the warfarin is discontinued. On the day of surgery, heparin should be discontinued as well. Anticoagulation may be restarted 12 hours after surgery with heparin and replaced with oral anticoagulants 1 to 2 days post surgery.[88] In the case of emergency surgery, the anticoagulant effects are readily reversed by administration of FFP and vitamin K.

Drug Interactions

Many drugs interact with warfarin, enhancing or diminishing its anticoagulant effects (Table 14–5). Cimetidine inhibits warfarin clearance in the liver and has been reported to be associated with clinical bleeding.[89] The use of aspirin concurrently with warfarin may result in severe gastrointestinal hemorrhage. Other drugs enhancing the anticoagulant effects of warfarin including cotrimoxazole,[90] metronidazole,[91] disulfiram,[92] allopurinol,[93] quinidine,[94] and amiodarone.[95] Barbiturates increase the activity of hepatic microsomal enzymes, which increase the metabolism of warfarin.[96] Warfarin dosages should be increased in patients receiving barbiturates and also need to be reduced when barbiturates are discontinued. Other drugs associated with diminishing the anticoagulant effect of warfarin include rifampin[97] and propanolol.[98] The volatile anesthetics may prolong the anticoagulation effect of warfarin by prolonging its elimination half-life.[99] Halothane, in particular, has also been shown to displace warfarin from protein binding sites resulting in increased plasma concentrations of free warfarin.[100]

Adverse Effects

Hemorrhage

As with heparin, hemorrhage is the most serious side effect of warfarin therapy. Gastrointestinal hemorrhage is most frequently encountered and is usually associated with undetected peptic ulcer disease and neoplasm. Warfarin therapy may also be associated with an increased incidence of intracranial bleeding following a cerebrovascular accident. Severe hemorrhage may occur in the face of a desired therapeutic PT value. Mild hemorrhage may be treated with 5 mg intravenous vitamin K over 5 minutes,

Table 14–5. Drugs that Interact with Coumarin Derivatives

Enhance Anticoagulant Effect	Diminish Anticoagulant Effect
Cimetidine	Barbiturates
Cotrimaxozole	Rifampin
Metronidazole	Propanolol
Volatile anesthetics	
Allopurinol	
Amiodarone	
Quinidine	
Disulfiram	

which generally returns the prothrombin time to normal within 6 to 24 hours. Immediate reversal of warfarin effects is done by administering FFP. As with heparin, use of major regional anesthetic techniques is best avoided in the presence of PT values greater than 15 seconds.

Teratogenicity

Warfarin crosses the placenta and is associated with serious teratogenic effects when used during the first trimester of pregnancy. Approximately one-third of infants exposed to warfarin are born with serious abnormalities, including blindness and nasal hypoplasia. Heparin does not cross the placenta and may be an alternative in parturients requiring anticoagulant therapy.

Major Organ System Disease

Hepatic Disease

Coagulation abnormalities have been reported in more than 70 percent of patients with hepatic failure, with nearly 30% having major hemorrhagic complications.[101] Most clotting factors are synthesized in the liver, including the vitamin K-dependent factors II, VII, IX, and X. Factors I, XI, XII, and XIII are also synthesized in the liver but are not dependent on vitamin K. Hepatic failure adversely affects hemostasis by both depressing the synthesis of coagulation factors and limiting the ability of the liver to clear activated clotting factors, plasma activators of the fibrinolytic system, and products of fibrinolysis from the circulation. In addition, damaged hepatocytes may release tissue thromboplastin triggering DIC. Consequently, the hemorrhagic diathesis of hepatic insufficiency is a multifactorial process with reduced levels of coagulation factors, uncontrolled fibrinolysis, and DIC all playing a role.

In biliary obstruction, only vitamin K-dependent factors are decreased because vitamin K-absorption is dependent on the presence of bile salts in the gastrointestinal tract. If biliary obstruction is the sole abnormality, parenteral vitamin K will replenish these factors. However, when hepatocellular disease is combined with an acquired vitamin K deficiency (e.g., antibiotic therapy, malnutrition), parenteral administration of vitamin K may not be effective (See vitamin K deficiency).

Hepatic failure is also associated with platelet abnormalities including defective platelet aggregation[102] and thrombocytopenia secondary to sequestration by an enlarged spleen (hepatosplenomegaly). Patients who are alcoholics often have thrombocytopenia associated with folic acid deficiency and the toxic effects of alcohol itself.[103]

Preoperative Evaluation

Coagulation abnormalities must be suspected in patients with hepatic insufficiency or jaundice. Preoperative laboratory studies should include a PT, APTT, and platelet count. A bleeding time is also useful if platelet dysfunction is suspected. Normally, only 20 to 30 percent coagulation factors are necessary to maintain normal hemostasis; however, when hepatic failure is severe, these factors

can reduce to critical levels quickly. If the PT is prolonged secondary to a vitamin K deficiency, parenteral vitamin K will normalize it within 48 hours. Persistent prolongation of the PT suggests hepatic failure, and preoperative transfusion of FFP is usually required. If PT and APTT are both elevated, evaluation for fibrinolysis and DIC should be done by measuring FDP and fibrinogen levels. Preoperative platelet transfusions should be administered to patients with hepatic disease who have platelet counts below 75,000/mm³ and increased bleeding times.

Perioperative Management

Surgery in patients with hepatic disease may be associated with excessive oozing from mucosal surfaces, poor capillary hemostasis, and poor clot formation. Administration of FFP and platelets is ideally guided by intraoperative coagulation tests; however, acute clinical bleeding may warrant empiric administration of blood products as coagulation tests are being performed (PT, APTT, platelet count, fibrinogen level, FDP). Desmopressin (DDAVP) may improve hemostatic function by improving platelet function and raising levels of circulating cofactors.[104,105] In addition, dilution of platelets and coagulation factors may aggravate the coagulopathy of hepatic failure during the massive transfusion of blood and fluids. Treatment is based on replacing blood products that are diluted, as well as treating preexisting deficits.

Major regional anesthetic techniques (e.g., spinal and epidural) should be performed cautiously in patients with hepatic failure. In the face of abnormal coagulation, major regional techniques are best avoided; however, preoperative normalization of PT, APTT, and bleeding time will minimize the potential of developing peridural hematomas.

Liver Transplantation

Liver transplantation is associated with major alterations in coagulation and fibrinolytic systems. There is a high risk of hemorrhage during this procedure, particularly in patients who have abnormal coagulation preoperatively.[106] During and after the anhepatic stage of the procedure, the concentration of many coagulation factors, including fibrinogen, decreases. Many of the these coagulation factors may have already been decreased preoperatively secondary to the liver disease. Intraoperative thrombocytopenia and transient increases in fibrinolytic activity are additional factors leading to uncontrolled hemorrhage. The pathogenesis of the increased fibrinolytic activity is complex, involving DIC, the release of tissue plasminogen activator (TPA), and loss of the ability of the liver to clear activated clotting factors.[107,108,109] Once circulation is established to the transplanted liver, transient excessive fibrinolysis occurs presumably secondary to TPA released from the vessels of the donor liver. This effect may be diminished by treating these patients with ε-aminocaproic acid.[110] Postoperatively, the titers of factors V, VIII, and vitamin K-dependent factors VII, IX, and X fall during the first hours of reperfusion but rise to normal levels a few days after surgery. Persistent thrombocytopenia during the first few days after transplantation may be due to platelet sequestration by the transplanted liver.[111] Survival after liver transplantation is adversely affected by excessive blood loss and massive transfusion. Although coagulation defects are of major concern during this procedure, much of the blood loss is likely to be of a mechanical nature rather than coagulation abnormalities.[112]

Renal Disease

Patients with renal failure frequently present with symptoms of abnormal hemostasis ranging from ecchymosis, purpura and epistaxis to severe gastrointestinal hemorrhage.[113] Although a number of factors are associated with this bleeding tendency, acquired platelet functional defects secondary to uremia are probably the most important.

Uremic patients have impaired platelet adhesion and aggregation. Although the mechanism for this is unknown, it is probably due to the accumulation of metabolic acids and their interference with von Willebrand factor and the subsequent aggregation of platelets. Clinically, the bleeding time is prolonged in the absence of thrombocytopenia. In vitro platelet function tests that assess adhesion and aggregation are also abnormal. In general, platelet dysfunction correlates with the degree of uremia. The frequency and severity of hemorrhagic symptoms are also related to the degree and duration of the uremic state. Although there is no recognized threshold blood urea nitrogen and creatinine level at which bleeding occurs, most patients with plasma creatinine less than 6 mg/dL exhibit normal platelet function. These platelet abnormalities return to normal after hemodialysis or renal transplantation,[114] confirming that these are reversible abnormalities that are a result of the uremic environment. Although hemodialysis corrects platelet abnormalities, systemic heparinization is often required to prevent clotting in the extracorporeal circulation and maintain patency of vascular shunts. The effects of heparin may persist post-dialysis contributing to the tendency for these patients to bleed.

Despite hemodialysis, some patients with renal failure continue to present with symptoms of abnormal hemostasis. There is evidence that anemia contributes to platelet dysfunction, as the bleeding time has been shown to shorten after red blood cell transfusions in uremic patients.[115,116] Prothrombin time and APTT are normal, as there are no abnormalities in the plasma coagulation system or fibrinolysis; however, vitamin K-dependent coagulation factors tend to be low in end stage renal disease. Other predisposing factors, including the ingestion of aspirin and antiplatelet medications, are likely to aggravate pre-existing hemostatic abnormalities.

Although bleeding is the most common hemostatic defect in renal failure, a thrombotic tendency is also associated with certain renal diseases. Thromboembolic phenomenon and renal vein thrombosis are common complications in patients with nephrotic syndrome.[117] Thrombotic thrombocytopenic purpura (TTP) and hemolytic-uremic syndrome (HUS) are two rare conditions characterized by renal failure, hemolytic anemia, thrombocytopenia, and fever. Hemolytic uremic syndrome usually occurs in infants, while TTP is often associated with neurologic deficits; however, these two conditions are closely related and often indistinguishable. In both conditions, platelet aggregates occlude small vessels, leading to multiple organ failure, including renal failure.

Preoperative Evaluation

Preoperative laboratory tests in patients with renal failure should include hematocrit, PT, APTT, platelet count, and bleeding time. The PT should detect any deficiencies in vitamin K-dependent coagulation factors, while the APTT will detect any residual effect from hemodialysis. The bleeding time may be prolonged beyond the upper limit of normal. Patients should undergo hemodialysis within 24 hours of elective surgery in order to maximize platelet function. In addition, transfusion of red blood cells to a hematocrit of 30 percent may also improve platelet function. Platelet transfusion is generally not effective in improving hemostasis, as normal platelets quickly become dysfunctional when transfused to uremic patients.[118]

Cryoprecipitate and desmopressin (DDAVP) can temporarily correct the bleeding tendency in patients with uremia. Cryoprecipitate has been shown to shorten the bleeding time for a duration of approximately 9 hours in patients undergoing major surgical procedures, resulting in significantly reduced blood loss.[119] However, the risk of transmission of blood-borne diseases and heterogeneity of preparations have minimized the use of cryoprecipitate. Desmopressin is a synthetic analogue of antidiuretic hormone that effectively improves platelet function and reduces clinical bleeding in uremic patients without the risk of transfusion therapy. Unlike antidiuretic hormone, DDAVP does not have vasoconstrictor activity and does not raise arterial pressure when administered. DDAVP appears to exert its effect by increasing circulating factors of von Willebrand factor.[120] An intravenous infusion of DDAVP (0.3 μg/kg) shortens the bleeding time significantly for at least 4 hours and can be repeated at 12 hour intervals. However, repeated infusions of DDAVP may lead to a progressively diminished response, hyponatremia, and water retention.[121]

The administration of conjugated estrogens has also been shown to effectively shorten prolonged bleeding times and prevent excessive postoperative hemorrhage in uremic patients.[122] When a cumulative dose of 3 mg/kg was infused over 5 days, normalization of bleeding times lasted up to 2 weeks without side effects. This long-lasting effect may make conjugated estrogens a useful adjunct too in the management of uremic patients undergoing major surgery. The mechanism of the estrogen effect is in part related to an increase in circulating von Willebrand factor.

Perioperative Management

Before undergoing major surgery, all patients should undergo preoperative hemodialysis. If bleeding times remain prolonged, red blood cells should be transfused. Desmopressin (0.3 to 0.4 μg/kg) should be administered one hour before surgery. If unexpected bleeding occurs during or after surgery, DDAVP and/or cryoprecipitate should be administered, depending on the severity of bleeding. As previously stated, conjugated estrogens may be useful for long-term therapy. As with liver failure, abnormal coagulation needs to be considered when performing regional anesthetic techniques on patients with chronic renal failure.

Patients undergoing renal transplantation may develop quantitative and qualitative changes in platelets after the procedure. Use of immunosuppressive drugs may result in thrombocytopenia secondary to bone marrow toxicity. Graft rejection is also associated with platelet aggregation and adhesion leading to thrombus formation. Platelet dysfunction may exist in patients with functioning transplants secondary, in part, to decreased intraplatelet concentrations of serotonin.[123]

Disseminated Intravascular Coagulation

Definition and Etiology

Disseminated intravascular coagulation is a thrombohemorrhagic disorder that occurs as a complication of a wide spectrum of clinical disorders including trauma, sepsis, and malignant neoplasms (Table 14–6). The clinical presentation of DIC is variable, as it exists as both an acute and chronic phenomenon. DIC is characterized by an inappropriate activation of the plasma coagulation system initially leading to a *hypercoagular state* and formation of microthrombi throughout the microcirculation. The microthrombi lead to vascular occlusion and ischemic damage of vital organs including the kidney, liver, adrenal glands, and central nervous system.[124] Platelets, fibrinogen, and other coagulation factors are rapidly consumed leading to a progressive bleeding diathesis. The presence of thrombin and microthrombi results in a secondary activation of the fibrinolytic system, further aggravating the hemorrhage. Fibrin degradation products produced in DIC inhibit coagulation, further exacerbating the bleeding tendency. Increased levels of fibrin/fibrinogen degradation products, or D-dimers that result from lysis of crosslinked fibrin, may assist in the diagnosis of DIC.

Pathogenesis

The main mechanisms responsible for triggering DIC involve the release of tissue thromboplastin into the circulation, widespread endothelial cell damage, and thrombin formation. Tissue thromboplastins activate the extrinsic pathway of the plasma coagulation and are released into the circulation following massive tissue destruction as seen with crush injuries, severe head trauma, significant burn injuries, and a variety of obstetrical complications. Endotoxins released by gram-negative bacteria release thromboplastins from endothelial and inflammatory cells, making DIC a frequent complication of sepsis. In addition to activating the extrinsic pathway, widespread endothelial injury results in platelet aggregation, activating the intrinsic pathway of the plasma coagulation system. Endothelial injury can be produced directly by microorganisms (e.g., meningococci, rickettsiae), viruses,

Table 14–6. Major Disorders Associated with Disseminated Intravascular Coagulation

Obstetric Complications
  Amniotic fluid embolism
  Intrauterine retention of a dead fetus
  Abruptio placentae
  Eclampsia
  Septic Abortion
Infections
  Bacterial: Gram-negative and gram-positive sepsis
                    (staphylococci, streptococci,
                    meningococcemia, pneumococci,
                    endocarditis, gram-negative bacilli)
  Viral: Herpes simplex, varicella, rubella, cytomegalic
                    viremia
  Parasitic: Malaria
  Mycotic: Candidiasis, histoplasmosis, aspergillosis
  Rickettsial: Rocky mountain spotted fever
  Other: Hepatitis, miliary tuberculosis
Massive tissue injury
  Traumatic shock
  Head injury
  Burns
  Extensive surgery
Malignancy
  Carcinomas of lung, prostate, and pancreas
  Acute promyelocytic leukemia
Miscellaneous
  Acute hemolytic process
  Hypothermia
  Malignant hyperthermia
  Liver disease
  Hemolytic uremic syndrome
  Aortic aneurysm
  Heat stroke
  Anaphylaxis

and disease-related antigen-antibody complexes (e.g., systemic lupus erythematosus, glomerulonephritis). Endothelial injury can also occur secondary to hypoxia, acidosis, hypothermia, and circulatory shock which commonly coexist with surgical and obstetric complications.

Clinical Presentation

The onset of DIC may be acute and fulminant as seen with gram-negative septic shock and massive trauma, or it may be chronic and insidious, as seen with malignant neoplasms.[126] In general, a hemorrhagic diathesis dominates the clinical picture of acute DIC, while thrombotic complications are associated with the chronic syndrome.

Disseminated intravascular coagulation is a systemic process, and bleeding can occur anywhere platelets and coagulation factors are consumed, including the respiratory and central nervous systems. In the acute syndrome, patients often present with bleeding from skin and mucous membrane surfaces. Hemorrhage from surgical incision, venipuncture, and catheter sites is also common. Occasionally, pre-gangrenous changes may be present in digits, genitalia, and the nose secondary to microthrombi and vasospasm. A hemolytic anemia is a common result of fragmentation of red blood cells as they move through narrowed microvasculature. Ischemic organ damage may ensue, with oliguria and acute renal failure dominating the picture. Patients with chronic DIC, or the low grade form such as that associated with malignancy, may have mild laboratory abnormalities present in the clinical picture.

Laboratory evidence of DIC includes thrombocytopenia and the presence of fragmented red blood cells secondary to damage within the microvasculature. Prothrombin time (PT), activated partial thromboplastin time (APTT), and thrombin time (TT) are prolonged secondary to consumption of coagulation factors. The fibrinogen level is reduced, and the level of fibrin degradation products (FDPs) are increased from primary, as well as secondary fibrinolysis. Of all laboratory measurements, a low plasma fibrinogen level most closely correlates with clinical evidence of bleeding.

Management

The treatment of DIC is directed at (1) attempting to correct the underlying disorder causing DIC and (2) controlling the major symptom of either hemorrhage or thrombosis. Treatment will vary depending on the underlying disorder. Bacterial sepsis and certain obstetric etiologies (e.g., abruptio placenta) may be relatively easy to correct, while chronic DIC associated with a malignancy may require long-term prophylactic measures to control symptoms. Improvement of DIC is associated with the stabilization of platelet counts and fibrinogen level, with decreased circulating levels of FDP.

Patients with bleeding as a major symptom should receive platelet concentrates and FFP as indicated by measurement of platelet count, PT and APTT. The use of heparin will prevent thrombin formation and has been recommended but the dose remains controversial. Although it is a reasonable way to reduce consumption of coagulation factors, heparin itself may induce bleeding when given at usual clinical dosages. Therefore, the use of heparin is generally reserved for patients with evidence of thrombosis or those who continue to bleed despite vigorous treatment. Antithrombin III concentrate infusions in patients with circulatory shock may be useful in reducing the severity of associated DIC.[127] Use of ε-aminocaproic acid and other inhibitors of fibrinolysis should be avoided, as fibrinolysis is a secondary protective mechanism and inhibition might be associated with unopposed thrombosis.

Patients with mild DIC may not be symptomatic until they undergo certain systemic stresses such as those associated with surgery. Most patients with mild presentations will be adequately controlled with platelet and plasma replacement. Patients with chronic DIC and thrombotic complications may require long-term heparin administration by intermittent subcutaneous injection or continuous infusion with a portable pump.

Massive Transfusion

The massive transfusion of blood equal to or greater than a patient's own blood volume (8 to 10 units in an adult) may lead to an acquired coagulopathy. The amount of blood transfused and the duration of hypotension and hypoperfusion are the factors that most closely correlate with the development of a hemorrhagic diathesis.[128] Large amounts of transfused blood are more likely to dilute platelets and coagulation factors to levels that are inadequate for hemostasis. Prolonged hypoperfusion can lead to regional ischemia and release of tissue thromboplastin, worsening any coexisting coagulopathy by producing DIC. In addition, associated conditions such as hypothermia and acidosis may alter platelet function and impair coagulation.[129,130]

Effects on Coagulation

Thrombocytopenia

Dilutional thrombocytopenia and altered platelet function, often in conjunction with DIC, is the most likely cause of a hemorrhagic diathesis in patients receiving massive blood transfusion.[131-133] Platelets are poorly preserved in banked blood, and platelet counts of less than $100,000/mm^3$ are common following massive transfusion. This reduction in circulating platelets correlates closely with the tendency to bleed, as bleeding is likely when platelet counts drop below $75,000/mm^3$ during surgery.[131] In addition, hypothermia, acidosis, drugs, and trauma can alter the function of existing platelets for days after the initial insult.[134]

In the past, these factors have motivated clinicians to empirically administer platelets in the absence of laboratory or clinical evidence of bleeding. Controlled clinical trials, however, have demonstrated that the prophylactic administration of platelets does not reduce transfusion requirements or coagulopathy during surgery.[135] Platelets should be administered only when indicated by laboratory evidence of thrombocytopenia or severe generalized coagulopathy. Because intraoperative platelet counts below $75,000/mm^3$ are frequently associated with clinical bleeding, platelet transfusions are indicated at that time.

Dilution of Coagulation Factors

Most coagulation factors are stable in stored blood with the exception of factors V and VIII. The levels of factor V and factor VIII are reduced below 50% of normal after 48 hours of storage and are even lower after 21 days. Only 5 to 20% of factor V and 30% of factor VIII are necessary for adequate hemostasis; these factors are rarely decreased to these low levels despite massive transfusion. Dilution of coagulation factors is rarely the sole cause of bleeding;[136] however, it may intensify bleeding stemming from dilutional thrombocytopenia and consumptive coagulopathy.

There is no scientific evidence supporting the routine use of FFP as replacement therapy during massive transfusion.[44,136] Before administering FFP, (1) thrombocytopenia should be ruled out as a cause of bleeding by ensuring that platelets are greater than $70,000/mm^3$ and (2) the activated partial thromboplastin time is at least 1.5 times greater than normal, suggesting low levels of factors V and VIII.

Diagnosis and Treatment

When a massive blood transfusion begins to approach a patient's blood volume (8 to 10 units); a blood specimen should be obtained and tested for platelet count, PTT, PT, and plasma fibrinogen level. Clinical observation becomes critical at this time, and the patient should be continuously evaluated for (1) evidence of a generalized bleeding tendency, (2) how much more blood replacement will be necessary, and (3) associated conditions that may contribute to a coagulopathy (i.e., trauma, hypotension, liver failure). If initial coagulation times are greater than 1.5 times normal and platelet count is less than 75,000/mm^3, one can assume that associated factors such as hypotension, organ failure, and trauma are contributing to the coagulopathy.[137] Fibrinogen is stable in banked blood, and a plasma level below 150 mg/100 ml strongly suggests DIC. When hypofibrinogenemia is associated with thrombocytopenia, DIC is the probable diagnosis. Coagulation studies should be repeated as justified by the clinical picture. The multifactorial nature of this coagulopathy may limit the usefulness of thromboelastography as a clinical monitor in this scenario. Treatment is ideally based on laboratory findings; however, in the face of severe uncontrollable bleeding, empiric administration of platelets and FFP may be warranted.

Cardiopulmonary Bypass

Cardiopulmonary bypass (CPB) is associated with multiple complex abnormalities affecting all aspects of the hemostatic mechanism. Platelet abnormalities are the most common cause of bleeding following CPB; however, activation of coagulation, fibrinolysis, and the effects of various cardiovascular drugs also play a role. These abnormalities lead to a bleeding diathesis in an estimated 5 to 20 percent of patients.[138,139] Approximately 5 percent of patients who undergo CPB procedures require reoperation for excessive bleeding.[140,141]

Cardiopulmonary bypass adversely affects both platelet count and platelet function. Immediately after initiating CPB, hemodilution reduces the platelet count to about 50 percent of preoperative levels but it usually remains above 100,000 μ/L.[142] A decreased platelet count often persists for several days following CPB and may be related to platelet sequestration in the liver.[143] Of greater significance is the progressive loss of platelet function induced by CPB. The bleeding time is prolonged and platelet aggregation studies are abnormal shortly after the initiation of CPB. Platelet dysfunction appears to be dependent on exposure of platelets to the extracorporeal circuit and hypothermia, while the degree of platelet dysfunction is directly related to the duration of CPB.[139,142]

The mechanism for this abnormality is unclear but may be related to a decrease in platelet synthesis of thromboxane A$_2$ (TxA$_2$),[129,144] transient platelet activation with impaired aggregation,[139,145] and depleted stores of ADP. Other co-existing factors having adverse effects on platelet function during CPB include the cardiotomy suction (destruction of platelets); filters; antiplatelet drugs and vasodilators; and protamine which produces a transient reduction in circulating platelets. The ingestion of aspirin by these patients is particularly associated with an increased risk of perioperative bleeding.[146] Platelet dysfunction is usually transient and returns to normal within 24 hours of surgery; however, prolonged dysfunction can exist. Aprotinin, a naturally occurring inhibitor of proteolytic enzymes, has been shown to preserve platelet function when given continuously during CPB resulting in reduced perioperative bleeding.[147]

Hemodilution associated with the initiation of CPB produces approximately a 40 percent reduction in most coagulation factors.[148] These reductions persist throughout CPB and usually return to normal levels within 24 to 48 hours of surgery. Although these reduced levels are generally still adequate for hemostasis, excessive hemodilution and pre-existing coagulation defects can lead to increased perioperative bleeding.

Primary fibrinolysis occurs when plasminogen is activated to plasmin, inducing lysis of fibrinogen and fibrin. Although heparin provides an anticoagulated state during CPB, it does not inhibit factor XII, an intrinsic activator of fibrinolysis. Primary or intrinsic fibrinolytic activity occurs with the initiation of CPB. In addition, secondary or extrinsic fibrinolysis is activated as CPB progresses.[149] Despite this, fibrinolysis is rarely a clinically significant cause of perioperative bleeding.[139,148]

Residual Heparin Effect

Heparin anticoagulation is necessary to avoid clotting that would otherwise occur when blood makes contact with the foreign surfaces of the extracorporeal circuit. Heparin is administered either through a central line or directly into the right atrium. A dose of 300 to 400 units/kg of heparin is used to initiate anticoagulation.

The ACT is the most widely used test to monitor the effectiveness of heparin. In routine CPB, an automated ACT above 400 seconds has been recommended to minimize the formation of fibrin monomers and consumption of coagulation factors.[150] Although recent studies suggest that an ACT less than 400 seconds may be clinically safe,[151] the safe lower limit of the ACT remains to be defined.

Heparin is neutralized at the conclusion of CPB by protamine, with the usual dose being approximately 1.0 mg of protamine for every 100 units of heparin used (see section about neutralization of heparin). The ACT is again used to monitor heparin neutralization. "Heparin rebound" refers to the recurrence of anticoagulation accompanied by an elevated ACT despite previous neutralization with protamine. Heparin rebound generally occurs 4 to 6 hours after protamine neutralization because the half-life of heparin is longer than that of protamine and responds to an additional dose of protamine. Occasionally, the ACT can not be returned to the baseline value despite adequate protamine, indicating the likelihood of a low plasma fibrinogen level.

Management and Treatment of Bleeding

After heparin has been neutralized by protamine, the surgical field should be meticulously inspected for bleeding and the appropriate hemostatic maneuvers should be employed the surgeon. If bleeding is significant and diffuse, a coagulation profile consisting of a PT, PTT, fibrinogen level, thrombin time, and platelet count should be performed. If residual heparin is suspected, the thrombin time will be prolonged. Thrombocytopenia should be treated with platelet transfusions in the face of excessive bleeding. Intrinsic impairment of platelet function should be assumed to be the primary hemostatic abnormality, while abnormalities of the plasma coagulation system are less likely. Use of FFP is rational treatment only after platelet abnormalities or excessive heparin have been corrected or ruled out.

Prophylactic Therapy

Fresh Frozen Plasma and Platelets

There is no evidence that the prophylactic administration of FFP or platelets have a positive clinical effect.[152,153] Fresh frozen plasma is indicated when the PT or APTT exceed 150 percent of the control value or when blood transfusion exceeds the patient's calculated blood volume. Transfusion of platelets is indicated when the platelet count is less than 50 to 75,000/mm^2 or when blood transfusion has exceeded the patient's calculated blood volume. If the patient is anemic, the transfusion of fresh whole blood has been shown to provide better hemostasis than when platelets are transfused alone.[154,155]

Desmopressin Acetate

The usefulness of desmopressin acetate (DDAVP, 1-desamino-8-D-arginine vasopressin) to reduce perioperative blood loss is a matter of debate. Desmopressin increases the level of circulating factors VIII:C and von Willebrand factor (vWF) and is associated with a shortening of the bleeding time. Although studies have shown that intravenous desmopressin (0.3 μg/kg) at the conclusion of CPB significantly reduces perioperative blood loss associated with CPB,[141,156] more recent studies have demonstrated no significant difference in blood loss and transfusion requirements in patients receiving DDAVP.[157,158] Because of these contradictory studies, DDAVP should not be given routinely, but rather reserved for those patients with excessive bleeding following CPB. The use of DDAVP is generally well tolerated, it may be associated with hypotension, antidiuresis, and activation of fibrinolysis. Tachyphylaxis to DDAVP has also been reported.

Natural and Synthetic Fibrinolytics

Although fibrinolysis is rarely a clinically significant cause of CPB related bleeding, the use of antifibrinolytic agents appear to be effective in both the treatment and prevention of excessive bleeding associated with cardiac surgery.[159,160] The exact mechanism by which natural (aprotinin) and synthetic antifibrinolytics (ϵ-aminocaproic acid (EACA) and tranexamic acid) exert their effects have been difficult to define but may be due to platelet preservation as well as inhibition of fibrinolysis. Both EACA and tranexamic acid (TA) are administered as a bolus dose followed by a continuous infusion. An intravenous bolus of 100 to 150 mg/kg of EACA followed by an infusion of 10 to 15 mg/kg-hr provides the desired plasma concentration in adults. Higher doses are avoided because EACA may inhibit fibrinogen binding to platelets resulting in platelet function abnormalities. Tranexamic acid is approximately 10 times as potent as EACA and a bolus of 10 mg/kg followed by an infusion of 1 mg/kg/hr. A bolus of two million KIU of aprotinin followed by an infusion of 500,000 KIU/hr, with an additional two million KIU added to the priming solution of the extracorporeal circuit has been used to reduce bleeding associated with CPB. Although use of antifibrinolytic therapy is theoretically associated with an increased risk of thrombosis, controlled studies employing prophylactic use of these agents have not demonstrated an increased incidence of venous, coronary, or cerebrovascular thrombosis.[160,161]

REFERENCES

1. Bennett E. J., Dalal F. Y.: Haemoglobin S and its clinical application. In Oxygen measurement in Biology and Medicine, Payne J. P., Hill DW, (Eds.), Butterworth, London, 1975.
2. Gibson Jr. J. R.: Anesthesia for the sickle cell diseases and other hemoglobinopathies. Semin Anesth 4:27, 1987.
3. Esseltine D. W., Baxter M., Bevan J. C.: Sickle cell states and the anesthetist. Can Anaesth Soc J 35:385, 1988.
4. Aldrete J. A., Guerra F.: Hematologic diseases. In Anesthesia and Uncommon Diseases, Katz J, Benumof, J Kadis, L. B. (Eds.), W. B. Saunders, Philadelphia, 1981.
5. Hathorn M.: Pattern or red cell destruction in sickle cell anemia. Br J Haematol 13:746, 1967.
6. Diggs W. W., Diggs L. W.: Hospital detection of sickle cell disease. Hosp Pract 9:109, 1972.
7. Green R. L., Huntsman R. G., Sergeant G. R.: The sickle cell and altitude. Br Med J 4:593, 1971.
8. Bullick F. G., Delage C., Frey N. S.: Sickle cell crisis associated with drugs. Arch Environ Health 26:221, 1973.
9. Lourie J. A., Kontopoulos I.: Sin and the sickle cell crisis. Lancet, 1:352, 1971.
10. Luban N., Epstein B., Watson S. P.: Sickle cell disease and anesthesia. In Advances in Anesthesia, Vol. 1, Gallagher TJ (Ed), Year Book Medical Publishers, Chicago, 1984.
11. Castro O.: Autotransfusion: A Management option for alloimmunized sickle cell patients? Prog Clin Biol Res 98:117, 1982.
11a. Eaton, W. A., Hofrichter, J.: The biophysics of sickle cell hydroxyurea therapy. Science 268: 1142,1995.
12. Holzman L., Finn H., Lichtman H. C., et. al: Anesthesia in patients with sickle cell disease. Anesth Analg 48:566, 1969.
13. Searle J. F.: Anesthesia in sickle cell states: a review. Anaesthesia 28:48, 1973.
14. Maduska A. L., Guince W. S., Henton J. A., et. al: Sickling dynamics of red blood cells during anesthesia. Anesth Analg 54:361, 1975.
15. Martin W. J., Green D. R., Dougherty N., et al: Tourniquet use in sickle-cell disease patients. J Am Podiatr Med Assoc 74:291, 1984.
16. Adu-Gyamfi Y., Sankarankutty M., Marwa S.: Use of a tourniquet in patients with sickle-cell disease. Can J Anaesth 40:1, 1993.
17. Koshy M., Burd L.: Management of pregnancy in sickle cell syndromes. Hematol Oncol Clin North Am 5:585, 1991.
18. Szentpetery S., Robertson L., Lower R. R.: Complete repair of tetrology associated with sickle-cell anaemia and G-6PD deficiency. J Thorac Cardiovasc Surg 72:276, 1976.
19. Hudson I., Davidson I. A., McGregor C. G. A.: Mitral valve

replacement using cold cardioplegia in a patient with sickle-cell trait. Thorax *36*:151, 1981.

20. Metras D., Coulibaly A. O., Ouattara K., et. al.: Open-heart surgery in sickle-cell haemoglobinapathies: report of 15 cases. Thorax *37*:486, 1982.

21. Niehius A. W.: Thalassemia Major: Molecular and clinical aspects. Ann Intern Med *91*:883–897, 1979.

22. Leon M. B., Borer J. J., Bacharach S. L., et al.: Detection of early cardiac dysfunction in patients with severe beta-thalassemia and chronic iron overload. N Engl J Med *301*:1143, 1979.

23. Waldenstrom J.: The porphyrias as inborn errors of metabolism. Am J Med *22*:758, 1957.

24. Silvay G.: Porphyrias. Anesthesiol Rev *6*:51, 1979.

25. Feldman D. S., Levere R. D., Lieberman J. S., et al.: Inhibition of the neuromuscular junction by porphobilinogen and porpholin as compared with uroporphyrins I and III. J Clin Invest *49*:28a, 1970.

26. Welland F. H., Hellman E. D., Goddes E. M., et al.: Factors affecting the excretion of porphyrin precursors by patients with acute intermittent porphyria: I. The effect of diet. Metabolism *13*:232, 1964.

27. Douer D., Weinberger A., Pinkhas J., Atsmon A.: Treatment of acute intermittent porphyria with large doses of propranolol. JAMA *240*:766, 1978.

28. Blum I. and Atsmon A.: Reduction of porphyrin excretion in porphyria variegate by propranolol. South Afr Med J *50*:898, 1976.

29. Watson C. J.: Hematin and porphyria. N Engl J Med *293*:605, 1975.

30. Peterson A., Bossenmaier I., Cardinal R., Watson C. J.: Hematin treatment of acute porphyria: Early remission in an almost fatal relapse. JAMA *325*:520, 1976.

31. Lamon J. M., Frykholm B. C., Hess R. A., Tschudy DP: Hematin therapy for acute porphyria. Medicine *58*:252, 1979.

32. Mustajoki P., Heinonen J.: General anesthesia in "inducible" porphyrias. Anesthesiology *53*:15, 1980.

33. McNeill M. J., Bennett A.. Use of regional anaesthesia in a patient with acute porphyria. Br J Anaesth *64*:371, 1990.

34. Rizk S. F., Jacobson J. H., Silvay G.: Ketamine as an induction agent for acute intermittent porphyria. Anesthesiology *46*:305, 1977.

35. Famewo C. E.: Induction of Anesthesia with etomidate in a patient with acute intermittent porphyria. Can Anaesth Soc J *32*:171, 1985.

36. Mitterschiffthaler G., Theiner A., Hetzel H., Fuith L. C.: Safe use of propofol in a patient with acute intermittent porphyria. Br J Anaesth *60*:109, 1988.

37. Dundee J. W., McCleery W. C., McLoughlin G.: The hazard of thiopental anesthesia in porphyria. Anesth Analg *41*:567–574, 1962.

38. Mees D. E., Jr, Frederickson E. L.: Anesthesia and the porphyrias. South Med J *68*:29, 1975.

39. Watson C. F.: The problem of porphyria. N Engl J Med *263*:1205, 1976.

40. Brenner D. A., Bloomer J. R.: The enzymatic defect in variegate porphyria. N Engl J Med *302*:765, 1980.

41. Becker P. S., Lux S. E.: Hereditary spherocytosis and related disorders. Clin Hematol *14*:15, 1985.

42. Valentine W. M., Tanaka K. R., Paglia D. E.: Hemolytic anemias and erythrocyte enzymopathies. Ann Intern Med *103*:425, 1985.

43. Shapley J. R., Wilson J. R.: Post-anesthetic jaundice due to glucose-6-phosphate dehydrogenase deficiency. Can Anaesth Soc J *20*:390, 1973.

44. National Institutes of Health: Fresh frozen plasma: indications and risks. JAMA *253*:551, 1985.

45. Webster M. W. I., Chesebro J. H., Fuster V: Platelet inhibitor therapy: Agents and clinical implications. Hematol/Oncol Clin North Am *4*:265, 1990.

46. Smith J. B., Willis A. L.: Aspirin selectivity inhibits prostaglandin production in human platelets. Nature *231*:235, 1971.

47. Bashein G., Nessly M. L., Rice A. L., et al: Preoperative aspirin therapy and reoperation for bleeding after coronary artery bypass surgery. Arch Intern Med *151*:89, 1991.

48. Horlocker T. T., Wedel D. J., Offord K. P.: Does preoperative antiplatelet therapy increase the risk of hemorrhagic complications associated with regional anesthesia? Anesth Analg *70*:631, 1990.

49. Shattil S. J., Bennett J. S.: Platelets and their membranes in hemostasis: physiology and pathophysiology. Ann Intern Med *94*:108, 1980.

50. Fass R. J., Copelan E. A., Brandt J. T., et. al.: Platelet-mediated bleeding caused by broad-spectrum penicillins. J Infect Dis *155*:1242, 1987.

51. Lichtenthal P. R., Rossi E. C., Louis G., et. al.: Dose-related prolongation of the bleeding time by intravenous nitroglycerine. Anesth Analg *64*:30, 1985.

52. Hines R., Barash P. G.: Infusion of sodium nitroprusside induces platelet dysfunction in vitro. Anesthesiology *70*:611, 1989.

53. Furlong B., Henderson A. H., Lewis M. J., Smith J. S.: Endothelium derived relaxing factor inhibits in vitro platelet aggregation. Br J Pharmacol *90*:687, 1987.

54. Moncada S., Palmer R. M. J., Higgs E. A.: The discovery of nitric oxide as the endogenous nitrovasodilator. Hypertension *12*:365, 1988.

55. Hines R.: Preservation of platelet function during trimethaphan infusion. Anesthesiology *72*:834, 1990.

56. Mehta J., Mehta P., Ostrowski N.: Influence of propranolol and 4-hydroxypropranolol on platelet aggregation and thromboxane A$_2$ generation. Clin Pharmacol Ther *34*:559, 1983.

57. Dale J., Landmark K. H., Myhr E.: The effects of nifedipine, a calcium antagonist, on platelet function. Am Heart J *105*:103, 1983.

58. Serneri G. G. N., Masotti G., Poggesi L., Morettini A.: Enhanced prostacycline production by dipyridamole in man. Eur J Clin Pharmacol *21*:9, 1981.

59. Dalsgaard-Nielssen J., Risbo A., Simmelkjaer P., Gormsen J.: Impaired platelet aggregation and increased bleeding time during general anesthesia with halothane. Br J Anaesth *53*:1039, 1981.

60. Fauss B. G., Meadows J. C., Bruni C. Y., Qureshi G. D.: The in vitro and in vivo effects of isoflurane and nitrous oxide in platelet aggregation. Anesth Analg *65*:1170, 1986.

61. Rosenberg R. D.: Actions and interactions of antithrombin and heparin. N Engl J Med *292*:146, 1975.

62. Shah M. C., Schwarz K. B.: Hazards of small amounts of heparin in a patient with subclinical vitamin K deficiency. J Parenteral Enteral Nutr *13*:324, 1989.

63. Owens E. L., Kasten G. W., Hessel E. A.: Spinal subarachnoid hematoma after lumbar puncture and heparinization. A case report, review of the literature, and discussion of anesthetic implication. Anesth Analg *65*:1201, 1986.

64. Odoom J. A., Sih I. C.: Epidural analgesia and anticoagulant therapy. Experience in one thousand cases of continuous epidurals. Anaesthesia *38*:254, 1983.

65. Matthews E. T., Abrams L. D.: Intrathecal morphine in open heart surgery (letter). Lancet *2*:543, 1980.

66. Rao T. L. K., El-Etr A. A.: Anticoagulation following placement of epidural and subarachnoid catheters. Anesthesiology 55:618, 1981.

67. Marciniak E., Gockerman J. P.: Heparin-induced decrease in circulating anti-thrombin III. Lancet 2:581, 1977.

68. Anderson E. F.: Heparin resistance prior to cardiopulmonary bypass. Anesthesiology 64:504, 1986.

69. Bell W. T., Royall R. M.: Heparin-associated thrombocytopenia: A comparison of three heparin preparations. N Engl J Med 303:902, 1980.

70. Becker P. S., Miller V. T.: Heparin-induced thrombocytopenia. Stroke, 20:1449, 1989, coagulation. Semin Thromb Hemostasis 15:347, 1989.

71. Walls J. T., Curtis J. J., Silver D., Boley T. M.: Heparin-induced thrombocytopenia in patients who undergo open heart surgery. Surgery 108:686, 1990.

72. Frame J. N., Mulvey K. P., Phares J. C., Anderson M. J.: Correction of severe heparin-associated thrombocytopenia with intravenous immunoglobin. Ann Intern Med 111:946, 1989.

73. Smith J. P., Walls J. T., Muscato M. S., et. al.: Extracorporeal circulation in a patient with heparin-induced thrombocytopenia. Anesthesiology 62:363, 1985.

74. Addonzio Jr V. P., Fisher C. A., Kappa J. R., Ellison N.: Prevention of heparin-induced thrombocytopenia during open heart surgery with Iloprost (ZK 36374). Surgery 102:796, 1987.

75. Kappa J. T., Cottrell E. D., Berkowitz H. D., et al: Carotid endarterectomy in patients with heparin-induced platelet activation: Comparitive efficacy of aspirin and iloprost (ZK36374). J Vasc Surg 5:693, 1987.

76. Casthely P. A., Goodman K., Fyman P. N., et. al.: Hemodynamic changes after administration of protamine. Anesth Analg 65:78, 1986.

77. Stoelting R. K., Henry D. P., Verburg K. M., et al: Haemodynamic changes and circulating histamine concentrations following protamine administration to patients and dogs. Can Anaesth Soc J, 31:534, 1984.

78. Horrow J. C.: Protamine: A review of its toxicity. Anesth Analg 64:348, 1985.

79. Sharath M. D., Metzger W. J., Richerson H. B., et. al.: Protamine-induced fatal anaphylaxis: prevalence of antiprotamine immunoglobin E antibody. J Thorac Cardiovasc Surg 90:86, 1985.

80. Campbell F. W., Goldstein M. F., Atkins P. C.: Management of the patient with protamine hypersensitivity for cardiac surgery. Anesthesiology 61:761, 1984.

81. Castaneda A. R., Gans H., Weber K. C., et al: Heparin neutralization: experimental and clinical studies. Surgery 62:686, 1967.

82. Lowenstein E., Johnston W., Lappas D., et al: Catastrophic pulmonary vasoconstriction associated with protamine reversal of heparin. Anesthesiology 59:470, 1983.

83. Morel D. R., Zapol W. M., Thomas S. J., et al: C5a and thromboxane generation associated with pulmonary vaso- and bronchoconstriction during protamine reversal of heparin. Anesthesiology 66:597, 1987.

84. Conzen P. F., Habzettl H., Gutmann R., et al: Thromboxane mediation of pulmonary hemodynamic responses after neutralization of heparin by protamine in pigs. Anesth Analg 68:25, 1989.

85. WHO Expert Committee on Biological Standardization. 28th Report: WHO Technical

86. Loeliger E. A.: ICSH/ISTH recommendations for reporting prothrombin time in oral anticoagulant control. Thrombo Haemostasis 53:155, 1985.

87. Tinker J. H., Tarhan S: Discontinuing anticoagulant therapy in surgical patients with cardiac valve prosthesis. Observations in 180 operations. JAMA 239:738, 1978.

88. Katholi R. E., Nolan S. P., McGuire L. B.: The management of anticoagulation during noncardiac operations in patients with prosthetic heart valves: a prospective study. Am Heart J 96:163, 1978.

89. Silver B. A., Bell W. R.: Cimetidine potentiation of the hypoprothrombinemic effect of warfarin. Ann Intern Med 90:348, 1979.

90. Hassall C., Feetam C. L., Leach R. H., et al: Potentiation of warfarin by cotrimoxazole (letter). Lancet 2:1155, 1975.

91. O'Rielly R. A.: The stereoselective interaction of metronidazole in man. N Engl J Med 295:354, 1976.

92. O'Rielly R. A.: Interaction of sodium warfarin and disulfuram (Antabuse) in man. Ann Intern Med 78:73, 1973.

93. Rawlins M. D., Smith S. E.: Influence of allopurinol on drug metabolism in man. Br J Pharmacol 48:693, 1973.

94. Koch-Weser J., Sellers E. M.: Drug interactions with coumarin anticoagulants. N Engl J Med 285:478, 1971.

95. Watt A. H., Stephens M. R., Buss D. C., et al: Amiodarone reduces plasma warfarin clearance in man. Br J Clin Pharmacol 20:707, 1986.

96. Udall J. A.: Clinical implications of warfarin: Interactions with five sedatives. Am J Cardiol 35:67, 1975.

97. O'Reilly R. A.: Interaction of sodium warfarin and rifampin: studies in man. Ann Intern Med 81:337, 1974.

98. Scott A. K., Park B. K., Breckenridge A. M.: Interaction between warfarin and propranolol. Br J Clin Pharmacol 17:559, 1984.

99. Ghoneim M. M., Delle M., Wilson W. R., Ambre J. J.: Alteration of warfarin kinetics in man associated with exposure to an operating-room environment. Anesthesiology 43:333, 1975.

100. Calvo R., Aguilera L., Suarez E., Rodriguez-Sasain J. M.: Displacement of warfarin from human serum proteins by halothane anesthesia. Acta Anaesthesiol Scand 33:575, 1989.

101. Kelly D. A., Tuddenham E. G. D.: Hemostatic problems in liver disease. Gut 27:339, 1986.

102. Owen J. S., Hutton R. A., Day R. C., et al: Platelet lipid composition and platelet aggregation in human liver disease. J Lipid Res 22:423, 1981.

103. Cowan D. H.: Effect of alcoholism on hemostasis. Semin Hematol 17:137, 1980.

104. Burroughs A. K., Matthews K., Quiri M.: Desmopressin and bleeding time in cirrhosis. Br Med J 291:1377, 1985.

105. Agnelli G., De Cunto M., Berretini M., et al: Desmopressin induced improvements of abnormal coagulation in chronic liver disease (letter). Lancet 1:645, 1983.

106. Botempo F. A., Lewis J. H., Van Thiel D. H., et al: The relation of preoperative coagulation findings to diagnosis, blood usage and survival in adult liver transplantation. Transplantation 39:532, 1985.

107. Owen Jr C. A., Rettke S. R., Bowie E. J. W., et al: Hemostatic evaluation of patients undergoing liver transplantation. Mayo Clin Proc 62:761, 1987.

108. Dzik W. H., Arkin C. F., Jenkins R. L., et al: Fibrinolysis during liver transplantation in humans: Role of tissue-type plasminogen activator. Blood 71:1090, 1988.

109. Palareti G., de Rosa V., Fortunato G., et al: Control of hemostasis during orthoptic liver transplantation. Fibrinolysis 2(suppl 3):61, 1988.

110. Kang Y. G., Lewis J. H., Novalgund A., et al: Epsilon-aminocaproic acid for treatment of fibrinolysis during liver transplantation. Anesthesiology 66:766, 1987.

111. Plevak D. J., Homls G. A., Forstrom L. A., et. al.: Thrombo-

cytopenia after liver transplantation. Transplant Proc, 20(suppl 1):630, 1988.

112. Iwatsuki S., Shaw Jr B. W., Starzl T. E.: Current status of hepatic transplantation, Semin Liver Dis 3:173, 1983.

113. Zuckerman G. R., Cornette G. L., Clouse R. E., et al: Upper gastrointestinal bleeding in patients with chronic renal failure. Ann Int Med 102:588, 1985.

114. Di Minno G., Martinez J., McKean M. L., et al: Platelet dysfunction in uremia: multifaceted defect partially corrected by dialysis. Am J Med 79:552, 1985.

115. Livio M., Gotti E., Marchesi D., et al: Uraemic bleeding: role of anaemia and beneficial effect of red cell transfusions. Lancet 2:1013, 1982.

116. Fernandez F., Goudable C., Sie P., et al: Low hematocrit and prolonged bleeding time in uraemic patients: Effect of red cell transfusions. Br J Haematol 59:139, 1985.

117. Llach F.: Hypercoagulability, renal vein thrombosis, and other thrombotic complications of nephrotic syndrome. Kidney Int 28:429, 1985.

118. Remuzzi G.: Bleeding in renal failure. Lancet 1:190, 1988.

119. Janson PA, Jubelirer SJ, Weinstein MJ, et al: Treatment of the bleeding tendency in uremia with cryoprecipitate. N Engl J Med 303:1318, 1980.

120. Gralnick H. R., McKeown L. P., Williams S. B., et al: Plasma and platelet von Willebrand factor defects in uremia. Am J Med 85:806, 1988.

121. Canavese C., Salomone M., Pacitti S., et al: Reduced response of uraemic bleeding to repeated doses of desmopressin. Lancet 1:867, 1985.

122. Livio M., Mannucci P. M., Vigano G., et al: Conjugated estrogens for the management of bleeding associated with renal failure. N Engl J Med 315:731, 1986.

123. Capitanio A., Mannucci P. M., Ponticelli C., et. al.: Detection of circulating released platelets after renal transplantation. Transplantation 33:298, 1982.

124. Fruchtamn S., Aledñt L. M.: Disseminated intravascular coagulation. J Am Coll Cardiol 8:159, 1986.

125. Carr J. M., McKinney M., McDoyagh J.: Diagnosis of DIC. Role of D dimer. Am J Clin Path 91:280–287, 1989.

126. Baker R.: Clinical aspects of disseminated intravascular coagulation. Semin Thromb Hemostasis 15:1, 1989.

127. Vinazzer H.: Therapeutic use of antithrombin III in shock and disseminated intravascular Report Series 610. World Health Organization Geneva 14:45, 1977.

128. Collins J. A.: Recent developments in the area of massive transfusion. World J Surg 11:75, 1987.

129. Valeri C. R., Feingold H, Cassidy G, et al: Hypothermia-induced reversible platelet dysfunction. Ann Surg 205:175, 1987.

130. Ferrara A., MacArthur J. D., Wright H. K., et al: Hypothermia and acidosis worsen coagulopathy in the patients requiring massive transfusion. Am J Surg 160:515, 1990.

131. Miller R. D., Robbins T. O., Tong M. J., et al: Coagulation defects associated with massive blood transfusion. Ann Surg 174:794, 1971.

132. Miller R. D.: Complications of massive transfusions. Anesthesiology 39:82, 1973.

133. Counts R. B., Haiseh C., Simon J. L., et al: Hemostasis in massively transfused trauma patients. Ann Surg 190:91, 1979.

134. Harrigan C., Lucas C. E., Ledgerwood AM: Primary hemostasis after massive transfusion injury. Ann Surg 48:393, 1982.

135. Reed R. L., Ciavarella D., Heimbach D. M., Baron L.: Prophylactic platelet administration during massive transfusion. A prospective, randomized, double blind clinical study. Ann Surg 203:40, 1986.

136. Martin D. I., Lucas C. E., Ledgerwood A. M., et al: Fresh frozen plasma supplement to massive red blood cell transfusion. Ann Surg 202:505, 1985.

137. Hewson J. R., Neame P. B., Kumar N., et al: Coagulopathy related to dilution and hypotension during massive transfusion. Crit Care Med 13:387, 1985.

138. Bick R. L., Arbegast N. R., Crawford L., et al: Hemostatic effects induced by cardiopulmonary bypass. Vasc Surg 9:28, 1975.

139. Harker L., Malpass T. W., Branson H. E., et al: Mechanism of abnormal bleeding in patients undergoing cardiopulmonary bypass: acquired transient platelet dysfunction associated with selective alpha-granule release. Blood 56:824, 1980.

140. Bachmann F., McKenna R., Cole E. R., et al: The hemostatic mechanism after open-heart surgery. I. Studies on plasma coagulation factors and fibrinolysis in 512 patients after extracorporeal circulation. J Thorac Cardiovasc Surg 70:76, 1975.

141. Czer L. S. C., Bateman T. M., Gray R. J., et al: Treatment of severe platelet dysfunction and hemorrhage after cardiopulmonary bypass: reduction of blood product usage with desmopressin. J Am Coll Cardiol 9:1139, 1987.

142. Woodman R. C., Harker L. A.: Bleeding complications associated with cardiopulmonary bypass. Blood 76:1680, 1990.

143. Hope A. F., Hcyns A. D., Lottcr M. G.: Kinctics and sites of sequestration of indium III-labeled human platelets during cardiopulmonary bypass. J Thorac Cardiovasc Surg 81:880, 1981.

144. Khabbaz K. R., Marquardt C. A., Wolfe J. A., et al: Reversible platelet dysfunction following cardiopulmonary bypass: a temperature dependent defect in platelet thromboxane A2 synthesis. Surg Forum 40:201, 1989.

145. Rinder C. S., Bohnert J., Rinder H. M., et al: Platelet activation and aggregation during cardiopulmonary bypass. Anesthesiology 75:388, 1991.

146. Ferraris V. A., Ferraris S. F., Lough F. C., et al: Preoperative aspirin ingestion increases operative blood loss after coronary artery bypass grafting. Ann Thorac Surg 45:71, 1988.

147. Harder M. P., Eijsman L., Roozendaal K. J., et al: Aprotonin reduces intraoperative and postoperative blood loss in membrane oxygenator cardiopulmonary bypass. Ann Thorac Surg 51:936, 1991.

148. Mammen E. F., Koets B. A., Washington B. C., et al: Hemostatic changes during cardiopulmonary bypass surgery. Semin Thromb Hemost 11:281, 1985.

149. Lijnen H. R., Collen D.: Interaction of plasminogen activators and inhibitors with plasminogen and fibrin. Semin Thromb Hemost 8:2, 1989.

150. Young J. A., Kisker C. T., Dory D. B.: Adequate anticoagulation during cardiopulmonary bypass determined by activated clotting time and the appearance of fibrin monomer. Ann Thorac Surg 26:231, 1978.

151. Metz S., Keats A. S.: Low activated coagulation time during cardiopulmonary bypass does not increase postoperative bleeding. Ann Thorac Surg 49:440, 1990.

152. Roy R. C., Stafford M. A., Hudspeth A. S., et. al.: Failure of prophylaxis with fresh frozen plasma after cardiopulmonary bypass. Anesthesiology 69:254, 1988.

153. Simon T. L., Ali B. F., Murphy W.: Controlled trial of routine platelet concentrates in cardiopulmonary bypass surgery. Am Thorac Surg 37:359, 1984.

154. Mohr R., Martinowitz V., Lavee J., et al: The hemostatic effect of fresh whole blood versus platelet concentrates after cardiac operations. J Thorac Cardiovasc Surg 96:530, 1988.

155. Lavee J., Martinowitz V., Mohr R.: The effect of fresh whole blood versus platelet concentrates after cardiac operations: a scanning electron microscopic study of platelet aggregation on extracellular matrix. J Thorac Cardiovasc Surg 97:204, 1989.

156. Salzman E. W., Weinstein M. J., Weintraub R. M., et al: Treatment with desmopressin acetate to reduce blood loss after cardiac surgery: a double-blind, randomized trial. N Engl J Med 314:1402, 1986.

157. Rocha E., Llorens R., Paramo J. A., et al: Does desmopressin acetate reduce blood loss after surgery in patients on cardiopulmonary bypass. Circulation 77:1319, 1988.

158. Hackmann, T., Gascoyne R. D., Naiman S. C., et al: A trial of desmopressin (1-desamino-8-d-arginine vasopressin) to reduce blood loss in uncomplicated cardiac surgery. N Engl J Med 321:1437, 1989.

159. Hardy J. F., Desroches J.: Natural and synthetic antifibrinolytics in cardiac surgery. Can J Anaesth 39:353, 1992.

160. Horrow J. C., Hlavacek J., Strong M. D., et al: Prophylactic tranexemic acid decreases bleeding after cardiac operations. J Thorac Cardiovasc Surg 99:70, 1990.

161. Del Rossi A. J., Cernaianu A. C., Botros S., et. al.: Prophylactic treatment of postperfusion bleeding using EACA. Chest 96:27, 1989.

Chapter 15

SHOCK: PATHOPHYSIOLOGY AND DIAGNOSIS

KENNETH D. CANDIDO

The state of shock, regardless of etiology, has as a basic perturbation poor perfusion of vital organs because of tissue hypoxia induced by oxygen supply and demand inequities. Shock is a dynamic syndrome that ultimately results in tissue damage as substrates required for aerobic metabolism are delivered at an insufficient rate by too little blood flow or maldistributed flow at the microcellular level. Inadequate perfusion of critical organs will lead to serious pathophysiologic consequences and eventually death. A basic defect common to shock types is that oxygen delivery to peripheral cells is delayed and these "sick" cells have a reduced capacity to extract oxygen from whatever little blood flow does arrive. With a change to anaerobic metabolism there is an accumulation of hydrogen ion in addition to lactate and pyruvate which are produced by the incomplete catabolism of glucose. The statistical probability of survival can actually be predicted by serum or arterial lactate levels. Reversal of the shock state demands early and aggressive therapy directed at restoration of organ blood flow and towards the elimination of the underlying cause. Pulmonary gas exchange may be inadequate in shock resulting from pulmonary venous congestion caused by increased capillary permeability. Cardiac output and the individual factors determining it (stroke volume; in turn composed of preload, afterload and contractility, and heart rate) may have to be evaluated separately to elicit both the etiology of shock as well as to plan appropriate treatment. Ventricular function curves based on Starling's law of the heart may be useful adjuncts to delineating treatment goals and planning appropriate regimens.

HISTORICAL ASPECTS

Major historical developments in shock diagnosis and treatment have occurred over the past four centuries. Some of the more significant discoveries to date are listed below:

1600s: The significance of blood loss in battle was recognized
1600s: Development of screw tourniquet by Petit and Mourand
1743: LeDran uses the word "secousse"; "jarring or shaking up of the patient by a gunshot"; unnamed English translator interprets this term as "shock"
1815: Guthrie uses term "shock" in relation to gunshot wounds of the extremities

1899: Crile publishes experimental results on shock work[1]
1908: Henderson describes the basic pathophysiology of shock
1930s: Blalock, Parsons, Phemister propose plasma as a shock remedy[2]
1930s: British resuscitate battle casualties with whole blood
1940s: Post-traumatic renal failure emerges as a syndrome as techniques of resuscitation improve
1949: Beecher describes resuscitation and anesthesia for wounded men in World War II.[3]
1950s: MASH units developed (Korean War); renal failure and death noted after apparently successful resuscitation from death
1960s: Shires uses balanced salt solutions as an important component of resuscitating traumatized patients
1960s: Vietnam: Uses of frozen blood and lactated Ringer's solution for resuscitation; respiratory distress syndrome[4]
1970s: Swan-Ganz catheter as adjunct to treatment
1970s: Decreased ATP in shocked cells recognized; damaged sodium pump mechanism
1980s: Research in clinical shock mostly geared toward septic shock
1990s: Newer drugs aimed at blocking specific mediators of shock undergoing evaluation

CLASSIFICATION

To be able to treat shock in any given patient the etiology or underlying insult must be identified. Each individual type of shock has as a final common pathway the inadequate delivery of substrates to vital organs, which if left unchecked results in death. Any of the subtypes of shock may coexist, emphasizing the need to aim treatment at vascular support and reversal of the primary process. For the purposes of this review, three broad categories of shock with many subclassifications have been developed (Table 15-1).

CLINICAL RECOGNITION

For practical purposes, we will consider as examples of the above listed shock types, hemorrhagic shock; hypovolemia with head injury; cardiogenic shock; and septic shock.

Table 15–1. Classification of Shock States

Hypovolemic shock

   Hemorrhagic shock, with and without head injury

   Traumatic shock (cervical spinal cord injury, for example)

      Nonhemorrhagic shock
         Gastrointestinal losses of fluid
            Vomiting (pyloric stenosis, intestinal obstruction)
            Diarrhea
         Renal losses of fluid
            Excessive diuresis
            Diabetes insipidus, diabetic ketoacidosis
            Hyperglycemia
            Salt-wasting nephritis
         Other
            Burns
            Peritonitis/perforated ulcer
            Pancreatitis
            Cirrhosis
            Adrenocortical-insufficiency
            Pheochromocytoma
            Bullous dermatologic disease
            Abdominal ascites
            Dehydration
            Villous adenoma

Cardiogenic shock

   Failure of the heart as a pump
      Left ventricular infarction; right ventricular infarction
      Congestive cardiomyopathy
      Secondary to cardiac surgery
   Ventricular-outflow impedance (LV-outflow obstruction)
      Compliance normal
         Aortic stenosis or coarctation of aorta
         Massive pulmonary embolism
         Pulmonary hypertension/cor pulmonale
         Aortic dissection
      Compliance decreased
         Idiopathic hypertrophic subaortic stenosis
         Cardiac amyloidosis

Ventricular-filling impaired (LV-inflow obstruction)

   Cardiac intrinsic
      Mitral stenosis
      Atrial thrombus or myxoma
   Cardiac extrinsic
      Pericardial tamponade
      Restrictive pericarditis
      Viral myocarditis

Valvular dysfunction as cause

   Regurgitant lesions
      Acute aortic regurgitation
      Acute mitral regurgitation
   Stenotic lesions
      Acute aortic stenosis
      Acute mitral stenosis

Failure to generate forward stroke volume

   Ventricular septal defect; left ventricular aneurysm, ruptured left-ventricular wall
   Due to dysrhythmias
      Tachydysrhythmias
      Bradydysrhythmias

Mixed shock

   Distributive shock states (abnormal distribution of intra-vascular volume)
      Septic shock
      Assorted others; neurogenic, drug overdose, anaphylaxis, acute renal failure, hyperosmolar non-ketotic coma, liver failure, hypothyroidism, endocrine failure, cyanide poisoning, ganglionic blockade, high spinal anesthesia, severe acidosis or alkalosis

The clinical recognition of the shock state depends on the cause of shock as well as severity of the syndrome (Table 15-2). In general, each individual type of shock as listed in Table 15–1 may present entirely different clinical pictures. This section presents generalizations of organ dysfunction associated with shock and proceeds to more specific changes associated with the individual types of shock.

Hypotension and vasoconstriction are present in hemorrhagic, hypovolemic and cardiogenic shock leading to decreased perfusion and vital organ dysfunction (Table 15-3). There are changes in regional vascular resistances which can compensate for modest decreases in perfusion pressure, thereby temporarily maintaining perfusion to vital organs. In general the skin is cool, clammy and mottled. Superficial veins are collapsed. The cerebral circulation is affected as well as the skin and other organs, resulting in classical signs of confusion and disorientation. Cerebral perfusion pressure is the difference between mean arterial pressure and intracranial pressure, or right atrial pressure, whichever is higher (CPP = MAP − ICP).

Autoregulation exists in the brain between mean arterial pressures of about 50 mm Hg and 150 mm Hg with this relationship being shifted to the right in chronic hypertensives. With hypotension which accompanies shock, there is a change in mental state manifested as anything from agitation to restlessness to clouding of the sensorium to frank coma as cerebral perfusion falls below critical levels. The reversal of the hypotensive state may be sufficient to reverse the changes in mentation. Indeed, a clearly lucid and appropriately responsive patient after resuscitative measures have been instituted may be an indication of improved hemodynamics in shock.

The heart is affected by shock. Coronary perfusion pressure, the difference between diastolic arterial blood pressure and left-ventricular end-diastolic pressure is reduced by hypotension and shock. Reflex tachycardia (or bradycardia),[5] which decreases diastolic filling of coronary arteries, may be present. The decrease in mean arterial pressure is usually due foremost to decreased systolic blood pressure; systemic vascular resistance is increased, and cardiac output is reduced.

In septic shock, however, there may be increased cardiac output and a decrease in systemic vascular resistance. Fever, rigors, and an increased white blood count are often noted in this situation. The pulse may be thready in shock. An increase in left-ventricular end-diastolic pressure can result in pulmonary edema and subsequent respiratory failure with concomitant hypoxemia. If diastolic arterial blood pressure falls, this will, if combined with an increased LVEDP, lead to coronary hypoperfusion and myocardial ischemia. Diastolic blood pressure correlates well with arterial vasoconstriction, while pulse pressure (systolic arterial blood pressure minus diastolic arterial blood pressure) is related to stroke volume and the rigidity of the aorta and larger aortic branches. The systolic arterial blood pressure reflects a combination of all of these factors.[6] In cardiogenic shock, there may be CHF, dyspnea, tachypnea, pulmonary edema with a decreased PaO_2 and an S_3 gallop auscultated.

The renal system also autoregulates to a degree, but with decreased perfusion from hypotension, glomerular filtration rate decreases which is recognized clinically as oliguria (less than 25–30 ml of urine output/hr/70 kg). There is a redistribution of renal blood flow from the cortex to the medulla, and urine becomes more concentrated. Urine sodium decreases to less than 10 mEq/L. The recognition of oliguria in the presence of other signs and symptoms of shock is of key importance to the successful resuscitation of the patient. Occasionally, high-output renal failure may be present and may confuse the initial diagnosis of these patients—especially the failure to recognize the presence of renal failure in the face of a normal or increased urine output.

The integument is also affected by both decreased perfusion and vasoconstriction. This is reflected by the skin becoming cold, with notable color changes (pale to dusky to cyanotic) Sympathetic nervous system activation results in increased sweating (sympathetic cholinergic response).

Metabolic acidosis almost invariably accompanies shock with the accumulation of lactic acid secondary to hypoxemia. Anaerobic metabolism is complicated by decreased hepatic function whereby the liver becomes unable to metabolize the lactate produced.

Shock, therefore, represents a perfusion abnormality due to a decrease from normal of cardiac output or maldistribution of the available cardiac output. It may also represent the inability of the tissues to utilize the supplied substrate, thereby mimicking a hypoperfusion state.[7] Since blood flow to organs reflects the relationship between perfusion pressure and vascular resistances of organs, any factor disturbing this relationship may result in shock.

PATHOPHYSIOLOGY

Shock is a dynamic syndrome affecting the entire patient, yet each individual type of shock is different in certain characteristic ways. Table 15–1 presents a generalized classification of the various shock types, yet even this is somewhat arbitrarily arranged.

As general criteria, shock may be said to exist when; (a) systolic arterial blood pressure is less than 80 mm Hg, (b) oliguria is present and not accountable for by mechanisms other than decreased renal blood flow, (c) metabolic acidosis is present, and (d) there exists evidence for poor tissue perfusion. Various hemodynamic patterns are present in the various shock states, and these are summarized in Table 15–4. Shock then, represents the failure of normal delivery systems bringing oxygen and substrates to tissues which results ultimately in diminished cellular function.

The three major determinants of oxygen delivery to tissues are cardiac output, defined as stroke volume times heart rate; oxygen saturation, defined as O_2 combined with Hgb/O_2 capacity $\times$ 100; and oxygen carrying capacity of blood, defined as O_2 content (ml/dl blood) = (Hgb) $\times$ 1.39 $\times$ O_2 sat% + 0.003 $\times$ PaO_2.

Any one or all three factors may be impaired so as to reduce oxygen delivery to critical tissue sites in vital organs. The resulting defects of these vital organs results in shock. Shock is, simply stated, an extremely severe form of dysfunction in the economy of oxygen supply and demand.

Hypovolemia causes an increase in activity in the carotid and aortic arch baroreceptors. Likewise, there is an increase in the activity of right atrial baroreceptors. Sympathetic nervous system activity is increased and results in cardiac stimulation and peripheral vasoconstriction. The pituitary gland releases ACTH and ADH, resulting in elevated cortisol levels, and sodium and water retention begins. The increases in adreno-cortical release of epinephrine and norepinephrine are soon apparent. Plasma renin-angiotensin-aldosterone increase with greater sodium and water retention and more peripheral vasoconstriction. As hypovolemia progresses, however, these compensatory mechanisms begin to fail and major organ dysfunction ensues.

Additional vasoactive hormones are released during the developing shock syndrome including various prostaglandins, histamine, bradykinin, serotonin, β-endorphin, MDF (myocardial depressant factor) and cachectin. These substances can affect intraorgan perfusion relationships and may promote increased vascular permeability as well as alter myocardial and platelet function.

Cellular Level

Shock is not necessarily the result of low flow per se, but rather may be due to persistent uneven vasoconstriction which results in maldistribution of blood flow. This in turn results in inadequate oxygen transport ($\dot{V}O_2$), decreased aerobic metabolism, and predominance of anaerobic metabolism. Lactic acid accumulates from pyruvate, and the result is less ATP production than via the pathway for aerobic metabolism.[9] Lactic acid levels greater than 2.5 mmol/L are associated with decreased O_2 delivery to tissues.[10]

At the cellular level there is failure of delivered substrate and inability to use the nutrients which are delivered or to produce energy from them as hypoperfusion persists. Production of ATP decreases and the mitochondrial endoplasmic reticulum swells from hypoxia; the mitochondria themselves swell and lysosomes rupture releasing enzymes which result in intracellular digestion.

Table 15–2. Clinical Recognition of Shock

Organ System	Clinical Sign/Symptom	Causes
CNS	Changes in Mentation	Decreased CPP
CVS	Tachycardia	Adrenergic stimulation
	Dysrhythmias	Coronary ischemia
	Hypotension	Decreased contractility 2° ischemia of MDF, or RVF; also, decreased SVR or preload
	Murmur	Valvular dysfunction
	Increased or decreased Jugular venous pulsations	Decreased volume/pre-load, or RV failure
Respiratory	Tachypnea	Pulmonary edema Resp. muscle failure Sepsis Acidosis Hypoxemia
Renal	Oliguria	Decreased perfusion, afferent arteriolar constriction
Skin	Cool, clammy, cyanosis, sweating	Vasoconstriction, sympathetic stimulation
Other	Lactic acidosis	Anaerobic metabolism
	Fever	Hepatic dysfunction infection

CNS = central nervous system; CVS = cardiovascular system; CPP = cerebral perfusion pressure; MDF = myocardial depressant factor; RVF = right ventricular failure; SVR = systemic vascular resistance.

Table 15–3. Clinical Presentation of Shock by Etiology

Shock Type	Clinical Presentation	Laboratory	Pathophysiology	Treatment
Hypovolemic/ hemorrhagic	Pallor, fainting, skin clammy, cold; tachycardia, hypotension & oliguria	Hct, Hgb ↓ ↓	blood volume ↓	Fluids Blood Control blood loss
Cardiogenic	Pallor, fainting, skin clammy, cold; dysrhythmias, oliguria, hypotension	CXR, ECG, cardiac enzymes	Decreased cardiac output	Antidysrhythmics Vasopressors Vasodilators Balloon support
Septic	Fever, chills, warm skin, tachycardia, oliguria, altered mental status	C & S	Decreased systemic vascular resistance	Antibiotics Fluids Drain abscesses

Table 15–4. Hemodynamic Patterns in Shock by Etiology

Cause of Shock	C.O.	S.V.R.	P.C.W.P.	C.V.P.	S$\overset{\circ}{V}O_2$
Hypovolemia (fluid lost from vascular space)	↓	↑	↓	↓	↓
Cardiogenic (heart fails as a pump)					
LV MI	↓	↑	↑	NL or ↑	↓
RV MI	↓	↑	NL- ↓	↑	↓
Pericardial tamponade	↓	↑	↑	↑	↓
Massive pulmonary embolism	↓	↑	±NL	↑	↓
Septic shock (blood sequestered and pooled in various vascular compartments)					
Early	↓, ↑	↑, ↓		NL or ↑	↓
Late	↓	↑	NL	NL	↓ (rarely ↑)

CO = cardiac output; SVR = systemic vascular resistance; PCWP = pulmonary capillary wedge pressure; CVP = central venous pressure; SVO₂ = mixed venous oxygen saturation; LV = left ventricle; RV = right ventricle; MI = myocardial infarction; NL = normal.

Hypoxia causes the destabilization of endothelial cell membranes and phospholipase A_2 activation which breaks down arachidonic acid to leukotrienes via the 5-lipooxygenase pathway; or prostaglandins and thromboxanes via the cyclooxygenase pathway (see section on pharmacological adjuncts to therapy). Thromboxane vasoconstricts and aggregates platelets, which in turn release serotonin. The leukotrienes stimulate the margination of white blood cells which release microsomal enzymes. Proteases and lipases produce oxygen-free radicals which cause tissue destruction and vasoconstriction. The complement system is also activated by the lipopolysaccharide fraction of endotoxins in either septic shock or the septic phase of other shock types. These then represent the basic changes at the cellular level in shock.[11]

The Neurohumoral Response

Low blood pressure causes a compensatory increase in activity of the carotid and aortic arch baroreceptors and the right atrial mechanoreceptors. Sympathetic nervous system activity increases as a result of released epinephrine and norepinephrine, and alpha-adrenergic activity predominates, leading to vasoconstriction.[12] All this is possibly the result of the hydrolysis of phosphatidylinositol with an ultimate increase in intracellular calcium leading to smooth muscle contraction. Cardiac output and peripheral vascular resistance are elevated as a result of this α-adrenergic response, and the pituitary releases increased quantities of ACTH and ADH. There is increased adrenocortical release of epinephrine and norepinephrine and the macula densa of the kidney is stimulated, producing[13,14] an outflow of renin-angiotensin which promotes the secretion of aldosterone.[13,14] This mechanism increases arterial pressure in addition to causing salt and water retention. Plasma renin activity and plasma renin concentration increase while angiotensin I degrading enzyme decrease significantly. The renin-angiotensin system may be activated at blood losses of about 3 ml/kg, and functions as a compensatory mechanism. The speed of hemorrhage may be an important factor regulating this response. In sheep, activation of the renin-angiotensin system occurred more rapidly in the fast hemorrhage group (as opposed to slowly hemorrhaged animals), while activation of the sympathetic nervous system did not differ between groups being increased in both slow and fast-hemorrhage groups.[14]

Increased renin results in increased levels of angiotensin I which is converted to angiotensin II, a potent vasoconstrictor. The so-called state of "cold shock" results, distinguished from distributive shock where release of endotoxin and endogenous vasodilators produce peripheral vasodilatation.

Hemorrhage also stimulates cortisol release, the production of which is augmented by vasopressin release in addition to ACTH stimulation. Vasopressin is released by a 10% reduction in circulating blood volume. The result is production of a concentrated urine, formed by a vasopressin concentration as low as 5 pg/ml. Vasopressin also increases smooth muscle contraction and causes an increase in arterial blood pressure.[11]

Catecholamines and vasopressin secretion are higher in hemorrhagic shock than in any other state except possibly during cardiac arrest or in those patients with very active pheochromocytomas. The hyperglycemic, lipolytic, ketogenic and glycolytic actions of epinephrine are present at levels greater than 125 to 150 pg/ml (approximately four times basal concentrations). Inhibition of insulin release does not occur until epinephrine levels reach at least 400 pg/ml, a mark easily surpassed during shock. Norepinephrine levels, however, must increase to 1800 pg/ml for changes in hemodynamics, i.e., pulse and blood pressure, to be apparent (ten times basal; easily surpassed in shock).[14]

Hyperglycemia is due to increased gluconeogenesis with increased lactate, pyruvate and alanine levels being noted. Insulin levels fall, further contributing to the increase in blood glucose concentration. Hyperglycemia results in increased cardiac output and heart rate, which may be blocked by calcium channel blockers but not beta blockers, implying a role for glucagon in reversing hypotension or shock induced by beta blockers. These changes are summarized in Figure 15-1.

As can be seen from Figure 15-1, cells become dependent on lipolysis and autodigestion of intracellular proteins for energy (ketones and amino acids). An increase in protein catabolism and decreased serum albumin result in decreased serum oncotic pressure and failure of or delayed wound healing. Hypoxia causes increased triglycerides and elevated levels of betahydroxybutarate and acetoacetate. Ultimately, lactic acidemia ensues with deleterious and often fatal results if not corrected.[11]

Other Biochemical Derangements

The role of vasoactive lipids as mediators of the shock state have been extensively reviewed.[16-18] Arachidonic acid undergoes two pathways of metabolism (Fig. 15-2).

Prostaglandins PGE_2 and PGF_2-alpha increase in hemorrhagic shock. It is unclear if using agents to inhibit production of these lipids would be beneficial in treating the hemodynamic effects associated with these agents, but use of cyclooxygenase-dependent inhibitor agents is a consideration. The other product of arachidonic acid metabolism using the cyclooxygenase enzyme is thromboxane A_2, an extremely potent vasoconstrictor substance. A metabolite of TxA_2 known as TxB_2 is found in shock states, and is also an extremely potent vasoconstrictor TxA_2, in addition to its vasoconstricting properties, is a potent platelet aggregating factor. This agent interferes with normal blood flow to organs, and may promote ischemia which is the reason that TxA_2-antagonists may be protective in shock. Leukotrienes have a role in acute anaphylaxis and are produced by enzymatic breakdown of arachidonic acid using lipoxygenase. Circulating levels of these substances cause cardiac output to decrease mostly by constricting blood vessels. Blockade of leukotriene-induced vasoconstriction may be produced by such substances as L-649,923.[18]

Bronchoconstriction also occurs with decreased lung compliance, increased pulmonary vascular resistance, platelet aggregation and activation of white blood cells. Antagonists to the leukotrienes may be protective in shock states.

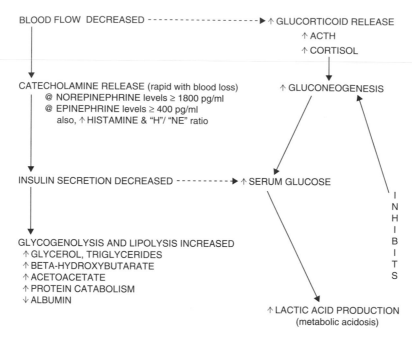

Fig. 15–1. Biochemical derangements in shock.

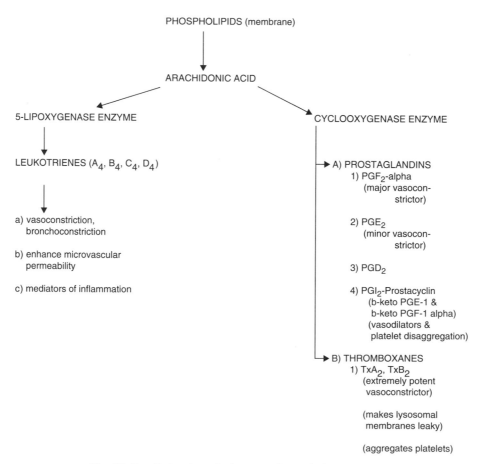

Fig. 15–2. Role of arachidonic acid metabolites in shock.

Platelet activating factor (PAF) may be associated with low blood pressure and shock secondary to increased peripheral vascular resistance due to platelet and white blood cell aggregation and possible right ventricular failure. PAF may also increase vascular permeability, cause bronchoconstriction, hypoxemia, coronary constriction and decreased myocardial contractility. Further work with these exciting substances may reveal whether they are the primary or simply secondary mediators of the various shock states.

That β-endorphin is increased in major trauma and shock is the subject of numerous reports, and the impetus for use of naloxone to try to reverse the deleterious effects of endorphins on the cardiovascular system.[19-21]

HYPOVOLEMIC/HEMORRHAGIC SHOCK

In hypovolemic shock due to hemorrhage, it is essential to characterize the percentage of blood volume lost as a guide to appropriate treatment. Generally, physical examination alone is inadequate to make this characterization; however the following schema is helpful in doing so.

Assuming normovolemia to indicate a 7.5 ml of blood per kilogram of body weight, hypovolemic shock may be divided into four groups based on estimated blood loss:[7]

I. Loss of 10 to 15% of EBV results in mild tachycardia and no shock.

II. Loss of 15 to 25% of EBV (1000 to 1250 ml loss per 70 kg) results in moderate shock, with tachycardia, decreased systolic and pulse blood pressure, slightly increased diastolic arterial blood pressure, sluggish capillary refill with blanching, and a positive table-tilt test. Urine output tends to remain close to normal at this level of blood loss.

III. Loss of 25 to 35% of EBV (1250 to 1750 ml loss per 70 kg) results in the patient having severe shock, with the following features; the skin is cold, clammy and pallid. The blood pressure is decreased by 30 to 40% (systolic blood pressure and pulse pressure), and there is increased diastolic arterial blood pressure by about 15 to 20%. Vasoconstriction is prominent, as is oliguria. The CNS is characterized by confusion progressing to stupor. Tachypnea results from metabolic acidosis secondary to hypoxemia, tissue hypoperfusion and anaerobic metabolism. Pulse rate is greater than or equal to 120 beats/minute.

IV. Loss of 35 to 45% of EBV (1750 to 2250 ml per 70 kg) results in profound shock, usually as a preterminal event. There is no palpable blood pressure, loss of peripheral pulses and possibly even loss of carotid arterial pulsations.

Data summarized by Beecher more than 40 years ago is still extremely useful in demonstrating the relationship between degrees of shock and derangements in blood factors in a previously normal 70 kg adult male (Table 15-5).[3]

Hemorrhagic shock is accompanied by hemodilution and re-expansion of plasma volume over an extended time period and therefore, hematocrit may not change for over three to four hours with acute hemorrhage.

Effect on the Cardiovascular System

Acute and uncompensated volume depletion results in an increased vascular resistance in several organs and redistribution of cardiac output to vital structures. Acute and uncompensated volume depletion of at least 10% estimated blood volume (EBV) results in redistribution of blood flow to the brain and heart at the expense of the skin, muscle, splanchnic bed and kidneys secondary to increased vascular resistance of these organs (Table 15-6). Though the brain and heart receive an increased fraction of total cardiac output, in actuality they receive less total blood flow. With mild to moderate shock, compensatory changes tend to support mean arterial pressure and mask the true extent of blood loss. As blood volume and cardiac output decrease, baroreceptors become activated quite rapidly (less than one minute later), resulting in increased sympathetic nervous system activity causing intense peripheral vasoconstriction as a result. Cardiac output tends to fall earlier than blood pressure and changes in MAP do not correlate well with the extent of hemorrhage or the decrease in cardiac output. Actually, CVP changes correlate more closely with a decrease in blood volume than do MAP changes. Following the trend of the CVP may be a more reliable indicator as to the severity of hemorrhage than is the MAP.

Diastolic arterial blood pressure increases early in hemorrhagic shock secondary to increased sympathetic nervous system activity; heart rate, systemic vascular resistance, and arterial-venous oxygen difference all increase. Pulse pressure decreases with decreased total blood volume, as does CVP. Left ventricular stroke work, oxygen delivery and oxygen consumption also fall. Later, with more extensive hemorrhage and failure of compensatory mechanisms, systolic blood pressure and diastolic blood pressure both decrease; there is redistribution of blood flow to the liver, heart and brain.

Urine output correlates well with renal blood flow, which depends upon cardiac output. With hemorrhage there is a shift of renal blood flow from the outer cortex to the inner medulla. In the inner medulla, there are less glomeruli and loops of Henle are longer than in the cortex. The shift in renal blood flow is accompanied by increased absorption of sodium and water, causing decreased urine sodium and increased urine osmolality.

The respiratory rate and minute ventilation are generally increased in hypovolemic shock causing respiratory alkalosis, especially if sepsis is superimposed on hypovolemia. Later, as metabolic acidosis complicates shock, the respiratory alkalosis acts as partial compensation for this acidosis, which is due to anaerobic metabolism and lactate production. Preterminally, there is a combined metabolic and respiratory acidosis with decreased pH, increased arterial carbon dioxide tension and decreased serum bicarbonate concentration. Airway resistance falls somewhat; pulmonary gas exchange is frequently inadequate due to pulmonary venous congestion or pulmonary edema that accompanies shock. Mixed venous oxygen

Table 15–5. Relationship Between Degree of Shock and Derangement in Blood Factors

Shock Grade	Blood Loss Volume % of normal	Hemoglobin % of normal	Hematocrit % cells	Plasma Protein grams %
I	14.4 ± 3.9	20.0 ± 5.2	42.5 ± 1.7	6.6 ± 0.1
II	20.7 ± 4.3	29.7 ± 4.1	38.4 ± 1.5	6.4 ± 0.1
III	34.3 ± 3.5	46.1 ± 3.4	34.6 ± 1.0	6.2 ± 0.1
IV	45.9 ± 4.7	54.4 ± 4.3	31.5 ± 1.5	6.0 ± 0.1

Data from Beecher, H. K.: The internal state of the severely wounded man on entry to the most forward hospital (World War II). Surgery, *22*:672, 1947; Beecher, H. K.: *Resuscitation and Anesthesia for Wounded Men (World War II)*. Springfield, IL, Charles C Thomas, 1949.

Table 15–6. Redistribution of Cardiac Output in Hypovolemic Shock

Regional Circulation	Normovolemic % Cardiac Output	S.V.R.	Blood Flow
Brain	13–15	sl. inc.	sl. decrease
Heart	4–6	no change	sl. decrease
Splanchnics	24–30	increase	decreased
Renal	22–24	marked inc.	marked decrease
Muscle	14–18	marked inc.	marked decrease
Cutaneous	7–9	marked inc.	marked decrease

SVR = systemic vascular resistance response to hemorrhage; sl = slight; inc = increase

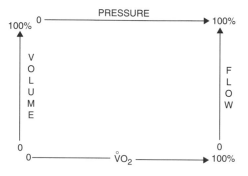

Fig. 15–3. Circulatory dynamics in shock.

decreases while oxygen extraction and alveolar to arterial oxygen differences increase. Pulmonary compliance increases as does dead space to tidal volume ratio (VD/VT) which correlates directly with decreases in pulmonary artery pressure. Even though $PaCO_2$ decreases as stated, there is increased carbon dioxide tension present at the tissue level. Base excess is often markedly reduced. Endotracheal intubation and mechanical ventilatory support are frequently required in shock.

Circulatory Dynamics

Shoemaker has idealized the circulatory dynamics of shock based upon four dimensions; pressure, volume, flow and function ($\dot{V}O_2$).[7] He has characterized each of the shock states as using these four parameters to increase or decrease by a certain percentage of normal. He then describes each shock state using this quadrangular approach as having a primary phase, a compensated phase, decompensated phase (preterminal), and a terminal phase. The terminal phase of all of the four shock states he characterizes, is the same; i.e., decreased volume, decreased pressure, decreased flow and decreased oxygen consumption (Fig. 15-3).

Oxygen Delivery and Oxygen Consumption

Overall in shock, there is a decrease in oxygen consumption by the total organism, or more appropriately, there is less oxygen consumption than is truly needed by the body to supply metabolic demand. The oxygen consumption deficit in shock may be expressed as : (CaO_2 − CvO_2) × C.I., in which CaO_2 is the content of oxygen in

arterial blood; CvO_2 is the content of oxygen in mixed venous blood; and C.I. is the cardiac index. In hemorrhaging animals, it was noted that greater than 140 ml/kg of oxygen consumption deficit was about 90% fatal.[22]

Oxygen transport is the major function of the circulation and oxygen has the greatest extraction ratio of any blood constituent. Oxygen is also the most flow-dependent of all blood constituents. There exists a relationship between the oxygen delivered at the tissue and cellular level and the oxygen consumed at these interfaces. In hemorrhagic shock, there is a decrease in the delivery of oxygen ($\dot{V}O_2$) which is significant, coupled with a moderate decrease in oxygen consumption ($\dot{V}O_2$); as compensation there is increased oxygen extraction.[22] In septic shock on the other hand, there is increased oxygen delivery initially, and decreased oxygen consumption as compensation. A supranormal $\dot{V}O_2$ (oxygen consumption) might be one of the best predictors of ultimate survival in septic shock.[23] Yet, even with an increased oxygen consumption, death can ensue rapidly in shock. A significant decrease in $\dot{V}O_2$ is a grave prognostic sign.

Other pulmonary complications and considerations in shock include the possibility of development of adult respiratory syndrome (ARDS), which is secondary to the activation of complement and blood neutrophils resulting in pulmonary vascular injury.[24] This is the subject of much interest in the critical care field, but is beyond the scope of this discussion.

The Role of the Thyroid Gland

Apparently, the thyroid is intimately associated with determining compensation to hemorrhagic shock states. Recent thyroidectomy with resultant hypothyroidism produces a reduction in cardiac output and a rise in PCWP in dogs during hemorrhagic shock, indicating reduced compensatory mechanisms to experimentally induced shock.[25] Likewise, dogs given TRH prior to experimentally induced shock had higher MAPs, cardiac outputs and SVRs than did control animals. Oxygen consumption was unchanged between groups in this one study.[26]

Hypovolemic Shock in Association with Head Injury

Shock itself may cause serious derangements of vital perfusion beds (e.g., the central nervous system and heart). While evaluation of these systems provides an indication of nutrient flow and aerobic metabolism via defined end points (i.e., level of consciousness, myocardial lactate extraction,[27] so may direct insults to these systems result in shock or exacerbate the pathophysiologic changes found in shock).

Head injury, in particular is important both as an etiologic concern in shock as well as for judging how patients with head injury and subsequent shock respond to resuscitative measures aimed at reversing shock. In an animal model, the combination of closed head injury with severe hypotension resulted in a significant reduction on phosphocreatine, ATP and intracellular pH in brain tissues when compared with either hypotension alone or head injury alone, respectively.[28] This has obvious implications for prognosis in cases in which brain injury complicates the shock state. Similarly, it has been noted that hemorrhagic lesions develop on the average within 1 hour of closed head injury in animals with resultant neurologic injury correlating with the size and severity of the lesion, becoming maximal at 18 hours.[29] From an anesthetic standpoint, it would seem prudent to consider employing agents or techniques for reducing intracranial pressure while simultaneously optimizing cerebral blood flow when head injury accompanies shock, if possible. Severe ischemia, however, may result in progressive brain hypoperfusion and irreversible neurologic damage if normal compensatory mechanisms are rendered ineffective in protecting the CNS from moderate hypoxia and ischemia.[30] Responsible factors in determining ischemic neuronal injury and ultimately cellular death may include astrocyte dysfunction, changes in calcium homeostasis, free radical metabolism, acidbase status and excitatory neurotransmitter release. Hypoxia itself only indirectly produces brain injury by impaired perfusion, since animals with arterial PO_2 values as low as 14 to 20 mm Hg only exhibit brain injury if concomitant hypotension exists.[31] Flow maldistribution from white blood cell plugging of capillaries further may exacerbate neurologic injury from hypotensive shock,[32] by reducing oxygen carrying-capacity and hence limiting brain tissue from maintaining aerobic metabolism.

The resuscitation from shock states associated with closed head injury might be complicated by the blood glucose levels on admission to the hospital or tertiary care setting. Several studies have indicated poorer neurologic outcomes following ischemic injury associated with closed head injury when serum glucose levels are elevated on admission.[33,34] It would be wise to monitor serial blood glucose levels during resuscitation from shock and head injury either intraoperatively, or in the intensive care setting. Resuscitation of shock complicated by the presence of an intracranial mass appears to be one situation where colloid resuscitation, at least initially, provides for significantly lower intracranial pressure when compared to resuscitation with lactated Ringer's solution.[35] Treatment regimens for resuscitation from shock commonly employ fluids as either crystalloid solutions or colloid solutions (see the section concerning resuscitation with intravenous fluid therapy in Chapter 16). It appears that from the standpoint of the brain injured shock patient resuscitation with either type of fluid results in similar efficacy of controlling brain injury[36] and minimizing cerebral edema.[37,38] However, with respect to effectiveness of resuscitation, smaller volumes of hypertonic saline solutions are equivalent to isotonic saline solutions and have the advantage of maintaining a lower intracranial pressure.[39] An agent such as mannitol, when given early in the brain-injured patient may be appropriate despite the presence of developing shock.[40]

In summary, head injury is frequently associated with the shock state, and must be considered in any resuscitative effort aimed at restoring blood flow to critical organs.

CARDIOGENIC SHOCK

Cardiogenic shock (CGS) is shock due to any factor disturbing normal cardiac function, or (specifically), factors affecting adversely on preload, afterload, contractility, heart rate or rhythm. Examples include right- or left-ventricular myocardial infarction, and any situation where the heart either fails as a pump, or ventricular filling or emptying are impaired (Table 15–1).

Many of the changes described above for hypovolemic/hemorrhagic shock are also found in cardiogenic shock (Tables 15–3 and 15–4). In cardiogenic shock caused by myocardial infarction, there are decreases in mean arterial pressure, cardiac output, stroke work index, left-ventricular end-diastolic pressure and volume and venous oxygen content. Heart rate, central venous pressure and arterial to venous oxygen content differences are increased, and systemic vascular resistance is also increased transiently as compensation.[41] The basic underlying problem is failure of the heart to pump blood to the peripheral tissues, whatever the cause. Treatment, as in all types of shock, is aimed at relieving the underlying insult while supporting the circulation using resuscitative measures. Of major importance is the salvaging of ischemic myocardium and the limiting of infarct size by correcting hemodynamic abnormalities and dysrhythmias. Myocardial revascularization, balloon angioplasty and thrombolytic therapies all have a place in the treatment scheme.

SEPTIC SHOCK

Incidence and Etiology

The final shock type to be discussed is septic shock. Shock complicates about 40% of cases of gram-negative bacteremia, carrying with it a mortality of about 40 to

90%.[42] Septic shock may be caused by bacteria, both gram-negative and gram-positive (endotoxins for Gm-[−], and exotoxins for Gm-[+]); for example, staphylococci, *S. pneumoniae, N. meningitidis, N. gonorrhea* or Clostridia, species; fungi, rickettsia or viruses. The lipopolysaccharide moiety of the gram-negative bacterial cell wall endotoxin may be a primary inciter of mediator release in this syndrome. Septic shock results from a sequestration or maldistribution of a normal or high cardiac output to different body compartments. Tumor necrosis factor (cachectin) has been shown to be a pivotal mediator of the clinical and humoral manifestations of shock induced by endotoxins (lipid-A and -O side chains) or by whole gram-negative bacteria.[43] Vasoactive mediators such as histamine, complement activation, kinin activation (especially prekallikrein), prostaglandins and possibly others produce vasodilatation not compensated for by augmented cardiac output. Leukocyte aggregation may cause capillary block with inadequate resultant blood flow through capillary beds. Microvascular thrombosis leads to consumption of platelets and coagulation factors, and stimulation of the fibrinolytic system manifest as DIC and resultant hemorrhage.[44] DIC caused by sepsis is associated with a decrease in factor XII, but endotoxins trigger both the intrinsic and extrinsic systems of blood coagulation.

One theory states that hemorrhagic shock progresses to septic shock as increased permeability of mucous membranes permits access of enteric bacteria into the blood stream.[45] In this model, severe cellular damage increases membrane permeability and shifts extracellular fluid into cells which is associated with breakdown in barrier function of membranes and intrusion of gram-negative or gram-positive bacteria into the blood stream. This cellular damage is reversed if successful resuscitation is undertaken, leaving bacteremia as a secondary phase. Survival may be improved if preshock treatment is instituted with broad spectrum antibiotics. Both gram-negative and gram-positive bacteria appear to induce the same cardiovascular abnormalities.

Clinical Characteristics

The cardiovascular system is affected by septic shock, both at the myocardial level as well as in the peripheral vasculature. Maldistribution of blood flow coupled with depressed myocardial performance is routinely present, with increased or normal cardiac output coupled with decreased SVR. Heart rate is increased, while mean arterial pressure, stroke volume, stroke work, oxygen consumption and arterial-to-venous oxygen content all decrease. As stated, cardiac output may be normal or increased. Patients with this condition have an enormous fluid requirement caused by peripheral vasodilatation. There is a decrease in left-ventricular ejection fraction (LVEF) and RVEF in addition to biventricular dilatation typically beginning two to four days after the onset of hypotension.[46] In survivors from septic shock states these hemodynamic values return to baseline by 7 to 10 days from the onset of septic shock. It has been noted that survivors of septic shock are more likely than non-survivors to have de-

creased LVEF and LV dilatation, suggesting a compensatory role of LV dilatation via the Frank-Starling mechanism. Nonsurvivors do not normalize heart rate, cardiac output or systemic vascular resistance (hyperdynamic state), whereas survivors tend to do so by 24 hours. The final common pathway to mortality appears to be irreversible hypotension from depressed SVR, and not necessarily a depression of cardiac output which is maintained at normal or above normal values almost until death. So, initially, there is a hyperdynamic state with high cardiac output and normal to low cardiac filling pressures, and a decreased systemic vascular resistance. Mixed venous oxygen saturation may be normal or low. Even with high cardiac outputs, there are abnormalities in systolic function (decreased stroke volume and decreased left-ventricular ejection fraction) and ventricular compliance. (The relationship between PCWP and LVEDV is not normal.) In later stages, the dynamics decrease and the picture resembles cardiogenic shock. Respiratory wise, there is an increased respiratory rate, hyperpnea, tachypnea and respiratory alkalosis. Antigen-antibody complexes activate the complement cascade. The entire process is outlined in Figure 15-4.[46]

Septicemia is frequently accompanied by and complicated by the Adult Respiratory Distress Syndrome (ARDS). Patients characteristically manifest dyspnea, hypoxemia, bilateral diffuse pulmonary infiltrates, reduced lung compliance and have pulmonary-capillary wedge pressures usually unchanged from baseline (especially if lung function was normal prior to the shock state).

Treatment

The therapy of human septic shock involves primarily eradicating the underlying cause, i.e., the infection, while temporizing the detrimental effects of bacterial toxins or endogenous host toxins and providing support for the cardiovascular and other involved systems.

A great deal of experimental research is currently underway to study agents for neutralizing the effects of toxins in septic shock. For the practicing anesthesiologist, however, most of these modalities are not of clinical importance, and are only mentioned for completeness sake. Current work involves monoclonal antibodies to parts of gram-negative bacteria, naloxone (see also section on pharmacologic adjuncts to treatment), prostaglandin inhibitors, Lipid X, antibodies to tumor necrosis factor (TNF), genetically engineered protease inhibitors and other recombinant or synthetic proteolytic inhibitors.

Cardiovascular support for the septic shock patient consists of fluids and vasopressors as needed. The general principles outlined herein are meant to supplement the guidelines delineated in other sections, particularly the section on hemorrhagic shock.

Fluid is required to optimize preload and cardiac output or even augment cardiac output above normal values so that MAP returns to baseline if possible or even initially to at least 60 mm Hg. Optimal PCWP appears to be about 12 to 15 mm Hg and obviously must be monitored by the invasive technique of pulmonary arterial flotation catheter. The type of fluid chosen does not appear to

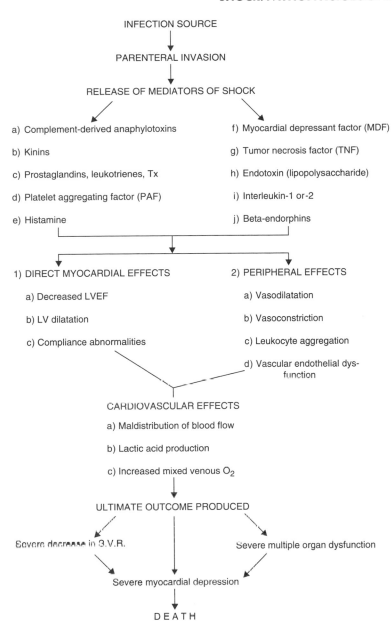

INFECTION SOURCE

PARENTERAL INVASION

RELEASE OF MEDIATORS OF SHOCK

a) Complement-derived anaphylotoxins

b) Kinins

c) Prostaglandins, leukotrienes, Tx

d) Platelet aggregating factor (PAF)

e) Histamine

f) Myocardial depressant factor (MDF)

g) Tumor necrosis factor (TNF)

h) Endotoxin (lipopolysaccharide)

i) Interleukin-1 or-2

j) Beta-endorphins

1) DIRECT MYOCARDIAL EFFECTS

a) Decreased LVEF

b) LV dilatation

c) Compliance abnormalities

2) PERIPHERAL EFFECTS

a) Vasodilatation

b) Vasoconstriction

c) Leukocyte aggregation

d) Vascular endothelial dysfunction

CARDIOVASCULAR EFFECTS

a) Maldistribution of blood flow

b) Lactic acid production

c) Increased mixed venous O_2

ULTIMATE OUTCOME PRODUCED

Severe decrease in S.V.R.

Severe multiple organ dysfunction

Severe myocardial depression

DEATH

Fig. 15–4. Pathophysiology of septic shock. Modified from Natanson, C., Hoffman, W. D., and Parrillo, J. F.: Septic Shock: The Cardiovascular Abnormality and Therapy. J Cardiothorac Anesth 3:215, 1989.

confer any particular advantage regarding outcome, although one recent study in an animal model of experimentally induced septic shock demonstrated significant improvement in cardiac output, PVR, extravascular lung water and venous admixture when Dextran-70 was used versus Ringer's lactate for resuscitation.[47] Fluid resuscitation has been shown to be effective in increasing both oxygen delivery ($\dot{V}O_2$) and oxygen consumption ($\dot{V}O_2$) in septic shock.[48]

Construction of ventricular function curves of the Frank-Starling variety and categorizing patients as to functional category or quadrant helps in deciding to add inotropes, diuretics and vasopressors to resuscitate patients. Optimizing oxygen transport by correcting anemia and also attaining serum albumin levels of at least 2 g/100 ml are important adjuncts to treatment. If volume alone does not correct hypotension, while maintaining PCWP at greater than or equal to 15 mm Hg, vasopressors may be cautiously added, beginning with low dose dopamine (1 to 3 μg/kg/min) and adding norepinephrine if larger doses of dopamine are ineffective in raising MAP or side effects become prominent (tachycardia, dysrhythmias). (Refer to section on pharmacologic adjuncts to treatment.) Epinephrine or dobutamine may be substituted for norepinephrine if the latter is ineffective or if low cardiac output necessitates the use of beta-mimetic adrenergic agonism.

MONITORING OF THE SHOCK STATE

Hemodynamic Monitoring

Patients in shock are critically ill and thus require the benefit of invasive hemodynamic monitoring, especially in those cases where vasoactive pharmacologic agents are employed for the resuscitation or support of their cardiovascular systems. In general, monitors may be classified as routine and extraordinary or non-routine. Routine monitors are those which should be employed in any critically ill patient receiving state-of-the-art care in an intensive care unit. Extraordinary or non-routine monitors are those which are specifically chosen for their use as adjuncts to routine monitors and which are not routinely found in the ICU setting, including means to measure extravascular lung water, for example.

While it is true that arterial blood pressure is an arbitrary way to measure shock because blood flow is determined by the relationship between cardiac output and systemic vascular resistance, nevertheless, in shock blood pressure must be measured using continuous techniques of monitoring beat-to-beat arterial pressures. Only rarely will the rapid cycling of an automated sphygmomanometer or Doppler blood pressure devices suffice in place of an arterial line. In addition, all patients should be monitored for heart rate and rhythm, respiratory rate, temperature, right- and left-sided heart pressures, electrocardiogram and hematocrit determinations. An indwelling arterial catheter permits the periodic sampling of arterial blood for determination of electrolytes and coagulation profiles, and arterial lactate levels as necessary. A thermistor-tipped pulmonary arterial flotation catheter may be invaluable for measurements of pulmonary arterypressures, pulmonary artery occlusion pressures, cardiac output, and many derived parameters including the vascular resistances. A pulmonary artery catheter with the capability of measuring mixed venous blood saturation may be especially useful in patients with cardiogenic shock. Central venous pressure monitoring is sometimes useful to determine or qualify blood loss, remembering that a 500 to 800 ml blood loss per 70 kilograms body weight will lower central venous pressure by about 7 cm of water.[49]

Those patients in shock who are also under general anesthesia may drop their arterial blood pressures faster than those not under anesthesia because compensatory measures to maintain sympathetic nervous system tone are blunted with anesthetics, and these patients certainly benefit from invasive continuous beat-to-beat monitoring of arterial blood pressure. Korotkoff sounds are diminished or absent with severe shock superimposed upon general anesthesia, and this is further support for placing invasive monitors in these patients.

The measurement of electrolytes and hematocrit by sampling arterial blood may provide important information during the resuscitation and management of shock states. Evaluation of blood volume and circulatory function are made with greater facility in those patients in whom serial laboratory measurements are possible. It takes about three to four hours for acute blood loss to be reflected by a significant change in hematocrit. A decreased capillary hydrostatic pressure with hemorrhage leads to increased absorption of interstitial fluid into the intravascular compartment. The intravascular compartment subsequently enlarges, and the hematocrit diminishes as the red cells form a smaller percentage of this compartment. It should be recalled that while treating shock and monitoring hemodynamic variables, no proof exists that simple correction of commonly evaluated parameters results in greater outcome or decreased morbidity.

Of the derived hemodynamic variables, two have received considerable attention as being of utmost importance in assessing shock; oxygen delivery and oxygen consumption.[41]

Oxygen delivery ($\dot{V}O_2$) is the product of the arterial oxygen content and the cardiac index. $\dot{V}O_2 = CaO_2 \times C.I. \times 10$, in which $CaO_2 = 1.39 \times Hgb \times \%$ Saturation + $(PaO_2 \times 0.003)$, and C.I. = cardiac output / body surface area. The normal values for $\dot{V}O_2$ are 520 to 720 ml/min/m^2.

Oxygen consumption ($\dot{V}O_2$ is the product of the arterial oxygen content minus the venous oxygen content and the cardiac index times 10 ($\dot{V}O_2 = CaO_2 - CvO_2 \times C.I. \times 10$). Normal values for $\dot{V}O_2$ are 100 to 180 ml/min/m^2. $\dot{V}O_2$ represents the sum of all oxidative metabolic reactions and is therefore a measure of the body's total overall metabolism.

Derived hemodynamic variables of interest also include the calculation of the shunt fraction Q_2 / Q_t, and the A-aDO$_2$, or alveolar to arterial oxygen difference. The flow-directed pulmonary artery catheter has revolutionized the treatment of shock patients by allowing them to be placed into functional categories based on modified Starling cardiac function curves. In general, it is useful to remember that mean pulmonary artery pressure is about 5 to 10 mm Hg higher than pulmonary capillary wedge pressure, and that pulmonary arterial diastolic pressure is about 0 to 3 mm Hg greater than PCWP. PCWP is about equal to left atrial pressure or left ventricular end-diastolic pressure except in cases of mitral stenosis, where the LVEDP cannot be determined or estimated from PCWP measurements. Also, cardiac output may be estimated using the thermodilution technique unless intracardiac shunts (left-to-right or right-to-left) are present.

Central Venous Pressure

Isolated CVP readings in shock are of little significance. The response of the central venous pressure to fluid challenges is, however, important as a guide to therapy. If the central venous pressure shows little or no change in the face of increased pulse pressure after fluid challenge, a second fluid challenge may be indicated. If CVP increases after the fluid bolus or challenge, the plan might be to not administer further fluids and to work towards achieving blood pressure augmentation by pharmacologic or other means.

Pulmonary Artery Diastolic Pressure

The PAdP is usually about 1 to 2 mm Hg greater than the PCWP, unless pulmonary hypertension is present. If the PAdP minus the PCWP is greater than 5 mm Hg, pulmonary hypertension is present. PAdP changes are useful for assessing the beneficial effects of fluid challenges in shock treatment.

Lactate Level

Arterial lactate level has been shown to be a valuable monitor of the shock state and has been correlated with prognosis.[50-56] In shock, lactate levels increase and the lactate to pyruvate ratio also increases. At greater than 2.5 mM/L of arterial blood lactate, the statistical probability

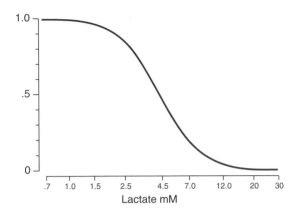

Fig. 15–5. The probability curve indicating the likelihood of survival based on a given value of arterial blood lactate in patients with circulatory shock. Redrawn from Weil, M. H. and Afifi, A. A.: Circulation 41:989, 1970.

of survival falls dramatically, and at 4.5 mM/L, the chance of survival is only about 50%. At greater than 7.0 mM/L, the chance of survival is less than 10%.

Survivors of the shock state seem to have lower lactate levels than do non-survivors and also seem to have lactate levels which fall by at least 10% per hour once treatment is instituted, whereas nonsurvivors have levels that do not fall even with treatment. Arterial lactate levels may be expressed as milligrams per milliliter or as millimoles per liter. Apparently, lactate levels may be measured from the arterial blood, or pulmonary artery central venous sites with equal degrees of accuracy.[55] One study showed no correlation between arterial blood lactate levels and changes in oxygen delivery in either septic shock or nonseptic shock.[56] Nevertheless, arterial lactate levels continue to serve as a valuable measurement of the presence and severity of the shock state (Fig. 15-5).[57]

EFFECTS ON THE LYMPHATIC SYSTEM

Major surgery is known to evoke endocrine stress responses in man, characterized by increased serum cortisol and elevated catecholamines including adrenaline and noradrenaline.[58] In addition, lymphopenia and granulocytosis in the peripheral blood are noted. These changes are also produced by an infusion of cortisol. Thus, surgical stress induces a redistribution of lymphocytes from the peripheral blood to the lymphatic system and tissues.[59] There is marked dilatation of the lymphatic vessels and increased lymph flow in the thoracic duct. This phenomenon is related to the increased capillary permeability in shock with plasma leakage into intercellular spaces.

REFERENCES

1. Crile, G. W.: Experimental research into surgical shock. Philadelphia, J.B. Lippincott Company, 1899.
2. Blalock, A.: Experimental shock: The cause of low blood pressure produced by muscle injury. Arch Surg 20:959, 1930.
3. Beecher, H. K.: The internal state of the severely wounded man on entry to the most forward hospital (World War II). Surgery 22:672, 1947; Beecher, H.K.: Resuscitation and Anesthesia for Wounded men (World War II). Springfield, Il, Charles C Thomas, 1949.
4. Blaisdell, F. W. and Lewis, F. R., Jr.: Respiratory distress syndrome of shock and trauma. Philadelphia, W.B. Saunders Company, 1977.
5. Jacobsen, J. and Secher N. H.: Slowing of the heart during anaphylactic shock—a report of five cases. Acta Anaesthesiol Scand 32:401–403, 1988.
6. Wilson, R. F.: Science and shock: A clinical perspective. Ann Emerg Med 14:714–723, 1985.
7. Shoemaker, W. C.: Circulatory mechanisms of shock and their mediators. Crit Care Med 15:787–794, 1987.
8. Shoemaker, W. C., et al., (eds.): Pathophysiology and therapy of shock syndromes. From "Textbook of Critical Care", W.B. Saunders, Co., Philadelphia, 1984, pp 52–72.
9. Rackow, E. C. and Weil, M.H.: Physiology of blood flow and oxygen utilization by peripheral tissue in circulatory shock. Clin Chem 36:1544, 1990.
10. Mavric, Z., Zaputovic, L., Zagar, D., et al.: Usefulness of blood lactate as a predictor of shock development in acute myocardial infarction. Am J Cardiol 67:565–568, 1991.
11. Woolf, P. D.: Endocrinology of shock. Ann Emerg Med 15:December, 1986.
12. Bond, R. F. and Johnson, III, G.: Vascular adrenergic interactions during hemorrhagic shock. Fed Proc 44:281–289, Feb 1985.
13. Michailov, M. L., Schad, H., Dahlheim, H., et. al.: Renin-angiotensin system responses of acute graded hemorrhage in dogs. Circ Shock 21:217–224, 1987.
14. Starc, T. J. and Stalcup, S. A.: Time course of changes of plasma renin activity and catecholamines during hemorrhage in conscious sheep. Circ Shock 21:129–140, 1987.
15. Roizen, M. F., Turkey, K., Ebert, P. A., et al: Blood flow, not low oxygen or pH, causes catechol response to shock in lambs. Anesth Analg 61:210–211, 1982.
16. Feuerstein, G. and Hallenbeck, J. M.: Prostaglandins, leukotrienes, and platelet activating factor in shock. Annu. Rev Pharmacol Toxicol 27:301–13, 1987.
17. Alemayehu, A., Sawmiller, D., Chou, B. S., et al: Intestinal prostacyclin and thromboxane production in irreversible hemorrhagic shock. Circ Shock 23:119–130, 1987.
18. Bitterman, H., Smith, B. A., Lefer, A. M.: Beneficial actions of antagonism of peptide leukotrienes in hemorrhagic shock. Circ Shock 24:159–168, 1988.
19. Shatnay, C. H., Cohen, R. M., Cohen, M. R., Imagawa, D. K.: Endogenous opioid activity in clinical hemorrhagic shock. Surg Gynecol Obstet 160:547–551, 1985.
20. Gurll, N. J., Vargish, T,, Reynolds, D. G., Lechner, R. B.: Opiate receptors and endorphins in the pathophysiology of hemorrhagic shock. Surgery 89:364–369, 1981.
21. Daly, T., Beamer, K. C., Vargish, T., Wilson, A.: Correlation of plasma beta-endorphin levels with mean arterial pressure and cardiac output in hypovolemic shock. Crit Care Med 15:723–25, 1987.
22. Kaufman, B. S., Rackow, E. C., Falk, J. L.: The relationship between oxygen delivery and consumption during fluid resuscitation of hypovolemic and septic shock. Chest 85:336–40, 1984.
23. Houtchens, B. A. and Westenskow, D. R.: Oxygen consumption in septic shock: Collective review. (review article). Circ Shock 13:361–384, 1984.
24. Ward, P. A., Johnson, K. J., Till, G. O.: Current concepts regarding adult respiratory distress syndrome. Ann Emerg Med Ang 14:724–728, 1985.
25. Gallick, H. L., Lucas, C. E., Ledgerwood Am, et al: Detrimental effect of recent thyroidectomy on hemorrhagic shock and resuscitation. Circ Shock 21:111–119, 1987.
26. Teba, L., Zakaria, M., Dedhia, H. V., et al.: Beneficial effect

of thyrotropin-releasing hormone in canine hemorrhagic shock. Circ Shock *21*:51-57, 1987.

27. Audio-Digest. Anesthesiology *30*: 1988.

28. Ishige, N., Pitts, L. H., Berry, I., et al.: The effects of hypovolemic hypotension on high-energy phosphate metabolism of traumatized brain in rats. J. Neurosurg *68*:129-136, 1988.

29. Shapira, Y., Shohami, E., Sidi, A., et al.: Experimental closed head injury in rats: Mechanical, pathophysiologic, and neurologic properties. Crit Care Med *16*:258-65, 1988.

30. Kaplan, J., Dimlich, R. V., Biros, M. H., et al: Mechanisms of ischemic cerebral injury. Resuscitation *15*:149-169, 1987.

31. DeCourten-Myers, G. M., Yamaguchi, S., Wagner, K. R., et al.: Brain injury from marked hypoxia in cats: Role of hypotension and hyperglycemia. Stroke *16*:1016-1021, 1985.

32. Yamakawa, T., Yamaguchi, S., Niimi, H., et al: White blood cell plugging and blood flow maldistribution in the capillary network of cat cerebral cortex in acute hemorrhagic hypotension: An intravital microscopic study. Circ Shock *22*:323-332, 1987.

33. Prough, D. S., Coker, L. H., Lee, S., et al.: Hyperglycemia and neurologic outcome in patients with closed head injury. Anesthesiology *XV*:Sept/Oct, 1988.

34. Contreras, F. L., Kadekaro, M., Eisenberg H. M.: The effect of hyperbaric oxygen on glucose utilization in a freeze-traumatized rat brain. J Neurosurg *68*:137-141, 1988.

35. Poole, G. V., Jr., Prough, D. S., Johnson, J. C., et al.: Effects of resuscitation from hemorrhagic shock on cerebral hemodynamics in the presence of an intracranial mass. J Trauma *27*:18-23, January, 1987.

36. Zornow, M. H., Oh, Y. S., Scheller, M. S.: A comparison of the cerebral and hemodynamic effects of mannitol and hypertonic saline in a rabbit model of brain injury. Anesthesiology *XV*: 1988.

37. Wisner, D., Busche. F., Sturm, J., et al.: Traumatic shock and head injury: Effects of fluid resuscitation on the brain. Surg Res *46*:49-59, 1989.

38. Sutin, K. M., Ruskin, K. J., Kaufman, B. S.: Intravenous fluid therapy in neurologic injury. Crit Care Clin *8*:367-408, 1992.

39. Gunnar, W. P., Merlotti, G. J., Barret, J., Jonasson, O,: Resuscitation from hemorrhagic shock: Alterations of the intracranial pressure after normal saline, 3% saline and dextran-40. Ann Surg *204*:686-692, 1986.

40. Feldman, J. A. and Fish, S.: Resuscitation fluid for a patient with head injury and hypovolemic shock. J Emerg Med *9*:465-8, 1991.

41. Shoemaker, W. C.: A new approach to physiology, monitoring and therapy of shock states. World J Surg Apr *11*:133-146, 1987.

42. Parker, M. M., Parrillo, J. E.: Septic shock: Hemodynamics and pathogenesis. JAMA *250*:3324-27, 1983.

43. Calandra, T., Baumgartner, J. D., Glauser, M. P.: Anti-lipopolysaccharide and anti-tumor necrosis factor/cachectin antibodies for the treatment of gram-negative bacteremia and septic shock. Prog Clin Biol Res *367*:141-159, 1991.

44. Colman, R. W.: The role of plasma proteases in septic shock. N Engl J Med *320*:1207-09, 1989.

45. Audio-Digest Anesthesiology *30*: 1988.

46. Natanson, C., Hoffman, W. D., Parrillo, J. E.: Septic shock: The cardiovascular abnormality and therapy (review article). J Cardiothorac Anesthes *3*:(2) (April): 215-27, 1989.

47. Modig, J.: Comparison of effects of dextran-70 and Ringer's acetate on pulmonary function, hemodynamics and survival in experimental septic shock. Crit Care Med *16*:(3):266-271, 1988.

48. Kaufman, B. S., Rackow, E. C., Falk, J. L.: The relationship between oxygen delivery and consumption during fluid resuscitation of hypovolemic and septic shock. Chest *85*:336-340, March, 1984.

49. Warren, J. V., Brannon, E. S., Stead, E. A., Jr., et al.: The effect of venesection and the pooling of blood in the extremities on arterial pressure and cardiac output in normal subjects with observations on acute circulatory collapse in three instances. J Clin Invest *24*(May):337, 1945.

50. Weil, M. H., Leavy, J., Rackow, E. C.: Prognosis in shock. Correspondence section; Anaesthesia *41*(1):80-82, 1986.

51. Cowan, B. N., Burns, H. J., Boyle, P., et al: The relative prognostic value of lactate and hemodynamic measurements in early shock. Anesthesia *39*(8):750-755, Aug, 1984.

52. Wiel, M. H. and Henning, R. J.: New concepts in the diagnosis and fluid treatment of circulatory shock. Anesth Analg *58*(2):124; Mar/Apr, 1979.

53. Vincent, J. L., Dufaye, P., Barre, J., et al.: Serial lactate determinations during circulatory shock. Crit Care Med *11*(6):449-451, Jun, 1983.

54. Shin, B., Mackenzie, C. F., Helrich, M.: Hypokalemia in trauma patients. Anesthesiology *65*(1):90-92, July, 1986.

55. Weil, M. H., Michaels, S., Rackow, E. C.: Comparison of blood lactate concentration in central venous, pulmonary artery and arterial blood. Crit Care Med *15*(5):489-90; May, 1987.

56. Groeneveld, A. B., Kester, A. D., Nauta, J. J.: Relation of arterial blood lactate to oxygen delivery and hemodynamic variables in human shock states. Circ Shock *22*(1):35053, 1987.

57. Weil, M. H. and Afifi, A. A.: Probability curve indicating likelihood of survival based on a given value of arterial blood lactate in patients with circulatory shock. Circulation *41*:989, 1970.

58. Selye, H.: The Physiology and Pathology of Exposure to Stress (1st Ed.) Aeta Inc Medical Publishers. Montreal, Canada. 1950.

59. Toft, P., Svendsen, P. Tonnesen, E., et al: Redistribution of lymphocytes after major surgical stress. Acta Anaesthesiol Scand *17*:245-249, 1993.

Chapter 16

MANAGEMENT OF SHOCK STATES

KENNETH D. CANDIDO

The goals of therapy should be to normalize hemodynamic parameters using whatever modalities are available to those performing resuscitation; however, simply restoring these variables to normal may not be equivalent to improving survival, and each patient presents a unique and individual set of problems that must be addressed. Table 16-1 provides a brief listing of some of the important parameters to be monitored in a shock state and the goals of therapy.

TREATMENT PLAN

The treatment of any of the shock types must be undertaken quickly, aggressively, and if possible, following a well-prepared and carefully written protocol. Basic life-support, followed by advanced life support as needed must be undertaken at once if survival is to be possible. Some of the major concerns include fluid therapy (both by volume loading with crystalloid and by RBC replacement or other colloid use), augmentation of preload and use of vasopressor substances as needed. The need for and expeditious use of tracheal intubation and mechanical ventilation must be implemented as assessed. Mechanical ventilation and supplemental oxygen therapy are required for almost all types of shock treatment to provide adequate oxygen delivery to cells. The respiratory mus-

Table 16-1. Therapeutic Goals of Shock Resuscitation

Mean arterial pressure (MAP)	>84 mm Hg
Central venous pressure (CVP)	>3 cm H_2O
Hemoglobin (Hgb)	>8g/dl
Pulmonary capillary wedge pressure (PCWP)	>9 mm Hg
Cardiac index (CI)	>4.5 L/min/m²
Left ventricular stroke work (LVSW)	>55 g · m/beat/m²
Heart rate (HR)	<100 beats/minute
Temperature (T)	98–101°F
Mixed venous oxygen tension ($P\bar{v}O_2$)	>35 mm Hg
Oxygen extraction	31%
Blood volume (EBV + 500 ml/70 kg)	(preferred in shock)
Lactate	.031 to 0.7 mg/ml
Oxygen delivery ($\dot{D}O_2$)	>600 ml/min · m² (sl. normal)
Oxygen consumption ($\dot{V}O_2$)	>170 ml/min · m² (30% normal)

Modified from Shoemaker, W. C.: A new approach to physiology, monitoring, and therapy of shock states. World J. Surg., *11*:133, 1987.

cles require a disproportionate share of the total cardiac output during shock.[1-3] Mechanical support allows blood flow to be redistributed and will decrease respiratory muscle oxygen requirements. Endotracheal intubation is also indicated for those patients with mental status changes that may make adequate protection of the airway uncertain.

The treatment of low arterial blood pressure and signs of vital organ dysfunction must be undertaken rapidly as alluded to throughout the previous chapter. End-points of this treatment include restoration of mental acuity, production of an adequate urine output; decrease of any signs of myocardial ischemia; and attempt at normalizing monitoring parameters including arterial blood pressure, pulmonary capillary wedge pressure, cardiac output, venous oxygen saturation, and oxygen consumption. Prognosis is related to whether the shock state is reversible or nonreversible. The severity, duration and underlying cause of the shock must be assessed. If preexisting vital organ dysfunction is present, this too must be assessed in its role in the etiology of the shock state.

RESUSCITATION WITH INTRAVENOUS FLUID THERAPY

The treatment of hypotension with signs of vital organ dysfunction must be aggressively undertaken; those signs include but are not limited to; mental obtundation, oliguria, pulmonary edema, angina, tachycardia or bradycardia, and cool and clammy skin. In shock states it is preferable to attain direct measurement of arterial blood pressure by means of an indwelling arterial cannula, which also assists one in obtaining blood samples for measurements of hematocrit and blood gases and electrolytes serially as indicated. In cases of non-cardiogenic shock states, the first line of resuscitative treatment is maintenance of blood pressure and cardiac output adequate to perfuse these vital organ beds, and vasopressors or intravascular volume expansion are the two currently acceptable methods of accomplishing this goal. Restoration of blood volume in shock is certainly of utmost importance in the treatment of hypovolemic shock. Prior to instituting fluid resuscitation, increases in the central venous return to the heart may be attempted by such measures as employment of the Trendelenburg position or the use of military antishock trousers (MAST); while realizing that MAST may actually worsen outcome in those patients with cardiac and thoracic trauma and vascular injury.[81] Several large bore intra-

Table 16–2. Fluids for Intravenous Resuscitation from Shock

	Na (mEq/L)	Cl (mEq/L)	Cations	Anions	Approx mOsm/L	Approx pH	Dextrose (mg/ml)
Lactated Ringer's (LR)	130	109	K-4, Ca-3	Lactate-28	273	6.5	0
D$_5$LR	130	109	K-4, Ca-3	Lactate-28	525	4–6.5	50
0.9% NaCl	154	154	NONE	NONE	308	5.0	0
D$_5$NaCl	154	154	NONE	NONE	560	4.0	50
Normosol-R or Polyionic-R	140	98	K-5, Mg-3	Acetate-27 Gluconate-23	295	6.4	0
Plasmalyte-148	140	98	K-5, Mg-3	Acetate-27 Gluconate-23	294	5.5	0

venous cannulae must be secured before beginning resuscitative efforts with intravenous fluids.

The choice of fluid type for resuscitation has been historically tainted by controversy as to whether crystalloid or colloid solutions result in better outcomes (Table 16-2). Fluid exchange in the normal lung[4] is described by: $Qf = k_w [(P_c - P_i) - \sigma_s (\pi_c - \pi_i)]$, where:

Qf = the net exchange of fluid across membranes
k_w = filtration coefficient of water
P_c = capillary hydrostatic pressure
P_i = interstitial hydrostatic pressure
σ_s = reflection coefficient of solute (0–1.0)
π_c = capillary osmotic pressure
π_i = interstitial osmotic pressure

Based on this theoretical model, some authorities suggest a role for colloid administration vs. crystalloids, since crystalloids could reduce oncotic pressure. However, studies show that there is no difference in lung water volumes in animals resuscitated with crystalloid or colloid.[5,6] Therefore, no choice of fluid can be deemed most appropriate without defining physiologic endpoints of therapy. Shoemaker claims that the efficacy of alternative fluid therapies is best evaluated by physiologic responses that are related to survival instead of by conveniently chosen, easily monitored variables.[7] The therapeutic agent used appears to be less important than is the achievement and maintenance of the desired physiologic goals. One treatment approach is to choose a fluid based on the type of fluid being lost from the body, in an attempt to restore both red cell mass in the case of hemorrhage and electrolytes in the case of non-RBC fluid loss. Basic goals of resuscitation should be established, including physiologic homeostatic parameters; expansion of vascular volume with improvement in cardiac index increased oxygen delivery; replenishment of interstitial fluids and adequate perfusion of the brain, heart and splanchnic and renal beds, respectively. Blood is excellent for resuscitation purposes as it provides oxygen carrying capacity, as well as volume, but blood supply is short and blood transfusion carries with it numerous risks which include transmission of disease and allergic reactions. Also, there is a certain irreducible time frame necessary before blood can be made available to any given patient if type and crossmatch procedures are deemed appropriate.[8-10]

With shock, metabolic acidosis occurs and the oxygen-hemoglobin dissociation curve is shifted to the right. The shift to the right is prolonged by an increased synthesis of 2,3-DPG. There is increased unloading of oxygen in tissues as well as increased aerobic metabolism as compensation. A depletion of purine-bases may occur if the supply made available by these compensatory mechanisms is not sufficient for oxidative phosphorylation. "Irreversibility" in hemorrhagic shock is related to loss of purine bases for restoration of cellular adenosine-triphosphate (ATP).[11] A lack of oxidative phosphorylation in hypoxic cells results in degradation of the purine compounds.

When instituting therapy based on physiologic parameters, one is frequently confronted with how to deal with laboratory variables to optimize therapy. In particular, when intravenous fluid therapy is instituted, a frequently asked question is at what hematocrit or below what hematocrit is blood necessary to afford the optimum oxygen-carrying capacity and cardiac output. This is an area of considerable debate, and for which numerous, mostly arbitrary limits have been suggested. One author suggests attaining a hematocrit of 30 as the minimal acceptable before instituting transfusion and the reasoning for this is as follows:[11] Oxygen consumption at rest is approximately equal to 250 ml per minute. If the alveolar to arterial oxygen difference is about 30% (A-aDO$_2$), total oxygen transport per minute is equal to 250 ml/.30 or 833 ml. Hemoglobin carries 1.39 ml of oxygen per gram, therefore, the amount of hemoglobin required to carry 833 ml of oxygen is 833/1.39 or 600 grams of hemoglobin. For a 75-kg person with an estimated blood volume (EBV) of 5.25 liters and a cardiac output approximately the same (5.25 L/min), the amount of hemoglobin per liter of blood to transport the above amount of oxygen is 600/5.25 or 114 grams of hemoglobin/liter which is equivalent to a hematocrit of about 33%. Therefore, based on analyses such as these, resuscitation from shock should commence with a non-RBC fluid and proceed to an RBC-containing solution upon reaching an estimated blood loss of about 30% of the EBV. Certainly, there are those who will contend that an adequate hematocrit is that which provides for sufficient oxygen to reach peripheral perfusion beds with normal functioning of the organs served, and this seems a logical way to approach therapy while avoiding overreliance on laboratory parameters as sole indicators of successful treatment. Critically ill patients with higher hemoglobins may maintain better intravascular volume, have a lower incidence of respiratory failure and may be more likely to survive.[12]

When data from multiple clinical trials is pooled to analyze it more reliably,[13] crystalloid treatment appears to be equal or more favorable to colloid with respect to mortality when shock accompanies trauma, whereas colloid proved more favorable in non-trauma shock and neither solution was better for treatment of adult-respiratory distress syndrome (ARDS) and sepsis; under these circumstances in fact colloid was deleterious. In any event, fluid therapy forms one of the cornerstones of the resuscitation and treatment of most forms of shock, the exception being cardiogenic shock, where vasopressors, vasodilators and antidysrhythmics are required to increase cardiac output. An excellent review of fluid therapy in shock has been written by Maier and Carrico,[14] and another by Virgilio et al.[15]

Crystalloid Solution Therapy

Advantages

Crystalloid solutions are cheap, easy to administer and replace deficiencies from total extracellular space losses (intracellular and interstitium).[16] There is no documented increase in morbidity or mortality when crystalloids are utilized in the treatment of hypovolemic shock states and no increased incidence of pulmonary or other organ dysfunction in patients resuscitated with balanced salt solutions (Table 16-2) as compared with albumin.[17-19] Massive volumes of isotonic salt solutions are necessary before severe changes in plasma oncotic pressure occur.

Crystalloids preserve renal function if normal hemodynamics are maintained. Myocardial efficiency may be improved after lactated Ringer's solution is utilized in the treatment of hemorrhagic shock.[20] Additionally, crystalloids are nonallergenic, and few side effects are associated with their use.

Disadvantages

One of the major disadvantages of the use of crystalloids for shock treatment is the large volume that must be used versus colloid solutions to enact the same effect. This is because balanced salt solutions rapidly equilibrate with the extravascular space.[8,21,22] There is also a drop in the serum concentration of proteins when this form of therapy is utilized versus colloids. Lactated Ringer's contains the anion, lactate in a concentration of 28 mEq/L; one-half of which is in the L-form and therefore which is converted to bicarbonate by the liver and may result in a rebound metabolic alkalosis (although this is really a trivial quantity of bicarbonate produced and anyway this would be a good thing if a concomitant metabolic acidosis is present, which invariably is the case. This would only be a bad thing if the liver is severely damaged by the shock state itself, which might result in a buildup of lactate with the subsequent worsening of the acidosis).

The use of crystalloids is also associated with a decrease in the colloid osmotic pressure, which, however is no problem if the pulmonary capillary wedge pressure (PCWP) is maintained at or near normal levels. Hematocrit also decreases, when this form of treatment of shock is implemented, with about 60% of the infused normal saline solution, when delivered as a bolus, diffusing out of the intravascular space within 20 minutes of administration.[16]

Colloid Administration

Advantages

The advantages of colloid solutions versus crystalloid include an increase in total protein and serum albumin levels when the former is used.[23] This results in an increased colloid osmotic pressure and there is no decrease in the COP-PCWP gradient following fluid resuscitation as there is when saline or salt solutions are used alone for resuscitation. Colloid is capable of larger acute and transient increases in plasma volume per unit volume versus balanced salt solutions.[24,25] Among others, hetastarch has been demonstrated to be very effective for resuscitation in hypovolemic shock.[26] At least one study reports lower incidences of pulmonary edema when colloids were utilized versus crystalloids,[21] although several others suggest that the opposite is true, that is, that pulmonary edema is more likely after large volume resuscitation using colloids versus crystalloids.

Disadvantages

Colloids are costly, greatly so when compared with the cost of crystalloids. Their value is transient because in severe shock there is an associated generalized disruption of the microvascular endothelium. Therefore colloids leak out of the vascular space into the interstitium within one to two hours of their administration.

Albumin may increase CVP, PCWP and impair oxygenation as reflected by the FiO_2 / PaO_2 ratio.[27] Colloids may prolong an impending renal insult by preferentially maintaining intravascular volume at the expense of a depleted interstitial volume.[28] Colloids may result in larger volumes of blood and saline requirements overall for successful resuscitation of the shock patient. With increased microvascular permeability, colloid extravasates into the interstitium, and therefore this is a relative contraindication for colloid utilization.[29]

Colloid use may be associated with decreased levels of free ionized calcium and a decreased free calcium to total calcium ratio. This theoretically could lead to a decreased inotropic effect. Trauma patients resuscitated with albumin have lower immunoglobulin levels when compared to trauma patients resuscitated with balanced salt solutions. Several studies have made the association between delayed organ dysfunction and the use of colloid solutions for resuscitation, especially pulmonary dysfunction.[29,30] Blood coagulation may be altered by albumin use. Water retention is increased as salt and water excretion are limited by albumin use.

Colloids are also associated with anaphylactic and anaphylactoid reactions and a recognized degree of antigenicity. Coagulopathies are possible with these solutions, and there may be interference with cross-matching results when these agents are employed prior to cross-matching.

Types of Fluids

As stated previously, several types of fluids are used in resuscitation from shock states (Table 16-2).

Hypertonic Saline

Hypertonic saline (7.5% NaCl; 2,400 mOsm/l) has been used successfully to reverse the hemodynamic changes associated with shock. Given intravenously, there is a transient increase in plasma volume with this agent, which also, however results in hemodilution.[31] There is an overall improvement in circulatory function with a decrease in total peripheral resistance. Tissue perfusion is improved as a result, and metabolic imbalances are reported to be resolved. This solution fills both the intravascular as well as the interstitial spaces. Cardiac output is increased to a greater degree than when the same volume of lactated Ringer's solution is used, as is urine output. Pulmonary arterial pressure is less than when lactated Ringer's solution is used for resuscitation.[32] In addition, mean arterial pressure and cardiac output are increased to a greater degree than when similar volumes of normal saline solution are used in the treatment of shock.[33,34]

Hetastarch

Hetastarch (Hydroxyethyl starch) is an artificial colloid, an amylopectin, prepared as a 6% solution in 0.9% NaCl with an average pH of 5.5 and osmolality of 310 mOsm/L. The average molecular weight of hetastarch is 69,000 and hetastarch has a longer intravascular half-life than albumin (24–36 hours; elimination 1/2-life is 17 days for 90% of the solution and 48 days for the other 10%).[35] Hetastarch results in a higher colloid osmotic pressure than albumin.[36] However, 6% hetastarch approximates albumin in colloidal properties. The overall hemodynamic effects may persist for approximately 24 hours. The average colloid osmotic pressure is 32 mm Hg. There are several reactions associated with the use of hetastarch, including anaphylactoid reactions (less than 0.011 to 0.006%). Several coagulopathies are associated with the use of hetastarch since hetastarch precipitates factors I, VIII and fibrin monomer and probably von Willebrand Factor. There may be an elevation of PTT and PT.[37] This coagulation effect is probably somewhere in between that produced by albumin and dextran.

The excretion of hetastarch is about 40% within 24 hours, primarily by renal mechanisms. The loading dose is 7.0 ml/kg; maintenance is 20 ml/kg/day, and the approximate cost at time of preparation of this report for replacing a 1-liter blood loss is from $150.00 to $200.00.

Dextran

Dextran is a polysaccharide, glucose polymer with two preparations in common use; high molecular weight (D-70, with a molecular weight of between 70,000 to 75,000), and a low molecular weight (D-40, with an average molecular weight of about 40,000). The high molecular dextran is a 6% solution in 0.9% NSS which tends to remain in the intravascular space for 12 to 24 hours. The low molecular dextran is a 10% solution in 0.9% NSS and which tends to remain in the intravascular space for only 2 to 4 hours and therefore is used primarily in the prevention of venous thrombosis and for thromboembolism. The dextrans lower blood viscosity, improve microcirculatory flow by preventing agglutination and sludging of blood.[38] The dextrans cost less than albumin or hetastarch. There is the risk of coagulopathy reactions with this preparation as well as the risk of anaphylactic/toid reactions with about a 0.008% incidence of severe reactions. Derangements in coagulation may occur due most likely to the precipitation of Factors I, VIII and fibrin monomer and probably von Willebrand Factor. Poor platelet function is a possibility as is an association with acute renal failure after use of this colloid, especially the low-molecular weight preparation. Certain plasma proteins are also depressed after the use of this solution. The approximate cost of replacing a one-liter blood loss using low molecular weight dextran is $80.00 to $100.00 and about $50.00 to $60.00 using the high molecular weight dextran.

Albumin

Albumin is prepared by heat treatment of pooled human sources at 60°C for 10 hours, therefore it carries little or no risk of disease transmission, if prepared properly. It comes as a 5% solution with an average molecular weight of 69,000. Albumin contains 100 to 160 mEq/L of sodium. Intravascular half-life is about 24 to 36 hours. The osmolality is 288 mOsm/L, and colloid osmotic pressure averages 20 mm Hg. Albumin has a pH of 7.0 and is associated with anaphylactoid reactions in about 0.085% of uses with severe reaction in only 0.003% of uses. The excretion of albumin is via renal mechanisms with 50% being excreted within 12 hours after its administration. The loading dose is 7.0 ml/kg and maintenance is to repeat the same dose as necessary. Albumin improves the colloid osmotic pressure and thereby redistributes water from the interstitial space into the intravascular space. Albumin also provides amino acids needed for nitrogen metabolism, which is essential for tissue repair and wound healing to occur.

Adverse effects associated with the use of albumin include chills, fever, urticaria and a variable effect on blood pressure, pulse, respiration, etc.[7] Albumin does not interfere with normal coagulation nor does it promote clotting. The average cost for replacing a one-liter blood loss using albumin is $250.00 to $300.00.[14]

One possible solution to the controversy concerning the use of fluids to resuscitate patients in shock is of course to utilize both types of solutions, that is, combine crystalloids with colloids to obtain the maximal benefit available from both modalities. In particular, small volumes of 7.5% NaCl in 6% Dextran-70 may be used, which was shown in at least one study to be superior to an equal volume of standard crystalloid in its ability to resuscitate animals from hemorrhagic shock if used early in resuscitation.[39] The same solution was shown to improve organ blood flow in animals, in another review.[40] In summary, when undertaking the resuscitation of patients in shock by fluid therapy, it helps to consider guidelines for treatment, including the use of discreet physiologic end-points. However as Shoemaker says, . . . "The quality of clinical management is exceedingly difficult to evaluate in emergency patients because resuscitation is often chaotic, disorderly and frantic", and . . . "The extreme urgency of life-threatening, multifactorial problems requires rapid administration of treatment with little or no time available to determine the physiological nature of problems or to measure the relative effectiveness of the various types of therapy."[41]

PHARMACOLOGIC ADJUNCTS TO TREATMENT OF SHOCK

There are numerous treatment modalities available as therapy of the myriad manifestations of the different shock states. There are commonly utilized resuscitative agents as well as several pharmacologic agents currently undergoing clinical trials for use as more specific receptors and endogenous peptides continue to be isolated and implicated in the pathophysiology of shock. For purposes of this review, two categories of pharmacologic treatment will be established; agents which are primarily utilized for their proven effectiveness as adjuncts to managing unstable circulatory states and agents whose effectiveness in managing critically ill patients continues to be elucidated. This review is not meant to be exhaustive, and the reader is urged to consult other chapters in this text for greater detail. Basic hemodynamic physiology must be appreciated and considered when instituting treatment measures. The following formulae assist one in determining how to approach the treatment of shock using these physiologic adjuncts:

Pressure = Flow × Resistance (from Ohm's Law)

$$\text{MAP} = \text{C.O.} \times \text{S.V.R.,}$$ where MAP = mean arterial pressure,
C.O. = cardiac output,
S.V.R. = systemic vascular resistance

$$\text{PAP} = \text{C.O.} \times \text{P.V.R.,}$$ where PAP = mean pulmonary arterial pressure,
P.V.R. = pulmonary vascular resistance

C.O. is a function of S.V. × H.R., where S.V. = stroke volume,
H.R. = heart rate

S.V. is composed of preload, afterload and contractility, which is estimated by the ejection fraction:

$$\left(\text{EF} = \frac{\text{EDV} - \text{ESV}}{\text{EDV}} \right)$$

$$\text{S.V.R.} = \frac{\overline{\text{M.A.P.}} - \text{R.A.P.}}{\text{C.O.}} \times 80$$

$$\text{P.V.R.} = \frac{\overline{\text{P.A.P.}} - \text{P.C.W.P.}}{\text{C.O.}} \times 80$$

C.P.P. = dBP − L.V.E.D.P., where C.P.P. = coronary perfusion pressure,
dBP = diastolic arterial blood pressure
L.V.E.D.P. = left ventricular end-diastolic pressure

With these considerations in mind, we can begin to plan our therapy as necessary and with rational, if somewhat arbitrary end-points to guide our thinking and planning.

Inotropes and Vasopressors

Positive inotropy is indicated when patients have low cardiac output and hypotension in the face of optimal or elevated preload. Table 16–3 lists most of the commonly used inotropes and vasopressors for use in the treatment of shock states and for critically ill patients.

Cardiac Glycosides

Digoxin is the prototypical cardiac glycoside, acting to increase the force and velocity of myocardial systolic contraction to increase cardiac output independent of a catecholamine response. It does so by blocking Na-K ATPase pump mechanisms, thereby facilitating the entry of calcium into myocardial cells resulting in positive inotropy. Its main utility is for rapid digitalization for CHF and for treatment of supraventricular dysrhythmias (atrial flutter, atrial fibrillation). Acutely, digoxin may cause the release of norepinephrine and angiotensin to increase, resulting in vasoconstriction. The onset of action is within 14 to 30 minutes after intravenous administration, which is considered relatively slow as inotropes go, with a peak effect seen in approximately 1.5 to 5 hours. Pharmacologic effect persists for 3 to 4 days after discontinuing therapy. Elimination half-life is 1.6 days which increases in patients with renal failure. Excretion of digoxin is 60 to 80% unchanged in the urine. For the treatment of CHF the dose of digoxin is 10 μg/kg.

Sympathomimetics

Actions of sympathomimetic agents are based on the drug's activity on alpha and beta receptors and various substances are classified as inotropes, vasopressors or mixed acting (see Table 16–3). Isoproterenol is an example of a pure inotrope, and phenylephrine is an example of a pure vasopressor. Agents may also be classified as to the mechanisms of producing clinically observed effects, i.e., as direct acting or indirect acting, relying on the release of endogenous humoral mediators to enact a response by the sympathetic nervous system. Agents are also divided into groupings based upon whether they are

Table 16–3. Inotropes and Vasopressors

| Agent | Sites of Action/Receptor Group Served | | | Usual IV Dose | Response Elicited | | | |
	β_1	β_2	Alpha-1		Cardiac Output	T.P.R.	B.P.	Renal Perfusion
Mostly inotropic								
Isoproterenol	+++	+++	0	0.5–4.0 μg/min	increase	decrease	inc./dec.	inc./dec.
Dobutamine	+++*	+	0 to +*	2.0–20.0 μg/kg/min	increase	decrease	increase	0
Dopamine	+++*	0 to +*	+ to +++*	1.0–20.0 μg/kg/min	increase	dec* or inc.	0 to inc.	increase
Epinephrine	+++	++*	+++*	1.0–4.0 μg/min	increase	decrease	inc./dec.	decrease
Mixed acting								
Norepinephrine	++	0	+++	2.0–8.0 μg/min	0 or dec.	increase	increase	decrease
Ephedrine	++	0 to +	+	10–25 mg bolus	increase	inc./dec.	increase	decrease
Mostly vasopressors								
Metaraminol	+	0	++	8.0–15.0 μg/kg/min	decrease	increase	increase	decrease
Methoxamine	0	0	+++	8.0–15.0 μg/kg/min	0 or dec.	increase	increase	decrease
Phenylephrine	0	0	+++	5.0–20.0 μg/min	decrease	increase	increase	decrease

B.P. = blood pressure; β = Beta; * = dose dependent; T.P.R. = total peripheral resistance.

naturally occurring or synthetically prepared (Table 16-4). Catecholamines are preferentially administered through a centrally placed venous access line to ensure their accurate delivery and to avoid the localized sloughing that can occur when they infiltrate the skin.

Isoproterenol

Isoproterenol is a synthetic, direct acting, pure beta agonist displaying immediate onset of action after intravenous administration. It increases cardiac output, heart rate and myocardial MVO$_2$. Peripheral vascular resistance is decreased. It is especially valuable for the shock patient who also has a decreased heart rate; if the heart rate is already greater than 120 beats per minute, isoproterenol may induce severe myocardial ischemia. The duration of action is 8 to 10 minutes but may be longer with increasing dosages. It is metabolized by COMT in the liver, lungs

Table 16–4. Adrenergic Agonists

Agent	Direct	Indirect	Dosage
Naturally occurring			
Norepinephrine	++++		0.05–0.3 μg/kg/min
Epinephrine	++++		0.05–0.2 μg/kg/min
Dopamine	++++		1–5 μg/kg/min
	+++	+	5–15 μg/kg/min
	+++	+	>15 μg/kg/min
Synthetic agents			
Isoproterenol	++++		0.01–0.2 μg/kg/min
Ephedrine	++	+++	0.2–1.0 mg/kg
Metaraminol	+	+++	10–100 μg/kg
Phenylephrine	++++		1–10 μg/kg/min
Methoxamine	++++		0.05–0.2 mg/kg
Dobutamine	++++		1–5 μg/kg/min

+ = slight stimulation; ++ = moderate stimulation; +++ = marked stimulation; ++++ = intense stimulation

and other tissues and by conjugation in the G.I. tract; 50% is excreted unchanged. Termination of activity of isoproterenol appears to be by uptake by adrenergic neurons. Dose is 0.01 to 0.2 μg/kg/min. Isoproterenol is prepared as an eight microgram per milliliter solution (2 mg in 250 ml of D$_5$W).

Dobutamine

Dobutamine is another pure beta agonist, with β-1 effects being greater than β-2 effects. Dobutamine has an onset of action of about one to two minutes and a peak effect after about 10 minutes. The duration of action is less than ten minutes after discontinuing the infusion. As compared with dopamine there may be less tachycardia, less increase in myocardial oxygen consumption and fewer dysrhythmias.[42,43] There is also the potential for a less intense increase in left-ventricular afterload, left-atrial pressure and systemic vascular resistance. Vasodilatation may occur as a result of β-2 stimulation.

The elimination 1/2-life is two minutes. Dobutamine is metabolized in the liver and other tissues by COMT and by conjugation with glucuronic acid. The dose is 1 to 5 μg/kg/min. Dobutamine is prepared as a 1 mg/ml solution (250 mg in 250 ml of D$_5$W).

Dopamine

Dopamine is a direct acting, beta-, alpha- and dopaminergic-receptor stimulating agent with effects determined by dose. The usual onset of effect is 2–5 minutes and dopamine has a duration of action of less than ten minutes after discontinuing the infusion. The elimination half-life is 2 minutes. It is metabolized in the liver, kidneys and plasma by MAO and COMT. The usual dose is 1 to 5 μg/kg/min for dopaminergic effects (increase in renal blood flow and urine output; little or no change in blood pressure or cardiac output). At 5 to 15 μg/kg/min there is predominance of beta effects (increase in blood pressure, cardiac output, stroke volume and myocardial contractility). At greater than 15 μg/kg/min there is predominance of alpha-mimetic actions with intense vasoconstriction occurring. Dopamine is prepared as a solution having a concentration of 0.8 mg/ml by adding 200 mg to 250 ml D$_5$W.

Epinephrine

Epinephrine is a naturally occurring, direct-acting agent with both alpha and beta-mimetic effects. Increases in systolic blood pressure, pulse pressure, heart rate and cardiac output occur. There is a modest decrease in diastolic blood pressure with vasodilation in skeletal muscle due to β-2 receptor stimulation. The overall change in MAP is not very profound. Cardiac output is preferentially redistributed to skeletal muscles. Hepatic glycogenolysis increases, and insulin release is inhibited. The action of epinephrine is terminated by uptake and metabolism in sympathetic nerve endings. In the liver and other tissues, metabolism is by MAO and COMT. Epinephrine is prepared as a solution having a concentration of 8 μg/ml by adding 2 mg per 250 ml D$_5$W. The normal dose for increasing cardiac output is about 0.05 to 0.2 μg/kg/min.

Norepinephrine

Norepinephrine (NE) is a naturally occurring, direct acting agent with both alpha and beta-mimetic effects. It is a very potent vasopressor, second only to angiotensin II on a per-weight basis. Onset of action is rapid, and duration of activity is about 1–2 minutes after discontinuing an intravenous infusion. The action of NE is terminated by uptake and metabolism in sympathetic nerve endings and by metabolism by the liver and other tissues by COMT and MAO. Norepinephrine is prepared as a solution with a concentration of 16 μg/ml by adding 4 mg/250 ml D$_5$W. The usual dose is 0.05 to 0.3 μg/kg/min. NE should only be used for short-term management since the incidence of adverse effects with prolonged usage is very high. As with all vasopressors, the use of this agent in shock is only for temporary treatment to restore cerebral perfusion pressure or coronary perfusion pressure after first administering a triad of fluids, ventilation with oxygen, and correction of acid-base abnormalities.[44] Inotropes should be the first-line treatment before vasopressors, and if possible, vasopressors should be reserved for those occasions where ventricular function curves of the Starling type may be first constructed.

Ephedrine

Ephedrine is both a direct and indirect-acting synthetic agent having both alpha and beta-mimetic effects. The duration of action of a bolus dose administered I.V. is about one hour. Metabolism is primarily by hepatic mechanisms. Ephedrine is administered in doses of 10 to 25 mg I.V. The cardiovascular effects of ephedrine approximate those of epinephrine, however, its blood pressure elevating effect is somewhat less prominent and also lasts significantly longer than that of epinephrine. Both systolic and diastolic blood pressure, heart rate and cardiac output are increased by ephedrine. Coronary and skeletal muscle blood flow increase, while renal and splanchnic blood flows are diminished, respectively.

Phenylephrine

Phenylephrine is a direct acting synthetic agent having an immediate onset after intravenous administration. Duration of activity is approximately 15 minutes after a bolus dose of 50 to 200 μg I.V. Phenylephrine stimulates primarily alpha-1 adrenergic receptors resulting in greater propensity to venoconstrict than produce arterial constriction. Phenylephrine approximates the effects of norepinephrine, however, it is less potent and longer lasting. Intravenous infusion dose is 1 to 10 μg/kg/min. The preparation is as a concentration of 40 μg/ml, made by adding 10 mg/250 ml D$_5$W.

Other, newer agents variably termed "ino-dilators", include amrinone and milrinone. These are bipyridine derivatives unrelated to cardiac glycosides or sympathomimetic agents which increase the force of myocardial contraction in systole. Heart rate remains unchanged or increases only slightly. The mechanism of action of these agents is by inhibiting cAMP phosphodiesterase activity which results in an increase in cAMP. Amrinone is also a direct-acting vasodilator, having greater propensity to do so than does dobutamine or dopamine. It is used in the short-term management of congestive heart failure and may be used in conjunction with cardiac glycosides as it produces additive inotropic effects without adverse cardiovascular effects. It may be instituted as therapy in those cases where there is minimal response to high dose sympathomimetic therapy. The onset of action of amrinone is within 2–5 minutes with a peak effect occurring within 10 minutes after intravenous administration. Duration of action is about 0.5 to 2 hours and the elimination $\frac{1}{2}$-life of amrinone is 3.6 hours. It is metabolized by hepatic mechanisms with 50% excreted unchanged in the urine. The dosage is initially as a bolus of 0.75 mg/kg over 2–3 minutes followed by an infusion of 5–10 μg/kg/min as maintenance, not to exceed a daily dose of 10 mg/kg. An infusion is prepared by adding 250 mg to 50 ml NSS.

Calcium

Calcium may be administered as the chloride or gluconate preparation. Its mechanism of action is related to an increase in the ionized calcium fraction facilitating the binding of actin and myosin resulting in an increase in myocardial muscle contractility.[45] Vasoconstriction also results from vascular smooth muscle arteriolar effects. The usual dose of CaCl$_2$ is as a 2 to 5 mg/kg IV bolus. An intact calcium-parathyroid apparatus or axis enhances resuscitation from shock. Interestingly, one study claimed efficacy of the calcium channel inhibitor, Verapamil, for improving hemodynamics during endotoxin shock states, but this remains to be proved.[46]

Other agents of potential benefit include glucose-insulin-potassium (GIK) and phosphodiesterase III inhibitors. GIK occasionally may increase cardiac function; 1000 ml NSS plus 100 to 200 g of glucose, 20 to 40 mEq KCl and 10 to 20 units of regular insulin are administered over about one to four hours, while monitoring serum levels of electrolytes and adjusting the infusion as indicated.

Phosphodiesterase III inhibitors increase myocardial contractility by increasing cAMP levels. However, vasodilatation also results since the level of cAMP also increases in smooth muscles.

Vasodilators

Vasodilator therapy is useful in shock states when afterload reduction is desired or deemed appropriate from ventricular function curves (Table 16-5). Alpha-adrenergic blocking or ganglionic blocking agents may be employed for this purpose. Cardiac output is improved as a result of a reduction in MAP or PAP. Efficacy is greatest in those situations where high vascular resistance accompanies low cardiac output. Vasodilators can improve organ perfusion, restore cellular integrity and prevent potentially deleterious effects of vasoconstriction. Among available modalities useful for attaining these means, alpha-adrenergic blocking drugs, angiotensin converting enzyme inhibitors (e.g., captopril), and selective inhibitors of the renin-angiotensin-aldosterone system all have proved efficacy. We will discuss only some of the more commonly employed agents.

NITROGLYCERIN

tNTG is a direct relaxant of vascular smooth muscle with a predilection for relaxing capacitance vessels. Preload and to a lesser extent afterload are reduced. The onset of action after starting an I.V. infusion is within 2 to 5 minutes and duration of pharmacologic action is 3 to 5 minutes. Elimination half-life is 1 to 4.4 minutes. tNTG is metabolized in the liver to less active metabolites. An infusion may be prepared by adding 200 mg/250 ml D_5W (0.8 mg/ml) or 50 mg/250 ml D_5W (0.2 mg/ml). The dosage is 0.1 to 10 $\mu g/kg/min$. Of importance is to bear in mind that tNTG may antagonize the effects of heparin if the latter is being used for anticoagulation. Glass bottles and non-PVC tubing must be used in the administration of tNTG.

Sodium Nitroprusside

SNP is a vasoactive agent structurally unrelated to other hypotensive agents and reduces arterial blood pressure more consistently and faster than nitroglycerin. Significant rebound hypertension frequently occurs after termination of SNP. The method of action of this substance is by a direct action on vascular smooth muscle. Onset of action is within 30 to 60 seconds from beginning an infusion with a peak in one to two minutes and a duration of 3 to 5 minutes. Metabolism os SNP is by interaction with sulfhydral groups in erythrocytes and tissues to cyanogen which is converted to thiocyanate in the liver by the enzyme rhodanase. Dosage of SNP is 0.5 − 10 $\mu g/kg/min$, not to exceed 10 $\mu g/kg/min$ or 10 mg/hour for any 24-hour period. SNP is prepared by adding 50 mg to 250 ml D_5W to make a 0.2-mg/ml concentration.

Hydralazine

Hydralazine is a direct-acting relaxant of arterial smooth muscle with an onset time of 10 to 20 minutes, and a duration of action of 2 to 6 hours after intravenous administration. The elimination half-life is 0.5 to 2.5 hours, increasing in patients with renal impairment. Vasodilatory effects are most notable on the coronary, cerebral, renal and splanchnic circulations than on other systems. The mechanism of action of hydralazine appears to be due to interference with calcium ion transport in vascular smooth muscle. Diastolic blood pressure is more often decreased than is systolic pressure. While SVR is reduced using this agent, there is a reflex increase in heart rate, stroke volume and cardiac output by baroreceptor mechanisms increasing sympathetic nervous system activity. Metabolism of hydralazine is extensive and is primarily by acetylation in the liver. Ten to 15% is excreted unchanged in the urine. The usual dose is 5 to 20 mg by IV bolus.

Trimethaphan Camsylate

This agent has a short duration of action, functioning as a peripheral vasodilator and ganglionic blocker. It lowers blood pressure by the dual mechanisms of decreasing cardiac output and by reducing systemic vascular resistance. It does this by directly relaxing capacitance vessels and by blocking autonomic nervous system reflexes. Preload, afterload and blood pressure are decreased; with cardiac output increasing or decreasing depending on initial hemodynamics. A usual dose is 10 to 200 $\mu g/kg/min$ as a continous infusion. Tachyphylaxis and side-effects of ganglionic blockade predominate at the higher doses (urinary retention, paralytic ileus, decreased visual accommodation). The usual preparation is as a 0.1% solution by adding 250 mg to 250 ml D_5W (1mg/ml) and running the infusion based upon individual patient response.

Whenever vasodilator therapy is utilized, several considerations must be realized and potential problems must be anticipated including coronary ischemia from diastolic hypotension, for example. Also, increased intracranial pressure and hypoxemia from reversal of hypoxic pul-

Table 16–5. Vasodilators Commonly Used in Resuscitation From Shock

Agent	Dosage	Site of Action	HR	MAP	PCWP	CI	SVR
Nitroglycerin	5–100 $\mu g/min$ I.V.	V, A	sl ↑, ↓	↓	↓	↑, ↓	sl ↓
Sodium Nitroprusside	15–400 $\mu g/min$ I.V.	A, V		sl ↓			
Hydralazine	50–100 mg p.o. q 6–8 hr		0		↓	↑	↓
	10–20 mg I.V.	A	0	sl ↓	sl ↓	↑	↓

A = arteries; V = veins

monary vasoconstriction are dangers associated with use of these agents. That these agents will continue to be important adjuncts to the treatment of shock states was reinforced by a recent study showing that in a canine model, the vasodilator felodipine when administered prior to an acute hemorrhage resulted in improved organ blood flow in situations of severe compromise.[47] Further research continues in the delineation of an expanded role for these chemicals in facilitating left ventricular forward stroke volume.

NEWER AND CONTROVERSIAL PHARMACOLOGIC ADJUNCTS TO TREATMENT OF SHOCK

Naloxone

Naloxone is an opiate receptor antagonist having both central and peripheral effects. Many of the signs of opioid overdose resemble those of circulatory shock[48] (Chapter 15). Endogenous opioid-like substances that are released might be in part responsible for the pathophysiology observed in shock, especially in septic and hemorrhagic types.[49] Naloxone binds preferentially to the μ receptor at low doses, but at higher doses appears to be a nonselective antagonist of μ, δ, and ϵ-receptors. At these larger doses, naloxone has been employed as an agent claimed to improve cardiovascular parameters in shock.[50] Naloxone administration for resuscitation during shock remains a controversial issue. The impetus for naloxone treatment began in the 1970's when Holaday and others proposed naloxone reversal of endotoxin hypotension as demonstrative of a role of endorphins in shock.[51] Work by Peters et al who successfully treated septic shock with 0.4 mg IV increments of naloxone in septicemic patients was followed by studies of naloxone use in hemorrhagic shock.[52,53] Several later studies, however, were either unable to reproduce the positive effects of this agent in shock, or showed absolutely no benefit of using naloxone versus placebo.[54,55,56] Other work showed no difference between naloxone and ibuprofen for treating the cardiovascular effects of septic shock.[57] Especially noted was that patients on prior glucocorticoid therapy before receiving the opioid antagonist had absolutely no response to it as regards hemodynamic parameters.[58]

Naloxone may prevent the development of shock into a progressive stage by several mechanisms including stimulation of ACTH secretion followed by an increase in glucocorticoid secretion or a direct effect on adrenocorticoid function.[59] There may also be stimulation of aldosterone secretion either directly or as a result of increased ACTH.

Thyrotropin-Releasing Hormone

Thyrotropin-releasing hormone (TRH), a tripeptide, has been hypothesized to be an endogenous opiate antagonist analogous to naloxone, and as such may have efficacy in reversing the shock state.[60,61] TRH reverses experimental hypovolemic and endotoxic shock in a rat model and in dogs,[62,63] in a dose-related manner. The actions of TRH are apparently centrally-mediated, having effect only when given in the ventricular system. An intact sympathetic nervous system appears to be necessary for TRH to exert its maximal therapeutic effect.[64] It has also been observed that recent thyrodectomy may decrease survival from shock.[65] Like naloxone, work with TRH is largely of academic interest and currently not applicable to daily anesthetic practice.

Corticosteroids

Steroids were once regarded as a cornerstone in the successful management of septic shock, but have fallen into a "select cases only" role.[66] One of best studies to date, a randomized, prospective one by Sprung, et al.,[67] showed that corticosteroids in high doses for patients in septic shock provided no difference in mortality or shock reversal unless given very early in the course of shock. These authors used approximately three times the dose of dexamethasone versus that of another study from the same year, which purported to demonstrate beneficial results for treating septic shock with steroids.[68] Two recent, multicenter studies demonstrated that the supposed benefit obtained by using glucocorticoids for treatment in septic shock probably involves the stabilization of lysosomal membranes, effects on the cellular and subcellular membranes with alterations of cellular mechanisms of metabolism, improvement in oxygen transport in peripheral tissues, and also a reduction in peripheral vascular resistance.[69,70] Probably their greatest efficacy is when used in those cases of shock superimposed on relative adrenal insufficiency, or hypothyroidism in patients with suppressed adrenal-pituitary function.

FUTURE RESEARCH EFFORTS

Pharmacologic Agents

Several agents are undergoing evaluation for a possible beneficial role in the management of various shock states.[71,72] Limited information is currently available regarding the cyclooxygenase inhibitors ibuprofen and indomethacin or the xanthine oxidase inhibitor allopurinol as adjuncts to the treatment of hypovolemic shock states. Other agents continue to receive attention as primary anesthetics for the resuscitation of patients in shock from various causes, and include ketamine, fentanyl and halogenated inhalation agents, particularly isoflurane. The interested reader is urged to consult the references under this subsection at the end of the chapter.[73-80]

Polyclonal antibodies to endotoxin and monoclonal antibodies to tumor necrosis factor for use in the treatment of septic shock from gram negative bacteremia continues to undergo therapeutic trials. Free radical scavengers are being studied as agents capable of blocking the biological effects of some of the mediators of septic shock.

MAST and the IABP

MAST is an acronym for military antishock trousers, a modality used as a temporary measure of treating the acutely injured shock patient. Briefly, the MAST increases afterload when inflated, but also decreases pulmonary vital capacity and results in compartment syndromes in a significant percentage of cases. Most importantly, there is no evidence to suggest that survival is increased in patients receiving this form of therapy when compared to a control population of injured patients in shock.[81] The MAST is generally used for patients who have received truncal injuries, penetrating abdominal wounds or penetrating thoracic wounds. It is only reserved for those situations where an acute increase in afterload cannot be accomplished by the use of other standard methods.

IABP stands for intra-aortic balloon counterpulsation, which is another temporary means to sustain certain patients in shock. This circulatory-assist device is programmed by the patients ECG with deflation of the balloon just prior to systole and inflation in diastole. The main utility of this device is for patients in cardiogenic shock, where at least 35 to 40% of the left ventricle is non-functional. Systolic arterial blood pressure is decreased by the presystolic deflation of the balloon which decreases afterload, in turn decreasing cardiac work and MVO_2. Diastolic blood pressure is increased by inflation of the balloon in diastole, which increases coronary perfusion pressure. Overall, there is a 10 to 20% reduction in systolic arterial blood pressure; a slight increase in mean arterial pressure; a 10 to 20% increase in cardiac output; a decrease in left-ventricular end-diastolic pressure and a decrease in myocardial oxygen consumption. The IABP may diminish the amount of mitral regurgitation present in the case of a ruptured papillary muscle and may decrease shunting through the intraventricular septum in the case of septal rupture.

Other devices of related interest include the LVAD, or left-ventricular assist device, the artificial heart and cardiac myoplasty, which may all buy some time in cases of shock associated with severe cardiac failure until cardiac transplantation becomes possible.

Glucose-ATP-MgCl2

In shock states there is a decrease in cellular ATP. ATP serves as the energy substrate for the maintenance of the normal transmembrane potential difference in both excitable as well as non-excitable tissues. The resting transmembrane potential difference relies upon energy-dependent sodium-potassium transport mechanisms. Mitochondrial depression results in less metabolism of both alpha-keto-glutarate and beta-hydroxybutarate. Recently, adenosine-triphosphate-magnesium chloride has been used to try to enhance the survival of ATP by rapidly entering injured cells.[82] However, exogenously aministered ATP is rapidly degraded in plasma, therefore this does not appear to prevent the depletion of liver ATP or skeletal muscle creatine phosphate.

ATP is a potent vasodilator and may be important as a means of decreasing oxygen consumption at the cellular level. Cardiac output increases as a result of the decreased peripheral resistance from ATP. There exists the distinct possibility that survival may be improved by the increased tissue or mitochondrial levels of magnesium. There is a progressive decrease in the rates of conversion of ADP to ATP in shock, as well as increased sodium-potassium ATP-ase enzyme activity. With these theoretical considerations in mind, it is no wonder that further research into the use of this combination continues. One

recent review suggested that this preparation may inhibit thromboxane A_2 which could result in an increased survival in septic shock states[83] (see section on pathophysiology of septic shock).

REFERENCES

1. Aubier M., Trippenbach T., Roussos C.: Respiratory muscle fatigue during cardiogenic shock. J Appl Physiol 51:499–508, 1981.
2. Hussain S. N., Graham R., Rutledge F., et al: Respiratory muscle energetics during endotoxin shock in dogs. J Appl Physiol 60:486–493, 1986.
3. Roussos C.: Diaphragmatic fatigue and blood flow distribution in shock. Can Anaesth Soc J 33:S-61-S-64, 1986.
4. Wisner D. H., Sturm J. A.: Controversies in the fluid management of post-traumatic lung disease. Injury 17:295–300, 1986.
5. Gabel J. C., Drake R. E.: Pulmonary capillary pressure and permeability. Crit Care Med 7:92–97, 1979.
6. Weil M. H., Henning R. J., Puri V. K.: Colloid oncotic pressure: Clinical significance. Crit Care Med 7:113–116, 1979.
7. Shoemaker W. C.: A new approach to physiology, monitoring and therapy of shock states. World J Surg 11:133–146, 1987.
8. Virgilio R. W., Rice C. l., Smith D. E., James D. R., Zarins C. K., Hobelmann C. F., Peters R. M.: Crystalloid versus colloid resuscitation: Is one better? A randomized clinical study. Surgery 85:129–139, 1979.
9. Audio-Digest. Anesthesiology 30: 1988.
10. Metildi L. A., Shackford S. R., Virgilio R. W., Peters R. M.: Crystalloid versus colloid in fluid resuscitation of patients with severe pulmonary insufficiency. Surg Gynecol Obstet 158:207–212, 1984.
11. Arturson, G., Thoren L.: Fluid therapy in shock. World J Surg 7:573–580, 1983.
12. Wilson R. F., Gibson D.: The use of arterial central venous oxygen differences to calculate cardiac output and oxygen consumption in critically ill surgical patients. Surgery 84:362–369, 1978.
13. Velanovich V.: Crystalloid versus colloid fluid resuscitation: A meta-analysis of mortality. Surgery 105:65–71, 1989.
14. Maier R. V., Carrico C. J.: Developments in the resuscitation of critically ill surgical patients. Adv Surg 19:271–328, 1986.
15. Virgilio R. W., Smith D. E., Zarins C. K.: Balanced electrolyte solutions: Experimental and clinical studies. Crit Care Med 7:98–106, 1979.
16. Greenfield R. H., Bessen H. A., Henneman P. L.: Effect of crystalloid infusion on hematocrit and intravascular volume in healthy, nonbleeding subjects. Ann Emerg Med 18:51–55, 1989.
17. Moss G. S., Lowe R. J., Jilek J., Levine H. D.: Colloid or crystalloid in the resuscitation of hemorrhagic shock: A controlled clinical trial. Surgery 89:434–438, 1981.
18. Gallagher T. J., Banner M. J., Barnes P. A.: Large volume crystalloid resuscitation does not increase extravascular lung water. Anesth Analg 64:323–326, 1985.
19. Layon J., Duncan D., Gallagher J. T., Banner M. J.: Hypertonic saline as a resuscitation solution in hemorrhagic shock: Effects on extravascular lung water and cardiopulmonary function. Anesth Analg 66:154–158, 1987.
20. Horton J., Landreneau R., Tuggle D.: Cardiac response to fluid resuscitation from hemorrhagic shock. Surg Gynecol Obstet 160:444–452, 1985.
21. Rackow E. C., Falk J. l., et al.,: Fluid resuscitation in circula-

tory shock: A comparison of the cardiorespiratory effects of albumin, hetastarch and saline solutions in patients with hypovolemic and septic shock. Crit Care Med *11*:839-850, 1983.

22. Modig J.: Effectiveness of dextran-70 versus Ringer's acetate in traumatic shock and adult respiratory distress syndrome. Crit Care Med *14*:454-457, 1986.

23. Lucas C. E., Weaver D., Higgins R. F., et al.,: Effects of albumin versus non-albumin resuscitation on plasma volume and renal excretory function. J Trauma *18*:564-570, 1978.

24. Kramer G. C., Perron P. R., Lindsey D. C., et al.,: Small-volume resuscitation with hypertonic saline dextran solution. Surgery *100*:239-247, 1986.

25. D'Angio R., Orlando R.: Fluid resuscitation: Colloid versus crystalloid? Conn Med *50*:689-91, 1986.

26. Puri V. K., Paidipaty B., White L.: Hydroxyethyl starch for resuscitation of patients with hypovolemia and shock. Crit Care Med *9*:833-837, December, 1981.

27. Lucas C. E.: Organ function after albumin resuscitation from hypovolemic shock. Resident Staff Physician 75-82, June, 1982.

28. Ramsay G., Ledinjham I. M.: Resuscitation in hemorrhagic shock-pulmonary and renal effects: An adverse effect of stabilised plasma protein solution on renal function? Circ Shock *22*:261-268, 1987.

29. Holcroft J. W., Trunkey D. D.: Extravascular lung water following hemorrhagic shock in the baboon: Comparison between resuscitation with Ringer's lactate and Plasmanate. Ann Surg *180*:408-417, 1974.

30. Hauser C. J., Shoemaker W. C., Turpin I., Goldberg S. J.: Oxygen transport responses to colloids and crystalloids in critically ill surgical patients. Surg Gynecol Obstet *150*:811-816, 1980.

31. Bitterman H., Triolo J., Lefer A. M.: Use of hypertonic saline in the treatment of hemorrhagic shock. Circ Shock *21*:271-283, 1987.

32. Nerlich M., Gunther R., Demling R. H.: Resuscitation from hemorrhagic shock with hypertonic saline or lactated Ringer's: Effect on the pulmonary and systemic microcirculation. Circ Shock *10*:179-188, 1983.

33. Nakayama S., Sibley L., Gunther R. A., et al., Small-volume resuscitation with hypertonic saline (2,400 mOsm/L) during hemorrhagic shock. Circ Shock *13*:149-159, 1984.

34. Peters R. M., Shackford S. R., Hogan J. S., Cologne J. P.: Comparison of isotonic and hypertonic fluids in resuscitation from hypovolemic shock. Surg Gynecol Obstet *163*:219-224, 1986.

35. Thompson W. L., et al.,: Intravascular persistence, tissue storage, and excretion of hydroxyethyl starch. Surg Gynecol Obstet *131*:965-972, Nov, 1970.

36. Haupt M. T., Rackow E. C.: Colloid osmotic pressure and fluid resuscitation with hetastarch, albumin and saline solutions. Crit Care Med *10*:159-162, 1982.

37. Lee W. H. Jr., Cooper N., Weedner M. G. Jr., et al.,: Clinical evaluation of a new plasma expander, hydroxyethyl starch. J Trauma *8*:381, 1968.

38. Messmer K., et al.,: Oxygen transport and tissue oxygenation during hemodilution with dextran. Adv Exp Med Biol *373*:669, 1973.

39. Maningas P. A., Bellamy R. F.: Hypertonic sodium chloride solutions for the prehospital management of traumatic hemorrhagic shock: A possible improvement in the standard of care? Ann Emerg Med *15*:1411-1414, 1986.

40. Maningas P. A.: Resuscitation with 7.5% NaCl in 6% dextran-70 during hemorrhagic shock in swine: Effects on organ blood flow. Crit Care Med *15*:1121-1126, 1987.

41. Shoemaker W. C., Schluchter M., Hopkins J. A., et al.,: Comparison of the relative effectiveness of colloids and crystalloids in emergency resuscitation. Am J Surg *142*:73-84, 1981.

42. Jardin F., Sportiche M., Bazin M., et al.,: Dobutamine: A hemodynamic evaluation in human septic shock. Crit Care Med *9*:329-332, 1981.

43. Vincent J. L., Van der Linden P., Domb M., et al.,: Dopamine compared with dobutamine in experimental septic shock: Relevence to fluid administration. Anesth Analg *66*:565-571, 1987.

44. Martin C., Saux P., Albanese J., et al: A new look at norepinephrine to treat human hyperdynamic septic shock. Anesthesiology *V-67*:A-648, 1987.

45. Denis R., et al.,: The beneficial role of calcium supplementation during resuscitation from shock. J Trauma *25*:594-600, 1985.

46. Kimura M., Hakoshima A., et al: The effect of verapamil on the spleen in the early stage of canine E. coli endotoxin shock. Anesthesiology *V-67*:A-128, 1987.

47. Saboun M., Hodge K., Jandhyala B. S.: Restoration of renal and mesenteric hemodynamics by felodipine in a canine model of hemorrhagic shock. Arch Pharmacol *337*:465-470, 1988.

48. Bernton E. W., Long J. B., Holaday J. W.: Opioids and neuropeptides: Mechanisms in circulatory shock. Fed Proc *44*:290-299, 1985.

49. Daly T., Beamer K. C., Vargish T., Wilson A.: Correlation of plasma beta-endorphin levels with mean arterial pressure and cardiac output in hypovolemic shock. Crit Care Med *15*:723-725, 1987.

50. Higgins T. L., Chernow B.: Pharmacotherapy of circulatory shock. Dis Mon *33*:309-361, 1987.

51. Holaday J. W., Faden A. I.: Naloxone reversal of endotoxin hypotension suggests a role of endorphins in shock. Nature *275*:450-451, 1978.

52. Peters W. P., Friedman P. A., Johnson M. W., Mitch W. E.: Pressor effect of naloxone in septic shock. Lancet *1*:529-532, 1981.

53. Salerno T. A., Milne B., Jhamandas K. H.: Hemodynamic effects of naloxone in hemorrhagic shock in pigs. Surg Gynecol Obstet *152*:773-776, 1981.

54. Groeger J. S., Carlon G. C., Howland W. S.: Naloxone in septic shock. Crit Care Med *11*:650-654, 1983.

55. DeMaria A., Craven D. E., Jeffernan J. J., et al.,: Naloxone versus placebo in treatment of septic shock. Lancet *1*:1363-1365, 1985.

56. Irei M., Davenport S., Traber L., et al.,: The effect of naloxone on an awake sheep model of hyperdynamic sepsis. Anesthesiology *65*:A-100, 1986.

57. Nishijima M., Breslow M., Miller C., Traystman R. J.: The effect of ibuprofen and naloxone on regional blood flow during endotoxin shock. Anesthesiology *65*:A-95, 1986.

58. Gurll N., Ganes E., Reynolds D. G.: Central nervous system is involved in the cardiovascular response to naloxone in canine endotoxic but not hemorrhagic shock. Circ Shock *22*:115-125, 1987.

59. Machuganska A., Zaharieva S.: Hormone changes and beta-endorphin in the pathogenesis of hemorrhagic shock. Acta Physiol Pharmacol Bulg *11*:26-33, 1985.

60. Faden A. I.: Opiate antagonists and thyrotropin-releasing hormone I. Potential role in the treatment of shock. JAMA *252*:1177-1180, 1984.

61. Bernton E. W.: Naloxone and TRH in the treatment of

shock and trauma: What future roles? Ann Emerg Med *14*:729–735, 1985.

62. Holaday J. W., D'Amato R. J., Faden A. I.: Thyrotropin-releasing hormone improves cardiovascular function in experimental endotoxic and hemorrhagic shock. Science *213*:216–218, 1981.

63. Teba L., Zakaria M., Dedhia H. V., et al.,: Beneficial effect of thyrotropin-releasing hormone in canine hemorrhagic shock. Circ Shock *21*:51–57, 1987.

64. Holaday J. W., D'Amato R. J., Ruvio B. A., et al.,: Action of naloxone and TRH on the autonomic regulation of circulation. Adv Biochem Psychopharmacol *33*:353–362, 1982.

65. Gallick H. L., Lucas C. E., Ledgerwood A. M., et al.,: Detrimental effect of recent thyroidectomy on hemorrhagic shock and resuscitation. Circ Shock *21*:111–119, 1987.

66. Chernow B., Roth B. L.: Pharmacologic manipulation of the peripheral vasculature in shock: Clinical and experimental approaches. Circ Shock *18*:141–155, 1986.

67. Sprung C. L., Caralis P. V., Marcial E. H., et al.,: The effects of high-dose corticosteroids in patients with septic shock: A prospective, controlled study. NEJM *311*:1137–1143, 1984.

68. Lucas C. E., Ledgerwood A. M.: The cardiopulmonary response to massive doses of steroids in patients with septic shock. Arch Surg *119*:537–541, 1984.

69. Bone R. C., Fisher C. J., Jr., Clemmer T. P., et al.,: A controlled clinical trial of high-dose methylprednisolone in the treatment of severe sepsis and septic shock. Sept. NEJM *317*:653–658, 1987.

70. Veterans Administration Systemic Sepsis Cooperative Study Group: Effect of high-dose glucocorticoid therapy on mortality in patients with clinical signs of systemic sepsis. NEJM *317*:659–665, 1987.

71. Beamer K. C., Daly T., Vargish T.: Hemodynamic evaluation of Ibuprofen in canine hypovolemic shock. Circ Shock *23*:51–57, 1987.

72. Bond R. F., Haines G. F., Johnson G. 3d: The effect of allopurinol and catalase on cardiovascular hemodynamics during hemorrhagic shock. Circ Shock *25*:139–151, 1988.

73. Longnecker D. E., Ross D. C., Silver I. A.: Anesthetic influence on arteriolar diameter and tissue oxygen tensions in hemorrhaged rats. Anesthesiology *57*:177–182, 1982.

74. Stanley T. H., Reddy P.: Fentanyl-oxygen anesthesia in septic shock. Anesthesiology *V51*:S-100, 1979.

75. Shin B., Mackenzie C. F., Helrich M.: Comparison of halothane versus droperidol-fentanyl in traumatic shock. Anesthesiology *V51*:S-101, Sept., 1979.

76. Idvall J.: Influence of ketamine anesthesia on cardiac output and tissue perfusion in rats subjected to hemorrhage. Anesthesiology *55*:297–304, Sept., 1981.

77. Worek F. S., Blumel G., Zeravik J., et al: Comparison of ketamine and pentobarbital anesthesia with the conscious state in a porcine model of Pseudomonas aeuroginosa septicemia. Acta Anaesthesiol Scand *32*:509–515, 1988.

78. Biber B., Fagraeus L., Schaeter C. F., et al: Dose-dependent superior mesenteric vascular effects of isoflurane during endotoxin shock in the rat. Anesthesiology *V65*:1986.

79. Newberg L. A., Michenfelder J. D.: Cerebral protection by isoflurane during hypoxemia or ischemia. Anesthesiology *59*:29–35, 1983.

80. Pfeiffer U., Massion W. H., Perker M., et al: Effect of anesthetic agents on survival time in a porcine septic shock model. Anesthesiology *63*:1985.

81. Pepe P. E., Bass R. R., Mattox K. L.: Clinical Trials of the pneumatic antishock garment in the urban prehospital setting. Ann Emerg Med *15*:1407–1410, 1986.

82. Harkema J. M., Chaudry I. H.: Magnesium-adenosine triphosphate in the treatment of shock, ischemia, and sepsis. Crit Care Med *20*:263–275, 1992.

83. Chaudry I. H., Clemens M. G., Bane A. E.: The role of ATP-magnesium in ischemic shock. Magnesium *5*:211–220, 1986.

Chapter 17

AUTONOMIC NERVOUS SYSTEM

VINCENT J. COLLINS

The thoraco-lumbar sympathetics are like the loud and soft pedals modulating all notes [functions] together; the cranio-sacral innervations are like separate keys.
WALTER CANNON, The Wisdom of the Body (Ref. 10), 1932

ANATOMIC CONSIDERATIONS

History[1,2]

Knowledge of the autonomic nervous system can be traced back to Galen. He spoke of the sympathy and consent of the body and was probably the first to describe the paravertebral nerve trunk. This notion persisted until the 16th century, when Etienne and Stephanos separated the ganglionic chain from the vagus. It was anatomically divorced from the brain by the careful dissections of Pourfour de Petit. Thomas Willis introduced the notion of involuntary movements. Robert Whytt recognized that adequate stimuli were necessary for visceral sensation and that all sympathy must be referred to the brain.

The system was called "sympathetic" by Jacob Winslow, who stressed its independence. At this time, Xavier Bichat divided the nervous system into two parts: a visceral nervous system (la vie organique) which functions continuously, and the somatic (la vie animal) which functions intermittently.

In 1852, Claude Bernard[3-5] described the fundamental role of the autonomic nervous system as that of maintaining homeostasis (la fixité du milieu interieur). Brown-Sequard published his experimental findings that sympathetic stimulation constricts blood vessels. Walter Gaskell described the white communicanti rami and recognized that the system contained two antagonistic sets of nerve fibers. John Langley,[6] in 1905, finally mapped three distinct divisions in the system, coined the term "autonomic," and declared that it was largely independent from the brain.

Definition[1,7]

Often called vegetative, visceral or involuntary nervous system, it consists of nerves, ganglia, and plexuses that innervate all viscera and tissue, except striated muscle.

The autonomic nervous system is primarily a peripheral efferent system. However, there are afferent fibers which travel in the autonomic system and central autonomic connections. In addition, there are supra-segmental centers with integrative action in the brain.

Visceral Afferent Fibers

Visceral afferent fibers are mostly nonmyelinated fibers carried into the cerebrospinal axis by the vagus, pelvic and other autonomic nerves. Cerebrospinal nerves also carry autonomic afferent fibers from blood vessels in the skeletal muscles and structures of the skin. The cell bodies of afferent fibers lie in the dorsal root ganglia of spinal nerves or in the sensory ganglia of some cranial nerves (nodose ganglion of vagus). Their proximal processes run through the dorsal spinal roots, entering the spinal cord and connecting (directly or through internuncial neurons) with cells lying in the intermediolateral columns. In this manner the afferent part of the autonomic reflex arc is completed.

Vasomotor, respiratory and visceromotor reflexes, visceral sensation (including pain and referred pain) and the interrelated visceral activities are mediated by autonomic afferent fibers.

Integration of the Autonomic Nervous System[8]

The integration of the autonomic nervous system above the spinal cord is located mainly at the medulla oblongata and the hypothalamus, but there are also supra-segmental levels of integration at the cerebral cortex. Autonomic centers of integration are closely correlated to somatic centers, anatomically and physiologically, in such a manner that somatic responses are always accompanied by visceral responses and vice versa.

Circulatory and respiratory centers of integration in the *medulla oblongata* are well known. The centers of regulation of body temperature, blood sugar, carbohydrate and fat metabolism, blood pressure, emotion and sleep are located in the *hypothalamus:* the posterior and lateral nuclei are sympathetic and their stimulation results in discharge of the sympatho-adrenal system, the midline and anterior nuclei are parasympathetic, the supraoptic nuclei also regulate the water metabolism through connections with the posterior lobe of the hypophysis (hypothalamic-neurohypophyseal system). The *cortex* is the site of correlation between somatic and autonomic functions. The activities of many of the body systems (cardiovascular, respiratory, gastrointestinal, etc.), conditioned reflexes and visceral processes related to mental states are partially regulated at this highest level.

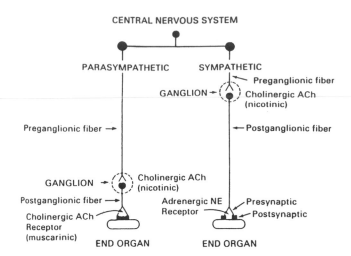

Fig. 17–1. Schematic diagram of the peripheral autonomic nervous system. Preganglionic fibers and postganglionic fibers of the parasympathetic nervous system and preganglionic fibers of the sympathetic nervous system release acetylcholine (ACh) as the neurotransmitter. Postganglionic fibers of the sympathetic nervous system release norepinephrine (NE) as the neurotransmitter (exceptions are fibers to sweat glands, which release ACh). (From Lawson and Wallfisch.)

Peripheral Autonomic System[9] (Fig. 17–1)

The effector or motor part of the autonomic system is divided into two components: the sympathetic or thoracolumbar outflow and the parasympathetic or craniosacral outflow. A schema for the entire system is illustrated (Fig. 17–2).

Sympathetic Nervous System

The sympathetic cell bodies are located at the intermedio-lateral columns of the spinal cord from the level of the eighth cervical to the second or third lumbar segment. Their axons follow the anterior spinal roots synapsing with neurons located in the sympathetic ganglia (Fig. 17–3).

There are three groups of sympathetic ganglia: vertebral, prevertebral, and terminal. The *vertebral ganglia* form two lateral chains on either side of the vertebral column, comprising 22 pairs connected with each other by nerve trunks and to the spinal nerves by rami communicanti. The white rami carry preganglionic myelinated fibers from the spinal cord and the gray rami carry postganglionic fibers back to the spinal nerves for distribution to the sweat glands, pilomotor muscles, and blood vessels of the skin and skeletal muscles. The *prevertebral ganglia,* located in the abdomen and pelvis, consist mainly of the coeliac, aorticorenal, superior and inferior mesenteric ganglia. The *terminal ganglia* are located near the organs they innervate, mainly the urinary bladder and the rectum. There are also small intermediate ganglia variable in number and location, usually close to the rami communicanti and the anterior spinal roots, but outside the main thoracolumbar vertebral chain.

The *cervical sympathetic chain* has its preganglionic fibers arising from the upper thoracic segments of the cord (no sympathetic fibers leave the central nervous system above the first thoracic level); its postganglionic fibers comprise all the sympathetic innervation of the head and neck (sudomotor, vasomotor, pilomotor, secretory and pupillo dilator). Postganglionic fibers of the *upper thoracic chain* form the cardiac, esophageal and pulmonary plexuses. The *splanchnic nerves* are formed by preganglionic fibers originating from the fifth to the last thoracic segment of the spinal cord that pass through the vertebral ganglia and do not synapse until they reach the coeliac ganglion. The postganglionic fibers of the coeliac ganglion, as well as of other prevertebral ganglia, ramify extensively innervating the smooth muscle and secretory glands of abdominal pelvic viscera.

Thus all the organs of the thorax, abdomen, and pelvis are innervated by postganglionic fibers coming from sympathetic ganglia. The trunk and the limbs are also supplied by vasomotor, sudomotor and pilomotor sympathetic postganglionic fibers carried in the spinal nerves. The *adrenal medulla* is the only exception; it acts as a sympathetic ganglion, and the gland cells receive direct innervation from preganglionic fibers.

Preganglionic sympathetic fibers may pass through several ganglia before synapsing, but they usually synapse in only one ganglion. At the ganglion they come into synaptic relationship with many postganglionic fibers (1 to 20 or more); thus their stimulation activates a large area and produces a massive sympathetic discharge throughout the body.

Parasympathetic Nervous System[1] (Figure 17–3)

The preganglionic fibers of this system arise from three locations in the nervous system: the midbrain or tectal outflow, the medulla oblongata or medullary outflow, and the sacral segment or sacral outflow. They usually travel a long way before synapsing in terminal ganglia, very close to the organs they innervate. Each preganglionic fiber enters into synaptic relationship with one or two short postganglionic fibers; thus the response to parasympathetic stimulation is restricted to a narrow region and very refined.

The *tectal outflow* originates in the Edinger-Westphal nucleus of the *third cranial nerve,* synapsing at the ciliary ganglion in the orbit. It innervates the muscle of the iris and the ciliary muscle.

The *medullary outflow* consists of the parasympathetic components in the seventh, ninth and tenth cranial nerves. In the facial nerve, the preganglionic fibers form two branches: (a) the *chorda tympani* which synapses in the submaxillary and sublingual glands and whose short postganglionic fibers innervate secretory cells of the glands, and (b) the *greater superficial petrosal nerve* which after joining the deep petrosal nerve to form the vidian nerve, synapses at the sphenopalatine ganglion—the postganglion fibers innervate the lachrymal gland.

The autonomic fibers of the *glossopharyngeal nerve* travel to the otic ganglion for synapsing and the postganglionic fibers innervate the parotid gland.

The preganglionic fibers of the *vagus nerve* are very long; they synapse in small ganglia that lie directly on or

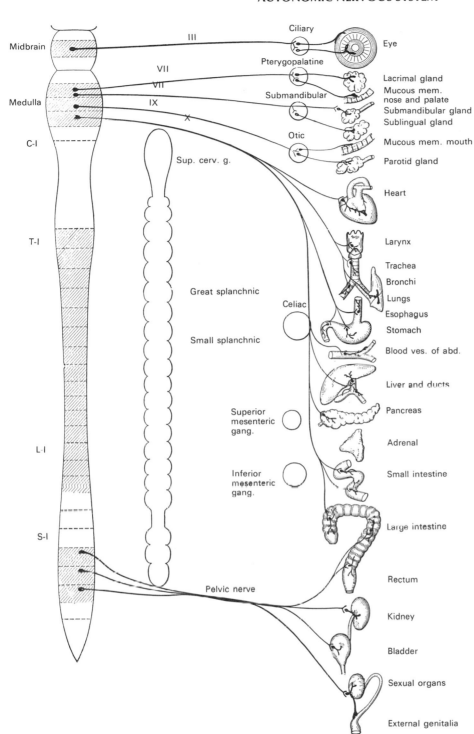

Midbrain
III — Ciliary — Eye
Medulla
VII — Pterygopalatine — Lacrimal gland
VII — Mucous mem. nose and palate
IX — Submandibular — Submandibular gland
Sublingual gland
X — Otic — Mucous mem. mouth
C-I — Parotid gland
Sup. cerv. g.
Heart
Larynx
Trachea
T-I — Bronchi
Lungs
Great splanchnic — Esophagus
Celiac — Stomach
Small splanchnic — Blood ves. of abd.
Liver and ducts
Pancreas
Superior mesenteric gang. — Adrenal
L-I — Small intestine
Inferior mesenteric gang. — Large intestine
S-I — Rectum
Pelvic nerve — Kidney
Bladder
Sexual organs
External genitalia

Fig. 17–2. Diagram of efferent autonomic nervous system. Cranial and sacral outflow, parasympathetic. Thoracolumbar outflow, sympathetic. Interrupted lines designate postganglionic fibers to spinal and cranial nerves to supply vasomotor innervation to head, trunk and limbs, motor fibers to smooth muscles of skin and fibers to sweat glands. Modified after Meyer and Gottlieb. This is only a diagram and does not accurately portray all the details of distribution. From Clemente, C.D.: Gray's Anatomy, 30th Ed. Philadelphia, Lea & Febiger, 1987.

in the viscera of the thorax and abdomen. In the heart they enter into intrinsic synapse in the muscle fiber. In the intestinal wall they form the plexus of Meissner and Auerbach. The vagus also carries afferent fibers—except pain fibers—which synapse in the nodose ganglion and mediate visceral reflexes.

The *sacral outflow* originates in the second, third and fourth sacral segments of the spinal cord. Preganglionic fibers form the *pelvic nerves* (nervis erigens) synapsing in terminal ganglia near the bladder, distal colon, rectum

and sexual organs. The vagus and pelvic nerves thus provide secretory vasodilator and motor fibers for the organs in the thorax, abdomen and pelvis.

Nerve Endings

Some organs receive one autonomic end fiber for each effector cell, as the ciliary muscle of the eye; whereas in the intestinal musculature only one cell in 100 receives a nerve ending. The nerve impulse is transmitted to the

Dorsal root & ganglion

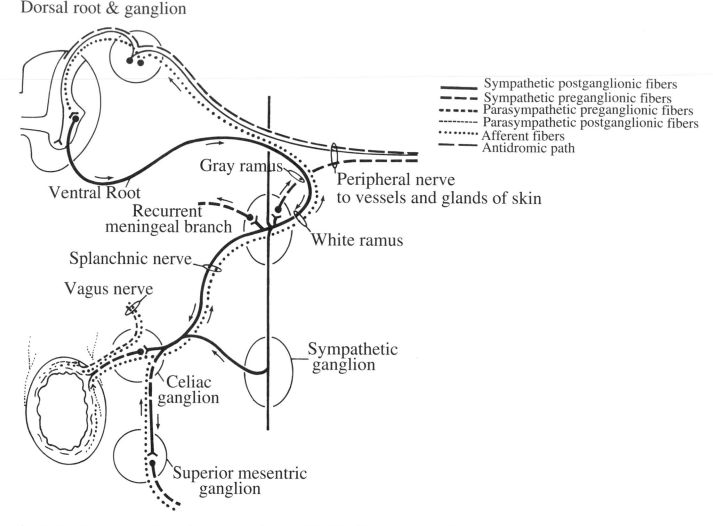

Fig. 17–3. Autonomic reflex pathways. From Netter, F.H.: The Ciba Collection of Medical Illustrations, Ciba Clinical Symposia, Ciba-Geigy Corp, Summit, NJ, April 1972. In Second Ed., Collins, Principles of Anesthesiology, Lea and Febiger, 1976.

cells that do not receive direct innervation by propagation from activated effector cells.

Autonomic nerve endings may terminate in the cytoplasm of effector cells, as in both cardiac and smooth muscle (Fig. 17–4), or they lie on the cell surface, as is the case in the adrenal, gastric and salivary glands. Although most of the organs receive innervation from both systems, sympathetic and parasympathetic fibers may innervate different effector cells.

PHYSIOLOGIC CONSIDERATIONS

Antagonistic Systems

Sympathetic and parasympathetic are considered antagonistic control systems; when one system inhibits a certain function, the other usually augments that function; homeostasis depends on the interaction of both systems. The balance, however, is far more complex than an on-and-off mechanical switch; when two impulses reach the effector cell at any one moment, the level of activity is the algebraic summation of the two component influences.[10]

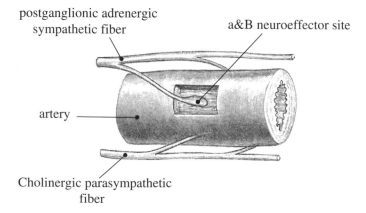

Fig. 17–4. Autonomic adrenergic nerve fibers terminate in the smooth muscle wall of an artery. Courtesy of Dr. D. LeRoy Crandell.

The sympathetic system is a compensatory, emergency, mechanism usually activated under conditions of stress, such as pain, fatigue, infection, hemorrhage, etc. It causes a burst of activity throughout the body and frequently discharges as a unit. However, it sustains some degree of activity at all times, to accomplish the finer adjustments to an environment that changes from minute to minute and from organ to organ in varying degrees.

The parasympathetic system, in contrast, is a protective mechanism, concerning itself with conservation and restoration of energy. It is most active when the body relaxes, being organized for a far more localized and discrete discharge.

Chemical Mediation

The history of chemical mediation is intimately associated with the autonomic nervous system.

After John Abel of Johns Hopkins isolated epinephrine in 1898, J. N. Langley[6] noted that extracts of the adrenal gland stimulated organs innervated by the sympathetic nerves (1901). On this basis he distinguished the sympathetic system, the parasympathetic and the somatic systems.

A student of Langley's at Cambridge, T. R. Elliott,[11] in 1902, injected epinephrine into animals and noted the responses to be similar to the stimulation of sympathetic nerves. He then suggested that epinephrine was released from nerves when stimulated and caused the response. Thus was enunciated the concept "of neural communication by means of chemical transmitters."

In 1907, Dixon[12] advanced the idea that the vagus nerve liberated a muscarine-like substance. In 1914, Sir Henry Dale,[13] after reinvestigating the properties of acetylcholine, introduced the term "Parasympathomimetic" to characterize its effects and postulated that its action was extremely brief due to rapid destruction by an esterase in the tissues in contrast to the relatively longer action of the chemical related to the sympathetic system.

The real proof of chemical transmission was established by Otto Loewi[14] in 1921, at the University of Graz in Austria who called the transmitter "vagusstoff" (vagus-substance). Dale and Feldberg (1934)[15] and many other investigators finally presented overwhelming evidence that Loewi's vagus-substance is acetylcholine and that the chemical is released peripherally after stimulation of the craniosacral autonomic nerves.

Walter Cannon and his associates in a series of experiments started in 1921, encouraged by Loewi's discoveries, reported the finding of a substance capable of increasing blood pressure and heart rate after sympathetic stimulation.[16] They called this substance "sympathin," to avoid confusion with epinephrine, and later they described an excitatory substance "sympathin E" and an inhibitory substance "sympathin I." Subsequent investigators, during the decade of 1930, repeatedly demonstrated that sympathin was probably a demethylated epinephrine. Finally, the Swedish physiologist, Ulf von Euler, in 1946 found a close resemblance between the sympathomimetic substance in highly purified extracts of sympathetic nerves and norepinephrine.[17] He proposed norepinephrine as the sympathetic chemical transmitter and stated that sympathetic nerve stimulation on some occasions may, in addition, liberate small quantities of epinephrine itself.

Principles of Chemical Mediation[18]

Neural communication is achieved by chemical transmitters. As nerve impulses reach the termination of a nerve, chemicals are released which then react with the surface membrane of another nerve cell or with an effector organ to cause depolarization and response.

Such interaction occurs at peripheral efferent nerve junctions; ganglionic synapses, postganglionic sympathetic and parasympathetic neuro-effector junctions; and neuro-muscular junctions. And a chemical interaction occurs at afferent nerve endings at central synapses in the spinal cord, brain stem and cerebrum.

Requisites for a Transmitter

To be classed as a true chemical transmitter four main criteria must be fulfilled:

1. Synthesis of the chemical must occur in the nerve and the enzymes required should be present.
2. The chemical should be released when the nerve is stimulated.
3. The chemical should react with a receptor at the postjunctional cell and cause a response.
4. Mechanisms should be available to terminate the action rapidly and to moderate the action.

On this basis two compounds are clearly established as neurotransmitters: acetylcholine in cholinergic nerves; and norepinephrine in adrenergic nerves; dopamine is probably a true transmitter in the central nervous system.

Certain nerve chemicals which do not meet all of the criteria are called "putative" transmitters. These include principally, serotonin, histamine, octopamine, gamma-amino-butyric acid, glutaric acid and glycine.

Synaptic and Parasympathetic Transmission

Acetylcholine is the chemical mediator at all the autonomic synapses, i.e., autonomic ganglia, at the end of postganglionic parasympathetic fibers and at the neuromuscular junction. It is also found all along the nerve fibers, bound to a protein, forming a physiologically inactive labile complex. It is resynthesized by choline acetylase. Acetylcholine is also a central transmitter and has been identified chemically and physiologically in the brain and spinal cord.[19,20]

Storage of acetylcholine is in synaptic vesicles of cholinergic nerve endings but is also distributed in the synaptoplasm. The latter accounts for 70% of the total acetylcholine. Synthesis by an acetyltransferase system occurs in two different pools: Principally in the synaptoplasm, but also in the synaptic vesicles which represent about 15% compared to amount formed in the synaptoplasm.[21,22]

When a nerve impulse reaches the synapses or the nerve endings, acetylcholine is liberated, crosses to and stimulates the receptors. After transmission the mediator is rapidly destroyed by cholinesterase; none is reutilized. However, there is a high level of choline acetylase at nerve terminals and the synthesis of acetylcholine is quickly accomplished.

Termination of Action

Cholinesterase is found in the blood and tissues where acetylcholine is released; its concentration is proportional to parasympathetic innervation. The enzyme splits acetylcholine into physiologically inactive choline and acetic acid. Cholinesterase is the generic name for a whole family of enzymes closely related. Two types of cholinesterases are most important in man: the true cholinesterase or acetylcholinesterase that has the highest affinity for acetylcholine and the nonspecific plasma or pseudocholinesterase that can also split acetylcholine, but whose normal physiological substrates are not yet clearly understood.[11]

Cholinergic Receptors[23]

The acetylcholine receptor is an oligomeric protein which mediates transmission of a nerve impulse by binding with the released transmitter (Table 17-1). This interaction causes a transient increase in membrane permeability to cations and reduces membrane potential. Membrane bound ACh receptors are large proteins of molecular size of 250,000 daltons; the receptor protein has four different polypeptide subunits.[24]

Acetylcholine activates the receptors by depolarizing its surface in the following sequence of events (Fig. 17-5)[25]:

1. In the resting state there are different concentrations of Na^+ outside the cell and K^+ inside the cell; thus the cell surface is polarized (90-94 millivolts).
2. With the arrival of a nerve impulse at a synapse, acetylcholine (ACh) is released from storage vesicles into a narrow cleft (200 Å) between the cells. A flux of ions across the cleft then carries Na^+ into the distal cell until the charges are balanced; stimulation then occurs.
3. Excess acetylcholine is immediately hydrolyzed by acetylcholine esterase (AChE), and K^+ ions leave the cell, reestablishing polarization.
4. Finally the ions return to their resting position by active transport and the cycle is completed.

Besides parasympathetic transmission acetylcholine is also the mediator at the endings of somatic nerves (myoneural junction),[20,26] central synapses[20,27] and postganglionic "sympathetic" fibers in the sweat glands.[28,29] The innervation of the sweat glands is anatomically sympathetic, but physiologically it must be considered parasympathetic.

Stimulation may result not only from the presence of acetylcholine, but from other choline esters or other direct stimulants; from the presence of AChE inhibitors (presuming the constant liberation of small amounts of ACh); or from other alteration of the electrical charge or ion concentration.[30]

Adrenergic Transmission[18,27,31]

Norepinephrine is the chemical mediator liberated at postganglionic sympathetic nerve endings, close to the effector cells (Fig. 17-6). Epinephrine is predominantly released by the adrenal medulla, discharged into the bloodstream, and exerts its effects when it is carried to all cells. During sympathoadrenal stimulation the actions of norepinephrine at the periphery are reinforced by those of epinephrine arriving in the circulation from the adrenal medulla.

Synthesis of Catecholamines[31,33,34]

In the synthesis of norepinephrine two phases are recognized. The *first* phase begins in the cell body of the nerve where the four enzymes needed for the production of norepinephrine are manufactured. These enzymes are carried down the axon by a natural flowing process dependent in part on concentration gradients to the nerve ending where the *second* phase or actual synthesis occurs (Fig. 17-7).[18]

Two of the enzymes act on the amino acid precursors phenylalanine and tyrosine to form dopamine. Two enzymes act now on dopamine to form norepinephrine and epinephrine.

Hydroxylase is the enzyme that acts on phenylalanine and also on the product tyrosine to form DOPA, a dihydroxy catechol product.[35] Next an aminoacid-decarboxylase removes the alpha-COOH group to form dopamine the first catecholamine. Dopamine is then converted by hydroxylation in the nerve axoplasm and in the adrenal medullary cells by the enzyme beta-oxidase to norepinephrine. In the adrenal medullary cells norepinephrine is methylated by N-methyl transferase to epinephrine.[36] Thus three enzymes are needed for the formation of norepinephrine and four enzymes for epinephrine synthesis.

The level of epinephrine, the rate of synthesis and stores in the adrenal medulla are dependent on the activity of tyrosine hydroxylase which appears to be the rate limiting factor. The activity of tyrosine hydroxylase and of dopamine beta hydroxylase (DBH) is greatly increased when glucocorticoid secretion is stimulated as by stress.[36]

The chemical steps are structurally represented in Figure 17-8.

Dopamine itself is a natural catecholamine, not simply an intermediate in the synthesis of norepinephrine. It is a true chemical transmitter in the brain where it functions between neurons which affect movement and behavior.

These catecholamines are formed in the sympathetic nerve fibers, in cells of the adrenal medulla and other chromaffin cells, and in the nerve cells in the brain. They are stored as granules that also contain ATP.

Storage of Epinephrine[18,33,37]

The adrenal medulla is the principle storage site for epinephrine. Adrenal stores amount to 0.25 to 1.0 mg per gram of tissue of the medullary catecholamines, 80% is epinephrine and the remainder is norepinephrine.

Table 17–1. Characteristics of Subtypes of Cholinergic Receptors*

Receptor	Agonists	Antagonists	Tissue	Responses	Molecular Mechanisms
Muscarinic					
M$_1$	Oxotremorine McN-A-343	Atropine Pirenzepine	Autonomic ganglia CNS[2]	Depolarization (late EPSP) Undefined	Stimulation of PLC with formation of IP$_3$ and DAG; increased cytosolic Ca^{2+}
M$_2$	—	Atropine AF-DX 115	Heart SA node	Slowed spontaneous depolarization; hyperpolarization	Activation of K$^+$ channels; inhibition of adenylyl cyclase
			Atrium	Shortened duration of action potential; decreased contractile force	
			AV node	Decreased conduction velocity	
			Ventricle	Slight decrease in contractile force	
M$_3$	—	Atropine Hexahydro-siladifenidol	Smooth muscle[3] Secretory glands[3]	Contraction[4] Increased secretion	Stimulation of PLC with formation of IP$_3$ and DAG; increased cytosolic Ca^{2+}
Nicotinic					
Muscle (N$_M$)	Phenyltrimethyl-ammonium	Tubocurarine α-Bungarotoxin	Neuromuscular junction	End-plate depolarization, skeletal muscle contraction	Opening of cation channel in N$_M$ receptor
Neuronal (N$_N$)[1]	Dimethylphenyl-piperazinium	Trimethaphan	Autonomic ganglia	Depolarization and firing of postganglionic neuron	Opening of cation channel in N$_N$ receptor
			Adrenal medula	Secretion of catecholamines	
			CNS	Undefined	

*This table provides examples of drugs that act on cholinergic receptors and of the location of subtypes of these receptors. Abbreviations are: excitatory postsynaptic potential (EPSP); phospholipase C (PLC); inositol-1,4,5-trisphosphate (IP$_3$); diacylglycerol (DAG).

[1]The nicotinic receptors of autonomic ganglia and the CNS contain a variety of different subunits; most of the subunits of receptors in the CNS are distinct from those in ganglia (see text).

[2]The CNS contains all known subtypes of muscarinic receptors.

[3]The subtypes in various smooth muscles or secretory glands have not been precisely determined, but are most likely to be mechanistically related to M$_3$ (or M$_1$) receptors.

[4]Relaxation occurs in sphincters in the urinary and gastrointestinal tracts, but this may result from the release of dilatory peptides from intrinsic ganglia or parasympathetic nerves; blood vessels relax as a consequence of release of factors from the endothelium (see text).

(From Gilman, A. G., et al. *Goodman and Gilman's The Pharmacological Basis of Therapeutics*, 8th Ed. New York, McGraw-Hill 1990.)

Storage of Norepinephrine[18,38]

The organ sites where norepinephrine is present and stored is noted (Table 17–2).

It is largely stored in adrenergic nerve endings. The stores amount to 5 to 10 μg/g of adrenergic nerve tissue. Tissues that are innervated by adrenergic nerves usually have a variable content of 0.1 to 2.0 μg/g^3 of norepinephrine.[38]

The norepinephrine appears to exist in three pools (Table 17–3) in adrenergic nerves somewhat similar to acetylcholine in cholinergic nerve terminals[37]: (1) a pool of norepinephrine concentrated about mitochondria where synthesis is achieved; (2) a storage pool consisting of vesicles containing packets or quanta of norepinephrine as well as the enzyme DBH; and (3) a readily releasable pool of vesicles close to the nerve membrane.

Release of Norepinephrine[33,38,39]

When a sympathetic nerve is stimulated, norepinephrine is released from vesicles into the synaptic cleft or

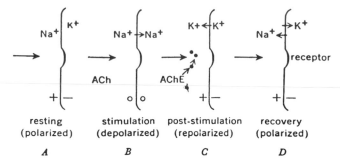

Fig. 17–5. Stimulation of a parasympathetic receptor. A. In the resting state the receptor mechanism is polarized (90 millivolts) because of different concentrations of Na^+ outside the cell and K^+ inside the cell. B. With the arrival of a nerve impulse, acetylcholine (ACh) is liberated and causes Na^+ to enter the cell until the charges are balanced; stimulation then occurs. C. Excess acetylcholine is immediately hydrolyzed by acetylcholine esterase (AChE), and K^+ ions leave the cell, re-establishing polarization. D, Finally, the ions are returned to their resting position by active transport and the cycle is complete. From Cutting, W: Handbook of Pharmacology, Meredith Publishing Co., 1962.

junctional gap. The vesicles close to the nerve membrane move to the terminal membrane of the nerve and fuse with it. This is followed by conformational changes and openings in the terminal membrane large enough to allow molecules of norepinephrine as well as DBH to be extruded. This mechanism is called exocytosis.[37]

Interior vesicles may also have their walls altered or deformed by a nerve impulse or by ionic changes, especially in the presence of calcium; the result is the release of molecules which migrate via neurotubules into the junctional gap. Calcium is of particular importance since it can activate microfilaments in many cells such as muscles to contract and form surface openings or pores.

Plasma Levels of Catecholamines (Table 17–4)

Resting plasma blood levels of epinephrine are low and approximate 0.06 μg/L. This translates into 6 nanograms/100ml of blood with a range of 4 to 10 ng/100 ml.

Norepinephrine blood levels at rest are higher and approximate 0.3 μg/L. This translates into 30 ng/100 ml in arterial blood, and 40 ng/100 ml in venous blood.

Various stresses and stimuli alter the plasma levels.[42] The concept of Cannon, that the autonomic sympathetic nervous system and these catecholamine secretions are designed for "fight or flight," is classic. Von Euler has shown gradations in catecholamine secretion due to various stresses including types of school examinations (Table 17–5). The least increase occurred with quizzes on sociological studies and highest with science examinations (mathematics). Coffee drinking may raise the epinephrine level three-four fold and norepinephrine twofold.[43]

Norepinephrine is less affected by emotions than is epinephrine but is more responsive to chronic stress.[44]

Receptor Classification[45,46]

There are two distinct types of receptors according to their responses to sympathetic transmitters: alpha and beta receptors (Table 17–6).

The alpha receptors are associated with increased contractility of all kinds of vascular smooth muscle, primarily in vasoconstriction (excitatory function), but also in one inhibitory function (intestinal relaxation).

The alpha adrenergic receptor consists of two distinct subtypes:[47] those receptors mediating postsynaptic and postjunctional responses to NE are the $alpha_{(1)}$-receptors; the second type is the prejunctional (presynaptic) $alpha_{(2)}$-receptor on the limiting membrane controlling the release of NE from adrenergic terminals at peripheral sympathetic junctions as well as at noradrenergic synapses in the central nervous system. Agonist action at $alpha_{(2)}$ is a type of feedback to the NE containing vesicles in the adrenergic nerve axoplasm inhibiting release of NE.[32] This autoregulation is to some extent accomplished by excessive NE in the synaptic cleft acting on the $alpha_{(2)}$-receptors.[49] A specific agonist of the $alpha_{(2)}$-receptor is the drug clonidine.[50]

The beta receptors are associated with most inhibitory functions, resulting in vasodilatation and relaxation of nonintestinal smooth muscle (bronchial, uterine) and one important excitatory function (myocardial stimulation).

The *beta receptor* (β) consists of two distinct subtypes.[51] Differences in response to sympathomimetic amines permits differentiation of one type of receptor (β_1) which is involved in cardiac stimulation and lipolysis, from a second type (β_2) which is involved in bronchiodilation, vasodepression and muscle glycogenolysis.[52,53]

A third type of receptor—beta 3 (gamma receptor)—has also been described; it is associated with glycogenolysis and other metabolic effects, responding promptly to epinephrine.[54]

Receptor-Transmitter Interaction[18,55]

Upon release, the adrenergic transmitter norepinephrine diffuses across the synaptic cleft to the effector cell. A response depends on the capacity of the receptor protein to selectively recognize the transmitter chemical and to combine with it. Once this chemical interaction oc-

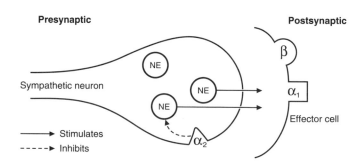

Fig. 17–6. Postganglionic sympathetic nerve ending showing presynaptic and postsynaptic receptors. Release of norepinephrine (NE) from the sympathetic neuron results in stimulation of the postsynaptic receptors with classic alpha-1, beta-1 and beta-2 effects.[27] The secretion of NE is accompanied by a feedback inhibition of subsequent norepinephrine release. Modified from Ram CVS, Kaplan NM: Alpha- and beta-receptor blocking drugs in the treatment of hypertension; and redrawn from Harvey WP, et al., eds. Current Problems in Cardiology. Chicago: Year Book Medical Publishers, 1979.

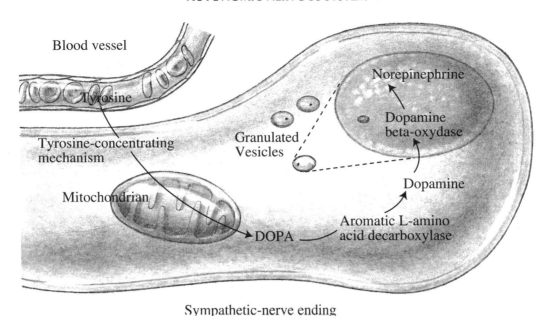

Blood vessel

Tyrosine

Tyrosine-concentrating mechanism

Mitochondrian

Granulated Vesicles

Norepinephrine

Dopamine beta-oxydase

Dopamine

DOPA

Aromatic L-amino acid decarboxylase

Sympathetic-nerve ending

Fig. 17–7. Intracellular movements of substrates in the biosynthesis of norepinephrine. From Wurtman, R. J.: Catecholamines. N. Engl. J. Med., *273*:637, 695, 746, 1965.

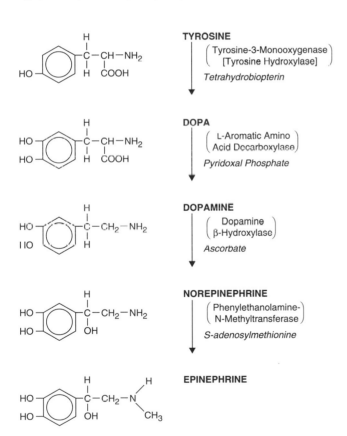

TYROSINE

(Tyrosine-3-Monooxygenase)
[Tyrosine Hydroxylase]

Tetrahydrobiopterin

DOPA

(L-Aromatic Amino)
Acid Decarboxylase

Pyridoxal Phosphate

DOPAMINE

(Dopamine)
β-Hydroxylase

Ascorbate

NOREPINEPHRINE

(Phenylethanolamine-)
N-Methyltransferase

S-adenosylmethionine

EPINEPHRINE

Fig. 17–8. Steps in enzymatic synthesis of norepinephrine and epinephrine. Modified from Goodman and Gilman.[23] Enzymes are shown in parenthesis.

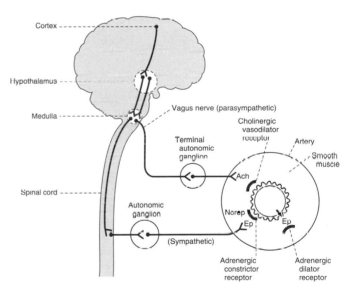

Fig. 17–9. The scheme of the adrenergic and cholinergic fiber system is shown. The sympathetic fiber is shown to have two adrenergic responses dependent on type of receptor: the alpha receptor is constrictor or stimulatory; the beta receptor is dilator or inhibitory. Courtesy of Dr. D. LeRoy Crandell.

sponses are "turned on" more slowly as when the receptor-transmitter interaction activates the machinery to synthesize intracellular enzymes (Fig. 17–9).

Termination of Action (Fig. 17–10)

Once the neurotransmitter reacts with the receptor of a post-junctional cell its action is terminated rapidly. This is accomplished principally through uptake by the nerve.[33] When radioactively labeled norepinephrine is injected, neuronal recapture of norepinephrine by sympathetic nerves is highly selective and accounts for 90% of the released transmitter.

curs, depolarization with ionic changes ensues and a series of responses are triggered. Most responses are "turned on" rapidly, as when alpha and beta receptors recognize and interact with norepinephrine or brain receptors recognize and interact with dopamine. Some re-

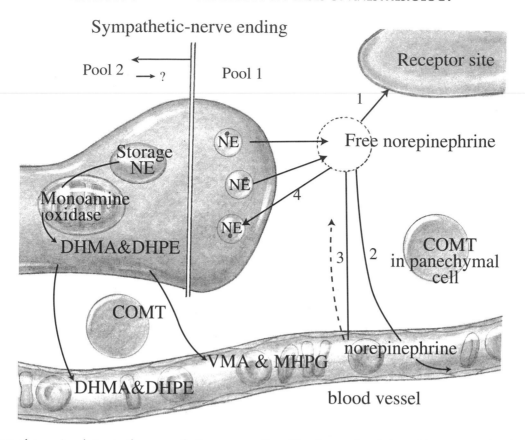

Fig. 17–10. Fate of norepinephrine in the sympathetic nerve ending. "Free" norepinephrine (1) interacts with adrenergic receptor sites, (2) is O-methylated by COMT, (3) is "washed out" by the circulation, or (4) is rebound within the sympathetic-nerve ending. Storage norepinephrine is deaminated by MAO within the sympathetic-nerve ending, and released as dihydroxymandleic acid (DHMA) or dihydroxyphenylglycol (DHPG). These compounds may subsequently be O-methylated to form 3-methoxy, 4-hydroxy-mandelic acid (vanillyl-mandelic acid, VMA) or methoxy-hydroxy phenylglycol (MHPG). From Wurtman, R. J.: Catecholamines. N. Engl. J. Med., *273*:637, 695, 746, 1965.

Table 17–2. Sites of Norepinephrine Storage in Tissue

Organ	Cell	Relative Amount	Present in Granulated Vesicle
Brain and spinal cord	Adrenergic neuron:		
	Cell body	Moderate	No
	Nerve ending	Very large	Partly
Sympathetic ganglia	Adrenergic neuron:		
	Cell body	Small	No
Organs with sympathetic innervation (i.e., heart, spleen, liver, kidney, muscle, salivary gland)	Adrenergic neuron: Sympathetic-nerve ending	Very large (most of the norepinephrine in the body)	Yes (adrenergic vesicle)
	Extraneural pool (in parenchymal cells)	Small	No
Adrenal medulla (and extramedullary chromaffin cells)	Chromaffin cell	Very large	Yes (chromaffin granule)
Uterus	Parenchyma (?)	Moderate	No

The concentrations of norepinephrine in the adrenergic cell body and nerve ending have been estimated to be 10–100 μg/g and 10,000 μg/g, respectively.

From Wurtman, R. J.: Catecholamines. N. Engl. J. Med., *273*:637, 695, 746, 1965.

Table 17–3. Pools of H^3-Norepinephrine in Sympathetic Nerve Endings

	Pool I	Pool II	Pool III
Anatomic localization	Probably within granulated vesicle in nerve ending	Same	Same
Rate of turnover, half-life	Approx. 2 hours	Approx. 24 hours	
Response to tyramine	Preferentially depleted	Refractory	Synthesis
Physiologic activity	Released upon sympathetic-nerve impulses	Storage pool	
Metabolic fate	O-Methylated outside the sympathetic-nerve ending	Deaminated within the sympathetic-nerve ending	Released to pool II

Modified from Wurtman, R. J.: Catecholamines. N. Engl. J. Med.,*273*:637, 695, 746, 1965.

Table 17–4. Plasma Levels—Catecholamines

	Mean	Range
Epinephrine	6.0 ng/100 ml	2.0–12.0
Norepinephrine	30.0 ng/100 ml	12.0–50.0

In venous blood from adrenal—average 40.0 ng/100 ml

Conversion to nanomoles:

$$\text{Nanomoles of epinephrine} = \frac{\text{Nanograms/L}}{180}$$

$$\text{Nanomoles of norepinephrine} = \frac{\text{Nanograms/L}}{165}$$

Nanograms per 100 ml arterial blood.

Table 17–5. Quantitation of Stress by Analysis of Blood Catecholamine Levels and Rate of Secretion

	Epinephrine (rate/min [ng])	Norepinephrine (rate/min)
1. Rest recumbent	2–3	10
2. Erect posture	6–7	(3X)30
3. Work (heavy muscular)	9–12	200–300
4. Excitation anger	12–24	
5. Hypoglycemia	5–20	
6. Transportation (air) metabolic stress	24	
7. Flying (Jumping)	18	
8. Mental stress of examinations:		
Biology	8	
Physics	15	
Math Advanced	21	
9. Pheochromocytoma		100 μg/24 hours

From von Euler, U.S.: Quantitation of stress by catecholamine analysis. Clin. Pharmacol. Ther., *5*:398, 1964.

A second mechanism for termination of action is the destruction of the catecholamines.[18] Excess molecules and those not recaptured are metabolized by two enzymes: catechol-o-methyl-transferase (COMT) and monamine oxidase (MAO). Both operate in peripheral nerves. But MAO which removes the amino group is important in the brain where it acts on a variety of compounds, including serotonin, dopamine and norepinephrine. It is also to be noted that the "transferase" degradation is a relatively slower process than the oxidase action.

Excretion

Catecholamines and metabolites are primarily excreted in the urine. About 5 to 30 μg of free epinephrine is excreted each day in the urine, and is derived from the adrenal gland. Intact norepinephrine is excreted at a rate of 10 to 80 μg per day and is derived largely from sympathetic nerve endings. Of the principal metabolites excreted, "VMA" (3 methoxy, 4 hydroxy, mandelic acid) makes up 80%; the methoxamines (metanephrines) about 15% and free catecholamines less than 1%. Of the metabolites, the methoxamine excretion ranges from 0.3 to 1.3 mg/day, and VMA 2.0 to 6.0 mg/day (Table 17–7).[44,55]

Regulation[49]

All neurotransmitters are in a state of flux and despite marked changes in activity in response to various stresses, the total amount of catecholamine in tissues remains constant. Depletion of norepinephrine results in increased formation of the appropriate enzymes, and enhanced norepinephrine production. Conversely, in the presence of large or excessive amounts of catecholamines there is both a greater metabolism of the NE and an inhibition of the enzymes for the synthesis of NE.

When a sympathetic nerve is stimulated and norepinephrine released, the conversion of tyrosine to norepinephrine is rapidly increased. A critical concentration itself specifically inhibits tyrosine hydroxylase and slows the formation of norepinephrine. Thus, norepinephrine and dopamine have a *negative feedback* on the machinery of their production. When stresses lower the level of norepinephrine the inhibition of the enzyme hydroxylase is reduced, and the enzyme converts more tyrosine to dopa and there is increased production of norepinephrine.

A further regulation of the level of norepinephrine in the axoplasm of sympathetic nerve endings is accomplished by the alpha$_1$ adrenergic receptor. When these receptors are occupied and/or the effector cells are activated, norepinephrine tends to accumulate in the synaptic cleft before being recaptured and these molecules then activate alpha$_2$ type receptors on the presynaptic membrane of the nerve terminal. In brief an increase in

Table 17–6. Characteristics of Subtypes of Adrenergic Receptors*

Receptor	Agonists	Antagonists	Tissue	Responses	Molecular Mechanisms[1]
Alpha-1 (α_1)[2] Excitatory	Epi ≥ NE >> Iso Phenylephrine	Prazosin Phentolamine Labetalol	Vascular smooth muscle	Contraction	Stimulation of PLC with formation of IP_3 and DAG; increased cytosolic Ca^{2+}
			Genitourinary smooth muscle	Contraction	
			Liver[3]	Glycogenolysis; gluconeogenesis	
			Intestinal smooth muscle	Hyperpolarization and relaxation	(Activation of Ca^{2+}-dependent K^+ channels)
			Heart	Increased contractile force; arrhythmias	(Inhibition of transient K^+ current)
Alpha-2 (α_2)[2] Inhibitory	Epi ≥ NE >> Iso Clonidine Dexmedetomidine	Yohimbine Phentolamine DH Ergot DH ergoleryptine	Pancreatic islets (β cells)	Decreased insulin secretion	Inhibition of adenylyl cyclase; activation of K^+ channels
			Platelets	Aggregation	
			Nerve terminals	Decreased release of NE	(Inhibition of neuronal Ca^{2+} channels)
			Vascular smooth muscle	Contraction	(Enhanced influx of Ca^{2+}; increased cytosolic Ca^{2+})
			CNS Postsynap	Potassium Increased conductance	

Adrenergic receptor	Agonists	Antagonists	Tissue	Responses	Mechanism
Beta-1 (β_1) Excitatory	Iso > Epi = NE; Dobutamine; Dopamine; Isoproterenol[b]	Metoprolol; Atenolol; Esmolol; Propranolol; Timolol; Labetalol; Acebutolol	Heart	Increased force and rate of contraction and AV nodal conduction velocity	Activation of adenylyl cyclase and Ca^{2+} channels
			Juxtaglomerular cells	Increased renin secretion	
Beta-2 (β_2) Inhibitory	Iso > Epi >> NE; Terbutaline; Albuterol; Ritodrine	Propranolol; Timolol; Labetalol	Smooth muscle (vascular, bronchial, gastrointestinal, and genitourinary)	Relaxation	Activation of adenylyl cyclase
			Skeletal muscle	Glycogenolysis; uptake of K^+	
			Liver[3]	Glycogenolysis; gluconeogenesis	
			Pancreas	Insulin secretion	
Beta-3 (β_3)[4]	Iso = NE > Epi; BRL 37344	ICI 118551; CGP 20712A	Adipose tissue	Lipolysis	Activation of adenylyl cyclase

*This table provides examples of drugs that act on adrenergic receptors and of the location of subtypes of adrenergic receptors. Abbreviations are: epinephrine (Epi); norepinephrine (NE); isoproterenol (Iso); phospholipase C (PLC); inositol-1,4,5-trisphosphate (IP₃); diacylglycerol (DAG).

[1] Entries in parentheses denote additional or alternative mechanisms that may be important in the responses of the tissue listed.

[2] At least two subtypes of α_1- and α_2-adrenergic receptors are known, but distinctions in their mechanism of action and tissue location have not been defined.

[3] In some species (e.g., rat), metabolic responses in the liver are mediated by α_1 receptors, whereas in others (e.g., dog) β_2 receptors are predominantly involved. Both types of receptors appear to contribute to responses in man.

[4] Metabolic responses in adipocytes and certain other tissues with atypical pharmacological characteristics may be mediated by this subtype of receptor. Most β-adrenergic antagonists (including propranolol) do not block these responses.

[a] Mixed alpha-1 and alpha-2 effects.

[b] Mixed beta-1 and beta-2 effects.

Modified from Goodman and Gilman's *Pharmacological Basis of Therapeutics*. Eighth Edition, Pergamon Press, New York 1990 and McGraw-Hill Book Co. With permission.

Table 17–7.   Daily Excretion of Catecholamines and Metabolites

Free epinephrine	5–30 μg
Free Norepinephrine	10–80 μg
Methoxamines	
Metanephrine adrenal source	100–200 μg
Nor-metanephrine adrenergic nerve	100–300 μg
"VMA" (3-meoxy-4 OH mandelic	
acid)	2–6 mg
Conversion to nanomoles:	

$$\text{Nanomoles of epinephrine} = \frac{\text{Nanograms/L}}{180}$$

$$\text{Nanomoles of norepinephrine} = \frac{\text{Nanograms/L}}{165}$$

From Kolle, G. E.: Functional anatomy of synaptic transmission. Anesthesiology, *29*:643, 1968.

norepinephrine concentration in the syneptic cleft is accompanied by an increase in number of active uptake sites and uptake is accelerated at the same time. This shuts off the further release of norepinephrine.[32]

Chronic stress and prolonged firing of sympathetic nerves evoke a slower regulatory process. When there is a greater and continuing need for neurotransmitters, there is a compensatory increase in the enzymes which synthesize the chemical. The manufacture of tyrosine hydroxylase and DBH are both increased. For example, the administration of reserpine releases norepinephrine and initially causes repetitive sympathetic nerve firing. But depletion of norepinephrine in the nerve ending has a positive feedback, and brings about an increase in the amount of the synthesizing enzymes.[56]

Another regulatory mechanism involves the influence of one nerve on another. If presynaptic nerves are cut and release of norepinephrine from the postsynaptic cell accomplished pharmacologically by reserpine, then the synthesizing enzymes of these isolated neurons are not increased. But the enzymes are greatly increased in nearly innervated postsynaptic nerves.

Sensitization Phenomena (Denervation)

Historical Aspects

In 1855, the German physiologist J.L. Budge noted that when nerves to a rabbit's eye were destroyed the pupil of that eye became more dilated than the innervated eye.[57,58] Cannon explained this phenomenon to be due to a greater responsiveness of effector cells and enunciated the "law of denervation supersensitivity."[59]

Supersensitivity Mechanism

Several procedures induce supersensitivity: destruction of an adrenergic nerve terminal, severance of an adrenergic nerve from its effector organ; depletion of the neurotransmitter NE stores or prolonged blockade of the receptors produces the phenomenon.[58,59]

Denervation supersensitivity is apparently due to two separate mechanisms.[60]

One is presynaptic and is immediate.[61] With destruction of an adrenergic nerve, there is diminished recapture of the neurotransmitter by the terminal membrane and a larger amount of the NE is available to react with receptors. This produces an exaggerated response. When the NE stores are depleted, the receptors are not stimulated and a short period of diminished responsiveness occurs.

Subsequently, a second or postjunctional mechanism develops involving changes in the degree of activity of the receptors.[62] This phenomenon can be induced particularly by prolonged receptor blockade. When the receptor on a postjunctional cell is deprived of its neurotransmitter for any period of time, it becomes avid for its chemical and there is increased binding. One packet of catecholamines is able to elicit a response that in the nondenervated organ requires 10 times as much.

A further postjunctional mechanism also occurs. Absence of the specific neurotransmitter induces the effector organ to increase the number of adrenergic receptor molecules.[61,62]

Desensitization Phenomenon[61]

Converse to the supersensitization process is the desensitization phenomenon due to exposure of an effector cell and its receptors to longterm stimulation. An abundance of transmitter molecules may tighten the receptor and diminish receptor affinity. More important is the evidence that longterm activation decreases the number of receptor molecules.[62] Thus, continued stimulation by NE as an agonist diminishes both alpha and beta-adrenergic receptors. On the other hand, stimulation of the beta-adrenergic system by the specific agonist isoproterenol diminishes the number of beta-receptors, but rapidly and reversibly increases the number of alpha receptors especially $alpha_2$ receptors at the central noradrenergic synapses.

Chemical Classification of Nerves (Fig. 17–11)

The better understanding of the mechanism of autonomic transmission and the parts played by acetylcholine, norepinephrine and epinephrine led to a new classification of nerves based on physiologic rather than anatomic findings.[18] The terms cholinergic and adrenergic are employed to describe the type of nerve ending at which the specific mediators, acetylcholine or norepinephrine, are respectively released to activate the effector organs. They are also used to refer to autonomic drugs and different types of effector cells and responses (Table 17–8).

The *cholinergic nerves* liberate acetylcholine at their terminals; the category includes postganglionic parasympathetic fibers, all the preganglionic nerves whether sympathetic or parasympathetic, the splanchnic preganglionic fibers to the adrenal medulla, the "sympathetic" fibers to sweat glands and the somatic motor nerves to the skeletal muscles.

The *adrenergic nerves* release norepinephrine or epinephrine at their endings, and consist exclusively of postganglionic sympathetic fibers.

The chemical classification of nerves explains some confusing data collected in experiments of nerve regener-

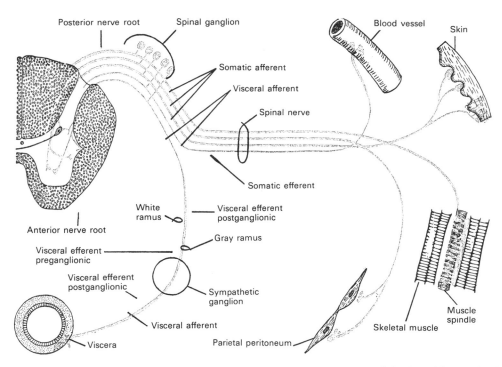

Fig. 17–11. Structure of a typical spinal nerve. Gray rami join all the spinal nerves, while the white rami arise only from the thoracic and first two lumbar segments. The gray ramus usually leaves the trunk at a ganglion near the same level as the spinal nerve, and in the thoracic and lumbar regions, where there are both gray and white rami, it is regularly proximal to the white. From Clemente, C.D.: Gray's Anatomy, 30th Ed. Philadelphia, Lea & Febiger, 1987.

ation. It became logical why the cross-suturing of adrenergic to cholinergic fibers would not result in functional activity to the effector organ. Only fibers of the same category (whether cholinergic or adrenergic) can be interchanged and establish a functional union to the effector organ; the two systems are exclusive.

Dopamine[23,64]

This is an endogenous catecholamine and is the first catecholamine formed in the synthesis of norepinephrine and epinephrine. In this regard it is a precursor of norepinephrine but has distinct pharmacologic actions on vascular beds, as a neurotransmitter in the brain and on endocrine organs. Biochemical techniques using specific ligands and the effects of agonist drugs have identified specific dopamine receptors and revealed an effect on neural adenyl cyclase. Two subtypes of dopamine receptors have been determined namely. DA_1 and DA_2.[64] Activation of D_1 receptors stimulates formation of adenyl cyclase, while activation of D_2 receptors results in inhibition of adenyl cyclase. and raises the cellular concentration of AMP (Table 17-9).

Activation of D_1 receptors occurs only at low concentrations of dopamine and at low rates of dopamine infusion such as 0.5 to 2.0 $\mu g/kg^{-1}/min^{-1}$, while larger doses activate $beta_1$ and alpha adrenergic receptors. All compounds activating the D_1 receptor system and subsequent beta and alpha receptors have a strict chemical structure with two OH groups occupying positions 3- and 4- of the benzene ring (Fig. 17-12).

Effects of low doses of dopamine are on the receptors of the vascular beds especially the renal as well as the mesenteric and coronary vasculature. Doses less than 3.0 $\mu g/kg^{-1}/min^{-1}$ produce vasodilatation and at these doses the secretion of aldosterone is inhibited to further promote vasodilatation with a significant redistribution of blood flow to the kidney.[66]

Effects of slightly higher concentrations of dopamine achieved by infusion doses between 3 to 10 $\mu g/kg^{-1}/min^{-1}$ exert a positive inotropic effect via $beta_1$ receptors. This dose rate also causes a release of norepinephrine from peripheral nerves.

High concentrations achieved by doses between 10 to 20 $\mu g/kg^{-1}/min^{-1}$ activate alpha adrenergic receptors and produce vasoconstriction. Infusion doses above these rates have an inhibitory action at the carotid body and thereby interfere with the ventilatory response to hypoxemia; the release of insulin is also inhibited.[67]

Location of DA_2 Receptors

These receptors are located on postganglionic fibers but specifically at the prejunctional site of the sympathetic nerve ending. When activated norepinephrine release from storage granules in the prejunctional nerve terminal is inhibited and sympathetic activity is minimized.

DA_2 receptors are also located in the brain and on endocrine tissues.[68] Particular sites are at the emetic center of the area postrema (CRTZ.); the anterior lobe of the pituitay gland. The parathyroid gland is endowed with these receptors.[69]

Table 17–8. Responses of Effector Organs to Autonomic Nerve Impulses

Effector Organs	Adrenergic Impulses[1]		Cholinergic Impulses[1]
	Receptor Type[2]	Responses[3]	Responses[3]
Eye			
Radial muscle, iris	α_1	Contraction (mydriasis) ++	—
Sphincter muscle, iris		—	Contraction (miosis) +++
Ciliary muscle	β_2	Relaxation for far vision +	Contraction for near vision +++
Heart[4]			
SA node	β_1	Increase in heart rate ++	Decrease in heart rate; vagal arrest +++
Atria	β_1	Increase in contractility and conduction velocity ++	Decrease in contractility, and shortened AP duration ++
AV node	β_1	Increase in automaticity and conduction velocity ++	Decrease in conduction velocity; AV block +++
His-Purkinje system	β_1	Increase in automaticity and conduction velocity +++	Little effect
Ventricles	β_1	Increase in contractility, conduction velocity, automaticity, and rate of idioventricular pacemakers +++	Slight decrease in contractility claimed by some
Arterioles			
Coronary	$\alpha_1, \alpha_2; \beta_2$	Constriction +; dilatation[5] ++	Constriction +
Skin and mucosa	α_1, α_2	Constriction +++	Dilatation[6]
Skeletal muscle	$\alpha; \beta_2$	Constriction ++; dilatation[5,7] ++	Dilatation[8] +
Cerebral	α_1	Constriction (slight)	Dilatation[6]
Pulmonary	$\alpha_1; \beta_2$	Constriction +; dilatation[5]	Dilatation[6]
Abdominal viscera	$\alpha_1; \beta_2$	Constriction +++; dilatation[7] +	—
Salivary glands	α_1, α_2	Constriction +++	Dilatation ++
Renal	$\alpha_1, \alpha_2; \beta_1, \beta_2$	Constriction +++; dilatation[7] +	—
Veins (Systemic)	$\alpha_1; \beta_2$	Constriction ++; dilatation ++	—
Lung			
Tracheal and bronchial muscle	β_2	Relaxation +	Contraction ++
Bronchial glands	$\alpha_1; \beta_2$	Decreased secretion; increased secretion	Stimulation +++
Stomach			
Motility and tone	$\alpha_1, \alpha_2; \beta_2$	Decrease (usually)[9] +	Increase +++
Sphincters	α_1	Contraction (usually) +	Relaxation (usually) +
Secretion		Inhibition (?)	Stimulation +++
Intestine			
Motility and tone	$\alpha_1, \alpha_2; \beta_1, \beta_2$	Decrease[9] +	Increase +++
Sphincters	α_1	Contraction (usually) +	Relaxation (usually) +
Secretion	α_2	Inhibition	Stimulation ++
Gallbladder and Ducts	β_2	Relaxation +	Contraction +
Kidney			
Renin secretion	$\alpha_1; \beta_1$	Decrease +; increase ++	—
Urinary Bladder			
Detrusor	β_2	Relaxation (usually) +	Contraction +++
Trigone and sphincter	α_1	Contraction ++	Relaxation ++
Ureter			
Motility and tone	α_1	Increase	Increase (?)
Uterus	$\alpha_1; \beta_2$	Pregnant; contraction (α_1); relaxation (β_2). Nonpregnant: relaxation (β_2)	Variable[10]
Sex Organs, Male	α_1	Ejaculation +++	Erection +++

(continued)

Table 17–8. Responses of Effector Organs to Autonomic Nerve Impulses (*Continued*)

Skin			
Pilomotor muscles	α_1	Contraction ++	—
Sweat glands	α_1	Localized secretion[11] +	Generalized secretion +++
Spleen Capsule	α_1; β_2	Contraction +++; relaxation +	—
Adrenal Medulla		—	Secretion of epinephrine and norepinephrine (nicotinic effect)
Skeletal Muscle	β_2	Increased contractility; glycogenolysis; K^+ uptake	—
Liver	α; β_2	Glycogenolysis and gluconeogenesis[12] +++	—
Pancreas			
Acini	α	Decreased secretion +	Secretion ++
Islets (β cells)	α_2	Decreased secretion +++	—
	β_2	Increased secretion +	—
Fat Cells	α; β_1 (β_3)	Lipolysis[12] +++	—
Salivary Glands	α_1	Potassium and water secretion +	Potassium and water secretion +++
	β	Amylase secretion +	
Lacrimal Glands	α	Secretion +	Secretion +++
Nasopharyngeal Glands		—	Secretion ++
Pineal Gland	β	Melatonin synthesis	—
Posterior Pituitary	β_1	Antidiuretic hormone secretion	—

[1]The anatomical classes of adrenergic and cholinergic nerve fibers are described. A dash signifies no known functional innervation. Subtypes of muscarinic cholinergic receptors are not indicated; most glands and smooth muscles appear to contain multiple subtypes, while the heart largely contains M_2 cholinergic receptors.

[2]Where a designation of subtype is not provided, the nature of the subtype has not been determined unequivocally.

[3]Responses are designated 1+ to 3+ to provide an approximate indication of the importance of adrenergic and cholinergic nerve activity in the control of the various organs and functions listed.

[4]Heart also contains α_1 and β_2 receptors, but they are less important for physiological responses.

[5]Dilatation predominates *in situ* due to metabolic autoregulatory phenomena.

[6]Cholinergic vasodilatation at these sites is of questionable physiological significance.

[7]Over the usual concentration range of physiologically released, circulating epinephrine, β-receptor response (vasodilatation) predominates in blood vessels of skeletal muscle and liver; α-receptor response (vasoconstriction), in blood vessels of other abdominal viscera. The renal and mesenteric vessels also contain specific dopaminergic receptors, activation of which causes dilatation (see review by Goldberg et al., 1978).

[8]Sympathetic cholinergic system causes vasodilatation in skeletal muscle, but this is not involved in most physiological responses.

[9]It has been proposed that adrenergic fibers terminate at inhibitory β receptors on smooth muscle fibers, and at inhibitory α receptors on parasympathetic cholinergic (excitatory) ganglion cells of Auerbach's plexus.

[10]Depends on stage of menstrual cycle, amount of circulating estrogen and progesterone, and other factors.

[11]Palms of hands and some other sites ("adrenergic sweating").

[12]There is significant variation among species in the type of receptor that mediates certain metabolic responses; α and β responses have not been determined in man. A β_3 receptor has been cloned and may mediate responses in fat cells in some species.

Modified from Goodman and Gilman's *The Pharmacological Basis of Therapeutics*, A. G. Gilman, T. W. Rall, A. S. Nies, P. Taylor, Editors. Eighth Edition, Pergamon Press, Elmsford, New York, 1990.

Table 17–9. Characteristics of Subtypes of Dopamine Receptors*

Receptor	Agonists	Antagonists	Tissue	Responses	Molecular Mechanisms[1]
Dopamine-1	Dopamine	Droperidol	Blood vessels	Dilation	Activation of adenylyl cyclase
Postjunctional vascular effector cell	Fenaldopam		Renal Mesenteric Coronary	Increased blood flow	
Dopamine-2	Dopamine	Domperidone	CNS Pituitary	Inhibition of norepinephrine release	Inhibition of adenylyl cyclase; activation of K^+ channels
Postganglionic (presynaptic) sympathetic nerve ending	Bromcriptine Dopa (oral) Ergot	Metoclopramide	CRTZ Parathyroid		

Information derived principally from Goldberg, L. I. and Rajfer, E. J.: Dopamine receptor applications in clinical cardiology. *Circulation*, *72*:245, 1985.

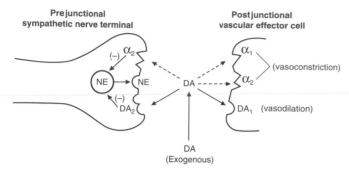

Fig. 17–12. Location of DA_1 receptors, α_1- and α_2-adrenoceptors on postganglionic vascular effector cells, and DA_2 receptors and α_2-adrenoceptors on the prejunctional sympathetic nerve terminal. When dopamine is administered, activation of DA_1 receptors causes vasodilation and activation of DA_2 receptors causes inhibition of norepinephrine (NE) release from storage granules. A larger dose of dopamine activates α_1- and α_2-adrenoceptors on the postjunctional effector cells to cause vasoconstriction and on α_2-adrenoceptors on the prejunctional sympathetic terminal to inhibit release of norepinephrine. Norepinephrine released from the prejunctional sympathetic terminal also acts on α_1- and α_2-adrenoceptors. Redrawn from Goldberg, L. I., Rajfer, E. J.: Dopamine receptor applications in clinical cardiology. Circulation *72*:245-248, 1985.

Significant stores of dopamine are found in the neural cells of the basal ganglia. Catecholamine metabolism occurs at the substantia nigra and passes to the corpus striatum. Dopamine receptors are present on the postsynaptic sites of the striatial neurones. When there is a critical reduction in dopamine synthesis due to degeneration of these nerves a Parkinsonian syndrome develops. In an attempt to ameliorate the condition there is a proliferation of dopamine receptors and an increased production of dopamine in surviving neurones.[70]

PHARMACOLOGIC CONSIDERATIONS

Definitions[23]

The drugs that act on the autonomic nervous system either stimulate or depress the response to the physiological mediators. According to their activity they are grouped as sympathetic and parasympathetic stimulants (-mimetic) or depressants (-lytic). Any drug that reproduces the same responses seen after stimulation of the nerve are known as "mimetic" agents—they mimic the natural response. These drugs may directly affect the receptor or affect the neurotransmitter thereby indirectly altering autonomic responses.

Any drug that blocks the responses ordinarily seen on stimulation of a nerve have a "lytic" effect. This may be direct or indirect. Any drug which influences the activity of an enzyme system connected with the removal of a mediator will interfere with the nerve transmission and will exhibit a "lytic" effect.

It must also be recalled that skeletal muscle endplates and autonomic ganglia do respond to some autonomic drugs, and that acetylcholine, nicotine, and anticholinesterases in small doses are excitatory, whereas in large doses they are depressants of ganglionic and myoneural transmission.

Specificity of Sympathomimetic Amines

Agents acting on distinct receptor sites clearly will cause specific responses. The excitatory or inhibitory activity of these various amines can range from pure alpha, combined alpha and beta, dual $beta_1$-$beta_2$ to pure $beta_2$.

Acetylcholine injected into the body acts directly on parasympathetic autonomic effector organs, ganglia and skeletal muscle. The action on smooth muscle, cardiac muscle and exocrine glands (visceral autonomic effector organs) is described as "muscarinic" because the alkaloid muscarine simulates these effects of parasympathetic stimulation. The action on ganglia and skeletal muscle is described as "nicotinic." Acetylcholine, as well as the alkaloid nicotine, in low concentrations stimulates these structures (depolarization of the postsynaptic membrane), whereas in large doses paralyzes them (persistent depolarization) (Fig. 17–13).

The nicotinic action of acetylcholine is blocked by nicotine itself (especially in ganglia) and by curare (especially in skeletal muscle). Nicotine causes persistent depolarization of the postsynaptic membrane; and curare competes with acetylcholine for the muscle end-plate receptors. The muscarinic action of acetylcholine is selectively blocked by atropine and related to alkaloids. They attach themselves to postganglionic receptors and thus prevent acetylcholine from interacting.

Sensitization to Amines

The removal of the nerve fibers to an effector organ sensitizes the effector cells to the action of autonomic drugs. When adrenergic postganglionic fibers are cut, the effector cells become more sensitive to both stimulation and depression by autonomic drugs. A classic example of this phenomenon is the "paradoxical pupillary reaction" described by Langendorff[57] in 1900: sympathetically denervated pupils become widely dilated under conditions of sympatho-adrenal discharge. Cholinergic structures also exhibit an increased responsiveness when deprived of their nerve supply.

Section of preganglionic fibers also causes an increased sensitivity of the ganglion cells to acetylcholine; at the

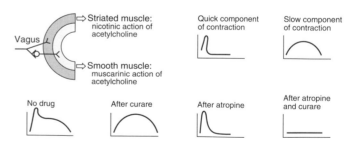

Fig. 17–13. Schematic representation of the nicotinic and muscarinic actions of acetylcholine. The two muscle coats of the intestinal wall of the tench are shown in the upper left diagram. The types of response elicited by vagal stimulation before and after administration of autonomic blocking agents are illustrated. From Goodman and Gilman: The Pharmacologic Basis of Therapeutics, Macmillan Co.

same time, the structures innervated by postganglionic fibers of a denervated ganglion show an increased responsiveness. This sensitization, however, is less marked than that caused by postganglionic denervation.

Nerve degeneration will similarly increase the response of skeletal muscle to acetylcholine. The myoneural junction and the ganglia exhibit many similitudes: they both receive medullated innervation, they have the same mediator—acetylcholine; they are affected by the same blocking agents—nicotine and curare; and each nerve supplies many effectors—1:20 or more postganglionic fibers and 1:20 or more muscle fibers.

There are certain drugs, which, like denervation, are capable of sensitizing effector cells to the action of the mediators. The ability of cocaine to potentiate the effects of norepinephrine on certain sympathetically innervated effector organs is well known since 1910.[58]

Many hypotheses have been advanced to explain the supersensitivity of effector cells under certain conditions; none has survived pharmacological and physiological testing. The current explanation connects supersensitivity with an increased permeability of the membrane or of the transfer sites to the mediators.[30,59]

Mechanisms of Drug Action

Drugs acting at neuroeffector junctions either increase or decrease the amount of the chemical neurotransmitter. Taking into consideration the neurotransmission system affected, drugs may be classified as adrenergic stimulants or adrenergic blockers (inhibitors). Aspects of cholinergic drug action will be described elsewhere and attention devoted to adrenergic drug activity (Table 17-4).

Drugs that act at adrenergic sites and modify the neurotransmitter norepinephrine levels are abundant. Certain drugs may increase the adrenergic response by increasing the release, or by increasing the receptivity of the transmitter. Other drugs depress the adrenergic response by depleting the transmitter, by decreasing its synthesis, by preventing its release, and by diminishing or blocking the receptivity of the receptor cell.

Increased Adrenergic Action

In 1910, O. Loewi[14] demonstrated that cocaine potentiates the effects of many sympathetically innervated effector organs. Axelrod, in 1960, showed that cocaine potentiates norepinephrine action and may even produce psychosis by its central action on central adrenergic or dopaminergic systems.[33] When administered in the experimental circumstances in the presence of radioactive norepinephrine, the uptake by the sympathetic nerve of the norepinephrine is inhibited and larger amounts are left to react with effector cells. Imipramine has the same effect and acts in the same manner.

Amphetamine stimulates noradrenergic nerves in two ways, by inhibiting uptake of norepinephrine and by increasing norepinephrine release. Large doses lead to psychosis manifested by repetitive and compulsive behavior and hallucinations.

MAO inhibitors prevent the breakdown of norepinephrine and permit a larger amount to act.[71]

Decreased Adrenergic Action

Reserpine releases norepinephrine and depletes the stores of adrenergic nerves. At the same time it inhibits recapture and the free norepinephrine is destroyed. This is the basis of its antihypertensive effect and of its depression of alpha-adrenergic effects.

Chlorpromazine among the phenothiazines is exemplary in that it significantly affects norepinephrine neurotransmission. This drug blocks the adrenergic as well as the dopaminergic receptors. Peripherally a norepinephrine-receptor interaction is prevented. At the same time there is an increased formation of catecholamines in adrenergic nerves and in the brain. The ability to block dopamine receptors is the basis of its antipsychotic effect and the capability of different drugs to block parallels their capacity to achieve schizophrenic symptoms.

An interesting mechanism is involved in the administration of "fake transmitters." Certain drugs such as alpha-methyl-dopa act as precursors and are transformed in the nerves into substances that resemble norepinephrine. These are stored and released along with norepinephrine and dilute the norepinephrine effect. They are also less potent in their action.

Role of Prostaglandins[72]

These naturally occuring substances are derived from essential fatty acids and are found in all tissues of the body. They are modulators of the ANS. They are synthetized by an enzyme synthetase from linolenic and arachidonic acid. There are no tissue stores and the plasma half-life is short (less than 3 minutes) and 90% degradation occurs in one passage through the liver and lungs. Physiologic action is widespread at the cellular level and appears to involve the regulation of cyclic AMP and cyclic GMP. Prostaglandins modify both sympathetic and parasympathetic neurotransmission and have antiarrhythmic properties. Prostaglandin PGE_1 modulates release of norepinephrine, but does not affect either synthesis or reuptake.[72] PGF_2-alpha does not have this effect. However, both PG groups have antiarrhythmic properties.[73]

Nonsteroidal anti-inflammatory agents such as indomethacin and aspirin inhibit PG synthesis; a greater release of norepinephrine may then ensue. Such agents might sensitize the heart to induced arrhythmias, but experimental studies do not support this hypothesis.[74]

Central Neurotransmission[75]

Advanced methodology for the study of catecholamines has elucidated brain chemical transmission and control.

Two main nerve tracts containing norepinephrine have been identified, known as the dorsal and ventral pathway. The cell bodies of these tracts are located in the lower brain stem levels in the area called the locus ceruleus or "blue place." These tracts extend to many parts including: (1) the cerebellum; (2) the hypothalamus; (3) the brain stem; and (4) the cortex.

The ventral tract appears to innervate in particular the hypothalamus and is concerned with visceral functions.

The dorsal tract neurons extend to the cerebellum and the cerebral cortex and are concerned with fine coordination of movement, alertness of the RAS and emotional responses of the limbic system.

Dopaminergic nerves are located in the brain stem at the substantia nigra. Axons course through the brain stem to the caudate nucleus which is concerned with the regulation of skeletal muscle movement.

In 1959, Carlsson[76] observed that reserpine given to rats reduced the dopamine content of the caudate nucleus and produced tremors; the administration of dopa that readily penetrated the blood-brain barrier prevents these tremors. It was soon determined that the dopamine brain content was low in patients who died of Parkinson's disease.[77]

Cotzias in 1960 treated Parkinsonian patients with l-dopa and found that the symptoms were effectively relieved.[70]

REFERENCES

1. White, J. C., Smithwick, R. H., Simeone, F. A.: The Autonomic Nervous System: Anatomy, Physiology and Surgical Application, 3rd ed. New York, The Macmillan Co., 1953.
2. Castiglioni, A.: A History of Medicine. Alfred A. Knopf Publishers, New York, 1941.
3. Bernard, C.: Lecons sur le phenomenes de la vie Communs aux animaux et aux vegetaux. (2 Vols.) Paris, J.B. Bailliere, 1878-1879.
4. Bernard, C.: Researches experimentales sur les fonctiones du nerf spinal. Memoires Vol X 1851. In An Introduction to the Study of Experimental Medicine. Henry Schuman Inc., New York 1949.
5. Fink, R. B.: Translation of Lectures on the Phenomena of Life by Claude Bernard. Published by Wood Library Museum an affiliate of the American Society of Anesthesiology (with concurrence of J.B. Baillere, Paris) 1989.
6. Langley, J. N.: On the reactions of cells and nerve endings to certain poisons, chiefly as regards the reaction of striated muscles to nicotine and curare. J Physiol 33:374, 1905.
7. Ranson, S. W., Clark, S. L.: The Anatomy of the Nervous System. 10th Ed. Philadelphia, W.B. Saunders Co., 1959.
8. Sherrington, C.: The Integrative Action of the Nervous System. Yale University Press 1947 Edition New Haven. First Edition Published by Charles Scribner's Sons, 1906.
9. Lawson, N. W., Wallfisch, H. K.: Cardiovascular pharmacology: A new look at the pressors. In: Stoelting R. K., Barash P. G., Gallagher T. J., eds. Advances in Anesthesia. Chicago, Year Book Medical Publishers 1986; 3:195-270.
10. Cannon, W. B.: The Wisdom of the Body. New York, W.W. Norton & Co., 1932.
11. Elliot, T. R.: The action of adrenalin. J Physiol 32:401, 1905.
12. Dixon, W. E.: On the mode of action of drugs. Med Mag 16:454, 1907.
13. Dale, H. H.: The action of certain esters and ethers of choline and their relation to muscarine. J Pharmacol Exp Therap 6:147, 1914.
14. Loewi, O.: Uber humorale ubertroybarkeit der herznervenwirkung. Arch fd ges Physiol 189:239, 1921.
15. Dale, H. H., Feldberg, W.: Chemical transmitter of vagus effect to stomach. J Physiol 81:320, 1934.
16. Cannon W. B., Rosenbleuth, A.: Studies on conditions of activity in endocrine organs; sympathin e and sympathin I. Am J Physiol 104:557, 1933.
17. von Euler, U. S.: A specific sympathomimetic ergone in adrenergic nerve fibers (sympathin) and its relation to adrenaline and nor-adrenaline. Acta Physiol Scand 12:73, 1946.
18. Wurtman, R. J.: Catecholamines. N Engl J Med 273:637, 695, 746, 1965.
19. Del Castillo, J., Katz, B.: Biochemical aspects of neuromuscular transmission. Prog Biophys Chem 6:121, 1956.
20. Eccles, J. C.: The Physiology of the Synapse. Oxford, Academic Press, 1964.
21. Katz, B., Miledi, R.: A study of spontaneous miniature potentials in spinal motoneurons. J Physiol 168:389, 1963.
22. Ritchie, A. K., Goldberg, A. M.: Vesicular and synaptoplasmic synthesis of acetylcholine. Science 169:489, 1970.
23. Gilman, A. G., et al (eds.): Goodman and Gilman's The Pharmacological Basis of Therapeutics, 8th Ed. New York, Mcgraw-Hill 1990.
24. Mendez, B., Martial, J. A., et al.: Cell free synthesis of acetylcholine receptor polypeptides. Science 209:695-697, 1980.
25. Cutting, W.: Handbook of Pharmacology: Appleton-Century-Crofts 7th Ed. Norwalk, Conn. 1984.
26. Symposium on neuro-humoral transmission (various authors). Pharmacol Rev 6:1, 1954.
27. Ram, C. V. S., Kaplan, N. M.: Alpha- and beta-receptor blocking drugs in the treatment of hypertension. In: Harvey W. P., et al., eds. Current Problems in Cardiology. Chicago, Year Book Medical Publishers 1979.
28. Koelle, G.: A new general concept of the neurohumoral functions of acetylcholine and acetylcholinesterase. J Pharm Pharmacol 14:65, 1962.
29. Dale, H. H., Feldberg, W.: Chemical transmission of secretory impulses to sweat glands of cat. J Physiol 81:320, 1934.
30. Furchgott, R. F., Kirpekar, S. M., Rieker, M., Schwab, A.: Actions and interactions of norepinephrine, tyramine and cocaine on aortic strips of rabbit and left stria of guinea pig and cat (the cocaine paradox). J Pharmacol Exp Therap 142:39, 1963.
31. von Euler, U. S.: Synthesis, uptake and storage of catecholamines in adrenergic nerves. The effects of drugs. In, Catecholamines. (Blaschko, H., and Muscholl, E., eds.) Handbuch der Experimentellen Pharmakologie, Vol. 33. Springer-Verlag, Berlin, 1972, pp. 186-230.
32. Langer S. Z.: Presynaptic regulation of catecholamine release. Biochem Pharmacol 23:1793, 1974.
33. Axelrod, J.: The formation, metabolism, uptake, and release of noradrenaline and adrenaline. In The Clinical Chemistry of Monoamines. Amsterdam, Elsevier, 1963, pp. 5-18.
34. Robinson, G. A., Butcher, R. W., Sutherland, E. W.: The Catecholamines. In Biochemical Actions of Hormones. Litwack, G., ed. Vol. II, pp. 81-111, 1972.
35. Weiner, N.: Tyrosine-3-monooxygenase (tyrosine hydroxylase). In Aromatic Amino Acid Hydroxylases: Biochemical and Physiological Aspects. Youdim, M.B.H., ed. John Wiley & Sons, Inc., New York, 1979b, pp. 141-190.
36. Weiner, N.: Control of the biosynthesis of adrenal catecholamines by the adrenal medulla. In. Adrenal Gland, Vol. 6. Sect. 7, Endocrinology. Handbook of Physiology. Blaschko, H., Sayers, G., Smith, A.D., eds. American Physiological Society, Washington, D.C. 1975, pp. 357-366.
37. Winkler, H., Fischer-Colbrie, F., Weber, A.: Molecular organization of vesicles storing transmitter: chromaffin vesicles as a model. In Chemical Neurotransmission—75 Years. Stjärne, L., Hedqvist, P., Lagercrantz, H., Wennmalm, Å., eds. Academic Press. Ltd., London, 1981, pp. 57-68.
38. Axelrod, J.: Noradrenaline: fate and control of its biosynthesis. Science 1973, 598-606, 1971.

39. Axelrod, J.: Multiple factors regulating the release of norepinephrine consequent to nerve stimulation. Fed Proc 38:2193-2202, 1979a.

40. Iverson L. L.: The catecholamines: biosynthesis (plasma levels). Nature (London) 214:8-14, 1967.

41. Blaschko, H.: Catecholamine biosynthesis. Brain Med Bull 29:105-109, 1973.

42. von Euler, U. S.: Quantitation of stress by catecholamine analysis. Clin Pharmacol Therap 5:398, 1964.

43. Robertson, D., Frolich, J. C., et al.: Effects of caffeine on plasma renin activity, catecholamines and blood pressure. N Engl J Med 298:181, 1978.

44. Elmajian, F., Hope, J. M., Lampson, E. T.: Excretion of epinephrine and norepinephrine in various emotional states. J Clin Endocrinol 17:608, 1957.

45. Ahlquist, R. P.: A study of the adrenotropic receptors. Am J Physiol 153:586, 1948.

46. Ahlquist, R. P.: Receptors of autonomic nervous system. J Pharm Sci 55:359, 1966.

47. Hoffman, B. B., Lefkowitz, R. J.: Alpha adrenergic subtypes NEJM 302:1390, 1980.

48. Kiowski, W., Hulthen, L., Ritz, R., Buhler, F. R.: Alpha 2 adrenoreceptor mediated vasoconstriction of arteries. Clin Pharmacol Ther 34:565-569, 1983.

49. Starke, K.: Regulation of noradrenaline release by presynaptic receptor systems. Rev Physiol Biochem Pharmacol 77:1-124, 1977.

50. Engelman, E., Lipszyc, M., Gilbert, E., et al.: Effects of clonidine on anesthetic drug requirements and hemodynamic response during aortic surgery. Anesthesiology 71:178-87, 1989.

51. Watanabe, A. M.: Recent advances in knowledge about beta-adrenergic receptors: Application to clinical cardiology. J Am Coll Cardiol 1:82-105, 1983.

52. Lands, A. M., Arnold, A., McAuliff, P. P., Ludnena, F. P., Brown, T. G.: Differentiation of receptor systems activated by sympathomimetic amines. Nature 214:597, 1967.

53. Minneman, K. P., Pittman, R. N., Molinoff, P. B.: Beta-adrenergic subtypes. Properties, distribution and regulation. Ann Rev. Neurosci 4:419-460, 1981.

54. Emorine, L. J., Maurullo, S., Briendsutren, M. M., et al.: Molecular characterization of the human Beta-3 adrenergic receptor. Science 245:1118-1121, 1989.

55. Kolle, G. E.: Functional anatomy of synaptic transmission. Anesthesiology 29:643-653, 1968.

56. Kandel, E., Schwartz, J. H.: Principles of Neural Science Elsevier, New York, 1985.

57. Langendorff, O.: Die Deutung der "paradoxen" Pupillnerveiterung. Klin Monatsbl f Auzenk 38:823, 1900.

58. Frohlich, A., Loewi, O.: Uber eine Steigerung der Adrenalinem f. kindlichkeit durch Cocain. Arch Exp Path Pharmak 62:160, 1910.

59. Cannon, W. B., Rosenbleuth, A.: The Supersensitivity of Denervated Structures: A Law of Denervation. New York, The Macmillan Co., 1949.

60. Sporn, J. R., Harden, T. K., et al: B-adrenergic receptor involvement in 6-hydroxy dopamine induced supersensitivity in rat cerebral cortex. Science 194:624-625, 1978.

61. U'Prichard, D. C., Bechtel, W. D., Snyder, S. H.: Multiple apparent alpha-adrenergic binding sites in rat brain: effect of 6-hydroxy dopamine. Mol Pharmacol 16:47-60, 1979.

62. Maggi, A., U'Prichard, D. C., Enna, S. J.: beta-adrenergic regulation of alpha$_2$ adrenergic receptors in the central nervous system. Science 207:645, 1980.

63. Dale, H. H.: Pharmacology and nerve endings. Proc Roy Soc Med 28:319, 1935.

64. Goldberg, L. I., Rajfer, E. J.: Dopamine receptor applications in clinical cardiology. Circulation 72:245-248, 1985.

65. Lawson, N. W., Wallfisch, H. K.: Cardiovascular Pharmacology: A new Look at the Pressors. In Advances in Anesthesia. Stoelting, R., ed. Year Book Medical Publishers Vol 3 (195-270) 1986.

66. Lokhandwala, M. F., Barrett, R. J.: Dopamine receptor agonists in cardiovascular therapy. Drug Review Res 3:299-310, 1983.

67. Higgins, T. L., Chernow, B.: Pharmacotherapy in circulatory shock. Dis Monit 33:309-361, 1987.

68. Leff, S. E., Creese, I. Dopamine receptors re-explained. Trends Pharmacol Sci 4:463-470, 1983.

69. Berkowitz, B. A.: Dopamine and dopamine receptors as target Sites for cardiovascular drug action. Fed Proc 42:3019-3025, 1983.

70. Severn, A. M.: Parkinsonism and the anaesthetist. Br J Anaesth 61:761-770, 1988.

71. Wells, D. G., Bjorksten, A. R.: Monoamine oxidase inhibitors revisited. Can J Anaesth 36:64-74, 1989.

72. Hedqvist P: Basic mechanisms of prostaglandin action on autonomic neurotransmission. Annu Rev Pharmacol Toxicol 17:259-279, 1977.

73. Zijlstra, W. G., Brunsting, J. R., Ten Hoor, F., et al: Prostaglandins E$_1$ and cardiac arrhythmia. Eur J Pharmacol 18:392-295, 1972.

74. Pace, N. L., Ohmura, A., Wong, K. C.: Epinephrine induced arrhythmias: Effect of exogenous prostaglandins and prostaglandin synthesis inhibition during halothane-O$_2$ anesthesia in dog. Anest Anal 58:401, 1979.

75. Bjorklund, A., Lindvall, O. Catecholaminergic brain stem regulatory systems. In Handbook of Physiology, vol IV, Sect 1. Bloom, F. E., ed. American Physiological Society, Bethesda, MD, 1986;155-236.

76. Carlsson, A., Lindquist, A., Magnusson, T., et al: On the presence of hydroxytyramine in the brain. Science 127:471-474, 1958.

77. Cotzias, G. C., Papavasiliou, P. S., Gellene, R.: Modification of Parkinsonism: chronic treatment with L-dopa. N Engl J Med 280:337-345 1969.

78. Ebert, T. J.: Preoperative evaluation of the autonomic nervous system. In: Stoelting RK, Barash PG, Gallagher TJ, eds. Advances in Anesthesia. St. Louis, Mosby-Year Book, 1993;10:49-68.

Chapter 18

DYSFUNCTION OF THE AUTONOMIC NERVOUS SYSTEM

KENNETH D. CANDIDO AND VINCENT J. COLLINS

The autonomic nervous system supplies and influences virtually every organ system in the body; disorders of it may have serious implications for anesthesia and surgery. The two major divisions of the autonomic nervous system (ANS), the sympathetic (or thoracolumbar) and parasympathetic (or craniosacral) nervous systems may be involved, with wide-ranging ramifications. This chapter will focus on specific disease entities or syndromes that are associated with ANS dysfunction, or dysautonomia. In cases of secondary dysautonomias, for example, that due to diabetes mellitus, only those features of the disease process relevant to the current topic will be presented.

Autonomic dysfunction may be due to lesions in single or multiple areas of the central or peripheral nervous system, resulting in a disorder either restricted to the ANS, or one involving other neurological systems, such as occurs in the Shy-Drager syndrome. Autonomic dysfunction may arise from disease processes which affect multiple organ systems, such as systemic amyloidosis or as mentioned, diabetes mellitus, or it may be a localized process.

The clinical problems in autonomic disorders, though often due to the failure of the ANS, might also be due to an increase in ANS activity, such as in hyperhidrosis or hypertension which occur in tetanus, the Guillain-Barré syndrome, or high spinal cord lesions.

In this chapter, basic disorders with a potential for causing difficult anesthesia management will be presented. Syndromes of generalized dysautonomia but not syndromes of restricted autonomic dysfunction (e.g., reflex sympathetic dystrophy) are discussed.

BASIC NEUROANATOMIC CONSIDERATIONS

The major brain areas that regulate autonomic function are located in the hypothalamus, the midbrain (Edinger-Westfall nucleus and locus ceruleus), and in the brainstem (nucleus tractus solitarius and vagal nuclei).

The sympathetic outflow is connected with major hypothalamic nuclei in the midbrain and brain stem. From these areas it descends through the cervical spinal cord at which point axons synapse with sympathetic neurons in the intermediolateral and intermediomedial cell masses. From the thoracic and upper lumbar spinal segments, myelinated axons emerge in the white rami of ventral roots and then synapse in the paravertebral sympathetic ganglia that are situated at some distance far from the target organs. The major ganglionic transmitter is acetylcholine (ACh) (Fig. 18-1). The postganglionic fibers are

unmyelinated. They rejoin the mixed nerve via the gray rami communicantes and innervate target organs after rejoining somatic nerve trunks except for the adrenal medulla (Fig. 18-2). The adrenal medulla receives only a preganglionic supply, via synapse on chromaffin cells.

The postganglionic neurotransmitter is norepinephrine (NE), except at sweat glands, which are sympathetic—cholinergic with Ach as the transmitter substance (Fig. 18-3).

The parasympathetic nervous system outflow consists of cranial and sacral efferents, including efferents accompanying cranial nerves III, VII, IX and X. The sacral outflow supplies the genitourinary tract and bladder, the large bowel and the reproductive system. The majority of parasympathetic ganglia lie close to target organs (Fig. 18-1). Acetylcholine is the major neurotransmitter at the ganglia and at post-ganglionic sites (Fig. 18-3).

Ganglionic block at nicotinic receptors prevents both parasympathetic and sympathetic activation. Atropine acts on muscarinic receptors at postganglionic parasympathetic and sympathetic cholinergic sites.

The efferent pathways of both the sympathetic and parasympathetic components of the ANS are formed by preganglionic nerve fibers, neurons grouped together in ganglia and postganglionic fibers.

In both the sympathetic and parasympathetic nerves, there are also visceral afferent fibers with cell bodies in the dorsal root ganglia or in the inferior ganglia of the glossopharyngeal and vagus nerves.

BASIC NEUROPHYSIOLOGY

The sympathetic nervous system and parasympathetic nervous system are functionally antagonistic. Whereas Table 18-1 represents the effects of selective adrenoreceptor stimulation of the sympathetic nervous system, the parasympathetic system acts as a check and balance system on those organs and functions innervated by both segments of the ANS.

Dysautonomic states may disrupt one or both of these main divisions of the ANS, with resulting physiologic changes apparent depending upon the integrity of residual sympathetic or parasympathetic function.

Table 18-2 lists the effects of some commonly employed autonomic agents. It is not intended to be all-inclusive, and simply represents a partial list of substances which might find clinical utility for treating autonomic hyper- or hypoactivity as seen in the dysantonomias.

PREGANGLIONIC FIBER	GANGLIA	POSTGANGLIONIC FIBER	TARGET ORGAN
Parasympathetic	ACh (nicotinic)	ACh (muscarinic)	Glands Smooth Muscle Heart
Sympathetic Noradrenergic	ACh (nicotinic)	NE	Blood Vessels Heart
Sympathetic Cholinergic	ACh (nicotinic)	ACh (muscarinic)	Sweat Glands
Sympathetic to Adrenal Medulla	ACh (nicotinic)	E, NE into Bloodstream	Adrenal Medulla

Fig. 18–1. Major neurotransmitters at autonomic ganglia and postganglionic sites on target organs: ACh = acetylcholine; NE = norepinephrine; E = epinephrine.

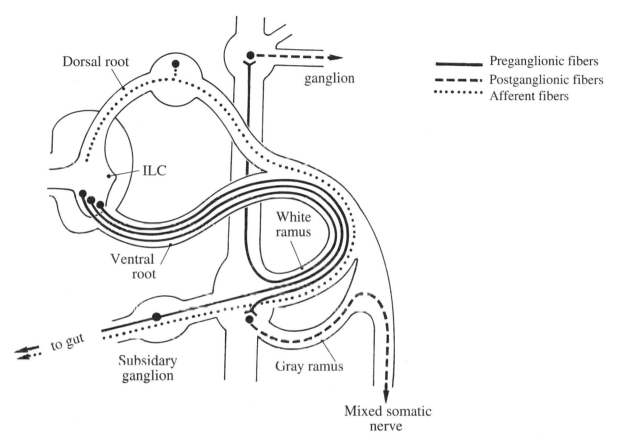

Preganglionic fibers
Postganglionic fibers
Afferent fibers

Fig. 18–2. Major peripheral pathways of the sympathetic nervous systems. ——————= preganglionic fibers; ----------------= postganglionic fibers; ··················= afferent fibers; ILC = intermediolateral cell column. Redrawn from Rosenberg, R. N., Grossman, R. G. (eds.): The Clinical Neurosciences. New York, Churchill Livingstone, 1983.

Because patients presenting for surgery and anesthesia and manifesting either a primary or secondary dysautonomic state are an enormous challenge, the anesthesiologist should have a fundamental appreciation of commonly used tests of autonomic function (Table 18–3). This will aid not only in a greater understanding of the extent of the problem, but may also guide the anesthesiologist in forming an intraoperative plan. Many of these examinations may have been done by other specialists caring for these patients, but some are so simple that a preoperative anesthesia visit would be an ideal time to verify the degree of say, orthostatic hypotension, or response to Valsalva's maneuver.

AUTONOMIC DYSFUNCTION

Classification of Dysautonomias

A generalized classification of the dysautonomias is provided (Table 18–4). The remainder of this chapter will deal with various syndromes and diseases with the anesthetic implications of each. Because of the exhaustive contents of the classification itself, it would not be possible in the scope of this work to give detailed descriptions of each syndrome causing dysautonomia. Likewise, many of the disease processes associated with altered autonomic function have wide-ranging implications for anes-

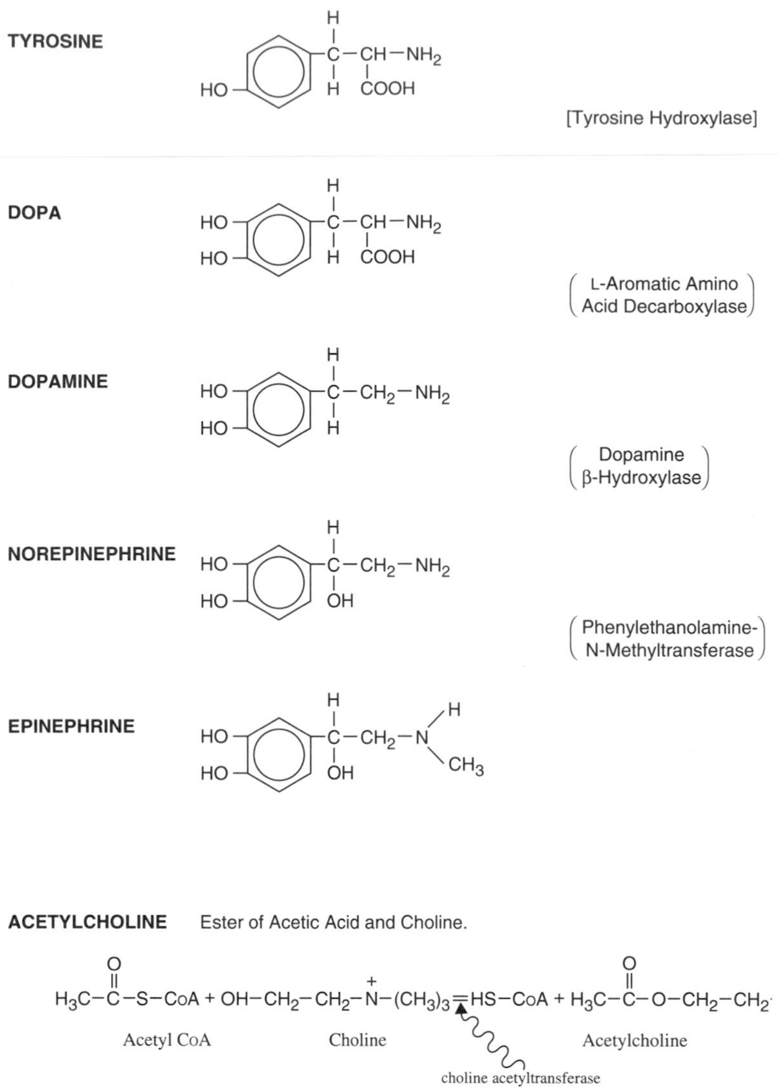

TYROSINE

DOPA

[Tyrosine Hydroxylase]

$\left(\begin{array}{c}\text{L-Aromatic Amino} \\ \text{Acid Decarboxylase}\end{array}\right)$

DOPAMINE

$\left(\begin{array}{c}\text{Dopamine} \\ \beta\text{-Hydroxylase}\end{array}\right)$

NOREPINEPHRINE

$\left(\begin{array}{c}\text{Phenylethanolamine-} \\ \text{N-Methyltransferase}\end{array}\right)$

EPINEPHRINE

ACETYLCHOLINE   Ester of Acetic Acid and Choline.

$$H_3C-\overset{O}{\overset{\|}{C}}-S-CoA + OH-CH_2-CH_2-\overset{+}{N}-(CH_3)_3 \rightleftharpoons HS-CoA + H_3C-\overset{O}{\overset{\|}{C}}-O-CH_2-CH_2$$

Acetyl CoA   Choline   Acetylcholine

choline acetyltransferase

Fig. 18–3. Chemical structure of major autonomic neurotransmitters; biosynthesis of norepinephrine and epinephrine from tyrosine. The enzyme converting norepinephrine to epinephrine is present only in the adrenal medulla and in a few neuronal pathways in the brainstem, but not in the postganglionic adrenergic nerve endings. From Iverson, L. I.: The catecholamines: biosynthesis (plasma levels). Nature *214*:8–14, 1967.

thesia and surgery aside from the autonomic component, and again, in the interest of continuity, those non-autonomic processes have generally not been included. The interested reader is urged to consult other chapters in this text for complete descriptions of anesthesia and diseases.

Diseases or syndromes associated with localized autonomic dysfunction, such as causalgia or reflex sympathetic dystrophy are not presented.

Clinical Syndromes

Shy-Drager Syndrome

The Shy-Drager syndrome is a primary dysautonomia that is associated with other neurological abnormalities. Disabling postural or orthostatic hypotension was first described by Bradbury and Eggleston in 1925[1]; and Shy and Drager in 1960 described the syndrome of autonomic failure associated with cerebellar ataxia, Parkinsonism, corticospinal and corticobulbar tract dysfunction and amyotrophy.[2] Their report was the first neuropathological examination of the syndrome.

Neuropathology

Parenchymatous degeneration of the CNS was noted, including degeneration of the intermediolateral columns, the dorsal nucleus of the vagus and other pigmented nuclei of the brainstem and cerebellar cortex. The sympathetic nervous system failure probably lies in the efferent limb of autonomic reflex arcs. There is a loss of preganglionic sympathetic cells and a depletion of substance P in the dorsal spinal cord and lateral horns, and in the CSF. The brain also has depleted norepinephrine and dopamine in areas where they normally have a high concentration.

Clinical Types

The Shy-Drager syndrome is manifested by at least three clinical subtypes:

1. Autonomic failure with mainly extrapyramidal features due to striatonigral degeneration and a loss of pigmented cells in the substantia nigra, locus ceruleus and putamen.
2. Autonomic failure with cerebellar and pyramidal

Table 18–1. Physiological Functions of Adrenoreceptors

Organ or Function	α-1 Postsynaptic	B^1 & B^2 Postsynaptic
Heart	—	Increase rate, force, automaticity (B-1)
Blood Vessels	Vasoconstriction	Vasodilation (B-2)
Bronchi	Bronchoconstriction	Bronchodilation (B-2)
Smooth Muscle		
Bladder	Contract sphincter	Relaxation
Iris	Mydriasis	—
Intestine	Relaxation	Relaxation (B2)
GI sphincters	Contraction	—
Uterus	—	Relaxation (B2)
Metabolism		
Gluconeogenesis	Promoted	—
Glycogenolysis	Promoted liver	Promoted (heart, skeletal muscle) (B2)
Lipolysis	—	Promoted (B2)
Miscellaneous		
Stimulation of α 2 presynaptic receptors $\longrightarrow$ inhibits (NE) release		
Stimulation of α 2 postsynaptic receptors $\longrightarrow$ platelet aggregation		
Stimulation of Dopamine—1 postsynaptic receptor $\longrightarrow$ vasodilation		
Stimulation of Dopamine—2 presynaptic receptors $\longrightarrow$ inhibits (NE) release		

Table 18–2. Autonomic Nervous System Drugs and Actions

Drug Type	Site of Action	Mechanism	Tissue/Organ	Result
Phenoxybenzamine	α-Adrenergic	Antagonism	Blood vessels	Vasodilatation
Phenylephrine Methoxamine	α_1-Adrenergic	Agonism	Blood vessels	Vasoconstriction
Prazocin	α_1-Adrenergic	Antagonism	Blood vessels	Vasodilatation
Yohimbine	α_2 Adrenergic	Antagonism	Blood vessels	Vasoconstriction
Clonidine; Dexmedetomidine	α_2-Adrenergic	Agonism	Blood vessels	Vasodilatation
Isoproterenol; Dobutamine	β-Adrenergic	Agonism	Heart	Increased rate and contractility
Metoprolol; Esmolol	β_1-Adrenergic	Antagonism	Heart	Decreased rate and contractility
Propranolol	β_1- and B_2 Adrenergic	Antagonism	Heart	Decreased rate and contractility
Terbutaline; Albuterol	β_2-Adrenergic	Agonism	Bronchi	Dilation
Atropine	Muscarinic, cholinergic	Antagonism	Pupil; Salivary gland; Bronchi; Heart	Mydriasis Dry mouth Dilation Tachycardia

manifestations due to atrophy of the olives, pons and cerebellum.

3. Autonomic failure with associated spinal cord gray column dysfunction.

Clinical Manifestations

The syndrome typically has onset between 40–75 years with an equal male: female incidence.

Early in the syndrome, signs and symptoms include orthostatic hypotension, worse upon arising, associated with blurred vision, dizziness on standing and fainting with walking. At this stage the multiple causes for syncope need to be reviewed. There may be genitourinary and bowel dysfunction (retention), including sexual impotence early on. Diminished sweating (sympathetic cholinergic system) and the loss of sinus arrhythmia may occur.

As the syndrome progresses, patients develop Parkinson-like features, including extrapyramidal rigidity, an atonic bladder with urinary retention, an intention tremor, ataxia, hyperactive tendon reflexes, fecal incontinence, iris atrophy, nocturia and decreased tearing and salivation (Table 18-5). Shy-Drager differs from true Parkinson's disease, however, because of its presentation with severe postural hypotension due to loss of vascular reflexes, as well as in its response to L-dopa and its prognosis.

Table 18–3. Tests of Autonomic Function

System Studied	Test	Normal Function	Autonomic Dysfunction
Cardiovascular	Head-up tilt >45°, standing (orthostatic challenge)	BP same as supine; BP diastolic falls <15 mm Hg, HR increases	Abnormal baroreceptor—vagus reflex. BP falls, no HR increase
	Sinus arrhythmia (deep breathing & HR)	HR varies >10 bpm; increase R-R interval	Abnormal baroreceptor—vagus reflex, no HR increase
	Carotid sinus massage	BP & HR fall	As above; no fall HR & BP
	Valsalva maneuver	Longest-to-shortest R-R interval, ratio normally is >1.4	Small HR change; BP drop not halted
	Atropine I.V. 1.0 mg	HR increases	Loss of vagal inhibitory influence; no change HR
	Immerse hand in ice	HR, BP both increase	Impairment of sympathetic vasoconstriction; no change HR, BP
	Measure serum NE, E from supine → erect	Increase 175–200% by position change	Minor or no increase with standing
	NE infusion 0.5 μg/min	Increase BP systolic, diastolic by <20%	Diastolic BP increases >20 mm Hg; = hypersensitivity, or BP systolic >40 mm Hg increase
	Tyramine I.V. 60–500 μg/min	Increase BP systolic >15 mm Hg at >300 μg/min	If no increase BP: severe postganglionic sympathetic damage if BP systolic increases >15 mm Hg at <300 μg/min: moderate hypersensitivity
Pupils	Local 4% cocaine; 1% hydroxyamphetamine	Pupils dilate	No pupillary dilation: reduced endogenous catecholamines
	Local 1% phenylephrine; 0.1% E	No dilation	Dilation: denervation super-sensitivity
	Local 2.5% methacholine	No constriction	Constriction: denervation supersensitivity
Sudomotor	Pilocarpine iontophoresis	Local sweating	Lack of sweating indicates a) abnormal sweat glands, or b) abnormal sudomotor fibers (sympathetic cholinergic denervation)
	Intradermal acetylcholine	Local sweating	As above
Genitourinary; rectal	Cremasteric reflex	Testicles retract with stroking skin of thigh	No testicular retraction
	Urinary sphincter electromyography	Normal 40–60 mm Hg	Reduced—less than 40 mm Hg leads to incontinence
Renin- angiotensin	Measure plasma renin activity (supine/upright)	Increases with head-up tilt	Reduced; no increase with head up tilt; aldosterone basal level also reduced

Table 18–4.   Classification of Dysautonomias

Primary

 Shy-Drager Syndrome
 Riley-Day Syndrome
 Idiopathic Orthostatic Hypotension
 Acute Dysautonomia

Secondary

 CNS Disorders
  Brain tumors
  Syringomyelia; syringobulbia
  Poliomyelitis
  Multiple sclerosis
  Tetanus
  Traumatic spinal cord transection
  Spinal tumors
  Parkinson's disease

 Peripheral Neuropathy
  Guillain-Barré syndrome
  Amyloid neuropathy
  Diabetic neuropathy
  Acute intermittent porphyria
  Tabes dorsalis
  Chronic renal failure
  Neoplasia
  HIV infection
  Autoimmune disorders

 Toxic Neuropathies
  Alcohol
  Thallium
  Arsenic
  Organic solvents
  Vincristine

 Secondary to Drugs
  Antihypertensives
  Phenothiazines
  L-Dopa
  Anesthetics

Table 18–5.   Signs and Symptoms: The Shy-Drager Syndrome[3, 4]

Cardiovascular
 Orthostatic hypotension
 Blurred vision
 Dizziness on standing
 Fainting with walking
 Loss of consciousness

Neurologic
 Intellect is intact
 Extrapyramidal rigidity
 Facial immobility
 Tremor
 Fasciculations
 Difficulty speaking, chewing, swallowing
 Stridor, apneic attacks
 Unequal pupils
 Iris atrophy
 External ocular palsies
 Nystagmus
 Wasting small hand muscles
 EMG evidence of neuropathy

Genitourinary
 Urinary incontinence
 Nocturia/polyuria at night
 Atonic bladder
 Penile impotence

Gastrointestinal
 Fecal incontinence
 Diarrhea/constipation
 Laxity of sphincters

Sudo-motor
 Heat intolerance
 Anhidrosis

Biochemical Abnormalities

Plasma norepinephrine is normal in the supine position as well as in the basal state. This is contrasted with idiopathic orthostatic hypotension, another primary dysautonomic stage, which has a low basal norepinephrine level. In Shy-Drager syndrome, norepinephrine levels fail to rise when the patient assumes an erect position. In idiopathic orthostatic hypotension detailed later on in the chapter, plasma norepinephrine levels are reduced even at rest secondary to postganglionic adrenergic failure.[5]

Clinical Course and Prognosis

The course of the Shy-Drager syndrome is steadily progressive, with death usually ensuing after 7–8 years. The usual cause of death is respiratory arrest from laryngeal obstruction due to atrophy of the vocal cord abductors, the cricoarytenoid muscles. Death may also occur from post-syncopal cerebral ischemia. Electromyography may be useful in determining which patients are suitable candidates for tracheostomy.[6]

Basic Management and Treatment

The basic management of this syndrome is detailed in Table 18–6, and the anesthetic approach is given in Table 18–7.

Anesthetic Management

The basic principles of anesthesia care for the patient with the Shy-Drager syndrome include monitoring and vigilance as well as a complete understanding of autonomic nervous system physiology and pharmacology. Regional or general anesthesia may be appropriate, depending on the nature and duration of the proposed procedure, the presence of concomitant systemic diseases and the wishes of the patient.

Intraoperative Hypotension

Because central blood volume becomes the primary determinant of blood pressure and cardiac output, obvious preloading with a balance salt-solution is of paramount importance before performing major conduction anesthesia. Of equal importance is the realization that blood pres-

Table 18–6. Basic Management of Shy-Drager Syndrome

Problem: Orthostatic Hypotension
  Physical Means
    Avoid sudden head-up position especially in A.M.
    Avoid straining during defecation
    Avoid ETOH or large carbohydrate and fat loads
    Avoid excessive heat/cold
    Use elastic stockings
    Use head-up tilt to sleep (reduces A.M. orthostasis plus
      hypertensive effects on brain)
    Use abdominal binders
  Chemical means[7]
    Salt supplementation
    Fludrocortisone (0.1 Mg p.o. TID for intravascular volume
      expansion
    Prostaglandin inhibitors (indomethacin 50 mg p.o. TID) to
      combat increased prostaglandin secretion 2° to
      decreased renin activity
    Dopamine receptor blockade (metaclopramide 30–60 mg
      p.o./day)
    Beta-blockade-propranolol
    Vasoconstrictors
      I.M. dihydroergotamine
      Ephedrine 25–50 mg p.o. TID
      Phenylephrine
      Clonidine
      Norepinephrine
      Tyramine plus MAO inhibitors
      Yohimbine, α-2 antagonists
Problem: urinary retention
  Chemical means
    Bethanechol 10 mg p.o. TID
    Desmopressin (to reduce nocturnal polyuria)

sure and cardiac output are intimately linked with depth of general anesthesia using potent inhalation agents, as well as to minute volume of controlled ventilation. Vasopressors and vasodilators must be used with extreme caution, and in dilute preparations.

Postoperative Autonomic Depression

These patients must be carefully observed in the post-anesthesia recovery unit for signs or symptoms of dysautonomia, especially related to depression of basic autonomic function that could be life-threatening.

Riley-Day Syndrome

The Riley-Day Syndrome is another primary dysautonomic syndrome. It is variably known as familial dysautonomia or hereditary sensory and autonomic neuropathy type III. The first description of the disorder was in 1949.[13] Almost all patients are Ashkenazi Jews. The disease is transmitted as an autosomal recessive with a 1:50 carrier rate among relatives of affected patients in the United States.

Neuropathology

Essentially, there is a congenital absence of autonomic and sensory ganglia manifest by neuronal depletion.[14] Although the brain and spinal cord are normal, there is denervation sensitivity of the pupils and other structures. A deficiency of neurons in the superior cervical ganglia and lateral horns of the spinal cord exists. A diminished neuronal population likewise exists in the parasympathetic sphenopalatine ganglia. Unmyelinated nerve fibers in the sural nerve have a reduced population. There is loss of small myelinated nerves with relative preservation of larger, myelinated axons. The parasympathetic ganglia are variably affected.

Clinical Manifestations

Affected babies may have a low birth weight and breech presentation. Diagnosis of postural hypotension at

Table 18–7. Anesthetic Management of Shy-Drager Syndrome[8,9,10,11,12]

Preoperative
  Detailed history and physical
  Patient reassurance
  Chest PT
  Prophylactic antibiotics
  Optimize gastric pH with cimetidine or ranitidine
  Pre-Med diazepam good (also treats dysautonomic crisis)
  Treat pre-op bradycardia with atropine (blunted response)
  Large bore intravenous access
Intraoperative
  Blood pressure sensitive to position changes, I.V. fluids. Use
    Trendelenburg and reverse to correct BP changes
  Avoid excessive decrease in cardiac output from volatiles or
    central neuraxial blockade (exaggerated hypotensive
    response)
  Avoid narcotics, especially histamine releasers (more
    sensitive)
  Avoid ganglionic blockers or neuromuscular blocking drugs
    which release histamine (curare, metubine, gallamine)
  Avoid droperidal as anti-emetic
  Use dilute direct-acting sympathometics e.g., phenylephrine
    10 µg/min—titrate or norepinephrine
  Be aware: Dopamine may be depressor, dysrhythmogenic as
    may epinephrine
  Metaraminol: not useful
  Routine monitors plus A-line; may need Swan-Ganz catheter
    for cardiac filling pressures; bladder catheter
  Treat hypertension with nitroglycerin
  Depressor effects noted with nitroprusside, isoproterenol,
    barbiturates, insulin
  Pupillary response to drugs is unreliable
  Hyperventilation causes respiratory depression
  Hypoventilation or rebreathing CO_2 will raise blood
    pressure
  Tendency to hypothermia
Postoperative
  Avoid head-up tilt suddenly
  Continue fludrocortisone in recovery room
  Watch for hypothermia, delayed respiratory depression
  Pupillary signs inadequate to assess neurologic status

birth associated with poor sucking ability, failure to thrive, unexplained fever, pneumonia and hyporeflexia are diagnostic. Repeated infections are common. Autonomic neuropathy may become more noticeable as time progresses. These patients have a constellation of signs and symptoms related to autonomic dysfunction (Table 18-8). Blood pressure lability is marked, with supine hypertension present due to elevated serum norepinephrine levels. Patients are exquisitely sensitive to sympathomimetic drugs often found in cold remedies. Faulty temperature regulation, hyperhidrosis, diminished hearing, blotchiness of the skin and emotional lability are cardinal findings. There may be a relative insensitivity to pain, while pressure and tactile senses are preserved. An absence of circumvallate and fungiform papillae on the tongue results in diminished capacity to distinguish sweet and salty tastes.[15,16]

Vomiting and poor swallowing of food with regurgitation, probably associated with elevated serum dopamine levels, is apparent. Esophageal and intestinal dilation occurs.

A lack of overflow tearing from absent corneal responses leads to corneal ulcerations. Dysautonomic crises occur after 3 years of age with elevated serum levels of dopamine and norepinephrine during attacks. These attacks are characterized by irritability, self mutilation, diaphoresis, tachycardia and hypertension, thermal instability and episodic vomiting. These children develop slowly, with stunted growth, cold hands and feet and delayed puberty. Those that survive may develop scoliosis. With advancing age, vomiting episodes decrease and adolescence is associated with fewer vasomotor crises.

However, as many as 40% have a seizure disorder. Because hypercapnia and hypoxemia are not associated with the expected increase in ventilatory effort in these individuals, coma has occurred at high altitudes.

Biochemical Abnormalities

Physiologically, serum shows reduced levels of dopamine-beta-hydroxylase (Fig. 18-3). Therefore there is no conversion of dopamine to norepinephrine. In urine,

levels of vanillymandelic acid (VMA) drop while homovanillic acid (HVA) rises, producing abnormal HVA/VMA ratios.[17]

Diagnostic Tests

The diagnosis of Riley-Day syndrome may be made by provocative tests such as intradermal injection of 0.03 to 0.05 ml of 1:1000 concentration of histamine (no pain, no axon flare) or intraocular installation of one drop of 2.5% methacholine or dilute pilocarpine (miosis results).

Symptomatic Management

There is no known treatment for this syndrome, and the longest-known survivors have reached the fifth decade of life.

Symptomatic measures of dealing with this process include anxiolytics, intravenous fluids and sedation.

Chlorpromazine, bethanecol and especially diazepam, are mainstays of treatment for dysautonomic crises. Diazepam increases GABA, which is probably effective by suppressing central dopamine release.

Anesthetic Management

The anesthetic management of patients with this syndrome is not unlike that for the Shy-Drager syndrome (Table 18-7).

Preoperative Preparation

Preoperative care includes an anesthetic visit to help allay anxiety and reduce psychological stress. Diazepam is a valuable adjunct and also is quite suitable as an induction agent, as is midazolam. Prior to surgery, chest PT and antibiotics to treat concurrent infections should be considered. Baseline SVR is low and since cardiac output is preload dependent, adequate hydration must be assured via loading of balance salt solutions using large-bore intravenous catheters. Vomiting tends to exacerbate the dehydration state and the use of invasive hemodynamic monitors, including arterial lines and pulmonary artery catheters, is indicated.

Choice of Anesthesia

Because there is a fixed chronotropy and inotropy and since significant hypotension may result from narcotics, thiobarbiturates or volatile anesthetics as well as from major conduction anesthesia, gentle implementation of anesthesia is essential. Regional or general anesthesia may be appropriate, depending upon the desires of the patient, the proposed surgery itself and the needs of the surgeon.

Sensitivity to Vasopressors

These individuals are sensitive to direct-acting vasopressors and exhibit erratic responses to indirect-acting ones. Therefore, dilute concentrations of direct-acting agents, titrated to effect, should be utilized to correct hypotensive episodes.

Table 18-8. Signs and Symptoms of Riley-Day Syndrome

Early Childhood	Later
Failure to thrive	Delayed puberty
Poor feeding	Scoliosis
Labile blood pressure	Seizure disorder
Pneumonia/recurrent infections	Muscle weakness
Hyporeflexia	Incoordination
Emotional lability	Increased salivation
Hyperhidrosis	GI motility
Stunted growth	problems
Insensitive to pain	
Orthostatic hypotension	
Recurrent vomiting	
Dysautonomic crises	
Corneal ulcerations	

Respiratory Considerations

Respiratory function should be optimized preoperatively realizing that these patients experience frequent episodes of aspiration pneumonitis and may have varying degrees of scoliosis and associated pulmonary disease. Additionally, there may be poor respiratory muscle function and a greater sensitivity to CNS depressants as both centrally and peripherally mediated responses to hypoxia and hypercarbia are diminished. Use of narcotics intraoperatively may further depress those patients undergoing general anesthesia.

General Considerations

As gastric emptying time may be reduced, it might be prudent to consider rapid-sequence induction and intubation for those patients requiring general anesthesia. Both depolarizing and nondepolarizing muscle relaxants have been used with similar consideration to histamine release as for Shy-Drager patients.

Postoperatively, delayed emergence requiring prolonged intubation, and controlled ventilation to prevent atelectasis may be necessary.[18-24]

Idiopathic Orthostatic Hypotension

The final primary dysautonomic state to be discussed is idiopathic orthostatic hypotension, also known as multisystem atrophy. By definition, there is a drop in systolic blood pressure by more than 30 mm Hg that results in near syncope when the affected individual stands. Paradoxically, in the supine position, hypertension may exist secondary to a loss of both the parasympathetic as well as the sympathetic nervous system regulation of the cardiovascular system.

There is no evidence of other neurological disorders or CNS involvement outside of the autonomic nervous system dysfunction.

Neurotransmitter and Receptor Derangement

The defect is a selective degeneration of postganglionic sympathetic neurons, as compared with the Shy-Drager syndrome where pre-ganglionic neurons are involved. There is depletion of norepinephrine from sympathetic nerve endings, and plasma levels of norepinephrine are reduced.[25] An increased number of beta-adrenoreceptors exists, and patients have exaggerated cardiovascular responses to such agonists as intravenous isoproterenol and phenylephrine.

The disease usually begins after the fifth decade of life with progression over 1 to 6 years as striatal nigral and/or olivopontocerebellar degeneration results in dysfunction of the cerebellum and extrapyramidal systems.

Clinical Manifestations

Signs and symptoms include postural hypotension with failure to develop compensatory tachycardia. Urinary and fecal incontinence with bladder, stomach and bowel atony are common. Impotence, loss of sweating, diminished salivation and tearing, Horner's syndrome and mydriasis with impaired visual accommodation, complete the clinical picture.

Neuropathology

Anatomically in this disorder there are a decreased number of neurons of the thoracic intermediolateral column, the final common pathway of autonomic outflow. Gliosis is prominent. Neurons may be reduced by up to 50%. Neuropeptide determinations in the dorsal spinal cord and lateral horns have demonstrated marked depletion of substance P and calcitonin gene-related peptide (CGRP).

The syndrome is not to be confused with orthostatic hypotension in the elderly. In this common syndrome (20% of persons older than 65 years) systolic blood pressure may fall by up to 20 mm Hg. These persons also have thermoregulatory impairment, impotence, and incontinence.

Treatment is symptomatic (Table 18-9).[28-30] Management of anesthesia in these individuals is as detailed previously for Shy-Drager syndrome, and Riley-Day syndrome (see earlier in chapter).

Secondary Dysautonomias

A host of diseases or disorders are associated with autonomic dysfunction (Table 18-4). Due to the voluminous nature of this list, it would not be possible in the course of one chapter to detail each separate condition. Therefore, selected syndromes will be mentioned with an emphasis on autonomic manifestations. Most anesthesia concerns are related to the cardiovascular, genitourinary, and gastrointestinal systems, as with the primary dysautonomias. Anesthetic management is complicated by the considerations attendant to the underlying disease process.

Parkinson's Disease

Parkinson's disease is diagnosed in about 1% of adults in the United States after the age of 50. The usual onset of the condition is between 40 to 70 years, and men are more affected than women.

The cause may be from drugs, toxins, viruses or CNS trauma.

Neurotransmitter Derangement

A relative deficiency of dopamine in the caudate nucleus and putamen results in an imbalance in inhibition

Table 18-9. Treatment Approach to Idiopathic Orthostatic Hypotension

Elastic stockings
Abdominal binders
Increase dietary salt and fluids
Fludrocortisone 0.1/mg/day up to 1.0 mg/day p.o.
NSAIDS; Indomethacin—inhibits prostaglandin-induced vasodilation.
Alpha-agonists ⎤ combination leads to unopposed alpha-
Beta-blockers ⎦ adrenergic peripheral constriction
MAO inhibitors[26]
Sub-Q dihydroergotamine plus caffeine[27]

(dopamine) and excitation (acetylcholine) as controlling influences of the basal ganglia.

Clinical Manifestations

As many as 90% of affected individuals may have autonomic dysfunction.[31,32] The most common symptom is postural dizziness (65%) as serum norepinephrine levels fail to rise with standing.[33,34] In decreasing order of frequency, other symptoms of dysautonomia, including constipation and GI dysfunction (60%), impotence or GU dysfunction (40%), diminished sweating (30%), sluggish pupillary reaction to light (30%), may occur. Unlike Shy-Drager syndrome, there is no abnormal Valsalva response[35] nor a higher basal heart rate than in normals. There is, however, a supersensitivity to intravenous pressors like norepinephrine,[36] frequent cardiac dysrhythmias and an abnormal sinus arrhythmia noted.[37] Some Parkinson's patients report dependent edema and livedo reticularis.[38] Orthostatic hypotension may be severe, especially postprandially, and may be exacerbated by levodopa.[39]

These patients frequently present for urologic, ophthalmologic, and orthopedic surgeries. Important considerations include preoperative continuance of pharmacotherapy up to and including the morning of surgery, realizing that L-dopa may produce dysrhythmias. Preoperative hypotension may be secondary to hypovolemia, norepinephrine depletion or autonomic dysfunction. Dilute direct acting vasopressors should be utilized to correct severe hypotension, such as phenylephrine.

Droperidol and other neuroleptic agents may antagonize the effects of dopamine in the basal ganglia and should be avoided.

Amyloidosis

Amyloidosis is a systemic disease associated with peripheral neuropathy. By definition, there is accumulation in tissues of various insoluble fibrillar proteins (amyloid) in quantities sufficient to produce impaired function.[10,28] (Greenfields Neuropathology.)

Of the various types of amyloidosis, familial amyloid polyneuropathy is associated with dysautonomia. It is associated with a genetic defect in chromosome 18. The disease is transmitted as an autosomal dominant trait with an equal male-to-female prevalence. It is variably named Portuguese or Andrade type amyloid, first characterized about 1939 when it was described as "foot disease," a chronic familial illness. Occasionally, it is called pseudosyringomyelia. (Alan S. Cohen, MD Boston City Hosp.)

The amyloid type is usually a transthyretin (prealbumin) molecule that has a single amino acid substitution from the parent molecule.

Clinical Manifestations

Onset of this disease is about 25 to 35 years of age, and it is slowly progressive with most deaths occurring within 10 to 15 years.

Symptoms and signs include numbness and paresthesias with pain in the lower legs and feet. There is minimal weakness, although deep tendon reflexes are blunted. A diminution of pain and thermal sense exists. Tactile, vibratory and position sense are intact. Walking is difficult and legs may be thin and appear wasted.

Autonomic dysfunction is manifest as a loss of pupillary light reflexes and miosis. Anhidrosis occurs, but most importantly from an anesthetic standpoint, orthostatic hypotension due to vasomotor paralysis may cause the same concerns as previously detailed for primary dysautonomias. Cranial nerve involvement is rare.

Impotence, and alternating diarrhea or constipation, may bring these patients to the attention of a physician.

Anesthetic Considerations

Besides orthostatic hypotension, considerations for the anesthesiologist include the possible existence of bundle branch block or AV block and cardiomegaly. Occasionally, severe amyloid heart with conduction abnormalities may pose a problem.

Patients may have severe dehydration and weight loss due to amyloid-induced malabsorption syndrome. Hepatomegaly and altered liver function may result in altered anesthetic drug metabolism. Death may occur from severe albuminuria, the nephrotic syndrome or uremia.

As there is no known cure, symptomatic treatment of the underlying problems is appropriate. Digitalis glycosides may precipitate dysrhythmias and should be avoided.

Syringomyelia

These two related conditions are chronic, slowly progressive degeneration of the spinal cord (syringomyelia) and medulla (syringobulbia).[10] Formation of an enlarged cerebrospinal fluid-filled central canal of the cervical spinal cord heralds the process. Reactive gliosis without associated acute inflammation or vascular compromise are noted. Cyst formation results from outflow obstruction of CSF from the fourth ventricle causing high CSF pressures directed into the central canal of the spinal cord.

Neuropathology

Destruction of the crossing spinothalamic tract fibers results in an asymmetrical loss of pain and temperature sensation of the upper extremities. Touch and position senses are left intact. A capelike sensory deficit over the shoulders and back results. Onset of symptoms is in the third to fourth decade of life. Later, lower motor neuron destruction causes atrophy and hyporeflexia of affected extremities. Paraspinal muscle weakness may produce scoliosis. The condition is frequently associated with spina bifida, Arnold-Chiari malformation, cervical rib, basilar impression, and platybasia. There may be paralysis of the palate, tongue and vocal cords of a loss of sensation over the face. There is no known treatment for syringomyelia/syringobulbia.

Anesthetic Considerations

These are similar to those for patients with spinal cord injury and include preparation for the management of sympathetic areflexia or autonomic hyperreflexia (Table 18-10).

Table 18–10. General Anesthetic Considerations for Syringomyelia

Preoperative
Pre-op visit and adequate pre-meds to allay anxiety.
Evaluate vocal cord function; protective airway reflexes.
PFTs for severe thoracic scoliosis; V/Q mismatch possible.

Intra-op
Monitors; A-line; possibly pulmonary artery catheter, bladder catheter, temperature probe
Prepare I.V. meds for treatment. Sympathetic areflexia or autonomic hyperreflexia
Warm rooms, I.V. fluids, circuit; bed (prone to poikilothermia)
Monitor ABGs; pulmonary function
Smooth I.V. induction (avoid coughing or bucking that raise ICP and can cause cord damage)
Muscle wasting: (impairment of corticospinal tracts of anterior horn cells at level of syrinx) depolarizers release K^+; susceptible to nondepolarizers (lower motor neuron disease)

Diabetes Mellitus

Autonomic neuropathy occurs in diabetics, primarily in patients with diabetic polyneuropathy, which is distal, symmetric and predominantly a sensory neuropathy. Diabetic lesions are found primarily affecting efferent nerves and nerve biopsies reveal predominant involvement of small myelinated and unmyelinated fibers.

Autonomic Disturbances

The most serious autonomic functions to be disturbed may involve the cardiovascular system and commonly are manifest as postural hypotension. Vasodilation or impaired vasoconstriction in the splanchnic, muscle and skin blood vessels may cause pooling of blood and diminished cardiac output in the upright position. The situation may be aggravated by dysfunction of baroreceptor reflexes. Inappropriate cardiac rate response to Valsalva's maneuver or on standing upright may signal vagal disturbances which precede disturbances of the cardiac sympathetic nerves.[40] Sinus arrhythmia is absent in affected individuals. Peripheral edema and erythema may be observed. Atrophy of skin and subcutaneous tissues with disordered sweating, from anhidrosis to reduced sweating distally in the limbs, to hyperhidrosis, may be present.[41,42]

The GI system may be involved with esophageal dysfunction, gastric atony or delayed gastric emptying, constipation or diarrhea and occasionally nocturnal fecal incontinence.

Impaired bladder function, impotence and retrograde ejaculation complete the genitourinary picture.

Anesthetic management for diabetics with dysautonomia is similar to that for the primary dysautonomias but is complicated by the pansystemic manifestations of the primary disease process. Readers should consult other chapters of this text for more detailed management plans for diabetics.

Guillain-Barré Syndrome

The Guillain-Barré syndrome, also known as acute idiopathic polyneuritis, is a rapidly progressive and occasionally fatal disorder of cell-mediated immunology but with an uncertain etiology. The annual incidence of the problem is about 0.75 to 2 cases per 100,000 population. Peripheral nerves are involved with inflammatory lesions scattered throughout the myelin sheath. Lymphocytic infiltration and macrophagic invasion produce segmental demyelination of peripheral nerves.

Neuropathology

Cranial nerves IX, and X and sympathetic nerve trunks and ganglia reveal lymphocytic infiltration and demyelination with secondary axonal degeneration. Involvement of preganglionic sympathetic fibers suggested by chromatolysis of neurons in the intermediolateral cell columns of the spinal cord produces sympathetic dysfunction.

Autonomic dysfunction

This is common and includes fluctuating and labile blood pressure, paroxysmal hypertension, orthostatic hypotension and sudden deaths. Cardiac conduction defects and persistent sinus tachycardia may be present in 50% of cases. Occasionally, atrial tachycardia, atrial fibrillation and episodes of asystole may be seen. Tachycardia that is not responsive to carotid sinus massage suggests parasympathetic hypoactivity of the vagal innervation of the heart. Other findings include hypo- or hyperhidrosis, urinary retention or incontinence (30%) and less frequently, fecal incontinence. Abnormal pupillary light reaction occurs and may interfere with clinical monitoring of autonomic drug effects. Inappropriate ADH secretion has been observed. No consistent changes in catecholamine excretion have been reported.[41]

Anesthetic Considerations

These include careful placement of invasive hemodynamic monitoring. Monitoring of respiratory or ventilatory status including arterial blood gas sampling plus monitoring of vital capacity should be undertaken. Blood pressure may be exquisitely sensitive to changes in operating room table position from flat. Dilute direct acting vasopressors and/or vasodilators may be necessary to control widely fluctuating blood pressures. Blood pressure may plummet by acute elevations of the head or using reverse Trendelenburg position, or by uncorrected blood loss or with positive airway pressure. Direct laryngoscopy and airway manipulation can produce severe hypertension. Succinylcholine should be avoided because this is a lower motor neuron disease. No unusual or abnormal responses to general or local anesthetics have been characteristic. A bladder catheter to assess urinary output is indicated. Pharyngeal muscle weakness predisposes patients to slow return of protective airway reflexes and to prolonged postoperative controlled ventilation.

Paraplegia and Quadriplegia

Spinal cord injury may be acute or chronic. Acute spinal cord transection, whether due to trauma, transverse myelitis, poliomyelitis or tumor infiltration, results in severe autonomic dysfunction related to the level of injury. Lesions above C_2 to C_4 are incompatible with survival. Lesions between T_5 and C_4 cause autonomic hypo- or hyperactivity. Below the level of the insult, flaccid paralysis with total loss of sensation results. A loss of temperature regulation and loss of spinal cord reflexes exist below the level of the lesion.

Soon after the injury a transient elevation in blood pressure is noted due to increases in systemic vascular resistance and myocardial contractility as well as the presence of dysrhythmias.[44]

Clinical Manifestations

Acute Spinal Cord Injury

In cervical spinal injury, blood pressure then falls due to interruption of spinal sympathetic tracts resulting in pooling of blood, bradycardia due to lack of competitive inhibition of the parasympathetic nervous system and a loss of the cardiac accelerator fibers from T_1 to T_4. Cardiac output may drop as compensatory vasoconstrictor mechanisms fail.[45]

In cervical spine lesions, spinal shock results after about 3 days to 6 weeks after the insult and is characterized as a generalized functional derangement of the thoracolumbar sympathetic and sacral parasympathetic neurons. There is also isolation of the spinal autonomic neurons from the hypothalamic and brain stem regulatory and reflex centers. Somatic and visceral sensation is lost and flaccid paralysis with absent deep tendon reflexes results. Retention of urine and feces may develop.

Chronic Phase

After the acute phase of cord injury resolves, a chronic stage sets in heralded by overactivity of the sympathetic nervous system and the phenomenon of autonomic hyperactivity as spinal cord reflexes return. As many as 85% of lesions occurring above T_6 may initiate this reflex,

Table 18–11.   Potential Causes of Autonomic Hyperreflexia

Cutaneous Stimuli	Visceral Stimuli
Burns	Ureteral calculus
Sores	Bladder distention
Infected toenails	Indwelling bladder catheter
Muscle spasms	Fecal retention
Bone fractures	Enemas
	Contractions in labor
	Gastric Ulcer
	Appendicitis
	Gallbladder disease
	Ejaculation
	Vaginal dilatation

Table 18–12.   Treatment Methods for Autonomic Hyperreflexia[46,47]

Afferent blockers
    Topical local anesthesia
Spinal cord blockers
    Spinal, epidural or general anesthesia
    Clonidine
    Reserpine
Sympathetic efferent
    Ganglionic blockers—trimethephan
    Nerve terminal: guanethidine
    Alpha receptors: phenoxybenzamine
Effectors
    Tri-nitroglycerine
    Sodium nitroprusside
    Hydralazine

which is produced by stimuli below the level of the spinal cord transection (Table 18–11). Lesions below T_{10} are not likely to produce autonomic hyperreflexia.

Mechanism of Autonomic Hyperreflexia

In summary, the mechanism of the autonomic hyperreflexia is denervation hypersensitivity of the sympathetic nervous system due to loss of supra-segmental control. Changes in total peripheral resistance are fundamental to the response. Increases in blood pressure are generally proportionate to the height of the lesion. Cardiac output is not significantly changed. Hypertensive crises are most common during surgery of the pelvic area. The mass response is characterized by hypertension and reflex bradycardia; piloerection, sweating and vasoconstriction occurring in areas below the lesion and flushing above the lesion. In patients with levels above T_2, tachycardia is prominent.

Management and Treatment

Agents utilized to treat autonomic hyperreflexia are listed in Table 18–12. Treatment is largely symptomatic and rehabilitative.

Anesthetic Considerations

These are related to the site of lesions and time from inciting event.[47] Cardiac reserve and output is generally diminished. Pulmonary ventilation is affected by weakened musculature. Above T_6 lesions, ventilation should be assisted or controlled to prevent alveolar hypoventilation. Because of the tendency to vasodilatation in areas above the cord lesion, there is often significant nasal congestion. Oropharyngeal secretions are greater than normal. With impaired cough mechanisms, aspiration and atelectasis are frequent problems. In quadriplegics, vital capacity may be reduced by 50%. ERV is diminished as is TLC and FEV_1. Expiratory force is reduced more than inspiratory force. Patients are acutely sensitive to changes in position. Sitting upright has an adverse effect on ventilation due to flaccidity of abdominal muscles. Uncontrolled muscle spasm due to spontaneous segmental reflex action may be present at 2 to 4 weeks of injury. Temperature control is abnormal, and patients are prone to hypothermia due to conductive heat loss in cool environments.

Preoperative Consideration

Preoperative medications should include anticholinergics to prevent bradycardia and control secretions. CNS depressants should be avoided, when possible. In chronic spinals, skin is fragile and bruising is frequent. Decubitus ulcers and chronic skin infections are common. Osteoporosis and fracture-dislocations may easily be produced. Positioning must be carefully done, and abrupt head-up positioning from flat must be avoided. Muscle spasms may interfere with proper positioning.

Administration of Anesthesia

Prevention of autonomic hyperreflexia is of paramount importance and can be undertaken using general or conduction anesthesia. Careful surgical manipulation is essential to prevent this dreaded complication.[49-53]

Large bore intravenous access must be assured and invasive hemodynamic monitoring including arterial lines and pulmonary artery catheters is indicated.

Dilute direct acting inotropes and vasopressors should be readily available when poor tissue perfusion results despite adequate fluid therapy. Isoproterenol is the pressor of choice.

Although nondepolarizing muscle relaxants may be used for general anesthesia cases, depolarizers are contraindicated due to the massive outpouring of potassium with hyperkalemia. This response is especially intense in the first 2-3 weeks from insult, but may continue for up to 12 weeks or even several months in paraplegics.

Endotracheal suctioning may produce bradycardia and cardiac arrest in quadriplegics due to unopposed vagal efferent activity. Great care is needed to manage the airway in these individuals.

Miscellaneous Dysautonomias

Many other syndromes or disease states can produce generalized dysautonomia. Porphyria, botulism, chronic renal failure, alcoholic neuropathy, neuritic beri beri, Fabry disease and paraneoplastic neuropathy or malignancy have all be associated with autonomic dysfunction.

A syndrome known as acute autonomic neuropathy has been described in a handful of cases over the past twenty years.[54] The etiology of the syndrome is unknown. High titers of Epstein-Barr virus have occasionally been found.[55] Course of the neuropathy is slowly progressive until a plateau is reached, after which resolution occurs over a period of several weeks. The clinical picture is not unlike previously described primary dysautonomias. Orthostatic hypotension, nausea and vomiting, constipation or diarrhea, bladder atony, impotence, anhidrosis, disorders of lacrimation and salivation and abnormal pupillary responses complete the physical findings.[56,57] EMG and nerve biopsies, conduction velocities, and CSF may all be normal.[58]

Anesthetic considerations are as for the primary dysautonomias.

Acute intermittent and coproporphyria are often associated with autonomic dysfunction. Cause is unknown, but axonal degeneration of somatic peripheral nerves is an associated finding. There are also abnormalities of the celiac ganglia, sympathetic trunks and vagus nerves.[59]

Sinus tachycardia, anhidrosis, nausea and vomiting, constipation, episodic hypertension, tachycardia and postural hypotension, possibly due to impaired adrenergic transmission, may mimic the Guillain-Barré syndrome or subacute autonomic neuropathy.

REFERENCES

1. Bradbury S., Eggleston C.: Postural hypotension: a report of three cases. Am Heart J *1*:73-86, 1925.
2. Shy G. M., Drager G. A.: A neurological syndrome associated with orthostatic hypotension: a clinical-pathologic study. Arch Neurol *2*:511, 1960.
3. Bevan D. R.; Shy-Drager syndrome: A review and a description of the anesthetic management. Anaesthesia *34*:866-873, 1979.
4. Schwartz G.: Orthostatic hypotension syndrome of Shy-Drager. Arch Neurol *16*:123, 1967.
5. Cohen J., Low P., Fealey R., et al: Somatic and autonomic function in progressive autonomic failure and multiple system atrophy. Ann Neurol *22*:692, 1987.
6. Guindi GM, Bannister R, Gibson WPR, et al: Laryngeal electromyography in multiple system atrophy with autonomic failure. J Neurol Neurosurg Psychiatr *44*:49, 1981.
7. Parks V. J., Sandison A. G., Skinner S. L., Whelan R. F.: Sympathomimetic drugs in orthostatic hypotension. Lancet *2*:1133-1136; 1961.
8. Cohen C. A.: Anesthetic management of a patient with the Shy-Drager syndrome. Anesthesiology *35*:95-97, 1971.
9. Malan M. D., Crago R. R.: Anaesthetic considerations in idiopathic hypotension and the Shy-Drager syndrome. Can Anaesth Soc J *26*:322-326, 1979.
10. Parris W. C. V., Goldberg M. R., Hollister A. S., Roberston D.: Anesthetic management in autonomic dysfunctions. Anesthesiol Rev *XI*:17-23, 1984.
11. Malan M. D., Crago R. R.: Anesthetic considerations in idiopathic orthostatic hypertension and the Shy-Drager syndrome. Can Anaesth Soc J *26*:322-326, 1979.
12. Saarnivaara L., Kautto U. M., Teravainen M.: Ketamine anaesthesia for a patient with the Shy-Drager syndrome. Acta Anaesthesial Scand *27*:123-125, 1983.
13. Riley C. M., Day R. L., Greely D. M., Langford, N. S.: Central autonomic dysfunction with defective lacrimation. I. Report of five cases. Pediatrics *3*:468-478, 1949.
14. Pearson J., Pytel B.: Quantitative Studies of Sympathetic ganglia and spinal cord intermediolateral gray columns in familial dysautonomia, J. Neurol Sci *39*:47-59, 1978.
15. Pearson J., Axelrod F., Dancis J.: Current concepts of dysautonomia: neuropathological defects. Ann NY Acad Sci *228*:228-300, 1974.
16. Brant B. W., McKusick V. A.: Familial dysautonomia, A report of genetic and clinical studies with a review of the literature. Medicine *49*:343-374, 1970.
17. Gitlin S. E., Bertani L. M., Wilk E., et al.; Excretion of catecholamine metabolites by children with familial dysautonomia. Pediatrics *46*:513-522, 1970.

18. Kritchman M. M., Schwartz M., Papper E. M.: Experience with general anesthesia in patients with familial dysautonomia. JAMA *170*:529-533, 1971.

19. McCaughey T. J.: Familial dysautonomia as an anesthetic hazard. Can Anath Soc J *12*:558, 1965.

20. Bartels J. M.: Familial dysautonomia. JAMA *212*:318, 1970.

21. Inlester J. S.: Anaesthesia for a patient suffering from familial dysautonomia. Br J Anaesth *43*:509-512, 1971.

22. Axelrod F. B., Danenfeld R. F., Danzier F., Turndorf H.: Anesthesia in familial dysautonomia. Anesthesiology *68*:631-635, 1988.

23. Beilin B., Maayan C. H., Vatashsky E., et al: Fentanyl anesthesia in familial dysautonomia. Anesth Analg *64*:72-76, 1985.

24. Sweeney B. P., Jones S., Langford R. M.: Anesthesia in dysautonomia: Further complications. Anaesthesia *40*:783-786, 1985.

25. Hui K. P., Connolly M. E.: Increased numbers of beta receptors in orthostatic hypotension due to autonomic dysfunction. NEJM *304*:1473-1476, 1981.

26. Schatz I. J : Orthostatic hypotension: I. Functional and neurogenic causes II. Clinical diagnosis, testing and treatment. Arch Intern Med *144*:773, 1037, 1984.

27. Hoeldtke R. D., Cavanaugh S. T., Hughes J. D., et al.; Treatment of orthostatic hypotension with dihydroergotamine and caffeine. Ann Intern Med *105*:168, 1986.

28. McLeod J. D., Tuck R. R.: Disorders of the autonomic nervous system: Part I. Pathophysiology and clinical features. Ann Neurol *21*:419-430, 1987.

29. McLeod J. D., Tuck R. R.: Disorders of the autonomic nervous system: Part II. Investigation and treatment. Ann Neurol *21*:419-529, 1987.

30. Thomas J. E., Schirger A.: Idiopathic orthostatic hypotension: A study of its natural history in 57 neurologically affected patients. Arch Neurol *22*:289-293, 1970.

31. Severn A. M : Parkinsonism and the anesthetist. Br J Anaesth *61*:761, 1988.

32. Turkka J. T., Juujarvi K. K., Lapinlampi T. O., Myllyla V. V.: Serum norepinephrine response to standing in patients with Parkinson's disease. Adv Neurol *45*:259-261, 1986.

33. Omaha E., Ikuta F.: Parkinson's disease: distribution of Lewy bodies and monoamine neuron system. Acta Neuropathol *34*:311-319, 1976.

34. Rosenthal T., Birch M., Osikowaska B., Sever O. S.: Changes in plasma noradrenaline concentration following sympathetic stimulation by gradual tilting. Cardiovasc Res *12*:144-147, 1978.

35. Camerlingo M., Aillon C., Bottacchi E., et al: Parasympathetic assessment in Parkinson's disease. Adv Neurol *45*:267-269, 1986.

36. Pollak P., Mallaret M., Gaio J. M., et al: Blood pressure effects of apomorphine and domperidone in Parkinsonism. Adv Neurol *45*:263-266, 1986.

37. Appelenzeller O., Goss J. E.: Autonomic deficits in Parkinson's syndrome. Arch Neurol *24*:50-57, 1971.

38. Aminoff M. J., Wilcox C. S.: Assessment of autonomic function in patients with a Parkinsonian syndrome. Br Med J *4*:80-84, 1971.

39. Korczyn A. D.: Autonomic nervous system disturbances in Parkinson's disease. Adv Neurol *53*:463-468, 1990.

40. Bennett T., Hosking D. J., Hampton J. R.: Baroreceptor sensitivity and responses in the valsalva manoeuvre in subjects with diabetes mellitus. J Neurol Neurosurg Psychiatr *39*:178-83, 1976.

41. Gunderson H. J. G, Neubauer B.: A long-term diabetic autonomic nervous abnormality. Diabetologia *13*:137-140, 1977.

42. Hilsted J.: Autonomic neuropathy: The diagnosis. Acta Neurol Scand *67*:193-201, 1983.

43. Yahr M. D., Frontera A. T.: Acute autonomic neuropathy: Its occurrence in infectious mononucleosis. Arch Neurol *32*:132, 1975.

44. Mackenzie C. F., Ducker T. B.: Cervical spinal cord injury. In Matjasko J, Katz J, eds. Neuroanesthesia and Neurosurgery, Orlando, Grune & Stratton, pp 77-134, 1986.

45. Bendo A. A., Giffen J. P., Cottrell J. E.: Anesthetic and surgical management of acute and chronic spinal cord injury. In Cottrell J. E., ed. Anesthesia and Neurosurgery. St. Louis. C. V. Mosby, pp 393-405, 1986.

46. Antognini J. F.: Anaesthesia for Charcot-Marie-Tooth Disease: A review of 86 cases. Can J Anaesth *39*:398-400, 1992.

47. Lambert D. H., Deane R. S., Mazuzan J. E.: Anesthesia and the control of blood pressure in patients with spinal cord injury. Anesth Analg *61*:344-8, 1982.

48. Babinski M. F.: Anesthetic considerations in the patient with acute spinal cord injury. Crit Care Clin *3*:619-634, 1987.

49. Stirt J. A., Marce A., Conklin D. A.: Obstetric anesthesia for a quadriplegic patient with autonomic hyperreflexia. Anesthesiology *51*:360, 1979.

50. Rocco A., Vandam L. D.: Problems in anesthesia for paraplegics. Anesthesiology *20*:348 (May, June), 1959.

51. Patel C., Miller S. M., Chalon J., Turndorf H: Anesthesia and spinal cord lesions. Bull NY Acad Med *54*:924, 1978.

52. Ciliberti B. J., Goldfern J., Rovenstine E. A.: Hypertension during spinal anesthesia in patients with spinal cord injuries. Anesthesiology *15*:273, 1954.

53. Thorn-Alquist A. M.: Prevention of hypertensive crises in patients with high spinal lesions during cystoscopy and lithotripsy. Acta Anaesth Scand *57*:79, 1975.

54. Young R. R., Asbury A K, Corbett J. L., Adams R. D.: Pure pandysautonomia with recovery. Brain *98*:613-636, 1975.

55. Fujii N., Tabira T., Shibasaki, et al: Acute autonomic and sensory neuropathy associated with elevated Epstein-Barr virus antibody titer. J Neurol Neurosurg Psychiatr *45*:656-657, 1982.

56. McLeod J. G., Tuck R. R.: Disorders of the autonomic nervous system. Ann Neurol *21*:419-430, 519-528, 1987.

57. Low P. A., Dyck P. J., Lambert E. H., et al: Acute panautonomic neuropathy. Ann Neurol *13*:412-417, 1983.

58. Appenzellar O.: The autonomic nervous system, 3rd ed. New York: Elsevier, 1982.

59. Laiwah A. C. Y., Mac Phee G. J. A., Boyle M. R., Goldberg A.: Autonomic neuropathy in acute intermittent porphyria. J Neurol Neurosurg Psychiatr *48*:1025-1030, 1985.

SUGGESTED READINGS

Adams J. H., Duchen L. W.: Greenfield's Neuropathology, Fifth Edition. Oxford University Press, New York, 1992.

Adams R. D., Victor M.: Principles of Neurology, Fifth Edition. McGraw-Hill, Inc., New York, 1993.

Davis R. L., Robertson D. M.: Textbook of Neuropathology, second edition. Williams & Wilkins, Baltimore, 1991.

Rosenberg R. N., Grossman R. G.: The Clinical Neurosciences, First Edition. Churchill Livingstone Inc., New York, 1983.

Rowland L. P.: Merritt's Textbook of Neurology, eighth edition. Lea & Febiger, PA, 1989.

Chapter 19

TEMPERATURE REGULATION AND HEAT PROBLEMS

VINCENT J. COLLINS

Living animals have been classified as regards their body temperature into two types[1]:

1. *Homothermic animals.* These animals are warm blooded, such as mammals and birds whose temperature remains constant though the surrounding temperature may vary from −30°F or below and 100°F or above.
2. *Poikilothermic animals.* These animals are cold blooded, such as frogs and turtles who take on the temperatures of their environments.

The human is a homothermic animal[2] whose temperature remains constant through a range of environmental changes. Core temperature varies only 0.3% over a range of 30°C (86°F) to −50°C. The average temperature of the human body, as determined by a thermometer placed in the mouth, is 37°C (98.6°F) with a range between 35°C (96.7°F) and 38°C (99°F). It appears as if evolution has set on this temperature as the optimum for humans and the mammalian class.

Variations in temperature are found with respect to different parts of the body, the time of day, activity, and age. At *the ankle*, the skin normal average temperature is 20°C (68°F); at *the waist*, 30°C (86°F) is the usual temperature (environmental 22.2°C or 72°F). Axillary temperature is about 1°F lower than the oral temperature, whereas rectal temperature is about 1°F higher than the oral temperature. The nasal temperature is −37.3°C (99°F); esophageal temperature is 37.7°C (100°F) and is the most reliable.

Tissue temperatures have been measured.[3,4] Of importance is the temperature of the hypothalamus. This area has been measured by sensor probes at the eardrum and at the forward wall of the ethmoid sinus. The temperature of internal organs is 2 or 3°F higher than oral.

Diurnal variations occur.[5] Temperature is low on rising (lowest at 4 AM) and reaches a maximum late in the day between 3 and 7 PM. Modification of the daily variations are due to activity or rest and to clothing. The highest body temperature that has been reliably recorded without a fatal result is 113°F (45°C) and the lowest 75.2°F (24°C.). Reduction of body temperature below 23°C results in loss of thermal regulatory control and is near the lethal limit. Death is by cardiac arrest. Lower temperatures, however, have been used during cardiopulmonary bypass without fatality. In children, the temperature is about ½ to 1°F higher. This may be an artifact due to observation of rectal temperatures.

Core temperature is defined as the temperature of blood perfusing vital major organ systems. It is 0.5°C higher than the oral temperature. Nasopharyngeal and esophageal temperatures are more representative of core temperature.

Infants have different thermoregulatory responses than adults, but there is little evidence that they are less efficient. In fact, infants maintain their temperature remarkably well in a cold environment, using nonshivering thermogenesis.[6] Even premature infants can mobilize nonshivering thermogenesis.[7] Infants below 6 months easily become hypothermic, whereas after 6 months and in children, the tendency is to become hyperthermic. In the older age group temperature tends to be subnormal.

TEMPERATURE BALANCE

Body temperature represents a balance between the heat produced by tissue metabolism plus that obtained from warmed food and the heat dissipated into the environment. Adjustments are made by generating heat and/or by altering heat loss mechanisms.[8] It is thus an open system so that body temperature normally is kept constant.

Heat Production

Heat production is mainly a chemical[9] process. Lavoisier showed that oxidative mechanisms furnish the body heat and the fuels of biological combustion are the foodstuffs. The process is an exothermic reaction and the quantity of heat produced varies from moment to moment but goes on continuously. The requirements can be expressed quantitatively in Newtonian formula concerning the cooling of warm bodies. It is calculated that to maintain body heat at −50°C (arctic) about 10 times as much heat must be generated than at 30°C (tropics).

As a measure of heat production, the rate of CO_2 production (CO_2 being the end product of combustion) furnishes a rough index. Each gram of fat combusted by tissues furnishes 9.3 calories of heat; each gram of carbohydrate furnishes 4.1 calories, and each gram of protein also furnishes 4.1 calories. Protein, furthermore, exerts a peculiar influence in enhancing overall metabolism, which capacity is termed the specific dynamic action of protein. Most of the body heat is furnished by burning of foodstuffs chiefly in skeletal muscles, and there appears to be a true thermal muscular tone furnishing basal heat.

In the absence of external work all metabolic energy appears as heat and this amounts to about 1 kcal/kg of body weight/hour.[8] Strenuous exercise increases the amount and may elevate the body temperature to 40°C exceeding the capacity of the heat loss mechanisms. Only one-fourth of the energy expended appears as work while three-fourths appears as body heat.

Brown Adipose Fat

A significant source[10,11] of fuel for the production of heat is the metabolic utilization of brown-adipose tissue (BAT). This is especially important in the neonate and infant. In the adult BAT is still present in the interscapular, perirenal, inguinal regions and in the posterior triangle of the neck. Nonshivering thermogenesis is not particularly important in adults.[12] Obese subjects maintain core temperature better than lean subjects because they lose less heat to the environment.[13]

Exposure to Cold[9]

On exposure to cold beginning at environmental temperatures below 28°C two processes are initiated: heat conservation mechanisms by limiting heat loss and increased heat production. The latter encompasses the following mechanisms:

1. Nonshivering Thermogenesis. Metabolic Thermogenesis. This is related to increased involuntary muscle tone and tension accompanied by enhanced combustion of foodstuffs. Mobilization of free fatty acids from fat deposits (FFA) mediated by increases in noradrenaline. Mobilization of some stores of brown fat due to increases in cyclic AMP.
2. Shivering. An autonomic mediated process controlled by the hypothalamus and limbic system. This process is initiated at temperatures below 28°C.
3. Voluntary muscle activity. Exercise causes a change in the hypothalamic set-point for temperature control.[14]

Heat Loss

Heat loss, on the other hand, is mainly a physical process. The body is a warm object in reference to its environment, and it is cooled by losing heat to the environment. However, if the surrounding temperature approaches that of the body, heat loss decreases. If the environmental temperature is between 82 to 95°F (28 to 35°C), effective avenues of heat loss and the approximate percentage loss from the human body are as follows:

1. Radiation conduction and convection 70%
   Radiation 50%
   Convection 15%
   Conduction 5%
2. Evaporation from skin (Each milliliter of water requires 580 calories) 14.5%
   Insensible perspiration
3. Heat in water of expired air 7.5%

4. Warming of inspired air 3.0%
5. Liberation of carbon dioxide 4.0%
6. Excreted (urine and feces) 2.0%
7. Sweating Variable

Associated with heat loss from the body certain variable factors must be considered: the environmental temperature and humidity; the artificial control imposed by clothing; the metabolic rate and the activity of the person; acclimatization; air currents, body insulation.

Radiation probably accounts for the major part of the body heat loss and the heat is transferred to the environment.[15] Whenever the discrepancy between body temperature and environmental temperature is great, the body will lose heat rapidly. The body is simply a radiator and as such it loses some of its heat energy as radiant energy. It is an infrared radiation with the wavelength (lambda) of the emissions averaging = 9 μ with a range of = 4-20 μ. The amount of radiation is related to the difference of the fourth power of the skin and environmental temperatures. The skin over neoplasms or over an abscess is 2-3°C higher than normal and the radiation thereabouts is proportionally higher.

As environmental temperature increases (i.e., the difference in temperature between the environment and body temperature decreases) the rate of heat loss by radiation decreases rapidly. As environmental temperature approaches the body temperature, little or no heat is lost by radiation. Loss of heat by radiation is also limited by a high water content of air, since humid air is more opaque to transmission of radiant energy than dry air.

About the body a layer of warm air 3 to 5 mm thick, saturated with water vapor, is formed.[8] Between this layer and the surrounding atmosphere (if it is cooler and has less water vapor) convection currents are set up serving to remove the warm layer of air from about the body. This process is obviously enhanced by wind and artificial air currents. Conduction of heat from the body to the surroundings such as touching cooler objects is ordinarily negligible as a means for losing heat.

Evaporation is the process whereby a liquid is changed to the gaseous state by absorbing heat. Evaporation from the skin and mucous membranes takes on increasing importance with rise in environmental temperature.[8] At 94.1°F (34.5°C) vaporization of water from the body accounts for all the heat loss from the body. Evaporation occurs without any change in temperature of the liquid and the heat absorbed by the liquid is called the heat of vaporization. The water for this process of vaporization is derived from:

1. Insensible water loss from the skin
2. Water vapor in expired air from the mucous membranes
3. Sweating

Changes in circulation to the skin alter the amount of heat brought to the skin surface. At a temperature of about 33°C, there is nearly complete vasodilatation of skin vessels and rapid volume rate of flow. Water passes from the subcutaneous capillaries of the skin and then to the skin surface by transudation. Regardless of the temperature a constant loss of about 800 ml (30 to 50 ml/hr.) of water per day occurs in the average adult in this way. Also since the mucosa of the tracheobronchial tree is moist, there is a constant daily insensible loss of water in the expired air by vaporization from the moist mucosal surface. This amounts to about 400 ml per day.

Sweating itself causes little heat loss from the body.[16] It is effective in cooling the body only when it vaporizes. For each ml of sweat that is vaporized, about 580 calories are absorbed from the body. If it drips, there is little benefit to be derived. Hence, humid environments are extremely unfavorable because of interference with vaporization. The other avenues of heat loss are self explanatory.

Primary Mechanism of Regulation[17]

Maintenance of a physical or chemical quantity at a constant level requires a servomechanism or a self-regulating chain of control.[1] This is true of all biological functions studied and one of the most exquisite is that of temperature constancy of the human body, despite a range of environmental temperatures.

The elements of a temperature servomechanism are three:[1,11,18]

1. A sense organ for measuring
2. A controller center for regulation
3. An effector

The Sense Organ

There is ample evidence that cells throughout the body have thermal sensitivity. Especially important are the spinal cord and the skin surface.[18,19] Temperature of the hypothalamus *per se* probably contributes only 20% of the total thermal input in mammals.

Regulatory responses to thermal perturbations are determined by mean body temperature (incorporating the skin surface, spinal cord, hypothalamus, other parts of the brain, and deep abdominal and thoracic tissues).

The intrathreshold range defined as the temperatures between sweating and vasoconstriction that do not initiate thermoregulatory responses is 0.2°C.[20] The "null zone" between sweating and shivering is 0.6°C.[21,22] In contrast, the skin surface is even more sensitive: an increase in skin temperature of 0.003°C can be detected by humans.[14] Thus makes a distinction between sensitivity of the receptors (very high) and tolerance of the regulatory system which is tight, but does allow core temperature to vary by several tenths of a degree.

Temperature sensitive cells, are also located in the hypothalamus and situated in the forward part of the hypothalamus (at the preotic region). These cells sample the temperature of blood flowing through the area from the internal carotid artery.[4] A measurement is integrated by the "controller" which compares it with a set-point. Elevation of blood temperature serves as the stimulus to the end-organ and the sensitivity is extremely fine. A rise of blood temperature of 0.01°C evokes heat dissipation mechanisms. Occlusion of the common carotid artery causes an elevation of the hypothalamic tissue tempera-

ture and causes a pronounced loss of heat from the body.[23] On the other hand, drugs which increase blood flow through the hypothalamus, such as pentobarbital, cause a reduction of hypothalamic tissue temperature and tend to raise body temperature. Serotonin injected into the brain causes hyperthermia while catecholamines so injected produce hypothermia.

Temperature-sense receptors in the skin (heat sensitive) are not the primary end-organs for regulation.[24] They do serve a particular function through a system which operates via centers of consciousness, thus bypassing the unconscious control center and temperature sensitive cells of the hypothalamus. Skin thermoreceptors also contribute to and regulate the skin temperature itself.[25]

Cutaneous temperature receptors do contribute substantially to behavioral regulation. However, they also contribute significantly to autonomic responses. The best evidence is that 30% of the total input comes from the skin's surface.

Peripheral Temperature Receptor Mechanism

Specific end-organ thermoreceptors have not been identified. However warm and cold sensations are mediated by two systems of uncapsulated "free nerve endings": one for warmth and the second for cold.[24] These thermoreceptors are responsible for impulse generation and by the rate of change in temperature with respect to intensity of cold. Warm sensation is dependent in a second population of receptor nerve endings independent of the cold receptors. Warm and cold spots have been identified in the skin by thermodes as have warmth fibers in nerve bundles by means of microelectrodes inserted percutaneously which are only activated by heat.[25] The skin temperature activating these units ranges between 33° to 35°C. Spontaneous activation of these units with skin temperatures above 35°C and up to 45°C shows a progressive increase in impulse frequency.

Transmitter factors of a chemical nature may also be involved in thermoregulation.[18] Such factors are released from the brain during changes in temperature. If the cerebrospinal fluid (CSF) of a cooled monkey is perfused through a normothermic monkey, a fever response occurs; a warm monkey's CSF, when so perfused, results in hypothermia.[26]

The Controller

The hypothalamus,[13] the controller, was identified by Aronsohn and Sachs in 1885, and has been verified by subsequent investigators. The hypothalamus functions as a thermostat to activate heat loss mechanisms or to inhibit heat loss mechanisms. It has a temperature set-point of 100°F (equivalent to an oral temperature of 98.4°F [36.9°C]). Women have slightly higher set-points than men.[27,28] The set-point is established or altered by tonic mechanisms.[26] An elevation of sodium in the posterior hypothalamus raises the set-point and in animal experiments the body temperature rises sharply. Conversely, increases in calcium ion produces a low set point and hypothermia.

Blood temperature changes which stimulate the sensitive end-organs also in the hypothalamus (anterior) are compared by the cells of the hypothalamus to the set-point.[28] Elevations of blood temperature evoke dissipation mechanisms as noted previously and an elevation of .01°C above the set-point will increase skin blood flow by 15 ml/min and will dissipate 1 cal/sec by sweating.[29,30] Electrical action potentials from the hypothalamus in response to temperature changes in the perfusing blood have been reported and parallel the temperature changes.[31]

Integration of visceral mechanisms that control heat loss and somatic mechanisms that govern heat production is controlled by the hypothalamus. Both the anterior and posterior hypothalamus are needed to provide protection against thermal changes. The role of each is not clear. At least the role may be more in induce behavioral somatic responses with increased skeletal muscle tension, changes in posture and shivering on the one hand and autonomic visceral responses on the other. It is clear that hypothalamic injury can lead to temperature misregulation. Rostral lesions may lead to hyperthermia with fever. Caudal lesions of the hypothalamus lead to hyperthermia if the environment is cool.

The Effector

These mechanisms of temperature control are primarily those of heat loss or heat conservation. In 1900 Max Rubiner demonstrated the role of skin vasodilatation and of sweating in dissipating body heat. Inhibition of loss mechanisms or heat conservation is the dominant way for maintaining or increasing body heat. Increasing metabolic rate is at best a relatively poor mechanism in adjustment to cold environment. Actual responses are a complicated function of skin and core temperatures, and are confounded by numerous other factors.[9,10]

Changes in the hypothalamic "set-point" are induced by a variety of conditions such as exercise[27] and sleep[32] as well as by drugs.[33-36]

Water Shifting Responses[2]

Certain shifts in body water take place in response to changes in environmental temperature.

In a warm environment hydremia occurs. This is denoted by an increase in blood volume and dilution of the blood with a relative decrease in the solids, salts, and proteins of the blood. To accomplish the above the following occurs:

1. Contraction of the spleen and discharge into the vascular system of whole blood.
2. Water passes from the intracellular compartment to the extracellular compartment. The major part of this extracellular fluid is drawn into the circulation. The chief sources of this fluid are the skin, muscle, liver, connective tissue, and kidney.

In a cold environment anhydremia occurs. There is a decrease in blood volume and hemoconcentration. The solids, salts, and proteins increase. This is accomplished by a shift of water from the circulation and extracellular compartment on an intracellular locus in tissues enumerated above as the sources of water.

Pyretic and Antipyretic Drugs

Certain drugs used by anesthetists have definite pyretic properties. Thus, the belladonna drugs, atropine and scopolamine produce hyperthermia by inhibiting sweating, by inhibiting postganglionic cholinergic responses, and by drying respiratory mucosa.

Morphine depresses the hypothalamus and disturbs water-shifting responses to changes in temperature. Sedatives such as phenobarbital and sodium amytal also act in a similar fashion. General anesthetics, by depressing hypothalamic function, also alter body responses to temperature changes. The amount of fluid shifted is relatively small and is not an important factor in thermoregulatory response.

Halothane and the other volatile anesthetics produce a specific thermoregulatory impairment: the intrathreshold range is increased, but maximum response intensity remains intact.[13] Thiopental produces a similar impairment, but has not specifically been tested. In the presence of these drugs, patients will become hyperthermic in a warm environment and hypothermic in a cold environment. By far the most important consequence is hypothermia. Pentobarbital has been reported to produce hyperpyrexia.[35]

Sympathetic stimulant drugs such as epinephrine and ephedrine raise body temperature by increasing muscle tone, decreasing skin circulation and increasing body metabolism as a whole.

Cocaine and other local anesthetics in toxic doses tend to raise body temperature through their central action. When absorbed, these drugs stimulate the cortex and thereby increase muscle tone and other body activities. Eventually, convulsions may result. The overall effect is to increase heat production and raise body temperature.

Other pyretic drugs[36] that need only be enumerated are as follows: tyramine; tetrahydronaphthalamine; methylene blue; toxins; dinitrophenol (increases oxygen consumption 10 times). Fever therapy has been carried out by injecting such substances as vaccines, turpentine, sodium nucleate, blood peptone, and milk. Also heat cabinets, by raising the environmental temperature about the body and preventing adequate loss, raises temperature.

Fever

Fever specifically refers to a regulated increase in core temperature; this is distinct from hyperthermia which is a term for an increase of any etiology. The belladonna drugs usually have no effect on core temperature. However, they do inhibit sweating and may result in hyperthermia (but not fever) during heat stress. Fever is not a failure of heat elimination but may be considered a positive heat balance.[37] Also body tissues undergo colloid change and become hydroscopic. There follows diminished blood volume and blood flow so that elimination is decreased.

Ether anesthesia is denoted by profuse sweating. Initially, a patient may exhibit signs of collapse. However, with dehydration and anhydremia, as well as hypothalamic depression, there may be an increase in body temperature and a state of hyperpyrexia.

Curare, and other non-depolarizing relaxants[13] by paralyzing muscles and decreasing the thermal muscular tone diminishes body heat production.

Regional anesthesia does alter thermoregulation by impairing afferent input.[13]

Prostoglandins act as pyrogens and may be the chemical intermediary for the production of fever. Inhibition of prostoglandin synthesis is considered the mechanism for the action of aspirin-like drugs.[38]

Adaptation to Cold[39]

Insulation either natural or artificial in the form of clothing is probably the most important means for adapting to cold. Humans generally become uncomfortable when the environment cools skin to a temperature 7°C or more below internal temperature.

An immediate response is to conserve heat.[9] The anterior hypothalamus is inhibited. Vasoconstriction of the skin vessels occurs and water shifts from the vascular compartment to the interstitial and cellular compartments.[40]

The mechanism of heat production by increasing metabolic rate begins when the air temperature falls to 28°C. At this time, there is a general increase in muscle tone and soon actual shivering may occur. Increasing metabolism is at best a limited affair and heat production may increase 300 to 400% readily, but this may be inadequate over a wide ambient temperature range of 60 to 80°F (15 to 30°C) when a 10-fold spread of heat loss or gain is required by Newtonian laws.

Adaptation to cold by both inhibiting loss and stimulating heat production is limited by hypoxia and hypercarbia.[24] Nerve desensitization also occurs with lowering temperatures.[41] The skin of the finger is only one-sixth as sensitive at 20°C as at 35°C. A stimulus to be appreciated must be 10 times greater.[41]

Adaptation to Heat[42]

Responses to a warm environment are summarized.
1. *Central Neural Excitation of Sweating.*
   a. Parallel vasodilatation, depends on—
   b. Increase in blood temperature. An 0.1°C rise increases loss by 10%.
2. *Central Inhibition of Heat Production*
   a. Increments of 0.1°C from set-point produces a 10% decrease in metabolism from basal.
   b. Shivering is totally abolished at 98.8°C.

Acclimatization[43]

This is a process whereby a man develops his capacity to perform efficiently a maximum amount of work in a new climatic environment to which he has not been previously exposed. The new climate may be either an extremely hot or cold one. Chief interest revolves about exposure to a new hot environment since accommodation to cold is more readily achieved by use of clothing and protection.

On exposure to a hot climate man cannot tolerate strenuous work at first. However, if the work load is light and short on the first day and progressively increased within the limits of tolerance, acclimatization is achieved by the end of the fourth day. If, after acclimatization a person changes to a different climate, this adaptation is retained for 1 to 2 weeks and is lost in 1 month.

Important rules and facts for acclimatization are as follows:[43]

Initial minimum work
Progressively increasing work schedule
Adequate and complete rest at night
Limited midday exposure
Alternating work and rest periods
Clothing light, loose and permeable
High carbohydrate diet

Water Requirements

At high temperature as much as 1 pint of water may be lost per hour by sweating while a man is at rest. This loss increases with work load. Hard work may increase the 8 hour water requirements to 3 gallons. Hydration may be considered adequate if at least 30 ounces of urine are eliminated each day. Water should be taken at short intervals in small amounts. The best guide is thirst.

Salt Requirements

There is an increased need during the first few days of acclimatization because of profuse sweating. Ordinarily, sweat is a weak solution (0.2 to 0.5%) of sodium chloride. During the first few days in a hot environment it is richer in salt. Thereafter, with adaptation, there is a decreased salt percentage than normally found. The food supplies a certain amount, but if total water intake approaches 1 gallon, there should be added salt. It is best supplied in solution or tablets. The daily requirement may be 5 to 50 grams each day. A solution of 0.1% salt in drinking water is efficient. The addition of lemon juice makes it somewhat more palatable and is called Wilder's solution. A 10 grain salt tablet in 1 pint of water is excellent. Direct ingestion with only an amount of water to aid in swallowing is not recommended. The salt is poorly absorbed and is nauseating.

Heat Syndromes (Table 19–1)[43,44]

Three syndromes that occur in man due to the adverse affects of heat are heat cramps, heat exhaustion, and heat retention (heat stroke). Heat cramps are essentially benign but heat exhaustion and retention are accompanied by an appreciable mortality. There is rarely a direct mortality in previously healthy persons. However, the aged, those suffering from debilitating or infectious diseases, children subject to prolonged exposure and alcoholics are vulnerable and succumb.[44] Usually, mortality incidence rises on the third or fourth day of a heat wave. Those who recover from exhaustion or retention are extremely susceptible to future attacks.[45,46]

Exhaustion is typified by peripheral circulatory failure due to vasomotor disturbance and decreased circulating blood volume.

Retention is the acute process of deranged hypothalamic function and is typified by failure of sweating mechanism due to prolonged excessive environmental temperature. Acute hepatitis may occur from hyperpyrexia.[47] Es-

Table 19–1. Differential Diagnosis

	Heat Cramps	Heat Exhaustion	Heat Retention
Skin:	Pale or normal. Dry. Not unduly warm; maybe cool.	Pale, cyanotic at times. Clammy (Shock). Cold.	Flushed (sunburn flush). Dry, except exposed parts. Hot.
Temperature:	Normal or slightly up.	Subnormal.	Hyperpyrexia.
Sensorium:	Slight changes. Mild vertigo, mild depress. Nausea sometimes.	Changes often marked. Vertigo, headache, visual. Apprehension-depression. Coma in extreme cases. Ataxia; nausea.	Changes often marked. Vertigo, headache, visual. Apprehension-delirium. Coma. Nausea.
Muscular:	Intermittent painful twitchings with digital flexors. Spasm of limbs and abd. Entire body sometimes 1 to 3 min.	Relaxation. Flaccidity in extreme. Sphincter relaxes.	Increase tone and twitch early, especially with delirium. Flaccidity follows. Sphincter relaxation. Reflexes absent in coma.
Respiration:	Rate increased. Hyperpnea during spasms.	Varies with degree depression. Usually rate increased, then depth. occ. sighing.	Hyperpnea the rule. Sighing; Kussmaul. Tachypnea.
Circulation:	Pulse rapid, strong. B.P normal or increased. Hemoconcent.	Pulse rapid, thready. B.P. depressed. Hemoconcent.	Pulse rapid, often thready. B.P. elevated; later depression.
Therapy:	I.V. hypertonic 1.5% saline. Water and salt by mouth. Cool environment M.S. rest.	Fluids by mouth. As shock: I.V. therapy. Saline 1.5% then normal. Avoid overheating. No stimulus. Cool shaded environment.	Reduce hyperpyres stat. Moist sheets; fans. Ice compresses to exposed parts. Alcohol sponges. I.V. therapy. Intubation S.O.S. Oxygen. Air temp. about 50°F.

Adapted from War Department TB 175 and Knochel 1974.

sential characteristics of these syndromes with suggested treatment is contained in the accompanying table.

It is important to emphasize that in the treatment of heat retention the use of cold tubs or ice application to the skin is drastic and detrimental. These measures tend to cause skin vessel constriction and drive blood to deeper areas of the body. It also fails to consider that if a patient is removed to a relatively cool environment heat loss will be the result of radiation and convection and is aided best by fans.

Syndrome of sclerema may occur in uncontrolled hypothermia in infancy. This consists of induration and rigidity of the skin and subcutaneous tissue—a leathery consistency. It is cold injury.[48]

OPERATING ROOM MANAGEMENT

Perioperative Hypothermia[49,50]

Hypothermia is a frequent problem in the infant and elderly adult, but is seen in other age groups as well. It usually develops during the first hour of anesthesia and surgery. Once hypothermia develops, it continues into the recovery and postoperative period and may be exaggerated (as the anesthesia is "worn off").

For the adult, assuming a normal core temperature of 37.0°C, it has been observed that 60% of the patients arriving in the recovery room have temperatures below 36.0°C by tympanic membrane measurement and 13% had temperatures below 35°C. Hypothermia as a problem may be considered to exist when core body temperature falls below 36.0°C. The lowest temperatures have been observed in patients following intra-abdominal or major vascular surgery (34.6°C). Patients having TURP show low temperatures. Elderly patients (over 60 years) usually have lower temperatures and hypothermia lasts longer, despite conservative warming; i.e., room temperature at 72°F and blankets. When hypothermia exists in patients on admission to the recovery room, shivering frequently ensues and the incidence is 18–20% at about 30 minutes after admission.[51]

In a study of nasopharyngeal temperatures during general anesthesia without humidification or heating, the mean temperature dropped from 36.2°C to 34.9°C. When the anesthetic inspired mixtures are heated (to 37°C) and humidifed (100% relative), patients remain normothermic.[52] Heating inspired air to 38° to 39°C, through the Y-connector of the anesthesia circle system by means of a two-stage heater humidifier at the inspiratory arm, provides for normothermia during the surgical period. In one study patients managed in this manner had an 0.5°C higher body temperature on recovery room admission. These patients maintained normothermia in the recovery room and appeared to have a 30% decreased recovery room time, or approximately a decrease by one hour of recovery room stay.[53]

Regional anesthesia is also associated with a similar significant incidence of hypothermia.[54] Administration of cold solutions into the epidural or subarachnoid space can cause a progressive fall in epidural temperature,[55] as measured by a small epidural thermistor, and accompanied by a high incidence of shivering. The incidence of shivering is greater with epidural than subarachnoid anesthesia. The injection of solutions at body temperature does not cause shivering. Koska[56] has demonstrated thermosensitive tissues in the spinal cord as being responsible. However, that is not the mechanism of shivering.[57] Shivering during epidural anesthesia is normal thermoregulatory shivering, and results from core temperature. The Koska studies are important for documenting that the hypothalamus is not the only important thermoreceptor in the body. However, it is not relevant to epidural anesthesia. In these physiological studies in animals the entire spinal cord was cooled aggressively. Furthermore, the cervical cord is far more sensitive to thermomanipulations than the lumbar region.[58]

Certain operations and conditions are associated with serious hypothermia.[59] An air-conditioned operating room with temperatures below 70°F (22°C) is a major contributor. Heat loss is particularly great during intra-abdominal and intra-thoracic surgery, where large visceral surface areas are exposed. It is compounded by prolonged surgery. Excessive fluid flushing of surgical incisions, puddling of solutions on the OR table, administration of cold blood, and prolongation of surgery are significant factors. The consequences of hypothermia, such as shivering, especially as the anesthetic wears off, must be controlled.

Another surgical situation accompanied by significant heat loss is in urologic cystoscopic surgery. Although heat-transfer is limited since bladder blood-flow is low, large volumes of fluid at room temperature used to irrigate the bladder and prostate bed may produce hypothermia.

Operating room temperatures lower than 72°F (22°C) may induce acute renal failure from the precipitation of cryoglobulins.[60] Cryoglobulinemia is a disorder in which circulating abnormal globulins precipitate in the presence of cold. These globulins may have a wide thermal amplitude and when precipitation occurs, it is associated with renal involvement in 20% of patients.[60]

In paralyzed patients, a decrease in core temperature is often observed and a decrease of 0.8°C induces a variety

of thermoregulatory mechanisms.[61] Jessen has shown that this is associated with the following: 1) a 40% increase in whole-body oxygen requirements; 2) a three-fold increase in circulating noradrenaline; 3) marked stimulation of lipolysis,[62] 4) an increase in myocardial oxygen requirements; 5) development of metabolic acidosis. Non-shivering thermogenesis does not occur during general anesthesia.[63,64]

Pattern of Temperature Change During General Anesthesia (Fig. 19–1)

The development of hypothermia during general anesthesia shows a stereotyped pattern.[65,66] Central body temperature is monitored by a tympanic membrane thermocouple, and shows a decrease of approximately 1.0° to 1.5°C during the first hour.[66] This is followed by a slower phase, during which heat loss exceeds heat production at a linear decrease of about 0.5°C per hour for 3 to 4 hours,[66] and then reaches a plateau without significant changes thereafter.[65]

The initial temperature seen after induction of anesthesia is due to a redistribution of cool peripheral blood to the central body tissues. Hypothermia develops when there is actual loss of heat that exceeds heat production. The heat production during anesthesia is at a basal level of 1.0 kcal/kg/hour. A loss of twice this amount will result in a decrease in body temperature of 1.0°C/hour.

Temperature Activation Thresholds for Central Thermoregulation

Normally, the response to cold is noted first by vasoconstriction at a core temperature of only 0.1° to 0.2°C below the normal central body temperature of 37°C, with

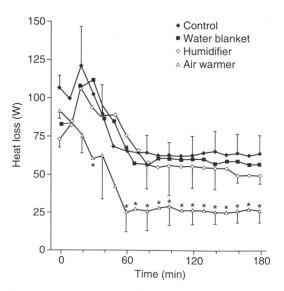

Fig. 19–1. Total cutaneous heat loss was greatest for all groups during the first 60 minutes, corresponding to the period when patients were mostly undraped. Total cutaneous heat loss subsequently was reduced by about 50% when patients were fully draped. Total cutaneous heat loss was about 35W less in the forced-air warmer group than in all the other groups. These differences were statistically significant at 30 minutes and at all times from 60 minutes on (indicated by *). Redrawn from J Clin Anesth 1992[66] with permission.

a fall in core temperature of 0.4° to 0.6°C below 37°C nonshivering thermogenesis (metabolic) is activated while at a temperature of 1.0°C below 37°C is induced.

General anesthesia inhibits the central thermoregulatory mechanism. That is, a greater reduction in the core temperature is needed to activate the centers in response to cold, as compared to the unanesthetized subject.[67] The threshold for response occurs when the core temperature falls by 2.5° below 37°C, or to about 34.5°. This reduced threshold is similar for the commonly used anesthetic agents[68] and is similar in infants, children, and adults.[69] It is noted that, for nonshivering thermogenesis in infants, there is uncoupling of the brown adipose tissue to provide part of the fuel for heat that does not ordinarily occur in adults.[63] In general, the thermoregulatory threshold is inversely related to the anesthetic concentration.[70]

On exposure to a warm environment, activation of heat loss mechanisms by vasodilitation and sweating occurs when the core temperature is increased by only 0.1°C above the normal core temperature. In the anesthetized subject, the threshold for activation of vasodilitation and sweating is about 38°C, or about 1.0° above normal core temperature. On exposure to a cold environment, the thermoregulatory mechanisms induce cutaneous vasoconstriction, and this in turn decreases cutaneous heat loss.[71] Furthermore, with muscular activity, there are pressure changes in intraocular pressure, with intraocular pressure rises to 4.8 mm Hg above normal.[72]

Intraoperative Control of Body Temperature (Table 19-2)

Among the specific strategies to control body temperature are the following: 1) maintain the operating room temperature at an appropriate level for adults, of 24 to 26°C (74 to 76°F)[73]; 2) use warmed inspired gases by means of attached humidifiers—this may reduce heat loss, but does not completely prevent it; 3) a convection warming system using forced warm air directly through a porous quilt is excellent; 4) a thermal or warming blanket is useful for adults, but if placed over the patient, the maintenance of body temperature by this means in in-

fants and children is far from effective. Indeed, there are some claims that it is of no value[74]; 5) to diminish heat loss, intravenous solutions and irrigating solutions should be warmed to above body temperature (intravenous solutions 40°C; irrigating solutions 40°C); 6) the use of an esophageal thermal tube has been proposed and has been found effective: in a study of patients undergoing abdominal surgery for three to four hours, results were falls in temperature to a mean of 35°C (95°F); in contrast, a companion group of patients—for whom heat was provided by means of the esophageal tube—had a median temperature at the end of the surgical procedure of 36.1-36.8°C (97-98°F)[75] (Fig. 19-2); 7) radiant heat systems should be directed to the "blush area" over the upper chest, face and neck where there is a high density of thermo-receptors.[75]

Intravenous Fluid Temperature

One overlooked mechanism for provoking shivering is the intravenous administration of crystalloid and other solutions that are at a temperature of 20-22°C (room temperature). For instance, in a study of parturient women, shivering occurred in 64% of patients[66]; when solutions were warmed to 30-33°C, fewer than 15% shivered. It is recommended that all solutions be warmed to 30°C for ordinary intravenous administration.[77]

Although intravenous solutions warmed to body temperature or above 30°C are a positive step, nevertheless, this may not represent the actual temperature of the solution as it is delivered at the venous site of the extension intravenous tubing.[78] Ordinarily, body heat production is about 2,500 kcal/day, or approximately 100 kcal/hour. When fluids are administered that are cool and differ by 1.0°C from the body temperature of 37°C, a burden is placed on metabolism to produce heat. For each 1,000 ml of fluid that is administered differing by 1.0 degree, the burden represents 1,000 cal or 1.0 kcal. Thus, the administration of 1,000 ml of a fluid at room temperature (22°C) means that the 15° difference in temperature between body heat and room temperature represents the need for expending 15 kcal to compensate for the cool fluids.

Table 19–2. General Strategies for Maintenance of Body Temperature and Prevention of Heat Loss

Passive insulators
  Cotton blankets
  Cloth or paper surgical drapes
  Disposable plastic drapes
  Plastic bags.
  A single layer of each type of covering material decreases heat loss by approximately 30%

Active warming systems.
  Convection Warming Systems (the most efficient)
  Warmed air is forced through a quilt-like porous blanket and passes over the skin warming it directly and also replaces the
    normal body "air-envelope" with a warm air envelope (Bair-Hugger Unit)

  Radiant Heat Systems
    Infra-red light
    Thermal ceiling lights

  Conductive Heating Systems
    Circulating warm water blankets at 37°C placed over the patient preferably. Heat exchange is limited
    Warmed inspired gases from a heater—humidifier

From Hynson and Sessler.[66]

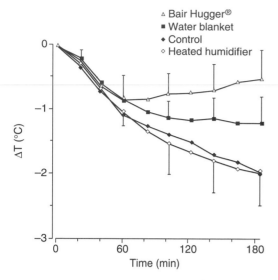

Fig. 19–2. Tympanic membrane temperature decreased uniformly during the first hour after induction of general anesthesia in each group. Temperature then increased over the remaining 2 hours in patients receiving forced-air warming, but remained nearly constant in those lying on a circulating-water blanket set at 40 °C. Patients in the control and heated-humidifier groups became progressively more hypothermic throughout surgery. The uniform initial hypothermia during the first hour of anesthesia results from internal redistribution of heat, and illustrates the difficulty of treating this temperature decrease. Core temperatures are presented as means ±SD. Differences between the forced-air warmer and the control and heated-humidifier groups achieved statistical significance after 100 minutes. Differences between the forced-air warmer and the circulating-water blanket groups were statistically significant at 160 minutes and beyond. ΔT = tympanic membrane temperature minus tympanic membrane temperature at the start of induction. Redrawn from Hynson and Sessler, J Clin Anesth, 1992.[11]

Since bag temperature and delivery temperature differ, it is suggested that fluids should be warmed to 40°C. If 1,000 ml of Ringer's solution is administered at the rate of 500 ml/hour, after 5.0 minutes the delivery temperature of the fluid at the end of an IV extension tubing would show a linear fall from about 37°C to 30°C after 1.0 hour and 26°C at 2.0 hours. It is suggested that when regulation of temperature is critical, another warmed container of fluid be used after 1.0 hour. In most hospitals today "fluid warmers" are used to provide a continuous flow of warm solutions.

Conversely, in the management of MH, containers of fluid should be cooled to 4.0°C and administered through short tubing. If the tubing is extensive, the temperature of the fluid during its progress through the tubing may rise at least 10°C on simple exposure to the room temperature. Hence, the full cooling effect on the body will not be realized.

Irrigating Solution Temperatures[24]

The problems of hypothermia have multiple etiologic factors. It is recognized that exposure of patients in operating rooms at temperatures of 70 degrees (20°C) is associated with falls in body temperature.[79] Shivering may occur when body temperature falls 0.6° to 0.7°C. There is in the elderly an age-related decline in thermoregulatory capacity. After the administration of most anesthetics, heat loss is increased by vasodilatation, especially during spinal anesthesia.

In transurethral resections, it has been found that the warming of irrigating solutions for the clearance of the endoscope visualization reduces both the fall in body temperature and the incidence of shivering.[80] When glycine solution 1.5% is heated to 37°C by a proper incubator and then utilized in the irrigation for transurethral procedures, there is a minimal loss of heat and marked decrease in the incidence of shivering. Generally the solutions achieve a temperature within the hour of approximately 33 degrees centigrade. In the study by Dyer, the heat loss was greater under general anesthesia than under spinal anesthesia.[80]

Shivering

Shivering and generalized muscle tremors are mechanisms, in addition to non-shivering thermogenesis, used by the body to increase core temperature.

Characteristically, shivering may show different degrees of intensity.[81] Fine fibrillary contractions may appear in the facial muscles, especially the masseter, and then spread into the neck, trunk and extremities. These contractions are fine and rapid and do not develop into convulsions.

Grading of Shivering

The severity of shivering can be graded clinically on a scale of 0 to 4: 0 = no shivering; 1 = intermittent mild tremors of jaw and neck muscles or minimal fasciculations of face; 2 = additional intense tremors of chest; 3 = intermittent vigorous generalized tremors; 4 = continuous violent generalized muscle activity. For more precise evaluation of shivering, oxygen consumption provides an index of the intensity[82] and electromyography provides information on the patterns of shivering.[81]

Incidence[26]

The incidence varies with the type of agent used, being most frequent following enflurane administration. However, it does occur with all of the other anesthetic agents during emergence.

When the average room temperature is between 62–65°F, a gross incidence for several agents is as follows: thiopental, 65%; ether, 31%; cyclopropane, 25%; halothane 20%; isoflurane and ethrane, 15%. Similarly, the severity of the process varies with premedication and the temperature of the environment. Thus, tremors are more pronounced and violent after thiopental and relatively mild after the volatile inhalation agents.

Causal Factors

Many factors contribute to the development of shivering, which is essentially an attempt to re-establish the basic core body temperature. Some factors have been assessed to understand the etiology: The lower the room temperature, the more severe the reaction. The depth of narcosis is important, since patients do not shiver when in surgical planes of anesthesia. The skin temperature, although increased on induction of anesthesia, shows some degree of cooling during maintenance. Stimulation of skin and organs by changes in temperature per se is the primary factor and patients are more likely to show some muscle rigidity than shiver. However, this is not frequent and shivering is not considered to be due to peripheral skin temperature changes during anesthesia.

Loss of heat during anesthesia plays a role. All patients lose heat through an enhanced surface loss and ventilatory loss. The ventilatory loss is probably less than 10% of metabolic loss and probably less than 5% of total loss during large operations.[83] The average fall in body temperature, however, is greater with those agents which produce some cutaneous vasodilitation.[63] Shivering is a reflex under hypothalamic control and this reflex is rapidly activated. Shivering is thus a true thermal phenomenon due to an increased sensitivity to cold.

Mixed Venous Oxygen Saturation Index[84]

An early indicator of increased oxygen consumption is a fall of mixed venous oxygen saturation (Fig. 19–3). S_{VO2} may fall when shivering begins from a normal value of 74 ± 6% to levels of 57 ± 12% as the shivering intensity increases. Simultaneously, an increase in oxygen consumption of over 100% occurs, while oxygen delivery may only increase by 20%.[84] This trend continues to the extent of a 3–4 fold increase in oxygen consumption. A gradual return to normal S_{VO2} values is seen with cessation of shivering.

Physiologic Effects

Shivering can be considered to have harmful effects. Because of the increased muscular activity, there is an enhanced oxygen demand of 200 to 400%. This imposes a risk of overutilization-hypoxia and and can be harmful in patients in poor physical condition—those who are anemic or have a variety of impaired cardiac actions.

It is associated with a significant increase in oxygen consumption of 300 or more percent.[85] This is paralleled by a similar increase in myocardial oxygen requirements and endangers patients with restricted myocardial reserve or in the elderly. Cardiac arrhythmia, failure and infarction are more postoperative complications.[86] Shivering is a frequent postanesthetic complication. The incidence varies quite widely and for the intermediate volatile inhalation anesthetics, varies between 60 to 70%. However, if a narcotic is part of preanesthetic medication, the incidence is reduced to 30%. Thus, the narcotic nitrous oxide balanced anesthesia technic is associated with an incidence of about 30 to 40% postanesthetic shivering.

When mild shivering occurs, the oxygen consumption is comparable to that required by light exercise.[87] However, when the shivering is severe, there may be a five-fold increase in the total body oxygen requirement. The usual method to control body temperature and, above all, to prevent shivering is first to *prevent heat loss* during the course of surgery and, secondly, to continue to pre-

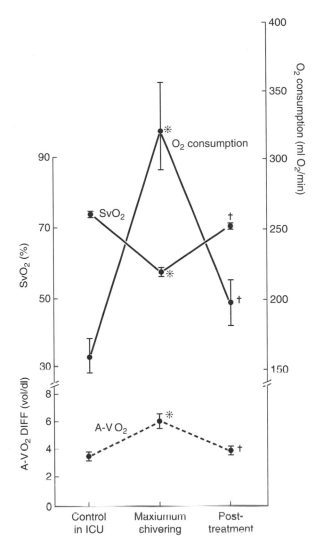

Fig. 19–3. Mixed venous oxygen saturation and A-V O_2 difference are compared with O_2 consumption at three points: (1) control, on arrival in ICU; (2) time of maximal shivering; and (3) after treatment. SvO_2 is at its lowest and oxygen consumption and extraction are greatest at the point of maximal shivering. All values are $\bar{x} \pm 1$ SE. Key: *P < .01 between 1 and 2: †P < .01 between 2 and 3. Redrawn from A. Guffin et al, J Cardiothoracic Anesth 1:24, 1987.[84]

vent heat loss by proper covering of the patient. It needs to be emphasized that the most important factor in preventing hypothermia is to maintain operating room temperatures at approximately 72°F (22°C). The recovery room temperature should be warmer and should be set at 75°F (23.5°C). For infants and children under two years of age, ambient temperature in the O.R. should be 88°F and, postoperatively, incubators are recommended.

Intraocular Pressure

Intraocular pressure is markedly increased when shivering occurs. Mahajan has determined increases of 5 to 8 mm Hg above preinduction values at 2 to 10 minutes postanesthesia. This can impose a risk on patient's ocular surgery.[72]

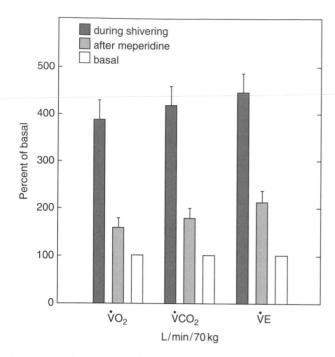

Fig. 19–4. $\dot{V}O_2$ (STPD), $\dot{V}O_2$ (STPD), and VE (BTPS) expressed as a percentage of expected basal values during shivering and after suppression of shivering by meperidine. Data presented as mean ± SEM. Redrawn from Anesth Analg 66:753, 1987. with permission of the authors (Dr. Pavlin)[89] and the International Anesthesia Research Society.

The overall effect of meperidine on the approximate 400% increase in metabolism is illustrated (Fig. 19–4).[89] Shivering is arrested within 5–10 minutes of the administration of 25 mg meperidine intravenously, and a repeat dose has been found successful in almost all patients. It has also been clearly found to be the most effective agent in spontaneously breathing patients.[90,91]

Metabolic Cost of Shivering[87]

Metabolic requirements are greatly increased during shivering after general anesthesia. Oxygen consumption and carbon dioxide production increases from 300–500% above base levels. Ventilation (V_E) increases in accordance with metabolic requirements. However, it has been shown that cardiac output may not increase in proportion to the metabolic demand.[85] Because of these changes, patients with diminished cardiopulmonary reserves may not be able to compensate effectively for the increased metabolic demand. In these patients, cardiac output may not increase when V_{O_2} is increased by shivering. Consequently, mixed venous oxygen saturation (SV_{O_2}) is reduced. During hypothermia there is increased oxygen solubility in blood RBC and a concomitant decrease by arterial P_{O_2}.[88] This should be appreciated in routine blood-gas analysis.

In a detailed study of the shivering patient[87] the oxygen requirement ($\dot{V}_{O_2}$) of 0.93 ± 0.36 L/min/70 kg and the carbon dioxide production ($\dot{V}_{CO_2}$) of 0.81 ± 0.34 L/min/70 kg represented a 380% increase above calculated basal values. Minute ventilation markedly increased during shivering and averaged about 25 L/min in 70 kg

subjects. This represents an increase of fourfold above the basal values. The arterial (P_{CO_2}) values were normal, indicating that the alveolar ventilation was adequate. However, the arterial P_{O_2} levels in shivering patients breathing room air were significantly below normal, at about 75 mm Hg. Many subjects had a Pa_{O_2} well below the 75 mm Hg level. Hence, a significant degree of hypoxemia and failing delivery of oxygen to tissues is evident.

In all patients, a metabolic acidosis was observed. Some patients exhibit arterial pH values of less than 7.3.

With the administration of meperidine,[89] marked improvement in the metabolic state was evident, although there was still a continued increase in metabolism, but only approximately 50% above basal values.

Prevention and Control [90,91]

Intraoperative shivering and non-shivering thermogenesis can be controlled by a comfortable room temperature, as already noted in the process of preventing heat loss.[92] For most adults a room temperature of 72°F is appropriate, while for the elderly a temperature of 74°F is preferred. For children, ages 4 through 12, a room temperature of 68° provides comfort.[93] A thermal blanket should also be used and placed on the table, since hyperthermia is more likely to occur in this age group. The thermal blanket can be a back-up for the control of hyperthermia. It is a standard of practice that for infants and those up to two years of age room temperature should be kept in the 80°F range (Table 19–3).

Postanesthetic Mechanisms[90,91]

Possible mechanisms for shivering after the conclusion of anesthesia may be divided into at least three categories: 1. The direct effect of anesthetic agents: This may be related to a change in central setpoint of temperature control. 2. The development of hypothermia and lowered core temperature during anesthesia as a result of significant heat loss: with recovery from anesthetic agents a progressive activation of thermoregulatory response mechanisms, both neural and metabolic, to environmental cold occurs. 3. Factors related to pyrogen release, type of surgery, tissue destruction and absorption of products.

Of these, it appears likely that shivering is essentially the result of cold stimulation of a lowered core temperature combined with the skin postanesthetically, evoking both heat production mechanisms and heat conservation (vasoconstriction).

The use of radiant heat to the skin, applied to the "blush area" of the face, neck, and upper chest where there is a high density of thermoreceptors, is revealing. Shivering is stopped within 60 seconds of its appearance, even while the body temperature remains low.[94] Shivering returns within 60 seconds on discontinuing the radiant heat.

It is not likely that a change in the central setpoint (hypothalamic thermostat) is an important mechanism. As core temperature approaches the normal preanesthetic temperature, shivering will diminish and then cease.

Mechanism of Nonshivering Thermogenesis[95,96]

Nonshivering as well as shivering thermogenesis is intimately related to the stress release by cold of cate-

Table 19–3.   Prevention of Hypothermia—Recommendations to Maintain Body Temperature

Perioperatively
    Comfortable operating rooms at 72°F (22°C) for patients[60]
    Humidification and warming of anesthetic inhaled mixtures[52]
    Use of low-flow or closed system anesthesia in critically ill patients and those at risk[51]
    Use of a forced air warming system[92]
    Use of warm intravenous crystalloid solutions[77,78]
        a. crystalloids for intravenous fluid balance
        b. solutions for irrigating surgical wounds
        c. solutions used in cystoscopic procedures
    Use of warm irrigating solutions in surgical field[51] and cystoscopic urologic procedures[80]
    Use of blood warmers for administration of blood, and warmed crystalloidal/colloidal solutions or blood fractions
    Avoidance of puddling of solutions on OR table
    Administration of small doses of narcotics during emergence for pain and to prevent shivering
    Meperidine is the most effective agent to deter shivering[91]
    Warm recovery room at 75°F (24°C)
    Enflurane anesthesia is least likely to be associated with postanesthetic shivering[93]
    Warm anesthetic solutions for epidural anesthesia may be used. However, the efficacy has not been proven.[54,55]

cholamines. In addition, cold stress activates the sympathetic adrenergic system, including the sympathetic activation of energy and heat production by brown adipose tissue. This tissue is an important energy buffer not only in infants but in adults. The characteristic multilocular brown adipose cells have been demonstrated in adults at all ages. Distribution includes inter scapular, subscapular and axillary deposits, and the nape of the neck (especially in outdoor workers). When stimulated by its intrinsic adrenergic innervation or by circulating norepinephrine, this tissue proceeds to oxidize its triglyceride stores with the production of heat.[95]

Since the mechanisms of response to cold are stimulated by incoming cold impulses through activation of hypothalamic and pituitary pathways, it appears that the cold stimuli can be overridden by radiant heat applied peripherally to the skin, even if the core or deep tissue temperature is below normal.[97] As core temperatures approach the pre-shivering levels, shivering will cease.

A pharmacologic approach has been proposed by Murphy. A central neurotransmitter, taurine (a monocarboxylic acid like GABA), is inhibitory to central heat production and conservation pathways.[98] In his group studies, intravenous administration of taurine to primates not only prevented shivering, even in the presence of a cold environment, but stopped shivering. Clinical studies of this drug are needed.[98]

Control of Postanesthetic Shivering

The control of shivering remains important. The most effective drug appears to be meperidine in small doses of 10–25 mg administered intravenously every 5–10 minutes.[90,91,99] Relief is attained in 90% of instances. Men tend to shiver more frequently than women. And women respond much more quickly to treatment. It is noteworthy that morphine relieves shivering in about 45% of occurrences and fentanyl in about 35%. These narcotics, thus, are less effective in controlling shivering than meperidine.[91]

In the event that 25–50 mg intravenous meperidine does not significantly control shivering, the administration of pancuronium has been found to accomplish the desired result.[84]

Radiant heat applied to a shivering patient stops the shivering in patients who are slightly hypothermic, within 1 minute. This is a rapidly effective method and noninvasive.[94] When the core temperature is below 35°C it is less effective. A radiant heat source can be simple: three 250-watt infrared heat lamps in a linear arrangement attached to an overhead stand can be centered over the thorax and abdomen.

Pediatric patients have a large surface area relative to body mass. When anesthetized, they are virtually poikilothermic. Under 6 months of age a significant reduction in temperature is common and spontaneous hypothermia occurs. If normal rectal temperature is taken as 37.5°C (99.6°F), then in the under-6-month group temperatures of 35°C (95°F) are common and lower temperatures of 32 to 34°C are frequent.[100]

Temperature Maintenance in Infants

Temperature maintenance in infants under six months of age undergoing anesthesia and surgery has been conducted with three different methods, and a comparison made of the effect of heat loss with a warming blanket, a humidifier and an overhead heater. The combination of all three is associated with significantly less heat loss than when a blanket is used alone. It is recommended that overhead heaters should be used during the induction and maintenance of anesthesia in infants.[101]

An additional method for the prevention of excessive heat loss is the use of a head-wrap with a thin insulate material. This provides a thermal insulation for babies exposed to unusual conditions.[102] It should be appreciated that the head surface area in the infant is approximately 20% of the total surface area.[103] This represents a very great area for heat loss. In addition, another biological factor is that the brain heat production represents 70% of the total body heat produced; thus limiting heat loss from the skin surface of the head is an important aspect of heat control. In the studies by Marks[102] with the use of a head-wrap, the mean skin temperature was maintained and there was a significant decrease in heat loss.

Postoperative Metabolic Stress

After anesthesia for major surgical procedures, there is a significant metabolic response of a catabolic type with an accelerated rate of nitrogen loss from the body. This is associated with muscle protein breakdown.

Several strategies have been used to minimize these metabolic effects with little success, including high dose narcotic anesthesia[104] and peridural analgesia.[105] Further studies of elderly patients undergoing large bowel surgery have revealed that heat conservation and maintenance of normothermia diminished muscle protein breakdown.[106] Both the excretion of the amino acid 3-methylhistidine (an indicator of muscle protein breakdown), as well as the excretion of urea nitrogen in the postoperative period are significantly decreased.[107] The patients who developed a 2.0°C fall in temperature had a urea nitrogen excretion of 6.5 mg per cent, while the perioperative normothermic patients had a normal excretion of 3.9 mg percent.

Monitoring Temperature[108]

Variations in temperature of patients in the operating room during anesthesia and surgery may be considerable. Monitoring the temperature is an integral part of vital sign observations and of the conduct of anesthesia.

Indications

Most patients should be monitored during general anesthesia and many during regional anesthesia.[108,109] There are specific situations, however, where it is necessary, particularly where heat loss may be great or the ability of the patient to produce heat or maintain a normal thermic state is deficient.[109] Specifically, the young patient, the neonate and the infant, as well as children, are not capable of good thermal balance. Similarly, the elderly are more likely to lose heat readily, but are subject to a definite inability for heat production. Situations that are mandatory for temperature monitoring include those patients who have an infectious process and who already have an elevated temperature or who are at risk for malignant hyperpyrexia.

Sites

Sites of monitoring include the tympanic membrane, the nasopharynx, the distal esophagus, and the pulmonary artery when a catheter is in place.[110] Of these sites the nasopharynx and the tympanic membrane are commonly used. It is noted that both these sites reflect brain temperature but that this does not differ from core temperature by more than 0.2°C. The esophageal site is currently the most commonly used one and is the most accurate utilizing an esophageal temperature probe. Tympanic thermometry has been associated with perforation of the tympanic membrane.[109]

MALIGNANT HYPERPYREXIA

Malignant hyperthermia was first described by Denborough in 1962,[111] and subsequently by Saidman[112] in 1964.

It is a clinical syndrome characterized by a rapid, precipitous rise in temperature during anesthesia in young adults.[113,114] The subjects at risk are usually healthy, well developed, and muscular. Males. predominate after 15 years of age in a ratio of 3 males to 1 female[115] (Table 19–4). The median age in collected reports is 21 years. Occurrence is unpredictable but can be diagnosed by vigilant continuous observation of the patient.

The incidence is set in the range of 1 in 6,800 to 38,000 and is fatal in 65 to 75% of patients. Generally, it occurs more often in older children and adolescents. With the incidence being 1 in 15,000 anesthetics. In adults the frequency is 1 in 50,000 to 1:100,000 anesthetics.[116]

The prevalence of susceptible individuals is estimated to be between 1-200 to 1 in 5000 of a population.[116] Most reports describe patients of Caucasian or African descent; however, many reports have appeared of malignant hyperthermia in Asian patients.[117,118]

Pharmacogenetics[119]

Malignant hyperthermia is evidently related to several phenotypic characteristics of the patients. In addition, there appears to be a genetic predisposition for these subjects to react adversely to certain pharmacologic agents. In an extensive study of familial distribution of malignant hyperthermia, McPherson and Taylor find no strong evidence for an MH gene or for simple mendelian patterns of inheritance. Instead, they provide evidence for the concept of heterogeneity. There is a contribution of many genes to form a mosaic of susceptibility. In a sense, MH is a non-specific symptom that may be caused by a variety of genetic, environmental and pharmacologic factors. About 20% of cases are sporadic, with autosomal dominant inheritance in one-half of the families.

Diagnosis

Patients are afebrile prior to induction. Tachycardia and hypertension are seen at the onset, but are succeeded by arrhythmias and hypotension. Such cardiovascular responses are due to rigor of heart muscle initially.[120] Decreased tissue O_2 plays a secondary role along with pH and $PaCO_2$ and electrolyte changes within the heart muscle cell.

Table 19–4. Sex and Age Distribution of MH Cases

Age (years)	Number of Patients		Ratio M/F
	Male	Female	
0–14	95	62	1.53
15–29	117	35	3.34
30–44	42	13	3.23
45–59	20	6	3.33
60	4	1	4.00

Britt, B. A., Kwong, F., and Endrenyi, L.: The Clinical and Laboratory Features of Malignant Hyperthermia Management. Henschel, E. O. ed.: Malignant Hyperthermia. Appleton-Century-Crofts, New York, 1977.

Tachypnea and hyperpnea are characteristic and often appear early. These respiratory changes are consequent to increased catabolism with over-utilization of oxygen and over-production of carbon dioxide.[121]

A wet sweaty skin may be seen early, but a hot dry skin is observed as often. Flushing and mottling of the skin is common. Cyanosis occurs because of increased utilization of oxygen and enhanced extraction. "Dark blood" is often noticed by the surgeon and may be the first indication of malignant hyperthermia, but is usually a later manifestation.[122]

A high, rapidly developing temperature is a dramatic characteristic of the syndrome.[121] A rapid rise greater than 1°F every 15 minutes (.55°C) or more than 2°C every hour may be seen and levels of 105 to 112°F can result. This explosive rise may be delayed for 1 to 3 hours after the appearance of other abnormal physiologic signs. A temperature of 107°F seems critical. In patients whose temperature exceeds this level, the mortality increases to 80 to 90%, although some patients with temperatures up to 112°F have survived. Patients with temperatures below the critical level of 107°F have a lower mortality between 50 to 60%.[123]

An unusual inability to produce muscle relaxation during induction of anesthesia, especially with succinylcholine is frequently encountered. Prolongation of the fasciculation phase of depolarizing drugs is seen, followed by actual muscle rigidity. Failure of jaw to relax for intubation is common.

Clinical Types[114]

Patients with hyperpyrexia may be divided clinically into two groups: those with obvious muscle rigidity (75%) and those without. The absence of rigidity may be real or may be due to failure to detect changes in skeletal muscle tone or pulmonary compliance. More often the syndrome is manifested by a true increase in muscle tone, leading to gross sustained muscle rigidity and chest wall stiffness. The onset may be rapid, accompanying induction or appearing shortly thereafter; on the other hand, a delay as long as several hours in the appearance of rigidity has been noted in some instances, though other signs are already manifest. Pronounced rigor mortis is usually present in patients who die.

Convulsions often occur as the temperature goes to higher levels and are seen in about 75% of patients with the syndrome. When convulsions occur later, they probably represent a complication of cerebral anoxia.

When the above cardiovascular and respiratory signs are accompanied by muscle contracture and elevation of temperature, the syndrome of malignant hyperpyrexia must be presumed.

Differential Diagnosis

The syndrome is an uncommon operating room experience and must be differentiated from fevers due to other causes. Ordinarily, a subject under general anesthesia has a decreased heat production and consequently reacts as a poikilothermic animal. Because of air conditioning, the use of narcotic drugs and autonomic adrenergic blocking agents, the body temperature tends to drift to the environmental temperature.

Neurolept Syndrome (NMS)[124,125]

The neurolept malignant syndrome (NMS) should also be considered in differential diagnosis. This is a rare idiosyncratic reaction to major tranquilizers and mimics to some degree the clinical characteristics of MH. Among the drugs commonly associated are the phenothiazines, butyrophenones; haloperidol, chlorpromazine and fluphenazine are commonly implicated. These drugs have a common central action in blocking dopaminergic pathways and dopamine receptors in basal ganglia and the hypothalamus. It may follow the administration of metoclopramide. Withdrawal of amantadine, levodopa and such preparations as used in Parkinsonism therapy will precipitate the syndrome. Ordinary doses of such drugs provoke the syndrome, which includes elevation of CPK. Muscle relaxation can be achieved by diazepam or pancuronium in this disorder, which is not likely to be seen in MH. It is also noted that during withdrawal from levodopa treatment of Parkinsonism the NMS may also appear.

Incidence[126]

The incidence of NMS in all patients taking neuroleptics has been estimated at 1.5%. Morbidity and mortality are due to respiratory failure; this is secondary to tachypneic hypoventilation from decreased chest wall compliance or pulmonary aspiration, infection and/or embolism. Acute renal failure may also occur from rhabdomyolysis and myoglobinuria. Seizure activity may develop. In Lavies' review, the mortality rate for the patients developing NMS was 9%. This syndrome can be successfully treated by dopaminergic agonists such as bromcriptine.[127]

Predisposing Factors

1. Loss of control of mechanisms contributing to heat loss combined with increased heat production.
2. Infections.
3. Dehydration.
4. Muscle activity—recent exercise.[128,129]

Muscular activity prior to the administration of triggering agents appears to increase the incidence of occurrence, the rapidity of onset and the intensity of the reaction.[130] Experimental studies confirm these clinical features: a short period of exercise in landrace pigs prior to halothane administration increases the incidence from 30% (non-exercised) to 100%. In the muscles phosphocreatine and ATP decrease to low values while lactate increases.[126]

5. CNS lesions, hypothalamic damage.
6. Biochemical derangements.[131,132]
7. A familial aspect—genetic abnormality with limited penetration.[111,128,133]
8. Metabolic disorders—denoted by high creatine phosphokinase (CPK), elevated serum pyrophosphate and increased total lactic dehydrogenase (LDH fraction).

Serum creatine phosphokinase is an important enzyme in diagnosing muscular and neurologic injury.[111,112] Three isoenzymes have been identified representing a) brain or nervous system injury (BB) type I isoenzyme; b) myocardial injury (M B) type II isoenzyme; c) skeletal muscle injury (MM) type III. Normal values for man are BB (0–2) IU/L: MB (0–3) IU/L: and MM (0–65) IU/L.[130] After myocardial infarction mean values may be of the order of 600 IU/L; in neurologic injury (meningitis, tumor) values are of the order of 100–300 IU/L for BB. In skeletal muscle disorders such as rhabdomyolysis extremely high values may be attained.[134]

9. Myopathies—disorders of musculoskeletal system exist in about 66% of patients who develop MH according to Britt.[133] The incidence of myopathy in relatives is 62% (1st to 3rd degree kinship) and 68% in probands. Patients with myotonia do not readily relax with succinylcholine, but few patients developing increased muscle tone after succinylcholine have pathologic muscle evidence of myotonia or other muscle disorders.

Of the common muscular dystrophies, Duchenne Muscular Dystrophy (DMD) is severe and rapidly progressive; malignant hyperpyrexia has been reported in such patients.[135] Myopathies such as the myotonias and central core diseases increase the susceptibility to MH.

Although physical and emotional stresses are often predisposing factors, it is important to emphasize that MHS individuals need not be restricted in their lifestyle activities.[129] Susceptible persons have been submitted to submaximal work by treadmill walking at 40% of maximal oxygen consumption without adverse effects. Measurements of body temperature, respiratory gas exchange, sweat evaporation rate, circulating catecholamines, as well as lactate, pyruvate, free fatty acid and plasma glucose were all in the same ranges as non-MHS subjects. The patients displayed the same thermoregulating plasma catecholamine and metabolic responses as normal subjects. It appears that noncompetitive, low intensity steady state exercise need not be contraindicated.

Preoperative Diagnosis of Risk

a. A high suspicion index.
b. Inquiry into family history.
c. Specific past anesthesia experiences.
d. Presence of neuromuscular disorders.
e. If clinical considerations are suspicious then laboratory tests should be considered.

Genetic History[117]

A personal history of anesthetic experiences and of untoward complications is of immediate importance. Do not ignore statements by a patient or of family members like "I had a high fever after anesthesia" or "my temperature went up during surgery." Details of family history are important and information indicating typical MH episodes and outcome are important. Information should be sought from hospital records, including experiences in other than the current hospital. A history of masseter nerve rigidity from succinylcholine is of importance.

Identification of subjects and relatives at risk is of major importance. A counseling program is recommended for the family that includes information gathering and interpretation of data from the personal history, family history, medical records, physical examination, and the laboratory (CPK measurements (3x) and the caffeine contracture test), as well as counseling regarding drugs and risk probability.

The risk of MH has been proposed on the basis of CPK values elevated above the 95th percentile, in accordance with Bayes' theorem.[117] If an individual, on the basis of history and physical, has a prior probability of 0.5 to be MH susceptible, an elevated CPR increases the risk to 0.94, while a normal CPK decreases risk to 0.17.

Prediction of Susceptibility[136]

A variety of adverse reactions noted clinically have been associated with the development of MH. These have been defined as otherwise unexplained, and include masseter spasm, generalized muscle rigidity, acidosis, hypercarbia and tachycardia (Table 19–5). All patients, mainly children, showed one or more of these reactions during an initial anesthetic experience. They were then submitted to muscle biopsy and exposure of the muscle to the halothane-caffeine contracture test.

In this series, the only predictor of MH susceptibility was found to be generalized muscle rigidity or masseter spasm during the anesthetic, which did include either halothane or succinylcholine or both. However, by itself, muscle rigidity was not an absolute predictor. About 25% of patients may have muscle rigidity associated with other adverse type reactions than that of MH. However, this muscle rigidity reaction, plus other evidence, such as myoglobinemia, elevated CK, or masseter rigidity together, do form a complex of clinical predictability.

Contracture Tests—Muscle Biopsy[137,138]

Tests presently available to determine susceptibility to MH rely on in vitro exposure of skeletal muscle to pharmacologic stimulants. Open biopsy of quadriceps or vastus lateralis muscle under local infiltration anesthesia is performed and the specimens preserved in Krebs-Ringer solution. Viability is confirmed by electrical stimulation and a length-tension curve plotted. The muscle is then exposed to particular stimulants in vitro:

Caffeine Contracture Test.

1) To sequential incremental concentrations of 0.25 to 32.0 mM of caffeine in Krebs-Ringer bath solution. MH susceptible subjects have a contracture threshold at 2.0 mM concentration of caffeine or less.

Exposure of Muscle-Preparation to Halothane.

2) To 2% halothane for 15 minutes; MH susceptible subjects show a *rapidly developing contracture tension*. Muscle from susceptible subjects or those who have an MH episode and survive have an enhanced contracture response.[139]

Table 19–5. Clinical Data Recorded During Initial Anesthetic and Relation to Biopsy Outcome

Type of Adverse Reaction	Biopsy Result						
	MH(+)		MH(−)		Equivocal	Total	
	No.	%	No.	%	No.	No.	%
Generalized muscle rigidity*	13	76	3	12	0	16	38
Masseter rigidity	10	59	11	46	0	21	50
Myoglobinuria	7	41	6	25	0	13	31
CK >100 U/l	17	100	15	62	1	33	79
CK 100 to 20,000	11	65	12	50	1	24	57
CK >20,000	6	35	2	8	0	8	19
Acidosis	5	29	4	17	0	9	21
Hypercarbia	4	24	0		0	4	10
Hypoxemia	1	6	1	4	0	2	5
Temperature elevation	4	24	9	38	1	14	33
Tachycardia	5	29	8	33	0	13	31
Arrhythmia	5	29	5	21	0	10	24
Total patients with adverse anesthetic reactions	17	100	24	100	1	42	100

*MH(+) group *vs.* MH(−) group, $P < 0.0001$, see text.
Larach, M. G., et al: Prediction of malignant hyperthermia susceptibility by clinical signs. *Anesthesiology 66*:546, 1987.

Regional anesthesia is recommended as a safe and non-interfering approach in biopsying a muscle bed. Gielen[140] reported on the safety of the 3-in-1 lumbar plexus block or psoas compartment block for biopsy of the vastus medialis muscle. Amide local anesthetics were employed and found safe.

Predisposition Tests[141] (Table 19–6)

Standardized Physical Stress Test[142]

The Bruce Protocol for continuous treadmill exercise is employed. This is a maximal exertion test and has been found to be one of the most satisfactory tests to estimate capacity for exercise.

In a comparison study of patients known to be MH susceptible and normal individuals it was found that MHS subjects developed generalized fatigue and exhaustion more rapidly with early maximal increases in heart rate and blood pressure (15 minutes vs 25 minutes). Pain in muscles also developed in MHS.

With the completion of exercise serial plasma cAMP concentrations were measured. It is noted that the before-exercise cAMP was consistently higher in MHS subjects than in normals. At the peak of exercise, concentrations of cAMP increased three-fold in contrast to a two-fold increase in normal subjects. After exercise the elevation in cAMP remained significantly elevated for two to four hours while the values in normals returned to baseline within 2 hours.

It is recommended that this test be added to other non-invasive tests for identification of MH susceptible individuals.[142]

Platelet-Halothane Bioassay Screening Test[144]

A relatively noninvasive screening technic has been proposed for assessing the effects of halothane in patients at risk for malignant hyperthermia. Platelets have meta-bolic characteristics similar to skeletal muscle, as well as contractile properties. On contraction, the platelet can lose its store of nucleotides. Halothane causes contracture of platelets and the released nucleotides can be measured. Patients at risk show a high free nucleotide profile and this assay correlates 100% with the contracture test for malignant hyperthermia.

Clinical Characteristics

A listing of the characteristics follows, but not in the order of their appearance.

1. *Hypertonia of skeletal muscle.*[19] Observable or masked; myoglobinuria denoting muscle damage is usually gross; present in 80% of cases.
2. *Hyperthermia.*[11] The rapid rise in temperature is consequent to deranged biological oxidation in

Table 19–6. Susceptibility Screening Tests

Stress exercise test (Stavec)[23]
   Increased cAMP

Muscle biopsy
   Calcium uptake[26]
   Caffeine-contracture[27, 60]
   Halothane challenge.

Platelet model
   Bioassay screen[25]
   Nucleotide plasma response (Solomon)[84]
   Requires large blood volume (45 ml)

Bone Calcium Index (Britt)[64]

Serum creatine kinase (CK) (Formerly known as creatine phosphokinase) (Gronent)[46]—Does not identify MH-susceptible patients (Paasuke).[65] As routinely determined, many false negative tests are observed.

skeletal muscle and liver leading to sustained muscle tension and heat production.[29]

3. *Hypercarbia and acidosis.*[115] Severe respiratory and metabolic acidosis develop due to an extraordinary rise in P_aCO_2 and lactic and pyruvic acid production with lowered pH. Therefore a base deficit of as much as 20 to 30 mEq. may occur.

   Initially hyperglycemia occurs and plasma noradrenaline is increased. In moderately severe reactions muscle glycogen is decreased and is moblized for heat production; in the violent reactions there is also an intense mobilization of liver glycogen.[149] Secondarily, hypoglycemia ensues and some changes in the membrane of the beta cells of the pancreas have been observed.

4. *Electrolytic changes.* A profound initial hypercalcemia occurs; presumably calcium is released from SR storage vesicles into both the myoplasm and extracellular fluid.[148] This is accompanied by hyperkalemia, hypermagnesemia, and hyperphosphatemia. During recovery hypocalcemia occurs and is accompanied by hypokalemia and hypophosphatemia.[150]

5. *Hydration.* Water balance is disturbed and a shift of fluid from the vascular and extracellular compartments occurs to the cells.[149] Tachypnea increases respiratory water loss (normally 60 mg H_2O per liter of expiration); as much as 1000 ml of H_2O may be lost per hour.

6. *Hypoxia.* A marked overutilization hypoxia occurs. Desaturation of hemoglobin results in cyanasis. There is an increased erythrocyte osmotic fragility in hyperthomic susceptible swine.[151]

7. *Damaged endothelium.*[152] Permits escape of fluid into tissue; and increased cutaneous blood flow diverts blood from central circulation; hypovolemia with a decreased plasma volume ensues.

Early Diagnostic Signs

Muscle Hypertonia

An inability to produce muscle relaxation during induction of anesthesia, especially with succinylcholine, is frequently encountered. Prolongation of the fasciculation phase of depolarizing drugs is seen, followed by actual muscle rigidity. Failure of the jaw to relax for airway insertion or intubation is not uncommon.

Masseter spasm, in fact, after succinylcholine administration, has been studied and is a well documented event, especially in children. Schwartz[153] has determined that such spasm occurs in one out of every 100 children who are anesthetized with halothane followed by intravenous succinylcholine. Some of his patients had associated cardiovascular changes and impressive increases in CPK levels of over 1000 IV and myoglobinemia. The biochemical changes were evident immediately after the appearance of masseter spasm, but were most marked after four hours. He suggests that the actual potential susceptibility in the general population, particularly of children, is more likely of the order of 1:100 and not 1:10,000. When masseter spasm occurs, it is recommended that the elec-

tive procedure be aborted. If emergency surgery is necessary, all potential triggering agents in susceptible patients should be discontinued or not employed. If halothane is administered, it is recommended that nondepolarizing muscle relaxants be employed.

Further evidence of the association of masseter spasm and MH susceptibility has been adduced by Flewellen.[154] By the halothane-caffeine contracture test of biopsied muscle fascicles, 60% of children had a positive response. These patients were classified phenotypically according to the spectrum of susceptibility of Nelson as phenotypes H and P (normal response to caffeine or halothane alone but abnormal contracture response to the combination).[155] A class of patients with an atypical response were classified as phenotype H and represented 40% of the patients. In all situations, it was considered that patients showing masseter spasm were MH susceptible and should not receive succinylcholine or halothane. A repeat exposure of these children to the halothane-succinylcholine anesthetic was considered unethical.

The rigidity and muscle hypertonia which develops with the onset of MH appears not to be related to a regular form of contractile activity but rather to a pronounced contracture caused by a continuous local depolarization other than that initiated by a propagated action potential. The accompanying increased body temperature reaching 43–44 degrees C is a consequence of the accelerated rate of energy metabolism of the muscle.[156]

Hypercarbia-CO_2 Monitoring[157]

One of the earliest signs of malignant hyperthermia is an increase in the end tidal CO_2 concentration. This is naturally related to the early onset of an increase in the metabolism in the muscle tissues. End tidal P_{CO2} may be monitored by a number of available devices connected to the endotracheal tube. A normal level should range between 34–40 mm Hg (between 4.5–5.3 kPa). It has been reported that within minutes of the development of malignant hyperpyrexia, there may be a dramatic and accelerated rise in the PE_{CO2}. In reported cases, the end tidal $PE_{CO}2$ was double within minutes and this occurred significantly. Other changes, such as those in temperature, lagged behind in changes in end tidal CO_2.

Histologic Aspects[152]

Muscle excised from patients or susceptible relatives shows several microscopic abnormalities.[39] Fiber diameter is quite variable. There are small angular fibers with clumps of pyknotic nuclei and large round fibers with multiple nuclei. Some cells are devoid of mitochondria or show degeneration and regeneration.[159]

In susceptible swine the liver shows abnormal mitochondria.[151]

Etiology[161]

Fulminant hyperpyrexia is due to disturbed biological oxidation. A pharmacogenetic disease of skeletal and cardiac muscle appears to exist which when appropriately stressed or triggered causes an acceleration of muscle and liver metabolism.[161]

The precise nature of the lesion is damage to the muscle cell plasma membrane causing excitation-contraction coupling dysfunction and or damage to the mitochondria.[162]

Triggering Agents

Clearly identified stressors or triggering agents are the fluorinated anesthetics. Halothane is the most frequently associated stressor in inducing MH. Similarly succinylcholine by itself is capable of significant precipitation of the syndrome. Other inhaled agents such as enflurane isoflurane and methoxyflurane have been implicated; but in these reports, succinylcholine has also been part of the anesthetic management.[163]

Isoflurane has been implicated as a precipitating cause of malignant hyperpyrexia particularly in MH-susceptible individuals. In the initial reports, isoflurane and succinylcholine were both employed when MH complication occurred. However, other reports, in which isoflurane alone was administered, did precipitate a full-blown picture of MH which had been successfully treated.[163]

The role of succinylcholine is well supported. Even apparently normal subjects given succinylcholine show some muscle damage and at least 30% show myoglobinuria.[164] Repeated doses are more harmful and increase the frequency of myoglobinuria.[164]

The consequence is marked increase in oxygen consumption, increased carbon dioxide and metabolic acid production, a release of potassium and passage of myoglobin into the urine (renal threshold of myoglobin is 15 to 20 mg/100 ml blood).

Inhibition of the development of myoglobin and of decreasing the levels of myoglobin can be accomplished to some extent by d-tubo-curarine.[165] This is in addition to dantrolene, both of which will reduce myoglobin and may be an adjunct in the management of MH. Other nondepolarizing relaxants may have similar action.

Normal production of heat by metabolism ranges from 40 kcal (at age 25 years) to 37 kcal (at age 50 years) per square meter of body surface per hour. This ordinarily amounts to 60 to 85 kcal per hour for a standard man. However, during vigorous muscular activity or in the condition of malignant hyperpyrexia the heat production may approach 600 kcal per hour. Simultaneously oxygen consumption is enormously accelerated to approximately 10 times the normal value.

The principal site of increase in whole body oxygen consumption ($\dot{V}O_2$) is the skeletal muscle. This site appears to account for 80% of the heat produced initially. The liver accounts for a considerable portion of the remainder heat.

Other sources of heat include glycolysis, hydrolysis of high-energy phosphates and neutralization of hydrogen ions.[146]

The mechanism of heat production in malignant hyperpyrexia appears to be aerobic metabolism in the initial phase and about 50% of the heat in the terminal phases. In the latter phase anaerobic metabolism is a mechanism.[166]

The body also has a large specific heat (.83 kcal per kg per degree), so that a rise in body temperature represents an increase in stored heat. Thus, a 70-kg man whose temperature increases 1°C will have an increase in body heat of 60 kcal. This storage may represent up to 2% of daily heat production.[166]

A genetic basis appears to exist in some patients.[161] Denborough first showed that the tendency to develop hyperpyrexia is inherited as an autosomal dominant.[111] However, the expression of an inheritable trait (penetrance) may be limited or not shown in individuals who have the primary genes. Other factors such as stresses, environment, vigorous exercise, epinephrine and drugs probably operate to cause the trait to emerge and be manifest clinically.

Experimental Studies

Studies of swine indicate a breed which develops malignant hyperthermia (MH) when stressed (Porcine stress syndrome).[167-169] These susceptible pigs develop the MH syndrome as a result of a wide variety of stresses: fighting, forced exercise, high environmental temperature, and drugs. It appears that heterozygous pigs (PTO) may be susceptible to halothane-triggering and resistant to succinylcholine. But homozygous pigs are apparently susceptible to triggering by either agent or more readily to combinations.[169]

In malignant hyperthermia syndrome (MHS)-susceptible pigs, the administration of althesin, a steroid anesthetic combination, blocks the initiation of the hyperpyrexia induced by halothane.[170] However, it has no effect on the established syndrome nor does it prevent the development of hyperpyrexia by succinylcholine.

Biochemical Changes

In acute malignant hyperpyrexia, the earliest detectable changes are to be observed in the venous blood from skeletal muscle. Due to the dramatic increse in both aerobic and anaerobic metabolism rapid biochemical changes occur: A marked increase in PCO_2 and lactate concentration and a concomitant decrease in pH and PO_2. The increased lactate is considered to be non-hypoxic and related to either a block in the transport of pyruvate from the sarcoplasm into the mitochondria preventing its oxidation or to loss of inorganic phosphate into extracellulr fluid.[156]

Biological Derangements

At the cellular level, two fundamental abnormalities are postulated to exist: either a mitochondrial defect resulting in uncoupling of oxidative phosphorylation[131] or an abnormality of the sarcoplasmic reticulum resulting in increased muscle metabolism due to a high concentration of myoplasmic intracellular calcium.[159,161]

Oxidative Phosphorylation

Uncoupling of oxidative phosphorylation in the cell can be experimentally produced by 2-4 dinitrophenol and results in a rapid rise in temperature.[131,132] Mitochondria from ATP from ADP plus inorganic phosphate (the energy for this reaction is supplied through the electron transport), and when the process of forming ATP is prevented, the ADP accumulates (especially when oxygen supply is limited) and heat is liberated.[132] However, in the average adult this mechanism does not account for the extraordinary heat production and temperature rise since the amount of heat liberated by this mechanism alone is small compared to that liberated by muscle activity. Indeed, the muscle mitochondria of susceptible humans shows a tightly coupled oxidative phosphorylation system even in the presence of triggering agents.[171,172]

Sarcoplasmic Reticulum (SR)

This cellular organelle plays a primary role in the regulation of myoplasmic free calcium.

It has been postulated by Britt[161,173] that a sarcolemmal defect may exist in the skeletal muscle cell. Specifically, an abnormality in cellular calcium metabolism appears to exist resulting in increased contracture of skeletal muscle when exposed to halothane, caffeine, succinylcholine and potassium in man (moulds).[171] The sarcoplasmic reticulum is less able and is slower than normal to accumulate or store calcium in M.H.S. humans.[132,173] Further there is a low threshold for the release of calcium from the SR and an increased rate of release.[174] This defect is further impaired by halothane which diminishes calcium uptake capacity by SR.[172] is apparent that the entry of calcium into the myoplasm from the sarcoplasmic reticulum is essential for myofibrillar contracture and for hyperpyrexia. There is concomitant reduction in concentrations of phosphocreatine, ATP and of the enzyme ATPase in the sarcoplasmic reticulum. Subsequently there is a failure to replenish the high energy storage compound phosphocreatine.[159]

Simultaneously, the excess free calcium accumulates in the myoplasm and stimulates several catabolic anaerobic and aerobic reactions.[175] Initially phosphorylase-kinase is activated. A rapid breakdown of glycogen and an increased glucose-6-phosphate ensues which is metabolized to lactate and carbon dioxide. Later myosin ATPase is stimulated and troponin is inhibited enabling contracture to occur.[176]

Studies by Denborough indicate that smooth muscle membranes are not affected by the abnormality evident in subjects susceptible to malignant hyperpyrexia.

Re-establishment of Normal Permeability

The myofibrillar elements of the muscle cell at the SR level, can be restored to normal permeability by the administration of procaine (or procainamide) as first reported by Beldavs in 1970[143] and confirmed by Kalow.[116] Tetracaine is also effective.[77] These agents in the ionized form accelerate transport of calcium out of the myoplasm and promote uptake and storage in the sarcoplasmic reticulum. Procaine and procainamide also block the caffeine-induced contractures in muscles exposed to halothane.[178] The preferred and specific agent is dantrolene (vida infra).

In contrast lidocaine and digitalis compounds extrude calcium from the terminal cisternae of the sarcoplasmic reticulum storage sites and should not be employed in this syndrome.

The difference between the ester and amide local anesthetics may be related to their pK_a's. It appears that the ionized form of a local anesthetic blocks the release of SR calcium. Since lidocaine has a low pK_a (7.8) in the range of physiologic blood pH there will be a large proportion of uncharged molecules which limits the drug effectiveness.

Molecular Mechanism

An abnormal mechanism for the release of calcium from SR has been identified in MH susceptible and MH patients. As noted by Endo there is a low threshold for the release and rapid rise in calcium release.[174] This process is enhanced by triggering agents; and the excessive concentration of the calcium in the myoplasm induces extraordinary catabolic anerobic and anaerobic metabolic reactions. This calcium excess represents the functional lesion of MH. This mechanism has been validated in MHS patients.[179]

Muscle Calcium-magnesium

Since defect in skeletal muscle specifically in the sarcoplasmic reticulum (SR) is presumed to exist in malignant hyperthermia and in susceptible individuals to malignant hyperthermia, attention has been focused on calcium regulation in the MH muscle cell. Many studies have been carried out, finding little or no difference in the calcium content of the skeletal muscle, differing from control normal human muscle. On the other hand, in a study by Nelson,[180] similarly no difference was found among the mean values for calcium content, whereas the magnesium (Mg^{2+}) content was significantly greater in MH muscle. In their study, more muscle fibers with calcium less than 12 umol/g were observed in MHS muscle, but the difference was not significant statistically. The study suggests that the distribution of calcium and magnesium values is different in MHS muscle as a result of unknown genetic factors associated with the disease.

Magnesium is involved in central and peripheral regulations of temperatures, and Britt and Kalow have suggested that its deficiency plays a role in hyperpyrexia.[145,173] Administration of magnesium protects animals from the uncoupling effects of thyroxine. In mammals, magnesium levels increase when temperature falls, but the actual role of magnesium in this M.H. syndrome is uncertain.

Bone-Calcium Index[145]

Patients who are MH susceptible have involvement of the cells of bone appendages as well as the muscles. By neutron activation analyses of bone, it has been found that there is a reduced calcium level in both non-rigid and rigid MH susceptible individuals. The reductions were marked in the non-rigid patients. Bone-calcium concentrations were also lower in males than in females and in those under 16 years and over 60 years of age. For the rigid MH patients, the bone-calcium index was not too significantly different from normal controls. However, in the non-rigid individuals, the significant reduction in bone-calcium index has represented a possible diagnostic use. It further provides evidence that malignant hyperthermia is based on a widespread defect affecting tissues and organs throughout the body.

Many of the non-rigid MH susceptible patients had an associated greater incidence of fractures than normal. Radiologically, the long bones are slightly thinner than the normal. Excessive numbers of caries, because of thin dental enamel, may also be present.

Role of Creatine Phosphokinase

Creatine is the physiologic substrate of the kinase enzyme CPK. Specifically the enzyme transfers energy-rich phosphorus groups from one substrate form to another. The energy donor for the reaction is ATP. Measurement of the activity of the enzyme can be accomplished readily (refer to Zsigmond).

Analysis of the structure of CPK reveals that it is a dimeric enzyme consisting of two monomers.[147] The (M) type monomer predominates in muscle and the (B) type in nerve tissue. Three combinations of the CPK monomers occur as isoenzymes: MM (CPK_3) is the skeletal muscle type (cathodal enzyme); BB (CPK_1) brain type (anodal enzyme); and MB (CPK_2) the cardiac muscle type.

Normal human tissue demonstrates each of the three isoenzymes, but one usually predominates. In adult brain BB is the dominant isoenzyme; in human heart muscle the MB is characteristic though MM predominates. In skeletal muscle, MM predominates with a smaller amount of MB. The ratio of MB to MM is 0.31 in adult skeletal muscle. The MM enzyme is identical to the M-band of the myofibril and binds to the myosin filaments. It represents about 75% of skeletal muscle, CPK enzyme with MB about 25% and BB absent.

Variations[181]

Fetal skeletal muscle contains BB primarily; by 4 years of age, the adult proportion is attained.[182] The amount of CPK parallels the degree of skeletal muscle specialization; the fast muscle has a higher CPK level and the cholinesterase activity is higher.

The pectoralis muscle and paravertebral muscles are an exception and show a pattern with all three isoenzymes.

In serum the MM enzyme is the only one present normally. In the following conditions the MB isoenzyme predominates: myocardial infarction, malignant hyperpyrexia, myotonia congenita and neurogenic atrophy. In myocardial infarction, this MB enzyme accounts for only 25–40% of myocardial CK.

In malignant hyperpyrexia, in contrast to most conditions, the BB isoenzyme is clearly demonstrated in the serum as well as significant amounts of the MB isoenzyme.

In myopathies and dystrophies, the MB enzyme is present in both sera and muscle tissues. Elevations of CK isoenzyme occur in various malignancies.[183] The isoenzyme CK-BB is commonly present in late stage prostate cancer with metastases and from other ectopic cancer states. In adenocarcinoma of the lung, the CK-MB may be elevated.

Screening Tests[181]

Many tests have been proposed to determine MH susceptibility (Table 19-7). Although CK isoenzymes (MB particularly) may be elevated in the presence of an ongoing hyperpyrexia episode, the use of CK levels does not identify MH susceptibility. In a large series of subjects submitted for muscle biopsy and in vitro contracture testing because of a family history, none had an elevation of CK. Yet about 30% had a positive contracture response. Routinely determined CK levels are not a predictor of MH susceptibility and false negatives are frequent.

Effect of Anesthetic Agents

Of the drugs used in anesthesia practice succinylcholine causes pronounced rises in serum CPK. This occurs regardless of the type of anesthetic induction and sequence.[164] The elevation is least following thiopental; slightly greater increases follow ether and methoxyflurane. The incidence and extent of CPK increases is greatest after halothane induction. The degree of elevation of CPK activity parallels the extent of visible muscle fasciculations. In brief, the highest rise in CPK activity is noted in the halothane-SCh sequence. Repeated doses of SCh are accompanied by further rises.

The administration of large doses of antagonists to nondepolarizing blocking drugs also results in rises in CPK activity.

Patients with predisposing factors to malignant hyperthermic myopathy and their relatives have an elevated CPK level.[181] Since they are candidates for the full blown complication it has been recommended that a routine preoperative serum CPK level be obtained and triggering agents be avoided.

Prophylaxis

1. Inquire about any history of pyrexia or difficulties during anesthesia in relatives. When noted, avoid succinylcholine and halogenated agents.
2. Identify patient at risk. Husky, young muscular males are more susceptible. Determine creatine phosphokinase (CPK)[39] aldolase and serum pyrophosphate (P-P) levels in suspects[68] to identify carriers. CPK is nonspecific but is elevated to 60 units or more in about 30% of asymptomatic M.H. carriers (relatives).[158] Normal value of CPK in males is 0 to 50 and females, 0 to 30. The value of CPK routine testing is good when positive. But 40 to 50% of those at risk may not have an abnormal value.

A reliable indicator of MHSV susceptibility is an abnormal caffeine contracture test (Britt) (vida infra method). This has been defined as the caffeine specific concentration (CSC) and is the concentration of caffeine required to induce a 1-g contracture in a strip of muscle. Control caffeine concentrations of 3.5 to 10.0 mM will induce a contracture in normal subjects.

Table 19–7. Summary of Tests for Malignant Hyperthermia

	Name of Test	Source of Tissue	References
Reliable	Halothane contracture*	Biopsied muscle	Rosenberg, H., Reed, S: Anesth. Analg. 62:417, 1983.[137]
	Caffeine contracture*	Biopsied muscle	Rosenberg, H., Reed, S: Anesth. Analg. 62:419, 1983.[137]
	Combined contracture* with hal + caff.	Biopsied muscle	European, M. H. Study Group: British J. Anesth. 58:646, 1986.[184]
	CPK elevation in families of MH probands	Serum	Gronert, G. A.: Anesthesiology 53:395–423, 1980.[166]
Promising	Ca uptake by lymphocytes with and without halothane	Blood	Klipp, A., Ramcal, T., Walker, D., Britt, B. A., Elliott, E.: Anesth. Analg. 66:381–385, 1987.[185]
	Platelet aggregation in response to epinephrine	Fresh blood	Zsigmond, E. K., Penner, J. Kothary, S. P. II: International Symposium on MH. Ed. Aldrete, J. A., Britt, B. A., New York, Grune and Stratton, 1978, pp 213–219.[186]
	Computerized electronmicroscopic platelet structural changes	Stored-fixed blood	O'Toole, E., Bonneville, M. A., Solomons, C. C., Zsigmond, E. K: J. Cell. Biol. 101:187, a., 1985.[187]
Unreliable	Pyrophosphate in serum	Serum	VanWormer, D. E., Armstrong, D. A., Solomons, C. C.: Malignant Hyperthermia. Martinus Nijhoff Publ., Boston, pp 261–266.[188]
	Muscle phosphorylase*	Biopsied muscle	Cheah, K. S., Cheah, A. M.: Experientia. 41:656, 1985.[189]
	Platelet ATP-depletion by halothane	Fresh blood	Solomons, C.: Acta Anesth. Scand. 28:185–190, 1984.[144]
	Ca uptake of muscle	Biopsied muscle	Blank, T. J. J., Gruener, R., Suffecool, S. L., Thompson, M.: Anesth. Analg. 60:492, 1981.[190]
	Se myoglobin levels	Serum	Zsigmond, E. K.: Unpublished data.

*Phosphorylase test. The *ratio* of muscle phosphorylase to total phosphorylase has been found elevated in muscle from subjects determined to be MH susceptible. This test only requires a needle biopsy sample.[191] However, a high number of false positive ratios makes this test unacceptable as a diagnostic tool.[192]
Prepared by Elemer K. Zsigmond, M. D., University of Illinois, Chicago, IL, 1987.[67]

Values of 2.5 mM of caffeine or less are indicative of susceptibility and can be used as diagnostic.[138]

3. For patients at risk to be given general anesthesia use a semi-open or semi-closed high flow circle system. This provides an additional avenue of heat loss.[193,194]

4. Acceptable agents[195] for patients at risk include: intravenous neurolept analgesia, thiopental, ketamine and althesin, droperidol, diazepam and procaine. Nitrous[196] oxide is safe as an inhalation agent.

Regional anesthesia is safe and avoids the hazard of disruptive biological oxidation.[195]

Midazolam has been found to be a safe agent.[197] Studies of biopsied muscle from MH susceptible patients have revealed the following: midazolam at maximum therapeutic concentrations (0.5 µg/ml^{-1}) had no detectable effect on muscle contraction from direct muscle stimulation. No interaction was found between midazolam and either halothane or caffeine on the directly stimulated muscle contracture. But, high concentrations of midazolam, well outside the human therapeutic range, permitted contracture in both control and MH muscle biopsies.

Non-depolarizing muscle relaxants are safe. Pancuronium or vecuronium actually inhibit the development of MH even after the use of succinylcholine and appear to be relaxants of choice.[198] In large doses pancuronium of vecuronium modify the response to halothane and afford protection against MH triggered by halothane.[199] Pancuronium also depresses or prevents halothane induced muscle contracture in muscle strips from MH susceptible patients.[195]

5. Depolarizing muscle relaxants, halothane and lidocaine are contraindicated. Fluorinated agents should be avoided or wisely chosen. Catecholamines and alpha-adrenergic agonists have been associated with fatal MH reactions in animals.[200] Contrariwise alpha-adrenergic antagonists have not been implicated. Experimentally bilateral adrenalectomy has been effective in preventing MH.[201] The false precursors to

the synthesis of catecholamines such as alpha-methyl tyrocine or alpha-methyl dopa can be used.

6. Continuous and vigilant observation of vital signs of all patients is essential. Temperature observations should be made throughout an anesthetic period. Early detection of increases in core body temperatures is necessary in suspects through use of esophageal thermister, tympanothermometry, or other electronic devices. Once any unusual or undetermined abnormality of cardiorespiratory physiology occurs, temperature observation and blood gas monitoring is mandatory.

7. Although dantrolene has been recommended for prophylaxis in MH susceptible subjects, no valid evidence has been adducted to confirm its value if the prime triggering anesthetic agents are avoided and a stress free state is achieved.[202] One exception may be where there is emergency surgery in conditions with massive muscle trauma, or other contributory conditions to MH. One study by J. Lerman (Toronto General Hospital) concludes that prophylactic dantrolene is unnecessary and the drug should be reserved for therapeutic purposes. Of 956 MH patients anesthetized with trigger-free agents and stress-free conditions for muscle biopsy, only 4 patients exhibited a reaction, or an incidence of 0.62%, and were treated successfully. It is also apparent that the reactions are more likely to occur in the recovery room.

In those instances of emergency surgery where the risk of MH is judged to exist, a prophylactic dose of 1.0 mg/kg of body weight should be administered intravenously just prior to induction of anesthesia.

Treatment

1. *Discontinue* administration of all anesthetic agents.[194]
   a. Remove and replace rubber goods.
   b. Employ any gas anesthetic machine without vaporizers.
   c. Change anesthesia machine if feasible.
2. *Treat Hypoxia.* Institute open or semiclosed, high flow inhalation system with oxygen and controlled hyperventilation. Artificial hyperventilation appears to enhance survival. Administer 10 to 20% dextrose intravenously to provide adequate substrate for brain metabolism.
3. *Initiate aggressive cooling.*
   a. Remove drapes.
   b. Apply ice chips to exposed body surface, especially to axilla and groin, and gently sponge all surfaces. This provides loss of heat by conduction. However, loss of heat by this method is low[203]; only 18 kcal are transferred from a warm surface to 500 ml of cold. Shivering must be prevented by alpha adrenergic blocking drugs such as chlorpromazine or dibenzyline.
   c. Promote convection currents of air at 70 °F by fans over nude patient (Knochel). This aids[203] in loss of heat by radiation by continuously remov-

ing the warm-air envelope surrounding the patient.[204] Heat loss increases with the square of the air velocity of the fan air (wind chill). If a fine mist of tepid water (80°F) is carried by the fan air and evaporated, then each ml will remove 537 calories.
   d. Intravenous iced Ringer's lactate solution (limited uptake of heat). Specific heat of 1 liter of Ringer's lactate solution is approximately 1 kcal. One liter at 0° raised to 37 °C will take up only 37 kcal of heat.
   e. Hypothermia blanket technic is effective.[205] Blanket should be in place prior to induction in patients at risk. (Makkah cooling unit).
   f. Immersion in a tub of ice has been recommended but impractical in most operating theaters. Furthermore, it is not necessarily the most effective cooling method since it relies on heat loss by conduction. It is difficult to sponge a patient with the ice; intense vasoconstriction occurs especially of surface vessels and limits the amount of heat brought to the surface by the blood.
   g. Intracavitary washing, with iced balanced salt solutions (during abdominal or thoracic surgery) has significant effect.
   h. Extracorporeal by-pass.[206]
   i. Temperature should be monitored at least every 5 minutes or, preferably, continuously. Do not let the temperature fall below 100°F (37.7°C) to prevent reactive hypothermia.
4. *Aggressive hydration* with Ringer's lactate solution (iced as noted) in volumes of 3 to 4 liters in 6 hours. CVP monitoring is mandatory in order to detect circulatory overload.
5. *Correct metabolic acidosis* with intravenous sodium bicarbonate. Base deficit (BD) × ECF volume = number mEq sodium bicarbonate. When blood gases are unavailable assume a base-deficit of 6 mmol.L^{-1} and administer an arbitrary dose of sodium bicarbonate; 10 mEq may be necessary. Hypernatremia may result and should be controlled by infusion of furosemide and/or mannitol. This will also assist in flushing out myoglobin through renal tubules. Mannitol also corrects the muscular and cerebral edema. (1.0 mg/kg)
6. *Treat tachycardia.* Small doses of beta-adrenergic blocking drugs are effective and safe. Do not move patient. Stimulation by movement incites or increases ventricular arrhythmias. Use intravenous procaine or procainamide for intractable arrhythmias.
7. Administer *intravenous procaine* (or procainamide) or tetracaine to stabilize the cell membranes, and calcium storage vesicles of skeletal muscles.[177] The dose of procaine is 0.5 to 1.0 mg/kg/minute (Procaine Unit). These agents in the ionized form promote uptake and storage of calcium in the sarcoplasmic reticulum. Procainamide has been used successfully to treat rigidity and an MH reaction.[207]
8. *Calcium Control.* High levels of sarcoplasmic cal-

cium increase the risk of initiating skeletal muscle contracture[208] in pig muscle, a critical level of free sarcoplasmic calcium is about 10^{-7}M. Lowering extracellular and plasma calcium and creating a gradient of calcium into sarcoplasmic reticulum minimizes contracture.[209]

Dantrolene is the key and specific drug available to slow the course of MH and even reverse the process. This drug acts directly and specifically within the skeletal muscle fiber.[210] It suppresses the release of calcium from the storage vesicles in the sarcoplasmic reticulum (SR).[137] For therapeusis in an established case of human MH, the dose is approximately 2.5 mg/kg of body weight.[202] This should be administered intravenously in divided doses of 1.0 mg/kg every 5 minutes until the total dose is given. Larger doses may be required up to a total dose of 10 mg/kg of body weight.

Calcium channel blockers have been found to be effective substitutes[211] Verapamil, nifedipine and diltiazem affect the cell surface of the slow channels to block the movement of calcium. The excitation-contraction coupling in skeletal muscle is also reduced by blocking the release of calcium from the sarcoplasmic reticulum and its transport into the sarcoplasm.

9. *Reduce the early hyperkalemia* by administration of insulin plus glucose (100 units regular in 500 ml of 10% dextrose), or put insulin in Ringer's lactate solution. Monitor serum potassium. When temperature subsides, stop insulin and be prepared to treat potassium depletion.

10. *Administer Glucocorticoids.* methylprednisolone has been effective in preventing contracture and valuable in treating MH.[196]

11. *Use alpha-blocking agents.* Chlorpromazine or dehydrobenzperidol provide skin vasodilatation and improve cutaneous blood flow. Shivering is inhibited. Thermogenesis is inhibited.

Experimental evidence indicates blocking the transmission of alpha adrenergic mediators can protect the triggering of MH. Reserpine and the prior administration of methyl-dopa are effective.[198] Phenoxybenzamine and prazosin are useful in this regard.

12. *Epidural Block.*[212] Experiments indicate that complete epidural block (use procaine) will prevent the triggering of M.H. by halothane. The nervous system is thus *one* important element in the precipitation of M.H.

Immediate Tests for MH on occurrence of reaction include blood for gases, electrolytes (K^+, Ca^{++}), and, after 4 hours, CPK and isoenzymes,[153] and urine for hemoglobin and myoglobin.

Delayed Complications

Hyperactive Bleeding (DIC)

Acute activation of clotting results from two mechanisms:

a. Endothelial damage is produced by hyperthermia and this activates the Hageman (XII) Factor.

b. Tissue hypoxia (oxygen over-utilization) causes mobilization of tissue thromboplastin and entry of this enzyme into the circulation.

Consequences include intravascular consumption of clotting factors: depletion of platelets, prothrombin, fibrinogen and Factors V, VII, and XII. This is the DIC syndrome.

c. Abnormal platelet aggregation appears to occur in susceptible patients which is increased by halothane.[144]

Erythrocyte Fragility[151]

Red blood cells show increased fragility. Hemoglobin is released from increased RBC breakdown. When levels higher than 200 mg/100 ml of blood are reached, hemoglobin then appears in the urine. The renal threshold for hemoglobin is 100 to 150 mg/100 ml of blood.

Liver Damage

Liver function tests during and immediately after acute crises are either normal or only slightly elevated, while liver enzymes are normal in all patients.[204] In patients who survive heat stroke, jaundice is common and liver damage is frequent.[203] In M.H. patients liver damage may be expected as a secondary effect of the hyperpyrexia, but no primary defect appears to exist. M.H. pigs whose livers are isolated and perfused with halothane do not become hyperthermic.[173] However, if there is skeletal muscle damage, liver metabolism may be elevated in the process of burning excessive lactic acid.

Hypothalamic Damage

Disturbed temperature regulation at the hypothalamus undoubtedly occurs but is not likely the initiating factor.[213] If the thermostat is raised, heat production will increase. For each 1°C. increase in body temperature there is a 13% increase in heat production.[214] This becomes a vicious cycle, especially if damage to the hypothalamic neurons occurs.

Dantrolene

In the management of malignant hyperthermia, the chemical dantrolene sodium has been accepted as a prophylactic and therapeutic agent in the management of human malignant hyperthermia. (Table 19–8).

Chemistry

Dantrolene is a lipid soluble hydantoin derivative. It is a complex imidazoline sodium salt, which is poorly soluble in water, but, because of its high lipid solubility, it crosses cell membranes readily. The structure and chemical name is represented in Figure 19-5. It structurally resembles diphenylhydantoin.

Preparation

A lyophylized formulation is available for parenteral use. The powder consists of 20 mg of dantrolene, 3 g of mannitol and sufficient sodium hydroxide to establish a pH of approximately 9.5 on being dissolved. When the

Table 19–8. Diagnostic Criteria for Dantrolene Sodium IV Administration

---

Tachyarrhythmias
Rigidity
Hyperpotassemia
Temperature rise during anesthesia
Increasing serum-CPK

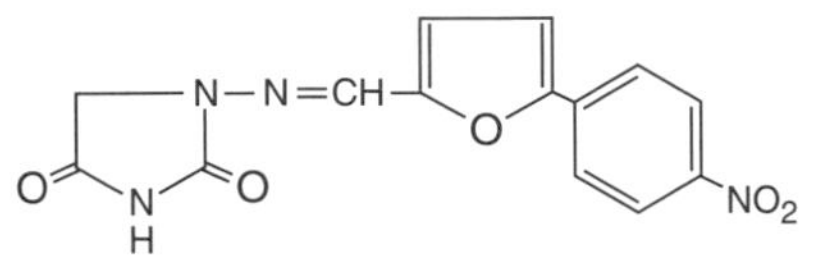

Dantrolene

Fig. 19–5. Dantrolene.

powder is dissolved by the addition of 60 ml of sterile distilled water, the resulting solution contains 0.33 mg/ml.[215] The drug has a short shelf-life and should be prepared fresh. At present, the drug is expensive. The reconstituted drug has a pH of 9.5.

Mechanism of Action

The site of action of dantrolene is within the skeletal muscle fiber and, thus, it may be considered an intracellular muscle relaxant. It appears to directly stabilize the sarcoplasmic reticulum membrane containing the vesicles of calcium and also acts on the transverse tubular membrane and the terminal cisternae of the sarcoplasmic reticulum.[216] Thus, the agent limits the availability of calcium ions by attenuating calcium release without affecting uptake. This limits the excitation-coupling reactions of the muscle contractile system.

In human volunteers, dantrolene causes subjective weakness and impairment of neuromuscular transmission. A 42% reduction in grip strength has been reported to occur after 2.2 mg/kg i.v. No significant recovery was noted 7 hours later.[217] A mean twitch depression of 75% has been achieved with doses of 2.4 mg/kg i.v.[218] At this time, the dantrolene blood level approximates 4.2 ug/ml.

On the other hand, in patients with myasthenia gravis, there appears to be a resistance to the effect of dantrolene on twitch depression. Twitch height may only be depressed by 60% with doses of 2.4 mg/kg. After 2–3 hours, there is a decrease in fade ratio. Recovery of grip strength is slow.[218]

Whether dantrolene has a role in improving the muscular condition in human myasthenia is a matter of speculation. In experimental auto-immune myasthenia gravis (EAMG), some improvement has been produced.[219]

Dosage

Careful experimental studies in susceptible MHS swine showed that an intravenous dose of 3.5 mg/kg of dantrolene was capable of maximal muscle depressant action to the extent of 95% and proved to be both prophylactic and therapeutic for halothane succinylcholine anesthetic challenge.[220]

A multicenter clinical study in the therapy of MH crisis showed that the dose of dantrolene needed to reverse a crisis was approximately 2.5 mg/kg of body weight. This was basically an empirical study.

Pharmacokinetics[217]

After the administration of dantrolene, blood levels decline according to first order kinetics. After a single rapid intravenous dose, there is an initial dilution in the vascular compartment and levels of approximately 3–4 ug/ml are achieved in 2–3 minutes. There then follows a rapid distribution and uptake of the drug by tissues. During this early distribution phase, the t $^{1}/_{2}$ alpha, a steady state exists for 2–3 hours with a mean blood dantrolene level of 3.6 ug/ml. This is followed by an elimination phase, t $^{1}/_{2}$ beta, approximately 12 hours. Thus, the administration of the recommended dose provides a continuing effective plasma level over a desirable period of time of 2–6 hours for the prophylaxis as well as the treatment of a crisis.

Other Pharmacologic Effects

Neuromuscular

Twitch tension depression occurs with the incremental intravenous doses of 0.1 mg/kg every 5 minutes until a cumulative dose of 2.5 mg/kg of body weight is reached when a maximal twitch depression of 75% is achieved. After each dose, the twitch depression stabilizes by 2–3 minutes.

Maximal depression of grip strength in awake volunteers was 42% after cumulative doses of 2.2 mg/kg.[221] Depression continues for 24 hours. All subjects complained of fatigue and muscle weakness for this period and did not feel recovery of normal strength until after 48 hours.[217]

Central Nervous System

Some subjective alterations of consciousness may occur. These altered sensations include dizziness, floating, light headedness, and a sleepy feeling is frequent. Nausea, vomiting, dysphagia, and mild motion sickness are side effects. All these symptoms clear by 48 hours.

Respiratory Effects

Respiratory changes and cardiovascular effects are insignificant.

Failures

Despite the prophylactic administration of dantrolene, MH susceptible patients may still be triggered with an MH crisis.[222]

Complications

No serious adverse reactions have been encountered. Kolb[9] has reported only two instances of superficial phlebitis in 5,000 administrations.[223] The alkaline pH of the reconstituted drug may account for irritation of the venous endothelium.

Interaction with calcium entry blockers[224] such as verapamil[225] and diltiazem with the administration of dantrolene in MH-susceptible or MH-treated patients may result in marked hyperkalemia and cardiovascular collapse.[226]

REFERENCES

1. West, John B., Ed: Best and Taylor's Physiologic Basis of Medical Practice. 12 Ed. Baltimore, The Williams and Wilkins Co., 1990, p 1061-1063.
2. Barbour, H. G.: The Heat Regulating Mechanism of the Body. Physiol Rev 1:295, 1921.
3. Good, A. L., Sellers, A. F.: Temperature Changes in the Blood of the Pulmonary Artery and Left Atrium of Dogs During Exposure to Extreme Cold. Am J Physiol 188:447, 1957.
4. Bazett, H. C. L., Love, M., Newton, L., Eisenberg, R. D., Forster, I.R.: Temperature Changes in Blood Flowing in Arteries and Veins in Man. J Appl Physiol 1:3, 1948.
5. Wakim, K. G.: The Physiologic Effects of Heat. JAMA 138:1091, 1948.
6. Dawkins, M. J. R., Scopes, J. W.: Non-shivering thermogenesis and brown adipose tissue in the human newborn infant. Nature 206:201-202, 1965.
7. Mestyan, J., Jarai, I., Bata, G., et al.: The significance of facial skin temperature in the chemical heat regulation of premature infants. Bio Neonat 7:243-254, 1964.
8. Machle, W., Hatch, T. F.: Heat: Man's Exchanges and Physiological Responses. Physiol Rev 27:200, 1947.
9. Hyndman, O. R., Wolkin, J.: The Automatic Mechanisms of Heat Conservation and Dissipation. Am Heart J 23:43, 1942.
10. Hey, E. N., Hatz, A.: Evaporated Heat Loss in the Newborn Baby. J Physiol 200:605-619, 1969.
11. Smith, R. E., Horowitz, B. A.: Brownfat Thermogenesis. Physiol Rev 49:330-425, 1965.
12. Jessen, K.: An assessment of human regulatory nonshivering thermogenesis. Acta Anaesthesiol Scand 24:138-143, 1980.
13. Jessen, K., Rabøl, A., Winkler, K.: Total body and splanchnic thermogenesis in curarized man during a short exposure to cold. Acta Anaesthesiol Scand 24:339-344, 1980.
14. Hardy, J. D., Oppel, T. W.: The thermal response of the skin to radiation. Physics 7:466-479, 1936.
15. Guyton, A. C.: Handbook of Medical Physiology. 4th Ed. W. A. Saunders, Philadelphia, 1971.
16. Hyndman, O. R., Wolkin, J.: Sweat Mechanisms in Man. Arch Neurol Psychiat 45:446, 1941.
17. Simon, E.: Temperature regulation: The spinal cord as a site of extrahypothalamic thermoregulatory functions. Rev Physiol Biochem Pharmacol 71:1-76, 1974.
18. Benzinger, T. H.: Heat regulation: Homeostasis of Central Temperature in Man. Physiol Rev 49:671-759, 1969.
19. Wyss, C. R., Brengelmann, G. L., Johnson, J. M., et al.: Altered control of skin blood flow at high skin and core temperatures. J Appl Physiol 38:839-845, 1975.
20. Lopez, M., Sessler, D. I., Walter, K., et al.: Rate- and gender-dependence of the sweating, vasoconstriction, and shivering thresholds in humans. Anesthesiology, in press.
21. Tam, H., Darling, R. C., Cheh, H., et al.: The dead zone of thermoregulation in normal and paraplegic man. Can J Physiol Pharmacol 56:976-983, 1978.
22. Mekjavic, I. B., Sundberg, C. J., Linnarsson, D.: Core temperature "null zone." J Appl Physiol 71:1289-1295, 1991.
23. McCook, R., Peiss, C. N., Randall, W. C.: Hypothalamic Temperatures and Blood Flow. Proc Soc Exp Biol Med 109:518, 1962.
24. Hensel, H.: Correlations of neural activity and thermal sensation in man. In: Sensory Function of the Skin edited by Y.Z. Herman, Oxford, UK. Pergamon Press, 331-353, 1976.
25. Torebjoerk, H. E., Ochoa, J. L.: Specific sensations evoked by activity in single identified sensory units in skin. Acta Physiol Scand 110:445-447, 1986.
26. Meyers, R. D., Sharpe, L. G.: Transmitter Factors Released from Brain During Thermo-regulation. Science 161:572, 1968.
27. Hardy, J. D.: The "set-point" concept in physiologic temperature regulation: In Physiological Controls and Regulations. Ed. Yamanibo, W.S. and Brobeck, J.R., Phila., W.B. Saunders, p98-116, 1965.
28. Washington, D., Sessler, D. I., Moayeri, A., et al.: Thermoregulatory responses to hyperthermia during isoflurane anesthesia in humans. J Appl Physiol 74:82-87, 1993.
29. Magoun, H. W., Harrison, W. F., Brobeck, J. R., Ranson, S.W.: Activation of Heat Loss Mechanisms by Local Heating of the Brain. J Neurophysiol 1:101-114, 1938.
30. Kunkel, P., Stead, E. A., Weiss, S.: Blood Flow and Vasomotor Reactions in the Hand, Forearm, Foot and Calf in Response to Physical and Chemical Stimuli. J Clin Invest 2:225, 1939.
31. Von Euler, U. S.: Adrenergic Neurotransmitting functions, Science 173:202-206, 1976.
32. Glotzbech, S. F., Heller, H. C.: Central Nervous Regulation of Body Temperature During Sleep. Science 194:537-539, 1976.
33. Sessler, D. I.: Perianesthetic thermoregulation and heat balance in humans. FASEB J 7:638-644, 1993.
34. Foregger, R.: Surface Temperature During Anesthesia. Anesthesiology 4:392, 1943.
35. Edmondson, R.E.: Case Reports: Hyperpyrexia Following the Administration of Pentobarbital. Anesthesiology 3:215, 1942.
36. Insel, P. A.: Analgesic-antipyretic and anti-inflammatory drugs: In Goodman & Gilman's The Pharmacologic of Therapeutics. Eighth Edition, Pergamon Press, New York, 1990.
37. Dinarello, C. A., Wolff, S. M.: Pathogenesis of Fever in Man. N Engl J Med 298:607-612, 1978.
38. Vane, J. R.: Inhibtion of Prostaglandin Synthesis as a Mechanism of Action of Aspirin-like Drugs. Nature New Biol 231:232-235, 1971.
39. Irving, L.: Adaptation to Cold. Science 161:94, 1966.
40. Irving, L.: Terrestrial Animals in Cold, Handbook of Physiology, Section 4, Adaptation to the Environment. Am Physiol Soc 1964.
41. Irving, L.: Effects of Temperature on Sensitivity of Fingers. J Appl Physiol 18:1201, 1963.
42. Dill, D. B.: Life, Heat and Altitudes: Physiological Effects of Hot Climates and Great Heights. Cambridge, Harvard University Press, 1951.
43. War Department Technical Bulletin, Washington, June, 1945. Prevention and Treatment of Adverse Effects of Heat. TD Med., 175.
44. Knochel, J. P.: Environmental heat illness. Arch Int Med 133:841, 1974.
45. Friedfeld, L.: Prophylaxis and Treatment of Heat Reaction States. N Engl J Med 240:1043, 1949.
46. Borden, D. L., Waddill, J.F., Grier, G.S.: Statistical Study of 265 Cases of Heat Disease. JAMA 128:1200, 1945.
47. Bragdon, J. H.: The Hepatitis of Hyperthermia. N Engl J Med 237:765, 1947.
48. Bower, B. D.: Cold injury in the newborn. Br Med J 1:303, 1960.
49. Sessler, D. I.: Perianesthetic thermoregulation and heat balance in humans. FASEB J 7:638-644, 1993.
50. Sessler, D. I.: Central thermoregulatory inhibition by general anesthesia (editorial). Anesthesiology 73:557-559, 1991.
51. Vaughan, M. S., Vaughan, R. W., Cork, R. C.: Postoperative

hypothermia in adults: Relationship of age, anesthesia, and shivering to rewarming. Anesth Analg 60:746, 1981.

52. Stone, D. R., Downs, J. B., Paul, W. L., Perkins, H. M.: Adult body temperature and heated humidification of anesthetic gases during general anesthesia. Anesth Analg 60:736, 1981.

53. Conahan, T. J., Williams, G. D., Apfelbaum, J. L., Lecky, J. H.: Airway heating reduces recovery room time. Anesthesiology 67:128-132, 1987.

54. Ponte, J., Collett, B. J., Walmsley, A. Anaesthetic temperature and shivering in epidural anaesthesia. Acta Anaesthesiol Scand 30:584-587, 1986.

55. Ponte, J., Sessler, D. I.: Extradurals and shivering: Effects of cold and warm extradural saline injections in volunteers. Br J Anaesth 64:731-733, 1990.

56. Kosaka, M., Simon, E., Thauer, R.: Shivering in intact and spinal rabbits during spinal cooling. Experienta 23:385, 1966.

57. Sessler, D. I., Ponte, J.: Shivering during epidural anesthesia. Anesthesiology 72:816-821, 1990.

58. Simon, E.: Temperature regulation: The spinal cord as a site of extraphypothalamic thermoregulatory functions. Rev Physiol Biochem Pharmacol 71:1-76, 1974.

59. Holdcroft, A., Hall, G. M.: Heat loss during anesthesia. Br J Anaesth 50:157, 1978.

60. Carloss, H. W., Tavassoli, M.: Acute renal failure from precipation of cryoglubulins in cool operating rooms. JAMA 244:1472, 1980.

61. Jessen, L.: An assessment of human regulatory non-shivering thermogenesis. Acta Anaesthesiol Scand 24:138, 1980.

62. Hall, G. M.: Body temperature and anaesthesia. Br J Anesth 50:39-44, 1978.

63. Sessler, D. I., McGuire, J., Moayeri, A., et al.: Isoflurane-induced vasodilation minimally increases cutaneous heat loss. Anesthesiology 74:226-232, 1991.

64. Hynson, J. M., Sessler, D. I., et al.: Absence of a non-shivering thermogenesis in anesthetized adults. Anesthesiology 79:695-703, 1993.

65. Belani, K., Sessler, D. I., Sessler, A. M., et al.: Leg heat content continues to decrease during the core temperature plateau in humans. Anesthesiology 78:856-863, 1993.

66. Hynson, J. M., Sessler, D. I.: Intraoperative warming therapies: a comparison of three devices. J Clin Anesth 4.194-199, 1992.

67. Sessler, D. I.: Central thermoregulatory inhibition by general anesthesia. (Editorial) Anesthesiology 73:557-559. 1991.

68. Sessler, D. I., Olofsson, C. I., Rubinstein, E. H., Beebe, J. J.: The thermoregulatory threshold in humans during nitrous oxide fentanyl anesthesia. Anesthesiology 69:357-360, 1988.

69. Bissonnette, B., Sessler, D. I.: The thermoregulatory threshold in infants and children anesthetized with isoflurane and caudal bupivicaine. Anesthesiology 73:1114-1118, 1990.

70. Stoen, R., Sessler, D. I.: The thermoregulatory threshold is inversely related to isoflurane concentration. Anesthesiology 72:811-822, 1990.

71. Sessler, D. I., Hynson, Moayeri, A., et al.: Thermoregulatory vasoconstriction decreases cutaneous heat loss. Anesthesiology 73:656-660, 1990.

72. Mahajan, P. P., Grover, V. K., Sharma, S. L., Singh, H.: Intraocular pressure changes during muscular hyperactivity after general anesthesia. Anesthesiology 66:419-422, 1987.

73. Morris, R. H.: Operating room temperature and the anaesthetized paralyzed patient. Arch Surg 102:95, 1971.

74. Goudsouzian, N. G., Morris, R. H., Ryan, J. F.: The effects of a warming blanket on the maintenance of body temperature in anesthetized infants and children. Anesthesiology 39:351, 1973.

75. Hensel, H.: Correlations of neural activity and thermal sensation in man. In Sensory Function of skin. Herman, Y.Z. (Ed) Oxford, UK. Pergamon Press 331-353, 1976.

76. Kristensen, G., Guldager, H., Graveson, H.: Prevention of perioperative hypothermia in abdominal surgery. Acta Anesthesiol Scand 30:314, 1986.

77. Workhoven, M. N.: Intravenous fluid temperature, shivering and parturient. Anesth Analg 65:496, 1986.

78. Norman, E. A., Ahmad, I., Zeig, N. J.: Delivery temperature of heated and cooled intravenous solutions. Anesth Analg 65:693, 1986.

79. Allen, T. D.: Body temperature changes during prostatic resection as related to temperature of the irrigation solution. J Urol 110:433, 1973.

80. Dyer, T. M., Heathcote, P. S.: Reduction of heat loss during transurethral resection of the prostate. Anesthes Intens Care 14:12, 1986.

81. Sessler, D. I., Rubinstein, E. H., Moayeri, A.: Physiological response to mild perianesthetic hypothermia in humans. Anesthesiology 75:594-610, 1991.

82. Just, B., Delva, E., Camus, U., et al.: Oxygen uptake during recovery following naloxone. Anesthesiology 76:60-64, 1992.

83. Bickler, P., Sessler, D. I.: Efficiency of airway heat and moisture exchangers in anesthetized humans. Anesth Analg 71:415-418, 1990.

84. Guffin, A., Girard, D., Kaplan, J. A.: Shivering following cardiac surgery: hemodynamic changes and reversal. J Cardiothorac Anesth 1:24, 1987.

85. Bay, J., Nunn, J., Prys-Roberts, C.: Factors influencing arterial PO_2 during recovery from anesthesia. Br J Anaesth 40:398, 1968.

86. Heymann, A. D.: The effect of incidental hypothermia on elderly surgical patients. J Gerentol 32:146, 1977.

87. Tølløfspud, S. G., Gunderson, Y., Andersen, R.: Perioperative hypothermia. Acta Anaesthesiol Scand 28:511, 1985.

88. Christoforides, C. and Hedley-White, J.: Effects of temperature on hemoglobin concentration and a solubility of oxygen in blood. J Appl Physiol 27:592-596, 1969.

89. MacIntyre, P. E., Pavlin, E. G., Dwersteg, J. F.: Effect of meperidine on oxygen consumption, carbon dioxide production and respiratory gas exchange. Anesth Analg 66:751-760, 1987.

90. Pflug, A. E., Aesheim, G. M., Foster, C., Martin, R. W.: Prevention of postanesthesia shivering in man. Acta Anaesthesiol Scand 28:138, 1984.

91. Pauca, A. L., Savage, R. T., Simpson, S., Roy, R. C.: Effect of pethidine, fentanyl and morphine on post-operative shivering in man. Acta Anaesthesiol Scand 28:138, 1984.

92. Hynson, J. M., Sessler, D. I., Moayeri, A., et al: Absence of nonshivering thermogenesis in anesthetized humans. Anesthesiology 79:695-703, 1993.

93. Stephen, C. R.: Body temperature regulation during anesthesia in infants and children. JAMA 174:1519-1522, 1960.

94. Sharkey, A., Lipton, J. M., Murphy, M. T., Giesecke, A. H.: Inhibition of post-anesthetic shivering with radiant heat. Anesthesiology 66:131, 1987.

95. Himms-Hagen, J.: Thermogenesis in brown adipose tissue as an energy buffer: Implications for obesity. Seminars in medicine of the Beth Israel Hospital, Boston. NEJM 311:1549, 1984.

96. Hall, G. M.: Brown fat: A thermogenic tissue of anesthetic importance. Br J Anaesth 54.:907, 1982.

97. Murphy, M. T., Lipton, J. M., Loughran, M. B., Giesecke,

Jr., A. H.: Postanesthetic shivering in primates: Inhibition by peripheral heating and β-taurine. Anesthesiology 63:161, 1985.

98. Harris, W. S., Lipton, J. M.: Intracerebroventricular taurine in rabbits: Effects on normal body temperature, endotoxin fever and hyperthermia produced by PGE₁ and amphetamine. J Physiol (London) 266:397, 1977.

99. Burks, L. C., Alsner, J., Fortner, C. L., Wiernik, P. H.: Meperidine for the treatment of shaking, chills, and fever. Arch Intern Med 140:483, 1980.

100. Stephen, C. R.: Body temperature regulation during anesthesia in infants and children. JAMA 174:1519–1522, 1960.

101. Gauntlett, I., Barnes, J., Brown, T. C. K., Bell, B. J.: Temperature and maintenance in infants undergoing anaesthesia and surgery. Anaesth Intens Care 13:304, 1985.

102. Marks, K. M., Devenyi, A. G., Bello, M. E., et al.: Thermal head wrap for infants. J Ped 107:956, 1985.

103. Cross, K. W., Stratton, D.: Aural temperature of the newborn infant. Lancet 2:1179, 1974.

104. Hall, G. M.: Fentanyl and the metabolic response to surgery. Br J Anaesth 52:561, 1980.

105. Brandt, M., Fernandes, A., Mordhurst, R., Kehlet, H.: Epidural analgesia improves postoperative nitrogen balance. Br J Anaesth 54:1023, 1982.

106. Carli, F., Clark, M. M., Woollen, J. W.: Investigation of the relationship between heat loss and nitrogen excretion in elderly patients undergoing major abdominal surgery under general anaesthetic. Br J Anaesth 54:1023, 1982.

107. Carli, F., Itiaba, K.: Effect of heat conservation during and after major abdominal surgery on muscle protein breakdown in elderly patients. Br J Anaesth 58:502, 1986.

108. Sessler, D. I., Rosenberg, H., Gronert, G. A., et al.: Statement on intraoperative temperature monitoring. American Society of Anesthesiologists.

109. Ilsey, A. H., Rutten, A. J., Runciman, W. B.: An evaluation of body temperature measurement. Anaesth Intens Care 11:31–39, 1983.

110. Ramsay, J. G., Ralley, F. E., Dellicolli, P., Wynads, J. E.: Site of temperature monitoring and prediction of afterdrop after open heart surgery. Can Anaesth Soc J 32:607–612, 1985.

111. Denborough, M. A.: Anesthetic Deaths in a Family. Br J Anaesth 34:395, 1962.

112. Saidman, L. T., Howard, E. S., Eger, E. I.: Hyperthermia During Anesthesia. JAMA 190:1029, 1964.

113. Editorial: Malignant Hyperpyrexia During General Anesthesia. Can Anesth Soc J 13:415, 1966.

114. Gordon, R. A., Britt, B. A., Kalow, W. (Editors): International Symposium on Malignant Hyperthermia. Springfield, Charles C. Thomas, 1973.

115. Britt, B. A., Kwong, F., and Endrenyi, L.: The Clinical and Laboratory Features of Malignant Hyperthermia in Henschel, E10. Ed: Malignant Hyperthermia, Appleton-Century-Crofts New York, 1977.

116. Kalow, W., Britt, B. A., Chan, F. Y.: Epidemiology and Inheritance of Malignant Hyperthermia. Intern Anesth Clin 17:119–139, 1979.

117. Murikawa, S.: Two Cases of Heat During Anesthesia in a Family. Jap J Anesth 10:895, 1970.

118. Iuchi, Y.: Two Cases of Malignant Hyperpyrexia. Jap J Anesth 21:487, 1972.

119. McPherson, E., Taylor, C. A.,: The Genetics of Malignant Hyperthermia. Am J Med Genet 11:273–288, 1982.

120. Gordon, R. A., Britt, B. A., Kalow, W.: International Symposium on Malignant Hyperthermia. Springfield, Charles C. Thomas, 1973.

121. Stephens, C. R.: Fulminant Hyperthermia During Anesthesia and Surgery. JAMA 202:178, 1967.

122. Daniels, J. C., Polayes, I. M., Villae, R., Hehre, F. W.: Malignant Hyperthermia with Disseminated Intravascular Coagulation During General Anesthesia. Anes Analg 48:877, 1969.

123. Wilson, R. D.: Malignant Hyperpyrexia with Anesthesia. JAMA 202:1983, 1967.

124. Smego, R., Durack, D.,: The Neurolept Malignant Syndrome. Arch Int Med 142:1183–1186, 1982.

125. Allsop, P., Twigley, A. J.: The Neurolept Malignant Syndrome. Anaesthesia 42:49–53, 1987.

126. Lavie, G. J., Olsmtead, T. R., et al.: Neuroleptic Malignant Syndrome. Postgrad Med 80:171–176, 1986.

127. Mueller, P., Vester, J., Fermaglich, H. J.: Neuroleptic Malignant Syndrome: successful treatment with bromocraptinea. JAMA 249:386–390, 1983.

128. Denborough, M. A., Ebiling, P., Krug, J. O., Zapt, P.: Myopathy and Malignant Hyperpyrexia. Lancet 1:1138, 1970.

129. Green, J. H., Ellis, F. R., Halsall, P. J., et al: Thermoregulation, plasma catecholamine and metabolite levels during submaximal work in individuals susceptible to malignant hyperpyrexia. Acta Anaesthsiol Scan 31:122, 1987.

130. Tobias, M. A., Miller, C. G.: Malignant Hypertonic Hyperpyrexia. Anaesthesia 25:253, 1970.

131. Wilson, R. D.: Disturbances of the Oxidative Phosphorylation Mechanism as a Possible Etiology Factor in Sudden Unexpected Hyperthermia. Anesthesiology 27:231, 1966.

132. Wang, J. K., Moffitt, E. A., Rosevear, J. W.: Oxidative Phosphorylation in Acute Hyperthermia. Anesthesiology 30:439, 1969.

133. Britt, B. A., Locher, W. G. and Kalow, W.: Hereditary Aspects of Malignant Hyperthermia. Can Anaesth Soc J 16:89, 1969.

134. Nevins, M. A., Sapan, M. Bright, M., et al.: Pitfalls in interpreting serum creative phosphokinase activity. JAMA 224:1382–1387, 1973.

135. Brownell, A. K. W. Malignant hyperthermia: Relationship to other diseases. Br J Anaesth 60:303–308, 1988

136. Larach, M. G., Rosenberg, H., Larach, D. R., Broennle, A. M.: Prediction of malignant hyperthermia susceptibility by clinical signs. Anesthesiology 66:547, 1987.

137. Rosenberg, H., Reed, S.: In vitro contracture tests for malignant hyperpyrexia. Anesth Analg 62:415–420, 1983.

138. Britt, B. A., Endrengi, L., Scott, E. W.: Effect of temperature, time and fascicle size in the caffeine contracture test. Can Anaesth Soc J 27:1–11, 1980.

139. Gronert, G. A.: Contracture responses and energy stores in quadriceps muscle from humans age 7–82 years. Hum Biol 52:43, 1980.

140. Gielen, M., Viering, W.: 3-in-1 lumbar plexus block for muscle biopsy in malignant hyperthermia patients. Amide local anaesthetics may be used safely. Acta Anaesthesiol Scan 30:581, 1986.

141. Aldrete, J. A., Padfield, A., Solomons, C. C., Rubright, M. W.: Possible Predictive Tests for Malignant Hyperthermia. JAMA 215:1465, 1971.

142. Stanec, A., Stefano, G: Cyclic AMP in normal and malignant hyperpyrexia susceptible individuals following exercise. Br J Anaesth 56:1243–1245, 1984.

143. Baldavs, J., Small, V., Cooper, D. A., Britt, V. A.: Postoperative Malignant Hyperthermia. Can Anaesth Soc J 18:202, 1971.

144. Solomons, C. C., Masson, N. C.: Platelet model for halothane-induced effects on nucleotide metabolism applied to malignant hyperthermia. Acta Anaesthesiol Scand 28:185–190, 1984.

145. Britt, B. A., Harrison, J. E., McNeill, K. G.: In-vivo neutron activation analysis for bone calcium in malignant hyperthermia susceptible patients. Can Anaesth Soc J 26:117, 1979.

146. Gronert, G. A., Heffron, J. A., Milde, J. H., Theye, R. A.: Porcine malignant hyperthermia. Role of skeletal muscle in increased oxygen consumption. Can Anaesth Soc J 24:103–107, 1977.

147. Paasuke, R. T., Brownell, A. K. W.: Serum creatine kinase level as a screening test for susceptibility to malignant hyperthermia. JAMA 225:769, 1986.

148. Van Winkle, W. B.: Calcium release from skeletal muscle sarcoplasmic reticulum. Site of action of dantrolene. Science 193:1130, (Sept.) 1976.

149. Harrison, G. G.: Recent Advances in the Understanding of Anaesthetic Induced Malignant Hyperpyrexia. Anaesthetist 22:373, 1973.

150. Pollack, R. A. and Watson, R. L.: Malignant Hyperthermia associated with Hypocalcemia. Anesthesiology 34:188, 1971.

151. Harrison, D. G. F. and Verburg, C.: Erythrocyte Osmotic Fragility in Hyperthermia Susceptible Swine. Br J Anaesth 45:131, 1973.

152. Isaacs, H., Frere, G., Mitchell, J.: Histological, Histochemical and Ultramicroscopic Findings in Muscle Biopsies from Carriers of the Trait for Malignant Hyperpyrexia. Br J Anaesth 45:860, 1973.

153. Schwartz, L., Rockoff, M. A., Koka, B. V.: Masseter spasm with anesthesia: Incidence and implications. Anesthesiology 61:772, 1984.

154. Flewellen, E. H., Nelson, T. E.: Halothane-succinylcholine induced masseter spasm: indicative of malignant hyperthermia susceptibility? Anesth Analg 63:693, 1984.

155. Nelson, T. E., Flewellen, E. H., Gloyna, D. F.: Spectrum of susceptibility to malignant hyperthermia—diagnostic dilemma. Anesth Anal 62:545, 1983.

156. Heffron, J. J. A. Malignant Hyperthermia: Biochemical aspects of the acute episode. Br J Anaesth 60:274–278, 1988.

157. Baudendistel, L.: Endtidal CO_2: Its use in the diagnosis and management of malignant hyperthermia. Anaesthesia 39:1000–1004, 1984.

158. Isaacs, H. I. and Barlow, M. B.: Identification of Asymptomatic Carriers of Malignant Hyperpyrexia. Br J Anaesth 42:1077, 1970.

159. Isaacs, H., Heffron, J. J. A.: Morphological and Biochemical Defects in Muscles of Human Carriers of the Malignant Hyperthermia Syndrome. Br J Anaesth 47:425, 1975.

160. Zsigmond, E.: Malignant hyperthermia—a misnomer. JAMA 243:513, 1980.

161. Britt, B. A.: Malignant Hyperthermia: A Pharmacogenetic Disease of Skeletal and Cardiac Muscle. N Engl J Med 290:1140, 1974.

162. Kelstrup, J., Reske-Nielsen, E., Haase, J., Jorni, J.: Malignant Hyperthermia in a Family. Acta Anaesth Scand 18:58, 1974.

163. Johannesson, G., Veel, T., Rogstadius, J.: Malignant Hyperthermia during Isoflurane Anesthesia. Acta Anaesth Scand 31:231–232, 1987.

164. Tammisto, J., Airaksinen, M.: Increase of Creatine Kinase Activity in Serum as a sign of Muscular Injury by Intermittently Administered Suxamethonium During Halothane Anesthesia. Br J Anaesth 38:510, 1966.

165. Asari, H.: Inhibitory effect of intravenous d-tubo curarine and oral dantrolene on halothane-succinylcholine myoglobinemia in children. Anesthesiology 61:332–335, 1984.

166. Gronert, G. A.: Malignant hyperthermia. Anesthesiology 53:395–423, 1980.

167. Jones, E. W., Nelson, T. E., Anderson, I. L.: Malignant Hyperthermia of Swine. Anesthesiology 36:42, 1972.

168. Kerr, D. D., Jones, E. W., Nelson, T. E., Gatz, E. E.: Treatment of Malignant Hyperthermia in Swine. Anesth Analg 52:734, 1973.

169. Nelson, T. E., Jones, E. W., Bedell, D. M.: Porcine Malignant Hyperthermia. A Study on the Triggering Effects of Succinylcholine. Anesth Analg 52:908, 1973.

170. Harrison, G. G.: Althesin and Malignant Hyperpyrexia. Br J Anaesth 45:1019, 1973.

171. Moulds, R. F. W., Denborough, M. A.: Biochemical basis of malignant hyperpyrexia. Br Med J 2:241–244, 1974.

172. Miller, R. N., Hunter, F. E.: Is Halothane a True Uncoupler of Oxidative Phosphorylation. Anesthesiology 35:256, 1971.

173. Britt, B. A., Kalow, W., Gordon, A., et al.: Malignant Hyperthermia—An Investigation. Can Anaesth Soc J 20:431, 1973.

174. Endo, M.: Calcium release from the sarcoplasmic reticulum. Physiol Rev 57:71–108, 1977.

175. Strobel, G. E.: Calcium, muscle and hyperthemia. Chap 7 in malignant hyperthermia. Current concepts. Ed E. O. Henschel. Appleton-Century Crofts, New York 1977.

176. Strobel, G. E., Bianchi, C. P.: An In-Vitro Model of Anesthetic Hypertonia, Hyperpyrexia, Halothane—Caffeine—Induced Muscle Contractures. Anesthesiology 35:465–473, 1971.

177. Harrison, G. G.: The effect of procaine and curare on the initiation of anesthetic-induced malignant hyperpyrexia. Chap. 23. Internat. Symposium on Malignant Hyperpyrexia. Gordon, R.A., Britt, B.A. and Kalow, W., Ed. Cleas C. Thomas, Springfield, IL, 1973.

178. Strobel, G. E.: Treatment of anesthetic induced hyperpyrexia. Lancet 1:40–43, 1971.

179. Horiuti, K., Matsumara, M., Matsui, R., Ilino, M. and Endo, M. (1986) The calcium induced calcium release mechanism in patients suspected of malignant hyperthermia. In Proceedings of the 4th International Malignant Hyperpyrexia Workshop (York, 1986), ed. by F.R. Ellis and P.J. Halsall, Biochemistry session, p. 7. Leeds: Leeds MH Investigation Unit. St. James University Hospital, 1986.

180. Nelson, T. E., Flewellen, E. H., Belt, M. W., Kennamer, D. L., et al: Calcium and magnesium content of skeletal muscle: Studies in subjects undergoing diagnostic testing for malignant hyperthermia Br J Anaesth 59:730, 1987.

181. Zsigmond, E.: Creatine Phosphokinase, Chap 13 in F. Foldes (Ed) Enzymes in Anesthesiology. Springer-Verlag, NY, 1978.

182. Solomons, C. C. and Myers, D. N.: Hyperthermia of Osteogenesis Imperfecta and Its Relation to Malignant Hyperthermia. Int. Symposium on M.H. Chap. 26. Springfield, Charles C. Thomas, 1973.

183. Gibson, G. R., Schnur, G. A.: Creatine kinase MB in a patient with adrenocarcinoma of the lung. JAMA 256:1035, 1986.

184. Ranklev, E., Fletcher, R., Blomquist, S.: Static v. dynamic tests in the in vitro diagnosis of malignant hyperthermia susceptibility. Br J Anaesth 58:646–648, 1986.

185. Klipp, A., Ramcal, T., Walker, D., Britt, B. A., Elliott, E.: Cytoplasmic calcium increase by anesthetic in pig lymphocytes. Towards a diagnosis of malignant hyperthermia. Anesth Analg 66:381–385, 1987.

186. Zsigmond, E. K., Penner, J., Kothary, S. P.: Normal erythrocyte fragility and abnormal platelet aggregation in M.H. families. A pilot study, Second International Symposium on Malignant Hyperthermia. Edited by J. A. Aldrete, B. A. Britt. New York, Grune and Stratton, pp 213–219, 1978.

187. O'Toole, E., Bonneville, M. A., Solomons, C. C., Zsigmond, E.K.: In vitro responses to halothane of human platelets in malignant hyperthermia. J Cell Biol 101:187a, 1985.

188. Van Wormer, D. E., Armstrong, D. A., Solomons, C. C.: Serum levels of inorganic pyrophosphate as a laboratory aid in assessing malignant hyperthermia risk, Second International Symposium on Malignant Hyperthermia. Edited

by J. A. Aldrete, B. A. Britt. New York, Grune and Stratton, pp 261–266, 1978.

189. Cheah, K. S., Cheah, A. M.: Malignant hyperthermia: Molecular defects in membrane permeability. Experientia 41:656, 1985.

190. Blanck, T. J. J., Gruener, R., Suffecool, S. L., Thompson, M.: Calcium uptake by isolated sarcoplasmic reticulum: Examination of halothane inhibition, pH dependence, and Ca^{2+} dependence of normal and malignant hyperthermic human muscle. Anesth Analg 60:492–498, 1981.

191. Willner, J. H., Wood, D. S., Cerri, C., Britt, B.: Increased myophosphorylase A in malignant hyperthermia. NEJM 303:138, 1980.

192. Traynor, C. A., Van Dyke, R. A., Gronert, G. A.: Phosphorylase ratio and susceptibility to malignant hyperthermia. Anesth Analg 62:324, 1983.

193. Allen, G.: A circle system is best when anesthetizing malignant hyperthermia susceptible patients. Anesthesiology 70:1025–1028, 1989.

194. Beebe, J. J., Sessler, D. I.: Preparation of anesthesia machines for patients susceptible to malignant hyperthermia. Anesthesiology 69:395–400, 1988.

195. Cain, P. A. and Ellis, F. R.: Anaesthesia for patients susceptible to malignant hyperthermia. Br J Anaesth 49:941–944, 1977.

196. Ellis, F. R. Clarke, I. M. C. et al. Malignant hyperpyrexia induced by nitrous oxide and treated by dexamethasone. Br Med J 4:270–276, 1974.

197. Fletcher, J. E., Rosenberg, H., Hilf, M.: Effects of midazolam on directly stimulated muscle biopsies from control and malignant hyperthermia positive patients. Can Anaesth Soc J 31:377–381, 1984.

198. Short, C. E., Paddleford, R., McGrath, C. J. and Williams, C. H.,: Preanesthetic evaluation and management of malignant hyperthermia experimental model. Anesth Analg 55:643–647, 1976.

199. Hall, G. M., Lucke, J.N., Liste, D.: Porcine malignant hyperthermia IV Neuromuscular blockade. Br J Anaesth 48:1135–1138, 1976.

200. Hall, G. M., Lucke, J. N., Lister, D.: Porcine malignant hyperthermia associated with infusion of alpha-adrenergic agonists. Br J Anaesth 49:855–860, 1977.

201. Lucke, J. N., Denny, H., Hall, R., et al.: Porcine MH: Effects of bilateral adrenalectomy and bretylium pretreatment. Br J Anaesth 50:241–246, 1978.

202. Flewellyn, E. H. and Nelson, T. E. (1984) Prophylactic and therapeutic doses of dantrolene for malignant hyperthermia. Anesthesiology 61:477–482, 1984.

203. Knochel, J. P.: Environmental Heat Illness. Arch Int Med 133:841, 1974.

204. Lloyd, E. L. and Scott, D. H. (1985) Cooling technique for malignant hyperthermia. Lancet 2:97.

205. Khogali, M: The Makkah body cooling unit. In Khogali M, Hales J. R. S., eds. Heat stroke and temperature regulation. London: Academic Press: 139, 1983.

206. Mort, T., Rintel, T., Altman, F.: Shivering in the cardiac patient: Evaluation of Bair-Hugger warming system. Anesthesiology 73:A 239, 1990.

207. Ryan, J. F., Donlon, J. V., Malt, R. A., Bland, J. H., Buckley, M. J., Streter, F., Lowenstein, E.: Cardiopulmonary Bypass in the Treatment of Malignant Hyperthermia. N Engl J Med 290:1121, 1974.

208. Noble, W. H.: Malignant Hyperthermia with Rigidity Successfully Treated with Procainamide. Anesthesiology 39:450, 1973.

209. Britt, B. A., Endrenyl, L., Cadman, D. L., Fan, H. M., Fung, H. Y-K.: Porcine Malignant Hyperthermia: Effects of Halothane on Mitochondrial Respiration and Calcium Accumulation. Anesthesiology 42:292, 1975.

210. Nelson, T. E., Bedell, D. M., Jones, E. W.: Porcine Malignant Hyperthermia: Effects of temperature and extra-cellular calcium concentration on halothane-induced contracture of Susceptible Skeletal Muscle. Anesthesiology 42:301, 1975.

211. Morgan, K. G., Bryant, S. H.: The mechanism of action of dantrolene sodium. J Pharmacol Exp Ther 201:138–141, 1977.

212. Iwatsuki, N., Koga, Y., Amaha, K.: Calcium channel blocker for treatment of malignant hyperthermia. Anesth Analg 62:861–2, 1983.

213. Kerr, D. D., Wingard, D. W., Gatz, E. E.: Prevention of Porcine Malignant Hyperthermia by Epidural Block. Anesthesiology 42:307, 1975.

214. Clark, R. E., Orkin, L. R. and Rovenstine, E. A.: Body temperature studies in anesthetized man: Effect on environmental temperature humidity and anesthesia system. JAMA 154:311–316, 1954.

215. Kubieck, W. G., Anderson, W. D., Gerber, W. F.: Effects of hypoxia on the course of reduced fever in dogs and monkeys. Am J Physiol 195:601–606, 1958.

216. Van Winkle, W. B.: Calcium release from skeletal muscle sarcoplasmic reticulum: Site of action of dantrolene. Science 193:1130, 1976.

217. Morgan, K. G., Bryant, S. H.: The mechanism of action of dantrolene sodium. J Pharmacol Exp Ther 201:138, 1977.

218. Flewellen, E. H., Nelson, T. E., Jones, W. P., Arens J. F., Wagner D. L.: Dantrolene dose response in awake man: implications for management of malignant hyperthermia. Anesthesiology 59:275, 1983.

219. Mora, C. T., Eisenkraft, J. B., Papatestas, A. E.: Intravenous dantrolene in a patient with myasthenia gravis. Anesthesiology 64:371, 1986.

220. Takamori, M., Sakato, S., Matsubara, S., Okumura, S.: Therapeutic approach to experimental autoimmune myasthenia gravis by dantrolene sodium. J Neurol Sci 58:17, 1983.

221. Flewellen, E. H., Nelson, T. E.: Dantrolene dose response in malignant hyperthermia susceptible (MHS) swine: Method to obtain prophylaxis and therapeusis. Anesthesiology 52:303, 1980.

222. Watson, C. B., Reverson, N., Norfleet, E. A.: Clinically significant muscle weakness induced by oral dautrolene sodium prophylaxes for MH. Anesthesiology 65:312–315, 1986.

223. Ruhland, G., Hinkle, A. J.: Malignant hyperthermia after oral and intravenous pretreatment with dantrolene in a patient susceptible to malignant hyperthermia. Anesthesiology 60:159, 1984.

224. Kolb, M. E., Horne, M. L., Martz, R.: Dantrolene in human malignant hyperthermia. Anesthesiology 56:254, 1982.

225. Iwatsuki, N., Koga, Y., Amaha, K.: Calcium channel blocker for treatment of malignant hyperthermia. Anes Analg 62:861, 1983.

226. Zeilani, M. R. Z., Al-Shanableh, J. S. H.: Verapamil and malignant hyperthermia. MEJ Anesth 8:37, 1985.

227. Rubin, A. S., Zablocki, A. D.: Hyperkalemia, verapamil, and dantrolene. Anesthesiology 66:246, 1987.

Chapter 20

IMMUNE RESPONSES AND HYPERSENSITIVITY REACTIONS DURING ANESTHESIA

MICHAEL F. ROIZEN, JERROLD H. LEVY, AND JONATHAN MOSS

By altering the immune function, anesthetic drugs and/or surgical manipulation can precipitate life-threatening situations for our patients. For example, the mortality from salmonella,[1] fecal peritonitis,[2] and anthrax[3] are increased substantially (doubled in one series) by halothane anesthesia alone. The data are insufficient to explain with certainty the occurrence of this impaired ability to ward off infection, or which steps in the normal non-specific or specific immune responses are inhibited by anesthesia and/or surgery.[4] For these reasons, this aspect of the impaired immunologic system will be addressed only briefly. On the other hand, life-threatening hypersensitivity or pseudoallergic reactions to exogenously derived and administered agents during anesthesia can be, and usually are, successfully treated by a prepared anesthetist.[5] These latter reactions are anaphylactic if immunologically-mediated, or anaphylactoid if chemically-mediated. Rapid recognition and treatment can prevent much of the morbidity and mortality that would otherwise occur.

IMMUNITY

The human body has the capacity to reject almost all damaging foreign organisms, substances, and toxins. This capacity, called immunity, exists in innate defense mechanisms (such as acid digestion of substances in the stomach, resistance to invasion by the skin, etc.), and in acquired immunity, which works through lymphocytes to form antibodies or activated lymphocytes.[6] The innate defense responses (non-specific immunity) are often altered by anesthesia and surgery. For example, many volatile and intravenous anesthetics,[7] as well as surgical incision, decrease mucociliary clearance. The other defense mechanism, acquired immunity (specific immunity), includes both cellular and humoral immunity.[6] In cellular immunity, the body produces activated lymphocytes called T cells, whereas humoral immunity relies on circulating antibodies secreted by B lymphocytes (B cells). Humoral immunity is thus called "antibody-mediated," or "B cell-mediated."

Cellular Immunity

In the embryo, lymphocytes that are destined to become activated lymphocytes migrate to, and receive instructions in the thymus gland (hence, "T cells"). In the cell membrane, these T lymphocytes gain surface receptor proteins (T cell markers) that are antigen specific. Little is known of the effect of anesthesia and/or surgery on the development of this process. Further, there are various types of T cells called T helper cells (T4 cells), T suppressor cells (T8 cells), and T killer cells (there are actually various forms of each of these T cell types, as well). The T helper cells, once activated by an antigen, secrete specific lymphokines which stimulate the B lymphocytes to reproduce, activate the B lymphocytes, or stimulate T killer cell production. Without the activity of T helper cells, B lymphocytes secrete only miniscule amounts of antibody to confront an antigenic challenge. For example, one of the lymphokines secreted by T helper cells is interleukin 2, which causes B cells to produce the intracellular organelles that produce antibodies. The AIDS virus (HIV) appears to alter immunity principally by depressing T helper cell function. Cytotoxic T cells (killer or natural killer cells) have receptors that bind to a foreign cell or organism, release cytotoxic substances (lysosomal enzymes) into it, and move on to repeat the process. The killer T cells, because they often have viral receptors, are especially attracted to cells that have been infected by viruses, since virus particles are often expressed or trapped in infected cell membranes. The killer T cells are also thought to be key to both destruction of cancer cells and transplant rejection.[6]

T suppressor cells suppress the functions of the T helper cells and T killer cells. They likely promote feedback regulation of the immune system and prevent it from excessive responses. This class of lymphocyte may also be important in suppressing autoimmune diseases.

Effect of Anesthetics on Acquired Immunity

Anesthetics have been tested for their effects on the cellular form of acquired immunity, but the results are at best equivocal.[4,8] Halothane decreases the cellular immune proliferation and toxicity between 1 and 2.5%, but only after 24 to 48 hours of exposure.[9,10] Five to seven hours of halothane or enflurane had no effect on these responses.[11] Others observed more immediate depression by halothane.[12] Balanced anesthesia caused no depression.[13] The intravenous agents thiopental, ketamine, droperidol, and lidocaine have also been reported to decrease lymphocyte proliferation and transfusion in response to an antigenic stimulus, but only at concentrations above those normally occurring during anesthesia.[14] On the other hand, these minor effects (20% inhibition) were at least additive when halothane and thiopental were added together to cultured cells in vitro.[15] The depth of anesthesia may profoundly alter levels of stress hormones, which may in turn alter acquired immunity. Therefore, it is important to separate effects of the agents per se from their indirect effects. This has been attempted by comparing light general to complete regional anesthesia (the underlinings represent the authors' interpretation of the methods). Light general anesthesia decreased proliferation and killer cell activity following TURP, hip pinning, or caesarian section to a greater degree than regional anesthesia in patients undergoing similar operations, though regional anesthesia would be expected to block the stress response.[16,17,18] Those studies did not determine the clinical significance of the effects. Thus, one cannot conclude from the available data whether anesthesia per se deranges cellular immunity, or whether we as anesthesiologists can do anything (such as administering stress-blocking doses of anesthetics or anesthetic adjuncts) to prevent such derangement if it does occur.

HUMORAL IMMUNITY

The other form of acquired immunity is humoral or B cell-mediated immunity.[19] In the embryo or shortly after birth, the lymphocytes that are destined to form antibodies are "instructed" (probably in the liver and bone marrow) to develop B lymphocytes. This type of cell was first discovered in birds where it occurs in the *bursa of Fabricius*, a structure not found in humans. Again, we know of no data regarding the effect of anesthesia and/or surgery on B cell development which would affect later immunity. B lymphocytes lie dormant until presented with a specific antigen. However, when challenged with a specific antigen, these B lymphocytes immediately enlarge and appear like lymphoblasts. These cells become incredible antibody production plants, producing over 2,000 molecules per second per plasma cell. The antibodies are in turn secreted into lymph. The enlargement of cells and antibody production is even further enhanced by a second challenge. This is one reason why vaccination is usually accomplished by injecting antigens at least twice, several weeks or months apart. Antibodies can engulf, lyse, or agglutinate when they combine with antigens, but their main function appears to be amplifying the effect of the complement system (see section of this chapter on hypersensitivity reactions—anaphylaxis).

While decreases in antibody production and B cell activation have been reported after heart surgery,[20] we have little data that speak to the question of whether the alterations in immunity induced by anesthesia and/or surgery are associated with humoral or B cell depression. Thus, the literature leads us to conclude that, while anesthesia and/or surgery may impair innate defense mechanisms, it may not significantly affect acquired immunity; however, if it does, life-threatening hypersensitivity (anaphylactic) reactions can occur during anesthesia.

LIFE-THREATENING HYPERSENSITIVITY REACTIONS DURING ANESTHESIA

Definitions and Clinical Spectra

Anaphylaxis is a life-threatening, allergic or immunologically-mediated reaction. The term "allergic" applies to immunologically-mediated reactions, as opposed to those caused by pharmacologic idiosyncracy, direct toxicity, drug overdose, or drug interactions.[21] Anaphylactoid reactions produce the same clinical syndrome, but are not immunologically-mediated. Vasoactive mediators of these reactions include histamine, eosinophilic chemotactic factors of anaphylaxis (ECF-A), slow reacting substance of anaphylaxis (SRS-A, a mixture of three leukotrienes, including a potent coronary vasoconstrictor), platelet activating factor (PAF), kinins, and prostaglandins. Symptoms usually occur within 15 minutes of parenteral injection of the causative agent, though they may be delayed. The net effect of these agents is a marked decrease in systemic vascular resistance and the leakage of fluid from the capillaries and postcapillary venules. This reduction in effective plasma volume can result in shock. Thus, volume replacement and administration of epinephrine are therapeutic mainstays. Common causes of such reactions are antibiotics, muscle relaxants, colloids, chymopapain, protamine, and radiocontrast materials.[22]

The recent introduction of chymopapain for use by the physician treating herniated nucleus pulposus has served as a model. Prior to the introduction of immunoglobulin E (IgE) screening, there was a relatively high incidence of anaphylactic reactions associated with chymopapain administration. We speculate that anesthesiologists could reduce by over 90% the morbidity and serious neurologic consequences associated with anaphylactic reactions if they understand the pathophysiology of such reactions. This speculation is based on the following data. In Australia and Britain, mortality rates from anaphylaxis are 3.4 and 4.35%, respectively, with an additional 5.6% of patients suffering irreversible brain damage.[22,23] In the United States, in a series of cases of anaphylaxis after chymopapain where physicians were aggressively educated and prepared for such reactions in advance, only 3 of 252 (less than 1.5%) patients died, or had permanent sequelae.[24] This aggressive education and preparation involved knowledge of immunology, inflammatory mediators, and the therapy for shock, as well as pretreatment with H_1 and H_2 antagonists. Such a therapeutic plan minimizes the consequences of anaphylactic reactions.

Classification of Allergic Reactions (According to Immune Mechanisms)

Gell et al divided immune mechanisms in allergic reactions into four types (Table 20–1).[25] "Immediate hypersensitivity" reactions (type I) are produced by the IgE-mediated release of pharmacologically active substances. These mediators in turn produce specific end-organ responses in the skin (urticaria), respiratory system (bronchospasm and upper airway edema), and cardiovascular system (vasodilation, changes in inotropy, and increased

Table 20-1. Classification of Allergic Reactions*

Type	Synonyms	Antibody	Complement	Effector cells	Chemical Mechanism	Examples
I	Anaphylactic Immediate hypersensitivity	IgE	Not involved	Mast cells Basophils	Antigen or allergen binds to IgE on the surface of mast cells and basophils with release of mast cell products.	Anaphylaxis Cutaneous wheal and flare Extrinsic asthma
II	Cytotoxic	IgG IgM	Fixed and activated	Polymorphonuclear cells	IgG or IgM binds to allergen on cell membranes; complement system is activated with cellular destruction.	Transfusion reactions Hemolytic anemia Rh disease
III	Immune complex	IgG IgM	Fixed and activated	Polymorphonuclear cells	IgG or IgM binds to allergen in the fluid phase and deposits in small blood vessels; complement system is activated with cellular destruction.	Serum sickness Glomerulonephritis Arthus reactions
IV	Delayed hypersensitivity/ Cell-mediated immunity	Not involved	Not involved	Thymus-derived lymphocytes	Sensitized cells bind to allergen and release, upon activation, effectors known as lymphokines.	Contact dermatitis Tuberculin immunity

*Classification by Gell et al. From Gell, P. G. H., Coombs, R. R. A., and Lachmann, P. J. (eds.): Clinical Aspects of Immunology. 3rd Ed. Oxford, Blackwell Scientific, 1975.

capillary permeability).[26,27] This clinical syndrome, first reported by Portier and Richet[28] as profound shock and death occurring in dogs in response to sea anemone toxin, was called "anaphylaxis." In contrast, biologic reactions that are not IgE-mediated, but produce a clinical syndrome indistinguishable from anaphylaxis, were called "anaphylactoid."[29]

Allergens in Anaphylactic Reactions

In anaphylactic reactions, the injected substance itself can serve as the allergen. Drugs of low molecular weight are believed to act as haptens which form immunogenic conjugates with host proteins. The offending substance, whether hapten or not, may be the parent compound, a nonenzymatically generated product, or a metabolic product formed in the patient. This hapten or drug protein complex (if the drug itself is the offending agent) induces a B lymphocyte to proliferate and differentiate into a clone of plasma cells capable of synthesizing and secreting thousands of identical IgE antibody molecules against that particular hapten-protein complex. Mast cells and basophils are studded with receptors for IgE, and the newly synthesized IgE antibody molecules bind to these receptors. When an antigen attaches to adjacent antibodies, it is thought to cause them to "bridge" the receptors on the cells together, probably altering the shape of the cell membrane. This complex causes the cells to release preformed histamine and ECF-A from the storage granules via a calcium- and energy-dependent process (Figure 20–1).[27,30,31] In model systems, steroids inhibit such a release.[32] Other chemical mediators, including SRS-A leukotrienes, other leukotrienes, kinins, platelet activating factors, and prostaglandins are rapidly synthesized and subsequently released in response to cellular activation.[26,27]

Clinical Syndrome of Anaphylaxis

The end-organ effects of the mediators produce the clinical syndrome, anaphylaxis. In a sensitized individual, the onset of the signs and symptoms caused by these mediators is usually immediate, but may be delayed 2 to 15 minutes, or, in rare cases, as long as $2\frac{1}{2}$ hours after the parenteral injection of the antigen (Figure 20–2).[33-35] After oral administration, manifestations may occur at unpredictable times.[26,27] True anaphylaxis requires immunologically-mediated release of some or all of these vasoactive mediators. In contrast, other mechanisms can liberate the vasoactive substances which produce this clinical syndrome. This nonimmunologically mediated, but clinically identical syndrome, is called an "anaphylactoid reaction" (see below systems that can generate anaphylactoid reactions). Patients with anaphylactic or anaphylactoid reactions may manifest some or all of the following signs and symptoms.[26,27,33-35]

Respiratory System

Patients may complain of nasal stuffiness or itching, difficulty in breathing, or retrosternal tightness. Coughing, wheezing, tachypnea, laryngeal stridor, and cyanosis are other manifestations, as are acute respiratory distress and pharyngeal, epiglottic, or glottic edema.

Cardiovascular System

Patients may report dizziness and/or changes in consciousness. They may also complain of chest tightness, sometimes due to myocardial ischemia. A total loss of pulse indicates profound hypotension. Electrocardiographic changes can vary from tachyarrhythmias and nonspecific changes of the S-T segment or T-wave, to ventricular fibrillation, dissociation of EKG electrical rhythm and the mechanical pumping power of the heart, and asystole.

Skin

Complaints may range from itching, warmth, and minor swelling of the face or an extremity, to itching of the eyes and nonpitting deep edematous processes in the cutaneous tissue. Patients may manifest the characteristic urticaria or flare of histamine release.

Other Indications of a Reaction

Perhaps most impressive in the awake patient is the patient's expression of a sense of doom. Thirteen of fifteen conscious patients experiencing an anaphylactic or anaphylactoid reaction have said something like, "I feel horrible," or "I'm going to die," before any hemodynamic or pulmonary symptoms or signs were evident.

Morbidity and Mortality Mechanisms

An anaphylactic or anaphylactoid reaction may involve any combination of these symptoms; however, the *sine qua non* of anaphylaxis is severe cardiovascular or respiratory compromise. Since this reaction includes vasodilation and translocation of fluid from capillaries and postcapillary venules (resulting in loss of fluid and colloid from intravascular spaces), there is a reduction in effective plasma volume, systemic vascular resistance, and shock. Thus, fluid resuscitation is first priority when treating this syndrome.

The most severe life-threatening reactions result from laryngeal edema, bronchospasm, and vascular collapse, probably end-organ responses secondary to the release of vasoactive substances. The full variety of vasoactive mediators of anaphylactic and anaphylactoid reactions is not known. However, understanding the known pharmacologic mediators helps explain the clinical manifestations and rationale for therapy of anaphylaxis.

MEDIATORS OF ANAPHYLACTIC REACTIONS

Histamine

Histamine is a low molecular weight amine stored predominantly in tissue mast cells and circulating basophils.[35] It dilates capillaries and venules and promotes vascular permeability. Its actions on the H_1 and H_2 receptors are thought to be responsible for both decreased systemic vascular resistence and increased permeability in venules.[36,37] Through H_1-mediated effects, histamine is

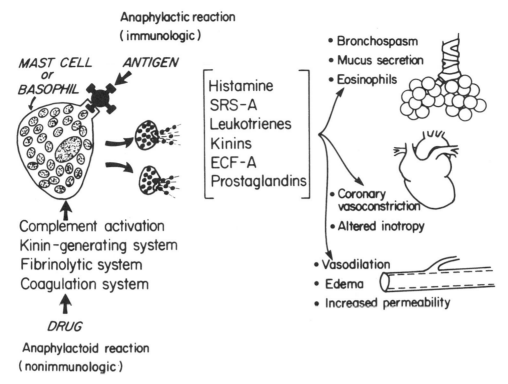

Fig. 20–1. A summary of the pathophysiologic changes in anaphylactic and anaphylactoid reactions. (Top) Anaphylactic reactions: The allergen enters the body, combines with IgE antibodies on the surface of mast cells and basophils. The mast cells and basophils degranulate, releasing mediators (histamine, slow reacting substance of anaphylaxis-leukotrienes, kinins, eosinophilic chemotactic factor, prostaglandins, platelet activating factors and others). The release of these substances is associated with the signs and symptoms of anaphylaxis—bronchospasm; pharyngeal, glottic, and pulmonary edema; vasodilation; hypotension; decreased cardiac contractility and dysrhythmias; subcutaneous edema; and urticaria. (Bottom) Anaphylactoid reactions: The offending agent enters the body and works by nonimmunologically activating systems that cause degranulation of mast cells and basophils. The systems that can be activated to cause release of mediators from basophils and mast cells include the complement system, the coagulation and fibrinolytic system, and the kinin-generating system. Activation of these systems can result in the release of the same mediators from basophils and mast cells, and in a syndrome that is clinically indistinguishable from anaphylaxis.

also a potent coronary vasoconstrictor.[38] Vascular responses of vasodilation and local cutaneous reactions (wheal and flare) are mediated by both H_1 and H_2 receptors.[37,38] H_2 receptors mediate chronotropic responses. Histamine is rapidly cleared across vascular beds, probably by the vascular endothelial cells.[39] Histamine increases levels of cyclic AMP, which probably helps terminate its release.[40]

Eosinophilic Chemotactic Factor of Anaphylaxis (ECF-A)

ECF-A is an acidic peptide with a molecular weight of 500–600 daltons,[41] stored in mast cell granules. It is chemotactic for eosinophils.[41] The exact role of the eosinophil in the allergic response is unclear. However, during phagocytosis, eosinophils release histaminase, phospholipase D, and arylsulfatase.[42] These enzymes can inactivate histamine and SRS-A.[42]

Platelet Activating Factor(s) (PAF)

Platelet activating factor (PAF) is acetylglyceryl ether phosphorylcholine. It causes platelet aggregation and bronchoconstriction, increases vascular permeability, and modulates leukocyte function.

Slow Reacting Substance of Anaphylaxis (SRS-A)

SRS-A is synthesized in response to antigens, and is not stored intracellularly. SRS-A is a mixture of products of the oxidative metabolism of arachidonic acid through the lipooxygenase pathway, and is composed of three mem-

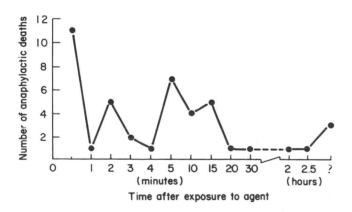

Fig. 20–2. Interval between exposure and reaction to the allergen in 43 cases of anaphylactic death. Adapted from Delage and Irey.[35]

bers of a class of compounds known as leukotrienes (leukotrienes C4, D4, and E4).[43,44] End-organ effects include potent constriction of bronchial smooth muscle. On a molar basis, SRS-A is 4,000 times as potent as histamine in causing bronchoconstriction in normal humans.[43] Other systemic effects of leukotrienes include provoking cutaneous inflammation, chemotaxis of polymorphonuclear leukocytes, and promotion of lysosomal enzyme release from leukocytes.[43,45] In sheep, leukotriene D4 is a potent coronary vasoconstrictor causing profound depression of myocardial contractility.[46]

Prostaglandins

Prostaglandins are unsaturated fatty acids synthesized at the time of the inflammatory stimulus.[43-45] They are also products of the metabolism of arachidonic acid, but through the cyclooxygenase pathway.[44] Their biologic activities are specific to the target organ on which they act. Prostaglandins are potent mediators of the inflammatory response and can increase capillary permeability, bronchospasm, pulmonary hypertension, and peripheral vasodilation.[44,47]

Kinins

Kinins are low molecular weight peptides which enhance capillary permeability, dilate certain blood vessels, contract certain smooth muscles, and are perhaps leukotactic.[48,49] Several processes independent of IgE can generate kinins.[48,50]

SYSTEMS THAT CAN GENERATE ANAPHYLACTOID REACTIONS

Histamine, ECF-A, SRS-A, prostaglandins, and kinins are the five known major pharmacologic mediators released by interactions between an antigen and IgE, i.e., true anaphylaxis. These vasoactive substances can be liberated by other mechanisms independently of IgE (i.e., anaphylactoid reactions) to produce the same clinical syndrome. There are multiple effector processes by which biologically active mediators can be generated to produce an anaphylactoid reaction; activation of the blood coagulation and fibrinolytic systems, the kinin-generating sequence, or the complement cascade can produce the same inflammatory substances as in an anaphylactic reaction (Fig. 20–1).

Coagulation and Fibrinolysis

Kinins can be generated in several ways involving the coagulation and fibrinolytic systems.[48,50] Factor XII of the intrinsic clotting system can be converted to XIIa by the effects of immune complexes (IgG or IgM), collagen, or phospholipids. Activation of XIIa leads to production of kallikrein from prekallikrein, which in turn can convert plasminogen to plasmin.[48] Plasmin, in addition to activating fibrinolysis, can activate the classical complement pathway.[48] Kallikrein can also generate bradykinin from kininogen precursors and manifest itself clinically as hypotension.[51] The Hageman factor and prekallikrein decrease, while bradykinin increases during hypotension associated with septicemia.[51,52]

Complement System

The complement system is an intricate system of multimolecular, self-assembling proteins. It can be activated by one of at least two triggering pathways.[53-55] Upon activation, the biologic effector proteins become humoral mediators of inflammation and tissue damage. The biologic sequence proceeds in an orderly, sequential fashion, comparable to activation of the clotting system. Fragments of native complement proteins are either released into the systemic circulation with ensuing anaphylactoid effects, or bind to other complement components to produce, eventually, membrane lysis of bacterial cells, red blood cells, or cells of other tissues.[53,54]

The two mechanisms known to activate the complement system are called "classical" and "alternative." The classical pathway can be activated through immune complexes of IgG or IgM (transfusion reactions), or plasmin.[48,50] The alternative pathway can be activated by lipopolysaccharides (endotoxin),[56] drugs (Althesin),[26,57,58] radiographic contrast media,[59,60] membranes (the nylon tricot membranes of bubble oxygenators,[61] the cellophane membranes of dialyzers),[62] vascular prostheses,[63] and perfluorocarbon artificial blood.[64,65] After activation of the complement system by either process, low molecular weight peptides of complement proteins C3 and C5 are released. These fragments, C3a and C5a, are both anaphylatoxins. They stimulate the release of mediators (including histamine) from mast cells and basophils,[53,66,67] contract certain smooth muscle, and increase vascular permeability. In addition, C5a interacts with specific high-affinity receptors on neutrophils to initiate cellular autoaggregation—an increase in adherence, chemotaxis, and lysosomal enzyme release.[45,68] These activated neutrophils liberate additional inflammatory mediators including leukotrienes.[44,45]

Generation of C5a may explain the neutropenia and hypoxia of dialysis,[62] cardiopulmonary bypass,[61,69,70] and adult respiratory distress syndrome.[68,71] Activation of complement by endotoxin has been invoked as the mechanism of vasodilation in gram-negative sepsis.[72]

Pharmacologic Release of Histamine

Histamine can be liberated independently of immunologic reactions.[29] Mast cells and basophils release histamine in response to chemicals or drugs.[73,74] Most narcotics in high doses can release histamine,[75] producing an anaphylactoid reaction. Radiographic contrast media[76] and d-tubocurarine[77,78] can also liberate histamine to produce anaphylactoid reactions. Why some patients are prone to histamine release in response to drugs is unknown, but hereditary and environmental factors may play a role.

DETERMINING THE CAUSE OF ANAPHYLACTIC REACTIONS

Frequently, several drugs are administered in a short time, making it difficult to ascertain which drug is responsible in an anaphylactic reaction. Obviously, the time course of events will often provide the answer. However, if more than one drug has been injected or absorbed, various tests are available to identify the allergen.

Skin Testing

Skin testing is the most widely used, least expensive, and easiest to perform technique for evaluating sensitivity to an allergen.[79-82] Allergists routinely perform skin tests on an outpatient basis. One of the problems associated with skin testing is false positive results.[83] In addition, reexposure to an agent that has produced serious adverse effects in the past may provoke another reaction. Thus, a small dose of the material is given, in dilutions of 1:1,000 to 1:1,000,000 of the initial strength.

Complement and Antibody Levels

Although complement level may be unchanged and IgE may decrease after an anaphylactic reaction,[84,85] these conditions do not prove immunologic involvement. As a test, patients have been given the suspected drugs intravenously, after which IgE levels have been observed.[85] This procedure, however, can be life-threatening.

The continuing problem with the skin test and provocative test (the two most commonly used tests) is exposing a possibly sensitized individual to an antigen. Ultimately, of course, one would like to be able to demonstrate a reaction to a suspected drug without incurring risk to the patient.

In Vitro Release of Histamine by Leukocytes

Histamine is released when leukocytes coated with IgE are exposed to immunospecific antigens.[79] The amount of histamine released thus depends on the degree and specificity of the IgE antibodies sensitizing the cells. However, some agents exert a direct, nonimmunologic effect on the cell that results in release of histamine.[75,88] The in vivo skin test assesses antigen-specific release of histamine from mast cells in the skin. The in vitro test provides the same information about specificity and sensitivity, and it avoids exposing a sensitized individual to a specific drug. This test has been used to demonstrate sensitivity to thiopental.[86] However, it is expensive and time-consuming.

RAST Testing

Antigen-specific IgE antibody can be measured using the radioallergosorbent tests (RAST).[87] In the RAST, a complex of a known antigen bound to an insoluble matrix is incubated with the patient's serum. The amount of immunospecific IgE antibody is determined by further incubation of the complex and serum with 125-labelled anti-IgE. Bound radioactivity reflects antigen-specific antibody and is compared with a reference system.

The RAST has demonstrated immunospecific IgE against such diverse agents as insulin, Hymenoptera extracts, and the penicilloyl derivatives of penicillin.[79,88] A positive RAST is rare, occurring in fewer than 0.5% of healthy, nonallergic humans.[88] Although the sensitivity and predictive positive value of RAST have been questioned, this relatively new test is promising. However, specific matrices for most drugs remain to be developed.

TEST INTERPRETATION

Several factors make interpreting test results difficult. First, anaphylaxis is a dose-independent response; therefore, it is almost impossible to determine the smallest effective test dose for assessing idiosyncratic allergic responses. Minute doses, including those used for skin testing, have caused anaphylaxis. For example, a patient who had an anaphylactic response was subsequently given a skin test with 1/4,000th of the normal intravenous dose. A wheal and flare developed over the injection site, followed by anaphylaxis which subsided after treatment.[89] Second, the immunologic mechanism of most clinically suspected allergic drug reactions is difficult to prove. Usually, such a mechanism is believed to exist only because the reaction occurs after the administration of a drug. Although some drugs are more frequently responsible for anaphylactic reactions than others, any drug has the potential for allergic, possibly fatal, reactions. Fortunately, most allergic reactions from drugs are not serious or life-threatening; they subside promptly when the drug is discontinued, or have easily suppressed clinical manifestations. Why some patients have localized cutaneous reactions while others have hypotension and bronchospasm is unclear. If a patient must have a drug that is likely to trigger an anaphylactic or anaphylactoid reaction, several steps should be taken. First, an allergist should be consulted. Second, repeated injections of small amounts of antigen or offending hapten may be given, as this procedure decreases the amount of specific IgE antibody produced, and may stimulate T suppressor cells. At the same time, this procedure usually increases the amount of competitive IgG antibody (i.e., blocking antibody). This blocking antibody can compete with IgE for receptors on the surface of basophils and mast cells to decrease the mediators released from these cells.

COMMON ANAPHYLACTIC AND ANAPHYLACTOID REACTIONS SEEN IN THE OPERATING ROOM

Chymopapain (Chymodiactin®)*

This agent was originally developed by Dr. Lyman Smith, an orthopedic surgeon (Northbrook IL). Baxter Laboratories took over the rights and the marketing of the agent about 1985. Production was discontinued soon after due to failure to receive approval from the FDA. It is now manufactured by BASF (Bandish, Analine, Soda, Farben) in Ludwigschaften, Germany and available in treatment kits. It is approved for clinical use in Great Britain, Canada, Germany, and other countries but not approved for use in the United States at this time.

Chymopapain, an agent used to treat herniated nucleus pulposus enzymatically, is associated with a 0.3 to 2% incidence of anaphylactic and anaphylactoid reactions. Women are three to ten times more likely to have such reactions (the incidence is 0.1-0.5% in men and 0.6-1.5% in women). Two of the 902 men and 11 of the 683

---

*This is a sulfhydroxy enzyme related to papain which acts on chrondromucoprotein as a component of the nucleus pulposus.

women in the phase II trial of chymopapain developed serious anaphylactic reactions. These reactions were manifested by bronchospasm in two subjects, severe hypotension in 13, laryngeal edema in two, and rash or pilometer changes in nine. Eleven of the 13 survived.[24]

From the release of Chymodiactin by the FDA in November 1982 to September 1983, the incidence of anaphylactic reactions had been similar to that in the phase II trial (i.e., approximately 0.4% in men and 1.3% in women for the first 30,000 patients treated).[24] Then the incidence dropped significantly (0.25% in men and 0.7% in women). The mortality rate from such anaphylaxis also dropped from two of 13 to three of 252. We believe that this successful outcome is due to knowledge of the pathophysiology of such reactions, vigilance when administering the drug, and pretreatment of the patient. Dr. McCulloch's series of 2,000 administrations of chymopapain also had successful outcomes after anaphylactic reactions.[90] Javid's review of six years of chymopapain use reveals that a large percentage of patients experience beneficial effects and few side effects.[91] Watts reviewed the reports of 13,700 patients given chymopapain and found sensitivity reactions occurred in 1.5%.[92] Eight deaths occurred, two resulting from anaphylactic shock, one from myocardial infarction two hours after the injection, and one from diskitis and subacute bacterial endocarditis 55 days after injection. The other four patients had pulmonary embolus, encephalitis, dissecting abdominal aortic aneurysm, and ruptured abdominal aneurysm; they died 99 days, 99 days, 4 days, and 72 days, respectively, after chemonucleolysis.

The decrease in mortality after anaphylaxis to chymopapain is not due to a decreased incidence of anaphylaxis, because mortality decreased during the period of 1982 to 1983 and anaphylaxis incidence decreased most dramatically from 1983 to 1984. Thus, while prophylactic administration of antihistamines may not significantly reduce the overall rate of anaphylaxis, their use may be a significant factor in reducing mortality attributable to anaphylactic reactions. Alternatively, better physician awareness about recognizing and treating anaphylaxis may be a significant factor in the dramatic decrease in mortality. In fact, the manufacturer of Chymodiactin® strongly emphasized physician education.

The factor that did change from 1982–1983 to 1983–1984 (the time when the incidence of anaphylaxis decreased most) was patient selection. Perhaps some reduction in the frequency of allergic reactions reflects patient selection. Patients with elevated levels of antibodies to chymopapain were often excluded from chemonucleolysis. However, immunologic tests were not widespread until September 1983, and thus could not have influenced the rate of anaphylaxis until after that date.[24,93–96] Subsequent use of such tests may have influenced overall reaction rates.

Another difference between the data from the clinical trials and the data from postmarketing surveillance questionnaires is that the former pertained to a limited geographic region (98% of the clinical trials occurred in the state of Illinois), whereas the postmarketing data were derived from 1,500 institutions throughout the U.S.[76] It ap-

pears that the overall rate of anaphylaxis to chymopapain varies significantly according to geography. Patients in Texas have a 10-fold increased chance of carrying the specific IgE than in Minnesota.[97] In the chymodiactin postmortuary survey, Agre et al.[97] found that while 28 of 967 patients undergoing chemonucleolysis in Texas had an anaphylactic reaction, only one of 1,155 patients undergoing the procedure in Minnesota had the reaction. The other states showed an intermediate incidence. The explanation for this geographic variability is unknown. It is not a factor in such allergies as reactions to penicillin or other compounds.

Thus, the survey of chymopapain anaphylaxis[24] documented a decrease in the incidence and severity of anaphylaxis after use of chymopapain. These decreases are independent of the type of anesthesia employed. In addition, there is no evident relationship between the incidence of anaphylaxis and the prophylactic use of antihistamines. However, the prophylactic use of antihistamines may account, in part, for the decreased mortality secondary to anaphylaxis. Other possible causes for the decreased mortality rate include vigorous preoperative fluid administration, patient selection (e.g., exclusion of high-risk patients by immunologic tests), and physician education. Comparison of these data with those of the earlier phase II trials and with reports from Australia and Britain has led us to conclude that 90% of the adverse outcomes after anaphylactic and anaphylactoid reactions can be avoided by proper physician and patient preparation.[4,22–24,90–92,94]

Narcotics

Most of the narcotics (with the possible exception of the fentanyl family) may cause direct release of histamine, urticaria along the vein of administration, and vasodilation. However, bronchospasm and angiodema have not been reported, even when large doses of these agents are used for anesthesia for cardiac procedures.[98] Although heroin may cause pulmonary edema and death in drug addicts, this appears to be due to injected impurities. Codeine has been implicated in several cases of anaphylactoid reactions; however, in all of these reported instances, more than one drug was used simultaneously. An anaphylactoid reaction to morphine and an inordinate sensitivity to histamine release have been reported, but skin testing in this patient produced negative results.[99] Meperidine is the only narcotic to which IgE antibodies have been demonstrated by RAST testing.[100]

Local Anesthetics

True allergy to the para-aminobenzoic ester agents, such as procaine, is well-documented, but documented allergic reactions to the amide local anesthetics are rare.[101–104] Methylparaben, a derivative of para-aminobenzoic acid, is a preservative used in many multidose vials of local anesthetics; it may well be the offending agent in anaphylactic reactions. If true allergy to one amide local anesthetic agent occurs, a potential for cross-reactivity exists. Although skin testing is used to identify which local anesthetic agents may be safe, there is no support for applying this technique to humans.[105] Clinical history appears a good discriminator. Most "reactions" in the dental chair appear to result from anxiety or epinephrine responses. For example, in a series of 71 patients having a history of possible allergic reaction to local anesthetics, only 15% had a history of clinical manifestations that indicated a hypersensitivity response (i.e., urticaria, wheezing, or facial swelling).[105]

Antibiotics

Of all parenteral medications, penicillin causes the highest incidence (0.7 to 10%[34]) of allergic reactions. However, the fatality rate from shock after administration of penicillin is 0.0015 to 0.002%.[14] Retrospectively, penicillin accounted for 75% of all fatal anaphylactic reactions.[35] For this reason, it should be administered carefully, and with full knowledge of allergic history to penicillin. In a study of 152 anaphylactic fatalities following penicillin administration, 14% of the patients had a history of a nonpenicillin allergy, 70% had received penicillin previously, and 33% had prior allergic reactions to penicillin.[34] In addition, patients who are allergic to penicillin have a 5 to 30% incidence of cross-reactivity with cephalosporins. Hypersensitivity to penicillin has been well-established as an IgE-mediated reaction to one of several moieties, the most common of which is the penicilloyl derivative of the molecule. Other antibiotics may cause anaphylactoid reactions. However, vancomycin, when administered rapidly, causes hypotension and flushing by a direct, pharmacologic effect.[106]

Volume Expanders

Colloid

Anaphylactoid reactions to the clinically used colloids have been studied extensively in Europe (Table 20–2).[107-110] Because of kinin contaminants, the purified protein fractions (PPF) are associated with a higher incidence of reactions than are other colloids. The complex polysaccharides can activate the complement system. These reactions do not depend on prior sensitization. The reported incidence of anaphylactoid reactions after PPF varies from 0.007 to 0.085% (Table 20–2).

Table 20–2. Incidence of Anaphylactoid Reactions to Colloid Volume Expanders

Colloid	Incidence (%)
Plasma protein	
Plasma protein derivative	0.019
Human serum albumin	0.011
Dextran	
Dextran 60/75	0.069
Dextran 40	0.007
Starch	
Hydroxyethyl starch	0.085

Adapted from Ring and Messmer.[107]

Blood Products

Transfusion reactions can be classified as hemolytic or nonhemolytic.[111,112] Hemolytic reactions result from ABO-antigen incompatible transfusions in which IgG or IgM antibodies from the donor or recipient react with red blood cells, complement is fixed and activated, and lysis of the cells and liberation of complement anaphylatoxins occur.[55,113] Urticaria, hypotension, and bronchospasm can occur in addition to activation of the clotting cascade.[113] In an anesthetized patient, bleeding or severe hypotension may be the only sign of a transfusion reaction.[112] The most common allergic reactions to transfusions are nonhemolytic, febrile reactions from leukoagglutinins.[113] Unlike red blood cells, leukocytes and platelets contain HLA antigens of the human histocompatibility system.[114] Antibodies of the IgG or IgM class to these antigens are known as leukoagglutinins.[92,93] The precise relationship of leukoagglutinins to anaphylactoid reactions remains unclear.[115] Patients who lack serum IgA will generate antibodies to IgA and may have a severe anaphylactoid reaction upon transfusion of IgA-replete normal blood.[116,117] In most cases of transfusion reaction, the magnitude of cell lysis, hypotension, bronchospasm, and increased capillary permeability probably relate directly to the rate and extent of complement activation.

Contrast Materials

Anaphylactoid reactions during radiographic contrast material infusions occur in 1 to 2% of procedures.[59,60,118] The mechanism of such reactions remains unknown.[59,60,76] These reactions have proved a futile ground for retrospective analysis of the benefits of premedicants. When repeated infusions of contrast materials are performed in patients with a history of an immediate anaphylactoid reaction to contrast materials, the incidence of repeat reactions is 17 to 35%.[118] In one study, pretreatment with prednisone and diphenhydramine was associated with subsequent hypotension in three of 415 previously reactive patients, pretreatment with prednisone, diphenhydramine and ephedrine with hypotension in none of 180, and pretreatment with prednisone, diphenhydramine, ephedrine and cimetidine in 0 of 100 previously reactive patients.[118] While these numbers are of necessity small, they seem to indicate that pretreatment with steroids, histamine receptor blocking drugs, and sympathomimetics decreases hypotension without a significant risk of adverse effects.

Protamine

A number of case reports and studies[119-128] have provided evidence that protamine reversal of heparin's effects can cause a severe life-threatening reaction with generation of anaphylatoxins (C5a) and thromboxane. It remains unclear whether or not these reactions are immune-mediated, or a combination of immune-mediated, and mediated by the freeing of vasoactive compounds by displacing vasoactive basic substances by protamine, or caused by some other mechanism. Protamine is derived from salmon sperm—thus, the theoretic possibility of antigenic crossover with fish allergy.[119,120] In addition, diabetics who have received protamine zinc insulin (PZI, 25 units contains 0.7 mg of protamine) appear to have an increased incidence of this reaction as well as antibodies to protamine.[123,125-128] One study indicates that perhaps more than one mechanism may be involved; production of C5a anaphylatoxins by any mechanism generates thromboxane A2, which causes pulmonary vaso-and bronchoconstriction and systemic hypotension.[125] Substitutes for both heparin and protamine are being developed so that patients with known risk factors will be able to undergo safe cardiopulmonary bypass. Until then, dose modification, obtaining hexadiomethine (polybrene) via investigational drug request from the FDA, or using prostaglandin I_2 for cardiopulmonary bypass remain options. Perhaps the routine use of calcium to treat hypotension after protamine should be abandoned (see "therapy" section).

PREVENTION AND TREATMENT

Sometimes a patient with a history of an anaphylactic or anaphylactoid reaction must receive a substance suspected of producing such a reaction (for example, iodinated contrast material). Also, some patients have a higher than average likelihood of a reaction, e.g., the atopic woman working in a meat tenderizer factory who is about to receive chymopapain. In such instances, pretreatment and therapy for possible anaphylactic and anaphylactoid reactions should be carefully planned (Table 20-3). Although virtually all "evidence" on these subjects is anecdotal, there is enough consistency throughout the literature to justify proposing an optimal approach to these problems.

First, predisposing factors should be sought, and the patient with a history of atopy or allergic rhinitis should be suspected as at risk. Because anaphylactic and anaphylactoid reactions to chymopapain occur five to ten times more frequently in women than in men, one might consider giving patients both H_1 and H_2 receptor antagonists for 16 to 24 hours before exposure to a suspected allergen.[94,129,130] Perhaps large doses of steroids (2 g hydrocortisone) should also be administered to women before exposure to agents associated with a high incidence of anaphylactic or anaphylactoid reactions.[32,131,132] Older patients present a special problem: they are more at risk of complications from both pretreatment (especially vigorous hydration and steroid administration) and therapy for anaphylactic reactions. Drugs likely to trigger anaphylactic or anaphylactoid reactions in this group should be avoided, and treatment protocols altered.

Second, and most important, the treatment plan for an anaphylactic or anaphylactoid reaction should be reviewed with other involved physicians and nurses, and specific tasks assigned in advance (e.g., who starts the second IV, who turns the patient supine). The slight probability of a serious reaction does not justify lack of planning. If the worst is expected and planned for, adverse outcomes of anaphylactic and anaphylactoid reactions can probably be reduced by more than 90% (see earlier section on "Chymopapain").

Although various drugs are used to treat anaphylactic and anaphylactoid reactions, cessation of the offending drug, maintenance of the airway, administration of oxygen, blood volume expansion, and administration of epinephrine are the mainstays of therapy (Table 3). These procedures are necessary to treat the sudden hypotension and hypoxia that result from vasodilation, increased capillary permeability, and bronchospasm. Establishing a plan beforehand for the successful therapy of these reactions

Table 20–3.   Possible Therapy for a 70-kg Individual if an Anaphylactic or Anaphylactoid Reaction is Likely to Occur

Prophylaxis
  Consider desensitization.
  Administer diphenhydramine, 50 mg, every 6 hours for 24 hours; cimetidine, 300 mg, every 6 hours for 24 hours, or ranitidine, 150 mg 9–12 hours for 24 hours; and hydrocortisone, 2 g IV, 1–6 hours before anticipated exposure.
  Establish large-bore IV and prehydrate patient with maintenance fluid and perhaps 500 ml more.
Protocol for action
  Plan for the worst and assign tasks in advance (e.g., who starts extra IV, who turns patient, who gets crash cart, who draws blood gases).
Initial therapy
  Stop administration of allergen.
  Maintain airway with 100% O_2.
  Stop negative inotropic and vasodilating anesthetics.
  Expand blood volume.
  If indicated, administer epinephrine, 0.05 to 0.1 mg (0.5 to 1 ml of 1:10,000 solution every 1–5 minutes up to a total of 1–2 mg over 1 hr).
Secondary therapy (if indicated)
  Administer antihistamines (50 mg of diphenhydramine, 300 mg of cimetidine).
  Administer aminophylline, 5–9 mg/kg, over 20–30 minutes.
  Drip infusion of catecholamines.
  Administer steroids (hydrocortisone, 2 g IV).
Evaluate airway for edema before extubating the trachea.

will diminish unfavorable outcomes. Although the data are not consistent enough to warrant a dogmatic treatment protocol, there is enough consistency to propose a treatment protocol. Even though anaphylactic and anaphylactoid reactions are triggered by different mechanisms, the mediators released and the treatment for these severe reactions are indistinguishable.

Management of Anaphylaxis

Initial Therapy

Discontinuation of Suspected Allergen

This prevents further recruitment of mast cells and release of mediators.

Airway Maintenance and Administration of 100% Oxygen

Severe mismatching of ventilation and perfusion may occur from bronchospasm, pulmonary hypertension, and pulmonary capillary leakage.[133-135] These changes can persist for several hours during anaphylactic reactions, thereby producing hypoxemia.[133,134] Therefore, the airway should be maintained and supplemental oxygen (we recommend 100%) administered until the situation improves. Intubation of the trachea should be considered if not already done.

Discontinuation of All Anesthetic Agents

Anesthetic agents may have negative inotropic properties and may decrease systemic vascular resistance. In addition, they often interfere with the body's compensatory response to cardiovascular problems. Thus, we believe that anesthetics should be discontinued to avoid hypotension. Halothane, enflurane, and/or isoflurane are not the bronchodilators of choice for anaphylaxis.

Blood Volume Expansion

Up to 40% of intravascular volume is rapidly lost into the interstitial spaces in an acute anaphylactic reaction during anesthesia.[136] Effective therapy consists of rapid replacement of blood volume.[137,138] Rapid fluid loss and successful treatment with fluid replacement have been documented with an anaphylactic reaction incidentally observed by transesophageal echocardiography[139] (Fig. 20-3). Evidence does not indicate that colloid is more effective than crystalloid. Rapid administration of 1 to 2 l of lactated Ringer's solution or normal saline is important in the initial therapy for these reactions. Further blood volume expansion may be necessary if hypotension persists.

Administration of Epinephrine

Epinephrine is a mainstay of therapy in acute anaphylaxis. Its alpha-adrenergic effects make it useful for treating hypotension. Its beta-adrenergic effects inhibit bronchoconstrictor effects and the release of mediators from stimulated mast cells or basophils, by stimulating the production of intracellular cyclic AMP.[140,141] For hypotension, 0.05 to 0.1 mg (0.5 to 1 ml of a 1/10,000 solution) of

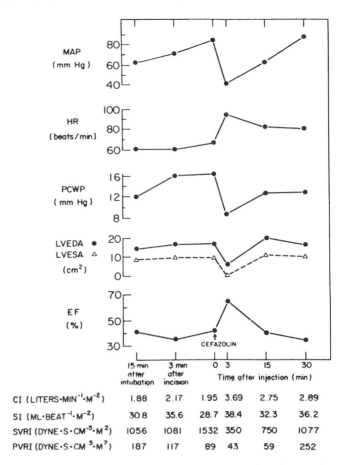

	15 min after intubation	3 min after incision	0	3	15	30
CI (LITERS·MIN^{-1}·M^{-2})	1.88	2.17	1.95	3.69	2.75	2.89
SI (ML·BEAT^{-1}·M^{-2})	30.8	35.6	28.7	38.4	32.3	36.2
SVRI (DYNE·S·CM^{-5}·M^2)	1056	1081	1532	350	750	1077
PVRI (DYNE·S·CM^{-5}·M^2)	187	117	89	43	59	252

Fig. 20-3. Hemodynamic and echocardiographic changes before, during, and after an anaphylactic reaction to cefazolin. MAP = mean arterial blood pressure; HR = heart rate; PCWP = pulmonary capillary wedge pressure; LVEDA and LVESA = left ventricular end-diastolic and end-systolic cross-sectional areas; EF = ejection fraction (LVEDA - LVESA)/LVEDA; CI = cardiac index; SI = stroke index; SVRI = systemic vascular resistance index; and PVRI = pulmonary vascular resistance index. Reprinted with permission from Beaupre PN, et al.[139]

epinephrine should be given initially as an intravenous bolus and repeated every 1 to 5 min up to 0.015 mg/kg (or 10 ml of a 1/10,000 solution) for a 70-kg patient, as needed. If cardiac arrest or a total loss of blood pressure or pulse occurs, full cardiopulmonary resuscitative doses (0.01 mg/kg, not to exceed 1.0 mg total) of epinephrine are indicated, along with rapid volume expansion. Intramuscular or subcutaneous administration of epinephrine may be unreliable in a hypotensive patient who requires immediate therapy. Interactions with propranolol are possible, and care must be taken not to overdose the patient with epinephrine to the point of severe hypertension (unopposed alpha-adrenergic effects) and its consequence.[142] Overdose can occur in the absence of propranolol, as well. However, the major threat from chronic beta-adrenergic blockade appears to be insufficient responses to epinephrine to terminate the reaction, and industrial doses of epinephrine may be required.[143] We believe that any amount of epinephrine is appropriate when titrated to effect, and the above mentioned doses solely provide a starting point.

Secondary Treatment

Antihistamines

Histamine is one of the major mediators of the acute manifestations of anaphylactic and anaphylactoid reactions. Because the vasodilatory effects are mediated by both H_1 and H_2 receptors, both receptor sites must be blocked if all potentially harmful cardiovascular effects of histamine are to be antagonized.[37,39,94,120] Studies involving the pretreatment of patients prior to histamine release demonstrate the effectiveness of preventing or blunting adverse cardiopulmonary responses when both H_1 and H_2 receptor antagonists are used.[94,129,130] Although histamine is only one of the mediators released in anaphylactic and anaphylactoid reactions, it may account for many of the initial adverse manifestations. No clinical evidence indicates that administration of antihistamines is effective in treating anaphylaxis once mediators have been released. Intact H_2 receptor blockade theoretically may facilitate the release of histamine and potentiate anaphylaxis. Administration of antihistamines is therefore recommended only as secondary treatment in acute anaphylactic and anaphylactoid reactions. (Suggested doses are diphenhydramine, 1 mg/kg; or chlorpheniramine, 0.1 mg/kg, as H_1 blockers; and cimetidine, 4 mg/kg, as an H_2 blocker.)

Aminophylline

If bronchospasm persists (and hemodynamic function is stable), aminophylline may be administered as a bronchodilator. Aminophylline inhibits phosphodiesterase, an enzyme that normally degrades cyclic AMP.[140,141] The intracellular accumulation of cyclic AMP restrains the release of mediators from mast cells and is a potent bronchodilator for histamine- or antigen-induced bronchospasm.[144] (The initial "loading" dose is 7 to 9 mg/kg, which should be given over 20 to 30 minutes.)

Catecholamines

Isoproterenol

If bronchospasm persists, isoproterenol may be useful as a pure beta-adrenergic agonist and bronchodilator. This drug may also prove useful when combined with epinephrine in the patient taking beta-adrenergic receptor blocking drugs.[142] The beta-2 adrenergic effects of isoproterenol cause vasodilation and possible hypotension, especially in patients already experiencing vasodilation or depletion of blood volume. Tachycardia is another possible unwanted effect. Because isoproterenol dilates the pulmonary artery, it may be useful in treating the increased pulmonary vascular resistance of severe anaphylactic reactions when oxygenation is a problem or right ventricular dysfunction occurs. (Starting doses for persistent bronchospasm are 0.5 to 1 μg/min/70 kg).

Epinephrine

When hypotension and bronchospasm persist, an intravenous epinephrine drip may be useful after blood volume expansion and the administration of boluses of epinephrine. The starting dose of epinephrine is 1 to 2 μg/min/70 kg and should be titrated to the desired effect.

Norepinephrine (Levophed)

Norepinephrine may be useful in maintaining blood pressure in a hypotensive patient until adequate volume expansion has been achieved.[33] Although theoretically, alpha-adrenergic drugs may potentiate the release of mediators,[140] hypotension is deleterious to both cerebral and coronary perfusion and must be treated aggressively.

Steroids

Although corticosteroids are important drugs to consider and should be given in severe reactions such as shock with refractory bronchospasm and hypotension,[145] there is no evidence as to what constitutes an appropriate dose or preparation.[131] However, we believe 2 g of hydrocortisone phosphate (or its equivalent) is appropriate for severe cardiopulmonary dysfunction. Large doses of methylprednisone (35 mg/kg) have been shown to inhibit complement-induced polymorphonuclear cell aggregation and lysosomal enzyme release in vitro.[132] Corticosteroids may decrease release of vasoactive mediators[32] and metabolites of arachidonic acid in anaphylaxis by stabilizing membrane phospholipids,[47] or by generating macrocortin, which inhibits phospholipid turnover.[43]

Sodium Bicarbonate

When hypotension is resistant to treatment, sodium bicarbonate, 0.5 to 1 mEq/kg, should be given and acid-base status monitored repeatedly.

Airway Evaluation

Laryngeal edema may occur in anaphylactic reactions, and swelling can persist.[146] If laryngeal edema has occurred, these structures can be examined upon extubation.

Calcium

Because release of mediators is a calcium-dependent process, theoretic and experimental evidence indicate that its administration may worsen an anaphylactic condition.[147]

In summary, a detailed and thorough drug history is usually obtained from all patients before any drug is administered. Management of the patient with a history of allergic reaction is described in Table 3. Patients given a parenteral drug should remain under close observation for at least 20 minutes.[35] If severe cardiovascular or respiratory symptoms occur, aggressive therapy must be instituted. Rapid volume replacement is important in treating profound hypotension, should it occur. Discontinuing the precipitating agent may prevent further recruitment of mast cells or basophils and release of mediators. Fully trained resuscitative staff must be available whenever parenteral medications are administered. If the patient has a history of allergic reaction to an agent, that drug should be strictly avoided. Although anaphylactic and anaphylactoid reactions are acute, potentially fatal events, their morbidity and mortality can probably be reduced at least 90% by anticipating, promptly recognizing, and aggressively treating these reactions.[24,33,90-94] Thus, altered immune responses can have important outcome implications for our patients, and can afford us, at least in hypersensitivity reactions, a place to demonstrate our mettle.

Operating Room Related Latex Reactions

Latex Allergic Reactions[148]

Three groups of high-risk individuals have been identified for allergic reaction to latex: myelodysplastic patients, health care workers, and patients with congenital urological anomalies.[149]

Screening of myelodysplastic patients reveals that 18% or more are latex-sensitive. The sources of the allergic response are proteins that are polymer extracts from the sap of the rubber tree, Hevea brasiliensis.[150] The current accepted means of diagnosing latex allergy is the skin scratch test, using a nonstandardized latex extract. Management is aimed at prevention. A prophylactic regimen should be used in high-risk and sensitized individuals, consisting of prednisone, diphenhydramine, and ranitidine. Avoidance of latex products is essential. IV tubing and angiocatheters should be flushed with sterile fluid prior to patient contact.[151] Safe gloves for both patients are made of Elastryn and vinyl products.

Further study is necessary to confirm the effects of surgery and anesthesia on immunity, and the mechanism of this alteration. For now we know that the perioperative period interferes with innate immunity (by mucous and skin membrane transgressions, for example) but it is not clear how much of a role altered acquired immunity plays. Our responses to the altered acquired immunity do, we believe, play a major role in patient outcome after such a reaction.

REFERENCES

1. Bruce, D. L.: Effect of halothane anesthesia on experimental salmonella peritonitis in mice. J Surg Res 7:180, 1967.
2. Duncan, P. G., Cullen, B. F., and Pearsell, N. N.: Anesthesia and the modification of response to infection in mice. Anesth Anal 55:776, 1976.
3. Snel, J. J.: Immunitat und narkose. Berlin Klin Wschrc 40:212, 1903.
4. Duncan, P. G., and Cullen, B. F.: Anesthesia and immunology. Anesthesiology 45:522, 1976.
5. Levy, J. H., Roizen, M. F., and Morris, J. M.: Anaphylactic and anaphylactoid reactions: A review. Spine 11:282, 1986.
6. Schwartz L. M. (ed): Compendium of Immunology. New York, Van Nostrand Reinhold, 1983.
7. Forbes, A. R., and Horrigan, R. W.: Mucociliary flow in the trachea during anesthesia with enflurane, ether, nitrous oxide, and morphine. Anesthesiology 46:319, 1977.
8. Moudgil, G. C.: Update on anaesthesia and the immune response. Can Anaesth Soc J 33:S54, 1986.
9. Bruce, D. L.: Halothane action on lymphocytes does not involve cyclic AM. Anesthesiology 44:151, 1976.
10. Cullen, B. F., Duncan, P. G., and Ray-Keil, L.: Inhibition of cell-mediated cytoxicity by halothane and nitrous oxide. Anesthesiology 44:386, 1976.
11. Duncan, P. G., Cullen, B. F., Calverly, R., Smith, N. T., Eger, E. I. II, and Bone R.: Failure of enflurane and halothane anesthesia to inhibit lymphocyte transformation in volunteers. Anesthesiology 45:661, 1976.
12. Doenicke, A., Grote, B., Suttmann, H., Graf, K.-J., Sprecht, U. V., Ott, H., Sarafoff, B., and Bretz, C.: Effect of halothane on the immunological system in healthy volunteers. Clin Research Reviews 1:23, 1981.
13. Salo, M.: The effect of anaesthesia and total hip replacement on the phytohaemagglutinin and concanavalin A responses of lymphocytes. Ann Chir Gynaecol 66:299, 1977.
14. Park, S. K., Brody, J. I., Wallace, H. A., and Blakemore, W.S.: Immunosuppressive effect of surgery. Lancet 1:53, 1971.
15. Duncan, P. G., Cullen, B. F., and Ray-Keil, L.: Thiopental inhibition of tumor immunity. Anesthesiology 46:97, 1977.
16. Hole, A.: Pre- and postoperative monocyte and lymphocyte functions: Effects of sera from patients operated under general or epidural anaesthesia. Acta Anaesthesiol Scand 28:287, 1984.
17. Whelan, P., and Morris, P. J.: Immunological responsiveness after transurethral resection of the prostate: General versus spinal anaesthetic. Clin Exp Immunol 48:611, 1982.
18. Ryhänen, P., Jouppila, R., Lanning, M., Jouppila, P., Hollmén, A., and Kouvalainen, K.: Natural killer cell activity after elective cesarean section under general and epidural anesthesia in healthy parturients and their newborns. Gynecol Obstet Invest 19:139, 1985.
19. Kehlet, H.: The stress response to anaesthesia and surgery: Release mechanisms and modifying factors. Clinics in Anesthesiology 2:315, 1984.
20. Eskola, J., Salo, M., Viljanen, M. K., and Ruuskanen, O.: Impaired B lymphocyte function during open-heart surgery: Effects of anaesthesia and surgery. Br J Anaesth 56:333, 1984.
21. Parker, C. W.: Drug allergy. N Engl J Med 292:511, 732, 957, 1975.
22. Fisher, M. M.: The epidemiology of anaesthetic anaphylactoid reactions in Australasia. Klin Wochenschr 60:1017, 1982.
23. Clarke, R. S. J., Dundee, J. W., Garrett, R. T., McArdle, G. K., and Sutton, J. A.: Adverse reactions to intravenous anaesthetics: A survey of 100 reports. Br J Anaesth 47:575, 1975.
24. Moss, J., Roizen, M. F., Nordby, E. J., Thisted, R., Apfelbaum, J. L., Schreider, B. D., and McDermott, D. J.: Decreased incidence and mortality of anaphylaxis to chymopapain. Anesth Analg 64:1197, 1985.
25. Gell, P. G. H., Coombs, R. R. A., and Lachmann, P. J. (eds): Clinical aspects of immunology. 3d ed. Oxford: Blackwell Scientific Publications, 1975.
26. Kelly, J. F., and Patterson, R.: Anaphylaxis: Course, mechanisms and treatment. JAMA 227:1431, 1974.
27. Austen, K. F.: Systemic anaphylaxis in the human being. N Engl J Med 291:661, 1974.
28. Portier, M. M., and Richet, C.: De l'action anaphylactique de certains venins. Société de Biologie 54:170, 1902.
29. Watkins, J.: Anaphylactoid reactions to I.V. substances. Br J Anaesth 51:51, 1979.
30. Mongar, J. L., and Schild, H. O.: The effect of calcium and pH on the anaphylactic reaction. J Physiol (Lond) 140:272, 1958.
31. Tanz, R. D., Kettelkamp, N., and Hirshman, C. A.: The effect of calcium on cardiac anaphylaxis in guinea-pig Langendorff heart preparations. Agents Actions 16:415, 1985.
32. Schleimer, R. P., MacGlashan Jr., D. W., Gillespie, E., and

Lichtenstein, L. M.: Inhibition of basophil histamine release by anti-inflammatory steroids. II. Studies on the mechanism of action. J Immunol 129:1632, 1982.

33. Smith, P. L., Kagey-Sobotka, A., Bleecher, E. R., Traystman, R., Kaplan, A. P., Gralnick, H., Valentine, M. D., Permutt, S., and Lichtenstein, L. M.: Physiologic manifestations of human anaphylaxis. J Clin Invest 66:1072, 1980.

34. Ids/e, O., Guthe, T., Willcox, R. R., and De Weck, A. L.: Nature and extent of penicillin side-reactions, with particular reference to fatalities from anaphylactic shock. Bull WHO 38:159, 1968.

35. Delage, C., and Irey, N. S.: Anaphylactic deaths: A clinicopathologic study of 43 cases. J Forensic Sci 17:525, 1972.

36. Beaven, M. A.: Histamine. N Engl J Med 294:30, 320, 1976.

37. Plaut, M.: Histamine, H1 and H2 antihistamines, and immediate hypersensitivity reactions. J Allergy Clin Immunol 63:371, 1979.

38. Bristow, M. R., Ginsburg, R., and Harrison, D. C.: Histamine and the human heart: The other receptor system. (editorial) Am J Cardiol 49:249, 1982.

39. Beaven, M. A., Robinson-White, A., Roderick, N. B., and Kauffman, G. L.: The demonstration of histamine release in clinical conditions: A review of past and present assay procedures. Klin Wochenschr 60:873, 1982.

40. Bourne, H. R., Melmon, K. L., and Lichtenstein, L. M.: Histamine augments leukocyte adenosine 3′,5′-monophosphate and blocks antigenic histamine release. Science 173:743, 1971.

41. Wasserman, S. I., Goetzl, E. J., and Austen, K. F.: Preformed eosinophil chemotactic factor of anaphylaxis (ECF-A). J Immunol 112:351, 1974.

42. Schatz, M., Wasserman, S., and Patterson, R.: The eosinophil and the lung. Arch Intern Med 142:1515, 1982.

43. Austen, K. F.: Tissue mast cells in immediate hypersensitivity. Hosp Pract 17:98, 1982.

44. Goetzl, E. J.: Mediators of immediate hypersensitivity derived from arachidonic acid. N Engl J Med 303:822, 1980.

45. Weissmann, G., Smolen, J. E., and Korchak, H. M.: Release of inflammatory mediators from stimulated neutrophils. N Engl J Med 303:27, 1980.

46. Michelassi F., Landa L., Hill R. D., Lowenstein E., Watkins W. D., Petkau A. J., Zapol W. M.: Leukotriene D4: A potent coronary artery vasoconstrictor associated with impaired ventricular contraction. Science 217:841, 1982.

47. Mathé, A.A., Hedqvist, P., Strandberg, K., and Leslie, C.A.: Aspects of prostaglandin function in the lung. N Engl J Med 296:850, 910, 1977.

48. Murano, G.: The "Hageman" connection: Interrelationships of blood coagulation, fibrino(geno)lysis, kinin generation, and complement activation. Am J Hematol 4:409, 1978.

49. Brocklehurst, W. E., and Lahiri, S. C.: The production of bradykinin in anaphylaxis. J Physiol (Lond) 160:15P, 1961.

50. Kaplan, A. P., and Austen, K. F.: Activation and control mechanisms of Hageman factor-dependent pathways of coagulation, fibrinolysis, and kinin generation and their contribution to the inflammatory response. J Allergy Clin Immunol 56:491, 1975.

51. Robinson, J. A., Klodnycky, M. L., Loeb, H. S., Racic, M. R., and Gunnar, R. M.: Endotoxin, prekallikrein, complement and systemic vascular resistance: Sequential measurements in man. Am J Med 59:61, 1975.

52. Mason, J. W., Kleeburg, U., Dolan, P., and Colman, R. W.: Plasma kallikrein and Hageman factor in gram-negative bacteremia. Ann Intern Med 73:545, 1970.

53. Ruddy, S., Gigli, I., and Austen, K. F.: The complement system of man. N Engl J Med 287:489, 545, 592, 642, 1972.

54. Måller-Eberhard, H. J.: Chemistry and function of the complement system. Hosp Pract 12:33, 1977.

55. Atkinson, J. P., and Frank, M. M.: Role of complement in the pathophysiology of hematolgic diseases. Prog Hematol 10:211, 1977.

56. Fearon, D. T., Ruddy, S., Schur, P. H., and McCabe, W. R.: Activation of the properdin pathway of complement in patients with gram-negative bacteremia. N Engl J Med 292:937, 1975.

57. Radford, S. G., Lockyer, J. A., and Simpson, P. J.: Immunological aspects of adverse reactions to althesin. Br J Anaesth 54:859, 1982.

58. Tachon, P., Descotes, J., Laschi-Loquerie, A., Guillot, J. P., and Evreux, J. C.: Assessment of the allergenic potential of althesin and its constituents. Br J Anaesth 55:715, 1983.

59. Lasser, E. C., Lang, J. H., Hamblin, A. E., Lyon, S. G., and Howard, M.: Activation systems in contrast idiosyncrasy. Invest Radiol 15(6 suppl): S2, 1980.

60. Lasser, E. C., Lang, J. H., Lyon, S. G., and Hamblin, A. E.: Complement and contrast material reactors. J Allergy Clin Immunol 64:105, 1979.

61. Chenoweth, D. E., Cooper, S. W., Hugli, T. E., Stewart, R. W., Blackstone, E. H., and Kirklin, J. W.: Complement activation during cardiopulmonary bypass: Evidence for generation of C3a and C5a anaphylatoxins. New Engl J Med 304:497, 1981.

62. Craddock, P. R., Fehr, J., Brigham, K. L., Kronenberg, R. S., and Jacob, H. S.: Complement and leukocyte-mediated pulmonary dysfunction in hemodialysis. N Engl J Med 296:769, 1977.

63. Roizen, M. F., Rodgers, G. M., Valone, F. H., Lampe, G. H., Benefiel, D. J., Smith, J. S., Cherry, K. P., Rapp, J., Oto, M., and Goetzl, E. J.: Anaphylactoid reactions to vascular graft material. (Abstract) Anesth Analg 64:276, 1985.

64. Vercellotti, G. M., Hammerschmidt, D. E., Craddock, P. R., and Jacob, H. S.: Activation of plasma complement by perfluorocarbon artificial blood: Probable mechanism of adverse pulmonary reactions in treated patients and rationale for corticosteroid prophylaxis. Blood 59:1299, 1982.

65. Vercellotti, G. M., Hammerschmidt, D. E., Jacob, H. S., and Craddock, P. R.: Activation of plasma complement (c) by perfluorocarbon artificial blood (fluosol-DA): Mechanism and prevention of resulting adverse pulmonary reactions. Clin Res 29:572A, 1981.

66. Vallota, E. H., and Müller-Eberhard, H. J.: Formation of C3a and C5a anaphylatoxins in whole human serum after inhibition of the anaphylatoxin inactivator. J Exp Med 137:1109, 1973.

67. Watkins, J., and Thornton, J. A.: Immunological and non-immunological mechanisms involved in adverse reactions to drugs. Klin Wochenschr 60:958, 1982.

68. Jacob, H. S., Craddock, P. R., Hammerschmidt, D. E., and Moldow, C. F.: Complement-induced granulocyte aggregation: An unsuspected mechanism of disease. N Engl J Med 302:789, 1980.

69. Haslam, P. L., Townsend, P. J., and Branthwaite, M. A.: Complement activation during cardiopulmonary bypass. Anaesthesia 35:22, 1980.

70. Jones, H. M., Matthews, N., Vaughn, R. S., and Stark, J. M.: Cardiopulmonary bypass and complement activation: Involvement of classical and alternative pathways. Anaesthesia 37:629, 1982.

71. Hammerschmidt, D. E., Weaver, L. J., Hudson, L. D., Craddock, P. R., and Jacob, H. S.: Association of complement activation and elevated plasma-C5a with adult respiratory distress syndrome. Lancet 1:947, 1980.

72. Sheagren, J. N.: Septic shock and corticosteroids. N Engl J Med 305:456, 1981.

73. Fisher, M. M.: Severe histamine mediated reactions to intravenous drugs used in anaesthesia. Anaesth Intensive Care 3:180, 1975.

74. Lorenz, W., Doenicke, A., Schöning, B., and Neugebauer, E.: The role of histamine in adverse reactions to intravenous agents. In Thornton, J.A., (ed.) Adverse Reactions of Anaesthetic Drugs. Amsterdam: Elsevier/North Holland Biomedical Press, 1981.

75. Rosow, C. E., Moss, J., Philbin, D. M., and Savarese, J. J.: Histamine release during morphine and fentanyl anesthesia. Anesthesiology 56:93, 1982.

76. Simon, R. A., Schatz, M., Stevenson, D. D., Curry, N., Yamamoto, F., Plow, E., Ring, J., and Arroyave, C.: Radiographic contrast media infusions: Measurements of histamine, complement, and fibrin split products and correlation with clinical parameters. J Allergy Clin Immunol 63:281, 1979.

77. Moss, J., Rosow, C. E., Savarese, J. J., Philbin, D. M., and Kniffen, K. J.: Role of histamine in the hypotensive action of d-tubocurarine in humans. Anesthesiology 55:19, 1981.

78. Moss, J., Philbin, D. M., Rosow, C. E., Basta, S. J., Gelb, C., and Savarese, J. J.: Histamine release by neuromuscular blocking agents in man. Klin Wochenschr 60:891, 1982.

79. Johansson, S. G. O.: In vitro diagnosis of reagin-mediated allergic diseases. Allergy 33:292, 1978.

80. Fisher, M. M.: Intradermal testing in the diagnosis of acute anaphylaxis during anaesthesia—results of five years experience. Anaesth Intensive Care 7:38, 1979.

81. Fisher, M. M.: The diagnosis of acute anaphylactoid reactions to anaesthetic drugs. Anaesth Intensive Care 9:235, 1981.

82. Fisher, M. M., and More, D. G.: The epidemiology and clinical features of anaphylactic reactions in anaesthesia. Anaesth Intensive Care 9:226, 1981.

83. Sage, D.: Intradermal drug testing following anaphylactoid reactions during anaesthesia. Anaesth Intensive Care 9:381, 1981.

84. Fisher, M. M.: Reaginic antibodies to drugs used in anesthesia. Anesthesiology 52:318, 1980.

85. Etter, M. S., Helrich, M., and Mackenzie, C. F.: Immunoglobulin E fluctuation in thiopental anaphylaxis. Anesthesiology 52:181, 1980.

86. Hirshman, C. A., Peters, J., and Cartwright-Lee, I.: Leukocyte histamine release to thiopental. Anesthesiology 56:64, 1982.

87. Wide, L.: Clinical significance of measurement of reaginic (IgE) antibody by RAST. Clin Allergy 3:583, 1973.

88. Berg, T. L. O., and Johansson, S. G. O.: Allergy diagnosis with the radioallergosorbent test: A comparison with the results of skin and provocation tests in an unselected group of children with asthma and hay fever. J Allergy Clin Immunol 54:209, 1974.

89. Royston, D., and Wilkes, R. G.: True anaphylaxis to suxamethonium chloride: A case report. Br J Anaesth 50:611, 1978.

90. McCulloch, J. A.: Chemonucleolysis: Experience with 2000 cases. Clin Orthopaed 146:128, 1980.

91. Javid, M. J.: Treatment of herniated lumbar disk syndrome with chymopapain. JAMA 243:2043, 1980.

92. Watts, C.: Complications of chemonucleolysis for lumbar disc disease. Neurosurgery 1:2, 1977.

93. Hall, B. B., and McCulloch, J. A.: Anaphylactic reactions following the intradiscal injection of chymopapain under local anesthesia. J Bone Joint Surg (Am) 65-A:1215, 1983.

94. Philbin, D. M., Moss, J., Akins, C. W., Rosow, C. E., Kono, K., Schneider, R. C., VerLee, T. R., and Savarese, J. J.: The use of H_1 and H_2 histamine antagonists with morphine anesthesia: A double-blind study. Anesthesiology 55:292, 1981.

95. Tsay, Y.-G., Jones, R., Calenoff, E., Sun, J., Arndt, L., Crispin, B., and Rock, H.: A preoperative chymopapain sensitivity test for chemonucleolysis candidates. Spine 9:764, 1984.

96. Bernstein, D. I., Gallagher, J. S., and Berstein, I. L.: Prospective evaluation of chymopapain sensitivity in patients undergoing chemonucleolysis. J Allergy Clin Immunol 73(suppl):180, 1984.

97. Agre K, et al: Chymodiactin postmarketing surveillance, demographic and adverse experience date in 29,075 patients. Spine 9:479, 1984.

98. Lowenstein, E., Hallowell, P., Levine, F. H., Daggett, W. M., Austen, W. G., and Laver, M. B.: Cardiovascular response to large doses of intravenous morphine in man. N Engl J Med 281:1389, 1969.

99. Fahmy, N. R.: Hemodynamics, plasma histamine, and catecholamine concentrations during an anaphylactoid reaction to morphine. Anesthesiology 55:329, 1981.

100. Levy, J. H., and Rockoff, M. A.: Anaphylaxis to meperidine. Anesth Analg 61:301, 1982.

101. Aldrete, J. A., and Johnson, D. A.: Allergy to local anesthetics. JAMA 207:356, 1969.

102. Fisher, M. M., and Pennington, J. C.: Allergy to local anaesthesia. Br J Anaesth 54:893, 1982.

103. Tannenbaum, H., Ruddy, S., and Schur, P. H.: Acute anaphylaxis associated with serum complement depletion. J Allergy Clin Immunol 56:226, 1975.

104. Brown, D. T., Beamish, D., and Wildsmith, J. A. W.: Allergic reaction to an amide local anaesthetic. Br J Anaesth 53, 435, 1981.

105. Incaudo, G., Schatz, M., Patterson, R., Rosenberg, M., Yamamoto, F., and Hamburger, R. N.: Administration of local anesthetics to patients with a history of prior adverse reaction. J Allergy Clin Immunol 61:339, 1978.

106. Newfield, P., and Roizen, M. F.: Hazards of rapid administration of vancomycin. Ann Intern Med 91:581, 1979.

107. Ring, J., and Messmer, K.: Incidence and severity of anaphylactoid reactions to colloid volume substitutes. Lancet 1:466, 1977.

108. Ring, J., Stephan, W., and Brendel, W.: Anaphylactoid reactions to infusions of plasma protein and human serum albumin. Clin Allergy 9:89, 1979.

109. Ellison, N., Behar, M., MacVaugh III, H., and Marshall, B. E.: Bradykinin, plasma protein fraction, and hypotension. Ann Thorac Surg 29:15, 1978.

110. Bland, J. H. L., Laver, B. M., and Lowenstein, E.: Vasodilator effect of commercial 5% plasma protein fraction solutions. JAMA 224:1721, 1973.

111. Milner, L. V., and Butcher, K.: Transfusion reactions reported after transfusions of red blood cells and of whole blood. Transfusion 18:493, 1978.

112. Schmidt, P. J.: Transfusion mortality; with special reference to surgical and intensive care facilities. J Fla Med Assoc 687:151, 1980.

113. Barton, J. C.: Nonhemolytic, noninfectious transfusion reactions. Semin Hematol 18:95, 1981.

114. Dubois, M., Lotze, M. T., Diamond, W. J., Kim, Y. D., Flye, M. W., and Macnamara, T. E.: Pulmonary shunting during leukoagglutinin-induced noncardiac pulmonary edema. JAMA 244:2186, 1980.

115. Thulstrup, H.: The influence of leukocyte and thrombocyte incompatibility on nonhaemolytic transfusion reactions. I. A retrospective study. Vox Sang 21:233, 1971.

116. Leikola, J., Koistinen, J., Lehtinen, M., and Virolainen, M.: IgA-induced anaphylactic transfusion reactions: A report of four cases. Blood 42:111, 1973.

117. Schmidt, A. P., Taswell, H. F., and Gleich, G. J.: Anaphylactic transfusion reactions associated with anti-IgA antibody. N Engl J Med 280:188, 1969.
118. Greenberger, P. A., Patterson, R., and Tapio, C. M.: Prophylaxis against repeated radiocontrast media reactions in 857 cases: Adverse experience with cimetidine and safety of β-adrenergic antagonists. Arch Intern Med 145:2197, 1985.
119. Caplan, S. N., and Berkman, E. M.: Protamine sulfate and fish allergy. N Engl J Med 295:172, 1976.
120. Knape, J. T.A., Schuller, J. L., DeHaan, P., DeJong, A. P., and Bovill, J. G.: An anaphylactic reaction to protamine in a patient allergic to fish. Anesthesiology 55:324, 1981.
121. Lakin, J. D., Blocker, T. J., Strong, D. M., and Yocum, M. W.: Anaphylaxis to protamine sulfate mediated by a complement-dependent IgG antibody. J Allergy Clin Immunol 61:102, 1978.
122. Cavarocchi, N. C., Schaff, H. V., Orszulak, T. A., Homburger, H. A., Schnell Jr., W. A., Pluth, J. R.: Evidence for complement activation by protamine-heparin interaction after cardiopulmonary bypass. Surgery 98:525, 1985.
123. Stewart, W. J., McSweeney, S. M., Kellett, M. A., Faxon, D. P., and Ryan, T. J.: Increased risk of severe protamine reactions in NPH insulin-dependent diabetics undergoing cardiac catheterization. Circulation 70:788, 1984.
124. Samuel, T.: Antibodies reacting with salmon and human protamines in sera from infertile men and from vasectomized men and monkeys. Clin Exp Immunol 30:181, 1977.
125. Morel, D. R., Zapol, W. M., Thomas, S. J., Kitain, E. M., Robinson, D. R., Moss, J., Chenoweth, D. E., and Lowenstein, E.: C5a and thromboxane generation associated with pulmonary vaso- and broncho-constriction during protamine reversal of heparin. Anesthesiology 66:597, 1987.
126. Doolan, L., McKenzie, I., Krafchek, J., Parsons, B., and Buxton, B.: Protamine sulfate hypersensitivity. Anaesth Intensive Care 9:147, 1981.
127. Moorthy, S. S., Pond, W., Rowland, R. G.: Severe circulatory shock following protamine (an anaphylactic reaction). Anesth Analg 59:77, 1980.
128. Stoelting, R. K.: Allergic reactions during anesthesia. Anesth Analg 62:341, 1983.
129. Kaliner, M., Sigler, R., Summers, R., Shelhamer, J. H.: Effects of infused histamine: Analysis of the effects of H-1 and H-2 histamine receptor antagonists on cardiovascular and pulmonary responses. J Allergy Clin Immunol 68:365, 1981.
130. Owen, D. A. A., Harvey, C. A., Boyce, M. J.: Effects of histamine on the circulatory system. Klin Wochenschr 60:972, 1982.
131. Schreiber, A. D.: Clinical immunology of the corticosteroids. Prog Clin Immunol 3:103, 1977.
132. Hammerschmidt, D. E., White, J. G., Craddock, P. R., Jacob, H. S.: Corticosteroids inhibit complement-induced granulocyte aggregation: A possible mechanism for their efficacy in shock states. J Clin Invest 63:798, 1979.
133. Smedegård, G., Revenäs, B., Lundberg, C., Arfors, K.-E.: Anaphylactic shock in monkeys passively sensitized with human reaginic serum: I. Hemodynamics and cardiac performance. Acta Physiol Scand 111:239, 1981.
134. Revenäs, B., Smedegård, G., Arfors, K.-E.: Anaphylaxis in the monkey: Respiratory mechanics, acid-base status and blood gases. Acta Anaesthesiol Scand 23:278, 1979.
135. Pavek, K., Wegmann, A., Nordström, L., Schwander, D.: Cardiovascular and respiratory mechanisms in anaphylactic and anaphylactoid shock reactions. Klin Wochenschr 60:941, 1982.
136. Fisher, M.: Blood volume replacement in acute anaphylactic cardiovascular collapse related to anaesthesia. Br J Anaesth 49:1023, 1977.
137. Fisher M. M.: The management of anaphylaxis. Med J Aust 1:793, 1977
138. Obeid, A. I., Johnson, L., Potts, J., Mookherjee, S., Eich, R. H.: Fluid therapy in severe systemic reaction to radiopaque dye. Ann Intern Med 83:317, 1975.
139. Beaupre, P. N., Roizen, M. F., Cahalan, M. K., Alpert, R. A., Cassorla, L., Schiller, N. B.: Hemodynamic and two-dimensional transesophageal echocardiographic analysis of an anaphylactic reaction in a human. Anesthesiology 60:482, 1984.
140. Winslow, C. M., and Austen, K. F.: Enzymatic regulation of mast cell activation and secretion by adenylate cyclase and cyclic AMP-dependent protein kinases. Fed Proc 41:22, 1982.
141. Ishizaka, T.: Analysis of triggering events in mast cells for immunoglobulin E-mediated histamine release. J Allergy Clin Immunol 67:90, 1981.
142. Foster, C. A., Aston, S. J.: Propranolol-epinephrine interaction: A potential disaster. Plast Reconstr Surg 72:74, 1983.
143. Jacobs, R. L., Rake Jr., G. W., Fournier, D. C., Chilton, R. J., Culver, W. G., Beckmann, C. H.: Potentiated anaphylaxis in patients with drug-induced beta-adrenergic blockade. J Allergy Clin Immunol 68:125, 1981.
144. Webb-Johnson, D. C., Andrews Jr., J. L.: Bronchodilator therapy. N Engl J Med 297:476, 1977.
145. Halevy, S., Altura, B. T., Altura, B. M.: Pathophysiological basis for the use of steroids in the treatment of shock and trauma. Klin Wochenschr 60:1021, 1982.
146. James Jr., L. P., Austen, K. F.: Fatal systemic anaphylaxis in man. N Engl J Med 270:597, 1964.
147. Tanz, R. D., Kettelkamp, N., Hirshman, C. A.: The effect of calcium on cardiac anaphylaxis in guinea pig Langendorff heart preparations. Agents and Actions 16:415, 1985.
148. Siegel, J. F., Rich, M., and Brock, W. A.: Latex allergy and anaphylaxis. Int Allergy Clin 31(1):141–145, 1993.
149. Swartz, J., Braude, B., Gilmour, R. Intraoperative anaphylaxis to latex. Can J Anaesth 37:589, 1990.
150. Slater, J. E., Mostello, L. A., and Shaer, C. Rubber-specific IgE in children with spina bifida. J Urol 146:578, 1991.
151. Shapiro, E., Kelly K. J., Setlock M. A., et al. Complications of latex Allergy. Dial Ped Urol 15:1, 1992.

Chapter 21

GASTROINTESTINAL PHYSIOLOGY AND PHARMACOLOGY: ASPIRATION OF GASTRIC CONTENTS AND POSTOPERATIVE NAUSEA AND VOMITING

PAULA A. CRAIGO

ASPIRATION

Significance in Anesthesia

Aspiration of matter or liquid into the respiratory passages is one of the most dreaded complications in anesthesia. With the adoption of modern anesthetic techniques, aspiration has become more rare, but the prevention of aspiration still dominates anesthetic preoperative evaluation and preparation in many patients. Patients are advised to remain "nil per os" for hours prior to their operation, and the procedure is cancelled or postponed if they eat or drink. Techniques of induction and intubation are frequently determined by the assessed potential for aspiration, or general anesthesia avoided altogether. When aspiration occurs it may be retrospectively assumed to have been predictable, entirely preventable,[1,2] and due to a lapse in technique or outright negligence, and the legal repercussions may be catastrophic.[3]

Most fatalities due to aspiration occur in patients who have not undergone any anesthetic care but lose protective reflexes secondary to illness or injury.[4] Aspiration in the perioperative period is the primary concern of the anesthesiologist, and this may occur even in the young and healthy when anesthetic administration depressed protective mechanisms. Hypoxic brain damage or death may result minutes after airway obstruction or massive alveolar filling (drowning), or follow days to weeks later when reactions to the aspirated matter culminate in adult respiratory distress syndrome. No technique is completely risk-free: significant aspiration has occurred during epidural and spinal anesthesia,[5] and monitored anesthesia care.[6]

Gastric contents are the chief offender in severe cases of aspiration (88% of cases in the ASA Closed Claims Study), although excessive salivary secretions, blood, pus, and teeth may be inhaled.[6] Iatrogenic materials, including antacids,[7] sucralfate,[8] enteral feeds, and barium[9] may also be aspirated. The volume and chemical composition of the gastric fluid, as well as its liquid or particulate character, determines the risk of significant pulmonary injury and the prognosis for recovery. Four major clinical syndromes are associated with aspiration: airway obstruction by particulate matter, chemical pneumonitis, infectious pneumonia, and drowning. Infectious sequelae to aspiration may eventually lead to necrotizing pneumonia, lung abscess, and empyema.[10,11]

Aspiration of gastric contents occurs far more frequently than does clinically significant pneumonitis.[2,12] Regurgitation, the passive reflux of gastric contents into the oropharynx and laryngeal inlet, is much more common than aspiration during anesthesia, and probably occurs frequently.[13] In Culver's study of unselected surgical patients undergoing general anesthesia, 26.3% regurgitated and 16.3% aspirated, but no clinically significant sequelae are mentioned. Eight percent of cases obviously vomited and 2/3 of these aspirated.[2] "Silent" regurgitation and aspiration have been of great concern but its clinical significance is unclear, and aspiration pneumonitis usually does not follow.

Incidence in Anesthesia

The incidence of death by aspiration perioperatively may have declined in the last thirty years. It is difficult to assess the real incidence of aspiration as it is most commonly reported as a fraction of anesthetic deaths, rather than the number of aspirations per anesthetic cases. Aspiration in the obstetric population has received special attention, and much of the data about aspiration comes from the more extensive records available from obstetric anesthesia complications (Table 21-1).

In Great Britain, 13 maternal deaths from aspiration were reported during 1973-75, and the number decreased in each biannual report, only 1 death being reported in 1985-87.[14] In Mendelson's report in 1946, 46 aspirations occurred during 44,016 obstetric *deliveries,* an incidence of 15 in 10,000 and a mortality rate of 0.45, with almost half the aspirations occurring during ether anesthesia for spontaneous vaginal delivery.[15] A computer-generated review of 185,358 anesthetics identified 87 cases of aspiration, for an incidence of 4.7 per 10,000. Five percent died, yielding a mortality of 0.2 per 10,000 anesthetics. In this same study, the incidence of aspiration during *cesarean section* was 15 per 10,000.[16] In Tiret's study of 198,103 regional and general anesthetics in France, there were 27 cases of aspiration (1.36/10,000), causing 6 deaths or persistent comas (0.3/10,000).[17] In another recent study, 262,850 anesthet-

Table 21–1. Deaths Due to Aspiration

Year	Author	Population Considered	Aspiration Cases (per 10,000)	Aspiration Deaths (per 10,000)
1946	Mendelson	Obstetric deliveries	15	0.45
1973	CIMD (in Cheek, 1993)	Maternal deaths	?	? (13 cases)
1985–87	CIMD (in Cheek, 1993)	Maternal deaths	?	? (1 case)
1986	Olsson	Mixed surgical	4.7	0.2
1986	Olsson	Cesarean-sections	15	0
1986	Tiret	Mixed surgical	1.36	0.3

Data from Cheek, T. D. and Gutsche, B. B: Pulmonary aspiration of gastric contents. *In* Anesthesia for Obstetrics. Edited by Shnider, S. M. and Levinson, G. Baltimore, Williams and Wilkins, 1993.
Mendelson, C. L.: Aspiration of stomach contents into lungs during obstetric anesthesia. Am. J. Obstet. Gynecol. *52*:191, 1946.
Olsson, G. L., Hallen, B. and Hambraeus-Jonzon: Aspiration during anaesthesia: a computer-aided study of 185,358 anaesthetics. Acta Anaesthesiol. Scand. *30*:84, 1986.
Tiret, L., Desmonts, J. M., Hatton, F. and Vourc'h, G.: Complications associated with anaesthesia—a prospective survey in France. Can. Soc. J. Anaesth. *33*:336, 1986.

ics generated 120 self-reported complications; aspiration of gastric contents accounted for only 2 of these reports and neither patient developed signs of pneumonitis postoperatively.[18]

Although anesthetic-related death is relatively rare, aspiration accounts for a significant number of these fatalities. In 1956, 1,000 deaths associated with anesthesia over a 5 year period were reported, and 10% of these were due to aspiration, while half the anesthetic-related obstetric deaths were due to aspiration;[19] by 1982, aspiration caused 12 out of 227 deaths (6%). In another study, six of the 46 anesthetic complications admitted to intensive care were aspirations.[20] Though examination of legal cases does not produce an accurate incidence of aspiration, it indirectly provides data about the role of aspiration in severe anesthetic outcomes. The American Society of Anesthesiologists Closed Claims Project found 3% of 2,046 litigation claims were related to aspiration. This is half the number of claims related to either difficult intubation or esophageal intubation and 1/4 the number following inadequate ventilation/oxygenation. However, these aspiration cases had catastrophic outcomes, as half died or had permanent brain damage, probably reflecting the greater tendency of the more severe outcomes to enter into litigation.[6]

Historical Background

Anesthetic techniques and drugs have changed dramatically since the 1940s, and changes in obstetric anesthesia practice clearly demonstrate the multiple developments related to management of patients at increased risk for aspiration. In contrast to practice at the time of Mendelson's report, current anesthetic methods for parturients avoid mask airway maintenance in the anesthetized patient; an increased utilization of regional anesthesia, rapid sequence endotracheal intubation when general anesthesia is indicated, and antacids and other prophylaxis has accompanied the reduced incidence of maternal death secondary to aspiration. Curiously, though mortality from aspiration pneumonitis is frequently cited as in excess of 50%, none of the 46 cases of acid aspiration reported by

Mendelson died. The two deaths he reported died on the delivery table from complete airway obstruction; another woman escaped that fate by coughing out a large plug of meat.[15] It has been suggested that this discrepancy in mortality indicates a worsening of outcome related to modern anesthetic techniques.[21] It is far more likely that Mendelson's patients aspirated only minute quantities of acid, represented some other clinical entity,[11] or that the mortality in milder forms of aspiration has been grossly over-estimated.

Cause of Pulmonary Dysfunction

Historically, the pulmonary dysfunction following aspiration was thought secondary to either the bacterial load, gastric enzymes or bile contained in the aspirate.[22] Winternitz studied the pulmonary pathology of phosgene poisoning and noted it to be identical to that caused by pulmonary instillation of hydrochloric acid. However, the role of acid in the pathophysiology of aspiration was not recognized until Mendelson's report of aspiration in obstetric patients, which was accompanied by animal experiments that established gastric acid as the agent of pulmonary damage.[15] Teabeaut confirmed these findings and demonstrated that a pH of 2.5 or less is required to produce the aspiration syndrome.[23]

Roberts and Shirley reported that 0.4 ml/kg of liquid with a pH of less than 2.5 caused severe respiratory dysfunction in an animal model, but their study was never subjected to peer review. These unpublished results were cited in a review article in 1974,[24] and established the widely quoted "critical" volume and pH of aspiration of 25 ml and 2.5 respectively. The only published information available concerning this study is in a letter to the editor in 1980,[25] which describes observations in a single monkey: almost immediately after 0.4 ml/kg of liquid with a pH of 1.5 had been instilled into the right mainstem bronchus, the animal developed acute pulmonary edema and cardiovascular collapse. Other investigators have not had such lethal results. In one recent animal study, *no* deaths occured from aspiration of liquid with a pH of 1 until a minimum volume of 0.8 ml/kg was given.

Aspiration of 1.0 ml/kg of liquid with a pH of 1.0 had a mortality of only 50%.[26] Regardless, the majority of studies of aspiration risk and prophylaxis use 0.4 ml/kg and a pH of 2.5 as end-points.

Determination of Risk

The risk of aspiration and efficacy of prophylaxis is usually inferred from measured gastric volume and pH, rather than the actual occurrence of aspiration. Because aspiration is so infrequent, randomized prospective studies would require prohibitively large patient populations, and retrospective studies are difficult to perform in the number needed and riddled with bias. In addition to questions regarding the validity of "critical volume and pH," other problems with this approach have been identified: faulty statistics; estimation of gastric volume by inaccurate means such as nasogastric suction; the unlikely assumption that a patient will regurgitate their entire gastric volume, then aspirate the whole;[27] and a perhaps misplaced emphasis on the role of gastric contents with little attention to the role of lower esophageal sphincter (LES) function.[28]

The majority of outpatients for elective surgery are at risk for aspiration pneumonitis by pH and volume criteria; 88% have a gastric pH less than 2.5, 56% have a gastric volume greater than 25 ml and pH greater than 2.5.[29] Despite finding that almost half of healthy elective surgical patients risked aspiration based on gastric volume and pH measurements, Hardy and co-workers found a very low incidence of gastroesophageal reflux.[30] The percentage of patients identified as at-risk for aspiration based solely on gastric pH and volume is probably falsely high.

Thus, most elective patients may be labeled "high risk," while the occurrence of significant pulmonary aspiration may be nearer 1 in 10,000 in elective inpatients, and death is "extremely rare."[28] In addition, while prophylaxis may alter gastric volume and pH, it is not possible to draw solid conclusions about the effect on aspiration itself. Still, aspiration may cause death through a number of mechanisms. Complete airway obstruction may prove impossible to remedy before hypoxic brain damage occurs, and treatment of ARDS is still primarily supportive. As the British anesthesiologist, J. Alfred Lee, said, "That which can not be easily treated had better be prevented."[31]

RISK FACTORS

Over 80% of patients who aspirate have some risk factor for it,[16] but it follows that 20% do not, and aspiration in those cases was not predictable. Loss or dysfunction of normal protective reflexes, secondary to altered mental status, muscular weakness or incoordination, loss of sensation or proprioception, incompetent upper or lower esophageal sphincters, or increased gastric pressure from vomiting, delayed emptying, gastrointestinal-bleeding or increased gastric acidity may predispose to aspiration of gastric contents, and worsen the sequelae of aspiration. In addition to these patient characteristics, certain surgical or anesthetic factors may increase the risk of aspiration, such as patient positioning, airway management, site of surgery and emergency status (Table 21–2).

Table 21–2. Risk Factors for Aspiration

Loss of protective reflexes
  Altered mental status
  Ineffective swallow or cough
  Sensory loss
  Motor weakness
  Motor incoordination
  Incompetent UES
  Incompetent LES

Decreased gastric emptying
  Drugs (narcotics, etc.)
  Stress and pain
  Medical illness
  Diabetes
  Scleroderma
  Achalasia
  Amyloidosis
  Hypothyroidism
  Renal failure
  Late pregnancy
  Small bowel obstruction
  Gastric outlet obstruction
  Symptomatic hiatal hernia

Increased gastric acidity
  Peptic ulcer disease
  Pregnancy

Difficult or esophageal Intubation

Emergency surgery

Abnormal Sphincteric and Gastric Function

Swallowing

Many "normal" people aspirate during deep sleep without significant clinical sequelae due to functional protective mechanisms and the relatively minimal quantities involved.[32] The complex activity required for normal swallowing suggests that relatively subtle defects may predispose to aspiration. It is frequently assumed that an active gag and cough reflex affords protection against aspiration, but the incidence of aspiration is not well correlated with the presence or absence of these reflexes in stroke patients.[33]

Normal deglutition has four phases: a preparatory phase, in which food is chewed and moved in the mouth; an oral phase, in which the tongue pushes food posteriorly, triggering the swallowing reflex; a pharyngeal phase, in which the bolus moves through the pharynx propelled by the swallow; and an esophageal phase, in which esophageal peristalsis moves the bolus down into the stomach.[34]

The preparatory and oral phases of swallowing require intact muscular strength and sensation for effective chewing and moving the bolus to the oropharynx without aspiration. The pharyngeal phase is complex; the soft palate elevates and retracts, closing the velopharyngeal port of entry to the nasopharynx, the bolus is propelled forward into the esophagus, and its safe passage ensured by coordinated elevation of the larynx, relaxation of the cricopharyngeal sphincter and laryngeal valving. Laryngeal valving affords physical protection of the larynx and involves the epiglottis, false vocal cords, and true vocal cords.[34]

In addition to adequate muscular strength and coordination, proprioception and sensory input are required. Abnormalities of the velar, pharyngeal, or laryngeal components of the pharyngeal phase may cause regurgitation through the nose, pooling in the vallecula and piriform sinuses, an incompletely protected laryngeal inlet, and aspiration.[34] Disordered swallowing may lead to aspiration even in the alert patient.[9]

Prolonged orotracheal intubation or tracheostomy tubes may cause swallowing disorders that may leave the extubated patient at risk for aspiration. In one study of patients after extubation, all eleven patients had a least one pharyngeal phase deficit during barium swallow with cideofluoroscopy. The deficits are temporary and may improve with swallowing therapy.[34]

Advancing age is associated with a progressive loss of protective airway reflexes,[35] and the elderly patient may be at greater risk for aspiration.

Upper Esophageal Sphincter (UES)

The sphincter is formed anteriorly by the lamina of the cricoid cartilage and posteriorly by the striated muscle of the lower part of the constrictor pharyngeus, the cricopharyngeus muscle. The cricopharyngeus originates from the lateral aspects of the cricoid cartilage and forms a sling around the constrictor pharyngeus. A pharyngeal-esophageal pressure zone about 4 cm long is created. The sphincter is innervated by the pharyngeal plexus, formed by pharyngeal branches from the superior cervical (sympathetic) ganglion as well as branches from the glossopharyngeal and vagus nerves. The muscle tone of the cricopharyngeus is reflexly modulated to prevent reflux into the oropharynx.

At rest in the awake state, the upper esophageal sphincter pressure (UESP) is about 40 mm Hg. The sphincter pressure increases slightly on inspiration (sealing the esophagus off from the airways), and increases significantly under emotional stress and arousal. Decreasing UESP from relaxation of the cricopharyngeus muscle normally occurs during swallowing, belching and vomiting. UESP decreases to a mean of 8 mm Hg during deep sleep, and with anesthesia and muscle relaxation without tracheal intubation averages 6 mm Hg. Tracheal intubation causes a rise in UESP. Cricoid pressure causes a rise in UESP, but this varies widely among patients. Elastic tissue pressure maintains a residual pressure level in the area, and so UESP does not fall to zero except when the larynx moves, fully opening the UES.[36] Complete opening of the UES (zero pressure) occurs during anterior movement of the larynx during swallowing, inflation of the lungs, and laryngoscopy.

Many anesthetic drugs affect the UESP in humans.[37] Ketamine appears to be the only intravenous anesthetic agent which maintains UESP in humans, increasing skeletal muscle tone and maintaining EMG activity of the upper airway muscles. Non-depolarizing muscle relaxants (curare) produce a fall in UES. Laryngeal reflexes are also depressed. The intravenous sedative drugs thiopental and midazolam decrease UESP to less than 10 mm Hg, and muscle relaxation with succinylcholine does not further lower the pressure. Induction with thiopental causes a fall in UESP which usually occurs before the loss of consciousness. The decrease in UESP occurs in two stages: first, an early decrease fluctuating with respiration, and second, a progressive decrease starting just before loss of consciousness and reaching its lowest level 30 seconds after loss of consciousness.[37] Cricoid pressure is used to counteract this decrease in UESP and prevent regurgitation prior to intubation; a pressure of at least 35 mm Hg should be effective.[38] Controversy has existed regarding at what point in induction cricoid pressure should be applied in order to avoid provoking vomiting or coughing while attempting to prevent passive reflux, but these observations suggest cricoid pressure should be applied before the patient loses consciousness.[37]

Lower Esophageal Sphincter (LES)

The LES represents a major barrier to gastroesophageal reflux, regurgitation, and vomiting. It is 2 to 5 cm long and extends above and below the diaphragm.[39] The sphincter is composed of both longitudinal and circumferential muscles and interdigitating folds of the lower esophagus, forming a valvular mechanism, not a true muscular sphincter. It has intrinsic tone and is richly innervated, with parasympathetics supplied by the vagal fibers, while spinal segments T6 through T10 supply sympathetic fibers. Reflux results not from the LESP itself, but from an inadequate barrier pressure. The barrier pressure (BrP) represents the integrity of the LES, and is the difference in pressure between that measured at the lower esophageal valve and the intragastric pressure. What barrier pressure is associated with reflux symptoms is not predictable, but a decrease in pressure would increase the risk of significant reflux. The LES probably remains competent when the intragastric pressure does not exceed 18 to 20 cm H_2O.[40] The LESP was 55 cm H_2O in nonpregnant controls and, in pregnant patients, 51 cm in those without heartburn and 45 cm in those with heartburn.[41]

The effects on the LES of drugs used in anesthesia practice have been studied with intraluminal esophageal manometry. Many of the drugs used in anesthesia cause a relaxation of this sphincter, and their effects may be additive[39,42] (Table 21-3). Drugs which lower LESP and increase the risk of reflux or regurgitation include antimuscarinics in doses used in anesthesia premedication and narcotic drugs with atropine-like effects. Drugs which raise LESP and decrease the risk of reflux or regurgitation include cholinomimetic drugs, anticholinesterases, metoclopramide and dromperidone. Succinylcholine raises LESP, but simultaneously also raises gastric pressure.[39]

Commonly used antiemetics have differing effects on LESP: cyclizine, prochlorperazine, and metoclopramide increase barrier pressure, while promethazine decreases it and droperidol has no effect. Promethazine decreases LESP perhaps due to its anticholinergic properties.[43]

The sphincter action of the lower and upper esophageal mechanism must be coordinated with other functions. Gastric reflux is a normal response to a full stomach because gastric distension causes reflex relaxation of the

Table 21–3. Effect on LES Tone of Drugs Used in Anesthesia

Increase LES Tone	Decrease LES Tone	No Change
Metoclopramide	Atropine	Propanolol
Domperidone	Glycopyrrolate	Oxprenolol
Prochlorperazine	Dopamine	Cimetidine
Cyclizine	Nitroprusside	Ranitidine
Edrophonium	Ganglionic blockers	Atracurium
Neostigmine	Pentothal	?Nitrous
Histamine	Tricyclic	oxide
Succinylcholine	antidepressants	
Pancuronium	B-adrenergic stimulants	
Metoprolol	Halothane	
A-adrenergic	Enflurane	
stimulants	Opiates	
Antacids	?Nitrous oxide	

With permission from Cotton, B. R. and Smith, G.: The lower esophageal sphincter and anesthesia. Br. J. Anaesth. *56*:37, 1984.

lower sphincter. During spontaneous reflux, the esophageal pressure rises abruptly by 5–10 mm Hg to equal gastric pressure and a common cavity is formed. The gastric pressure in the supine position may reach levels of 25 mm Hg. However, regurgitation into the pharynx does not occur in the awake subject unless the upper esophageal pressure falls below 25 mm Hg.[36]

Gastric Contents

As discussed, processes that increase gastric volume or delay emptying, or increase the production of gastric acidity, may predispose to aspiration or else worsen its consequences.

Gastric emptying and motility have been studied by a variety of methods, beginning with the direct observations made by William Beaumont in 1833 through the gastric fistula left by a gunshot wound. Beaumont noted that solid food required up to five hours to be processed, while clear liquids were quickly emptied. Estimation of gastric volume has been an important way to detect changes in the rate of gastric emptying. Nasogastric tubes or the Salem sump tube have been used to empty the stomach contents and thereby determine gastric volume, but the amount recovered may not be complete and the volume underestimated.[44] Other methods measure passage of radioactive tracers or the rate of drug absorption. Drugs which pass through the stomach and are absorbed in the upper small intestine provide an index of gastric emptying. Paracetamol is not absorbed in the stomach, but is readily absorbed in the upper intestine and measurement of the change in its concentration is a common technique for investigation of gastric emptying.

Besides the volume and pH of gastric fluid, the particulate matter and bacterial content of gastric fluid has a major influence on the severity of the pulmonary response. Small food particles can cause severe pulmonary damage, even when pH and volume do not reach critical values. In addition, food particles of sufficient size may obstruct a mainstem or segmental bronchus. An atelecta-

sis distal to this obstruction may follow, causing right-to-left pulmonary shunting and severe hypoxemia. Complete airway obstruction can result in death from hypoxia in minutes.[15] Particulate matter may also produce bronchoconstriction and bronchospasm through vagally mediated irritant reflexes. Nonparticulate antacids are probably safer to use perioperatively.[45]

Several factors that affect gastric contents are described as follows.

Age

Although high gastric acidity and increased gastric contents before induction of anesthesia have been reported in all age groups, generally, gastric acidity and volume decrease with age. Mean gastric pH was 1.99 in pediatric patients, 2.40 in adults, and 3.32 in geriatric patients. Only 60% of geriatric patients had a pH of less than 2.5, while 92% of pediatric patients were below the critical pH of 2.5. Mean gastric volumes showed a highest value (0.5 ml/kg) in children, and 0.25 ml/kg in adults over 65 years old.[46] Children admitted for emergency surgery had a median gastric volume of 0.6 ml/kg. When data were analyzed further according to age, the highest gastric volumes are reported for the 6–10 year age group. The pH values obtained were higher (median pH of 3.0) in the 0–5 year age group than in the older children.[47] In one large study of adults and pediatric patients, those aged 0–9 years had the highest incidence of aspiration.[16] Despite their relative lesser acidity and gastric volume when compared to younger patients, the risk of regurgitation and aspiration in the geriatric patient may be increased in certain situations. The presence of symptomatic hiatal hernias, gastroesophageal reflux, and decreased gastric motility in the geriatric patient may increase the risk of aspiration, and pre-existing cardiopulmonary dysfunction may make the insult of aspiration poorly tolerated.

Cigarette Smoking

Smokers have a higher gastric volume and higher acidity than non-smokers, and recent abstinence may be beneficial. Patients who smoke on the day of surgery, although NPO, have been found to have gastric volumes of 20 ml, twice that found in non-smokers (9.0 ml).[48] However, another study found no difference between aspirated gastric volume and pH in non-smokers compared with smokers deprived of cigarettes overnight.[49]

Miscellaneous Conditions

Medical illness may delay gastric emptying. Gastroparesis may be associated with gastric tumors, hypothyroidism, amyloidosis, connective tissue diseases such as scleroderma and diabetes mellitus. Aspiration pneumonitis has occurred after electroconvulsive therapy in patients with gastroparesis.[50] In the ASA Closed Claims Study, 29% of cases of aspiration occurred in obstetric patients, compared to 12% of the overall data base.[6] Opioids, surgery, traumatic injuries, stress, pain, anxiety, and even minor surgery under regional anesthesia[51] may be associated with a decrease in gastric emptying.

Anesthetic and Surgical Factors

Intensive Care Unit Management

In the intensive care setting, aspiration is a common occurrence due to the large proportion of patients at increased risk for aspiration due to diminished levels of consciousness, disordered swallowing, depressed gag reflexes, slowed gastric emptying or gastrointestinal motility, and tracheal intubation.[52] Endotracheal intubation is not completely protective: though it may prevent large-volume or obstructive aspirations, "microaspiration" with pulmonary colonization and infection is common. Gastric contents contaminate the pulmonary tree in at least 30 to 40% of intubated ICU patients, as shown by microbiologic and direct detection methods.[53] Enteral feedings are frequently aspirated, and gastrostomy does not guarantee protection.

Emergency Surgery

In the ASA Closed Claims Study, nearly half of the cases of aspiration occurred during emergency surgery, while emergency surgical cases accounted for only 19% of the database.[6] Emergency cases frequently have recent food ingestion and delayed gastric emptying; in addition, fatigue or inexperience of anesthetists may play a role.[16]

Patient Positioning

The effect of patient position on risk of aspiration is unclear, and the data are from early studies of dye contamination of respiratory passages during anesthesia, rather than quantification of the incidence of significant aspiration in various surgical positions. Surgery in the Trendelenburg and lateral positions was found to be more hazardous than in the supine position in one study,[2] but in another, the head-down position carried no more risk of aspiration and regurgitation than did the supine position.[12] Blitt found an increased incidence of "silent" regurgitation and aspiration in the prone position.[13]

Airway Management

Aspiration in the ASA Closed Claims study usually occurred during general anesthesia (95%). Maintenance of the airway by mask was a major risk factor, accounting for 41% of the total.[6] Of 58 patients who aspirated, 4 (6.9%) did so despite a cuffed endotracheal tube.[6] In a study in which adults were intubated with an uncuffed endotracheal tube, regurgitation occurred in 25% of those patients intubated and 14% of the total aspirated.[12]

Phase of Anesthesia

The initiation and termination of anesthesia are generally assumed to be the highest risk periods for several anesthesia complications, including aspiration. In the ASA Closed Claims Study, 34% of aspirations occurred during induction prior to intubation and 18% during emergence.[6] Of 6 cases of aspiration admitted to intensive care in one study, two occurred during induction, one during maintenance, and three during recovery.[20] In Tiret's study, 22%

occurred at induction, 30% during maintenance, and 48% postoperatively. Of the 6 cases of persistent coma or death in this study, 2 resulted from aspiration during induction, and 4 from aspiration in the postoperative period; none occurred during maintenance. However, 50% of patients were returned directly to the general wards from the operating room and the lack of recovery care may have contributed to the relatively high incidence and severity of outcome in this period.[17]

Induction is particularly high-risk because of the possibility of airway-management difficulties, as well as vomiting during induction, before the endotracheal tube is in place. Of the six patients who vomited during induction in one study, 4 had dye in the lungs.[54] In the age of inhalation inductions in adults, during "difficult" inductions, defined as a prolonged second stage of anesthesia, excitement, or retching, 24% vomited and 12% aspirated, while in "smooth" inductions, regurgitation occurred in 11% and aspiration in 6%. Contamination of the oropharynx or respiratory passages with dye was used as an end-point.[12] Airway problems such as esophageal intubation and difficult intubation were the outstanding risk factors for aspiration in the ASA Closed Claims Study.[6] When difficulties related to airway management occurred, the risk of regurgitation and aspiration was greatly increased, even in elective cases.

Regional Anesthesia

Regional anesthesia is frequently chosen for poor risk patients who are elderly, frail, and may have significant cardiopulmonary disease, but such techniques are not a guarantee against vomiting or aspiration.[5] Aspiration may occur during decreased consciousness due to a high spinal, local anesthetic toxicity-induced seizures, hypotension, aortocaval compression (in pregnancy), or excessive sedation. Nausea is less frequent during spinal anesthesia with use of supplemental oxygen and use of vasopressor agents to maintain systolic blood pressure.[55]

Practitioner Experience

Culver found that there was no difference in the incidence of regurgitation in patients cared for by inexperienced versus experienced anesthetists, but that 80% of aspirations occurred during care by inexperienced anesthetists.[2] In one article stating that experienced practitioners had less aspirations, "experience" was not defined.[54] The incidence of aspiration at night is six times greater than during daytime working hours, possibly due to less experienced staff, fatigue, or increased percentage of emergency cases.[16]

Gastric Suctioning

Decompression of the stomach via a gastric tube affords some protection against aspiration when there is marked distension of the stomach. It is difficult to separate the effect of the clinical syndrome requiring the gastric tube from the effect of the gastric tube itself on the risk of aspiration.[12,13] It is contended that such tubes disrupt the patency of the LES and increase the chance of re-

Table 21–4. Techniques of Avoiding Aspiration

Preoperative assessment
  Risk factors predisposing to aspiration
  Difficult airway identification
Prophylaxis
  Gastric suction in obstructed patients
  Drug therapy to decrease volume and acidity
Anesthetic techniques
  Regional anesthesia when appropriate
  Awake intubation if difficult airway
  Rapid sequence induction
  Plan for failed intubation/ventilation
  Extubation when airway reflexes returned
Postoperative observation until recovered

gurgitation. Though the tubes are probably effective at decreasing excess intragastric pressure in obstructed patients, complete emptying of the stomach is not guaranteed and significant quanitites of acidic gastric fluid may remain.[44,56]

PREVENTION (TABLE 21–4)

Preoperative Management

Preoperative assessment identifies risk factors for aspiration, airway difficulties, and assesses the relative risk-benefit ratios of the available anesthetic techniques. "Risk" is relative, and the conflicting dictates of various factors must be mediated by informed judgement, as when the patient at risk for aspiration has concomitant coronary artery disease and diminished left ventricular function.

Fasting Guidelines

"The purpose of the preoperative fast is to allow sufficient time for gastric emptying of ingested food and liquid ..."[57] Fasting is used to decrease gastric volume and acidity, though results after prolonged fasting are variable,[24] and even after 12 hours of fasting significant quantities of fluid may remain in the stomach. In addition, more prolonged fasting appears to increase gastric acidity.[58]

Despite fasting, the majority of outpatients for elective surgery are at risk for aspiration pneumonitis by pH and volume criteria.[29] If only clear liquids have been taken previously by healthy patients for elective surgery, the gastric fluid pH and volume are not changed further after fasts of more than 2 hours duration. After this point, gastric secretion determines the character of gastric contents.[57] In addition, ingestion of 150 ml of water reduces residual gastric volume and pH.[59] Clear fluid up to three hours before surgery increases neither gastric volume or acidity in healthy children aged 2 to 12 years.[60-62] Patients who have received water 2 hours prior to surgery may safely receive morphine 1 hour preoperatively, without any significant increase in gastric volume or acidity.[63]

Based on this evidence the common practice of fasting 6, or even 8 to 12 hours prior to surgery, is giving way to a more relaxed attitude in many centers. It has been suggested that for healthy patients, avoidance of solid foods, with ingestion of unrestricted clear liquid until 3 hours before the scheduled time of surgery is a reasonable approach. Oral medication may be taken with 30 ml of water up to 1 hour before surgery, and H2 receptor blockers given to patients at risk for aspiration.[57]

There has also been a loosening of NPO policies for laboring women, and the lay press has further advanced the idea that NPO may excessively interfere with "natural functions."[64] Policies regarding oral intake of liquids and solid food during labor vary widely among labor units. The majority allow some form of intake, but frequently stratify patients loosely by perceived risk, though there is little consensus or consistency in risk evaluation of the patients, or correlation between the perceived risk and recommended oral intake.[65]

Pain and apprehension decrease gastric emptying and increase gastric acidity, and most emergency patients should therefore be considered "full stomachs" regardless of the length of time they have spent "NPO."[66]

Recognition of the Difficult Airway

When appropriate, regional techniques may greatly simplify anesthetic management of patients with expected airway difficulties.

When faced by a patient at risk for aspiration who has a difficult airway and requires general anesthesia, consideration should be given to awake intubation, by direct laryngoscopy or fiberoptic technique. Nine of the 56 cases of aspiration noted in the ASA Closed Claims Study occurred during difficult intubations.[6] Of the 21 cases of aspiration reported to the Society for Obstetric Anesthesia and Perinatology, 14 occurred during "difficult" endotracheal intubation.[67]

The safe execution of awake direct laryngoscopy has been well described,[68,69] and less than 5% of patients expressed the experience to be "quite unpleasant."[68] After identical preparation of the patient and airway mucosa, fiberoptic-assisted intubation has been shown to be more often successful and to cause a slightly less increase in blood pressure than direct laryngoscopy.[70] Fiberoptic-assisted intubation of a large group of patients has been described, and the average maximal increase in heart rate was 14 beats per minute, though mean arterial pressure increased more than 20 mm Hg in 32% of intubations and more than 30 mm Hg in 11.5%.[71] This technique does require special equipment and training, is not available in all centers, and has limited applicability in true airway emergencies.

Recognition of Prior Aspiration

Most fatal cases of aspiration are unrelated to anesthesia.[4] Clinical scenarios producing aspiration include depressed laryngeal reflexes due to muscular incoordination or altered levels of consciousness. Drug or alcohol intoxication, head injury, or coma from other CNS event or fulminant systemic process such as sepsis, respiratory, renal or hepatic failure may blunt or inactivate the sensory and motor responses necessary to detect and remove material entering the tracheobronchial tree. Neuromuscular problems such as amyotrophic lateral sclerosis and multiple sclerosis may render a patient unable to swallow saliva, much less expectorate regurgitated gastric contents or generate a cough.

Aspiration occurs in up to 70% of patients with uncuffed tracheostomy tubes. Prolonged orotracheal intubation or tracheostomy tubes may cause swallowing disorders that may leave the extubated patient at risk for aspiration.[34] Subclinical aspiration of nasogastric feeding appears to be associated with nosocomial pneumonia in mechanically ventilated patients.[72] While nasogastric tubes help in preventing gastric distention, draining gastric contents and administering drugs or feedings, reflux and oropharyngeal colonization may be increased, with an increased risk of pneumonia.[52] Chronic aspiration in patients with hiatal hernia may cause pulmonary fibrosis.[73]

Patients at risk for aspiration who present for surgery and evidence signs or symptoms possibly related to aspiration, such as tachypnea, dyspnea, wheezing, or hypoxemia, should, at the minimum, have their preoperative status documented.

Drug Prophylaxis

Drugs may be given perioperatively to decrease gastric volume and acidity, increase gastric emptying and increase LES tone. Administration of these drugs to patients at increased risk for aspiration perioperatively is widely accepted, but routine prophylaxis of all patients remains controversial: benefits are undemonstrated and the risk not quantified.[74] Although anxiety may decrease gastric emptying and increase acid production, there was no difference in gastric pH and volume in patients treated with diazepam, meperidine, hydroxyzine or prochlorperazine compared to patients not pretreated.[29,75] Various antacids and anticholinergic regimens, as well as H1 and H2 blocking agents and gastric emptying agents such as metochlopramide are used in aspiration prophylaxis. The prokinetic agents, antacids, H2 receptor blockers, proton pump inhibitors have important roles in aspiration prophylaxis and will be discussed in some detail.

Anticholinergics

Administration of anticholinergic agents to decrease gastric secretions and volume of gastric fluid is no longer first-line therapy, because the effects on gastric contents are not dependable, and other agents are available.[76] Side effects of these agents include tachycardia and dry mouth, as well as decreased protective sphincter tone and slowed gastric emptying. Children frequently receive anticholinergic agents preoperatively to lessen secretions and prevent bradycardia. A majority of atropine-treated children had a gastric pH of less than 2.5 and gastric volume greater than 0.4 ml/kg, while administration of IV glycopyrrolate at induction of anesthesia led to less gastric volume and stomach acidity.[77]

Antacids

Preanesthetic antacids reduce gastric acidity[24] but do not protect against particulate aspiration. Particulate antacids are no longer used because of potential pulmonary damage if aspirated.[7,45] A survey of obstetric anesthetic practices in Great Britain showed the combination of ranitidine and sodium citrate was routinely used in 56% of departments for emergency cesarean section while the use of particulate antacids (magnesium trisilicate) had declined to 10% of patients.[78]

Citrate solutions offer nonparticulate neutralization of acid. 30 ml of sodium citrate solution may be given 15–45 minutes before induction of anesthesia. Bicitra is a commercial preparation of sodium citrate and citric acid in a clear liquid solution. An oral dose of 30 ml can raise pH above 2.5 in over 85% of patients. At the same time, over 80% of the patients receiving this dose had a gastric volume greater than 25 ml. Manchikanti[79] found that metoclopramide 10 mg IV in addition to the Bicitra reduces the gastric volume to less than 25 ml in 70% of patients. Twenty ml of sodium bicarbonate administered immediately before induction of anesthesia in 48 patients undergoing emergency cesarean section raised pH above 2.5 in all but four women; 36 received ranitidine 150 mg every 6 hours plus bicarbonate: all these patients had pH above 2.5. There were no significant differences in gastric volumes.[80]

Thus, prophylaxis of aspiration aims to reduce gastric volume to 25 ml or less and to raise the pH above 2.5. There is evidence that a relationship exists between pH and volume such that it is less damaging to aspirate a larger volume of liquid of higher pH than a smaller volume of a more acid liquid.[81] However, preanesthetic alkali therapy must not lead to a false sense of security, and other protective measures must be utilized, as alkali aspirate may also cause severe pulmonary damage, and may cause aspiration pneumonitis in humans.[7] In an animal model 0.1 N sodium hydroxide solution was as harmful to the lungs as hydrochloric acid.[82]

Chronic use of antacids in the intensive care setting to prophylax against gastric and duodenal ulcers may predispose to nosocomial pneumonias. Gastric fluid is normally sterile at an acid pH because of the potent antibacterial activity of hydrochloric acid.[83] In addition to the bacterial growth-promoting effect of the alkaline gastric pH when antacids are used to protect against UGI bleeding, antacids also contribute significantly to gastric volume, particularly if a 2 hour regimen is used, which may contribute 480 ml per day into the stomach through the NG.[84] Sucralfate is as efficacious in prophylaxing stress ulcers as antacid or H2 blocker therapy while associated with less incidence of pneumonia,[85-87] though it appears to slow gastric emptying.[88]

Histamine Antagonists

Histamine receptor blockers are used to decrease the production of gastric acid. The histamine molecule contains an imidazole ring and an ethylamine side chain. The H2 receptor blockers are analogs of the histamine molcule that have a bulky side chain replacing the ethylamine group, and compete with the parent molecule at the histamine receptor. Cimetidine retains the imidazole ring, but in ranitidine the ring is replaced by a furan and in famotidine it is replaced by a thiazole structure.

These drugs have limited access to the central nervous system due to their hydrophilic nature, and are highly specific for the H2 receptor. There is little effect on physiologic function except the decrease in gastric acid production, but the other effects of histamine are blocked. In addition to the dose-dependent competitive antagonism of the effects of histamine on gastric acid production, stimulation of gastric acid secretion by gastric and muscarinic agonists is inhibited. Both basal and stimulated acid levels are decreased, and the volume of gastric secretions is diminished. Gastrin and intrinsic factor secretion fall. There is no effect on gastric emptying, pancreatic secretion, or LESP.

Oral administration leads to rapid absorption, and plasma levels peak within 2 hours. Cimetidine, ranitidine, and famotidine are subject to hepatic first-pass metabolism and thus their bioavailability is about 50%, while that of nizatidine is 90%. The elimination half-life of the former group is 2 to 3 hours, while that of nizatidine is slightly longer than 1 hour. The drugs are secreted largely unchanged in the urine; liver dysfunction prolongs the half-life of ranitidine.

Adverse effects are infrequent and relatively minor, due to the narrow function of H2 receptors and their inability to penetrate the blood-brain barrier. Some CNS side effects, such as sedation or delirium, may occur with cimetidine, particularly in the aged or patients with limited renal function, and dosing intervals should be longer in these persons. Drug interactions result from two phenomena: altered gastric absorption due to altered pH, and altered drug metabolism by hepatic mixed-function oxidases due to inhibition of cytochrome P-450. Drug-induced hepatitis has been reported with all histamine-2 antagonists, but may be more frequent with ranitidine.[89]

Cimetidine

The short term use of cimetidine has few serious adverse effects. More chronic use may lead to altered hepatic metabolism of certain drugs. Cimetidine inhibits microsomal drug oxidative action, and this inhibition is not related to its H2 antagonist efficacy.[90] Cimetidine prolongs elimination of lidocaine, diazepam, aminophylline, phenytoin, coumadin and propanolol, although ranitidine apparently does not.[91] It impairs tubular secretion of procainamide by competition. Cimetidine significantly increases the serum levels of epidurally administered lidocaine, but levels measured were still well within the therapeutic limits for lidocaine drips used to treat ventricular ectopy.[92,93] There is no significant increase in maternal venous local anesthetic concentration in women undergoing caesarean section with epidural lidocaine or bupivacaine anesthesia who receive one dose of cimetidine or ranitidine.[91,94]

Cimetidine was superior to the antacid in reducing gastric acidity and volume in women scheduled for elective cesarean-section. After cimetidine, gastric volume averaged 11.5 ml and gastric pH 6.3; patients treated by antacid alone had a gastric volume of 35.0 ml and a pH of 5.5. No adverse maternal or fetal effects were noted following cimetidine, and the Apgar and neurobehavioral scores were not depressed.[95] Antacids inhibit the absorption of cimetidine.[96]

Ranitidine

The pharmacokinetics of ranitidine differ little from those of cimetidine: the half-life is almost 40 minutes and the elimination half-life is 3 hours. However, the drug is 5 times as potent and in equivalent doses induces a long suppression of both basal and food-stimulated gastric acid secretion.

Ranitidine is oxidatively metabolized in the liver and subject to first-pass kinetics.[97] Ranitidine has much less affinity for cytochrome P-450 than cimetidine has,[97] however, enzyme induction may increase the affinity of ranitidine significantly.[98] Ranitidine does not impair oxidative or conjugative metabolism, thus does not significantly alter the half-life of drugs undergoing oxidative metabolism in the liver as does cimetidine. In usual doses the clearance of oxidatively metablized drugs such as antipyrine,[90] theophylline, diazepam and propanolol are not affected.[98] However, plasma concentrations of metoprolol increased.[99]

In subjects with a 50% decrease in renal function, the beta elimination half-life increases from 3 to 5 hours, primarily due to reduced clearance. In subjects with less than 50% normal renal function, dosing intervals of 18 to 24 hours are appropriate.

Perioperatively, intravenous administration may be preferable. The agent is administered 30 to 60 minutes before induction at a dose of 0.5 to 1.0 mg/kg. Studies by Brock-Utne demonstrate that ranitidine increases LES tone by 21 cm H_2O, and counteracts the sphincter relaxation that normally accompanies clinical doses of atropine.[100] Ranitidine 150 mg orally on the night before and the morning of surgery achieved gastric volume less than 25 ml and pH more than 2.5 in 90% of patients, and a single morning dose was effective in 76%.[101] Adverse reactions are infrequent: urticarial rashes have been reported as well as moderate upper airway stridor, and headache and mental confusion occasionally occur.

Famotidine

Famotidine inhibits basal gastric acid secretion in a dose-dependent manner for at least 12 hours after oral intake. Gastric emptying times are not affected. Little effect is seen on hepatic blood flow, induction of drug metabolizing enzymes or hemodynamic variables.[102] It is at least 20 times more potent than cimetidine in inhibiting stimulated gastric acid secretion.[103] The usual oral dose is 20 to 40 mg. Two oral doses of 20 mg in the evening and morning will raise the pH values to 5.0, while 40 mg will raise it to 6.4. Maximal effects are attained with 40 mg doses and this provides a more uniform response. Peak antisecretory response is reached within 1-2 hours and lasts 10-12 hours. A dose of 20 mg intravenously produces plasma concentrations of 30 ng/ml, with the onset of action in 10-15 minutes and a peak within 30 minutes.

Famotidine is minimally protein-bound, has a relatively short half-life and rapid elimination time. After oral intake by normal subjects, the plasma distribution half-life is 2.5-3.5 hours and the elimination half-life is 8-10 hours. It is partly metabolized in the liver and partly excreted renally; 65-70% of the drug appears in the urine unchanged by 8 hours. Elimination half-life may increase to 20 hours in renal dysfunction, and the dose should be halved for patients with end-stage renal disease, it does not impair the excretion of procainamide, a drug that is eliminated by tubular secretion.[103]

Famotidine does not inhibit the hepatic mixed function oxidase system and the metabolism of diazepam,[103] phenytoin, theophylline or aminopyrine is not affected. Epidural administration of lidocaine after famotidine, unlike cimetidine, does not result in a significantly increased serum level.[92] When given to elective surgical patients, famotidine significantly reduced the gastric volume compared with ranitidine, but there was no significant difference between the effects of ranitidine and famotidine on gastric pH.[75] In pediatric patients, gastric pH is significantly increased after a single oral dose of famotidine, but gastric volume did not differ from that found after placebo.[102]

PROTON PUMP INHIBITORS

Parietal cells secrete gastric acid in response to stimulation of cholinergic, gastrinergic and histaminergic receptors: the final common pathway involves cAMP formation to activate the proton pump. Gastric H+,K+-ATPase, the proton pump, exchanges luminal potassium for cellular hydrogen ions at the apical membrane of the parietal cell, and gastric acidity is decreased by inhibiting this enzyme. Omeprazole, one of the substituted benzimidazoles, irreversibly inhibits this enzyme. After absorption from the duodenum it is rapidly cleared from plasma and concentrated in the gastric parietal cell, where it may remain for up to 24 hours.[104] The action of omeprazole requires generation of an active form that depends on the acid environment found in the parietal cell, and with its short plasma half-life and rapid elimination, its effects are limited to gastric acid secretion. Little effect on gastric volume, intrinsic factor or pepsin secretion is seen, and gastric motility is essentially unchanged.

Orally ingested omeprazole is rapidly absorbed, but to a variable extent dependent upon gastric pH and dose. Highly protein-bound, it is metabolized by the liver and has a half-life of 30 to 90 minutes, and metabolites are subsequently excreted in the urine. Twenty to 40-mg doses effectively reduces gastric acidity for 12 to 24 hours, and the drug may be successful in treating peptic ulcer disease refractory to H2 antagonists. However, when given to patients presenting for elective cesarean section, 20% still had a gastric pH below 2.5.[105] In nonpregnant surgery patients who received 40 mg omeprazole the night prior to operation, 21 of 22 patients had a gastric pH greater than 2.5; volume was not significantly affected.[106] A single intravenous dose of 80 mg omeprazole significantly increased the pH when compared to controls, but the average pH in the group treated 3 hours before surgery was 2.25; the drug was more efficacious in reducing acidity and volume when given 1 hour prior to surgery rather than 3.[104] Oral omeprazole given to women the night before and again on the morning of surgery was effective in reducing gastric volume and acidity, without any adverse drug reactions in mothers or neonates.[107]

Large daily doses have been administered with little adverse effect. Nausea, diarrhea, and abdominal cramps are reported in a small percentage. In vitro studies show interaction with cytochrome P-450 and hepatic metabolism of other drugs may possibly be affected. The drug is metabolized by the liver to inactive metabolites; no adjustment of dose or dosing interval is needed in renal failure.

PROKINETIC AGENTS

Metoclopramide

Metoclopramide is a benzamide similar in structure to procainamide though devoid of useful antiarrhythmic or local anesthetic properties. Blockade of central dopaminergic receptors may potentially cause extrapyramidal symptoms,[108,109] drowsiness, and anxiety, though no therapeutic antipsychotic effects are seen. Apomorphine-induced emesis is blocked. Metoclopramide increases gastric emptying by increasing smooth muscle motility from the esophagus through the proximal small bowel; the prokinetic effect may occasionally cause abdominal cramps on rapid intravenous administration, and bowel obstruction is a contraindication. The more rapid transit through the bowel may decrease bioavailability of concurrently ingested medications; diabetics may require changes in insulin regimen to offset the diminished absorption of foods.

Its primary use in aspiration prophylaxis is to decrease gastric volume and increase LESP. It is useful in diabetic gastroparesis, as an antiemetic and in treating the gastric hypomotility seen with achlorhydria or after gastric surgery. There is little effect on gastric secretion or colonic activity. Interestingly, the prokinetic effects are antagonized by antimuscarinic drugs, but vagotomy does not negate its effects.

Domperidone

Domperidone is a benzimidazole derivative that blocks dopamine receptors and acts as a prokinetic and antiemetic with effects on gastrointestinal motility much like those of metoclopramide. Unlike metoclopramide, the effects of domperidone are not antagonized by atropine. Extrapyramidal side effects are rare and only limited travel across the blood brain barrier occurs. Like metoclopramide, it blocks apomorphine-induced vomiting. Domperidone increased lower esophageal sphincter tone in pregnant patients and increased barrier pressure in both nonpregnant controls and pregnant patients with and without heartburn.[41] The effect on LESP lasts at least 60 minutes.[41] It has also been tried in the therapy of postoperative vomiting.[41,110]

Cisapride is another benzamide that acts like metoclopramide to increase motility of the stomach and small bowel, but also stimulates colonic motility and may cause diarrhea. These actions are abolished by atropine. There is no dopaminergic antagonism. It has some efficacy in treating nausea.[111]

Anesthetic Techniques

Historical Evolution

In current practice, anesthetic techniques to prevent the risk of aspiration may be divided into two groups: techniques maintaining laryngeal reflexes and those using general anesthesia in which the trachea is protected by means of a endotracheal tube. Anesthetic techniques have evolved considerably, and avoidance of mask ventilation in patients at risk for aspiration, rapid sequence induction with thiopental and succinylcholine,[112] and application of cricoid pressure[113] may account for the decrease in aspiration deaths. Recognition of problems associated with the difficult airway has led to increased emphasis on airway evaluation and awake intubation in selected patients, and use of regional techniques when appropriate.

Although the use of regional anesthesia is not completely protective, certain procedures, especially those on the extremities, can be performed safely and successfully: brachial plexus block for hand and arm surgery; block of nerves of lumbar plexus for lower extremity; in obstetric practice, pudendal or lumbar epidural anesthesia. A high incidence of nausea and vomiting in the patient undergoing spinal anesthesia has been documented, and may be prevented with supplemental oxygen and careful avoidance of hypotension,[55] but excessive sedation or loss of consciousness due to hypotension[5] may place these patients at risk for aspiration.

Induction and Maintenance of Anesthesia

The most critical periods in anesthetic management are induction-intubation and emergence. In early studies, intubation with a cuffed endotracheal tube in patients at risk lowered the incidence of aspiration in those who did regurgitate.[12,13] Although 41% of cases of aspiration in the ASA Closed Claims Study occurred during maintenance of anesthesia, 20 of these 23 cases occurred during mask ventilation.[6]

As instrumentation of the airway is extremely stimulating, excellent mucosal anesthesia is usually necessary in even the most cooperative patient unless they are markedly weakened or debilitated. Topical anesthesia or nerve blocks may hamper protective reflexes and controversy exists regarding what degree of anesthesia is safe in the patient at risk for aspiration. It is generally agreed that topicalization of the tongue and pharynx, with loss of gag, is acceptable.[114] Opinion varies as to the wisdom of blocking sensation in the laryngeal inlet or trachea, but some feel that the awake patient is unlikely to aspirate significantly no matter how numb their mucosa. Judicious sedation is helpful, and amnesia beneficial. Intravenous administration of fentanyl (100 μg) and droperidol (5 mg) had no effect on glottic closure response to inhaled ammonia, while transtracheal block with 2 ml of 4% lidocaine markedly altered the response.[115]

The laryngeal mask airway (LMA) is less stimulating to place, acts as a conduit for the fiberoptic bronchoscope, and its placement in awake patients to facilitate fiberoptic intubation has been described.[116] "Anterior" placement of the larynx frequently compromises visualization of the vocal cords by direct laryngoscopy, but may make placement of the LMA easier.[117] It is, however, not recommended for definitive airway management in patients at risk for aspiration.[118]

Though the LMA is gaining in popularity, being used in over half of cases in some areas of Great Britain,[118] its use does not protect against aspiration,[119] and near-fatal consequences have occurred.[120] The two problems with using the LMA in patients at risk for aspiration include the lack of an air-tight seal, and variability in positioning that is not detectable in routine care.[118] The proper positioning brings the laryngeal inlet entirely within the rim of the mask, while the epiglottis and esophagus are outside, but this positioning is seen only 50 to 60% of the time. In 6 to 15% of cases, the esophagus is within the rim, and this malposition remains undetected as respirations may be adequate and placement appear appropriate clinically.[118,119] In this situation, positive pressure ventilation may cause gastric dilatation. Should vomiting or reflux occur during any point of anesthetic management, the LMA with the cuff inflated prevents escape of fluid from the pharynx.[119] If vomiting is suspected, the LMA should be removed immediately,[120] and the wisdom of leaving LMAs in place to be removed by recovery room staff has been questioned.[119]

Awake fiberoptic intubation in the patient at risk for aspiration may be safely performed.[121] Inability to intubate or ventilate the anesthetized patient may require needle cricothroidotomy and transtracheal jet ventilation. In one animal model, transtracheal jet ventilation appeared to provide protection against aspiration similar to that of insertion of a cuffed endotracheal tube, as cephalad flow of gas tends to expel fluid and material from the trachea.[122]

Historically, induction of anesthesia by nitrous oxide-oxygen and ether was done in parturients on the theory that vomiting usually occurred during induction, and the mother should be able to protect her airway. Chloroform was advocated by some because its smoother induction was thought to cause less vomiting.[112] The "crash induction" technique with pentothal and muscle relaxant was viewed as contraindicated in patients with full stomachs in early writings.[123]

Patient positioning may be modified. A head-down tilt of 10 to 20 degrees has been recommended to prevent passive flow of gastric contents into the trachea. However, this position increases intragastric pressure and the volume of vomitus and may make endotracheal intubation more difficult. The head-up tilt may reduce reflux and intragastric pressure, but make pulmonary aspiration in the event of vomiting more likely, while increasing the risk of hypotension. Because of these multiple factors, the supine position has been recommended.[14] A good "sniffing" position to optimize visualization of the cords should be verified prior to induction, to limit fumbling with the head of an unconscious patient. Induction in the lithotomy position may predispose to regurgitation and aspiration during induction due to increased intragastric pressure and should be avoided in patients at increased risk of aspiration. Obviously, this position cannot always be avoided, as when emergent induction is required for uterine relaxation for delivery of the entrapped after-coming head during breech delivery.[124]

A naso- or orogastric tube may be inserted to decrease intragastric volume and pressure, though one must assume that the stomach is not completely empty.[44,56] Blood pressure and heart rate responses to the insertion of nasogastric tubes may be seen in either the awake patient or during general anesthesia. If the NG tube is inserted with the aid of laryngoscopy rather than blindly, there is a higher incidence of increased heart rate, elevated systolic blood pressure, and ventricular extrasystoles. The systolic blood pressure elevation usually declines during the following 3 minutes. These cardiovascular responses occur in the absence of any hypoxia or hypercarbia.[125]

Controversy exists over whether or not the nasogastric tube should remain in place for induction, and if cricoid pressure is efficacious with it in place. Salem found cricoid pressure efficacious in infants with nasogastric tubes in place.[126] The presence of a gastric tube further complicates the induction of anesthesia since it is difficult to secure a snug mask fit, adding to the difficulties of induction and intubation. One approach is that the distended stomach be decompressed and the gastric tube removed just prior to induction. The tube may then be replaced after endotracheal intubation.

While decompression of the distended stomach with a nasogastric rube is helpful, emptying the stomach by this method is unsatisfactory, because large particles will not pass through the tube and even liquids are not reliably removed. More rigid larger-bore orogastric tubes are more effective, and have been used for gastric lavage in drug overdose, but are poorly tolerated by the awake patient and are not part of anesthetic practice. Historically, emetics such as apomorphine or epiglottic stimulation were given preoperatively to induce gastric emptying by vomiting, but this is no longer commonly done, due to patient discomfort and relative rarity of aspiration. In addition, past techniques included placing cuffed tubes in the esophagus or a balloon in the stomach to obstruct passage of gastric contents from the stomach to the esophagus, but consistent blockade is questionable due to the marked distensibility of the esophagus and relaxation of its muscular wall during vomiting.[22,127]

Rapid Sequence Induction (RSI)

Intubating awake patients under topical anesthesia is not always appropriate, and the rapid-sequence induction technique has developed as an alternative. Historically, inhalation induction was done in the patient with a full stomach but by the early 1960s the popularity of this technique had declined in favor of rapid intravenous induction and intubation.[128] The technique utilized a head-up position, preoxygenation, administration of thiopental and succinylcholine, and expeditious intubation, avoiding positive pressure ventilation until the airway was secured. However, protection against aspiration was inadequate, and in 3 patients gastric contents refluxed into the pharynx during the muscle fasciculations induced by succinylcholine.

The development of the technique of cricoid pressure by Sellick[113] made supine induction of anesthesia, with greater hemodynamic stability, safe in patients with increased risk for aspiration. Stept and Safar described safe induction of 80 patients with full stomachs without aspiration with this technique.[129]

In brief, after preoxygenation, RSI begins with a rapid injection of an IV induction agent followed immediately, without testing the ability to mask ventilate, by IV administration of a rapid-acting muscle relaxant and application of cricoid pressure. After optimum relaxation for intubation is obtained, the trachea is quickly intubated by direct laryngoscopy. The patient is not ventilated by mask nor stimulated in any way prior to this. Cricoid pressure is maintained until tracheal intubation is verified.

Although a simple technique, safe and successful execution of RSI requires attention to detail. Prior to induction, thorough denitrogenation with 100% oxygen increases the period of apnea that will be tolerated without hypoxemia, lessening the need for mask ventilation and providing a margin of safety if any airway difficulty occurs. The adequacy of suction should be rechecked, and a rigid, large-bore suction placed close at hand. An assistant must be present and if unfamiliar to the anesthesiologist, his/her understanding of their actions verified, as removal of cricoid pressure prior to verifying that the endotracheal tube is in the trachea is a common error.[130]

The patient may be supine or with a slight head-up tilt. The position for intubation should be optimized prior to induction, so that a "sniff" position is seen, with the neck flexed on the chest and extended at the atlantoaxial joint,[25] and a "pyramid" of blankets built under the head and shoulders of obese patients.[131] A styleted endotracheal tube, one-half to one size smaller than routinely used, with a functional cuff and a laryngoscope with a strong, unwavering, firmly-attached light should be used. Alternate types and sizes of blades should be available.

The induction agent and muscle relaxant chosen must be dependable and rapid-acting, and a short duration of action may be life-saving in the event of an unexpected difficult intubation and inability to mask ventilate. The ultra short-acting thiobarbiturates thiopental and thiamylal or propofol or ketamine are useful induction agents. Benzodiazepines are not generally used due to their slower onset and longer duration, and high dose narcotics are seldom used alone for rapid induction but may be added to the induction agents to blunt cardiovascular responses to laryngoscopy and intubation.

Succinylcholine is a frequent choice for muscle relaxation, though it may be contraindicated in certain patients. Its fasciculations increase intragastric pressure[40] as well as LES tone, but the overall effect probably does not increase risk of regurgitation. Intracranial and intraocular pressure[132] are also increased and prior "defasciculation" with small doses of nondepolarizing relaxants do not dependably block the increase.[133] Dysrhythmias may occur. Vecuronium is an alternative in patients for whom succinylcholine is contraindicated. A priming dose of 0.01 mg/kg followed by 0.2 mg/kg may provide intubating conditions within 90 seconds. However, the duration of paralysis achieved with this drug make careful airway evaluation and patient selection imperative.

Attempts at laryngoscopy and intubation before full relaxation is achieved may cause abdominal straining and coughing in a significant proportion of patients, increasing risk of regurgitation and elevations in intraocular and intracranial pressure, as well as making intubation more difficult.[134] The dose of succinylcholine should be 1.5 mg/kg after a small "defasciculating" dose of a nondepolarizing muscle relaxant to ensure that the cords are relaxed and the patient motionless during laryngoscopy and intubation, as 1 mg/kg may be inadequate.[135]

Firm pressure on the cricoid ring as the patient loses consciousness is used to occlude the esophagus to prevent reflux of gastric and esophageal contents into the oropharynx.[113] Though the rapid-sequence induction technique with cricoid pressure has certainly decreased the incidence of aspiration, aspiration still can occur with this technique, as seen in 6 of the 56 cases of aspiration in the ASA Closed Claims Study.[6] The majority of anesthesiologists surveyed in one study had seen the inadvertent release of cricoid pressure at an inappropriate time and 10% had witnessed regurgitation during the application of cricoid pressure.[130]

The force required to occlude the esophagus is the same whether the patient is male or female.[38] The technique is also effective in infants, and in one study, was not impeded by the presence of a nasogastric tube.[126]

At first, cricoid pressure should be gentle, at about 20 N (2 kg), and then increased to about 40 N (4 kg) as the patient loses consciousness. 40 N generated a UESP above 32 mm Hg in all patients in one series. An UESP of over 35 mm Hg should prevent passive regurgitation.[36] Studies in cadavers showed that cricoid compression can provide protection from intraesophageal pressures of at least 50 cm H_2O or more.[136] In fasting patients, intragastric pressures are about 10 cm H_2O, during vomiting pressure may exceed 60 cm H_2O, and succinylcholine-induced fasciculations may increase pressure to more than 40 cm H_2O. Theoretically, esophageal rupture during vomiting while cricoid pressure is being held is possible, but has not been reported.[131]

RSI produces a light anesthetic and cardiovascular and bronchospastic responses to laryngoscopy and intubation will not be prevented. In a series of 100 patients, systolic blood pressure rose more than 20% in 19 patients, and fell more than 20% in 9 patients.[134] In twelve patients without cardiopulmonary problems, RSI with thiopental 5 mg/kg followed by succinylcholine 1.5 mg/kg was associated with a 46% increase in mean arterial blood pressure (85 to 124) and 46% increase in heart rate (68 to 99). Left ventricular ejection fraction decreased from 70% to 48% after laryngoscopy.[137] Additionally, the bolus administration of thiopental may be associated with cardiovascular collapse, particularly in volume depleted or frail

patients.[134,138] Adding alfentanil 100 μg/kg immediately before 5 mg/kg thiopental and 1 minute before laryngoscopy and intubation in healthy patients blocks the hypertensive and tachycardiac response, the decrease in left ventricular ejection fraction and activation of plasma catecholamines, though not without lowering the mean arterial pressure by 25% from pre-induction values.[137]

Esophageal intubation may occur, and cricoid pressure must be maintained until tracheal placement of the endotracheal tube and adequate inflation of the protective cuff is verified: A series of several waveforms of CO_2 exhalation is the best method, as other methods are not as dependable, and one or two CO_2 waveforms mimicking tracheal gases may be seen after esophageal intubation.[139,140] Esophageal intubation should be recognized as soon as possible in order to avoid further gastric dilatation. Four of the 56 cases of aspiration in the ASA Closed Claims Study occurred during esophageal intubation.[6]

The rapid-sequence technique is a safe method of induction and intubation for the relatively healthy patient with a normal airway who is at increased risk for aspiration.[134,135] In the ASA Closed Claims Study, one-third of aspirations during induction had a rapid-sequence technique, one-third should have had but did not in the opinion of the reviewer, and one-third did not have a RSI but it was not required in the opinion of the reviewers.[6]

The "failed intubation drill" initially aimed at prevention of death by aspiration, and the inability to ventilate the lungs was not a fear:[141] the patient is turned onto the left side in head-down tilt and lungs ventilated with cricoid pressure held until consciousness returns. If ventilation is difficult, complete or partial release of the cricoid pressure may improve it.[142] The initial failed intubation drill stressed immediate assumption of the left lateral position, but others note that this is frequently impractical and may further complicate attempts to maintain ventilation.[143]

Bernhard et al found that a minimum intracuff pressure of 25 cm H_2O appeared necessary to prevent aspiration of dye past large-diameter, thin walled cuffs during either controlled or spontaneous ventilation.[144] This was not affected by use of neuromuscular blocking agents or mode of ventilation. Inflating the cuff till there is no audible air leak may not protect against aspiration, and some advocate inflating the cuff to 25 cm H_2O.[145] Pavlin documented aspiration past a high-volume, low-pressure cuff until the intracuff pressure was increased to 50 cm H_2O. The thicker the wall of the cuff, the more pressure is required to conform the cuff to the trachea and diminish channeling of liquid down along the folds of the cuff material.[144,146,147] A change in position or deep inspiration may have the effect of lowering the effective pressure at the tracheal wall of the cuff from 30 to 5 cm H_2O.[148]

Aspiration of dye has been documented in 31.2% of patients intubated with a Mallinckrodt Hi-Lo endotracheal tube, but no mention of any clinically significant pulmonary insult was made.[148] A study of pediatric intensive care unit patients showed that 77% of patients with uncuffed endotracheal tube aspirate dye, while 11% of patients with cuffed tubes aspirated, and 2 mm Hg CPAP did not affect the incidence.[147] Recently, a decrease in colonization of tracheal aspirates and nosocomial pneumonia was seen with use of a special endotracheal tube with a special lumen that permitted subglottic drainage of secretions pooled above the cuff.[84]

Emergence

The stomach should be decompressed by a naso- or orogastric tube while an appropriate depth of anesthesia exists. The patient with a full stomach is extubated only when awake and after adequate laryngeal-tracheal reflexes are present. After thorough oropharyngeal suctioning, the patient is extubated at the point of full inspiration so the following exhalation will help mobilize pooled secretions out of the trachea where they may be suctioned or coughed out. The oropharyngeal airway may be removed before the gag reflex becomes active as the patient should be able to maintain a patent airway. It is frequently recommended that patients with depressed protective reflexes be maintained in a lateral position to permit oral contents to drain to the side.

RECOGNITION AND MANAGEMENT OF ASPIRATION SYNDROMES

Presentation and Differential Diagnosis

As discussed, the aspiration of material into the tracheobronchial tree may have the following serious consequences: airway obstruction by particulate matter, drowning due to alveolar filling, chemical pneumonitis, and infectious pneumonitis.[10] Airway obstruction and massive alveolar filling are relatively uncommon, and when they occur, are usually clinically obvious, and may result in death from hypoxia in a matter of minutes,[11] or a reflex cardiovascular collapse. Mendelson noted airway obstruction in five patients; three had complete airway obstruction and two of these died on the delivery table, the other woman surviving after coughing out a piece of meat.[15]

As Mendelson reported, aspiration of liquid gastric contents often initially escaped recognition, and subclinical aspiration may initially be misdiagnosed as an exacerbation of asthma or bronchospasm. Respiratory distress, bronchospasm, laryngospasm, tachypnea and hypoxemia may be initial features in the awake or sedated patient. During general anesthesia presentation may include increasing inspiratory pressure, bronchospasm with a diagnostic up-ramping of the end-tidal CO_2 curve, and hypoxia. Physical examination reveals wheezes, rales, rhonchi, tachycardia and possibly cyanosis. There may be evidence of cardiac failure and occasionally pulmonary edema. Acute respiratory decompensation signals that significant amounts of fluid have entered the lung.[11] Whether or not the material is acid, neutral, particulate or nonparticulate may not influence the initial presentation, but recovery from the insult may be more rapid when the pH is more than 2.5, and the aspirate is nonparticulate and not hypertonic.[11] Aspiration of neutral liquid is accompanied by a similar clinical picture of bronchospasm and hypoxemia, but it resolves relatively rapidly.[15]

No specific diagnostic criteria exist, and clinical suspicion in the proper setting generally leads to the diagnosis.

Hypoxemia, new pulmonary infiltrates on chest x-ray, fever and leukocytosis after an episode clinically consistent with aspiration generally cinches the diagnosis; the presence of obvious gastric contents in endotracheal aspirate is unusual but verifies the diagnosis.[149] On bronchoscopy, erythema and petechiae mark the respiratory mucosa affected by gastric acid.[150]

In Mendelson's series[15] and in animal models and patient studies, aspiration enters the right main stem bronchus unless it is massive, in which case both sides are contaminated.[2] The x-ray findings in cases of chemical pneumonitis reveal generalized irregular soft mottled densities in the involved areas, which are determined by patient positioning at the time of the aspiration. Lateral positioning causes drainage into the posterior segments of the superior lobe on the dependent side, supine position is associated with infiltrates in the superor (apical) segments of the inferior lobes, while aspiration in the sitting position involves the basal segments of the inferior lobes bilaterally.[151] In the event of airway obstruction, other x-ray findings may include atelectasis of a segment, lobe, or entire lung, accompanied by mediastinal shift and elevation of the diaphragm. Obstructive emphysema due to a ball-valve effect may cause hyperlucency of the affected areas.

Pathophysiology

Hypoxia quickly occurs, due to four factors: reflex airway closure as an immediate response to inhaled material; a decrease in surfactant activity, whether diluted or destroyed; interstitial and alveolar edema due to potentially massive transudation of fluid and protein; alveolar hemorrhage and consolidation.[11] Acid distributes rapidly throughout the lung, and damage is immediate. Mendelson demonstrated the similarity of clinical gross and pathologic presentation of aspiration of acid and gastric contents. Rapid development of cyanosis and respiratory distress is followed in minutes or hours by frothy pulmonary edema fluid. On anatomic examination, the trachea contains copious pink frothy material, there are pleural effusions and large subpleural hemorrhages, with areas of doughiness and increased lung weight. Microscopic exam shows intact epithelium, a wavy bronchiolar pattern consistent with smooth muscle spasm, peribronchiolar hemorrhage, areas of necrotic bronchiolar epithelium, marked perivascular edema, and congestion and edema.[15]

Acid damage causes pulmonary vasculature to become leaky; administration of furosemide decreased leakage of protein and water, but albumin did not.[152] Aspiration is followed by pulmonary edema with subsequent noncompliant lungs and increased work of breathing. This may occur even at normal filling pressures, and increasing vascular oncotic pressure does not improve this. Lowering filling pressures with plasmapheresis in a canine model decreased aspiration-induced pulmonary edema.[153] The increase in venous admixture may prevent resolution with the administration of 100% oxygen. Initially, pulmonary hypertension occurs, but resolves as cardiac output subsequently falls with intravascular volume depletion.[11] Pulmonary vascular resistance will remain increased, while pulmonary artery pressure is low or normal.[11]

Pathophysiologic changes include a large alveolar/arterial oxygen gradient, pulmonary shunting, pulmonary hypertension[154] and severe hypoxemia. The capillary endothelium injury increases vascular permeability. Chemotactic factors are generated and neutrophils and other inflammatory cells accumulate in the alveoli, triggering release of oxygen radicals and lysosomal proteases. Hydrochloric acid from the stomach acts on the respiratory mucosa, producing a marked mucosal edema and congestion of the bronchopulmonary segments with extensive exudative reactions. Necrosis of the mucosal cell lining is followed by fibroblastic changes and regeneration of mucosa if the patient survives. Interstitial edema and exudation also occurs.

Histologically, diffuse alveolar capillary damage is seen. Destruction of surfactant results in alveolar instability and collapse. Alveolar flooding with plasma and erythrocytes from the capillaries is usual. There is both a rapid transudative process and a developing exudative response. Fluid is present in the interstitium and in the alveoli, with scattered alveolar hemorrhages.

Acid aspiration stimulates 15-lipoxygenase activity and alters eicosanoid activity in the lung which may have a role in inflammatory responses, cell chemotaxis, and development of pulmonary edema. Systemic corticosteroids may decrease release of pulmonary eicosanoids.[155] However, little efficacy in treating the syndrome with steroids is seen. The pulmonary edema fluid that follows aspiration in rabbits has been demonstrated to inhibit surfactant activity,[156] and administration of surfactant may be a potential treatment.

During the ensuing few hours, bronchial epithelium degenerates and there is pulmonary edema and hemorrhage. Type I alveolar cells die. Polymorphonuclear cells infiltrate within 4 hours. Alveolar type II cells begin to degenerate. The extensive polymorphonuclear infiltration over the next 24 to 36 hours causes alveolar consolidation. The airway mucosal may delaminate. The lungs are heavy, edematous, and hemorrhagic. Repair begins at 72 hours, and regeneration of epithelium and proliferation of fibroblasts is seen.[11]

Aspiration of nonacid liquid is characterized by minimal neutrophilic infiltration or alveolar cell death. Pulmonary edema and congestion rapidly follows aspiration of significant amounts of any liquid, including saline or water. However, acid aspiration is much slower to resolve. After nonacid aspiration, fluid shift into the lungs is less rapid, occuring 3 to 4 hours after aspiration and being relatively limited, but small food particles may cause a marked hemorrhagic pneumonia, and the alveoli and bronchi fill with erythrocytes, granulocytes and macrophages.[11] The late cellular reaction is mononuclear. Food particles may cause a significant lasting inflammatory response characterized by granuloma formation.[11]

The aspiration of sucrafate has been studied in rats, and compared to saline and the particulate antacid, Mylanta.[8] Sucralfate, a basic aluminum salt of sulphated sucrose, is frequently used to prophylax against stress ulceration in critically ill patients, as it is effective without alkalinizing the gastric milieu, does not encourage gastric colonization with gram-negative organisms, and does not increase risk of nosocomial pneumonia.[85] In the rats studied, large-volume aspiration caused significant acute pneumonitis that was similar in degree to that caused by Mylanta, and associated pulmonary hemorrhage greater than that seen with Mylanta.[8]

Barium sulfate is frequently ingested for diagnostic radiology examination, and may be aspirated into the lungs. Though initial reports were that there was minimal pulmonary response to the aspiration, and barium was felt to be one of the safest agents for bronchography, the solutions used in these studies were quite dilute. Aspiration of more concentrated solutions may cause an acute inflammatory infiltrate, copious mucus production and acute pulmonary edema. In patients at risk for aspiration, safer substances include low osmolar contrast media; gastrografin may cause fatal pulmonary edema.[9]

Infectious complications following aspiration tend to be of two types. The aspiration of a heavily infected, though small quantity of matter probably is the first step in the development of lung abscess, empyema, or necrotizing pneumonitis.[11] The infection in these patients may be slow to develop, but is the first indication that aspiration has occurred. This is classically seen in the medical patient with disorganized swallowing, a seizure disorder or chronic drug or alcohol ingestion, and infected teeth. The second type of infection follows a large aspiration, and may be the development of infection in lungs damaged by the aspiration.[11] The pulmonary edema fluid of the aspiration syndrome may itself provide a breeding ground for bacteria.

MANAGEMENT

One approach to the immediate management of evident aspiration, whether of large particles or liquid gastric materials, is as follows:

Although cricoid pressure is not always effective, immediate application of cricoid pressure may "convert a flood to a trickle."[157] Head-down tilt and immediate suction limits aspiration of gastric contents. Placing the patient on the side is recommended if possible, to prevent soiling the opposite lung.[157] Placing the table in a head-down position of 15 to 20 degrees may enlist gravity to prevent further passive aspiration but is best done by an assistant while the airway is suctioned and cleared of debris. Largyngoscopy and thorough laryngeal and tracheal suctioning is performed followed by endotracheal intubation and ventilation with 100% oxygen. Bronchoscopy is warranted only to remove particulate matter but should not take precedence unless the patient cannot be ventilated due to major airway obstruction; in this situation, a Heimlich manuever[158] may be required, but there are no reports of its use intraoperatively.

Bronchial lavage is no longer recommended, as it serves to spread the chemical burn from the acid contents throughout the respiratory tree, and the damage from the acid is almost instantaneous, as is buffering of the acid.[11,82] Lavage with water, bicarbonate or saline or steroids is not helpful but may increase the extent of lung damage.[82,159] However, an animal model has suggested that lavage to dilute possible surfactant inhibiting substances followed by administration of surfactant may be of benefit.[156]

Beta-2 agonists such as albuterol or terbutaline may be given by nebulized solution or metered dose inhaler treat bronchospasm. Prophylactic antibiotics may be given if the aspirate is feculent, but are otherwise not usually indicated,[1] and may increase the risk of subsequent infection with resistant organisms or confusing the results of bacterial cultures. 36% of patients aspirating required antibiotics a mean of 4.4 days after aspiration.[149] Bronchial brushings by a protected specimen brush may be used to guide antibiotic therapy.[149] In animal models, parenteral hydrocortisone appeared to limit the extent of pulmonary damage from aspiration.[82] Intratracheal, intramuscular or systemic corticosteroids have not been demonstrated to be beneficial[11,160] and are associated with known adverse effects, including immune suppression.

Ventilatory support is indicated in patients with continued respiratory insufficiency or altered mental status. Positive end-expiratory pressure (PEEP) is used to improve oxygenation by redistributing pulmonary extravascular water in both increased permeability and hydrostatic pulmonary edema from the alveoli to the perivascular cuffs.[161] Significant amounts of PEEP may be required to maintain oxygenation, with negative effects on cardiac output, and insertion of a pulmonary artery catheter may be helpful. Attempts to support cardiac output with volume expansion may worsen alveolar transudate, and fluid restriction is recommended; cardiac function may be improved with dobutamine. In addition to decreasing cardiac output, high levels of PEEP may worsen ventilation with ensuing hypercarbia and respiratory acidosis.[162] PEEP thus may render end-tidal carbon dioxide monitoring of ventilation misleading, and frequent arterial blood gas analysis necessary.

Fluid management of these patients has been controversial. The rapid development of hypotension as fluid poured into the alveolar spaces was treated by albumin or crystalloid volume expansion.[163] The frequent occurrence of pulmonary edema has led to volume restriction, digitalization and use of inotropes to support cardiac output, in hopes of keeping filling pressures and low and limiting transudation of fluid across the leaky capillary membrane.

Low mortality of 7.5% was achieved in one retrospective study in which adequate fluids to maintain clinical perfusion were given, and inotropic agents added as needed after PCWP reached 18 to 20.[149] If the patient will require ventilation for some time, appropriate sedation, pain therapy and amnestic agents are indicated. Extracorporeal CO_2 removal has been used.[149]

Though most clinical studies have shown a high mortality (40 to 90%) when massive aspiration and subsequent pneumonia occurs,[1] one retrospective study of patients with aspiration severe enough to required mechanical ventilation revealed a mortality of 7.5% directly attributable to the aspiration, and a mortality of 21% from all causes.[149] There were no deaths in patients with three or fewer lobes of the lung involved on X-ray.[149] The alveolar-arterial oxygen gradient may be more predictive of outcome than findings.[154]

As mentioned, there were no deaths from acid aspiration in the original report by Mendelson.[15] In Olsson's study, 5% of perioperative aspirations died.[16] Tiret found death or persistent coma in 22% of the aspirations that occurred, though a significant proportion of these may have been unwitnessed, with a higher risk of significant hypoxia prior to rescue.[17] Of 178 patients with severe pneumonia admitted to intensive care, 28 (15.7%) were due to aspiration. 14% of these died, a much lower incidence than was seen with the other types of pneumonia.[164] Severe aspiration pneumonia requiring admission to intensive care has a high rate of survival when compared to other types of severe pneumonia or ARDS,[164,165] and aspiration may not be the "death sentence" it is frequently assumed to be.

Still, once aspiration occurs, efforts to control the quantity and quality of aspirated material and the severity of subsequent pulmonary damage are of limited efficacy, and treatment of the pulmonary lesion is essentially supportive, with no effective means of undoing the damage that has been done. Careful preoperative assessment for aspiration risk, with appropriate prophylaxis and alteration of anesthetic technique, and the immediate ability to respond appropriately to aspiration when it occurs, are still important parts of the anesthesiologist's commitment to the safety of the patient in his or her care.

VOMITING

Nausea and vomiting are common postanesthetic problems that may be intensely distressing to patients even when causing no lasting harm. Rarely, more serious effects occur, and may include suture line disruption and wound dehiscence, intraocular bleeding, Mallory-Weiss or Boerhaave's syndromes, volume and electrolyte abnormalities, and aspiration of gastric contents. While emesis after opiate premedication and prolonged ether anesthesia occurred in as many as 75 80% of patients, the incidence of postoperative nausea and vomiting (PONV) appears to have been reduced by almost 50% with the use of modern anesthetic agents.[166] PONV occurs in 10% of patients in the post-anesthesia care unit and 30% during the first 24 hours of anesthesia.[166] However, the current increase in ambulatory surgery potentiates the impact of PONV on patient comfort, convenience and economics. Emesis has been called the "big little problem" in anesthesia for ambulatory surgery[167] because it may delay discharge from the post-anesthetic care unit and may cause unplanned admission for 0.1 to 1% of ambulatory surgery patients.[168-170] PONV was found to be the most important factor in determining the length of stay after ambulatory anesthesia.[171]

The specific mechanism of PONV is unclear, and therapies shown effective for better-understood types of emesis are applied in hopes they will prove effective in PONV. As anesthesia has been delivered for over 100 years, and the problem identified soon after its institution, why is the mechanism not better defined? Andrews indicates four factors that have complicated study in this area: the complexity of the interaction of surgical, anesthetic, and patient factors; inadequate quantification of the phenomena of nausea and vomiting; inadequately controlled antiemetic regimens and the lack of a suitable animal model.[172]

Underlying these four factors, in addition to the complexities of the perioperative environment, is the complicated and partly understood nature of emesis itself. A remarkable range of clinical conditions may be associated with nausea and vomiting, from intracranial hypertension, labyrinthitis and pregnancy to intestinal obstruction, renal failure and myocardial infarction. In addition, therapeutic interventions such as surgery, anesthesia, radiation and chemotherapy, and drugs such as opiates, levodopa, digoxin and aminophylline may provoke the same syndrome. Although the causes of emesis are legion and without common thread, the sensations, behaviors and coordinated muscular and physiologic response of nausea and vomiting are stereotypical. Two questions are central to research in this area: how do all these various stimuli bring about identical vomiting, and how does the central nervous system organize the vomiting response?[173] Answers to these questions may lead to the development of more effective treatment and prophylaxis of PONV.

Development of an animal model has been difficult and application of the results to humans tenuous. Compared to other species, humans are among the most sensitive to emetic stimuli.[174] Vomiting seems to be a more highly developed reflex in carnivores, and the carnivorous cat, dog, and ferret are among the most dependable research animals.[173] However, PONV is unusual in animal models and does not really mimic the experience undergone by a human patient in a hospital. Species vary in their sensitivity to emetic stimuli, and may respond to the same stimuli with differing physiological reactions, so it is difficult to extrapolate the findings to humans. Further, differing species may have the same response to an emetic stimulus but by a different mechanism.

Overview

Pre-ejection Phase

Vomiting or emesis is the forceful expulsion of gastric contents, in contrast to the passive reflux or regurgitation of gastric contents that occurs when the lower esophageal sphincter relaxes in the comatose or infant human.[175] The complex muscular activation seen with emesis does not occur with regurgitation.[172] Emesis may be divided into three stages: pre-ejection, ejection, and post-ejection. The pre-ejection phase is dominated by nausea and its associated autonomic and gastrointestinal changes. Prodromal symptoms in humans include heavy salivation, swallowing, sweating, pallor and tachycardia.[175] Nausea, derived from the Greek word for "ship,"[173] is an unpleasant sensation presumed to arise from the same pathways and structures involved in vomiting; it has been suggested that low-level stimulation of vomiting pathways may result in nausea without vomiting. It may occur in "waves" and may be relieved by vomiting. The autonomic manifestations often precede active

vomiting and may result from the proximity of vomiting centers to vagal and regulatory nuclei. The pre-ejection phase may last minutes, hours, or even days, as seen with chemotherapy, space sickness and pregnancy,[173] and may never culminate in actual vomiting. Conversely, vomiting may occur with minimal nausea, as in intracranial hypertension.[175]

Gastrointestinal changes during the pre-ejection phase include relaxation of the proximal stomach and changes in gut motility. Two distinct motor events have been defined as the gastrointestinal motor correlates of vomiting and consist of a retrograde giant contraction (RGC) that begins in the small intestine and moves retrograde through the antrum, followed by post-RGC phasic contractions, moderate amplitude phasic contractions in the distal small intestine.[176] Antral contents move orad because of the proximal relaxation and retrograde contraction. Gastric motility is decreased, while abnormal peristalsis in the small bowel is marked, although less effective in propelling contents distally. The RGC causes reflux into the stomach,[177] but does not appear to be directly involved in vomiting as it occurs well before expulsion of gastric contents.[176]

Vagal efferents appear to initiate the gastrointestinal motor correlates of vomiting but the control mechanisms of the RGC and post-RGC phasic contractions differ. Anticholinergics block the RGC but not the post-RGC contractions.[176] The RGC is vagally mediated and acetylcholine is the involved transmitter.[172] Vagal non-adrenergic, non-cholinergic (NANC) fibers appear to mediate the relaxation of the proximal stomach, probably utilizing vasoactive intestinal polypeptide (VIP) or nitric oxide as a neurotransmitter,[172] while ATP is an unlikely candidate.[176] The motor patterns of retroperistalsis and proximal gastric relaxation are detected by vagal afferents and transmitted to higher CNS functions via the nucleus tractus solitarii. In humans a relationship exists between nausea and antral dysmotility. Though the abnormal motility patterns may not cause nausea, they may intensify the sensation and thus account for the anti-emetic efficacy of gastrokinetic agents with little activity at the chemoreceptor trigger zone (CTZ).[111]

Ejection Phase

The ejection phase consists of retching and vomiting. Marked retching with limited vomiting may be seen with some stimuli such as apomorphine and cisplatin,[173] but retching need not always terminate in vomiting. The esophagus and stomach do not eject gastric contents; they have a passive role in the emetic reflex and emesis is achieved by the action of the diaphragmatic, thoracic and abdominal muscles.[177] Retching is the act of rhythmic inspiratory movements against a closed glottis. Rocking inspiratory movements of chest wall and diaphragm with expiratory efforts of the muscles of the abdominal wall are seen, identical to vomiting. While the glottis remains closed, the abdominal and external intercostal muscles and diaphragm contract rhythmically, causing a rapid decrease in intrathoracic pressure as intra-abdominal pressure increases. This "thoracic suction pulse" differentiates retching from vomiting and is due to efforts to expand the thoracic cage and contract the diaphragm while keeping the glottis closed.[178] Gastric contents may oscillate between the stomach and esophagus, with the upper esophageal sphincter (UES) relaxing during the retch, but contracting in between retches. Retching may function to overcome the antireflux mechanisms of the lower esophagus and cardia.[179]

In *vomiting* the contraction of the rectus abdominis and external oblique muscles overlying the stomach expells gastric contents. In contrast to retching, actual vomiting is accompanied by diaphragmatic ascent and a positive thoracic pressure wave.[178] The rectus abdominis and external oblique muscles generate the positive pressure seen in both the thorax and abdomen, while the thoracic expiratory muscles are inactive during both retching and vomiting.[180] The UES and esophagus relax, the abdominal muscles and diaphragm contract, and the intrathoracic and intra-abdominal pressures both increase to about 100 mm Hg. The relaxation of the hiatal (periesophageal) portion of the diaphragm during vomiting allows transmission of the abdominal pressure up into the thorax and expulsion of the gastric contents. This relaxation is also seen during eructation and regurgitation[181] but not during retching.[176] During vomiting, animals assume a characteristic posture that permits maximal compression of the stomach by abdominal musculature.[173] Characteristically, a widely opened mouth, spine held in flexion, and the forceful expulsion of upper gastrointestinal contents are observed.

Post-ejection Phase

The post-ejection phase is characterized by recovery from emesis and the sequelae of vomiting. Emesis may occur again and again, cycling through the pre-ejection and ejection phases. The immediate consequences of vomiting include loss of fluid and electrolytes, lethargy, muscular weakness and possibly body heat loss;[173] More prolonged vomiting may lead to an increased risk of those rare serious consequences previously discussed.

NEUROPHYSIOLOGY OF NAUSEA AND VOMITING

Integrative Mechanisms

Vomiting is a complex integrated reflex act with three major components: emetic detectors, integrative mechanisms, and autonomic and somatic outputs.[172] The central nervous system (CNS) integrates the afferent (sensory) and efferent (effector) limbs of the vomiting reflex and closely orchestrates the interaction between the autonomic and somatic motor systems. As an example of this coordination, retching does not begin until the RGC has reached the stomach, and the RGC does not begin until the proximal stomach has relaxed.[176]

The existence of a vomiting center was postulated near the turn of the century in an attempt to explain how this careful coordination might be achieved. The traditional understanding of the neurophysiologic mechanisms involved is based on the classic studies of Borison and

Wang, who in 1953 explored the mechanism of vomiting.[182] Stimulation of the lateral medullary reticular formation of animals produced retching, vomiting, and prodromal signs such as salivation and licking. This area of the medulla oblongata, close to centers regulating visceral and somatic components of emesis, was termed the "vomiting center."

Although electrical stimulation of this area causes vomiting, and its destruction blocks certain types of vomiting, no evidence exists that emetic substances act by direct effect on this center. Instead, the vomiting center acts as a relay and integrating center. It receives imput from the chemoreceptor trigger zone (CTZ) (see below), the vestibular structures, cortical and brain stem structures and visceral afferents originating in the heart, testes, GI tract and other viscera.[182] A discrete group of neurons regulating all aspects of nausea and vomiting has not conclusively been identified. As Borison and Wang wrote, "The claim for a center must be held in abeyance until the structures in question are demonstrated both physiologically and morphologically to have an integrating function. Most arguments advanced in support of an emetic center on the basis of ablation or even stimulation experiments can very well apply to receptor elements. An hypothesis for a neural center can be considered valid only if it encompasses all aspects concerned in the regulation of the given function, and when it has stood the test of time and trial."[182]

In a more recent study, electrical stimulation of the brain stem was not so successful in provoking emesis, and it was concluded that a discretely localized center does not exist and the neurons involved in emesis are more diffusely distributed.[183] The parvicellular reticular formation (PCRF) was shown to have some of the neuroanatomical connections required of a "vomiting center," but the researchers concluded that, regardless of whether it constitutes the "vomiting center" per se, "the PCRF is of primary importance as the structural substrate of the final coordinating mechanism in the elucidation of the vomiting reflex."[184]

An alternative model consists of several neuronal centers acting in concert to produce nausea and vomiting. This is consistent with the observation that all the involved motor nuclei subserve other functions, and their synchronization into nausea and emesis requires a unique pattern of activation. This also explains why, in experimental models, it has been easier to evoke single components of the emetic act rather than the entire complex. Thus, the "vomiting center" is short-hand terminology for the central vomiting coordinating mechanism[172] which has also been called "the emetic central pattern generator".[176]

This emetic central pattern generator activates gastrointestinal and somatomotor responses in an independent and apparently parallel fashion. The gastrointestinal motor patterns do not themselves cause vomiting or associated cardiorespiratory changes; the cardiorespiratory changes prior to vomiting occur even when the gastrointestinal motor changes are blocked by vagotomy; and the gastrointestinal motor correlates of vomiting elicited by

CCK-8 are not associated with increases in heart or respiratory rate.[176]

The Emetic Detectors

Higher CNS and Miscellaneous Detectors

The major detectors of emetic stimuli include the abdominal visceral afferents, the area postrema, and the vestibular system, though higher cerebral centers, as well as miscellaneous inputs from taste, smell and vagal and glossopharyngeal stimulation may provoke vomiting. Davis and co-workers have proposed the "hierarchical hypothesis" that suggests several classes of stimuli act to protect the organism. The senses of taste and smell and the gag reflex provide early attempts to remove the offending substance, while visceral efferents may provoke the emetic reflex to rid the organism of toxins when the first level of defense fails; if the first two levels of detectors fail, a blood bathed sensor in the brain acts to protect the CNS by sensing the toxin and activating the vomiting reflex.[185]

The efficacy of smell and taste in provoking nausea and vomiting enhances learned avoidance of emetic substances and may be related to early defense of the organism against toxins. Although vomiting may be a learned response, the cortex is not a necessary part of the arc. Stimuli applied to the area postrema, vagus or vestibular apparatus, will elicit vomiting even in decerebrate animals.

Visceral Receptors

A second level of defense against ingested toxins are the gastrointestinal chemoreceptors and mechanoreceptors. Chemical or mechanical stimulation of the mucosal receptors may evoke retrograde duodenal and antral contractions.[186,187] The vagus is the primary innervation of the abdominal visceral afferents, and electrical stimulation of this portion of the nerve causes emesis.[188] The fibers of the abdominal portion of the vagus are 80–90% afferent. Specific chemoreceptors for glucose, amino-acids and osmotic (hyper- or hypo-) stimuli have been identified in animal species. These chemoreceptors may be activated by acid or alkali, and irritants such as copper sulfate. The nausea and vomiting following gastric irritation with hypertonic sodium chloride, copper sulfate or mustard require intact mucosal innervation. Most studies demonstrate a major involvement by vagal afferents, which appear to be polymodal, and respond to various stimuli. Vagal denervation blocks the emetic response to gastric irritants such as copper sulfate but ablation of the area postrema has no effect. If the visceral detectors are destroyed then vomiting is only delayed, but prior area postrema destruction prevents emesis in this model.

Mechanical stimulation causes readily observable changes in motor and secretory function. Contraction and distention of the gut activates mechanoreceptors in the gut wall[189] that relay information to the dorsal vagal motor nucleus. The central neurons are then either stimulated or inhibited by the two major vagal motor pathways: the excitatory cholinergic pathways and the inhibitory NANC pathways.[190] The receptors may activate vagal afferents that relax the proximal stomach via non-adrenergic, non-cholinergic, inhibitory neurons in the wall of the stomach.

Distention of the antrum, small intestine, colon and biliary ducts may cause vomiting, and this is blocked by denervation of the involved organ. Distention of the antrum evokes vagally mediated vomiting but distention of the fundus of the stomach does not. Due to the muscle characteristics and non-adrenergic, non-cholinergic inhibitory innervation of the gastric body, it tolerates large volumes. The antral muscle is thicker and less able to relax; increases in antral volume cause greater changes in wall tension and a continuously distended antrum will cause continuous afferent discharge and trigger vomiting.

The majority of evidence shows that viscerally evoked vomiting is vagally mediated, but splanchnic afferents may be involved in certain types of vomiting, such as the response to noxious stimuli. The vascular system also contains emetic detectors, and their stimulation leads to the same nausea and gastrointestinal motor changes described, and may constitute a third level of defense against toxins. Cardiac fibers may cause nausea and vomiting associated with myocardial infarction.[191]

The Chemoreceptor Trigger Zone

The receptors and afferent connections of the CTZ are better characterized than those of the vomiting center. The CTZ lies in the floor of the fourth ventricle near the surface of the medulla oblongata, in the area postrema. The area postrema is well-vascularized by the posterior inferior cerebellar artery. Because the capillaries are fenestrated, essentially no barrier exists between the circulating blood and CSF, and agents in the blood and cerebrospinal fluid have ready access to the area postrema.[192]

This area was identified when it was noted that application of apomorphine to the caudal end of the floor of the fourth ventricle has the same emetic effect as when systemically administered. Unlike electrical stimulation of the lateral reticular formation, electrical stimulation of the CTZ does not cause vomiting. Damaging the CTZ decreases the response to systemic emetics, but only slightly alters the response to agents acting directly in the gut.[182] Ablation of the CTZ does not affect the emesis caused by oral copper sulfate, but transection of the abdominal vagal fibers and sympathetic nerves does. It was proposed that circulating agents are detected at the CTZ in the area postrema which then stimulates the vomiting center, while those agents that irritate visceral afferents act directly through the vomiting center. In addition to blood-borne stimuli, the CTZ receives vagal and glossopharyngeal input. A functional vomiting center is required for CTZ-mediated vomiting, as the CTZ does not itself regulate vomiting, but acts as a trigger by stimulating the vomiting center.

The CTZ appears to be intimately involved in the vomiting associated with opiates and dopaminergic agonists (apomorphine, L-DOPA, bromocriptine). Ablation of the

CTZ alone, leaving the vomiting center intact, blocks the emetic effect of apomorphine, an opiate and dopamine agonist, and prevents vomiting from motion sickness,[193,194] uremia and the early phase of radiation sickness.[195]

The nucleus tractus solitarius (NTS) is the main receptor site for vagal and sympathetic afferent neurons.[196] From the NTS information is transmitted to the dorsal motor nucleus which mediates parasympathetic responses, to the nucleus ambiguus to cause glottic closure and to the medullary reticular formation. Involvement of the diaphragm and abdominal muscles results from reticular formation input into the spinal cord. The dorsal motor vagal nucleus and nucleus ambiguus receive outputs from the area postrema,[173] which may coordinate the motor changes in the GI tract seen with emesis.

If the emetic action of an agent is inhibited by abolition of the area postrema this is considered evidence that the agent acts through a central mechanism; however, the area postrema may be a part of the afferent pathway, and be a product of abdominal vagal afferents.

In addition to dopamine, the mammalian CTZ contains other possible transmitters, and the CTZ may cause vomiting in response to endogenous neurotransmitters and neuropeptides as well as drugs and toxins. Neurochemical studies of the area postrema reveal the presence of possible transmitters: 5-HT, dopamine, norepinephrine, somatostatin, VIP, substance P, enkephalins, oholecystokinin, GABA. In addition, receptors or binding sites have ben identified for dopaminergic, histaminergic, alpha2-adrenergic, CCK, ENK, muscarinic agents; synthetic or degradative enzymes present in the area and important in the synthesis or degradation of possible transmitters include acetylcholinesterase, choline acetyltransferase, decarboxylase, histidine decarboxylase, enkephalinase, tyrosine hydroxylase, and dopamine beta-hydroxylase.[173] The function of the emetic regions of the reticular formation of the cat brain stem is subserved by catecholaminergic and 5-hydroxytryptaminergic elements.[197]

The area postrema has two main roles in provoking emesis: it responds to vagal afferents, directly or indirectly, and it detects emetic chemicals in the circulation or CSF. Emetic agents may be endogenous (dopamine, acetylcholine, and enkephalin) or exogenous chemicals (cisplatin, copper sulfate, and emetine).[173] Stress-induced emesis may be due to overspill of epinephrine in the CSF, activating the area postrema to induce emesis. Intracerebroventricular administration of catecholamines has been shown to induce vomiting.[197] Also, endogenous agents may accumulate in blood or CSF during pathologic states, such as uremia, that are associated with nausea and vomiting.

VESTIBULAR SYSTEM

A vestibular component may be involved in several factors causing PONV, including emesis related to movement, opiates, nitrous oxide and ear surgery (see below), thus the receptors and pathways involved in motion sickness are of some concern in the neurophysiology of PONV. It has been suggested that motion sickness results from conflicting input from sensory modalities that normally supply orientation in space and awareness of being in motion.[193] The visual system detects motion of the environment, while the vestibular system detects rotatory movement and gravitational forces. Rotatory movement (angular acceleration) causes movement of endolymphatic fluid and stimulation of receptors in the semicircular canals. Gravitational forces and linear acceleration in the horizontal plane are detected by the utriculus, while vibration and linear acceleration in the dorsoventral plane stimulate the sacculi.[198] The utricule and saccule are also known as otolith organs.[184] The vestibular nerve fibers terminate in the vestibular nuclei in the floor of the fourth ventricle, while some fibers go directly to the flocculonodular lobe of the cerebellum.[198] Information from one sensory system that is contradicted by another may trigger motion sickness. Such sensory conflict may occur during turning of an automobile, in which the otoliths perceive a change in gravitational pull while the semicircular canals perceive no change as the head has not rotated. Similarly, when an aircraft turns, the banking of the airplane stimulates the semi-circular canals but the otoliths note no change in the directional pull of gravity, as the rotation of the plane leaves the axis of the gravitational force perpendicular to the floor of the craft.[193] Pathologic states that may result in nausea and vomiting due to vestibular stimuli include labyrinthitis, Meniere's disease, and unilateral labyrinthectomy.

A functional vestibular system is required for motion sickness. Removal of the cerebellar nodulus and uvula block motion sickness in dogs,[199] but autonomic innervation of the gut is not involved.[193,200] An intact CTZ is required for motion-induced emesis.[194]

The emesis associated with opiates appears to have a vestibular component, as the emetic effect appears to be increased with vestibular stimulation,[201] motion or ambulation. The emetic response to apomorphine is more intense when certain head/body positions are assumed.[202]

Autonomic and Somatic Output in the Emetic Reflex

Heavy salivation is a frequent prodrome of vomiting, and may cause increased swallowing; the salivary glands are innervated by the facial and glossopharyngeal nerves, which have their cell bodies in the PCRF. Airway secretions are also increased, and this may originate from either vagal fibers from the nucleus ambiguus or sympathetic fibers from the spinal cord. Tachycardia is usually seen during nausea, but it is not clear whether this is a direct effect or secondary to stress. Bradycardia is the characteristic response to retching and vomiting, but this may be secondary to intrathoracic pressure changes as described above, and be vagally mediated. Although gastric acid secretion is decreased, the primary effect of nausea and vomiting is on gastric motility.[173]

As discussed previously, the proximal stomach relaxes and retroperistalsis and gastric motility abnormalities occur. Tonic activity in the vagal efferents to the intramural cholinergic excitatory neurons is inhibited and the vagal efferent nerves supplying the intramural, non-adrenergic, noncholinergic inhibitory neurons become more active. Retroperistaltic waves begin in the lower small intestine and pass over the distal stomach prior to vomiting, perhaps accounting for bilious and (rarely) feculent vomiting. During the pre-ejection phase the proximal stomach relaxes; slow wave activity in the antrum, duodenum and upper jejunum is inhibited as is the superimposed spiking seen with contraction.[173]

Causes of Postoperative Nausea and Vomiting

PONV is a common problem in the Post-Anesthetic Care Unit (PACU) and is important both for its negative effect on patients' comfort as well as additional unplanned hospital admissions and delayed discharge from the PACU. Factors involved in PONV include pain and the opiates used to treat it, anesthetic agents or techniques, positional changes and movement, especially ambulation, surgery site, and patient factors including prior history of motion sickness or PONV, obesity, and female sex, as well as day of menstrual cycle.[203] These interacting and complex factors will be considered through the phases of the surgical experience.

Preoperative Factors

Fasting

The ingestion of food in the preoperative period may increase the risk of emesis during the postoperative period, although fasting prior to anesthesia is more for reduction of risk of aspiration. However, fasting does not have absolutely predictable effects on gastric contents as gastric emptying varies among individuals and depends also on the substance ingested, as, for example, fatty foods are cleared at a slower rate. However, food ingestion does not normally stimulate emesis, so why should it do so under anesthesia? The ferret will vomit after anesthetized with intraperitoneal urethane unless previously fasted for at least 12 hours.[172] It is suggested that food ingestion stimulates release by the gut of hormones including gastrin, motilin, and peptide YY, and perhaps these sensitize the area postrema to emetic stimuli. Likewise, the postprandial release of hepatic portal vein 5-HT may sensitize gastrointestinal afferents. Further complicating an already complex situation, fasting itself may cause nausea.[172] In one small study of healthy volunteers, the majority of women reported nausea after a fast of 7 hours; while slightly over one-third of men did so after a slightly longer fast.[204]

Apprehension

Anxiety may predispose to vomiting but sedation does not appear effective in diminishing its incidence. Fear and pain may mediate emesis through the release of catecholamines by the adrenal medulla.[204] Intracerebroventricular injection of catecholamines provokes emesis in the cat.[197] The importance of preoperative anxiety in inducing PONV is unclear. Aerophagia associated with anxiety also may worsen gastric distention and increase PONV.[166]

Pre-existing Surgical/Medical Conditions

The indications for surgery may include a condition that renders the patient more prone to emesis, such as intracranial hypertension or small bowel obstruction. Uremia, diabetic gastropathy and other illnesses that chronically decrease gastric emptying and cause vomiting are likely to do so in the postoperative period.[166]

Patient Factors

Korttila identifies background factors that modify the incidence of PONV and must be controlled in clinical studies (Table 21-5): patient age and sex, history of motion sickness, history of PONV after previous anesthesia, administration of antiemetics before the operation and the phase of the menstrual cycle in female patients.[205]

Uncontrolled variables make analysis of the effect of age on the incidence of PONV difficult. It is the most likely reason for unplanned admission after ambulatory surgery in children.[170,206] PONV is likely to be lowest in infants less than 12 months of age,[207] maximum in school age children (34-51%)[206,208] then may decrease with age.[209] The incidence of PONV in adults may be 5% or less.[207] Advancing age appears to make the incidence of PONV more equal between the sexes.[209]

Adult women have two to three times the incidence of PONV seen in adult males.[209,210] The greatest incidence occurs in the third and fourth week of the menstrual cycle.[210] Two recent retrospective studies studied PONV and menstrual cycle in women undergoing gynecological laparoscopy, but had contradictory results; however, interpretation of the results is complicated by one study examining PONV during the first 2 hours while the other examined the incidence during the first 24 hours, and serum concentrations of female sex hormones were not measured.[211,212] The predilection of females to have increased PONV is not seen in the elderly.[210]

Pregnancy termination in the first trimester is associated with a higher incidence of nausea and vomiting; during this trimester morning sickness is common. As mentioned, fasting may have a slightly greater nauseant effect in women than in men.[204]

A history of motion sickness or prior PONV may increase the risk of PONV for subsequent procedures.[213]

Table 21-5. Background Factors That May Modify PONV and Must Be Controlled in Clinical Studies

Patient age and sex
History of motion sickness
History of PONV after previous anesthesia
Administration of antiemetics before operation
Phase of menstrual cycle

With permission from Korttila, K.: The study of post-operative nausea and vomiting. Br. J. Anaesth. *69*:20, 1992.

Obesity has been suggested to increase the incidence of PONV.[210,214] However, a large, controlled study failed to find a relationship between the body mass index and the incidence of PONV.[209] In this study, patients were not ventilated by mask prior to ventilation;[209] it is possible that the difficulties with mask ventilation that occur in the obese patient may increase the risk of vomiting.[166]

Perioperative Factors

Premedication

Preoperative medications usually include analgesics and/or antiemetics. Atropine in a dose of 0.6 mg IM can slow gastric emptying, and may therefore contribute to PONV. Morphine has either stimulatory or inhibiting effects on emesis depending on the dose used, and an opioid-activated antiemetic center has been postulated.[215] The emetic effect of opioids may be due to mu receptor stimulation in the area postrema, as ablating this area blocks the emetic effect. Fentanyl in addition has a broad antiemetic effect in higher doses, blocking the emesis induced by morphine, apomorphine, copper sulfate and cisplatin, and this effect is antagonized by naloxone.[216] This wide range of activity suggests an action beyond the area postrema.[216] The inability to define a discrete vomiting center led to the theory that many different effectors summate to trigger the emetic reflex,[185] and this would involve the area postrema, dorsal vagal motor nucleus, nucleus tractus solitarius and reticular formation.[216] Higher doses of morphine do not induce emesis in the ferret, and prevent the emesis induced by cisplatin.[217] Loperamide-induced emesis in the ferret appears to be mediated by the area postrema, possibly through mu receptors, and D2 receptor antagonism with domperidone or 5-HT3 receptor antagonism with ondansetron do not block this emesis.[218] 5-HT3 receptor blockade does not prevent morphine—or loperamide induced vomiting in the ferret,[217,218] though it is effective in the treatment of emesis related to radiation and chemotherapy. The emetic side-effects of morphine appear to be due to the actions of morphine itself rather than one of its metabolites, though morphine 6-glucuronide has a more potent emetic effect than the parent compound.[217]

Effects of Anesthesia and Surgery

Endocrine Effects

Although the endocrine effects of anesthesia and surgery have been studied, their role in vomiting is unclear. Many peptides have been demonstrated to be emetics either systemically or after intracerebroventricular injection, and act via stimulation of the area postrema.[219]

Cardiovascular Effects

Hypotension is associated with nausea and vomiting,[210] whether it be due to anesthetics, regional anesthesia with vasodilation, hemorrhage, or other etiology. The mechanism of this is not well-established. One possibility is that a sympathetic discharge related to adrenal medullary release of epinephrine may act on the area postrema to stimulate emesis. The ventricles of the heart have unmyelinated axons that when strongly stimulated may activate vagal afferent mechanoreceptors resulting in the vomiting associated with inferior myocardial infarction and vasovagal fainting.[191] Tachycardia secondary to hypovolemia also may occur post-operatively when the patient attempts to move or sit upright, which may also stimulate these fibers. The cardiac afferents also may activate vagal efferent NANC inhibitory neurons causing gastric relaxation which may increase gastric stasis.[172] The incidence of emesis during spinal anesthesia increases when the systolic blood pressure falls below 80 mm Hg but is lessened by inhalation of 100% oxygen,[55] and by keeping systolic blood pressure above 80 mm Hg with fluids and/or methoxamine.[55]

Gastrointestinal Effects

The ability of surgery to reduce gastrointestinal motility is more profound and longer-lasting than that of anesthesia. The effect of surgery on motility may be measured by the effect on the migrating motor complex (MMC). The MMC has been called the "housekeeper of the bowel," and acts to move contents distally during fasting. In terms of inhibition of the MMC, the effect is least with skin incision (in order of increasing effect) muscle division, laparotomy, and gut manipulation decrease MMC. Sympathectomy limits the length of time that MMC is reduced after surgery but does not prevent its inhibition.[220] Stasis leads to accumulation of fluids and air or gas which can activate GI visceral afferents by distending the stomach. Although emesis may not be seen at the time of surgery, multiple factors may culminate in emesis in the postoperative period. The CNS pathways involved in emesis may be sensitized and more susceptible to other nausea-provoking stimuli such as movement. The gut motility disturbance persists postoperatively so that a patient may vomit after ingestion of food or liquid.[172] Opiates also have a well-established inhibitory effect on gastric motility that is reversed by naloxone.[221]

Physical Effects of Volatile Agents

Volatile agents may act through changes in middle ear pressure,[222,223] but it is more likely that they encourage emesis through their action on the gut. Ventilation by mask may force gas into the stomach, causing distention and vomiting through activation of abdominal, vagal, and splanchnic afferents. This may be more likely in the obese patient who is prone to be difficult to ventilate by mask. The level of experience of the anesthesiologist performing mask ventilation may also have an effect on vomiting, with the incidence being greater among the less experienced practitioners, possibly due to a greater tendency to force air into the stomach.[210,224] It has been suggested that avoidance of positive pressure ventilation prior to intubation may decrease vomiting.[204] In the case of nitrous oxide, diffusion into the gut may occur during the course of anesthesia and surgery and increase distention.

In general, the anesthetic volatile agents suppress gastric and small intestinal motility. The mechanism commonly thought involved has been peripheral, either the release of ACh from the myenteric plexus or an increase in sympathetic discharge that acts directly or indirectly. However, recent evidence suggests a vagal mechanism, perhaps a reduction in vagal cholinergic tone, or an increase in vagal NANC inhibitory activity.[172]

Nausea and vomiting is associated with a relaxation of gastrointestinal activity and some of the motor effects of anesthetics may be part of a generalized emetic activation. 5-HT release may be triggered by opioids, epinephrine, ischemia and mechanical stimulation of the gut.

The use of neostigmine is associated with an increase in PONV,[225] due perhaps to its stimulation of gastric motility, or through direct activation of central cholinergic pathways.[172]

Though some investigators find a lower incidence of PONV with halothane others see no significant difference among the modern inhalational agents.

Direct Effects of Agents on the Emetic Reflex

The older volatile agents such as cyclopropane and ether were associated with a significantly higher incidence of nausea and vomiting than are the newer agents; it was hypothesized that those agents such as cyclopropane and diethyl ether that are associated with the release of circulating catecholamines have a particularly high incidence of PONV. Alpha-adrenergic stimulation via intracerebroventricular injection of norepinephrine stimulates emesis in the cat, apparently through its action at alpha-2 receptors in the area postrema.[197] Ablation of the area postrema inhibited cyclopropane induced vomiting in dogs. This does not demonstrate that area postrema stimulation is the immediate cause of anesthetic-induced vomiting, as stimulation could cause release of a mediator and thus act indirectly.

An alternative mechanism is blockade of the antiemetic center.[215] PONV could be related to some inhibitory effect of anesthetics on this center in combination with its other emetic-potentiating actions.[172]

The role of visceral afferents in PONV is unclear; if they are involved, it is possibly through signalling to the brain that alterations in gastric motility secondary to anesthesia and surgery have occurred.

Many anesthetics alter 5-HT metabolism in the brain. Thus, anesthetics could induce emesis by altering neurotransmitter handling at the forebrain sites associated with emesis or by acting at brain stem sites that are stimulated by the area postrema and vagal afferents.

Effects of Specific Anesthetic/Techniques

Nitrous Oxide

Nitrous oxide has been reported to increase the incidence of nausea and vomiting. Literature supporting this thesis has included studies of children undergoing strabismus surgery,[226] women who had minor gynecologic surgery,[227] or pelvic laparoscopy,[228,229] On the other hand, there was no increase in PONV with the use of nitrous oxide to maintain anesthesia in pediatric outpatients undergoing tonsillectomy-adenoidectomy,[230] or

women undergoing gynecologic laparoscopy,[231] or adults undergoing various procedures.[209] The studies in which the patients were women have been criticized for not controlling for menstrual phase, which may confound results.[214]

Theories that could explain an emetic effect of nitrous oxide include its effect on middle ear pressure, which might be emetic through a vestibular mechanism; diffusion into gases in the stomach and intestine which might distend the gut and provoke vomiting; and a possible opiate agonist effect. It has been suggested in addition that the decreased concentration of oxygen mandated by use of a significant concentration of nitrous oxide might increase PONV, but Pandit found no effect of differing oxygen concentrations.[230] The increased sympathetic activity associated with nitrous oxide is a possible contributor to postoperative emesis.

Gastric Suction

Evacuation of the stomach may reduce the incidence of PONV in certain patients, but an indwelling tube postoperatively may increase the incidence of nausea and retching by pharyngeal stimulation.[204] The use of gastric evacuation may be helpful in preventing PONV after laparoscopic gynecological surgery,[232] but other reports are equivocal.[233,234] It has been suggested that the use of gastric decompression may be most reasonable and effective when used in patients in whom gastric distention may exist (upper abdominal surgeries, or prolonged or difficult mask ventilation, for example), but that nausea related to other factors, such as vestibular stimulation or opiate administration, would not be prevented.[204]

Propofol

Propofol may be appropriate to use as an anesthetic in patients with an increased risk of PONV, particularly in shorter procedures when its pharmacokinetic properties are most useful. Induction of anesthesia with propofol, followed by maintenance with a volatile agent, may or may not[171] decrease the incidence of PONV. Continuing an infusion of propofol for the first 25 minutes of maintenance appears to decrease PONV.[171] Total intravenous anesthesia with alfentanil and propofol, when compared to anesthesia with nitrous oxide and enflurane, had a significantly lesser incidence of postoperative nausea, vomiting, and unscheduled hospital admission.[235] Addition of nitrous oxide to a propofol anesthetic has been shown to significantly increase PONV compared to propofol alone.[226] Children undergoing strabismus surgery had a lower incidence of postoperative vomiting, a shorter recovery time, more perioperative bradycardia, and more postoperative anxiety when anesthetized with propofol-fentanyl than with thiopental-halothane.[236]

Airway Management

Mask ventilation may increase the risk of PONV[210] through increasing gastric distention. Some studies show no significant difference among airway management techniques[233] and the experience of the anesthetist may be a factor.[224]

Table 21–6. Factors Related to Operation and Anesthesia That May Modify PONV

Type and duration of operation
Type of premedication
Type of induction agent
Type of maintenance agent
Reversal of muscle relaxation
Postoperative pain and its treatment
Movement of patient

With permission from Korttila, K.: The study of post-operative nausea and vomiting. Br. J. Anaesth. 69:20, 1992

Miscellaneous

Other perioperative problems have been suggested to contribute to PONV, including hypoxemia, hypercapnia, and hypotension, but only significant decrease in blood pressure is well-documented as a contributor.[55,210]

Surgical and Anesthetic Risk Factors for PONV

Korttila defined several factors related to operation and anesthesia that may affect the incidence of PONV and may complicate interpretation of the literature, as it is difficult to separate the contribution of all these factors (Table 21–6). The type and duration of operation, type of premedication, type of induction agent, maintenance agent, reversal of muscle relaxation, postoperative pain and its treatment, and movement of the patient all may affect the occurrence of vomiting.[205]

Of the various surgical factors that may influence the incidence of PONV, the surgical site most likely has the determining effect, but the medical literature contains a myriad of studies in which confounding variables complicate this evaluation. Intra-abdominal procedures appear to have a distinctly higher risk of PONV than non-abdominal procedures.[166] Outpatient laparoscopic surgery patients may have PONV more than 50% of the time.[231,237–239] In children, the case mix is different, and the surgical site associated most commonly with an increased risk of PONV is strabismus surgery.[240]

Eye Surgery

There is high incidence (up to 80%) of PONV in both adults and children after this type of surgery,[241–244] but not all types of ocular surgery are affected: strabismus surgery is associated with a two-fold increase in PONV when compared to other types of ocular surgery.[245] PONV is the most common type of complication after strabismus surgery, but it is less frequent in the first 2 hours after surgery.[208] Two types of emesis are described; the early form which occurs in the operating room at termination of the procedure or in the PACU, and delayed emesis, which occurs later, up to 48 hours after surgery. In one study 41% of children vomited while at the hospital while 50 to 56% vomited while at home, primarily during the first day.[242] Another study shows a significant, though lesser, contribution of post-discharge PONV.[243] Yentis and Bissonnette showed a 17 to 27% incidence of

vomiting before and a 34 to 45% incidence after discharge from the hospital.[246] Others have failed to show a higher incidence in younger patients, though female sex increased the incidence of PONV.[245,247]

Several theories have been suggested to account for this high incidence of PONV in certain opthalmic procedures: traction on extraocular muscles, postoperative fluid ingestion, and stimulation of vestibular mechanisms by visual distortion. In addition to the proposed oculo-emetic reflex, which may be related to the known vagal effect of the oculo-cardiac reflex,[245] interocular mismatch between the normal and corrected eye may cause vestibular stimulation initiating a motion-sickness like syndrome.[172] The incidence of vomiting does not appear to be dependably related to the number of muscles operated,[248] spontaneous vs controlled ventilation,[248] acupuncture,[246] lidocaine,[244,249] gender,[248] use of codeine versus acetaminophen,[243] or duration of anesthesia.[248]

Because of the frequency of PONV, strabismus surgery may be an instance in which therapy or prophylaxis are appropriate.[166] Droperidol has been used successfully as prophylaxis but is associated with delayed recovery in usual doses, though smaller doses (75 µg/kg) also offer some decrease in PONV.[241,243] Metoclopramide, dixyrazine and transdermal scopolamine have been used successfully and have less risk of prolonging the recovery period.[247,250,251] The effect of lidocaine is variable.[243,249] Propofol maintenance after halothane induction results in a more rapid recovery and less PONV than halothane-N2O-O2 plus droperidol 75 µg/kg, but propofol-N2O had the same or greater incidence of PONV as did maintenance with a volatile agent.[226] The incidence of a significant oculocardiac reflex is significantly higher with propofol than with halothane-N2O.[226] Metoclopramide, droperidol and dixyrazine have been used successfully after the surgical procedure,[241,247,250] though it has been suggested that antiemetic prophylaxis may be more successful when given prior to the emetic stimulation.[251] However, Yentis and Bissonnette found no significant difference in PONV after strabismus surgery in children when comparing acupuncture, droperidol, or combined therapy, and found a high incidence of restlessness in patients treated with droperidol.[246]

ENT Surgery

The incidence of PONV after tonsillectomy and adenoidectomy in children is high, up to 76%.[230,252–254] Three reasons for the high incidence have been suggested: blood irritates gastrointestinal chemoreceptors;[233] trigeminal nerve afferents may be stimulated during surgery; and postoperative opioid administration.

Surgery of the middle ear is associated with a high incidence of PONV perhaps due to stimulation of the vestibular afferent paths involved in motion sickness; the auricular branch of the vagus may also be involved in emesis related to tympanic stimulation. The Roman practice of tickling the tympanum with a feather to provoke vomiting after gastronomic excess illustrates the efficacy of stimulation of the auricular branch of the vagus nerve.[172]

Stimulation of the pharynx readily causes gagging, retching and emesis via glossopharyngeal afferents that relay to the brain stem.

Abdominal Surgery

Intra-abdominal procedures appear to be associated with more PONV than abdominal procedures performed outside the abdominal cavity.[204] Mechanical stimulation of the gut is unavoidable during abdominal procedures, and causes discharge of vagal and splanchnic afferents that signal the CNS. In addition to afferent stimulation, increased release of 5-HT due to mechanical stimulation may activate afferents and sensitize the emetic pathways to other stimuli.[173]

Gynecologic Surgery

As mentioned, women are more sensitive than men to the emetic stimuli of the perioperative period, and thus gynecologic surgery could be expected to result in a high incidence of PONV. In addition, stimulation of the uterus, broad ligament and vaginal cervix have demonstrated afferents projecting to the spinal cord along the hypogastric and pelvic nerves. Vomiting may be more common in operations in which the vagina is packed or the cervix dilated.[204]

Although the incidence of PONV is high after diagnostic and therapeutic laparoscopy,[231,237,239,255,256] and major gynecologic surgery and hysterectomy,[238] dilation and curettage does not have this same high incidence.[213,227,257]

Postoperative Factors

Time Course

PONV dissipates within 24 hours, and is usually most intense in the initial 2 hours. However, a significant proportion of PONV occurs after discharge from the hospital in outpatient surgery patients, and failure to detect this "late" emesis may lead to misleading conclusions.

Prolonged disruption of gut function may occur after anesthesia or surgery, and the resumption of oral intake prior to return of completely normal function may provoke nausea and vomiting. This altered function is probably best described in studies of postoperative ileus. The uncomplicated postoperative ileus would be expected to resolve with 2 to 3 days; if it does not, and persists past 3 days, it may be termed paralytic postoperative ileus.[220] Postoperative ileus is most likely caused by disruption of extrinsic motility regulation, particularly in the colon; paralytic ileus involves all parts of the bowel and is probably due to disruption of local intrinsic contractile systems.[220]

Pain

Pain may provoke nausea and vomiting, perhaps through an increase in circulating catecholamines secondary to stress. It has also been suggested that pain has an arousing function that may not increase PONV so much as facilitate its expression.[172] Disagreement has existed over what role unrelieved pain may assume in

causing PONV, but one author feels that the opiates themselves probably have more of a provocative than a preventive effect on vomiting.[166]

Postoperative Fluid Intake

Postoperative fluid intake may stimulate vomiting and the mandatory intake of fluid prior to discharge from the PACU is currently controversial.[208] Mandatory fluid intake after surgery has a small but statistically significant effect on increasing the incidence of PONV and prolongation of hospital stay.[208] It is possible that withholding fluids until the child requests them may halve the incidence of PONV but this is not yet well-established. The number of readmissions for vomiting in this group is very small.

Movement

Vestibular stimulation has been shown to potentiate the emesis associated with apomorphine and morphine administration.[201,202] A history of motion sickness may increase the risk of PONV, and a significant proportion of patients who vomit after anesthesia report that movement, whether passive or active, provoked the emesis.[213]

Drug Therapy of PONV

Receptors have been identified in several regions of the brain involved in the emetic reflex, including those for acetylcholine (muscarinic), dopamine (D2), histamine (H1) and serotonin (5HT-3). Action at these receptors is the mechanism of effect of many of the antiemetic drugs. However, some drugs, such as the cannabinoids and dexamethasone, have mechanisms of action that remain obscure.[196] The action of the antiemetics is frequently not simple, as, in addition to the multiple factors that may act simultaneously to stimulate emesis, the antiemetic drugs commonly have effects at more than one type of receptor, and may have peripheral as well as central effects that contribute to the efficacy of their antiemetic action.

Because of the multitude of factors that may contribute to PONV, some drugs may be more effective in certain patients than others, but it is at present difficult to determine the primary etiology involved in a specific patient. Many drugs may have emesis as a side effect due to quite different mechanisms, such as aminoglycoside-induced emesis being related to its ototoxicity and treated with antihistamines, while cisplatin-induced nausea responds to the 5-HT3 antagonist, ondansetron.

Knowing the pathways and types of receptors involved in the process of nausea and vomiting enables one to select appropriate antiemetic agents; the lack of detailed knowledge of many of the portions of the emetic reflex involved in PONV make that rational selection more difficult. It has been proposed that a combination of drugs to block multiple types of receptors would be more effective than a higher dose of a single agent.

Prophylaxis versus Treatment

The routine prophylactic use of antiemetics to control postoperative nausea and vomiting is difficult to justify.

Since serious vomiting occurs in about 4% of patients postoperatively, over 95% of the patients would be receiving one or more drugs with admittedly little risk but less benefit and significant cumulative cost. Prophylaxis of selected patients who are at particularly high risk for PONV due to patient or procedural characteristics is more acceptable to many practitioners. Particular procedures, such as delicate eye surgery or oral surgery requiring wiring together of the jaws, may have an increased risk of significant complications when vomiting occurs, and prophylaxis may be universally indicated for these procedures.[258] The prevention of nausea and vomiting is at best only partially effective.

Antiemetic Drugs

Antimuscarinic Drugs

Scopolamine

Scopolamine is an effective antiemetic whose usage has been limited by a short duration of antiemetic effect[259] and troublesome side effects, in particular CNS disturbances including sedation, agitation and delirium. The development of a transdermal patch has offered a means to maintain low but consistent serum levels for up to three days.[237] The patch consists of an impermeable layer and a microporous membrane that holds a reservoir of the drug in mineral oil and polyisobutyline. A loading dose of 140 μg of scopolamine is in contact with the skin to achieve rapid blood levels. The patch contains a total of 1.5 mg of scopolamine and is expected to deliver the drug at a constant rate of 5 μg/hour.[237] Side effects include dry mouth, somnolence, amblyopia, mydriasis, and dizziness.[237] It may be contraindicated in patients with glaucoma or urinary obstruction.[237]

Though it is clearly effective prophylaxis for motion sickness, the efficacy of transdermal scopolamine in preventing PONV is less clear. When applied several hours preoperatively, it reduced by 50% the incidence of nausea and vomiting in outpatients undergoing laparoscopic procedures, but over a third of patients still experienced PONV.[237] Prophylactic use of the patches decreased the nausea and vomiting associated with the postoperative use of epidural morphine,[260] but was ineffective in pediatric patients undergoing ophthalmic surgery.[261] In addition, the patch had to be removed because of delirium in 5 of 21 children, one of whom was combative and hallucinating preoperatively, causing cancellation of the surgery.[261]

Antihistamines

Antihistaminic drugs may be used in the treatment of PONV and, particularly in combination with opiates, as a premedication. Common drugs with antihistaminic effects include the piperazines hydroxyzine (Vistaril), meclizine (Antivert) and cyclizine (Marezine), the ethanolamines diphenhydramine (Benadryl) and dimenhydrinate (Dramamine), and the phenothiazine promethazine (Phenergan). Hydroxyzine (Vistaril, Atarax), may be used in the perioperative period in combination with opi-

ates for potentiation of sedation and as an antiemetic; it may also be used in patients with allergic-related pruritus, as well as liver and renal failure patients with chronic itching. Less commonly used in the perioperative period, meclizine is a piperazine with minimal anticholinergic effects that is used in the treatment of vertigo and motion sickness. Diphenhydramine is used primarily to treat allergic reactions, but also for the prophylaxis of motion sickness; sedation may occur, and the elderly may have an increased risk of dizziness, sedation or hypotension. It also has significant affinity for muscarinic receptors.[262] Dimenhydrinate is the salt of diphenhydramine, and exerts a depressant effect on overly stimulated labyrinthine function and thereby inhibits the emetic effects of motion.

Dopamine Receptor Antagonists

Neuroleptic Drugs

Major tranquilizers used in the treatment of psychotic symptoms and related drugs have antiemetic effects most likely due to central dopaminergic blocking effects at the CTZ, though antihistaminic and anticholinergic effects may also be seen. Included in this group of drugs are the phenothiazines, thioxanthenes and butyrophenones. While dopamine receptor antagonists are frequently more effective antiemetics than the antihistamines, they are associated with a higher incidence of distressing CNS side effects. Most of the effective antipsychotic drugs have extrapyramidal side effects that can be very distressing to patients, and thus are as a group no longer first-line therapy in the treatment of PONV. Of this group, the butyrophenone droperidol is still frequently used in the perioperative period for its antiemetic properties, and some phenothiazines with lesser antipsychotic effects (such as promethazine and prochlorperazine) may also be useful.

Phenothiazines

The phenothiazines include prochlorperazine (Compazine), promethazine (Phenergan), thiethylperazine (Torecan), perphenazine (Trilafon) and chlorpromazine (Thorazine). Most phenothiazines have antihistaminic, anticholinergic, and antiemetic effects, but vary in antiemetic effectiveness. The antiemetic effect appears to be due to D2-receptor blockade in the CTZ, as apomorphine-induced vomiting is prevented, though motion sickness is not.[196] These drugs may cause extrapyramidal symptoms and sedation, potentiating CNS depressants. Extrapyramidal side effects (EPS) include motor restlessness, dystonias, torticollis, extensor rigidity of trunk muscles, carpopedal spasm trismus, oculogyric crises and tongue protrusion. Tardive dyskinesia is possible, but associated with chronic use, and rarely a perioperative concern. Anticholinergic effects of these agents may cause problems in patients with glaucoma, bladder neck obstruction and thermoregulatory mechanisms may be impaired. Neuroleptic malignant syndrome may occur. In general, these drugs lower the seizure threshold.

Prochlorperazine is usually well-tolerated, but has multiple potential side effects and a higher risk of EPS, especially in children or when administered parenterally. It may diminish the effect of anticoagulants; orthostatic hypotension can occur secondary to alpha-blockade. It may decrease the antihypertensive efficacy of guanethidine and related compounds. Though the seizure threshold may be lowered, Dilantin levels tend to increase EPS as do propanolol levels. Hypotension and sedation may occur. Doses for adults are 5 to 10 mg po every 4 to 6 hours, 5 to 10 mg IM every 4 hours, or 2.5 to 10 mg IV slowly every 4 hours. Suppositories and oral tablets are available.

Promethazine has less potential for EPS side effects than prochlorperazine. It has more affinity for histamine and muscarinic receptors than for dopamine receptors.[262] The primary side effect is sedation, and CNS depressants are potentiated. It can be given IM or IV in doses of 12.5 to 25 mg. Extrapyramidal symptoms may occur with higher doses.

Droperidol

Droperidol is one of the most effective drugs blocking the D2 receptor but has relatively little affinity for the H1 and muscarinic receptors.[262] Like haloperidol, it is a butyrophenone.

Complications associated with the use of droperidol are dose-related and may include hypotension, postoperative drowsiness and delayed recovery, dysphoria and extrapyramidal symptoms. One study found a significantly higher incidence of restlessness (63%) in children receiving 75 μg/kg of droperidol after induction for strabismus surgery.[246]

While very low doses of 5 μg/kg may be effective in adults and children over 11, low doses of droperidol do not seem to lower the incidence of PONV in children under the age of 11 from 54% to 27%.[263] A prophylactic dose of 75 μg/kg significantly reduced PONV in strabismus surgery with some slight prolongation of PACU stay[241,249] and 50 μg/kg in an earlier study did not.[242] However, another study found no difference between acupuncture, droperidol or combination therapy in preventing the PONV associated with strabismus surgery.[246] In adult women, droperidol 2.5 mg at the close of surgery was more effective than domperidone or metoclopramide in preventing PONV.[238] However, another study found neither droperidol or metoclopramide to be an effective prophylaxis in female outpatients.[264] Higher doses of 100 μg/kg may be associated with extrapyramidal syndromes in children,[265] and there appears to be a significant number of outpatients who develop anxiety or restlessness after discharge when droperidol 1.25 mg IV was given immediately before induction of anesthesia.[266]

It is has been suggested that it may be more efficacious to administer intravenous droperidol prior to ocular manipulation soon after induction for strabismus surgery, rather than at the end of the procedure.[243]

Domperidone

Domperidone is a benzimidazole derivative that does not cross the blood-brain barrier to a significant extent, but blocks D2 receptors in the CTZ, thus having an antiemetic effect.[110] Drowsiness is less likely and there is a very low incidence of EPS. It increases lower esophageal sphincter tone in pregnant women[41] and appears to increase peristaltic motility, but, unlike metoclopramide, this latter effect is variable and blocked by antimuscarinic agents. Its short duration of action appears to hamper its effectiveness in treating PONV.[175] Primary indications are vomiting associated with therapy for Parkinsonism and cytotoxic chemotherapy. Due to cardiac toxicity ascribed to intravenous administration, it is no longer available for that use.[196] Domperidone 20 mg IV at the end of operation was not as effective as droperidol 2.5 mg in preventing PONV in women.[238]

Metoclopramide

Metoclopramide is a dopaminergic antagonist that has central antiemetic actions and in higher doses also blocks 5-HT3 receptors.[196,262] In addition, it increases gastric emptying and LES tone, and anticholinergic agents and opiates may block its promotility effect. Metoclopramide has little effect on colonic motility. Its antiemetic action is not associated with sedation, and it is less likely than the phenothiazines to cause extrapyramidal symptoms, though these have been reported, particularly at higher doses and in children. Metoclopramide blocks emesis induced by levodopa or apomorphine, and appears to be effective in treating most types of emesis, except that associated with motion sickness. It triggers prolactin release and a temporary increase in aldosterone levels, which may result in fluid retention. It is effective in treatment of emesis following chemotherapy and in the perioperative period, but not as treatment or prophylaxis of motion sickness.

It should be avoided in patients in whom stimulation of gastrointestinal motility is contraindicated, including those with mechanical obstruction or perforation, and theoretically may increase tension on suture lines following gut anastomosis. Patients with pheochromocytoma may respond with hypertensive crisis. Metoclopramide may potentiate CNS depressants. Rapid intravenous administration may cause a transient though intense sensation of anxiety and restlessness. A usual dose in adults is 10 to 20 mg IM or IV, though much higher doses are used in prophylaxis of chemotherapy-associated emesis.

Metoclopramide 0.15 mg/kg significantly reduces the incidence and severity of PONV after strabismus surgery in children from 59% to 37% compared to placebo and significantly shortens the PACU stay.[250] In another study, this dose of metoclopramide did not significantly decrease PONV compared to placebo, while a dose of 0.25 mg/kg did significantly decrease PONV and PACU stay to a degree similar to that of droperidol 75 μg/kg; there were no cases of extrapyramidal side effects.[251] A dose of 10 mg of metoclopramide IV at the end of surgery was not as effective as 2.5 mg of droperidol in women undergoing gynecologic surgery.[238] At higher doses such as used to treat chemotherapy related emesis (1.5 to 3.0 mg/kg) it also appears to antagonize 5-HT3 receptors, which may account for some of its efficacy in this patient group.

5-HT3 RECEPTOR ANTAGONISTS

The 5-HT3 receptor antagonists include ondansetron, granisetron, and tropisetron. This group of drugs appears effective in treating the nausea and vomiting associated with cytotoxic chemotherapy, and ondansetron has been studied for its effects on PONV. In the dog, apomorphine-induced emesis is not inhibited.[267] Cytotoxic drugs and radiation cause release of serotonin from mucosal enterochromaffin cells because of damage they do to the gastrointestinal mucosa. The released serotonin may stimulate 5-HT3 receptors triggering vagal afferents that activate the vomiting reflex.[188] Vagotomy in the ferret inhibits this type of vomiting.[268] It is suggested that such serotonin release may be secondary to anesthetic effects on the gut mucosa, gastrointestinal distention related to stasis or nitrous oxide diffusion, or laparatomy with manipulation and irritation of the gut. It is theorized that an anesthetic substance could stimulate the area postrema and provoke vomiting via a pathway involving 5-HT.[268]

Ondansetron

Ondansetron (Zofran) is effective in ameliorating the emesis induced by radiation or chemotherapy, has some effectiveness in PONV but is not effective in treating motion sickness in humans, or intragastric irritants or morphine in animal models.[188,218] Thus ondansetron may be effective in abdominal surgery where 5-HT may be released but not so effective in nonabdominal surgery or in opiate-induced nausea and vomiting. Ondansetron 8 mg IV administered to women complaining of vomiting or persistent nausea after nitrous oxide-alfentanil anesthesia for gynecologic laparoscopy decreased further PONV to 51% compared to 92% for placebo.[269] Preoperative administration of ondansetron 8 mg appeared to be superior to droperidol 1.25 mg or metoclopramide 10 mg IV.[270]

Side effects of 5-HT3 antagonists reported include headache, dry mouth, diarrhea and sedation. Its lack of effect at dopaminergic, cholinergic, or histaminergic receptors should make drowsiness, dysphoria and dystonias much more uncommon than after administration of other antiemetics.[167]

Granisterone

Granisterone is another selective antagonist of 5 HT type 3 receptors and a blocker of serotonin release. It has been found more potent and longer lasting than ondansterone against cisplantin induced emesis. After general anesthesia it has a significant antiemetic action when single doses of 3.0 mg are administered intravenously. This action has been studied in a comparison with metoclopramide and found to be superior. The effect needs to be compared to ondansterone in a controlled study.[171]

Miscellaneous

Benzquinamide (Emete-con) is not related to the phenothiazines and other antiemetics, but has antiemetic, antihistaminic, and mild anticholinergic and sedative actions. It is indicated for the prevention and treatment of PONV. The usual dose is 0.5 to 1.0 mg/kg. The IM route is preferred because of reports of cardiac arrhythmias and hypertension with IV administration, so caution is advised in patients with a cardiac history.

Trimethobenzamide (Tigan) is available as capsules, suppositories, and in injectable form. Its antiemetic effects probably result from an effect at the CTZ, as the emetic effect of intragastric copper sulfate is not inhibited. It should not be administered intravenously. The usual dose in adults is 200 mg tid or qid.

Combination Therapy

Use of a combination of antiemetic agents acting at different receptors to maximize efficacy while decreasing the dose-related side effects of specific agents has been suggested by several authors and has an obvious rationale. This is commonly practiced in prophylaxing against cytotoxic-induced vomiting. Thus, in the postoperative patient who fails to respond to one emetic agent, administration of another agent with a different mechanism of action, rather than using unusually high doses of the first drug, is intuitively beneficial.

Overview

PONV is a common problem that seldom causes major complications, but increases patient distress, slows recovery and increases medical costs, and may lead to increased anxiety when further surgery and anesthesia are necessary in patients with a prior history of PONV. In a few cases, such as especially delicate surgery in critical sites, or when airway protection is compromised, emesis can lead to significant postoperative complications. Very rarely, significant trauma may follow directly from emesis, with volume depletion, electrolyte disturbances, or gastrointestinal injury resulting. Universal prophylaxis is probably not indicated because of costs and increased risk of drug reactions, but high-risk patients and procedures may be identified with increased benefit to be gained from alteration of anesthetic technique or emetic prophylaxis. However, no anesthetic technique or prophylactic regimen affords any absolute guarantee that vomiting can be prevented. For the actively vomiting patient, multiple avenues of treatment are available. Adequate treatment of pain, maintenance of intravascular volume, avoidance of sudden motion, and selection of appropriate antiemetic drugs based on knowledge of drug mechanisms can decrease the incidence, severity and complications related to recurrent postoperative vomiting. The gaps in knowledge of the particular mechanisms operant in PONV limit the efficacy of therapy for this condition, but future research advances in this area can be expected to offer further improvement in perioperative patient care and satisfaction.

REFERENCES

1. Cheek, 1987 #4541. Stewardson, R. H. and Nyhus, M. L.: Pulmonary aspiration. Arch. Surg. *112*:1192, 1977.

2. Culver, G. A., Makel, H. P. and Beecher, H. K.: Frequency of aspiration of gastric contents by lungs during anesthesia and surgery. Ann. Surg. *133*:289, 1951.
3. Boysen, P. G.: Pulmonary disease. *In* Risk and Outcome in Anesthesia. 2d Ed. Edited by D. L. Brown. Philadelphia, J. B. Lippincott Company, 1992.
4. Haleen, M. A.: Aspiration pneumonia as a cause of death. Br. J. Clin. Pract. *44*:398, 1990.
5. Endler, G. C., Mariona, F. G., Sokol, R. J. and Stevenson, L. B.: Anesthesia-related maternal mortality in Michigan, 1972 to 1984. Am. J. Obstet. Gynecol. *159*:187, 1988.
6. Cheney, F. W., Posner, K. L. and Caplan, R. A.: Adverse respiratory events infrequently leading to malpractice suits. Anesthesiology *75*:932, 1991.
7. Taylor, G.: Acid pulmonary aspiration syndrome after antacids. Br. J. Anaesth. *471*:615, 1975.
8. Shepherd, H. E., Faulkner, C. S. and Leiter, J. C.: Acute histologic effects of simulated large-volume aspiration of sucralfate into the lungs of rats. Crit. Care Med. *18*:524, 1990.
9. Gray, C., Sivaloganathan, S. and Simpkins, K. C.: Aspiration of high-density barium contrast medium causing acute pulmonary inflammation—report of two fatal cases in elderly women with disordered swallowing. Clin. Radiol. *40*:397, 1989.
10. Lode, H.: Microbiological and clinical aspects of aspiration pneumonia. J. Antimicrob. Chemother. *21*:83, 1988.
11. Wynne, J. W. and Modell, J. H.: Respiratory aspiration of stomach contents. Ann. Intern. Med. *87*:466, 1977.
12. Berson, W. and Adriani, J.: "Silent" regurgitation and aspiration during anesthesia. Anesthesiology *15*:644, 1954.
13. Blitt, C. D., *et. al.:* "Silent" regurgitation and aspiration during general anesthesia. Anesth. Analg. *49*:707, 1970.
14. Cheek, T. D. and Gutsche, B. B.: Pulmonary aspiration of gastric contents. *In* Anesthesia for Obstetrics. 3d Ed. Edited by S. M. Shnider and G. Levinson. Baltimore, Williams and Wilkins, 1993.
15. Mendelson, C. L.: Aspiration of stomach contents into lungs during obstetric anesthesia. Am. J. Obstet Gynecol. *52*:191, 1946.
16. Olsson, G. L., Hallen, B. and Hambraeus-Jonzon: Aspiration during anesthesia: a computer-aided study of 185,358 anaesthetics. Acta. Anaesthesiol. Scand. *30*:84, 1986.
17. Tiret, L., Desmonts, J. M., Hatton, F. and Vourc'h, G.: Complications associated with anaesthesia—a prospective survey in France. Can. Anaesth. Soc. J. *33*:336, 1986.
18. Wang, L. P. and Hagerdal, M.: Reported anesthetic complications during an 11-year period: a retrospective study. Acta. Anaesthesiol. Scand. *36*:234, 1992.
19. Edwards, G., Morton, H. J. V., Pask, E. A. and Wylie, W. D.: Deaths associated with anesthesia. Anaesthesia *11*:194, 1956.
20. Leigh, J. M. and Tytler, J. A.: Admissions to the intensive care unit after complications of anaesthetic techniques over 10 years: the second 5 years. Anaesthesia *45*:814, 1990.
21. Scott, D. B.: Mendelson's syndrome (editorial). Br. J. Anaesth. *50*:977, 1978.
22. Bannister, W. K. and Sattilaro, A. J.: Vomiting and aspiration during anesthesia. Anesthesiology *23*:251, 1962.
23. Teabeaut, J. R.: Aspiration of gastric contents: an experimental study. Am. J. Pathol. *28*:51, 1952.
24. Roberts, R. B. and Shirley, M. A.: Reducing the risk of acid aspiration during cesarean section. Anesth. Analg. *53*:859, 1974.
25. Roberts, R. B. and Shirley, M. A.: Antacid therapy in obstetrics (letter). Anesthesiology *53*:83, 1980.
26. Raidoo, D. M., *et al.:* Critical volume for pulmonary acid aspiration: reappraisal in a primate model. Br. J. Anaesth. *65*:248, 1990.
27. Gorback, M. S.: Cut-off values and aspiration risk. Anesth. Analg. *69*:417, 1989.
28. Maltby, J. R. and Shaffer, E. A.: Measurement of gastric contents. Can. J. Anaesth. 597, 1990.
29. Manchikanti, L., Canella, M. G., Hohlbein, L. J. and Colliver, J. A.: Assessment of effect of various modes of premedication on acid aspiration risk factors in outpatient surgery. Anesth. Analg. *66*:81, 1987.
30. Hardy, J. F., Lepage, Y. and Bonneville-Chouinard, N.: Occurrence of gastroesophageal reflux on induction of anaesthesia does not correlate with the volume of gastric contents. Can. J. Anaesth. *37*:502, 1990.
31. Cheek, T. G. and Gutsche, B. B.: Pulmonary aspiration of gastric contents. *In* Anesthesia for Obstetrics. 2d Ed. Edited by S. M. Levinson and G. Levinson. Baltimore, Williams and Wilkins, 1987.
32. Huxley, E. J., Viroslav, J., Gray, W. R. and Pierce, A. K.: Pharyngeal aspiration in normal adults and patients with depressed consciousness. Am. J. Med. *64*:564, 1978.
33. Horner, J. and Massey, E. W.: Silent aspiration following stroke. Neurology *38*:317, 1988.
34. DeVita, M. A. and Spierer-Rundback, L.: Swallowing disorders in patients with prolonged orotracheal intubation or tracheostomy tubes. Crit. Care Med. *18*:1328, 1990.
35. Pontoppidan, H.: Progressive loss of protective reflexes in the airway with the advance of age. JAMA *174*:2209, 1960.
36. Vanner, R. G., O'Dwyer, J. P., Pryle, B. J. and Reynolds, F.: Upper oesophageal sphincter pressure and the effect of cricoid pressure. Anaesthesia *47*:95, 1992.
37. Vanner, R. G., Pryle, B. J., O'Dwyer, J. P. and Reynolds, F.: Upper esophageal sphincter pressure and the intravenous induction of anaesthesia. Anaesthesia *47*:371, 1992.
38. Wraight, W. J., Chamney, A. R. and Howells, T. H.: The determination of an effective cricoid pressure. Anaesthesia *38*:461, 1983.
39. Cotton, B. R. and Smith, G.: The lower esophageal sphincter and anaesthesia. Br. J. Anaesth. *56*:37, 1984.
40. La Cour, D.: Rise in intragastric pressure caused by suxamethonium fasciculations. Acta Anaesthesiol. Scand. *13*:255, 1969.
41. Brock-Utne, J. G., *et al.:* Effect of domperidone on lower esophageal sphincter tone in late pregnancy. Anesthesiology *52*:321, 1980.
42. Tweedle, D. and Nightingale, P.: Anesthesia and gastrointestinal surgery. Acta Chir. Scand. Suppl. *550*:131, 1988.
43. Brock-Utne, J. G., *et al.:* The action of commonly used antiemetics on the lower esophageal sphincter. Br. J. Anaesth. *50*:295, 1978.
44. Adelhoj, B., Petring, O. U. and Hagelsten, J. O.: Inaccuracy of peranesthetic gastric intubation for emptying liquid stomach contents. Acta Anaesthesiol. Scand. *30*:41, 1986.
45. Gibbs, C. P., *et al.:* Antacid pulmonary aspiration in the dog. Anesthesiology *51*:380, 1979.
46. Manchikanti, L., Colliver, J. A., Marrero, T. C. and Roush, J.R.: Assessment of age-related acid aspiration risk factors in pediatric, adult, and geriatric patients. Anesth. Analg. *64*:11, 1985.
47. Schurizek, B. A., Rybro, L., Boggild-Madsen, N. B. and Juhl, B.: Gastric volume and pH in children for emergency surgery. Acta Anaesthesiol. Scand. *30*:404, 1986.
48. Wright, D. J. and Pandya, A.: Smoking and gastric juice volume in outpatients. Can. Anaesth. Soc. J. *26*:328, 1979.
49. Adelhoj, B., *et al.:* Influence of cigarette smoking on the

risk of acid pulmonary aspiration. Acta Anaesthesiol. Scand. *31*:7, 1987.

50. Zibrak, J. D., Jensen, W. A. and Bloomingdale, K.: Aspiration pneumonitis following electroconvulsive therapy in patients with gastroparesis. Biol. Psychiatry *24*:812, 1988.

51. Adelhoj, B., Petring, O. U. and Frosig, F.: The effect of spinal analgesia and surgery on peroperative drug absorption and gastric emptying in man. Acta Anaesthesiol. Scand. *31*:165, 1987.

52. Craven, D. E., Steger, K. A., Barat, L. M. and Duncan, R. A.: Nosocomial pneumonia epidemiology and infection control. Intensive Care Med. *18*:S3, 1992.

53. Tryba, M.: The gastropulmonary route of infection—fact or fiction? Am. J. Med. *91 (Suppl. 2A)*:135, 1991.

54. Weiss, W.: Regurgitation and aspiration of gastric contents during inhalation anesthesia. Anesthesiology *11*:102, 1950.

55. Ratra, C. K., Badola, R. P. and Bhargava, K. P.: A study of factors concerned in emesis during spinal anesthesia. Br. J. Anaesth. *44*:1208, 1972.

56. Brock-Utne, J. G., Rout, C., Moodley, J. and Mayat, N.: Influence of preoperative gastric aspiration on the volume and pH of gastric contents in obstetric patients undergoing caesarean section. Br. J. Anaesth. *62*:397, 1989.

57. Goresky, G. V. and Malty, J. R.: Fasting guidelines for elective surgical patients. Can. J. Anaesth. *37*:493, 1990.

58. Hutchinson, B. R., Merry, A. F. and Wild, C. J.: The relationship of duration of fast to the volume and pH of gastric contents. Anaesth. Intensive Care *14*:128, 1986.

59. Maltby, J. R., Sutherland, A. D., Sale, J. P. and Shaffer, E. A.: Preoperative oral fluids: is a five-hour fast justified prior to elective surgery? Anesth. Analg. *65*:1112, 1986.

60. Crawford, M., Lerman, J., Christensen, S. and Farrow-Gillespie, A.: Effects of duration of fasting on gastric fluid pH and volume in healthy children. Anesth. Analg. *71*:400, 1990.

61. Schreiner, M. S., Triebwasser, A. and Keon, T. P.: Ingestion of liquids compared with preoperative fasting in pediatric outpatients. Anesthesiology *72*:593, 1990.

62. Splinter, W. M., Schaefer, J. D. and Zunder, I. H.: Clear fluids three hours before surgery do not affect the gastric fluid contents of children. Can. J. Anaesth. *37*:498, 1990.

63. Agarwal, A., Chari, P. and Singh, H.: Fluid deprivation before operation: the effect of a small drink. Anaesthesia *44*:632, 1989.

64. Dalton, C. and Gudgeon, C. W.: Fasting or feeding during labor (letter). Med. J. Aust. *147*:625, 1987.

65. Michael, S., Reilly, C. S. and Caunt, J.A.: Policies for oral intake during labour. Anaesthesia *46*:1071, 1991.

66. Bricker, S. R. W., McLuckie, A. and Nightingale, D. A.: Gastric aspirates after trauma in children. Anaesthesia *44*:721, 1989.

67. Gibbs, C. P., Rolbin, S. H. and Norman, P.: Cause and prevention of maternal aspiration (letter). Anesthesiology *61*:111, 1984.

68. Kopman, A. F., Wollman, S. B., Ross, K. and Surks, S. N.: Awake endotracheal intubation: a review of 267 cases. Anesth. Analg. *54*:323, 1975.

69. Thomas, J. L.: Awake intubation. Indications, techniques and a review of 25 patients. Anaesthesia *24*:28, 1969.

70. Schrader, S., Ovassapian, A., Dykes, M. H. M. and Avram, M.: Cardiovascular changes during awake rigid and fiberoptic laryngoscopy. Anesthesiology *67*:A28, 1987.

71. Ovassapian, A., Yelich, S. J., Dykes, M. H. M. and Golman, M. E.: Blood pressure and heart rate changes during awake fiberoptic nasotracheal intubation. Anesth. Analg. *62*:951, 1983.

72. Kingston, G. W., Phang, P. T. and Leathley, M. J.: Increased incidence of nosocomial pneumonia in mechanically ventilated patients with subclinical aspiration. Am. J. Surg. *161*:589, 1991.

73. Pearson, J. E. G. and Wilson, R. S. E.: Diffuse pulmonary fibrosis and hernia. Thorax *26*:300, 1971.

74. Editorial, L.: Routine H2-receptor antagonists before elective surgery. Lancet *1*:1363, 1989.

75. Escolano, F., *et al.*: Comparison of the effects of famotidine and ranitidine on gastric secretion in patients undergoing elective surgery. Anaesthesia *44*:22, 1989.

76. Manchikanti, L., Kraus, J. W. and Edds, S. P.: Cimetidine and related drugs anesthesia. Anesth. Analg. *61*:595, 1982.

77. Randell, T., Saarnivaara, L., Oikkonen, M. and Lindgren, L.: Oral atropine enhances the risk for acid aspiration in children. Acta Anaesthesiol. Scand. *35*:65, 1991.

78. Tordoff, S. G. and Sweeney, B. P.: Acid aspiration prophylaxis in 288 obstetric anaesthetic departments in the United Kingdom. Anaesthesia *1990*:776, 1990.

79. Manchikanti, L., Grow, J. B. and Collivier, J. A.: Bicitra (sodium citrate) and metoclopramide in outpatient anesthesia for prophylaxis against aspiration pneumonitis. Anesthesiology *63*:378, 1985.

80. Mathews, H. M. I. and Moore, J.: Sodium bicarbonate as a single dose antacid in obstetric anaesthesia. Anaesthesia *44*:590, 1989.

81. James, C. F., *et al.*: Pulmonary aspiration—effects of volume and pH in the rat. Anesth. Analg. *63*:665, 1984.

82. Bannister, W. K., Sattilaro, A. J. and Otis, R. D.: Therapeutic aspects of aspiration pneumonitis in experimental animals. Anesthesiology *22*:440, 1961.

83. Giannella, R. A., Broitman, S. A. and Zamcheck, N.: Gastric acid barrier to ingested microorganisms in man: studies in vivo and in vitro. Gut *13*:251, 1972.

84. Mahul, P., *et al.*: Prevention of nosocomial pneumonia in intubated patients: respective role of mechanical subglottic secretions drainage and stress ulcer prophylaxis. Intensive Care Med *18*:20, 1992.

85. Driks, M. R., *et al.*: Nosocomial pneumonia in intubated patients given sucralfate as compared with antacids or histamine type 2 blockers. N. Engl. J. Med. *317*:, 1987.

86. Kappstein, I., *et al.*: The incidence of pneumonia in mechanically ventilated patients treated with sucralfate or cimetidine as prophylaxis for stress bleeding: bacterial colonization of the stomach. Am. J. Med. *91 (Suppl 2A)*:125, 1991.

87. Tryba, M.: Risk of acute stress bleeding and nosocomial pneumonia in ventilated intensive care unit patients: sucralfate versus antacids. Am. J. Med. *83 (suppl 3B)*:117, 1987.

88. Hurwitz, A., *et al.*: Prolongation of gastric emptying by sucralfate in man. Gastroenterology *82*:1088, 1982.

89. Lewis, J. H.: Hepatic effects of drugs used in the treatment of peptic ulcer disease. Am. J. Gastroenterol. *82*:987, 1987.

90. Henry, D. A., *et al.*: Cimetidine and rantidine: comparison of effects on hepatic drug metabolism. BMJ *281*:775, 1980.

91. Dailey, P. A., *et al.*: Effect of cimetidine and rantidine on lidocaine concentrations during epidural anesthesia for cesarean section. Anesthesiology *69*:1013, 1988

92. Kishikawa, K., Namiki, A., Miyashita, K. and Saitoh, K.: Effects of famotidine and cimetidine on plasma levels of epidurally administered lignocaine. Anaesthesia *45*:719, 1990.

93. Singh, B. N., Opie, L. H. and Marcus, F. I.: Antiarrhythmic agents. *In* Drugs for the Heart. 3d Ed. Edited by L. H. Opie. Philadelphia, W. B. Saunders, 1991.

94. Flynn, R. J., Moore, J., Collier, P. S. and McClean, E.: Does pretreatment with cimetidine and ranitidine affect the disposition of bupivacaine? Br. J. Anaesth. *62*:87, 1989.

95. Hodgkinson, R., Glassenberg, R. and Joyce, T. H.: Safety and efficacy of cimetidine and antacid in reducing gastric acidity before elective cesarean section. Anesthesiology 57:A408, 1982.

96. Steinberg, W. M., Lewis, J. H. and Katz, D. M.: Antacids inhibit absorption of cimetidine. N. Engl. J. Med. 307:400, 1982.

97. Zeldis, J. R., Friedman, L. S. and Isselbacher, K. J.: Ranitidine: a new H2-receptor antagonist. N. Engl. J. Med. 309:1368, 1983.

98. Hoensch, H. P., Hutzel, H., Kirch, W. and Ohnhaus, E. E.: Isolation of human hepatic microsomes and their inhibition by cimetidine and ranitidine. Eur. J. Clin. Pharmacol. 29:199, 1985.

99. Spahn, H., et al.: Influence of ranitidine on plasma metoprolol and atenolol concentrations. BMJ 286:1546, 1983.

100. Brock-Utne, J. G., Downing, J. W. and Humphrey, D.: Effect of ranitidine given before atropine sulphate on lower esophageal sphincter tone. Anaesth. Intensive Care 12:140, 1984.

101. Andrews, A. D., Brock-Utne, J. G. and Downing, J. W.: Protection against pulmonary acid aspiration with ranitidine. Anaesthesia 37:22, 1982.

102. Jahr, J. S., et al.: Effects of famotidine on gastric pH and residual volume in pediatric surgery. Acta Anaesthesiol. Scand. 35:457, 1991.

103. Klotz, U., Arvela, P. and Rosenkranz, B.: Famotidine, a new H2-receptor antagonist, does not affect hepatic elimination of diazepam or tubular secretion of procainamide. Eur. J. Clin. Pharmacol. 28:671, 1985.

104. Cruickshank, R. H., Morrison, D. A., Bamber, P. A. and Nimmo, W. S.: Effect of IV omeprazole on the pH and volume of gastric contents before surgery. Br. J. Anaesth. 63:536, 1989.

105. Moore, J., et al.: Effect of single-dose omeprazole on intragastric acidity and volume during obstetric anaesthesia. Anaesthesia 44:559, 1989.

106. Ng Wingtin, L., Glomaud, D., Hardy, F. and Phil, S.: Omeprazole for prophylaxis of acid aspiration in elective surgery. Anaesthesia 45:436, 1990.

107. Gin, T., Ewart, M. C., Yau, G. and Oh, T. E.: Effect of oral omeprazole on intragastric pH and volume in women undergoing elective cesarean sections. Br. J. Anaesth. 65:616, 1990.

108. Bateman, D. N., Rawlins, M. D. and Simpson, J. M.: Extrapyramidal reactions with metoclopramide. BMJ 293:930, 1985.

109. Kris, M. G., et al.: Extrapyramidal reactions with high-dose metoclopramide. N. Engl. J. Med. 309:433, 1983.

110. Fragen, R. J. and Caldwell, N.: A new benzimidazole antiemetic, domperidone, for the treatment of postoperative nausea and vomiting. Anesthesiology 49:289, 1978.

111. Creytens, G.: Effect of the non-antidopaminergic drug cisapride on postprandial nausea. Current Therapeutic Research 36:1063, 1984.

112. Hodges, R. J. H., Bennett, J. R., Tunstall, M. E. and Knight, R. F.: General anesthesia for operative obstetrics, with special reference to the use of thiopentone and suxamethonium. Br. J. Anaesth. 31:152, 1959.

113. Sellick, B. A.: Cricoid pressure to control regurgitation of stomach contents during induction of anesthesia. Lancet 2:404, 1961.

114. Walts, L. F.: Anesthesia of the larynx in the patient with a full stomach. JAMA 192:705, 1965.

115. Claeys, D. W., Lockhard, C. H. and Hinkle, J. E.: The effects of translaryngeal block and Innovar on glottic competence. Anesthesiology 38:485, 1973.

116. Asai, T.: Use of the laryngeal mask for tracheal intubation in patients at increased risk of aspiration of gastric contents. Anesthesiology 77:1029, 1992.

117. Brain, A. I. J.: Three cases of difficult intubation overcome by the larygneal mask airway. Anaesthesia 40:353, 1985.

118. Benumof, J. L.: Laryngeal mask airway: indications and contraindications. Anesthesiology 77:843, 1992.

119. Koehli, N.: Aspiration and the laryngeal mask airway. Anaesthesia 46:419, 1991.

120. Nanji, G. M. and Maltby, J. R.: Vomiting and aspiration pneumonitis with the laryngeal mask airway. Can. J. Anaesth. 39:69, 1992.

121. Ovassapian, A., Krejcie, T. C., Yelich, S. J. and Dykes, M. H. M.: Awake fibreoptic intubation in the patient at high risk of aspiration. Br. J. Anaesth. 62:13, 1989.

122. Yealy, D. M., et al.: Manual translaryngeal jet ventilation and the risk of aspiration in a canine model. Ann. Emerg. Med. 19:1238, 1990.

123. Editorial. Anaesthesia 6:189, 1951.

124. Morgan, M.: Anaesthetic contribution to maternal mortality. Br. J. Anaesth. 59:842, 1987.

125. Fassoulaki, A. and Athanassiou, E.: Cardiovascular responses to the insertion of nasogastric tubes during general anesthesia. Can. Anaesth. Soc. J. 32:651, 1985.

126. Salem, M. R., Wong, A. Y. and Fizzotti, G. F.: Efficacy of cricoid pressure in preventing aspiration of gastric content in pediatric patients. Br. J. Anaesth. 44:401, 1972.

127. Wycoff, C. C.: Aspiration during induction of anesthesia. Anesth. Analg. 38:5, 1959.

128. Elliott, C. J. R.: A study in regurgitation. Anaesthesia 18:324, 1963.

129. Stept, W. J. and Safar, P.: Rapid induction/intubation for prevention of gastric-content aspiration. Anesth. Analg. 49:633, 1970.

130. Howells, T. H., Chamney, A. R., Wraight, W. J. and Simon, R. S.: The application of cricoid pressure. An assessment and a survey of its practice. Anaesthesia 38:457, 1983.

131. Davies, J. M., Weeks, S., Crone, L. A. and Pavlin, E.: Difficult intubation in the parturient. Can. J. Anaesth. 36:668, 1989.

132. Lincoff, H. A., et al.: The effect of succinylcholine on intraocular pressure. Am. J. Ophthalmol. 40:501, 1955.

133. La Cour, D.: Prevention of rise in intragastric pressure due to suxamethonium fasciculations by prior dose of d-tubocurarine. Acta Anaesthesiol. Scand. 14:5, 1970.

134. Barr, A. M. and Thornley, B. A.: Thiopentone and suxamethonium crash induction. An assessment of the potential hazards. Anaesthesia 31:23, 1976.

135. Khawaja, A. A.: A rapid intubation technique for prevention of aspiration during induction of anaesthesia. Br. J. Anaesthesia 43:980, 1971.

136. Fanning, G. L.: The efficacy of cricoid pressure in preventing regurgitation of gastric contents. Anesthesiology 32:553, 1970.

137. Chraemmer B., et al.: Does alfentanil preserve left ventricular pump function during rapid sequence induction of anaesthesia. Acta Anaesthesiol. Scand. 36:362, 1992.

138. Marx, G. F., et al.: Hazards of "crash" induction-intubation techniques. N.Y. State J. Med. 68:1957, 1968.

139. Birmingham, P. K., Cheney, F. W. and Ward, R. J.: Esophageal intubation: a review of detection techniques. Anesth. Analg. 65:886, 1986.

140. Ping, S. T. S.: Letter. Anesth. Analg. 66:483, 1987.

141. Tunstall, M. E.: Failed intubation in the parturient (editorial). Can. J. Anaesth. 36:611, 1989.

142. Lyons, G.: Failed intubation: six years' experience in a teaching maternity unit. Anaesthesia 40:759, 1985.

143. Rosen, M.: Difficult and failed intubation in obstetrics. *In* Difficulties in Tracheal Intubation. Edited by Latto, I.P. and Rosen, M. East Sussex, England, Bailliere Tindall, 1985.

144. Bernhard, W. N., *et al.*: Adjustment of intracuff pressure to prevent aspiration. Anesthesiology *50*:363, 1979.

145. MacRae, W. and Wallace, P.: Aspiration around high-volume, low-pressure endotracheal cuff (letter). BMJ *283*:1220, 1981.

146. Pavlin, E. G., Van Nimwegan, D. and Hornbein, T. F.: Failure of a high-compliance low-pressure cuff to prevent aspiration. Anesthesiology *42*:216, 1975.

147. Browning, D. H. and Graves, S. A.: Incidence of aspiration with endotracheal tubes in children. J. Pediatr. *102*:582, 1983.

148. Petring, O. U., *et al.*: Prevention of silent aspiration due to leaks around-cuffs of endotracheal tubes. Anesth. Analg. *65*:777, 1986.

149. Hickling, K. G. and Howard, R.: A retrospective survey of treatment and mortality in aspiration pneumonia. Intensive Care Med. *14*:617, 1988.

150. Wolfe, J. E., Bone, R. C. and Ruth, W. E.: Diagnosis of gastric aspiration by fiberoptic bronchoscopy. Chest *70*:458, 1976.

151. Merrill, R. B. and Hingson, R. A.: Study of incidence of maternal mortality from aspiration of vomitus during anesthesia occurring in major obstetric hospitals in United States. Anesth. Analg. *30*:121, 1951.

152. Grimbert, F. A., Parker, J. C. and Taylor, A. E.: Increased pulmonary vascular permeability following acid aspiration. Am. J. Physiol. 335, 1981.

153. Long, R., Breen, P. H., Mayers, I. and Wood, L. D. H.: Treatment of canine aspiration pneumonitis: fluid volume reduction vs. fluid volume expansion. Am. J. Physiol. 1736, 1988.

154. Bynum, L. J. and Pierce, A. K.: Pulmonary aspiration of gastric contents. Am. Rev. Resp. Dis. *114*:1129, 1976.

155. Nagase, T., *et al.*: Intravenous bolus of prednisolone decreases 15-hydroxyeicosatetraenoic acid formation in the rat model of acid aspiration. Crit. Care Med. *19*:950, 1991.

156. Kobayashi, T., *et al.*: Lung lavage and surfactant replacement for hydrochloric acid aspiration in rabbits. Acta Anaesthesiol. Scand. *34*:216, 1990.

157. Cormack, R. S. and Lehane, J.: Difficult tracheal intubation in obstetrics. Anaesthesia *39*:1105, 1984.

158. Heimlich, H.: A life-saving manuever to prevent food-choking. JAMA *234*:398, 1975.

159. Taylor, G. and Pryse-Davies, J.: Evaluation of endotracheal steroid therapy in acid pulmonary aspiration syndrome (Mendelson's syndrome). Anesthesiology *29*:17, 1968.

160. Bernard, *et al.*: High-dose corticosteroids in patients with the adult respiratory distress syndrome. N. Engl. J. Med. *317*:1565, 1987.

161. Barrowcliffe, M. P. and Jones, J. G.: Pulmonary clearance of 99mTc-DTPA in the diagnosis and evolution of increased permeability pulmonary edema. Anaesth. Intens. Care *17*:422, 1989.

162. Chapman, R. L., *et al.*: Effect of continuous postive pressure ventilation and steroids on aspiration of hydrochloric acid (pH 1.8) in dogs. Anesth. Analg. *53*:556, 1974.

163. Toung, T. J. K., *et al.*: Aspiration pneumonia: experimental evaluation of albumin and steroid therapy. Ann. Surg. *183*:179, 1976.

164. Polgieter, P. D. and Hammond, J. M. J.: Etiology and diagnosis of pneumonia requiring ICU admission. Chest *101*:199, 1992.

165. Suchyta, M. R., *et al.*: The adult respiratory distress syndrome: a report of survival and modifying factors. Chest *101*:1074, 1992.

166. Lerman, J.: Surgical and patient factors involved in postoperative nausea and vomiting. Br. J. Anaesth. *69 (Suppl. 1)*:24, 1992.

167. Kapur, P. A.: Editorial: The big "little problem." Anesth Analg *73*:243, 1991.

168. Gold, B. S., Kitz, D. S., Lecky, J. H. and Neuhaus, J. M.: Unanticipated admission to the hospital following ambulatory surgery. JAMA *262*:3008, 1989.

169. Meridy, H. W.: Criteria for selection of ambulatory surgical patients and guidelines for anesthetic management: a retrospective study of 1553 cases. Anesth. Analg. *61*:921, 1982.

170. Patel, R. I. and Hannallah, R. S.: Anesthetic complications following pediatric ambulatory surgery: a 3-year study. Anesthesiology *69*:1009, 1988.

171. Green, G. and Jonsson, L.: Nausea: the most important factor determining length of stay after ambulatory anesthesia. Acta Anaesthesiol. Scand. *37*:742, 1993.

172. Andrews, P. L. R.: Physiology of nausea and vomiting. Br. J. Anaesth. *69 (Suppl. 1)*:2, 1992.

173. Andrews, P. L. and Hawthorn, J.: Neurophysiology of vomiting. Baillieres Clin. Gastroenterol. *2*:141, 1988.

174. Harding, R. K.: Concepts and conflicts in the mechanism of emesis. Can. J. Physiol. Pharmacol. *68*:218, 1990.

175. Clarke, R. S. J.: Nausea and vomiting. Br. J. Anaesth. *56*:19, 1984.

176. Lang, I. M.: Digestive tract motor correlates of vomiting and nausea. Can. J. Physiol. Pharmacol. *68*:242, 1990.

177. Smith, C. C. and Brizzee, K. R.: Cineradiographic analysis of vomiting in the cat. Gastroenterology *40*:654, 1961.

178. McCarthy, L. E. and Borison, H. L.: Respiratory mechanics of vomiting in decerebrate cats. Am. J. Physiol. *226*:738, 1974.

179. McCarthy, L. E., Borison, H. L., Spiegel, P. K. and Friedlander, R. M.: Vomiting: Radiographic and oscillographic correlates in the decerebrate cat. Gastroenterology *67*:1126, 1974.

180. Brizzee, K. R.: Mechanics of vomiting: a minireview. Can. J. Physiol. Pharmacol. *68*:221, 1990.

181. Tan, L. K. and Miller, A. D.: Innervation of periesophageal region of cat's diaphragm: implication for studies of control of vomiting. Neurosci. Lett. *68*:339, 1986.

182. Borison, H. L. and Wang, S. C.: Physiology and pharmacology of vomiting. Pharmacol. Rev. *5*:193, 1953.

183. Miller, A. D. and Wilson, V. J.: "vomiting center" reanalyzed: an electrical stimulation study. Brain Res. *270*:154, 1983.

184. Brizzee, K. R. and Mehler, W. R.: The central nervous connections involved in the vomiting reflex. *In* Nausea and Vomiting: Mechanisms and Treatment. Edited by Davis, C. J., Lake-Bakaar, G. V. and Grahame-Smith, D. G. Berlin, Springer-Verlag, 1986.

185. Davis, C. J., Harding, R. K., Leslie, R. A. and Andrews, P. L. R.: The organization of vomiting as a protective reflex. *In* Nausea and Vomiting: Mechanisms and Treatment. Edited by Davis, C. J., Lake-Bakaar, G. V. and Grahame-Smith, D. G. Berlin, Springer-Verlag, 1986.

186. Lee, K. Y., Park, H. J. and Chey, W. Y.: Studies on mechanism of retching and vomiting in dogs. Dig. Dis. Sci. *30*:22, 1985.

187. Azpiroz, F. and Malagelada, J.-R.: Pressure activity patterns in the canine proximal stomach: response to distension. Am. J. Physiol. *247*:G265, 1984.

188. Andrews, P. L. R., *et al.*: The abdominal visceral innervation and the emetic reflex: pathways, pharmacology, and plasticity. Can. J. Physiol. Pharmacol. *68*:325, 1990.

189. Blackshaw, L. A., Grundy, D. and Scratcherd, T.: Vagal af-

ferent discharge from gastric mechanoreceptors during contraction and relaxation of the ferret corpus. J. Auton. Nerv. Syst. *18*:19, 1987.

190. Blackshaw, L. A., Grundy, D. and Scratcherd, T.: Involvement of gastrointestinal mechano- and intestinal chemoreceptors in vagal reflexes: an electrophysiological study. J. Auton. Nerv. Syst. *18*:225, 1987.

191. Sleight, P.: Cardiac vomiting. Br. Heart J. *46*:5, 1981.

192. Borison, H. L.: Anatomy and physiology of the chemoreceptor trigger zone and area postrema. *In* Nausea and vomiting: mechanisms and treatment. Edited by Davis, C. J., Lake-Bakaar, G. V. and Grahame-Smith, D. G. Berlin, Springer-Verlag, 1984.

193. Stott, J. R. R.: Mechanisms and treatment of motion illness. *In* Nausea and vomiting: mechanisms and treatment. Edited by Davis, C. J., Lake-Bakaar, G. V. and Grahame-Smith, D. G. Berlin, Springer-Verlag, 1986.

194. Wang, S. C. and Chinn, H. L.: Experimental motion sickness in dogs: functional importance of chemoreceptive emetic trigger zone. Am. J. Physiol. *178*:111, 1954.

195. Young, R. W.: Mechanisms and treatment of radiation-induced nausea and vomiting. *In* Nausea and vomiting: mechanisms and treatment. Edited by Davis, C. H., Lake-Bakaar, G. V. and Grahame-Smith, D. G. Berlin, Springer-Verlag, 1986.

196. Mitchelson. F.: Pharmacological agents affecting emesis: a review (part I). Drugs *43*:295, 1992a.

197. Beleslin, D. B. and Strbac, M.: Noradrenaline-induced emesis: alpha 2 adrenoceptor mediation in the area postrema. Neuropharmacology *26*:1157, 1987.

198. Gilman, S. and Winans, S. S.: The vestibular system. *In* Essentials of Clinical Neuroanatomy and Neurophysiology. Sixth. Edited by Philadelphia, F. A. Davis, 1982.

199. Wang, S. C. and Chinn, H. I.: Experimental motion sickness in dogs: importance of labyrinth and vestibular cerebellum. Am. J. Physiol. *185*:617, 1956.

200. Wang, S. C., Chinn, H. I. and Renzi, A. A.: Experimental motion sickness in dogs: role of abdominal visceral afferents. Am. J. Physiol. *190*:578, 1957.

201. Rubin, A. and Winston, J.: The role of the vestibular apparatus in the production of nausea and vomiting following the administration of morphine to man. J Clin Invest *29*:1261, 1950.

202. Isaacs, B.: The influence of head and body position on the emetic action of paomorphine in man. Clin. Sci. *16*:215, 1957.

203. Wetchler, B. V.: Postoperative nausea and vomiting in daycase surgery. Br. J. Anaesth. *69 (Suppl. 1)*:33, 1992.

204. Palazzo, M. G. A. and Strunin, L.: Anesthesia and emesis. I: etiology. Can Anaesth Soc J *31*:178, 1984.

205. Korttila, K.: The study of post-operative nausea and vomiting. Br. J. Anaesth. *69*:20, 1992.

206. Cohen, M. M., Cameron, C. B. and Duncan, P. G.: Pediatric anesthesia morbidity and mortality in the perioperative period. Anesth Analg *70*:160, 1990.

207. Cohen, M. M., Duncan, P. G., Pope, W. D. B. and Wolkenstein, C.: A survey of 112,000 anesthetics at one teaching hospital (1975–83). Can Anaesth Soc J *33*:22, 1986.

208. Schreiner, M. S., Nicolson, S. C., Martin, T. and Whitney, L.: Should children drink before discharge from day surgery? Anesthesiology *76*:528, 1992.

209. Muir, J. J., *et al.*: Role of nitrous oxide and other factors in postoperative nausea and vomiting: a randomized and blinded prospective study. Anesthesiology *66*:513, 1987.

210. Bellville, J. W., Bross, I. D. J. and Howland, W. S.: Postoperative nausea and vomiting IV: factors related to postoperative nausea and vomiting. Anesthesiology *21*:186, 1960.

211. Beattie, W. S., Lindblad, T., Buckley, D. N. and Forrest, J. B.: The incidence of postoperative nausea and vomiting in women undergoing laparoscopy is influenced by the day of menstrual cycle. Can J Anaesth *38*:298, 1991.

212. Honkevaara, P., Lehtinen, A.-M., Hovorka, J. and Korttila, K.: Nausea and vomiting after gynecological laparoscopy depends upon the phase of the menstrual cycle. Can J Anaesth *38*:876, 1991.

213. Kamath, B., *et al.*: Anesthesia, movement and emesis. Br. J. Anaesth. *64*:728, 1990.

214. Watcha, M. F. and White, P. F.: Postoperative nausea and vomiting. Anesthesiology 77:162, 1992.

215. Costello, D. J. and Borison, H. L.: Naloxone antagonizes narcotic self-blockade of emesis in the cat. J. Pharmacol. Exp. Ther. *203*:222, 1977.

216. Barnes, N. M., Bunce, K. T., Naylor, R. J. and Rudd, J. A.: The actions of fentanyl to inhibit drug-induced emesis. Neuropharmacology *30*:1073, 1991.

217. Thompson, P. I., *et al.*: Morphine 6-glucuronide: a metabolite of morpine with greater emetic potency than morphine in the ferret. Br J Pharmacol *106*:3, 1992.

218. Bhandari, P., Bingham, S. and Andrews, P. L. R.: The neuropharmacology of loperamide-induced emesis in the ferret: the role of the area postrema, vagus, opiate and 5-HT3 receptors. Neuropharmacology *31*:735, 1992.

219. Carpenter, D. O.: Neural mechanisms of emesis. Can J Physiol Pharmacol *68*:230, 1990.

220. Livingstone, E. H. and Passaro, E. P.: Postoperative ileus. Dig. Dis. Sci. *35*:121, 1990.

221. Nimmo, W. S., Heading; R. C., Wilson, J. and Prescott, L. F.: Reversal of narcotic-induced delay in gastric emptying and paracetamol absorption by naloxone. BMJ 1189, 1979.

222. Montgomery, C. J., Vaghadia, H. and Blackstock, D.: Negative middle ear pressure and postoperative vomiting in pediatric outpatients. Anesthesiology *68*:288, 1988.

223. Davis, I., Moore, J. R. M. and Lahiti, S. K.: Nitrous oxide and the middle ear. Anaesthesia *34*:147, 1979.

224. Hovorka, J., Korttila, K. and Erkola, O.: The experience of the person ventilating the lungs does influence postoperative nausea and vomiting. Acta Anaesthesiol. Scand. *34*:203, 1990.

225. King, M. J., Milazkiewicz, R., Carli, F. and Deacock, A. R.: Influence of neostigmine on postoperative vomiting. Br J Anaesth *61*:403, 1988.

226. Watcha, M. F., Simeon, R. M., White, P. F. and Stevens, J. L.: Effect of propofol on the incidence of postoperative vomiting after strabismus surgery in pediatric outpatients. Anesthesiology 75:204, 1991.

227. Melnick, B. M. and Johnson, L. S.: Effects of eliminating nitrous oxide in outpatient anesthesia. Anesthesiology 67:982, 1987.

228. Alexander, G. D., Skupski, J. N. and Brown, E. M.: The role of nitrous oxide in postoperative nausea and vomiting. Anesth Analg *63*:175, 1984.

229. Sengupta, P. and Plantevin, O. M.: Nitrous oxide and daycase laparoscopy: effects on nausea, vomiting and return to normal activity. Br. J. Anaesth. *60*:570, 1988.

230. Pandit, U., *et al.*: Nitrous oxide does not increase postoperative nausea/vomiting in pediatric outpatients undergoing tonsillectomy-adenoidectomy. Anesthesiology 73:A1245, 1990.

231. Hovorka, J., Korttila, K. and Erkola, O.: Nitrous oxide does not increase nausea and vomiting following gynecological laparoscopy. Can J Anaesth *36*:145, 1989.

232. McCarroll, S. M., Mori, S. and Bras, P. J.: The effect of gastric intubation and removal of gastric contents on the inci-

dence of postoperative nausea and vomiting. Anesth Analg 70:S262, 1990.

233. Dent, S. J., Ramachandra, V. and Stephen, C. R.: Postoperative vomiting: incidence, analysis, and therapeutic measures in 3,000 patients. Anesthesiology 16:564, 1955.

234. Heyman, H. J., Salem, M. R. and Joseph, N. J.: Does gastric suction enhance the efficacy of droperidol prophylaxis of post-operative nausea and vomiting? Anesthesiology 73:A19, 1990.

235. Raftery, S. and Sherry, E.: Total intravenous aneaesthesia with propofol and lafentanil protects against postoperative nausea and vomiting. Can J Anaesth 39:37, 1992.

236. Larsson, S., Ageirsson, B. and Magnusson, J.: Propofol-fentanyl anesthesia compared to thiopental-halothane with special reference to recovery and vomiting after pediatric strabismus surgery. Acta Anaesthesiol. Scand. 36:182, 1992.

237. Bailey, P. L., et al.: Transdermal scopolamine reduces nausea and vomiting after outpatient laparoscopy. Anesthesiology 72:977, 1990.

238. Madej, T. H. and Simpson, K. H.: Comparison of the use of domperidone, droperidol and metoclopramide in the prevention of nausea and vomiting following major gynaecological surgery. Br J Anaesth 58:884, 1986.

239. Pataky, A. L., Kitz, D. S., Andrews, R. W. and Lecky, J. H.: Nausea and vomiting following ambulatory surgery: are all procedures created equal? Anesth Analg 67:S163, 1988.

240. Rowley, M. P. and Brown, T. C. K.: Postoperative vomiting in children. Anaesth Intensive Care 10:309, 1982.

241. Abramowitz, M. D., et al.: The antiemetic effect of droperidol following outpatient strabismus surgery in children. Anesthesiology 59:579, 1983.

242. Hardy, J. F., Charest, J., Girourard, G. and Lepage, Y.: Nausea and vomiting after strabismus surgery in preschool children. Can Anesth Soc J 33:57, 1986.

243. Lerman, J., Eustis, S. and Smith, D. R.: Effect of droperidol pretreatment on postanesthetic vomiting in children undergoing strabismus surgery. Anesthesiology 65:322, 1986.

244. Warner, L. O., et al.: Intravenous lidocaine reduces the incidence of vomiting in children after surgery to correct strabismus. Anesthesiology 68:618, 1988.

245. Van den Berg, A. A., Lambourne, A. and Clyburn, P. A.: The oculo-emetic reflex. Anaesthesia 44:110, 1989.

246. Yentis, S. M. and Bissonnette, B.: Ineffectiveness of acupuncture and droperidol in preventing vomiting following strabismus repair in children. Can J Anaesth 39:151, 1992.

247. Larsson and Jonmarker, C.: Postoperative emesis after pediatric strabismus surgery: the effect of dixyrazine compared to droperidol. Acta Anaesthesiol. Scand. 34:227, 1990.

248. Walsh, C., Smith, C. E., Polomeno, R. C. and Bevan, J. C.: Postoperative vomiting following strabismus surgery in paediatric outpatients: spontaneous versus controlled ventilation. Can J Anaesth 35:31, 1988.

249. Christensen, S., Farrow-Gillespie, A. and Lerman, J.: Incidence of emesis and postanesthetic recovery after strabismus surgery in children: a comparison of droperidol and lidocaine. Anesthesiology 70:251, 1989.

250. Broadman, L. M., et al.: Metoclopramide reduces the incidence of vomiting following strabismus surgery in children. Anesthesiology 72:245, 1990.

251. Lin, D. M., Furst, S. R. and Rodarte, A.: A double-blinded comparison of metoclopramide and droperidol for prevention of emesis following strabismus surgery. Anesthesiology 76:357, 1992.

252. Grunwald, Z., et al.: Droperidol decreases vomiting after tonsillectomy and adenoidectomy in children. Anesth Analg 70:S138, 1990.

253. Puttick, N. and Van der Walt, J. H.: The effect of premedication on the incidence of postoperative vomiting in children after E.N.T. surgery. Anaesth Intensive Care 15:158, 1987.

254. Yentis, S. M. and Bissonnette, B.: P6 acupuncture and postoperative vomiting after tonsillectomy in children. Br J Anaesth 67:779, 1991.

255. Lindblad, T., Forrest, J. B., Buckley, D. N. and Beattie, W. S.: Anesthesia decreases a hormone mediated threshold for nausea and vomiting. Anesth Analg 70:S242, 1990.

256. Metter, S. E., et al.: Nausea and vomiting after outpatient laparoscopy: incidence, impact on recovery room stay and cost. Anesth Analg 66:S116, 1987.

257. Gold, M. I.: Postanesthetic vomiting in the recovery room. Br. J. Anaesth. 41:143, 1969.

258. Palazzo, M. G. A. and Strunin, L.: Anesthesia and emesis II: prevention and management. Can. Anaesth. Soc. J. 31:407, 1984.

259. Clarke, R. S. J., Dundee, J. W. and Love, W. J.: Studies of drugs given before anesthesia VIII: morphine 10 mg alone and with atropine or hyoscine. Br. J. Anaesth. 37:772, 1965.

260. Loper, K. A., Ready, L. B. and Dorman, B. H.: Prophylactic transdermal scopolamine patches reduce nausea in postoperative patients receiving epidural morphine. Anesth Analg 68:144, 1989.

261. Gibbons, P. A., et al.: Scopolamine does not prevent postoperative emesis after pediatric eye surgery. Anesthesiology 61:A435, 1984.

262. Peroutka, S. J. and Snyder, S. H.: Antiemetics: neurotransmitter receptor binding predicts therapeutic actions. Lancet 1:658, 1982.

263. Rita, L., Goodarzi, M. and Seleny, F.: Effect of low dose droperidol on postoperative vomiting in children. Can Anaesth Soc J 28:259, 1981.

264. Cohen, S. E., Woods, W. A. and Wyner, J.: Antiemetic efficacy of droperidol and metoclopramide. Anesthesiology 60:67, 1984.

265. Dupre, L. J. and Stieglitz, P.: Extrapyramidal syndromes after premedication with droperidol in children. Br. J. Anaesth. 52:831, 1980.

266. Melnick, B., et al.: Delayed side effects of droperidol after ambulatory general anesthesia. Anesth Analg 69:748, 1989.

267. Bermudez, J., Boyle, E. A., Miner, W. D. and Sanger, G. J.: The anti-emetic potential of the 5-hydroxytryptamine$_3$ receptor antagonist BRL 43694. Br J Cancer 58:644, 1988.

268. Bunce, K. T. and Tyers, M. B.: The role of 5-HT in postoperative nausea and vomiting. B J A 69:60, 1992.

269. Bodner, M. and White, P. F.: Antiemetic efficacy of ondansetron after outpatient laparoscopy. Anesth Analg 73:250, 1991.

270. Alon, E. and Himmelseher, S.: Ondansetron in the treatment of postoperative vomiting: a randomized, double-blind comparison with droperidol and etoclopramide. Anesth Analg 75:561, 1992.

271. Fujii, Y., Tanaka, H., Toyooka, H.: Reduction of postoperative nausea and vomiting with granisteron. Can J Anaesth 41:291, 1994.

Chapter 22

HEPATOBILIARY DISEASE AND ANESTHESIA

DENNIS W. COALSON

The liver is the largest organ in the body and plays an essential role in many of the body's most vital physiologic functions. Its strategic position between the splanchnic and the systemic circulations is a location well suited for its function. It receives blood relatively low in oxygen content but rich in materials absorbed from the splanchnic circulation via the portal vein and an alternate more highly oxygenated source of blood from the hepatic artery. Substances absorbed by the gastrointestinal tract, hormones secreted by the intestine and pancreas, as well as solutes delivered via the hepatic artery, will be exposed to the liver for uptake and biotransformation. The fundamental role of the liver is to regulate the concentration of substances that will reach distant organs via the systemic circulation and bile. The liver performs this task by modulating the uptake of incoming substances as well as the rate of secretion of biotransformed or synthesized substances into sinusoidal blood and bile.

Modulation of the supply of substrates by the liver is accomplished by several processes or functional capacities of liver cells. These encompass: (a) removal of substances from sinusoidal blood via uptake, (b) intracellular modification of uptaken substances, (c) intracellular de novo synthesis and storage of new products, and (d) secretion of manufactured and biotransformed substances into bile and into sinusoidal blood. Each of these processes is the subject of complex regulation involving changes in blood flow, afferent neural input, availability of substrates and cofactors, distribution of transport systems, and activity of rate-limiting enzymes, among other factors. In addition the liver participates in the immune protective system, and can serve as a reservoir for blood during periods of hypovolemia.

ANATOMY

The liver in an adult weighs 1200 to 1500 g. It constitutes approximately 2% of the body weight in the adult, but is proportionately larger (5% of the body weight) in the newborn. The greater part of the liver lies under cover of the ribs and costal cartilage. It is in contact with the diaphragm which separates it from the pericardium and from the right pleural cavity and lung. The liver has two distinct surfaces: (1) the diaphragmatic surface and (2) the postero inferior or visceral surface. The most obvious anatomic landmark of the liver is the fold of peritoneum along the anterior diaphragmatic surface called the falciform ligament. This structure carries the umbili-

cal vein during fetal development. Although this ligament is frequently described as the anatomical structure dividing the left from the right lobe of the liver, this division by the falciform ligament is a morphologic one and does not conform with a functional division. When the vascular supply and drainage of the liver are defined it becomes clear that the falciform ligament does not correlate with blood supply or biliary drainage.

Divisions of the Liver

The liver is divided into two hemi-livers determined by their blood supply from the right and left branches of the hepatic artery and portal vein. There is no visible mark that permits individualization of true lobes. The main dividing line goes from the middle of the gallbladder fossa anteriorly to the left side of the vena cava posteriorly. The right and left hemi-livers individualized by the main portal division are independent in regards to the portal and arterial vascularization and the biliary drainage. Although the portal vein and hepatic artery vessels branch together and become the basis for dividing the liver into sectors and segments, the hepatic veins may cross these planes at right angles.[1] Thus, there are no avascular planes which can be dissected through during liver resection. A functional anatomical classification allows interpretation of radiological data[2] and is of importance to the surgeon planning a liver resection.

Blood Supply to the Liver

The portal vein supplies approximately 65 to 75% of the liver's total blood flow with the hepatic artery supplying the remaining 25 to 35%. The portal venous system drains the intestine (except the lowest part of the rectum and anal canal), the spleen, pancreas, and gallbladder. The portal vein communicates with the systemic venous system at the gastroesophageal junction through the esophageal veins; at the umbilicus through the paraumbilical veins; and in the rectum through the superior rectal vein. These communications become dilated in the presence of portal hypertension and can lead to significant hemorrhage and morbidity. The common hepatic artery originates as a branch of the celiac trunk. It then gives off the right gastric, gastroduodenal, and cystic arteries before bifurcating into the left and right branches of the hepatic artery and entering the liver.

The liver is perfused by the right and left branches of the portal vein and hepatic artery. Branches of bile ducts accompany the vascular plexus. Terminal vascular branches representing the vascular core of the hepatic acinus originate from small portal spaces called preterminal portal tracts. There is an extensive network of capillaries surrounding bile ducts in portal spaces. This system which is perfused by branches of the hepatic artery, has been called the peribiliary plexus.

MICROANATOMY

For many years, it was maintained that the microcirculatory unit of liver was the hepatic lobule. The lobule consisted of the central hepatic venule with the hepatic parenchymal plates radiating out in a circular fashion with several portal triads lining the circumference of the lobule. Rappaport proposed that the structural and functional unit of hepatic parenchyma was the liver acinus rather than the hepatic lobule.[3]

Following Rappaport's description, hepatocytes within the liver are organized in tridimensional microvascular units or hepatic acini. *The simple hepatic acinus represents the structural and functional unit of the liver parenchyma.* It is at the level of this microvascular unit that liver function is performed. Within the hepatic acinus, blood flows from the terminal portal venule and hepatic arteriole at the acinar core to the terminal hepatic venules at the periphery. The perfusion of hepatocytes in an individual hepatic acinus, therefore, proceeds in a sequential manner from those hepatocytes surrounding the terminal portal venules to those surrounding the terminal hepatic venules. Based on this microcirculatory pattern, the hepatic acinus has been arbitrarily divided into three zones: zone 1 represents hepatocytes located around the terminal portal venule and receives blood containing the largest solute load; zone 2 represents hepatocytes intermediate between those of zones 1 and 3; zone 3 represents hepatocytes surrounding the terminal hepatic venule.

Given its location and capabilities, the liver establishes a link between substances ingested and absorbed and the needs of other organs. This can be accomplished because the structure of the liver allows a wide interaction between blood and hepatocytes. Each of the liver acinar units consists of a three-dimensional mass of one-cell thick plates of hepatic cells perfused unidirectionally by blood flowing in specialized capillaries called hepatic sinusoids. The length of these three dimensional plates vary in size but average about 20-25 hepatocytes in length. Bile secreted by hepatic cells runs in the opposite direction, from the periphery to the core of the acinus. Two characteristics of the liver function are critical: (a) incoming substances are progressively modified within the hepatic acinus due to the sequential perfusion of hepatocytes, and (b) hepatocytes located in different positions within the liver acinus have distinct functional capabilities or heterogeneity[4,5] (Fig. 22-1).

Hepatic Sinusoids

Hepatic sinusoids can be seen as conduits connecting the core of the acinus (terminal portal venule and terminal hepatic arteriole) with the hepatic venules. Specially adapted endothelial-type cells line the sinusoids in single layer and because of their unique properties allow easy passage of solutes from the sinusoidal lumen to the luminal side of the hepatocytes. In contrast to other endothelial lined capillaries, the liver sinusoids possess a much less developed basement membrane (an extracellular supporting stroma with primary constituents of glycoproteins, and collagens). The continuity of the endothelial mass of sinusoids is interrupted by pores or fenestrae. A fenestration is an area of cell wall where the inner and outer plasma membranes are fused, so that a molecule can pass directly through the cell without entering the cytoplasm. The size of the these fenestrae in the fixed

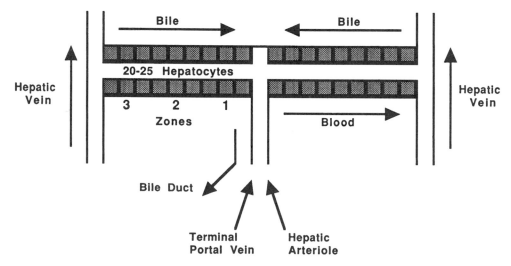

Fig. 22–1. Schematic representation of the hepatic acinus. The acinus is a three-dimensional mass of hepatocytes possessing a vascular core that perfuses all cells and is drained by hepatic venules at the periphery. The core is formed by the terminal portal venule and the terminal hepatic arteriole carrying blood into the acinus and by bile ducts carrying bile in the opposite direction into the main bile ducts and gallbladder. The periphery of the acinus is demarcated by two or more hepatic venules. There are about 20–25 hepatocytes between the core and the peripheral hepatic veins. (Modified from Kaplowitz N.: Liver and Biliary Diseases, Baltimore, 1992, Williams & Wilkins.)

liver is such that most solutes, except for large complexes, should have free access to the space of Disse (i.e., the space between the sinusoidal calls and the hepatocyte).

The terminal branches of the hepatic arteriole also enter directly into sinusoids. There is controversy whether the arterioles enter only near the vascular core or zone 1 or enter the sinusoids throughout the acinus. A single entry would mean that, as oxygen is removed by hepatocytes first exposed to the incoming blood, oxygen concentration in sinusoidal blood would progressively decrease. Hepatocytes located downstream may then be exposed to blood with a relatively lower oxygen content. In contrast, multiple entry points would tend to maintain a more homogeneous concentration of oxygen throughout the acinus. Whether the oxygen concentration in zone 3 reaches a critical point influencing either function or susceptibility to injury of these hepatocytes has been difficult to measure. However, it has been demonstrated that hepatocytes located in zone 3 are particularly susceptible to hypoxia.[6]

Nonhepatocyte Cells

There are other cells within the liver that are not hepatocytes. Sinusoidal cells with their bodies and cytoplasmic extensions form the walls of the hepatic sinusoids enclosing the sinusoidal vascular space. Another cell type is the Kupffer cell. This cell is located within the sinusoidal vascular space and plays an important role in the removal of large particles from the circulation. Kupffer cells have been described as the largest group of fixed macrophages in the body. A fourth cell type is the Ito, or fat-storing cell. This cell is located in the perisinusoidal space and is characterized by the presence of fat droplets in the cytoplasm. Fat-storing cells seem to play an important role in the storage of vitamin A in liver, and may be the source of collagen formation during fibrogenesis in cirrhosis. Biliary epithelial cells represent about 3–5% of the liver nuclear population. These cells form conduits carrying bile into the gallbladder and small intestine. The hepatocyte population accounts for approximately 80% of the liver tissue volume, whereas cells that are not hepatocytes constitute about 6% (3% endothelial cells, 2% Kupffer cells, and 1% fat-storing cells). The extracellular space represents about 16% of the liver tissue volume.

Perisinusoidal Space of Disse

Between the hepatocyte plasma membrane and the endothelial cells forming the walls of the hepatic sinusoids, there is a space called perisinusoidal space or space of Disse. The microvilli of the sinusoidal side of the hepatocyte plasma membrane protrude into the space of Disse. Solutes traverse from the vascular space into the space of Disse mainly through the sinusoidal fenestrae. Contact is established with hepatocytes, and this may result in the total or partial removal of a solute.

Formation of Hepatic Lymph

The formation of hepatic lymph is still not clearly defined. It is presumed that lymph is formed at the level of the space of Disse. Excess solutes and water in this space are believed to contribute to hepatic lymph formation. Since lymphatic capillaries have not been seen accompanying hepatocytes, it has been proposed that most of the fluid flows from the space of Disse into the space of Mall (space between the limiting plate and the connective tissue surrounding small portal tracts) and from there into larger lymphatics, which leave the liver via the hepatic hilum and finally empty into the thoracic duct.

Hepatic Nerves

The liver is predominantly innervated by two plexuses. The anterior plexus surrounds the hepatic artery and is made out of fibers from the celiac ganglia and anterior vagus nerve. The posterior plexus surrounds the portal vein and bile duct and is formed from branches of the right celiac ganglia and posterior vagus nerve. The vast majority of nerve fibers terminate in plexuses in the adventitia around hepatic arterioles and venules. Small fibers from these plexuses then end on smooth muscle cells in the media of these vessels. Within the hepatic acinus the majority of nerve fibers are observed in periportal regions. A minority of nerve fibers also terminate on the endothelial cells, Kupffer cells, fat-storing cells, and on hepatocytes. Extensive innervation of hepatocytes may not be necessary since stimulation of one hepatocyte may be conveyed to distant hepatocytes through gap junctions.[7]

Stimulation of sympathetic fibers causes an increase in vascular resistance and a decrease in hepatic blood volume. Activation of the periarterial nerves results in rapid increases in serum levels of glucose. This increment in glucose level is under alpha-adrenergic control. The resulting efflux of glucose is dependent on glycogenolysis. In contrast parasympathetic stimulation promotes glucose uptake and utilization.

HEPATIC CIRCULATION

The liver in an average size adult weighs approximately 1500 g. Hepatic blood flow is approximately 100 ml/100 g of tissue. This 1500 ml/min blood flow represents approximately 25% of the cardiac output. The portal vein delivers about 65 to 75% of the total hepatic blood flow but because it is partially deoxygenated by splanchnic oxygen uptake it provides only 50 to 55% of the oxygen delivered to the liver. The hepatic artery delivers the remaining 25 to 35% of the hepatic blood flow and because it has systemic arterial content of oxygen it provides 45 to 50% of the liver's oxygen.

Blood flow through the portal vein is regulated primarily by arterioles in the preportal splanchnic organs. Portal vein pressure, normally 7 to 10 mm Hg is determined by the portal vein flow and resistance to flow within the liver. The pressure within the sinusoids is determined by the tone of presinusoidal and postsinusoidal sphincters and blood flow. Presinusoidal sphincters permit relatively uniform distribution of flow through the liver and play a limited role in the regulation of portal flow. The major site of venous resistance within the liver is at the postsinusoidal sphincters.

Venous compliance is regulated by smooth muscles in the wall of the venules and is predominantly controlled by the sympathetic innervation mediated through alpha-adrenergic receptors. Changes in the hepatic venous compliance contribute in the total body venous return and regulation of cardiac output. The liver can serve as a substantial reservoir of blood volume during periods of hypovolemia and or hemorrhage. Patients with chronic liver disease have a decreased sensitivity to catecholamines, probably because of an increase in the concentration of glucagon and other vasodilating compounds. The sympathetic nervous system responses to hypovolemia and hemorrhage are constriction of resistive vessels in the musculature and splanchnic areas and constriction of capacitance vessels to direct blood volume to the systemic circulation. These responses are attenuated in the presence of chronic liver disease.

The major site of resistance in the hepatic arterial vasculature is at the level of the arterioles. Hepatic arteriolar tone is partially determined by portal vein blood flow and is primarily achieved by local and intrinsic mechanisms. The consequence is an increase in hepatic arterial flow when portal flow decreases.[8,9] This increase in arterial flow is an attempt to maintain total hepatic blood flow and hepatic oxygen delivery. This autoregulation of hepatic artery blood flow is dependent on neural, metabolic, and myogenic factors.[8,10] The "washout theory" maintains that a vasodilating substance, probably adenosine, is released by liver cells.[11] When portal vein blood flow decreases, less of this vasodilating substance is removed and it therefore accumulates leading to hepatic arterial vasodilation. With an increase in portal vein blood flow, more effective washout of this compound occurs resulting in decreased vasodilation in the hepatic arterial system.

Effects of Anesthetics and Surgery on Hepatic Circulation

Hepatic blood flow is altered by general anesthetics and surgical interventions. Anesthesia and surgery (or surgical preparations in experimental models) affect the hepatic circulation, including the interaction of hepatic arterial and portal venous blood flow, and may cause reduction in total hepatic blood and oxygen supply. Surgical intervention plays a predominate role in splanchnic circulatory disturbances, while anesthetic agents play a less significant role.

The majority of anesthetic agents used to produce general anesthesia decrease portal blood flow in association with a decrease in cardiac output. However, hepatic arterial blood flow can be unchanged, decreased; or increased depending on the anesthetic agent administered and its influence on hemodynamics. The increase in hepatic arterial blood flow, when it occurs usually does not fully offset the decrease in portal blood flow and therefore total hepatic blood flow is usually decreased during general anesthesia.

Anesthetics can alter the hepatic circulation by different mechanisms. These include: direct effects of anesthetics on the splanchnic vasculature; changes in systemic hemodynamics (cardiac output, vascular resistance, blood pressure); and neural and humoral mechanisms (including the release of "stress" hormones and mediators such as ACTH, cortisol, catecholamines, antidiuretic hormone). The majority of anesthetic agents decrease total splanchnic blood flow. Many anesthetics also decrease total splanchnic and hepatic oxygen consumption, however, usually to a lesser extent than the decrease in total splanchnic blood flow.[12]

Inhalation Anesthetics

Halothane

This drug decreases portal blood flow in animals and humans. The decrease closely parallels the decrease in blood pressure and particularly cardiac output.[13-19] Cardiac output is the main determinant of portal blood flow during halothane anesthesia. The direct effect of halothane on the intestinal vasculature is vasodilation. However, in intact animals, halothane causes a decrease in blood flow through preportal organs and tissues which is due to the indirect effects mediated through alterations in sympathetic nervous tone and systemic hemodynamics, mainly cardiac output.

The changes in hepatic arterial blood flow during halothane anesthesia reveals marked variation between studies. The methodology employed appears to dramatically affect the results. In animal studies where laparotomy was performed and (or) a barbiturate was used as a base-line anesthetic, hepatic arterial blood flow decreased. In the majority of studies where laparotomy was not performed, hepatic arterial blood flow increased or did not change, provided halothane anesthetic did not reduce blood pressure and (or) cardiac output by more than 30%.[12,15,17,20-23]

In a canine study, the clearance of indocyanine green (ICG) decreased during halothane anesthesia and was unchanged during isoflurane anesthesia. The degree of decrease in the clearance of ICG during halothane anesthesia did not correlate with the level of anesthesia or the decrease in total hepatic blood flow. These results suggest that not only is ICG clearance during halothane anesthesia related to a decrease in hepatic blood flow, but in addition, or even mainly, to a decrease in the liver's metabolic capacity.[20]

Enflurane

In intact animal studies, enflurane reduced portal vein blood flow.[17,24,25] This reduction was related to changes in the systemic circulation (mainly a decrease in cardiac output), and possibly to a decrease in oxygen requirement in the preportal area. The percentage of the cardiac output going to hepatic arterial flow was usually increased during enflurane anesthesia.[17,18] This suggests that, when used in equipotent doses, enflurane may preserve splanchnic blood flow and liver oxygen supply better than halothane.

Isoflurane

In isolated intestinal loop preparations, isoflurane, as well as halothane and enflurane, decreased intestinal vascular resistance and intestinal oxygen requirement and uptake.[26] However, in intact animals, isoflurane decreased blood flow through the preportal areas, as did the other inhalation agents.[15,20,27] This decrease in blood flow through the preportal area is related probably to both a reduction in cardiac output and a reduction in oxygen requirement. Hepatic arterial blood flow was substantially increased at low to moderate levels of isoflurane.[13,20,27] This increase in hepatic artery blood flow may represent the preserved autoregulatory ability of the hepatic arterial vasculature to increase flow in response to a reduction in portal blood flow. Total hepatic blood flow was unchanged or even slightly increased during isoflurane anesthesia.[13,15,20,27]

Nitrous Oxide

Inhalation of nitrous oxide is usually not accompanied by substantial changes in blood pressure and cardiac output. Hepatic circulation was not disturbed significantly when nitrous oxide was used in trained animals without any base-line anesthesia or surgical preparation.[27] However, a significant decrease in both portal and hepatic artery blood flows was observed when nitrous oxide was used in conditions of barbiturate anesthesia and laparotomy.[28]

Comparing inhalation agents, it appears that all the volatile agents have a direct dilatory effect on the intestinal vasculature. However, in intact animals, splanchnic and thus portal blood flow is reduced. This reduction is associated with a decrease in cardiac output and partially with a reduction in intestinal oxygen requirement. Isoflurane and enflurane appear to facilitate oxygen delivery to the liver much better than halothane, mainly by a more effective preservation of hepatic arterial blood flow.[12]

Intravenous Anesthetics

Although the effect of barbiturates on hepatic blood flow has been examined in several animal studies, the results vary considerably. The discrepancies may be related to many different factors, including the animal model used, the depth of anesthesia, and involvement of respiratory depression with a subsequent increase in sympathetic discharge. The changes reported in hepatic blood flow include; a decrease in flow though preportal organs;[29-33] increased splanchnic blood flow;[34] significant deceases in portal vein, hepatic artery, and total hepatic blood flow;[35] and decreased portal flow accompanied by an increase in hepatic arterial flow.[36-38]

Ketamine has been shown to increase, decrease or have little effect on the splanchnic and hepatic artery blood flow depending on the animal model and methodology of the study.[18,39-41] Etomidate in dogs, caused a decrease in portal flow and hepatic artery flow that corresponded to a decrease in arterial pressure and cardiac output.[42]

The effects of **morphine** on the splanchnic circulation and hepatic blood flow have been variable depending on the study. Morphine has caused splanchnic vasodilation and increased hepatic blood flow in low dosages with higher doses leading to splanchnic arteriolar vasoconstriction.[43-46] In experiments on isolated intestinal loop preparations with maintained perfusion pressure, fentanyl lead to a dose-related vasodilation of the intestinal vasculature with a substantial decrease in oxygen requirement and

uptake.[43] In intact animals fentanyl does not decrease cardiac output and may therefore preserve portal blood flow, and with a decrease in intestinal oxygen uptake may lead to an improved hepatic oxygen supply.[47] Alfentanil in conditions of halothane anesthetized dogs decreased hepatic arterial blood flow to a greater extent than it reduced mean arterial pressure or cardiac output.[48]

Muscle Relaxants

Of the neuromuscular blocking agents studied, pancuronium and vecuronium did not significantly affect the splanchnic circulation, while d-tubocurarine induced arterial hypotension, increased blood flow to the stomach, but reduced flow to the spleen, intestines, and hepatic artery.[49-51]

Surgical Intervention

Irrespective of the background anesthetic, surgical intervention induces certain splanchnic circulatory disturbances. Most studies demonstrate that laparotomy alone reduces splanchnic blood flow. When a surgical procedure is superimposed on an anesthetic which decreases splanchnic blood flow, liver blood flow is further decreased. The degree of the decrease varies with the type of surgical intervention. Minor peripheral procedures are accompanied by a small decrease in hepatic blood flow, while major procedures such as laparotomy are associated with a substantial decrease in liver blood flow. The degree of blood flow reduction suggests that surgical intervention, rather than anesthesia, is the main determinant of the alterations in the splanchnic circulation.

The decrease in portal blood flow which accompanied laparotomy was associated with increased hepatic arterial blood flow.[30,52,53] Traction and manipulation of the splanchnic organs may play a certain role in these disturbances. The release of hormones in response to surgical stress seems to be important. Acute hypophysectomy abolished the marked mesenteric vasoconstriction and reduction in gastrointestinal blood flow during laparotomy.[54]

Continuous positive pressure ventilation, especially with large tidal volumes or with increased end expiratory pressure, decreases splanchnic blood flow.[55-57] Controlled positive pressure ventilation reduces mesenteric arterial flow and portal blood flow approximately to the same magnitude it decreases cardiac output.[58-60] Conventional and high frequency ventilation at high airway pressure were equivalent in their 65 to 70% reduction in hepatic arterial blood flow.[61]

The effects of CO_2 concentration on hepatic blood flow has resulted in varying and contradictory results from many investigators and this is due to the complex mechanisms of hepatic blood flow control and the difference in experimental design, including the presence of surgical manipulation and the presence of different baseline anesthetics.

Hypocarbia in most animal studies has been associated with a reduction in portal blood flow and a reduction in total hepatic blood flow. However, if cardiac output and blood pressure are maintained there is an incomplete compensatory increase in hepatic artery blood flow.

Hypercarbia is usually accompanied by a substantial increase in blood flow through the portal vein. Hypercarbia has been associated with a depression of hepatic function, demonstrated by an increased indocyanine green half-life in the presence of the increased portal vein and total hepatic blood flow.[62]

Regional Anesthesia

Regional anesthesia can also modulate hepatic circulation. High spinal anesthesia has been demonstrated to decrease hepatic blood flow in parallel with a decrease in arterial blood pressure.[63] In dogs, high epidural block reduced hepatic blood flow by lowering the portal venous blood flow without change in hepatic arterial blood flow.[64] Intravenous ephedrine restored splanchnic hemodynamics by increasing portal venous blood flow to preanesthetic values.[65] Nakayama demonstrated, in humans, that the decrease in indocyanine green clearance during spinal anesthesia could be prevented with intravenous ephedrine given as an infusion maintaining arterial blood pressure at baseline levels.[66]

DRUG METABOLISM AND ELIMINATION

The liver is a major site for drug metabolism. The metabolism of drugs and environmental toxins by hepatocytes is called biotransformation. Many drugs are lipid soluble and circulate in plasma bound to plasma proteins. The ultimate goal of the process of biotransformation is the metabolic transformation of drugs, rendering them inactive and water soluble. This allows the excretion of the metabolic products into the water medium of either bile or urine.

A series of reactions participate in these modifications. These have been classified into phase I and phase II reactions.

Phase I reactions, represents oxidation or reduction reactions, mostly catalyzed by the cytochromes P-450. These reactions cause minor modifications of the parent compound with limited effects on aqueous solubility. Phase I reactions may add or expose a functional group, such as an hydroxyl radical, which then can serve as a structural locus for phase II conjugation. The product of phase I transformation can be an inactive or an active metabolite.

Partially polar metabolites can now react with phase II enzymes, which conjugate metabolites, increase polarity and, thus, water solubility, and transform them into inactive products. Phase II reactions produce a large change in size and solubility of drugs by adding, or conjugating, with a charged molecule, such as glucuronic acid, sulfate, or glutathione.

Some drugs are directly or mainly metabolized by phase II reactions. The sequence or relative importance of either route of handling is critical in certain situations. For example, in advanced liver disease, phase I reactions are impaired, whereas phase II reactions may be better preserved. Thus, the handling of diazepam, a P-450 substrate, is severely impaired in cirrhosis;[67] whereas the benzodiazepine oxazepam, is handled normally by glucuronyltransferase.[68] Acetaminophen is metabolized mainly by phase II (glucuronidation and sulfation), yielding polar, non-toxic metabolites. However, a small percentage is oxidized to a reactive metabolite.

Most of the phase I reactions involve the participation of a family of integral proteins named cytochromes P-450 which are located in the membranes of the smooth endoplasmic reticulum. There are several families of P-450, each one with several members. The families have been grouped according to the degree of amino acid or nucleic acid homology. Also, a substance metabolized by a cytochrome P-450 can induce an increase in content and activity of these enzymes.

Components of Drug Metabolism

The drug metabolizing function of the liver consists of three important components: (1) membrane transport of organic substances, (2) intracellular metabolism or biotransformation, and (3) release back into the sinusoids or secretion into bile of these metabolized compounds. Therefore, their ultimate elimination often requires bile secretion. However, excretion in bile is not an inevitable consequence of all hepatic biotransformation. In some instances, the polar products of biotransformation are transported into plasma via the sinusoids and hepatic venules and then are eliminated in urine.

Biotransformation is the intermediate step between hepatic uptake and excretion of a wide variety of endogenous substance and drugs. Since the liver takes up a variety of organic chemicals of limited aqueous solubility, it is critical to process these chemicals into more polar forms. There are two major advantages in producing more aqueous soluble metabolites of lipophilic parent compounds: (a) the ability of a substance to leave the hepatocyte by carrier-mediated transport in most cases depends on the transporter in the canalicular or sinusoidal membrane recognizing highly charged groups, and (b) the removal of the metabolite in bile or plasma and subsequent excretion in feces or urine depend on aqueous solubility in these excretory fluids.

Hepatocytic Enzymes

Hepatocytes contains a wide variety of enzymes that can process drugs or foreign chemicals. Each enzyme represents a large family of distinct gene products, all of which share a common cofactor or endogenous co-substrate. Specific gene products may be induced by different xenobiotics. There is considerable redundancy in the substrate specificity of the individual components of any enzyme family.

The cytochromes P-450 system has a broad substrate specificity due to its multiplicity of isoenzymes. Numerous oxidative reactions are catalyzed by these isoenzymes, including aromatic and aliphatic hydroxylation, epoxidation, N-demethylation, O-dealkylation, and N-oxidation.

Many factors influence drug metabolism including nutrition and cofactor availability in addition to genetics, induction, and disease. Another feature of hepatic biotransformation that may have important consequences is the zonation (lobular heterogeneity) of enzymes, cofactors, cofactor synthesis, and induction.

Multiple apoproteins of P-450 are under separate genetic control. Exposure to specific substrates leads to the induction of certain forms of P-450, usually the form(s) that metabolizes those substrates. Induction may be especially important in promoting liver toxicity if the form induced is also largely responsible for the activation of a hepatotoxin. For example, chronic ethanol exposure induces a form of P-450 that can oxidize acetaminophen to an electrophilic product. The mechanism of induction can vary between induction agents. Some agents like polycyclic hydrocarbons modulate gene transcription. Ethanol has a post-transcriptional regulating effect.

Genetic variations in the expression of the P-450s known as genetic polymorphism can influence the metabolism of xenobiotics and result in increased toxicity from a decreased metabolism of the drug or from increased production of a toxic metabolite.

LIVER DISEASE

Liver disease can by separated into parenchymal disease or cholestatic disease. Either form of liver disease may be acute or chronic. Parenchymal liver disease may be the result of variety of insults including chronic alcohol ingestion, viral infection, acute toxicity such as from acetaminophen and halothane, inborn errors of metabolism, and autoimmune diseases. The end result of all these causative insults include a decrease in metabolic capacity of the hepatocytes leading to a decrease in biotransformation of endogenous and exogenous compounds and a decrease in synthetic function. With chronic liver disease the architecture of the liver acinus is altered with fibrotic tissue increasing coinciding with the loss of hepatocytes. With progression of the disease, hallmark signs of liver disease appear and include portal hypertension with enlargement of collateral venous channels, ascites, jaundice, hypoalbuminemia, CNS alteration and coagulopathy.

CHRONIC HEPATIC FAILURE

Etiology

Chronic hepatic failure can be caused by chronic alcohol ingestion (most common etiology in the United States), exposure to toxins, autoimmune disorders, or chronic viral infection from hepatitis B, hepatitis C, CMV, or coinfection with the hepatitis Delta virus. Regardless of the etiology the end result is architectural changes within the liver. The liver may be enlarged, normal size or small during late phases of cirrhosis. Common clinical signs of cirrhosis are splenomegaly, jaundice, esophageal varices, ascites, spider nevi, and asterixis. Clinical symptoms include fatigue, weakness, anorexia, nausea, vomiting, and abdominal pain. All organ systems are affected in the patient with advanced parenchymal hepatic disease.

Effect on Cardiovascular System

Cirrhotic patients with portal hypertension have a hyperdynamic cardiovascular system with high cardiac output and low systemic vascular resistance, with usually normal cardiac filling pressures and normal or increased heart rate. Low vascular resistance results from pulmonary and systemic arteriovenous fistulas and increased systemic concentrations of endogenous vasodilators, such

Table 22–1. Hemodynamic Changes in Cirrhosis

Increased
  Blood volume
  Cardiac output
  Pulmonary, splanchnic, muscle, and skin blood flow
  Venous O_2 content
Decreased
  Systemic vascular resistance
  Portal vein blood flow to liver
  Response to catecholamines
  Albumin and oncotic pressure
  Arteriovenous O_2 content difference
Normal
  Arterial pressure (maintained until end-stage disease)
  Heart rate (maintained until end-state disease)
  Ventricular filling pressures (maintained until end-stage disease)
  Renal blood flow (cortical blood flow decreased in late stages)
  Hepatic artery blood flow (may be increased)

as glucagon, and vasoactive intestinal polypeptide.[69-71] Plasma volume may be increased, although venous filling pressures may be within the normal range. Resting ventricular function is usually normal, and ventricular ejection fraction, both left and right, are often elevated. However, decreased myocardial contractility may be seen in patients with alcoholic liver disease, hemochromatosis, or Wilson's disease. The circulating blood volume is usually increased, with decreases in arteriovenous difference in oxygen content resulting in increased oxygen content in the peripheral and mixed venous blood (Table 22–1).

Effect on Pulmonary System

Most patients with advanced liver disease have one or more types of lung function abnormalities. These include intrapulmonary arteriovenous shunts, ventilation-perfusion imbalances, abnormal diffusion capacity, impaired hypoxic pulmonary vasoconstriction, restrictive lung disease, and pulmonary hypertension. Using contrast echocardiography intrapulmonary right-to-left shunting was demonstrated in 47% in patients with severe liver disease.[72] Evaluating pulmonary function tests and chest X-rays in patients being evaluated for liver transplantation, Hourani et al found a reduced carbon dioxide diffusing capacity DL_{CO} to be the single most common functional defect occurring in 48 to 71% of patients depending on previous smoking histories. A widened alveolar-arterial oxygen gradient was noted in 45% of all patients, ventilatory restriction in 25%, and airflow obstruction in only 3%.[73] To a large degree the pulmonary dysfunction is reversible after liver transplantation and thus a reversible hepato-pulmonary syndrome has been described.[74,75] Pulmonary artery hypertension in individuals with liver disease is well recognized, but rare.[76]

Effect on Renal System

Primary liver disease can give rise to a host of abnormalities in renal function, ranging from salt retention to the two azotemic syndromes, acute tubular necrosis and hepatorenal syndrome. The hepatorenal syndrome is defined as the occurrence of renal failure without any obvious cause in a patient with liver disease. It is most commonly seen in patients with alcoholic cirrhosis, but may complicate other liver disease, including acute hepatitis, fulminant hepatic failure, and hepatic malignancy.

HEPATORENAL SYNDROME

Hepatorenal syndrome usually occurs in the setting of severe liver disease, i.e., decompensated cirrhosis or fulminant hepatitis. Almost all patients with HRS have ascites and other clinical signs of hepatic dysfunction and portal hypertension, including some degree of hepatic encephalopathy and jaundice. Because of decreases in muscle mass secondary to poor nutrition and hepatic failure, measurements of serum creatinine frequently overestimates the glomerular filtration rate. GFR can decrease markedly without a concomitant change in serum creatinine. Azotemia often occurs suddenly without any apparent trigger, and it almost always develops after the patient with liver disease is hospitalized. Although recovery is uncommon it does occur and usually appears following a dramatic improvement in liver function. The renal failure is usually only one aspect of a more general deterioration.

Both acute tubular necrosis and hepato-renal syndrome HRS present as acute renal failure, but the biochemical features and the prognosis differ. The diagnosis of HRS is essentially one of exclusion. The abrupt onset of oliguria and azotemia in a cirrhotic patient does not necessarily imply the onset of the hepatorenal syndrome. It is important to consider prerenal causes, particularly because they constitute reversible conditions if recognized and treated in the incipient phase. Volume contraction or cardiac pump failure must be ruled out as the cause of oliguria.

Pathogenesis

This is incompletely understood. Much evidence suggests that the renal failure is functional and has a prominent hemodynamic component. The pathologic findings are minimal and inconsistent. Several investigators have demonstrated that the underlying abnormality is severe renal vasoconstriction. Angiographic studies have demonstrated severely impaired renal circulation and vasomotor instability. Using radioactive isotopes, renal blood flow measurements have shown marked renal hypoperfusion, with the reduction in blood flow greatest in the cortex, where filtration takes place.[77] The functional nature of the renal lesion in the syndrome has been demonstrated by normal function of transplanted kidneys from donors who have died from liver failure with concomitant hepatorenal syndrome.[78] Conversely, patients with this syndrome have had return of normal kidney function after undergoing orthotopic liver transplantation.

Renal Hypoperfusion

Renal hypoperfusion with preferential renal cortical ischemia has been shown to underlie the renal failure of HRS, but the factors responsible for sustaining cortical is-

chemia and suppression of glomerular filtration have not been fully elucidated. At least two major theories have been proposed to explain the genesis of HRS. The traditional concept, the "underfill" theory, holds that a contraction of the effective blood volume (the portion of total circulating volume that stimulates volume receptors) constitutes a pivotal event predisposing to HRS. The overflow hypothesis suggests that a primary event within the kidney results in sodium avidity.

Diminished Effective Vascular Volume

Strong support for the concept that a diminished effective intravascular volume is a major determinant of renal hypoperfusion in cirrhotic patients is given by the results of water immersion studies. In these studies, patients with liver disease and renal dysfunction are immersed in a tank of water to investigate the effects of fluid redistribution on renal function. The clinical effect of water immersion on the cirrhotic patient with ascites who is avidly retaining salt and water is dramatic. Immersion induces a striking normalization of renal excretory function characterized by a marked diuresis and natriuresis. Thus, the marked antinatriuresis of cirrhosis is promptly reversed by a manipulation that alters the distribution of plasma volume without increasing total plasma volume.

Neuro-hormonal Factors

Several hormonal or neural mechanisms have been proposed to mediate such renal changes, including alterations of the renin-angiotensin system, an increase in sympathetic nervous system activity, alteration in the endogenous release of renal prostaglandins, deficiency of atrial natriuretic factor, and endotoxemia. Patients with decompensated cirrhosis frequently have elevated plasma renin levels, and those with impaired renal function manifest the most profound elevations.

Role of Prostaglandins

Considerable evidence indicates that local prostaglandins act as critical modulators of renal function during states of volume contractions. Drugs that impair renal prostaglandin synthesis reduce GFR and renal plasma flow. Cirrhotic patients without ascites do not seem to be susceptible to this side effect. In a study with cirrhotic patients with ascites pretreatment with indomethacin caused an 82% decrease in furosemide induced natriuresis.[79] Urinary excretion of vasodilatory prostaglandins have been shown to be decreased in patients with HRS. Furthermore, urinary excretion of prostaglandins is increased in cirrhotic patients during water immersion studies.[80,81]

HEPATIC ENCEPHALOPATHY

Hepatic encephalopathy is a clinical syndrome characterized by abnormal mental status occurring in patients with severe hepatic insufficiency. It is a neuropsychiatric disorder associated with characteristic but nonspecific histologic lesions in the central nervous system. The clinical manifestations range from a slightly altered mental status to coma (Table 22–2).

Table 22–2. Classification of Hepatic Encephalopathy

Grade I:	Mild lack of awareness, shortened attention span, impairment on arithmetic testing
Grade II:	Lethargic, disoriented, clear personality change; asterixis
Grade III:	Somnolent, continuous suppression of consciousness level, and responsive to painful stimuli
Grade IV:	Coma, unresponsive to painful stimuli, decorticate or decerebrate posture

Hepatic encephalopathy is commonly considered secondary to accumulation in extracellular fluid of toxic products that have not been metabolized by the liver. This has been shown to occur in patients with end-stage liver disease in whom collateral portal-systemic circulation secondary to increased portal venous pressure has developed. Other important mechanisms may also be involved. These include changes in the blood-brain barrier, abnormal neurotransmitter balance, disturbed cerebral metabolism, and impairment of the sodium-potassium-ATPase activity in neuronal membranes.

Elevated plasma ammonia is a common occurrence both in patients with cirrhotic liver disease or hepatic coma. The production of ammonia in the gastrointestinal tract occurs as a result of ingestion of meat, or other protein, as well as gastrointestinal bleeding. Ammonia is generated in the gut primarily by the action of colonic bacteria and mucosal enzymes acting on these substrates. After ammonia is generated, it is transported through the portal circulation to the liver, where it is normally converted to urea through the urea cycle. In patients with hepatic failure, ammonia is not completely metabolized, so it enters the systemic circulation without being converted into urea. The excess ammonia can then enter the central nervous system. However, it is uncertain to what extent these changes contribute to the development of hepatic encephalopathy. Hepatic coma cannot unequivocally be equated with ammonia toxicity. In hepatic encephalopathy, 10% of blood ammonia values are within the normal range regardless of the depth of coma.

The syndrome of hepatic encephalopathy is marked by profound neuro-inhibition which might be induced by effects on neurotransmitter systems. GABA is the principal inhibitory neurotransmitter of the brain. Increased GABA levels have been confirmed in the plasma of patients with liver disease and hepatic encephalopathy[82] and increased permeability of the blood-brain barrier to GABA has been shown in experimental hepatic coma.[83] Also an increased number of binding sites for GABA have been shown in the brain of a fulminant hepatic failure animal model.[84]

Other substances which may have a role in hepatic encephalopathy include the aromatic amino acids tyrosine, phenylalanine, and tryptophan.[85] Also implicated are mercaptans and free fatty acids which have both been shown to interfere with brain detoxification of ammonia. Together, mercaptans and free fatty acids can act synergistically with ammonia to produce encephalopathy at lower concentrations than are usually required individually.

Hematologic Effects of Chronic Liver Disease

Chronic liver disease is usually accompanied by multiple hematologic alterations. Plasma volume is frequently increased in patients with cirrhosis, especially with ascites and also with long-standing obstructive jaundice or hepatitis. This hypervolemia may partially account for a low peripheral hemoglobin level. Bone marrow of chronic hepatocellular failure is hyperplastic and macronormoblastic. Nevertheless, erythrocyte volume is depressed and the marrow therefore does not seem able to compensate completely for the anemia. Increased red cell destruction occurs with hepatocellular failure and jaundice of all types.

Abnormalities in platelet numbers, structure and function[86,87] are common in patients with all forms of liver disease. The thrombocytopenia of chronic liver disease is extremely common and is largely due to hypersplenism. Qualitatively, the platelets may be inadequate. Disseminated intravascular consumption may be present in severe liver failure.[86,88-90]

Disturbed blood coagulation in patients with hepatobiliary disease is particularly complex. The liver is the principal site of synthesis of all the coagulation proteins with the exception of the von Willebrand factor and the fibrinolytic proteins. The liver also synthesizes protease inhibitors which modulate the coagulation cascade such as antithrombin III, protein C, and heparin cofactor II. Inadequate vitamin K absorption as a result of failure of bile salt secretion into the intestine may also contribute to the coagulopathy associated with liver disease.

The liver synthesizes fibrinogen and the vitamin K-dependent factors, II, VII, IX and X, also labile factor V, factor VIII, contact factors XI, and XII, and fibrin stabilizing factor XIII. The half-life of all these clotting proteins is very short and hence reductions in the circulating amounts of these factors can occur very rapidly during acute hepatocellular necrosis.

In hepatic disease, the factors most likely to be affected are VII, followed by II and X. Factor IX is the last to be reduced. Synthesis of factors V and fibrinogen may be decreased but are less easily depressed than the others.[91]

Fulminant Hepatic Failure

Fulminant hepatic failure is an acute catastrophic event that occurs in patients without pre-existing liver disease and is characterized by the sudden onset of hepatocyte necrosis and the development of encephalopathy within 8 weeks of the onset of initial symptoms or jaundice. FHF is associated with high mortality (range 80 to 94%) when only supportive treatment is used.

Etiology

This can be subdivided into five categories: (1) infection, (2) toxin, (3) drug-induced, (4) ischemic, and (5) metabolic. Hepatitis viruses are responsible for three-fourths of all reported cases of fulminant hepatitis. The second most common etiology for FHF is chemical-related hepatitis. This classification includes idiosyncratic drug reactions as well as direct cellular toxicity from therapeutic drug overdoses, such as acetaminophen overdose. The most frequent cause of FHF are viral hepatitis A, B, and C. The proportion of the different types varies on the geographical location. Other viruses can cause a fatal hepatic necrosis especially in an immunocompromised individual. These include herpes simplex, cytomegalovirus, adenoviruses, Epstein-Barr, and varicella (Table 22-3).

Prognosis

For fulminant hepatitis A the prognosis is better than for other forms of viral hepatitis, with a survival rate of approximately 40%. Hepatitis B is responsible for approximately three-fourths of cases of fulminant viral hepatitis in the US. In about 50% of hepatitis-B-positive patients, the fulminant course is precipitated by another factor usually acute or superinfection with the delta virus. The development of fulminant hepatitis is seen in less than 1% of cases of acute hepatitis B. Acute hepatitis C is responsible for greater than 90% of transfusion-associated hepatitis.[92-94] Also, acute hepatitis C is responsible for greater than 50% of cases of sporadic non-A, non-B hepatitis.[95] The incidence of fulminant hepatitis developing in patients with hepatitis C infections is not known but is thought to be low. The prognosis of fulminant hepatitis C seems poorer than other forms of viral hepatitis, with a survival rate of about 10%.

Pathophysiology

This is not completely understood, but is likely to be as variable as the various etiologies. The one final mechanism that all these etiologies share is massive hepatocellular necrosis. The major cause of death in patients with FHF is cerebral edema, which is found in 60 to 80% of the patients who die. Clinical findings in patients presenting

Table 22-3. Major Causes of Fulminant Hepatic Failure

Viral infection
  Hepatitis A
  Hepatitis B
  Hepatitis C
  Delta hepatitis
    Coinfection with hepatitis B
  Hepatitis E
Drugs, chemicals, poisons
  Acetaminophen
  Ethyl alcohol
  Idiosyncratic drug reactions
  Amanita mushroom poisoning
  Industrial poisons
Miscellaneous
  Acute, fatty liver of pregnancy
  Reye's syndrome
  Wilson's disease
  Ischemia
  Budd-Chiari syndrome
  Malignancy

in FHF may include jaundice, encephalopathy, and fetor hepaticus. Notably absent on physical examination should be the stigmata of chronic liver disease. Therefore, a lack of (a) a history of pre-existing liver disease, (b) marked hepatomegaly, (c) splenomegaly, (d) spider nevi are all consistent with the acute presentation of fulminant hepatitis. The presence of encephalopathy, by definition, must be present within 8 weeks from the onset of liver dysfunction. Hepatic encephalopathy is graded from I to IV. Other complications frequently contributing to death include bacterial and fungal infections, GI hemorrhage, and hepatocellular failure.

COMPLICATIONS

There are many medical complications that commonly occur in FHF (Table 22-4). Cerebral edema is reported to occur in up to 80% of patients with FHF and is the leading cause of mortality in these conditions.[96] Cerebral edema is frequently associated with stage IV coma and a high intracranial pressures (>25 mm Hg). The goal of treatment of cerebral edema is to prevent life-threatening neurologic complications. At some institutions ICP monitoring is utilized to evaluate patients for the development of cerebral edema. This is the most direct and best method of measuring changes in ICP, but it carries an increased risk of bleeding and infection. Newer extradural monitors have decreased the rate of infection but the risk of hemorrhage remains a consideration. Prolonged elevation of ICP above 30 mm Hg should be aggressively treated with intravenous boluses of 20% mannitol.[97] Repeat doses can be given in patients with normal renal function or serum osmolality less than 320 mOSM. Corticosteroids and prolonged controlled hyperventilation have not proven to be of any benefit in controlling or preventing increased ICP in FHF.[97,98]

Coagulopathies

The complex coagulopathy seen in FHF is, in part, due to decreased hepatic synthesis of clotting factors. In addition to the decrease in factor synthesis, increase consumption of clotting factors by a low-grade disseminated intravascular coagulation process in FHF is common.[89] Also, platelet counts, morphology, and function are all adversely affected in this condition.

Table 22-4. Extrahepatic Complications of Fulminant Hepatic Failure

Hepatic encephalopathy
Complex coagulopathy
Cerebral edema
Cardiovascular abnormalities
Acid-base disturbances
Gastrointestinal bleeding
Electrolyte imbalances
Renal failure
Pulmonary complications
Hypoglycemia
Sepsis
Pancreatitis

Cardiovascular Effects

Cardiovascular changes seen in FHF are characterized by a decreased systemic vascular resistance and a compensatory rise in cardiac output. There is no evidence of an abnormal pressor response to tyramine or catecholamines in FHF as in chronic liver disease.[99] Hypotension is a common finding in patients with advanced coma. Arrhythmias, including sinus tachycardia, are common in FHF being reported in over 90% of cases. Underlying hypoxia, acidosis, and electrolyte imbalances can contribute to the initiation and propagation of cardiac arrhythmias.

Renal Failure

Renal failure is a common complication of FHF, occurring in 30% to 75% of cases, depending on the etiology.[100] As with renal failure associated with cirrhosis and chronic liver disease, functional renal failure or hepatorenal syndrome makes up most of the cases of renal failure in FHF[101] The pathophysiology of HRS remains obscure but the final pathway of the renal failure seems to be renal hypoperfusion with preferential renal cortical ischemia. Decreased renal prostaglandin synthesis occurs as it does in renal failure associated with cirrhotic liver disease.[102]

Pulmonary Complications

Pulmonary complications include hypoxemia, aspiration, and high incidence of low pressure pulmonary edema or adult respiratory distress syndrome (ARDS).[103] Other complications include acid-base and electrolyte imbalances, sepsis, and pancreatitis.

Mortality

The survival of a patient with FHF depends on the massiveness of hepatic destruction, the ability of the remaining liver cells to regenerate, and the management of medical complications that may arise during the clinical course. The availability of orthotopic liver transplantation as a therapeutic option for those patients who would not survive makes the need for early prognostic parameters even more crucial. A patient with FHF should be treated in a medical center where there is a liver transplantation program or be transferred to one at the first signs of encephalopathy.

The survival rate of FHF varies according to the etiology. In one series from the Liver Unit, King's College, the authors included among those with a better survival rate; Hepatitis A (survival 66.7%); hepatitis B (38.9%), and acetaminophen overdose (52.9%). A worse survival rate was observed in presumed non-A, non-B hepatitis (20%) and for halothane or drug hepatotoxicity in general (12.5%).[104]

Other prognostic factors include age, coma, hepatic size, and laboratory tests. The survival rate in patients less than 14 years of age was 35%; between 15 and 45 years, the rate was 22%; and in those who were more than 45 years of age, it was 5%.[105,106] Various groups have observed an association between the maximum degree of hepatic encephalopathy and survival. The use of liver and abdominal CT scan has given support to the clinical impression that a decrease in liver size is a bad prognostic finding.[107] Laboratory studies have found that survival correlated with the variables of arterial blood pH, prothrombin time, and serum creatinine in patients with acetaminophen-induced failure.[108] In patients with non acetaminophen-associated FHF serum bilirubin greater than 300 μmol/L and prothrombin time greater than 50 seconds were associated with a poor prognosis.[104]

Cholestatic Diseases

Diagnosis

Impaired bile formation or drainage is the hallmark of cholestasis. Bile is a complex fluid, iso-osmotic with plasma, composed primarily of water, inorganic electrolytes, and organic solutes, such as bile acids, phospholipids, cholesterol, and the bile pigments. Cholestatic liver disease can be categorized as either a functional defect in bile formation at the level of the hepatocyte (intrahepatic cholestasis) or a structural or mechanical impairment on bile secretion and flow (extrahepatic cholestasis) (Table 22–5). Clinically, cholestasis is reflected by the appearance in blood of several solutes, including bilirubin, bile acids, and cholesterol, that are preferentially excreted into bile under normal conditions.

Intrahepatic cholestasis occurs at the level of the hepatocytes or the intrahepatic biliary ducts. The initial symptoms of pruritus and jaundice occur from the increase in blood of solutes normally found in bile. Following prolonged cholestasis biliary cirrhosis occurs; the time taken for its development varies from months to years.

Extrahepatic cholestasis is most commonly due to structural or mechanical obstruction of the bile ducts by choledocholithiasis, pancreatic and periampullary cancer, or biliary strictures. Biochemical features are similar to those observed in patients with intrahepatic cholestasis, with striking elevations in serum bilirubin and alkaline phosphatase.

Table 22–5. Cholestatic Syndromes

Intrahepatic	Extrahepatic
Acute hepatocellular injury	Choledocholithiasis
Viral hepatitis	Biliary strictures
Alcoholic fatty liver and/or hepatitis	Sclerosing cholangitis
	Cholangiocarcinoma
Drugs	Pancreatic carcinoma
Chronic hepatocellular injury	Pancreatitis (acute or chronic)
Primary biliary cirrhosis	Periampullary carcinoma
Sclerosing cholangitis	Biliary atresia
Drugs	Choledochal cysts
Total parenteral nutrition	Metastatic tumor
Systemic infection	
Pregnancy	
Benign recurrent disorders	

Signs and Symptoms of Extrahepatic Cholestasis

Cholestasis may be associated with many extrahepatic manifestations. Fat malabsorption secondary to diminished delivery of bile salts to the intestinal lumen may lead to deficiencies in the fat-soluble vitamins A, D, E, and K. Prolongation of the prothrombin time may respond to administration of vitamin K for 3 days, and thereafter as dictated by the prothrombin time. Cardiovascular responses are abnormal and peripheral vasoconstriction in response to hypotension is impaired. Sinus node dysfunction resulting in clinically significant bradycardia has been associated with obstructive jaundice. The mechanism appears to be mediated via stimulation of the vagus nerve, although the stimulus for enhanced vagal tone has not been identified. Obstructive jaundice also has adverse effects on renal function, particularly in the postoperative patient. The mechanism of suppression of normal renal function in patients with extrahepatic biliary obstruction has not been established. Impaired cell-mediated immunity and interleukin production by circulating mononuclear cells has been linked to hyperbilirubinemia and may account for the increased risk of infectious complications observed in patients with extrahepatic cholestasis. Two major forms of metabolic bone disease osteomalacia and osteoporosis are associated with cholestatic liver disease.

CLINICAL LABORATORY TESTS

Liver chemistry tests are used to determine the presence of liver disease. However, no single chemical test is able to establish the diagnosis of a particular type of liver disease. And although some of the values on liver chemistry tests may allow a degree of severity assessment, they have proven less than reliable prognostic indicators.

Serum Bilirubin

A raised serum bilirubin level is an indicator for the presence of liver disease, although patients with hemolytic anemia may also have elevated levels. Therefore, the test lacks specificity. And an occasional patient with cirrhosis or other hepatic disease has normal values. The clinical value of serum bilirubin is considerably enhanced by measuring the conjugated and unconjugated bilirubin (Table 22-6).

Increased Unconjugated Bilirubin

An increase in the level of unconjugated bilirubin may be due to overproduction, decrease in hepatic uptake, or a decrease in hepatic binding and conjugation. Disorders of overproduction are characterized by a proportional increase in the unconjugated and conjugated serum bilirubin levels. Hemolytic anemia is the most frequent cause. Patients with blood in tissues or body cavities due to trauma or surgery may also have proportional increases in the conjugated and unconjugated serum bilirubin. In the disorders characterized by a decrease in hepatic uptake, the unconjugated serum bilirubin usually increases to a greater degree than the conjugated serum bilirubin. The other liver chemistry tests are generally normal. Some drugs, such as rifampin and some radiocontrast agents

Table 22–6. Causes of Hyperbilirubinemia

Mainly unconjugated
- Overproduction
  - *Hemolysis*
  - *Extravasation*
  - *Shunt hyperbilirubinemia*
- Reduced uptake
  - *Portosystemic shunt*
  - *Drugs*
  - *Gilbert Syndrome (some cases)*
- Conjugation defect
  - Acquired
    - *Neonatal*
    - *Maternal milk*
    - *Lucey-Driscoll*
    - *Drugs*
    - *Hyperthyroidism*
    - *Chronic persistent hepatitis*
  - Inherited
    - *Crigler-Najjar I*
    - *Crigler-Najjar II*
    - *Gilbert syndrome*

Both conjugated and unconjugated
- Biliary obstruction
  - *Common duct stones*
  - *Tumors*
- Intrahepatic cholestasis
  - *Steroids*
  - *Allergic*
  - *Hepatitis (occasional)*
- Hepatocellular injury
  - Acute
  - Chronic
- Hepatocellular defects of canalicular excretion
  - *Dubin-Johnson*
  - *Rotor syndrome*

may be competitive inhibitors of bilirubin uptake and can lead to elevated levels of unconjugated bilirubin. Gilbert's syndrome is a benign familial disorder which results in increased levels of unconjugated bilirubin.

As with defects in hepatic uptake of bilirubin, abnormalities of binding and conjugation generally result in a disproportional increase in the unconjugated serum bilirubin level. Gilbert's syndrome may fit into this category also; the Crigler-Najjar syndrome in which hepatic glucuronyltransferase is absent.

Decreased Levels of Bilirubin

In disorders due to decreased canalicular excretions both the unconjugated and conjugated serum bilirubin levels rise, but there is a disproportional increase in the conjugated serum bilirubin level. Some drugs such as chlorpromazine and sulfonamides, mainly produce canalicular injury. Extrahepatic obstruction of bile flow will result in elevated conjugated hyperbilirubinemia.

Patients with hepatobiliary diseases such as acute and chronic hepatitis, prolonged biliary tract obstruction, alcoholic and nonalcoholic cirrhosis, and metabolic disorders such as Wilson's disease and alpha$_1$-antitrypsin deficiency often have raised serum bilirubin levels. Several abnormalities of bilirubin metabolism are usually present in such patients, but the conjugated serum bilirubin is usually disproportionately raised. Decreased hepatic excretion is probably the major factor, because it is the rate-limiting step in hepatic bilirubin metabolism. Shortened red cell survival is associated with liver disease and may account for an increased pigment load. Hepatic bilirubin uptake and glucuronyltransferase activity appear to be preserved in most liver diseases, but increasing levels of unconjugated bilirubin in fulminant hepatic failure may reflect decreased bilirubin uptake and decreased glucuronyltransferase activity. All steps in bilirubin metabolism may be impaired as functional hepatic mass declines in end-stage liver disease.[109]

Serum Alkaline Phosphatase

Serum alkaline phosphatase is the name applied to a group of enzymes that catalyze the hydrolysis of phosphate esters at an alkaline pH. This enzyme is widely distributed in human tissue, including liver, bone, placenta, intestine, kidney, and leukocytes. In the liver, the enzyme is mainly bound to canalicular membranes. Liver and bone isoenzymes are the major fractions of the serum alkaline phosphatase in healthy adults. Serum alkaline phosphatase level is most useful in detecting cholestasis. Most patients with some form of cholestasis have a value more than three times the upper limit of normal. Thus, a markedly elevated serum alkaline phosphatase suggests the possibility of disorders such as extrahepatic bile duct obstruction, primary biliary cirrhosis, primary sclerosing cholangitis, or cholestasis due to drugs. Unfortunately, the level of the serum alkaline phosphatase is not helpful in differentiating extra- from intrahepatic cholestasis. Disorders such as viral hepatitis, chronic hepatitis, alcoholic hepatitis, and cirrhosis are usually associated with milder increases in the serum alkaline phosphatase.

5'-Nucleotidase and gamma-glutamyl transferase are both enzymes found in canalicular membranes and plasma membranes of hepatocytes. The main clinical use for the measurement of these two enzymes is to determine the source of a raised serum alkaline phosphatase. Both enzymes are quite specific for liver disease and may be normal in clinical situations where alkaline phosphatase is elevated for nonhepatic causes such as rapid bone growth in children and adolescents and increased alkaline phosphatase production by the placenta during pregnancy.

Enzymes Reflecting Hepatocellular Injury

The aspartate aminotransferase (AST or SGOT) and alanine aminotransferases (ALT or SGPT) catalyze the transfer of the alpha amino group from aspartate or alanine to alpha-ketoglutarate with the release of pyruvate, oxalacetate, and glutamate. Aspartate aminotransferase (AST) is located in both the cytosol and mitochondria of the liver cell. There are individual isoenzymes, and the main serum component is from the cytosolic fraction. This enzyme is

also located in cardiac muscle, skeletal muscle, brain, kidney, pancreas, and leukocytes. Alanine aminotransferase (ALT) can also be found in several tissues throughout the body, but the concentration in liver is considerably higher than elsewhere.

The aspartate and alanine aminotransferases often exceed 500 IU/L in conditions associated with acute hepatocellular injury, such as viral hepatitis, drug hepatitis, and exposure to hepatotoxins. Markedly raised values are also seen with hepatic ischemia due to acute congestive heart failure or following orthotopic liver transplantation. Occasionally, patients with acute biliary tract obstruction due to passage of a common duct stone may have markedly raised aminotransferases.[110] In these conditions, the aminotransferases often return to normal in a few days, whereas the decline is slower in patients with viral and drug-induced hepatitis. In contrast, patients with other forms of liver disease generally have aminotransferases that do not exceed 10 times the upper limit of normal.[111] Such conditions include alcoholic hepatitis and cirrhosis, postnecrotic cirrhosis, primary biliary cirrhosis, obstructive jaundice, Wilson's disease, and fatty infiltration of the liver. The aminotransferases generally begin to increase late in the prodrome of viral hepatitis and are often already decreasing when jaundice appears.

In patients with alcoholic hepatitis and cirrhosis, the aminotransferases rarely exceed 300 IU/L, and the ratio of aspartate aminotransferase to alanine aminotransferase is usually greater than 2.[112,113] The depressed alanine aminotransferase level is probably due to nutritional deficiency of pyridoxal phosphate. Administration of this nutrient to alcoholics results in a rapid increase in aspartate aminotransferase.[114]

Aspartate aminotransferase may be elevated in a number of non hepatic conditions as well. These include cerebrovascular accident, myocardial infarction, and acute muscle injury, such as rhabdomyolysis. In addition, heavy physical exercise may sometimes account for a mild increase in the aspartate aminotransferase.

Lactic dehydrogenase (LDH) is distributed in many human tissues, particularly the liver, red blood cells, cardiac muscle, and kidney. Five isoenzymes have been described. Isoenzyme 5, represents the liver's contribution. The clinical importance of this test in liver disease is limited. It lacks both sensitivity and specificity, even when isoenzyme measurements are performed. Values are generally higher in acute hepatocellular injury than in other types of liver disease, but the aminotransferases are more sensitive and specific.

Serum Proteins in Liver Disease

Serum albumin is the main export protein synthesized by the liver and is the single most important factor in maintaining plasma oncotic pressure. Serum albumin also provides an important vehicle for the transport of many drugs and xenobiotics. Up to 500 g are present in healthy subjects, and approximately 10 g are synthesized daily. Synthesis is influenced by liver injury, nutritional status, and catabolic states such as infections and burns.

Serum albumin and globulin measurements lack sensitivity and specificity for the detection of liver disease.

However, patients with chronic liver disease, particularly cirrhosis, often have a depressed serum albumin level and a raised serum globulin level. Occasionally, a patient with cirrhosis may display only this liver chemistry test abnormality.

A depressed serum albumin level in a patient with cirrhosis used to be taken as evidence of impaired albumin synthesis. More recent studies show that patients with cirrhosis often have normal albumin production rates, but the explanation for low serum levels is uncertain. Because of the multiple factors that affect the serum albumin level, this test is less useful in establishing a prognosis than the prothrombin time.[115]

The liver makes a major contribution to normal blood coagulation. Most of the proteins involved in blood coagulation are synthesized in the liver, including factors I (fibrinogen), II (prothrombin), V, VI, IX, and X. Only major injury to the liver produces a clinically important fall in the concentration of these factors and an increase risk of bleeding, because they are present in a large excess. Vitamin K is essential for normal blood coagulation. Vitamin K activates factors II, VII, IX, and X for coagulation by carboxylating glutamine residues at the gamma position.

The prothrombin time is not a sensitive indicator of liver disease, because damage is usually severe before abnormal values are detected. The prothrombin time is generally normal in most patients with acute hepatocellular injury and in many patients with mild chronic liver disease. The test also lacks specificity. Disorders besides liver disease may cause abnormalities, including congenital deficiency of coagulation factors, nutritional deficiency, malabsorption, and suppression of the intestinal bacterial flora by antibiotics.

Most of the conditions that result in a prolonged prothrombin time can usually be distinguished from parenchymal damage by parenteral administration of 10 mg of vitamin K daily for 3 days. If the prothrombin time improves 30% or more 24 hours after an initial injection of vitamin K, vitamin K deficiency due to obstructive jaundice rather than to severe parenchymal liver disease is the likely explanation.

The prothrombin time is the only standard liver chemistry test that provides useful information about the prognosis of liver disease. Patients with acute hepatitis who develop fulminant hepatic failure often have marked prolongation of the prothrombin time prior to clinical evidence of severe hepatic injury. However, many patients with acute hepatitis may have a mildly prolonged prothrombin time early in their course and yet have a benign outcome.

Functional Liver Tests

Substrates with a low extraction ratio, generally 20–30%, have been used to measure functional hepatic mass or hepatic metabolic capacity. Changes in hepatic blood flow exert little effect on the clearance of such substrates, but changes in hepatic enzymes that metabolize the drug exert major effects on clearance. Antipyrine clearance or plasma half-life has been widely studied by assaying the test substrate in plasma or salivary samples. Clearance is decreased and half-life prolonged in patients with cirrhosis compared to healthy subjects.

The aminopyrine breath test is a measure of hepatic microsomal function and N-demethylation. For this test radiolabeled aminopyrine substrate is administered orally, and the radiolabeled carbons are removed by a rate-limiting, hepatic microsomal enzyme. Radiolabeled carbon ultimately equilibrates in exhaled CO_2, and samples of exhaled gases are collected. The isotope enrichment of the samples reflects hepatic microsomal enzyme activity. The values are markedly depressed in patients with cirrhosis compared with those from healthy subjects. It is a sensitive and quantitative indicator of liver dysfunction.[116,117]

Indocyanine green (ICG) is an organic anionic dye which is taken up by the liver. ICG does not undergo extrahepatic removal, intrahepatic conjugation, or interohepatic circulation and therefore serves as a measure of hepatic protein receptor mass. The maximal rate of uptake correlates closely with functional liver mass when administered in doses of 1.0 to 5.0 mg/kg body weight. When given in smaller doses receptor uptake may not be maximal and the limiting factor in removal is liver blood flow rather than hepatocellular function. Measurement of indocyanine green clearance after injection of 0.5 mg/kg body weight through a peripheral vein provides a reasonable approximation of hepatic blood flow when compared to constant infusion methods of measurement.

Studies suggest that the use of tests that measure hepatic metabolism may be useful in following the progress of liver disease and may add new prognostic information to those already available using the standard Child-Turcotte-Pugh classifications.[118]

Markers of Specific Liver Diseases

a. **Serum ferritin** is often useful in establishing a diagnosis of idiopathic hemochromatosis, a genetic disorder of iron metabolism with injury to several parenchymal organs including the liver. The concentration of ferritin is proportional to body iron stores. It is of value in assessing uncomplicated iron overload, but can be unreliable in early diagnosis of the pre-cirrhotic stage. A normal value does not exclude iron storage disease.[119,120]

b. **Ceruloplasmin** is the major copper-binding protein synthesized by the liver and secreted into the bloodstream of healthy subjects. The absence or deficiency of ceruloplasmin per se is unlikely to be primarily involved in the pathogenesis of Wilson's disease. Nonetheless, it is a useful test for Wilson's disease, and values in most homozygotes are markedly decreased.[121] Measurement of copper excretion in a 24-hour urine specimen may be helpful in diagnosis of these patients.

c. **Alpha-fetoprotein** is a major circulating plasma protein during fetal development and remains markedly elevated at birth. Values decline to the usual adult level by 1 year of age. Markedly raised serum alpha-fetoprotein levels are fairly sensitive and specific for the presence of hepatocellular carcinoma. In adults, up to 70% of patients with hepatocellular carcinomas have levels above 500 ng/ml. Some patients have less elevated values, and tumors in some patients do not produce this protein. Pediatric patients with hepatoblastomas usually have markedly raised values.

Other acute and chronic liver diseases may also be associated with raised alpha-fetoprotein levels, but the values are generally not as high as in most patients with hepatocellular carcinomas.[122] Raised serum alpha-fetoprotein levels in patients with chronic hepatitis, alcoholic hepatitis, and fulminant hepatic failure probably reflect hepatic inflammation and regeneration. Elevated values often decline in these conditions as hepatic inflammation subsides, but values generally rise progressively in patients with hepatocellular carcinomas. Thus, this test may be helpful in the early detection of hepatocellular carcinoma in high risk groups, such as patients with chronic hepatitis B, hepatitis C, alcoholic cirrhosis, and hemochromatosis.[123,124]

    d. **Alpha$_1$-Antitrypsin deficiency** should be considered as a potential cause of neonatal hepatitis, but it is an uncommon etiology for liver disease in children and adults. The main function of alpha$_1$-antitrypsin is to inhibit serum trypsin activity. Alpha$_1$-antitrypsin is the major component of serum alpha$_1$-globulin, so a depressed alpha$_1$-globulin level suggests the diagnosis of alpha$_1$-antitrypsin deficiency.

LIVER DISEASE AND DRUGS

In patients with liver disease, handling of drugs by the liver may be disturbed greatly by several mechanisms, including altered absorption, distribution, and elimination. Drug elimination is influenced by many factors in patients with liver disease, the most important of which are abnormal (usually reduced) liver blood flow, portal-systemic shunting and impaired metabolic capacity.

Drugs may be classified according to their dependence on liver blood flow for drug metabolism.

High Extraction Drugs

The disposition of drugs which have a high hepatic extraction, normally more than 60% of available drug in a single pass, is highly dependent upon liver blood flow, with first-pass elimination limiting systemic availability of orally administered drug. In patients with liver disease, liver blood flow in general, although not invariably, is reduced and portal-systemic shunting allows blood draining from the splanchnic circulation to bypass the liver. Both of these factors may effect drug pharmacokinetics, leading to high peak drug concentrations with less effect on drug half-life. If such drugs are to be prescribed, particularly by oral administration, the dose to be administered should be reduced, without change in dosing frequency.

The pharmacokinetic profiles of high extraction drugs after parenteral administration (which reduces the effect of high first-pass extract by allowing drug access to the systemic circulation without passing through the portal vein) might be expected to be relatively unchanged in patients with hepatic disease. In reality, factors such as decreased hepatic uptake of drugs and intrahepatic shunting complicate the situation.

Low Extraction Drugs

These have an extraction of less than 30% in a single pass through the liver depend much less on liver blood flow and more on the metabolic capacity of the liver. Systemic bioavailability of these agents, after oral administration, is much greater than for high extraction drugs. Low extraction drugs, although more dependent on the metabolic capacity of the liver rather than its blood flow, may demonstrate variable rates of metabolism in patients with liver disease depending on the metabolic pathways involved.

Oxidation of drugs (a phase I reaction) is carried out principally by the cytochrome P-450 enzymes, which are situated predominantly in zone 3 (perivenous) of the hepatic acinus. In contrast, enzymes responsible for conjugation (phase II reactions), such as the glucuronyltransferases, are plentiful in zone 1 (the periportal area). Enzymes situated in zone 3, appear to be affected more in liver disease than those in zone 1. There is evidence that glucuronidation, a phase II reaction, is relatively well preserved in patients with liver disease, unlike phase I reactions. In patients with liver disease caused by ethanol, enzyme induction may be present and influence drug metabolism. The metabolic capacity impairment of the liver is not a homogeneous entity in patients with liver disease, but depends upon the metabolic pathways involved.

The **pharmacokinetic profiles** of low extraction drugs tend not to show particularly high peak blood concentrations, but rather increased half-life. Therefore, it should be the frequency between drug administrations that should be increased, rather than the dosage.

Absorption of drugs and distribution within the body may be altered in liver disease, leading to abnormal bioavailability. Because of associated hypoalbuminemia, drug binding may be reduced in liver disease, increasing the proportion of free drug available for metabolism. This tends to normalize pharmacokinetics in patients with reduced metabolic capacity. Reduced plasma protein binding also influences penetration of drugs into tissues and drug distribution. The increase in total body water found in liver disease, particularly in those with ascites, increases the volume of distribution of hydrophilic substances such as the neuromuscular blocking agents.[125]

Opioids

Morphine is normally an intermediate-high extraction drug (extraction ratio 0.5 to 0.8), with a low plasma binding (15 to 30%), and is detoxified by conjugation with glucuronic acid. In a study evaluating the extraction ratio of morphine in control and cirrhotic patients, the extraction ratio was reduced by 25% in the cirrhotics. This reduction was due to impaired enzyme capacity rather than reduced hepatic blood flow. The effect of cirrhosis is less than that reported in similar studies of high clearance oxidized drugs and this lends support to the concept that glucuronidation may be relatively spared in cirrhosis.[126]

Patwardhan et al demonstrated that, even in the presence of decreased liver blood flow, morphine clearance is similar in humans with normal liver function and in those with cirrhosis.[127] More recent studies have demonstrated that morphine elimination and clearance are impaired in patients with severe liver disease.[128,129] The bioavailability of orally administered morphine was increased in individuals with severe cirrhosis.[129] Whether cirrhotic patients have an increased pharmacodynamic response to morphine is still uncertain.[127,130]

Meperidine and pentazocine had higher bioavailability when given orally in cirrhotics and a decreased systemic blood clearance.[131] The elimination of meperidine was prolonged in cirrhotic patients after a single intravenous injection.[132]

Fentanyl given as a single intravenous dose had pharmacokinetic values not altered in surgical patients with cirrhosis.[133] Sufentanil also given in a single bolus dose to anesthetized patients had similar pharmacokinetics when given to patients with uncomplicated cirrhosis and in control patients.[134]

Alfentanil had decreased clearance and an increased free fraction in cirrhotic patients when given as a single bolus dose during general anesthesia.[135] This could result in a pronounced and prolonged effect from alfentanil in these patients. However, Bower et al demonstrated that the disposition of alfentanil can be altered differently in cirrhotics depending on the etiology of the liver disease. Patients with non-alcoholic liver disease had a lower plasma clearance of alfentanil than the group of patients with alcoholic liver disease.[136]

Benzodiazepines

The clearance of diazepam and midazolam were decreased in cirrhotic patients.[67,137,138] Kraus et al demonstrated an increase in elimination half life of lorazepam in patients with cirrhosis which was secondary to a increase in volume of distribution.[139] Oxazepam, an active metabolite of diazepam which requires only conjugation for biotransformation, had unaltered elimination in humans with acute viral hepatitis and in those with cirrhosis.[68] In addition to the altered pharmacokinetics of most benzodiazepines, patients with cirrhosis demonstrated increased CNS sensitivity to benzodiazepines.[67,137,140]

Barbiturates

Thiopental given as a single induction dose showed a significant increase in free fraction in cirrhotic patients.[141,142] There was a linear correlation between the free fraction and the plasma albumin level. The clearance was not altered in the cirrhotics from normal. These findings could result in enhanced pharmacologic activity and acute toxicity of thiopental in cirrhotics but little alteration in the prolonged effect from decreased elimination.[142]

Propofol

Propofol has a very high clearance and is hydroxylated and conjugated by the liver. However, in patients with uncomplicated cirrhosis propofol pharmacokinetics and protein binding following a single intravenous bolus dose were not markedly affected.[143] The pharmacokinetics of propofol given by infusion to maintain general anesthesia was not affected markedly by moderate cirrhosis. However the recovery times were increased in the cirrhotic patients.[144,145]

Muscle Relaxants

An increased requirement for d-tubocurarine in patients with liver disease was noted by Dundee and Gray 1953.[146] This increased requirement has been correlated with levels of gamma globulin which can be in increased in patients with liver disease.[147] However other studies have not demonstrated and increase in protein binding of d-tubocurarine.[148,149] With pancuronium, a two-fold increase in both the distribution half-life (T 1/2 alpha) from 11 to 24 min and in the elimination half-life (T 1/2 beta) from 114 to 208 min was observed in patients with cirrhosis. In these individuals, the total apparent volume of distribution of pancuronium was increased by 50%. Plasma clearance of pancuronium was decreased by 22%. These results suggest that there is a risk of prolonged duration of action of pancuronium in patients with cirrhosis. In these patients, the initial dose to achieve adequate muscle relaxation is high and simultaneously there is slow disappearance of pancuronium from plasma. These alterations are mainly a consequence of the increase in the distribution volume of pancuronium in patients with cirrhosis.[150]

Arden et al demonstrated that alcoholic liver disease does not affect the pharmacokinetics or duration of action of vecuronium when an intravenous bolus dose of 0.1 mg/kg was administered.[151] In a study using higher doses of vecuronium, 0.15 mg/kg was found to have a similar duration of action in both normal and cirrhotic patients, and vecuronium 0.2 mg/kg had a significantly longer action in the cirrhotic group.[152] In patients with cholestatic liver disease the plasma clearance of vecuronium was decreased, elimination half-life increased and a longer duration of effect was observed.[153]

Because atracurium's elimination is determined mainly by Hofmann decomposition it should be relatively independent of hepatic and renal function. This has been demonstrated in adult and pediatric patients with liver disease.[154-158] Although the pharmacokinetics of atracurium are not altered in patients with liver disease the elimination half life and the total volume of distribution of the metabolite laudanosine are increased.[154,157]

TREATMENT OF PORTAL HYPERTENSION

Etiology

In patients with cirrhosis, esophageal variceal hemorrhage is a common event associated with often catastrophic consequences. It is the leading cause of death in patients with portal hypertension. The treatment modalities are aimed at both preventing variceal hemorrhage and achieving acute hemostasis. The therapies include, the use of pharmacologic agents, endoscopic techniques, surgical techniques and recently non-operative portal-systemic shunt procedures.

Although varices can be found throughout the gastrointestinal tract in patients with portal hypertension, only those varices located in the distal esophagus and proximal stomach are likely to bleed. Approximately 50% of patients found to have esophageal varices will eventually bleed from those varices. Clinical studies suggest that large esophageal varices are more likely to bleed than small ones.

Mortality rates of initial esophageal varices hemorrhage range from 40 to 70%.[159] The cause of death is often multifactorial, primarily due to complications of liver failure and less often due to frank exsanguination. Recurrence of bleeding during the initial hospital admission is 60% and long-term mortality is 60% after 2 years. The severity of the underlying liver disease is one of the most important determinants of mortality rates in patients with variceal hemorrhage.[160]

Management of Acute Hemorrhage

Variceal hemorrhage may present subacutely with melena or acutely with massive hematemesis, hematochezia, or shock. If a patient suffers sustained hypotension, any preexisting hepatocellular disease may be aggravated. Therefore, aggressive but judicious replacement of lost blood volume is essential. Overzealous expansion of blood volume may provoke recurrent variceal hemorrhage, presumably by increasing portal vein pressures.

Emergency therapies include: pharmacologic agents, balloon tamponade, endoscopic sclerotherapy or ligation, transhepatic variceal embolization, surgical portal-systemic shunt procedures, and radiographically placed transhepatic portal-systemic shunts.

Pharmacologic Therapy

Vasopressin is an endogenous peptide at pharmacologic dosages, acts directly on mesenteric vascular smooth muscle, increasing vascular resistance, decreasing splanchnic flow, and ultimately decreasing portal and variceal flow and pressure. At present, vasopressin has not been conclusively shown to control acute variceal hemorrhage or improve survival any better than placebo.[161-163] Vasopressin's major complications include myocardial ischemia and gastrointestinal symptoms of diarrhea and abdominal cramping. Nitroglycerin has been administered with vasopressin in attempts to reduce the cardiac complications.[164-166]

Synthetic somatostatin selectively reduces splanchnic blood flow by vasoconstriction and is thought by some to also reduce portal pressure and flow.[167-169] Somatostatin has less vasoconstrictive effect on the systemic circulation.

Mechanical Therapy

Esophageal balloon tamponade therapy has been used for the past four decades, the Sengstaken-Blakemore tube being the most commonly used device. Balloon tamponade therapy of hemorrhaging varices, although intuitively appealing, has unfortunately had only variable clinical success (40–90% initial hemostatic rate) with often unacceptably high rates of complications.[170-173]

Endoscopic Therapy

Endoscopic injection sclerotherapy has become the treatment of choice for esophageal variceal hemorrhage. The goals of sclerotherapy are acute hemostasis and long term variceal obliteration. Several randomized trials have shown that sclerotherapy more effectively controls acute esophageal variceal hemorrhage than do combinations of balloon tamponade, vasopressin, and vasopressin plus nitroglycerin.[170,171,173,174] Bleeding is controlled in about 90% of patients treated with sclerotherapy as compared to approximately 60–70% with medical therapy. Patients treated with sclerotherapy were also less likely to suffer fatal variceal hemorrhage.[170-173]

Endoscopic ligation of bleeding varices has been recently explored and long term results appear comparable to those of endoscopic sclerotherapy.[175]

Most patients who survive a variceal hemorrhage will rebleed. With the exception of emergency shunt surgery, all the emergency therapies do not decrease the risk of recurrent variceal bleeding. Emergency shunt surgery, although resulting in negligible rebleeding, unfortunately has a discouragingly high operative mortality rate.[176-178]

Long-term pharmacologic therapy has been mostly concentrated on the use of nonselective beta adrenergic receptor antagonist. They have the ability to decrease portal pressure by splanchnic vasoconstriction and by decreasing cardiac output. However, even with these characteristics the results confirming the efficacy of beta blockers in decreasing recurrent variceal hemorrhage and mortality are conflicting.[179-182] Propranolol continues to be used and studied alone and in combination with sclerotherapy in the hope of further reducing recurrent bleeding.[183]

Elective Shunt Surgery

There are randomized controlled prospective trials that have compared elective portal-caval shunts to supportive medical management (without sclerotherapy). These studies reported a significant reduction in recurrent variceal bleeding in the surgically treated groups. Portal-systemic shunt surgery is extremely effective at preventing variceal rebleeding, but is often complicated by encephalopathy and enhanced progression of liver disease. This potential deterioration in the patient's quality of life must be weighed against the risks and benefits of other nonsurgical procedures, most of which require multiple treatment sessions, chronic surveillance, a high degree of patient compliance, and continue to have higher rebleeding rates. No studies have shown significantly prolonged survival with surgical shunting.

TIPS-Intrahepatic Portal-Systemic Shunt

Transjugular intrahepatic portal-systemic shunts (TIPS) is a non-operative therapeutic alternative for the treatment of variceal bleeding as a consequence of portal hypertension. First described in animals in 1969, intraparenchymal portal decompression is achieved through a percutaneously created channel between a hepatic vein and the portal vein.[184] Shunt occlusion limited the clinical application originally but after the introduction of metallic stents in the 1980s many investigators have demonstrated that prolonged shunt patency can be achieved.[185-188] The procedure is performed by interventional radiologists and can performed with local anesthetics and intravenous sedation or general anesthesia necessitating the involvement of anesthesia providers. A technique for administration of local anesthetic to the area of the transparenchymal tract has been described.[189]

TIPS has been used for an effective short-term therapy for esophageal variceal hemorrhage which has failed to be controlled with endoscopic sclerotherapy. It offers advantages over surgically created portal-systemic shunts of shorter recovery periods, and less operative distortion and scarring of right upper quadrant anatomic structures which could inhibit or impede subsequent liver transplantation. Operative portal-caval shunts result in periportal adhesions that substantially increase the difficulty and blood loss of subsequent liver transplantation. In contrast, TIP shunts are constructed entirely within the liver and do not interfere with subsequent transplantation surgery.

Investigators have reported high stent patency rates. However, the 30 day mortality rate remain high (15 to 45%).[185-188] A recent study demonstrated high mortality rates particularly in the urgent cases with active variceal bleeding.[188] Their 56% mortality rate observed in patients undergoing TIPS urgently is similar to that reported for surgical portal-systemic shunt procedures in acutely bleeding patients and suggests that every effort should be made to control bleeding and to stabilize and resuscitate the patient before performing TIPS.

LIVER TRANSPLANTATION

Liver transplantation has become a well accepted treatment of end-stage liver disease from multiple etiologies. The liver can be transplanted as an extra (auxiliary) organ at an ectopic site, or in the orthotopic location after the removal of the host liver. The orthotopic location is used almost exclusively and auxiliary procedures used rarely, usually in cases of inborn errors of metabolism.

Indications

The most common underlying hepatic disease making transplantation necessary differs in adult and pediatric patients. In adults postnecrotic cirrhosis is the most common indication for liver transplantation. Within this category, cirrhosis may result from chronic active viral hepatitis and autoimmune hepatitis. Cirrhosis due to alcohol abuse or resulting from chronic toxic injuries are also within this group. The next largest group of diseases treated by liver transplantation are cholestatic disorders including primary biliary cirrhosis, secondary biliary cirrhosis, and sclerosing cholangitis. Metabolic disorders including Wilson's disease and hemochromatosis constitute another group. Fulminant hepatic failure from toxin ingestion, such as acetaminophen, as a result of metabolic disorder, such as acute Wilson's crisis, or resulting from viral hepatitis has frequently been treated by liver transplantation despite the somewhat poorer results in the group. Generally, tumors of the liver are no longer considered a prime indication for liver transplantation be-

cause of the high rate of early recurrence. Nevertheless, for some special tumor types, liver transplantation provides satisfactory therapy. Vascular disorders, primarily Budd-Chiari syndrome, comprise a final category of indications. Half or more of the pediatric recipients have biliary atresia, with inborn metabolic errors a distant second (Table 22-7).

The first human liver transplant was performed in 1963 by Starzle.[190] In the following 17 years, the progress of liver transplantation grew slowly as organs were scarce and the technique was imperfect. The introduction in 1979 of cyclosporine, coincided with a revolution in liver transplantation.[191] Finally, the acceptance of liver transplantation as a preferred therapy for end-stage liver disease permitted the application of the procedure to less desperately ill patients, contributing to an additional increment in success. Liver transplantation once seemed so drastic that it was used only as a last resort treatment for critically ill patients with end stage hepatic failure. Every patient with primary progressive liver disease or fulminate hepatic failure should receive early evaluation for potential liver transplantation surgery. Allowing a patient's condition to deteriorate to the point at which life-support systems are required before considering liver transplantation should be avoided. A problem in the timing of transplantation surgery exists due to the heterogeneity of liver diseases and the variable rates of progression. In addition to the estimated duration of survival the patient's quality of life is an important consideration in the timing of transplantation. In some patients the liver disease, although advanced, is stable or slowly progres-

Table 22-7. Possible Candidates for Liver Transplantation

Parenchymal
    Postnecrotic cirrhosis
    Alcoholic cirrhosis
    Fulminant hepatic failure
    Congenital hepatic fibrosis
    Cystic fibrosis
    Neonatal hepatitis
    Hepatic trauma
Cholestatic
    Biliary atresia
    Primary biliary cirrhosis
    Sclerosing cholangitis
    Secondary biliary cirrhosis
    Familial cholestasis
Inborn errors of metabolism
    Alpha$_1$-Antitrypsin deficiency
    Wilson's disease
    Tyrosinemia
    Glycogen storage diseases
    Crigler-Najjary type I
    Hemochromatosis
Vascular
    Budd-Chiari syndrome
    Veno-occlusive disease
Tumors
    Benign
    Primary malignant

sive, but the quality of life is unacceptably poor. As an example, the fatigue and pruritus experienced by patients with primary biliary cirrhosis may become intolerable even though synthetic liver function remains acceptable.

Selection of Patients[192–194]

Patients accepted for transplantation should have advanced, irreversible liver disease that is refractory to all appropriate medical therapy. While the presence or threat of a fatal complication argues strongly in favor of liver transplantation, it is often in the best interest of the patient to consider and to perform liver transplantation before the appearance of such a decompensation of liver function. Careful consideration of remote and recent history, the present level of general fitness and liver function, as well as surgical considerations will maximize the potential benefit and minimize the surgical and postoperative risk for each patient and allow optimum timing of transplantation.

Preoperative Evaluation

The evaluation of the fitness of the potential recipient for transplantation should include a careful evaluation of the **cardiovascular system.** In a young patient without a history of cardiac disease, an ECG is the only additional study required. In older patients, or if cardiac impairment is suggested by history, examination, or ECG, then echocardiography, stress testing, or more invasive cardiac evaluation may be indicated. Patients with alcoholic liver disease or cirrhosis secondary to hemochromatosis should have more careful cardiac evaluations.

Pulmonary function is evaluated to detect significant decrements in function and the presence of hepatopulmonary syndrome that may interfere with oxygenation in the perioperative period. Most patients with advanced liver disease have one or more types of abnormality in lung function, a reduced diffusing capacity to carbon dioxide DL_{CO} being the single most common functional defect.[73] Mechanisms accounting for the abnormality in gas transfer may include intrapulmonary vascular dilatation, diffuse interstitial lung disease, restrictive lung disease secondary to ascites, and/or ventilation-perfusion imbalance.[192]

Renal function may be difficult to assess because of altered urea metabolism and diminished creatinine production due to a decrement in muscle mass. However, reversible causes of oliguria and azotemia must by identified and treated before labeling the renal failure as hepatorenal syndrome. In a retrospective study, baseline preoperative serum creatinine level provided the best indication of the short-term prognosis after liver transplantation.[193]

Neurologic evaluation includes a general examination to evaluate the presence and stage of hepatic encephalopathy and to seek focal findings that may suggest an intracranial lesion. The essentially reversible nature of the cerebral disturbance, at least in the early stages, and the diffuse involvement suggest that the change is a metabolic one. If patients have not had an intracranial hemorrhage or prolonged periods of intracranial hypertension the encephalopathic CNS impairment is largely reversible with resolution of the hepatic failure. At many centers intracranial pressure monitoring is used in the perioperative period to facilitate monitoring and initiate treatment of elevated intracranial pressure.

Survival Rates

The development of liver transplantation has paralleled the expansion of transplantation of other organs such as kidney, heart and bone marrow. The current success of liver transplantation can be attributed to critical selection of recipients, modern anesthetic and surgical techniques, improved perioperative care, accurate diagnosis of rejection and superior immunosuppression with cyclosporine. The 1 year survival rate is 70–90%[194–196] These patients have an excellent prospect of long-term survival. Children under 1 year of age or less weighing less than 10 kg have 1 year survival of approximately 70%. The emerging evidence indicates that the rehabilitation and quality of life of most liver recipients are good.[196]

Preparation for Anesthesia

Choice of Anesthesia

Liver transplantation surgery is performed with the aid of general anesthesia. Central axis anesthesia or analgesia to supplement general anesthesia are not employed since the majority of the patients have a pre-existing coagulopathy and those with a normal coagulation profile will demonstrate some degree of impaired coagulation during the anhepatic stage.

The operating room must be equipped with patient warming devices which may include, warming mattress, forced air warmers, active breathing circuit warmers, and fluid warmers. Since these surgeries may involve large volumes of blood loss and massive fluid and blood product replacement, IV access should include multiple large caliber intravenous sites and appropriate fluid warming equipment. Lower extremity IVs are avoided as venous return will be impeded during periods of surgery when the inferior vena cava is surgically occluded.

Monitoring

All patients will require arterial catheter placement for hemodynamic monitoring and serial evaluation of pulmonary and metabolic status. Upper extremity arterial pressure monitoring is preferred as aortic occlusion clamps may be placed by the surgeons during the anastomosis of the donor hepatic artery to the aorta. In most cases the arterial catheters may be inserted after the induction of general anesthesia. Central vein access is crucial as a reliable intravenous access for administration of rapid fluid therapy and for hemodynamic monitoring. The choice between central venous pressure monitoring and the use of a pulmonary artery catheter should be made based on the cardiac function of each individual patient. Transesophageal echocardiography (TEE) can be used intraoperatively to evaluate left ventricular volume, ventricular function and evidence of ventricular ischemia. However, in patients with dilated esophageal varices, the risk of bleeding from trauma associated with the insertion and manipulation of the TEE must be considered. The use of oral gastric suction sumps rather than the more common nasal route should be considered because of the risk of significant hemorrhage with placement via the nasal route in the presence of a coagulopathy.

Blood Requirements

The improvement in surgical techniques and performance of liver transplantation surgery in patients with less advanced disease has led to a decrease in the average amount of blood product replacement required. However, the potential for massive hemorrhage exists for every case and adequate supplies of immediately available blood products should be verified prior to initiation of the surgery. The use of blood salvage devices has also lead to a decreased need for homologous red blood cells.[199-200]

Anesthetic Procedure

Induction

Intravenous premedication with midazolam is recommended 1 hour prior to establishing catheters and monitors. Most patients require only a peripheral intravenous catheter and routine monitors prior to induction. Hepatic disease may have pulmonary manifestations resulting in decreased PaO$_2$ levels secondary to elevated diaphragms and decreased FRC from ascites, pulmonary V/Q mismatching and or increased pulmonary shunt. All patients should be fully pre-oxygenated prior to induction as rapid arterial desaturation may occur. Because of the ascites raising intra-abdominal pressure and the delayed gastric transit time due to general poor health, a rapid sequence induction to prevent passive regurgitation of gastric contents may be indicated.

Intravenous agents and induction with a barbiturate or midazolam is common practice.

Hypoalbuminemia is commonly present and may result in higher percentages of unbound drugs which normally bind to albumin such as barbiturates. This may necessitate decreases in the induction dose of barbiturates. Patients with ascites have an increased volume of distribution for hydrophilic drugs such as the neuromuscular blocking agents. This may require a larger initial dose to achieve adequate intubating conditions in equivalent time. If succinylcholine is to be used attention should be focused on the potential impaired renal function and the plasma level of potassium.

Maintenance

This is accomplished with an agent such as isoflurane or desflurane, and supplemented by intravenous fentanyl as indicated.

Surgical Procedure

Liver transplantation surgery can be divided into three phases: 1) prehepatic stage, in which the recipient hepatectomy is performed; 2) the anhepatic stage, during which the vascular anastomosis between donor and transplanted liver are made; 3) and the hepatic stage, during which the allograft is reperfused, hemostasis is achieved, and biliary anastomosis is made.

Prehepatic Phase

During the prehepatic phase a midline and bilateral subcostal incision is made, followed by mobilization of the diseased liver. The infra- and supra-hepatic inferior vena cava, hepatic veins, portal vein, hepatic artery, and biliary system are identified and mobilized in preparation for vascular occlusion. This stage may be prolonged in cases of repeat transplantation occurring more than several weeks after initial transplantation or in cases with previous abdominal surgeries. The presence of scar tissue or adhesions from previous surgeries also leads to increased blood loss.

Anhepatic Phase

During the anhepatic phase the portal vein and lower body venous circulation is interrupted by occlusion clamps placed on the infra- and supra-hepatic inferior vena cava, portal vein, and hepatic artery. Cardiovascular changes at this time include decreases in systolic arterial pressure, decreased pulmonary artery pressure, decreased pulmonary artery occlusion pressure, and decreased cardiac output. There are compensatory increases in systemic vascular resistance. These occluded vessels are then ligated and the diseased liver is removed.

Extracorporeal venovenous-bypass may be used during the anhepatic phase to decompress the splanchnic and lower body venous systems, and increase venous return to the heart thereby increasing cardiac output and arterial blood pressure. Venovenous-bypass requires cannulation of the portal vein and femoral vein for venous inflow and axillary vein for return of the diverted blood to the patient's venous circulation (Fig. 22–2). If bypass flow is maintained above 1,000 ml/min clot formation or platelet aggregation within the bypass circuit is unlikely to occur and systemic heparinization is not required. As much as 40 to 50% of the cardiac output can be returned to the heart from the lower body and viscera via the bypass. Although the use of venovenous bypass does attenuate the metabolic and hemodynamic changes that occur with hepatic vascular occlusion and reperfusion, the claimed advantages of decreased blood loss and increased renal perfusion with a subsequent decrease in postoperative renal dysfunction has not been conclusively demonstrated in randomized trials. At many centers the patient's cardiovascular hemodynamics will be observed after a trial of volume loading and occlusion of the hepatic vasculature. Venovenous bypass is then selectively instituted only if sufficient arterial blood pressure and cardiac output cannot be maintained.

Transplantation for acute hepatic failure will result in more severe cardiovascular changes with occlusion of the vena cava and portal vein due to absence of a well developed collateral venous system and will likely require venovenous bypass. Venovenous bypass is too cumbersome to use in very small infants, and low bypass flow may result in thrombus formation. Also, infants and young children have less hemodynamic changes in response to vascular occlusion of the liver.

To complete the anhepatic phase the following anastomoses are then made with the donor liver: suprahepatic inferior vena cava, infrahepatic inferior vena cava, celiac truck or aorta graft to common hepatic artery or aorta of recipient, and portal vein. Before completion of the anastomosis, 500–1000 cc of Lactated Ringer's or 5% albumin is flushed through the allograft and then suctioned from the operative field. This flushing is to remove organ preservation solution which contains intracellular concentrations of potassium ions and entrapped air within the allograft. Reperfusion of the newly implanted liver is now instituted via the portal vein and hepatic artery and marks the beginning of the hepatic phase.

Hepatic Stage

The reperfusion period is the intraoperative period associated with the greatest cardiovascular instability. After the infra- and supra-hepatic vena cava, and portal vein occlusion clamps are released, hyperkalemia, dysrhythmias, hypotension, decreased cardiac output, and cardiac arrest may be seen. Despite prior flushing of the allograft, the sudden bolus of cold, hyperkalemic, acidotic blood from the liver and lower body may cause hemodynamic disturbances. Hypotension often with bradycardia is frequently seen in 1 to 5 minutes after unclamping of the vena cava

and portal vein. This is associated with an increased CVP, increased PAOP, decreased cardiac output, decreased systemic vascular resistance, and decreased mixed venous oxygen saturation. Investigators using transesophageal echocardiography have observed right heart dysfunction, regional contractile abnormalities and the presence of air and thrombotic emboli. Several factors contribute to these hemodynamic changes including (1) increase in venous return from splanchnic and lower extremities, (2) high potassium levels, low pH, low temperature, and low hematocrit of the returning blood, (3) residual preservation solution incompletely flushed from the donor liver, (4) reflex vasodilation after reperfusion and (5) embolic material including air. Clinically significant venous air embolism can occur during transplantation, particularly during the reperfusion stage with incomplete flushing of the liver. These hemodynamic changes may require immediate treatment with $CaCl_2$ to counteract the effects of the high levels of potassium ions, $NaHCO_3$ to raise pH and shift potassium ions intracellularly, and vasoconstrictor or inotropic support to counteract cardiac dysfunction and raise SVR. Glucose and insulin may be required if potassium remains high after initial redistribution.

Assessment of Graft

During the hepatic phase the vascular anastomoses are examined and hemostasis is accomplished. The biliary tract is then reconstructed by connecting either the donor's and recipient's common ducts end to end over a T-tube stent or the common duct of the homograft to a limb of the jejunum in a Roux loop anastomosis (Fig. 22–3).

Administration of large amounts of blood products results in a substantial delivery of the anticoagulant citrate.

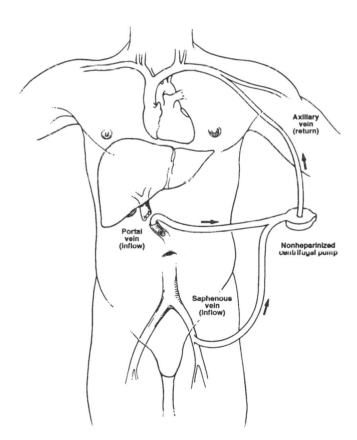

Fig. 22–2. Venovenous bypass. The portal vein is divided and the devascularization of the liver is completed. The portal vein is cannulated and a second cannula is placed into the iliac vein via the saphenous vein. The blood is pumped by a centrifugal pump in a nonheparinized system and returned to the patient via a cannula placed in the axillary vein. Flows of 2–5 liters/minute are commonly attained. Flow must be maintained above 700–1000 ml/minute to prevent thrombosis. (Modified from Kaplowitz N.: Liver and Biliary Diseases, Baltimore, 1992, Williams & Wilkins.)

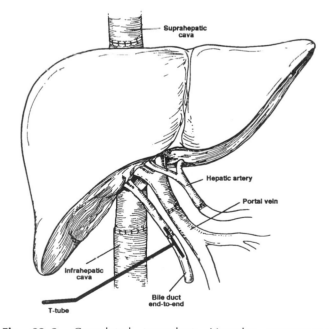

Fig. 22–3. Completed transplant. Vascular anastomoses include the suprahepatic vena cava, the infrahepatic vena cava, the portal vein, and the hepatic artery. An end-to-end bile duct anastomosis is depicted. (Modified from Kaplowitz N.: Liver and Biliary Diseases, Baltimore, 1992, Williams & Wilkins.)

Citrate is metabolized by the liver and therefore the removal of citrate is compromised during the mobilization phase and absent during the anhepatic phase of the operation. Thus, citrate accumulates, decreasing the levels of ionized calcium which may result in depression of myocardial performance. The ionized calcium level should be measured frequently during the operation and calcium chloride given when hypotension not responding to appropriate preload occurs with documented low ionized calcium ion levels.

Retransplantation Risk

The rate of retransplantation in the first three postoperative months is 10 to 20%. There are four general reasons for graft failure: a technically imperfect operation, unrecognized liver disease in the donor, an ischemic injury in the graft, and accelerated rejection. Technical complications account for less than 10% of the primary graft failures in adults but 30% of those in infants and children. The risk in infants is inversely related to the patient's size, and complications are mainly attributable to vascular thrombosis.

REFERENCES

1. Bismuth H.: Surgical anatomy and anatomical surgery of the liver. World J Surg 6:3, 1982
2. Mukai J. K., Stack C. M., et al.: Imaging of surgically relevant hepatic vascular and segmental anatomy. Am J Roentgenol 149:287, 1987
3. Rappaport A. M., Borowy Z. J., et al.: Subdivision of hexagonal liver lobules into a structural and functional unit: role in hepatic physiology and pathology. Anat Rec 119:11, 1954
4. Traber P. G., Chianale J., et al.: Physiologic significance and regulation of hepatocellular heterogeneity. Gastroenterology 95:1130, 1988
5. Gumucio J. J.: Functional and anatomic heterogeneity in the liver acinus: impact on transport. Am J Physiol 244:G578, 1983
6. Shingu K., Eger E., et al.: Hypoxia per se can produce hepatic damage without death in rats. Anesth Analg 61:820, 1982
7. Bioulac-Sage P., Lafon M. E., et al.: Nerves and perisinusoidal cells in human liver. J Hepatol 10:105, 1990
8. Lautt W. W.: Mechanism and role of intrinsic regulation of hepatic arterial blood flow: hepatic arterial buffer response. Am J Physiol 249:G549, 1985
9. Gelman S. I.: The effect of enteral oxygen administration on the hepatic circulation during halothane anaesthesia: experimental investigations. Br J Anaesth 47:1253, 1975
10. Gelman S., Ernst E. A.: Role of pH, PCO$_2$, and O$_2$ content of portal blood in hepatic circulatory autoregulation. Am J Physiol 233:E255, 1977
11. Lautt W. W., Legare D. J., et al.: Adenosine as putative regulator of hepatic arterial flow: the buffer response. Am J Physiol 248:H331, 1985
12. Gelman S.: General anesthesia and hepatic circulation. Can J Physiol Pharmacol 65:1762, 1987
13. Goldfarb G., Debaene B., et al.: Hepatic blood flow in humans during isoflurane-N$_2$O and halothane-N$_2$O anesthesia. Anesth Analg 71:349, 1990
14. Gelman S., Rimerman V., et al.: The effect of halothane, isoflurane, and blood loss on hepatotoxicity and hepatic oxygen availability in phenobarbital-pretreated hypoxic rats. Anesth Analg 63:965, 1984
15. Gelman S., Fowler K. C., et al.: Regional blood flow during isoflurane and halothane anesthesia. Anesth Analg 63:557, 1984
16. Seyde W. C., Longnecker D. E.: Anesthetic influences on regional hemodynamics in normal and hemorrhaged rats. Anesthesiology 61:686, 1984
17. Tranquilli W. J., Manohar M., et al.: Systemic and regional blood flow distribution in unanesthetized swine and swine anesthetized with halothane + nitrous oxide, halothane, or enflurane. Anesthesiology 56:369, 1982
18. Miller E. Jr., Kistner J. R., et al.: Whole-body distribution of radioactively labelled microspheres in the rat during anesthesia with halothane, enflurane, or ketamine. Anesthesiology 52:296, 1980
19. Hursh D., Gelman S., et al.: Hepatic oxygen supply during halothane or isoflurane anesthesia in guinea pigs. Anesthesiology 67:701, 1987
20. Gelman S., Fowler K. C., et al.: Liver circulation and function during isoflurane and halothane anesthesia. Anesthesiology 61:726, 1984
21. Lees M. H., Hill J., et al.: Regional blood flows of the rhesus monkey during halothane anesthesia. Anesth Analg 50:270, 1971
22. Gelman S. I.: The effect of enteral oxygen administratihepatic circulation during halothane anaesthesia: experimental investigations. Br J Anaesth 47:1253, 1975
23. Wyler F.: Effect of general anesthesia on distribution of cardiac output and organ blood flow in the rabbit: halothane and chloralose-urethane. J Surg Res 17:381, 1974
24. Hughes R. L., Campbell D., et al.: Effects of enflurane and halothane on liver blood flow and oxygen consumption in the greyhound. Br J Anaesth 52:1079, 1980
25. Irestedt L., Andreen M.: Effects of enflurane on haemodynamics and oxygen consumption in the dog with special reference to the liver and preportal tissues. Acta Anaesthesiol Scand 23:13, 1979
26. Tverskoy M., Gelman S., et al.: Intestinal circulation during inhalation anesthesia. Anesthesiology 62:462, 1985
27. Lundeen G., Manohar M., et al.: Systemic distribution of blood flow in swine while awake and during 1.0 and 1.5 MAC isoflurane anesthesia with or without 50% nitrous oxide. Anesth Analg 62:499, 1983
28. Thomson I. A., Hughes R. L., et al.: Effects of nitrous oxide on liver haemodynamics and oxygen consumption in the greyhound. Anaesthesia 37:548, 1982
29. Ericsson B. F.: Effect of pentobarbital sodium anesthesia, as judged with aid of radioactive carbonized microspheres, on cardiac output and its fractional distribution in the dog. Acta Chir Scand 137:613, 1971
30. Bond J. H., Prentiss R. A., et al.: The effect of anesthesia and laparotomy on blood flow to the stomach, small bowel, and colon of the dog. Surgery 87:313, 1980
31. Svanvik J., Lundgren O.: Gastrointestinal circulation. Int Rev Physiol 12:1, 1977
32. Forsyth R. P., Hoffbrand B. I.: Redistribution of cardiac output after sodium pentobarbital anesthesia in the monkey. Am J Physiol 218:214, 1970
33. Becker H., Manganaro A., et al.: Limitations of studying splanchnic blood flow during anesthesia. Surg Forum 30:347, 1979
34. Manders W. T., Vatner S. F.: Effects of sodium pentobarbital anesthesia on left ventricular function and distribution of cardiac output in dogs, with particular reference to the mechanism for tachycardia. Circ Res 39:512, 1976

35. Ahlgren I., Aronsen K. F., et al.: Hemodynamics during superficial thiopental anesthesia in the dog. Acta Anaesthesiol Scand 22:76, 1978

36. Katz M. L., Bergman E. N.: Simultaneous measurements of hepatic and portal venous blood flow in the sheep and dog. Am J Physiol 216:946, 1969

37. Sjostrom B., Wulff K. E.: Influence of long-term anesthesia on regional blood flow distribution and hemodynamics in the dog. Eur Surg Res 7:1, 1975

38. Tuma R. F., Irion G. L., et al.: Age-related changes in regional blood flow in the rat. Am J Physiol 249:H485, 1985

39. Idvall J., Aronsen K. F., et al.: Tissue perfusion and distribution of cardiac output during ketamine anesthesia in normovolemic rats. Acta Anaesthesiol Scand 24:257, 1980

40. Dhasmana K. M., Saxena P. R., et al.: A study on the influence of ketamine on systemic and regional haemodynamics in conscious rabbits. Arch Int Pharmacodyn Ther 269:323, 1984

41. Bell G. J., Hiley C. R., et al.: The effects of four general anaesthetic agents on the regional distribution of cardiac output in the rat. Br J Pharmacol 61:126, 1977

42. Thomson I. A., Fitch W., et al.: Effects of certain i.v. anaesthetics on liver blood flow and hepatic oxygen consumption in the greyhound. Br J Anaesth 58:69, 1986

43. Tverskoy M., Gelman S., et al.: Influence of fentanyl and morphine on intestinal circulation. Anesth Analg 64:577, 1985

44. Priano L. L., Vatner S. F.: Morphine effects on cardiac output and regional blood flow distribution in conscious dogs. Anesthesiology 55:236, 1981

45. Leaman D. M., Levenson L., et al.: Effect of morphine on splanchnic blood flow. Br Heart J 40:569, 1978

46. Miller R. L., Forsyth R. P., et al.: Morphine-induced redistribution of cardiac output in the unanesthetized monkey. Pharmacology 7:138, 1972

47. Stanley T. H., Webster L. R.: Anesthetic requirements and cardiovascular effects of fentanyl-oxygen and fentanyl-diazepam-oxygen anesthesia in man. Anesth Analg 57:411, 1978

48. Kien N. D., Reitan J. A., et al.: Hemodynamic responses to alfentanil in halothane-anesthetized dogs. Anesth Analg 65:765, 1986

49. Johnstone M., Mahmoud A. A., et al.: Cardiovascular effects of tubocurarine in man. Anaesthesia 33:587, 1978

50. Saxena P. R., Dhasmana K. M., et al.: A comparison of systemic and regional hemodynamic effects of d-tubocurarine, pancuronium, and vecuronium. Anesthesiology 59:102, 1983

51. Varma Y. S., Sharma P. L., et al.: Comparative evaluation of cerebral and hepatic blood flow under d-tubocurarine and pancuronium in dogs. Indian J Med Res 66:317, 1977

52. Gelman S.: Use of microspheres for gut blood flow determination. Surgery 89:526, 1981

53. Gelman S. I.: Disturbances in hepatic blood flow during anesthesia and surgery. Arch Surg 111:881, 1976

54. McNeill J. R., Pang C. C.: Effect of pentobarbital anesthesia and surgery on the control of arterial pressure and mesenteric resistance in cats: role of vasopressin and angiotensin. Can J Physiol Pharmacol 60:363, 1982

55. Manny J., Justice R., et al.: Abnormalities in organ blood flow and its distribution during positive end-expiratory pressure. Surgery 85:425, 1979

56. Halden E., Jakobson S., et al.: Effects of positive end-expiratory pressure on cardiac output distribution in the pig. Acta Anaesthesiol Scand 26:403, 1982

57. Johnson E. E.: Splanchnic hemodynamic response to passive hyperventilation. J Appl Physiol 38:156, 1975

58. Bredenberg C. E., Paskanik A. M.: Relation of portal hemodynamics to cardiac output during mechanical ventilation with PEEP. Ann Surg 198:218, 1983

59. Bonnet F., Richard C., et al.: Changes in hepatic flow induced by continuous positive pressure ventilation in critically ill patients. Crit Care Med 10:703, 1982

60. Bredenberg C. E., Paskanik A., et al.: Portal hemodynamics in dogs during mechanical ventilation with positive end-expiratory pressure. Surgery 90:817, 1981

61. Gioia F. R., Harris A. P., et al.: Organ blood flow during high-frequency ventilation at low and high airway pressure in dogs. Anesthesiology 65:50, 1986

62. Fujita Y., Sakai T., et al.: Effects of hypocapnia and hypercapnia on splanchnic circulation and hepatic function in the beagle. Anesth Analg 69:152, 1989

63. Kennedy W. Jr., Everett G. B., et al.: Simultaneous systemic and hepatic hemodynamic measurements during high spinal anesthesia in normal man. Anesth Analg 49:1016, 1970

64. Greitz T., Andreen M., et al.: Haemodynamics and oxygen consumption in the dog during high epidural block with special reference to the splanchnic region. Acta Anaesthesiol Scand 27:211, 1983

65. Greitz T., Andreen M., et al.: Effects of ephedrine on haemodynamics and oxygen consumption in the dog during high epidural block with special reference to the splanchnic region. Acta Anaesthesiol Scand 28:557, 1984

66. Nakayama M., Kanaya N., et al.: Effects of ephedrine on indocyanine green clearance during spinal anesthesia: Evaluation by the finger piece method. Anesth Analg 77:947, 1993

67. Branch R. A., Morgan M. H., et al.: Intravenous administration of diazepam in patients with chronic liver disease. Gut 17:975, 1976

68. Shull H. J., Wilkinson G. R., et al.: Normal disposition of oxazepam in acute viral hepatitis and cirrhosis. Ann Intern Med 84:420, 1976

69. Sherlock S.: Vasodilatation associated with hepatocellular disease: relation to functional organ failure. Gut 31:365, 1990

70. Lunzer M., Newman S. P., et al.: Skeletal muscle blood flow and neurovascular reactivity in liver disease. Gut 14:354, 1973

71. Lee S. S., Moreau R., et al.: Glucagon selectively increases splanchnic blood flow in patients with well-compensated cirrhosis. Hepatology 8:1501, 1988

72. Hopkins W. E., Waggoner A. D., et al.: Frequency and significance of intrapulmonary right-to-left shunting in end-stage hepatic disease. Am J Cardiol 70:516, 1992

73. Hourani J. M., Bellamy P. E., et al.: Pulmonary dysfunction in advanced liver disease: frequent occurrence of an abnormal diffusing capacity. Am J Med 90:93, 1991

74. Eriksson L. S., Soderman C., et al.: Normalization of ventilation/perfusion relationships after liver transplantation in patients with decompensated cirrhosis: evidence for a hepatopulmonary syndrome. 1350, 1990

75. Stoller J. K., Moodie D., et al.: Reduction of intrapulmonary shunt and resolution of digital clubbing associated with primary biliary cirrhosis after liver transplantation. Hepatology 11:54, 1990

76. Hadengue A., Benhayoun M. K., et al.: Pulmonary hypertension complicating portal hypertension: prevalence and relation to splanchnic hemodynamics. Gastroenterology 100:520, 1991

77. Kew M. C., Brunt P. W., et al.: Renal and intrarenal blood-flow in cirrhosis of the liver. Lancet 2:504, 1971

78. Koppel M. H., Coburn J. W., et al.: Transplantation of ca-

daveric kidneys from patients with hepatorenal syndrome. Evidence for the functional nature of renal failure in advanced liver disease. N Engl J Med 280:1367, 1969

79. Mirouze D., Zipser R. D., et al.: Effect of inhibitors of prostaglandin synthesis on induced diuresis in cirrhosis. Hepatology 3:50, 1983

80. Epstein M., Lifschitz M. D., et al.: Relationship between renal prostaglandin E and renal sodium handling during water immersion in normal man. Circ Res 45:71, 1979

81. Epstein M., Lifschitz M., et al.: Characterization of renal prostaglandin E responsiveness in decompensated cirrhosis: implications for renal sodium handling. Clin Sci 63:555, 1982

82. Levy L. J., Leek J., et al.: Evidence for gamma-aminobutyric acid as the inhibitor of gamma- aminobutyric acid binding in the plasma of humans with liver disease and hepatic encephalopathy. Clin Sci 73:531, 1987

83. Zaki A. E., Ede R. J., et al.: Experimental studies of blood brain permeability in acute hepatic failure. Hepatology 4:359, 1984

84. Baraldi M., Zeneroli Z. L.: Experimental hepatic encephalopathy: changes in the binding of gamma- aminobutyric acid. Science 216:427, 1982

85. Grippon P., Le Poncin Lafitte M., et al.: Evidence for the role of ammonia in the intracerebral transfer and metabolism of tryptophan. Hepatology 6:682, 1986

86. Rubin M. H., Weston M. J., et al.: Platelet function in chronic liver disease: relationship to disease severity. Dig Dis Sci 24:197, 1979

87. Jorgensen B., Fischer E., et al.: Decreased blood platelet volume and count in patients with liver disease. Scand J Gastroenterol 19:492, 1984

88. Hillenbrand P., Parbhoo S. P., et al.: Significance of intravascular coagulation and fibrinolysis in acute hepatic failure. Gut 15:83, 1974

89. Rake M. O., Flute P. T., et al.: Intravascular coagulation in acute hepatic necrosis. Lancet 1:533, 1970

90. Carr J. M.: Disseminated intravascular coagulation in cirrhosis. Hepatology 10:103, 1989

91. Kelly D. A., Summerfield J.A.: Hemostasis in liver disease. Semin Liver Dis 7:182, 1987

92. Aach R. D., Stevens C. E., et al.: Hepatitis C virus infection in post-transfusion hepatitis. An analysis with first- and second-generation assays. N Engl J Med 325:1325, 1991

93. Alter H. J., Purcell R. H., et al.: Detection of antibody to hepatitis C virus in prospectively followed transfusion recipients with acute and chronic non-A, non-B hepatitis. N Engl J Med 321:1494, 1989

94. Miyamura T., Saito I., et al.: Detection of antibody against antigen expressed by molecularly cloned hepatitis C virus cDNA: application to diagnosis and blood screening for posttransfusion hepatitis. Proc Natl Acad Sci U S A 87:983, 1990

95. Hopf U., Moller B., et al.: Long-term follow-up of posttransfusion and sporadic chronic hepatitis non-A, non-B and frequency of circulating antibodies to hepatitis C virus (HCV). J Hepatol 10:69, 1990

96. Ede R. J., Williams R. W.: Hepatic encephalopathy and cerebral edema. Semin Liver Dis 6:107, 1986

97. Hanid M.A., Davies M., et al.: Clinical monitoring of intracranial pressure in fulminant hepatic failure. Gut 21:866, 1980

98. Ede R. J., Gimson A. E., et al.: Controlled hyperventilation in the prevention of cerebral oedema in fulminant hepatic failure. J Hepatol 2:43, 1986

99. Trewby P. N., Chase R. A., et al.: The role of the false neurotransmitter octopamine in the hypotension of fulminant hepatic failure. Clin Sci Mol Med 52:305, 1977

100. O'Grady J. G., Williams R.: Management of acute liver failure. Schweiz. med. Wschr 116:541, 1986

101. Ring-Larsen H., Palazzo U.: Renal failure in fulminant hepatic failure and terminal cirrhosis: a comparison between incidence, types, and prognosis. Gut 22:585, 1981

102. Guarner F., Hughes R. D., et al.: Renal function in fulminant hepatic failure: haemodynamics and renal prostaglandins. Gut 28:1643, 1987

103. Trewby P. N., Warren R., et al.: Incidence and pathophysiology of pulmonary edema in fulminant hepatic failure. Gastroenterology 74:859, 1978

104. O'Grady J. G., Alexander G. J., et al.: Early indicators of prognosis in fulminant hepatic failure. Gastroenterology 97:439, 1989

105. Speizer F. E., Trey C., et al.: The uses of multiple causes of death data to clarify changing patterns of cirrhosis mortality in Massachusetts. Am J Public Health 67:333, 1977

106. Trey C.: The fulminant hepatic failure surveillance study: Brief review of the effects of presumed etiology and age of survival. Can Med Assoc J 26:Suppl:525, 1972

107. Komori H., Hirasa M., et al.: Concept of the clinical stages of acute hepatic failure. Am J Gastroenterol 81:544, 1986

108. Bihari D., Gimson A. E., et al.: Lactic acidosis in fulminant hepatic failure. Some aspects of pathogenesis and prognosis. J Hepatol 1:405, 1985

109. Muraca M., Fevery J., et al.: Analytic aspects and clinical interpretation of serum bilirubins. Semin Liver Dis 8:137, 1988

110. Fortson W. C., Tedesco F. J., et al.: Marked elevation of serum transaminase activity associated with extrahepatic biliary tract disease. J Clin Gastroenterol 7:502, 1985

111. Hultcrantz R., Glaumann H., et al.: Liver investigation in 149 asymptomatic patients with moderately elevated activities of serum aminotransferases. Scand J Gastroenterol 21:109, 1986

112. Cohen J. A., Kaplan M. M.: The SGOT/SGPT ratio{md}an indicator of alcoholic liver disease. Dig Dis Sci 24:835, 1979

113. Matloff D. S., Selinger M. J., et al.: Hepatic transaminase activity in alocholic liver disease. Gastroenterology 78:1389, 1980

114. Diehl A. M., Potter J., et al.: Relationship between pyridoxal 5'-phosphate deficiency and aminotransferase levels in alcoholic hepatitis. Gastroenterology 86:632, 1984

115. Rothschild M. A., Oratz M., et al.: Serum albumin. Hepatology 8:385, 1988

116. Galizzi J., Long R. G., et al.: Assessment of the (14C) aminopyrine breath test in liver disease. Gut 19:40, 1978

117. Baker A. L., Kotake A. N., et al.: Clinical utility of breath tests for the assessment of hepatic function. Semin Liver Dis 3:318, 1983

118. Merkel C., Gatta A., et al.: Prognostic value of galactose elimination capacity, aminopyrine breath test, and ICG clearance in patients with cirrhosis. Comparison with the Pugh score. Dig Dis Sci 36:1197, 1991

119. Prieto J., Barry M., et al.: Serum ferritin in patients with iron overload and with acute and chronic liver diseases. Gastroenterology 68:525, 1975

120. Batey R. G., Hussein S., et al.: The role of serum ferritin in the management of idiopathic haemochromatosis. Scand J Gastroenterol 13:953, 1978

121. Gibbs K., Walshe J. M.: A study of the caeruloplasmin concentrations found in 75 patients with Wilson's disease, their kinships and various control groups. Q J Med 48:447, 1979

122. Taketa K.: Alpha-fetoprotein: reevaluation in hepatology. Hepatology 12:1420, 1990

123. Lok A. S., Lai C. L.: alpha-Fetoprotein monitoring in Chi-

nese patients with chronic hepatitis B virus infection: role in the early detection of hepatocellular carcinoma. Hepatology 9:110, 1989

124. Lee H. S., Chung Y. H., et al.: Specificities of serum alpha-fetoprotein in HBsAg+ and HBsAg− patients in the diagnosis of hepatocellular carcinoma. Hepatology 14:68, 1991

125. Hayes P. C.: Liver disease and drug disposition. Br J Anaesth 68:459, 1992

126. Crotty B., Watson K. J., et al.: Hepatic extraction of morphine is impaired in cirrhosis. Eur J Clin Pharmacol 36:501, 1989

127. Patwardhan R. V., Johnson R. F., et al.: Normal metabolism of morphine in cirrhosis. Gastroenterology 81:1006, 1981

128. Mazoit J. X., Sandouk P., et al.: Pharmacokinetics of unchanged morphine in normal and cirrhotic subjects. Anesth Analg 66:293, 1987

129. Hasselstrom J., Eriksson S., et al.: The metabolism and bioavailability of morphine in patients with severe liver cirrhosis. Br J Clin Pharmacol 29:289, 1990

130. Laidlaw J., Read A. E., et al.: Morphine tolerance in hepatic cirrhosis. Gastroenterology 40:389, 1961

131. Neal E. A., Meffin P. J., et al.: Enhanced bioavailability and decreased clearance of analgesics in patients with cirrhosis. Gastroenterology 77:96, 1979

132. Klotz U., McHorse T. S., et al.: The effect of cirrhosis on the disposition and elimination of meperidine in man. Clin Pharmacol Ther 16:667, 1974

133. Haberer J. P., Schoeffler P., et al.: Fentanyl pharmacokinetics in anaesthetized patients with cirrhosis. Br J Anaesth 54:1267, 1982

134. Chauvin M., Ferrier C., et al.: Sufentanil pharmacokinetics in patients with cirrhosis. Anesth Analg 68:1, 1989

135. Ferrier C., Marty J., et al.: Alfentanil pharmacokinetics in patients with cirrhosis. Anesthesiology 62:480, 1985

136. Bower S., Sear J. W., et al.: Effects of different hepatic pathologies on disposition of alfentanil in anaesthetized patients. Br J Anaesth 68:462, 1992

137. MacGilchrist A. J., Birnie G. G., et al.: Pharmacokinetics and pharmacodynamics of intravenous midazolam in patients with severe alcoholic cirrhosis. Gut 27:190, 1986

138. Trouvin J. H., Farinotti R., et al.: Pharmacokinetics of midazolam in anaesthetized cirrhotic patients. Br J Anaesth 60:762, 1988

139. Kraus J. W., Desmond P. V., et al.: Effects of aging and liver disease on disposition of lorazepam. Clin Pharmacol Ther 24:411, 1978

140. Bakti G., Fisch H. U., et al.: Mechanism of the excessive sedative response of cirrhotics to benzodiazepines: model experiments with triazolam. Hepatology 7:629, 1987

141. Ghoneim M. M., Pandya H.: Plasma protein binding of thiopental in patients with impaired renal or hepatic function. Anesthesiology 42:545, 1975

142. Pandele G., Chaux F., et al.: Thiopental pharmacokinetics in patients with cirrhosis. Anesthesiology 59:123, 1983

143. Servin F., Desmonts J. M., et al.: Pharmacokinetics and protein binding of propofol in patients with cirrhosis. Anesthesiology 69:887, 1988

144. Servin F., Cockshott I. D., et al.: Pharmacokinetics of propofol infusions in patients with cirrhosis. Br J Anaesth 65:177, 1990

145. Servin F., Desmonts J. M., et al.: Pharmacokinetics of propofol administered by continuous infusion in patients with cirrhosis. Preliminary results. Anaesthesia 43: 23, 1988

146. Dundee J. W., Gray T. C.: Resistance to d-tubocurarine chloride in the presence of liver damage. Lancet 2:16, 1953

147. Baraka A., Gabali F.: Correlation between tubocurarine re-

quirements and plasma protein pattern. Br J Anaesth 40:89, 1968

148. Ghoneim M. M., Kramer E., et al.: Binding of d-tubocurarine to plasma proteins in normal man and in patients with hepatic or renal disease. Anesthesiology 39:410, 1973

149. Duvaldestin P., Henzel D.: Binding of tubocurarine, fazadinium, pancuronium and Org NC 45 to serum proteins in normal man and in patients with cirrhosis. Br J Anaesth 54:513, 1982

150. Duvaldestin P., Agoston S., et al.: Pancuronium pharmacokinetics in patients with liver cirrhosis. Br J Anaesth 50:1131, 1978

151. Arden J. R., Lynam D. P., et al.: Vecuronium in alcoholic liver disease: a pharmacokinetic and pharmacodynamic analysis. Anesthesiology 68:771, 1988

152. Hunter J. M., Parker C. J., et al.: The use of different doses of vecuronium in patients with liver dysfunction. Br J Anaesth 57:758, 1985

153. Lebrault C., Duvaldestin P., et al.: Pharmacokinetics and pharmacodynamics of vecuronium in patients with cholestasis. Br J Anaesth 58:983, 1986

154. Brandom B. W., Stiller R. L., et al.: Pharmacokinetics of atracurium in anaesthetized infants and children. Br J Anaesth 58:1210, 1986

155. Ward S., Weatherley B. C.: Pharmacokinetics of atracurium and its metabolites. Br J Anaesth 58:6, 1986

156. Bell C. F., Hunter J. M., et al.: Use of atracurium and vecuronium in patients with oesophageal varices. Br J Anaesth 57:160, 1985

157. Parker C. J., Hunter J. M.: Pharmacokinetics of atracurium and laudanosine in patients with hepatic cirrhosis. Br J Anaesth 62:177, 1989

158. Leroy B., Baclet L., et al.: Atracurium and cirrhosis: clinical study of the curariform action. Ann Fr Anesth Reanim 4:489, 1985

159. Fleig W. E., Stange E. F.: Esophageal varices: current therapy in 1989. Endoscopy 21:89, 1989

160. Kleber G., Sauerbruch T., et al.: Prediction of variceal hemorrhage in cirrhosis: a prospective follow-up study. Gastroenterology 100:1332, 1991

161. Fogel M. R., Knauer C. M., et al.: Continuous intravenous vasopressin in active upper gastrointestinal bleeding. Ann Intern Med 96:565, 1982

162. Mallory A., Schaefer J. W., et al.: Selective intra-arterial vasopression infusion for upper gastrointestinal tract hemorrhage: a controlled trial. Arch Surg 115:30, 1980

163. Conn H. O., Ramsby G. R., et al.: Intraarterial vasopressin in the treatment of upper gastrointestinal hemorrhage: a prospective, controlled clinical trial. Gastroenterology 68:211, 1975

164. Bosch J., Groszmann R. J., et al.: Association of transdermal nitroglycerin to vasopressin infusion in the treatment of variceal hemorrhage: a placebo-controlled clinical trial. Hepatology 10:962, 1989

165. Gimson A. E., Westaby D., et al.: A randomized trial of vasopressin and vasopressin plus nitroglycerin in the control of acute variceal hemorrhage. Hepatology 6:410, 1986

166. Tsai Y. T., Lay C. S., et al.: Controlled trial of vasopressin plus nitroglycerin vs. vasopressin alone in the treatment of bleeding esophageal varices. Hepatology 6:406, 1986

167. Jenkins S. A., Baxter J. N., et al.: A prospective randomised controlled clinical trial comparing somatostatin and vasopressin in controlling acute variceal haemorrhage. Br Med J 290:275, 1985

168. Burroughs A. K., McCormick P. A., et al.: Randomized, double-blind, placebo-controlled trial of somatostatin for variceal bleeding. Emergency control and prevention of early variceal rebleeding. Gastroenterology 99:1388, 1990

169. Kravetz D., Bosch J., *et al.*: Comparison of intravenous somatostatin and vasopressin infusions in treatment of acute variceal hemorrhage. Hepatology *4*:442, 1984

170. Barsoum M. S., Bolous F. I., *et al.*: Tamponade and injection sclerotherapy in the management of bleeding oesophageal varices. Br J Surg *69*:76, 1982

171. Paquet K. J., Feussner H.: Endoscopic sclerosis and esophageal balloon tamponade in acute hemorrhage from esophagogastric varices: a prospective controlled randomized trial. Hepatology *5*:580, 1985

172. Moreto M., Zaballa M., *et al.*: A randomized trial of tamponade or sclerotherapy as immediate treatment for bleeding esophageal varices. Surg Gynecol Obstet *167*:331, 1988

173. Soderlund C., Ihre T.: Endoscopic sclerotherapy v. conservative management of bleeding oesophageal varices. A 5-year prospective controlled trial of emergency and long-term treatment. Acta Chir Scand *151*:449, 1985

174. Larson A. W., Cohen H., *et al.*: Acute esophageal variceal sclerotherapy. Results of a prospective randomized controlled trial. Jama *255*:497, 1986

175. Stiegmann G. V., Goff J. S., *et al.*: Endoscopic sclerotherapy as compared with endoscopic ligation for bleeding esophageal varices. N Engl J Med *326*:1527, 1992

176. Osborne D. R., Hobbs K. E.: The acute treatment of haemorrhage from oesophageal varices: a comparison of oesophageal transection and staple gun anastomosis with mesocaval shunt. Br J Surg *68*:734, 1981

177. Resnick R. H., Iber F. L., *et al.*: A controlled study of the therapeutic portacaval shunt. Gastroenterology *67*:843, 1974

178. Cello J. P., Grendell J. H., *et al.*: Endoscopic sclerotherapy versus portacaval shunt in patient with severe cirrhosis and acute variceal hemorrhage. Long-term follow-up. N Engl J Med *316*:11, 1987

179. Garden O. J., Mills P. R., *et al.*: Propranolol in the prevention of recurrent variceal hemorrhage in cirrhotic patients. A controlled trial. Gastroenterology *98*:185, 1990

180. Lebrec D., Poynard T., *et al.*: A randomized controlled study of propranolol for prevention of recurrent gastrointestinal bleeding in patients with cirrhosis: a final report. Hepatology *4*:355, 1984

181. Villeneuve J. P., Pomier-Layrargues G., *et al.*: Propranolol for the prevention of recurrent variceal hemorrhage: a controlled trial. Hepatology *6*:1239, 1986

182. Burroughs A. K., Jenkins W. J., *et al.*: Controlled trial of propranolol for the prevention of recurrent variceal hemorrhage in patients with cirrhosis. N Engl J Med *309*:1539, 1983

183. O'Connor K. W., Lehman G., *et al.*: Comparison of three nonsurgical treatments for bleeding esophageal varices. Gastroenterology *96*:899, 1989

184. Rosch J., Hanafee W. N., *et al.*: Transjugular portal venography and radiologic portacaval shunt: an experimental study. Radiology *92*:1112, 1969

185. Gordon J. D., Colapinto R. F., *et al.*: Transjugular intrahepatic portosystemic shunt: a nonoperative approach to life-threatening variceal bleeding. Can J Surg *30*:45, 1987

186. LaBerge J. M., Ring E. J., *et al.*: Transjugular intrahepatic portosystemic shunts: preliminary results in 25 patients. J Vasc Surg *16*:258, 1992

187. Ring E. J., Lake J. R., *et al.*: Using transjugular intrahepatic portosystemic shunts to control variceal bleeding before liver transplantation. Ann Intern Med *116*:304, 1992

188. Helton W. S., Belshaw A., *et al.*: Critical appraisal of the angiographic portacaval shunt (TIPS). Am J Surg *165*:566, 1993

189. Pulido-Duque J. M., Reyes R., *et al.*: Intraparenchymal anesthesia infiltration during transjugular intrahepatic portosystemic shunting. Radiology *185*:903, 1992

190. Krowka M. J., Tajik A. J., *et al.*: Intrapulmonary vascular dilatations (IPVD) in liver transplant candidates. Screening by two-dimensional contrast-enhanced echocardiography. Chest *97*:1165, 1990

191. Cuervas-Mons V., Millan I., *et al.*: Prognostic value of preoperatively obtained clinical and laboratory data in predicting survival following orthotopic liver transplantation. Hepatology *6*:922, 1986

192. Busuttil R. W., Seu P., *et al.*: Liver transplantation in children. Ann Surg *213*:48, 1991

193. Salt A., Noble-Jamieson G., *et al.*: Liver transplantation in 100 children: Cambridge and King's College Hospital series. Bmj *304*:416, 1992

194. Gonwa T. A., Morris C. A., *et al.*: Race and liver transplantation. Arch Surg *126*:1141, 1991

195. Cox K., Nakazato P., *et al.*: Liver transplantation in infants weighing less than 10 kilograms. Transplant Proc *23*:1579, 1991

196. Tarter R. E., Switala J., *et al.*: Quality of life before and after orthotopic hepatic transplantation. Arch Intern Med *151*:1521, 1991

197. Van Voorst S. J., Peters T. G., *et al.*: Autotransfusion in hepatic transplantation. Am Surg *51*:623, 1985

198. Dzik W. H., Jenkins R.: Use of intraoperative blood salvage during orthotopic liver transplantation. Arch Surg *120*:946, 1985

199. Carmichael F. J., Lindop M. J., *et al.*: Anesthesia for hepatic transplantation: cardiovascular and metabolic alterations and their management. Anesth Analg *64*:108, 1985

200. Shaw B. Jr., Martin D. J., *et al.*: Venous bypass in clinical liver transplantation. Ann Surg *200*:524, 1984

201. Veroli P., el Hage C., *et al.*: Does adult liver transplantation without venovenous bypass result in renal failure? Anesth Analg *75*:489, 1992

202. Taura P., Beltran J., *et al.*: Hemodynamic prediction of the need for venovenous bypass in orthotopic liver transplantation. Transplant Proc *23*:1951, 1991

203. Taura P., Beltran J., *et al.*: The need for venovenous bypass in orthotopic liver transplantation. Transplantation *52*:730, 1991.

204. Steltzer H., Blazek G., *et al.*: Two-dimensional transesophageal echocardiography in early diagnosis and treatment of hemodynamic disturbances during liver transplantation. Transplant Proc *23*:1957, 1991.

205. Ellis J. E., Lichtor J. L., *et al.*: Right heart dysfunction, pulmonary embolism, and paradoxical embolization during liver transplantation. A transesophageal two-dimensional echocardiographic study. Anesth Analg *68*:777, 1989.

206. Prager M. C., Gregory G. A., *et al.*: Massive venous air embolism during orthotopic liver transplantation. Anesthesiology *72*:198, 1990.

207. Todo S., Nery J., *et al.*: Extended preservation of human liver grafts with UW solution. Jama *261*:711, 1989.

208. Starzl T. E., Demetris A. J., *et al.*: Liver transplantation (1). N Engl J Med *321*:1014, 1989.

209. Starzl T. E., Iwatsuki, S., Klintmclm, G. *et al.*: Liver transplantation with the use of cyclosporin A and prednisone. N Engl J Med *305*:266, 1981.

Chapter 23

RENAL PHYSIOLOGY, PHYSIOPATHOLOGY, AND PHARMACOLOGIC EFFECTS ON KIDNEY FUNCTION

RAHIM BEHNIA

The kidneys are regulatory organs that selectively conserve and excrete water and various chemical compounds. They both eliminate waste liquids and potentially harmful end products of metabolism, such as urea, sulfate, uric acid, and phosphates and conserve the substances that are essential to life such as water, sugar, amino acids, sodium, potassium, chloride, and bicarbonate. The kidneys also regulate blood pressure-volume homeostasis, acid-base and sodium-potassium balance, as a result, improve microcirculation, tissue perfusion as well as cell nutrition.[1-18] Because anesthetic agents and the accompanying stress of surgical procedures can affect renal function and drug clearance, the anesthesiologist should have a working knowledge of renal physio-pharmacology for the proper administration of anesthesia in healthy and critically ill patients. This chapter will briefly focus on the following areas:

1) renal anatomy; 2) renal physiology; 3) physiology of bladder and micturation reflex; 4) renal pharmacology; 5) renal pathology; 6) evaluation of renal function; and 7) medical management of renal failure patients.

RENAL ANATOMY

Gross anatomy of the mammalian kidney consists of cortical and medullary substances and a pelvis that connects with the ureter and bladder. The cortex has two types of nephron, the outer cortical nephron arises in the more superficial parts of the cortex and the juxtamedullary nephron arises from the deep cortical region. The inner medulla has one or two papillae (tips) depending upon the species, and the outer medulla is further divided into an outer and inner stripe (Fig. 23-1).

Renal Circulation

The renal artery enters the kidney alongside the ureter, branches off into the interlobar, the arcade artery, the interlobular artery, the afferent artery leading to the glomerular capillary network. As this capillary network becomes enclosed in Bowman's capsule, it loses its spiraled coat of smooth muscle and rapidly divides into coiled capillary loops to form the *glomerular tuft*. A regrouping of these capillaries forms the efferent arteriole. This anatomical arrangement is designed for outward filtration. Blood enters the afferent arterioles, spreads over a large area (1 to 1.5 square meter) of thin-walled capillaries in the glomerulus, and then makes its exit through the efferent arteriole. This arrangement of two arterioles on each side of the filtering bed allows for delicate pressure adjustments and close control of filtration. The venous system similarly subdivides, forming the renal vein alongside the ureter (Fig. 23-1).

The Nephron

The functional unit of the kidney consists of a glomerular capillary network that is surrounded by Bowman's capsule, a proximal tubule, a loop of Henle, a distal tubule, and a collecting duct. Adult human kidneys have roughly two million nephrons. Two types have been described: 1) The outer cortical nephron, located in the superficial part of the cortex, has a short loop of Henle that reaches varying distance into the outer medulla. Its efferent arterioles branch into their own and another peritubular capillary network. This capillary network nourishes the tubular cells, transports substances to the tubules for secretion, or reabsorbs materials from the tubules. 2) The juxtamedullary nephron, arising from the deep cortical area, has a larger glomerulus and its loop of Henle extends to the inner medulla. Its efferent arteriole extends to the peritubular network and also makes a series of vascular loops called *vasa recta* that surround the collecting ducts and ascending limbs of Henle. Blood returns to the cortex in the ascending *vasa recta* that run within the venous system (Figs. 23-1, 23-2).

Juxtaglomerular Apparatus (JGA)

JGA is a combination of specialized secretory cells at the vascular pole where the afferent and efferent arterioles enter and leave the glomerulus and specialized epithelial cells in the thick ascending limb of Henle (*macula densa cells*) (Fig. 23-3). The JGA secretes renin and its physiologic significance will be described later.

Innervation of Urogenital Apparatus

Table 23-1 provides a brief description of sensory and motor pathways for innervation of urogenital apparatus.[19-23] Rich plexus renalis sympathetic constrictor fibers are derived from the T4 to L1 spinal cord segments through the celiac plexus. The kidney's blood vessels are richly innervated by both alpha (α_1 and α_2)- and beta (β_1

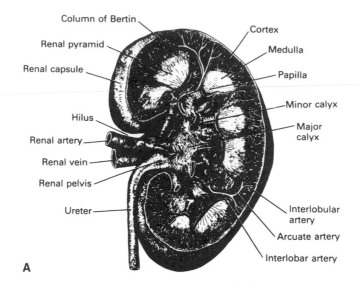

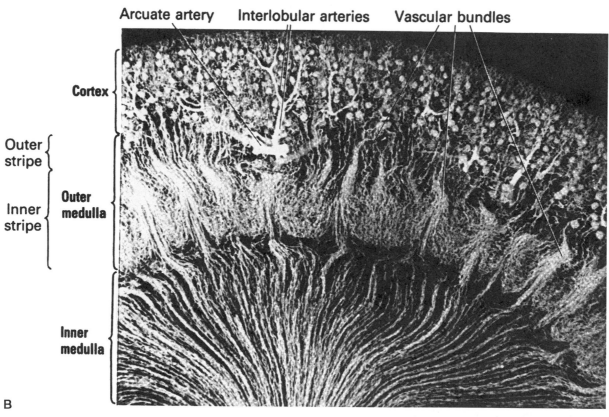

Fig 23–1.   A. Sagittal section of a human kidney showing the major gross anatomical features. The renal columns are extensions of cortical tissue between the medullary areas. Not shown is the adrenergic nerve supply, not only to the large renal vessels but also to the vascular and tubular components of the nephron. Redrawn and very slightly modified from Braus, H. *Anatomie des Menschen*, Vol. 2. Berlin: Springer, 1924. B. Vasculature of the kidney from a desert rodent (Meriones), showing: the cortex with numerous glomeruli; the outer medulla, containing capillary networks, and vascular bundles with vasa recta; and the inner medulla, containing vasa recta. The vessels were filled with silicone rubber (Microfil) by arterial injection. Courtesy of Lise Bankir. Reproduced with permission from Valtin, H. Renal function: Mechanisms Preserving Fluid and Solute Balance in Health. Little Brown Company: Boston 1983.

and β_2)-adrenergic fibers. Stimulation of these fibers induced by surgical stress, general anesthesia, hypoxia, hypotension, pain, severe bleeding, and strenuous exercise, can lead to renal vasoconstriction and the reduction in both renal blood flow (RBF) and glomerular filtration rate (GFR).[16-18, 24-29] While administration of epinephrine and norepinephrine in low concentrations increases systemic blood pressure, it also can result in a decreased total RBF.

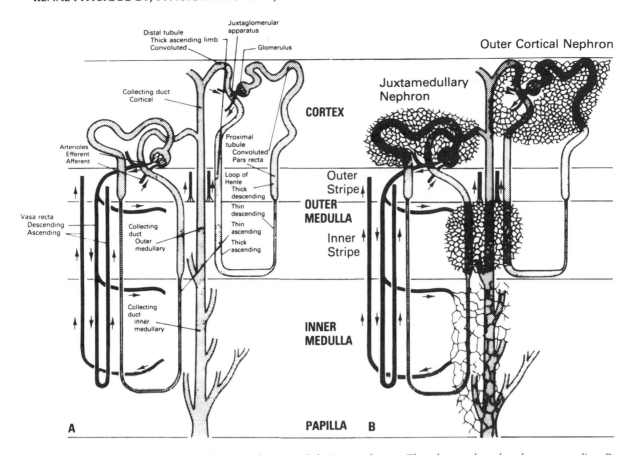

Fig. 23–2. A. Outer cortical and juxtamedullary nephrons and their vasculature. The glomerulus plus the surrounding Bowman's capsule are known as the "renal corpuscle." There is some overlapping nomenclature; for example, the loop of Henle consists of the pars recta, the descending and ascending thin limbs, and the ascending thick limb, even though the first and the last parts are also considered to belong to the proximal and distal tubules, respectively. The beginning of the proximal tubule—the so-called urinary pole—lies opposite the vascular pole, where the afferent and efferent arterioles enter and leave the glomerulus. The ascending thick limb of the distal tubule is always closely associated with the vascular pole belonging to the same nephron; the juxtaglomerular apparatus is located at the point of contact. B. Capillary networks have been superimposed on the nephrons illustrated in (A). Both diagrams are highly schematic (for a more accurate portrayal, see Beeuwkes, R., III, and Bonventre, J.V. *Am J. Physiol,* 229:695, 1975), and they do not accurately reflect some relationships that probably have functional meanings. In the rat, for example, long thin descending limbs of Henle are located next to collecting ducts, and short thin descending limbs are closely associated with the vascular bundles made up of descending and ascending vasa recta in the outer medulla. The drawings are based mainly on Kriz, W. *Am J. Physiol,* 241 (Regulatory Integrative Comp. Physiol. 10):R3, 1981. Reproduced with permission from Valtin, H. Renal function: Mechanisms Preserving Fluid and Solute Balance in Health. Little Brown Company: Boston 1983.

The termination of these nerves on renal tubule cell and their influence on sodium transport has been reported.[30-31] Both α_1 and α_2 receptors have been identified in renal juxtaglomerular cells, where they mediate renin release and sodium reabsorption.[32] Dopamine (D_1 and D_2) receptors have a specific effect on intra-renal vessels leading to redistribution of blood flow under various conditions. Dopamine agonists and their effect on RBF and natriuresis will be discussed later.

RENAL PHYSIOLOGY

Five aspects of renal physiology will be reviewed in this section. 1) the physiology of renal blood flow, 2) physiology of urine formation, 3) measurement of glomerular filtration rate, 4) tubular function (reabsorption, secretion and synthesis), and 5) hormonal and humoral factors affecting renal physiology.

Renal Blood Flow (RBF)

Although kidneys weigh only 300–400 grams representing 0.4% of total body mass, they receive 20 to 25% of cardiac output, indicating very low intrarenal resistance. This high RBF phenomenon leads to a very low arteriovenous oxygen content difference of 1.5 ml%. RBF in the adult is approximately 1250 ml/minute making the kidney the prime organ involved in maintaining volume-pressure homeostasis during hemodynamic instability. Of this 1250 ml of RBF, in normal conditions, about 1249 ml/min of RBF leave through the renal vein, and 1 ml/min is filtered as urine. Renal plasma flow (RPF) is the amount of plasma that transfers through the renal vasculature. If hematocrit is 45%, RPF will be 55% of RBF.

RBF is autoregulated when renal arterial pressure is between 80–180 mm Hg. Although the mechanism of au-

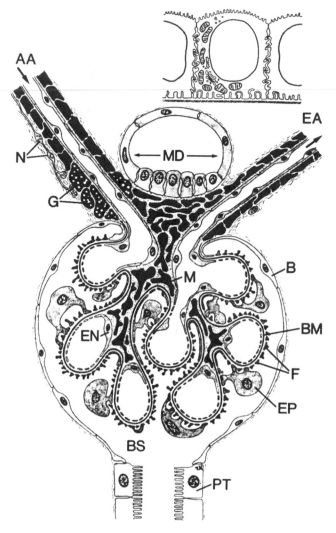

Fig. 23–3. An overview of a renal corpuscle and JGA. At the vascular pole, an afferent arteriole (AA) enters and an efferent arteriole (EA) leaves the glomerulus. At the urinary pole, Bowman's space (BS) becomes the tubular lumen of the proximal tubule. The epithelial cells comprising Bowman's capsule (B) enclose Bowman's space. Smooth muscle cells proper of the arterioles and all cells derived from smooth muscle are shown in black, including the granular cells (G). The afferent arteriole is innervated by sympathetic nerve terminals (N). The extraglomerular mesangial cells are located at the angle between AA and EA and continue into the mesangial cells (M) of the glomerular tuft. The glomerular capillaries are outlined by fenestrated endothelial cells (EN) and covered from the outside by the epithelial cells (EP) with foot processes (F). The glomerular basement membrane (BM) is continuous throughout the glomerulus. At the vascular pole, the thick ascending limb touches with the macula densa (MD) the extraglomerular mesangium. The *inset* shown at the top depicts the ultrastructural organization of the macula densa epithelium. Reproduced with permission from Koushanpour, E., Kritz, W. Renal Physiology. Principles, Structures, and Function (Second Edition) New York: Springer Verlag 1986.

toregulation is not understood fully, it has been attributed to the intrinsic property of arterial smooth muscle and tubuloglomerular feedback. Indeed, renal autoregulation persists even when the kidney is totaly denervated, when α-adrenergic blockers such as phentolamine and phenoxibenzamine are used, and when the isolated kidney is perfused in vitro. Intrarenal tissue pressure, accumulation of vasoactive metabolites, myogenic processes, and macula densa feedback mechanism between afferent arteriole and distal tubular lumen, have also been said to contribute to autoregulation of RBF. Because, RBF and glomerular filtration rate (GFR) are closely correlated, RBF and GFR autoregulation has been attributed to changes in afferent arteriolar resistance.[33]

Total RBF may be measured by relatively direct techniques such as electromagnetic flow meter or ultrasound Doppler flow.[33-35] RBF can also be indirectly estimated by the Fick principle. For example, effective renal plasma flow (ERPF) can be determined by using the *p-aminohippurate* (PAH) extraction technique and RBF can be calculated from RBF=ERPF/(1 − Htc). By applying radioactive markers such as ^{85}Kr and ^{133}Xe, it has been shown that renal cortex receives 93%, outer medulla 6%, and the inner medulla about 1% of the total renal blood flow.[33] Due to the heterogeneous distribution of blood flow, severe local tissue hypoxia may develop in spite of adequate RBF. This heterogeneous oxygen delivery can be a potential source of localized injury during renal hypoperfusion. The medullary thick ascending limb of Henle's loop (mTAL) is selectively vulnerable to this hypoxic injury.

Urine Formation

Filtration, reabsorption, and secretion are three major physiologic functions of the kidneys. Even though, kidneys filter approximately 180 liters every 24 hours, 99 percent of the filtered solute is reabsorbed. Approximately 27,000 mEq of sodium, and 20,000 mEq of chloride are filtered through the glomeruli of normal humans and a major portion of these substances is also reabsorbed through tubular cells. The daily urinary volume is only 1–2 liters per day. Capillaries in the *glomerular tuft* are unique because they sustain a head pressure of about 75 mm Hg compared to other 25 to 30 mm Hg of capillary pressure elsewhere. Glomerular capillary hydrostatic pressure is opposed by plasma oncotic pressure (30 mm Hg) and intracapsular pressure (20 mm Hg). Net filtration pressure is about 25 mm Hg.

GFR is described by the following equation:

$$GFR = K_f (P_{gh} - P_{ic} - P_\pi)$$

Where: K_f is glomerular filtration coefficient
P_{gh} is glomerular hydrostatic pressure
P_{ic} is intracapsular pressure
P_π is plasma oncotic pressure

In patients undergoing intra-abdominal surgery, mechanical blockage of the ureters by abdominal pack, retractor, or kinked Foley catheter can increase P_{ic} and re-

Table 23–1. Innervation of Urogenital Apparatus

Sensory Nerves	Organ	Motor Nerves
Lower splanchnics Regional sympath. ganglia $T_{10} - L_1$	Kidney	
Renal and urethral plexuses $T_{11} - L_1$	Ureter	
Somatic and sympathetic nerves of lower thoracic segments	Bladder Fundus	Sacral parasympathetics $S_2 - S_4$
Pelvic nerves $S_2 - S_4$	Trigone Prostate Urethra	Hypogastric sympathetics $T_{11} - L_1$
Sacral nerves $S_2 - S_4$ Genitofemoral $L_1 - L_2$ Spermatic plexus T_{10}	Testicle	
Plexus along ovarian artery T_{10}	Ovaries	
Super hypog. plexus $T_{11} - L_1$	Uterine fundus	
Pelvic nerves $S_2 - S_4$	Cervix and upper vagina	

duce urine output, thereby making diuretic or fluid therapies ineffective.

Measurement of GFR

GFR is determined from the plasma clearance of low molecular weight markers, i.e., completely removing these markers from theoretical plasma volume within a defined period of time. An ideal filtration marker as described by Homer Smith[37] is one that is freely and completely filtered at the glomerulus, not undergo metabolism by the kidney, not be reabsorbed or secreted by the tubules, lacking significant protein binding, and physiologically inert and not interfering with renal function. Inulin, a 5200 dalton fructose polymer, meets all these criteria, and is considered to be a "gold standard" for determination of GFR.

GFR is described by the following equation:

$$GFR = \frac{[U]_x \cdot V}{[P]_x} = \text{(Inulin clearance is 132 ml/min)}$$

Where: GFR is ml/min
[U]$_x$ is urinary concentration of marker x
V is urine volume (ml/min)
[P]$_x$ is plasma concentration of marker x.

GFR is reduced in conditions of hypotension, reduced cardiac output and decreased RBF, renal vasoconstriction, reduced K_f due to a tightening of endothelial junction, intratubular obstruction, and back leakage of filtrate to circulation through the cell membrane of damaged tubular cell.

In clinical practice, plasma creatinine and creatinine clearance are used as simplified alternative methods to assess GFR. The creatinine clearance measurement has two major assumptions: (1) it assumes that endogenous creatinine is produced at constant a rate and (2) it assumes that creatinine is solely excreted via glomerular filtration. It is widely recognized that creatinine clearance varies according to changes in muscle mass and alterations in dietary intake. Creatinine clearance tends to over estimate GFR.[37] Therefore, both plasma creatinine and creatinine clearance are insensitive indicators of reduced GFR. Due to difficulties associated with the measurement of inulin clearance and limitations of plasma creatinine and creatinine clearance, radioisotopic filtration markers have been used for accurate measurement of GFR.[38] The ratio of GFR to renal plasma flow is called the filtration fraction (FF) and its normal value is 20%.

Occasionally, during patient care, it becomes necessary to calculate osmolar and free water clearance using the following equations:

$$C_{osmo} = \frac{U_{osmo} \cdot V}{P_{osmo}}$$

$$C_{H_2O} = V - C_{osmo}$$

where: C_{osmo} is osmolar clearance
U_{osmo} is urine osmolality
V is urine volume (ml/min)
P_{osmo} is plasma osmolality
C_{H_2O} is free water clearance

Tubular Function

Renal tubules are known to perform three functions: (1) reabsorption of water and certain substances from the glomerular filtrate; (2) excretion of foreign substances from the peritubular capillaries into the filtrate; and (3) synthesis of ammonia and like substances, thereby, in part, regulating the acid-base balance.

The reabsorption process is selective. Substances useful to the body such as water, glucose, and basic ions are actively absorbed. Most substances have a limit beyond which they are not absorbed. The maximal capacity of tubules to absorb such substances can be measured. This type of reabsorption is called an "obligatory process" (Fig. 23–4).

Proximal Tubule

About 80-88% of the glomerular filtrate is absorbed from the proximal convoluted tubules. The major function of the proximal tubule is sodium reabsorption. Sodium is actively transported out of the proximal tubular cells as capillary side by membrane-bound Na^+-K^+-AT-Pase. As a result, low intra cellular concentration of Na^+ allows passive movement of Na^+ from tubular fluid into epithelial cells following its concentration gradient. Sodium reabsorption is coupled with other solutes such as phosphate, all glucose, all proteins, a greater portion of bicarbonate, and most of the water.

An exchange of 3 K^+ for 2 K^+ causes a net loss of intracellular positive charge leading to absorption of other cations such as Ca^{2+} and Mg^{2+}. Thus, $Na^+-K^+-ATPase$ at the tubular cells provides the energy for the reabsorption of most solutes. Sodium reabsorption at the luminal membrane is also coupled with the secretion of H^+ and reabsorption of 90% of the filtered bicarbonate ions. Unlike other solutes, chloride can diffuse through the tight junction between adjacent tubular epithelial cells. Therefore, chloride reabsorption is mostly passive and follows

its concentration gradient. Proximal tubules secrete organic cations such as creatinine, cimetidine and quinidine. Organic anions such as urate, keto acids, penicillins, cephalosporins, diuretics, salicylates and x-ray dye contrasts also are secreted by proximal tubules.

Loop of Henle

The loop of Henle consists of descending and ascending segments. The thin descending portion is a continuation of the proximal tubule. The ascending portion consists of a thin and a thick segment. The loop of Henle reabsorbs 15-20% of filtered sodium load. With the exception of the ascending thick segment, water and solute reabsorption in the loop of Henle is passive and follows osmotic and concentration gradients. In the ascending thick segment, Na^+ is actively reabsorbed due to $Na^+-K^+-ATPase$ activity on the capillary side of the epithelial cells. The thick part of the ascending limb is impermeable to water. As a result, the interstitium surrounding the loop of Henle is hypertonic and tubular fluid flowing out of the loop of Henle is hypotonic (100-200 mosmol/L). The thick ascending loop of Henle also reabsorbs calcium and magnesium. The parathyroid hormone regulates calcium reabsorption at this site.

Distal Tubule

About 5% of filtered sodium load is actively reabsorbed in the distal tubule by the energy driven from Na^+-K^+-AT-pase. The distal tubule also is the major site of parathyroid hormone and vitamin D-mediated calcium reabsorption.

Collecting Tubule

The cortical part of the collecting tubule is a continuation of the distal tubule and is the principal site of the aldosterone-mediated Na^+ reabsorption. Sodium reabsorption is governed by the level of aldosterone. The release of aldesterone, in turn, is regulated by the effects of plasma sodium on adrenal glomerulosa cells, renin-angiotensin system and atrial natriuretic peptide (Figs. 23-5, 23-6). The medullary collecting tubule is the principal site of action for antidiuretic hormone (ADH). Both cortical and medullary collecting tubules contain a H^+-secreting ATPase on their luminal membrane. This pump mediates reabsorption of HCO_3^- in the distal tubule and plays a major role in regulating acid-base balance. The H^+ is excreted in urine in the form of titratable acids, such as phosphates, and as ammonium ions. Metabolic acidosis and aldosterone secretion enhance H^+ secretion at this site.[19-23,39] The distal segment of both the distal convoluted tubule and collecting ducts reabsorbs an additional amount of water as well as electrolytes with the production of either hypotonic or hypertonic urine. This reabsorption of water is governed primarily by ADH. Also ADH plays a major role in recycling of urea within the kidney (Fig. 23-7). Eventually, all but 1% of the glomerular filtrate is absorbed, resulting in an average urine volume 1-1.5 liters per day.[19-23,39]

Net reabsorption for all nephrons combined, is calculated using the following formula:

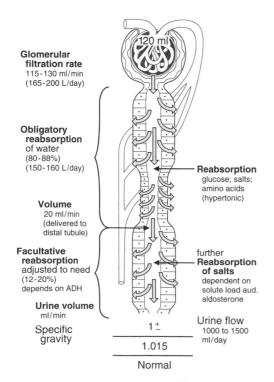

Glomerular filtration rate
115-130 ml/min
(165-200 L/day)

Obligatory reabsorption of water
(80-88%)
(150-160 L/day)

Volume
20 ml/min
(delivered to distal tubule)

Facultative reabsorption
adjusted to need
(12-20%)
depends on ADH

Urine volume
ml/min

Specific gravity

Reabsorption
glucose; salts;
amino acids
(hypertonic)

further
Reabsorption of salts
dependent on
solute load aud.
aldosterone

Urine flow
1000 to 1500
ml/day

$$\frac{1 \pm}{1.015}$$

Normal

Fig. 23–4.   Normal renal function.

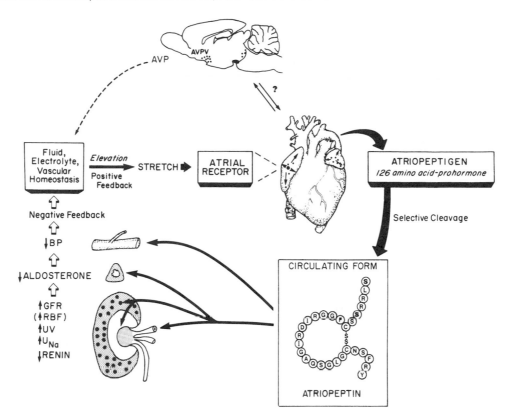

Fig. 23–5. Schematic Diagram of the Atriopeptin Hormonal System. The 126-amino acid prohormone, atriopeptigen, is stored in granules in perinuclear atrial cardiocytes. Elevated vascular volume results in the release of atriopeptin, which acts on the kidney (glomeruli and papilla) to increase the glomerular filtration rate (GFR), renal blood flow (RBF), urine volume (UV), and sodium excretion (U_{Na}), and to decrease plasma renin activity. Natriuresis and diuresis are also facilitated by the suppression of aldosterone and the release of arginine vasopressin (AVP). Diminution of vascular volume provides a negative feedback that suppresses circulating levels of atriopeptin. Reproduced with permission from Needleman and Greenwald[18] N. Engl. J. Med. 314:829, 1986.

Quantity reabsorbed

$$= \text{Quantity filtered} - \text{Quantity excreted}$$

For example, sodium reabsorption is calculated by:

$$\text{Sodium reabsorbed} = (\text{GFR} \cdot P_{Na}) - (U_{Na} \cdot V)$$

where GFR is glomerular filtration rate
       P_{Na} is plasma sodium concentration
       U_{Na} is urine sodium concentration
       V is urine volume (ml/min)

The cost of active reabsorption of sodium into the interstitium against an osmotic gradient is about 1μMol oxygen for every 28 μEq of sodium reabsorbed. Thus tubular oxygen consumption can be roughly calculated from sodium reabsorption capacity.

Countercurrent Multiplication and Countercurrent Exchange

Glomerular fluid is isotonic as it enters the descending limb and passes toward the medullary part of the kidney. In the medulla, the surrounding interstitial fluid becomes increasingly concentrated with sodium from the cortex

to the papilla by a countercurrent mechanism. This mechanism consists of countercurrent multiplication, which takes place in the loop of Henle, and countercurrent exchange, which occurs in the *vasa recta*. Similarly, concentrated (hyperosmotic) urine is created via a passive reabsorption of water by this countercurrent mechanism. Countercurrent multiplication of the reabsorbed Na^+ and Cl^-, (without reabsorption of water), from the ascending limb of Henle results in a progressive hyperosmolality of the interstitium. This phenomenon is called corticopapillary osmotic gradient. Dissipation of this gradient by medullary blood flow is minimized by the countercurrent exchange function of the *vasa recta* (Figs. 23-2, 23-6).

Urea, the end product of protein catabolism in mammals, has a unique role in the countercurrent system and water conservation. Urea indirectly enhances the concentration of nonurea solutes in urine, possibly, through *passive* countercurrent multiplication in the inner medulla (Figs. 23-6, 23-7).

In all parts of the nephron except the thin loop of the Henle, the transport of Na^+ (and its anions) is active, while water reabsorption is passive. Although passive reabsorption of water follows reabsorption of Na^+, water balance is primarily regulated by blood concentration of ADH or vasopressin. ADH adjusts the amount of water

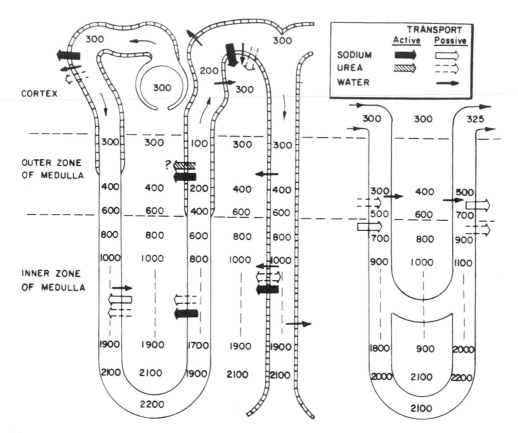

Fig. 23–6. Simplified model for the operation of the countercurrent multiplication system in a nephron with a long loop and in the vasa recta. The numbers represent hypothetical osmolality values. No quantitative significance is to be attached to the number of arrows, and only net movements are indicated. As is the case with the vascular loops, not all the loops of Henle reach the tip of the papilla, and hence the fluid in them does not become as concentrated as that of the final urine, but only as concentrated as the medullary interstitial fluid at the same level. Reproduced with permission from Koushanpour, E., Kirtz, W. Renal Physiology. Principles, Structure, and Function (Second Edition) New York: Springer Verlag, 1986. Adapted from Gottschalk, C.W. and Mylle, M. Micropuncture studies of the mammalian urinary concentrating mechanisms: evidence for the countercurrent hypothesis. Am. J. Physiol. 196: 927–936, 1959.

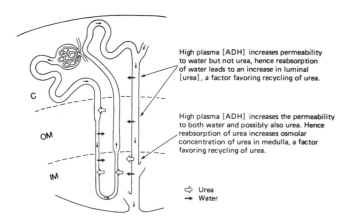

Fig. 23–7. Recycling of urea within the kidney. Reproduced with permission from Koushanpour, E., Kirtz, W. Renal Physiology. Principles, Structure, and Function (Second Edition) New York: Springer Verlag, 1986.

that is reabsorbed from the late distal tubules and collecting ducts. With a high concentration of ADH and resultant high water permeability, water reabsorbs passively in response to the osmotic gradient between the late distal tubules and collecting ducts and the surrounding interstitium, and hypertonic urine as high as 1200 mOsm/kg H_2O is formed. Conversely, a low concentration of ADH reduces the water permeability of late distal tubules and collecting ducts, which leads to the formation of hypotonic urine as low as 50 mOsm/kg H_2O (water diuresis).

Hormonal and Humoral Factors

Kidney and Renin-Angiotensin-Aldosterone-Axis

The renin-angiotensin-aldosterone system is important for the simultaneous regulation of blood pressure-volume homeostasis and sodium-potassium balance. The system has two effector hormones, angiotensin 2 (ANG2) and aldosterone.[1] ANG2 promotes arteriolar constriction, sodium retention and an increase in aldosterone secretion, and aldosterone plays a major role in regulating Na^+

and K[+] homeostasis.[2,3,5-7] The activity of this system is coupled with those of atrial natriuretic peptide, arginine-vasopressin, prostaglandins, and other neurovascular, humoral and local cellular mechanisms.[8-18] Available evidence also suggests that the intracellular concentration of calcium is necessary for both the release of renin and angiotensin stimulation of aldosterone biosynthesis.[41-47] Theories of the pathophysiology of essential hypertension, pulmonary hypertension and congestive heart failure are directly based on measurements of these factors.[1-9,48-54]

Renin Secretion

Three mechanisms operate to stimulate the secretion of renin:

1) Volume flow reduction or decrease in afferent arteriole pressure activates JGA (baroreceptor);
2) Plasma sodium reduction activates the macular densa in the walls of the distal convoluted tubules (osmoreceptors);
3) Direct adrenergic stimulation of the beta-receptors at JGA.

Reduction in blood flow or pressure at the JGA stimulates renin output. Decreased venous return, negative/positive pressure breathing, upright posture, bleeding, and any reduction of renal perfusion are specific potent stimuli producing high levels of renin.

Renin secretion is regulated by the overall state of sodium balance. This is accomplished at the macula densa, the specialized group of cells in the wall of the distal convoluted tubule located in apposition to the JGA. These are chemoreceptors (osmoreceptor type). A lowering of plasma sodium activates these cells and stimulates renin secretion followed by aldosterone production.

The sympathetic adrenergic nervous system modulates the production of renin. Beta-adrenergic agonists activate renin secretion. Beta-adrenergic receptor cells located on the JGA cells may be stimulated by stress to cause renin secretion.

With low plasma levels of renin angiotensin II stimulates preferentially the secretion of aldosterone by the adrenal gland; but with high plasma levels of renin, the angiotensin II acts as a vasoconstrictor.

Inhibition of Renin Secretion

Renin secretion may be inhibited by volume expansion and sodium loading; by atrial natriuretic peptide and by arginine-vasopressin.[1-4,9-11,14-18,55-58] These conditions are commonly seen in patients with advanced cardiopulmonary, renal and liver disease and during major surgical procedures under various anesthetic agents.[28,29,59-66] Renin secretion may be blocked by beta-adrenergic antagonists such as propranolol and metoprolol.

Role of Renin

The action of renin, an enzyme, is on its substrate, the circulating plasma protein designated as angiotensinogen. This is necessary for the production of angiotensin I (ANG I), an inactive decapeptide. This peptide in turn is converted to angiotensin II (ANG II), an octapeptide, in the presence of hydrolase enzyme ACE, a converting enzyme mainly found in the lungs and produced by the endothelial cells of the pulmonary capillaries (Fig. 23-8). In view of the major role of pulmonary conversion, it is conceived that certain pulmonary disorders may be associated with faulty production of ANG 2.[67-69] Convertase is also present in tissue macrophages, alveolar cells and in granulomata (Sarcoidoses); it is higher in smokers than non-smokers.

The converting-enzyme hydrolase is identical to kinase II which degrades bradykinin. If hydrolase is blocked then both an antihypertensive effect occurs due to decreased angiotensin II and there is a concomitant accumulation of bradykinin so that vasodilation ensues. Further bradykinin releases vasodepressor prostaglandins.[12,70]

Role of Angiotensin II

Angiotensin II acts on receptors sites in: a) vascular smooth muscle causing vasoconstriction; b) in the adrenal cortex (glomerulosa) causing aldosterone secre-

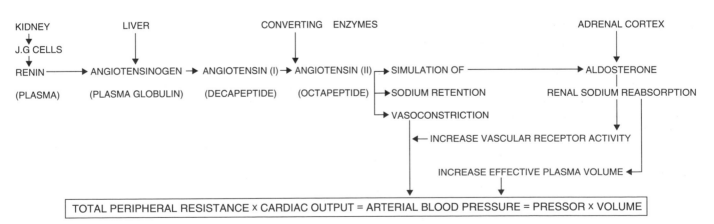

Fig. 23–8. The renin-angiotensin aldosterone system in the regulation of sodium, fluid volume and blood pressure (Based on Laragh, J:H., and Sealy, J.F. In: Handbook of Physiology. Renal Physiology, Am Physiological Soc. 1973, pp 831–908)

tion; c) in the kidney at the distal tubules and collecting ducts for reabsorption of sodium; d) receptors in the central nervous system for the regulatory process in thirst.

Effects of Anesthetics on Renin Angiotensin Axis

None of the conventional anesthetics appear to exert an effect on renin activity in the production of Angiotensin I or the conversion to Angiotensin II. In animals anesthetized with halothane and enflurane, there is a decrease in arterial pressure. No fall in pressure occurs during ketamine or fluroxene administration. Halothane and enflurane blunt vascular reactivity directly and also attenuate sympathic influence whereupon Angiotensin assumes the role of blood pressure maintenance.[58]

During halothane anesthesia the pressure response to administration of either Angiotensin I or II is depressed. Ketamine accentuates pressor activity of Angiotensin I and Angiotensin II.

Kidney and Atrial Natriuretic-Arginine Vasopressin Peptides Axis and Blood Pressure Electrolyte Homeostasis

The ANP hormone is primarily secreted by atrial myocytes in response to local wall stretch (i.e., volume expansion) and in pulmonary hypertension.[9,11,14,18] Through its effect on renal microvasculature, adrenal glomerulosa cells, and tubular epithelium, NAP inhibits Na^+ transport, suppresses renin, and inhibits aldosterone biosynthesis either by reducing renin or through direct action on adrenal glomerulosa cells (Fig. 23–5).[47,48] ANP also inhibits secretion of aldosterone by adrenal glomerulosa cells. Both acutely and chronically the various effects of ANP, decrease systemic blood pressure, intravascular volume and cardiac output. While sectioning of bilateral vagi does not alter the renal mediated hemodynamic effects of ANP[79] its natriuretic effect is prevented following cardiac denervation which indicates that stimulation of the sympathetic efferent nerve to the right atrial appendage is responsible for ANP release.

Studies in both isolated perfused and intact animals and humans indicate that ANP increases GFR. This effect is remarkable since it can occur even with reduction of both arterial blood pressure and RBF. Increased GFR has been attributed to decreased afferent arteriolar tone, increased efferent arteriolar tone, and increased filtration coefficient, K_f. NAP enhances natriuresis by decreasing sodium reabsorption in the ascending limb of Henle's loop, thereby disrupting load-reabsorption balance in the distal nephron which leads to an increase in GFR.

ANP can also function as a neuropeptide in suppressing the release of arginine-vasopressin (AVP).[46] AVP or ADH is secreted from the posterior pituitary gland. Blood concentration of ADH is regulated by osmolality of blood and blood volume. One hand, increased blood osmolality stimulates osmoreceptors that generate afferent signals calling for the secretion of ADH. On the other hand, increased blood volume stimulates volume receptors located in the low pressure portion of the circulation, as in the left atria or in the pulmonary veins leading to a reduction of ADH (Fig. 23–5).

ADH has been shown to have two receptor types: V_1 receptors located in the vascular wall whose stimulation leads to vasoconstriction; and V_2 receptors located in the renal tubule whose stimulation increases absorption of free water, using cyclic AMP as the intracellular messenger.[8] Suppression of ADH by ANP may modulate V_1 and V_2 receptors and alter pressure volume homeostasis and $Na^+ - K^+$ balance. Other factors such as drugs, anesthetic agents, alcohol, catecholamines, changes in intrathoracic pressure, upright position, lower body immersion in water, and hemorrhage can modulate the blood concentration of ADH, leading to hypertonic or hypotonic urine formation.

Kidney and Endothelin and Endothelium-Derived Relaxing Factor

The physiologic function of the vascular endothelium in the regulation of local vascular smooth muscle and organ blood flow has been well established. Several biochemical and mechanical stimuli induce the release of endothelin and endothelial-derived relaxing factor (EDRF).[80-83] An expanding array of biological activities has been attributed to endothelin, which has been reported to cause potent renal vasoconstriction and decreased GFR. Micropuncture studies determine that decreased GFR by endothelin is related to increased vas-cular resistance and decreased glomerular capillary ultrafiltration coefficient (K_f). There is growing evidence that endothelin may initiate various pathophysiologic conditions such as hypertension, renal injury, cardiogenic shock, gastric ulceration and inflammation.[84]

While more than one EDRF is released from vascular endothelium, nitric oxide (NO) is considered an important EDRF.[85] NO is formed by vascular endothelial cells from the terminal guanido nitrogen atom of the amino acid, L-arginine. NO, sodium nitroprusside, glyceryl trinitrates and other organic nitrate esters are potent vasodilators that stimulate guanylate cyclase. Several reports provide evidence that EDRF/NO produced in renal endothelial cells can have significant physiologic effect in the regulation of renal hemodynamic and glomerular function. Thus, dysfunction of the endothelium and decreased EDRF/NO release have been attributed to development of vasculo-occlusive pathology.[80]

Prostaglandin E_2 (PGE_2)

Prostaglandins are fatty acids found in the lung, brain, renal medulla, and pancreas. Prostaglandin E_2 (PGE_2), a potent renal vascular dilator, is intimately involved in the physiologic regulation of RBF. Prostaglandins play a major role in the preservation of blood flow distribution within the kidney. Experimental evidence demonstrates that treatment with PGE_2 after ischemic insult to the kidneys significantly improves RBF and GFR during the post ischemic period.[86] PGE_2 increases medullary blood flow, and decreases tubular oxygen consumption through inhibition of active transport in the medullary thick ascending limb of the loop of Henle (mTAL) cells.[87] PGE_2 opposes the vasoconstrictive effect of angiotensin and results in increased cortical blood flow, increased sodium excretion independent of GFR, and reduced medullary blood flow.[88] The reported toxicity of nonsteroidal anti-inflammatory drugs such as indometocin, ibuprofen, naproxin, fanoprofen, and aspirin, has been attributed to their inhibition of prostaglandin synthesis.[89]

PHYSIOLOGY OF BLADDER AND MICTURATION REFLEX

Adequate stimulus for voiding is distention of the bladder with the development of an increased wall tension. This is essentially a stretch receptor mechanism and the stretch sensory cells are proprioceptive end organs in the wall of the bladder.[90]

The afferent pathway is over the visceral afferent fibers through the pelvic nerves to the spinal reflex center at S2 through S4.[20] Impulses are carried from the bladder wall over this pathway. From the spinal reflex center, impulses are further carried to the fasciculus gracilis in the posterior columns to the micturation center in the brain stem located in the pons. The sensation is then carried to the voluntary center for micturation in the paracentral lobule of the cerebral cortex. Integration of the stimulus and modulation is carried out both here and in the pontile center.

The efferent pathway is parasympathetically mediated.[21] Impulses pass from the spinal reflex center by the parasympathetic nerves of the sacral outflow to the pelvic plexus and plexus in the bladder wall. At this point the impulse is carried by postganglionic fibers from these plexi directly to the muscle. Efferent impulses from S2 to S4 also pass through the pudendal nerve to the external urethra.

The spinal reflex micturation center is normally inhibited by corticoregulatory tracts, which inhibit efferent impulses to the bladder and to the urethra. Removal of this inhibition by proper sensory stimulation of the bladder results in contraction of the bladder and opening of the urethra.

Compliance of the Bladder[91]

As bladder volume gradually increases with urine, the cavitary radius increases and the bladder wall is stretched. However, intravesicule pressure remains constant and is generally equal to the intraabdominal pressure. This adaptation of the smooth detrusor muscle and the accommodation of intraventricular volume is not dependent upon neurogenic mechanisms, but rather upon the gradual stretching of the proprioreceptors imbedded in the bladder wall.

There is a very small and gradual increase in the intravesicular pressure and at a filling capacity of 400 ml, the pressure is approximately 10 cm of water. The first sensation of filling of the bladder occurs at a volume of 100–150 ml in the adult. The urge to void occurs generally at filling volume of 150–250 ml. A maximum volume of 250–450 ml may be achieved without undue discomfort. The normal capacity of the bladder is usually twice that volume at which there is an urge to void. However, when the volume of the bladder reaches approximately one liter, it may rupture.[92]

Urethral Coordination

Once the bladder detrusor tone reaches a level of urge and the spinal cord center efferent impulses are permitted to affect detrusor action, there is a simultaneous and coordinated relaxation of the bladder sphincter and an opening of the membranous, bulbous and penile urethras, all of which are determined by parasympathetic influences.

When voiding contraction is initiated, urine is discharged from the urinary bladder, facilitated by impulses from the brain stem. Once the bladder and the posterior urethra are emptied, the external sphincter closes, the detrusor muscle relaxes and then the posterior urethra closes. The perineal muscles very often are involved in a voluntary contraction along with the external sphincter to arrest the voiding stream. Any urine that is still in the membranous urethra may be forced back into the bladder, since there is collapse of the posterior urethra. Under general, spinal or epidural anesthesia, micturation is interrupted, thereby altering the emptying reflex.[88-90] In addition distention of the bladder beyond its capacity can cause changes in blood pressure and heart rate. Because sudden emptying of an overdistended bladder may cause hypotension, it must be emptied gradually. During prolonged surgical procedures, patients thus require urinary catheterization.

RENAL PHARMACOLOGY

In this section we will briefly discuss: 1) the pharmacology of diuretics; 2) the effect of deliberate hypotension on renal hemodynamics; 3) the pharmacology and renal effect of modern antihypertensive drugs; 4) the effect of vasopressors on the renal hemodynamics; 5) the effect of anesthetic agents and techniques on renal function; and 6) muscle relaxants and renal physiopathology.

Diuretics

Diuretics greatly enhance the efficacy of blood pressure lowering drugs such as β-adrenoreceptor blockers, calcium channel blockers, and angiotensin converting enzyme inhibitors. Therefore, diuretics are commonly used before, during and after anesthetic management of patients suffering from hypertension, chronic heart failure, peripheral edema, acute or chronic renal insufficiency, and those undergoing renal transplantation.

However, diuretics are not without their complications. Diuretic-induced hypokalemia, is associated with an increased incidence of arrhythmias in hypertensive patients. Furthermore, long-term diuretic therapy also can promote increased glucose tolerance and elevated plasma cholesterol, thereby creating further cardiovascular complications. The anesthesiologist should be familiar with the pharmacology and side effects of this class of drugs. A detailed discussion of the chemistry and pharmacology of diuretics is beyond the scope of this text, and those interested readers are referred to an excellent book by Reyes.[93]

Diuretics have been classified according to chemical structure, to their site of action within the nephron (Fig.

23-9), or on the basis of their mechanism of action and their efficacy (Table 23-2).[94]

Osmotic Diuretics

Osmotic diuretics do not belong to any one specific chemical group. Among their common characteristics are their ability to filter freely from the glomeruli, their lack of metabolization, and their slow reabsorption from renal tubules. In the presence of non-reabsorbable osmotic agents, the reabsorption of water is reduced relative to that of sodium. Thus, urine flow increases albeit a smaller increment of the electrolyte excretion.

Mannitol, the most widely used osmotic diuretic, is a metabolically inert hexose sugar that permeates poorly into the cell and is distributed mainly in the extracellular compartment. It is used during neurosurgery to reduce cerebral edema, and is also used to prevent acute renal failure. A drawback to the use of mannitol is the possibility that it can precipitate pulmonary edema in patients with early congestive heart failure and limited cardiac reserve. Other osmotic diuretics include urea which is rarely used, and glycerin and isosorbid administered orally to reduce intraocular pressure.[93]

Dopaminergic Agonists

Recent research on peripheral dopaminergic drugs that would produce vasodilation, increase renal blood flow, and natriuresis have produced two type of diuretics. The first is pro dopamine drug ibopamine, the disobutyryl ester of N-methyldopamine which causes diuresis mediated by arteriolar vasodilation. The second is N-allyl substituted fenoldopam, which demonstrates D_1 and D_2 agonist activity. Fenoldopam is a new selective dopamine D_1 receptor agonist which increases renal plasma flow decreases sodium reabsorption in proximal and distal tubules, and has no effect on GFR.[94]

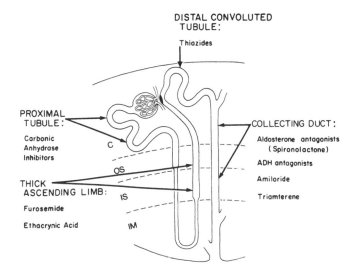

Fig. 23–9. Sites of action of the commonly used diuretics along the nephron. Reproduced with permission from Koushanpour, E., Kirtz, W.[34] Renal Physiology. Principles, Structure, and Function (Second Edition) New York: Springer Verlag, 1986.

Administration of dopamine at very low doses (1 to 3 μg/kg/min) reduces renal vascular resistance leading to an increase in RBF, GFR, and sodium excretion. Higher doses of 4 to 6 μg/kg/min produces an extra β-adrenergic effect, causing an increase in heart rate and myocardial contractility. At even higher doses (7 to 10 μg/kg/min.) dopamine resembles norepinephrine and reduces renal blood flow due to vasoconstriction.[95]

Diuretics and Renal Insufficiency

The kidney's response to diuretics in patients with renal and liver diseases is different from that in healthy individuals. For example, carbonic anhydrase inhibitors has very little use in patients with renal and hepatic diseases because of the lower magnitude of their effect. Thiazide diuretics as single agents have no clinical efficacy in renal insufficiency when GFR is below 30–40 ml/min. Potassium-retaining diuretics similarly are ineffective and should not be used because of the risk of hyperkalemia.[96] Other diuretics may have positive effects. For example, spironolactone is particularly useful in patients with cirrhosis and secondary hyperaldosteronism. While, osmotic diuretics are rarely used in chronic renal insufficiency because of the risks associated volume expansion and hyponatremia, monitol is used in patients with acute oliguria to prevent renal failure or convert oliguric to non-oliguric renal failure.

Although, renal clearance of all loop diuretics are decreased in patients with renal insufficiency, the response of remaining nephrons to these drugs is normal. In patients with renal insufficiency because of kinetic changes and delayed time appearance of these drugs in the urine, the total amount of drug reaching the site of action relative to dose is decreased. The objective of therapy is to administer a dose of diuretic that is delivered to the remaining nephrons. Voelker and associates[97] have shown that furosemide dose should be about five fold higher in patients with endstage renal disease than doses used in patients with normal function.

Effect of Deliberate Hypotension on Renal Hemodynamic

Deliberate hypotension induced by sodium nitroprusside, trimethaphan, nitroglycerine, and adenosin affect renal function, renal tissue oxygen, and RBF in different ways, but these parameters return to normal limits following restoration of blood pressure.[98–99]

Effect of Modern Antihypertensive Drugs

Angiotensin, Converting Enzyme (ACE) Inhibitors

Within the last decade, ACE-inhibitors (ie, Captopril, Enalapril) have been used for treatment of arterial hypertension. ACE-inhibitors are particularly effective in patients with high plasma renin and associated excessive angiotensin II. ACE-inhibitors also have been effectively used in low plasma renin hypertensive patients, indicating that these agents block both systemic formation and local intracellular metabolism of angiotensin II.[100,101] ACE-inhibitors are the drug of choice in the treatment of hypertension associated with congestive heart failure.[102] Be-

Table 23–2. Urinary Electrolyte Composition Relative to Naturietic Potency of Some Commonly Used Diuretics

Diuretics	Class of Diuretic	Volume (ml/min)	Sites of Action	Effects on Excretions (mM)					Filtered Sodium % Excreted Max. Fraction
				pH	Na$^+$	K$^+$	Cl$^-$	HCO$_3^-$	
Control		1		6	50	15	60	1	3
Mannitol	Osmotic	10	Filtered at glomerulus limited reabsorption	6.5	90	15	110	4	5
Acetazolamide	Inhibitors of carbonic anhydrase	3	Proximal tubule and distal tubule	8.2	70	60	15	120	5
Benzothiadiazides (thiazides)	Selective proximal tubule and early distal tubulae chloride excretion	3	Proximal tubule and distal tubule	7.4	150	25	150	25	8
Ethacrynic and furosomide	Loop diuretics "high ceiling"	8	Thick ascending loop of Henle	6	140	10	155	1	25
Spironolactone	Aldosterone antagonist	2	Collecting duct and distal tubule	7.2	130	5	110	15	3
Amiloride	Potassium sparing								
Triameterene	Potassium sparing								

From data of Golberg, Martin M. Renal tubular sites of action of diuretics, pp. 99–119. In Fisher, J. W. and Cafruny, E. J., Eds., Renal Pharmacology, 1971. Appleton Century Crofts, New York, 1971. Now (1993) Appleton Lang, Norwalk, CT. Weimer, I. M. Diuretics and other agents in the mobilization of edema fluid, Chap. 28, in Goodman and Gilman's, The Pharmacological Basis of Therapeutics, Eighth Edition. Pergamon Press, Elmsford, New York, 1990.[93]

cause of a possible deterioration in renal function owing to decreased GFR, the use of ACE-inhibitors in patients with bilateral renal artery stenosis or a solitary kidney with renal artery stenosis is contraindicated.[103] In contrast, ACE-inhibitors have nephroprotective properties in conditions of high intraglomerular pressure such as glomerular sclerosis. Captopril has a half-life of approximately 2 hours, while the others have half-lives ranging from 10–12 hours.

These agents are also the drug of choice in diabetic hypertension because they slow down the process of glomerulosclerosis, thereby preventing the development of chronic renal failure.[104,105] Since the plasma renin activity is suppressed in primary aldosteronism, ACE inhibitors are not effective in patients with Conn's syndrome. Side effects of ACE inhibitors include transient hypotension, neutropenia, angioedema, hyperkalemia, urticaria and rashes.

Captopril

A relatively specific competitive inhibitor of angiotensin-converting enzyme is an effective antihypertensive agent. It is orally active and taken about one hour before meals. Treatment is accompanied by a marked increase in renin but a major reduction in angiotensin II production.[70]

The hypotension action is largely due to the inhibition of angiotensin II production. However, bradykinin, normally inactivated by the converting-enzyme, increases in the plasma and produces vasodilatation and venodilitation. Further, bradykinin releases vasodepressor prostaglandins from various organs enhancing hypotension. Baroreceptor responses remain intact and there are

normal responses to norepinephrine, hence no orthostatic hypotension. Serum potassium is retained. If administered during diuretic therapy the administration of a potassium supplement is generally obviated.[70]

Enalapril

This is a long-lasting inhibitor of the angiotensin-converting enzyme (ACE) and is effective when taken orally. It is a pro-drug, being the ethyl ester of the active agent, enalaprilat. It is bioactivated by the hydrolysis of ester to enalaprilat, which itself is poorly absorbed from the gut. Peak serum concentrations of enalapril occur in one hour, while the peak concentration of the hydrolyzed agent enalaprilat occurs in 3–4 hours. The elimination half-life is approximately 12 hours.

Only about 60% of the enalapril is absorbed.[102]

Excretion of the parent and active drug is primarily renal. The principal component in the urine is enalaprilat and represents 40% of the absorbed drug, while 20% of the urinary drug is enalapril. No metabolites have been identified. The drug not absorbed is excreted in the feces; and, thus, renal plus gut excretion accounts for 95% of the oral dose. The oral dosage is 5.0 mg daily. It is useful in the management of hypertension and in the presence of diuretics the effect is additive.

Adverse Effects

Severe hypotension may occur in up to 2% of patients. It is likely to be more frequent in surgical patients under anesthesia, and it is especially likely in salt or volume depleted subjects. This can be corrected by volume expansion.

Angioedema has been reported with the ACE inhibitor

drugs. This may include edema of the face, tongue and/or glottis. Laryngeal stridor may be noted. Hyperkalemia may occur and rise to levels greater than 5.7 mEq/L, as observed in 1% of patients. This should be noted since high levels of potassium may antagonize non-depolarizing muscle relaxants. Contrariwise, succinylcholine may enhance K$^+$ release to dangerous levels. It is recommended that this depolarizing agent be avoided.

Impaired renal function may be evident by increases in blood urea nitrogen and serum creatinine. This may occur when the glomerular filtration rate is <30 ml/min or the urine output is <0.5 ml/kg of body weight. Blood components may be affected. Hemoglobin and hematocrit decrease may be seen of 0.3g and 1.0% volume, but are usually inconsequential. However, neutropenia does occur.

Calcium Channel Blockers

Calcium channel blockers used for the treatment of hypertension cardiac arrhythmia and renal protection, exert natriuretic and diuretic action in experimental animals, in healthy subjects and in patients suffering from essential hypertension. The natriuretic effect of calcium channel blockers depends upon sodium intake, central hemodynamics and the state of renal circulation.[106,107]

Beta-Adrenergic Blockers

A detailed study of the renal effect of Beta-adrenergic blockers used for treatment of hypertension and cardiac arrhythmia is beyond the scope of this text, and the reader is referred to a review by Beaufils.[108] This class of drugs may have different actions on the kidney depending on whether they block β_1 or β_2 adrenergic receptors. For example, while propranolol, a non-selective beta-adrenergic blocker with no intrinsic sympathetic activity, decreases renal blood flow and GFR, tertatolol, another β_1 and β_2 adrenergic blocker, increases renal blood flow. However, atenolol, which is a selective β1 adrenergic blocker has no effect on RBF and GFR.

β-adrenergic blocking drugs can be used intra- and postoperatively for blood pressure control. They are especially effective because secretion of renin in part is mediated by β1-adrenergic receptors. Esmolol because of its short half-life and titratability is a drug of choice for treatment of renin-mediated hypertensive crisis.

Effect of Vasopressors on Renal Hemodynamics

Most vasopressors markedly reduce in renal blood flow. The only exceptions are the isoproterenol and dopaminergic drugs which allow an increased renal blood flow in smaller concentrations.

Norepinephrine, through its severe renal vasoactive effect causes reduction in RBF and urine flow. Administration of epinephrine to severely hypotensive patients, on the other hand, may temporarily increase RBF by supporting general hemodynamics and head pressure. However, continued use for more than a few hours results in renal ischemia and tubular necrosis. Epinephrine, methoxamine, metaraminol and phenylephrine also depress renal hemodynamic and tubular function.[109-111]

Effect of Anesthetic Agents and Techniques on Renal Function

The reported effects of various anesthetics on renal function are dependent on the experimental protocols used, premedication, fluid regimen, depth of anesthesia, body temperature, and surgical stress. The depressant effect of anesthetics on renal function is direct, indirect, or a combination of both. Through its indirect effect on circulatory, sympathetic, and endocrine systems, an anesthetic can modify RBF, oxygen demand and supply, GFR, and tubular function. The anesthetic can also directly affect tubular transport.

General anesthetics can cause myocardial depression, peripheral vasodilation, and hypotension. These effects are exaggerated with positive pressure ventilation, body positioning and hypovolemia. Anesthetics also can cause an increased level of catecholamines in the blood, renal vasoconstriction, reduced RBF, and marked depression of renal function. Anesthetics also can modify humoral factors, such as those mediated by renin-angiotensin-aldosterone axis, parathyroid hormone, ADH, prostaglandins, ANF, and endothelial-derived relaxing factor.

The following is a brief summary of the effects of inhaled, intravenous, epidural and spinal anesthesia on renal function.

Inhaled Anesthetics

Older Agents

Although these agents are not used in clinical anesthesia, their renal effect is both of physiologic and historical interest. Both *cyclopropane* and *diethyl ether* cause a decrease in renal plasma flow, GFR, and urine output.[113-115] *Chloroform* may cause tubular epithelial damage.[116] *Vinethene* at higher concentrations produces a progressive decrease in kidney function leading to anuria, oliguria, congestion of glomeruli and cloudy swelling of tubular epithelium.[117] *Ethylene* has little effect on renal function.[118] *Methoxyflurane* produces typical generalized depression of renal function and causes postanesthetic high output renal failure.[119]

Newer Agents

Commonly used inhalation anesthetics produce a decline in renal function that returns to normal with termination of use. Halothane and enflurane reduce GFR and urine output.[120-123] At low concentrations, halothane does not appear to change the autoregulation of RBF even when administered during acute bleeding and hypovolemia. Isoflurane reduces GFR and urine output but has little effect on renal blood flow.[124] Nitrous oxide, when added to halothane, potentiates a reduction in urine output, but this combination does not appear to adversely affect the autoregulation of RBF.[125]

Sevoflurane

Sevoflurane is an experimental, nonflammable, fluorinated inhalation anesthetic that has been clinically used during surgical procedures in Japan and Germany. With its relatively minimal effect on hemodynamic parameters along with no significant change in heart rate, sevoflurane is advantageous for use during outpatient surgery.[126]

However, there have been some problems reported with its use. Sevoflurane at 1.0 MAC has not changed renal blood flow in spontaneously ventilated rats. Sevoflurane is metabolized in human and experimental animals to inorganic fluoride ion and organic fluorine metabolites which may cause renal toxicity. Fluoride levels in excess of 50 μM have been reported in clinical studies.[127,128] Thus, the risk of renal toxicity remains to be ruled out.[129]

Desflurane (I-653)

This agent is a new volatile anesthetic with low blood/gas partition coefficient of 0.42, leading to a rapid induction and recovery period. It is stable in moist soda lime and has been reported to be nontoxic to hypoxic enzyme-induced rats.[130] Volunteers following 90 minutes exposure to desflurane showed no evidence of renal dysfunction or of significant elevation of serum fluoride levels.[131-132] The renal effect of desflurane nonetheless requires further investigation.

Intravenous Induction Agents

In the normal kidney, thiopental, even at higher doses does not have significant effect on RBF. Ketamine increases systemic arterial pressure, RBF and renal vascular resistance.[133] Volume of distribution of fentanyl is increased, but no alteration in protein binding and its kinetics have been reported. Although a small dose of fentanyl has minimal effect on renal function, larger doses increase intrarenal resistance and reduce GFR, ERPF, and urine output.[134] Meperidine is metabolized to normeperidine which is then eliminated by urine. A marked cumulation of normeperidine in end stage renal disease (ESRD) can cause seizures which is reversible by naloxone.[135,136]

In the normal kidney, morphine, even at higher doses, has no effect on RBF.[137] Morphine and barbiturates bind to plasma protein, a phenomenon which limits the amount of a pharmacologically available free drug. In patients with chronic renal failure who have lower concentrations of plasma protein, pharmacologically active drugs become easily available.[138] In addition, in chronic renal patients as a result of metabolic acidosis, proteins bind to organic acids, leading to an increased pharmacologically active drug. In uremic patients, the blood-brain barrier becomes more permeable to morphine which causes greater than expected central nervous system depression. Because the morphine molecule is relatively large and not readily dialyzable, its use in anephric patients should be carefully monitored. In addition, morphine is metabolized to morphine-3 glucuronide and morphine-6β glucuronide. Morphine-6β glucuronide is an active metabolite and is a potent analgesic.[139] This high potency of morphine-6β glucuronide strongly suggests a significant role in morphine's action. Since morphine-6β glucuronide is excreted by the kidney, administration of large doses of morphine should be avoided in chronic renal patients.[140] The adverse effects of opioid analgesics include respiratory depression, hypotension, and mental abtundation. Prolonged narcosis following administration of morphine, dihydrocodeine, and codeine in patients with renal failure has been reported.[135]

In the normal kidney, a combination of alfentanil and midazolam anesthesia has no effect on creatinine clearance, osmolar clearance, plasma renin activity and plasma aldosterone concentration, but can increase ADH and reduce free water clearance and urine output.[141] Midazolam, a short acting water-soluble benzodiazepam, is hydroxylized in the liver to inactive metabolites and has minimal renal elimination.

Clearance and elimination half-life of a single dose of midazolam in end stage renal disease (ESRD) is similar to normal volunteers.[142] In ESRD, the half-life of diazepam increases while its single dose clearance decreases.[143] In uremic patients, combination of available free drugs and increased permeability through the blood-brain barrier, require that hypnotics and narcotics be used sparingly.

Epidural and Spinal Anesthesia

The renal effect of epidural and spinal anesthesia depends upon intravascular volume and preanesthesia administration of intravenous fluid. In general, spinal or epidural anesthesia does not have a significant effect on RBF and GFR in humans.[144] Epidural anesthesia does not improve renal function nor does it affect the outcome of ischemic insult.[145-146]

Hypothermia

A reduction in body temperature produces a parallel reduction in renal function. At 27°C there is 32% reduction in RBF and 69% reduction in GFR. However, as a result of central effect of hypothermia on ADH, tubular reabsorption of water is reduced to a proportionally greater degree so that urine output is actually increased. Likewise the clearance of the substances normally reabsorbed by the tubules, such as water, sodium and chloride, is increased.[147]

Positive Pressure Ventilation

Positive pressure ventilation reduces GFR, RBF, and urine output. Salem reports that in patients on ventilator CPPV at +10 cm H_2O urine flow is reduced from about 30 ml/hour to 10 ml/hour while negative pressure breathing (−10 cm H_2O) increases urine flow to 50 ml/hr.[148-149]

Muscle Relaxants and Renal Physiopathology

Succinylcholine

Because ultrashort acting nondepolarizing muscle relaxants are unavailable, succinylcholine is the drug of choice for rapid sequence induction and tracheal intubation. In patients with ESRD and uremia, serum cholinestrase level is about 45 percent of normal value because of increased plasma volume and impaired hepatic synthesis of serum cholinestrase.[150] However, this decrease in pseudocholinesterase activity does not prolong the action of succinylcholine.

Following administration of 1 mg/kg of succinylcholine, serum potassium increases by 0.2 to 0.5 mEqu/lit/min. in normal subjects and in patients with renal failure.[151-152] A second dose of succinylcholine in patients with ESRD has been reported to cause a massive increase in serum potassium levels leading to cardiac arrhythmia, ventricular tachycardia, and cardiac arrest.[152-155] Hypocalcemia, hyponatremia, hypermagnesemia, and acidosis can prolong the action of both depolarizing and nondepolarizing muscle relaxants.

D-tubocurarine

Even though ESRD patients are not sensitive to d-tubocurarine its elimination half-life is increased in this group of patients. Therefore, the duration of action of repeated dose of d-tubocurarine is progressively prolonged in patients with renal insufficiency. Nonetheless, d-tubocurarine is an undesirable agent for patients with ESRD. Because of its potential to cause marked hypotension from histamine release and ganglionic blocking effect.[156]

Pancuronium

Pancuronium is deacetylated at either the 3 position or the 17 position or both, to give metabolites. These metabolites not only have neuromuscular blocking activity but also contribute to the elimination of pancuronium. Elimination half-life of pancuronium is increased in patients with renal disease. Repeated or high doses of pancuronium in patients with ESRD can cause prolonged neuromuscular blockade. In addition, as a result of its vagolitic and sympathomimetic effect pancuronium may cause tachycardia. Therefore, the use of pancuronium in combination with isoflurane in patients with ESRD and who are suffering from coronary artery disease is not desirable.[157]

Vecuronium

Although pancuronium and vecuronium have the same onset of action, the duration of action of vecuronium is shorter. Vecuronium is primarily eliminated by the bile with only 10 to 25 percent excreted by the kidney. Because of this rapid hepatic uptake and biliary excretion, vecuronium has faster clearance and shorter elimination of half-life than pancuronium in patients with and without ESRD.[158-160] A single dose of vecuronium used during kidney transplant did not have significant increase in onset, duration of action, and recovery. However, elimination half-life of vecuronium in patients with ESDR was reported to have increased 32 percent as compared to a 500 percent increase with pancuronium.[158-161] Because vecuronium has minimal effect on hemodynamic parameters, it is an ideal muscle relaxant in patients with renal insufficiency. With intraoperative neuromuscular blockade monitoring, it should be easily reversible.

Atracurium

Both spontaneous degradation by Hofmann elimination[162] and ester hydrolysis[163] have been reported to play a major role in the elimination and excretion of atracurium. Multiple doses of atracurium in patients with ESRD has no apparent cumulative effect. Hepatorenal failure does not prolong its plasma elimination half-life.[164-165] However, a high dose of atracurium produces a significant histamine release, leading to hypotension, and tachycardia.[166-167] The metabolic breakdown product of atracurium, laudanosine, can cross the blood-brain barrier, thereby creating the possibility of seizure following repeated doses or prolonged infusion of atracurium.[168-169] However, massive production of laudanosine following atracurium is unlikely.[170-171]

Recuronium Bromide (ORG 9426)

Recuronium bromide is a new nondepolarizing monoquaternary steroid neuromuscular drug with a rapid onset and an intermediate duration of action. This drug produces good to excellent conditions for tracheal intubation within 60–90 seconds. Recuronium bromide is five to six times less potent than vecuronium and has minimal adverse effects on cardiovascular system. Its total plasma clearance and volume of the central compartment is similar in patients with normal kidneys as well as in renal transplant patients. However, its volume of distribution is greater and elimination half life is longer in patients with renal failure. Thus renal failure alter the distribution but not the clearance of recuronium.[172,173]

Doxacurium

Doxacurium is a potent long-acting benzylisoquirolinium nondepolarizing neuromuscular blocking agent, primarily excreted by the kidney. Therefore, the clearance of doxacuronium in patients with renal dysfunction is slower and its duration of action is longer than normal patients.[174]

Pipecurium Bromide (Arduran)

Pipecurium bromide is a long-acting nondepolarizing neuromuscular blocking drug; with a structure similar to pancuronium but with no cardiovascular effects. Due to the unpredictable response and possibility of prolonged blockade, pipecurium is less suitable for use in patients with renal failure than vecuronium and atracurium.[175]

Reversal Agents

Edrophonium, neostigmine, and pyridostigmine all are eliminated by renal excretion. As a result, the half-lives of these drugs in patients with renal disease are prolonged.

RENAL PATHOLOGY

Occasionally the anesthesiologist is involved in the anesthetic and medical management of patients suffering from varying degrees of preexisting renal insufficiencies. Some critically ill patients will develop renal failure in the operating room or during the postoperative period. Certain patients will develop renal insufficiency as a result of the administration of anesthetic agents, nephrotoxic antibiotic therapy, use of dye contrast for radiologic procedures, trauma, hemorrhage, and major surgical procedures such as abdominal aneurysm, organ transplants, and open heart surgery.[119,120,176] A detailed description of renal pathology is beyond the scope of this text. However, because the anesthesiologist should be familiar with preoperative, intraoperative, and postoperative management of these patients, the clinical and laboratory signs and common causes of acute and chronic renal failure are discussed below.

Acute Renal Failure (ARF)

The causes of ARF are categorized as pre-renal (renal hypotension), intrinsic (renal medical disease), and postrenal (urinary obstruction).[176-179] The most common cause of ARF is summarized in Table 23–3. As a result of a rich blood supply and medullary hypertonicity, kidneys can be exposed to high concentrations of toxic substances leading to acute or chronic renal failure. The degree of renal damage will depend on the concentration and protein bonding of toxin and the duration of exposure.[177] If blood supply to the kidney is interrupted for more than 30 to 60 minutes, ischemic hypoxia will injure pars recat and proximal tubules, resulting in irreversible cell damage and ARF. In the human, the medullary thick ascending limb of the loop of Henle (mTAL) is very vulnerable to ischemia because of high oxygen demand as a result of active reabsorption of sodium and chloride. Because of an increasing number of patients undergoing advanced cardiovascular and abdominal surgeries, the chance of iatrogenic causes of ARF has increased.[178]

Clinical symptoms of ARF can be manifested by oliguria, annuria, or polyurea. The mortality rate of ARF is very high, reaching 60 to 90 percent in oliguric and 40 to 50 percent in nonoliguric patients.[176]

An anesthetic can directly cause toxic renal damage or precipitate renal damage induced by other drugs or toxins. Methoxyflurane causes renal toxicity as a result of its transformation to inorganic fluoride ion *in situ*. Clinical symptoms of renal damage induced with methoxyflurane are: polyuria (unresponsive to ADH administration and fluid deprivation), marked weight loss, hypernatremia, serum hyperosmolality, increased BUN and serum creatinine, increased serum uric acid, decreased in uric acid clearance, and delayed return of preoperative concentrating ability. The inability of the kidney to concentrate urine may be related to F^- induced intrarenal vasodilation and interference with the countercurrent mechanism. Alternatively, F^- induced inhibition of adenylate cyclase activity necessary for physiologic function of ADH on distal convoluted tubules may be responsible for polyuria. Serum F concentrations that exceed 50 $\mu M/l$ have been shown to cause renal toxicity.[123] Increased urinary oxalic acid excretion and serum inorganic fluoride concentration and the presence of oxalic acid crystals in renal biopsy are laboratory characteristics of methoxyflurane nephrotoxicity.[119]

Table 23–3. Representative Causes of Acute Renal Failure

I. Prerenal
  Hypotension (e.g., trauma, myocardial infarction, septicemia)
  Hemorrhage, external or internal (e,.g., obstetric, traumatic, surgical)
  Contraction of body fluid volumes, especially extracellular volume (e.g., severe gastronteritis, "third space" effect)
  Major surgical procedures (e.g., operations on the heart, biliary tract, and major vessels)

II. Renal Initial damage to tubular epithelium
  Ischemia
  Prerenal causes if sufficiently severe and prolonged
  Trauma ("crush syndrome")
  Burns
  Obstetric disorders
  Transfusion reactions
  Sepsis
  Thrombosis or embolization of major renal vessels
  Toxins
  Heavy metals (e.g., mercuric chloride)
  Organic solvents (e.g., carbon tetrachloride, methanol)
  Drugs (e.g., methoxyflurane, cytolytic agents, diphenylhydantoin, gentamicin, amphotericin)
  Pesticides (e.g., chlorinated hydrocarbons)
  Others (e.g., uric acid, mushrooms, snake bites, radiographic contrast agents, non-traumatic rhabdomyolysis)

  Initial damage to glomeruli and small renal vessels
  Acute glomerulonephritides
  Polyarteritis nodosa
  Lupus erythematous
  Hemolytic-uremic syndrome
  Goodpasture's syndrome
  Serum sickness
  Malignant hypertension

III. Postrenal
  Lower urinary tract obstruction (e.g., benign or malignant hypertrophy of the prostate)
  Upper urinary tract obstruction (e.g., uterine tumor pressing on both ureters, renal stone in the ureter of a single kidney)

Enflurane and sevoflurane can also release small amounts of fluoride ion and potentially cause renal damage in the presence of precipitating factors and in patients with preexisting renal disease.

Diabetic Nephropathy

Diabetic nephropathy accounts for 25 percent of end-stage renal disease. Clinically, diabetic nephropathy has three manifestations: persistence proteinuria, arterial hypertension and falling GFR. Diabetic patients also can have associated complications such as retinopathy, peripheral neuropathy, autonomic neuropathy, neurogenic bladder, coronary artery disease, cerebrovascular disease and peripheral artery disease. Despite insulin therapy, diabetes remains a devastating disease in over five million people in the United States. Many of these patients will have various surgeries including vascular procedures. During surgery, they may develop hypotension and low renal perfusion, and also receive nephrotoxic aminoglycoside antibiotics or dye contrast for angiography, all which may precipitate or worsen renal insufficiency.[29] Diabetic patients with end-stage renal failure have been routinely accepted for kidney transplantation since 1968.

Nephrotic Syndrome

Clinical signs of the nephrotic syndrome are increased urinary excretion of albumin and other proteins of similar size, hypoproteinemia, hyperlipidemia and edema formation.[179] These patients have poor tolerance to blood loss and a high tendency to hypotension and hemodynamic instability. Disturbed acid-base, anemia, increased abdominal pressure from ascites, and compromised oxygenation from generalized edema are commonly seen in these patients. Medical and anesthetic management of these patients require delicate fluid administration and hemodynamic and acid-base balance monitoring.[180]

Glomerulonephritis

In this disease, renal plasma flow, GFR, and clearance values are all depressed, and oliguria, fever, and sepsis may be present. As a result of glomerular lesion, there is an excessive leakage of protein. Gross hematuria occurs and leukocytes, casts and desquamated epithelium appears. Consequently, this group of patients suffers from anemia, low plasma protein, azotemia, metabolic acidosis and hypertension. A rise in serum acid phosphate is frequently accompanied by a fall in calcium and this may be sufficient to produce tetany. Serum potassium may also fall.

Essential Hypertension

This disease is basically renal in origin and is characterized by endarteritis and arteriolar necrosis and reduced RBF. Chronically diminished renal circulation may further increase plasma renin activity, leading to an increase in systemic arterial pressure and a permanent impairment of renal function and nephrosclerosis.[181] In addition, these patients may have anemia, myocardial hypertrophy and

heart failure. The primary cause of the inadequate red cell production in chronic renal failure and uremic subjects has been attributed to impaired production of erythropoietin. Many patients are on antihypertensive therapy, and care must be taken to avoid profound hypotension or marked fluctuation in blood pressure.

Pyelonephritis

This and other suppurative diseases of the kidney including pyelitis and hydronephrosis are often accompanied by signs of sepsis with fever and leukocytosis.

EVALUATION OF RENAL FUNCTION

Urine Output

Measurement of urine output during perioperative and postoperative periods provides a good estimate of the adequacy of renal perfusion. However, intraoperative urine output is not an accurate predictor of postoperative outcome.[174] The most common cause of low urine output in the operating room is mechanical obstruction of the foley catheter. Urine volume can also be pathologically reduced from dehydration, severe burn, low blood volume, hypotension, trauma, septic shock, intravascular hemolysis, myoglobinurea, obstruction of urinary tract, drug induced renal vasoconstriction, onset of acute renal failure, or preexisting chronic renal failure.

Urine Analysis

Clinically, urine is analyzed for clarity, pH, specific gravity, osmolarity, blood cells, concentrations of electrolytes, presence of glucose or protein. Urine analysis is a good guide for anesthetic and medical management of patients suffering from preexisting kidney disease, diabetes, and ARF. For example, while low urinary concentrations of sodium (<10 to 20 mEq/L) and high urinary osmolarity (>450 mOsmol/L) are possible indications of hypovolemia, high sodium excretion (40 mEq/L) and low urinary osmolarity (<300 mOsmol/L) may suggest tubular lesion. While the presence of protein in urine indicates renal parenchymal disease, glucosuria without hyperglycemia indicates proximal tubular damage. Urine pH and microscopic evaluation of urinary sediment can also be used as diagnostic and treatment tools during management of patients suffering from kidney disease.

GFR

Precise measurements of GFR can be determined with standard techniques described previously. Although serum levels of creatinine and BUN are not abnormal until 70% of renal function is lost, traditionally these substances have been used to estimate GFR under the following equation:

$$\text{GFR} = \frac{(140 - \text{Age}) \times \text{Body Weight (kg)}}{72 \times \text{Serum Creatinine in mg\%}}$$

For women, the result is multiplied by 0.85. If GFR ceased completely, serum concentration of creatinine could increase 1 to 3/dl/day and BUN could rise as high as 10–20 mg/dl/day. Clinically, the ratio of BUN/serum creatinine can provide useful information for estimation of renal function. The normal value for this ratio is in the order of 10:1. A low renal tubular flow rate increases urea reabsorption but has no effect on creatinine elimination. As a result, ratio of BUN/serum creatinine increases above 10:1. Increased BUN/serum creatinine ratio can be seen in patients with volume depletion, heart failure, nephrotic syndrome, cirrhosis, increased protein catabolism, and obstration of the urinary tract.

Renal Blood Flow

As explained earlier, RBF can be measured by PAH clearance, and by magnetic or ultrasound Doppler techniques, washout of inert gas, and radioactive microspheres.

Renal Plasma Flow (RPF)

RPF is a function of the urinary excretion rate of the substance in question and arteriovenous concentration difference. If a substance is excreted in one passage through the kidney, then renal vein concentration of that substance will be near zero. Therefore, the RPF multiplied by the plasma concentration will equal urine volume times urine concentration. Diodrast and p-amino hippuric acid are such substances and can be used to measure RPF. These substances are in part filtered, but chiefly secreted by tubules. It must be appreciated that clearance tests are in part dependent on RPF. Over 87% of PAH at low plasma concentration is cleared in passage by filtration and excretion. As a result, RPF is commonly measured by PAH clearance and RBF is calculated from:

$$RBF = \frac{RPF}{1\text{-Hematocrit}}$$

The PSP test or phenolsulfonphthalein is a commonly used test to assess renal plasma flow and tubular secretory function. This dye is primarily secreted by the tubules and about 94% is removed in one passage. Since 80% of this substance is bound to protein, only about 5% is filtered. As the excretion of the dye is affected both by RBF and tubular secretion, a reduction may indicate a combined impairment.

PSP clearance, particularly the fractional 15 minute clearance, bears some relationship with GFR and urea clearance. It has been found that excellent PSP clearance parallels excellent urea clearance. However, a poor PSP test cannot be related necessarily to GFR. Nonetheless, PSP test indicates renal tubular function and a depressed urea clearance is always associated with a depressed PSP test (Table 23–4).

Proximal Tubular Function

Proximal tubular function is twofold: One is reabsorption of glucose and second is its secretory ability. Complete reabsorption of glucose takes place in this segment when the plasma glucose level is within normal limits or the capacity of the tubular cells to reabsorb is not ex-

Table 23–4. Standard Tests of Renal Function

Modality	Quantitative Test	Semiquantitative Test
Renal blood flow	p-Aminohippurate clearance	(Fractional PSP excretion)
Glomerular filtration	Inulin clearance	Urea clearance (and blood urea)
Tubular reabsorptive capacity	Urine concentration test	Urine concentration test
Tubular excretory capacity	p-Aminohippurate excretion	(Fractional PSP excretion)

ceeded. When the plasma glucose level reaches 280 mg percent, the maximal reabsorptive capacity is reached. However, glucose begins to appear in the urine when tubules reach only three-fourths of their reabsorptive capacity and glucosuria occurs at a plasma level of 180–220 mg, percent. In absolute amounts the normal kidney can reabsorb 350 to 400 mg of glucose per minute.

The capacity of glucose absorption may be used as an indicator of proximal tubular function. Application of these data provide valuable detailed information but is not practical in clinical work. Because diodrast and p-amino hippurate are completely secreted by proximal tubules, these agents, even at lower plasma levels, can be used to measure their maximal secretory capacity. At certain levels the capacity to secrete is reached and some material remains in the venous blood. The maximal tubular rate for diodrast is 42 to 52 mg per minute and for PAH the capacity ranges from 60–80 mg per minute.

Distal Tubular Function and Urinary Concentration Ability

The function of the distal tubule is to reabsorb water. This part of the nephron can be assessed by a urine concentration test. After passage through the proximal tubule the glomerular filtrate has a specific gravity of 1.010. With water *deprivation*, active reabsorption occurs within 6 hours and specific gravity may rise to 1.028 to 1.034. Values below 1.027 are suspicious and if below 1.020, there may be impaired function of the distal segment. In advanced renal hypertensive disease, the concentrating capacity is lost and specific gravity becomes fixed at 1.010. The concentrating capacity of the kidney can be determined rapidly by injecting 5–10 units of vasopressin intramuscularly, and measuring the specific gravity of the urine voided 1–2 hours later. Osmolality may also be determined. A summary of standard renal function tests are shown in Table 23-4.

MEDICAL MANAGEMENT OF RENAL FAILURE

Due to limitations in venous access, the presence of hemodialysis arteriovenous shunt and the risks of infection, the management of chronic or acute renal failure should be conservative. However, in some occasions such as coronary artery disease, congestive heart failure, volume overload, uremic pericarditis and negative inotropism

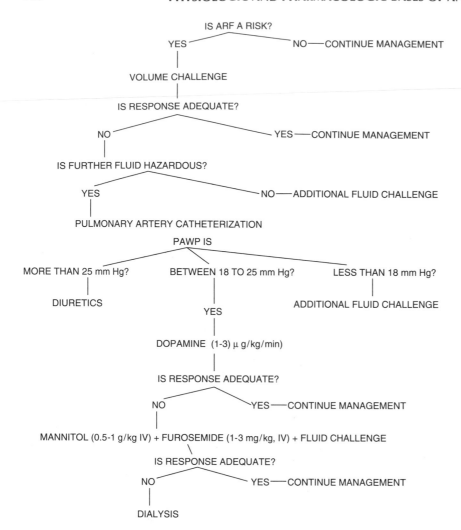

Fig 23–10. A Suggested Algorithm and Guideline for Treatment of Oliguria.

from acidosis, hyperkalemia and hypermagnesemia may necessitate invasive hemodynamic monitoring such as measurement of central venous pressure, pulmonary capillary wedge pressure and direct arterial pressure. Although loop diuretics may help to prevent ARF, their use for treatment of ARF might be counterproductive. The osmotic diuretic monitol is the treatment of choice due to its favorable effect of renal microcirculation. As explained earlier, activation of DA_1 receptors with dopamine at very low doses (1 to 3 μg/kg/min) reduces renal vascular resistance which leads to an increase in RBF, GFR, and sodium excretion. Activation of DA_2 receptors also decrease intrarenal norepinephrine release leading to improved RBF. Since the beneficial effect of dopamine can be blocked with cyclooxygenase inhibitor (indomethacin) which reduces prostaglandin synthesis, dopamine's vasodilation effect is possibly mediated through its modification of prostaglandins.[181] Therefore, dopamine is a useful drug for treatment of ARF. In some patients, an inotropic drug such as digitalis might be used to improve myocardial performance and urine output.

Although most patients suffering from ARF and chronic renal failure can be managed by conservative methods, some patients will need peritoneal dialysis or hemodialysis. In oligoric patients prior to or following surgery or

trauma, maintaining solute and water balance becomes difficult. In such patients, production of ketoacids and release of the K^+ and water from the cells will lead to a severe alteration in acid-base balance and electrolytes. Conservative treatment will not prevent these life threatening conditions.

Briefly, dialysis is indicated if one of the following conditions are met: 1) uncontrollable hyperkalemia; 2) high serum creatinine concentration of 10–13 mg/100 ml; 3) severe uremia with clinical signs of nausea, vomiting and neuromuscular irritability; 4) severe ascites; and 5) acute poisoning. Patients on dialysis have decreased cardiac output and hypovolemia which can cause postural hypotension and associated symptoms. Therefore, medical and anesthetic management of these patients require delicate hemodynamic monitoring.[182] A suggested algorithm for treatment of oliguria is shown in Figure 23–10.

REFERENCES

1. Laragh, J. H., and J. F. Sealey.: The Renin-Angiotensin-Aldosterone Hormonal System and Regulation of Sodium, Potassium, and Blood Pressure Homeostasis. In: Handbook of Physiology: Renal physiology. Washington, DC: Am Physiol Soc 1973, pp. 831–908.
2. Ehrlich, E. N. Electrolyte Metabolism: Adrenal Regulation

of Electrolyte and Water Metabolism. In: Endocrinology. edited by L.J. Degroot. W. B. Saunders, Philadelphia: 1989, pp. 1582-1597.

3. De Wardner, H. E. The Control of Sodium Excretion. In: Handbook of Physiology. Renal physiology. Washington DC: Am Physiol Soc 1973, pp. 677-720.

4. Sealy, J. E.: Plasma Renin Activity and Plasma Prorenin Assays. Clinical Chem., *37*, 1811-1819, 1991.

5. Laragh, J. H., and Sealy, J. H.: Abnormal Sodium Metabolism and Plasma Renin Activity (Renal Renin Secretion) and the Vasoconstriction Volume Hypothesis: Implications for Pathogenesis and Treatment of Hypertension and its Vascular Consequences (Heart Attack, Stroke). Clinical Chem., *37*, 1820-1827, 1991.

6. Biglieri, E. G., and Kater, C. E.: Steroid Characteristics of Mineralocorticoid Adrenocortical Hypertension. Clinical Chem., *37*, 1843-1848, 1991.

7. Carey, R. M., and Sen, S.: Recent Progress in the Control of Aldosterone Secretion. Recent Progress in Hormone Research, *42*, 251-296, 1986.

8. Gavras, H.: Role of Vasopressin in Clinical Hypertension and Congestive Cardiac Failure: Interaction With Sympathetic Nervous System. Clinical Chem., *37*, 1828-1830, 1991.

9. Needleman, P., Adams, S. P., Cole, B. R., Currie, M. G., Geller, D. M., Michener, M. L., Saper, C. B., Schwartz, D., and Standaert, D. G.: Atriopeptins as Cardiac Hormones. Hypertension *7*, 469-482, 1985.

10. Brenner, B. M., Ballermann, B. J., Gunning, M. E., and Zeidel M. I.: Diverse Biological Actions of Atrial Natriuretic Peptide. Physiological Rev., *70*, 665-699, 1990.

11. de Bold, A. J.: Atrial Natriuretic Factor: an Overview. Federation Proc., *45*, 2081-2085, 1986.

12. McGiff, J. C., Crowshaw, K., and Itskovitz, H. D.: Prostaglandins and Renal Function. Federation Proc., *33*, 39-47, 1974.

13. Lee, J. B., Patak, R. V., and Mookerjee, B. K.: Renal Prostaglandins and the Regulation of Blood Pressure and Sodium and Water Homeostasis. Am J Med., *60*, 798-816, 1976.

14. Laragh, J. H.: Atrial Natriuretic Hormone, the Renin-Aldosterone Axis, and Blood Pressure-Electrolyte Homeostasis. N Engl J Med., *313*, 1330-1340, 1985.

15. Maack, T., Marion, D M., Camargo, M. J. F., Kleinert, H. D., Laragh, J. H., Vaughan, E. D. Jr., and Atlas, S. A.: Effects of Auriculin (Atrial Natriuretic Factor) on Blood Pressure, Renal Function, and Renin-Aldosterone System in Dogs. Am J Med., *77*, 1069-1075, 1984.

16. de Bold, A. J. Atrial Natriuretic Factor: A Hormone Produced by the Heart. Science., *230*, 767-770, 1985.

17. Sonnenberg, H.: Mechanism of Release and Renal Tubular Action of Atrial Natriuretic Factor. Federation Proc., *45*, 2106-2110, 1986.

18. Needleman, P., and Greenwald, J. E.: Atriopeptin: A Cardiac Hormone Intimately Involved in Fluid, Electrolyte, and Blood-Pressure Homeostasis. N Eng J Med., *314*, 828-834, 1986.

19. Valtin, H.: *Renal Function: Mechanisms Preserving Fluid and Solute Balance in Health.* Boston, Little Brown & Co., 1983.

20. Fletcher, T. F., Bradley, W. E.: Neuroanatomy of the bladder and urethra. J. Urol. *119*, 152-160, 1978.

21. Clemente, C. D. (editor): The Urogenital System. In *Gray's Anatomy of the Human Body, 30th Ed.* Philadelphia, Lea & Febiger, 1935.

22. Kluck, P.: The autonomic innervation of the human urinary bladder, bladder neck, and urethra: a histochemical study. Anat. Rec. *199*, 439-447.

23. Koushanpour, E., and Kritz, W.: *Renal Physiology: Principles, Structure and Function.* Second Edition. New York, Springer Verlag, 1986.

24. Brody, M. J., and Kadowitz, P. J.: Prostaglandins and Modulators of the Autonomic Nervous System. Federation. Proc., *33*, 48, 1974.

25. Behnia, R., Siqueira, E. B., and Brunner, E. A.: Sodium Nitroprusside-Induced Hypotension: Effect on Renal Function. Anesth Analg., *57*, 521, 1978.

26. Behnia, R., Martin, A., Koushanpour, and E., Brunner, E. A.: Trimethaphan-Induced Hypotension: Effect on Renal Function. Can Anaesth Soc J., *29*, 581-586, 1982.

27. Behnia, R., Koushanpour, E., Goldstick, T. K., Linde, H. W., and Osborn, R.: Renal Tissue Oxygenation Following Induced Hypotension in Dogs. Br J Anaesth., *56*, 1037-1043, 1984.

28. Behnia, R. Deliberate Hypotension. In Dripps, R. D., Eckenhoff, J. E., Vandam, L. D., ed. *Introduction to Anesthesia. The Principle of Safe Practice.* Philadelphia, W.B. Saunders, 1988, pp. 380-387.

29. Behnia, R.: Arterial Hypotension During Anesthesia. In Dripps, R. D., Eckenhoff, J. E., Vandam, L. D., ed. *Introduction to Anesthesia. The Principle of Safe Practice.* Philadelphia, W.B. Saunders, 1988, pp. 389-402.

30. Muller, J., and Barajas, L.: Electron Microscopic and Histochemical Evidence for a Tubular Innervation in Renal Cortex of Monkey. J Ultrastruct Res., *41*, 533-549, 1972.

31. Slick, G. L., Aguilera, A. J., Zambraski, E. J., DiBona, G. F., and Kaloyanides, G. J.: Renal Neuroadrenergic Transmission. Am J Physiol., *229*, 60-65, 1975.

32. Struyker-Boudier, H. A. J., Janssen, B. J. A., and Smith, J. F. M.: Adrenoceptors in the Kidney: Localization and Pharmacology. Clin Exp Hypertens., *A9 (Suppl. 1)*, 135-150, 1987.

33. Valtin, H.: *Renal Function: Mechanisms Preserving Fluid and Solute Balance in Health.* Second Edition. Boston, Little Brown & Co, 1983, pp. 106-108.

34. Haywood, J. R., Shaffer, R. A., Fastenow, C., Fink, G. D., and Brody, M. J.: Regional Blood Flow Measurement with Pulsed Doppler Flowmeter in Conscious Rat. Am J Physiol., *241* (Heart Circ. Physiol. 10), H273-H278, 1981.

35. Solomon, A., Wiencek, J. G., Feinstein, S. B., et al.: Assessment of Renal Blood Flow with Contrast Ultrasonography. Anesth. Analg., *76*, 964, 1993.

36. Koushanpour, E., and Behnia, R.: Partition of Carotid Baroreceptor Response in Two-Kidney Renal Hypertensive Dogs. Am. J. Physiol., *253* (22), R568, 1987.

37. Smith, H. W.: Measurement of Filtration Rate. *The Kidney: Structure and Function in Health and Disease.* New York, Oxford University Press, 1951, pp 39-62.

38. Mulhern, J. G., and Perrone, R. D.: Accurate Measurement of Glomerular Filtration Rate. In Andreucci VE, Fine LG, ed. *International Yearbook of Nephrology 1991.* Boston, Kluwer Academic Publishers, 1991, pp 277-290.

39. Koushanpour, E., Kritz, W.: *Renal Physiology, 2nd Ed.* New York, Springer-Verlag, 1986.

40. Cogan, M. G.: *Fluid and Electrolytes: Physiology and Pathophysiology.* Norwalk, Appleton & Lang, 1991.

41. Standaert, D. G., Cechetto, D. F., Needleman, P., and Saper, C. B.: Inhibition of the Firing of Vasopressin Neurons by Atriopeptin. Nature Lond., *329*, 151-153, 1987.

42. Maack, T., Atlas, S. A., Camargo, M. J. F., and Cogan, M. G.: Renal Hemodynamic and Natriuretic Effects of Atrial Natriuretic Factor. Federation Proc., *45*, 2128-2132, 1986.

43. deBold, A. J.: Atrial natriuertic factor: an overview. Fed. Proc. *45*, 2081-2085, 1986.

44. Ackermann, U.: Cardiovascular Effects of Atrial Natriuretic

Extract in the Whole Animal. Federation Proc., *45,* 2111-2114, 1986.

45. Blaine, E. H., Seymour, A. A., Marsh, E. A., and Napier, M. A.: Effects of Atrial Natriuretic Factor on Renal Function and Cyclic GMP Production. Federation Proc., *45,* 2122-2127, 1986.

46. Atlas, S. A., Volpe, M., Sosa, R. E., Laragh, J. H., Camargo, M. J. F., and Maack, T.: Effect of Atrial Natriuretic Factor on Blood Pressure and Renin-Angiotensin-Aldosterone System. Federation Proc., *45,* 2115-2121, 1986.

47. Samson, W. K.: Atrial Natriuretic Factor Inhibits Dehydration and Hemorrhagic-Induced Vasopressin Release. Neuroendocrinology, *40,* 277-279, 1985.

48. Hara, H., Ogihara, T., Shima, J., Saito, H., Rakugi, H., Iinuma, K., Kumahara, Y., and Minamino, T.: Plasma Atrial Natriuretic Peptide Level as an Index for the Severity of Congestive Heart Failure. Clin Cardiol., *10,* 437-442, 1987.

49. Rascher, W., Tulassay, T., and Lang, R. E.: Atrial Natriuretic Peptide in Plasma of Volume-Overloaded Children with Chronic Renal Failure. Lancet, 303-305, 1985.

50. Akimoto, K., Miyata, A., Kangawa, K., Matsuo, H., Koga, Y., Matsuoka, Y., and Hayakawa, K.: Plasma and Right Auricular Concentrations of Atrial Natriuretic Polypeptide in Children with Cardiac Disease. Eur J Pediatric., *147,* 485-489, 1988.

51. Cody, R. J., Altas, S. A., Laragh, J. H., Kubo, S. K., Covit, A. B., and Ryman, K. S.: Atrial Natriuretic Factor in Normal Subjects and Heart Failure Patients. J Clin Invest., *78,* 1362-1374, 1986.

52. Bates, E. R., Shenker, Y., and Grekin, R. J.: The Relationship Between Plasma Levels of Immunoreactive Atrial Natriuretic Hormone and Hemodynamic Function in Man. Circulation, *73,* 1155-1161, 1986.

53. Pickering, T. G.: The Role of Laboratory Testing in the Diagnosis of Renovascular Hypertension. Clinical Chem., *37,* 1831-1837, 1991.

54. Mary, E. E., and Goodfriend, T. L.: Inhibition of Aldosterone Synthesis by Atrial Natriuretic Factor. Federation Proc., *45,* 2376-2381, 1986.

55. Zakheim, R. M., Molteni, A., Mattioli, L., and Myung, P.: Plasma Angiotensin II Levels in Hypoxic and Hypovolemic Stress in Unanesthetized Rabbits. J Appl Physiol., *41,* 462-465, 1976.

56. Horky, K., Gutkowska, J., Garcia, R., Thibault, G., Genest, J., and Cantin, M.: Effect of Different Anesthetics on Immunoreactive Atrial Natriuretic Factor Concentrations in Rat Plasma. Biochem Biophys Res Comm., *129,* 651-657, 1985.

57. Haber, E.: Renin Inhibitors N Eng J Med, *298,* 1023, 1978.

58. Miller, E. D. Jr., Gianfagna, W., Ackerly, J. A., and et al.: Converting Enzyme Activity and Pressor Responses to Angiotensin I and II in the Rat Awake and During Anesthesia. Anesthesiology, *50,* 88, 1979.

59. Haber, E.: Renin and Vascular Homeostasis During Anesthesia. Anesthesiology, *50,* 83, 1979.

60. Michaels, E. K., Chin, S. K. B., Fowler, J., Jr., Behnia, R., Linde H. W., and Moss, J.: Hemodynamic and Adrenal Response to Shock Wave Energy. J Endourology, *5,* 345-50, 1991.

61. Hynynen, M., Tikkanen, I., Salmenpera, M., Heinonen, J., and Fyhrquist, F.: Plasma Natriuretic Peptide Concentrations During Induction of Anesthesia and Acute Volume Loading in Patients Undergoing Cardiac Surgery. J Cardiothoracic Anesth., *1,* 401-407, 1987.

62. Behnia, R., Moss, J., Graham, J. B., Linde, H. W., and Roizen, M. F.: Hemodynamic and Catecholamine Re-

sponses Associated with Extracorporeal Shock Wave Lithotripsy. J Clin Anesth., *2,* 158-162, 1990.

63. Hirose, M., Hashimoto, S., and Tanaka, Y.: Effect of the Head-Down Tilt Position During Lower Abdominal Surgery on Endocrine and Renal Function Response. Anesth Analg., *76,* 40, 1993.

64. Blake, D. W., Way, D., Trigg, L., Langton, D., and McGrath, B. P.: Cardiovascular Effects of Volatile Anesthesia in Rabbits: Influence of Chronic Heart Failure and Enalaprilat Treatment. Anesth Analg., *73,* 441-448, 1991.

65. Flezzani, P., McIntyre, R. W., Xuan, Y. T., Su, Y. F., Leslie, J. B., and Watkins, W. D.: Atrial Natriuretic Peptide Plasma Levels During Cardiac Surgery. J Cardiothoracic Anesth., *2,* 274-280, 1988.

66. Behnia, R., Shanks, C. A., Ovassapian, A., and Wilson, L. A.: Hemodynamic Response Associated with Lithotripsy. Anesth Analg., *66,* 354-6, 1987.

67. Kay, J. M., Keane, P. M., Suyama, K. L., and Gauthier, D.: Angiotensin Converting Enzyme Activity and Evolution of Pulmonary Vascular Disease in Rats with Monocrotaline Pulmonary Hypertension. Thorax, *37,* 88-96, 1982.

68. Keane, P. M., Kay, J. M., Suyama, K. L., Gauthier, D., and Andrew, K.: Lung Angiotensin Converting Enzyme Activity in Rats with Pulmonary Hypertension. Thorax, *37,* 198-204, 1982.

69. Mattioli, L., Zakheim, R. M., Mullis, K., and Molteni, A.: Angiotensin-I-Converting Enzyme Activity in Idiopathic Respiratory Distress Syndrome of the Newborn Infant and in the Experimental Alveolar Hypoxia in Mice. J Ped., *87* (1), 97-101, 1975.

70. Vidt, D. G., Bravo, E. L., Fouad, F. M.: Drug Therapy: Captoril. N Eng J Med., *306,* 214, 1982.

71. Atarashi, K., Mulrow, P. J., and Franco-Saenz, R.: Effect of Atrial Peptides on Aldosterone Production. J Clin Invest., *76,* 1807-1811, 1985.

72. Campbell, W. B., Currie, M. G., and Needleman, P.: Inhibition of Aldosterone Biosynthesis by Atriopeptins in Rat Adrenal Cells. Circ Res., *57,* 113-118, 1985.

73. Ledsome, J. R., Wilson, N., Courneya, C. A., and Rankin, A. J.: Release of Atrial Natriuretic Peptide by Atrial Distension. Can J Physiol Pharmacol., *63,* 739-742, 1985.

74. Ballermann, B. J., and Brenner, B. M.: Biologically Active Atrial Peptides. J Clin Invest., *76,* 2041-2048, 1985.

75. Ballermann, B. J., and Brenner, B. M.: Role of Atrial Peptides in Body Fluid Homeostasis: Circ Res., *58,* 619-630, 1986.

76. Salazar, F. J., Romero, C. J., Burnett, Jr., J. C., Schryver, S., and Granger, J. P.: Atrial Natriuretic Peptide Levels During Acute and Chronic Saline Loading in Conscious Dogs. Am J Physiol., *251* (Regulatory Integrative Comp Physiol 20), R499-R503, 1986.

77. Akimoto, K., Miyata, A., Hayakawa, K., Kangawa, K., and Matsuo, H.: Plasma and Atrial Level of Atrial Natriuretic Peptide (ANP) in Pulmonary Hypertensive Rats. Life Sci., *43,* 1125-35, 1988.

78. Huang, Chou-Long., Lewicki, J., Johnson, L. K., and Cogan, M. G.: Renal Mechanism of Action of Rat Atrial Natriuretic Factor. J Clin Invest., *75,* 769-773, 1985.

79. Veress, A. T., and Pearce, J. W.: Effect of Vagotomy on Renal Response to Blood Volume Expansion in the Rat. Can J Physiol Pharmacol., *50,* 463-466, 1972.

80. Takahashi, K., Katoh, T., and Badr, K.: Endothelin and Endothelium-Derived Relaxing Factor in the Control of Glomerular Filtration and Renal Blood Flow. In Andreucci VE, Fine LG, ed. *International Yearbook of Nephrology 1991.* Boston, Kluwer Academic Publishers, 1991, pp 3-19.

81. Yanagisawa, M., Kurihara, H., Kimura, S., Tombe, Y., Kobayashi, M., Mitsui, Y., Yazaki, Y., Goto, K., and Masaki, T.: A Novel Potent Vasoconstrictor Peptide Produced by Vascular Endothelial Cells. Nature (Lond.), *332*, 411–415, 1988.

82. de Nucci, G., Thomas, R., D'Orleans-Juste, P., Antunes, E., Walder, C., Warner, T. D., Vane, J. R.: Pressor Effects of Circulating Endothelin are Limited by its removal in the pulmonary circulation and by the releases of prostacycline and endothelium-derived relaxing factor. Proc Natl Acad Sci USA., *85*, 9797–9800, 1988.

83. Badr, K. F., Murray, J. J., Breyer, M. D., Takahashi, K., Inagami, T., Harris, R.: Mesangial Cell, Glomerular and Renal Vascular Responses to Endothelin in the Rat Kidney. J Clin Invest., *83*, 336–342, 1989.

84. Cernacek, P., and Stewart, D. J.: Immunoreactive Endothelin in Human Plasma: Marked Elevations in Patients in Cardiogenic Shock. Biochem Biophys Res Commun., *161*, 562–567, 1989.

85. Palmer, R. M. J., Ferrige A. G., and Moncada, S.: Nitric Oxide Release Accounts for the Biological Activity of Endothelium-Derived Relaxing Factor. Nature (London), *327*, 524–526, 1987.

86. Neumayer, H. H., Wagner, K., Groll, J., Schudrowitsch, L., Schultze, G., Molzahn, M.: Beneficial Effect of Long-Term Prostaglandin E2 Infusion on the Course of Postischemic Renal Failure. Renal Physiol. (Basel), *8*, 159, 1985.

87. Brezis, M., Rosen, S. N., Epstein, F. H.: The Pathophysiological Implications of Medullary Hypoxia. Am J Kid Dis., *13*, 253, 1989.

88. Terragno, N. A., Terragno, D. A., McGiff, J. C., Contribution of Prostaglandins to the Renal Circulation in Conscious, Anesthetized, and Laparotomized Dogs. Cir Res., *40*, 590, 1977.

89. Kimberly, R. P., Bowden, R. E., Keiser, H. R., and Plotz, P. H.: Reduction of Renal Function by Newer Nonsteroidal Anti-Inflammatory Drugs. Am J Med., *64*, 804, 1978.

90. Lapides, J.: Neuromuscular vesicule and Urethral Dysfunction. *Urology*. Third edition. M. F. Cambell and J. H. Harrison, ed. Philadelphia, W.B. Saunders, pp 1343–1378, 1970.

91. Brobeck, J. R., ed.: *Best & Taylor's Physiological Bases of Medical Practice*. Tenth edition. Baltimore, Williams & Wilkins, 1981.

92. Axelsson, K., Möllefors, K., Olsson, J. O., Lingardh, G., Widman, B.: Bladder Function in Spinal Anaesthesia. Acta Anaesthesiol. Scand., *29*, 315, 1985.

93. Reyes, A. J., Ed.: *Diuretics: Clinical Pharmacology and Use in Cardiovascular Medicine, Nephrology and Hepatology*. New York, Gustav Fischer, 1990.

94. Allison, N. L., Dubb, J. W., Ziemniak, J. A., Alexander, F., and Stote, R. M.: The Effect of Fenoldopam a Dopaminergic Agonist, on Renal Hemodynamics Clin Pharmacol Ther., *41*, 282–288, 1987.

95. Miller, E. D.: Renal Effects of Dopamine. Anesthesiology, *61*, 487, 1984.

96. Brater, D. C.: Use of Diuretics in Chronic Renal Insufficiency and Nephrotic Syndrome. Semin Nephrol., *8*, 333–341, 1988.

97. Voelke, J. R., Cartwright-Brown, D., Anderson, S., Leinfelder, J., Sica, D. A., Kokko, J. P., and Brater, D. C.: Comparison of Loop Diuretics in Patients with Chronic Renal Insufficiency: Mechanism of Difference in Response. Kidney Int., *32*, 572–578, 1987.

98. Sperry, R. J., Monk, C. R., Durieux, M. E., and Longnecker, D. E.: The Influence of Hemorrhage on Organ Perfusion During Deliberate Hypotension in Rat, *77*, Anesthesiology, 1171, 1992.

99. Zäll, S., Edén, E., Winsö, I., Volkmann, R., et al.: Controlled Hypotension with Adenosine or Sodium Nitroprusside During Cerebral Aneurysm Surgery: Effect on Renal Hemodynamics, Excretory Function, and Renin Release. Anesth. Analg., *71*, 631, 1990.

100. Swartz, S. L., Williams, G. H., Hollenberg, N. K., Moore, T. J., and Dluhy, R. G.: Converting Enzyme Inhibition in Essential Hypertension: The Hypotensive Response Does Not Reflect Only Reduced Angiotensin II Formation. Hypertension, *1*, 106–111, 1979.

101. Dzau, V. J.: Implications of local angiotensin production in cardiovascular physiology and pharmacology. Am J Cardiol., *59*, 59A–65A, 1987.

102. The Consensus Trial Study Group.: Effects of Enalapril on Mortality in Severe Congestive Heart Failure: (Consensus) Results of the Cooperative North Scandinavian Enalapril Survival Study. N Engl J Med., *316*, 1429–1435, 1987.

103. Packer, M., Lee, W. H., Medina, N., Yushak, M. Kessler, P. D.: Functional Renal Insufficiency During Long-Term Therapy with Captopril and Enalapril in Severe Chronic Heart Failure. Ann Intern Med., *106*, 346–354, 1987.

104. Keane, W. F., Anderson, S., Aurell, M., de Zeeun, D., Narins, R. G., Povar, G.: Angiotensin Converting Enzyme Inhibitors and Progressive Renal Insufficiency. Current Experience and Future Directions. Ann Intern Med., *111*, 503–516, 1989.

105. Merck Sharp & Dohme.: Vasotec (Brochure). Summary of Pharmacology. December, 1985.

106. Epstein, M.: Calcium Antagonists and the Kidney: Implications for Renal Protection. Am J Hypertens., *4*, 482S–486S, 1991.

107. Woolley, J. L., Barker, G. R., Jacobsen, W. K., Gingrich, G. A., et al.: Effect of Calcium Entry Blocker Verapamil on Renal Ischemia. Crit. Care. Med., *16*, 48, 1988.

108. Beaufils, M.: Alterations in Renal Hemodynamics During Chronic and Acute Beta-Blockade in Humans. Am J Hypertens., *2*, 233S–236S, 1989.

109. Churchill-Davidson, H. C., Wylie, W. D., Miles, B. E., and de Wardener, H. E.: The Effects of Adrenalin, Noradrenalin, and Methedrine on the Renal Circulation During Anesthesia. Lancet, *2*, 803, 1951.

110. Marson, F. G. W.: Effect of Noradrenalin on Urine and Blood Flow. Brit. J. Pharmacol., *11*, 431, 1956.

111. Mac Cann, R.: Renal Hemodynamic Response to Vasopressors. Texas State J. Med., *50*, 346, 1954.

112. Mills, L. C., Voudoukis, I. J., Moyer, J. H., and Heider, C.: Treatment of Shock with Sympathomimetic Drugs. Arch. Int. Med., *106*, 816, 1960.

113. Habif, D. V., Papper, E. M., Fitzpatrick, H. E., Lawrence, P., Smyth, McC. C., and Bradley, S. E.: The Renal and Hepatic Blood Flow, Glomerular Filtration Rate, and Urinary Output of Electrolytes During Cyclopropane, Ether and Thiopental Anesthesia Operation and Immediate Postoperative Period. Surgery, *30*, 241, 1951.

114. Waters, R. M., and Schmidt, E. R.: Cyclopropane Anesthesia. J.A.M.A., *103*, 975, 1934.

115. Burnett, C. H.: Comparison of Effects of Ether and Cyclopropane Anesthesia on Renal Function of Man. J. Pharmacol. & Exper. Therap., *96*, 380, 1949.

116. Adams, R. C. and Lundy, J. S.: Anesthesia in Cases of Poor Surgical Risk. Surg. Gynec. & Obst., *74*, 1011, 1942.

117. Orth, O. S., Slocum, H. C., Stutzman, J. W., and Meek, W. J.: Studies on Vinethene as an Anesthetic Agent. Anesthesiology, *1*, 246, 1940.

118. Walton, P. R.: Effect on Kidney Function of Ether, Ethylene, Amytal, and Avertin. J. Pharmacol. and Exper. Therap., *47*, 141, 1933.

119. Mazze, M. I., and Cousins, C. J.: Renal Toxicity of Anesthetics: With Specific Reference to the Nephrotoxicity of Methoxyflurane. Canad. Anaesth. Soc. J., *20*, 64, 1973.

120. Mazze, R. I., Schwartz, F. D., Slocum, H. C., and Barry, K.G.: Renal Function During Anesthesia and Surgery. Anesthesiology, *24*, 279, 1963.

121. Bastron, R. D., Perkins, F. M., Pyne, J. L.: Autoregulation of Renal Blood Flow During Halothane Anesthesia. Anesthesiology, *46*, 142, 1977.

122. Priano, L. L.: Effect of Halothane on Renal Hemodynamics During Normovolemia and Acute Hemorrhagic Hypovolemia. Anesthesiology, *63*, 357, 1985.

123. Cousins, M. J., Greenstein, L. R., Hill, B. A., Mazze, R. I.: Metabolism and Renal Effect of Enflurane in Man. Anesthesiology, *44*, 44, 1976.

124. Gelman, S., Fowler, K. C., and Smith, L. R.: Regional Blood Flow During Isoflurane and Halothane Anesthesia. Anesth. Analg., *63*, 557, 1984.

125. Hill, G. E., Lunn, J. K., Hodges, M. R., et al.: N₂O Modification of Halothane-Altered Renal Function in the Dog. Anesth. Analg., *56*, 690, 1977.

126. Crawford, M. W., Lerman, J., Saldivia, V., and Carmichael, F. J.: Hemodynamic and Organ Blood Flow Responses to Halothane and Sevoflurane Anesthesia During Spontaneous Ventilation. Anesth. Analg., *75*, 1000, 1992.

127. Kobayashi, Y., Ochiai, R., Takeda, J., Sekiguchi, H., and Fukushima, K.: Serum and Urinary Inorganic Fluoride Concentration After Prolonged Inhalation of Sevoflurane in Human. Anesth. Analg., *74*, 753, 1992.

128. Frink, E. J., Jr., Ghantous, H., Malan, T. P., Morgan, S., Fernando, J., Gandolfi, A. J., and Brown, B. R.: Plasma Inorganic Fluoride with Sevoflurane Anesthesia: Correlation with Indices of Hepatic and Renal Function. Anesth. Analg., *74*, 231, 1992.

129. Mazze, R. I.: The Safety of Sevoflurane in Human. Anesthesiology, *77*, 1062, 1992.

130. Egger, E. I. II., Johnson, B. H., Strum, D. P., Ferrell, L. D.: Studies of the Toxicity of I-653, Halothane, and Isothane in Enzyme-Induced, Hypoxic Rats. Anesth. Analg., *66*, 1227, 1987.

131. Jones, R. M., Koblin, D. D., Cashman, J. N., Egger, E. I., II., Johnson, B. H., and Damask, M. C.: Biotransformation and Hepatorenal Function in Volunteers After Exposure to Desflurane. Br. J. Anaesth., *64*, 482, 1990.

132. Jones, R. M.: Desflurane and Sevoflurane: Inhalation Anesthetics for This Decade?. Br. J. Anaesth., *65*, 527, 1990.

133. Priano, L. L.: Alteration of Renal Hemodynamic by Thiopental, Diazepam, and Ketamine in Conscious Dogs. Anesth. Analg., *61*, 853, 1982.

134. Hunter, J. M., Jones, R. S., and Utting, J. E.: Effect of Anesthesia with Nitrous Oxide in Oxygen and Fentanyl on Renal Function in the Artificially Ventilated Dogs. Br. J. Anaesth., *52*, 343, 1980.

135. Chan, G. L. C., and Matzke, G. R.: Effect of Renal Insufficiency on the Pharmacokinetics and Pharmacodynamics of Opioid Analgesics. Drug Intelligence and Clinical Pharmacy, *21*, 773, 1987.

136. Gelman, S.: *Anesthesia and Organ Transplantation.* Philadelphia, W.B. Saunders Co., 1987, pp. 61.

137. Bidwai, A. V., Stanley, T. H., Bloomer, H. A., Blatnick, R. A.: Effect of Anesthetic Doses of Morphine on Renal Function in Dog. Anesth. Analg., *54*, 357, 1975.

138. Brater, C.: Drug Use in Renal Disease. ADIS Press, Australia: 1982, pp. 4.

139. Paul, D., Standifer, K. M., Inturrisi, C. E., and Pasternak, G. W.: Pharmacological Characterization of Morphine-6β Glucuronide, a Very Potent Morphine Metabolite. J. Pharm. Exper. Therapeutics., *251*, 477, 1989.

140. Bennett, W. M., Aronoff, G. R., Morrison, G., et al.: Drug Prescribing in Renal Failure: Dosing Guidelines for Adults. Am. J. Kidney Dis. *3*, 155, 1983.

141. Brizio-Molteni, L., Behnia, R., Molteni, A., Jalali, N.: Do Midazolam and Alfantanyl Affect Renal Function? FSEB, A59, 1993.

142. Vinik, H. R., Reyes, J. G., Greenblatt, D. J., et al.: The Pharmacokinetics of Midazolam in Chronic Renal Failure Patients. Anesthesiology, *59*, 390, 1983.

143. Ochs, H. R., Greenblatt, D. J., Kaschell, H. J., et al.: Diazepam Kinetics in Patients with Renal Insufficiency or Hyperthyroidism. Br. J. Clin. Pharmacol., *12*, 829, 1981.

144. Kennedy, W. F., Jr., Sawyer, T. K., Gerbershagen, H. U., Gutler, R. E., Allen, G. D., and Bonica, J. J.: Systemic Cardiovascular and Renal Hemodynamic Alterations During Peridural Anesthesia in Normal Man. Anesthesiology, *31*, 414, 1969.

145. Gamulin, Z., Forster, A., Simonet, F., Aymon, E., and Favre, H.: Effects of Renal Sympathetic Blockade on Renal Hemodynamics in Patients Undergoing Major Aortic Abdominal Surgery. Anesthesiology, *65*, 688, 1986.

146. Baron, J.-F., Bertrand, M., Barre, et al.: Combined Epidural and General Anesthesia versus General Anesthesia for Abdominal Aortic Surgery. Anesthesiology, *75*, 611, 1991.

147. Moyer, J. H., Morris, G. C., and Debakey, M. E.: Renal Function Response to Hypothermia and Ischemia in Man and Dog. Physiology of Hypothermia. Publication 431 Nat. Acad. Sci. Nat. Res. Council Wash., 1956.

148. Drury, D. R., Henry, J. P., and Goodman, J.: The Effect of Continuous Pressure Breathing on Kidney Function. J. Clin. Investig., *26*, 945, 1947.

149. Salem M. R., Ginsberg, D., Rattenberg, C. G., and Holaday, D.A.: The Effect of Continuous Positive and Negative Pressure Breathing on the Urine formation. Fed. Proc., *23*, 362, 1964.

150. McArdle, B.: The Serum Cholinesterase in Jaundice and Diseases of the Liver. Q. J. Med., *33*, 107, 1940.

151. Miller, R. D., Way W. L., Hamilton, W. K., and Layzer, R. B.: Succinylcholine-Induced Hyperkalemia in Patients with Renal Failure?, Anesthesiology, *36*, 138, 1972.

152. Koide, M., and Waud, B. E.: Serum Potassium Concentrations after Succinylcholine in Patients with Renal Failure. Anesthesiology, *36*, 142, 1972.

153. Roth, F., and Wuthrich, H.: The Clinical Importance of Hyperkalemia Following Suxamethonium Administration. Br. J. Anaesth., *41*, 311, 1969.

154. Powell, J. N.: Suxamethonium-Induced Hyperkalemia in a Uremic Patient. Br. J. Anaesth., *42*, 806, 1970.

155. Walton, J. D., and Farman, J. V.: Suxamethonium Hyperkalaemia in Uraemic Neuropathy. Anesthesia, *28*, 666, 1973.

156. Miller, R. D., Matteo, R. S. Benet, R. Z., et al.: The Pharmacokinetics of d-tubocurarine in Man with and without Renal Failure J. Pharmacol. Exp. Ther., *202*, 1, 1977.

157. Miller, R. D., Stevens, W. C., and Way, W. L.: The Effect of Renal Failure and Hyperkalemia on the Duration of Pancuronium Neuromuscular Blockade in Man. Anesth. Analg., *52*, 661, 1973.

158. Fahey, M. R., Morris, R. B., Miller, R. D., et al.: The Pharmacokinetics of Org Nc 45 (Norcuron) in Patients With and Without Renal Failure. Br. J. Anaesth., *53*, 1049, 1981.

159. Meistalman, C., Lienhart, A., Leveque, C. et al.: Pharmacology of Vecuronium in Patients with End Stage Renal Failure. Anesthesiology, *59*, A293, 1983.

160. Bevan, D. R., Donati, F., Gyasi, H., and Williams, A.: Vecuronium in Renal Failure. Can. Anaesth. Soc. J., *31*, 491, 1984.

161. Lynam, D. P., Cronnelly, R., Castagnoli, K. P., Canfell, P.

C., et al.: The Pharmacodynamics and Pharmacokinetics of Vecuronium in Patients Anesthetized with Isoflurane with Normal Renal function or with Renal Failure. Anesthesiology, *69,* 227, 1988.

162. Stenlake, J. B., Waigh, R. D., Urwin, J., et al.: Atracurium: Conception and Inception. Br. J. Anaesth., *55,* 3S, 1983.

163. Nigrovic, V., Auen, M., and Wajskol, A.: Enzymatic Hydrolysis of Atracurium In Vivo. Anesthesiology, *62,* 606, 1985.

164. de Bros, F. M., Lai, A., Scott, R., et al.: Pharmacokinetics and Pharmacodynamics of Atracurium Under Isoflurane Anesthesia in Normal and Anephric Patients. Anesth. Analg., *64,* 207, 1985.

165. Hunter, J. M., Jones, R. S., and Utting, J. E.: Use of Atracurium in Patients with No Renal Function. Br. J. Anaesth., *54,* 1251, 1982.

166. Hunter, J. M., Jones, R. S., Utting, J. E.: Comparison of Vecuronium, Atracurium and Tubocurarine in Normal Patients and in Patients with No Renal Function. Br. J. Anaesth., *56,* 941, 1984.

167. Miller, R. D., Rupp, S. M., Fisher, D. M., et al.: Clinical Pharmacology of Vecuronium and Atracurium. Anesthesiology, *61,* 444, 1984.

168. Cato, A. E., Lineburg, C. G., Macklin, A. W.: Concerning Toxicity Testing of Atracurium. Anesthesiology, *62,* 94, 1985.

169. Fahey, M. R., Rupp, S. M., Fisher, D. M., et al.: The Pharmacokinetics and Pharmacodynamics of Atracurium in Patients With and Without Renal Failure. Anesthesiology, *61,* 699, 1984.

170. Ward, S., Boheimer, N., Weatherley, B. C., Simmonds, R. J., and Dopson, T. A.: Pharmacokinetics of Atracurium and its Metabolites in Patients with Normal Renal Function and in Patients in Renal Failure. Br. J. Anaesth., *59,* 697, 1987.

171. Ingram, M. D., Sclabassi, R. J., Stiller, R. L., et al.: Cardiovascular and Electroencephographic Effects of Laudanosine in "Nephrectomized" Cats. Anesth. Analg., *64,* 232, 1985.

172. Szenohradszky, J., Fisher, D. M., Segredo, V., Caldwell, J. E., et al.: Pharmacokinetics of Recuronium Bromide

(ORG9426) In Patients with normal Renal Function or Patients Undergoing Cadaver Renal Transplantation. Anesthesiology, *77,* 899, 1992.

173. Foldes, F. F., Nagashima, H., Nguyen, H. D., Schiller, W. S., et al: The Neuromuscular Effects of ORG9426 in Patients Receiving Balanced Anesthesia. Anesthesiology, *75,* 191, 1991.

174. Cook, R. D., Freeman, J. A., Lai, A. A., Robertson, K. A., et al.: Pharmacokinetics and Pharmacodynamics of Doxacurium in normal Patients and in Those with Hepatic or Renal Failure. Anesth. Analg., *72,* 145, 1991.

175. Caldwell, J. E., Canfell, P. C., Castagnoli, K. P., Lynam, D. P., et al.: The Influence of Renal Failure on the Pharmacokinetics and Duration of Action of Pipecurium Bromide in Patients Anesthetized with Halothane and Nitrous Oxide. Anesthesiology, *70,* 7, 1989.

176. Valtin, H. Renal Dysfunction: Mechanisms Involved in Fluid and Solute Imbalance. Boston, Little, Brown and Co., pp 227–256, 1979.

177. Murray, K. M., Pharm, D., and Keane W. R.: Review of Drug-Induced Acute Interstitial Nephritis. Pharmacotherapy, *12* (6), 462, 1992.

178. Mcnashe, P. I., Ross, S. A., and Gotlieb, J. E.: Acquired Renal Insufficiency in Critically Ill Patients. Critical. Care. Med., *16,* 1106, 1988.

179. Roxe, D. M.: Toxic Nephropathy from Diagnostic and Therapeutic Agents: Review and Commentary. Am. J. Med., *69,* 759, 1980.

180. Alpert, R. A., Roizen, M. F., Hamilton, W. K., Stoney, R. J., et al.: Intraoperative Urinary Output Does Not Predict Postoperative Renal Function in Patients Undergoing Abdominal Aortic Revascularization. Surgery, *95,* 707, 1984.

181. Yeyati, N. L., Altenberg, G. A., Rainoldi, F. A., and Greco, J.: Reversal by Indomethacin of Renal Effects of Dopamine in Subjects with Normal Function. Acta. Physiol. Pharmacol. Lestinoam., *36,* 127, 1986.

182. Myers, B. D., and Moran, M. S.: Hemodynamically Mediated Acute Renal Failure. New. Engl. J. Med., *314,* 97, 1986.

Chapter 24

ANESTHESIA FOR GENITOURINARY SURGERY

RAHIM BEHNIA

With advances in immunosuppressive and surgical techniques, kidney transplantations are increasing. With the increase in the elderly population, helped by preventive medicine, diet, and health care, more prostate and other radical surgeries are performed using newer and better techniques. To meet these new challenges, the anesthesiologist should have a working knowledge of anatomy, physiology, pharmacology, and the pathology of the urogenital system. The anesthesiologist must also be familiar with advanced sophisticated laboratory tests and monitoring devices for proper medical and anesthetic management of patients with both normal and diseased kidneys.

In this chapter, I discuss anesthetic management in (1) kidney transplants, (2) miscellaneous surgical procedures in patients with chronic renal failure, and (3) miscellaneous urogenital procedures.

KIDNEY TRANSPLANTATION

What follows is a brief discussion of anesthetic management of the living related donor, the cadaveric donor, and the kidney recipient. Gelman[1] discusses in detail anesthetic management in kidney transplant procedures.

Living Related Donor

In the preoperative visit, the living related donor is expected to be free of systemic disease. Preoperatively, the living related donor should be hydrated with 5% dextrose in 0.45% sodium chloride at the rate of 10 to 15 ml/kg. Routine monitoring parameters such as electrocardiogram (ECG), intermittent blood pressure, body temperature, oxygen saturation, and end-tidal CO_2 must be determined. In the preinduction area, patients should be sedated with fentanyl and midazolam or another sedative of the physician's choice. Anesthesia is generally induced with thiopental and nondepolarizing muscle relaxants and then maintained with isoflurane in oxygen and air and supplemented with fentanyl. When the patient has a difficult airway, the trachea should be intubated using fiberoptics when the patient is awake or asleep. Care should be given to prevent corneal abrasion and brachial plexus palsy. As kidney rest is raised, hemodynamic parameters should be closely monitored and hypotension treated with intravenous fluid and lightening of the anesthesia. Vasopressors should be avoided if at all possible. Before the ureter is cut, mannitol and furosemide are given. Before wound closure, pleural leaks must be

checked for possible pneumothorax. After extubation, bilateral breath sound is auscultated. When the patient emerges from anesthesia, a chest roentgenogram is performed to rule out pneumothorax.

Cadaveric Donor

Before surgery, the chart should be checked for proper consent forms and death certificate. Throughout surgery, anesthesia personnel should support the cadaveric donor until the aorta is cross clamped. The systemic arterial pressure and arterial PO_2 should be above 100 mm Hg, and urine output should be more than 100 ml/hr (the rule of 100s).[1] If crystalloid is insufficient to maintain blood pressure, volume expanders such as hetastarch or albumin may be used. Dopamine also can be used to support blood pressure and to increase urine output.

Transplant Recipient

Patients with end-stage renal disease (ESRD) suffer from gastrointestinal, neurologic, psychiatric, cardiovascular, pulmonary, hematologic, musculoskeletal, metabolic, and electrolyte disorders. During the preoperative visit, the anesthesiologist should search for signs of uremic neuropathy. Patients may experience nausea, vomiting, hiccup, and delayed gastric emptying time. Many dialysis patients are chronic carriers of hepatitis B surface antigen.

Some of these patients have abnormal autonomic nervous system function, decreased baroreceptor sensitivity, and reduced response to Valsalva's maneuver. Certain patients may become hypotensive from extracellular volume depletion, excessive antihypertensive medication, or anesthetic agents. In patients who develop hypertensive crises, the treatment of choice is direct vasodilators such as sodium nitroprusside (SNP) and nitroglycerin. Metabolism of SNP yields cyanide (CN) in presence of sulfhydril groups in erythrocytes and in other tissue. Approximately two thirds of the CN is converted enzymatically in presence of thiosulfate to thiocyanate by liver and tissue rhodnase, and thiocyanate is then excreted by the kidney. Because both CN and thiocyanate are toxic, administration of excess amounts of SNP in patients with ESRD can cause histotoxicity.[2] Intravenous esmolol can also be an effective treatment for hypertensive crises.

Patients with ESRD are anemic as a result of decreased erythropoietin production and iron and folic acid deficiency. In patients with ESRD, increased levels of 2,3-

diphosphoglycerate (2,3-DPG) are lower than in nonrenal anemic patients. However, the increased 2,3-DPG improves oxygen delivery to tissue and compensates for a decreased oxygen carrying capacity.

Twelve to 36 hours before renal transplantation, the patient is dialyzed to control blood pressure and potassium. All this time, laboratory facilities are essential for the rapid determination of electrolyte, glucose, blood gas, and hematocrit levels. In patients in whom peripheral venous access presents a problem, a triple-lumen catheter can be inserted for administration of fluid and drugs and for measurement of central venous pressure. The arteriovenous fistula should be protected intraoperatively, and the presence of bruit should be noted before and after surgery. A blood pressure cuff and an intravenous catheter should not be placed on any extremity with a functioning dialysis shunt. Throughout this time, routine monitoring parameters such as ECG, intermittent arterial blood pressure, pulse oxymeter, body temperature, and end-tidal CO_2 must be determined. Some anesthesiologists have advocated spinal or epidural anesthesia to avoid tracheal intubation and the risks associated with a full stomach and cardiac arrhythmias secondary to hyperkalemia. Because of the risks of epidural hematoma from heparin, uremic neuropathy, infection, and marked hypotension, however, many anesthesiologists prefer general anesthesia.

Before induction of anesthesia, patients should be oxygenated. Thiopental is a good choice of induction agent. In a study that compared kidney transplant patients with patients with normal kidney function, no difference was noted in the required thiopental dose, nor was a significant change in stroke volume and cardiac output seen during the first 5 minutes following induction of anesthesia.[3] In cases of delayed gastric emptying and full stomach following cricoid pressure, thiopental and succinylcholine should be used for rapid sequence induction and endotracheal intubation. In patients with minimal cardiac reserve, etomidate, 0.2 to 0.4 mg/kg, is a suitable alternative. Furthermore, fiberoptic intubation while the patient is awake may also be performed in patients with full stomachs and in those who have a difficult airway.

Although halothane and enflurane have been used for maintenance of anesthesia, isoflurane in oxygen and air is the preferred agent because isoflurane releases insignificant amounts of fluoride ion and causes minimal myocardial depression. Isoflurane may result in tachycardia if used with pancuronium or anticholinergic drugs, however. Intravenous narcotics such as fentanyl or alfentanil can be used to decrease heart rate, isoflurane concentration, and postoperative pain. Vecuronium and atracurium are the preferred muscle relaxants.[4,5] Neuromuscular function should be monitored to assess the degree of neuromuscular blockade. When large doses of atracurium are administered, histamine release, hypotension, and tachycardia can occur. Hence, frequent monitoring of hemodynamic parameters is necessary. Ventilation should be controlled to keep arterial PCO_2 within normal limits. The transplanted kidney is usually anastomosed to the right or left iliac fossa of the recipient patient. Before revascularization, the transplant patient should be adequately hy-

drated. The patient's hemodynamic status must be supported before vascular clamps are released. If necessary, packed cells are given to increase the hematocrit to 24 to 25%.[1,6]

If volume loading and lightening of general anesthesia were inadequate to keep systemic blood pressure, dopamine infusion (4 to 6 μg/kg/min) can be used to support blood pressure and to improve urine output.[7] After removal of vascular clamps, the transplanted kidney should turn from gray to pink. The patient's blood pressure then must be carefully monitored to avoid hypotension. Urine output must be replaced with half-normal saline in 5% dextrose. At the conclusion of surgery, the effect of the muscle relaxant is reversed, ventilatory parameters are evaluated, and the trachea is extubated. In patients with inadequate ventilation, an endotracheal tube remains to support ventilation. Some patients may develop severe hyperkalemia, which should be treated with diuretics, insulin, and glucose infusion, kayexalate, or dialysis.

Immunotherapy

Although different centers use various regimens for immunotherapy, most use Cyclosporin A concomitantly with other immunosuppressive agents such as azathioprine (Imuran), prednisone, OKT3, or Minnesota antilymphocyte globulin.

Cyclosporine

Cyclosporine is isolated from fungi and acts selectively on helper T lymphocytes. The initial daily dose of cyclosporine is 150 mg/m^2, which is adjusted to obtain true blood levels of 200 to 400 ng/ml. Cyclosporine is said to induce nephrotoxicity, hypertension, and hyperkalemia.[8] Some report that calcium channel blockers (verapamil, diltiazem) have some protective effect against cyclosporine nephrotoxicity.[9] One in vitro study has shown, however, that verapamil potentiates the effect of cyclosporine and enhances its nephrotoxicity.[10]

Corticosteroids

High doses of corticosteroids have remained the cornerstone of antirejection therapy for the last quarter century. Corticosteroid action is nonspecific, however, and inhibits lymphocytes, granulocytes, and monocytes. These agents have several side effects, including infection, hyperglycemia, poor wound healing, myopathy, avascular necrosis of bone, and Cushing's syndrome.

OKT3 (muromonab-CD3)

OKT3 is a murine IgG$_{2a}$ monoclonal antibody and was first tested and approved for treatment of allograft rejection. OKT3 is directed against the CD3 molecular complex, present on the surface of all mature, post-thymic T lymphocytes. The CD3 molecular complex appears to be involved in the transduction of signals from the cell surface antigen receptor to the intracellular activation process. Following the initial dose of OKT3 and antibody binding to the CD3 complex, T cells in the peripheral blood rapidly disappear. After several days, T cells begin to reappear, but they do not express the CD3 antigen and are immunologically incompetent.[11]

The use of OKT3 has been associated with aseptic meningitis and the development of anti-OKT3 antibodies. The first injection of OKT3 causes a series of complex symptoms such as fever (70 to 90%), rigors (30 to 60%), respiratory symptoms such as dyspnea, wheezing, chest pain, and tightness (10 to 20%), and gastrointestinal symptoms such as nausea, vomiting, and diarrhea (10 to 20%). These symptoms are thought to result from a release of pyrogenic and vasoactive mediators from T lymphocytes following opsonization of OKT3-coated cells. Those patients who receive a second course of OKT3 treatment should be monitored carefully, with either serum anti-OKT3 antibody levels or peripheral blood $CD3^+$ cell numbers, for evidence of a developing anti-OKT3 response.[12]

Azathioprine (Imuran)

Azathioprine is an immunosuppressive antimetabolite used as an adjunct to the prevention of rejection in renal transplantation. This agent can produce hematologic toxicity, nausea and vomiting, and occasional hepatotoxicity. Hematologic toxicity manifestes as leukopenia and thrombocytopenia. This substance must be monitored to guide its therapeutic dose. Prophylactic therapy is usually initiated with a daily dose of 3 to 10 mg/kg, and the usual maintenance dose is 1 to 3 mg/kg.

Administration of immunosupressive drugs during kidney transplantation varies in different centers and among individual transplantation teams. The following are general guidelines for administration of commonly used drugs:

1. Methyprednisone sodium, 1000 mg, IV, before induction of anesthesia.
2. OKT3, 2.5 mg (for patient under 30 kg) and 5 mg (for patient over 30 kg), IV, to follow azathioprine 3 to 5 mg/kg, IV, 20 minutes after induction of anesthesia.
3. Furosemide, 400 mg, in 500 ml 20% mannitol immediately after kidney transplantation.
4. At the end of procedure, a second dose of methyprednisone, 1000 mg, IV.

MISCELLANEOUS SURGICAL PROCEDURES IN PATIENTS WITH RENAL INSUFFICIENCY

Patients with renal failure may require various emergency or elective surgical procedures. Preoperative preparation, monitoring techniques, anesthetic management, and postoperative care of these patients are essentially similar to those in patients receiving kidney transplants. These patients, however, unlike transplant patients, do not need immunosuppressive drugs.

Some of these surgical procedures can be performed under local anesthesia with monitored anesthesia care. Before administration of regional anesthesia, peripheral neuropathy should be ruled out. Bleeding time, platelet count, fibrinogen levels, prothrombin time, and partial thromboplastin time also should be determined. Spinal anesthesia with 0.75% bupivacaine in patients with chronic renal failure may be associated with rapid spread of sensory blockade, higher level of block, and rapid recovery of motor blockade.[13]

MISCELLANEOUS UROGENITAL PROCEDURES

Many patients undergoing urologic surgery are either elderly or pediatric. Because geriatric patients may suffer from cardiovascular or pulmonary diseases, the primary principles of anesthesia in such patients must be emphasized. These include avoidance of hypoxia, hypotension, and hypoventilation. Maintenance of the airway and a slow and minimal administration of drugs are essential for anesthetic management of these patients. Blood pressure fluctuation is undesirable and should be treated accordingly, to avoid its cardiovascular and central nervous system (CNS) side effects.

Radical Prostate or Renal Surgery

If renal function is disturbed by urologic disease, as is most likely, consideration must be given to agents that have a minimal effect of renal physiology. The effects of anesthetics are outlined in Chapter 23, and these theoretic discussions should form the basis for the practical selection of an anesthetic agent.

In older patients, emphysema is usually present. Hence, premedication with sedative drugs should be curtailed. In addition, the problem of renal or prerenal tumors should be mentioned separately. Cysts are prone to invade the abdominal cavity and induce mechanical disturbances. Intra-abdominal pressure may increase and may alter venous blood flow. Mobilization of the tumor mass causes rapid decompression with splanchnic pooling and circulatory collapse. Tumors should be mobilized slowly, deep anesthesia should be avoided, and vasopressor therapy should be immediately available.

The size or position of tumors may limit ventilation. Specifically, lateral kidney and lithotomy positions interfere with circulatory and respiratory physiology by diminishing venous return and vital capacity. An exaggerated position should only be used for a portion of the procedure when necessary. In poor-risk patients, tolerance to the position should be tested by frequent blood pressure measurement. Pressure points should be protected with soft padding to avoid peripheral nerve damage, and peripheral arterial pulses following positioning should be verified. Deep vein thrombosis is a common complication in patients undergoing genitourinary surgery. Epidural anesthesia and application of compression boots may reduce incidence of venous thrombosis.[14] Respiration should be controlled to keep end-tidal CO_2 within normal limits.

Patients undergoing radical prostatectomy or total or partial nephrectomy can have severe intraoperative bleeding. Typed and cross-matched blood should be available. In selected patients, autologous blood transfusion and hemodilution techniques reduce transfusion reaction and eliminate transmission of blood-borne diseases. Measurement of direct arterial pressure and central venous pressure or pulmonary arterial pressure may be necessary for on-line monitoring of hemodynamic changes and fluid shift. Geriatric patients should be closely monitored in the recovery room to avoid hemodynamic instability and respiratory depression. In some patients, postoperative chest radiography and ECG may be required. Critically ill patients may need to be transferred to the hospital's intensive care unit.

Cystoscopy and Transurethral Resection

The performance of cystoscopy procedures in a darkened room can be problematic because observation of the patient may be limited. If general anesthesia is used, routine monitors should be applied, and indirect lighting must be available.

Irrigating Solution

During cystoscopic procedures, and particularly during a transurethral resection procedure (TURP), irrigating solutions under mild pressure are used to distend the prostatic urethra and to clear visual field by washing away blood and dissected tissue. Irrigating solution should be clear, translucent, nontoxic, nonionized, and isotonic. During TURP surgery, irrigating fluid can enter the vascular system. The extend to which fluid enters depends on the following factors: the hydrostatic pressure of the irrigating solution, the number of venous sinuses opened, the time of exposure, and excessive venous bleeding.

The following irrigating solutions have been used during cystoscopy and TURP:

1. Distilled water.
2. Cytal: 10% mannitol and sorbitol.
3. Urea 0.9%.
4. Dextrose 4%.
5. Plavolex.
6. Glycine 1.5%.

Associated Problems

The anesthesiologist may face several problems associated with TURP and cystoscopic procedures. These conditions are discussed in the following paragraphs.

Intravascular Hemolysis with Use of Distilled Water

Water has been used for irrigation during transurethral cystoscopic procedures. Significant intravascular hemolysis may occur, however. Low hydrostatic fluid pressure (less than 75 cm above pubis), frequent emptying of the bladder, restricting the operating time to 1 hour, and limiting dissection to the superficial fibers of the surgical capsule can reduce the amount of intravascular hemolysis.[15,16] Isotonic or isosmotic solutions remove the hazard of intravascular hemolysis.

Hyperglycemia

With 4 to 5% dextrose, blood glucose level can increase up to 100%. This condition is hazardous for diabetic patients.

Dilutional Hypervolemia

The clinical picture of fluid absorption and dilution hypervolemia is often called the TURP syndrome. Initially, the time of onset is slower during regional, spinal, or epidural anesthesia than during general anesthesia.[17] The gravity of TURP syndrome depends on the volume of solution absorbed into the circulation from the surgical prostate bed and the type of solution used for irrigation.

Regardless of type of the solution used, large volumes, as much as 2000 ml in 1 hour, may enter the circulation and may cause overload and hemodilution.[18] Radioisotope techniques have demonstrated that, during a single TURP, 3 to 4 L of fluid can be absorbed and can cause noncardiac pulmonary edema.[16]

Clinical Signs

Manifestations of the absorption of large amount of fluid vary with the type of anesthesia.[19] Generally, a picture of hypertension develops. During regional block, the following tetrad appears: (1) a rise in systolic blood pressure with a lesser rise in diastolic pressure; (2) a slowing of the pulse; (3) changes in nervous system activity with mental confusion, semicoma, restlessness, headache, nausea; and (4) pulmonary congestion in the form of dyspnea, cyanosis, and wheezing.

During general anesthesia, varying signs of hypervolemia are seen. CNS symptoms are absent until patients are taken to the recovery room, however. Respiratory signs are usually masked by assisted or controlled ventilation and the high concentrations of oxygen used during anesthesia. Clinical signs of dilutional hypervolemia should not be attributed to hypercarbia, light anesthesia, drug effects, heat retention, and endocrine abnormalities. Distended neck veins, wheezing, crackling breath sounds, and abnormal arterial blood gases are early signs of severe fluid overload. When patients emerge from general anesthesia, they can be sleepy, confused, or comatose as a result of brain-water intoxication and increased ammonia from glycine metabolism. To prevent water intoxication, the height of irrigating solution should be between 60 and 90 cm above the prostatic bed. In patients with severe cardiopulmonary disease, direct arterial pressure, central venous pressure, or pulmonary capillary pressure should be monitored. The use of spinal or epidural anesthesia with minimal sedation may facilitate early diagnosis of fluid overload.

Glycine Solution and Its Potential Toxicity

Glycine is an amino acid that has many characteristics of a CNS inhibitory transmitter. The locus of its action is predominantly in the brain stem and spinal cord and results from hyperpolarization of the postsynaptic membrane by increasing chloride conductance. This is in contrast to the inhibitor τ-aminobutyric acid (GABA) acting in the cortical and subcortical areas. To this extent, glycine mimics the benzodiazapines.

A 1.5% glycine solution was introduced by Nesbitt for irrigation of the bladder during cystoscopy and TURP. Like other solutions used for irrigation of the prostatic bed, glycine is absorbed into the vascular compartment and undergoes hepatic metabolism. It then is broken down by oxidative deamination and forms two products: ammonia and oxylate. Hyperoxaluria may also occur.[20-22]

Besides simple fluid overload and water intoxication, glycine can cause CNS disturbance. CNS changes may be related to certain metabolites of glycine such as ammonia or to glycine itself.[23,24]

Clinical signs of ammonia toxicity are CNS depression or postoperative somnolence, and ammonia toxicity may occur despite correction of fluid and electrolyte abnormalities.[25] The signs and symptoms begin with nausea, followed by vomiting and muscular twitching. Confusion, agitation, convulsion, stupor, and coma may occur. The onset of symptoms and of coma occurs when serum blood levels of ammonia reach between 11 and 35 nmol/L.[22] Symptoms usually occur quickly, but they can be delayed as long as 10 hours postoperatively.

Treatment of this condition is largely symptomatic, and high levels of ammonia usually are cleared within 24 to 48 hours. The use of L-arginine decreases the peak ammonia level once toxicity is evident, and it speeds the return of blood ammonia levels to normal.[23] Visual disturbance and temporary blindness have been reported following administration of glycine irrigating solution. Visual disturbances have been attributed to elevated ammonia and not to cerebral edema.[24,25]

Hahn proposed that 1.5% glycine prepared in water containing 2% ethanol can enable one to detect the presence and the degree of absorbed irrigating solution.[26] This solution is commercially produced by Travenol AB (Sweden) and is available for clinical use. During the procedure, expired breath testing of ethanol is continuously monitored by Detax gas analyzer or is monitored by an alcohol meter every 5 minutes. Because end-tidal ethanol concentration is directly related to serum glycine level, the cumulative absorbed volume of the irrigating solution can be estimated.

Electrolyte Changes

Electrolyte disturbances can be in the form of hyponatremia or hypocalcemia.

Hyponatremia

Dilutional hypervolemia and water intoxication lead to dilutional hyponatremia. The increased intravascular hydrostatic pressure and decreased oncotic pressure cause massive movement of fluid into the interstitial space. Such fluid flux into the interstitial space also carries significant amounts of sodium and causes hyponatremia.[18] If the serum sodium concentration drops below 130 mmol/L, one may see the CNS sign of hyponatremia: disorientation, excitation, muscle twitch, focal or generalized seizures, and coma.[19] The ECG reveals wide QRS complex and a T-wave depression.

Hypocalcemia

Many patients undergoing TURP are frequently treated with digitalis, calcium antagonists, and β blockers. A significant decrease in total serum calcium and whole blood ionized calcium have been reported during epidural anesthesia and hemodilution.[27] Alteration in serum calcium level in elderly patients may lead to altered cardiac function or reduced effectiveness of digitalis compounds.

Hypothermia

Heat loss during anesthesia and TURP is a common problem. Generally, preoperative heat loss arises more rapidly in elderly patients. Indeed, an average of 370 kJ may be lost during the first hour of surgery. Irrigating solution kept refrigerated or at room temperature facilitates the development of hypothermia. Regardless of the anesthetic technique, core temperature may decrease an average of 1° to 1.5°C by the end of surgery. Nonetheless, heat loss is greater under general anesthesia.[28] A patient with marked hypothermia may develop shivering, increased oxygen consumption, metabolic acidosis, and cardiac arrhythmia. Hypothermia should be prevented and treated during the operation and recovery period. The use of a low-flow semiclosed anesthesia system, a warming blanket, and a fluid warmer is recommended.

Organ Perforation

Organ perforation may occur into the space of Retzius or into the peritoneal cavity. In the first instance, mild lower abdominal pain is the main symptom. Peritoneal irritability, epigastric pain, and shoulder pain accompany organ perforation. This complication is readily recognized when spinal anesthesia is used. If spinal anesthesia is higher than the T10 sensory level, however, the diagnosis of peritoneal perforation is masked. A slow return of irrigating solution and distention of lower abdomen may also lead to the diagnosis of peritoneal perforation.

Autonomic Hyperreflexia

Quadriplegic or paraplegic patients often require repeated cystoscopies and removal of bladder stones. Depending on their level of spinal lesion and degree of sensory pain, this group of patients can be managed by monitored anesthesia care or with spinal or general anesthesia. If the spinal cord is injured above T5, these patients may develop autonomic hyperreflexia, which is manifested as hypertension, bradycardia, cardiac dysrhythmias, and sweating. This acute sympathetic hyperreflexia syndrome occurs in 66 to 85% of quadriplegics and in those with high spinal cord lesions from interruption of the spinal and central inhibitory pathways. Autonomic hyperreflexia is severe if spinal cord injury is above the splanchnic outflow. In patients with spinal lesions between T5 and T10, clinical signs are mild. Sympathetic hyperreflexia syndrome should be treated immediately with direct vasodilators such as SNP, nitroglycerin, or the short-acting ganglionic blocker trimethaphan.[29,30]

Septicemia

During cystoscopy, TURP, or infected stone manipulation, some patients may develop septicemia, fever, chills, tachycardia, and hypotension. If such problems are not treated, life-threatening conditions related to septic shock may occur. Infectious conditions should be treated preoperatively with broad-spectrum antibiotic therapy to prevent septic shock syndrome.[31]

Disseminated Intravascular Coagulopathy (DIC syndrome)

Some patients may develop DIC syndrome from dilutional hypervolemia, septicemia, or combination of both conditions. Consultation with a hematologist is required for proper treatment of this syndrome. This is discussed in detail in Chapter 13.

Blood Loss in TURP

In general, blood loss during TURP depends on the vascularity of the prostate gland, the experience and surgical skills of the surgeon, and the length of the operation.[32-34] Levin and associates[34] have shown a fairly constant 15-ml blood loss for each gram of resected tissue. Because blood is diluted with irrigating fluid, it is difficult to assess blood loss during TURP. A visual estimation of blood loss is inaccurate, and dilutional hypervolemia often masks hemodynamic changes associated with blood loss. Blood transfusions may be required after assessing the degree of blood loss, the patient's hemoglobin, hemodynamic conditions, and coagulation profile.

Urodynamic Studies

The average man first senses a full bladder at a volume of 300 to 400 ml. When this occurs, maximal detrusor contraction strength is 50 to 60 cm H_2O pressure, and urethral pressure is approximately 30 to 50 cm H_2O. Cystometric examination of bladder function, neurologic control, and the mechanical elements of micturation can be carried out with either CO_2 or a saline distending fluid under spinal anesthesia. Following administration of spinal anesthesia, when somatosensory block is at L5 or above, bladder analgesia and micturation reflex are lost within 30 to 60 seconds. Some patients have a continuing dull tension that usually disappears within 2 to 3 minutes. When the somatic sensory level reaches T10 or above, all components of afferent sense to void, micturation sensory, and voluntary micturation are blocked. At a sensory level of T10, the bladder may be distended beyond the capacity noted before the administration of spinal anesthesia without discomfort. Urethral pressure is reduced by about 50% with the development of bladder paralysis.

Once skeletal muscle motor block partially recovers from spinal anesthesia, some detrusor strength may return as determined by cystometry. With the onset of peripheral somatic sensation and response to pin prick, the development of some bladder sense and the afferent arc of the micturation reflex can be noticed. Once bladder sensation appears, the full strength of detrusor is present, and the efferent arc of the micturation reflex rapidly recovers.

External Genitalia Operations

Anesthesia for circumcision, penile prostheses, and orchiopexy may be performed with the patient under general anesthesia or spinal, caudal, or penile blockade. The somatic sensory innervation of the penis is mediated by the dorsal nerves of the penis through the perineal and pudendal nerves to the posterior sacral spinal roots at S2, S3, and S4. Parasympathetic fibers also pass from the sacral anterior roots by the nerves from the pelvic plexus to innervate blood vessels of the penis (dilator).

Caudal anesthesia blocks the sacral parasympathetic outflow from the spinal cord, as well as somatic afferent nerve conduction. During caudal blockade, bladder function and micturation are often disturbed. Patients who have a dorsal nerve block have a low incidence of postoperative nausea and vomiting and may return to normal activity in the early postoperative period.[35] In children, general inhalation anesthesia is followed by either a caudal block or a block of the dorsal nerves. These blocks provide postoperative pain relief for 4 to 6 hours. Caudal anesthesia can also cause delayed micturation and some inability to stand, however.[36] Pain responses are present in the neonate, and it is now preferred practice to provide some analgesia or anesthesia for circumcision of the newborn.[36a]

Treatment of Priapism

Penile erection is a reflex phenomenon peculiarly related to the vascular and structural pattern of the penis. Blood is supplied to the penis from the internal pudendal artery (branch of the hypogastric artery), which consists of three paired penile arteries: the dorsal arteries, the corporal arteries, and the ventral spongiosal arteries. The corporal arteries are responsible for tumescences of the corpora cavernosa. Ordinarily, blood flow is directed through open arteriovenous anastomoses into the deep venous plexus and away from the spongy corpora cavernosa. During tumescence, these shunts are largely closed, and blood flows into the corpora. The corpora of the penis consist of sponge-like tissue that is potentially cavernous and ordinarily contains little blood.

With appropriate physical or psychic stimuli, afferent impulses pass from the glans penis and frenulum through the dorsal nerve of the penis over the pudendal somatic nerves to a reflex erection center in the sacral spinal cord. The erection is mediated by parasympathetic efferent impulses from this center of the sacral cord by the fibers coursing in the pudendal nerve that serve as a motor path. The efferent impulses to the penis act on the penile vascular system and result in marked arterial dilation.

Engorgement of the penis occurs by blood flow through dilated corporal penile arteries into a series of convoluted branches called helicine vessels in the arterial tree, which empty into the corpora cavernosa. Erection is considered primarily an arterial event. At the same time, the venous drainage diminishes and thereby traps the blood and enhances the engorgement. Diminished venous return is related to venoconstriction and mechanical compression of the outflow veins by the engorged corpora. At the time of maximal penile distention and rigidity, the pressure at the corpora reaches a level approximating that of the carotid artery. Detumescence depends on the opening of arterial venous shunts, with a redirection of blood away from the corpora cavernosa and dilatation of the penile vein. This is mediated, in part, by sympathetic stimulation.[37]

Occasionally, patients are admitted for the treatment of persistent and painful priapism, or treatment is required if temporary penile turgescence occurs during cystoscopic procedures. As described later, numerous techniques for detumescence have been used; however, no one agent or technique has been effective completely.[38-48]

Suggested Treatment of Penile Turgescence

The following treatments, alone or in combination, have been used for treatment of penile turgescence:

1. Ketamine.[38-42]
2. Inhalation of amyl nitrate.[43]
3. Intravenous nitroglycerin with an effect usually shorter than 2 minutes.
4. Topical application of 2% nitroglycerin paste to the shaft of the penis.[44]
5. Intravenous administration of hydralazine.[45]
6. Intravenous infusion of magnesium sulfate.[46]
7. Intravenous administration of dextran 40 (200 to 400 ml).[47]
8. Induction of hyponatremia with D-arginine vasopressin (ADH).[48]
9. Low spinal anesthesia (block only sacral nerve).
10. Surgical evacuation of corpora.

Laser Procedures

Laser, specifically the neodymium-YAG laser, is used increasingly to treat bladder tumors and other benign and malignant external genitalia lesions. Depending on the extent of the surgical procedure and the patient's condition, local infiltration of local anesthetic, epidural or spinal block, or general anesthesia can be used for anesthetic management of laser surgery.

Lithotripsy

Percutaneous ultrasonic lithotripsy and extracorporeal shock wave lithotripsy (ESWL) have been used to treat urinary stones. Anesthetic management for these procedures includes general anesthesia, epidural or spinal block, and regional field block.

Percutaneous Ultrasonic Lithotripsy

During this technique, the patient is placed in a lateral position, and a nephroscope is introduced through a small flank incision. A hollow metal probe is inserted through the nephroscope to contact the calculus. The ultrasonic energy delivered through this metal probe fractures renal or upper ureteral stones. The crushed stone is then flushed out by irrigating normal saline solution.[31] Possible complications of this procedure include organ perforation, diaphragmatic rupture, air embolism, acute hypotremia, hyperkalemia, and acute hemolysis.[49]

Extracorporeal Shock Wave Lithotripsy (ESWL)

ESWL is a newer and widely used noninvasive treatment of kidney and ureteral stones. This technique is superior to open surgery and percutaneous nephrolithotripsy because of lower mortality and morbidity rates, a higher success rate, lower costs, and shorter hospital stays. Most patients resume normal activities within 24 hours after the procedure.

Destruction of urinary stones by high-energy shock waves was first proposed by Russian engineers in 1955. After 25 years, an aerospace company in Germany (Dornier) developed ESWL for noninvasive disintegration of urinary stones.

The ESWL technique has three major components. The first component is a shock wave generator, which works by discharging a spark plug using 18- to 24-kV current (Fig. 24-1). The initiation of the spark causes the transmission of high-pressure waves radiating equally from the original focal point of the explosion. A brass ellipsoid is used to reflect the emergent pressure wave back to the second point of the ellipsoid (F_2), generating the maximum shock force (Fig. 24-2). The second component is an x-ray image intensifier that locates the stone in a three-dimensional axis for the F_2 foci. The third component is a computer-assisted remote control panel to focus on the kidney stone in the center of the high-power shock wave (Fig. 24-3). To reduce the potential for the development of cardiac arrhythmia, the ESWL shock wave generator is triggered by the R wave of an ECG and is delivered to the kidney during the refractory period of the myocardium.[50,51]

With the older generation of Dornier lithotriptors, patients are immersed in a water bath to the level of their clavicles at a temperature of 37°C. The stones are located by a computer-assisted image intensifier and are then disintegrated by high-energy shock waves. During and after treatments, patients are hydrated, and the remaining small particles are passed in the urine. Because the physical properties and acoustic densities of biologic tissues and solid abdominal organs are similar to those of water, immersion in water permits ultrashort high-energy wave to reach the urinary stones without damaging the tissues.[51]

Lithotripsy using the older generation of Dornier lithotriptors was painful and required general or epidural anesthesia. With technologic advances, however, the newer spark gap with less painful stimuli has been developed. In addition, piezoelectric devices using ceramic crystals to generate shock wave from ultrasonic waves and electromagnetic devices, such as the Siemens Lithostar, have been introduced for treatment of kidney stones. These newer devices emit a less powerful shock wave than early-generation water bath machines. The newer machines also use a dry table, conducting shock waves through a water pillow, which allows patients to be treated with minimal or no anesthesia.[52-54]

Anesthetic Techniques

General anesthesia, regional techniques (spinal or epidural, intercostal block), intravenous sedation, and local infiltration of the entry site have been used for ESWL. Many anesthesiologists prefer continuous epidural anesthesia because some patients require cystoscopy and stone manipulation just before ESWL, and the same epidural catheter can be used for both surgical proce-

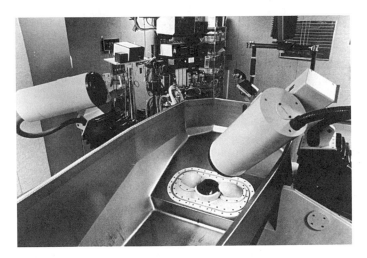

Fig. 24–1. View of shock wave generator.

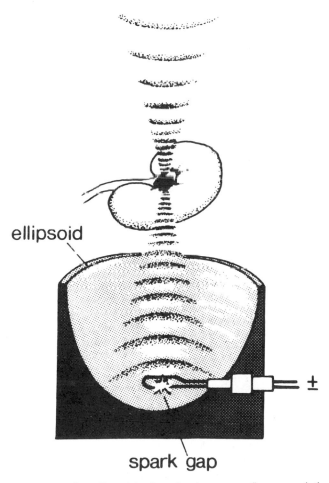

ellipsoid

spark gap

Fig. 24–2. The ellipsoid of a shock wave reflector and the area of maximal energy density. From Gravenstein, J. S., Peter, K. (eds.). Extra Corporeal Shockwave Lithotripsy for Renal Stone Disease: Technical and Clinical Aspects. Boston, Butterworth, 1986.

dures. Moreover, patients are awake and may be hemodynamically more stable during transfer from the cystoscopy table to the ESWL chair. If an epidural anesthetic is used, the catheter site must be covered with sterile waterproof adhesive dressing to prevent possible infection. A sensory level of T6 is required. Because a sympathetic blockade under spinal anesthesia is both more profound than epidural anesthesia, and because it can cause severe circulatory changes during positioning, epidural anesthesia is preferred.

Patients undergoing lithotripsy under general anesthesia are either placed in a lithotripsy chair before induction of anesthesia or are anesthetized on the cystoscopy table for cystoscopy and stent placement and are then transferred to the lithotripsy chair. Following induction of anesthesia with thiopental or propofol or other short-acting hypnotic drugs, the trachea is intubated with an intermediate muscle relaxant. Ventilation must be controlled to keep end-tidal CO_2 within normal limits. A small tidal volume and higher respiratory rate is used to minimize diaphragmatic movement and displacement of kidney stone on the image intensifier's screen. Some centers have advocated high-frequency jet ventilators or high-frequency positive-pressure ventilation, with a tidal volume of 3 ml/kg and a respiratory rate of 80/min using a conventional anesthesia machine, as a method of keeping the stone in focus.[55,56] Anesthesia is maintained with halothane, enflurane, or isoflurane, in nitrous oxide and oxygen. Because ESWL is triggered by the R wave of the ECG tracing, waterproof ECG pads are properly positioned on the patient's chest wall to produce strong R-wave signals and to prevent burn. Pulse oximetry is mandatory, and an ear or nose probe should be used to avoid electrical shortage and interference. An esophageal stethoscope with a temperature probe is placed to monitor temperature and cardiopulmonary sounds.

Epidural Anesthesia

Continuous lumbar epidural anesthesia has many advantages in providing anesthesia for ESWL.[57] It is relatively less reliable and the results are abnormal when lum-

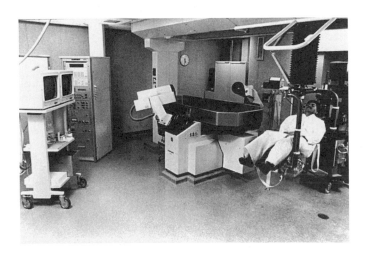

Fig. 24–3. Extracorporeal shock wave lithotripsy equipment, with computer-assisted remote control panel.

bar epidural anesthesia is repeated, however. Among the complications frequently noted include pain in the back and posterior thighs during the injection of local anesthetics at the time of repeat administration of epidural anesthesia. One has an impression that, in injecting the anesthetic solutions after a catheter is in place, compliance in the epidural space is decreased. Aspiration of bloody local anesthetic solution from the epidural needle or catheter has been observed.

The pain on injection of the anesthetic solution is related directly to the speed of the injection. It is probably related to an inflammatory process, whereas an epidural hematoma could explain the decreased compliance of the epidural space.

Another explanation for many of the problems may be related to the effect of lithotripter shock waves on the epidural space. The shock wave path is apparently wide, as evidenced by the distribution of tenderness and bruises on the patient's back after ESWL. Some of the shock wave apparently must travel through the epidural space. The energy of such a shock wave into surrounding tissues can be greatly increased by the presence of an air-fluid interface.[58] If in the administration of epidural anesthesia a loss of resistance technique is used with the introduction of a small volume of air, then the conditions are set for the development of an extraordinary amount of energy directed at the nerve tissues. Air bubbles in the epidural space may cause epidural tissue damage as well as pitting of the nerve tissue. Korbon's report recommended that the injection of air for the identification of the epidural space be avoided.[58]

Repeated administration of epidural anesthesia is associated with a significant failure rate, to the extent of 40 to 50%; another 50% of the patients may present abnormal problems and complications related to the epidural anesthesia.

Effects on Organ Functions

Anesthesia, a head-up semisitting position, immersion in water, and ESWL can significantly affect the cardiovascular system, pulmonary function, and the kidney.[59,60] Cardiac arrhythmia, myocardial ischemia and infarction, hypertension and hypotension, cerebrovascular accidents, and renal subcapsular hematoma and demarcation of the cortimedullary region have been reported after ESWL.[61] Behnia and associates, using a transesophageal Doppler ultrasonic cardiac output monitor, demonstrated a reduction in cardiac output with a concomitant increase in mean arterial pressure and systemic vascular resistance in patients under general anesthesia for ESWL.[62] These ESWL-associated hemodynamic changes were not mediated by epinephrine or norepinephrine, but they may be modulated by the renin-angiotensin system.[63,64] Hemodynamic instability, severe systemic hypertension, and pulmonary edema have been reported after ESWL in patients with histories of high blood pressure and poor cardiac reserve.[65] Invasive monitoring through a radial arterial line, central venous pressure measurements, pulmonary artery capillary pressure determinations may be indicated in these patients. Because of possible hemody-

namic changes, extra caution should be taken in transferring the patient in and out of the water bath and into the lithotripsy chair.

Kaude and associates,[66] using magnetic resonance imaging and radionuclide renal function testing, showed a loss of corticomedullary differentiation, subcapsular hematomas, and a partial parenchymal obstruction pattern after ESWL. Thomas and co-workers,[67] using a quantitative scintillation τ camera, demonstrated a reduction in renal function and estimated renal plasma flow following ESWL treatment. Acute destruction of renal parenchyma and tubular epithelium in the renal cortical region, along with hemorrhage into glomeruli, tubules, juxtaglomerular apparatus, and interstitium 1 to 24 hours after ESWL have been reported in dogs.[68] A direct correlation was seen between the severity of these changes and the number of shock waves applied. Severe retroperitoneal hematomas requiring blood transfusion also have been reported following ESWL.

ESWL is contraindicated in the presence of spinal cord hemangioma, abdominal aortic aneurysm, pregnancy, coagulation disturbance, artificial cardiac pacemaker implants, and lumbar orthopedic implants.[50]

Temperature Changes of Patients During ESWL

Both hyperthermia and hypothermia have been reported as complications of ESWL and can follow either epidural anesthesia or general anesthesia.[69] The cause of the temperature changes is related to the temperature of the water in which the patient is immersed. The recommended temperature is 35° to 37°C. Frequently, temperatures of the water have been found to be in excess of 40°C or below 34°C. Immersion in water, of course, is related to a much more accelerated conduction of heat away from the patient's body, or to the body by a factor of 32 times, as opposed to air temperatures.

The tub water should always be tested by the anesthesiologist with his or her hand. This should be done whether or not the recording thermometer of the tub water itself appears to be within the proper range. Too often, warm water is allowed to run into a bath at a higher temperature than is desired, assuming that heat will be lost because of the temperature of the room. A second preventive measure is to maintain the room temperatures where the lithotripsy is performed in the neighborhood of 80° to 85°F rather than at the recommended temperature of the standard operating room of 72°F.

Pain Management Supplement During ESWL: Topical Anesthesia

The pain during ESW lithotripsy originates in part from the shock wave entry at the skin level and at the more deeply situated visceral and musculoskeletal structures.[70] Using an unmodified Dornier HM3 lithotripter (Dornier Medical Systems, Berlin) in patients orally premedicated with 75 mg of meperidine and 5 mg of diazepam, Tiselius found that cutaneous anesthesia with a local anesthetic cream of lidocaine and prilocaine (EMLA Cream)[71] was sufficient to provide adequate anesthesia in over 70% of patients. Additional analgesia was provided with 25 mg of meperidine administered intramuscularly if pain was reported. The generator voltage at the start of the procedure was 14 kV and could be increased to 20 kV if necessary. Additional analgesia was needed most often in patients with stones in the upper caliceal system.

The anesthetic cream is applied on a skin area 15 × 15 cm corresponding to the entry site of the shock wave. For stones in the kidney and the proximal ureter, the cream is applied to the patient's back; for stones in the midureter, the cream is applied to the abdominal region. The amount of cream applied is 30 g. The cream layer is then covered with a plastic dressing. This is done about 60 minutes before the ESWL.

REFERENCES

1. Gelman, S.: Anesthesia and Organ Transplantation. Philadelphia, W.B. Saunders, 1987, p. 61.
2. Smith, R. P., Kruszyna, H.: Nitroprusside produces cyanide poisoning via a reaction with hemoglobin. J Pharmacol Exp Ther 191:557, 1974.
3. Christensen, J. H., Andreasen, F., Jansen, J.: Pharmacokinetics and pharmacodynamics of thiopental in patients undergoing renal transplantation. Acta Anaesth Scand 27:513, 1983.
4. Lynam, D. P., et al.: The pharmacodynamics and pharmacokinetics of vecuronium in patients anesthetized with isoflurane with normal renal function or with renal failure. Anesthesiology 69:227, 1988.
5. Fahey, M. R., et al.: The pharmacokinetics and pharmacodynamics of atracurium in patients with and without renal failure. Anesthesiology 61:699, 1984.
6. Diethelm, A. G., et al.: Large volume diuresis as a mechanism for immediate maximum renal function after transplantation. Surg Gynecol Obstet 138:869, 1974.
7. Miller, E. D.: Renal effects of dopamine. Anesthesiology 61:487, 1984.
8. Soon-Shiong, P., Lanza, R. P., Mendez, R.: Renal and pancreas transplantation in diabetic chronic uremic patients. In Andreucci, V.E., Fine, L.G. (eds.). International Yearbook of Nephrology 1991. Boston, Kluwer Academic Publishers, 1991, p. 259.
9. Nagineni, C. N., Misra, B. C., Lee, D. B. N, Yanagawa N.: Cyclosporin A-calcium channel interaction: a possible mechanism for nephrotoxicity. Transplant Proc 19:1358, 1987.
10. McMillen, M. A., et al.: Potentiation of cyclosporine by verapamil in vitro. Transplantation 40:444, 1985.
11. David, C. J.: Monoclonal antibodies in the treatment of transplant rejection. In Andreucci, V. E., Fine, L. G., Hatano, M., Kjellstrand, C. M. (eds.). International Yearbook of Nephrology. Boston, Kluwer Academic Publishers, 1989, p. 325.
12. Shield, C. F., Norman, D. J.: Immunologic monitoring during and after OKT3 therapy. Am J Kidney Dis 11:120, 1988.
13. Orko, R., PitKänen, M., Rosenberg, P. H.: Subarachnoid anesthesia with 0.75% bupivacaine in patients with chronic renal failure. Br J Anaesth 58:605, 1986.
14. Hendlin, H., Mattila, M. A. K., Poilkolainen, E.: The effect of lumbar epidural analgesia on the development of deep vein thrombosis of the legs after open prostatectomy. Acta Chir Scand 147:425, 1981.
15. Filman, E. M., Hanson, O. L., Gilbert, L. O, Kan, T.: Radioisotopic study of effects of irrigating fluid in transurethral prostatectomy. JAMA 171:1488, 1959.
16. Madsen, P. O., Naber, K. G.: The importance of the pressure in the prostatic fossa and absorption of irrigating fluid during transurethral resection of the prostate. J Urol 109:446, 1973.
17. Marx, G. F., Orkin, L. R.: Complications associated with transurethral surgery. Anesthesiology 23:802, 1962.
18. Tylor, R. O., et al.: Volumetric, gravimetric and radioisotope determination of fluid transfer in transurethral prostatectomy. Urology 79:490, 1958.
19. Zimmerman, B., Wangensteen, O. H.: Observation in water intoxication in surgical patients. Surgery 31:654, 1952.
20. Alexander, J. P., Polland, A., Gillespie, I. A.: Glycine and transurethral resection. Anaesthesia 41:1189, 1986.
21. Stephenson, T. P., et al.: Comparison between continuous flow and intermittent flow transurethral resection of 40 patients presenting with acute retention. Br J Urol 52:523, 1980.
22. Fahey, J. L.: Toxicity and blood ammonia rise resulting from intravenous amino acid administration in man: the protective effect of L-arginine. J Clin Invest 36:1647, 1957.
23. Nathans, D., Fahey, J. L., Ship, A. G.: Sites of origin and removal of blood ammonia formed during glycine infusion: effect of L-arginine. J Lab Clin Med 51:124, 1958.
24. Ovassapian, A., Joshi, C. W., Brunner, E. A.: Visual disturbances: an unusual symptom of transurethral prostatic resection reaction. Anesthesiology 57:332, 1982.
25. Roesch, R. P., et al.: Ammonia toxicity resulting from glycine absorption during a transurethral resection of the prostate. Anesthesiology 58:577, 1983.
26. Hahn, R. G.: Ethanol monitoring of irrigating fluid absorption in transurethral prostatic surgery. Anesthesiology 68:867, 1988.
27. Kancir, C. B., Petersen, P. H., Wandrup, J.: The effect of plasma volume variations on the calcium concentration during epidural anaesthesia. Acta Anaesthesiol Scand 31:338, 1987.
28. Stjernstrom, H., et al.: Thermal balance during transurethral resection of the prostate: a comparison of general anesthesia and epidural analgesia. Acta Anaesthesiol Scand 29:743, 1985.
29. Guttmann, L., Whitteridge, D.: Effect of bladder distention on autonomic mechanisms after spinal cord injuries. Brain 70:361, 1947.
30. Lambert, D. H., Deane, R. S., Mazuzan, J. E.: Anesthesia and the control of blood pressure in patients with spinal cord injury. Anesth Analg 61:344, 1982.
31. Whitfield, H. N., Hendry, W. F.: Endoscopic surgery. In Textbook of Genito-Urinary Surgery, Vol. 2. New York, Churchill Livingstone, 1985, p. 1373.
32. Abrams, P. H., et al.: Blood loss during transurethral resection of the prostate. Anaesthesia 37:71, 1982.
33. Lambardo, L. J.: Fibrinolysis following prostate surgery. J Urol 77:289, 1957.
34. Levin, K., Nyren, O., Pompeius, R.: Blood loss tissue weight and operating time in transurethral prostatectomy. Scand J Urol Nephrol 15:197, 1981.
35. May, A. E., Wandless, J., James, R. D.: Analgesia for circumcision in children. Acta Anaesth Scand 26:331, 1982.
36. Vater, M., Wandless, J.: Caudal or dorsal nerve block? A comparison of two local anesthetic techniques for postoperative analgesia following day case circumcision. Acta Anaesthesiol Scand 29:175, 1985.
36a. Anand, K.: Pain and its effects in the human neonate and fetus. N Engl J Med 317:1321, 1987.
37. Krane, F. J., Siroky, M. B.: Neurophysiology of erection. Urol Clin North Am 8:91, 1981.
38. Gale, A. S.: Ketamine prevention of penile turgescence. JAMA 219:1629, 1972.
39. Van Arsdalen, K. N., Chen, J. W., Smith, V. M. H. J.: Penile

erections complicating transurethral surgery. J Urol 129:374, 1983.

40. Pietras, J. R., Cromie, W. J., Duckett, J. M.: Ketamine as a detumescence agent during hypospadias repair. J Urol 121:654, 1979.

41. Benzon, H. T., Leventhal, J. B., Ovassapian, A.: Ketamine treatment of penile erection in operating room. Anesth Analg 62:457, 1983.

42. Roy, R.: Cardiovascular effects of ketamine given to relieve penile turgescence after high doses of fentanyl. Anesthesiology 61:610, 1984.

43. Welti, R. S., Brodsky, J. B.: Treatment of intraoperative penile tumescence. J Urol 124:924, 1980.

44. Snyder, A. R., Ilko, R.: Topical nitroglycerin for intraoperative penile turgescence. Anesth Analg 66:1022, 1987.

45. Noguchi, C. T., Schechter, A. V.: NIH reports medical news. JAMA 247:1543, 1982.

46. Hugh-Jones, K., Lehmann, H., McAlister, J. M.: Some experience in managing sickle cell anaemia in children and young adults using alkalis and magnesium. Br Med J 2:226, 1964.

47. Carey, J. S., et al.: Circulatory response to low viscosity dextran in clinical shock. Surg Gynecol Obstet 121:563, 1965.

48. Rosa, R. M., et al.: A study of induced hyponatremia in the prevention and treatment of sickle cell crisis. N Engl J Med 303:1138, 1980.

49. Bennett, M. J., Smith, R. W., Fuchs, E.: Sudden cardiac arrest during percutaneous ultrasonic nephrostolithotomy. Anesthesiology 60:245, 1984.

50. Drach, G. W., et al.: Report of the United States Cooperative Study of Extracorporeal Shock Wave Lithotripsy. J Urol 135:1127, 1986.

51. Gravenstein, J. S., Peter, K. (eds.): Extra Corporeal Shockwave Lithotripsy for Renal Stone Disease: Technical and Clinical Aspects. Boston, Butterworth, 1986, p. 9.

52. Graff, J., et al.: Newer generator for low pressure lithotripsy with the Dornier HM3: preliminary experience of two centers. J Urol 139:904, 1988.

53. Rassweiler, J., et al.: Extracoporeal piezoelectric lithotripsy using the Wolf Lithotripter versus low energy lithotripsy with the modified Dornier HM3: a cooperative study. World J Urol 5:218, 1987.

54. Gravenstein, J. S.: Anesthesia for lithotripsy: an update. Curr Rev Clin Anesth 12:181, 1992.

55. Schulte am Esch, J., Kochs, E., Meyer, W. H.: Improved efficiency of extracorporeal shock-wave lithotripsy during high frequency jet ventilation. Anesthesiology 63:A177, 1985.

56. Perel, A., et al.: High frequency positive pressure ventilation during general anesthesia for extracorporeal shock wave lithotripsy. Anesth Analg 65:1231, 1986.

57. Korbon, G. A., et al.: Repeated epidural anesthesia for extracorporeal shock-wave lithotripsy is unreliable. Anesth Analg 66:669, 1987.

58. Chaussey, C.: Extracorporeal Shock Wave Lithotripsy: New Aspects in the Treatment of Kidney Stone Disease. Augsburg, Karger, 1982, p. 78.

59. Gauer, O. H., Thorn, H. L.: Postural changes in circulation. In Hamilton, W.F., Dow, P. (eds.). Handbook of Physiology. Baltimore, Williams & Wilkins, 1965, p. 2409.

60. Arborelius, M., Balldin, U. L., Lija, B., Lundberg, C. E. G.: Hemodynamic changes in man during immersion with the head above water. Aerospace Med 43:592, 1972.

61. Goldsmith, M. F.: Stones Are crushed and many patients elated by results of new ESWL therapy. JAMA 256:437, 1986.

62. Behnia, R., Shanks, C. A., Ovassapian, A., Wilson, L. A.: Hemodynamic response associated with lithotripsy. Anesth Analg 66:354, 1987.

63. Michaels, E. K., et al.: Hemodynamic and adrenal response to shock wave energy. J Endourol 5:345, 1991.

64. Behnia, R., et al.: Hemodynamic and catecholamine responses associated with extracorporeal shock wave lithotripsy. J Clin Anesth 2:158, 1990.

65. Michaels, E. K., Behnia, R., Fowler, J. E., Jr.: Extracorporeal shock-wave lithotripsy in hypertensive patients: importance of pretreatment cardiac evaluation. Urology 40:41, 1992.

66. Kaude, J. V., et al.: Renal morphology and function immediately after extracorporeal shock wave lithotripsy. AJR Am J Roentgenol 145:305, 1985.

67. Thomas, R., Roberts, J., Sloane, B., Kaack, B.: Effect of extracorporeal shock wave lithotripsy on renal function. J Endourol 2:141, 1988.

68. Jaeger, P., Redha, F., Uhlschmiid, G., Dauri, D.: Morphologic changes In canine kidneys following extracorporeal shock wave treatment. J Endourol 2:205, 1988.

69. Malhortra, V.: Hyperthermia and hypothermia as complications of extracorporeal shock wave lithotripsy. Anesthesiology 67:448, 1987.

70. Tiselius, H.-G.: Cutaneous anesthesia with lidocaine-prilocaine cream: a useful adjunct during shock wave lithotripsy with analgesic sedation. J Urol 149:8, 1993.

71. Bjerring, P., Arendt-Nielsen L.: Depth and duration of skin analgesia to needle insertion after topical application of EMLA cream. Br J Anaesth 64:173, 1990.

Chapter 25

THEORETIC MECHANISMS OF GENERAL ANESTHESIA

MARK V. BOSWELL AND STUART R. HAMEROFF

General anesthetics render patients unconscious, amnestic, and insensible to pain in a rapid, reversible, and predictable manner. Modern surgery would be impossible without the use of the general anesthetics that we have come to regard as commonplace. Indeed, the safety of surgery today is due in part to the relative safety of modern anesthetics. Precisely how anesthetics render patients unconscious remains unknown, however. Whether different general anesthetics have a common mechanism of action or a common site of action is also unclear.[1-3] The development of safer anesthetics requires a better understanding of how and where they work.

Understanding mechanisms by which anesthetic drugs act is of interest beyond the practice of anesthesiology. Because anesthetics appear to inhibit consciousness selectively while sparing more vegetative functions such as breathing and autonomic regulation, the key to anesthetic action may unlock the mysteries of the highest levels of brain function: consciousness. The currently accepted paradigm for understanding the brain and mind is as an array of 40 billion parallel neurons laterally connected by adaptive synapses: "neural nets." Computers and artificial intelligence designs are based on neural net models; thus, understanding anesthetic mechanisms has implications for neuroscience, cognitive science, computer science, and philosophy. Because synapses are particularly sensitive to general anesthetics at clinically relevant concentrations,[4,5] effects on synaptic activity may be a common link in the brain-mind connection.

For many years, the terms anesthesia and narcosis were synonymous. Discovery of opioid receptors and endogenous peptide opioids has demonstrated mechanistic differences from inhalation anesthetics, however. Subpopulations of opioid receptors (μ, δ, κ, σ) have selective effects,[6-8] and unlike inhalation anesthetics, a receptor-mediated mechanism is clear. At extremely high doses, however, opioids may also have nonspecific effects on membranes.[9] Ketamine, another intravenous anesthetic, may act through opioid receptors,[10] although this action has been disputed.[11] Ketamine and related compounds such as phencyclidine have been shown to block non-competitively neural excitation induced by the amino acid N-methyl-D-aspartate.[12]

Evidence for receptor-mediated effects of benzodiazepines[13,14] and barbiturates,[15-17] involving a τ-aminobutyric acid (GABA) receptor-chloride ion channel complex is substantial. The receptor complex is composed of at least four receptor sites that interact allosterically and modulate chloride ion conductance, which, in turn, mediates inhibitory neuronal activity. The sedative and anticonvulsant properties of these drugs appear to result from enhanced GABA-ergic activity. Whether this accounts for their hypnotic effects is uncertain, however.[16] Also unclear is how benzodiazepines cause amnesia. Although barbiturates are not considered analgesics, mild antinociceptive effects have been attributed to benzodiazepines, which may result from enhanced sedation or interactions with endogenous opioids.

Thus, distinct differences exist between drugs that have selective hypnotic, amnestic, or analgesic effects through actions on specific receptors and inhalation anesthetics, which have no apparent structure-activity relationship, yet provide all aspects of general anesthesia. This chapter emphasizes inhalation anesthetics, although this distinction may eventually prove arbitrary.

Inhalation (gaseous and volatile) anesthetics do not comprise a single chemical class and include compounds as diverse as xenon, a nonreactive noble gas under physiologic conditions, nitrous oxide, cyclopropane, diethyl ether, and halothane. Because of this structural diversity, most theories of anesthesia have attempted to relate potency to some physical property of anesthetics. Meyer (1899)[18] and Overton (1901)[19] observed what has proved to be a remarkable correlation between anesthetic potency and anesthetic solubility in olive oil. This relationship, the Meyer-Overton rule, is the basis for the unitary hypothesis of anesthesia, which proposes that all anesthetics act at membrane sites with identical molecular structure, although these sites may be widely distributed throughout the nervous system. The potency-solubility relationship predicts that anesthetics exert their effects when a specific number of molecules have reached the anesthetic "site of action." It also tells us something about the site of action: it is similar to olive oil. This has been interpreted to mean that the anesthetic site of action is a lipid with specific hydrophobic properties, but proteins have hydrophobic regions as well. Although describing a property of the anesthetic site of action, the Meyer-Overton rule does not provide a mechanistic explanation of general anesthesia.

The question of anesthetic mechanism may be approached from several levels. Where do general anesthetics act anatomically? That is, what part of the brain is most susceptible to anesthetics, and can this account for global interruption of consciousness? Is it within hippocampal regions where information is entered into memory, the reticular activating system, which regulates wakefulness, or synapses widely distributed throughout the cortex whose collective effects are cognitive awareness? The prefrontal cortex appears to have an executive function in retrieving information from storage memory sites and in acting on this information.

Some evidence suggests that anesthetics alter the balance between ascending and descending pathways in the reticular activating system, and this imbalance may induce unconsciousness.[20] We really do not know at what anatomic level general anesthetics act, however. What types of fiber tracts are involved? Are monosynaptic or polysynaptic pathways preferentially affected? Polysynaptic pathways, such as the reticular activating system, appear to be more sensitive to general anesthetics. Where do anesthetics act at the neuronal level? The answer to this question may depend largely on the doses of anesthetics used. At clinically relevant concentrations, general anesthetics inhibit excitatory synaptic transmission at both presynaptic and postsynaptic sites. At higher concentrations, axonal conduction block[21] (as with local anesthetics), inhibition of axonal transport, and depolymerization of microtubules may occur.

General anesthetics do not appear to inhibit synaptic transmission by depleting neurotransmitters; neither halothane nor enflurane affects acetylcholine levels in brain.[22] On the other hand, halothane and cyclopropane may increase levels of norepinephrine in specific regions of rat brain, such as the locus ceruleus of the brain stem reticular formation.[23] Enflurane has also been reported to increase whole-brain levels of dopamine.[24] In contrast, ablation of areas in the brain stem that secrete norepinephrine and dopamine appear to decrease halothane and cyclopropane minimum alveolar concentration (MAC) in rats, but only by about 35%.[25] The physiologic significance of these observations is unclear, because changes in neurotransmitter levels do not distinguish cause from effect. Measurable neurotransmitter levels may change because of alterations in production, metabolism, release, or other factors. Accordingly, experimental results often appear contradictory, and specific effects depend on the particular nerve preparation, neurotransmitter, and anesthetic studied.

Potentiation of inhibitory neuronal transmission may also occur.[26,27] For example, halothane and enflurane inhibit catabolism of GABA in rat brain synaptosomes in a dose-dependent fashion.[28] More recent work suggests that volatile anesthetics enhance inhibitory transmission in rat hippocampus, but probably by a mechanism other than $GABA_A$ potentiation.[29] Dluzewski and associates[30] have reviewed anesthetic effects on neuronal activity at the anatomic and cellular levels, and effects on synapses have been extensively reviewed by Wann and Macdonald.[31] Alteration of synaptic activity fits nicely with the neural net concept but does not address the question of how anesthetics work at a molecular level.

HISTORICAL REVIEW OF THEORIES OF ANESTHESIA

Efforts to understand anesthesia go back nearly a century and a half. Many were simply correlative and attempted to relate anesthetic potency to a physical property of the drug. Several of the more outstanding of these are briefly reviewed. Although some of these early theories are naive by today's standards, they are the forerunners of modern molecular theories of anesthesia.

1847: Cell Fat Dissolution Theory

Von Bibra and Harless[32] established a correlation between anesthetic action and relative solubility of anesthetics in lipid and nonlipid constituents of brain cells. They believed that ethers and ethyl chloride dissolved fat-like substances from the brain and deposited them in the liver, thereby causing anesthesia. In this belief they erred, but the lipid-solubility factor was the precursor of the work of Meyer and Overton in 1899 to 1901.

1875: Colloid Theory

Claude Bernard[33] believed that a reversible coagulation of cell colloids produced or accompanied anesthesia. His belief was based on observations of anesthetic-induced cessation of protoplasmic streaming in slime mold. The colloid theory may best be remembered as the first suggesting that anesthetics act by a common mechanism; this was probably the first statement of a unitary hypothesis of anesthesia.

Today, we have a much greater understanding of the nature and dynamics of protoplasm. Cytoskeletal proteins (microtubules, actin, and intermediate filaments, for example) organize protoplasmic activities and are susceptible to anesthetics. A modern view of the colloid theory was suggested by Allison and Nunn,[34] who showed that halothane depolymerized microtubules (an effect also produced by high pressure). Depolymerization, however, occurred at higher than clinical concentrations of halothane. Nonetheless, cytoskeletal activities, which have been implicated in cognitive functions,[35] may be inhibited by clinically relevant anesthetic concentrations. Another possibility is that membrane proteins (ion channels and receptors) anchored to the cytoskeleton may be rendered dysfunctional because of cytoplasmic-cytoskeletal disruption.

1899 to 1901: Lipid-Solubility Theory

Based on the earlier work of von Bibra and Harless, Meyer[18] and Overton[19] independently proposed a theory of anesthesia based on the solubility of anesthetics in lipid. Three postulates governed this theory:

1. Any chemical soluble in fat or fat-like substances must exert an anesthetic action, insofar as it can become distributed in it.
2. The effect must manifest itself first and most markedly in those cells in which lipids are crucial to function, e.g., nerve cells.
3. The relative potency of anesthetics must correlate with their lipid solubility.

Meyer and Overton assessed potency by determining concentrations of anesthetics necessary to anesthetize tadpoles in water and measured anesthetic oil/gas and oil/water partition coefficients. They concluded that anesthetic concentrations in lipid (olive oil) were the same whether administered in the gas or aqueous phase, and thus potency of an anesthetic was dependent only on its lipid solubility. The relation of anesthetic potency to lipid solubility holds true today and is a correlation that must be accounted for by all modern theories of anesthesia.

1907: Alteration of Cell Membrane Permeability

In 1907, Hober[36] suggested that absorbed anesthetics decrease the permeability of the cell. In 1909, Lillie[37] brought forth his view that anything that made the cell membrane less permeable or less capable of undergoing electrical depolarization had an inhibitory effect on the cell. Anesthetics were thought to decrease normal cell permeability, whereas stimulants had an opposite effect.

This theory is of more than historical interest because it presaged a modern theory of general anesthesia. Gage and associates[27] have proposed that general anesthetics alter the stability of receptor-channel complexes, either decreasing ionic channel open time at excitatory synapses or increasing channel open time at inhibitory synapses. The net result would be depression of excitatory synaptic transmission. The potency of anesthetics (ether, enflurane, halothane, and chloroform) in shortening the duration of postsynaptic end-plate potentials in mouse diaphragm preparations increases with increasing lipid solubility, in accordance with the Meyer-Overton rule.[38] Again, the molecular basis for these effects is uncertain. Whether inhalation anesthetics block ion channels directly (the open channel blocking model), alter ion channel conductance by increasing surrounding membrane fluidity, or interact with the channel complex at the lipid-protein interface is not clear. Anesthetic binding to hydrophobic regions of transmembrane channel proteins may alter kinetics of channel opening and closing without directly blocking ion conductance pathways.[39]

1954: Membrane Volume Expansion

Mullins[40] reexamined the relation between olive oil solubility and anesthetic potency and suggested that potency correlated better with the volume than with the number of anesthetic molecules dissolved in the oil phase of the membrane. He speculated that anesthetics filled voids in the membrane rather than adding to membrane volume. The observation that general anesthetic potency was reduced by high hydrostatic pressure,[41,42] however, suggested that anesthetics do increase membrane volume. This led Miller and colleagues[43] to propose the critical volume hypothesis, which states that anesthesia occurs when absorbed anesthetics expand membrane volume beyond a critical amount. Pressure is thought to reverse the anesthetic effect by compressing the membrane back to its original volume, trapping anesthetic molecules in membrane target sites. This theory is discussed in greater detail later in this chapter.

1957: Anesthetic Potency and van der Waals Constants

Wulf and Featherstone[44] identified a qualitative correlation between potency of anesthetics and their van der Waals constants. The van der Waals equation modifies the ideal gas law ($p\overline{V} = RT$) to take into account the influence of molecular size and weak intermolecular forces on the pressure of a gas.

$$P = [RT/(\overline{V} - b)] - a/\overline{V}^2$$

is the van der Waals equation, where P is pressure, T is temperature, $\overline{V}$ is molar volume, R is the gas constant, and "a" and "b" are constants. "a" ($liter^2 \times moles^{-2}$) is a positive constant roughly proportional to the energy of vaporization of a liquid and is a measure of weak attractive forces between molecules; "b" (liters/mole) is the molar volume of a gas at $0°K$; as pressure becomes infinite, the molar volume of a gas approaches the limiting value of b. Thus, the van der Waals equation gives qualitative reasons for deviations from ideal behavior of real gases.[45] Koski and colleagues[46] examined this relationship more closely and demonstrated a linear relationship between the log of anesthetic partial pressure (potency) and $a^{1/2}$. Such a plot divides the anesthetics into three categories: (1) those that form nearly ideal solutions, e.g., inert gases such as argon and xenon; (2) hydrogen-bonding molecules such as the ethers; and (3) fluorinated anesthetics, which have an excess electronegative charge. Biologic potency may arise from various physical properties of anesthetic molecules, such as charge distribution and ability to form hydrogen bonds, which affect their ability to interact with the active site. That the van der Waals constants, like solubility, correlate with potency is reasonable because solubility depends not only on temperature and pressure, but also on attractive forces between solute (gas) and solvent (active site).

The significance of Wulf and Featherstone's work is that it began to provide a mechanistic explanation, in molecular terms, of how a physical property such as lipid solubility may account for anesthetic potency. An updated version of their correlation suggests that anesthetics bind to hydrophobic sites by hydrogen bonding or by weaker, reversible van der Waals forces. This interaction, in turn, may alter the binding site. Using a nonbiologic model, Hameroff and Watt[47] showed that the potent inhalation anesthetics halothane, enflurane, isoflurane, and trichloroethylene strongly inhibit free electron mobility. These investigators speculated that, whereas hydrophobic solubility determines anesthetic binding at the site of action, inhibition of electron mobility therein may determine anesthetic effects by preventing electron dipole-related conformational changes of proteins required for neuronal activity.

PHYSICAL AND CHEMICAL PROPERTIES OF INHALED ANESTHETICS

The bewildering array of molecules with anesthetic effects has prompted attempts to relate anesthetic activity to general physical properties of these drugs. Before discussing various theories further, it is worthwhile to review some of the physical and chemical properties of inhalation anesthetics.

Although at least 15 inhalation anesthetics have been introduced into clinical practice since diethyl ether was first used,[48] only nitrous oxide, halothane (a halogenated alkane), and enflurane and isoflurane (isomers of a halogenated ether) are in common use today. Desflurane, a substituted derivative of isoflurane (fluorine for chlorine) was introduced into clinical use in 1992, and experience with the agent is still not widespread. Sevoflurane, another agent with a promising clinical profile, has not yet been released for general clinical use. Although all the obsolete agents produced anesthesia, most were abandoned because they were flammable or had undesirable cardiac or toxic side effects. Chemical structures of various inhalation anesthetics are shown in Figure 25-1, and some physical and chemical properties are listed in Table 25-1. Chemical structures do not correlate well with anesthetic activity; however, they do have a relation to various unwanted side effects. In this regard some generalizations on structure-activity relationships can be made[54-56]:

1. Although halogenation of hydrocarbons and ethers increases anesthetic potency, it also increases the potential for inducing cardiac arrhythmias in the following order: F < Cl < Br.
2. Ethers that have an asymmetric halogenated carbon tend to be good anesthetics (such as enflurane).

3. Halogenated methyl ethyl ethers (enflurane and isoflurane) are more stable, are more potent, and have better clinical profiles than halogenated diethyl ethers.
4. Fluorination decreases flammability and increases stability of adjacent halogenated carbons.
5. Complete halogenation of alkanes and ethers or full halogenation of end methyl groups decreases potency and enhances convulsant activity. Flurothyl ($CF_3CH_2OCH_2CF_3$) is a potent convulsant, with a median effective dose (ED_{50}) for convulsions in mice of 0.00122 atm.[55]
6. The presence of double bonds tends to increase chemical reactivity and toxicity.

These comments are just a few of the generalizations that can be made about the relation of chemical structure of anesthetics to clinical profiles and are largely empiric. Nonetheless, they have served as useful guidelines for the development of new anesthetics. Terrell[48] and Halsey[56] reviewed the physical and chemical properties of the inhalation anesthetics in detail.

ANESTHETIC POTENCY AND LIPID SOLUBILITY

Theories of anesthetic mechanisms of action (as well as clinical utility) require a measure of relative anesthetic potencies. Traditionally, the pharmacologic term ED_{50}, the concentration of a drug that produces a specific effect in 50% of animals tested, has served as a measure of

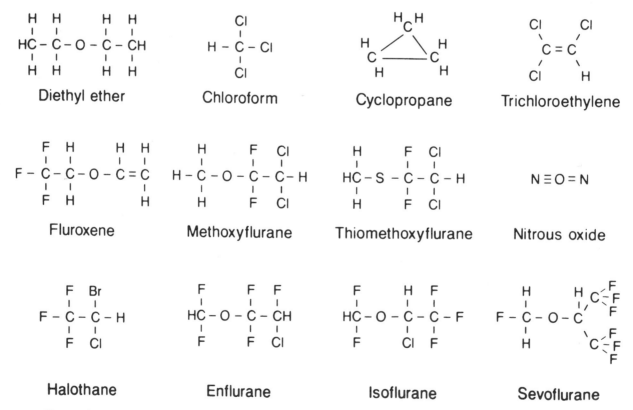

Fig. 25-1. Chemical structures of inhaled anesthetics. Desflurane, the newest agent released into clinical practice, has the same structure as isoflurane, except that the chlorine atom is replaced by fluorine.

Table 25-1. Physical and Chemical Properties of Inhaled Anesthetics

Name	Chemical Formula	Fist Clinical Use	Mol. Wt. (g/mol)	BP* (°C)	VP† (mmHg at 20°C)	Oil/Gas Partition Coefficient (at 37°C)
Nitrous oxide	N_2O	1844	44.0	−88.5	—	1.4
Diethyl ether	$(C_2H_5)O$	1842 1846	74.1	34.6	440	65
Chloroform	$CHCl_3$	1847	119.4	61.2	160	265
Cyclopropane	$C\text{-}C_3H_6$	1933	42.1	−32.9	—	11.8
Trichloroethylene	CCl_2CHCl	1935	131.4	87.2	64.5	200–250
Halothane	$CF_3CHClBr$	1956	197.4	50.2	243	224
Fluroxene	$CF_3CH_2OCHCH_2$	1960	126.0	43.2	369	47.7
Methoxyflurane	$CH_3OCF_2CHCl_2$	1962	165.0	104.8	23	970
Thiomethoxyflurane	$CH_3SCF_2CHCl_2$	—	180.0	—	6 (25°C)	7,230
Enflurane	CHF_2OCF_2CHFCl	1972	184.5	56.5	175	96.5
Isoflurane	$CHF_2OCHClCF_3$	1981	184.5	48.5	239	90.8
Sevoflurane	$CH_2FOCH(CF_3)_2$	—	200.1	58.5	157	55
Desflurane	$CHF_2OCHFCF_3$	1992	168.0	23.5	664	18.7

Values were obtained from references 48, 49, 50, 51, 52, and 53.
*Boiling point.
†Vapor pressure.

Table 25-2. Lipid Solubilities and Potencies of Inhaled Anesthetics

Anesthetics	Oil/Gas Partition Coefficient (37°C)	MAC Dogs (atm)*	MAC Humans (atm)
Thiomethoxyflurane	7,230	.00035	—
Methoxyflurane	970	.0023	.0016
Chloroform	265	.0077	—
Halothane	224	.0087	.0077
Enflurane	96.5	.0267	.0168
Isoflurane	90.8	.0141	.0115
Ether	65	.0304	.0192
Sevoflurane	55	.0236	.0205
Fluroxene	47.7	.0599	.034
Desflurane	18.7	—	.072
Cyclopropane	11.8	.175	.092
Xenon	1.9	1.19	.71
Nitrous oxide	1.4	1.88	1.04
Sulfur hexafluoride	0.293	4.9	—
Carbon tetrafluoride	0.073	26	—

*To convert from atmospheres to percent inspired gas, multiply by 100.
Values were obtained from references 48 to 53.
MAC = minimum alveolar concentration.

anesthetic potency. When comparing inhaled anesthetics, a more convenient way of expressing potency was provided by Merkel and Eger,[57] who introduced the concept of MAC, or minimal alveolar concentration. MAC is the alveolar concentration of an anesthetic, expressed in atmospheres, partial pressure, or percentage of total alveolar gases, that prevents movement in 50% of subjects in response to skin incision or some other noxious stimulus. MAC is determined after equilibration of inspired and end-tidal (alveolar) anesthetic has occurred, which assumes an equal anesthetic partial pressure (not concentration, which varies with solubility) in alveoli, blood, and brain. Potency is the reciprocal of MAC; i.e., the higher the potency, the lower the MAC. Table 25-2 shows MAC values for certain inhaled anesthetics. Values are highly reproducible within a species and correlate well among species (Fig. 25-2).

The physical property of inhalation anesthetics that correlates best with potency is lipid solubility.[50] As shown in Figure 25-3, a log-log plot of experimentally derived MAC values in dogs versus solubility in olive oil yields a straight line with a slope of −1 over a 100,000-fold range of anesthetic partial pressures and oil/gas partition coefficients.[49] This relationship predicts that all anes-

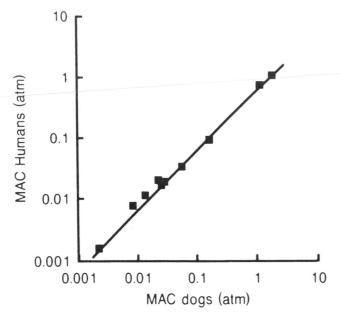

Fig. 25–2. Correlation of minimum alveolar concentration (MAC) values for dogs and humans (data from Table 25–2).

thetics exert their action when an equal number of molecules have reached the anesthetic site of action.[50] Stated another way, all anesthetics are equally potent at the lipid-like site of action.[1] The relationship between anesthetic potency and concentration at the anesthetic site of action can be demonstrated by mathematic manipulation of the relationship depicted graphically in Figure 25-3:

$$\log MAC = -\log S + A \qquad (1)$$

where S is the oil/gas solubility coefficient (the ratio of anesthetic concentrations in oil and gas; i.e., the volume

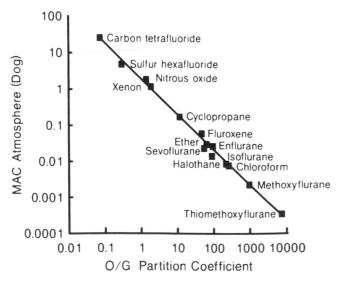

Fig. 25–3. Log-log plot of oil/gas (O/G) partition coefficients and minimum alveolar concentration (MAC) values for dogs (data from Table 25–2).

of anesthetic gas absorbed per volume of oil versus the volume of anesthetic per volume of total gas) and A is a constant that varies among species.

Equation 1 may be rewritten as follows:

$$\log MAC = \log 1/S + A \qquad (2)$$

and accordingly:

$$10^{(\log MAC)} = 10^{(\log 1/S + A)}$$
$$10^{(\log MAC)} = 10^{(\log 1/S)} \times 10^A \qquad (3)$$

and:

$$MAC = 1/S \times 10^A$$

thus:

$$MAC \times S = 10^A \qquad (4)$$

Letting 10^A (a constant) = K, then:

$$MAC \times S = K \qquad (5)$$

S is simply the ratio of anesthetic concentrations in an olive oil-like site and in the gas phase, however. At MAC, it may be rewritten as follows:

$$S = C_{50}/MAC \qquad (6)$$

where C_{50} is the concentration of anesthetic at the active site when 50% of organisms are anesthetized.[58]

Rewriting equation 5 yields:

$$MAC \times C_{50}/MAC = K \qquad (7)$$

and:

$$C_{50} = K \qquad (8)$$

Therefore, the concentration of any anesthetic at such a site is constant at MAC. In this derivation, K (or C_{54}) is expressed in atmospheres, and is equivalent to the volume (in liters) of anesthetic gas absorbed (per liter of oil) at the "olive oil-like" site. It is a relatively simple matter to convert from atmospheres (vapor volume) to moles. From Avogadro's law, we know that the volume of 1 mol of gas at 0°C and 1 atm (STP) is 22.4 L and at 37°C is 25.4 L (obtained by multiplying 22.4 × 310°/273°). An average value of K for 18 inhaled anesthetics in dogs determined by Koblin and Eger[50] is 2.12 ± 0.13 (SD) atmospheres (atm). To convert to moles, divide this number by 25.4 L of anesthetic gas/mole. This yields a theoretic concentration of anesthetic at the olive oil-like site of about 80 mmol/L. For humans, the concentration is about 50 mmol/L, based on a mean value of K for 10 inhaled anesthetics of 1.35 ± 0.09 atm.[50] In fact, these theoretic concentrations are probably too large. As Seeman[59] pointed out, experimentally determined erythrocyte membrane/buffer partition coefficients for certain inhaled anesthetics are about 7 to 15 times less than their corresponding oil/water coefficients. Accordingly, based on the foregoing calculations, the theoretic concentration of anesthetic at the membrane active site may be closer to 5 mmol/L. (Seeman suggested a value of 3 mmol/L anesthetic/kg dry membrane.)

This concentration is still high when one considers that many drugs are effective in the nanomolar to micromolar range. Thus, it is not really surprising that inhalation anesthetics have so many side effects (e.g., cardiac arrhythmias, toxicities, etc.) unrelated to apparent anesthetic activity. In this regard, each anesthetic has its own clinical profile of associated circulatory, pulmonary, and cerebral blood flow effects that must be appreciated by the anesthesiologist. Much of the clinical research on anesthetics necessarily focuses on these issues, because the principal factor that now determines the acceptability of a general anesthetic is the incidence of adverse side effects.[60]

The remarkably good correlation of anesthetic potency with solubility in olive oil holds true only when considering the inhaled anesthetics. The correlation is not as good for other anesthetic agents, such as the alcohols. When the slightly more polar solvent octanol is used, however, an excellent correlation for all anesthetics and all animals is obtained.[61] In contrast, a nonpolar solvent such as hexadecane gives a poor correlation. This suggests that the active site is more like octanol than olive oil and is amphiphilic in nature, having both polar and apolar characteristics.[1]

Despite this generally good correlation, apparent exceptions to the rule exist, such as with the poorly soluble gases (e.g., hydrogen). Another is the so-called "cutoff effect," in which a loss in anesthetic potency occurs with higher members of a homologous series of anesthetic agents, such as with the n-alcohols and n-alkanes. Activity disappears at about C_{13} with the alcohols[62] and at about C_{10} with the alkanes.[63] This phenomenon has been attributed to the low aqueous solubilities of the larger compounds, which prevents anesthetizing concentrations from being achieved in membranes.[64] Alternatively, it has been suggested that larger members of these series are simply too big to fit into the membrane site of action.[63,65]

Another apparent deviation from the Meyer-Overton rule is the ability of some anesthetics to cause convulsions.[50] Enflurane, for example, has weak convulsant effects, whereas flurothyl is a potent convulsant. Koblin and associates[55] compared the convulsant and anesthetic activities of flurothyl in mice and demonstrated that the ED_{50} for convulsions is 0.00122 atm, tenfold lower than the ED_{50} for its anesthetic effect. The product of the ED_{50} for loss of the righting reflex, 0.0122 atm, and the oil/gas partition coefficient, 46.9, equals 0.57 atm, a value that falls within the range of K values determined for other anesthetics in mice.[55] This indicates that anesthetics may have properties that are antagonistic to their anesthetic effects, which become apparent at different concentrations. This finding is consistent with the observations of Richter and colleagues,[66] who showed, using isolated crab neuromuscular junction preparations, that methoxyflurane (0.1 mmol/L) selectively blocked excitatory (glutamate) synaptic transmission, whereas flurothyl (0.1

mmol/L) specifically blocked inhibitory (GABA) transmission. At higher concentrations (1 mmol/L), both drugs inhibited excitatory and inhibitory transmission. This type of phenomenon may explain why enflurane, an isomer of isoflurane with about the same lipid solubility, has a MAC approximately 50% higher than that of isoflurane.

Because the potency-solubility relationship implies that the number, rather than the type of molecules, determines anesthetic action, one would predict that the effects of anesthetics should be additive; 0.5 MAC of one agent plus 0.5 MAC of a second agent should be roughly equivalent to 1.0 MAC of either agent alone. In general, this appears to be true. For example, 70% nitrous oxide (0.67 MAC) lowers halothane MAC by about 60%[67] and enflurane MAC by about 70%.[68]

Again, exceptions to the rule exist. For example, sulfur hexafluoride and argon appear to be antagonistic in mice, in which the cumulative effect is less than would be expected, based on the potencies of the individual agents alone.[69] The reason for this effect is not clear, but as Wardley-Smith and Halsey[3] pointed out, nonadditivity was seen only at high pressures, when sulfur hexafluoride (ED_{50} in mice of about 5 atm) was combined with argon (ED_{50} of about 16 atm), a gas of low solubility. This brings up the issues of pressure reversal of anesthesia (discussed later in the chapter) and effects of high pressure, which are themselves controversial. High pressure induces the high-pressure neurologic syndrome (HPNS) in animals, which may obscure or antagonize anesthetic effects. Pressure reversal of anesthesia may be caused by activation of separate physiologic processes in the central nervous system, unrelated to anesthetic action, that override anesthetic effects.[31]

That opioids such as morphine and fentanyl have a "ceiling effect" in reducing enflurane MAC, however, is not surprising, because opioids clearly have a receptor-mediated basis of action. Even at extremely high doses, morphine (5 mg/kg) and fentanyl (270 μg/kg) only reduce enflurane MAC in dogs by a maximum of about 65 percent.[70,71]

Several points can be made in summarizing this section. The Meyer-Overton rule implies a unitary molecular site of action of inhaled anesthetics.[50] Additivity of inhaled agents adds further support for this hypothesis. A logarithmic plot of anesthetic potencies and lipid solubilities tends to obscure deviations from the rule, such as the differing potencies of enflurane and isoflurane, however, despite their similar solubilities. Deviations from the Meyer-Overton rule lend credence to alternate theories, e.g., the multisite hypothesis of anesthesia,[3] although confounding factors arising from experimental technique may cloud the issue.

MOLECULAR MECHANISMS OF GENERAL ANESTHESIA

The question of how inhalation anesthetics act at a molecular level can be approached from two general directions: (1) anesthetic-induced effects on bulk membrane lipids, including alterations in membrane physical state; and (2) effects on membrane proteins. Both may include effects at the lipid-protein interface. The rapid and reversible actions of anesthetics tend to discount long-term biochemical alterations as a viable explanation of anesthetic action, although short-term biochemical mechanisms have not been excluded. These have been reviewed be Ueda and Kamaya[72] and are not discussed further here.

Anesthesiologists generally agree that anesthetics ultimately affect membrane proteins. Whether anesthetics act directly on proteins or affect them indirectly by first altering membrane lipids is unclear, however. The Meyer-Overton rule has been used to support both points of view. Effects on membrane lipids are considered first, after a brief review of membrane structure.

Structure of Cell Membranes

Every cell has a boundary membrane about 80 Å thick that plays an active role in controlling the flow of molecules into and out of the cell. Membranes are composed of phospholipids with interspersed protein units. The phospholipid components have a hydrophilic phosphorus group head and a long, hydrophobic fatty acid tail. Such molecules are arranged in a bilayer formation with the hydrophilic polar heads outward and the hydrophobic tails inward, parallel to each other in the membrane interior. Proteins are embedded in the lipid matrix. Some span the membrane and function as ion channels, which may be activated by ligand-receptor interactions or by changes in membrane potential (voltage-dependent channels). Activation results in a conformational change in channel proteins that allows ions to flow across the membrane. The resultant current generates an action potential.

Critical Volume Hypothesis

Most lipid theories of anesthesia assume that general anesthetics are dissolved in the lipid components of the membrane and thus exert their primary effects on lipid moieties. A major clue to how anesthetics may affect membranes was provided by the phenomenon of pressure reversal of anesthesia, in which simple hydrostatic pressure, on the order of 100 to 150 atm, was shown to reverse anesthetic inhibition of light emission by luminous bacteria.[73] Pressure reversal of anesthesia was subsequently confirmed in higher organisms, which led Miller and colleagues[43] to propose the critical volume hypothesis. This theory postulates that anesthesia occurs when absorbed anesthetics expand membrane volume beyond a critical amount. Pressure is thought to reverse the anesthetic effect by compressing membrane hydrophobic sites back to their original volume, trapping anesthetic molecules in the target site, or perhaps squeezing them out. This theory predicts that more anesthetic is required in the presence of higher pressures, to counteract the pressure-induced reduction in volume of the active site. This prediction agrees well with pressure reversal data for inhaled anesthetics in newts and mice.

The critical volume hypothesis also predicts that gaseous anesthetics in the clinical range should expand the membrane by about 0.2%, if olive oil is used as a model of membrane lipids.[43] This hypothesis is in agreement with measurements obtained with artificial lipid bilayers.[2] Confirmation of this with biologic membranes has been a technically difficult problem. Franks and Lieb[74] reexamined this issue by measuring solution densities of membrane suspensions. This procedure allowed them to make direct measurements of the volume occupied by general anesthetics in biologic membranes. Red cell membranes, which are about 50% protein, were found to expand considerably less than previously thought, only about 0.1%. Although anesthetics such as halothane did increase membrane volume, the expansion was attributed almost entirely to the van der Waals volume of the anesthetic molecules themselves; the volume occupied by a halothane molecule is the same in membranes, water, and liquid halothane. Anesthetic molecules did not appear to create a large additional volume in membranes that can then be compressed by high pressure. The small increase that was seen is equivalent to that caused by a rise in temperature of only 1° or 2°C. Clearly, increasing body temperature by a few degrees does not induce anesthesia in cold-blooded animals or humans. Franks and Lieb concluded from their study that membrane volume expansion is irrelevant to the mechanism of anesthesia.[74]

Ueda and Kamaya[72] criticized the critical volume hypothesis on thermodynamic grounds, because it ignores certain thermodynamic parameters, including thermal expansibility, compressibility, and partial molar volumes of other components of the system (in addition to the anesthetic and membrane target site). These investigators argued that the hypothesis would hold only when all other factors that contribute to the volume of the entire system remained constant under high pressure.

Alterations in Lipid Bilayer Fluidity

In 1968, Metcalf and co-workers[75] demonstrated that benzyl alcohol increased mobility of membrane components in erythrocytes. This finding led to the hypothesis that general anesthetics act by increasing membrane lipid fluidity, which indirectly perturbs membrane protein function. Halothane causes a dose-related increase in the mobility of fatty acid chains in phospholipid bilayers, at clinically relevant concentrations.[76] High pressure in the range of 100 atm does have a weak ordering effect on membranes, consistent with pressure reversal data. Changes in fluidity are extremely small, however; equivalent increases in fluidity occur when lipid bilayers are warmed by less than 1°C.

Phase-Transition Theory

Problems with the fluidization theory led Trudell[77] to speculate that anesthetics may produce small alterations in membrane physical state that are subsequently amplified, producing a larger change in some other property of the membrane. He proposed that phospholipid bilayers are poised at a temperature-dependent transition between liquid and gel states. This coexistence of fluid and gel domains in a membrane is termed lateral phase separation, because it occurs laterally in the plane of the membrane. Trudell speculated that, during membrane excitation, ionic channel proteins undergo a conformational change that increases lateral dimensions of the protein and opens the ionic channel. Expansion of the channel protein is accommodated by transition of adjacent lipid from the disordered fluid phase into the more compact gel phase. As noted previously, anesthetics increase lipid fluidity, which would tend to prevent conversion to the gel phase. A small increase in membrane fluidity may result in a large decrease in lateral compressibility of the bilayer. It is hypothesized that this prevents conformational changes in ionic channel proteins and thus inhibits membrane excitation. A small, nonspecific change in lipid physical state could conceivably result in a physiologically important change in ion channel function. The same criticisms involving temperature apply to the lateral phase separation theory, however. Although the phase-transition temperature (from gel to fluid) of lipid bilayers is decreased several degrees by clinical concentrations of anesthetics, an effect that can be reversed by small amounts of pressure (around 20 atm), an equivalent fluidization can be produced by an increase in membrane temperature of less than 1°C.[78] This theory also has been criticized because anesthetic potencies do not correlate with anesthetic-induced phase transition temperature changes.[62]

An enormous amount of research has accumulated on the interaction of anesthetics with lipids. This subject has been reviewed in detail by Miller,[2] Dluzewski and associates,[30] Wann and Macdonald,[31] and Ueda and Kamaya.[72] In general, lipid theories imply a nonspecific, physicochemical basis for anesthetic effects, rather than a selective interaction of anesthetic molecules with a specific molecular target. The interaction is presumed to be nonspecific because of the structural and chemical diversity of anesthetic molecules. How perturbation of membrane lipids can alter specific membrane proteins, such as ion channels, remains unclear, however.

Protein-Anesthetic Interactions

In spite of the large amount of research devoted to lipid theories, there is a growing consensus that anesthetics act directly on proteins. For years, Franks and Lieb[1,61,65,74] have pointed out inconsistencies in lipid hypotheses. A major criticism has been that lipid perturbations are exceedingly small at clinical concentrations of anesthetics. By a process of elimination, these investigators suggested that the anesthetic site must be, at least in part, protein. This led them to reconsider whether olive oil is a good model of the anesthetic target site. They suggested that octanol is a better model,[61] thereby implying that, although the site is hydrophobic, it also has polar characteristics. Such a site could reside on membrane proteins or at the lipid-protein interface.

Numerous reports note that anesthetics can interact directly with proteins, such as the acetylcholine receptor, and induce conformational changes that alter binding equilibria of ligands.[79] The most convincing evidence is provided by anesthetic inhibition of the purified light-emitting enzyme luciferase.[80-83] Firefly luciferase, a 100,000-molecular weight soluble protein, emits a photon of light when it combines with its substrate luciferin (280 mW), in the presence of adenosine triphosphate,

magnesium, and oxygen. Anesthetics are thought to inhibit luciferase activity by competing with luciferin for the enzyme active site.

To determine whether anesthetic potencies correlate with enzyme inhibiting activity, Franks and Lieb[83] studied many anesthetics, including diethyl ether, chloroform, halothane, and methoxyflurane. These investigators found that anesthetic potencies over a 100,000-fold range correlated almost exactly with anesthetic ED_{50s} for inhibition of luciferase. Analysis of these data provided an estimate of the dimensions of the target site; it can accommodate 2 halothane molecules but only 1 molecule of decanol (or 1 molecule of the natural substrate luciferin). From analysis of equilibrium data, Franks and Lieb calculated that the dissociation constant for halothane (the aqueous concentration that half-saturates the binding sites) is 0.54 mmol/L. The luciferin-anesthetic binding site appears to be a hydrophobic pocket in the luciferase protein. If it extends to the water-protein surface, then it should have both polar and apolar characteristics. Indeed, chloroform and hexanol, which show nearly equipotent inhibition of luciferase, have almost identical octanol/water coefficients.[84] Thus, the anesthetic binding site on luciferase is similar to that of octanol, and inhibition of luciferase by general anesthetics appears to obey the Meyer-Overton rule. Moreover, anesthetic binding to luciferase demonstrates definite cutoff effects, similar to those found for general anesthesia, which may be attributed to the circumscribed dimensions of the binding site.[65]

Luciferase appears to be a good model of the anesthetic site of action. Clearly, however, luciferase has no relation to anesthesia. What, then, are the implications of this model for possible molecular mechanisms of anesthesia? Franks and Lieb[84] speculate that, because hydrophobic pockets have been found on certain soluble proteins, similar sites will likely be found on membrane receptors in the nervous system. Anesthetics may act by competing with endogenous ligands, such as neurotransmitters, for these active sites.

Given that proteins may satisfy the physical and functional requirements of an anesthetic binding site, does evidence indicate that such sites actually exist in the central nervous system? An initial report by Evers and co-workers[85] generated considerable interest because halothane appeared to bind selectively to sites in whole rat brain that became saturated at clinical concentrations of the anesthetic. Using nuclear magnetic resonance spectroscopy, halothane concentrations in brain appeared to plateau at an inspired concentration of about 2.5%; half-maximal "saturation" occurred at 1.2%, a value close to the MAC of halothane in rats. In a subsequent, carefully conducted study, however, Lockhart and colleagues[86] showed that this lack of correlation between inspired and brain concentrations of halothane was actually due to respiratory depression caused by the anesthetic, rather than to saturation of cerebral binding sites. Similar results were obtained with isoflurane. Thus, at present, little evidence of saturable binding sites for inhalation anesthetics exists.

In molecular terms, how might anesthetics alter neuronal activity? Gage and associates[27] have suggested that general anesthetics interfere with the stability of membrane receptor channel proteins, thereby decreasing ionic conductance. Brett and colleagues[39] studied the effects of isoflurane on the functional properties of a well-characterized membrane ion channel, the acetylcholine receptor channel. Using the extremely sensitive patch clamp technique, they were able to record acetylcholine-induced electrical currents through single ion channels on muscle cells in culture. Kinetic properties of the channels were rapidly and reversibly altered by isoflurane concentrations as low as 0.45 mmol/L. In the presence of isoflurane, the channels were observed to "flicker" rapidly, in a burst-like pattern between open and closed states. Open channel time tended to shorten, and closed time to lengthen, in a dose-dependent fashion. The mean amplitude of ionic currents was unchanged, indicating that partial occlusion of channels did not occur. Although some of these effects were consistent with the open channel blocking model, these investigators that the kinetics of channel activity failed to support that hypothesis. They also believed their data tended to exclude non-specific effects on membrane lipids as a cause of altered channel activity. For example, according to the membrane fluidity hypothesis, warming of the membrane by several degrees should alter channel activity. Although warming did enhance channel closing rates, raising membrane temperature by up to 15°C did not reproduce the flickering activity caused by isoflurane. The authors concluded that the most probable sites of action of isoflurane are at or near the lipid-protein interface. They speculated that isoflurane may alter channel kinetics by an allosteric mechanism, perhaps by binding to hydrophobic domains on transmembrane channel proteins.

Finally, a promising new approach to investigating anesthetic action should be mentioned. The complexity of the nervous system in higher organisms has made it difficult to relate anesthetic-induced changes in membranes to disruption of neurologic function in whole animals. This prompted Morgan and Cascorbi[87] to search for a simpler animal model with which to study anesthetic action. They proposed that the small, free-living nematode *Caenorhabditis elegans* is such a model. The hermaphrodite always consists of 959 cells, of which exactly 302 are neurons. Every synapse in the nervous system has been mapped, along with all cell lineages. In addition, large parts of the organism's genome have been sequenced, and it is possible to clone these genes and to manufacture their protein products.

Most important, *C. elegans* responds to volatile anesthetics in a manner similar to that of mammals, in accordance with the Meyer-Overton rule.[87] In addition, two mutant strains of the organism have been identified that are two to three times more sensitive to the highly lipid-soluble anesthetics halothane, chloroform, methoxyflurane, and thiomethoxyflurane than the wild-type strain.[88,89] Responses of these mutants to volatile anesthetics with oil/gas partition coefficients equal to or larger than halothane deviate sharply from the Meyer-Overton rule. These strains may represent the first animals that exhibit a documented deviation from this correlation.[89] Morgan and associates[89] believe that these mutants have a geneti-

cally altered site of action for volatile anesthetics. They speculate that the corresponding wild-type forms of the mutant genes may code for enzymes in a common metabolic pathway; the products of this pathway somehow control anesthetic sensitivity.

Morgan and colleagues[90] extended their observations to include nine volatile anesthetics and characterized mutations in three other genes that act as indirect suppressors of the two mutant genes that increase sensitivity to the highly lipid-soluble anesthetics. These investigators suggest the existence of multiple classes of volatile anesthetics, which have similar but distinct molecular sites of action within the membrane. Because of their similarities, the different membrane sites are susceptible to anesthetic effects, but at slightly different concentrations. Small deviations from the Meyer-Overton rule may not be apparent on a log-log plot of potencies and lipid solubilities.

What are the anesthetic sites of action? They may be a family of structurally similar ion channels or regions in cell membranes. By cloning genes in *C. elegans* that alter anesthetic sensitivity and by sequencing their products, investigators may possibly be able to identify specific molecular targets for volatile anesthetics. If control of anesthetic responses can be analyzed at the molecular level in a simple animal such as *C. elegans,* basic principles may emerge that apply to other species.

SUMMARY

Efforts to understand mechanisms of action of anesthetics go back nearly 150 years. The wide range of molecules that cause anesthesia suggests that function must relate to some physical property of these drugs. The property of inhaled anesthetics that correlates best with potency is lipid solubility. This correlation has led to the widespread belief that anesthetics interact with lipid components of membranes. Because of the structural and chemical diversity of anesthetic molecules, most lipid theories imply a nonspecific, physicochemical basis for anesthesia, rather than a selective interaction with a known molecular target. Most agree that anesthetics ultimately affect membrane proteins, however.

A problem with lipid theories is that it remains unclear how nonspecific perturbations of membrane lipids can alter membrane protein function. The result is a growing consensus that anesthetics must somehow interact directly with proteins. The luciferase model demonstrates that anesthetics can directly alter protein function in a manner consistent with the physical and functional constraints that have been defined for the anesthetic site of action.

The Meyer-Overton rule has been taken as evidence supporting a unitary hypothesis of anesthesia, which proposes that all inhalation anesthetics induce the anesthetic state by acting at membrane sites with identical membrane structure, although these sites may be widely distributed throughout the nervous system. More recent evidence lends renewed support for a multisite hypothesis, however, in which, for example, different classes of anesthetics act at structurally similar but distinct sites of action, each with slightly different anesthetic sensitivities.

These small differences in sensitivities may be obscured by a log-log plot of potencies and lipid solubilities.

Clinically, anesthetics have numerous side effects, which vary among agents. This variation suggests that they do have multiple sites of action, many of which may be unrelated to the mechanism of anesthesia. On the other hand, some anesthetics have dose-related effects that appear to antagonize their anesthetic action. Enflurane, for example, has convulsant properties that may reduce its anesthetic potency.

How inhalation anesthetics alter membrane function at a molecular level is speculative. In addition to possible effects on lipids, they may compete with endogenous ligands, such as neurotransmitters, for binding sites on receptors or induce conformational changes in ion channels. Possible membrane sites of action are summarized in Figure 25-4.

Although predicting how a better understanding of molecular mechanisms of anesthesia may eventually apply to the practice of medicine is difficult, we cannot advance far in our clinical use of anesthetics while our theoretic grasp of their mode of action is so primitive (M.M. Sedensky, personal communication). The many nonspecific and often undesirable side effects of our current anesthetics may be avoided in the future if anesthetic molecules can be designed for a specific target site, in a manner similar to the evolution of synthetic opioids following the discovery of opioid receptors. Ultimately, this knowledge may provide a basis for understanding the range of clinical responses exhibited by individual patients to our anesthetics.

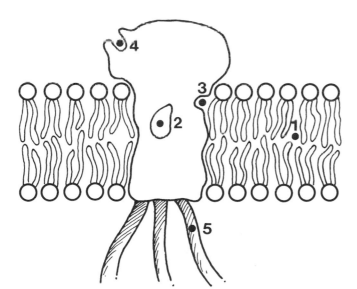

Fig. 25–4. Possible membrane sites of action of general anesthetics: (1) nonspecific interaction with bulk lipids at hydrophobic core of membranes may indirectly affect protein function; (2) binding to channel protein within ion-conducting pathway may alter permeability of channel; (3) binding to a hydrophobic domain on channel protein at lipid-protein interface may interfere directly with protein function by an allosteric mechanism; (4) binding to a receptor site on channel protein may prevent binding of an endogenous ligand; (5) interaction with cytoskeletal elements that anchor channel protein to cytoplasm may alter activity of protein. Modified from Franks, N.P., Lieb, W.R.: Anaesthetics on the mind. Nature *328*:113, 1987.

REFERENCES

1. Franks, N. P., Lieb, W. R.: Molecular mechanisms of general anesthesia. Nature *300*:487, 1982.
2. Miller, K. W.: The nature of the site of general anesthesia. Int Rev Neurobiol *27*:1, 1985.
3. Wardley-Smith, B., Halsey, M. J.: Mixture of inhalation and I. V. anaesthetics at high pressure: a test of the multisite hypothesis of general anesthesia. Br J Anaesth *57*:1248, 1985.
4. Richards, C. D.: The action of anesthetics on synaptic transmission. Gen Pharmacol *9*:287, 1978.
5. Gage, P. W., Hamill, O. P.: Effects of anesthetics on ion channels in synapses. Int Rev Physiol *25*:1, 1981.
6. Maze, M.: Clinical implications of membrane receptor function in anesthesia. Anesthesiology *51*:160, 1981.
7. Thorpe, D. H.: Opiate structure and activity: a guide to understanding the receptor. Anesth Analg *63*:143, 1984.
8. Vaught, J. L., Rothman, R. B., Westfall, T. C.: Mu and delta receptors: their role in analgesia and in the differential effects of opioid peptides on analgesia. Life Sci *30*:1443, 1982.
9. Dodson, B. A., Miller, K. W.: Evidence for a dual mechanism in the anesthetic action of an opioid peptide. Anesthesiology *62*:615, 1985.
10. Smith, D. J., et al.: Ketamine interacts with opiate receptors as an agonist. Anesthesiology *53*.85, 1980.
11. Fratta, W., et al.: Failure of ketamine to interact with opiate receptors. Eur J Pharmacol *61*:389, 1980.
12. Robinson, M. B., Coyle, J. T.: Glutamate and related acidic excitatory neurotransmitters: from basic science to clinical application. FASEB J *1*:446, 1987.
13. Richter, J. J.: Current theories about the mechanism of benzodiazepine and neuroleptic drugs. Anesthesiology *54*:66, 1981.
14. Olsen, R. W.: GABA-benzodiazepine-barbiturate receptor interactions. J Neurochem *37*:1, 1981.
15. Olsen, R. W., Fischer, J. B., Dunwiddie, T. V.: Barbiturate enhancement of gamma-aminobutyric acid receptor binding and function as a mechanism of anesthesia. *In* Roth, S. H., Miller, K. W. (eds.). Molecular and Cellular Mechanisms of Anesthetics. New York, Plenum Medical Book, 1986, p. 165.
16. Ticku, M. J., Rastogi, S. K.: Barbiturate-sensitive sites in the benzodiazepine-GABA receptor-ionophore complex. *In* Roth, S. H., Miller, K. W. (eds.). Molecular and Cellular Mechanisms of Anesthetics. New York, Plenum Medical Book, 1986, p. 179.
17. Eldefrawi, A. T., Eldefrawi, M. E.: Receptors of gamma-aminobutyric acid and voltage-dependent chloride channels as targets for drugs and toxicants. FASEB J *1*:262, 1987.
18. Meyer, H. H.: Zur Theorie der Alkoholnarkose. I Mitt. Welche Eigenschaft der Anesthetika bedingt ihre narkotische Wirkung? Arch Exp Pathol Pharmakol *42*:108, 1899.
19. Overton, E.: Studien uber die Narkose zugleich ein beitrag zur allgemeinen Pharmakologie. Jena, G. Fischer, 1901.
20. Angel, A.: Effects of anaesthetics on nervous pathways. *In* Gray, T. C., Nunn, J. F. Utting, J. E. (eds.). General Anesthesia, 4th Ed. London, Butterworth, 1980, p. 117.
21. Larrabee, M. G., Posternak, J. M.: Selective action of anesthetics on synapses and axons in mammalian sympathetic ganglia. J Neurophysiol *15*:91, 1952.
22. Ngai, S. H., Cheney, D. L., Finck, D. L.: Acetylcholine concentrations and turnover in rat brain structures during anesthesia with halothane, enflurane, and ketamine. Anesthesiology *48*:4, 1978.

23. Roizen, M. F., et al.: The effects of two anesthetic agents on norepinephrine and dopamine in discrete brain nuclei, fiber tracts, and terminal regions of the rat. Brain Res 110:515, 1976.

24. Rosenberg, P. H., Klinge, E.: Some effects of enflurane anesthesia on biogenic amines in the brain and plasma of rats. Br J Anaesth 46:708, 1974.

25. Roizen, M. F., White, P. F., Eger, E. I., II, Brownstein, M. L.: Effects of ablation of serotonin or norepinephrine brain stem areas on halothane and cyclopropane MACs in rats. Anesthesiology 49:252, 1978.

26. Nicoll, R. A.: The effects of anesthetics on synaptic excitation and inhibition in the olfactory bulb. J Physiol 223:803, 1972.

27. Gage, P. W., McKinnon, D., Robertson, B.: The influence of anesthetics on postsynaptic ion channels. In Roth, S. H., Miller, K. W. (eds.). Molecular and Cellular Mechanisms of Anesthetics. New York, Plenum Medical Book, 1986, p. 139.

28. Cheng, S. C., Brunner, E. A.: Effects of anesthetic agents on synaptosomal GABA disposal. Anesthesiology 55:34, 1981.

29. Pearce, R. A., Stringer, J. L., Lothman, E. W.: Effect of volatile anesthetics on synaptic transmission in the rat hippocampus. Anesthesiology 71:591, 1989.

30. Dluzewski, A. R., Halsey, M. J., Simmonds, A. C.: Membrane interactions with general and local anaesthetics: a review of molecular hypotheses of anaesthesia. Mol Aspects Med 6:459, 1983.

31. Wann, K. T., Macdonald, A. G.: Actions and interactions of high pressure and general anaesthetics. Prog Neurobiol 30:271, 1988.

32. von Bibra, E., Harless, E.: Die Wirkung des Schwefeläthers in Chemische und Physikologische Bezighung. Erlangen, Germany, 1847.

33. Bernard, C.: Leçons sur les anesthésiques et sur l'asphyxsie. Paris, J.B. Bailliere et Fils, 1875.

34. Allison, A. C., et al.: The effect of inhalational anaesthetics on the microtubular system in Actinosphaereium nucleofilum. J Cell Sci 7:483, 1970.

35. Hameroff, S. R.: Ultimate computing: Biomolecular Consciousness and Nanotechnology. Amsterdam, Elsevier North-Holland, 1987.

36. Little, D. M.: Classical Anesthesia Files. Baltimore, Waverly Press, 1985, p. 147.

37. Lillie, R. S.: On the connection between changes of permeability and stimulation and on significance of changes in permeability to carbon dioxide. Am J Physiol 24:14, 1909.

38. Gage, P. W., Hamill, O.: Effects of several inhalation anaesthetics on the kinetics of postsynaptic conduction changes in mouse diaphragm. Br J Pharmacol 57:263, 1976.

39. Brett, R. S., Dilger, J. P., Yland, K. F.: Isoflurane causes "flickering" of the acetylcholine receptor channel: observations using the patch clamp. Anesthesiology 69:161, 1988.

40. Mullins, L. J.: Some physical mechanisms in narcosis. Chem Rev 54:289, 1954.

41. Johnson, F. H., Flagler, E. A.: Hydrostatic pressure reversal of narcosis in tadpoles. Science 112:91, 1950.

42. Lever, M. J., Miller, K. W., Paton, W. D. M., Smith, E. B.: Pressure reversal of anaesthesia. Nature 231:368, 1971.

43. Miller, K. W., Paton, W. D. M., Smith, R. A., Smith, E. B.: The pressure reversal of general anesthesia and the critical volume hypothesis. Mol Pharmacol 9:131, 1973.

44. Wulf, R. J., Featherstone, R. M.: A correlation of van der Waal's constants with anesthetic potency. Anesthesiology 18:97, 1957.

45. Castellan, G. W.: Physical Chemistry, 2nd Ed. Reading, MA, Addison-Wesley Publishing, 1971, p. 29.

46. Koski, W. S., Wilson, K. M., Kaufman, J. J.: Correlation between anesthetic potency and the van der Waal's a constant. In Fink, B. R. (ed.). Molecular Mechanisms of Anesthesia. Progress In Anesthesia, Vol. 1. New York, Plenum Press, 1975, p. 277.

47. Hameroff, S. R., Watt, R. C.: Do anesthetics act by altering electron mobility? Anesth Analg 62:936, 1983.

48. Terrell, R. C.: Physical and chemical properties of anaesthetic agents. Br J Anaesth 56(Suppl):3s, 1984.

49. Tanifuji, Y., Eger, E. I., II, Terrell, R. C.: Some characteristics of an exceptionally potent inhaled anesthetic: thiomethoxyflurane. Anesth Analg 56:387, 1977.

50. Koblin, D. D., Eger, E. I., II: How do inhaled anesthetics work. In Miller, R. D. (ed.). Anesthesia, 2nd Ed. New York, Churchill Livingstone, 1986, p. 581.

51. Firestone, L. L., Miller, J. C., Miller, K. W.: Tables of physical and pharmacological properties of anesthetics. In Roth, S. H., Miller, K. W. (eds.). Molecular and Cellular Mechanisms of Anesthetics. New York, Plenum Medical Book, 1986, p. 455.

52. Scheller, M. S., Saidman, L. J., Partridge, B. L.: MAC of sevoflurane in humans and the New Zealand white rabbit. Can J Anaesth 35:153, 1988.

53. Rampil, I. J., et al.: Clinical characteristics of desflurane in surgical patients: minimum alveolar concentration. Anesthesiology 74:429, 1991.

54. Rudo, F. G., Krantz, J. C.: Anaesthetic molecules. Br J Anaesth 46:181, 1974.

55. Koblin, D. D., et al.: Are convulsant gases also anesthetics? Anesth Analg 60:464, 1981.

56. Halsey, M. J.: A reassessment of the molecular structure-functional relationships of the inhaled general anesthetics. Br J Anaesth 56(Suppl 1):9s, 1984.

57. Merkel, G., Eger, E. I., II: A comparative study of halothane and haloprane anesthesia. Anesthesiology 24:346, 1963.

58. Morgan, P. G.: Personal communication.

59. Seeman, P.: The membrane actions of anesthetics and tranquilizers. Pharmacol Rev 24:583, 1972.

60. Marshall, B. E., Wollman, H.: General Anesthetics. In Gilman, A. G., et al. (eds.). The Pharmacological Basis of Therapeutics, 7th Ed. New York, Macmillan, 1985, p. 276.

61. Franks, N. P., Lieb, W. R.: Where do general anaesthetics act? Nature 274:339, 1978.

62. Pringle, M. J., Brown, K. B., Miller, K. W.: Can the lipid theories of anesthesia account for the cutoff in anesthetic potency in homologous series of alcohol? Mol Pharmacol 19:49, 1981.

63. Mullins, L. J.: Anesthetics. In Lajtha, A. (ed.). Handbook of Neurochemistry, Vol. 6. New York, Plenum Press, 1971, p. 395.

64. Janoff, A. G., Pringle, M. J., Miller, K. W.: Correlation of general anaesthetic potency with solubility in membranes. Biochim Biophys Acta 649:125, 1981.

65. Franks, N. P., Lieb, W. R.: Mapping of general anaesthetic target sites provides a molecular basis for cutoff effects. Nature 316:349, 1985.

66. Richter, J., Landau, E. M., Cohen, S.: Anaesthetic and convulsant ethers act on different sites in the crab neuromuscular junction in vitro. Nature 266:70, 1977.

67. Saidman, L. J., Eger, E. I., II: effect of nitrous oxide and of narcotic premedication on the alveolar concentrations of halothane required for anesthesia. Anesthesiology 25:302, 1964.

68. Torri, G., Damia, G., Fabiani, M. L.: Effect of nitrous oxide on the anaesthetic requirement of enflurane. Br J Anaesth 46:468, 1974.

69. Clarke, R. F., et al.: Potency of mixtures of general anaesthetic agents. Br J Anaesth 50:979, 1978.

70. Murphy, M. A., Hug, C. C.: The enflurance sparing effect of

morphine, butorphanol and nalbuphine. Anesthesiology *57*:489, 1982.

71. Murphy, M. R., Hug, C. C.: The anesthetic potency of fentanyl in terms of its reduction of enflurance MAC. Anesthesiology *57*:485, 1982.

72. Ueda, I., Kamaya, H.: Molecular mechanisms of anesthesia. Anesth Analg *63*:929, 1984.

73. Johnson, F. H., Brown, D. E., Marsland, D. A.: Pressure reversal of the action of certain narcotics. J Cell Comp Physiol *20*:247, 1942.

74. Franks, N. P., Lieb, W. R.: Is membrane expansion relevant to anaesthesia? Nature *292*:248, 1981.

75. Metcalfe, J. C., Seeman, P., Burgen, A. S. V.: The protein relaxation of benzyl alcohol in erythrocyte membranes. Mol Pharmacol *4*:87, 1968.

76. Mastrangelo, C. J., Trudell, J. R., Edmunds, H. N., Cohen, E. N.: Effect of clinical concentrations of halothane on phospholipid-cholesterol membrane fluidity. Mol Pharmacol *14*:463, 1978.

77. Trudell, J. R.: A unitary theory of anesthesia based on lateral phase separations in nerve membranes. Anesthesiology *46*:5, 1977.

78. Kamaya, H., Ueda, I., Moore, P. S., Eyring, H.: Antagonism between high pressure and anesthetics in the thermal phase-transition of dipalmitoyl phosphatidyl choline bilayer. Biochim Biophys Acta *550*:131, 1979.

79. Young, A. P., Sigman, D. S.: Allosteric effects of volatile anesthetics on the membrane-bound acetycholine receptor protein. I. Stabilization of the high-affinity state. Mol Pharmacol *20*:498, 1981.

80. Ueda, I., Kamaya, H.: Kinetic and thermodynamic aspects of the mechanisms of general anesthesia in a model system of firefly luminescence in vitro. Anesthesiology *38*:425, 1973.

81. Ueda, I., Shieh, D. D., Eyring, H.: Disordering effects of anesthetics in firefly luciferase and in lecithin surface mono-layer. *In* Fink, B.R. (ed). Molecular Mechanisms of Anesthesia. Progress in Anesthesia, Vol. 1. New York, Raven Press, 291, 1975, p. 291.

82. White, D. C., Wardley-Smith, B., Adey, G.: Anesthetics and bioluminescence. *In* Fink, B. R. (ed). Molecular Mechanisms of Anesthesia. Progress in Anesthesia, Vol. 1. New York, Raven Press, 1975, p. 583.

83. Franks, N. P., Lieb, W. R.: Do general anaesthetics act by competitive binding to specific receptors? Nature *310*:599, 1984.

84. Franks, N. P., Lieb, W. R.: Do direct protein/anesthetic interactions underlie the mechanism of general anesthesia. *In* Roth, S. H., Miller, K. W. (eds). Molecular and Cellular Mechanisms of Anesthetics. New York, Plenum Medical Book, 1986, p. 319.

85. Evers, A. S., Berkowitz, B. A., d'Avignon, D. A.: Correlation between the anaesthetic effect of halothane and saturable binding in brain. Nature *328*:157, 1987.

86. Lockhart, S. H., et al.: Absence of abundant binding sites for anesthetics in rabbit brain: an in vivo NMR study. Anesthesiology *73*:455, 1990.

87. Morgan, P. G., Cascorbi, H. F.: Effect of anesthetics and a convulsant on normal and mutant *Caenorhabditis elegans* Anesthesiology *62*:738, 1985.

88. Sedensky, M. M., Meneely, P. M.: Genetic analysis of halothane sensitivity in *Caenorhabditis elegans*. Science *236*:952, 1987.

89. Morgan, P. G., Sedensky, M. M., Meneely, P. M., Cascorbi, H. F.: The effect of two genes on anesthetic response in the nematode *Caenorhabditis elegans*. Anesthesiology *69*:246, 1988.

90. Morgan, P. G., Sedensky, M., Meneely, P. M.: Multiple sites of action of volatile anesthetics in *Caenorhabditis elegans*. Proc Natl Acad Sci USA *87*:2965, 1990.

91. Franks, N. P., Lieb, W. R.: Anaesthetics on the mind. Nature *328*:113, 1987.

Chapter 26

PRINCIPLES OF PHARMACOKINETICS AND PHARMACODYNAMICS

COLIN A. SHANKS

The intensity and duration of any drug effect depend on its concentration at the sites of action and drug concentration-response relationships at that site, termed the *pharmacodynamics*. The time-course of drug action is easily appreciated for a rapidly acting drug administered intravenously. The observed dose-response relationships also depend on the delivery of drug from the point of administration, characterized as the plasma *pharmacokinetics* (Fig. 26–1).

The utility of kinetic-dynamic models is to allow predictions of drug concentrations at the sites of action, to project the time-course of effect with different dosing regimens or for various disease states. These mathematic models are seldom simple and require nomograms or computer programs to simplify their use, especially when the clinician wishes to achieve and maintain a desired drug concentration range in the plasma or at the effect site. The majority of the information of intravenous drugs is obtained from analysis of their plasma concentrations, measured in blood sampled over a specific time period. Statistical assessment of the plasma concentration-time curve then provides the best fit to characterize these data, the resultant mathematic model describing the curve. Such models should be viewed from the standpoint of plasma concentrations, because they seldom show kinship to anatomic or physiologic reality, but they are a convenient way to lump tissues and organs together as if they acted as a group.

This chapter outlinse pharmacokinetic principles, attempting condensation of its mathematic basis, depicting results largely in graphic terms. Those wishing to review multicompartmental modeling will find only the graphic solutions of drug disposition, because this review endeavors to provide the clinician with a feel for drug movement without the distraction of detailed mathematic equations. Readers who desire greater detail are referred to the standard texts.[1,2] Many drugs associated with anesthesia are administered intravenously, usually as a single bolus dose, and this chapter focuses on the fate of such a drug in the body, particularly the pharmacokinetic variables of distribution and elimination. Because few of these drugs have the plasma as the primary site of action, it is appropriate then to explore the range of therapeutic concentrations in a hypothetic effect compartment and the pharmacodynamics, represented as a second black box in Figure 26–1. Pharmacokinetic-pharmacodynamic modeling is an area likely to receive increasing attention,[3] because it enables exploration of the relationships among dosing, plasma concentrations, and the time-course of drug activity.

CALCULATING PHARMACOKINETICS: AN EXAMPLE WITH PANCURONIUM

Volumes of Distribution

The amount of drug administered can be considered in units of mass. Its concentration is similarly expressed in terms of mass per unit volume. If none of the drug has been removed from the system, then volume is derived with division of the dose by measured concentration: mass divided by mass cancels, and the volume term (a double reciprocal) is all that remains.

For example,

Pancuronium:	Amount	Concentration	Volume
	5 mg	1 mg/ml	5 ml
Comment:	Clinical dose		Syringe

Inherent in such a calculation is the assumption that the drug is mixed completely and evenly throughout the volume. Because this assumption is usually untrue in pharmacokinetics, calculations from plasma concentra-

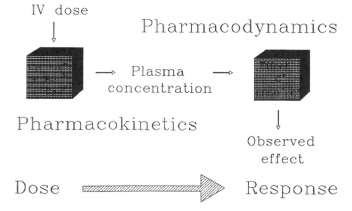

Fig. 26–1. Dose-response relationships are based on the two black boxes: pharmacokinetics, what the body does to the drug, and pharmacodynamics, what the drug does to the body.

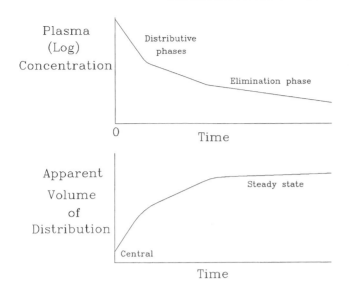

Fig. 26–2. Above, a schematic of a triexponential plasma concentration-time curve. The central volume, the apparent volume of distribution at time 0, is calculated as the dose divided by the concentration at time 0. Thereafter, drug in the body appears to redistribute into an increasingly large volume.

tions are termed *apparent volumes of distribution.* Worse, the dose administered is assumed to have mixed instantaneously throughout a back-extrapolated volume at the moment of injection, a volume often similar to that of the blood. The volume calculated at the concentration intercept, time 0 (Fig. 26–2), is often called the central volume. Thereafter, the drug is distributed by processes of flow, mixing, and diffusion to its eventual, larger, steady-state volume of distribution. For a highly polarized molecule such as pancuronium that does not easily cross membranes, this resembles the volume of the extracellular fluid. Not all drugs are so convenient in their distribution. When the assumption of perfect mixing throughout the body is violated, as with drugs having high ratios for protein binding or lipid solubility, then calculated volumes can be large, sometimes multiples of the body weight.

The schematic in Figure 26–2 shows a plasma concentration-time curve typical for most drugs administered as an intravenous bolus dose during anesthesia. The log concentration-time curve has two inflections, suggesting a likely need for it to be characterized by a three-compartment model. Figure 26–2 also depicts the nonlinear changes in the apparent volume of distribution across time. These are calculated from the amount of drug remaining in the body at any time and from the plasma concentration at that time. Three selected points on a concentration-time curve are shown in Table 26–1.

In Table 26–1, the plasma concentrations of pancuronium decrease much more rapidly in the first 2 hours than in the subsequent 2 hours, reflecting the increase in its apparent volume of distribution. The rate of increase in apparent distribution volume may be multiexponential, reflected in the shape of the concentration-time curve associated with a bolus dose (see Fig. 26–2).

Table 26–1. Sample Values for Concentrations and Amounts of Pancuronium in the Body

Time (hours)	Amount (mg)	Concentration (mg/L)	Volume (L)
0	5.0	1.0	5.0
2	1.4	0.1	14.0
4	0.7	0.05	14.0

Half-life and Clearance

Assuming the redistribution of pancuronium to be complete after 2 hours (Table 26–1), then the decrease in plasma concentrations from the second to the fourth hour, from 0.1 to 0.05 mg/L, gives an elimination half-life of 2 hours. Looked at another way, had an imaginary molecular sieve swept through the 14-L volume during these 2 hours, crowding the pancuronium molecules together until their concentration is again 0.1 mg/L, these would now be compressed into a 7-L volume. The other 7 L has had all pancuronium molecules removed in this same 2 hours, giving a plasma clearance for pancuronium of 3.5 L/hour for this example. This does not imply that clearance does not exist for the first 2 hours, but that its effects are overshadowed by redistribution.

PHARMACOKINETIC AND HYDRAULIC MODELS

The upper graph in Figure 26–2 shows three linear portions in the (log) concentration-time curve, implying the need for three distinct volumes in a model that characterizes this (triexponential) curve. Figure 26–3 shows two related models, each with three compartments: central, fast, and slow. In the pharmacokinetic model, the size of the circles is proportional to the respective compartmental volumes. For the hydraulic model, these become the bases of three cylinders, their cross-sectional areas. The central volume is that into which the drug is administered and from which it is eliminated. The elimination clearance (Cl_e) is indicated by an exit arrow. Intercompartmental clearance for the two peripheral compartments $(Cl_f$ and $Cl_s)$ is represented in the hydraulic model by conducting tubes. Pharmacokinetic models seldom show concentrations in the peripheral compartments, but these are easily represented in a hydraulic model by the height of fluid in each cylinder (Table 26–2). The pharmacodynamic effect compartment does not remove sufficient drug mass to affect the pharmacokinetic model.

BOLUS DOSING

The three-compartment hydraulic model provides insights into drug disposition. With a single intravenous bolus dose administered into the central compartment, the cylinder is assumed to be filled completely and instantaneously to the appropriate concentration at time 0 (Fig. 26–4). Immediately, fluid levels in the central cylinder fall rapidly, as drug is both eliminated and distributed to the two peripheral cylinders. At time 1 (Fig. 26–5), drug ceases to enter the fast compartment because levels in

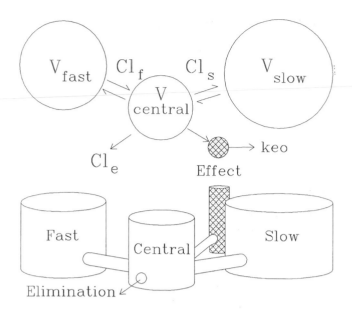

Fig. 26–3. Pharmacokinetic and hydraulic renditions of a three-compartment model. Drug administered into the central volume is removed by the elimination clearance (Cl_e) and redistributed by intercompartmental clearances (Cl_f and Cl_s). The pharmacokinetic model is the forcing function for the "effect compartment" (shaded).

Table 26–2. Correspondences for the Pharmacokinetic and Hydraulic Models

Pharmacokinetic	Hydraulic
Compartmental volume	Cross-sectional area
Drug concentration	Fluid height
Elimination clearance	Exit hole dimensions
Intercompartmental clearance	Conducting tube dimensions
Amount of drug	Fluid volume
Infusion rate	Fluid volume added per unit time
Drug elimination rate	Fluid volume lost per unit time

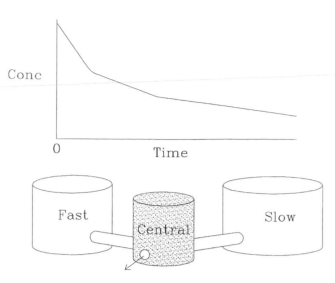

Fig. 26–4. The concentration-time curve associated with a bolus dose into the central compartment. This is depicted in the hydraulic model as completely filling the central cylinder at time 0.

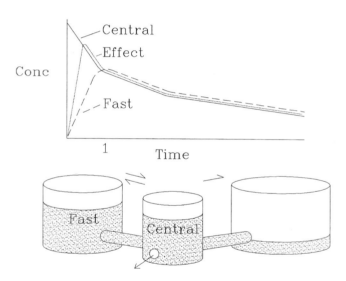

Fig. 26–5. Concentration-time curves for the central compartment (solid line) and the fast compartment (dashed line). At time 1, one sees a pseudoequilibrium between these two compartments, shown in the hydraulic model as equality of their fluid levels. After this time, concentrations in the fast compartment exceed those in the central compartment. Concentrations in the effect compartment (dotted) reach an early pseudoequilibrium with those in the central compartment, then follow them closely.

the fast and central cylinders are now equal; thereafter, drug returns from the fast compartment, and the rate of decrease of concentrations in the central compartment is reduced. Figure 26-6 shows a similar pseudoequilibrium point for the slow compartment; at time 2, there is as much drug entering as is leaving, and distribution to the periphery is complete. The concentration-time curve for the bolus dose then reaches the elimination phase, and its slope provides the elimination half-life (see Fig. 26-2). Although the elimination half-life is always reported in papers on the pharmacokinetics of any new drug, it is the least useful of these parameters, mainly because this slope is seldom relevant to the therapeutic range of concentrations. Most drugs administered intravenously during anesthesia have a rapid onset of effect, implying that pseudoequilibrium in the effect compartment (see Figs.

26-5 and 26-6) occurs earlier than the fast compartment. Thereafter, analogous to concentrations in the fast compartment, concentrations in the effect compartment decrease in parallel with those in the central compartment.

Spontaneous recovery from drug is related to concentrations in the effect compartment, and Figure 26-7 uses an example with a nondepolarizing neuromuscular block-

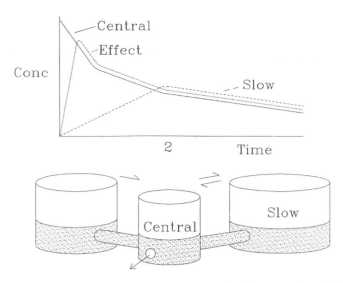

Fig. 26–6. Concentration-time curves for the central (solid line) and slow (dashed line) compartments. At time 2, a pseudoequilibrium has been achieved, analogous to that in Figure 26–4.

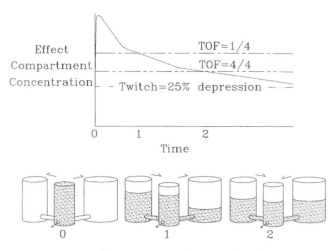

Fig. 26–8. Concentrations with a large bolus dose. The time required for spontaneous recovery to each end point is increased out of proportion for the dose ratio with that in Figure 26–7. TOF = train of four.

ing agent. This schematic includes the count of responses to a train-of-four stimulation, responses familiar to every clinician. Other drugs, such as narcotics, have less clear concentration-effect relationships, and the concept of "context-sensitive" half-lives has been introduced.[4] The schematic in Figure 26–7 shows concentrations of a relaxant given as a single dose insufficient to ablate the first response to train-of-four stimulation. The range of concentrations associated with both adequate surgical relaxation and countable responses lies between the two upper dashed lines. The lower two dashed lines represent 25 and 75% twitch depression, in which the time interval required for the concentration-time curve to pass through this range is the "recovery index." In Figure 26–7, the

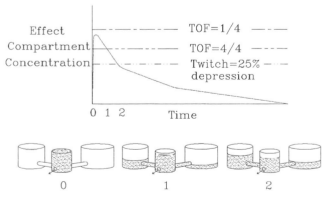

Fig. 26–7. Concentrations in the effect compartment with a bolus dose of a neuromuscular blocking agent suppressing all but one of responses to train-of-four (TOF) stimulation. Spontaneous recovery to reappearance of all four twitches (time 2) is due largely to redistribution. The recovery index, the time taken for concentrations to traverse the range between the lower dashed lines, is also related to rapid redistribution.

time interval for spontaneous recovery from 75% twitch depression (also equivalent to reappearance of four-of-four responses) and 25% twitch depression is related to the phase of fast redistribution.

Figure 26–8 depicts a larger, "intubating" dose of relaxant, indicated by an increased height of the central cylinder at time 0. The concentration-time curve for the central compartment has the same shape as that in Figure 26–7, but transposed upward. This upward transposition now places the range of concentrations associated with surgical relaxation (less than four responses) later on the concentration-time curve, resulting in a longer time interval for spontaneous recovery between reappearance of ¼ and reappearance of ¾: the recovery index is dose-dependent. One would see no further increase in this interval once the dose produced sufficient upward transposition for the concentration range to intersect only with the elimination phase; doses larger than that in Figure 26–8 would exhibit the same recovery index. For a relaxant with small central and fast compartment volumes, the range of concentrations associated with spontaneous recovery would always be represented in the elimination phase, and there would be no change in the recovery index with increasing dosage. The nonlinearity of the concentration-time curve can produce nonlinearity in the relationship between increase in the dosed amount and the duration of effect. For example, three times the dose could have more than three times the duration.

The concentrations associated with the desired effect are, as shown in Figures 26–7 and 26–8, consistent in the effect compartment, remaining the same for both onset and offset of drug action. Concentrations in the central and effect compartments are equal at the time of pseudoequilibrium (see Figs. 26–5 and 26–6), or at steady state. Concentrations in the plasma and effect compartments are reasonably congruent after the time of peak effect, during spontaneous recovery. Before this, the relationship is not intuitively obvious, being related to the effect compartment rate constant, k_{eo} (see Fig. 26–3). The value of this rate constant is determined by the pattern of the changing responses across time, including the time delay before peak effect is observed.

MULTIPLE BOLUS DOSING

The concentration-time curves of serial bolus doses build on each other; that is, the concentrations are additive. Following the initial dose, the repeat dose needs to replace both that drug lost by elimination clearance and that redistributed by the incremental increase in the distribution volume (see Fig. 26-2)—the latter dominates when the dosing interval is shortest. In Figure 26-9, the concentration-time curve of each separate dose is continued as a dashed line, whereas concentrations in the effect compartment increase to a new peak with each repeat dose. Figure 26-9 represents a small initial dose of relaxant, insufficient to ablate the twitch response, with further relaxant added on reappearance of the fourth response to train-of-four stimulation. Redistribution of the initial dose is followed by a rapid decrease in plasma and effect compartment concentrations. The duration of the first repeat dose is also brief. The second repeat dose in Figure 26-10 is added when the redistribution with the initial dose into the fast compartment is complete, and its duration is longer than that of the first. The hydraulic representation of the second maintenance dose indicates a greater peak concentration than that achieved by either of the previous doses.

The third dose is added at a later point on the concentration-time curves, and the result is a further increase in the peak concentration and in duration of effect. The observer notes the increasing duration of repeat doses 1 to 4 and reports cumulation of the relaxant, as noted with pancuronium.[5] If a larger initial dose is administered, as in Figure 26-10, all four of the responses vanish for a time, and the interval for recovery between the return of the first and the fourth responses is longer than in Figure 26-9. All repeat doses in Figure 26-10 are now required later, at the same part of the concentration-time curve as for the fifth dose in Figure 26-10, and the dosing interval

dose not change—cumulation is a dose-dependent observation.

Differences in spontaneous recovery after multiple bolus dosing can be inferred from Figures 26-9 and 26-10. Recovery after the first three doses in Figure 26-9 would be more rapid than that after the fifth dose, or any dose in Figure 26-10, based purely on the shape of the concentration-time curve produced by each dose and the sum of its predecessors. Barely adequate bolus doses, as in Figure 26-7, are associated with considerable redistribution, resulting in rapid recovery; larger or repeated doses (see Figs. 26-8 and 26-10) are associated with hardly any redistribution, and the concentration-time curve intersects with the concentration range at a lesser slope, and thus a slower recovery.

CONTINUOUS INFUSION

Drugs are administered by continuous infusion to produce prolonged action while retaining the ability for closely controlled intensity of effect. The alternatives to infusion are the administration of large doses, or multiple bolus doses, attempting to keep concentrations within the therapeutic range, below the toxic and above the minimum acceptable levels. The effective concentration is usually described for the plasma, although attention should really be focused on effect compartment concentrations. Once steady state has been reached, the final infusion rate is that necessary to maintain the desired concentration, the product of this concentration, and the rate of drug removal, its clearance from the body. A single constant rate of infusion suitable for maintenance of the desired concentration is much too slow (Fig. 26-11, infusion alone), necessitating a loading dose at time zero. The major problem with an infusion is the initial establishment of a safe, effective concentration.

Drugs with a small therapeutic margin have a narrow range between those concentrations necessary for the desired effect and those producing toxicity. Too large a bolus dose produces toxicity, whereas an adequate non-

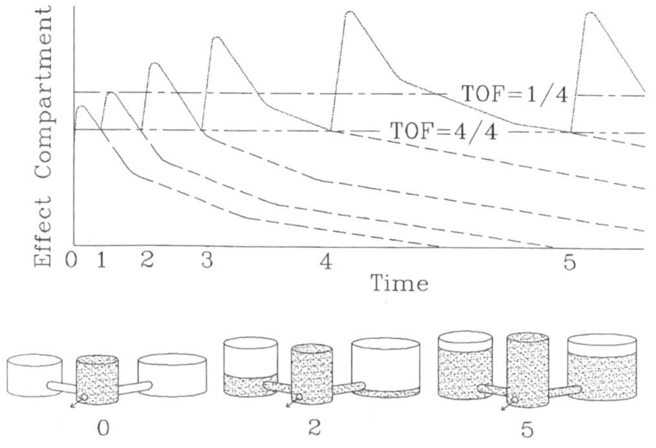

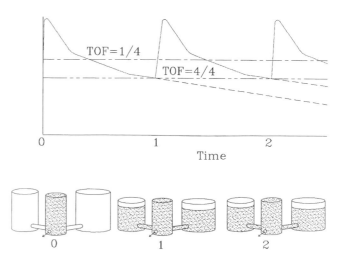

Fig. 26-9. Blockade with a small initial dose of relaxant, with redosing whenever the fourth response returned. The time interval for repeat dosing increases until the fifth dose, but remains constant thereafter. TOF = train of four.

Fig. 26-10. Blockade observable after a larger initial dose than in Figure 26-9. The time interval between redosing does not alter, for the same relaxant as in Figure 26-9. TOF = train of four.

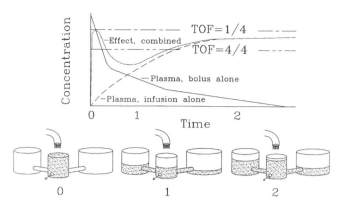

Fig. 26–11. The small bolus dose administered in Figure 26–7 has been combined with an infusion at a rate that will eventually provide the desired concentration at steady state, showing a need for additional drug to prevent reduction of concentrations below an acceptable level. TOF = train of four.

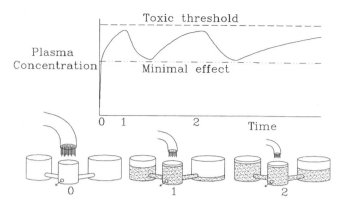

Fig. 26–12. A three-stage infusion, in which the three infusion rates are calculated to attain the effective concentration range as rapidly as possible after time 0, with reductions at times 1 and 2 to avoid reaching toxic levels. The maintenance rate achieves steady state, calculated to maintain a concentration in the therapeutic range.

toxic dose has an evanescent duration of effect. As shown in Figures 26–7 and 26–9, a small dose achieves the required concentrations, but its duration is short. The initial bolus dose is calculated by multiplication of the desired concentration (either in the plasma or in the effect compartment) and a volume, often the initial distribution volume (time 0). Simultaneous commencement of the infusion at its maintenance rate is too slow to prevent a reduction in concentrations below the therapeutic range (see Fig. 26–11), as the distribution volume enlarges (see Fig. 26–2). For each increment in time, the distribution volume becomes greater, and a further incremental bolus dose is needed to fill this additional volume; if the increments are small enough, this becomes a supplementary infusion. For a three-compartment model, plasma concentrations are maintained in the desired range by the combination of a biexponentially decreasing infusion added to the maintenance infusion rate.[6] The bolus dose calculated for Figure 26–11 (bolus alone) to give a peak effect with barely appreciable ¼ responses is based on that volume appropriate to the drug at the time of that peak effect, focusing on concentrations in the effect compartment. Figure 26–2 indicates that this would be larger than at time 0, but it may still require a supplementary infusion to prevent a period of suboptimal concentrations (see Fig. 26–11).

Alternatively, the initial bolus is replaced with a rapid infusion, which, with concentrations entering the therapeutic range, is reduced to a selected intermediate rate to avoid toxic levels.[7] Eventually, the rate of administration is reduced to the maintenance rate (Fig. 26–12). For drugs with a large margin of safety, the problem of toxic levels is ignored, and an initial bolus dose can be calculated using the steady-state distribution volume (Fig. 26–13) or the volume based on the area under the concentration-time curve.[8] Although this produces an overdose in the early going, it allows time for the maintenance rate of infusion to reach therapeutic concentrations.

Any one of the concentration-time curves in Figure 26–11 could be redesigned, superimposing them on a constant-rate infusion. Such a schematic would show

that, when an increase in intensity of effect is necessary during an infusion, a small bolus dose is more rapidly effective than an increase in the infusion rate. Although a combination of the two may be followed by seeming recovery, this is followed by a continuing increase in concentrations as the increased infusion rate proceeds to a new steady-state concentration.

RECOVERY FOLLOWING CONTINUOUS INFUSION

Spontaneous recovery following cessation of a continuous infusion depends both on the magnitude of the interval between the concentration at that time and the mini-

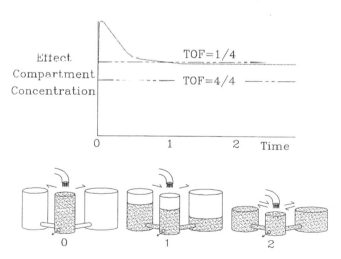

Fig. 26-13. Effect compartment concentrations with a large bolus dose administered concomitantly with a continuous infusion of neuromuscular blocking agent. The infusion is designed to maintain a steady-state concentration related to one response to the train of four (TOF), matching drug administration rate with clearance (time 2). This approach is suitable only for drugs with a high therapeutic threshold and may be associated with prolonged absence of all twitch responses early in the procedure.

mal effective concentration and on the shape of the concentration-time curve as it crosses this interval. Figure 26-2 indicates that the apparent volume of distribution is a function of time and that drug has spread out into the peripheral compartments. Recovery after an infusion is similarly time-dependent, a function of the duration of the infusion. When an infusion is discontinued after a short time, the peripheral compartments have concentrations less than that of the central compartment (Fig. 26-14). The gradient between the central and peripheral compartments results in a rapid reduction in central concentrations, perhaps through the effective range.

During a prolonged infusion that has reached steady state, the concentrations in the peripheral compartments have asymptotically approached that in the central compartment. At one extreme, when intercompartmental clearance is high, decrease in central concentrations is related only to the elimination phase, and recovery rate is related to the elimination half-life. A more rapid decrease after cessation depends on the relative influences of the summed intercompartmental clearances versus the elimination clearance (see Fig. 26-3). At the other extreme, if transfer from the periphery is relatively slow, the a gradient develops between the peripheral and the central compartments, and production of this gradient by central elimination results in an initially rapid reduction in central concentrations (Fig. 26-15).

DOSE-RESPONSE RELATIONSHIPS

Figure 26-1 illustrates pharmacokinetics and pharmacodynamics as two black boxes between the known variables: dose, plasma concentrations, and responses across time. Plasma pharmacokinetics instigates changes in the effect compartment concentrations (top, Fig. 26-16). The concentration-effect relationship should be consistent for both onset and offset and is often assumed to have a sigmoid shape (bottom, Fig. 26-16); its log-linear plot is linear in the 20 to 80% range of effect. For a response in

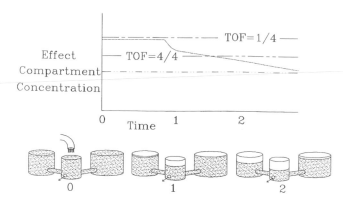

Fig. 26-15. Concentrations at termination of a steady-state infusion, a continuation of Figure 26–13. Despite achievement of steady state, the decrease in concentrations in the central compartment is not always the slope of the elimination phase. This is seen when drug elimination exceeds drug return to the central compartment from the periphery (time 1). This may produce more rapid clinical recovery than would be predicted from the elimination half-life. TOF = train of four.

which the maximal response can be defined for any subject, the midpoint of the sigmoid curve is that concentration at which one sees half the maximum response, the EC_{50}. Some workers factor in the zero-response baseline, the concentration associated with threshold response.

When responses are quantal, yes/no, such as movement/no movement, the effect axis can represent only that proportion of the population affected by a particular concentration. This midpoint value is best known to clinicians for the inhalation agents as MAC, the minimum alveolar concentration that produces immobility in 50% of patients; it is only the midpoint, and users of multiples of

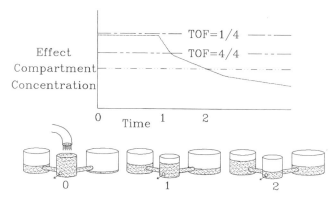

Fig. 26-14. Concentrations with early termination of an infusion, when equilibrium has not been reached with either peripheral compartment. Initially, concentrations in the central compartment decrease rapidly because of continuing redistribution, as a result of a gradient from the central to both peripheral compartments (time 0). Drug reenters from the periphery only with reversal of this gradient (times 1 and 2). TOF = train of four.

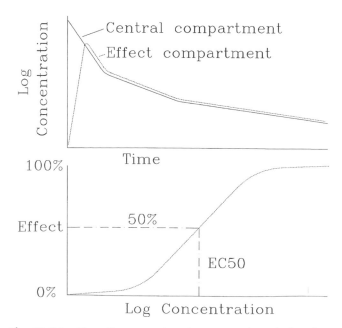

Fig. 26-16. Top, Concentration-time curve for a bolus dose. Bottom, Concentration-effect curve for the effect compartment. Combined modeling allows prediction of the time-course of effect.

MAC assume homogeneity of curve slopes among these agents. Such homogeneity was not observed in all patient groups in one study reporting cumulative frequency dose-response curves for loss of consciousness with thiopental.[9]

The concentration-effect curve in Figure 26-16 implies that the same dosing pattern should produce congruent concentration-time curves, with the amount administered altering only the range of concentrations achieved (for example, the two bolus doses in Figs. 26–7 and 26–8). Pooling of peak responses to a range of bolus doses then results in a sigmoid dose-response curve. The chief pharmacokinetic factor affecting these peak response to a given dose is the apparent volume of distribution at the time of peak concentration in the effect compartment. Distribution volumes may be altered in disease, resulting in changed dose-response relationships.

The classic dose-response relationship in pharmacologic reports is for a tissue in an organ-bath, in which the concentrations are held constant for each response measurement. This is approximated clinically during prolonged infusion of the drug. Under these circumstances, the chief pharmacokinetic factor affecting response to an infused dose is the clearance, with reduced clearance resulting in a more intense effect.

Some responses are not only dose-dependent, but also time-dependent. For example, a dose of a drug that produces histamine release is less likely to do so if the rate of intravenous administration is slowed. Classic pharmacokinetics is unable to account for this phenomenon, assuming complete mixing at time 0, as in Figure 26–4. Figure 26–17 is based on a more complex model[10] than the simple three-compartment model, a model incorporating time delays to account for the time necessary for the circulation to deliver drug and for recirculation during its mixing within the blood. Figure 26–17 contrasts differences in the concentrations during the first 2 minutes with a bolus dose versus administration of the same dose over 30 seconds. The maximum concentrations attained with the 1-second dose are almost double those with the 30-second dose; from 2 minutes onward, the concentration-time curves do not differ. Drugs that produce histamine release do so when a sufficiently large dose is administered sufficiently rapidly. Figure 26–17 suggests that the initial peak arterial concentrations are modified by a slower injection rate and that fewer mast cells would be triggered with the lesser peak.

SUMMARY

This chapter presents the principles of pharmacokinetics for three-compartment models, which are the most common in the anesthesia literature. The majority of textbooks present the concepts and equations for one-compartment systems; the three-compartment equations are considerably more daunting, but are readily available in the literature of clinical pharmacokinetics. This complexity prompted a graphic approach, assuming that clinicians comprehend characterization of data with graphs better than with complex equations. The pharmacokinetic and kinetic-dynamic models are shown as schematics, illustrating details of single and multiple bolus intravenous dosing and continuous infusion. Several of the examples are for neuromuscular blocking agents, because their intraoperative end points can be clearly identified with train-of-four stimulation. Use of hydraulic models emphasizes the importance of relative concentrations in the various compartments, and these models are used ex-

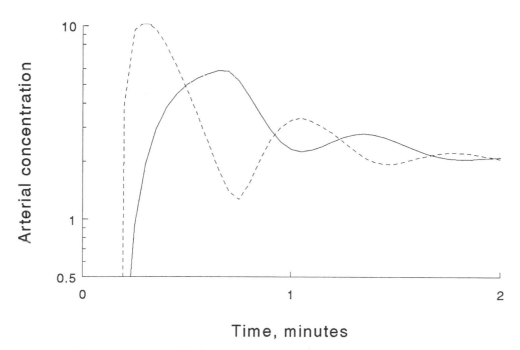

Fig. 26-17. Arterial concentrations in the first 2 minutes with two rates of administration. The delay in initial appearance and recirculation require more complex modeling than that in Figure 26–3.

tensively to demonstrate the mechanisms underlying the time course of both pharmacokinetics and pharmacodynamics.

REFERENCES

1. Gibaldi, M., Perrier, D.: Pharmacokinetics: Drugs and Pharmaceutical Sciences, 2nd Ed. New York, Marcel Dekker, 1982.
2. Rowland, M., Tozer, T. N.: Clinical Pharmacokinetics: Concepts and Applications, 2nd Ed. Philadelphia, Lea & Febiger, 1989.
3. van Boxtel, C. J., Holford, N. H. G., Danhof, M.: The in Vivo Study of Drug Action. Amsterdam, Elsevier, 1992.
4. Shafer, S. L., Varvel, J. R.: Pharmacokinetics, pharmacodynamics, and rational opiod selection. Anesthesiology 74:53, 1991.
5. Fahey, M. R., et al.: Clinical pharmacology of ORG NC45 (Norcuron): a new nondepolarizing muscle relaxant. Anesthesiology 55:6, 1981.
6. Krüger-Thiemer, E.: Continuous intravenous infusion and multicompartmental accumulation. Eur J Pharmacol 4:317, 1968.
7. Vaughan, D. P., Tucker, G. T.: General theory for rapidly establishing steady state drug concentrations using two consecutive constant rate intravenous infusions. Eur J Clin Pharmacol 9:235, 1975.
8. Mitenko, P. A., Ogilvie, R. I.: Rapidly achieved plasma concentration plateaus, with observations on theophylline kinetics. Clin Pharmacol Ther 13:329, 1972.
9. Avram, M. J., et al.: Determinants of thiopental dose requirements. Anesth Analg 76:10, 1993.
10. Henthorn, T. K., et al.: Minimal compartmental model of circulatory mixing of indocyanine green. Am J Physiol 262:H903, 1992.

Chapter 27

PHARMACOLOGY OF OXYGEN AND EFFECTS OF HYPOXIA

VINCENT J. COLLINS

"Anoxia not only stops the machine but wrecks the machinery"—J.S. Haldane.

HISTORICAL BACKGROUND[1]

Oxygen is one of the three basic essentials for the maintenance of life. Deprivation of oxygen leads most rapidly to death. The cells and tissues of the body must be continually supplied with oxygen by the circulation, especially given that they have no oxygen reserve.

Stephen Hale may have prepared oxygen in 1727, but the identification and discovery that oxygen was a normal constituent of air was the work of Joseph Priestley in 1774. Priestley noted that oxygen might be useful in certain diseases but thought that our lives would "burn out" faster if only oxygen were breathed.

In the same year, Scheele prepared oxygen, and, in the following year, it was prepared by Lavoisier by slightly different techniques. Lavoisier demonstrated that oxygen is taken up into the body through the lungs, is in metabolism, and is eliminated as carbon dioxide and water.

Oxygen therapy was introduced by Beddoes in 1794. His work, which was published in collaboration with James Watt and entitled "Considerations on the Medicinal Use and Production of Factitious Airs," might be considered the beginning of inhalation therapy. Beddoes established a pneumatic laboratory at Bristol, England. In his overenthusiasm for oxygen therapy, in which he treated all kinds of diseases, including scrofula, leprosy, and paralysis, he naturally had many failures, and much of his work fell into disrepute. Some 125 years later, in 1917, oxygen therapy was placed on a sound physiologic basis by such men as Haldane and Barcroft in England, who observed the favorable results in treating war gas poisoning and pneumonia, and Yandell Henderson in the United States, who reported favorable results of oxygen use for resuscitation. As a consequence, oxygen is recognized as an excellent therapeutic agent when not used indiscriminately.[2,3]

PROPERTIES OF THERAPEUTIC GASES

Oxygen[4]

Oxygen is a tasteless, colorless, odorless gas. The specific gravity is 1.105 (air = 1). The critical temperature of oxygen is $-118°C$. (155° absolute), and at this temperature, a pressure of 50 atm is required to liquefy the gas. At temperatures warmer than the critical temperature such as room temperature, no amount of pressure can compress the gas into a liquid. The gas also condenses to a liquid at $-183°C$ at ordinary atmospheric pressure. Oxygen possesses some solubility in water, and at 20°C about 3.1 ml will dissolve in 100 ml of water. The solubility of oxygen in arterial blood of a subject breathing air is 0.24 ml per 100 ml. Oxygen is highly reactive and combines with many substances.

Preparations of oxygen for medicinal purposes must have a minimum of 99.5% oxygen as required by U.S.P. standards. The modern commercial method of preparing oxygen is by fractional distillation of liquid air. Because nitrogen is more volatile and boils at a lower temperature (centigrade) than oxygen, liquid oxygen is be left as a residue (78° absolute for nitrogen or $-195°C$) (90° absolute or $-183°C$ for oxygen).

Liquid Oxygen

When large amounts of oxygen are required, it is efficient to store the oxygen as a liquid.

Large, insulated, double-walled steel cylinders are kept upright and are housed outside a hospital building or other facility. The oxygen in these cylinders is compressed to a resting pressure of 120 to 140 psi or an average of 10 atm (10 bar). Because the critical temperature of oxygen is $-116°C$, it cannot be liquified by any amount of pressure above this temperature level. At or below this critical temperature, however, it can be liquified by a pressure of 50 atm (50 bar) or 740 psig. To maintain the liquid state, the oxygen must be continually cooled. This is accomplished by evaporation of some of the oxygen liquid at the surface, which removes an enormous amount of heat from the liquid interior to do this. The containers are vented to the outside so the vaporized oxygen is exhausted from the container. About 5% of the liquid oxygen is lost each day by the process of vaporization.

The resting pressure prevents excessive evaporation. The container pressure during use of the oxygen is usually between P 100 and P 75. The piping system to the risers in the hospital has a delivery pressure of P 75 and a bedside pressure of P 50 or approximately twice atmospheric pressure.

Actually, oxygen may be liquified by markedly reducing its molecular motion by further cooling through more rapid evaporation of the surface oxygen. If the temperature is reduced to $-183°C$, the gaseous oxygen will liquify at a pressure of 1 atm. This is also the boiling point of oxygen.

Mixture of Gases

The quantitative determination of oxygen in a mixture of gases is accomplished by the Orsat type of apparatus. Certain chemicals in the apparatus combine with oxygen and remove it from the gas mixture. Three types of chemical reagents are employed:

1. Pyrogallic acid (1,2,3-trihydroxy benzene). This is readily oxidized to quinones.
2. Copper compounds. These are widely used clinically, metallic copper in the form of a screen immersed in an ammonium hydroxide. Ammonium chloride solution is readily oxidized to cupric oxide on exposure to oxygen. The ammonium hydroxide dissolves the oxide from the surface of the screen to form complex copper ammonium compounds.
3. Sodium hydrosulfide. This is converted to sulfate in the presence of oxygen. The difference between the original and final volume represents the oxygen volume.

OXYGEN TOXICITY[5,6]

Etiology

Supplemental oxygen should be considered a drug, and its administration involves risks. Complications from administration of ordinary therapeutic concentrations of oxygen under 50% are almost unknown.[7] Oxygen in high concentrations inhaled for prolonged periods may be considered a pulmonary intoxicant. Under these circumstances, adverse physiologic effects and pulmonary damage may result.

Symptoms and Signs[8,9]

In humans, the inhalation of 100% oxygen for periods in excess of 14 hours produces the following symptoms:

1. Substernal distress and dyspnea.[10]
2. Cough, sore throat, nasal congestion, and nasopharyngeal infections.
3. Eye irritation and conjunctivitis.
4. Earache, probably due to absorption of nitrogen from the middle ear.
5. Paresthesias: tingling in the extremities.
6. Muscular pain, especially in the legs.
7. Cerebral symptoms of dizziness, lightheadedness, and convulsions.[11,12]
8. Hemodynamic effects.[13]

Among the signs are the following:

1. Lower respiratory tract pathologic conditions.[11,14,15]
   a. Pulmonary congestion.[16]
   b. Edema.
   c. Tracheobronchitis.
2. Inhibition of ciliary activity and inhibition of mucus transport.[17]

3. Accumulation and inspissation of secretions.
4. Reduced vital capacity, functional residual capacity (FRC), and compliance; early airway closure.[18]
5. Reduced PaO_2 with a large $A-aO_2$ difference.[19]
6. Changes in ventilation and perfusion patterns and ratio.
7. Increasing pulmonary physiologic shunt fraction, a reliable early diagnostic sign.
8. Depression of erythropoiesis.[20]
9. Cardiovascular effects of hyperoxia.

Significant hemodynamic effects of high oxygen concentrations occur. The following pressor breathing responses are noted[13]:

Mean arterial pressure (MAP) elevated by 78%
Diastolic pressure increased by 10%
Systemic vascular resistance increased by 22%
Stroke volume unchanged
Heart rate decreased by 5%
Cardiac index decreased by 12%

These pressor changes may persist for 40 minutes after discontinuing the oxygen. The mechanism is probably a major effect on constriction of the microcirculation, including the capillary bed. The response is noted after sympathetic blockade.

Lambertsen noted that breathing high oxygen concentrations increased cerebrovascular resistance and that an increase in cerebral tissue carbon dioxide levels occurred.[6]

Types of Tissue Damage

Oxygen has a histotoxic effect, and three particular pathologic changes may develop from use of high concentrations. These are as follows: (1) primary pulmonary cell injury; (2) bronchopulmonary dysplasia; and (3) retinopathy of prematurity, or retrolental fibroplasia (RLF) in infants.

Primary Pulmonary Cell Damage[15]

At some critical arterial oxygen tension and duration of oxygen exposure, pulmonary tissue injury is inevitable and pursues a typical pathogenetic course.[21,22] *First stage* is the transudation phase with capillary congestion, capillary leakage, and perivascular edema. *Second stage* is the exudative phase with fibrinous material and blood cells appearing in the extravascular spaces and intra-alveolar hemorrhages. Cellular changes in type II alveolar cells and endothelial cells and necrosis occur, followed by the *third stage* or proliferative phase, with continued but more extensive interlobular edema, alveolar edema, fibroblastic proliferation, and fibrosis. Postmortem studies of lungs of adults who have died after prolonged ventilation with oxygen reveal morphologic changes in the pulmonary tissue. The following are significant: alveolar septal edema; fibroblastic proliferation; hyperplasia of alveolar lining cells; and hyaline alveolar membranes of fibrinous-type material.

Bronchopulmonary Dysplasia

During oxygen therapy of newborns, dysplasia of the pulmonary epithelium occurs in respiratory distress syndromes (RDS). The degree of damage is dose-related and can be diagnosed during life by radiography and by exfoliative cytology and correlated with the clinical picture. Four phases of development can be identified:

Stage I spans 1 to 3 days of age. It is denoted by hyperemia and alveolar collapse; it resembles RDS, but includes evidence of excessive mucosal necrosis. Some cuboidal epithelial cells appear in the secretions, but the majority of shed cells are squamous.

Stage II spans 4 to 10 days. One sees accelerated desquamation of mucosal cells with the appearance of atypical and immature cells. This reflects both increased necrosis and enhanced attempt at repair.

Stage III is seen between 10 and 20 days. Cell metaplasia, thick secretions, and casts of respiratory mucosal cells are present.

Stage IV is the period of chronicity. The lungs become noncompliant, and a type of centrolobular emphysema is noted. One sees continued metaplasia, mild fibrosis, and hypertrophy of the smooth muscle of small pulmonary and bronchial arteries.

Retinopathy of Prematurity

This acute form of vascular retinopathy occurs in premature infants. Its appearance in such infants was first recognized in 1942,[23] and in 1951 hyperoxia was implicated as one of the causes by Campbell.[24] A prospective, randomized study in the early 1950s of otherwise healthy premature infants showed that the administration of high concentrations of oxygen in incubators (50%) produced retrolental fibroplasia (RLF) in 37% of these subjects.[25] The incidence of the acute form of the disorder is inversely proportional to birth weight.[26] The damage occurs during the development of the retinal vessels.[27] High concentrations of oxygen experimentally result in an increase in the vascularity of the retinal vessels: one sees dilatation, tortuosity, and retinal hemorrhages. Subsequently, cicatricial changes occur.

Lanman and co-workers[28] compared the administration of high oxygen concentrations of 70% for 2 weeks to premature infants weighing less than 1.5 kg, with the administration of low concentrations of 38% intermittently and only for indications such as cyanosis. The differences in survival and in the development of vascular changes were dramatic: 61% of infants on high oxygen developed vascular changes, which progressed to fibroplasia in 22%. In the low-oxygen group, 7% had vascular changes, and none developed RLF.

Thus, one should not administer oxygen therapeutically to premature infants at concentrations greater than 40%. Oxygen at higher concentrations should be given only when a definite indication exists. In the stages of resuscitation and in the course of administration of oxygen for anesthesia, larger concentrations are permissible. These represent, of course, temporary emergency measures and should not be confused with continuous therapy in spontaneously breathing infants.

Risk Factors

Multiple factors other than hyperoxia have been identified and analyzed by Flynn.[29] An actual increase in RLF of the severe form in the premature infant appears to have occurred, despite the curtailment of excessive oxygen therapy. At the present time, many more low-weight infants are surviving, and RLF is prevalent in this group to the extent of 50 to 90%, despite the lack of high oxygen administration. Hence, the oxygen risk factor becomes less important than prematurity.[30]

Risk in multiple births is increased, even in infants who are not underweight or premature. The risk is three times greater than in single births. The duration of exposure to supplemental oxygen, even at low concentration of oxygen, increases the risk.[30] Clinical variables include low gestational age, occurrence of apnea, artificial ventilation, blood transfusions, and sepsis. Correlation of RLF also occurs when the $PACO_2$ is elevated and when hypotension or hypoxia occurs from any cause. Treatment with aspirin, a prostaglandin synthesis inhibitor, increases the severity of retinopathy.[31] Prostaglandins are vasodilators, and the decrease in availability of the specific prostaglandin by the administration of aspirin enhances the risk of retinopathy. As yet, the occurrence of blindness does not correlate entirely with hyperoxia, and restriction of oxygen supplements has not eliminated the occurrence of RLF.[31]

Coma During Oxygen Therapy

Delirium stupor and coma may develop in certain patients with chronic hypoxemia when treated with the inhalation of 50 to 100% oxygen.[32] This is particularly so in patients with emphysema. The cause is uncertain, but it is likely due to carbon dioxide excess causing narcosis.[33,34] The events leading to high arterial PCO_2 are probably as follows: The hypoxemic emphysematous patient receives a much of the respiratory drive from the stimulation of carotid and aortic body chemoreceptors. When the anoxemia stimulus is withdrawn by administering high concentrations of oxygen, respiration becomes shallow, and minute volume exchange diminishes. Elimination of carbon dioxide is decreased; an accumulation of 10% or more of carbon dioxide is within the narcotic range. Another operative mechanism may be the removal of the cortical stimulant effect of anoxia by administration of high oxygen concentrations, whereas a third mechanism may be due to a direct depression of cerebral metabolism by high arterial oxygen concentrations.

Mechanism of Toxicity[9,12]

The inciting of oxygen toxicity is related to the arterial oxygen tension and not to the inspired oxygen concentration. At some critical oxygen arterial tension and after exposure to this oxygen tension for 1 to 2 days, toxic physiologic effects occur. After 2 to 3 days, morphologic changes are likely.

A reduction in bronchial blood flow with a decrease in pulmonary surfactant is a significant element in pathophysiology. A vasoconstrictor agent appears to be elaborated locally from pulmonary chromaffin bodies. Accompanying this are decreased lung volume and reduced pulmonary compliance combined with an increased capillary physiologic shunting. In addition, ciliary activity is markedly reduced, so secretions easily accumulate and the mucus transport system is inhibited.

In the early course of intoxication, these physiologic effects are reversible.[18]

Experimentally, dogs may be regularly killed by 70% oxygen, and desquamation of pulmonary epithelium is seen.[35] High oxygen arterial tensions may increase bleeding.[23] Stadie[36] has indicated that high oxygen pressure interferes with the oxidative enzyme system of the body. Succinic dehydrogenase and cytochrome oxidase are depressed. Most of the enzymes inhibited contain sulfhydryl groups involved in the intermediate metabolism of carbohydrate.

Experimentally, elevation of cerebral arterial PO_2 also results in impairment of oxidative metabolism.[9,36] This was shown to result from "poisoning the catalyst," with oxidation of enzyme sulfhydryl bonds, reduction in oxygen consumption, and decrease in cerebral adenosine triphosphate (ATP).[12] Indeed, acute oxygen toxicity is manifested by convulsions, as well as by the lung lesions of RDS. For rats subjected to hyperbaric oxygen, both the neural and pulmonary impairment were prevented by anesthesia. That the damage to the lung is not attributable solely to exposure of the pulmonary tissue to high-inspired FIO_2, but parallels elevated arterial PO_2, has been demonstrated. When the lungs of a dog are intubated differentially, while one lung breathes air and the other breathes 100% oxygen, the lesions appear in both.[14] Ventilation of a small fraction of the pulmonary mass with hyperbaric oxygen without elevation of arterial oxygen tension failed to produce the lesions locally or remotely.[15]

Hyperbaric oxygen causes a decrease in ATP and a reduction of intracellular ionic gradients in slices of cerebral cortex. An increase of intracellular lipid peroxides occurs, as does an increase in inorganic phosphates.[37]

Molecular Mechanisms

Ordinarily, oxygen is a stable molecule, but a powerful oxidizing agent. The molecule can undergo subtle modifications and can be transformed into free radicals and various toxic substances, however. Among the more reactive substances are superoxide anions, hydrogen peroxide, and the hydroxyl free radicals. The main molecular targets of oxygen toxicity are DNA lipids and sulfhydroxyl-containing proteins.[38]

Prevention and Treatment

The use of the lowest concentration of oxygen for the shortest period of time consistent with sustaining life functions is the principle of safe oxygen therapy. Patients who receive oxygen concentrations over 60% ($FIO_2 > 0.6$) for 2 to 3 days are at risk.

In clinical practice, concentration of oxygen over 60% should be reserved for resuscitation and early management of respiratory insufficiency.[39] When ventilatory therapy is stable, FIO_2 should be reduced to levels below 0.5 FIO_2; that is, an FIO_2 should be selected that will provide an acceptable normal PaO_2 for that patient. If continued administration of a lowered FIO_2 is not tolerated, then intermittent lowering of FIO_2 to 0.3 to 0.4 for half an hour is frequently helpful. Early use of positive end-expiratory pressure to reduce large shunt fractions is effective in recruiting collapsed alveoli and in improving the ventilation-perfusion ratio. If a shunt QS/QT above 20 to 30% continues on an FIO_2 above 50% with a continued low PaO_2, one may be required to settle for a hypoxemic range of PaO_2. The use of breathing mixtures with an inert gas such as nitrogen (20%) reduces atelectasis.

Reduction of oxygen consumption is essential. Eliminating anxiety, sedating the patient, reducing metabolism by morphine, reducing fever, and reducing skeletal muscle activity are all desired.

The toxic effects of oxygen may be inhibited at least experimentally by three types of compounds[38]: (1) sulfhydryl compounds; (2) metabolic agents and antioxidants (vitamin E); and (3) acid-base buffers. Suppression of adrenal and thyroid function appears to limit the injury. Conversely, the administration of corticosteroids enhances the damage to pulmonary tissue:

1. Sulfhydryl compounds provide a reducing environment that diminishes the effect of high oxygen tensions. Cysteine and reduced glutathione, combined with succinate, provide protection in animals. The onset of convulsions is delayed, and the incidence of abnormal muscular activity is reduced fourfold.
2. Metabolic agents stimulate the production of ATP for cellular energy. Succinate belongs to this category, as does vitamin E. In the presence of high ATP, oxygen toxicity is minimized.
3. Acid-base buffers balance possible pH changes due to elevated carbon dioxide concentrations.

SPECIAL USES OF OXYGEN[39,40]

1. *Coronary occlusion.*[41] The use of high concentrations of oxygen in this pathologic state ameliorates dyspnea. Coronary arterioles may be released from spasm to some extent, and the collateral circulation may be improved. Eckenhoff[42] studied the effect of inhalation of 100% oxygen on coronary vessels of a dog, however, and found a consistent decrease of about 11% in coronary blood flow.

Russek and associates[43] also questioned the utility of oxygen administration in coronary occlusion from their clinical experience.

The inhalation of oxygen-rich gas mixture exerts a beneficial effect in humans on the ischemic myocardium. The inhalation of 100% oxygen for 60 minutes in patients with myocardial ischemic injury reduces the ST-segment elevation, and one sees a reduction in infarct size. The increased arterial oxygen tension also enhances the gradient of oxygen and enhances tissue diffusion.

2. *Vasospastic diseases.* Freeman has demonstrated that the use of oxygen releases peripheral vessels from spasm, such as occurs in Buerger's disease, and increases peripheral blood flow.

Topical oxygen also promotes healing of leg ulcers from phlebitis, arteriosclerosis, trauma, and lupus erythematosus. One technique consists of using a plastic bag enclosing an extremity and allowing 3.4 L/min of oxygen to flow into the bag, which provides an atmosphere of about 12 mm of Hg of oxygen above atmosphere. Tissue fluid oxygen tension 1 mm below the skin surface is significantly increased. Initial tissue PO_2 values have been determined to be about 50 mm Hg, whereas during oxygen exposure in the bag the average tissue oxygen it about 450 mm Hg.[44]

3. *Acute pulmonary disease, pneumonia.*

4. *Cardiac decompensation.*

5. *Chronic pulmonary diseases.* These disorders include chronic bronchitis, emphysema, and fibrosis, in which an interference exists in the actual flow and diffusion of gases and air from the exterior into the alveolar sacs.

6. *Pulmonary edema.*[45] Oxygen is used to treat edema such as occurs as a complication of pneumonia and as a manifestation of cardiac insufficiency, postoperative pulmonary edema, and the pulmonary edema of gas poisoning. When pulmonary edema is diagnosed, oxygen should be administered, but under positive pressure. This can be done with an anesthetic machine, with an iron lung or a resuscitator, and the amount of pressure is about 3 to 4 mm Hg.

7. *High-altitude flying.*[46] The dangers of aeroembolism are well known to flight surgeons. The cause is that nitrogen dissolved in the blood tends to come out of solution at high altitudes or low pressures and forms bubbles. When such bubbles strike important vital centers, death often ensues. This condition of air embolism is often prophylactically overcome by preoxygenation of aviators for half an hour to 3 hours before they are scheduled to go on high-altitude missions. Cramps and air sickness are other conditions occurring in aviators that are treated with oxygen.

8. *Postoperative excitement and delirium* are controlled by oxygen.

9. *Distention,* a common postoperative complication and due chiefly to swallowing air, is successfully treated and prevented by administration of oxygen.[47] The nitrogen of the air is diluted and its partial pressure in the blood diminished, so intestinal nitrogen is better absorbed. Moreover, because the air that is swallowed once oxygen administration has begun consists mostly of oxygen and only a small percentage of nitrogen, this mixture will be better absorbed if swallowed than air.

10. *Migraine.*

PATHOLOGIC OXYGENATION

Classification of Hypoxia

Originally Barcroft divided pathologic oxygenation into three categories: anoxic, anemic, and stagnant anoxia. Peters and Van Slyke added histotoxic anoxia. A simpler and more logical classification is based on etiology, according to Comroe and Dripps[48] and modified as follows:

I. Disturbances of oxygen loading
  A. Defective oxygenation of normal lung
    1. Atmospheric hypoxia
    2. Obstructive hypoxia
    3. Respiratory hypoxia
  B. Defective oxygenation due to abnormal lungs
    1. Insufficient pulmonary tissue
    2. Improper gas mixing: nonuniform
    3. Improper alveolar membrane gas diffusion
II. Disturbances of oxygen delivery
  A. Defective transportation of oxygen
    1. Lowered oxygen capacity (anemic anoxia)
    2. Deficient circulation
    3. Incomplete circulation of blood (venous-arterial shunt)
  B. Defective tissue oxygenation (histotoxic anoxia)
    1. Histotoxic hypoxia (including tissue overutilization)
    2. Abnormal intracellular transport
    3. Mitochrondeal disorders: increased utilization
      a. Luft disease of muscle
      b. Thyrotoxicosis
      c. Polycythemia vera
    4. Hyperoxia
    5. Various poisons: iron, salicylate, dinitrophenol
    6. Decreased utilization: hypothyroidism, cyanide poisoning, cellular edema

Atmospheric Hypoxia[49]

This type is characterized by lowered oxygen tension in the inspired air. Such a condition may be brought about by ascent to high altitudes, by dilution with inert gases, or by dilution with anesthetic inhalation agents.

At sea level, the partial pressure of oxygen is 159 mm Hg. At 10,000 feet, the partial pressure of oxygen is about 110 mm Hg and blood arterial oxygen saturation is 85%. Unacclimatized persons usually have some definite handicap, and the reduction in blood oxygen is sufficient to cause an increase in rate and depth of respiration through stimulation of the carotid body. Oxygen supplements are needed.

At 18,000 feet, the partial pressure of oxygen is 79 mm Hg or half that at sea level, and arterial oxygen saturation is 70%, with a serious handicap. At Mount Everest, with an elevation of 29,028 feet (8845 m), the mean barometric pressure is 236 mm Hg. When the water vapor pressure is considered, the mean barometric pressure is reduced to about 189 mm Hg and the partial pressure of oxygen then becomes 40 mm Hg. Above these levels, supplemental oxygen is required, 100% oxygen must be breathed, and/or the respired atmosphere must be under pressure.

Above 35,000 feet, the pressure of 100% oxygen falls below the partial pressure at sea level, whereas at 40,000 feet, the oxygen pressure decreases to the point where not enough is absorbed by the blood. At this point, 100% oxygen must be respired under pressure.

Dilution of the atmosphere by inert gases may likewise

diminish the oxygen content and positive pressure sufficiently to decrease the arterial blood oxygen. In mines, a variety of conditions are sometimes found in which the oxygen is diluted. Diluents are methane (fire damp), nitrogen (flat damp), carbon dioxide (after damp). Carbon monoxide asphyxia is partially due to the diluting effect of the partially combusted carbon on the atmosphere.

Obstructive Hypoxia

Obstruction in the respiratory passages prevents the free flow of oxygen into the lungs. This is particularly seen in comatose patients, in whom "falling back" of the tongue and relaxation of the pharyngeal tissues are common. Edema of the tissue, foreign bodies, and tumors may encroach on the tracheobronchial lumen to cause obstruction and diminished oxygenation. Paralysis of vocal cords acts similarly.

Respiratory Hypoxia

Defects in the neuromuscular mechanism of respiration cause hypoxia. Such defects include central depression of the respiratory center (drugs and trauma with raised intracranial pressure) on the one hand and impairment of muscle action on the other (poliomyelitis, myasthenia gravis, curare overdose).

Insufficient Pulmonary Tissue

A diminution in the amount of functioning of pulmonary tissue is seen in a variety of pathologic states including atelectasis, pneumonia, tumors, tuberculous cavitation, and infarction; it is seen in heart failure, pneumothorax, and hydrothorax, in which encroachment on the compressible pulmonary parenchyma occurs. Occasionally, extensive surgical removal of lung tissue leaves an insufficient quantity of pulmonary tissue.

Improper Gas Mixing

Poor mixing of inspired gases in all alveoli, as occurs in emphysema, results in low arterial oxygen tensions.

Improper Alveolar Membrane Diffusion

Inspired gases may fail to diffuse readily through the alveolar-capillary partition. This occurs in pulmonary edema, exudative pulmonary infection, fibrosis, and capillary sclerosis.

Lowered Oxygen Capacity

This condition is essentially anemic hypoxia and is due to diminution in amount of active hemoglobin or of the red cells. Such a condition exists in various anemias as well as in methemoglobinemia and carbon monoxide poisoning.

Deficient Circulation

This condition is essentially stagnant hypoxia. The circulation is slowed, and the necessary blood volume flow per minute is diminished. Conditions causing this state include hemorrhage, shock, heart failure, vasoconstriction, and cerebral thrombosis.

Incomplete Circulation of Blood

This disorder is essentially a condition of deficient circulation but is more specifically due to venous arterial shunting of blood. It is seen particularly in certain congenital heart diseases.

Defective Tissue Oxygenation

This condition may be due to deficient transfer of oxygen from the blood to the tissues because of inadequate gradient of oxygen partial pressure. Edema of tissues may also interfere with the diffusion of oxygen to cells.

Variations in tissue metabolic needs and oxygen utilization may result in histotoxic hypoxia. Poisoning of enzyme systems, as from cyanide, may prevent uptake of available oxygen by cells. Hypermetabolism from fever or hyperthyroidism may create an abnormal oxygen demand, especially in tissues with a high metabolic rate (heart, liver, brain).

HYPOXIA

Causal Factors

Survey of Hypoxia Potential

In reviewing any clinical setting for the potential for the development of hypoxia, the following checklist is useful:

   I. Assessment of general patient factors
  II. The atmospheric breathing mixture (estimate both the FIO_2 and $PATMO_2$)
 III. Ventilatory efficiency (measured by $PaCO_2$)
 IV. Efficiency of oxygen uptake (denoted by saturation of hemoglobin-SaO_2)
  V. Transport profile: hemoglobin and blood volume
 VI. Cardiac output
VII. Degree of shunting: PaO_2; $DAaO_2$
VIII. Tissue uptake: oxygen consumption and arteriovenous oxygen difference

Predisposing Clinical Factors

Many physiologic and pathologic conditions may limit the oxygenation process.

The age factor must be considered because PaO_2 values progressively decrease normally with advancing years (Fig. 27–1). Accepted ranges (Sorbini[40a]) are as follows:

Age in Years	PaO₂ (mmhg)
10 – 30	97 – 91
30 – 40	90 – 85
40 – 60	85 – 75
60 – 90	80 – 70

The rate of arterial desaturation is also faster in the aged subject. Hence the saturation process or oxygen loading of venous blood in the lung is more demanding.

Obese patients have is a reduction in PaO_2 value. The reduction is proportional to the degree of obesity.[50]

Mechanical factors restricting chest movement reduce oxygen tension, increase the effort required for breathing, and increase oxygen needs. Position influences PaO_2

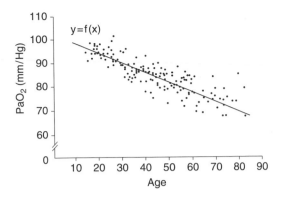

Fig. 27–1. Arterial oxygen tension in relation to age. The points represent duplicate estimations of PaO_2 in 152 normal supine adult subjects. The regression line is shown. The arterial oxygen tension may be approximated by the equation $PaO_2 = 109 - 0.43 \times$ (age in years) $\pm$ 4 mm Hg. (Courtesy of Sorbini.)

values, which are lower in supine as compared with upright posture.

Preexisting cardiopulmonary disease not only limits uptake of oxygen, but *prevents compensation* when demands are increased. The following are circulatory limitations: inability to increase cardiac output; diminished myocardial reserve; and inability to dilate coronary vessels. Pulmonary disease reduces ventilatory reserve.[42]

Deficient transport mechanisms predispose to hypoxia. A significant deficiency is lack of hemoglobin: 12.0 g/100 ml of blood reduces oxygen transport per unit volume by 20%, whereas a 9.0-g value reduces transport by 40%. Low blood volumes limit transportation efficiency.

Trauma, shock, and burns lead to circulatory stagnation and a serious handicap to compensation for any subsequent hypoxia. In burns, the decrease in PaO_2 is proportional to the surface extent of the injury. Intravascular coagulation leads to serious impairment of oxygen transport.

Depressant drugs limit the capacity for compensation.

Factors During Anesthesia

In surveying factors during anesthesia, many clinical conditions may lead to hypoxia:

I. Impaired preanesthetic oxygenation system
1. Poor physical status
2. Drug intake, premedication, decreased compensatory mechanisms
II. Decreased partial pressure and concentration of inspired oxygen in anesthetic breathing mixture: mechanical factors
1. Flow meter defects
2. Inaccurate readings at low flows
3. Pressure gauge defects
4. Exhausted oxygen cylinders (unlikely with failsafe system)
5. Obstructed delivery tubes
III. Impaired ventilatory efficiency
1. Airway obstruction: upper and lower
2. Hypoventilation: decreased effective alveolar ventilation
3. Increased shunting

4. Obstructive diseases
5. Type of operation
   a. Thoracic operation: 50% shunt
   b. Abdominal operation: 35% shunt
6. Poor patterns of ventilation
7. Lack of periodic hyperinflation (artificial sighing)
IV. Impaired ventilation-perfusion relations
1. Increased shunting
2. Increased dead space
V. Deficient oxygen loading
1. Acidosis
2. Low hemoglobin
3. Pulmonary edema
VI. Decreased transport: hypovolemia (blood loss; fluid loss)
VII. Cardiocirculatory instability
1. Preexisting compensatory disability
2. Decreased cardiac output
3. Myocardial disease
4. Acidosis
5. Negative inotropic drugs
6. Arrhythmias
7. Myocardial depression: drugs, acidosis
8. Interference with venous return (i.e., retractors on vena cava)
9. Circulatory depression: blood loss, sympatheticoparalysis
10. Excessive pressure
11. Positive means airway
VIII. Impaired tissue delivery
1. Impaired regional blood flow
2. Increased utilization; acidosis
3. Hypocarbia and decreased cerebral blood flow (CBF)
4. Excess tissue lactate

Clinical Factors after Anesthesia

The immediate postanesthetic period is one of maximal danger. Relaxation of supervision and observation of the patients is frequent, and the need for specialized postanesthesia recovery units and specially trained anesthesia personnel is evident.

A checklist of some causes of postanesthesia and postoperative hypoxia is provided:

I. General patient factors: continuation of preoperative conditions predisposing to hypoxia continue and need to be appreciated: obesity, excessive age, cardiopulmonary diseases; these must be assessed and treatment continued where necessary
II. Diminished inspired oxygen
1. Lack of oxygen supplements
2. Excessive suctioning[51]
3. Diffusion hypoxia after nitrous oxide anesthesia[52]
III. Impaired ventilatory efficiency
1. Obstructed upper airway: tongue; uvula
2. Obstructed lower airway: secretions; bronchospasm; atelectasis
3. Musculoskeletal weakness
4. The pharmacologic "shadow": residual effects of respiratory depressant anesthetics, narcotics, residual neuromuscular paralysis

    5. Surgical factors: binders; wounds
    6. Pain
    7. Excessive analgesic medication
 IV. Abnormal ventilation-perfusion relations
    1. Exaggerated shunting
    2. Loss of sigh mechanism[53]
    3. Increased dead space effect
  V. Deficient oxygen loading
 VI. Diminished transport
    1. Extension of preoperative factors
    2. Continuation of uncorrected surgical factors
VII. Cardiovascular instability
    1. Uncorrected acid-base abnormalities
    2. Electrolyte and fluid imbalance
    3 Cardiac depression from drugs and acidosis
VIII. Impaired tissue delivery
    1. Capillary stasis
    2. Loss of tissue perfusion
    3. Tissue lactate
    4. Cellular drug effects

Clinical Signs

Symptoms of Oxygen Want[48]

The signs and symptoms of oxygen want are similar to those of drunkenness and inebriation. In other words, the effects of oxygen lack and of alcohol are similar. In regard to the central nervous system, one first notes a mild exhilaration often manifested by argumentativeness and boisterousness. There then follows emotional impairment and later impairment in judgment, which sometimes finally results in complete delirium. Similarly, one sees incoordination, particularly psychomotor incoordination (Table 27–1).

An interesting psychologic experiment has been conducted by the United States Army Air Corps. This consists in testing future pilots in atmospheres of 12% oxygen.[54] In the pretest period, candidates are selected who are considered anxious personalities and are segregated for statistical purposes from the group of normal individuals. When the anxiety-prone subjects were exposed for a pe-

riod of about 12 minutes to an atmosphere of 12% oxygen, approximately 25% collapsed, and approximately an equal number showed some impairment in emotional stability and judgment. Of the normal group or of those considered normal by usual psychic tests, none collapsed, and only 18% showed any impairment in judgment.

Sensory symptoms exhibited are as follows: Most patients exhibit mild to severe headaches. Often, precordial pain is present, typical of the type that occurs in anginal patients. Finally, lassitude and malaise are common features in the anoxic patient.

Gastrointestinal symptoms consist essentially of nausea, retching, and vomiting.

Respiratory Signs[48,54]

Contrary to common belief, the respiratory response to hypoxia is neither marked nor significant. Not until a 16% oxygen atmosphere is breathed does respiration increase, and the minute volume then increases 7%; while breathing an atmosphere of 10% oxygen, the minute volume increases only 17%. Only in the presence of severe active hypoxia does a vigorous hyperpnea occur. The change in minute volume is brought about through an increase in both rate and depth. Initially, the rate shows a periodic increase, but after prolonged hypoxia, depression in rate occurs. Amplitude is irregularly increased at first but later shows a slight but constant increase (Table 27–2).

The mechanism of respiratory stimulation is the chemoreceptor system of the carotid and aortic bodies. These receptors respond only to hypoxemia when the tension of the oxygen (the Pa_{O_2}) is reduced below normal. Thus, low arterial *oxygen content*, which would occur in hemorrhage, anemia, or carbon monoxide poisoning, does not stimulate chemoreceptors and increase respiratory exchange.

Cardiovascular Signs[48,55]

The pulse rate offers a more accurate index of hypoxemia. The increase in pulse rate occurs in circumstances either of lowered arterial oxygen tension (Pa_{O_2}) or of lowered oxygen content. Hence pulse responses differ from the respiratory response to anoxemia. The pulse rate also increases at reduced arterial oxygen tensions, which do not cause a respiratory response. Usually, the degree of

Table 27–1. Symptoms of Hypoxia

General	Similar to drunkenness
Psychic	Higher centers first impaired
	Psychomotor and emotional
	Judgment poor
	Boisterous, argumentative—
	delirious
Sensory	Headache, malaise, lassitude
	Precordial pain
Gastrointestinal	Nausea, retching, vomiting
Muscular	Incoordination, convulsions, flaccidity
Experimental	12% oxygen
	Normals—
	18% impairment, no collapse
	Anxiety cases—
	50% impairment
	25% collapse

Table 27–2. Respiratory Signs of Hypoxia

Oxygen percent	Minute volume
16	7% increase
10	17% increase

Pattern of Response
  Increase in both rate and depth
  First rate increases but later is slowed
  Amplitude is irregularly increased at first but later is constant

Mechanism
  Chemoreceptors

Stimulus
  Lowered Pa_{O_2} (oxygen tension)
  Lowered oxygen content (shock-anemia); no changes

tachycardia is directly proportional to the reduction of arterial oxygen saturation.

As hypoxemia becomes severe (levels not encountered clinically) and is prolonged, the pulse may slow and become full and bounding. This sign, however, is neither constant nor reliable, except in the late stages.

The diagnosis of hypoxemia may often be substantiated by the therapeutic test. This relies on the observation that the pulse rate will decrease by 10 or more beats per minute within a minute or two of the start of oxygen therapy.

The mechanism of pulse changes due to hypoxemia is probably twofold.[48] When *oxygen tension* is low, the chemoreceptors are probably stimulated to produce reflex tachycardia. This does not preclude direct stimulation of cardiac centers by hypoxemia, which may also occur. When *oxygen content* decreases but tension is normal, the tachycardia that occurs is probably produced through changes in circulation. Specifically, peripheral vasodilatation occurs as a result of tissue hypoxia followed by lowered peripheral resistance and lowered arterial blood pressure. Tachycardia is then produced as a reflex through pressoreceptor mechanisms (Table 27–3).

Blood pressure changes are relatively insignificant in clinical situations of hypoxemia.[55] Generally, one sees a slight increase in both systolic and diastolic pressures with moderate hypoxemia (arterial saturation 80% or better). Exposure of a vein to a 10% oxygen atmosphere produces systolic changes of 6 to 12 mm Hg and diastolic changes of 0 to 3 mm Hg, however. In many individuals, blood pressure falls. With severe hypoxemia (arterial oxygen saturation less than 80%), greater elevations in systolic pressure may occur, but diastolic invariably falls.[56] Such changes may occur promptly, but if the hypoxemia is prolonged, the blood pressure falls markedly and shock supervenes.

Effect of Hypoxia on Pulmonary Circulation[57]

Breathing 10% oxygen mixtures in normal individuals produces a rise in pulmonary artery pressure, but pulmonary capillary pressure is unchanged. Acute hypoxia is considered to cause vasoconstriction of pulmonary precapillary vessels. Patients with chronic pulmonary disease have an exaggerated rise in pulmonary artery pressure. The hypoxia probably increases pulmonary blood flow (increased rate) and/or direct increased vascular resistance.

Table 27–3. Cardiocirculatory Signs of Hypoxia

Mechanism of Pulse Changes

Law Oxygen Tension
  Stimulates chemoreceptors
  Response is reflex tachycardia

Law Oxygen Content
  Causes tissue hypoxia → vasodilation
  Lowered peripheral resistance → stimulates
    pressoreceptors
  Response is reflex tachycardia

Possible Stimulation at Cardiac Centers

Biochemical Changes

In the presence of partial or complete airway obstruction, hypoxemia and a respiratory acidosis ensue. A two-stage effect occurs, with a release of epinephrine initially. Together with an increase in blood sugar, it produces a reduction in concentration.[58]

Clinical Stages

During progressive increase in hypoxemia, three stages may be defined with respect to vital signs (Fig. 27–2):

1. *Precrisis stage*:
   Inhalation of 10 to 12% oxygen atmosphere.
   Arterial oxygen saturation 80% or better.
   Arterial blood oxygen content 12 to 14 vol per 100 ml of blood.
   Respiration: increase in both rate and depth.
   Blood pressure: increase in systolic; slight or no elevation in diastolic.
   Pulse: tachycardia and reduced peripheral resistance.

2. *Circulatory crisis stage*:
   Inhalation of 8 to 10% oxygen.
   Arterial oxygen saturation less than 80%.
   Arterial blood oxygen content 10 ml or less per 100 ml of blood.
   Respiration: minute volume increased about 17 to 20%.
   Blood pressure: systolic pressure may be sharply elevated but soon falls; diastolic pressure falls.
   Pulse: bradycardia for a brief period followed by gradual increase in rate.

3. *Terminal stage*:
   Continuation of 8 to 10% oxygen inhalation for 20 minutes or less than 8% oxygen inhalation for 10 minutes or less.
   Blood arterial oxygen content 4 ml or less per 100 ml of blood.
   Apnea.
   Blood pressure: rapid fall of pressure to zero.
   Pulse: terminal slowing developing into ventricular fibrillation or asystole.

Neuromuscular Signs

Incoordination and twitchings of the muscles are early signs of oxygen lack. These gradually progress to the states of convulsion, which may be local or generalized and show the typical features of the epileptic state, namely, clonic-tonic contractions of the muscles and then clonic convulsions. After a short period of this type of stimulation, the muscles completely relax and are flaccid.

Cyanosis

The color of the skin is a misleading sign to follow in determining the need for oxygen. In the normal person, cyanosis is defined as a blueness of the skin due to changes in color of capillary blood. It is evident only when the patient has approximately 5 g of reduced hemoglobin per 100 ml of capillary blood. Furthermore,

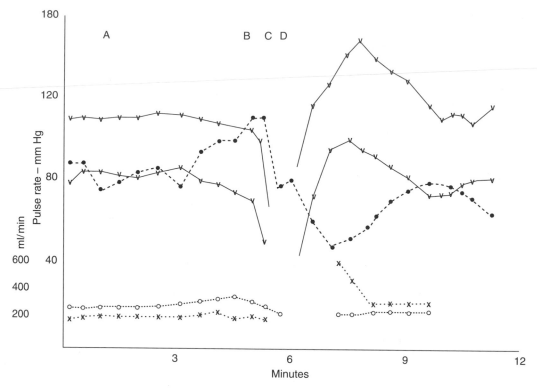

Fig. 27–2. Record of changes accompanying acute oxygen want. Blood pressure = v-v; pulse rate = closed circles-closed circles; respiratory rate = o-o; tidal volume = x-x. The column of figures on the extreme left represents tidal volume in milliliters. The second column of figures represents blood pressure in millimeters of mercury, and pulse and respiratory rates per minute. After a 25-year-old woman had been under nitrous oxide anesthesia for 35 minutes, she was given pure nitrous oxide to inhale through an endotracheal airway from a recording spirometer for approximately 5 minutes (A to D). At B, the pulse was weak and the color only slightly cyanotic. At C, the blood pressure could not be read; at D, the respiration had almost ceased. The chest was then inflated twice with pure oxygen. After the period of apnea lasting 30 seconds, note rise in blood pressures and tidal volume and decrease in pulse rate. Premedication (morphine sulfate, 8.1 mg; scopolamine hydrobromide, 0.3 mg and paraldehyde, 31 g) frequently modifies the typical "oxygen crisis" in laboratory animals subjected to acute oxygen want. Redrawn from Rovenstine, E. A.: Fundamentals of Anesthesia. Chicago, American Medical Association, 1954.

cyanosis is masked by such conditions as heavy skin pigmentation, racial pigmentation, icterus, or the presence of argyria.

Effects on Cerebral Physiology[59]

A critical reduction in available oxygen to cerebral cells is due either to *hypoxemia,* indicating a reduction in PaO_2, or to *ischemia,* signifying a decrease in cerebral blood flow. The critical values are those levels that are insufficient to maintain normal function and may lead to cell damage.

Basic supply and energy requirement of the brain have been noted (see Chapter 8). Some special metabolic characteristics that increase the vulnerability of the brain to oxygen lack are summarized.[60,61]

1. A high resting oxygen consumption: 20% of total body oxygen consumption for 2% of body weight.
2. Continuous and unvarying oxygen consumption during the waking state and sleep.
3. Sole dependence on glucose as the nutritional substrate (normal adult) and dependence on aerobic degradation to carbon dioxide and water. Anaerobic

degradation by glycolytic paths to lactic acid yields insufficient energy for maintenance.

4. No oxygen or energy stores (glycogen) or preformed high-energy phosphate compounds (ATP). Complete interruption of circulation exhausts oxygen in 10 seconds and uses up the available glucose in 2 minutes.

Metabolism in Hypoxemia

A reduction of arterial PO_2 results in a diminished oxygen delivery to brain per unit time. To maintain a constant cerebral metabolic rate $(CMR)O_2$, either the oxygen extraction must increase or CBF must increase.

When oxygen extraction increases, that is, arteriovenous DO_2 increases, the end-capillary venous PO_2 decreases, so the gradient of some parts may not be sufficient for oxidative phosphorylation. A fall in venous PO_2 from a normal of 35 to 25 mm Hg elicits a reactive hyperemia, which is called "reaction" threshold and is accompanied by electroencephalographic changes changes. A further fall of venous PO_2 to 19 to 17 mm Hg is critical and causes unconsciousness, whereas a fall to 10 to 12 mm Hg is the "lethal threshold" and usually results in brain cell damage and/or cardiac arrest.

Cerebral arterial PO_2 reduced below 45 mm Hg is usually accompanied by a homeostatic decrease in vascular resistance resulting from the lactic acidosis. In circumstances of hypoxemia, acidosis has a salutary effect, and if blood pressure is maintained, energy requirements may be met. Blood pressure in states of anoxemia is, therefore, of critical importance to the brain if cell necrosis is to be prevented.

Metabolism in Ischemia

The sequence of homeostatic responses to ischemia differs from that to anoxemia. Ischemia results from a reduction in perfusion pressure to brain tissue either from lowering mean arterial pressure or from vascular obstruction due to luminal narrowing or compression (i.e., raised intracranial pressure). When perfusion pressure is reduced to a level of 50 to 70 mm Hg, a detectable decrease in CBF ensues. Until this critical level is reached, autoregulatory mechanisms with dilation of vessels usually maintain flow, and this can occur independent of local tissue acidosis. Energy utilization and production continue to be adequate without cell damage until perfusion pressure reaches 30 to 40 mm Hg or until CBF is lowered below 50%, as from hyperventilation.

When CBF is reduced to a level where the capillary tissue PO_2 gradient reaches the "critical threshold" denoted by venous PO_2 of 17 to 19 mm Hg, anoxic changes may occur. Apparently, lowering PO_2 values alone does not necessarily produce energy alterations, but brain anoxia is more closely related to a fall in CBF. The regional maldistribution of circulation must also be emphasized, rather than the overall CBF. If acidosis is permitted within circumstance, other areas of the brain may be deprived of adequate circulation. Acidosis in ischemic states is likely to be harmful. Therefore, in clinical conditions of ischemia, the correction of acidosis is of prime importance.

In conclusion, in hypoxic states, the prevention of brain dysfunction and cerebral tissue damage requires that both the arterial pressure be maintained above "reaction" threshold and that acidosis be vigorously corrected.

Encephalopathy

Ischemic and cellular hypoxia may be of four types: (1) focal ischemia, as in cardiovascular accidents (strokes); (2) global ischemia, from respiratory or cardiac arrest; (3) head injury with direct cell damage or ischemia from increased intracranial pressure; and (4) acute metabolic or infectious processes producing raised intracranial pressure and ischemia. In all instances, cerebral hypoxia produces varying degrees of dysfunction or disintegration. The neurologic signs and symptoms are referred to as a syndrome of hypoxic "encephalopathy."

Pathology

Tolerance to Hypoxia[54]

The ability of a tissue or organ to maintain its functional capacity despite inadequate oxygen supply, or to survive a period of complete oxygen deprivation without irreversible damage, is defined as tolerance.

All tissues and organs have a degree of vulnerability; the most vulnerable organs are the brain, heart, and adrenal glands. Periods of oxygen deprivation of 2 to 6 minutes may seriously impair function of these organs, and varying degrees of cell damage may occur. In all tissues, function is initially impaired; following such impairment, persistence of the stress usually produces organic changes. In the brain, the highest centers show the least tolerance to oxygen lack and are the first to cease functioning and the first to show structural changes. Function may cease in less than 1 to 2 minutes, and damage may occur within 2 to 4 minutes.

The age factor is recognized as of great importance. The fetus is more tolerant of hypoxia and is less likely to be damaged than is the newborn. In turn, the newborn has a greater tolerance than the adult, whereas children in the active growing periods have diminished tolerance and greater likelihood of damage.

Metabolic factors play a role, and it is recognized that in periods of high metabolism, the susceptibility to damage is greater. This susceptibility to hypoxia is correlated with the metabolic rate. Moreover, in hypermetabolic states such as thyrotoxicosis, the organism is more vulnerable.

When severe hypoxia is imposed on the organism, anaerobic pathways of metabolism are stimulated. In newborns, such pathways are available, but they are not effective in the adult brain. This alternate pathway represents the ability to metabolize substrates to lactic and pyruvic acids.

Obesity plays an important role, and correlated with increasing overweight is a decreasing tolerance to hypoxia. Thus, obese individuals cannot tolerate severe degrees of oxygen lack.

Correlated with metabolism is the effect of temperature. Extremes of temperature decrease tolerance to oxygen lack. In periods of fever, the organism is much more vulnerable.

Tissue Pathology

Haldane succinctly delineated the effect of hypoxia on the body when he stated "Anoxia not only stops the machine but wrecks the machinery."[62]

After disintegration of function, the tissues and organs may undergo cellular disorganization. The fundamental structural changes seen are stereotyped for all organs and are briefly outlined and illustrated (Fig. 27-3).[63]

Hemorrhage

Punctate hemorrhages are particularly found in the cerebral cortex. They are also found in the epicardium and the adventitia of the aorta.

Congestion

Congestion is seen in the pulmonary and systemic circuits. Pulmonary congestion occurs in all cases. In the systemic circulation, the kidneys and submucosal layer of stomach and intestines are involved. The portal circulation is congested markedly, as is the liver.

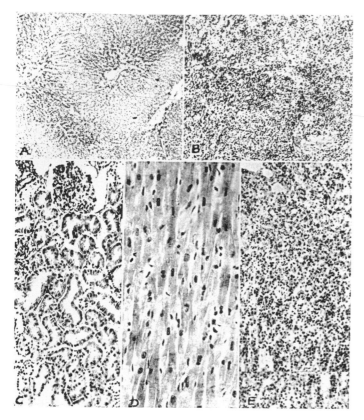

Fig. 27–3. General pathology of anoxia. Autopsy No. 7-258. Survival for 5 days after anoxemic episode under nitrous oxide anesthesia. A, Perivenous necrosis of the liver. H & E, × 45. B, Cellular infiltration of spleen ("acute splenitis"). H & E, × 95. C, Degenerative changes in epithelium of renal tubules. H & E, × 130. D, Minimal brown atrophy of cardiac muscle. E, focal hemorrhage into adrenal cortex. H & E, × 105. From Courville, C. B.: Cerebral Anoxia. Los Angeles, San Lucas Press, 1953.

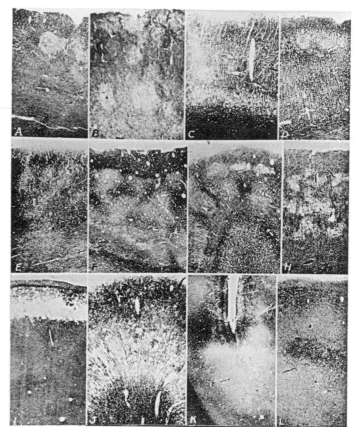

Fig. 27–4. Alterations in cerebral cortex consequent to anoxia of nitrous oxide etiology. Variable pattern of necrosis and its irregular distribution is noteworthy. With progression of the lesion, multiple isolated foci of necrosis coalesce to form laminar or multiple laminar necroses leading to subcortical cortical necrosis (bottom row of figures). In less severe cases, focal or laminar loss of nerve cells or formation of focal scars may also occur resulting in an irregular atrophy of the cerebral cortex. All these photomicrographs were taken from reduced silver preparations under low magnifications. From Courville, C. B.: Cerebral Anoxia. Los Angeles, San Lucas Press, 1953.

Edema

Swelling of endothelial cells, of capillaries, of renal medulla, and of renal tubules occurs.

Vacuolization

Fat and glycogen vacuoles appear in the liver and heart.

Necrosis

This process occurs in brain, liver, and kidney.

Severity of Damage[64] (Fig. 27–4)

The *brain* is particularly vulnerable to oxygen lack. The cellular changes seen after a bout of hypoxia depend first on the severity and duration of the hypoxia and second on the period of survival.

If *survival is of short duration,* that is, less than 40 hours, the following changes are usually observed:

1. Brain: pial vessels are congested; congestion is present in cortex, in gray areas, and in the basal ganglia.

2. Lungs and heart: congestion, thickening of alveolar walls, hemorrhage, and interstitial infiltration with leukocytes; the heart muscle may show brown atrophy.
3. Liver: middle and central lobular necrosis.
4. Kidney: tubular necrosis.

If *survival is beyond 40 hours,* brain damage is extensive, including architectural, cellular, and interstitial changes. The various parts of the brain, in the order of their susceptibility, are the cortex, where both large and small pyramidal cells are affected, the basal ganglia, especially the globus and putamen (lenticular nuclei), and the caudate and thalamic nuclei, which show only the general effects of hypoxia, that is, local dilatation of vessels.

In the cortex, one sees degeneration of individual cells and areas of focal necrosis. The various zonal layers of pyramidal cells show degeneration. In the early stages,

4.2 mm Hg for every 100 mm Hg drop in pressure. Bicarbonate excretion in the urine increases, lowering the alkaline arterial pH to normal values within a few weeks.

Both residual and total lung volumes are increased, but vital capacity changes little. Pulmonary vascular engorgement occurs as a result of both increased total blood volume and a 5% increase in the volume of blood distributed to the lungs (12 to 15% of the total blood volume is in lungs at sea level, against 20% at high altitude.)

Maximal diffusing capacity of the lungs is increased as a result of an increase in the number of pulmonary capillaries. Alveolar-arterial oxygen differences are essentially zero (as compared with 8 to 12 mm Hg at sea level). Exhaled oxygen concentrations are markedly decreased, pointing to an increased oxygen extraction from alveolar air.

The pulmonary vasculature in adults shows a typical hypertrophy of the muscularis, mainly at the arteriolar level, resembling the findings in newborns at sea level. An increased pulmonary vascular resistance occurs and is accompanied by a mild pulmonary artery hypertension (mean 24 mm Hg as compared with 12 mm Hg at sea level).

Chronic hypoxia, pulmonary artery hypertension, and a decrease in systemic blood pressure may account for a high incidence of patent ductus arteriosus (15 times higher than at sea level).

Cardiovascular Changes

Cardiovascular adaptation is characterized by bradycardia, mild hypotension, and a slight increase in venous pressure.

Total blood volume is considerably higher, primarily because of an increase in the number of red cells. Plasma volume (in ml/kg) remains unchanged. Hypervolemia and polycythemia are important factors in increasing the oxygen-carrying capacity of the blood. The increase in hemoglobin concentration is approximately 10% for every 100-mm Hg drop in pressure; erythropoietic activity is enhanced. Six to 8 weeks are required to produce maximal polycythemia. The higher the altitude, the longer the time required. The oxyhemoglobin dissociation curve is slightly shifted to the right at constant plasma pH, showing a slightly decreased affinity of hemoglobin for oxygen. One sees a small reduction in tension with a given decrease in oxygen content and saturation.

Perfusion of the kidneys is decreased, as evidenced by a decrease in renal plasma flow and filtration index. The adrenal glands are less responsive to adrenocorticotropic hormone.

Endocrine Effects

Observations on pituitary and thyroid function at high altitudes compared with sea level values have been reported.[70] A progressive rise occurs at 5400 m (17,700 feet) and at 6300 m (20,700 feet) in serum thyroxine (T_4) concentrations, and a persistent elevation is seen in serum triiodothyronine (T_3) concentrations. Serum levels of thyroid-stimulating hormone, elaborated from the pituitary, are also increased. This curious finding suggests altered regulation of the pituitary and the usual feedback inhibition by increased T_4 levels as normally occurs at sea level. No alteration of the capacity of the pituitary to respond to the administration of thyrotropin-releasing hormone occurs. No significant increase in thyroglobulin has been noted. Because the ratio of T_4 to T_3 is increased, it is suggested that conversion of T_4 to T_3 is impaired. In brief, high altitude causes a hyperthyroxemic state in euthyroid subjects.

Complications of High-Altitude Exposure

The healthy sea-level resident transferred to high altitude may develop signs of "acute mountain sickness": mental excitement or torpidity, headache, nausea, vomiting, dyspnea, gastrointestinal hypermotility, and considerable tachycardia following even minimal exercise.

Sudden exposure to high altitude may induce acute pulmonary edema. It becomes apparent 6 to 26 hours after reaching altitudes above 10,000 feet. Continuous oxygen administration and transfer to lower levels constitute effective treatment. The mechanisms of acute high-altitude pulmonary edema" are not well understood. The following possibilities, based on actual case studies, have been suggested: (1) increased capillary permeability due to hypoxia; (2) left-sided myocardial insufficiency; (3) increased pulmonary venous resistance; and (4) acute increase in pulmonary blood flow volume.

High-altitude residents and natives show an unusual incidence of certain disease states: gallbladder disease (with or without cholesterol calculi), right bundle block, intestinal adhesions, megacolon with volvulus, pulmonary silicosis (mine workers), fibrosing pulmonary tuberculosis (subnutrition), and keloid formation in wound healing. An appreciably low incidence of coronary occlusion is noted.

A small percentage of high-altitude residents may develop a peculiar syndrome known as "chronic mountain sickness" that seems to be an exacerbation of the normal polycythemia and other acclimatizing mechanisms. Characteristics are extreme cyanosis, congestion of the mucous membranes, severe dyspnea, cephalalgia, pulmonary rales, acute pulmonary edema, and death. Laboratory studies show an excessive polycythemia (15 million/mm^3 red cells and 4 million/mm^3 leukocytes) and hematocrit values up to 93.8%. Blood volumes of the order of 155 and 122 ml/kg and cardiac indexes from 4 to 5 L/min/m^2 have been measured. Pulmonary function is impaired: $PaCO_2$ rises and PaO_2 falls. Oxygen-diffusing capacity and oxygen saturation are markedly decreased below levels that are normal for that altitude. Arterial hemoglobin oxygen content as low as 56% and venous saturations of 31% suggest a decreased oxygen extraction.

The treatment of this syndrome consists of 100% oxygen with intermittent positive-pressure breathing, tracheobronchial toilet, bronchodilators, and phlebotomy when necessary. Digitalization is justified. Rapid transport to sea level is indicated. Occasional spontaneous remission of this syndrome has been reported.

Anesthesia Problems at High Altitudes

See James' Chapter 17, on climate and anesthesia, in Volume 1 of *Principles of Anesthesiology.*[69]

REFERENCES

1. Gilman, A. G., et al. (eds.): Goodman and Gilman's The Pharmacological Basis of Therapeutics, 8th Ed. New York, McGraw-Hill, 1990.
2. Comroe, J. H., Dripps, R. D.: The Physiological Basis of Oxygen Therapy. Springfield, IL, Charles C Thomas, 1950.
3. Barach, A.: Inhalational Therapy. Philadelphia, J.B. Lippincott, 1994.
4. Adriani, J.: The Chemistry and Physics of Anesthesia, 2nd Ed. Springfield, IL, Charles C Thomas, 1972.
5. Comroe, J.H., Jr., et al.: Oxygen toxicity. JAMA 128:710, 1945.
6. Lambertson, C. J., et al.: Oxygen toxicity: effects in man of oxygen inhalation at 1 and 3:5 atmospheres upon blood transport cerebral circulation and cerebral metabolism. J Appl Physiol 5:471, 1953.
7. Cheney, F. W., Jr., Huang, T. W., Gronka, R.: The effects of 50% oxygen on resolution of experimental lung injury. Am Rev Respir Dis 122:373, 1980.
8. Lambertson, C. J.: Effects of hypoxia on organs and their tissues. In Robin, E. D. (ed.). Extrapulmonary Manifestations of Respiratory Diseases. Vol. 8. Lung Biology. New York, Marcel Dekker, 1978, p. 234.
9. Moss, G.: Shock, cerebral hypoxia and pulmonary vascular control: the centrineurogenic etiology of the respiratory distress syndrome. Bull NY Acad Med 49:689, 1973.
10. Van deWater, J., et al.: Response of the Lung to six to twelve hours of 100% Oxygen Inhalation in Man. N Engl J Med 283:621, 1970.
11. Bean, J. W., Kee, D., Thom, B.: Pulmonary changes with convulsions induced by drugs and O₂ at high pressure. J Appl Physiol 21:865, 1966.
12. Chance, B., Jamieson, D., Coles, H.: Energy linked pyridine nucleotide reduction: inhibitor effects of hyperbaric oxygen in vitro and in vivo. Nature 206:243, 1966.
13. Eggers, G. W. N.: Personal communication, 1977.
14. Motlaugh, F. A., et al.: Electron microscopic appearance and surface tension properties of the lungs ventilated with dry or humid air or oxygen. Surg Forum 20:219, 1969.
15. Suga, T., Tait, J. L., Reich, T.: Pathogenesis of pulmonary oxygen toxicity. Surg Forum 21:210, 1979.
16. Davis, W. B., et al.: Pulmonary oxygen toxicity. N Engl J Med 309:878, 1983.
17. Balentine, J.: Pathologic effects of exposure to high oxygen tensions: a review. N Engl J Med 275:1038, 1966.
18. Clark, J. M.: Pulmonary limits of oxygen tolerance in many. Exp Lung Res 14:887, 1988.
19. Clark, J. M., Lambertson, C. J.: Alveolar arterial oxygen difference in man during exposure to oxygen pressure. J Appl Physiol 30:753, 1971.
20. Tinsley, J. C., Jr., et al.: Role of oxygen in regulation of erythropoiesis. J Clin Invest 28:1544, 1949.
21. Wiebel, E. R.: Oxygen effect on lung cells. Arch Intern Med 128:54, 1971.
22. Robin, E. D.: Dysoxia: abnormal tissue oxygen utility. Arch Intern Med 137:905, 1977.
23. Apgar, V.: Principles of anesthesia in plastic surgery. Surg Clin North Am 24:474, 1944.
24. Campbell, K.: Intensive oxygen therapy as a possible cause of retrolental fibroplasia. Med J Aust 2:48, 1951.
25. Kinsey, V. E.: Retrolental fibroplasia: cooperative study of retrolental fibroplasia and the use of oxygen. Arch Ophthalmol 56:481, 1956.
26. American Academy of Pediatrics Committee on Fetus and Newborn: History of oxygen therapy and retrolental fibroplasia. Pediatrics 57(Suppl 2):591, 1976.
27. Campbell, F. W.: Influence of low atmospheric pressure on the development of retinal vessels in the rat. Trans Ophthalmol Soc (UK) 71:287, 1952.
28. Lanman, J. T., Guy, L. P., Davis, J.: Retrolental fibroplasia and oxygen therapy. JAMA 155:223, 1954.
29. Flynn, J. T.: Oxygen and retrolental fibroplasia: update and challenge. Anesthesiology 60:397, 1984.
30. Alper, M.: Acute proliferative retrolental fibroplasia: multivariate risk analyses. Trans Am Ophthalmol Soc 81:549, 1983.
31. Silverman, W. A.: Retinopathy of prematurity: oxygen dogma challenged. Arch Dis Child 57:731, 1982.
32. Barach, A. L.: Oxygen therapy. Med Clin North Am 1:704, 1944.
33. Comroe, J. H., Jr., Bahnson, E. R., Coates, E. O.: Mental changes occurring in chronically anoxemic patients during oxygen therapy. JAMA 143:1044, 1950.
34. Seevers, M.: The narcotic properties of carbon dioxide. NY State J Med 44:597, 1944.
35. Paine, J. R., Lynn, D., Keys, A.: Observation on the effects of prolonged administration of high oxygen concentrations in dogs. J Thorac Surg 11:151, 1941.
36. Stadie, W. C., Hangaard, N.: Oxygen poisoning: effects of high oxygen pressure upon enzymes (succinic dehydrogenase and cytochrome oxidase). J Biol Chem 161:153, 1945.
37. Joanny, P., Corriol, J.: Hyperbaric oxygen: effects on metabolism and ionic movement in cerebral cortex slices. Science 167:1508, 1970.
38. Halliwell, B., Gutteridge, J. M. C.: Free Radicals in Biology and Medicine. Oxford, Clarendon Press, 1985.
39. Saklad, M.: Inhalation Therapy and Resuscitation. Springfield, IL, Charles C Thomas, 1953.
40. Seal, M. S.: Advances in inhalation therapy with reference to cardio-respiratory disease. N Engl J Med 231:553, 1944.
40a. Sorbini, C. A.: Recent progress. Medica 77:587, 1986.
41. Gilber, N. C.: Coronary thrombosis. Bull Chicago Med Assoc 18:321, 1942.
42. Eckenhoff, J. E., Hafkenschiel, J. H., Laudmesser, C. M.: The coronary circulation of the dog. Am J Physiol 148:582, 1947.
43. Russek, H. I., et al.: One hundred per cent oxygen in the treatment of acute myocardial infarction and severe angina pectoris. JAMA 144:373, 1950.
44. Safar, P.: Respiratory Therapy. Philadelphia, F.A. Davis, 1965.
45. Barach, A.: The treatment of pulmonary edema due to gas poisoning in war and civilian life. N Engl J Med 230:216, 1944.
46. Kritzler, R. A.: Acute high altitude anoxia. War Med 6:369, 1944.
47. Fine, J., Banks, B. M., Sears, J. B., Hermanson, L.: The treatment of gaseous distention of the intestine by inhalation of 95% oxygen. Ann Surg 103:375, 1936.
48. Comroe, J. H., Jr., Dripps, R. D.: The Physiologic Basis of Oxygen Therapy. Springfield, IL, Charles C Thomas, 1950, p. 63.
49. Weaver, R. H., Virtue, R. W.: Blood oxygenation as affected by tidal volume and tension of nitrous oxide-oxygen inhaled at one mile altitude. Anesthesiology 16:57, 1955.
50. Cherniack, R. M.: Respiratory effects of obesity. Can Med Assoc J 80:613, 1959.

51. Rosen, M., Hillard, E. K.: The use of suction in clinical medicine. Br J Anaesth 32:486, 1960.

52. Fink, B. R.: Diffusion anoxia. Anesthesiology 16:511, 1955.

53. Egbert, L. O., Laver, M. B., Bendixen, H. H.: Intermittent deep breaths and compliance during anesthesia in man. Anesthesiology 24:57, 1963.

54. Dripps, R. D., Comroe, J. H., Jr.: The effect of the inhalation of high and low oxygen concentrations. Am J Physiol 149:277, 1947.

55. Sands, J., DeGraff, A. C.: The effects of progressive anoxemia on the heart and circulation. Am J Physiol 74:416, 1925.

56. Rovenstine, E. A.: Fundamentals of Anesthesia. Chicago, American Medical Association, 1954.

57. Doyle, J. T., Wilson, J. S., Warren, J. O.: Effects of hypoxia on pulmonary circulation. Circulation 5:265, 1952.

58. Cohen, P.: The metabolic function of oxygen and biochemical lesions of hypoxia. Anesthesiology 37:148, 1972.

59. Cohen, P. J., et al.: Effects of hypoxia and normocarbia on cerebral blood flow and metabolism in conscious man. J Appl Physiol 23:183, 1967.

60. Siesjo, B. K., Plum, F.: Pathophysiology of anoxic brain damage. In Gaull, G. (ed.). Biology of Cerebral Dysfunction. New York, Plenum Press, 1972, p. 319.

61. Siesjo, B. K., Wieloch, T.: Cerebral metabolism in ischemia: neurochemical bases for therapy. Br J Anaesth 57:47, 1985.

62. Haldane, J. S.: Respiration. New Haven, CT, Yale University Press, 1922.

63. Morrison, L. R.: Histopathologic effects of anoxia on central nervous system. Arch Neurol Psychiatry 55:1, 1946.

64. Courville, C. B.: Cerebral Anoxia. Los Angeles, San Lucas Press, 1953.

65. Meitchenfelder, J.: A valid demonstration of barbiturate brain protection in man: at last. Anesthesiology 64:140, 1986.

66. Secher, O., Wilhjelm, B.: The protective action of anesthetics against hypoxia. Can Anaesth Soc J 15:423, 1968.

67. Stullken, E. H.: Effect of nimodipine and vasodilators in cerebral aneurysm clipping. Anesthesiology 62:346, 1985.

68. Safar, P., Tenicela, R.: High altitude physiology in relation to anesthesia and inhalation therapy. Anesthesiology 25:515, 1964.

69. James, M. F.: Climate and anesthesia. In Collins, V. J. (ed.). Principles of Anesthesiology, Vol. 1. Philadelphia, Lea & Febiger, 1993.

70. Mordes, J. P., et al.: High altitude pituitary-thyroid dysfunction on Mount Everest. N Engl J Med 308:1135, 1983.

Chapter 28

PHYSIOLOGY AND PHARMACOLOGY OF CARBON DIOXIDE

THEODORE C. SMITH AND VINCENT J. COLLINS

Carbon dioxide (CO_2) can be found in distant galactic dust clouds, in the depths of the earth and ocean, and in the air we breathe. Next to oxygen, it is perhaps our most important gas and hence has always been of interest to scientists, and of particular interest to anesthesiologists. Plants depend on the atmospheric content to produce carbohydrate for their structure and our food. Animals depend on its ionized hydration product to regulate many physiologic processes. It adds zest to our beverages, safety to fire-hazardous areas (in extinguishers), power for instruments and pellet guns (as compressed gas), and cold for food and organ preservation (as dry ice), for example.

It is strange that, almost as a conditioned reflex, anesthesiologists think that "CO_2 IS BAD." In fact, a modest increase in CO_2 improves the fraction of cardiac output going to heart and brain while decreasing the fraction going to skin and resting muscle, a good idea in shock. It improves oxygen unloading in tissues while stimulating oxygen delivery to the lungs, a good idea in exercise. It does cause acidosis, but slowly: any doubling of P_{CO_2} only lowers pH 0.2 units, while at the same time stimulating homeostatic processes that may be lifesaving, another good idea.

On the other hand, respiratory alkalosis is not the benign condition one might assume. It decreases oxygen delivery both by mechanical effects on venous return and by autoregulatory effects of hypocapnia. It decreases oxygen unloading by a left upward shift of the oxyhemoglobin dissociation curve. It reduces concentration of electrolytes, on whose balance muscle membranes (including those of the heart) depend for excitation-contraction coupling, notably calcium (Ca^{++}), magnesium (Mg^{++}), and potassium (K^+). It partially uncouples adenosine triphosphate (ATP) production from oxidative phosphorylation, raising body oxygen consumption for any needed energy expenditure. It increases airway resistance, and if large tidal volumes are employed, it decreases total compliance. Perhaps none of these ills offer a major insult for minor degrees of alkalosis, but combined and maximized, they give pause for thought. One cannot blindly accept hyperventilation without a good overriding justification, such as control of intracranial pressure.

The anesthesiologist can manipulate CO_2 by affecting its production and (more important) its elimination. Therefore, much of what is touched on in other chapters

of this work is collected here, to facilitate the application of essential knowledge.

HISTORY

Humankind had long noticed the production of CO_2 gas, in fermentation of fruit or grain, but Priestly first identified it as a compound in the late eighteenth century,[1] and shortly thereafter, Lavoisier studied its relation to breathing in humans and animals.[2] Lavoisier also described the three elements of the basic chemical reaction of fire and combustion: (1) a fuel, (2) an oxidizer (oxygen), and (3) heat to a proper temperature (ignition).[3]

In the next century, the presence of small concentrations in air (0.03%!) were found to be absolutely essential for plant life and of paramount importance in regulatory activity in animal physiology. The explosion of biologic and medical information in the twentieth century has only added to the importance of understanding CO_2 cycles and balance. Atmospheric CO_2 percentage is not affected by altitude, but the partial pressure decreases. Slight geographic changes occur such as a decrease in CO_2 content in seawater and in air as one progresses from tropical to northern seas.

The earth as a whole has huge stores of CO_2 in carbonate minerals, as well as smaller but still large stores in the form of fossil fuels and biomass.[4] A significant store is found in seawater, both dissolved and as bicarbonate and carbonate compounds.[5] A large volume may be temporarily trapped in the depths of some lakes and released cataclysmically, as at Lake Nyos, with lethal effects on human and animal life.[6]

The usual amount in the air is quantitatively minuscule, but it represents a balance between production of CO_2 (burning fuels, metabolizing biomass, venting volcanic gasses, etc.) and uptake of CO_2 (solution in water, growth of biomass, both plant and animal, and fixation as limestone precursors, largely by marine organisms). Yet this minute atmospheric concentration is as important to life as are ozone and oxygen, not only as metabolites, but also as a trap for infrared radiation from the earth, warming the surface thereby. In ancient ages, the concentration of CO_2 has varied up and down two to threefold, with important effects on contemporaneous climate and life forms. At present, we seem to be experiencing a secular increase, with predicted doubling of the CO_2 level in the next few decades or centuries, depending on the model chosen for examination. Predictions include coastal flooding, desert expansion, and mass extinction of plants, particularly trees. The immediate effects of a doubling or halving of CO_2 in patients is, by contrast, nonspeculative, more important, and susceptible to control by informed anesthesiologists.

CHEMISTRY[7]

CO_2 has a molecular weight of about 44, almost identical with that of nitrous oxide (of importance in mass spectroscopy). Structurally, it consists of a central carbon atom with two stable double bonds to oxygen. It is a gas at room temperature, but can be liquified by 750 psi pressure at room temperature, or solidified by cooling to $-78.5°C$, from which it sublimes to a gas at atmosphere pressure. It was first described in 1757 by Black.[8,9]

It dissolves readily in water: 1 L of water at body temperature dissolves about 0.5 L of CO_2 at 1 atm of CO_2 pressure. Blood solubility is also high.[12] At $36°C$ and 1 atm pressure, 100 ml of arterial blood contains 50 ml of CO_2 distributed as follows: 3.0 ml physically dissolved; 3.0 ml in carbamino form; and 44 ml as bicarbonate. At the capillary, 5.0 ml CO_2 is added to each 100 ml of capillary blood in the resting subject (250 ml/min) (Table 28–1). Of greater importance is that CO_2 reacts in the aqueous fluids of our bodies to produce bicarbonate and carbamate (reaction with H_2O and amino acids, respectively), which permit both transportation from sites of production to sites of elimination and control of hydrogen ion and hence pH. The latter is accomplished by the reaction:

$$CO_2 + H_2O \; H_2CO_3 \; H^+ + HCO_3 2H^+ + CO_3 \quad (1)$$

The last step, to carbonate, is uncommon at body pH. The carbonate can be incorporated by bone in the mineral hydroxy appetite formation, and represents a relatively stable store of CO_2. But more important is the buffering effect of hydrogen ion production/neutralization, with a pK of about 6.1. Still more important is the reaction with amino acids of protein, particularly hemoglobin in blood and myoglobin is muscle, to form carbamates with a pK of about 7.4. The reaction can be summarized as reaction of unionized amino acid (R-NH$_2$) with either hydrogen ions (H+) or molecular (dissolved) CO_2:

$$\underset{\text{unionized amino acid}}{R—NH_2} + H^+ \rightarrow \underset{\text{ionized amino acid}}{R—(NH_3)^+} \quad (2)$$

Table 28–1. Typical Values of Body Carbon Dioxide

(70 · kg man)	Conscious (Basal) Respiration Spontaneous	Anesthetized Ventilation Artificial	Ventilation Spontaneous
CO_2 output ml/m^2 BTPS	230		195
Arterial P_{CO_2} mm Hg	39	36	63
Venous P_{CO_2} mm Hg	45	45	68
Alveolar P_{CO_2} mm Hg	40	40	62

$$\underset{\text{unionized amino acid}}{R—NH_2} + CO_2 \rightarrow \underset{\text{amino carbamate}}{R—NH\text{-}COOH} \quad (3)$$

The greater relative importance of the ionization of carbonic acid over the reaction of protein with CO_2 is due to our ability to measure each of the reactants in equation 1) and by use of the Hassalbach transform (logarithmic) of Henderson's relationship:

$$pH = pKa' + \log [\text{base/acid}] \quad (4)$$

separate metabolic from respiratory events. CO_2 diffuses readily in gas and tissue, but bicarbonate does not (it is charged!). Near-equilibrium of P_{CO_2} results across cell membranes, with nearly the same P_{CO_2} in cells and extracellular fluid. Bicarbonate and hence pH may be quite different on either side of a cell membrane, however.

PHYSIOLOGY[10,11]

CO_2 is the end product of metabolism of all foodstuffs, carbohydrate, protein, and fat. It fluctuates with the rate of metabolism. The tissues of resting awake humans produce 112 to 118 ml CO_2/min/m^2 body surface area, when a normal diet is taken. For the same energy production (and hence oxygen consumption), metabolism of carbohydrate can increase that number about 20%, whereas starvation with fat utilization can reduce it 12% approximately. Anesthesia with spontaneous ventilation (and a P_{CO_2} of 50 to 55 mm Hg!) decreases the CO_2 production and oxygen consumption only 5 to 10%. Concomitant hyperventilation, however, with absent oxygen cost of breathing and mild alkalosis, and the fall in body temperature commonly associated with anesthesia to 33 to 35°C, may lower metabolic rate by an additional 15 to 25%.

For quick estimates, the CO_2 production is often approximated as 200 ml/min in an awake and 160 ml/min in a paralyzed anesthetized man of average size (Table 28–1). During sustained work (600 cal/h), about 90 to 100 L may be produced, transported, and excreted per hour (an eightfold increase).

BIOCHEMICAL MECHANISMS OF COMBUSTION[11]

Three complex processes provide the mechanism for the combustion of organic molecules in the body. They are cyclic in nature: (1) glycolysis (Embden-Meyerhoff); (2) the pentose-phosphate cycle; and (3) the citric acid cycle (tricarboxylic acid or Krebs cycle). The first two are actually devices used to convert glucose and other stuffs to intermediates that can enter the citric acid cycle. This last named is the key mechanism for cellular combustion. In this cycle, pyruvic acid is converted to CO_2 and water in five oxidative steps. CO_2 is produced primarily by the decarboxylation of the α-ketoacids at this stage.

Preparation of the macromolecules of these substances involves the breaking of their chemical bonds and the production of small moieties.

The organic molecules that are specifically combustible are acid and are as follows: pyruvic acid; acetic acid; citric acid; succinic acid; fumaric acid; malic acid; and oxaloacetic acid.

In the case of proteins, this represents the breaking of peptide links and the production of component amino acids. These are then altered to a form that is directly combustible.

In the case of lipids, preparation for combustion involves the hydrolysis of the ester bonds and eventually a breaking up of the original molecule to the basic components, namely, the fatty acids, glycerol, and nitrogenous parts. Oxidation produces acetic acid, a combustible product. Carbohydrates are broken up by enzymes into monosaccharides and are degraded ultimately to pyruvic acid.

SITE OF CO_2 PRODUCTION[11]

CO_2 is produced primarily by the ATP-generating Krebs cycle, at mitochondrial membrane surfaces. Fat, protein, and glycogen are converted to carbohydrate before energy production. The pressure of physiologic P_{CO_2} at this site offers negligible back pressure to production, so metabolism can be considered as a constant flow generator of CO_2, appearing as a dissolved gas in cells, diffusing through cells and extracellular fluid to capillaries.

In the capillary plasma, CO_2 undergoes hydration, neutralization (buffering), and other reactions. As a result, CO_2 is transported to the lungs in several physical forms: dissolved gaseous CO_2, bicarbonate ion, carbamate on plasma proteins, and (especially important because of the high concentration) red blood cell carbamate-hemoglobin. The reactions are facilitated by several processes: plasma and cellular carbonic anhydrase speed the CO_2-H_2O reaction in both directions. The back-to-CO_2 direction is important in pulmonary unloading. Mixing is augmented by turbulence and red cell uptake by a short plasma path length in capillaries. Red cell capacity is augmented by shift of chloride across the red cell membrane through special mechanisms. CO_2 transport in blood is considered in Chapter 5.

DISSOCIATION BLOOD CO_2 CURVE[12]

The total amount of CO_2 in blood is a log function of CO_2 tension (Table 28-2). On a linear plot of CO_2 content versus CO_2 tension, it is reasonably approximated by a straight line from 40 to 100 mm Hg. Below that, it curves to intersect the origin (Fig. 28-1). This graph is called the CO_2 dissociation curve and is similar to the oxyhemoglobin dissociation curve when the ordinate is expressed as O_2 content. Figure 28-1 shows typical O_2 and CO_2 curves for a normal hemoglobin. The straight lines at the bottom are the dissolved CO_2 and O_2 stores. Notice that because the arteriovenous content of CO_2 is only 80% of the O_2 arteriovenous content, and because the dissociation curve is appreciably steeper, the normal partial pressure arteriovenous difference of oxygen is much larger (circa 60) than that of CO_2 (circa 6).

TISSUE DISTRIBUTION AND STORAGE[12,13]
(Table 28-3)

The CO_2 content of any tissue depends on three factors: (1) its intrinsic metabolic rate (high for heart and

Table 28-2. Stores of Body Carbon Dioxide

70-kg: $P_{ACO_2} = 40$ mm Hg Basal Values—CO_2 Volumes	
Lung gas dioxide —	130 ml
Arterial blood —	672 ml
Venous blood —	2,184 ml
Tissue (soft) —	16,000 ml

Data derived from Table 28-3.

brain, low for skin and fat); (2) its organ blood flow (similarly high for heart and brain and low for thermoneutral skin and fat); and (3) its capacity to store CO_2, measured by the solubility factor, which is essentially the slope of the CO_2 dissociation curve in millimeters per kilogram per millimeters of mercury (lower for heart and skin, higher for brain and muscle and extremely high for fat). The interaction of these factors accounts for the kinetics of CO_2 where change in respiration alters CO_2 elimination (see later), or less frequently and to a smaller extent, where change in production occurs.

Analogous to the earth's CO_2 stores, the bulk of extractable human CO_2 is tightly bound in bone minerals, amounting to about 110 to 120 L. At normal CO_2 tension, 12 to 18 L are dissolved in tissue and body fluids. Any change with these stores is proportional to change in CO_2 tension. The storage capacity varies from tissue to tissue from 0.3 to 12 ml CO_2/kg/mm Hg P_{CO_2}.[14] At normal tension, the lung alveoli contain about 130 ml CO_2 (5.2% × 2.5 L functional residual capacity [FRC]). The arterial and venous blood contain about 2.8 L and the soft tissues about 14 L (see Table 28-2). The skeletal muscle has the most, 8 to 12 L, depending on muscularity. Fat contains

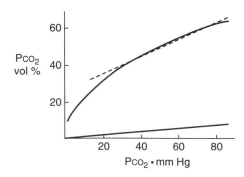

Fig. 28-1. The continuous line represents the CO_2 dissociation curve of blood. The dotted line is a straight line having a slope of 0.45 vol. %/mm Hg P_{CO_2}. This is the storage capacity of blood, and for arterial blood it is defined as the additional amount that can be stored for each increment of pressure. The error is introduced by assuming this to be a constant slope of the blood curve between 30 and 80 mm Hg. P_{CO_2} is small compared with the variations in other biologic parameters used. Redrawn from Farhi, L. E., Rahn, H.: Dynamics of changes in carbon dioxide stores. Anesthesiology *27*:604, 1960.

Table 28–3. Carbon Dioxide Stores of the Body by Compartments

Electronic Equivalent: B = Intensity, H = Potential, L = Charge, P = Capacitance, Q = Resistance, R = Time Constant.

Compartment	A Weight, kg.	B CO_2 Production, ml/mm	C Blood Flow (ml/mm)	D Blood Flow (% of Total)	E Equil. Blood Volume (ml)	F (Cv–Ca) CO_2 (ml/ml)	G $CvCO_2$ (ml/ml)	H $PvCO_2$ (mm)	I CO_2 Content: Tissue (ml/kg)	J CO_2 Content: Tissue L/organ	K CO_2 Content: Equil. Blood (liters)	L CO_2 Content: Total (liters)	M Slope of Dissociation Curve, (ml/kg/mm)	N Slope of Dissociation Curve, (ml/organ/mm)	O Slope of Dissociation Curve, Equil. Blood Vol (ml/mm)	P Slope of Dissociation Curve, Equil. Blood Vol (ml/mm)	Q Resistance (mm/ml/min)	R Time Constant (min)
Alveoli		240			2,400		.480	40		.160	1.15	1.31		4.0	10.8	14.8	.167	2.47
Heart	.30	26	210	4	180	.124	.604	67	487	.146	.109	.225	2.4	.7	.8	1.5	1.08	1.62
Brain	1.35	68	730	14	630	.093	.573	61	401	.542	.360	.902	2.9	3.9	2.8	6.7	.31	2.07
Muscle	28.0	40	850	16	720	.047	.527	50	542	9.600	.380	9.98	4.2	117.0	3.2	120.2	.25	30.0
Bone	2.2								12,500	113.0		113.0						
Fat	18.0								50	.900		.900						
Other	6.0	70	3,100	51	2,300	.023	.503	45	355	2.160	1.150	3.310	3.0	18.0	10.3	31.4	.10	
Total	70	240	5,200	100	6,000					126.5	3.150	130.0*		165.2		174.6		1.98

*If bone is excluded, the "total labile CO_2 store" (soft tissue) is 16.6L.
Columns (A), (C), and (D) were obtained from the Handbook of Biological Data. Columns (B), (I), and (M) were obtained from Rahn. Column (E) indicates the amount of blood equilibrated with a tissue or organ present in the venous circulation. It is assumed to be proportional to the perfusion of the organ and is calculated as 4500 × (D). Column (F) is calculated as (B)/(C). Column (G) is derived by adding (F) to 0.480, which is assumed to be the arterial blood CO_2 content. Column (H) is obtained by multiplying (F) by 0.0045 (which is assumed to be the slope of the blood dissociation curve), and adding the figure obtained to the arterial PcO_2, assumed to be 40. Column J is calculated as (I) × (A). Column K is equal to $(E) \times (G) \times \frac{1}{1000}$. Column L is the sum of (J) plus (K). Column N is derived by multiplying (M) × (A). Column O is .0045 × (E). Column P is the sum of (N) + (O). Column Q is $\frac{1}{.0045 \times (C)}$. Column R is (P) × (Q).

From Farhi, L. E., Rahn, H.: Dynamics of changes in carbon dioxide stores. Anesthesiology 27:604, 1960.

0.8 to 4 L (thin to obese—even more with morbid obesity), but this CO_2 is only slowly mobilizable, because of the low blood flow of fat.

ALTERATION OF STORES[13]

The body stores of CO_2 may be altered by anything that affects the ratio of production (metabolism) to elimination (alveolar ventilation) or the storage capacity of any tissues. The last may be dismissed readily by anesthetists. Only a massive gain or loss of body mass can do this, slow processes by our time scale. It is true that the capacity of all tissues, like blood, depends on the current acid-base status in part. The slope of the CO_2 dissociation curve is always lower at low P_{CO_2} and higher at high (refer to Fig. 28-1 for blood as an example), but the change is not great.

Reduction of metabolic rate lowers CO_2 stores, all other factors held constant. Autoregulatory tissues, however, particularly heart and brain, reduce their demand on the cardiac output, pari pasu with reduced metabolism. In fact, the cardiac output is, to a good first approximation, regulated by total body metabolism, to keep venous blood contents of oxygen and CO_2 nearly constant in metabolic states ranging from coma or deep sleep, through basal state, ordinary activity, to maximal exertion. Despite what is taught cardiac anesthetists, that cardiac output is regulated by rate and stroke volume, the sum of tissue conductance of blood flow sets cardiac output, by a complex variety of controls and feedbacks. Similarly, ventilation is set to balance pulmonary secretion of CO_2 to production. The anesthetist may lower metabolic rate to half of normal by total body hypothermia of 28 to 30°C and to one quarter of normal at temperatures below 22°C (the Q10 of the whole body—the ratio of metabolism at two temperatures 10°C apart—is about 2.3). De Backer and associates[15] provide an illuminating study mimicking a step fall in ventilation by hemodialysis-induced CO_2 unloading. A marked fall in spontaneous ventilation was seen, followed by periodic breathing, and apnea intervals, all attesting to the innate link of metabolic load with breathing.

Conversely, the anesthesiologist may see the rate rise in malignant hyperpyrexia to 5 to 10 times normal resting values, with rise in body stores. The rate of fall or rise depends on the current balance between production and elimination, but the two are not exactly mirror images of each other. The most common circumstances altering body stores, and the one discussed in detail here, are those associated with sudden changes in ventilation with little or no change in metabolism: apnea and a threefold rise in ventilation are used as examples.

Rise During Apnea[16,17]

Several rules of thumb are often proposed to explain the rise in the first minute (more rapid) and the constant, slower rise thereafter. The difference in the two rates is due to two distinctly different processes with different times courses: specifying an artificial difference in rates occurring at 1 minute only confuses understanding (Fig. 28-2).

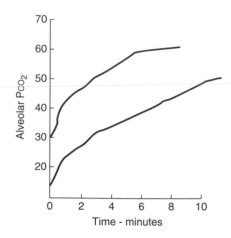

Fig. 28–2. Average rates of rise of P_{CO_2} before (upper graph) and after (lower graph) hyperventilation. The length of each graph is determined by the number of minutes during which points are present from all five subjects. Redrawn from Eger, E. I., Severinghaus, J. W.: The rate of rise of $PaCO_2$ in the apneic anesthetized patient. Anesthesiology 22:419, 1961.

Equilibration of alveoli with mixed venous CO_2 tension is the first process. Mixed venous blood, with a tension of 47 mm Hg, normally delivers 200 ml of CO_2 for diffusion into the lungs, which have an average alveolar volume of 2.4 L. When apnea stops pulmonary excretion, the alveolar $PaCO_2$ rises toward the venous. With each 1-mm Hg rise, however, the original 7-mm Hg diffusion gradient from venous to alveolar tension falls and so does the diffusion of CO_2 into alveoli. A process that goes at a rate proportional to the driving force is called an exponential or first-order process. It is described quantitatively by its time constant. In the case of a volume being filled by a flow, the time constant (called α) is given by

$$x = \text{volume divided by ventilation} \qquad (5)$$

The volume here is the change in CO_2 in the lung from a tension of 40 to 47 mm Hg, about 1% of the FRC or 24 ml. The "ventilation" is the production of CO_2, VCO_2, normally about 200 ml/min. Therefore,

$$x = 24 \text{ ml/min } 200 \text{ ml/min} \times 60 \text{ sec/min} = 7 \text{ sec}$$

If the metabolic rate is 160 ml (during anesthesia) and the FRC is 2.4 L, then α is a bit longer, 9 seconds. In first-order processes, the reaction has gone 99% of the way in 5 time constants. In our example, between 35 and 45 seconds after apnea, alveolar gas would have reached venous tension, and so would arterial tension. CO_2 exchange would stop if venous tension stayed constant, but it does not.

The second process follows as a result of the rise in arterial CO_2 tension and content from the first process. When the tissues begin to "see" a rising arterial tension, they ignore it as far as CO_2 production is concerned. The same amount of CO_2 continues to be put into capillary blood each minute. So the venous blood tension starts to rise, just as fast as the arterial tension, but it is delayed by the circulation time from lung to tissue, a matter of tens of seconds. After a bit more time (the transit time from tissue to lung), the venous blood tension entering pulmonary capillaries starts to rise, at a rate determined by the dissociation curve (see Fig. 28–1) and the CO_2 production. A normal production with an arteriovenous content difference of 4 vol% causes a rise of about 4 mm Hg per minute at normal tension, a bit less if P_{CO_2} is initially low, and a bit more if it is high.

The actual rate of rise of CO_2 with apnea is the sum of these two processes, one falling exponentially to zero within the first minute, the second about constant after a slow start. With long periods of apnea, hours or more, the latter would be expected to decline slightly, because poorly perfused fat with a large capacity can begin to store significant amounts of CO_2 if its arterial-to-cell difference rises appreciably.

The rate of rise of CO_2 with apnea has been studied by Eger and Severinghaus[17] and by Frumin and colleagues[16] (see Fig. 28–2). Stock and colleagues[18] point out that critically ill awake patients, receiving mechanical ventilation, who perhaps are febrile, may be more active metabolically than the patients studied by Eger and Frumin. In these patients, CO_2 rises at a rate of 6 mm Hg/min after the first minute or so.[19] Further, as pointed out by Mertzlufft and associates, hyperoxygenation, especially of venous blood, also increases the $P_{a-v_{CO_2}}$.[20]

Mertzlufft and colleagues found a steady rise of nearly 4 mm Hg/min for anesthetized patients, but a rising arteriovenous pressure difference they attributed to the Christiansen-Douglas-Haldane effect of reduced hemoglobin versus oxygenated.[21,22]

Initial hyperventilation before apnea produces a minor difference: the arteriovenous P_{CO_2} difference is a bit smaller, so the lungs' capacity to store CO_2 at the venous tension is less, lowering the time constant. Further, because of the increased slope of the CO_2 dissociation curve (see Fig. 28–1) at lower tension, a given CO_2 load raises the P_{CO_2} less. The result is a rise of CO_2 during apnea of closer to 3 than 4 mm Hg/min after the initial rise of 6 to 8 mm Hg in the first minute.

Fall During Hyperventilation[14]

Hyperventilation over a period of 2 to 4 minutes to reduce the Pa_{CO_2} to 30 mm Hg or less reduces the body tissues stores (Table 28–4). Several practical factors affect the changes due to hyperventilation seen in the $P_{ET_{CO_2}}$ or Pa_{CO_2}. Here the model is the washout of all lung CO_2, at a rate dependent on the alveolar ventilation, modified by

the continued input of CO_2 from venous blood. The first process can be modeled by the washout of N_2 during O_2 breathing. A normal person washes out 95% of the N_2 in about 3 minutes in a nearly pure first-order process. An emphysematous patient with a large "slow space" may take two or more times that long.

One could thus describe P_{CO_2} fall in lung air and hence in arterial blood fall as exponential with a time constant of about 40 seconds. During that 40 seconds, however, the lung is partially refilled with nearly 140 ml CO_2 (from continued ingress of venous blood at 47 mm Hg Pv_{CO_2}, unloading at an ever lower PA_{CO_2} and higher Pv-a differences). This slows the CO_2 fall in alveoli with blood. In a few minutes, the body's blood and rapidly perfused tissues reach a quasisteady state, in which pulmonary excretion only slightly exceeds tissue production of CO_2. The small difference comes from body CO_2 stores, which fall slowly for up to 1 hour thereafter.

For illustration,[23] a resting person at V_{CO_2} of 0.2 L/min and VE of 6 L/min is suddenly subjected to a step change in VE of 20 L/min by mechanically augmenting breathing. Approximately a threefold increase in alveolar ventilation results (increased alveolar dead space accounts for the rest). From the ventilation-CO_2 hyperbola:

$$V_A \times F_{A_{CO_2}} = V_{CO_2} \qquad (6)$$

one calculates that the $F_{A_{CO_2}}$ will plateau at a value of one third of normal or 13 mm Hg. It will get there in a curvilinear fashion, however: the $P_{ET_{CO_2}}$ will fall rapidly for a few minutes only, to about 25 mm Hg, and then slowly thereafter. Think of it this way: when hyperventilation lowers the alveolar P_{CO_2} to 33 from 40 mm Hg, it effectively doubles the $Pv-a_{CO_2}$, doubling the CO_2 transport to the lung, even with constant tissue metabolism. This extra CO_2 transportation lowers tissue stores of CO_2. In a few minutes, however, the lowered Pa_{CO_2} effects a lowering of Pv_{CO_2}, restoring the initial $Pv-a_{CO_2}$ difference. The additional factors, cardiac output, alveolar dead space, various tissue perfusion rates, blood CO_2 content, and so on, add a degree of complexity that modeling has not been able to match experimentally. Nonetheless, the anesthesiologist should feel confident that he or she can effect a halving of P_{CO_2}, with its concomitant rise in 0.2 pH units, more rapidly than the same alkalotic effect could be produced by bicarbonate or intravenous administration. After a threefold step increase in ventilation, however, blood gases and tissue stores may not reach a final steady state for 20 to 120 minutes.[23]

USES OF CARBON DIOXIDE

The average person may be aware of the use of gaseous CO_2 as a propellant when ordering a draft beer, or the use of solid CO_2 (dry ice) to produce special effects at Halloween parties. CO_2 is further used commercially as a chemical reactant or regulator, largely through its ability to buffer pH in aqueous solution, or as an oxygen excluder in certain chemical engineering applications.

Anesthesiologists find uses for CO_2 in the operating room. English anesthetists, not so indoctrinated in the

Table 28–4. Effect of Hyperventilation on Carbon Dioxide Stores

	At Pa_{CO_2} of 40 mm Hg (ml)	At Pa_{CO_2} of 20 mm Hg (ml)
Muscle	10,000	7,700
Venous blood	2,000	1,500
Fat	1,000	1,000

"CO_2 IS BAD" refrain, vote to include CO_2 flowmeters and cylinders on anesthesia trolleys.[24] Used intelligently, CO_2 facilitates induction, blind nasal intubation, and shortens emergence from anesthesia.[25,26] Endoscopy employing CO_2 has been reported by many. In knee arthroscopy, it improves visualization compared to fluid media.[27] In laparoscopy, it causes an easily managed rise in arterial CO_2 tension,[28] and it avoids the risk of nitrous oxide-bowel gas fire but not without some slight risk: CO_2 pneumothorax has occurred.[29] Reacting with soda lime it gives water, mole for mole, to aid humidification in breathing circuits. In the physiology laboratory, CO_2 can be used to assess cardiac output noninvasively.[30] It has been used to dissect plaque in endarterectomy.[31] Inhaled 5% CO_2 in oxygen is used to treat acute mountain sickness, and it raises tumor cell-normal cell susceptibility to x-ray therapy.[32]

HYPERCAPNIA AND HYPOCAPNIA

The short-term variation in CO_2 experienced by anesthesiologists may be extreme. A P_{CO_2} of 254 mm Hg due to failure to place valve disks in a breathing circuit has been reported.[33]

Other extremes in blood gases have been reported, such as pH of 7.85 and P_{CO_2} of 11 mm Hg during cardiopulmonary bypass weaning and warming, resulting from gas flow of 42 L/min to the oxygenator. These patients had uneventful recoveries from anesthesia and surgery, attesting to the benign nature of acute respiratory acid-base alterations. In both cases, the patient was well oxygenated, and effects of mechanical ventilation were slight or absent.[34]

Much of the fear that anesthetists manifest over hypercarbia comes from two separate historical circumstances not applicable in todays' anesthetic practice.[35] First, breathing air, with an increase in CO_2, causes an even greater decrease in arterial oxygen tension, because of the respiratory quotient effect on the alveolar air equation and physiologic shunt. A hypoventilation-induced rise to 60 mm Hg Pa_{CO_2} drops arterial Pa_{O_2} to below 70 mm Hg in a normal patient whose P_{O_2} was originally 95 mm Hg. Administration of oxygen to raise the F_{IO_2} to merely 25% will completely compensate for this, however. Anesthesiologists rarely use so little O_2 today.

Second, older anesthetic agents, notably ether, cyclopropane, and fluroxene, actively stimulated the autonomic nervous system, increasing the likelihood of arrhythmia. Newer halogenated agents have progressively offered increasing cardiac stability, however.

PHYSIOLOGIC EFFECTS

In arbitrary fashion, any changes in an organ or system function when CO_2 tension changes from the normal values are ascribed to the pharmacologic effects of CO_2. In a variety of studies of awake and anesthetized patients, CO_2 at these nonphysiologic levels produces effects on the central nervous system (CNS), the cardiovascular system, the respiratory system, and other systems.

Central Nervous System[36]

The major interest of anesthesiologists in CNS effects of CO_2 involve the interaction of cerebral blood flow regulation, metabolism, and the state of anesthesia. CO_2 does have other CNS effects, however. It produces subjective effects when inhaled, it augments inhalation anesthesia, and it is anesthetic itself, albeit unpleasant. It activates the sympathetic nervous system and thereby produces secondary effects. Its most striking effect is manifest by changes in the neural control of breathing. Chapter 3 is devoted to this topic. The CNS is also important in cardiovascular control, as discussed later in this chapter.

Subjective Effects[36]

Inspired air at normal atmospheric pressure containing 3 to 5% CO_2 produces a feeling of discomfort in conscious subjects. This percentage is about the maximum that can be tolerated. A breathing mixture of 6% causes acute distress with disorientation, dyspnea, anxiety, and erratic behavior.

Concentrations greater than 8% cause depression of the cerebral cortex.[37] At 8%, a narcotic action is noted[38]; a concentration of 10% or better is intolerable and toxic and causes unconsciousness. Concentrations of 11% no longer exert a respiratory stimulant action, but actually depress the respiratory center and show a general anesthetic effect, particularly if hypoxia coexists.[39] Concentrations of 20 to 30% may cause convulsions.

Effects on Consciousness and Sensory Modalities

In the unanesthetized subject, CO_2 has a direct effect on the level of consciousness.[40] The alerting mechanism is maintained, and the pain response is directly related to the arterial P_{CO_2} values up to a critical level of 70 mm Hg.

Conversely, when P_{CO_2} values fall below 25 mm Hg, sedative effects appear. The electroencephalogram (EEG) shows slow-sleep waves, and the reticular activating system is depressed.[41] The pain threshold is elevated, and the patient loses mental acuity and visceral sensation. Hyperventilation is recognized as having a quieting and sedative effect, and it is considered to be effected through decreased P_{CO_2} levels.

The mechanism of this effect has been disputed. A decrease in cerebral blood flow with cerebral hypoxia has been proposed.[42] The work of Robinson and Gray,[43] however, showed that the simultaneous administration of amyl nitrate (to promote cerebral blood flow), when combined with hyperventilation and lowered Pa_{CO_2}, still gave a sedative response.

Anesthetic Modification

Hypocapnia diminishes the potency of nitrous oxide, and hypercapnia enhances it. CO_2 and nitrous oxide have additive effects; both act as inert anesthetic gases. With each 10-mm rise in Pa_{CO_2}, the nitrous oxide may be decreased by 6%.[44] This finding agrees with the long-known anesthetic effects of inhalation of 25% CO_2.[45,46] During states of narcosis of unconsciousness produced by CO_2, cerebral oxygen consumption is lowered; however, when convulsions are produced oxygen consumption is greatly increased.

Cerebral Blood Flow Regulation[47]

In a normal awake person, the cerebral blood flow is closely related to cerebral metabolic rate. The control is accomplished largely by change in arterial and arteriolar resistance with change in local CO_2 tension or hydrogen ion concentration, which is proportional to PCO_2. Local hypoxia is an almost equally effective stimulus to dilation, however. Flow is higher in metabolically active gray matter and lower in white matter. Major changes in cerebral perfusion pressure can alter regulated flow, especially at mean pressure below 50 mm Hg, in a normal person, or at proportionally higher mean pressures in patients with untreated chronic hypertension.

Age does not seem to affect cerebral blood flow, but diseases associated with aging may. Atherosclerosis of the carotid and basilar systems does not reduce cerebral blood flow until it becomes impossible for distal (downstream) vasodilation to compensate for increasing atheromatous obstruction. Stroke and dementia decrease cerebral metabolic activity, and flow decreases proportionately. Areas adjacent to infarcted areas may lose autoregulation and vasodilate, giving "luxury perfusion" and perhaps stealing blood flow from adjacent compromised areas. Vasculature in areas ischemic from thrombosis or hemorrhage, or adjacent to tumor, may already be maximally dilated and unreactive to additional CO_2. The effects of altering blood flow by manipulating $PaCO_2$ (as described later) may not be predictable, and trials in specific patients may be necessary to decide whether altered $PaCO_2$ is of value. The ability of $PaCO_2$ to control vascular flow appears to be mediated by extracellular, and not intracellular, fluid pH or PCO_2. Extremes of PCO_2, 20 to 80 mm Hg, can alter extracellular fluid pH from 7.6 to 7.2, whereas intracellular pH is more nearly constant, 7.1 to 7.0. Autonomic regulation of cerebral blood flow is apparently negligible, because vasopressors and sympathetic block do little to change flow.[48]

In the case of carotid surgery for atheromas, these considerations have led to suggestions to hypoventilate or add CO_2, to block sympathetic activity with local anesthetic techniques, and to maintain a modest hypertension. No convincing evidence for any of these has accumulated, but marked hypotension and hypocarbia are generally best avoided.[49]

Hypocarbia can restrict cerebral blood flow so severely that inadequate oxygen or substrate delivery ensues.[50] Further hypocarbia induces hypoxic vasodilation, resulting in little or no further fall in flow. With an arterial blood oxygen content of 20 vol%, a minimal cerebral blood flow of about 20 ml/min/100 g tissue results from a $PaCO_2$ of about 20 mm Hg. Both subjective and measurable metabolic consequences result. Metabolic alkalosis has been found to be slightly vasodilatory when added to marked respiratory alkalosis. A bicarbonate-induced pH change from 7.6 to 7.8 with $PaCO_2$ held at 20 mm Hg raises cerebral blood flow from 26 to 31 ml/min/100 g tissue.

Conversely, respiratory acidosis causes a linearly increased cerebral blood flow of about 1 ml/min/100 g for each 1 mm Hg until maximum vasodilation results, usually well above 60 mm Hg $PaCO_2$.

Cerebral perfusion pressure changes can, in the extreme, affect blood flow. Mean perfusion pressure is calculated by subtracting the higher of cerebral venous pressure or cerebral spinal fluid pressure from mean arterial pressure, all measured with the same zero reference. Below perfusion pressures of 50, blood flow decreases as a function of the hypotension and may stop altogether at 10 to 20 mm Hg if hemodynamics and blood vessel mechanics result in a critical closing pressure. Probably, a slight increase in flow occurs over a mean pressure range of 50 to 150 mm Hg, as a result of vascular distention. Patients with severe hypotension may have marked vasodilation due to accumulation of CO_2 and metabolites, but insufficient to maintain oxygen delivery and CO_2 elimination. This may be the case in ineffective cardiopulmonary resuscitation.

The regulation of cerebral blood flow by CO_2 has one clinical application: the regulation of intracranial pressure. Increased blood flow increases the volume of blood in the calvarium, largely by increases in venous blood volume, less by increases in arterial volume. Normally, this has little effect on intracranial pressure, especially if the changes are slow, because of compensating changes in cerebral spinal fluid volume. In the case of tumor or brain edema, however, the cerebral spinal fluid volume may already be low, giving rise to decreased "compliance" in the skull. In such patients, flow may improve with modest hyperventilation, because the fall in intracranial pressure raises cerebral perfusion pressure and flow more than the fall in $PaCO_2$ lowers it.

Effect of Inhalation Anesthetics

Inhalation anesthetics, in general, increase cerebral blood flow and increase the CO_2 responsiveness. This is a dose-related increase in flow and responsiveness until maximum vasodilation results, at flows approaching a 2.5-fold increase. Differences exist between agents. Clinically, one may see more than just potentiation of CO_2-induced vasodilation: effects produced by hemodynamic change in cerebral perfusion pressure as well as by change in metabolic rate of the brain must be considered.

Halothane increases cerebral blood flow with little or no decrease in cerebral metabolic rate. The PCO_2 responsiveness is also greater than in an awake person. Enflurane is perhaps less vasodilating, and less potentiating for CO_2 vasodilation, but it can markedly increase metabolic rate, especially with hypocapnia-induced electrical seizures, markedly secondarily increasing cerebral blood flow to maintain brain oxygenation normal. Isoflurane is the least effective of the common inhalation agents in causing direct vasodilation, although some occurs, and in potentiating CO_2 vasodilation, although again some is reported. Isoflurane has two properties that recommend it, however: it can reduce cerebral metabolic rate significantly, largely by reduction in the electrical activity of the brain, and it maintains systemic blood pressure with cardiac output better than other agents at equivalent minimum alveolar concentration (MAC) multiples. Sevoflurane and desflurane are not well studied clinically, but in animal work, we have no reason to suspect that these agents will prove superior to isoflurane.

Nitrous oxide offers a problem in deciphering the data: apparently contradictory results can only in part by explained by different experimental designs. In early but careful studies, a person breathing 70% nitrous oxide had cerebral blood flow and CO_2 responsiveness similar to that of an awake person.[51-53]

None of these were comparisons of pure nitrous oxide effect at anesthetic levels, however: thiopental, morphine, severe hyperventilation, and hypocarbia were involved.[54] In more recent reports, nitrous oxide-activated brain activity (presumably with increased metabolic rate) decreased arterial venous oxygen content across the brain. The effects of nitrous oxide are additive to anesthesia with halothane.[55]

Some investigators have suggested that nitrous oxide may increase cerebral blood flow by increasing cerebral metabolic rate, an effect probably blocked with intravenous agents.[55] Use of nitrous oxide in neurosurgery is declining, possibly because of fear of its effects in closed air spaces, which is more rational than fear of increases in intracranial pressure or cerebral blood flow.

Action on Autonomic Nervous System[56]

CO_2 produces an excitation of the sympathoadrenal system and simultaneously provokes multiple responses. Under any specific set of circumstances, the net effect may be either sympathetic or parasympathetic. Primarily parasympathetic responses are promoted or augmented.

The sympathetic response is mediated by (1) central medullary nervous system pathways and (2) direct action on adrenal medulla. The parasympathetic response is mediated by (1) central nervous action and (2) peripheral inhibition of acetylcholinesterase.

Sympathetic Systems[57]

Many of the sympathetic effects of CO_2 are directly related to its action on the medullary centers. Low concentrations are capable of evoking this action. Especially evident is stimulation of vasomotor centers. In addition is stimulation of chemoreceptor areas of carotid and aortic bodies. The efferent pathways from these centers is over the sympathetic system.

High concentrations of CO_2 cause the release of catecholamines from the adrenal medulla and other chromaffin tissue.[57] Epinephrine is released, and the plasma concentrations of norepinephrine and epinephrine are raised two- to threefold.[58] Norepinephrine levels may go from 25 to 75 $\mu g/dl$; epinephrine levels increase from 5 to 30 $\mu g/dl$ to a range of 60 to 70 $\mu g/dl$.[59] The chemical mechanism involved is not clearly defined, but both the CO_2 as well as the induced changes in pH are interrelated. Nevertheless, the action is not direct because the integrity of the medullary centers and, to some extent, of the spinal cord is necessary. Thus, the response of the adrenal gland occurs consequent to intense stimulation of appropriate medullary centers by CO_2 levels and the transmission of impulses to the adrenal tissue.[60]

Once epinephrine is released, certain secondary effects are to be noted. In addition to the usually recognized effects, one must recognize the action on the anterior pituitary directly[61] and via the hypothalamus with the secretion of adrenocorticotropic hormone.[62] Evidence also indicates that CO_2 directly activates the hypothalamus.[63,64]

An equally important action of CO_2 is its influence on potassium balance.[63] In the presence of high PCO_2 levels, the liver cells lose potassium, and other cells, especially the heart, gain potassium. Simultaneously, hormonal factors such as the epinephrine levels tend to raise serum potassium. These two actions must summate in any given situation.

In summary, four systems related to sympathetic effects are activated by high CO_2 values: (1) direct effect on cells; (2) effects on the sympathetic nervous system; (3) release of adrenal medullary hormones; and (4) release of adrenal cortical hormones.

Parasympathetic Systems

In the synthesis of acetylcholine, a critical concentration of CO_2 is essential for optimal results. The specific enzyme choline acetylase-transferase acetyl groups from coenzyme A to choline.[65] CO_2 catalyzes this process. In addition, acetylcholine appears to exist in a protein-bound form in tissues. Many factors are capable of converting the acetylcholine to a free effective ion. Because hydrogen ion concentration is one, it can be assumed that CO_2 is also influential.

Studies have shown that the rate of disappearance of acetylcholine is a direct function of pH over the range of pH 5.6 to 8.4. In acid media, one notes inhibition of acetylcholinesterase and slow hydrolysis of acetylcholine. Therefore, any acidifying effect is expected to inhibit acetylcholinesterase further and to prolong the action of acetylcholine.

The effects of vagal stimulation on the heart when the subject is breathing 10 to 20% CO_2 is one of augmentation.[66] In animals,[66] the period of asystole is prolonged. The mechanism may be direct or through a change in pH because inhalation of these concentrations of CO_2 lowers pH to 7.0 to 7.2.

Cardiovascular System[67,68]

Under carefully controlled conditions in awake persons, the net cardiovascular responses to the administration of CO_2 have been detailed.[68] When exogenous CO_2 is added to a breathing mixture during either controlled or spontaneous respiration to produce a $PaCO_2$ range of 39 to 50 mm Hg, the following responses have been determined:

Increased:	Cardiac output
	Cardiac index
	Heart rate
	Stroke rate
	Myocardial contractility
	Forearm blood flow
Decreased:	Total peripheral resistance
	Ejection time

Table 28–5. Cardiovascular Effects of Carbon Dioxide

	Controlled Respiration	Spontaneous Respiration
	Percent Change with 10 mm Hg Increase in Pa_{CO_2}	Percent Change with 10mm Hg Increase in Pa_{CO_2}
Cardiac output (L/min)	39 ± 5	32 ± 4
Cardiac index (L/min)	39 ± 5	32 ± 4
Stroke volume (ml)*	10 ± 2	11 ± 2
Stroke index (ml/m²)	11 ± 2	11 ± 2
Heart rate (beats/min)	28 ± 4	26 ± 3
Mean arterial pressure (mm Hg)	9 ± 1	10 ± 2
Mean right atrial pressure (mm Hg)	0	0
Total peripheral resistance (dynes/sec/cm^{-3})	−17 ± 4	−14 ± 3
Erection time (msec)	−0.544 ± 0.77	−3 ± 2
Mean rate ventricular ejection (ml/sec)	3 ± 4	8 ± 3
Left ventricular stroke work (kg · m)	12 ± 3	25 ± 10
Left ventricular work (kg · m/min)	54 ± 11	46 ± 5
Tension-time index	10 ± 2	65 ± 2
Forearm blood flow (ml/100 g tissue/min)	30 ± 11	44 ± 10
Forearm vascular resistance (dynes/sec/cm^{-3})	−6 ± 9	−10 ± 10
Forearm venous compliance (ml/mm Hg)	0	0

*There was no significant difference comparing the circulatory responses to CO_2 during spontaneous respiration with those during controlled respiration.
Modified from Cullen, D. J., Eger, E. I., II: Cardiovascular effects of carbon dioxide in man. Anesthesiology *41*:345, 1974.

These careful determinations are summarized in Table 28–5 and may serve as reference data for other cardiovascular studies.

The cardiovascular system consists of (1) a pump, the myocardium with both contractility and rhythmicity that may be affected by CO_2, (2) the conducting vessels, which have the ability to contract or dilate, and (3) blood, which buffers the effects of CO_2 in hydrogen ion production. Most of the cardiovascular effects of CO_2 are due to pH changes in blood, but these are confounded by the accompanying CNS effects mediated both by altering neurogenic control of the circulation and by the action of catecholamines (humoral). Further, acute and chronic effects may differ.

The difference between acute and chronic effects may be illustrated by the relationship between P_{CO_2} and pH in blood; when P_{CO_2} is expressed on a log scale, this relation is described by a straight line. The line is appreciably steeper (better buffering) in chronic conditions, however. Progressive acidosis progressively activates adrenergic mechanisms. In extreme acidosis, however, adrenergic compensation fails. This decrease in adrenergic compensation has a threshold at about 7.2, with progressive inactivation of adrenergic reflexes, failing completely at 6.6 to 6.8 units.

In isolated hearts and in animal preparations, the effects of both increased and decreased CO_2 appear to be a consequence of the pH change alone,[67] with acidosis (a fall of 0.5 pH units) halving the contractile force of the heart and alkalosis giving a much less marked increase in force. Cardiac rhythm is not directly affected until extreme changes are produced. In intact humans and animals, autonomic nervous system activation is involved. Cullen and Eger[68] found that heart rate increased 26% and cardiac output increased 32% with a 10-mm Hg rise in P_{CO_2}.

Myocardial Oxygen Consumption

Indirect measurements of myocardial oxygen requirements reveal a significant increase. One sees a rise in time-tension index and a shortening of the diastolic filling time. From systolic time interval studies there is a shortening of preejection period and left ventricular ejection fraction. Mild elevations of CO_2 do not affect the heart rate. At levels of 56 to 65 mm Hg Pa_{CO_2}, however, systolic blood pressure rises greatly along with heart rate. Therefore, the myocardium is directly depressed,[67] although overall myocardial oxygen consumption is increased.[59]

Peripheral Blood Flow

More peripheral vascular areas are estimated to be dilated than constricted. The direct effect of increased plasma tension of CO_2 on blood vessels is *generally* to cause vasodilatation. Noteworthy are the effects on cerebral vessels previously described.[47] Also to be noted is the increase in coronary blood flow and the decreased renal resistance due to P_{CO_2} elevation. The increased blood flow in skin vessels on inhalation of CO_2 is frequently observed.[67]

Exceptions to the rule of vasodilatation due to increased P_{CO_2} or to acidosis are the effects on blood vessels of the muscle and those of the pulmonary bed. In the isolated lung, increased CO_2 tension appears to cause constriction, but in intact persons, vasodilatation occurs.

In limb vessels, CO_2 inhalation causes a more pronounced dilatation on postarteriolar beds than in the arteries or arterioles. Because the vascular capacity of the entire circulation is chiefly in the veins (60%) and capillaries (20%), pooling at these sites significantly diminishes venous return. One may conclude that anatomically the vessels most affected are the capillaries and veins.[67,68]

Hooker has shown that CO_2 decreases directly the tone of both mammalian arteries and veins.[69]

Mechanism of Effect on Vasculature

The effect of CO_2 on the vasculature is similarly the net effect of direct and indirect (neurogenic) actions of altered CO_2. Total peripheral resistance falls 14%, and muscle-skin flow increases 44% with a 10-mm Hg increase in P_{CO_2}.[68] Major increases in both plasma epinephrine and norepinephrine are associated with exogenously administered CO_2.[57]

The effect on blood pressure results from the interaction of increased cardiac output and decreased peripheral resistance. The usual effect is a minor increase in mean blood pressure, but the magnitude may vary from slight hypotension to marked hypertension. With sympathectomy and adrenalectomy, CO_2 produces a striking fall in pressure.[60,66]

Coronary Circulation

Coronary arteries are dilated by increases in Pa_{CO_2}. If perfusion pressure remains constant, coronary blood flow increases.[70]

Coronary blood flow is also autoregulated much like cerebral blood flow, matched to local tissue metabolism by a pH-dependent mechanism. Although respiratory or metabolic acidosis increase coronary blood flow as they do cerebral blood flow, anesthetic-induced augmentation is not prominent, however, probably because of associated anesthetic depression of contractility and of cardiac work, reducing coronary blood flow by the resultant change in autoregulation.

Myocardial Effects

Cardiac effects of increased arterial CO_2 tension on the heart are both direct and indirect. These two actions are in fact antagonistic.[68,71]

The *direct effect* is to reduce the contractile force of the myocardium and to slow the rate of contraction.[74] The ability of CO_2 to act in this manner may be through changes in pH that are induced, leading to acidosis. In the isolated dog heart, a decrease of one-half unit in the pH of arterial blood reduces the contractile force about 50%.[67] The mechanism is apparently at the cellular level. That is, elevated P_{CO_2} levels enhance the relaxation process in muscle. The rephosphorylation of adenosine diphosphate bound to contractile protein is a key chemical step in the relaxation process, and this is increased by elevated P_{CO_2}.[71-73]

The chief *indirect effect* is to elevate cardiac output. In normal unanesthetized persons breathing mixtures high in CO_2 (5 to 7%), cardiac output may increase about 60%, whereas the increase in oxygen consumption is elevated only 10 to 20%.[59] This response is probably due to two mechanisms: (1) the effect of CO_2 causing hyperventila-tion and increasing venous return; and (2) the effect of the CO_2 in increasing sympathetic nervous system discharge and the release of catecholamines.[57]

The net result of the direct and indirect effects is actually an increased cardiac output. These responses are attenuated in the anesthetized subject. The reactivity of the respiratory center and of the contiguous vasomotor center is enhanced by CO_2, but the response is diminished during general anesthesia.[28] This indicates that one part of the mechanism of action of CO_2 is on the CNS.

Cardiac Rhythm

In unanesthetized subjects, high levels of CO_2 are needed to influence cardiac rhythm.[57] The response to P_{CO_2} levels twice normal and to pH of arterial blood of 6.9 is not appreciable (Sechzer), and the following electrocardiographic effects have been observed:

The PR interval is unchanged.
Atrioventricular nodal beats may appear.
ST-segment elevation or depression occurs.
T waves are occasionally inverted.
QRS changes are not observed.

Arrhythmias

The threshold level of Pa_{CO_2} that produces arrhythmias is high but may be modified by various anesthetic agents.[75] The effect of CO_2 alteration on production of cardiac arrhythmias is generally not of importance unless accompanying electrolyte changes affect the electrical activity of pacemaker and conducting cardiac tissue. Acidosis can elevate potassium ions in plasma, and alkalosis can reduce them. Intracellular potassium does not change as much, because of water movement out of or into cells.[76] More important are adrenergic changes, especially with chloroform and cyclopropane, which increase arrhythmogenesis. Newer agents seem to be less prone to sensitize the heart to either CO_2 or epinephrine-increased dysrhythmia. After severe hypercarbia, arrhythmias may be more serious during correction of the acidosis.

Respiratory System

The most striking effect of CO_2 on this system is mediated through central respiratory control and is discussed in Chapter 3. Three minor effects are noted here: on smooth muscle of the airway, on striated muscles of respiration, and on pulmonary blood flow and vasculature.

Both the direct effect of CO_2 on bronchial smooth muscle and the induced effect by CO_2-activated adrenergic mechanism (both neural and humoral) are dilatory. On the other hand, respiratory alkalosis does cause some increase in tone of airway muscle, but in mechanically ventilated persons, this is countered by the positive pressure and lung volume increase. In asthmatic subjects, one can see a marked hypocapnic contribution to airway obstruction.[77] Anesthetic vapors are themselves bronchodilating and may further block the alkalotic constriction of asthmatics.[78,79]

Direct Effects of Hypercapnia on Muscle

Skeletal muscle, like smooth and cardiac muscle, may be depressed by extreme respiratory acidosis. Juan and colleagues[80] found that 54- to 60-mm Hg end-tidal P_{CO_2} caused both decreased contractility (10 to 30%) and earlier fatigue of the diaphragm of a normal person. The ability of the diaphragm to generate pressure, as shown by the time-tension index and electromyographic changes, is curtailed during hypercapnia (breathing 7.5% CO_2).[80] Respiratory alkalosis (end-tidal CO_2 of 25 mm Hg) had little effect.

Pulmonary Blood Flow and Distribution in the Lungs

Pulmonary blood flow, essentially cardiac output, is increased by adrenergic mechanisms when CO_2 is inhaled.[81] The distribution of that flow within the lung is not uniform even in normal persons, however, and it becomes nonuniform with mechanical ventilation (during anesthesia). Both physiologic shunt and physiologic dead space changes reflect the nonuniformity. Mitchenfelder[82] found that alkalosis increased shunt by about 8% and that adding CO_2, without altering ventilation, decreased it. Prolonged respiratory alkalosis during anesthesia has been reported to cause progressive alveolar dead space increase in some,[83] but not all, reports.[84] What is clear is that alkalosis gives a progressive blunting of the hypoxic pulmonary vasoconstrictive response, abolishing it at a pH of 7.8 (P_{CO_2} at 20 acutely).

Other Organ Systems

Gastrointestinal, Hepatic, and Renal Systems

As in the cardiovascular and respiratory systems, effects of CO_2 may be mediated by direct effects or by neurogenic (indirect effects). In general, little is known, and perhaps little is to be known, of CO_2-mediated changes in organ physiology metabolism or function (see Chapters 21 to 23).

Changes Related to Respiratory Alkalosis

One may presume that the cardiocirculatory responses to respiratory alkalosis are the reverse of excessive CO_2 levels. This is essentially correct, and one may summarize the effects of lowered P_{CO_2} as follows:

1. Direct enhancement of cardiac contractility.
2. A tendency to reduction in systolic blood pressure.
3. Regional circulatory effects.
   a. Cerebral vasoconstriction to the point of ischemia when P_{CO_2} values are 20 mm Hg.
   b. Constriction of skin vessels.
   c. Dilatation of muscle vessels.
4. Respiratory changes.
   a. Increased diaphragmatic muscle strength.[80]
   b. Blunting of hypoxic pulmonary vasoconstriction.[85]
5. Maintenance of plasma phosphate[86] (hypophosphatemia decreases muscle strength).

Toxic Action[87] in Diving

The P_{CO_2} in the alveolar air is about 40 mm Hg in an individual at rest and breathing normally. The P_{CO_2} present in arterial blood is in equilibrium with that of the alveolar air. Venous blood, however, on its return from the tissues, has a P_{CO_2} of about 46 mm. This slight excess is sufficient to allow rapid elimination by diffusion into the alveoli when the blood reaches the lung, and equilibrium is reached as the blood becomes arterialized; 40 mm Hg pressure of CO_2 in the alveoli at atmospheric conditions are exerted by about 5.6% CO_2: [40 = (760 − 47 P_{H_2O} vapor pressure) × 5.6]. This percentage is actually present in the alveolar air under normal conditions.

In addition to the toxic effects of CO_2 alone, investigators have also found that CO_2 accumulation within the body enhances the toxicity of oxygen and the narcotic effect of nitrogen.[87] With respect to work under compressed air, a higher incidence of "bends" has also been associated with a rise in the CO_2 level. The term nitrogen narcosis may be a misnomer, and the condition is better described as "nitrogen-CO_2 narcosis."[88]

Analyzing the alveolar air of a diver having adequate air supply and exposed to 3 atm of absolute pressure (66 feet water depth), a CO_2 percentage of about 1.8% is found in alveolar air.[89] By calculation, this percentage exerts a partial pressure identical to that present on the surface: 0.018 × [(760 × 3) − 47] = 40. This example is cited to convey the importance of keeping the CO_2 content of the inspired air down to an absolute minimum. To accomplish this, the air within a diver's breathing system must be constantly cleared of the CO_2 given off by the diver—in other words, adequate ventilation by abundant air supply must be maintained. If, for instance, some CO_2 were allowed to accumulate in the breathing system, the result would be a higher percentage of CO_2 in the air breathed, and consequently, its partial pressure in the alveoli would be correspondingly increased. The diver would attempt to remove this CO_2 by rapid or labored breathing, but if more contaminated air were inspired, these efforts would be useless. Under such conditions, the diver would become exhausted, not only from labored breathing, but also from the toxic effects of CO_2 accumulated within the body tissues. Any attempt to work under such conditions would only aggravate the diver's condition because more CO_2 is produced by the exercise involved.[90,91]

When the inspired air at normal atmospheric pressure contains 3% CO_2, the breathing begins to be noticeably increased; 6% causes distress, and 10% or more unconsciousness.[89] Because 3% CO_2 at ambient conditions is about the maximum that can be tolerated without respiratory distress, this level must not be reached or exceeded in closed rebreathing systems. To keep the CO_2 content of the helmet within this maximum permissible percentage, a minimum air supply of 1.5 cubic feet per minute (measured at the absolute pressure to which the dive is made) is necessary.[92] According to Boyle's law, the air supply measured at the surface must be increased in proportion to the absolute pressure if adequate ventilation is to be provided. Because each 33 feet of seawater exerts a pressure of 1 atm, the air supply measured at the surface must be increased by one thirty-third (1/33) for each foot of dive.[93] Using the reciprocal 0.0303, the minimum air supply for any depth can be calculated by the equation S = 1.5 [1 + F (0.0303)], in which S is the required air supply in cubic feet measured at the surface and F is the number of feet the diver is below the surface. Better ventilation than this is imperative, particularly if hard work is performed by the diver, and allowances should be made to supply three times this quantity of air per minute. An attempt is always made to keep the CO_2 concentration within the diver's helmet to a value equivalent to 0.1 or 0.2% at 1 atm.

Effects in Laparoscopy[94,95]

Kelling introduced laparoscopy in 1902. Through the years, improvements in technique and the introduction of the fiber optiscope has established the procedure as an important diagnostic and therapeutic method.

After the patient receiving general endotracheal anesthesia is stabilized, a Verres-type needle is inserted in the midline below the umbilicus and is directed toward the uterus. Pneumoperitoneum is created by the installation of 4.0 to 6.0 L of 100% CO_2 from an automatic pressure regulator.[95]

The effects of exogenous gas volumes in body cavities are often considerable, both mechanically and physiologically. Eventually, all gases must be resorbed and an equilibrium established. The rate of absorption is determined by the following:

1. Solubility of gas in tissues.
2. Pressure gradient across containing membranes of the cavity.
3. Diffusion constant of the gas.
4. Blood flow about the area.

CO_2 is soluble in body fluids, much more so than oxygen, the ratio being 23:1, and much more than nitrogen, 35:1.[7] In laparoscopy, considerable elevation of blood CO_2 occurs. $Paco_2$ values may increase from 8 to 20 mm Hg.[95] Complications of restricted ventilation, respiratory acidosis, and arrhythmias do occur. Anesthetic management requires a general agent, endotracheal technique, good relaxation, and vigorous hyperventilation.[96] If one begins with a respiratory alkalosis and a $Paco_2$ value of 27 to 30 mm Hg, the average rise of Pco_2 may still be 9 to 10 mm Hg in spite of continued hyperventilation.

THERAPEUTIC USES[98]

In most instances where CO_2 has been suggested, other more effective therapies are available. A few special circumstances remain:

1. Management of carbon monoxide poisoning.
2. Treatment of hiccoughs.
3. Use in petit mal seizures.
4. Stimulation of respiration to accelerate the uptake or elimination of volatile agents; acceleration of blood flow through CNS and aid in clearing the tissues of the anesthetic agent.
5. Questioned use to offset the tendency to atelectasis during quiet breathing.

6. Counteraction of the deleterious effects of low oxygen levels on intellectual function (Gibbs), and improvement of the abnormal EEG patterns associated with hypoxemia.
7. Use in laparoscopy.
8. In normalizing $Paco_2$ during mechanical ventilation (instead of adding dead space).

ANALYSIS OF CARBON DIOXIDE

The CO_2 values of interest to anesthesiologists may be either in gas mixtures (e.g., end-tidal CO_2) or in body fluids (e.g., arterial CO_2). In either case, CO_2 may be quantitated by either of two different determinations, the content or the partial pressure of CO_2 in the sample.[97] The value of monitoring CO_2 allows one to assess the adequacy of ventilation and in calculating acid-base disturbances.

For gases, we usually talk about the content as CONCENTRATION, for which the physiologic abbreviation is F_I, to remind us that it is fraction, written chemically or as per hundred (%). Alternately, we may speak of the partial pressure as TENSION, in units of mm Hg (or kPa with the SI usage). The two are directly related: partial pressure of CO_2 equals concentration times the sum of all partial pressures excluding water vapor:

$$Pco_2 = Fco_2 \times (P_{Barometric} - P_{H_2O}) \qquad (7)$$

This convention, with the exclusion of water vapor, is inherited from days when measurements were made by volumetric chemical analyses over aqueous reagents and produced the same answer for the same sample in Aberdeen, Scotland at 12°C room temperature and Hyderabad, India at 36°C.

Methods of Analysis

Gas Carbon Dioxide[98]

In anesthesia, we may employ infrared gas analysis, mass spectrometry, Ramon spectrometry or (rarely) Severinghaus electrodes. All are sensitive to the number of CO_2 molecules in the sample chamber and are thus measures of partial pressure at the conditions of temperature and pressure in the chamber. They are, however, "calibrated" with a sample of known concentration (and hence calculable tension) at ambient conditions and may be adjusted to read out either CO_2 concentration (%) or tension (mm Hg). The latter is usually adjusted to read correctly a sample saturated with water at body temperature and is in error to a small degree with a cooler or dryer sample.

Content in Liquids

In liquids, we may speak of the CO_2 content of a sample, measured volumetrically after strong acidification to push all carbonate and bicarbonate to carbonic acid and thence to molecular CO_2, for example:

$$H^+ + HCO_3 \rightarrow H_2CO_3 \rightarrow CO_2 + H_2O$$
$$\text{in the presence of strong acid} \qquad \text{water}$$

More commonly, however, in the presence of strong acid, we speak of the bicarbonate concentration, which is usually calculated from the Henderson-Hasselbalch equation after measurement of sample pH and P_{CO_2} with electrodes:

$$pH = 6.1 + \log \frac{(HCO_3)}{P_{CO_2}} \qquad (8)$$

In either case of gas or liquid sample, obtaining the correct value by analysis depends on proper sample handling. In the case of gases, it is relatively simple to avoid leaks and air contamination, but care must be taken to calibrate the analyzer with the same procedures used with the sample: in the case of respiratory monitoring, the same sample flow through the same sample tube length must be used in calibration so the sample chamber has the same internal pressure. In the case of liquids (usually blood), one must avoid contamination and metabolic changes before analyses. This means discarding samples with air bubbles, using minimal anticoagulant (less then 0.1 ml heparin per milliliter of sample—heparin is acidic) and analyzing immediately or cooling the sample in ice slush. The latter does *not* mean resting the syringe on a few ice cubes: it means immersing the syringe in water and ice at 0°C, so the whole barrel is cooled quickly. In practice, a small bubble of less the 0.1 ml expelled from the barrel within 30 seconds of blood sampling gives results clinically acceptable. If the liquid sample is cerebrospinal fluid, urine, or other liquids without the buffering effect of concentrated hemoglobin, however, even such a small bubble will distort the analysis unacceptably. Blood in plastic syringes must be analyzed more quickly than in glass because CO_2 and especially O_2 diffuse in or out of the blood through plastic and rubber.[99]

Capnographic Analysis

Gas samples analyzed for CO_2 are usually taken continuously from the airway. The analogue display as a function of time is a *capnogram*. The analytic instruments are generically called *capnometers* and may sample, digitize, and display the minimum CO_2 tension within one respiratory cycle, usually labeled inspired CO_2, and the maximum, termed end-tidal CO_2. The analytic chamber may be a portion of the airway itself, a segment inserted between endotracheal tube and breathing circuit, for example. This is called a mainstream analyzer.[100] Newer instruments have reduced the volume and weight of these to acceptably low values, and they offer theoretic advantages in sampling the whole expirate in real time. Many other instruments in use sample the gas at or within the airway through a small plastic tube, drawn at a flow rate of 100 to 300 ml/min. This permits a more sophisticated sample chamber, such as smaller size, temperature controlled, with multiple gas analysis capability, at a cost of some delay, danger of mixing inspired gas with the expirate at low patient expiratory flows, and plugging from mucus or water condensate.[100]

Evaluation of the Capnogram[101,102]

The capnogram should be displayed, and little reliance should be placed on digitized values alone, because the morphology of the capnogram contains useful information. A typical form has four segments of interest, labeled a, b, c, and d. The first, a, represents inspired gas, and in most cases, including Mapleson's circuits with adequate fresh gas flow, should be at or near the zero level. The second, b, represents the washout of dead space and should be a nearly vertical stroke, slurring into the next segment. This, c, is a slightly up-sloping segment representing alveolar gas. It slopes upward 1 to 2 torr per breath, as a result of at least two factors: the later emptying of lower V/Q lung units and the continued delivery of CO_2 to the decreasing lung volume during exhalation. If there is an end-expiratory pause in exhalation, it may be horizontal briefly, showing continued sampling of an unchanged gas mixture.

Ideally, the segment d is nearly a vertical segment like b. If the sample flow exceeds expiratory flow, fresh gas may be aspirated in the latter part of segment c, slurring to an early representation of washout of alveolar gas with inspired (fresh) gas.

Abnormalities of the Capnogram[102]

A variety of abnormalities have been described in each segment and have been published in atlases of capnography or reviews. Important cautions and criteria should be familiar to the user. The inspired CO_2 may rise with failure of CO_2 absorption, stuck expiratory valves, analyzer drift, or inadequate sampling; the last usually gives markedly slurred b and d segments.

Use During Anesthesia

The capnometer can be used in several ways during anesthesia: monitoring the ratio of alveolar ventilation to CO_2 production is but one. The so-called anatomic dead space can be estimated, roughly as the volume exhaled when the trace reaches half the height of the alveolar plateau. The mixed expired CO_2 F_{ECO_2} can be measured from a mixing chamber, for which the anesthesia bag or ventilator bellows may be a good approximation—but not from mixing a continuously drawn sample before analyzing it. Such a sample is time weighed and not volume weighted. Mixed expired CO_2 is used to compute physiologic dead space, CO_2 excretion, and other variables.[101,103,104]

Utility of Blood Sampling[98]

Blood samples taken to determine arterial P_{CO_2} tension (Pa_{CO_2}) are almost always analyzed for a variety of other variables as well. The medical student may know that 5.3 pKa (or 40 mm Hg) is a normal value and may slavishly sample blood and adjust ventilators to arrive at and keep that value. A good anesthetist evaluates that value in the light of other data, including the simultaneous P_{O_2} and pH values, as well as other clinical data from history and concurrent observation. For example, a Pa_{CO_2} of 50 mm Hg is "high" but should not be lowered if pH is 7.42. A Pa_{CO_2} of 44 mm Hg with F_{IO_2} of 0.5 and P_{O_2} of 150 should be recognized as an increase in physiologic shunt and V_T increased before $\dot{V}_E$ is increased. Positive end-expiratory pressure may be tried before increasing F_{IO_2} OR $\dot{V}_E$. A consultant anesthesiologist may recognize presence or absence of factors contributing to an arterial-alveolar difference for CO_2 and may sample Pa_{CO_2} less often when P_{ETCO_2} and other data are stable, or the consultant anesthesiologist may elect to manage acid-base balance differently, in hypothermia, using α-stat theory and uncorrected blood gas values. Other circumstances may impinge on simple alteration of ventilation for P_{CO_2} changes.[105]

Estimation of Pulmonary Dead Space

The anatomic dead space may be readily *estimated* as a fraction of the total volume, using capnography and mixed expired air as well as airway analysis from:

$$\frac{V_D}{V_T} = \frac{P_{ET} - P_E}{P_{ET} - P_I} \quad (9)$$

Usually, P_I is zero, of course.

Physiologic dead space is calculated similarly: simply replace P_{ET} WITH Pa_{CO_2}. The elimination of CO_2 from the lung is also readily calculated after measure of P_{ECO_2}. First display or convert capnometer values to concentration (C_{ECO_2}) by:

$$C_E CO_2 = P_E CO_2/(P_{Barometer} - P_{Water\ vapor})$$

The tension of water vapor is about 23 mm Hg in the breathing bag, saturated water vapor at room temperature. Next multiply by ventilation to get CO_2 production:

$$\dot{V}_{CO_2} = \dot{V}_E \times C_E CO_2 \text{ at ATPS} \quad (10)$$

Conventionally, $\dot{V}_{CO_2}$ is usually quoted at standard temperature and pressure (STPD) and can be estimated as $\frac{1}{8}$ less than calculated at ambient temperature and pressure, saturated (ATPS).

This segment of the text is intended to stimulate inquisitive thought, further study, and more detailed patient care procedures. The reader is directed to more detailed monographs.[98,106] Inquisitive and curious anesthetists will find increasing value in our soon-to-be ubiquitous capnometers.

Application of CO_2 Determinations

One should probably consider P_{ETCO_2} as a useful but different variable than Pa_{CO_2}. It is a ventilation-weighted measure of alveolar CO_2 tension, whereas arterial blood is a perfusion-weighted average. Like the Dow Jones and Value Line averages, neither is "correct": they measure different things. In patients with extremely slow respiratory frequency, and slow expiratory flow, P_{ET} may exceed Pa! With increasing "alveolar dead space," Pa exceeds P_{ET}. Certain circumstances, such as carbonic anhydrase inhibition, may cause the CO_2 tension in end-pulmonary capillary blood (by convention considered identical to alveolar CO_2 tension) to rise measurably as blood flows through pulmonary veins to the heart.

Sudden pulmonary hypotension can be detected by a rapid decrease in end-tidal CO_2 due to the alveolar dead space effect. Cardiac arrest stops CO_2 delivery, and continued ventilation gives P_{ETCO_2} exponentially approaching zero in a few minutes. Mixed venous (oxygenated) CO_2 tension can be measured by the method of Hackney and associates,[107] permitting the capnometer to reduce the frequency of arterial sampling because, although the aAD_{CO_2} is variable, the a-vco_2 tension is constant, varying from 5 to 7 mm Hg over usual ranges of Pa_{CO_2} encountered clinically.

Role of Arterial to Alveolar Tension Difference

Of particularly overlooked value is the arterial to alveolar difference for CO_2, aAD_{CO_2}. Many have dismissed it because it changes, and they have not bothered to inquire why. It may be small, less than 1 mm Hg in certain normal patient circumstances.[108,109] The aAP_{CO_2} divided by the arterial CO_2 gives the ratio of alveolar dead space to tidal volume. It rises with increasing pressure used in mechanical ventilation and with pulmonary arterial hypotension.[110]

REFERENCES

1. Fulton, J. F., Peters, C. H.: An introduction to a bibliography of the educational and scientific works of Joseph Priestley. Papers Bibliogr Soc Am *30:*150, 1936.
2. Lavoisier, A.: Elements of Chemistry. Book I, 1787. Translation by Robert Kerr. Chicago, Henry Regnery (Great Books Foundation), 1949.
3. Long, M.: The heart of the flame. Yale Alumni Mag *57:*38, 1994.
4. Henderson, Y.: Adventures in Respiration. Baltimore, Williams & Wilkins, 1988.
5. Eckenhoff, J. E.: Introduction to symposium: carbon dioxide and man. Anesthesiology *21:*585, 1960.
6. Baxter, P., Jaskapila, M., Mfonfu, D.: Lake Nyos disaster, Cameroon 1986: the medical effects of large-scale emission of carbon dioxide. Br Med J *298:*1437, 1989.
7. Adriani, J.: The Chemistry and Physics of Anesthesia, 2nd Ed. Springfield, IL, Charles C Thomas, 1962, p. 199.
8. Black, J.: Experiments Upon Magnesia Alba 1755, Reprint No. 1, Alembic Club. Named "Fixed Air" in 1757. See: Cartwright, F.F.: The English Pioneers of Anaesthesia. Baltimore, Williams & Wilkins, 1952.
9. Foregger, R.: Identification of carbon dioxide. Anesthesiology *18:*257, 1957.
10. Steinberg, D.: Metabolism. *In* West, J. B. (ed.) Best and Taylor's Physiological Basis of Medical Practice, 12th Ed. Baltimore, Williams & Wilkins, 1990.
11. Fleischer, S.: The metabolic production of carbon dioxide. Anesthesiology *21:*497, 1960.
12. Farhi, L. E., Rahn, H.: Gas stores of body and unsteady state. J Appl Physiol *7:*472, 1955.
13. Farhi, L. E., Rahn, H.: Dynamics of changes in carbon dioxide stores. Anesthesiology *27:*604, 1960.
14. Vance, J. W., Fowler, W. S.: Adjustment of stores of carbon dioxide during hyperventilation. Dis Chest *37:*304, 1960.
15. De Backer, W. A., et al.: Ventilation and breathing patterns during hemodialysis induced carbon dioxide unloading Am Rev Respir Dis *136:*408, 1987.
16. Frumin, J. M., Epstein, R. M., Cohen, G.: Apneic oxygenation in man. Anesthesiology *20:*789, 1959.
17. Eger, E. I., Severinghaus, J. W.: The rate of rise of Pa_{CO_2} in the apneic anesthetized patient. Anesthesiology *22:*419, 1961.

18. Stock, M. C., Downs, J. B., McDonald, E. T.: The carbon dioxide rate of rise in awake apneic patients. J Clin Anesth 1:96, 1988.

19. Stock, M., Schisler, J. Q., McSweeney, T. D.: The $PaCO_2$ rate of rise in anesthetized patients with airway obstruction. J Clin Anesth 1:328, 1989.

20. Mertzlufft, F. O., Brandt, L., Stanton-Hicks, M., Dick, W.: Arterial and mixed venous blood gas: proof of the Christiansen-Douglas-Haldane effect in vivo. Anaesth Intensive Care 17:325, 1989.

21. Christiansen, J., Douglas, C. G., Haldane, J. S.: The absorption and dissociation of carbon dioxide by human blood. J Physiol (Lond) 48:244, 1914.

22. Haldane, J. S., Priestley, J. G.: Respiration. New Haven, Yale University Press, 1935.

23. Henneberg, S., et al.: Carbon dioxide production during mechanical ventilation. Crit Care Med 15:8, 1987.

24. Nunn, J. F.: Carbon dioxide cylinders on anaesthesia apparatus (Editorial). Br J Anaesth 65:155, 1990.

25. Coleman, S. A., McCrory, J. W., Vallis, C. J., Boys, R. J.: Inhalation induction of anaesthesia with isoflurane: effect of added carbon dioxide. Br J Anaesth 67:257, 1991.

26. Razis, P.: Carbon dioxide: A survey of its use in anaesthesia in the United Kingdom. Anaesthesia 44:348, 1989.

27. Riddell, R. R.: Carbon dioxide arthroscopy of the knee. J Clin Orthop 252:92, 1990.

28. Liu, S.-Y., et al.: Prospective analysis of cardiopulmonary responses to laparoscopic cholecystectomy. J Laparoendosc Surg 1:241, 1991.

29. Gabbatt, D. A., Dunkley, A. B., Roberts, F. L.: Carbon dioxide pneumothorax occurring during laparoscopic cholecystectomy. Anaesthesia 47:587, 1992.

30. Reybrouck, T. E., Fragen, R.: Assessment of cardiac output at rest and during exercise by carbon dioxide rebreathing method. Eur Heart J 11(Suppl):21, 1990.

31. Taylor, R. S.: Gas (CO_2) endarterectomy. Am Heart J 76:436, 1968.

32. Brown, J. M.: Carbogen and nicotinamide: Expectations too high? Radiother Oncol 24:75, 1992.

33. Cooper, J. B., Newbower, R. S., Kitz, R. J.: An analysis of major errors and equipment failures in anesthetic management. Anesthesiology 60:34, 1989.

34. Smith, T. C.: Commentary on elevated carbon dioxide. Personal communication, 1994.

35. Don, H.: Hypoxemia and hypercapnia during and after anesthesia. In Orkin, F.K., Cooperman, L.H. (eds.). Complications in Anesthesia. Philadelphia, J.B. Lippincott, 1983, p. 183.

36. Brazier, M.: Physiological effects of CO_2 on activity of CNS in man. Medicine 22:205, 1943.

37. Seevers, M. H.: The narcotic properties of carbon dioxide. NY State J Med 44:597, 1944.

38. Eisele, J. H., Eger, E. I., Muallem, M.: Narcotic properties of carbon dioxide. Anesthesiology 28:856, 1967.

39. Eastman, N. J.: Fetal blood studies. Bull Johns Hopkins 50:39, 1932.

40. Bonvallet, M., Hugelin, A., Dell, P.: Sensibilité comparée du système reticule activateur ascendant et du centre respiratoire aux gaz du sang et à l'adrénaline. J Physiol (Paris) 47:651, 1955.

41. Bonvallet, M., Dell, P.: Reflections on mechanism of action on hyperventilation upon the EEG, electroencephalography. J Physiol (Montreal) 48:170, 1956.

42. Clutton-Brock, J.: Cerebral effects of overventilation. Br J Anaesth 29:111, 1957.

43. Robinson, J. S., Gray, T. C.: Observations on cerebral effects of passive hyperventilation. Br J Anaesth 33:62, 1961.

44. McAleavy, J. C., et al.: The effect of PCO_2 on the depth of anesthesia. Anesthesiology 22:260, 1961.

45. Dundee, J. W.: Influence of controlled respiration on dosage of thiopentone and D-tubocurarine chloride required for abdominal surgery. Br Med J 2:893, 1952.

46. Hickman, H. H.: From ironbridge letters (1824). In Keys, T.E. (ed.). History of Surgical Anesthesia. New York, Dover, 1963.

47. Sokoloff, L.: The effects of carbon dioxide on the cerebral circulation. Anesthesiology 21:664, 1960.

48. Jensen, K. E., Thomsen, C., Henrickson, O.: In vivo measurement of intracellular pH in human brain during different tensions of CO_2 in arterial blood. Acta Physiol Scand 134:295, 1988.

49. Rapela, C. E., Green, H. D., Dennison, A. B., Jr.: Baroreceptor reflexes and autoregulation of cerebral blood flow in dogs. Circ Res 21:559, 1967.

50. Wollman, H., et al.: Effects of extremes of respiratory and metabolic alkalosis. J Appl Physiol 24:60, 1968.

51. Alexander, S. C., et al.: Cerebral carbohydrate metabolism during hypocarbia in man. Studies during nitrous oxide anesthesia. Anesthesiology 26:624, 1965.

52. Wollman, H., et al.: Cerebral circulation during general anesthesia and hyperventilation in man: thiopental induction to nitrous oxide and d-tubocurarine. Anesthesiology 26:329, 1965.

53. Smith, A. L., Neigh, A. L., Hoffman, J. C., Wollman, H.: Effects of general anesthesia on autoregulation of cerebral blood flow in man. J Appl Physiol 23:665, 1970.

54. Jobes, D. R., et al.: Cerebral blood flow and metabolism during morphine-nitrous oxide anesthesia in man. Anesthesiology 47:16, 1977.

55. Pelligrino, D. A., et al.: Nitrous oxide markedly increases cerebral cortical metabolic rate and blood flow in the goat. Anesthesiology 60:405, 1984.

56. Tenney, S. M.: Effect of carbon dioxide on neuro-humoral and endocrine mechanisms. Anesthesiology 21:674, 1960.

57. Sechzer, P. H., et al.: Effect of carbon dioxide inhalation on arterial pressure, electrocardiogram and plasma concentration of catecholamines and 17-OH corticosteroids in normal man. J Appl Physiol 15:454, 1960.

58. Staszewska-Barczak, J., Dusting, G. J.: Importance of circulating angiotensin II for elevation of arterial pressure during acute hypercapnia in anesthetized dogs. Clin Exp Pharmacol Physiol 8:189, 1981.

59. Rasmussen, J. P., et al.: Cardiac function and hypercarbia. Arch Surg 113:1196, 1978.

60. Pinkston, J. O., Parkington, P. E., Rosenbleuth, A.: Study of reflex changes in blood pressure in completely sympathectomized animals. Am J Physiol 115:711, 1936.

61. Langley, L. L., Nims, L. F., Clarke, R. W.: Role of CO_2 in the stress reaction to hypoxia. Am J Physiol 161:331, 1950.

62. Long, C. N. H.: Regulation of ACTH secretion. Horm Res 7:75, 1952.

63. Nunn, J. F.: Carbon dioxide. In Applied Respiratory Physiology, 3d Ed. London, Butterworth, 1987, p. 207.

64. Carey, C. R., Schaefer, K. E., Delgado, S. M. R.: Influence of various concentrations CO_2 on activity of the brain in the walking monkey. Fed Proc 14:25, 1955.

65. Foldes, F. F.: Enzymes in Anesthesiology. New York, Springer, 1978.

66. Young, W. C., Sealy, W. C., Harris, J., Botwin, A.: Effects of hypercapnia and hypoxia on responses of heart to vagal stimulation. Surg Gynecol Obstet 93:51, 1951.

67. Price, H. L.: Effects of carbon dioxide on the cardiovascular system. Anesthesiology 21:652, 1960.

68. Cullen, D. J., Eger, E. I., II: Cardiovascular effects of carbon dioxide in man. Anesthesiology 48:345, 1974.
69. Hooker, D. R.: Effect of carbon dioxide and of oxygen upon musculature in blood vessels and alimentary canal. Am J Physiol 31:47, 1912.
70. Feinberg, H., Geroki, A., Katz, L. N.: Effect of changes in blood CO_2 levels on coronary blood flow and myocardial oxygen consumption. Am J Physiol 238:H54, 1980.
71. Patterson, S. W.: The antagonistic action of carbon dioxide and adrenaline on the heart. Proc R Soc Med 85:371, 1988.
72. Etsten, B.: Effects of respiratory acidosis upon cardiac output, blood pressure and total peripheral resistance during cyclopropane anesthesia in man. J Pharmacol Exp Ther 119:144, 1957.
73. Foex, P., Prys Roberts, C.: Effect of CO_2 on myocardial contractility and input impedence. Br J Anaesth 47:669, 1975.
74. Boniface, K. J., Brown, J. M.: Effect of carbon dioxide excess on the contractile force of the heart. Am J Physiol 172:752, 1953.
75. Price, H. L., et al.: Cyclopropane anesthesia: epinephrine and norepinephrine in initiation of ventricular arrhythmias by carbon dioxide inhalation. Anesthesiology 19:619, 1958.
76. Spurr, G. B., Lambert, H.: Cardiac and skeletal muscle electrolytes in acute respiratory alkalemia and acidemia. J Appl Physiol 15:459, 1960.
77. Van den Elshout, F. J. J., van Herwaarden, C. L. A., Folgering, H.T.: Effects of hypercapnia and hypocapnia on respiratory resistance in normal and asthmatic subjects. Thorax 46:28, 1991.
78. Duane, S. F., Weir, E. K., Steward, R. M., Niewoehner, D.E.: Distal airway response to changes in oxygen and carbon dioxide tensions. Respir Physiol 38:303, 1979.
79. Lau, H.-P., Sayiner, A., Warner, D. O., Rehder, K.: Halothane alters the response of isolated airway smooth muscle to carbon dioxide. Respir Physiol 87:255, 1992.
80. Juan, G., et al.: Effect of carbon dioxide on diaphragmatic function in human beings. N Engl J Med 310:874, 1984.
81. McArdle, L., Roddie, J. C.: Vascular responses to carbon dioxide during anesthesia. Br J Anaesth 30:358, 1958.
82. Mitchenfelder, J.: CO_2 levels and pulmonary shunting in anesthetized man. J Appl Physiol 21:1471, 1966.
83. Askrog, V. F., Pender, J., Smith, T. C., Eckenhoff, J.: Changes in respiratory dead space during halothane, cyclopropane and nitrous oxide. Anesthesiology 25:342, 1964.
84. Lumley, J., Morgan, M., Sykes, M.: Changes in alveolar-arterial oxygen tension difference and physiological dead space during controlled ventilation. Br J Anaesth 40:803, 1968.
85. Fitts, R. H., Holloszy, J. O.: Lactate and contractile force of frog muscle during development of fatigue recovery. Am J Physiol 231:430, 1976.
86. Aubier, M., Murcians, D., Lecocguic, Y.: Effect of hypophosphatemia on diaphragmatic contractility in patients with acute respiratory failure. N Engl J Med 313:420, 1985.
87. Lambertsen, C. J.: Harmful effect of oxygen, nitrogen, carbon monoxide. In Bard, P. (ed.). Medical Physiology, 11th Ed. St. Louis, C.V. Mosby, 1961.
88. Bean, J. W.: Tensional changes of alveolar gases in reaction to rapid compression and decompression and the question of nitrogen narcosis. Biol Abstr 24:324, 1950.
89. Lambertsen, C. J.: Basic requirements for improving diving depth and decompression tolerance. In Underwater Physiology. Baltimore, Williams & Wilkins, 1966.
90. Strauss, R. H., Prockop, L. D.: Decompression sickness among scuba divers. JAMA 223:637, 1973.
91. Empleton, B. E.: The New Science of Skin and Scuba Diving, 3rd Ed. New York, Association Press, 1968.
92. United States Navy: U.S. Navy Diving Manual. Washington, D.C., Navy Department NAVSHIPS 0994-001-9010, 1970.
93. Schaefer, K. E., et al: Pulmonary and circulatory adjustments determining the limits of depths in breathhold diving. Science 162:1020, 1968.
94. Kelling, G.: Uber Oesophagoskopie Gastroskopie und Colioskopie. Munchen Med Wochnschr 49:21, 1902.
95. Siegler, A. M., Berenyi, K. J.: Laparoscopy in gynecology. Obstet Gynecol 34:572, 1969.
96. Berenyi, K. J., Fujita, T., Siegler, A. M.: Carbon dioxide laparoscopy: anesthetic management and determination of acid base parameters. Acta Anaesthesiol Scand 14:77, 1970.
97. Smith, T. C.: Carbon Dioxide and Anesthesia. ASA Refresher Course No. 83. Park Ridge, IL, American Society of Anesthesiologists, 1976.
98. Shapiro, B., Harrison, R. A., Cane, R. D., Templin, R.: Clinical Application of Blood Gases, 4th Ed. Chicago, Year Book Medical Publishers, 1989.
99. Harsten, A., Berg, B., Inerot, S., Muth, L.: Importance of correct handling of samples for the results of blood gas analysis. Acta Anesthesiol Scand 32:365, 1988.
100. Block, F. E., McDonald, J. S.: Sidestream versus mainstream carbon dioxide analyzers. J Clin Monit 8:139, 1992.
101. Bhavani-Shanker, K., Moseley, H., Kumar, A. Y., Delph, Y.: Capnometry and Anaesthesia. Can J Anaesth 39:617, 1992.
102. Liu, S.-Y., Lee, T.-S., Bongard, F.: Accuracy of capnography in nonintubated surgical patients. Chest 102:1512, 1992.
103. Fretscher, R., Warth, H., Deusch, H., Kloss, T.: Kapnometrie in der Kinderanasthesie: Einfluss von Messort und Atemfrequenz. Anaesthesist 41:463, 1992.
104. Gravenstein, J. S., Paulus, D. A., Hayes, T. J.: Capnography in Clinical Practice. Boston, Butterworth, 1989.
105. Patel, P. M.: Hyperventilation as a therapeutic intervention: do the potential benefits outweigh the known risks? J Neurosurg Anesthesiol 5:62, 1993.
106. Saidman, L. J., Smith, N. T.: Monitoring in Anesthesia, 3rd Ed. Boston, Butterworth-Heineman, 1993.
107. Hackney, J. D., Sears, C. H., Collier, C. R.: Estimation of arterial CO_2 tension by rebreathing technique. J Appl Physiol 12:425, 1958.
108. Pansard, J. L., et al.: Variation in arterial to end-tidal CO_2 tension differences during anesthesia in the "kidney rest" lateral decubitus position. Anesth Analg 75:506, 1992.
109. Garfield, B. R., Graybeal, J. M., Strout, J. C.: Stability of arterial to end-tidal carbon dioxide gradients during postoperative cardio-respiratory support. Can J Anaesth 37:560, 1990.
110. Brampton, W. J., Watson, R. J.: Arterial to end-tidal carbon dioxide tension differences during laparoscopy: magnitude and effect of anaesthetic technique. Anaesthesia 45:210, 1990.

Chapter 29

SEDATIVE AND HYPNOTIC DRUGS: BARBITURATES

VINCENT J. COLLINS

HISTORICAL BACKGROUND[1]

The barbiturates are the most versatile of all the depressant drugs. The whole spectrum of depression can be produced from mild sedation to deep anesthesia. In 1864, Adolf van Bayer in Ghent made the parent compound by combining urea (an animal waste product) and malonic acid (derived from the acid of apples) to obtain a synthetic compound called "barbituric acid." For this, which laid the foundations for subsequent derivatives, he received the Nobel Prize in Chemistry in 1905.

The source of this name is apocryphal. On the day Bayer discovered his new drug, he went to the local tavern with his fellow chemists to celebrate. At the same time, the town's artillery garrison was celebrating the feast of Saint Barbara, the patron saint of artillerists, and in the same tavern. One of the artillery officers, hearing of the new chemical, is said to have christened the substance by combining the words Barbara and urea.

Many derivatives of barbituric acid were produced in the ensuing years. In 1903, Fischer and von Mering discovered that one of the compounds, diethyl barbituric acid, was effective in putting dogs to sleep.[2] This compound was called veronal (barbital) in honor of the City of Verona, the most peaceful city Van Mering knew. The second oldest hypnotic barbiturate was phenobarbital and was introduced in 1912. Then followed feverish chemical and pharmacologic activity, so at present, over 2500 barbiturates have been synthesized and over 750 analogues have been tested. Of these, less than 2 dozen have achieved a place in medicine.

PHYSIOCHEMICAL FACTORS[3]

The barbiturates are white powders with melting points between 100° and 200°C. Barbituric acid is insoluble in water, but the basic salts are soluble. Solutions, however, are unstable. The salt preparations are stabilized in an organic solvent of propylene glycal, alcohol, and water.

Barbituric acid, which forms the essential structure for the barbiturates, is produced by a condensation of urea and malonic acid (Fig. 29–1). The derivatives are acidic and form salts with alkali. All barbiturates are weak organic acids.

STRUCTURE AND ACTIVITY[2]

The two hydrogen atoms encircled in the formula are very reactive, and when they are substituted by aliphatic aromatic radicals, various agents are produced, varying in activity. When both hydrogen atoms are replaced by short aliphatic groups, long-acting compounds are produced; if one hydrogen is replaced by a short radical and one by a long radical, short-acting barbiturates are produced. When both aliphatic groups are over five or six carbon atoms long, no hypnotic activity is found, but convulsive properties appear. As the molecular weight of the radical is increased, potency increases, as does toxicity, until the molecular weight of the radical reaches 250.

Modification of barbiturate molecule may be made according to the following, to alter effects:

1. Hydrogen atoms at position (5). Both must be replaced to produce hypnotic action. (R_1) and (R_2) may be replaced by aliphatic, aromatic, and/or heterocyclic groups. Optimum activity results when one chain is short and the other is long or is a ring structure.
2. Oxygen replaced by sulfur results in drugs of short duration due to altered distribution (not due to destruction). Plasma protein binding is greater. Equilibration with brain tissue is rapid.
3. Hydrogen atoms on the nitrogen (position 1). Replacement with methyl or ethyl groups increases rapidity of onset and recovery but accompanied by some convulsant action.

CHEMICAL CLASSIFICATION[1,3]

In the structure of the barbiturate nucleus are three principal sites for chemical alteration. Substitution at positions (1) and (2) produces four large chemical groups. These are the oxybarbiturates and their methylated derivatives and the thiobarbiturates and their methylated derivatives (Table 29–1). In addition, substitution at position

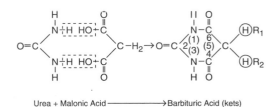

Urea + Malonic Acid ⟶ Barbituric Acid (kets)

Fig. 29–1. Structure of barbituric acid.

Table 29–1. Chemical Classification of Barbiturates (Shows the barbiturate nucleus and the sites of substitution; members of each group are listed with the chemical radicals substituted at the appropriate site)

GENERAL STRUCTURE

Chemical Group	(1) R_3	Structural Positions		
		(2) X	(5) R_1	(5) R_2
I. Oxybarbiturates				
Barbital	H	0	Ethyl	Ethyl
Phenobarbital	H	0	Ethyl	Phenyl
Pentobarbital	H	0	Ethyl	Methyl-butyl
Amobarbital	H	0	Ethyl	Isopentyl
Secobarbital	H	0	Allyl	Methyl-butyl
Butabarbital	H	0	Ethyl	Methyl-propyl
II. Methylated Barbiturates				
Hexobarbital	CH_3	0	Methyl	Cyclohexenyl
Methohexital	CH_3	0	Allyl	1-Methyl-2-pentynyl
III. Thiobarbiturates				
Thiopental	H	S	Ethyl	Methyl-butyl
Thiamylal	H	S	Allyl	Methyl-butyl
Thialbarbital (See intravenous barbiturates)	H	S	Allyl	Cyclo-hexenyl
IV. Methylated Thiobarbiturates				
Methylthiobutabarbital	CH_3	S	Ethyl	Methyl-propyl

(5) produces drugs with significant differences in pharmacologic effects.

CLINICAL CLASSIFICATION

The historic classification of barbiturates, as formalized by Tatum in 1939, is based on the duration of action as observed principally in animals. Four groups are recognized:[4]

This terminology is scientifically unsound when applied to human subjects.[5] The spectrum of effects of all barbiturates is stereotyped and extends in a dose-dependent fashion from *sedation* → hypnosis → anesthesia → poisoning → death. Any of these effects may be obtained with an appropriate dose (Table 29-2). Clinically, the intravenous barbiturates are not ultra short-acting, and although there is an apparent return to consciousness, mental clouding and central depression persist for many hours. In contrast, the short-acting drugs can cause sedation for as many hours as the "long-acting" drugs. Studies on the time and degree of hypnotic action of 100-mg doses of secobarbital and phenobarbital do not permit a distinction. Mark[5] has therefore proposed to classify the order of barbiturate drugs into two clinical families:

1. Sedative-hypnotic barbiturates or "basal hypnotics."
2. Anesthetic barbiturates.

Differences in physiochemical properties and pharmokinetic behavior do confer some degree of specialization on individual barbiturates in the therapeutic range.

ADMINISTRATION AND DOSAGE[6]

These drugs may be given by all routes: oral, rectal, intravenous, intramuscular, and intraperitoneal.

The oral administration results in a significantly variable effect because of the "first-pass effect" with the removal of drug by the liver and less reaching the circulation.

The intramuscular injection of short-acting barbiturates is superior to the oral administration. Such injections are frequently accompanied by pain at the injection site even

Table 29–2. Dose Schedule

Action	Time of Action (hours)	Sleep Dose Range (grams)
Long	15–20	0.3–0.6
Medium	10–15	0.2–0.4
Short	5–10	0.1–0.2
Ultra-short	½–2	up to 1.0

Table 29–3. Half-Lives, Dosage Forms, and Oral Dosages of Sedative-Hypnotic Drugs

Drug Classes, Nonproprietary Names, and Trade Names	Half-Life (hours)	Dosage Forms*	Adult Oral Dosage (mg)	
			Sedative†	Hypnotic
Barbiturates				
Amobarbital (sodium) (Amytal)	8–42	C.T.I.P	30–50, 2–3×d	65–200
Aprobarbital (Alurate)	14–34	E	40, 3×d	40–160
Butabarbital (sodium) (Butisol. sodium, others)	34–42	C.T.E	15–30, 3–4×d	50–100
Butalbital ‖	—	M ‖	—	—
Mephobarbital (Mebaral)	11–67	T	32–100, 3–4×d	—
Pentobarbital (sodium) (Nembutal)	15–48	C.E.I.S	20, 3–4×d	100
Phenobarbital (sodium) (Luminal sodium, others)	80–120	C.T.E.I	15–40, 2–4×d	100–320
Secobarbital (sodium) (Seconal sodium)	15–40	C.T.I	30–50, 3–4×d	50–200
Talbutal (Lotusate)	—	T	15–40, 2–3×d	120

*C = capsule; E = elixir; ERC = extended-release capsule; 1 = injection; L = liquid; P = powder; S = suppository; T = tablet.
†Dose, number per day: dosages do not apply for extended-release forms.
‖ Marketed only in mixture.
Modified from Rall, R. W.: Hypnotics and sedatives. *In* Goodman, L. S., et al. (eds.). The Pharmacologic Basis of Therapeutics, 8th Ed. New York, McGraw-Hill, 1990, p. 357.

when in aqueous solution, however. Preparations stabilized with organic solvents produce a higher incidence of pain that is more severe and persistent.[7]

Administration by the intramuscular route should be deep into the muscle bed; otherwise, pain and tissue necrosis may occur if deposit is superficial. The intraperitoneal route is especially good for animal anesthesia (Table 29-3).

In small doses, these drugs are sedative and reduce emotional turmoil and anxiety.[8] At three to five times the sedative dose, the same drug produces sleep. In still larger doses, unconsciousness is produced from which the patient cannot be aroused to a coordinate rational state. Further increase in dose produces anesthesia; spinal cord reflexes are reduced. Relaxation of muscles does not occur, however, and surgical manipulation or stimulation produces tensing and spasm. In excessive doses, muscular relaxation may be produced, but this is at the expense of good physiology.

PHARMACOKINETICS AND DISPOSITION[9,10]

Absorption readily occurs through the mucosa of the small intestine and rectum. When large doses are given, small amounts may be absorbed from the stomach. In the blood, these drugs are distributed to the tissues in amounts related to the regional circulation. Varying fractions are then taken up by the tissues (Table 29-4).

The placenta offers no barrier to the passage of barbiturates, which readily cross the placenta to the fetus.[11]

In the blood, binding to plasma proteins is a function of lipid solubility. Thiopental has highest lipid solubility of the barbiturates, and about 65% is bound. Benzodiazepines are bound to the extent of 70 to 99% (diazepam).

The half-life[6] of the sedative-hypnotic barbiturates ranges from 8 to 15 hours for amobarbital and secobarbital[12,13] to over 80 hours for phenobarbital (see Table 29-3).

Disposition of the barbiturates depends on renal or hepatic mechanisms. The sedative-hypnotic or longer-acting drugs are usually processed by the kidney, whereas the shorter-acting and anesthetic barbiturates are largely processed by the liver (Table 29-5).

Metabolism

Short- and intermediate-acting barbiturates are metabolized by the liver. Two hepatic processes are involved: hepatic mixed-function oxidases and hydroxylation. Amobarbital is of particular interest because two hydroxylation products have been identified, namely, 3-hydroxy amobarbital and N-hydroxy amobarbital. In addition, a glucose-conjugate is formed (N-glucose pyramidsyl amobarbital). Of radiolabeled amobarbital, about 80 to 90% appears in the urine as metabolites; less than 1% of the parent drug is so excreted. About 5% is excreted in the bile and appears in the feces. The elimination in humans is a first-order process, and some of the mechanisms appear to be under genetic control.[12]

Besides the mixed-function oxidase system two hydroxylation pathways appear to exist. The half-life of amobarbital is approximately 23 hours. Pretreatment with phenobarbital speeds up the transformation.

Drug Interactions

During liver metabolism, the barbiturates act as enzyme inducers[14] and increase the amount of liver acetaldehyde dehydrogenase.[15] This enzyme plays a role in

Table 29–4. Barbiturates: Relation Between Physicochemical Factors, Distribution, and Fate

Barbiturate	Partition Coefficient*	Plasma Protein Binding†	Brain Protein Binding‡	Delay in Onset of Activity§	Excreted by Kidney¶	Degradation by Liver Slices#	pK_a**
Barbital	1	0.05	0.06	22	65–90	—	7.8
Phenobarbital	3	0.20	0.19	12	27–50	—	7.3
Pentobarbital	39	0.35	0.29	0.1	—	0.21	8.0
Secobarbital	52	0.44	0.39	0.1	—	0.28	7.9
Thiopental	580	0.65	0.50	—	—	0.38	7.4

*(Concentration in methylene chloride):(concentration in aqueous phase) of the nonionized form at approximately 25°C (Bush, 1963).
†Binding of 0.001 M barbituric acids by 1% bovine serum albumin in M/15 phosphate buffer at pH 7.4; fraction bound (Goldbaum and Smith, 1954).
‡Fraction of barbiturate bound by rabbit brain homogenates (Goldbaum and Smith, 1954).
§Minutes until anesthesia after intravenous injection in mice (Butler, 1942).
¶Approximate percentage of total dose excreted unchanged in urine of man.
#Fraction degraded *in vitro* by liver slices in 3 hours (Dorfman and Goldbaum, 1947).
**Ionization exponent at 25°C (Bush, 1963). The values have not been corrected thermodynamically.
From Goodman, L. S., Gilman, A. and Harvey, S. C. (eds.): In The Pharmacological Basis of Therapeutics, 5th Ed. New York, Macmillan, 1975.

enhanced breakdown of ethanol metabolites and explains tolerance to some degree. Conversely, alcohol intake results in an enhanced breakdown of barbiturates and explains the tolerance of alcoholics to barbiturates.

Antihistamines alter the permeability of the blood-brain pathway. Following the administration of such medication, the barbiturate levels in the brain are always higher.[16]

Chlorpromazine and other phenothiazines have additive effects with the barbiturates.[7] Antianalgesic drugs such as promethazine and scopolamine increase the incidence of excitatory effects of barbiturates, however.

Atropine-like compounds and drugs for treatment of Parkinson disease have a prolonging effect on the barbiturates.

Rate of Biotransformation[17]

Studies on biotransformation of the barbiturates also demonstrate that the rate of change is a relatively slow process. Initial recovery from intravenous barbiturate anesthesia is due primarily to redistribution of the drug and not to drug destruction. In human subjects, thiopental is transformed at a rate of only 15% per hour, whereas methohexital is metabolized at a rate of 20% per hour.[17] A newer drug, thiohexital, is transformed in humans at a rate of 25% per hour. This thioderivative of methohexital without the methyl side chain is rapidly metabolized. When the sedative-hypnotic barbiturates, so-called short-acting drugs, are injected intravenously, the rate of metabolism is slower.

Table 29–5. Disposition of Barbiturates

Action	Detoxified by Kidney	Detoxified by Liver
Long	80%	20%
Medium	20%	80%
Short	0%	100%
Ultra-short	Rapidly distributed in body tissues and then detoxified by liver and by enzymes in the blood.	

Three ranges in the rates of biotransformation of barbiturates are evident. This represents a more precise classification of barbiturates according to rate of destruction:[18] a relatively slow rate of 2 to 3% per hour *per day*, characteristic of the long-acting drugs; 5 to 15% for medium-acting barbiturates; and 5.0 to 20% per hour, characteristic of the anesthetic and short-acting barbiturates.

Locus of Action

Barbiturates act throughout the entire central nervous system. Good evidence indicates that the depression and inhibition are active processes and that the site of action is in large part due to a block of transmission of impulses at the brain stem reticular formation, thereby reducing reticulocortical activation.[19]

MECHANISM OF ACTION[20]

Many theories have been advanced to explain the mechanism of action of barbiturates on the central nervous system as well as the peripheral nervous system. Investigators have postulated that these drugs owe their depressant action to their ability to inhibit the action of lactic acid dehydrogenase in brain cell metabolism. One effect is a reduction in the overall oxygen requirement of cerebral cells;[21] this may be due to impedence of adenosine triphosphate (ATP) synthesis and the uptake of phosphate. Finally, this may cause a reduction in the oxidation of glucose the primary fuel for cell function.[22] Production of ATP is thus essential for the activity of brain activity and for the synthesis of the brain neurotransmitter acetylcholine. Although this change does not prevent the access of oxygen to the brain cells, it produces changes in cellular metabolism, in the electrical impedance of cell walls, and in the frequency of electroencephalograms.

Effect on Synaptic Neurotransmission

Much evidence exists that barbiturates act to block excitatory transmitter action at both central and ganglionic synapses. Studies[23] of pentobarbital as a representative agent indicate that barbiturates have multiple neuronal effects. Nonanesthetic barbiturate doses preferentially block polysynaptic responses, so decreased facilitation and enhanced inhibitory effects are seen. Inhibition occurs mainly at synapses where neurotransmission is mediated by τ-aminobutyric acid (GABA).[24] *Postsynaptic* inhibition occurs at central sites: at the cortex and at cerebellar pyramidal cells; at the substantia nigra; and at the thalamic relay neurons.[25]

At sympathetic ganglia, pentobarbital depresses only the fast nicotinic excitatory postsynaptic potential.[25] The mechanism appears to be due to a decrease in sodium conductance.[24] On the other hand, slow excitatory and inhibitatory potentials are not blocked because these actions depend on a presynaptic release of acetylcholine. At the spinal cord level, presynaptic inhibition occurs.

Stereoisomerism plays a significant role.[26] Thus, the dextro(+) isomer has predominantly excitatory action on membrane properties and the levo isomer has predominantly inhibitory effects. The levo isomer potentiates the inhibitory response of the transmitter GABA.[27]

Molecular Mechanisms

Hypnotic-anesthetic and anticonvulsant barbiturates potentiate GABA inhibition by increasing chloride conductance and decreasing sodium conductance, thereby reducing glutamide-induced depolarization in spinal neurons.

High concentrations of barbiturates not only enhance chloride conductance, but also depress Ca^{2+}-dependent action potentials and reduce the Ca^{2+}-dependent release of neurotransmitter. This can occur in the absence of GABA, and thus barbiturates also appear to have intrinsic GABA-mimetic effects.[28] Pentobarbital has a more potent action than phenobarbital in this regard.

The chloride currents appear to result from prolonged periods of channel openings, instead of increased frequency of bursts of channel openings.[24] Anticonvulsant barbiturates are considered to have a lower capacity to produce profound depression of neuronal function, as compared with the hypnotic and anesthetic barbiturates.

The capacity of barbiturates to enhance GABA-inhibition is similar to the mechanism of action of benzodiazepines.[26] Barbiturates do not displace benzodiazepines at their binding sites, however, but they actually increase the binding of benzodiazepines and enhance GABA binding.

PHYSIOLOGIC EFFECTS

Central Nervous System

Barbiturates are hypnotic and antispasmodic. They have a low degree of selectivity, except for phenobarbital and its congeners. Thus, a broad range of central depression exists. These agents are not analgesic and do not allay pain except in anesthetic doses; however, analgesics are potentiated. Administration of a sedative in the presence of pain results in delirium.

The time of maximal depressant effect and the duration of action of the more commonly used drugs are diagrammed in Figure 29–2.

Any degree of depression is possible with barbiturates, ranging from calmness, sedation, and hypnosis to anticon-

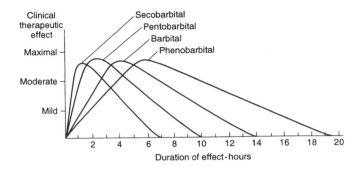

Fig. 29–2. Barbiturate action. Diagram of onset of action and duration of effect with barbiturates of the short, intermediate, and long-acting group.

vulsant activity and anesthesia. Sleep, when produced, is pleasant and approaches physiologic sleep.[29] The barbiturates reduce the amount of time spent in the rapid eye movement (REM) phase of sleep, however. If deprived of REM sleep for several nights, a rebound may be exhibited with increased REM sleep. This is also seen after withdrawal of barbiturates.[30]

Much evidence indicates a subcortical locus of action on the vegetative and sleep centers and that selective depression of the brain stem occurs before cortical depression.[19]

The presence of phenyl group, as in phenobarbital, however, results in selective depression of the motor cortex and diminution of electrical excitability.

Pain perception and response are relatively unimpaired. Low doses of these barbiturates may increase the responses to pain and produce delerium. Only with large doses and production of unconsciousness are pain responses obtunded.[7]

Studies of effects of barbiturates on cerebral hemodynamics have been done in humans (Table 29-6).[31] Large therapeutic doses of all barbiturates lower the mean arterial blood pressure and the cerebral flow. Cerebral vascular resistance is generally increased except with amobarbital. Oxygen utilization may be decreased as much as 50%.

Hypothalamic temperature regulating centers are depressed. Large doses cause the release of antidiuretic hormone from the pituitary gland and produce an antidiuretic effect.[7]

Peripheral Nervous System

Monosynaptic spinal reflexes are depressed.[25] The excitatory postsynaptic potential is decreased. This action occurs in doses that do not affect the membrane properties and is probably due to a decreased response of the effector organ to the transmitter chemical or to a decrease in the amount of transmitter released.

The synapses in multineuronal networks are depressed. Polysynaptic pathways seem to be more depressed than monosynaptic. Impulses over corticospinal paths, however, are initially facilitated.

Protective reflexes are often exaggerated with therapeutic doses. Thus, coughing, sneezing, hiccoughing, and laryngospasm are not infrequent.

Table 29–6. Effects of Barbiturates on Cerebral Hemodynamics

	Mean Arterial Blood Pressure	Anteriovenous Oxygen Diffusion	Cerebral Blood Flow	Cerebral Vascular Resistance
Thiopental	Lowered	Slight decrease	Definite reduction	Increased
Amobarbital	Lowered	Decreased	Reduction	Not altered
Phenobarbital	Lowered	No change	Slight reduction	Not altered

Respiratory System[32]

Direct depression of medullary centers occurs only with large hypnotic doses, and then both rate and depth of respiration are decreased. The mechanisms depressed are the neurogenic, the chemical, and the hypoxic "drives." Mechanisms in the pons and vagal system for rhythmic respiration are also depressed, but only slightly.

Bronchoconstriction occurs with most barbiturates and laryngospasm is likely. Ciliary activity of the tracheobronchial tree is decreased. Phenobarbital and amytal do not increase bronchomotor tone.

Gastrointestinal Tract[7]

Intestinal tone and motility are generally decreased with large or anesthetic doses. The amplitude of rhythmic contractions is decreased. This is most evident with the oxybarbiturates. With hypnotic doses, gastric emptying is not delayed.

Liver

The microsomal drug metabolizing system is inhibited. The barbiturates combine with cytochrome P-450 and interfere with the biotransformation of many drugs.[7]

With long-term administration, however, enzyme induction[14] occurs. This increase in the mixed oxidase P-450 system results in increased metabolism of many other drugs metabolized by the liver.[33] (Note that P-450 is *not* a single enzyme but a complex mixture of enzymes.) The barbiturates are also more rapidly metabolized and provide a basis for tolerance.[34]

Liver glycogen is depleted and liver function is depressed, as evidenced by dye tests with the ultra short-acting and short-acting drugs.

Cardiovascular System[35]

Hypnotic doses have little effect on the cardiovascular system. Large doses, however, depress the vasomotor center, resulting in peripheral vasodilatation. Cerebral vessels are generally dilated. By a direct effect on the musculature of the finer blood vessels and capillaries, dilatation occurs with increased permeability.

Genitourinary System

Large and anesthetic doses have an antidiuretic effect because of central inhibition of the hypothalamic-pituitary system. Oliguria also results from hypotension. Anesthetic doses decrease the force and frequency of uterine contractions.

Synaptic Transmission at Neuromuscular Junction

Transmission across the neuromuscular junction is inhibited by barbiturates.[36] The postsynaptic membrane is insensitive to the action of acetylcholine; similarly, the action of succinylcholine is diminished. The effects of *d*-tubocurarine and decamethonium are enhanced, however.[36]

Selective depression of transmission in sympathetic ganglia occurs with small concentrations of barbiturates.

At adrenergic endings near vascular smooth muscle, norepinephrine is released by thiopental.

At parasympathetic ganglia, transmission is also depressed. Stimulation of the cardiac vagus in the presence of a barbiturate produces a diminished response. Amytal is particularly effective.

Miscellaneous Effects

The barbiturates may generally be considered as having parasympathomimetic activity.

The basal metabolic rate is decreased with anesthetic doses and oxygen consumption is definitely lowered.

Large doses tend to depress all smooth muscle.

Temperature-regulating centers are depressed.

Barbital is habit forming and tends to accumulate.

Blood sugar varies with the barbiturate used; however, the level is not significantly altered, and the drugs are not contraindicated in diabetes mellitus. Amytal and thiotothal raise blood sugar.

Plasma volume is increased with amytal, and red cells usually decrease in number.

Cerebrospinal fluid pressure is increased.

General efficiency is reduced for 6 to 8 hours. Mental and memory tests are impaired for as long as 18 to 24 hours.[37]

Hirschfelder and Haury[38] have shown that nephrectomy prolongs the action of the intermediate and long-acting barbiturates. Renal dysfunction with accumulation of nitrogenous products and elevation of blood urea prolongs and intensifies the action of barbiturates.[39,40]

Clinical Uses

1. Sedation
2. Insomnia
3. Anticonvulsion
4. Epilepsy

5. Psychologic exploration
6. Pylorospasm
7. Vomiting of pregnancy
8. Poisoning—cocaine, strychnine

Barbiturates are not used to treat anxiety and are poor agents for sedation in the elderly. Among the adverse effects on sleep are paradoxic excitement, suppression of REM sleep, rebound dreaming, and insomnia. The therapeutic ratio is low, and the risk of overdose is greater in the elderly patient.[41]

Chloral hydrate is recommended as an excellent sedative for the elderly. Dreaming, disorientation, and delerium are rare. One sees few adverse effects on the sleep cycle and limited habituation. Interaction with other drugs, such as those of an acidic nature—warfarin and diphenylhydantoin—that are displaced from plasma protein, represents the only significant caution.[42]

Antihistamines are used as sedatives, but in the elderly patient, greater disorientation and even delerium occur.

Addiction[43]

If barbiturates are taken on a long-term basis in large doses, tolerance and physical dependence develop, and a characteristic abstinence syndrome appears when the drug is abruptly discontinued. This differs from the reaction following opiate withdrawal. The symptoms that appear may be classified as minor or major.

The minor symptoms, according to their order of appearance, include anxiety, involuntary muscle twitching, coarse intention tremors of hands and fingers, progressive weakness, dizziness, distorted visual perception (curved walls), nausea, vomiting, insomnia, weight loss, and postural hypotension.

The major symptoms are convulsions of grand-mal type and a delirium, as in alcoholic delirium tremens. Patients have one to several convulsions, and the delirium may last one to several days.

After withdrawal of the barbiturates, dramatic electroencephalographic changes appear. These consist of either high-voltage paroxysmal discharges or high-voltage paroxysmal activity of a slow type (6 cps). Untreated patients usually recover in 8 to 14 days.

A minimal addictive dose exists for the various barbiturates.[10] To produce physical dependence of a clinical degree, a sufficiently high dose is required.[43] Thus, the dose of phenobarbital is about 0.4 g daily; barbital, 1.2 g daily; amobarbital, more than 0.18 g daily; and secobarbital or pentobarbital, 0.4 g daily. Persons taking less than these doses do not develop dependence of a significant degree. They may have psychic dependence and may require psychiatric treatment, however.

The intensity of the dependence increases with the dose ingested. The most severe states develop in patients who are chronically and continuously intoxicated with high doses. The period of time necessary to develop a state of dependence appears to be at least a month. After 90 days of intake, independence is invariable.

Treatment of the addictive state must be gradual and careful. The abstinence syndrome is more lethal than the narcotic withdrawal syndrome. Gradual reduction in dosage is a key feature. Wulff has stated that, for most barbiturates, "phenobarbital substitution is an effective approach."

Poisoning[44]

Most systems are depressed—the respiratory more than the circulatory. In acute poisoning, a profound sleep occurs; mental confusion, nausea, weakness, incoordination, and stupor first appear, followed by cyanosis, cold skin, coma, and respiratory failure. With the short-acting barbiturates, respiratory depression is marked, and the pharyngeal reflex is obtunded, resulting in obstruction from the tongue falling into pharynx; pulmonary edema and asphyxia usually ensue.[45]

In chronic poisoning, the commonest signs and symptoms are erythematous rashes, foul breath, constipation, emotional instability, hallucinations, and poor memory.[46]

Urine Test

Urine can be tested by the cobalt acetate reaction as follows: extract a volume of urine with 10 vol of chloroform. To 1 ml of the extract add 0.1 ml of 5% isopropylamine in absolute methyl alcohol. Then add 1.0 ml of cobalt acetate in absolute methyl alcohol. A violet red reaction is positive for barbiturates.

Treatment

First aid measures are as follows:

1. Secure and maintain an adequate airway.
2. Clear the airway.
3. Administer oxygen and provide artificial respiratory support.
4. Transport the patient to a hospital and to the intensive care unit.
5. Consultation with anesthesiologist on arrival; establish diagnosis.
6. See details of management described later in this chapter.

PREANESTHETIC MEDICATION

The barbiturates are a useful group of drugs in preanesthetic medication. The full range of effects from mild sedation to basal hypnosis can be produced by judicious doses. As a class, these drugs possess common fundamental actions, as presented earlier. Certain qualitative differences are of importance in choosing a barbiturate for preanesthetic medication, however, and these are outlined.

Appreciation of the method of detoxification is the first consideration.[47] The long-acting barbiturates and, to some extent, the intermediate-acting members, such as amobarbital, are handled by kidney elimination.[12,13] Thus, renal disease poses a relative contraindication to their use. On the other hand, the short-acting agents are detoxified chiefly by hepatic mechanisms and are therefore undesirable in the presence of liver disease.[17]

Barbiturates decrease respiratory exchange, and, with the short-acting agents, this is most pronounced approximately 1 hour after oral intake. Respiratory volume may be depressed as much as 22% at this time but lessens later.[48] Thus, the optimum time for barbiturate medication is at least 1½ to 2 hours preoperatively.

Barbiturates also decrease the general tonus of intestinal musculature and the amplitude of contractions. Because it is possible theoretically for rupture of an obstructed gut to occur after spinal anesthesia, barbiturates then should have a beneficial action by minimizing this possibility. Furthermore, spinal anesthesia does increase intestinal tone and cramps; amobarbital and phenobarbital, by decreasing vagal activity, especially decrease this gastrointestinal action.

Indications and Administration[49]

For the suppression of overactivity of the cortical segment of the central nervous system, the barbiturates are keystones. Emotional reactions are quieted; apprehension and anxiety are effectively allayed. Irritability of the subject is decreased. The effects of concomitantly administered narcotics are enhanced. The toxic effects of local anesthetic agents are diminished; thus, if a barbiturate is given before procaine or another local agent, three times as much agent can be administered without untoward stimulation reactions.

The commonly used barbiturates are secobarbital, pentobarbital, and amobarbital.[50] For sedation, they are administered orally in doses of 100 mg for adults. The dose of sodium amobarbital is 200 mg to achieve comparable effects to secobarbital or pentobarbital. All are given 1½ to 2 hours preceding the anesthetic.

In children, the oral sedative dose is based on 0.5 mg per pound and may be administered in various elixirs. More cooperative children take a capsule readily. Administration by rectum is also effective, and the dose is approximately twice the oral dose. The rectal route is preferred in children, and the dose is based on a rate of 1 mg per pound. When a greater depression is desired, such as basal hypnosis, the dose scale is about 10.0 mg per pound. Studies with rectal secobarbital have demonstrated its effectiveness.[51] This agent is more rapidly detoxified in the body and in children provides a wider margin of safety. Capsules containing the desired dose are pierced at both ends and are inserted into the rectum in the manner of a suppository.

Intramuscular Administration of Thiobarbiturate[52,53]

The technique of intramuscular administration of the rapid-acting barbiturate (thiopental) is of utility in patients under 4 years of age. Accessibility of veins and the technical difficulties of venipuncture in anxious children are a challenge. Adequate sedation, hypnosis, or unconsciousness can be produced simply by intramuscular injection. The agent is prepared as a 5% solution in distilled water and is injected deep into the buttocks. The dose of thiopental sodium is adjusted to the metabolic rate. This varies from 5 to 10 mg per pound of body weight. In older children over 2 years of age, the dose is closer to 5 mg, and in children under 2 years, the dose is closer to 10 mg per pound. In anemic, debilitated, or cyanotic patients, a trial injection at the lower dose level is recommended.

Induction time to sleep varies from 5 to 15 minutes. It can be shortened by use of hyaluronidase. Usually, 15 TR units of this "spreading agent" are added to each 1 ml of 5% thiopental.

As with thiopental administered by other routes, the same complications can be anticipated, and laryngospasm is seen.

Differences

Different actions of the short-acting compounds exist, particularly with respect to the autonomic nervous system.[10,25] One may conveniently compare amobarbital and pentobarbital.[7,12,13] The former inhibits the cardiac action of the vagus and may cause a slight elevation in pulse rate. Because of an apparent vagal blocking effect, amobarbital also diminishes bronchomotor tone and hence is well tolerated by patients with asthma or other bronchospastic disease. When amobarbital is administered, the overnight fasting gastric secretion is diminished. Thus, this agent is preferable to the other short-acting barbiturates in patients with gastroduodenal ulcers. Evaluation of barbiturate effects in toxemias of pregnancy reveals that amobarbital is accompanied by lowering of cerebrovascular resistance and increased cerebral blood flow.[31]

In contrast, pentobarbital and secobarbital tend to have parasympathomimetic properties.[32] The cardiac rate is slowed from enhanced vagal action. Bronchomotor tone is increased, and hence these drugs are not desirable in asthma or emphysema. Measurement of overnight gastric secretion reveals that the volume is significantly increased over control values. Therefore, these drugs are not recommended for sedation in the presence of gastric disorder. The aforementioned studies on toxemias indicate that cerebral blood flow is diminished. This agrees with the observation that, in the older age group, pentobarbital particularly often results in disorientation and uncooperative behavior.

Side Effects

Although the barbiturates provide fairly good physiologic sleep, certain poor effects must be noted.[41,42] Hangover is common; it is particularly found in women. The overall incidence varies from 5 to 20%.[10] Pentobarbital is accompanied by a higher rate of this complication and amobarbital by the lowest rate. The sense of dullness and mental impairment following hypnotic doses has been found to persist for 6 to 12 hours following a night's sleep aided by pentobarbital. Efficiency is reduced, and both mental and memory tests are poorly performed.[37]

MANAGEMENT OF BARBITURATE POISONING

Intoxication with hypnotic drugs[54,55] is a modern medical problem in patients with either a suicidal or an accidental intent; less than 10% are accidental. It is a serious problem to which both the community and the physician should be constantly alert.

Barbiturates account for 20% of acute poisonings in patients admitted to hospitals. Mortality rates vary in different parts of the world. In the United States, these drugs are responsible for about 24% of accidental and suicidal deaths, an incidence greater than for any other poison.

In 1964, 2200 registered deaths in Great Britain were due to barbiturate poisoning. For the period 1957 to 1963, 166 fatalities occurred each year in New York City alone. At the Copenhagen Center, more than 1500 cases of coma due to poison are treated each year, of which about 75% are the result of hypnotic drugs. At this center, the collective mortality for all hypnotic drugs was 1 to 2%; for barbiturates alone, it was between 5 and 8%.[55]

The overall mortality rate since 1980 has been about 2% for patients hospitalized with a diagnosis of barbiturate intoxication in an intensive care unit.

The *lethal dose* of a barbiturate varies with many clinical factors and with the type of drug. Short-acting derivatives are more toxic than long-acting agents.

Plasma levels likely to produce death range from 10 to 20 µg/ml for the shorter-acting barbiturates such as secobarbital; 30 to 40 µg/ml for intermediate-acting barbiturates such as amobarbital and pentobarbital; and 60 to 100 µg/ml of plasma for phenobarbital and barbital.[10,56] To produce these blood levels, the minimal potentially fatal amount of ingested drug ranges from 2 to 3 g secobarbital; 4 to 6 pentobarbital and amobarbital; and 6 to 10 g for long-lasting agents such as phenobarbital and barbital.[57]

Until the 1940s, the basis of treatment was massive gastric lavage, often with suspensions of powdered carbon together with intensive use of central analeptics.[58] The results of this treatment showed no improvement over those during the previous 20 years, and the central analeptics did not fulfill the promise indicated by animal experiments.[59] In 1942, Harstad, Möller, and Simesen showed that gastric lavage was not entirely without risk and that its therapeutic value was doubtful.[60] The quantities of barbiturate that could be removed in this way were small compared with the amount ingested, and patients were usually admitted after the greater part of the barbiturate had passed on into the small intestine. Not infrequently, in fatal cases carbon particles were found in the lungs at autopsy. The aspiration pneumonia often found in such cases must, therefore, be considered one of the results of treatment.[57]

Intensive central stimulation therapy by analeptics during this era did not reduce the mortality below 20%. This therapy also confused the clinical picture, and it was difficult to estimate the patient's condition. Patients exhibited a mixture of symptoms partly due to the poison, partly a sequela of the comatose condition, and partly a result of the stimulating drug.[59]

Animal experiments also showed that central analeptics may cause complications in the form of convulsions, reduced cerebral oxygen tension, and postconvulsion episodes of hypoxia.

In 1955, Shaw reported on the effects of a presumed true antidote.[61] Bemegride (Megimide) was supposed to lighten the coma of even deeply unconscious patients, shorten the duration of coma, and hasten the elimination of the barbiturates.[62] Careful investigations in 1956 by Pedersen[63] and by Kjaer-Larsen[64] *failed to confirm* these findings. Attempts to enhance drug elimination apparently are usually not effective or indicated.

A conspicuous conclusion from this experience is that no antagonist exists at present for barbiturates.

Basis of Modern Treatment (The Scandinavian Method)

In 1946, Kirkegaard showed that one of the most important pathophysiologic features was peripheral circulatory collapse.[65] The therapeutically important result of Kirkegaard's work was the introduction of effective measures to combat the associated shock. When the further significance of a free and continuously patent airway, together with the prevention of long periods of hypoxia by adequate continuous mechanical ventilation, was pointed out by Nilsson in 1951, the way was opened for a more effective approach to treatment.[66]

By eliminating central analeptics or stimulants from the treatment and by carefully observing physiologic principles in therapy, the mortality rate has been reduced markedly. By providing antishock measures, by establishing a free airway, by using antibiotics to prevent pulmonary complications (pneumonia, atelectasis), and by using forced diuresis or dialysis to speed up the elimination of the drug, therapy is effectively accomplished.

Role of Physostigmine[67]

This agent readily crosses the blood-brain barrier and increases acetylcholine at the central synapses, particularly at the reticular activating system (RAS) where arousal is induced. Physostigmine is a specific key to the management of poisoning due to overdoses of drugs possessing anticholinergic action, such as scopolamine, antidepressants, and antiparkinsonian drugs. Partial reversal of coma from overdoses of drugs without anticholinergic action such as benzodiazepines and barbiturates has been reported, however. This action is nonspecific. An important observation is that the administration of physostigmine induces pupillary dilatation in all patients in coma from nonanticholinergic drugs. The dose schedule approximates 1.0 mg per minute to a dose of 4 mg. If no response occurs, another bolus dose is administered in the same manner approximately 20 minutes after the first dose (this sequence can be continued).

Simultaneous improvement in blood pressure and increase in heart rate occur. An increase in the level of consciousness is apparent in many patients poisoned with these depressant drugs. Such effects together with dilatation of the pupil indicate increased sympathetic activity. The mechanism appears to be related to enhanced cholinergic transmission centrally at the RAS and peripherally at the sympathetic ganglia.

Role of Naloxone

To determine whether a narcotic drug is present and masked by the overriding presence and history of barbiturate ingestion, a small test dose of naloxone may be administered (5.0 mg intravenously) to rule out a concomitant narcotic depression.

Classification

The clinical signs of depth of anesthesia should be used to classify the state of coma of patients. Reed and associates classified patients in coma from barbiturate intoxication into four groups (Table 29-7).[68] Other coma scales have been proposed, but all rely on the stages and signs of anesthesia.

One significant consideration is the blood level of short-acting barbiturates at different depths of sedation, unconsciousness, and coma.[45] This correlated with studies of drug levels at the different depths of anesthesia. In alert, awake individuals after an ordinary oral dose of a short-acting barbiturate (secobarbital or pentobarbital), blood levels are less than 6 µg/ml; a drowsy patient has an average of 8 to 10 µg/ml, whereas a stuporous patient has a level of 14 to 18 µg/ml.

An unconscious patient has a blood level of 18 to 22 µg/ml; a patient in the stages of beginning anesthesia (group 2 of Reed) has a barbiturate level of 22 to 26 µg/ml. Anesthetic levels from oral short-acting barbiturates are 28 to 34 µg/ml or more, which compares with thiopental levels of 30 µg/ml or more at stage III clinical depths.

General Measures

1. Isolate the patient in a quiet, air-conditioned room.
2. Place air mattress (alternating pressure pad) under the patient.
3. Prepare a hypothermia machine in the room; in case of fever, the patient should be cooled to normal temperature.
4. Start intravenous fluids; keep running throughout a 24-hour period. If there is difficulty in finding a vein, a cut-down should be done.
5. Provide oropharyngeal suction and suction patient frequently by aseptic technique.
6. Place electrodes on patients for monitoring electrocardiogram and electroencephalogram.

7. Turn patient every 2 hours to avoid hypostasis.
8. Check vital signs (respiration, blood pressure, pulse, temperature) every 15 minutes and record.
9. Insert an indwelling catheter and measure hourly urinary output.
10. Record fluid intake and urinary output carefully.
11. Draw blood daily for electrolytes and for barbiturate levels, as well as for renal clearance and liver function tests.
12. Collect urine for daily barbiturate level determination and creatinine clearance.
13. Keep endotracheal intubation and tracheotomy sets ready in the room.
14. Use a mechanical ventilator when indicated.
15. Insert a gastric tube if indicated. Consider gastric lavage if less than 4 hours have elapsed since ingestion. If more than 4 hours have elapsed, little barbiturate can be recovered from the stomach.[69] Barbiturates can reduce gastrointestinal motility, and much of the drug may be retained. Lavage should be attempted only if precautions are taken to avoid aspiration. After lavage, activated charcoal and/or a cathartic (Sorbital) may be administered. In 1982, the use of activated charcoal instilled by nasogastric tube was reviewed and was reported as a treatment of phenobarbital oral overdose. It appeared that the serum concentration was more quickly reduced to levels below the toxic level of deep coma (stage III anesthesia) of 60 to 80 µg/ml.[70] As much as 300 to 400 mg of most barbiturates can be absorbed by 1 g of the activated charcoal.[71] Repeated doses of charcoal may shorten the half-life of phenobarbital but not other barbiturates. Charcoal shortened the half-life from 100 to 20 hours.[70] Treatment should be undertaken if bowel sounds are present.[72]

Respiratory Care

Airway Management

1. Oropharyngeal airway or bite block. If the patient is classified in group 1 or 2 and respiratory exchange is adequate, the airway is patent, no obstruction is

Table 29-7. Signs and Symptoms of CNS Intoxication from Depressant Drugs: Classic Reed Classification

Degree of Severity	Characteristics
0 No Depression	Subject asleep, arousable, answers questions
Group I (Mild) Stage II of anesthesia	Patients who are comatose but withdraw from painful stimuli; circulatory embarrassment is not present; all reflexes are intact
Group II (Moderate) Stage III Plane i of Surgical Anesthesia	Patients who do not withdraw from painful stimuli; somatic reflexes are obtunded; no respiratory or circulatory depression, most or all of the autonomic or protective reflexes are intact
Group III (Intermediate) Stage III Plane ii to iii	Patients whose reflexes are all or almost all absent; respiratory and circulatory systems are depressed
Group IV (Severe) Stage III Plane iii and iv	Patients whose reflexes are all absent and who have evidence of severe respiratory depression of circulatory failure, shock and renal complications

present, oropharyngeal airway or bite block can be used with nasopharyngeal insufflation.

2. Endotracheal tube. This is indicated when coma is deeper and depression greater (class 3 or 4).
3. Tracheostomy. After the initial use of endotracheal tube for 24 to 72 hours, tracheostomy should be done *routinely* unless, after consultation, decision is made to continue airway management with endotracheal tube. The otorhinolaryngology service is to be called to perform the tracheostomy.

Tracheobronchial Toilet

1. Endotracheal tube.
   a. Change the endotracheal tube every 12 hours.
   b. Perform aspiration as described under routine tracheostomy care.
2. Routine tracheostomy care.
   a. Have two suction catheters, one for oropharyngeal suction and one for tracheal suction.
   b. Keep suction catheters in 70% solution (in pint jar). Before aspirating, rinse catheters in sterile normal saline solution (keep in quart jar).
   c. Aspirate trachea and oropharynx at 20 minute intervals. *First* clean the oropharynx, *then* clean the trachea. Before aspiration of trachea, instill 2 to 8 ml of sterile normal saline solution into the tracheostomy tube.
   d. Take out and clean the inner tracheostomy cannula every 60 minutes, more frequently if indicated.
   e. Complete change of the tracheostomy tube should be done every 48 hours by a physician, unless otherwise indicated.
   f. If patient is on a ventilator, be sure that it is properly connected to the tracheostomy tube after aspiration.
   g. Change suction catheters every 6 hours.
   h. Clean skin around the tracheostomy tube with 1:750 benzalkonium (Zephiran) solution and change dressing and tape as necessary.
   i. Plastic Flo-Trol suction catheters are provided in sizes 10, 14, and 18 French.
3. Send secretions for bacteriologic examination once a day if atelectasis or pneumonitis develops.
4. Obtain chest x-ray films every other day or as indicated by clinical signs.

Ventilation

1. Respiratory assistance or control.
   a. Assisted respiration. Intermittent positive pressure breathing (IPPB) devices are used as ventilatory assisters. These devices can be adjusted to assist respirations, and in the event of apnea, the machine will take over and control the patient's respiration.
   b. Controlled respiration. Mechanical ventilators are used to breathe for patients who have no spontaneous effort. *It is absolutely essential* that either distilled water or some medication be placed in the nebulizer while this device is in use to provide humidification. DRY OXYGEN UNDER PRESSURE SHOULD *NEVER* BE ADMINISTERED TO THE PATIENT.
   c. The routine administration of oxygen by inhalation (patient breathing).
      (1) To the adult tracheostomized patient, administration is accomplished by the use of a special partial rebreathing type mask.
      (2) To children, the routine administration of oxygen and aerosol is accomplished by the use of a head tent or oxygen hood.
2. Humidification. Increased moisture in the inspired air is provided by the use of a large reservoir nebulizer and special tracheostomy aerosol mask. *Distilled water only is used for this purpose.*
3. Wetting agents and other aerosols.
   a. When the patient's secretions are tenacious and difficult to raise, the aerosol administration of wetting agents is provided. The agents of this purpose used are Alevaire, Tergemist, and normal saline solution. These are administered via nebulizer and tracheostomy aerosol mask.
   b. Before the administration of the wetting agents, it is sometimes advisable to administer a bronchodilator. For this purpose, 0.5 ml. phenylephrine (Neo-Synephrine) 1/2% is used.
4. Medications.
   a. Penicillin to be given routinely, either 400,000 U aqueous penicillin in the IV solution, tid., or 600,000 U procaine penicillin IM once a day.
   b. Broad-spectrum antibiotics are also given for control or prevention of complication infections.
   c. The choice of antibiotics for secondary infections may be modified as indicated by culture and sensitivity studies (culture tracheobronchial secretions).

Cardiovascular System Care

An overdose of barbiturate can lead to a primary fall in blood pressure, which is a feature of the drug's effect on the vasomotor center. Later comes a secondary fall in pressure, the result of the barbiturate's effect on the myocardium. The patient, thus, develops a typical shock syndrome consisting of both vasogenic shock and cardiogenic shock. Treatment should be started at once.

1. Vasopressors. Effective vasopressors drugs that increase cardiac output through direct effect on the myocardium and have a peripheral vasoconstrictive effect without limiting renal blood flow are used:
   a. Desoxyephedrine HCl (Methedrine)
      Dosage: 40 mg in 600 ml 5% D/W IV or 15 mg IM
   b. Metaraminol (Aramine)
      Dosage: 20 to 40 mg in 600 ml 5% D/W IV or 10 to 20 mg IM
   c. Ephedrine sulfate
      Dosage: 25 mg IV or IM
2. Blood or plasma. In serious cases, classified as group IV, blood or plasma transfusions may be given. The purpose of this is to combat the severe shock and for nutrition in patients who are in coma more than 4 days. Blood or plasma transfusions should be de-

cided individually on each case; it is not a routine treatment in all cases.

3. Corticosteroids. Water-soluble corticosteroid preparations for intravenous use are available. Their anti-stress properties are utilized in barbiturate poisoning.
   a. Solu-Medrol (methylprednisolone)
   Dosage: 40 to 80 mg in 600 ml 5% D/W daily
   b. Solu-Cortef (hydrocortisone)
   Dosage: 100 to 200 mg IV daily

Diuresis versus Dialysis and Renal Complications[73]

Kidney failure is a serious complication, because the elimination of the long-acting, and to some extent the short-acting, barbiturates and their detoxification products are dependent on excretion by this organ (Fig. 29-3). Anuria and uremia are encountered not only in comatose patients, but also in those who at a later stage have regained consciousness.

In attempting to avoid this complication, which likely is the sequela of irreversible shock and hypotension together with prolonged hypoxia, management proceeds along the following lines:

1. Alkalinization and forced diuresis. Increased diuresis can be obtained by pushing the pH of the blood toward alkalinity.[74] A significant increase in barbiturate excretion is accomplished by this means.[75,76] Furthermore, alkalinization of the blood brings about a rise in blood barbiturate levels, signifying a mobilization and transfer of the drug from cell to plasma. All barbiturates are weak organic acids with

pK ranges from 7.2 for phenobarbital to 8.0 for pentobarbital and secobarbital. Those drugs close to the physiologic pH are less ionized in biologic fluids than when at a higher pH. At the pH of 7.5, about 5% of phenobarbital is nonionized, but at 7.2 pH, it is only 50% nonionized. Secobarbital (pK 7.9) at 7.4 pH is nonionized to 98%.[77]

To accomplish forced diuresis, the Lassen technique is followed (Table 29-8).[73] A special intravenous solution containing urea is administered by the hour, around the clock for 2 to 6 days, depending on the individual case.

The removal rate of phenobarbital is between 90 and 100 mg/hr. The elimination rate for intermediate and short-acting barbiturates is slower. The range is 30 to 60 mg/hour for intermediate drugs and 10 to 40 mg/hour for secobarbital and pentobarbital.

Diamox (acetazolamide) increases urine flow and alkalinizes the urine.[78] It increases renal elimination of phenobarbital. THAM has been used as an alkalizing agent.[79]

2. Dialysis. Success with hemodialysis requires access to and cooperation with a specialized artificial kidney unit. It is a most effective form of therapy. The removal rate for phenobarbital is from 100 to 350 mg/hr. Peritoneal dialysis may occasionally be used in selected patients. A removal rate of 50 to 90 mg/hr is possible.

Because of the excellent results with forced diuresis, dialysis with artificial kidney has been used infrequently; and peritoneal dialysis is considered the least effective method.

Conclusion

The foregoing routine management of barbiturate intoxication has been referred to as the "Scandinavian

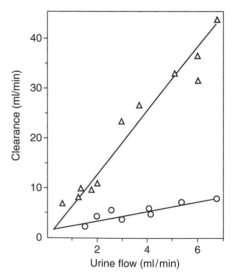

Fig. 29–3. Renal clearance of phenobarbital in the dog as it is related to urinary pH and the rate of urine flow. The values designated by circles are from experiments in which diuresis was induced by administration of water orally or Na_2SO_4 intravenously and the urinary pH was below 7.0. The values designated by triangles are from experiments in which $NaHCO_3$ was administered intravenously and in which the urinary pH was 7.8 to 8.0. Redrawn from Waddell, W. J., Butler, T. C.: The distribution and excretion of phenobarbital. J Clin Invest 36:1217, 1957.

Table 29–8. Barbiturate Intoxication. Osmotic Diuresis Program and Preparation of Solutions (Modified Scandinavian Technique)

1. Initial fluids for osmotic diuresis as follows:
   a. 300 ml/hr electrolyte solution = 1,200 ml in 4 hours
   b. First 2 hours include 80 ml 50% urea solution = 40 g
   c. Second 2 hours include 40 ml 50% urea solution = 20 g

2. Maintenance Fluids:
   a. 600 ml/hr electrolyte solution
   b. Urea solution (50%)   40 ml for 2 h 20 g
                                 30 ml for 2 h 15 g
                                 20 ml for 2 h 10 g
                                 10 ml for 2 h 5 g

3. Hourly fluid intake 400 to 600 ml/hr

4. Output desired: 12 to 14 L/day

5. How to prepare the urea solution:
   Add to urea solution (Ureaphil 40 g in 30 ml)
   50 ml of 5% D/W to make 80 ml of solution
   Each ml will contain 0.5 g (155 mEq)
   i.e., 80 × 0.5 g = 40 mg

6. Composition of electrolyte solution:
   25 g glucose
   40 mEq sodium lactate   } 1 L
   12 mEq potassium chloride
   12 mEq sodium chloride

method." It requires an organization and a staff capable of carrying out treatment along the lines indicated previously and demands intensive, around-the-clock effort.

Such management can be carried out in the medical therapy section (intensive care section) of the hospital.

REFERENCES

1. Dundee, J. W., McIlroy, D. A.: The history of barbiturates. Anaesthesia 37:726, 1982.
2. Fisher, E., Mering, J.: Ubereine neue Classe von Schlafmittein. Ther Gegenw 5:97, 1903.
3. Goodman, L., Gilman, A.: The Pharmacologic Basis of Therapeutics, 5th Ed. New York, Macmillan, 1975.
4. Tatum, A. L.: The present status of the barbiturate problem. Physiol Rev 19:472, 1939.
5. Mark, L. C.: Archaic classification of barbiturates: commentary. Clin Pharmacol Ther 10:287, 1969.
6. Rall, T. W.: Hypnotics and sedatives. In Gilman, A.G., et al. (eds.). Goodman and Gilman's The Pharmacologic Basis of Therapeutics, 8th Ed. New York, McGraw-Hill, 1990.
7. Dundee, J. W., Wyant, G. M.: Intravenous Anesthesia, 2nd Ed. Edinburgh, Churchill Livingstone, 1988.
8. Parsons, T. W.: Clinical comparison of barbiturates as hypnotics. Br Med J 2:1035, 1963.
9. Breimer, D. D.: Clinical pharmacokinetics of hypnotics. Clin Pharmacokinet 2:93, 1977
10. Harvey, S. C.: Hypnotics and sedatives: the barbiturates. In Goodman, L. S., Gilman, A. (eds.). The Pharmacological Basis of Therapeutics, 5th Ed. New York, Macmillan, 1975.
11. Morgan, P. J., Blackman, G. L., Paull, J. D., Wolff, L. J.: Pharmacokinetics and plasma binding of thiopental. II. Studies in caesarean section. Anesthesiology 54:474, 1981.
12. Tang, B. K., Inaba, T., Kalow, W.: N Hydroxyamobarbital, the second major metabolite of amobarbital in man. Clin Pharmacol Ther 20:439, 1976.
13. Kalow, W., et al.: Destructive patterns of amobarbital metabolism. Clin Pharmacol Ther 24:576, 1978.
14. Conney, A. H.: Pharmacological implications of microsomal enzyme induction. Pharmacol Rev 19:317, 1967.
15. Redmond, G., Cohen, G.: Induction of liver acetaldehyde dehydrogenase: possible role in ethanol tolerance after exposure to barbiturates. Science 171:387, 1971.
16. Winter, C. A.: Potentiating effect of antihistaminic drugs upon the sedative actions of barbiturates. J Pharmacol Exp Ther 94:7, 1948.
17. Mark, L. C.: Metabolism of barbiturates in man. Clin Pharmacol Ther 4:504, 1963.
18. Andrews, P. R., Mark, L. C.: Structural specificity of barbiturates and related drugs. Anesthesiology 57:314, 1982.
19. Magoun, H. W.: Brain mechanisms for wakefulness. Br J Anaesth 33:183, 1961.
20. Ho, I. K., Harris, R. A.: Mechanism of action of barbiturates. Annu Rev Pharmacol Toxicol 21:83, 1981.
21. Quastel, J. H., Wheatley, A. H. M.: Narcosis and oxidation of brain. Proc R Soc Lond (Biol) 112:60, 1932.
22. Quastel, J. H.: Biochemical aspects of narcosis. Curr Res Anesth Analg 31:151, 1952.
23. Macdonald, R. I.: Anticonvulsant drugs: mechanisms of action. Adv Neurol 44:713, 1986.
24. Twyman, R. E., Rogers, C. J., Macdonald, R. I.: Differential regulation of τ-aminobutyric acid receptor channels by diazepam and phenobarbital. Ann Neurol 25:213, 1989.
25. Nicoll, R. A.: Pentobarbital: differential postsynaptic actions on sympathetic ganglion cells. Science 199:451, 1978.
26. Huang, L. M., Barker, J. L.: Pentobarbital: stereospecific actions of (+) and (−) isomers revealed on cultured mammalian neurons. Science 207:195, 1980.
27. Olsen, R. W.: GABA drug interactions. Prog Drug Res 31:224, 1987.
28. Macdonald, R. I., McLean, M. J.: Cellular basis of barbiturate and phenytoin anticonvulsant drug action. Epilepsia 23(Suppl):S7, 1982.
29. Kay, D. C., Blackburn, A. B., Buckingham, J. A., Karacan, I.: Human pharmacology of sleep. In Williams, R. I., Karacan, I. (eds.). Pharmacology of Sleep. New York, John Wiley and Sons, 1976.
30. Mendelson, W. B., Gillen, J. C., Wyatt, R. J.: Human sleep and its disorders. New York, Plenum Press, 1977.
31. McCall, M., Taylor, H.: Barbiturates in toxemias of pregnancy. JAMA 149:51, 1952.
32. Brown, C. R., Forrest, W. H., Jr., Hayden, J. H.: The respiratory effects of pentobarbital and secobarbital in clinical doses. J Clin Pharmacol 13:28, 1973.
33. Remmer, H.: Drug intolerance. In Mongar, J. L., de Reuck, A.V.S. (eds.). Enzymes and Drug Action. London, Churchill, 1962.
34. Pantuck, E. L., et al.: Effects of nutritional regimens on oxidative drug metabolism. Anesthesiology 60:534, 1984.
35. Price, H. L.: General anesthesia and circulatory homeostasis. Physiol Rev 40:187, 1960.
36. Thesleff, S.: The pharmacological properties of succinylcholine iodide. Acta Physiol Scand 26:103, 1952.
37. Lasagna, L., Beecher, H. K.: The persistence of mental impairment following a hypnotic dose of a barbiturate. J Pharmacol Exp Ther 109:284, 1953.
38. Hirschfelder, A. D., Haury, V. G.: Effect of nephrectomy on duration of action of barbital. Proc Soc Exp Biol Med 30:1059, 1932.
39. Dundee, J., Richards, R. K.: Effect of azotemia upon the action of intravenous barbiturate anesthesia. Anesthesiology 15:333, 1954.
40. Dundee, J. W.: Alterations in response to somatic pain associated with anesthesia: thiopentone and pentobarbitone. Br J Anaesth 32:407, 1960.
41. Kales, A., Kales, J. D.: Sleep disorders: recent findings in the diagnosis and treatment of disturbed sleep. N Engl J Med 280:487, 1974.
42. Greenblatt, D. J., Miller, R. R.: Rational use of psychotropic drugs. I. Hypnotics. Am J Hosp Pharm 31:990, 1974.
43. Fraser, H. I., Wikler, A., Essig, C. F., Isbell, H.: Degree of physical dependence induced by secobarbital or pentobarbital. JAMA 166:126, 1958.
44. Smith, D., Wesson, D. R.: A new method for treatment of barbiturate dependence. JAMA 213:294, 1970.
45. McCarron, M. M., et al.: Short-acting barbiturate overdosage. JAMA 248:55, 1982.
46. Isbell, H., et al.: Chronic barbiturate intoxication. Arch Neurol Psychiatry 64:1, 1950.
47. Smith, S. E., Rawlins, M. D.: Variability in Human Drug Response. London, Butterworth, 1973.
48. Burdick, O. I., Rovenstine, E. A.: Picrotoxin in barbiturate poisoning. Ann Intern Med 22:819, 1945.
49. Waters, R. M.: A study of morphine, scopolamine, and atropine and their relation to preoperative medication. Tex State J Med 34:304, 1938.
50. Hawk, M. H., Wangeman, C. P.: The effects of Nembutal and scopolamine on human subjects. Anesthesiology 4:238, 1943.
51. Poe, M. F., Karp, M.: Seconal as a basal anesthetic agent in children. Anesth Analg 25:152, 1946.
52. Kamikulio, Y., Onchi, Y.: Anesthetic management of car-

diac catheterization in children using intramuscular thiopental sodium. Far East J Anes 2:17, 1957.

53. Onchi, Y., Stringham, J., Smith, S. M.: Studies in Intramuscular Use of Thiopental. University of Utah Postgraduate Course, 1960.

54. Gary, N. E., Tresnewsky, O.: Clinical aspects of intoxication: barbiturates and a potpourri of other sedatives, hypnotics, and tranquilizers. Heart Lung 12:122, 1983.

55. Essig, C.: Chronic abuse of sedative hypnotic drugs. In Zarafonetis, J. D. (ed.). Drug Abuse. Philadelphia, Lea & Febiger, 1972.

56. Lous, P.: Barbituric acid concentration in serum from patients with severe acute poisoning. Acta Pharmacol Toxicol 10:261, 1954.

57. Isbell, H.: Acute and chronic barbiturate intoxication. Veterans Admin Tech Bull 10-76:1, 1956.

58. Clemensen, C., Nilsson, E.: Therapeutic trends in the treatment of barbiturate poisoning: the Scandinavian method. Clin Pharmacol Ther 2:220, 1962.

59. Eckenhoff, J. D., Dam, W.: Treatment of barbiturate poisoning with or without analeptics. Am J Med 20:912, 1956.

60. Harstad, E., Möller, K., Simesen, M.: Über den Wert der Magenspölung bei der Behandlung von akuten Vergiftungen. Acta Med Scand 112:478, 1942.

61. Shaw, F. H., et al.: Barbiturate antagonism. Nature 174:402, 1954.

62. Clemensen, C.: Effect of Megimide and amiphenazole on respiratory paresis. Lancet 2:966, 1956.

63. Pedersen, J.: Arousing effect of Megimide and amiphenazole in allylpropymal poisoning. Lancet 2:965, 1956.

64. Kjaer-Larsen, J.: Delirious psychosis and convulsions due to Megimide. Lancet 2:967, 1956.

65. Kirkegaard, Å.: Den Svaere Akutte barbitursyre-forgiftning. Thesis, University of Copenhagen, 1951.

66. Nilsson, S. E. H.: Treatment of acute barbiturate poisoning: a modified clinical approach (Thesis). Acta Med Scand Suppl 253, 1951.

67. Nilsson, E.: Physostigmine treatment of various drug induced intoxications. Ann Clin Res 14:165, 1982.

68. Reed, C. E., Briggs, M. F., Foote, C.: Acute barbiturate intoxication. Ann Intern Med 37:290, 1952.

69. Matthew, H., Mackintosh, T. F., Thomsett, S. L., Cameron, J. C.: Gastric aspiration and lavage in acute poisoning. Br Med J 1:1333, 1966.

70. Goldberg, M., Berlinger, W. G.: Treatment of phenobarbital overdose with activated charcoal. JAMA 247:2400, 1982.

71. Mann, J. B., Sandberg, D. H.: Therapy of sedative overdosage. Pediatr Clin North Am 17:617, 1970.

72. Pond, S. M., Olson, K. R., Osterloh, J. D., Tong, T. G.: Randomized study of treatment of phenobarbital overdose with activated charcoal. JAMA 251:3104, 1984.

73. Lassen, N. A.: Treatment of severe acute barbiturate poisoning by forced diuresis and alkalinisation of the urine. Lancet 2:338, 1960.

74. Waddell, W. J., Butler, T. C.: The distribution and excretion of phenobarbital. J Clin Invest 36:1217, 1957.

75. Klaassen, C. D.: Principles of toxicology. In Gilman, A. G., et al. (eds.). Goodman and Gilman's The Pharmacological Basis of Therapeutics, 8th Ed. New York, McGraw-Hill, 1990.

76. Mollaret, P., Rapin, M., Pocidalo, J., Monsallier, J. F.: Le Traitement de l'intoxication barbiturique aiguë. Presse Med 67:1435, 1959.

77. Arena, J. M.: Poisoning: Toxicology, Symptoms and Treatment, 4th Ed. Springfield, IL, Charles C Thomas, 1979.

78. Kelley, W. N., Richardson, A. P., Mason, M. F., Rector, F. C.: Acetazolamide in phenobarbital poisoning. Arch Intern Med 117:64, 1966.

79. Balabot, R. C.: Use of Tham in the treatment of barbiturate intoxication. JAMA 178:1000, 1961.

Chapter 30

BENZODIAZEPINES

J. LANCE LICHTOR AND VINCENT J. COLLINS

Compounds of this chemical class were synthesized in the early 1930s and were found by Randall 30 years later to have a "taming" effect on animals. Clinical trials in humans revealed an antianxiety effect.[1,2]

Ten derivatives have found clinical utility in anesthesia practice.[2] Chlordiazepoxide, diazepam, oxazepam, and chlorazepate are essentially tranquilizers and are particularly effective as antianxiety agents, whereas lorazepam, midazolam, flurazepam, nitrazepam, temazepam, and triazolam have significant hypnotic action. All these compounds also have a singular characteristic of inducing muscle hypotonia and of decreasing rigidity due to central nervous system (CNS) disease, such as cerebral palsy (Table 30-1).[3]

PHYSIOCHEMICAL CHARACTER

All benzodiazepines consist of lipid-soluble molecules. Hence, the volume distribution is much greater than total body water.

The first four of these compounds have a high lipid solubility.[2,3] Consequently, they are extensively bound, because binding correlates with lipid solubility: diazepam is 99% bound to plasma albumin. With these drugs, the duration of action depends more on drug distribution and uptake at peripheral sites such as adipose tissue and less on elimination factors. Second, these agents behave according to a three-compartment model. Compounds such as lorazepam, flurazepam, nitrazepam, midazolam, temazepam, and triazolam have a lower lipid solubility and a greater water solubility. Binding to plasma protein is less than for the compounds with high lipid solubility, and their pharmacokinetic behavior is according to a two-compartment model. Chlorazepate and diazepam have significant anticonvulsant effects, whereas chlorazepate is largely used as an anticonvulsant[2,4] (Table 30-2).

PHARMACOKINETICS

Absorption

Rates of absorption are related both to the physiochemical properties of the drug and to the pharmaceutical formulation of the drug, as well as the site of administration. Taken orally, these drugs dissolve in the gastric contents, and absorption then depend on their solubility characteristics. All the benzodiazepines have varying degrees of lipophilicity. Highly lipophilic congeners, such as diazepam, flurazepam, and triazolam, are almost completely and rapidly absorbed. The agents with a low lipophilicity are more slowly absorbed from the gastrointestinal tract.

After intramuscular injection, absorption of those agents with a high lipophilicity is variable and unpredictable. Such drugs include diazepam and chlordiazepoxide. Plasma levels are achieved more slowly than after oral intake. Diazepam, when injected into muscles, causes pain and discomfort. It is variably absorbed, and crystallization occurs at the site of injection; prolonged pain ensues, lasting 2 to 3 weeks. For these drugs, the site of injection is also critical. Diazepam, when injected into the deltoid muscle, is fairly well absorbed, but plasma levels are slow to be achieved. In contrast, injection into the gluteal or vastus lateralis muscle is unpredictable, and the drug is not adequately absorbed.[5]

Reliable effects are found after intravenous administration of diazepam, flunitrazepam, and midazolam. Diazepam, when injected intravenously, causes burning and some instances of phlebitis. Midazolam has a low lipid solubility and a high aqueous solubility; it is readily distributed and may be injected intravenously without discomfort.[5]

Biotransformation

Most benzodiazepines are converted to inactive metabolites by hepatic mechanisms. Two principal pathways are involved in biotransformation (Fig. 30-1):[2,6,7]

1. Hepatic microsomal oxidation, by n-dealkylation or by aliphatic hydroxylation.
2. Glucuronide conjugation.

The hepatic oxidative pathway is known as a "susceptible" path, because it is impaired in the elderly, in disease states affecting the liver, in malnutrition, and by coadministration of other drugs (cimetidine, estrogens, isoniazid). Conjugation is designated as "nonsusceptible," far less impaired by illness.[6]

Variable Factors

Age

Age has been demonstrated to have a major effect on the benzodiazepine agents degraded by oxidative mechanisms. Clearance is impaired in the elderly by about 50%. Other drugs have also been identified, and these may compete for the pathway of microsomal oxidative reactions.

Table 30–1. Commonly Used Benzodiazepines: Predominant Effects, Onset of Action, and Rapidity of Elimination

Generic Name	Commercial	Predominant Use/Effects	Onset (Oral Dose)	Elimination
Chlordiazepoxide	Librium	Anxiolytic	Intermediate	Slow
Chlorazepate	Tranxene	(Anxiolytic (Anticonvulsant (Alcohol withdrawal	Rapid	Slow
Diazepam	Valium	(Tranquilizer (Anxiolytic (Anticonvulsant (Short amnesia (Muscle relaxant	Rapid	Slow
Oxazepam	Serax	Anxiolytic	Intermediate to slow	Intermediate
Lorazepam	Ativan	(Mild tranquilizer (Anxiolytic	Intermediate	Intermediate
Flurazepam	Dalmane	(Hypnotic (Mild tranquilizer	Rapid to intermediate	Slow
Temazepam	Restoril	(Hypnotic (Sedative	Intermediate	Intermediate to rapid
Nitrazepam (flunitrazepam)	Mogadon	Hypnotic	Intermediate	Intermediate
Triazolam	Halcion	(Hypnotic-S (Sedative (insomnia)	Intermediate to rapid	Rapid
Midazolam	—	(Intravenous (Tranquilizer (Anxiolytic (Anticonvulsant (Short-term amnesia	Rapid	Rapid

Data from Greenblatt, D. J., Koch-Weser, J.: Intramuscular injection of drugs. N. Engl. J. Med. *309*:354, 1983; and Greenblatt, D. J.: Pharmacokinetics of midazolam. Sleep *5* (Suppl #1), 1982.

Smoking

Controlled studies showed no significant induction effect on the metabolism of the following congeners: midazolam, diazepam, triazolam, and lorazepam. Smoking does apparently influence many of the other benzodiazepines, however.

Lipophilicity and Duration of Action

The in vivo volume of distribution does affect the duration of action. A reduced lean body mass is concurrent with a relative increase in adipose tissue. An altered body habitus occurs in the elderly and, as previously noted, one sees an increase in duration of effect. The altered

Table 30–2. Half-Lives and Oral Dosages of Selected Benzodiazepines

Drug Classes, Nonproprietary Names, and Trade Names	Half-Life (hours)	Adult Oral Dosage (mg)	
		Sedative	Hypnotic
Chlordiazepoxide (Librium, others)	5–15	15–100, 1–3×d	—
Chorazepate (dipotassium) (Tranxene, others)	50–80 §	3.75–20, 2–4×d	—
Diazepam (Valium, others)	30–60	5–10, 3–4×d	—
Flurazepam HCl (Dalmane, others)	50–100 §	—	15–30
Lorazepam (Ativan, others)	10–20	—	2–4
Oxazepam (Serax, others)	5–10	15–30, 3–4×d	—
Temazepam (Restoril, others)	10–17	—	15–30
Triazolam (Halcion)	2–4	—	0.125–0.5
Midazolam	2–5	5–10	10–20

Modified from Rall, T. W.: Hypnotics and sedatives. In Gilman, A. G., et al. (eds.). Goodman and Gilman's Pharmacologic Basis of Therapeutics, 8th Ed. New York, McGraw-Hill, 1990, p. 357.

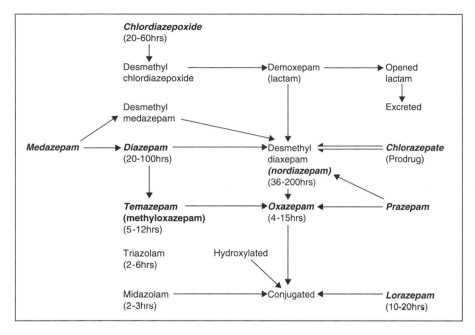

Fig. 30–1. Biotransformation pathways for some benzodiazepines. Italic indicate compounds marketed as separate drugs. Prepared from reports of Greenblatt, D. J., Shader, R. I., Abernethy, D. R.: Drug therapy: current status of benzodiazepines (first of two parts). N Engl J Med *309:*354, 1983; Greenblatt, D. J., Shader, R. I., Abernethy, D. R.: Drug therapy: current status of benzodiazepines (second of two parts). N Engl J Med *309:*410, 1983; and Greenblatt, D. J.: Pharmacokinetics of midazolam. Sleep *5(Suppl 1),* 1982.

Biotransformation pathways of some benzodiazepines. Italics indicates compound marketed as separate drug.

habitus influences drug disposition, depending on the lipophilicity of the drug. Lipid solubility partly determines the extent of benzodiazepine distribution. The more lipid soluble the drug, the longer the duration of action.

Drug Interactions

Oral contraceptives, low-dose estrogen, and other drugs inhibit the metabolism of those benzodiazepines managed by oxidation, such as triazolam and alprazolam, and increase the elimination time.[8] Those conjugates such as temazepam and lorazepam have a decreased elimination time with increased clearance and accelerated metabolism.[9]

CLINICAL CLASSIFICATION

A useful classification of benzodiazepines is based on their duration of action and elimination half-lives (Table 30-3).

Diazepam, flurazepam, and chlordiazepoxide are considered "long-acting" drugs with elimination half-lives $(T^{1}/_{2}\text{-}\beta)$ of 24 hours or longer. They are metabolized by oxidation, and the metabolites are active. The metabolites accumulate for days, so by 1 week, the plasma level may be four to six times as high as after the first night.[10] These long-acting agents are able to induce their own metabolism and are affected by liver disease.

Oxazepam, midazolam, and lorazepam are exceptions; they are primarily conjugated with glucuronic acid and may be safer or more appropriate than oxidized benzodiazepines in elderly and sick patients. These three drugs are considered short-acting and are not affected by liver disease.[9] They do not induce their own metabolism.

Flurazepam (Dalmane) is represented specifically as an hypnotic, but in fact it has no unique hypnotic properties that are not possessed by most other benzodiazepines.[11] After oral administration, the agent is almost immediately metabolized in the gastrointestinal tract and in the liver. The principal metabolite is desalkylflurazepam, which is active and accounts for the drug's effect. The metabolite is long lasting (72 hours) and accumulates during long-term therapy for 7 to 10 days.

MOLECULAR MECHANICS

Receptors[12]

A receptor unit was demonstrated by Mohler and Okada in 1977 in the CNS, in various areas of the brain with which the benzodiazepines combine.[13] Because τ-aminobutyric acid (GABA) appears to be the natural mediator at these sites and also combines with this receptor

Table 30–3. Clinical Classification of Benzodiazepines Based on Their Elimination Half-Lives

Long-acting: Half-life of 24 hours or more
  Diazepam
  Nitrazepam
  Chlordiazepoxide
  Flunitrazepam
  Flurazepam

Moderate-acting: Half-life of 6 to 24 hours
  Lorazepam
  Oxazepam
  Temazepam

Short-acting: Half-life less than 5 hours
  Midazolam
  Triazolam

substance, investigators have postulated that GABA is the physiologic agonist[14] with inhibitory actions and that the benzodiazepines facilitate this action. The affinity of benzodiazepines for the receptor is enhanced by pentobarbital.[15]

Binding Sites

Specific cellular membrane binding sites were determined by Young in 1981.[16] These sites are confined to the CNS and are predominately localized in neuronal surface membranes. The distribution within the CNS is extensive, with concentrations in every brain region.[13,16]

The order of receptor densities from highest to lowest is as follows:

High: cerebral > limbic forebrain > subcortical nuclei > thalamus
Low: brain stem > spinal cord > corpus callosum

MECHANISM OF ACTION

The exact biochemical basis of anxiety is imprecise.[17] Several neurophysiologic effects are seen following the administration of benzodiazepines, however, effects that indicate an antianxiety action[18,19]: (1) electroencephalographic arousal from activity of the reticular activating system is blocked; (2) electrical afterdischarges from the limbic system are depressed; (3) the amygdala is blocked and the seizure threshold is raised.

The action of benzodiazepines, as previously noted, is probably mediated through a facilitation of the GABA-ergic transmission at specific receptor sites.[14] This is an inhibitory system to the noradrenergic and dopaminergic wakeful and alerting systems. Hence, the benzodiazepines are able to produce sleep. A direct blocking action on the noradrenergic and dopaminergic systems may also be considered. The principal site of action is the noradrenergic cell system of the locus ceruleus complex.[20]

Benzodiazepines do not act by blocking any natural neurotransmitter. Electrophysiologic studies show an augmentation of the action of GABA, the inhibitory neurotransmitter acting at sensory presynaptic areas and also at many postsynaptic sites. Intracellular-extracellular studies indicate that GABA lowers membrane potential away from threshold, so neuronal excitability is lost at the molecular level. This effect is achieved by opening two-state channels that are permeable to chloride ions; a widening of the channels, with an increase in ion conductance, occurs to alter the membrane potential and to prevent an action potential.[14]

Benzodiazepines act by increasing the frequency of openings of the GABA-modulated chloride channels.[17] Some increase in the time during which the channels stay open also occurs. Barbiturates also potentiate GABA[15] action, but they do so principally by keeping the chloride channels open for a longer period of time, while simultaneously decreasing the frequency of channel opening.

The major site of these molecular actions is most likely an alteration of postsynaptic responses to GABA.[12]

PREMEDICATION[21]

Consistent with the aim of preanesthetic medication to reduce anxiety—both situational and trait (fear)—the use of benzodiazepines is a variable procedure. These agents are particularly effective in patients with trait or neurotic anxiety and may be given orally or parenterally (maladaptive, pathologic anxiety).[22]

The highly lipid-soluble derivatives are almost completely and rapidly absorbed after oral intake, and reliable effects are observed in 30 to 60 minutes.[23] For rapid control of a panic state, diazepam, chlordiazepoxide, flunitrazepam, and midazolam, administered intravenously, are useful drugs.

PHYSIOLOGIC EFFECTS

At least five distinct human behavioral effects are seen[24]: anxiolysis, sedation-hypnosis, amnesia, muscle relaxation (centrally mediated), and anticonvulsion.[2,3,25]

Anxiolysis

Anxiety is frequent in patients before anesthesia and surgery. It is likely present in all patients in varying degrees, but it is significant in trait-type personalities and borders on fear in 40 to 60%.[26]

Relief of anxiety provides several advantages: induction of anesthesia is easier; the amount of anesthetic is lessened; and a reduction in stress responses occurs, that is, catecholamine and steroid release is diminished. Minimizing anxiety means safer stress-free anesthesia and surgery.

Trait and neurotic anxiety is best relieved by tranquilizers, and the benzodiazepines are effective. In this regard, they are superior to the barbiturates.

Oral lorazepam, diazepam, midazolam, and oxazepam provide good relief from anxiety in adults.[27] In children, barbiturates appear to be better anxiolytic drugs.[28]

Sedation[22,24]

In the instance of benzodiazepines, the appearance of sedation is the consequence of the lack of anxiety. Larger than usual doses appear to increase sedation, but they do not further alleviate apprehension. The quality of night sleep following oral benzodiazepines has been analyzed: flunitrazepam, lorazepam, and midazolam appear to provide good sleep in 90% of patients at oral doses of 2.0, 2.5, and 3.0 mg, respectively. This is about equal to the classic barbiturate sedatives and is superior to the antihistamines. Unlike the barbiturates, these drugs usually do not suppress rapid eye movement (REM) sleep and are less commonly associated with hangover. Flunitrazepam (30 mg) is associated with REM suppression, however.[29] The shorter-acting benzodiazepines have excellent hypnotic-sedative action. Temazepam, with a 5- to 10-hour therapeutic effect, is a good choice for night sedation. The ultrarapid agent triazolam provides an excellent sedative effect for 5 hours and has less of a carry-over into the morning of surgery.

Benzodiazepines are useful in treating the sleep latency-insomnia disorders, especially in addicts.[30] Flurazepam and perphenazine are excellent in this regard. Also effective are the following: chloral hydrate > chlorpromazine > diphenhydramine.

Amnesic Action

Amnesic action is significant and compares with that of scopolamine. Oral diazepam at 10 and 20 mg shows a dose-dependent effect: 10 mg provides 120 minutes of amnesia, whereas 20 mg limits recall of the entire operative day.[31] In children, two dosage schedules of diazepam have been used to modify recall: 0.25 or 0.5 mg/kg as an oral syrup. Neither dose dependably produces amnesia or eliminates recall.[28] No correlation between plasma levels and answers could be determined. Lorazepam by mouth seems to be the most potent derivative, producing long-lasting amnesia. The onset is slow, it but is accompanied by sedation and superior antegrade amnesia.[32]

Muscle Relaxation

This effect was first described by Randall and appears to be selective.[33] This is a centrally mediated, independent effect rather than a peripheral effect.[34]

Other Actions

Important additional actions are noted: antiemesis is good; prolongation of tubocurarine neuromuscular block is observed; no independent analgesia occurs, but potentiation of narcotic analgesia is seen. A decrease in plasma cortisol has been reported with benzodiazepines.[35]

CLINICAL DIFFERENCES

All the benzodiazepines have similar pharmacologic profiles. Clinical differences in potency are quantitative and are related to individual pharmacokinetics of absorption, distribution, and metabolism. All these drugs have common features of anxiolysis, sedation, hypnotic action, and anticonvulsion in ascending order of dose and brain concentrations.

Subtle pharmacodynamic differences among various benzodiazepine derivatives have been summarized by Kanto (Table 30–4).[21]

Besides the antianxiety and anti-insomnia effects, these agents have muscle relaxant effects related to a central upper motoneuronal action. Diazepam is effective in relieving spasticity and athetosis in cerebral palsy.

SELECTION OF BENZODIAZEPINES[25]

The benzodiazepines have similar dynamic profiles, with some subtle differences with regard to the effects on behavioral elements. Much of the process of selection is related to the large differences in pharmacokinetics, and, thus, one significant classification of these drugs is based on the duration of action. In anesthesia practice, four injectable benzodiazepines are usually selected. The chemical structures of these agents are illustrated (Fig. 30-2).

Midazolam

This is the most commonly used benzodiazepine perioperatively. Unlike diazepam, it is water soluble. Chemically, it is an imidazo-benzodiazepine derivative. The nitrogen in the imidazole ring confers a higher basicity to the molecule and a greater water solubility. This occurs at pH values under 4.0. Solubility is actually pH dependent, and in the condition of low pH, the imidazole ring is reversibly open.[36] The commercial preparation of midazolam maleate or chloride salt is freely water soluble and is buffered to a pH of 3.5, and the stability of the aqueous midazolam is maintained. At higher pH values and at the pH of the plasma of 7.4, however, the ring is closed, conferring a higher degree of lipid solubility. The closed ring is the effective structure, and the process takes about 5 to 10 minutes to be completed (Fig. 30-3).[37]

Table 30–4. Some Differences Between Benzodiazepine Derivatives Estimated in the Operating Room Just Before Induction of Anesthesia

Sedation
  Flunitrazepam > lorazepam = oxazepam = diazepam = nitrazepam midazolam >> placebo; temazepam = triazolam = flurazepam >> placebo

Apprehension + excitement (anxiolysis)
  Flunitrazepam >> placebo < diazepam = oxazepam = lorazepam = nitrazepam = chlorazepate

Dizziness
  Flunitrazepam >>> placebo << nitrazepam = lorazepam > oxazepam = diazepam > temazepam > triazolam

Headache
  Nitrazepam > placebo = diazepam = oxazepam = lorazepam > flunitrazepam > short-acting benzodiazepines

Cardiovascular changes
  Flunitrazepam < placebo = diazepam = oxazepam = nitrazepam = lorazepam
  Nitrazepam < no premedication

Assessments were made after two oral doses (the night before, and morning of, operation) using the method of Dundee, Moore and Nicholl (1962), with minor alterations (diazepam 10 + 10 mg, nitrazepam 5 + 5 mg, flunitrazepam 1 + 1 mg or 2 + 2 mg, oxazepam 25 + 25 mg or 30 + 30 mg, lorazepam 2.5 + 2.5 mg).
Modified from Kanto, J.: Benzodiazepines as oral premedicants. Br J Anaesth 53:1179, 1981.

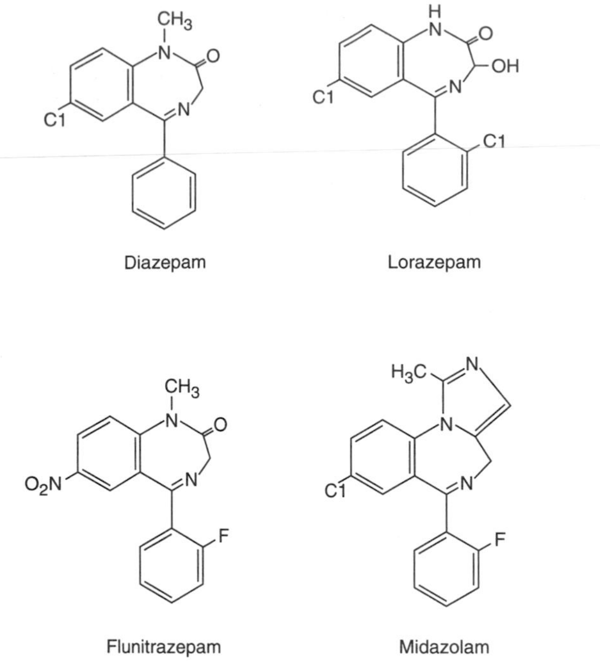

Fig. 30–2. The chemical structures of four injectable benzodiazepines commonly used in anesthesia.

The potency of midazolam is about 1½ to 2 times that of diazepam.

Administration

Oral

Oral administration of midazolam is a particularly effective manner of producing sleep in infants and children. The drug is prepared by dissolving the parenteral preparation (5 mg/ml) in an equal volume of a chocolate-cherry syrup or an equal volume of simple syrup NF flavored with oil of peppermint.[38] A palatable preparation acceptable to most children is a solution constituted as follows: to 15 ml of midazolam parenteral preparation (5.0 mg/ml) add 14.5 ml of simple syrup NF mixed with 0.5 ml of peppermint oil. This provides a final concentration of 2.5 mg/ml of midazolam.

A slightly more concentrated solution can be prepared in a similar manner so that there is 3.0 mg/ml of midazolam. These solutions are stable for up to 14 days in amber glass bottles at room temperature.[39]

Doses of 0.5, 0.75, and 1.0 mg/kg of body weight have been demonstrated to produce excellent sedation and anxiolysis within 15 minutes.[38] For children 1 to 6 years of age, an oral dose of 0.5 mg/kg (5.0 to 15 ml of solution) permits separation of a child from the parent as early as 10 minutes later.[40] One may wish to use a larger dose for more robust children and older patients and to provide a more rapid onset of sedation with doses up to 1.0 mg/kg.[40] Absorption is relatively rapid, and onset of sedation is seen in 15 minutes and a peak effect in about 30 minutes. Extensive first-pass metabolism in the liver leads to a bioavailability of about 50% of the dose.[41,42]

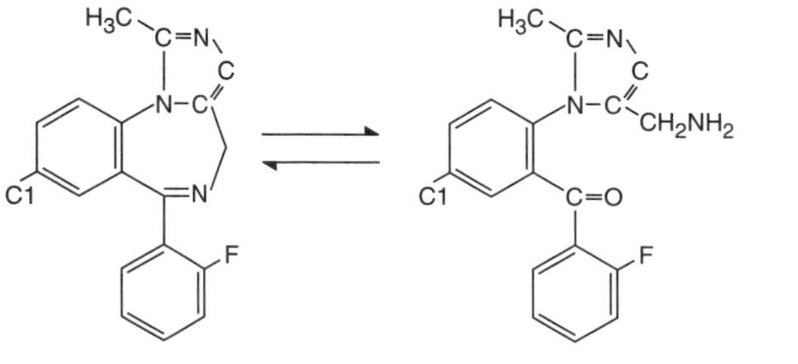

Intramuscular[43]

Because the drug is water soluble, it is rapidly absorbed and 90% is bioavailable. Onset of action is within 15 minutes after a dose of 0.1 mg/kg. The dose for sedation and anxiolysis is 0.1 mg/kg.[43] The peak sedative effect is achieved between 30 and 45 minutes, which corresponds to the mean time of plasma maximal concentration. The preferred site of injection is into the vastus lateralis muscle. Pain is noted in about 10% of patients. The plasma concentration is about half that following the same dose intravenously.

Intravenous

On entrance into the circulation, the drug is immediately subject to pharmacokinetic variables. A slight delay in pharmacodynamic responses occurs from the conversion from the open ring structure to the effective closed ring. The use of midazolam as an intravenous induction agent is presented in detail elsewhere.[43a] The dose for the production of unconsciousness is 0.2 to 0.25 mg/kg.[44] Unlike diazepam, this benzodiazepine does not produce thrombosis or thrombophlebitis, and the metabolites have no sedative effects.[45]

Pharmacokinetics (Table 30–5)[46–49]

The behavior follows a two-compartment model. The initial dilution phase in the vascular compartment is short, requiring less than 2 minutes; this is followed by the initial distribution to vascular-rich tissues with a half-life of 7.2 minutes. The elimination half-life is short, with an average of 2.5 hours (range 2.1 to 3.4 hours). The principal elimination processes are related to metabolism and excretion. In elderly patients, the elimination half-life increases to 5.6 hours, and in obese patients it inceases to 8.4 hours (Table 30–6).[50]

Metabolism[50]

The liver is the main site of metabolism (Fig. 30–4), and nearly all the drug undergoes hydroxylation at the methyl group on the imidazole ring to either α-hydroxymidazo-

Fig. 30–3. The unique midazolam ring structure. Solubility is pH dependent. At pH less than 4.0, the midazolam is an open ring structure (2), which is the water-soluble configuration present in commercial preparations. At a pH above 4.0, the ring closes and becomes lipid soluble: (1) the active lipid-soluble ring configuration in blood; (2) the inactive water-soluble configuration open ring. Modified from Stanski, D. R., Watkins, W. D.: Drug Disposition in Anesthesia. New York, Grune & Stratton, 1982.

Table 30–5. Physicochemical and Pharmacokinetic Properties of Diazepam and Midazolam

Property	Diazepam	Midazolam
Physicochemical		
Solubility	Insoluble in water	Solubility in water because of hydrophilic
	Available in organic solution or lipid emulsion	imidazole group
Form of IV presentation	Organic solvent Emulsion	Aqueous solution
pKa	3.4	6.2
Lipophilicity		
Octanol: buffer partition ratio	309	34
Pharmacokinetics		
Plasma protein binding	97–99%	94–98%
Volume of distribution (V_D (1 kg^{-1}))	0.7–1.6	0.8–1.6
Elimination half-life (h) ($T_{1/2}$-β)	20–70	1.5–5
Clearance		
Total body (ml min^{-1} kg^{-1})	0.24–0.53	6.4–11.1
Plasma (ml min^{-1})	20–47	268–630
Metabolism	To desmethyldiazepam and oxazepam	Active metabolite α-hydroxymidazolam, which is very rapidly conjugated to inactive form($T_{1/2}$-β < 1 h)
	Both hypnotically active	
Second peak	Present at 6–8 h due to enterohepatic recirculation and is of clinical significance	If present, is small and not clinically significant
Pharmacodynamics		
Onset (minutes)	10	2–12
Duration (hours)	4–5	2.5
Effective concentration	300–400 ng/ml	40–50 ng/ml sedation
	600 ng/ml (sleep)	50–100 ng/ml sleep

From Dundee, J. W. Wyant, G. M.: Intravenous Anaesthesia, 2nd Ed. Edinburgh, Churchill Livingstone, 1988.

lam or to 4-hydroxymidazolam, both of which are rapidly conjugated in the liver. Both the initial metabolites may also undergo further hydroxylation to the dihydroxy α,4 form and then are conjugated to glucoronides. The main metabolite is α-hydroxymethylmidazolam, which has some pharmacologic activity, but this is rapidly conjugated and is of no clinical significance. Hepatic elimination is flow dependent. Changes in hepatic blood flow can alter clearance. Extrahepatic metabolism may also occur.[51]

Clearance from the blood of midazolam is rapid and is 10 times faster than for diazepam. About a half-liter of plasma is cleared per hour per kilogram.

Excretion[52]

All the metabolites as glucuronides are detected in the urine. The main metabolite, α hydroxymethylmidazolam, represents almost 45 to 50% of the conjugated urinary glucuronides.[49,53] Less than 1% of intact midazolam is excreted.[52,53]

Plasma Binding[54]

Midazolam is highly bound to plasma protein to the extent of about 94% of the injected drug. The binding is to the albumin fraction. Hypoalbuminemia can diminish the

Table 30–6. Midazolam: Pharmacokinetic Data

Availability (Oral) (%)	Urinary Excretion (%)	Bound in Plasma (%)	Clearance (ml · min^{-1} · kg^{-1})	Vol. Dist. (L/kg)	Half-Life (h)	Effective Concentrations
44 ± 17	56 ± 26	95 ± 2	6.6 ± 1.8	1.1 ± 0.6	2.5 ± 0.6	Sedation: 40–50 ng/ml
↑ Cirrhosis	⟷ Smokers, Aged	↓ Aged, Uremia	↑ Uremia*	↑ Obesity	↑ Aged, Obesity	Sleep: 50–100 ng/ml
		⟷ Smokers, Cirrhosis	↓ Cirrhosis	⟷ Cirrhosis	Cirrhosis	
			⟷ Obesity, Smokers		⟷ Smokers	

*Owing to increased free fraction; unbound clearance is unchanged.
From Garzone, P. D., Kroboth, P. D.: Pharmacokinetics of the newer benzodiazepines. Clin Pharmacokinet 16:337, 1989.

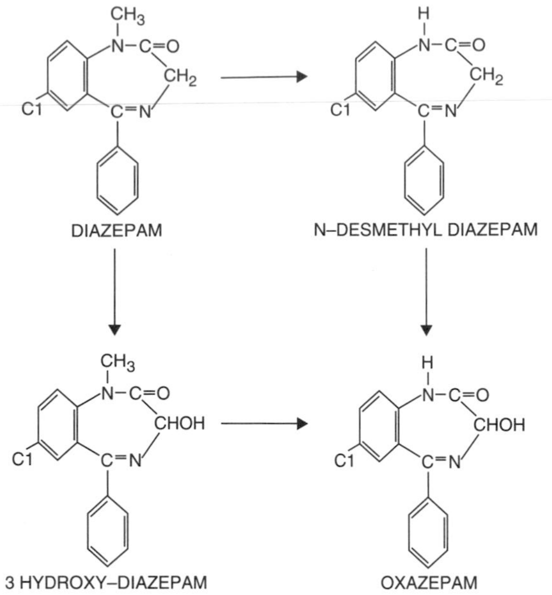

DIAZEPAM → N–DESMETHYL DIAZEPAM

3 HYDROXY–DIAZEPAM → OXAZEPAM

Diazepam and its metabolites.

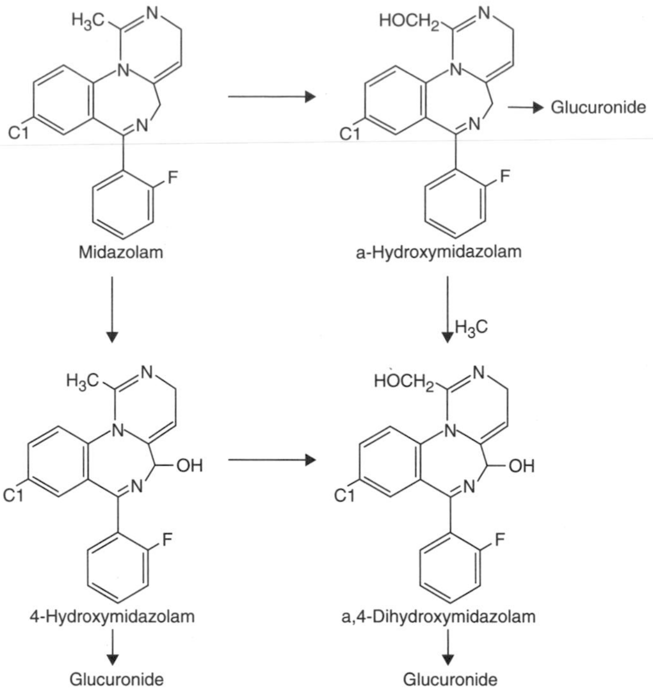

Midazolam → a-Hydroxymidazolam → Glucuronide

4-Hydroxymidazolam → Glucuronide

a,4-Dihydroxymidazolam → Glucuronide

Midazolam and its metabolites.

Fig. 30–4. Comparative biotransformation and the principal metabolites of diazepam and midazolam. From Dundee, J. W., Wyant, G. M.: Intravenous Anaesthesia, 2nd Ed. Edinburgh, Churchill Livingstone, 1988.

bound fraction and can result in large changes in the fraction of the free drug.

Plasma Levels[49,53]

After administration intravenously of a dose of 0.1 mg/kg of midazolam, one notes an immediate peak of the drug to about 300 ng/ml, followed by a decline in a biexponential manner. An initial rapid decline to 100 ng/ml is related to the distribution to vascular-rich tissues and represents the α phase, with a half-life of 12 minutes. This is followed by a slower decline to 30 ng/kg representative of the β phase, with a half-life of about 2.5 hours. This decline is due to elimination processes.

Variations in Dose

The dose of midazolam required to produce sedation decreases approximately 15% per decade of life (Fig. 30–5). Midazolam should therefore be used carefully in the elderly.[55,56]

Diazepam

Diazepam is available in oral and intravenous forms both in the United States and in Europe, although with the advent of midazolam, the use of the intravenous form has greatly decreased. Because the drug can be given orally, it is a popular drug for reduction of preoperative anxiety when patients can be seen earlier than 1 day before surgery.

Pharmacokinetics

After intravenous administration, diazepam's distribution half-life is 1 hour and the excretion half-life is 32.9 ± 8.8 hours[54] (see Table 30–5). The drug is 99% bound to plasma albumin. The duration of action of the drug de-

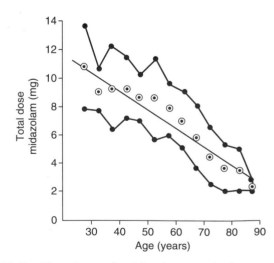

Fig. 30–5. The dose of midazolam required to provide sedation adequate for upper gastrointestinal endoscopy is inversely related to the age of the patient. Redrawn from Scholer, S. G., Schafer, D. F., Potter, J. F.: The effect of age on the relative potency of midazolam and diazepam for sedation in upper gastrointestinal endoscopy. J Clin Gastroenterol *12*:145, 1990.

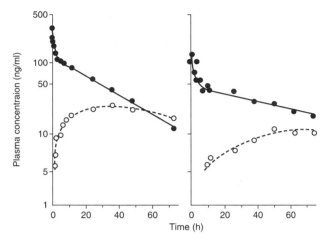

Fig. 30–6. Plasma concentration versus time curves for diazepam (solid line) and desmethyldiazepam (broken line) after intravenous injection of diazepam (0.1 mg/kg) in two asymptomatic adults having no laboratory evidence of disease: a 20-year-old (A) and a 67-year-old (B). The elimination half-life of diazepam was 21.6 hours for the younger person and 51.9 hours for the older person. Redrawn from Klotz, U., et al.: The effects of age and liver disease on the disposition and elimination of diazepam in adult man. J Clin Invest 55.347, 1975.

pends more on drug distribution and uptake at peripheral sites, such as adipose tissue, and less on elimination factors. Its elimination half-life is longer in older individuals than in young individuals, primarily because of an increased volume of distribution (Fig. 30–6)[57] (Table 30–7).[58]

Absorption

Orally administered diazepam is well absorbed from the intestine, and plasma levels peak after 60 minutes.[59] Delayed gastric emptying seen, for example, when narcotics or atropine are administered simultaneously with oral diazepam, results in a lower plasma concentration of diazepam. This can be reversed by metoclopramide.[60] Conversely, serum levels of diazepam may increase if food is ingested 5 hours after intravenous administration, possibly because diazepam is excreted in the bile and is reabsorbed from the intestine.[61] Injection of diazepam into the gluteal region, particularly in areas of fat rather than muscle, produces low plasma levels of the drug.[62]

Metabolism (see Fig. 30–4)

Because diazepam requires microsomal nonconjugative pathways for degradation and elimination,[63] it should not be used for patients with acute hepatitis. A major metabolite of diazepam is desmethyldiazepam. Desmethyldiazepam can be detected after 2 hours, decreases only after 36 hours, and has pharmacologic properties similar to those of diazepam. The long action of diazepam is attributable not only to its own long excretion half-life, but also to the long half-life of its metabolite. With increasing age, individuals become progressively more sensitive to midazolam. Until age 60 years, diazepam is one half to one fourth as potent as midazolam, after which time the relative potency of diazepam increases[63] (Fig. 30-7).

Administration

Injection of diazepam intramuscularly or intravenously is associated with pain and thrombophlebitis. Venous thrombosis is more frequent in older than in younger patients (Fig. 30-8) and when diazepam is injected into smaller veins rather than larger veins. Propylene glycol, which is used to promote solubility of the injectable form of diazepam, produces both pain on injection and thrombophlebitis.[64]

In animals, diazepam has been shown to reduce seizure threshold and to protect against seizures caused by local anesthetics.[65,66] No study of patients undergoing regional anesthesia has demonstrated that diazepam specifically and the benzodiazepines in general reduce the incidence of seizures, however. In fact, in one clinical study, diazepam, 0.14 mg/kg, did not blunt the degree of severity of the number of CNS symptoms after lidocaine, 1 mg/kg.[67] A few convulsions have also been associated with midazolam.[68]

Table 30–7. Diazepam: Pharmacokinetic Data

Availability (Oral) (%)	Urinary Excretion (%)	Bound in Plasma (%)	Clearance (ml · min⁻¹ · kg⁻¹)	Vol. Dist. (L/kg)	Half-Life (h)	Effective Concentrations
100 ± 14	<1	98.7 ± 0.2 ↓ Uremia, cirrhosis, NS, pregnancy, neonates, albuminemia† ⟷ Aged, HTh	0.38 ± 0.06* ↑ Albuminemia, epilepsy‡ ↓ Cirrhosis, hepatitis ⟷ Aged, smokers HTh	1.1 ± 0.3 ↑ Cirrhosis, aged, albuminemia ⟷ Uremia, HTh	43 ± 13* ↑ Aged, cirrhosis, hepatitis ↓ Epilepsy‡ ⟷ HTh	300–400 ng/ml§ >600 ng/ml‖

*Active metabolites, desmethyldiazepam and oxazepam; *see also* listing for those compounds. Genetic variability in clearance related to hydroxylation phenotype.
†Alcoholics.
‡Due to administration of other drugs that induce metabolic enzymes.
§Anxiolytic.
‖For control of seizures.
From Greenblat, D. J., Allen. M. D.; Harmatz, J. S., Schader, R. I.: Diazepam disposition determinants. Clin Pharmacol Ther, *27*:301, 1980.

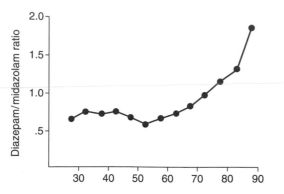

Fig. 30–7. Patient age affects the potency ratio of diazepam to midazolam regarding doses required to provide sedation adequate for upper gastrointestinal endoscopy. Above age 60 years, subjects become progressively more sensitive to midazolam. Redrawn from Scholer, S. G., Schafer, D. F., Potter, J. F.: The effect of age on the relative potency of midazolam and diazepam for sedation in upper gastrointestinal endoscopy. J Clin Gastroenterol 12:145, 1990.

Lorazepam

The potency of lorazepam is approximately four times that of diazepam.[69] Oral, intramuscular, and intravenous routes are reliable for absorption. Administration of 2.5 mg orally is equivalent to 10 mg of diazepam.[69]

Pharmacodynamics[70]

Onset of action is slower than that of diazepam. The full effect is achieved in 30 to 60 minutes, and the duration of action is three to four times longer than diazepam and extends for 4 to 6 hours.

Pharmacokinetics[71]

After administration, the plasma level attained by 30 minutes is about 30 ng/ml and reaches 90 ng/ml by 60 minutes. After 4 hours, the level begins to fall and contin-

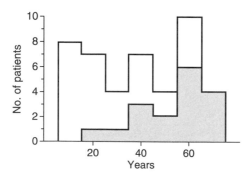

Fig. 30–8. The incidence of venous thrombosis 7 to 10 days after intravenous injection of 10 mg of diazepam increases with age. The clear outline represents the total number of patients given diazepam. The cross-hatched outline represents the number of patients having venous thrombosis. Redrawn from Hegarty, J. E., Dundee, J. W.: Sequelae after the intravenous injection of three benzodiazepines—diazepam, lorazepam and flunitrazepam. Br Med J 1:1384, 1977.

ues progressively; by 6 hours, the plasma level reaches 10 ng/ml, which does not provide an adequate effect. The mean elimination half-life, the $T_{1/2}$-β, is 12 to 16 hours.[72]

Because the drug is less lipid soluble than diazepam and its congeners, its pharmacokinetic pattern tends to follow a one-compartment model. A large fraction is bound to plasma protein, about 90% to albumin. This is decreased in patients with cirrhosis.[7]

Metabolism and Excretion[7]

Like midazolam but unlike diazepam, the metabolites of lorazepam are not active.[73]

Metabolism is partly by hepatic microsomal oxidation, but the major part of the drug is simply conjugated with glucuronic acid. The glucuronide is eliminated by the kidney, and the β phase ($T_{1/2}$-β) is 12 to 16 hours. Little drug is excreted unchanged.

Dosage

Dosage by mouth is of the order of 2.0 mg for patients under 60 kg of weight and 3.0 mg for those up to 80 kg; over 80 kg, the dose is 4.0 mg. For preanesthetic medication, the drug may be administered intramuscularly at a dosage of 50 µg/kg 1.5 to 2.0 hours before induction of anesthesia for maximum effect; 2.0 mg is about equal to 10 mg of diazepam.[69]

With intravenous administration, the dosage is 40 µg/kg and the onset of a hypnotic state is slow: up to 30 to 40 minutes, compared with diazepam, which takes 60 to 90 seconds. Hence, it is not suitable for anesthetic induction.[70]

In open heart surgery, the plasma concentration of lorazepam, after an oral premedicant dose, falls to levels that do not provide amnesia. Therefore, additional doses must be given intravenously before cardiopulmonary bypass.[74]

Physiologic Effects

As with other benzodiazepines, the three principal effects are anxiolysis, sedation consequent to the antianxiety effect, and amnesia.[75] Antianxiety effects and amnesia do not coincide. Small doses of 2 to 2.5 mg preoperatively provide anxiolysis and some sedation, but little amnesia.[76] The amnesic effect is thus dose-dependent and is achieved with doses of 3 to 4 mg. Antegrade antirecall is evident in 15 to 30 minutes. Ordinary nonpainful stimuli and antegrade events are not recalled.[77] Disturbing and painful auditory stimuli are recalled. Overdose is reversible with aminophylline (1.0 mg/kg).[78]

Uses and Advantages

- Lorazepam is useful for management of anxiety in the preoperative period and for hypnotic effect the evening before operation.
- The drug is effective as a basal tranquilizer and sedative during regional anesthesia when given by mouth 30 minutes preanesthetically.
- Combined with a narcotic preanesthetically, anxiolysis and amnesia are provided with modest pain relief for invasive monitoring procedures.

- The incidence of venous sequelae are fewer than after diazepam[73] (15% versus 69%, respectively).

Temazepam

This benzodiazepine hypnotic has a time course that is appropriate for night sleep and insomnia.[79] It is administered orally and is well absorbed.

Chemical Description

The chemical name is 7-chloro-1,3-dihydro-3-hydroxyl-1-methyl-5-phenyl-28-1,4-benzodiazepine-2-0.N.E. This is a metabolite of diazepam.[80]

Dose and Administration

As a relatively shorter-acting benzodiazepine with respect to diazepam, temazepam provides approximately 9 to 10 hours' sleep. The dose is 15 to 30 mg, taken orally.

Pharmacokinetics

After a single dose of 15 to 30 mg approximately, absorption is rapid, and a steady state plasma concentration is usually achieved within 1 hour. Throughout the period of activity, the plasma level is approximately 382 ng/ml at 2.5 hours after a 30-mg dose. At 24 hours following a single dose, the plasma level is approximately 26 ng/ml. The α half-life is estimated at 2.5 hours, whereas the β or elimination phase approximates 10 hours. Cumulative effects are not seen.[81]

Disposition

Temazepam is completely metabolized, and approximately 80 to 90% of the dose appears in the urine as metabolites. The major metabolite is an orthoconjugate, which represents 90% of the biotransformed drug. A second metabolite has been identified as N-dimethyl temazepam and represents approximately 7% of the degraded parent drug. No active metabolites have been identified.

Clinical Pharmacology

This drug is useful in terms of providing tranquilization in anxious patients and, with it, hypnosis and sedation. Multiple doses do not show major accumulation, and no evidence of enzyme induction exists.

Indications

This drug is a safe night sedative and antianxiety agent, taken on the night before anesthesia and surgery. It is slowly absorbed and is not ideal in patients with prolonged sleep latency. It should be administered 1 to 2 hours before bedtime. A 15-mg dose may be administered at approximately 9:00 P.M., and, if insufficient, a repeat of 15 mg to a total of 30 mg can be accomplished if the second dose is given before midnight. The patient usually shows great ease of falling asleep and does not have any complaints about nocturnal awakening. In the morning, patients are relaxed. Fewer residual effects on psychomotor and cognitive function are noted.[29]

Precautions

As with other benzodiazepines, this drug may cause some fetal damage during first trimester pregnancy. As with diazepam, a risk of congenital malformation exists. Transplacental passage causes neonatal CNS depression if the drug is administered during the last weeks of pregnancy. Thus, temazepam is relatively contraindicated in pregnant women.

Adverse Reactions

The most common adverse reactions are continued drowsiness, some dizziness, and lethargy in the early morning hours, but these effects wane later in the morning.

Abuse potential and dependence do exist, but they are usually evident in patients who are receiving prolonged benzodiazepine therapy. In hospital surgery and anesthesia practice over a short period of time, this phenomenon, including that of the withdrawal phenomenon of convulsions, is not seen.

Flurazepam (Dalmane)[11]

The kinetics of flurazepam are unusual. After a single oral dose of 15 mg, only trace amounts of the parent drug have been detected in the plasma in the early 2-hour period ($T_{1/2}\beta$) after administration. The drug is essentially a pro-drug because only the desalkyl metabolite is found in appreciable amounts and continues to be the only substance found thereafter. It appears that much of the tranquilizing and hypnotic effects of this compound are due to the metabolite. The maximum concentration of this metabolite is reached in about 16 hours. The elimination half-life is long and is approximately 70 hours in men and 100 hours in women.[11] The metabolite is degraded in the liver. The clearance of the metabolite desalkylflurazepam is $4.5 + 2.3$ ml^{-1}min^{-1}kg^{-1} This drug is a well-known sedative and hypnotic used primarily in the control of insomnia.

PHARMACOLOGIC EFFECTS

Allergic reactions associated with the benzodiazepines are extremely rare.[82] Unusual perception, including fantasies or hallucinations, is more common, but it is still rare.[83,84] Unusual perception has included sexual fantasies, at times with subsequent allegations of sexual assault.[85] This fact emphasizes the importance of always having another person present when sedating patients.

Cardiovascular Function

Benzodiazepines can cause both respiratory depression and hypotension. This finding was made particularly apparent with the introduction of midazolam, when adverse publicity was generated in the lay press because of deaths in elderly patients, in part due to hypotension and respiratory depression.[86,87] This publicity and a better appreciation of proper dosing resulted in several reductions in recommended dosing.[88,89] More recent data suggest, in fact, that midazolam places patients at no additional risk than diazepam.[90] The drop in blood pressure in normal

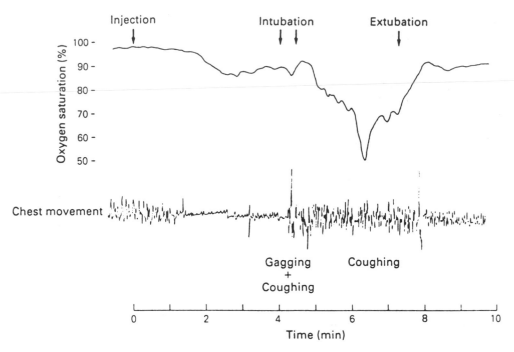

Fig. 30–9. Oxygen saturation and chest wall movements decreased in a patient after injection of midazolam during gastroscopy. After introduction of the gastroscope, the patient coughed and oxygen saturation decreased even more. Redrawn from Bell, G. D., et al.: Intravenous midazolam: a study of the degree of oxygen desaturation occurring during upper gastrointestinal endoscopy. Br J Clin Pharmacol 23:703, 1987.

individuals is trivial (10%).[91,92] In older patients, however, particularly in those with heart disease, blood pressure may drop as much as 20 to 35% and may be associated with apnea.[93] The benzodiazepines interact with other drugs (e.g., alfentanil, methohexital, morphine, thiopental, and the inhaled agents) to produce greater drops in blood pressure.[94-101] The drop in blood pressure is further accentuated if the patient has cardiac disease.[100,102-104] Loss of baroreflex control of heart rate also occurs after benzodiazepines,[105] although this loss is greater after the inhalation agents.[106]

Respiratory Function

The benzodiazepines depress respiratory function. Oxygenation after midazolam can fall, even to the point of cardiorespiratory arrest and death.[107] This is most evident during endoscopic procedures or during regional conduction block, particularly without the use of supplemental oxygen (Figs. 30–9 and 30–10).[108-110] Oxygen supplementation obviously can greatly improve oxygenation during sedation with benzodiazepines. Therefore, routine administration of supplemental oxygen, with or without continuous monitoring of arterial oxygenation, is recommended whenever benzodiazepines are given.[111,112] Although the respiratory response to carbon dioxide is also blunted by the benzodiazepines, this response is greater after narcotics.[113,114] The benzodiazepines potentiate the respiratory depression seen with narcotics, however (Fig. 30–11).[115] This is important because, in over 50% of the respiratory deaths associated with midazolam, narcotics were also administered.[115] The response to carbon diox-

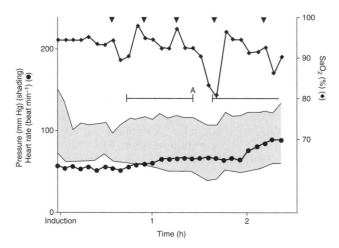

Fig. 30–10. Blood pressure, heart rate, and arterial oxygen saturation (SaO_2) in a patient given incremental doses of midazolam are shown at various times (arrows) during regional anesthesia. The horizontal lines indicate administration of oxygen, 2 L/min. At point A, the patient removed the oxygen catheter. Redrawn from Smith, D. C., Crul, J. F.: Oxygen desaturation following sedation for regional analgesia. Br J Anaesth 62:206, 1989.

ide after midazolam administration is also much more profound in patients with chronic obstructive pulmonary disease.[116] Finally, the risk of respiratory failure may also be increased when intravenous benzodiazepines are given to sedate patients with neurologic injuries.[117]

Psychomotor impairment in volunteers is seen for up to 7 hours after diazepam administration and up to 3

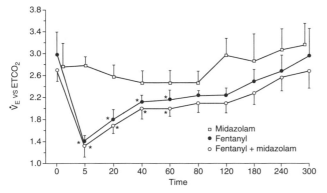

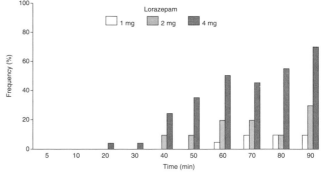

Fig. 30–11. Slope of the ventilatory response to carbon dioxide ($\dot{V}_E$ versus $ETCO_2 1 \cdot min^{-1} \cdot mm\ Hg^{-1}$ before (time 0) and minutes after midazolam, fentanyl, and midazolam plus fentanyl (*$p < 0.05$). In addition (not seen in graph), apnea occurred in 6 of 12 subjects receiving both midazolam and fentanyl, but not in individuals who received either midazolam or fentanyl. Redrawn from Bailey, P. L., et al.: Frequent hypoxemia and apnea after sedation with midazolam and fentanyl. Anesthesiology 73:826, 1990.

Fig. 30–12. Amnesia after oral administration of 1, 2, or 4 mg of lorazepam, expressed as the frequency of failure (as a percentage) to recognize a previously seen stimulus (picture postcard), shown at the times indicated. Recall was assessed 6 hours after surgery. The card shown at 90 minutes after lorazepam 4 mg was not recognized in over 75% of patients. Redrawn from McKay, A. C., Dundee, J. W.: Effect of oral benzodiazepines on memory. Br J Anaesth 52:1247, 1980.

hours after midazolam administration.[118,119] Pain and nausea may also affect recovery, so these differences in patients are not as apparent.[120-122] As expected, impairment of psychomotor function after lorazepam administration is present for a longer time than after diazepam or midazolam administration, and the drug is probably not appropriate for ambulatory surgery.[123,124]

Amnesia that occurs after premedication with benzodiazepines can be problematic. In one report, patients given midazolam, 2 mg intravenously, did not remember seeing the surgeon and anesthesiologist before surgery and wondered whether these physicians had been present for the operation.[125] In controlled studies, amnesia

is present after benzodiazepine administration, but retrograde amnesia has not been demonstrated to occur.[91,121,126-130] In fact, amnesia may occur without premedication. For example, in one study, after placebo, most patients could not remember induction of anesthesia.[131] Amnesia after lorazepam can last for up to 4 hours and is more intense than after diazepam (Figs. 30-12 and 30-13).[132]

The benzodiazepines are useful in controlling preoperative anxiety: oral diazepam for advance treatment and intravenous midazolam immediately before surgery. Amnesia that is seen with these drugs can also be useful.[54]

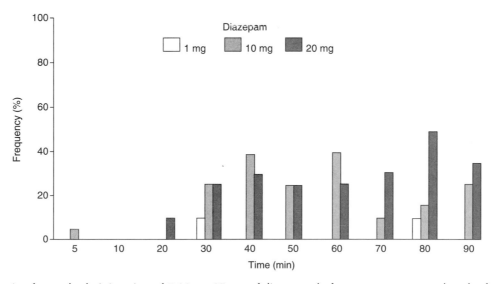

Fig. 30–13. Amnesia after oral administration of 5.10, or 15 mg of diazepam before surgery expressed as the frequency of failure (as a Percentage) to recognize a previously seen stimulus (picture postcard) shown at the times indicated. Recall was assessed 6 hours after surgery. Note that only 30% of patients had amnesia to the stimulus shown at 90 minutes after the largest dose of diazepam. Redrawn from McKay, A. C., Dundee, J. W.: Effect of oral benzodiazepines on memory. Br J Anaesth 52:1247, 1980.

Toxicity

Adverse responses to benzodiazepines are minimal.[133] The prolonged duration of a somnolent action is undesirable.[134] Occasionally, the depressant action in the postoperative period and situations of overdose need to be reversed.[135]

Physiologic Antagonism

Two drugs have been found effective in antagonizing overdoses or excessive benzodiazepine sedation. These are physostigmine and aminophylline. Physostigmine has been found effective in antagonizing diazepam and producing arousal.[136,137]

The effective dose is 1.0 mg.[138] A generalized arousal effect is produced by inhibiting acetylcholinesterase. This enzyme is concentrated at those cholinergic neurons located in the reticular activating system, which also corresponds to the location of benzodiazepine receptors.[13] The benzodiazepines block the excitatory cholinergic mechanisms and thereby produce somnolence. Physostigmine allows cholinergic activity to be unimpeded and thereby produces arousal.[136]

Large doses of physostigmine greater than 2.0 mg may produce a variable reaction.[135] Greater sedation may occur, along with slurred speech, slowed thinking, and impaired memory. Lower doses alone may enhance the storage of information into long-term memory.

Aminophylline is an antagonist to the excessive sedative and depressant effects of several benzodiazepines. It has been effective in reversing the effects of diazepam,[139] flurazepam,[140] and lorazepam, as well as other congeners.[78]

Specific Antagonist

An imidazodiazepine agent, flumazenil (Romazicon), has been found to be a potent competitive inhibitor of the specific binding of midazolam and other benzodiazepines.[141,142] It appears selectively to reverse impaired psychomotor performance without altering anxiolytic action or mood changes.[143]

Chemical Nature

This compound is ethyl-8-fluoro-5.6-dihydro-5-methyl-6-oxo-4H-imidazo-[1.5a]-[1.4]-benzodiazepine-3-carboxylate (Fig. 30–14).[144]

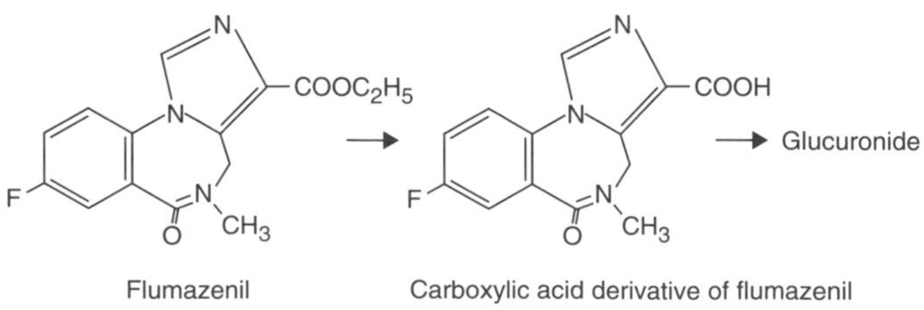

Fig. 30–14. Flumazenil and its metabolism. The only known metabolite in humans is the inactive carboxylic acid derivative, which is immediately glucuronized. From Amrein, L., et al: Clinical pharmacology of Dormicum (midazolam) and Anexate (flumazenil). Resuscitation *16:*S5, 1988.

Use

Flumazenil is used to reverse overdoses and to terminate the effects of benzodiazepines (diazepam; midazolam) rapidly at the termination of surgery or in the anesthesia recovery room.[145,146]

Dosage[146]

An initial dose of 0.2 mg of the drug is administered intravenously. This is followed by doses of 0.2 mg/minute until a satisfactory awakening end point is achieved. A total dose of 1.0 to 2.0 mg may be given. The usual total dose is 0.5 mg.

Pharmacokinetics[147]

Onset of action is prompt. Patients are usually awake and responsive within 3 minutes and are fully awake by 5 to 6 minutes.

The duration of action is between 1 and 3.5 hours. The elimination phase has a $T_{1/2}\text{-}\beta$ of 50 to 60 minutes.

Pharmacodynamics[148]

This drug produces complete antagonism and reversal of many of the behavioral effects, neurologic effects, and electrophysiologic changes resulting from the administration of benzodiazepines.

Sedation is readily reversed.[148] One sees an immediate improvement in orientation as to time and space and in comprehension and an ability to respond to commands. The degree of antigrade amnesia is also diminished. The drug does not appear to affect arterial pressure, heart rate, or ventilatory rate, and it does not leave the patient with an unusual anxiety state.[149]

Comment

The antegrade amnesic action of midazolam is greatly attenuated. In comparison, the amnesic action of diazepam and its sedative-tranquilizing effects are abolished.[150] The anxiolytic effect is not affected, however.[150] This finding emphasizes the presence of several benzodiazepine receptors, each apparently affecting different pharmacodynamic responses.[151]

REFERENCES

1. Sternbock, L. H., Randall, L. O., Gustatson, S. R.: Benzodiazepines. *In* Gordon, M. (ed.). Psychopharmacological Agents. New York, Academic Press, 1964.
2. Greenblatt, D. J., Shader, R. I., Abernethy, D. R.: Drug therapy: current status of benzodiazepines (first of two parts). N Engl J Med *309:*354, 1983.
3. Greenblatt, D. J., Koch-Weser, J.: Intramuscular injection of drugs. N Engl J Med *295:*542, 1976.
4. Rall, T. W.: Hypnotics and sedatives. *In* Gilman, A. G., et al. (eds.). Goodman and Gilman's The Pharmacological Basis of Therapeutics, 8th Ed. New York, McGraw-Hill, 1990.
5. Kortilla, K., Linnoila, M.: Absorption and sedative effects of diazepam after oral and intramuscular administration into vastus lateralis muscle and deltoid muscle. Br J Anaesth *47:*857, 1975.
6. Greenblatt, D. J., Shader, R. I., Abernethy, D. R.: Drug therapy: current status of benzodiazepines (second of two parts). N Engl J Med *309:*410, 1983.

7. Greenblatt, D. J.: Clinical pharmacokinetics of oxazepam and lorazepam. Clin Pharmacokinet 6:89, 1981.

8. Stoehr, G. P., et al.: Effect of oral contraceptives on triazolam, temazepam, alprazolam, and lorazepam kinetics. Clin Pharmacol Ther 36:683, 1984.

9. Sellers, E. M., et al.: Chlordiazepoxide oxazepam disposition cirrhosis. Clin Pharmacol Ther 26:240, 1979.

10. Linnoila, M.: Efficacy and side effects of flurazepam and a combination of amobarbital and secobarbital in somniac patients. J Clin Pharmacol 20:117, 1980.

11. Jochemsen, R., Van Boxtel, C. J., Hermans, J., Breimer, D. D.: Kinetics of five benzodiazepine hypnotics in healthy subjects. Clin Pharmacol Ther 34:42, 1983.

12. Tallman, J. R., Paul, S. M., Skolnick P, Gallagher, D. W.: Receptors for the age of anxiety: pharmacology of the benzodiazepines. Science 207:274, 1980.

13. Mohler, H., Okada, T.: Benzodiazepine receptor: demonstration in the central nervous system. Science 198:849, 1977.

14. Baraldi, M., Guidotti, A., Schwartz, J.P., Costa, E.: GABA receptors in clonal cell lives: a model for study of benzodiazepine action at molecular level. Science 205:821, 1979.

15. Skolnick, P.: Pentobarbital: Dual actions to increase brain benzodiazepine receptor affinity. Science 211:1448, 1981.

16. Young, W. S., et al.: Multiple benzodiazepine receptor localization by light microscopic radiohistochemistry. J Pharmacol Exp Ther 216:425, 1981.

17. Study, R. E., Barker, J. L.: Cellular mechanisms of benzodiazepine action. JAMA 247:2147, 1982.

18. Costa, E., et al.: New concepts on the mechanism of action of benzodiazepines. Life Sci 17:167, 1975.

19. Goodman, L., Gilman, A.: The Pharmacological Basis of Therapeutics, 6th Ed. New York, MacMillan, 1980.

20. Fuxe, K., Aquati, A., Bolme, P.: The possible involvement of GABA mechanisms in action of benzodiazepines. Psychopharmacol Bull 11:55, 1975.

21. Kanto, J.: Benzodiazepines as oral premedicants. Br J Anaesth 53:1179, 1971.

22. Rosenbaum, J. F.: The drug treatment of anxiety. N Engl J Med 306:401, 1982.

23. Greenblatt, D. J., et al.: In vitro quantitation of benzodiazepine lipophilicity: relation to in vivo distribution. Br J Anaesth 55:985, 1983.

24. Zbinden, G., Randall, L. O.: Behavioral effects of benzodiazepines. Adv Pharmacol 5:213, 1967.

25. Greenblatt, D. J., Divoll, M., Abernethy, D. R., Shader, R. I.: Benzodiazepine hypnotics: kinetic and therapeutic options. Sleep 5:S18, 1982.

26. Norris, W., Baird, W. L. M.: Preoperative anxiety: incidence and etiology. Br J Anaesth 39:503, 1967.

27. Greenblatt, D. J., Sellers, E. M., Shader, R. I.: Drug disposition in old age. N Engl J Med 306:1081, 1982.

28. Fell, D., Gough, M. B., Northan, A. A., Henderson, C. O.: Diazepam premedication in children. Anaesthesia 40:12, 1985.

29. Roth, T., et al.: Effects of temazepam, flurazepam and quinalbarbitone on sleep: psychomotor and cognitive function. Br J Clin Pharmacol 8(Suppl):47S, 1979.

30. Roth, T., et al.: Effects of benzodiazepines on sleep and wakefulness. Br J Clin Pharmacol 11(Suppl):31, 1981.

31. George, K. A., Dundee, J. W.: Relative amnesic actions of diazepam, flunitrazepam and lorazepam in man. Br J Clin Pharmacol 4:45, 1977.

32. Wilson, J.: Lorazepam as a premedicant for general anesthesia. Curr Med Res Opin 1:308, 1973.

33. Randall, L. O., et al.: Behavioral effects of benzodiazepines: muscle relaxation. J Pharmacol Exp Ther 129:163, 1960.

34. Ngai, S. H., Seng, D. T. C., Wang, C.: Muscle relaxation of benzodiazepines: a central effect. J Pharmacol Exp Ther 153:344, 1966.

35. James, M., Fisher, A.: Nitrazepam as a premedicant in minor surgery. Anaesthesia 25:264, 1980.

36. Gerecke, M.: Chemical structure and properties of midazolam compared to other benzodiazepines. Br J Clin Pharmacol 16:11S, 1983.

37. Stanski, D. R., Watkins, W. D.: Drug Disposition in Anesthesia. New York, Grune & Stratton, 1982.

38. McMillan, C. O., et al.: Premedication of children with oral midazolam. Can J Anaesth 39:545, 1992.

39. Gregory, D. F., Koestner, J. A., Tobias, J. D.: Stability of midazolam prepared for oral administration. South Med J 89:771, 1993.

40. Levin, M. F., et al.: Oral midazolam premedication in children: the minimum time interval for separation from parents. Can J Anaesth 40:726, 1993.

41. Heizmann, P., Eckert, M., Ziegler, W. H.: Pharmacokinetics and bioavailability of midazolam in man. Br J Clin Pharmacol 16:43S, 1983.

42. Greenblatt, D. J., et al.: Clinical pharmacokinetics of the newer benzodiazepines. Clin Pharmacokinet 8:233, 1983.

43. Reinhart, K.: Comparison of midazolam, diazepam and placebo intramuscularly as premedication for regional anaesthesia. Br J Anaesth 57:294, 1985.

43a. Collins, V. J. (ed.): Principles of Anesthesia, 3rd Ed. Philadelphia, Lea & Febiger, 1993.

44. Reves, J. G., Kissin, I., Smith, I. R.: The effective dose of midazolam. Anesthesiology 55:82, 1981.

45. Dundee, J. W.: New I. V. anaesthetics. Br J Anaesth 51:641, 1979.

46. Dundee, J. W., Wyant, G. M.: Intravenous Anaesthesia, 2nd Ed. Edinburgh, Churchill Livingstone, 1988.

47. Greenblatt, D. J., Locniskar, A., Ochs, H. R., Lauven, P. M.: Automated gas chromatography for studies of midazolam pharmacokinetics. Anesthesiology 55:176, 1981.

48. Greenblatt, D. J., et al.: Effect of age, gender, and obesity on midazolam kinetics. Anesthesiology 61:27, 1984.

49. Greenblatt, D. J.: Pharmacokinetics of midazolam. Sleep 5(Suppl 1), 1982.

50. Garzone, P. D., Kroboth, P. D.: Pharmacokinetics of the newer benzodiazepines. Clin Pharmacokinet 16:337, 1989.

51. Park, G. R., Manara, A. R., Dawling, S.: Extra-hepatic metabolism of midazolam. Br J Clin Pharmacol 27:634, 1989.

52. Smith, M. T., Eadie, M. T., Brophy, T.O'R.: The pharmacokinetics of midazolam in man. Eur J Clin Pharmacol 19:271, 1981.

53. Allonen, H., Ziegler, G., Klotz, U.: Midazolam kinetics. Clin Pharmacol Ther 30:653, 1981.

54. Klotz, U., Antonin, K-H., Bieck, P. R.: Pharmacokinetics and plasma binding of diazepam in man, dog, rabbit, guinea pig and rat. J Pharmacol Exp Ther 199:67, 1976.

55. Bell, G. D., et al.: Intravenous midazolam for upper gastrointestinal endoscopy: a study of 800 consecutive cases relating dose to age and sex of patient. Br J Clin Pharmacol 23:241, 1987.

56. Scholer, S. G., Schafer, D. F., Potter, J. F.: The effect of age on the relative potency of midazolam and diazepam for sedation in upper gastrointestinal endoscopy. J Clin Gastroenterol 12:145, 1990.

57. Klotz, U., et al.: The effects of age and liver disease on the disposition and elimination of diazepam in adult man. J Clin Invest 55:347, 1975.

58. Greenblatt, D. J., et al.: Diazepam disposition determinants. Clin Pharmacol Ther 27:301, 1980.

59. Gamble, J. A. S., Gaston, J. H., Nair, S. G., Dundee, J. W.: Some pharmacological factors influencing the absorption

of diazepam following oral administration. Br J Anaesth 48:1181, 1976.

60. McNeill, M. J., Ho, E.T., Kenny, G. N. C.: Effect of I.V. metoclopramide on gastric emptying after opioid premedication. Br J Anaesth 64:450, 1990.

61. Linnoila, M., Korttila, K., Mattila, M. F.: Effect of food and repeated injections on serum diazepam levels. Acta Pharmacol Toxicol 36:181, 1975.

62. Gamble, J. A. S., Dundee, J. W., Assaf, R. A. E.: Plasma diazepam levels after single dose oral and intramuscular administration. Anaesthesia 30:164, 1975.

63. Williams, R. L.: Drug administration in hepatic disease. N Engl J Med 309:1616, 1983.

64. Hegarty, J. E., Dundee, J. W.: Sequelae after the intravenous injection of three benzodiazepines—diazepam, lorazepam and flunitrazepam. Br Med J 1:1384, 1977.

65. de Jong, R. H., Bonin, J. D.: Benzodiazepines protect mice from local anesthetic convulsions and deaths. Anesth Analg 60:385, 1981.

66. Ausinsch, B., Malagodi, M. H., Munson, E. S.: Diazepam in the prophylaxis of lignocaine seizures. Br J Anaesth 48:309, 1976.

67. Haasio, J., Hekali, R., Rosenberg, P. H.: Influence of premedication of lignocaine-induced acute toxicity and plasma concentrations of lignocaine. Br J Anaesth 61:131, 1988.

68. Engstrom, R. H., Cohen, S. E.: A complication associated with the use of midazolam (Letter). Anesthesiology 70:719, 1989.

69. Dundee, J. W., et al.: Comparison of the actions of diazepam and lorazepam. Br J Anaesth 51:439, 1979.

70. Dundee, J. W., Lilburn, J. K., Nair, S. G., George, K. A.: Studies of drugs given before anaesthesia. XXVI: Lorazepam. Br J Anaesth 49:1047, 1977.

71. Bradshaw, E. G., Ali, A. A., Mulley, B. A., Rye, R. M.: Plasma concentrations and clinical effects of lorazepam after oral administration. Br J Anaesth 53:517, 1981.

72. Greenblatt, D. J., et al.: Pharmacokinetics and bioavailability of intravenous, intramuscular, and oral lorazepam in humans. J Pharm Sci 68:57, 1979.

73. Korttila, K., Tarkkanen, J.: Comparison of diazepam and midazolam for sedation during local anaesthesia for bronchoscopy. Br J Anaesth 57:581, 1985.

74. Boscoe, M. J., Dawling, S., Thompson, M. A., Jones, R. M.: Lorazepam in open-heart surgery: plasma concentrations before, during and after bypass following different dose regimens. Anaesth Intensive Care 12:9, 1984.

75. Pandit, S., Heisterkamp, A. V., Cohen, P. J.: Further studies of the anti-recall effect of lorazepam. Anesthesiology 45:495, 1976.

76. Fragen, R. J., Caldwell, N.: Lorazepam premedication: lack of recall and relief of anxiety. Anesth Analg 55:792, 1976.

77. Paymaster, N. J.: Lorazepam (WY 4036) as a preoperative medication. Anaesthesia 28:521, 1973.

78. Wangler, M. A., Kilpatrick, D. S.: Aminophylline is an antagonist of lorazepam. Anesth Analg 64:834, 1985.

79. Fuccella, L. M., et al.: Study of physiological availability of temazepam in man. Int J Clin Pharmacol 6:303, 1972.

80. Nicholson, A. N., Stone, B. M.: Effect of metabolites of diazepam, 3-hydroxydiazepam (temazepam), on sleep in man. Br J Clin Pharmacol 3:543, 1976.

81. Schwartz, H. J.: Lack of accumulation of temazepam after consecutive daily doses. Br J Clin Pharmacol 8:23, 1979.

82. Gosh, J. S.: Allergy to diazepam and other benzodiazepines. Br Med J 1:902, 1977.

83. Dundee, J. W.: Unpleasant sequelae of benzodiazepine sedation (Letter). Anaesthesia 45:336, 1990.

84. Lurie, Y., Gottesfeld, F., Bass, D. D.: Benzodiazepines and fantasy (Letter). Lancet 336:576, 1990.

85. Brahams, D.: Benzodiazepine sedation and allegations of sexual assault. Lancet 1:1339, 1989.

86. U.S. is asked to sharply limit use of sedative. New York Times, Feb. 14, 1988, p. I37.

87. Leary, W. E.: House report faults F.D.A. approval of sedative. New York Times, Oct. 18, 1988, p. C11.

88. Physicians' Desk Reference, 41st Ed. Oradell, NJ, Medical Economics, 1987, p. 1685.

89. Physicians' Desk Reference, 42nd Ed. Oradell, NJ, Medical Economics, 1988, p. 1754.

90. Arrowsmith, J. B., Gerstman, B. B., Fleischer, D. E., Benjamin, S. B.: Results from the American Society for Gastrointestinal Endoscopy/U.S. Food and Drug Administration collaborative study on complication rates and drug use during gastrointestinal endoscopy. Gastrointest Endosc 37:421, 1991.

91. Forster, A., Gardaz, J. P., Suter, P. M., Gemperle, M.: I.V. midazolam as an induction agent for anaesthesia: a study in volunteers. Br J Anaesth 52:907, 1980.

92. Sunzel, M., Paalzow, L., Berggren, L., Eriksson, I.: Respiratory and cardiovascular effects in relation to plasma levels of midazolam and diazepam. Br J Clin Pharmacol 25:561, 1988.

93. Samuelson, P. N., et al.: Hemodynamic responses to anesthetic induction with midazolam or diazepam in patients with ischemic heart disease. Anesth Analg 60:802, 1981.

94. Vinik, H. R., Bradley, E. L., Jr., Kissin, I.: Midazolam-alfentanil synergism for anesthetic induction in patients. Anesth Analg 69:213, 1989.

95. Kissin, I., Vinik, H. R., Castillo, R., Bradley, E. L., Jr.: Fentanyl potentiates midazolam-induced unconsciousness in subanalgesic doses. Anesth Analg 71:65, 1990.

96. Tverskoy, M., et al.: Midazolam acts synergistically with methohexitone for induction of anaesthesia. Br J Anaesth 63:109, 1989.

97. Tverskoy, M., et al.: Midazolam-morphine sedative interaction in patients. Anesth Analg 68:282, 1989.

98. Lauven, P. M.: Pharmacology of drugs for conscious sedation. Scand J Gastroenterol 25(Suppl 179):1, 1990.

99. Short, T. G., Galletly, D. C., Plummer, J. L.: Hypnotic and anaesthetic action of thiopentone and midazolam alone and in combination. Br J Anaesth 66:13, 1991.

100. Hartke, R. H., Gonzalez-Rothi, R. J., Abbey, N. C.: Midazolam-associated alterations in cardiorespiratory function during colonoscopy. Gastrointest Endosc 35:232, 1989.

101. Smith, D. C., Crul, J. F.: Oxygen desaturation following sedation for regional analgesia. Br J Anaesth 62:206, 1989.

102. Spiess, B. D., Sathoff, R. H., El-Ganzouri, A. R. S., Ivankovich, A. D.: High-dose sufentanil: four cases of sudden hypotension on induction. Anesth Analg 65:703, 1986.

103. West, J. M., Estrada, S., Heerdt, M.: Sudden hypotension associated with midazolam and sufentanil (Letter). Anesth Analg 66:693, 1987.

104. Heikkilä, H., et al.: Midazolam as adjunct to high-dose fentanyl anaesthesia for coronary artery bypass grafting operation. Acta Anaesthesiol Scand 28:683, 1984.

105. Marty, J., et al.: Effects of diazepam and midazolam on baroreflex control of heart rate and on sympathetic activity in humans. Anesth Analg 65:113, 1986.

106. Kotrly, K. J., et al.: Baroreceptor reflex control of heart rate during isoflurane anesthesia in humans. Anesthesiology 60:173, 1984.

107. Taylor, J. W., Simon, K. B.: Possible intramuscular midazolam-associated cardiorespiratory arrest and death. Ann Pharmacother 24:695, 1990.

108. Bell, G. D., et al.: Intravenous midazolam: a study of the degree of oxygen desaturation occurring during upper gastrointestinal endoscopy. Br J Clin Pharmacol 23:703, 1987.

109. O'Connor, K. W., Jones, S.: Oxygen desaturation is common and clinically underappreciated during elective endoscopic procedures. Gastrointest Endosc 36:S2, 1990.

110. Smith, D. C., Crul, J. F.: Oxygen desaturation following sedation for regional analgesia. Br J Anaesth 62:206, 1989.

111. Gross, J. B., Long, W. B.: Nasal oxygen alleviates hypoxemia in colonoscopy patients sedated with midazolam and meperidine. Gastrointest Endosc 36:26, 1990.

112. Jones, R. D. M., et al.: Effect of premedication on arterial blood gases prior to cardiac surgery. Anaesth Intensive Care 18:15, 1990.

113. Forster, A., Gardaz, J.-P., Suter, P. M., Gemperle, M.: Respiratory depression by midazolam and diazepam. Anesthesiology 53:494, 1980.

114. Knill, R., Cosgrove, J. F., Olley, P. M., Levison, H.: Components of respiratory depression after narcotic premedication in adolescents. Can Anaesth Soc J 23:449, 1976.

115. Bailey, P. L., et al.: Frequent hypoxemia and apnea after sedation with midazolam and fentanyl. Anesthesiology 73:826, 1990.

116. Gross, J. B., et al.: Time course of ventilatory depression after thiopental and midazolam in normal subjects and in patients with chronic obstructive pulmonary disease. Anesthesiology 58:540, 1983.

117. Eldridge, P. R., Punt, J. A.: Risks associated with giving benzodiazepines to patients with acute neurological injuries. Br Med J 300:1189, 1990.

118. Korttila, K., Linnoila, M.: Recovery and skills related to driving after intravenous sedation: dose-response relationship with diazepam. Br J Anaesth 47:457, 1975.

119. Galletly, D., Forrest, P., Purdie, G.: Comparison of the recovery characteristics of diazepam and midazolam. Br J Anaesth 60:520, 1988.

120. Korttila, K., Tarkkanen, J.: Comparison of diazepam and midazolam for sedation during local anaesthesia for bronchoscopy. Br J Anaesth 57:581, 1985.

121. White, P. F., et al.: Comparison of midazolam and diazepam for sedation during plastic surgery. Plast Reconstr Surg 81:703, 1988.

122. Clyburn, P., Kay, N. H., McKenzie, P. J.: Effects of diazepam and midazolam on recovery from anaesthesia in outpatients. Br J Anaesth 58:872, 1986.

123. Thomas, D., et al.: Triazolam premedication: a comparison with lorazepam and placebo in gynaecological patients. Anaesthesia 41:692, 1986.

124. Stoller, K. P., Belleville, J. P., Belleville, J. W.: Visual tracking following lorazepam or pentobarbital. Anesthesiology 45:565, 1976.

125. Philip, B. K.: Hazards of amnesia after midazolam in ambulatory surgical patients (Letter). Anesth Analg 66:97, 1987.

126. O'Boyle, C. A., et al.: Comparison of midazolam by mouth and diazepam I.V. in outpatient oral surgery. Br J Anaesth 59:746, 1987.

127. Liu, S., Miller, N., Waye, J. D.: Retrograde amnesia effects of intravenous diazepam in endoscopy patients. Gastrointest Endosc 30:340, 1984.

128. McKay, A. C., Dundee, J. W.: Effect of oral benzodiazepines on memory. Br J Anaesth 52:1247, 1980.

129. Clark, M. S., Silverstone, L. M., Coke, J. M., Hicks, J.: Midazolam, diazepam, and placebo as intravenous sedatives for dental surgery. Oral Surg Oral Med Oral Pathol 63:127, 1987.

130. Barclay, J. K., Hunter, K. M., McMillan, W.: Midazolam and diazepam compared as sedatives for outpatient surgery under local analgesia. Oral Surg Oral Med Oral Pathol 59:349, 1985.

131. Raeder, J. C., Brejvik, H.: Premedication with midazolam in outpatient general anesthesia: a comparison with morphine-scopolamine and placebo. Acta Anaesthesiol Scand 31:509, 1987.

132. McKay, A. C., Dundee, J. W.: Effect of oral benzodiazepines on memory. Br J Anaesth 52:1247, 1980.

133. Greenblatt, D. J., Allen, M. D., Noel, B. J., Shader, R. I.: Acute overdosage with benzodiazepine derivatives. Clin Pharmacol Ther 21:497, 1977.

134. Lawton, M. P., Cahn, B.: The effects of diazepam (Valium) and alcohol on psychomotor performance. J Nerv Ment Dis 136:550, 1963.

135. Davis, J. M., Bartlett, E., Termini, B. A.: Overdosage of psychotropic drugs: a review. Dis Nerv Syst 29:157, 1968.

136. Bidwai, A. V., et al.: Reversal of diazepam-induced postanesthetic somnolence with physostigmine. Anesthesiology 51:256, 1979.

137. DiLiberti, J., O'Brien, M. L., Turner, T.: The use of physostigmine as an antidote in accidental diazepam intoxication. J Pediatr 86:106, 1975.

138. Ghoneim, M. M., Mewaldt, J. P., Berie, J. L., Hinrichs, J. V.: Memory and performance effects of single and three week administration of diazepam. Psychopharmacology 73:147, 1981.

139. Stirt, J. A.: Aminophylline is a diazepam antagonist. Anesth Analg 60:767, 1981.

140. Phillis, J. W., et al.: Theophylline antagonizes flurazepam-induced depression of cerebral cortical neurons. Can J Physiol Pharmacol 57:917, 1979.

141. Lauven, P. M., Schwilden, H., Stoeckel, H., Greenblatt, D. J.: The effects of a benzodiazepine antagonist Ro 15-1788 in the presence of stable concentrations of midazolam. Anesthesiology 63:61, 1985.

142. Darragh, A., et al.: Investigation in man of the efficacy of a benzodiazepine antagonist, Ro 15-1788. Lancet 2:8, 1981.

143. Dodgson, M. S., et al.: Antagonism of diazepam-induced sedative effects by Ro 15-1788 in patients after surgery under lumbar epidural block: a double-blind placebo-controlled investigation of efficacy and safety. Acta Anaesthesiol Scand 31:629, 1987.

144. Amrein, L., et al.: Clinical pharmacology of Dormicum (midazolam) an Anexate (flumazenil). Resuscitation 16:S5, 1988.

145. Forster, A., Rouiller, M., Morel, D., Gemperle, M.: Double-blind randomized study evaluating a specific benzodiazepine antagonist. Anesthesiology 59:A375, 1983.

146. Wolff, J., Carl, P., Clausen, T. G., Mikkelsen, B. O.: Ro 15-1788 for postoperative recovery: a randomised clinical trial in patients undergoing minor surgical procedures under midazolam anaesthesia. Anaesthesia 41:1001, 1986.

147. Klotz, U., Ziegler, G., Reimann, I. W.: Pharmacokinetics of the selective benzodiazepine antagonist Ro 15-1788 in man. Eur J Clin Pharmacol 27:115, 1984.

148. Sage, D. J., Close, A., Boas, R. A.: Reversal of midazolam sedation with anexate. Br J Anaesth 59:459, 1987.

149. Louis, M., Forster, A., Suter, P. M., Gemperle, M.: Clinical and hemodynamic effects of a specific benzodiazepine antagonist after open heart surgery. Anesthesiology 61:A61, 1984.

150. O'Boyle, C., et al.: Ro 15-1788 antagonizes the effects of diazepam in man without affecting its bio-availability. Br J Anaesth 55:349, 1983.

151. Whitman, J. G.: Benzodiazepines (Editorial). Anaesthesia 42:1255, 1987.

Chapter 31

OPIATE AND NARCOTIC DRUGS

VINCENT J. COLLINS

"Among the remedies which it has pleased Almighty God to give to man to relieve his sufferings, none is so universal and so efficacious as opium."—Sydenham, 1680

OPIUM DRUGS

The natural plant product opium has played a role in the relief of pain and the production of sleep for centuries. "Opium" is a Greek word designating a drug obtained from the milky exudate of the unripe seed capsule of the opium poppy native to Asia Minor. Crude extracts were employed until the nineteenth century, when the German apothecary, Serturner, isolated the principal alkaloid and named it morphine (1803).

Chemistry of Opium[1]

Opium powder contains several ingredients, but the pharmacologically active constituents are alkaloids. These comprise about 25% of the weight of opium. About 25 alkaloids have been identified, and these may be divided into two groups: (1) the *phenanthrene group*, which yields the narcotics; and (2) the *isoquinoline group*, which yields papaverine and other related substances.

Morphine constitutes 10% of the opium powder and is the most important member of the phenanthrene alkaloids. The major natural biosynthetic steps leading to morphine in the opium poppy have been elucidated.[2] Tracer experiments using radioactive carbon in the amino acid tyrosine reveals the following sequence of chemical transformations[2]: tyrosine—norlaudanosine—reticuline—salutaridine—thebaine—codeine—morphine.

Structure of Morphine

The chemical structure of morphine was determined in 1925 by Gulland and Robinson.[3] This structure was verified by Gates and Tschudi in 1952,[4,5] who proceeded to effect the first total synthesis of morphine (Fig. 31–1).

In the formula, one notes chemical groups of fundamental importance. First is the phenanthrene nucleus; second are two hydroxyl groups important from the standpoint of pharmacologic action; third, the tertiary nitrogen renders the compound basic in reaction and capable of forming salts; fourth, the ethenamine bridge containing the nitrogen is necessary for its central nervous system (CNS) activity.

Regarding chemical structure and activity certain generalizations may be made:

1. Narcotic action is dependent on an intact nitrogen ring. Opening the nitrogen ring abolishes narcotic activity.
2. Narcotic potency depends on the phenolic hydroxyl. Actions dependent on this group include analgesia, hypnosis, respiratory depression, enhanced smooth muscle tone (action on myenteric plexus and bronchiolar muscle), and ureteral and biliary tract spasm. Masking of this "OH" (as by methylation) decreases the foregoing effects.
3. The alcoholic hydroxyl is responsible for central stimulant effects. The phenolic depressant effects are counteracted by this group. The emetic attribute is dependent on this hydroxyl. If this "OH" is masked by acetylation, however, the narcotic and respiratory depressant actions are enhanced.
4. Removal of the double bond adjacent to the alcoholic hydroxyl increases analgesic activity as well as the depressant effects.

Analgesic activity depends on the presence of a τ-phenyl-N-methyl piperidine group (Fig. 31–2). The piperidine ring has a chair shape and is not in the same plane as the phenyl ring.[6] This special grouping is common to all morphine, benzmorphan, and meperidine derivatives, and the methadone compounds also assume this structure. Morphine has two water-repelling surfaces at right angles to each other. The quarternary N-ion is able to form ionic bonds.

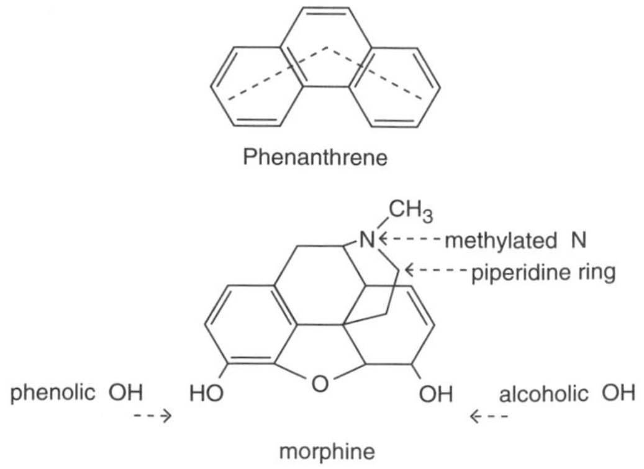

Fig. 31–1. The structure of morphine.

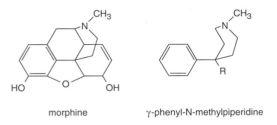

morphine   γ-phenyl-N-methylpiperidine

Fig. 31–2. The active moiety for analgesia in morphine is the τ-phenyl-N-methyl piperidine group.

Analgesic activity of opiates is also highly stereoscopic. Almost all activity resides in those isomers with a configuration analogous to that of D (—) morphine (levorotatory).[7]

Opiate Receptors

Locations

Opiate receptors were first identified in 1973 by Pert and Snyder.[8] Receptors have been demonstrated in several CNS locations, they are discretely distributed in subcellular fractions of synaptic membranes, and the greatest binding occurs in the microsomal fraction.[7] High-affinity areas are strikingly related to the paleospinothalamic pathway and the medial portion of the thalamus. This latter area subserves dull, chronic, and poorly localized pain[8] (Fig. 31–3).

An abundance of receptors also exist in the *limbic system,* the amygdala, the corpus striatum, and the hypothalamus. These areas are related to emotional components of the pain experience and are involved in euphoric responses to opiate administration. The amount of such receptors is far less in the cortex.

The order of distribution of opiate receptors from the highest concentration to the lowest in the CNS is as follows: globus pallidus—periaqueductal gray—medial thalamus—amygdala—pontile areas—medulla—caudate—putamen—lateral thalamus—hypothalamus—cerebellum—hippocampal gyrus.

In the spinal cord, clusters of receptors are located in the substantia gelatinosa,[9,10] where significant concentrations are found in lamina I and lamina V. The administration of morphine intrathecally produces analgesia and modification of operant behavior.[11] Moreover, serotonin injected intrathecally produces an antinociceptive effect, but the receptors for serotonin appear to be different than the opiate receptor.[12]

Studies by Yaksh at the Mayo Foundation show two distinct subpopulations of opiate receptors, μ and δ, which mediate analgesia. The opioid alkaloids, as well as 31-amino acid polypeptide β-endorphin, preferentially bind to μ receptors, small peptides, all analogues of enkephalin; and particularly, two pentapeptides—leu-enkephalin and metkephamid—interact with the δ receptor.[13-15]

Enkephalinergic terminals are numerous in this part of the spinal cord, and the small interneurons may serve to regulate the activity of primary sensory afferents.[15]

Enkephalin-containing nerve terminals and appropriate receptors of the opiate type are also found in the nerve terminals in the duodenum. Specifically, these terminals are found in Meissner's plexus. Enkephalin is probably a neurotransmitter, affecting the motility of the gastrointestinal tract.

Other areas of concentration of the receptor protein include solitary nuclei and the periventricular gray areas along the midline of the brain stem.

Endogenous Pain Control[16]

Enkephalinergic nerve terminals are also prevalent in areas rich in opiate receptors and wherever sensory pain traffic is heavy.[17]

The periaqueductal gray matter is a well-recognized area for sensory and pain traffic. The neurons contain significant quantities of enkephalin. Stimulation of this area produces analgesia. Generally, stimulation of the midbrain nucleus, raphe magnus, produces analgesia and pain relief. If naloxone is administered, however, no analgesia is produced. Furthermore, if the dorsal lateral funiculus in the spinal cord, which passes through the periaqueductal gray matter, is cut, no analgesia ensues. This funiculus is a descending pathway to the spinal cord, and the transmitter at the terminations of the neurons of the axon is serotonin. If serotonin is blocked (by lysergic acid diethylamide or by chlorphenylalanine), no analgesia ensues.

Drugs that stimulate serotonin mechanisms enhance analgesia,[12] and drugs that deplete catecholamines and increase plasma levels diminish analgesia. So long as the noradrenergic neurons contain a full complement of catecholamines that is not released, analgesia continues. Thus, noradrenergic receptor blocking agents (action at postsynaptic membrane) that permit reuptake by α-adrenergic fibers enhance analgesia.

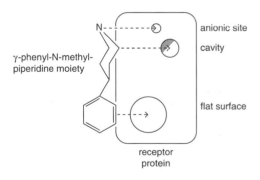

γ-phenyl-N-methyl-piperidine moiety

anionic site

cavity

flat surface

receptor protein

Fig. 31–3. Receptor attachment of morphine and its analogues is related to the piperidine group, as illustrated. The positively charged N of the piperidine moiety, in the same plane as the aromatic (phenyl) ring, is attracted by the anionic site; the chair form of the piperidine ring fits into the cavity at a different plane; the aromatic ring is attached at a cationic site and held flat to the surface by van der Waal's forces (from Cutting). From Beckett, N., Casey, A. F.: Receptor attachment of morphine to the piperidine group. J Pharm Pharmacol 6:986, 1954.

Nature of the Receptor

The nature of the receptor is that of a proteolipid, and this binding substance is most abundant in the brain and the corpus striatum.[8] Studies on brain tissue for the opiate receptor on neurons show that the greatest binding occurs in the microsomal fraction especially of the corpus striatums.[8] At least two different conformations are possible, and the same receptor is capable of binding with either the agonist or the antagonist.[18] The binding between the proteolipid and morphine, with respect to analgesia and respiratory depression, is prevented by naloxone, but not by other antagonists.[7] Sodium ions alter the extent of the binding of the agonist. The agonist form of the receptor is thus a minimum sodium receptor.[10] On this basis, a sodium index has been developed that correlates with potency. The index is a ratio of concentration of the opiate required to inhibit the antagonist naloxone in the presence of sodium over concentration in the absence of sodium. Naloxone has an index of 1; morphine has a weak index of 12; benzomorphan has an index of 3 to 7.

According to Jacquet,[19] two separate classes of opioid receptors exist in the CNS: (1) an endorphin receptor, which has stereospecific affinity for opiates, mediates analgesic and catatonic effects, and is naloxone sensitive—this has been designated the μ receptor; (2) a second receptor, which shows nonstereospecific affinity for opiates, is naloxone insensitive, and mediates the behavioral hyperexcitability effects of morphine (explosive motor behavior). It has been designated as the δ receptor by Lord and Kosterlitz and their associates.[20,21] The first receptor has affinity for morphine and endorphins. This receptor, when occupied by an opiate, appears to have an inhibitory action on the second; if it is unoccupied or is occupied by the antagonist, explosive behavior similar to abstinence syndrome ensues.[22] The second receptor has affinity for adrenocorticotropic peptide hormones. Administration into the periaqueductal gray matter of ACTH produces an abstinence syndrome. Metkephamid, an analogue of methionine enkephalin, has potent opioid δ receptor activity.[23,24]

The presence of two types of opiate receptors may explain the studies on induced pain and on mood by Goldstein.[24,25] Human subjects who are submitted to ischemic pain when given naloxone do not have any change in their pain ratings. The pain is not accentuated. After the induction and establishment of pain, however, naloxone does provide a significant elevation of mood and a decrease in anxiety.

Type of Receptor Binding[25]

On the basis of observed structure of enkephalin-type receptors and the structure of known agonists, investigators have proposed five intermolecular binding arrangements. The receptor seems to conform to three hydrophilic regions of the agonist molecule and to two hydrophobic groups. The hydrophilicity involves an intermolecular hydrogen binding at the amino group, the hydroxyl group, and the carboxyl groups.[24]

Endogenous Opioids[25]

Endogenous morphine-like substances have been isolated from various brain structures where opiate receptors exist. These were termed endorphins by Lord and associates.[20] They represent a class of physiologically active long-chain peptides from which small peptide chain fragments, the pentapeptides, called "enkephalins," are derived that have a molecular weight of less than 1000.[25] These pentapeptides are discretely concentrated, not randomly distributed, and appear to act as *neuromodulutors* or inhibitory *neurotransmitters* at enkephalinergic nerve terminals.[24,26]

The highest concentrations are at the very sites where the opiate receptors are prevalent,[27] as well as (especially the endorphins) in the pituitary gland. It appears that endogenous plasma opioid peptides follow a diurnal rhythm: low plasma levels in early morning hours (4 A.M. to 12 noon) and high levels from 12 noon to midnight.

Balagot has demonstrated that the administration of D-phenylalanine (PA) increases synthesis as well as the plasma levels of enkephalins. The increase in levels produced by phenylalanine is in part due to the ability of this amino acid to inhibit two enzymes, carboxypeptidase and leucine amino peptidase, which function to destroy enkephalins. The oral dose of PA is of the order of 1.0 g per day.

Stress-Induced Analgesia

Studies in animals and humans show that repetitive stress raises the pain threshold and the level of plasma endorphins.[28] Either anticipation of pain or repetitive sural nerve stimulation raises the human threshold to a nociceptive stimulus for a flexion reflex of lower limb. Also demonstrable is that naloxone completely antagonizes this type of analgesia and indeed produces hyperalgesia.[29]

Naloxone has also been shown to antagonize the analgesia of general anesthesia.[29]

Pain Neurotransmitter

Substance P, next to enkephalin, is the most carefully studied brain peptide and resembles the distributions of neurotensin and enkephalin. Its role as a sensory transmitter is well supported[28]:

- It occurs in 20% of dorsal root ganglion cells; these cells have processes extending into lamina I and the substantia gelatinosa (lamina II), where noxious stimuli are received.
- Cutting the dorsal root causes degeneration of terminals in the gray matter of the posterior gray horns, especially lamina I and II.
- Spinal cord neurons excited by substance P are the same as those responding to painful stimuli.
- This substance also regulates axon reflexes causing vasodilatation in injured areas.
- The release of substance P in the spinal dorsal horns is blocked by opiates.
- Neurons containing enkephalin and those containing substance P are juxtaposed in many areas.

- In striatonigral pathways, the τ-aminobutyric acid (GABA) system parallels the P fiber system.
- Areas with a rich content include amygdala, periaqueductal gray, and raphe nuclei. Cells projecting to preoptic area are rich in substance P.

Bradykinin is also a pain-provoking substance. It appears to be the most potent pain-producing substance. The principal group of cells producing bradykinin is in the hypothalamus.

Pituitary Opiate Receptors[25]

Evidence has accumulated that the hypophysis plays a role in pain perception and pain inhibition. This involves an endorphinergic mechanism. In animals, naloxone produces hyperalgesia, whereas in the hypophysectomized animal, naloxone does not produce this effect. Severe stress has been shown to produce analgesia, which appears to be associated with an increase in *endorphin* activity in the pituitary, with the simultaneous release of ACTH and β-endorphin.[30] Hypophysectomy eliminates these responses, however.

Enkephalinergic cell bodies have been demonstrated in the nuclei of the hypothalamus. In turn, enkephalinergic nerve fibers have also been demonstrated to project from the hypothalamus into the pars nervosa of the pituitary.[31] Further, opiate receptors have been demonstrated in the pituitary gland itself.[32]

Thus, an anatomic basis for central pain mechanisms is available. A painful stress stimulus reaching the CNS and stimulating the hypothalamus increases endorphins and acts on the receptors in the pituitary to relieve pain. Similarly, an exogenous opioid also relieves pain by block at the pituitary receptor level.

In a study measuring evoked potentials in the pituitary and the somatosensory cortex by stimulating tooth pulp, Trouwborst has demonstrated the involvement of the hypophyseal-pituitary complex in pain and opiate analgesia.[33] After the administration of fentanyl, tooth pulp-evoked potentials at the pituitary were facilitated with a simultaneous increase in endorphins, whereas the evoked potentials from the primary somatosensory cortex were markedly inhibited.

Classification of Opioid Receptor Systems (Table 31–1)

Opioids may be classified by type of receptor binding.[34-36] Clinical evidence, dissimilar pharmacologic profiles of various opioid agents, different sensitivity to naloxone, and changes in seizure threshold in animals by different opioids have permitted the opioids to be subdivided into four receptor groups[37,38]:

1. Group 1 (μ agonist receptor)
   Prototype: morphine
   Others: methadone, levorphanol, and phenazocine
   Effect attenuated by naloxone; tolerance develops
2. Group 2 (σ agonist receptor)
   Prototype: cyclazocine
   Effect not attenuated by naloxone

Table 31–1. Multiple Opioid Receptor Systems

μ Receptor	Medullary MS receptor; nalbuphine to some extent
σ Receptor	Agonist-antagonist class; dysphoria
κ Receptor	Spinal and supraspinal locus; MS acts here to a lesser extent Agonist-antagonist group acts to great extent; may be selection for spinal-epidural anesthesia to avoid delayed respiratory depression
δ Receptor	Enkephalins; reciprocates with μ receptor

MS = morphine sulfate.
Gilbert, P. E., Martin, R. W.: Multiple opioid receptor systems. J. Pharmacol. Exp. Ther. *198*:66, 1976.

3. Group 3 (κ agonist receptor)
   Prototype: normorphine; naloxone itself
   No consistent dose-related effect on seizures
4. Group 4 (δ designation?)
   Prototype: pentazocine
   Others: meperidine, enkephalins
   Effects on seizure potentiated by naloxone

MORPHINE

For the alleviation of pain and to provide freedom from anxiety, morphine is the classic and dependable agent. It furnishes the primary desirable attributes of a narcotic, namely, analgesia, euphoria, or more important, dissociation and subjective depression. The various psychologic effects and sedation outlast the simple analgesic effect by many hours. Many opiates have been refined and synthesized, but most substitutes have not been an improvement over morphine and at the same time have introduced their own undesirable side effects.

Locus of Action

The action of morphine on the CNS appears to be diffuse; all levels of integration are affected. Selective action occurs at the cortical level at the diencephalic centers, at corpus striatum, at the brain stem, and at the spinal level. Both depressant and stimulant actions occur at all levels of neuraxis, apparently at interneurons. Analgesics appear to have five principal sites of action[39]:

1. Synapses between receptor neurons and connector neurons of pain afferents in the spinal cord (substantia gelatinosa).
2. At the interneurons medial to the posteroventral nucleus of the thalamus.
3. At the hypothalamus.
4. At the thalamic projection system and amygdala.
5. At the interneurons of the cortex.

Mechanism of Action

Data on decorticate and spinal preparations indicate that analgesic effects are produced by two mechanisms:

1. Depression of supraspinal facilitatory centers.
2. Direct depression of spinal reflex centers.

In regard to the most important therapeutic effect, relief of pain, it appears that the elevation of pain threshold at the thalamic nuclei plays a lesser role, whereas alterations in reaction to pain stimuli are of major importance.

Biochemical evidence indicates that morphine does affect cerebral oxidative activity and acetylcholine metabolism. The esterase of acetylcholine is inhibited.[40] Probably, if the opiate receptor is associated with a neurotransmitter, then acetylcholine is the agent.[40]

Doses

Morphine may be safely administered by the subcutaneous, intramuscular, or intravenous route. The dose should be based on physiologic age plus a consideration of those factors influencing metabolic rate. Safety in the use of this and other drugs depends on the ability to prescribe a proper dose. Doses ordinarily should not exceed 0.2 mg/kg of body weight.

The optimal dose of morphine for pain relief in the average adult male (70 kg) is about 10 mg.[41] Comparison of different doses reveals that a 10-mg dose affords 74% pain relief, whereas 15 mg merely increases the extent of relief to 84%. The administration of morphine before the onset of pain is much more effective than administration in the presence of pain.

In addition, morphine provides unique relief from the anxiety attached to the anticipation of pain.[42]

The initial dose of morphine in the presence of pain is less effective than subsequent doses. The better response to second doses is thought to be due to a "priming" effect, but it may merely mean that the pain was of greater severity initially.

The use of a narcotic as part of preanesthetic medication delays the onset of postoperative pain.[43] The need for analgesics is significantly delayed when morphine is part of the preanesthetic medication. Thus, patients receiving a placebo or a barbiturate preoperatively require an analgesic 2½ hours sooner than patients treated with morphine. Moreover, morphine relieves moderate pain longer, i.e., about 5½ hours, as compared with 4 hours in the presence of severe pain.[44]

To achieve the objective of good preanesthetic medication, the following average doses are recommended for adults:

Adult male dose (70 kg): 10 mg
Adult female dose (60 kg): 8 mg (or about 75% of male dose)

If a dose greater than 15 mg is to be administered in a short period, it should be given in divided doses. In general, the onset of action of some important morphine effects after subcutaneous injection are maximal respiratory

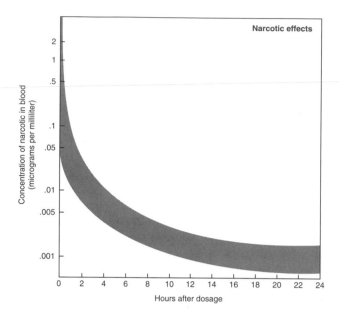

Fig. 31–4. Pharmacokinetics as related to analgesic effects of morphine. Redrawn from Vincent Doyle, 1978.

depression (30 minutes), maximal analgesia and reduction of basal metabolism (60 minutes), and maximal sedative effect (90 minutes) (Fig. 31–4).

Some of the undesirable effects of morphine are partly counteracted by combination with a belladonna drug.[45] This subject of balanced doses is discussed elsewhere.[45a]

Children are proportionately more sensitive to morphine and narcotics than adults. This is probably due to greater permeability of infant brain.[46] A general rule for determining dose is as follows:

For first 20 lb or 1 year of age: 1 mg
For each additional 10 lb: 1 mg
  OR
For each additional 1 lb: 0.1 mg

Diurnal Rhythm Analgesic Effect

A diurnal rhythm in the analgesic activity of morphine has been observed. During early and morning hours, the analgesic response to administered morphine is diminished. Painful stimuli produce a heightened response. Later, during the hours of noon to midnight, an increased effect of morphine coincides with the circadian increase in blood levels of endogenous opioids. At these times, especially in the late afternoon and early evening hours, one sees a diminished response to painful stimuli, and analgesics have an enhanced effect. From noon to midnight, the circadian rhythm of glucocorticoids is at progressively lower levels when the opioids are at higher levels[47] (Fig. 31–5).

Effect of Age on Analgesic Response[48]

Age has been found to alter the response to morphine.: after 40 years, an increasing analgesic effect is seen with a given dose of morphine of about 10 to 15% per decade.[48]

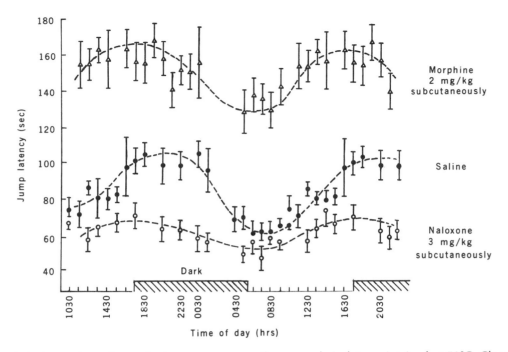

Fig. 31–5. Diurnal rhythm in latencies to the jump response on the mouse hot plate maintained at 52°C. Closed circles refer to animals treated with saline, subcutaneously, 15 minutes before testing. Open circles refer to animals treated with naloxone at 3 mg/kg, subcutaneously, 15 minutes before testing. Open triangles refer to animals treated with morphine at 2 mg/kg, subcutaneously, 30 minutes before testing. The latencies (mean ± S.E., N = 10 to 100) in seconds are plotted as a function of the time of day. The datum points at each half-hour are the means of values collected over a 1-hour period. For example, the points plotted at 0930 hours are the means of measurements made from 0900 to 1000 hours. Lights were off during the time period marked by the hatched bars. Several points are repeated beyond 24 hours to better illustrate the rhythm. From Frederickson, R. C.: Diurnal rhythm in response to pain and to action of morphine: hyperalgesic induced by naloxone. Science 198:756, 1977.

Hormonal Effects[49]

Release of growth hormone and prolactin is stimulated, whereas release of leuteinizing hormone (LH) is blocked. Antidiuretic hormone (ADH) release is stimulated. These effects are secondary to a pronounced action on the hypothalamus.

Pharmacokinetics

Absorption[50]

Differences in rate of absorption depend on the route of administration. All the opium alkaloids are poorly absorbed from the gastrointestinal tract, but the process is unpredictable. Orally administered morphine is effective but variable. The parenteral to oral dose ratio is one fourth to one sixth the subcutaneous dose; that is, 40 to 60 mg orally is about effective as 10 mg subcutaneously. Rectal absorption occurs, and morphine as well as other opioids can be administered by suppository. Absorption from subcutaneous sites is variable and depends on state of circulation. The only assured route of administration is the intravenous route. This is the choice in states of cardiocirculatory impairment (shock, vasoconstriction).

Pharmacokinetic Data

After intravenous administration of 10 mg, the disappearance of morphine from plasma generally follows a triexponential function[51,52] (Table 31-2 and Fig. 31-6). The initial disposition of morphine is rapid and appears to be complete within an average of 3.0 minutes. The apparent distribution is extensive, and the total volume averages about 3.0 L/kg. This is due to high lipid and tissue uptake. After 3.0 minutes, when the plasma level varies between 30 and 40 ng/ml, the disappearance from plasma proceeds more slowly, and the half-life of this phase averages slightly less than 3.0 hours.[51] At 3 hours, the plasma level ranges from 5 to 10 ng/ml.[52] The mean total clearance has been determined at about 15 ml/min/kg (14.7), consistent with an hepatic extraction ratio of 0.7. This assumes that hepatic biotransformation accounts for nearly all morphine clearance and a hepatic blood flow of 21 ml/min/kg. Age influences the plasma morphine concentrations, which fall more rapidly in the elderly than in the young,[54] but the duration of analgesia is longer at lower administered doses in the elderly[55,56] (Fig. 31-7).

On the basis of extensive hepatic clearance, about 70% of orally administered morphine is biotransformed on first pass through the liver, and only 30% reaches the systemic circulation. Within 12 hours, plasma levels fall to less than 2.5 ng/ml. Terminal elimination time extends from 18 to 60 hours, however[57] (Table 31-3).

After intramuscular injection, absorption is rapid and complete. A mean peak plasma level of 5.6 ng/ml is reached between 7.5 and 20 minutes after injection. The apparent first-order absorption half-life ranges between 3 and 12 minutes, and total absorption is usually complete in 45 minutes.

Table 31–2. Pharmocokinetic Variables Following Intravenous Morphine

	Spector*	Stanski†	Dahlstrom‡ (perioperative)
Dilution phase II (minutes)	1.8	1.25	1.4 ± 0.4
$T_{1/2}$-α (minutes)	5–10	7.7(± 1.6)	16 ± 7
$T_{1/2}$-β (hours)	3.1	2.9	3.8 ± 2.3
Total elimination (Hours)	10–44	—	12–24
Volume Distribution	—	3.2 L/kg	6.3 ± 3 L/kg
Clearance (ml/min/kg)	—	14.7(± 0.9)	20 ± 7.0
		(healthy volunteers)	
Extraction Ratio	—	0.7	—

*Data from Spector, S.: Disposition of morphine sulfate in man. Science *174*:421, 1972.
†Data from Stanski, D. R., Greenblatt, D. J., Lowenstein, E.: Kinetics of intravenous and intramuscular morphine. Clin Pharmacol Ther *24*:52, 1978.
‡The perioperative and postoperative study by Dahlstrom and associates of effects of anesthesia and surgery. Some significant alteration of clearance occurred; i.e., it is more rapid. It slowed if shock or protracted surgery occurred. Postoperative dynamics showed a severalfold variation in morphine analgesic needs.
Data from Dahlstrom, B., Tamsen, A., Paalzow, L., Hartvig, P.: Patient-controlled analgesic therapy. Part IV. Pharmacokinetics and analgesic plasma concentrations of morphine. Clin Pharmacol Ther *7*:266, 1982.

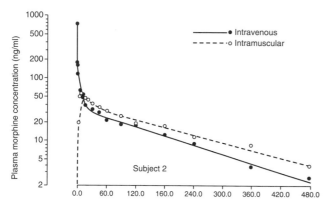

Fig. 31–6. Plasma morphine concentrations following intravenous and intramuscular administration of morphine. Redrawn from Stanski, D. R., Greenblatt, D. J., Lowenstein, E.: Kinetics of intravenous and intramuscular morphine. Clin Pharmacol Ther *24*:52, 1978.

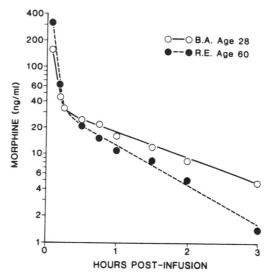

Fig. 31–7. Plasma morphine concentration-time curves for an elderly and a young individual representative of each group. Morphine concentrations are expressed as nanograms of morphine base per milliliter of plasma. From Owen, J. A., et al.: Age-related morphine kinetics. Clin Pharmacol Ther *34*:365, 1983.

The elimination half-life and clearance are similar to those after intravenous administration. After 12 hours, the plasma levels fall to less than 2.5 ng/ml. After large intravenous doses of morphine (45 to 80 mg infused at a rate of 5 mg/min), the apparent elimination half-life of about 4 to 5 hours is longer than after smaller doses.[58]

Uptake

After absorption, morphine is distributed to all the parenchymatous tissues of the body. This has been demonstrated by means of radioactive tagging techniques. A great part of the injected drug is found in skeletal muscle, but the concentration is a lower level than in other tissues. Although the chief site of action is in the CNS, only small quantities of morphine pass the blood-brain barrier under normal physiologic conditions.[59]

According to the pH partition hypothesis, an alkaline medium increases the availability of uncharged base and increases not only lipid solubility but also penetrability.[60] Uptake by brain areas and binding by gray matter have been studied by radioactive 14C morphine. In the brain tissue, a two- to threefold entry and an increase in brain concentration during metabolic or respiratory alkalosis occur.[61] These effects coincide with clinical reports on enhanced morphine and meperidine analgesia in the presence of alkalosis.[62] The binding to certain brain regions is definitely enhanced and demonstrates an increase in the usual concentrations in the amygdala nucleus area, in the periaqueductal gray, and the thalamus. The binding is related to lipophilicity, and this is pH dependent and in accordance with the pH partition hypothesis.

Table 31–3. Pharmacokinetic Data: Morphine*

Availability (Oral) (%)	Urinary Excretion (%)	Bound in Plasma (%)	Clearance (ml · min⁻¹ · kg⁻¹)	Vol. Dist. (L/kg)	Half-Life (h)	Effective Concentrations
24 ± 12	6–10	35 ± 2 ↓ AVH, Cirr, Alb	24 ± 10 ⟷ Aged, Cirr, Urem, Child ↓ Neo	3.3 ± 0.9 ⟷ Cirr, Urem	1.9 ± 0.5 ⟷ Cirr, Urem, Child ↑ Neo	65 ± 80 ng/ml†

*Active metabolite, morphine-6-glucuronide; $T_{1/2}$ = 4.0 ± 1.5 hours (50 ± 37 hours in uremia).
†To achieve surgical analgesia.
From Gilman, A. G., et al.: Goodman and Gilman's The Pharmacological Basis of Therapeutics, 8th Ed. New York, McGraw-Hill, 1990.

Plasma Protein Binding

About 36% is bound to protein. Most of the morphine (80 to 90%) is "bound" to plasma albumin and to a lesser extent to the plasma globulin, but not to any of the lipoproteins. The binding is increased in addicts and is decreased in patients with hepatic or renal failure.

Metabolism and Excretion

Morphine is almost completely metabolized in the liver, principally by glucuronidation by hepatic glucuronal transferase.[63] About 10% is destroyed by demethylation with the formation of inactive normorphine. Two chief compounds are produced by conjugation with glucuronide and are more water soluble than the parent compound.

In humans, 85% is eliminated as the morphine glucuronide metabolites and 5% as normorphine in the urine along with less than 5% unchanged morphine. A portion of the morphine glucuronide metabolites, about 8%, is eliminated in the bile. Approximately 90% of all morphine compounds are excreted (cleared from the body) in 12 to 24 hours.[64]

Morphine-3-glucuronide is the major metabolite. In animal studies, it exhibits some analgesic activity.[65] The other metabolite, 6β-morphine-glucuronide, has great analgesic potency and has been detected in humans in small amounts.[65,66]

Extrahepatic metabolism of morphine has been suggested in humans from a study of total body clearance of morphine. Total body clearance is about 38% greater than the hepatic clearance. An extrahepatic, extraintestinal metabolism of morphine is suggested to occur via the kidney.[67]

Pharmacokinetics in Infants[68]

In infants less than 10 weeks old, morphine has a longer elimination half-life and a lower clearance value than in older infants and children. In the newborn and in infants up to 4 days old, the elimination half-life is about 6.8 hours, versus 4.0 hours in older infants (2 weeks to 2 months). This compares with the adult value of about 2.0 hours.

The clearance in early infancy is about one third that seen in older infants and is represented as about 6.3 versus 2.4 ml/kg/min. The clearance in infants over 1 month old using steady-state infusion methods is about 19 ml/kg/min, which is comparable to children from 1 to 17 years of age. In the unanesthetized adult, the clearance rate is about 12 ml/kg/min. Early maturation of morphine clearance occurs by 1 year of age and continues through childhood. Processes of elimination in older infants and children appear to approach (or surpass) those of the adult at an early age.[69]

Pharmacokinetics in Cirrhosis

Morphine has a longer terminal half-life in patients with cirrhosis of the liver than in normal subjects.[70] The rate of metabolism is also decreased. Studies of unchanged morphine, using a highly specific immunoassay, show the terminal half-life to be 201 ± 39 minutes in cirrhotic patients, compared with 111 ± 32 minutes in normal subjects.[71] This prolongation is related to a lower total body clearance. In normal subjects, clearance is of the order of 33.5 ± 8 ml · min⁻¹ · kg⁻¹ whereas in the cirrhotic patients without ascites but impaired function, the clearance is lower, at 21 ± 7.5 ml · min⁻¹ · kg⁻¹. Two mechanisms probably cause this slower elimination: a decrease in the hepatic extraction ratio and a decrease in hepatic blood flow. Cirrhosis is usually associated with significant decreased blood flow.[72] Other factors such as volume of distribution at steady state (V_{ss}), the volume of central compartment, and the volume of distribution do not differ significantly from normal versus cirrhotic subjects.

Pharmacokinetics in Renal Failure

In chronic renal failure, unchanged morphine is readily metabolized by hepatic glucuronyl transferase to morphine glucuronides. The elimination half-life of morphine and plasma clearance in these patients are similar to the values in patients with normal renal function ($T_{1/2}\beta$ = 185 min; $CL_{ml/min/kg}$ = 17 versus 21). In patients with chronic renal failure the central compartment is significantly smaller than normal (0.3 ± 0.2 L/kg versus 0.8 ± 0.4 L/kg), however, as is the volume of distribution at steady state (2.8 ± 1.0 L/kg versus 3.7 ± 1.2 L/kg).[73]

The metabolites reach an almost identical peak in both patients with renal failure and normal subjects. After 2 hours, the plasma concentration in normal subjects decreased to less than 100 ng/ml and continued to decline to an undetectable level at 12 hours. In the patients with renal failure, however, the plasma concentration of the metabolites at 2 hours was about 100 ng/ml and continued at a plateau for 24 to 36 hours at plasma levels of 80 ng/ml.[73]

Pharmacologic Effects

Central Nervous System

The effects are chiefly thalamic as well as cortical. The locus of action is subcortical; analgesia is prominent, the pain threshold being elevated. This effect occurs without first producing sleep and appears highly selective. If the drug is administered before the pain stimulus, the appreciation of the pain sense is markedly diminished, whereas if given after pain has been induced, the sensation is not so completely obtunded. In either case, the pattern of reaction alters so the patient may be comfortable, yet still perceive the pain sense. This dissociation or "chemical lobotomy" has been achieved by surgical lobotomy in cases of intractable pain. Many of these effects on pains are comparable to transection of the corticothalamic tracts.[42]

Sedation is also accomplished. Sleep produced with ordinary doses of morphine and the onset of the sedative action occur later than the analgesic effect. The patient has a decrease in time sense, and when morphine is used alone, some minimal *amnesia* occurs.

Spinal cord excitation is seen frequently, especially in women. The pupils are constricted.

Cerebrospinal fluid pressure is raised. This is due to the increased carbon dioxide (CO_2) content of plasma resulting from the respiratory depressant effect of morphine (Fig. 31–8). Increased Pa_{CO_2} levels are instrumental in raising intracranial pressure.[74]

Action on the hypothalamic centers results in depression of heat-regulating mechanisms and decreased re-

sponsiveness of autonomic reflexes. High doses taken on a long-term basis may lead to increases in body temperature.[34]

Respiratory System

A summary of the effects on the respiratory system is as follows:

1. Depression of respiratory center directly.[75,76]
2. Decreased response of carotid body and aortic chemoreceptors to anoxia.[77]
3. Decreased ciliary action in bronchial tree.[78]
4. Increased bronchial tonus.[78]

After intravenous injection, maximal respiratory depression (decrease in *respiratory minute volume*), evidenced by *decrease in both* rate and depth, occurs in majority of cases between 3 and 7 minutes. Average depression has been placed at 13.6%. At 30 minutes, average depression was 11.6%, and subsequent observations at longer intervals did not differ much. After intramuscular injection, depression occurred maximally at about 20 minutes and was about 12.4%. This is achieved mostly by decrease in rate. After an initial period of depression of rate and some depth, one sees a return to normal and even an increase in tidal volume.[79] The data indicate that respiratory depression is not significantly different whether morphine is given intravenously or intramuscularly. Formerly, it was considered that intravenous morphine depressed respiration dangerously.

After subcutaneous injection, maximal respiratory depression occurs in 30 to 45 minutes. Again, the depression is achieved mostly by a decrease in rate.

Age As a Factor in Response

After intramuscular or intravenous morphine administration, both young and old healthy subjects show a similar depression of respiration.[80] Dripps evaluated intravenous morphine with respect to respiratory frequency (f) and minute ventilation ($\dot{V}E$) and concluded that elderly subjects did not possess a greater sensitivity. A study of end-tidal CO_2 tension (PET_{CO_2}) before and after either subcutaneous or intravenous morphine showed a similar elevation. The ventilatory response of elderly men to breathing a CO_2-enriched mixture is about equal after morphine in the young and the elderly.[81]

After intravenous morphine (10 mg/70 kg adult), both young and elderly patients have a significant but similar depression of respiration, as evidenced by a reduction in the slope of the CO_2 response curve, a rise in resting PET_{CO_2}, and a rise in the CO_2 threshold. The last represents the PET_{CO_2} value at which ventilation begins to rise from the basal level.[82]

The minute ventilation at a given PET_{CO_2} (5.5% = 7.3 kPa) was found to be reduced in both groups of subjects. The young group (18 to 30 years) showed a 28% decrease, and the elderly had a greater average decrease of 39%, but the difference was not determined to be significant.

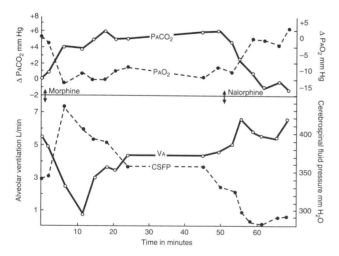

Fig. 31–8. Effect of morphine and nalorphine on the cerebrospinal fluid pressure. The alveolar gas tensions are represented as PA_{O_2} and PA_{CO_2}. Changes in gas tension, alveolar ventilation, and spinal fluid pressure are simultaneously compared after a dose of the antagonist nalorphine. Redrawn from Keats, A. S., Mithoefer, J. C.: The mechanism of increased intracranial pressure induced by morphine. N Engl J Med *252*:1110, 1955.

Carbon Dioxide-Response Curve

To study the respiratory effects of opiates and other drugs, Eckenhoff introduced the Carbon Dioxide-Respiratory Center Challenge Method.[83] It is a rebreathing technique that is simple, inexpensive, accurate, and reproducible. The respiratory response in terms of RMV (respiratory minute volume in liters per minute) to endogenously accumulated CO_2, as represented by the alveolar CO_2 tension is determined. The RMV is plotted against the $Paco_2$[84] (Fig. 31–9). A flattening of the slope from the normal progression line indicates a diminishing response and respiratory depression.

The basic method has been modified by Bellville using an analog computer so that a respiratory response curve is plotted automatically and a point obtained for each breath.[84]

Interpretation

In revealing depression of respiratory control and ventilation, two features of the CO_2 response curve are observed: (1) a shift in the response curve, which is manifested by a shift to the right in the presence of CNS depressants; the extent of this shift is dose related; (2) a change in the slope, this may reflect two different sites of action of the different drugs, the first of which may be mediated by opiate receptors in the brain stem and the second by depressing the generalized sensory alerting mechanisms.

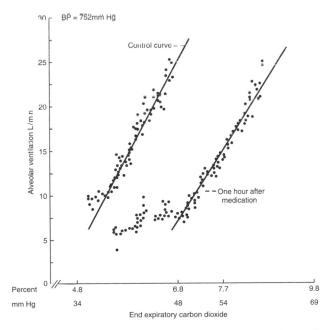

Fig. 31–9. Respiratory response curves before and 1 hour after 10 mg morphine plus 10 mg nalorphine. Alveolar ventilation is plotted versus end-expiratory carbon dioxide for each breath by a special-purpose analogue computer while the subject rebreathes in a closed-circuit system. Calibration of the x-axis with known CO_2-O_2 mixtures is shown. Redrawn from Bellville, J. W., Fleischli, G.: The interaction of morphine and nalorphine on respiration. Clin Pharmacol Ther *9*:152, 1968.

Narcotics and opiates in the analgesic dose range characteristically shift the ventilatory CO_2 response curve to the right, whereas the slope of the curve is unchanged and remains parallel to the resting ventilatory CO_2 response.[85] Generally, there continues to be a proportional response to increasing levels of CO_2. A condition of metabolic alkalosis may enhance the respiratory depression of opioids.[86]

Other CNS depressant drugs that decrease the level of consciousness and responsiveness shift the curve to the right but invariably cause a decrease in the slope of the CO_2 response curve. Such agents include the inhalational agents,[87] nitrous oxide,[88] isoflurane,[89] halothane, cyclopropane,[90] large-dose opioid balanced anesthesia,[91] barbiturates,[92] and benzodiazepines.[93]

One exception to the rule that drugs that produce unconsciousness cause a flattening of slope is ketamine.[93] This drug shifts the curve to the right, but the slope remains unchanged. Thus, ketamine's curve demonstrates the character of narcotics and confirms the agent's recognized analgesic effect.

Effect of Epidural Morphine[94]

Following surgery, the CO_2 response curve is shifted to the right and the slope of the curve, $Ve/Petco_2$, is decreased. This may be related to the residual anesthetic effect to pain or the surgical trauma. The administration of morphine via an epidural catheter to provide postoperative analgesia in children results in depressed ventilatory response to CO_2, both the slope and the Ve at 35 mm Hg CO_2 tension. This depression was found to continue for the $Ve/Petco_2$ for 22 hours and for Ve for 10 hours. Hence, these patients must be monitored for at least 24 hours.[94]

Effect of β-Adrenergic Blockers[95]

Some reports suggest that propranolol depresses the ventilatory response to CO_2 rebreathing in normal subjects. A careful study by Twum-Barima, Ahmad, Hamilton, and Carruthers,[95] however, demonstrates clearly that single or cumulative doses of the most common β_1 or β_2 blockers are not effective in altering the central sensitivity to increasing CO_2 concentration.

Cardiocirculatory System

A summary of effects is as follows:

1. Depression of vasoconstrictor center.[96]
2. Decreased arteriolar tone and peripheral resistance; reduced afterload.[97]
3. Depressed circulatory compensation to postural changes.[96]
4. Reduced venous tone; increase in venous pooling and decrease in venous return to the heart.
5. Decreased cardiac output from diminished venous return with large doses.[98]
6. Depressed circulatory responses to asphyxia (masking signs of asphyxia).[99]

Morphine produces changes in circulatory system that are revealed usually when a stress is placed on the system.[96] Thus, some patients given morphine faint when they assume the upright posture. Usually, 8% of healthy males show some symptoms of collapse on change of posture from horizontal to 75° head-up position, and after morphine administration this increases to 44%. Peripheral vasodilatation is probably the important factor because the incidence of fainting can be diminished by wrapping the legs and thighs with elastic bandages. The pulse is usually increased and cardiac output is increased; however, in doses used clinically, cutaneous vasodilatation may be produced with little effect on the skeletal muscle circulation.[100,101]

Cardiac Effects[102]

Some mild myocardial effects have been noted with the administration of large doses of morphine. A reduction in left ventricular dimensions and diminished intracavitary wall stresses occur. The result is a reduction in ventricular work and attenuation of myocardial oxygen demands. In the acute phase of a myocardial infarction, these effects of morphine are enhanced and, together with a reduction in the afterload, are of significant benefit. The left ventricular end-diastolic pressure may be reduced in these patients by 20% and the work index by 8%.

In an experimental study of the effects of morphine on cat papillary muscle, low doses showed some positive inotropism. An increase in the extent of shortening, the velocity of shortening, the rate of tension development was observed. Augmentations in cardiac work and cardiac power were demonstrated. Meperidine and fentanyl in low doses showed no positive effects. The doses of morphine were 20 to 200 times lower than those of meperidine. With large doses of morphine, greater than those compared with clinical analgesic doses, a dose-dependent decrease in inotropic values was noted.[103]

Cerebral Hemodynamics[104]

Morphine affects cerebral hemodynamics and metabolism.[104] Cerebral blood flow is not significantly altered even after a dose of 60 mg intravenously. Any response is usually related to the systemic hemodynamic changes. Oxygen consumption and cerebral metabolic rate are decreased with morphine.[105]

Gastrointestinal Tract[105]

The smooth muscle is stimulated; muscular tone is enhanced and all movements of the intestinal tract are inhibited, including propulsive and segmenting movements. In the large intestine, tone is increased to the point of spasm and sphincters are contracted. Propulsive movements are diminished to the point of absence. The anal sphincter tone is greatly increased. Thus, retention of contents as well as constipation can be expected. Secretions are generally decreased. Gastric hydrochloric acid is decreased; biliary, pancreatic, and intestinal secretions are all decreased. These effects of morphine and other opioids are mediated by μ and δ receptors in the bowel wall.

The incidence of nausea and vomiting varies from 4 to 40% after therapeutic doses, whereas the average incidence is 25%.[106] If a patient remains supine after morphine administration, the incidence of nausea and vomiting is diminished.

Gastric Emptying[107]

Gastric emptying in human subjects is prolonged by narcotics. This has been studied in volunteers who have received a radioactive test meal and who have had the changes in radioactivity monitored by τ camera scans. Following an intravenous injection of saline, gastric emptying was nearly complete at the end of 1 hour. Morphine, on the other hand, in 80% of patients showed gastric emptying times of about 2 hours. In comparison, nalbuphine, 5 mg intravenously, prolonged gastric emptying and only about one third of such patients had gastric emptying half-times less than 2 hours. The administration intravenously of 10 mg nalbuphine prolonged gastric emptying for up to 7 or more hours.

Small Intestinal Transit Times

Following the saline placebo, small intestinal transit times were completed by 4 hours. The morphine (5.0 mg) transit time was approximately 4 hours; and nalbuphine, 5.0 mg, similarly had a slightly prolonged transit time, but only 80% of patients had a similar transit time as those who had received morphine. Nalbuphine, 10 mg, markedly prolonged the transit time to over 7 hours.

Biliary Physiology

Biliary pressure is increased 2 to 4 times by therapeutic doses of morphine.[108] A subcutaneous dose of 10 mg of morphine increases the biliary tract pressure from a resting normal pressure of 20 mm H_2O to levels of 200 to 300 mm H_2. Reduction in the caliber of the common bile duct and a spasmolytic effect have been demonstrated by direct ultrasonographic technique after the administration of analgesic doses of morphine.[109]

Other Smooth Muscle[110]

In general, morphine exerts a vagomimetic action on smooth muscle and hence the effects of its administration qualitatively duplicate stimulation of the parasympathetic system.

	Tone
Ureter and urinary bladder	++
Vesical sphincter	++
Biliary tract	++
Bronchial musculature	++
Uterus	+
Pregnancy, full-term	0
Pregnancy and oxytocic	Normal
Menstruating	—

Kidney

Decreased glomerular filtration and renal plasma flow are observed after morphine administration. Because of the indirect release of ADH from stimulation of hypothalamic-hypophyseal system,[104] there is a proportionate reduction in urine volume, depending on the amount of hormone released and consequent increased tubular reabsorption of water. In patients suffering from chronic renal failure, prolonged narcosis and ventilatory depression may be observed on administration of morphine.[111,112] Evidence of accumulation of metabolites appears to be responsible for this effect, because morphine elimination half-life and plasma clearance are similar to those in patients with normal renal function[113] (see the section of this chapter on pharmacokinetics).

Metabolic Effects

The peripheral vasodilatation increases heat loss and, combined with depression of temperature-regulating centers, may cause a fall in body temperature.

Morphine tends to stimulate supraspinal autonomic centers to cause sympathoadrenal discharge. Hyperglycemia occurs from the enhanced liver glycogenolysis.[114]

Administration of morphine stimulates the elaboration of ketosteroids from the adrenal cortex. A single dose of morphine reduces the adrenal stores of corticosteroid by 35%[115] and increases the plasma levels. Thereafter, adrenal cortical suppression occurs. This is likely due to depression of ACTH elaboration[116] because the adrenal glands show normal responsiveness to exogenous ACTH.

Neuroendocrine Systems[117]

Most of the effects on the peripheral endocrine mechanisms are related to a primary direct action of morphine on the hypothalamus. Inhibition of the secretion of releasing factors occurs (Fig. 31–10):

Corticotropin-releasing hormone (CRH) in hypothalamic-ACTH-cortisol axis
Gonadotropin-releasing hormone (GnRH) in hypothalamic-pituitary-gonad axis

As a result, the pituitary is not stimulated to release the trophic hormones, corticotropin (ACTH) and gonadotropin. Specifically, in the first axis, the synthesis and secretion of ACTH and β-endorphin (released in equimolar quantities) in the pituitary are reduced when CRH is inhibited. In the second axis, the pituitary synthesis and secretion of LH and follicle-stimulating hormone (FSH) are reduced. In addition, CRH activates the sympathetic nervous system, and this action is also inhibited[118] (Table 31–4).

FSH and LH also regulate gonadal function in the male, and when their release is inhibited, levels of testosterone are reduced.

Thyroid-releasing hormone is not inhibited by morphine, so secretion of thyrotropin (TSH) is not affected.

Growth hormone synthesis and secretion are not affected by morphine or by μ agonists, although other opioids enhance its secretion.

ADH is secreted by the posterior pituitary to act on collecting ducts of the kidney and to conserve body water. Morphine promotes the release of ADH, as do other μ-

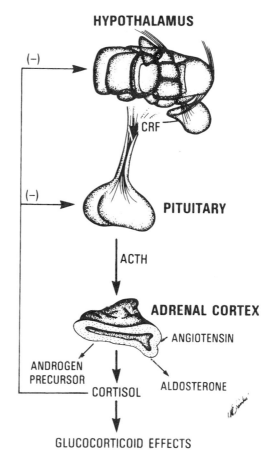

Fig. 31–10. Hypothalamic-pituitary-adrenocortical axis. From West, J. B. (ed.): Best and Taylor's Physiologic Basis of Medical Practice, 12th Ed. Baltimore, Williams & Wilkins, 1990.

opioid agonists. On the other hand, κ-agonists such as normorphine and naloxone inhibit the release of ADH. Prolactin release is stimulated.

In response to stress is progressive activation of the sympathetic nervous system. Stores of catecholamines in the adrenal gland are depleted, and considerable norepinephrine is released. Morphine obtunds this process by inhibiting the release of CRH from the hypothalamus, however.[100]

Miscellaneous Effects

Acute Abdominal Pain

A board-like rigidity with cramps may occur in persons addicted to opium and to morphine. In an addict, this is sometimes confused with the surgical abdomen.

Feline Reaction

An agitated state with hyperactive spinal reflexes represents this type of reaction. It may be seen in women in the preovulatory estrogen phase of the menstrual cycle.

Dependence

Although the ancients were aware of the addicting property of opium, it was Thomas DeQuincey who first

Table 31–4. Production Rates and Plasma Concentrations of Major Adrenocortical Hormones*

Class	Steroid	Production Rate (mg/day)	Plasma Concentration (ng/ml)
Glucocorticoid	Cortisol	8–25	40–180
	Corticosterone	1–4	2–4
Mineralocorticoid	Aldosterone	0.05–0.15	0.15
	Deoxycorticosterone	0.6	0.15
Androgenic	DHEA	7–15	5
	DHEA-S		1,200
	Androstenedione	2–3	1.8

*Concentrations vary with time of day, sex and stage of menstrual cycle for particular steroids.
From West, J. B. (ed.): Best and Taylor's Physiologic Basis of Medical Practice, 12th Ed. Baltimore, Williams & Wilkins, 1990.

described in detail the manifestations of addiction. DeQuincey was a brilliant man of letters who became addicted to laudanum. In *Confessions of an English Opium Eater*, published in a magazine in 1821, he described both the psychologic and physiologic signs and the symptoms of withdrawal. The development of addiction has been a disadvantage to the use of opiates, and investigators have searched for analgesic drugs as potent as morphine but without addiction liability.

Physiologic dependence is a complex phenomenon.[119] When withdrawal symptoms appear, the drug level in the body is waning, and only traces are present at 36 to 48 hours. Yet the intensity of reaction continues for 10 to 16 days.[119] Effects on cell membranes are important. Morphine alters cell penetration by ions and alters the calcium-phospholipid relationship at the membrane interface.[120] Calcium appears to be bound strongly by morphine at the membrane, and if calcium is increased, morphine withdrawal effects are diminished. It thus appears that calcium has an antagonistic effect in the production of the addiction state by morphine.[121]

Neuromuscular Transmission

In studies on grip strength induced by subclinical doses of *d*-tubocurarine, Bellville and colleagues[122] reported that morphine in doses of 10 mg or less did not affect grip strength. On the other hand, some animal studies[123] demonstrated that morphine significantly decreased the indirectly elicited repetitive twitch responses in frog sciatic nerve sartorius preparations and in the rat phrenic nerve hemidiaphragm preparation. In their study, these investigators demonstrated a decrease in the amount of acetylcholine released per nerve impulse in the presence of morphine.[123]

A newer study on the effect of morphine on human neuromuscular transmission utilized a high-frequency nerve stimulation technique.[124] Although the tetanic phase did not change during a 1-hour period after the infusion of morphine, nevertheless post-tetanic depression of single twitch responses occurred. This depression increased progressively over a 1-hour period. This was in contrast to control subjects, in which either no change or a slight increase in post-tetanic facilitation was reported. Morphine may exert a presynaptic action whereby intraterminal mobilization of acetylcholine is impaired by the opiate drug.

Potentiation Drug Interactions

Nearly all CNS-acting depressant drugs increase the sedative and analgesic effects of morphine and some other opioids.[49] The depressant effect is exaggerated and prolonged by the following drugs: phenothiazines; monoamine oxidase inhibitors; tricyclic antidepressants; and most sedatives and hyonotics. Antihistamines have a modest sedative enhancement of morphine and increase the analgesic action of morphine. Hydroxyzine enhances the analgesic action of low doses of morphine and other opiates.[125] Most phenothiazines reduce the amount of opioid needed to produce a given level of analgesia; at the same time, the respiratory depressant effect of morphine and other opioids is increased, and hypotensive effects are more prominent. Some phenothiazines enhance the sedative action of morphine but have an antianalgesic effect, so a greater amount of morphine or other opioid is needed to produce satisfactory pain relief.[126]

Of the antidepressants, desipramine is able to enhance morphine analgesia postoperatively. Small doses of amphetamines augment the euphoriant and analgesic effect of morphine and decrease the sedative action. For example, a dose of 10 mg of morphine accompanied by 10 mg of dextroamphetamine doubles the analgesic effect and generally offsets undesirable actions such as somnolence and alertness. This has been a successful combination in the management of postoperative pain.[127]

Physostigmine has been found to offset the somnolence and sedative actions of several sedative and hypnotic drugs.[128] As a result of this action, physostigmine, in a dose of 1.0 mg per minute up to four doses, has been used to antagonize the sedative effects of morphine without affecting the analgesia, and it has been demonstrated thereby to antagonize a significant part of the respiratory depression induced by morphine.[129]

Histamine Release

In human subjects, morphine causes the release of histamine. This has long been accepted on the basis of the indirect evidence of flushing and urticaria. Measurements of plasma histamine by Fahmy and Philbin and their colleagues[130,131] provided direct evidence of histamine release; rapid elevations of plasma histamine follows the administration of morphine intravenously. This effect can be blocked by histamine antagonists.[131]

Fahmy measured histamine levels following ordinary doses of morphine of 0.2 to 0.3 mg/kg in human subjects.[130] From control levels of about 1.0 ng/ml, a two- to four-fold increase in histamine was reported within 2 to 5 minutes to levels of 3.0 to 4.0 ng/ml. Simultaneously, plasma epinephrine increases by four- to eightfold from 50 to 60 pg/ml to 200 pg/ml at 5 minutes and 400 pg/ml at 20 minutes. These changes occurred soon after the peak elevation in histamine, indicating that histamine releases epinephrine from the adrenal gland. No significant changes in norepinephrine occurred.

Hemodynamic responses were also observed.[132] Systolic pressure, mean arterial pressure, and systemic vascular resistance decreased. Cardiac output, however, increased, and this was related to both the increased heart rate and an increased stroke volume. These changes all correlated with the increased levels of histamine-epinephrine release.

When morphine is administered in larger intravenous doses, as in neurolept narcotic anesthesia techniques, one sees a significant increase in plasma histamine.[133] Doses of 0.6 mg/kg intravenously produce increases from a baseline plasma level of 0.1 ng/ml to 0.3 ng/ml within 1.2 minutes, and this remains elevated for 6.0 minutes, but it returns to baseline in about 25 minutes. An occasional patient may have a great rise in histamine to 12 ng/ml in 1.2 minutes and continues elevated at 0.55 ng/ml at 6.0 minutes.[133] At 25 minutes, the level returns to baseline.

Anesthetic Doses and Histamine Blood Levels

Large doses of morphine—1 mg/kg administered intravenously by infusion at a rate of 100 μg/kg/min—produces elevations of histamine from control levels of about 1000 pg/ml (1.0 ng/ml) to levels of 8000 pg/ml within 2 to 4 minutes. These levels of histamine decrease over the following 15 minutes to approximately 2000 pg/ml, but they continue above control values for over 1 hour. Accompanying the histamine release is a significant fall in mean arterial pressure and a fall in systemic vascular resistance. The fall in systemic vascular resistance is proportional to the increase in the plasma histamine level.

This effect of morphine contrasts with fentanyl, which, when administered in a comparable large dose manner, does not produce changes in plasma histamine.[134]

Because histamine release is activated by both H_1 and H_2 stimulation, *both* H_1 and H_2 blockers attenuate histamine release and prevent anaphylactoid reactions to morphine.[132,135]

Morphine Pruritus[136]

Many patients experience an itch at the corner of the nose or mouth and lips. It is more frequent in females and is seen in many facial areas after spinal morphine. This reaction is considered to be an enkephalinergic reflex and not due to histamine release. An "itch center" has been proposed in the medullary area and in the floor of the fourth ventricle. It appears to be related to the spinal nucleus of the trigeminal nerve, which is rich in opiate receptors. The itch can be eliminated, if disturbing, by naloxone administration.[136]

PREPARATIONS AND RELATED SUBSTITUTES FOR MORPHINE

Pantopon (Papaveritum BPC)

This is a mixture of purified opium alkaloids of which approximately 50% is morphine. It is standardized so 50% is anhydrous morphine and the other 50% consists of codeine, papaverine, thebaine, narcotine, and others. The basic effect of this preparation is due to morphine content. The dose is 20 mg (gr. ⅓) and this is equivalent to morphine sulfate 10 mg (gr. ⅙). The original claim of lesser respiratory depression and of lesser nausea and vomiting was purely an impression. Administration of a dose of morphine equal to the amount in a given Pantopon dose achieves the same result; in equivalent doses, the incidence of nausea and respiratory depression is about equal. Because the expense of Pantopon is several times that of morphine, its use is not warranted. This preparation is not available in the United States, but is available in United Kingdom, as papaveritum or Omnopon. [49a]

Long-Acting Preparation—Duramorph[137]

Duramorph is a microcrystalline preparation of morphine, containing a morphine base of 64 mg in 1.0 ml; approximately 3.0 mg is present as free morphine, and the remainder is in crystals of varying sizes from 50 to 250 μm in diameter, from which the drug is slowly released over 9 to 12 hours. The dose is 1.0 ml every 12 hours. This agent is preservative free and can be used epidurally and intraspinally.

Pharmacodynamics

Significant analgesia is evident within 1.0 hour after the intramuscular administration of 1.0 ml Duramorph. One sees a progressive increase in pain relief and an optimal relief at 3.0 hours at the time of peak plasma concentrations. Pain relief continues for 8.0 hours at an optimal level. Patients rarely require further injections until after 12 hours, which thus represents the duration of analgesic effect.

Pharmacokinetics

Progressive increases in plasma concentrations, to a level of about 65 ng/ml, occur at 3.0 hours. Thereafter, plasma concentrations decline to levels of approximately 16 ng/ml at 8.0 hours. The level continues to be in the range of 10 ng/ml up to 12 hours. The analgesia continues to the 12-hour period.

Comment[138,139]

Intramuscular Duramorph thus represents a significant advance in postoperative analgesia. The lipid solubility of morphine is relatively low, compared with that of other opiate analgesics. Morphine also equilibrates slowly with the CNS. After the administration of intramuscular Duramorph, significant concentrations of morphine in plasma remain for 12 hours and are associated with prolonged and enhanced analgesia. In general, the plasma concentrations by this preparation and the method of intramuscular administration are usually greater than those produced by conventional intramuscular doses (every 4 hours) of morphine. Moreover, the use of this method is associated with a small percentage of patients complaining of moderate nausea and vomiting. A small proportion (10 to 20%) of patients experience sedation. No evidence of cumulation has been adduced when Duramorph is given every 8 hours for a period up to 48 hours, or a total of six injections.[137]

Slow-Release Morphine (MST)

An oral preparation of morphine for slow release designated as MST Contin is available in doses of 30 g and MS Contin in doses of 60 mg. The morphine sulfate is mixed with inactive ingredients of cellulose, methylcellulose in cetosteryl alcohol plus lactose, talc, magnesium stearate, and others.[140]

Absorption

After oral administration, presystemic elimination occurs in the gut wall and liver in which a fraction is demethylated and a larger fraction is metabolized to morphine-3-glucuronate, so the bioavailability is only 35 to 50% reaching the systemic circulation.[141]

Pharmacokinetics

It takes about 30 minutes for the drug to reach the central compartment. The peak plasma concentration is reached in T_{max} of 2 to 2.5 hours. The concentration C_{max} at this time is about 14 ng/ml.[142] The volume of distribution is 40 L/kg. The terminal half-life is 2 to 4 hours.

Dosage

For long-term use, as in cancer patients, the dose is established by first determining the daily oral dose with conventional morphine administered in a regimen of every 4 to 6 hours to provide 24 hours of pain relief. If less than 60 mg is required, then the MST tablet containing 15 mg is administered twice a day; if 60 to 120 mg is required for pain relief, the 60-mg tablet of MST is administered twice a day. The peak effect and plasma concentration of the morphine are higher with this regimen, and the trough of concentration and effect is lower than with the 4- to 6-hour regimen.[142]

Pharmacodynamics

The onset of drug action is slow and initially is not seen for 30 to 60 minutes. The duration of effect is variable but lasts for 8 and up to 12 hours.

Usage

This preparation is principally of use in patients with chronic pain such cancer pain. Although effective for postoperative pain, it is not recommended for the first 24 hours, but conventional morphine dosage can be converted to the MST dose form carefully after 12 hours.[143] For preanesthetic medication, it was not found satisfactory in the study by Simpson and associates. Nausea and emesis were more frequent than after conventional morphine.

Hydromorphone (Dilaudid)

This is a synthetic alkaloid obtained by altering naturally occurring morphine to dihydromorphinone. The average adult dose is approximately ¼ that of morphine or 2 to 4 mg for parenteral injection available in solutions of 1 to 4 mg/ml. Tablets of 1 to 4 mg each and suppositories are available.

Analgesia on a weight-for-weight basis is 10 times greater than morphine, whereas its hypnotic effect is only 4 times greater. Pain may thus be relieved without producing sleep. Adequate pain relief occurs with plasma concentrations of 4.0 ng/ml.[144]

Respiratory center depressant effects follow the administration of hydromorphone. The CO_2-response curve shows that 1.25 mg of this drug is equivalent to 10.0 mg of morphine.[145]

Side effects are less pronounced than with morphine, but the margin of safety is no greater. The duration of action is shorter than with morphine.

Levorphanol (Levorphan or Dromoran)
Chemistry

This is a morphine analogue synthetized by Schneider and Grussner.[146] The chemical name is 3-hydroxyl-N-methyl morphinan. It differs from morphine in lacking the alcoholic OH and the oxygen bridge. It is a highly active and long-lasting analgesic in man.

Central Nervous System Actions[147]

A definite central sedative effect is denoted by drowsiness in patients receiving therapeutic doses. The outstanding effect is that of analgesia, however. The effective dose is 5 mg, and this compares with 10 mg of morphine. The relation between minimal effective dose and median lethal dose is low, so the drug affords a wide margin of safety. The onset of action after a subcutaneous injection is about 30 minutes, and peak action occurs in 60 to 90 minutes. The duration of analgesic effect is about 4 to 6 hours.

Postoperative pain is relieved in 75% of the cases.[145] In general, levorphanol compares with morphine and is superior to meperidine, but it less effective than hydromorphone. Like morphine, levorphanol is useful in cutaneous-type pain.

Cardiovascular Effects

Some hypotension is manifested when stresses are applied. This response is little different from the effects of morphine.

Respiration

Although experimental studies indicated that equieffective doses produce less respiratory depression than morphine, this is not supported clinically.

Uses

This agent has been used in premedication in the following approximate dose schedule: children 1 to 5 years = 1 to 1.5 mg; children 5 to 10 years = 2.5 mg; adolescents 10 to 16 years = 2.5 mg; adolescents 10 to 16 years = 3.0 mg; adults = 3.5 to 5.0 mg. This scale is usually satisfactory. Patients are mentally at ease, without pain or anxiety, and, although drowsy, responsive to questions.[148]

Levorphanol has been used to supplement nitrous oxide-oxygen anesthesia.[149] It is administered either by intermittent intravenous injections of 0.5 to 1.0 mg as indicated by patient responses to pain, or it may be used in continuous-drip infusion of 25 mg in 500 ml 5% dextrose in water. The needs of the patient are met by changing the rate of drip.

Heroin[150]

Chemically, heroin is diacetylmorphine (Fig. 31-11). From pharmacokinetic and pharmacodynamic studies, heroin may be considered a prodrug.[150] Parenteral administration (intramuscular or intravenous) results in measurable blood levels of heroin and metabolites. The heroin is rapidly biotransformed to 6-mono-acetylmorphine and

HEROIN
(Diacetylmonphine)

HYDROMOPHONE HTDROCHLORIDE
(Dilaudid)

OXYMORPHONE HTDROCHLORIDE
(Numorphan)

LEVORPHANOL TARTRATE
(Levo-Dromoran)

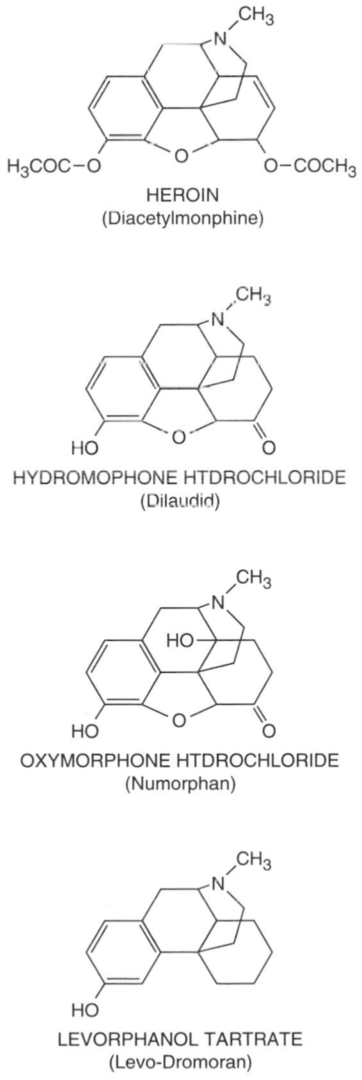

Fig. 31–11. Structural formulas for morphine derivatives.

then to morphine, both of which have potent opioid activity. Most human tissues transform heroin. Organ clearance is the main determinant of rapid disappearance from systemic circulation, although the blood also contributes to the degradation. The mean half-life of heroin after intravenous administration is only 3.0 minutes, whereas the clearance of heroin at steady state was determined at about 30 ml/kg body weight/min. Morphine levels rise more gradually.[151]

From pharmacokinetic studies, it is evident that heroin and acetylmorphine are present in the blood during the first 10 to 15 minutes after intravenous injection. At this time, the onset of pain relief occurs, although no morphine is present in plasma.[152]

The mono-acetylmorphine appears to be the key effective agent. At any rate, heroin induces faster pain relief and has greater potency but shorter duration of effect than morphine.[152]

Oral heroin is converted to morphine slowly but not to acetylmorphine, and it is an inefficient means of producing morphine.[151]

Oxymorphone Hydrochloride (Numorphan)

Oxymorphone is a synthetic morphine derivative that is 10 times more potent than morphine. The duration of action is slightly longer (6 hours) than that of morphine, but tolerance may develop more rapidly to repeated doses. The therapeutic subcutaneous dose is 1.5 mg.[49]

Chemically, the drug is 14-hydroxydihydromorphinane. Pharmacologic actions are similar to those of morphine. Oxymorphone is able to relieve severe pain, and it also provides a sedative-euphoric action. It is less constipating than morphine and appears to have little antitussive effect.

Central respiratory depression by equianalgesic doses is quantitatively similar to morphine, although claims have been made to the contrary. In young subjects, the respiratory rate is not significantly changed and the resting minute ventilation is reduced only about 6 to 10%. In older and debilitated subjects, clinically evident respiratory depression is readily seen and minute ventilation at rest may be reduced 15 to 35%.

Codeine

In the treatment of postoperative pain,[153] 30 mg of codeine is inferior to 10 mg of morphine, whereas 60 mg of codeine affords significant relief. Even 120 mg of codeine failed to equal the pain-relieving performance of 10 mg of morphine, however.

The respiratory depressant effects of codeine have been compared to those of morphine. Intramuscular codeine has a potency ratio of 0.1 as compared with morphine. Oxycodone is about 5 times as potent as codeine. Oral codeine is about 0.7 as potent as intramuscular codeine in analgesic effects.[154]

Codeine Combination

Combinations of codeine with other agents, such as aspirin, result in increased analgesic effect. Usually, the effect is additive.[155] Caffeine combinations also significantly enhance the analgesic potency. Lasha has studied various formulations: the addition of caffeine (65 mg) to either aspirin (650 mg) or codeine (32 mg) results in enhanced analgesic effect.[156] The aspirin-caffeine combination particularly gives added analgesia to the extent of increased relative potency from 1.0 to 1.4. Thus, codeine-aspirin and aspirin-acetaminophen-caffeine and codeine-aspirin-caffeine are useful effective combinations.

Dextropropoxyphene (Darvon)

This drug is an effective non-narcotic analgesic when administered orally (30 to 60 mg). It does cause some respiratory depression. Clinical studies show the relative respiratory depressant effect to be 0.33 as potent as codeine.[157] That is, 180 mg of dextropropoxyphene orally produces respiratory depression equal to that of 60 mg of codeine orally.

MEPERIDINE AND ANALOGUES

Modification of the morphine molecule has yielded many active drugs, but in 1939 a totally synthetic analgesic was introduced by Eisleb and Schaumann in Germany.[158] It is a synthetic piperidine derivative and, therefore, differs in its basic nucleus from morphine (Fig. 31-12). Originally, the drug was introduced as an antispasmodic because of the structural similarity to atropine. The initial tests demonstrated that it had the same effect on mice as morphine in causing erection of their tails (Straub phenomenon), however. This indicated that meperidine was analgesic, and subsequent application verified this effect and the utility of meperidine.[159] In general, two actions of this drug are outstanding, namely, spasmolysis and analgesia.[160]

Pharmacologic Actions

Central Nervous System

Analgesia is the outstanding effect. The locus of action is chiefly subcortical. A dose of 50 to 75 mg intramuscularly raises the pain threshold about 50%, or the equivalent of 10 mg of morphine. A dose of 100 to 125 mg raises the threshold about 75% or the equivalent of 15 mg of morphine (radiant heat technique of Wolff-Hardy).[161]

The analgesic effect lasts between 2 to 4 hours and is briefer than that of morphine. As with other narcotics, when pain is severe, the duration is shorter.[162]

Pain of all types is satisfactorily relieved; however, visceral-type pain is singularly obtunded. This is particularly true of the gastrointestinal and urinary tracts.[163]

Sedation is apparent only with large doses. It is possible, therefore, to achieve good pain relief without producing sleep.[164] If sleep is desired, the drug should be combined with a barbiturate, and under these circumstances, the hypnotic action of the barbiturate is enhanced.

Cerebrospinal Fluid Pressure

Elevations of 25 to 50% follow the administration of therapeutic doses.[165] This is unrelated to blood pressure changes but is related to decreased ventilation and increases in blood CO_2; therefore, the drug should be used cautiously in patients with raised cerebrospinal fluid pressure or intracranial lesions.[166]

Respiration

Depression of human respiration occurs following therapeutic doses.[167] One sees an initial depression of both rate and depth, especially after intravenous administration. After 15 minutes, the respiratory rate returns to normal or above normal values. Tidal volume remains reduced, however,[167] and minute volume is measurably depressed for as long as 4 hours.[168-170] The degree of this depression is variable and may be extensive. It is also more evident when meperidine medication is followed by potent anesthetic agents; in the presence of raised intracranial pressure, this depression is also marked. The normal response of the respiratory center to inhalation of CO_2 is also diminished following therapeutic doses of meperidine.[168]

Profound depressions during anesthesia in patients premedicated with meperidine have been reported.[171] Note is made, too, of the marked and unpredictable depression when thiopental anesthesia is employed. This combination is also known to provoke edema of the pharyngeal and laryngeal membranes.

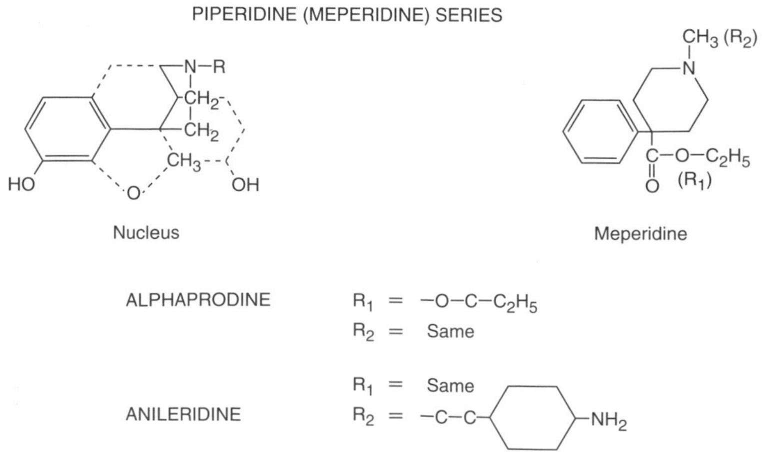

PIPERIDINE (MEPERIDINE) SERIES

Nucleus

Meperidine

ALPHAPRODINE R_1 = —O—C—C$_2$H$_5$
R_2 = Same

ANILERIDINE R_1 = Same
R_2 = —C—C— —NH$_2$

Fig. 31–12. Shows basic structure of meperidine series. Alteration of the morphine molecule is shown on the left: The oxygen bridge is removed; the alcoholic ring structure is eliminated and the center ring has been broken. The τ-phenyl-N-methyl piperidine structure is retained. The residue is the essence of the meperidine series of agents.

Little effect on the normal bronchial musculature is apparent after meperidine. In the presence of agents or diseases producing bronchospasm, however, relaxation occurs. The drug is thus recommended in the presence of bronchospastic diseases because of its anticholinergic action.

Heart

Intravenous meperidine produces an increased heart rate.[172] Some investigations indicate that meperidine exerts a protective action against the arrhythmias occurring during halothane administration.

The mechanism may be a direct sedative or quinidine-like effect on the myocardium or the vasolytic effect of meperidine balancing the parasympathomimetic effects of the halothane.[173]

In the presence of atrial tachyarrhythmias, the atropine-like action of meperidine is a disadvantage.[174] When administered to patients with atrial flutter or atrial fibrillation, an elevation of pulse rate or ventricular rate ensues. The removal of the vagal influence allows more atrial impulses to reach the ventricle; thus, a 6:1 or 4:1 block may be converted to a 2:1 block. The subsequent increased ventricular load can result in failure.

A direct depressant action on the myocardium has been determined.[174] In the intact subject, this effect is minimized or masked by compensatory sympathoadrenal discharge. Thus, blood pressure and cardiac contractility remain adequate under these circumstances and can be correlated with elevated norepinephrine blood levels. Meperidine appears to exert some direct nervous system action on the sympathetic system. If the sympathetic system is blocked by epidural anesthesia, however, then the myocardial depression is evident. Furthermore, this depression is enhanced by barbiturate anesthesia.

Advantage should be taken of the depressant action under those circumstances involving an irritable myocardium. Here, the drug is a cardiac sedative and possesses antiarrhythmic properties. It synergizes with such drugs as quinidine, procaine, and procainamide. Care should be exercised to avoid toxicity.[175]

These findings suggest that meperidine is a poor agent for use in the following situations: (1) patients with myocardial disease with or without failure and those in whom digitalis is needed; (2) patients with atrial arrhythmias.

On the other hand, the drug is most effective in the following instances: (1) in the presence of ventricular arrhythmias and an irritable myocardium; (2) preliminary to anesthesia.

Circulatory System[172]

Some slight fall in blood pressure may be seen following therapeutic doses. Approximately 5% of ambulatory patients exhibit a syncopal reaction.[176] Similarly, hypotension and syncope are observed frequently following intravenous administration of single therapeutic doses. In brief, the central compensatory mechanisms to circulatory stress are impaired. This is probably consequent to specific depression of the vasomotor center.

Gastrointestinal Tract

Meperidine has a pronounced quiescent effect on gastric contractile waves. This effect persists for 2 hours.[160] On both the intestinal and colon musculature, a marked relaxing occurs, as well as spasmolytic effect: peristaltic waves, segmental contractions, and large tonal waves are inhibited,[162] as observed by measurement of intraluminal pressure changes through ileostomy and colostomy openings.

On the biliary tract, as well as the duodenum, however, the drug has a significant spasmogenic effect. The mean baseline pressures in common ducts of man, as measured through a T-tube drain by Gaensler and associates,[108] varied between 25 and 55 mm H_2O, with an average of 44 mm H_2O. When a dose of meperidine or morphine is administered, sudden rises in pressure to 100 and 140 mm H_2O occur, with morphine producing higher pressures. This could be counteracted by amyl nitrate and by aminophylline. Thus, meperidine apparently may also increase biliary pressure and should be accompanied by a modest dose of atropine.

Most studies indicate that the effect of morphine is[109] about twice that of meperidine in raising biliary pressure in the absence of biliary disease, however. In the presence of biliary spasm, the administration of meperidine results in a significant fall in biliary pressure.[163]

Local Anesthetic Action

Meperidine has been shown to have local anesthetic properties by Way.[177] This narcotic has been used in spinal and epidural anesthesia, and its ability to relieve pain has been amply demonstrated.[178]

Antimicrobial Action[179]

Grimmond has demonstrated a significant antimicrobial action of meperidine on a variety of bacteria and other pathogens. This is similar to the action of several local anesthetics.

Miscellaneous Actions[1]

Two unusual actions are of importance to anesthesiologists. After systemic administration, corneal anesthesia is produced and the corneal reflex abolished. Second, some depression of autonomic ganglia may occur.

Electroencephalographic Effects[1]

Small single doses of meperidine have no significant electrical cortical effect. Administration of large doses or frequent administration of small doses at short intervals produces the following changes: appearance of slow waves after a few days that become progressively slower and of increased amplitude. These abnormal slow waves persist for as long as 48 hours after drug withdrawal.

Histamine Release

Intravenous meperidine in doses of 5.0 mg/kg induces a severalfold increase in plasma histamine.[133] From a baseline of about 0.12 ng/ml, the plasma level may rise to levels of 20 to 30 ng/ml within 1.2 minutes and may continue high for 6.0 or more minutes at levels of 7.0 ng/ml. Such increases occur in about 50% of subjects. At 25 minutes, the level is still high at 0.28 ng/ml in all patients. Meperidine apparently has a much greater capacity to induce histamine release than morphine.[180]

Drug Interactions[49]

Many of these interactions are similar to those with morphine. Most of the phenothiazines, particularly chlorpromazine, and the tricyclic antidepressants increase the respiratory depressant action and induce significant sedation. The benzodiazepines appear not to potentiate the depressant effects of meperidine; this is true of diazepam.

Concomitant administration of phenobarbitol or phenytoin increases the clearance rate of meperidine; if these drugs are administered with oral meperidine, one sees a decrease in bioavailability. Associated with these actions is an elevation of the metabolite normeperidine.[170]

Of singular importance are the reactions of patients receiving monoamine oxidase inhibitors. Two clinical syndromes have been recognized: (1) severe respiratory depression; and (2) a syndrome of excitation manifested by delerium, hyperpyrexia, and convulsions.

Administration of amphetamines, as with morphine, enhances the analgesic effect but decreases the sedative effect of meperidine and related derivatives.[127]

Excitatory symptoms may also be produced in subjects tolerant to the depressant effects of meperidine. These consist of tremors, muscle twitches, hyperactive reflexes, dilated pupils, and convulsions. Large doses of meperidine administered at short intervals precipitate the syndrome. The mechanism is due to the accumulation of the metabolite normeperidine. In patients with decreased hepatic and/or renal function, these toxic symptoms are frequently seen.[181] An occasion for the reaction is in the postoperative period following kidney transplantation when meperidine is administered for analgesia.

Parkinsonian-Type Reactions[182]

A parkinsonian-type reaction may be seen in elderly patients after large doses of meperidine in the postoperative period. Neurologic examination shows a masked face, low voice, drooling, flexed neck, rigidity of muscles, resting tremor, and festinating gait. Carbidopa-levodopa (Sinemet) treatment readily reverses the process. The reaction may be due to a byproduct of meperidine synthesis as a contaminant or as a metabolite, or it may be caused by the actual illicit use of MPTP (1-methyl-4-phenyl-1,2,3,6-tetrahydropyridine).[182]

Pregnant Patient and the Fetus

Meperidine is one of the most widely used analgesics for relief of labor pains. It appears to have a degree of spasticity for the visceral-type pain associated with uterine contractions, as does one of its analogues, alphaprodine. A metabolite of the meperidine, normeperidine is an active derivative, whereas the degraded product, meperidinic acid, is inactive.[183]

The parent meperidine drug crosses the placenta and enters the fetal circulation. When administered to the mother, intramuscularly, it is readily absorbed and soon appears in the fetus.[184] The highest level in the fetus is reached between 2 and 3 hours after administration to the mother.[185] O'Donoghue demonstrated that the neonate, when given meperidine, can metabolize the narcotic within 24 hours and produce normeperidine.[186] Both meperidine and the metabolite have been identified in umbilical cord blood and in neonatal urine.

Although the highest levels of meperidine are reached in the fetus soon after administration to the mother, an increasing blood level of normeperidine is seen in the fetus as the interval between drug administration and delivery time increases.[187] This is designated as DDT (drug to delivery time). Thus, neonatal depression can continue into the postdelivery period for 1 to 2 days.[188] The half-life of meperidine in the neonate is about 13 hours, but the half-life of normeperidine is set at 62 hours. When a woman in labor is given meperidine, both the unchanged drug and its metabolite are recoverable from the plasma and urine of the neonate, and metabolite is still present after the first day of life. The levels of these drugs are higher when delivery is delayed, when multiple doses of the narcotic are given to the mother, or when the drug is given 2 to 3 hours before delivery. These factors are associated with respiratory depression, low Apgar scores, neonatal acidosis, electroencephalographic abnormalities, abnormal reflexes, and low behavioral scores.[188] Both the Scanlon[189] test and the Brazelton[190] behavioral assessment are decreased.[191] All these factors are associated with greater neonatal morbidity and mortality.

Such adverse effects are minimized by administration of meperidine to the mother within 2 hours of anticipated delivery; the use of low doses; avoidance of drug combinations; and avoidance of combining inappropriate timing with epidural and other anesthetics.

Pharmacokinetics

Absorption

Meperidine is absorbed by all routes of administration.[49] After oral administration, absorption from the intestinal tract is appreciatively rapid, with an onset of action at about 15 to 20 minutes, but a peak effect that is delayed. Only 50% of the oral dose reaches the systemic circulation because of the first-pass metabolism of the drug in the gut wall and in the liver. The effectiveness of oral meperidine is better than for morphine, however, but it is not as good as for codeine.

Absorption from the subcutaneous and intramuscular routes is erratic, and the onset and peak concentrations may vary widely. Administration by the subcutaneous route especially is unpleasant, and local tissue irritation and tissue induration occur with both routes.

Blood and Plasma Binding[192]

Meperidine is reversibly bound to plasma protein by the α_1-acid glycoprotein and by association with red blood cells. The amount so bound is about 60%, of which

Table 31–5. Pharmacokinetic Data: Meperidine

Availability (Oral) (%)	Urinary Excretion (%)	Bound in Plasma (%)	Clearance (ml · min^{-1} · kg^{-1})	Vol. Dist. (L/kg)	Half-Life (h)	Effective Concentrations
52 ± 3 ↑ Cirrhosis	1–25*	58 ± 9† ↓ Aged, Uremia ←→ Cirrhosis	17 ± 5 ↓ AVH, Cirrhosis, Uremia ←→ Aged, Pregnancy, Smoking	4.4 ± 0.9 ↑ Aged ←→ Cirrhosis, Pregnancy, Uremia	3.2 ± 0.8‡ ↑ AVH, Cirrhosis, Aged, Uremia ←→ Pregnancy	0.4–0.7 µg/ml§

*Meperidine is a weak acid (pK_a = 9.6) and is excreted to a greater extent in the urine at low urinary pH and to a lesser extent at high pH.
†Correlates with the concentration of α_1-acid glycoprotein.
‡A longer half-life (7 hours) is also observed.
§Postoperative analgesia.
From Gilman, A. G., et al.: Goodman and Gilman's The Pharmacological Basis of Therapeutics, 8th Ed. New York, McGraw-Hill, 1990.

49% is bound to the protein and 20% is attached to the red cells. Some variations in binding are to be noted. After intramuscular intravenous injections in patients over 70 years of age, about twice as much of meperidine is bound to protein than in patients under 30 years of age; that is, with increasing age, an increasing fraction of drugs is found in the plasma and a larger fraction of this is also unbound.

Alcoholic consumption influences both plasma distribution and plasma clearance.[193] The levels are lowest in social drinkers, whereas in nondrinkers and in heavy drinkers, clearance is good. Initial plasma concentrations of meperidine are lower in heavy drinkers, but the volume of distribution is greater, probably because of an expanded vascular bed.

Pharmacokinetic Data (Table 31–5)

The kinetics of meperidine in healthy human volunteers and in surgical patients has been studied.[194] Doses of 1.0 mg/kg (range of 0.7 to 1.4 mg/kg) when administered intravenously appear to be disposed into a two-compartment system, in which plotting of plasma concentration against time shows a biphasic decay. This occurs after an initial dilution period in the blood volume, lasting about 1.6 minutes (P phase) First, a rapid decline in plasma concentration occurs as a result of distribution to vascular-rich tissues and receptor uptake (Fig. 31-13). The drug is extensively localized in tissues where the concentration is six times higher than in the plasma.[192] This α phase is short, with a $T_{1/2}$-α of 4.0 minutes. A second, slower phase of decline in plasma occurs in the ensuing 2 to 4 hours because of redistribution to liver and kidney. Thus, β elimination phase follows, whose half-life ($T_{1/2}$-β) is between 3.1 and 3.9 hours.[195] This depends on hepatic metabolism of meperidine and its renal elimination. The total plasma clearance is calculated at a rate of about 0.85 L/min. The volume of distribution at steady state is relatively large, with a $V_{D_{ss}}$ of 200 L.

High doses of 5.0 mg/kg have been administered to surgical patients and the kinetics determined.[196] The β phase is slightly longer, with a $T_{1/2}$-β of 4.4 hours. Plasma clearance is slightly less, at 0.08 ± 0.33 L/min, and the apparent volume of distribution is larger and is determined at

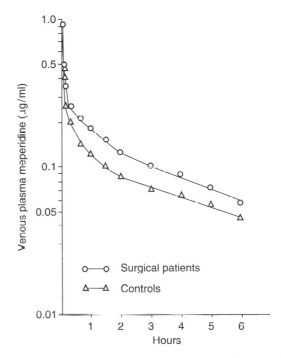

Fig. 31–13. Mean plasma concentrations following intravenous injection of 50 mg meperidine HCl over 1 minute. Redrawn from Mather, L. E., et al.: Meperidine kinetics in man: intravenous injection in surgical patients and volunteers. Clin Pharmacol Ther *17*:21, 1975.

280 L.[196] The results show that larger doses do not saturate metabolic mechanisms of degradation, nor do they alter elimination of the drug.

Kinetic Variables

Alcohol consumption tends to increase the volume of distribution. In nondrinkers, the $V_{D_{ss}}$ is about half that of heavy drinkers. The $T_{1/2}$-β is about twice as long as in nondrinkers (3.2 hours versus 1.7 hours).[195] The larger volume of distribution with a lower plasma concentration probably accounts for decreased drug effect often seen in chronic alcoholics with cirrhosis. The bioavailability after oral administration is increased as much as 80%, however, and the half-life of meperidine and normeperidine is increased.[193]

Age influences plasma binding of meperidine in a positive manner. From age 20 to 80 years, the free fraction in plasma increases from 0.25 to 0.65.[197]

Clearance is almost completely related to metabolic degradation. The renal excretion of unchanged meperidine amounts to only about 7% (2 to 10%) of an administered dose. If acidification of urine (ammonium chloride) is pursued (to a pH < 5), the elimination of intact meperidine may be increased to 20 to 30% of the dose, whereas alkalization reduces the amount excreted intact to about 1.0% of administered dose.[198]

Induction of anesthesia is associated with a rise in venous plasma concentration. This effect is immediately seen and is probably related to the redistribution of blood from the viscera to the peripheral pool. This hemodynamic change results in a washout of drug from the tissue compartment.[199]

After the bolus dose alone, blood levels are initially higher than necessary and fall into the subtherapeutic range after 20 to 40 minutes.[195] With the continuous infusion of 0.4 mg/min alone, it takes slightly more than 2 hours to reach the lowest analgesic concentrations.[200] By combining the two methods of administration, blood levels of meperidine remain within the analgesic range. The use of a priming infusion of higher concentration would limit the peak concentration and minimize the depth of the concentration trough. A concentration of 0.7 μg/ml was estimated to provide pain relief in 95% of cases and gave no evidence of clinically significant respiratory depression (or toxicity).[201] These techniques reduce fluctuations in plasma concentration and in analgesic effect.[202]

Effective Analgesic Blood Concentrations[200]

In the treatment of pain, an analgesic response is related to the blood concentration (Fig. 31-14). The minimum effective analgesic concentration has been determined to be about 0.50 μg/kg. In the study by Austin and colleagues,[201] the value is reported as 0.46 μg/ml (S.D. = 0.18). Moreover, a blood concentration as high as 0.41 μg/ml apparently may still be associated with severe

pain. On the contrary, a blood concentration of 0.6 μg/ml appears to provide relief from severe pain in 84% of individuals, whereas a blood level of 0.7 μg/ml offers relief from severe pain in 95% of individuals.[202]

Metabolism[203]

Meperidine is largely destroyed in the body to the extent of about 90%. This is accomplished principally by the liver and occurs at a rate of 10 to 22% per hour, with an average rate of 17% per hour.[192] Two hepatic metabolic routes are involved. In one, hydrolysis produces meperidinic acid. The second route is one of demethylation to form a metabolite, normeperidine. Normeperidine is then further handled by hydrolysis to normeperidinic acid (Fig. 31-15). Excretion of both normeperidine and normeperidinic acid is primarily renal. The acid metabolites are pharmacologically inert; however, normeperidine has significant pharmacologic activity.[204] The elimination half-lives of meperidine and normeperidine are 3.0 to 6.0 hours and 15 to 40 hours, respectively. Many of the toxic effects of meperidine are related to the presence of normeperidine.[205]

Normeperidine Toxicity

The toxicity of this metabolite was first described in 1977.[206] This degradation product of meperidine can accumulate under circumstances of continuous administration of high doses of meperidine or as a result of impaired renal excretion.

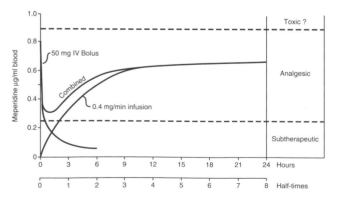

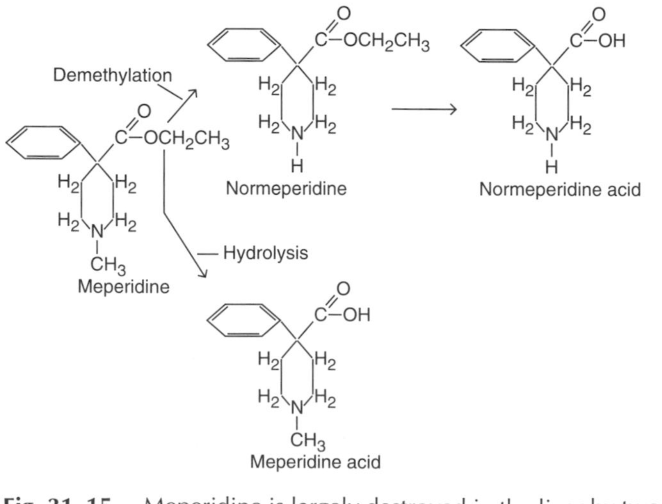

Fig. 31-15. Meperidine is largely destroyed in the liver by two metabolic routes of hydrolysis and demethylation. Hydrolysis produces meperidinic acid, whereas demethylation produces normeperidine, which is further hydrolyzed to normeperidinic acid. The de-esterification process to yield normeperidine is the more important pathway; the demethylation pathway is a minor route, and the methyl group is removed as formaldehyde and is not catabolized by the liver microsomal enzyme system. None of the metabolites appear to have analgesic action. From Burns, J. J., et al.: The physiological disposition and fate of meperidine in man and a method for its estimation in plasma. J Pharmacol Exp Ther *114*:289, 1955.

Fig. 31-14. Blood levels of meperidine associated with an analgesic effect. (A composite by Hug of data by Mather, Austin, and Stapleton; see text). Redrawn from Hug, C. C.: Improving analgesic therapy. Anesthesiology *53*:441, 1980.

The metabolite itself has some analgesic action. Symptoms of CNS excitation such as restlessness, discomfort, and tremors are not to be interpreted as pain, however. At plasma levels of 0.8 μg/ml, myoclonus and grand mal seizures may occur.[173]

Biotransformation Mechanisms[192]

Meperidine degradation is accomplished by the liver. Fractions are handled as follows: demthylation (3 to 8%); de-esterification (3 to 8%); conjugated (8 to 15%); oxidized (3 to 8%); and hydrolyzed (20%).

Excretion[192]

Meperidine is largely excreted in the form of various metabolites. Only 2 to 10% of the dose of the parent drug is excreted unchanged under normal urinary pH conditions. Under conditions of forced acidity of the urine, that is, a pH less than 5.0, the fraction of whole meperidine excreted may be increased to 20 to 30% of the administered dose.

Dosage and Administration[164]

Dosage in children approximates 0.5 mg/kg body weight. If accompanied by a barbiturate, this dose should be reduced by about one third. Adult doses range from 50 to 150 mg for single doses or 1.0 mg/kg. On a milligram weight basis, this is approximately 10 times the therapeutic dose of morphine. Caution must be exercised in prescribing a dose for the elderly patient, and in these patients, the recommended range is 20 to 50 mg as a single dose.

Although the drug is absorbed from the intestinal tract and from all parenteral sites of injection, it is recommended that it be administered either intramuscularly or intravenously. If administered subcutaneously, it is irritating.

Useful in producing a basal narcotic state is the intravenous administration of meperidine in dilute solution.[207] A 0.02 to 0.04% solution is prepared for this purpose. The rate of administration is balanced against clinical signs of hypnosis, unconsciousness, and anesthesia. This technique provides an even level of narcosis on which surgical anesthesia can be established with nitrous oxide or ethylene.[208]

Pharmacodynamics (Fig. 31–16)[194]

The time of maximal analgesic effect corresponds to the peak serum concentration and is related to the route of administration. After oral adiministration, analgesic effects are noted in about 15 minutes; they reach a peak in 2 hours and subside over the following 2 to 4 hours. The total analgesic effect is about half that after parenteral administration. Bioavailability is 40 to 60% of the oral dose.

Following subcutaneous or intramuscular administration, the onset of analgesia is faster, occurring within 10 minutes, and reaches a peak in 30 to 60 minutes corresponding to peak serum concentration. The duration of effect is between 3 and 5 hours.

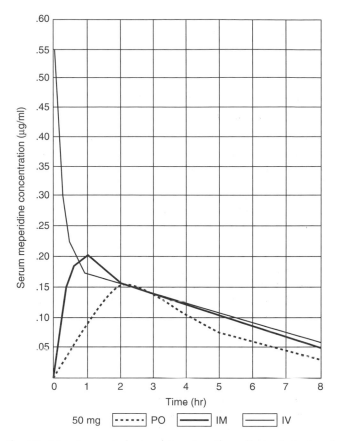

50 mg · · · · · PO ▬▬ IM ▭ IV

Fig. 31–16. In a study to determine the effect of route of administration on the serum level of meperidine, it was found that while the initial concentration was higher when the drug was given intravenously, at about 30 minutes, the intramuscular-derived concentration was equal to that after intravenous injection, and at 2 hours—and thereafter—oral administration provided equal levels. Redrawn from Shambaugh, H. E., Wainer, I. W., Sanstead, J. R., Hemphill, D. M.: The clinical pharmacology of meperidine: comparison of routes of administration. J Clin Pharm Ther 16:245, 1976.

Uses in Anesthesia[164]

Meperidine is widely used in preanesthetic medication and in postoperative pain management; however, its application should be selective. It is recommended in the following circumstances:

1. As medication preliminary to halothane administration.
2. In patients with asthma, emphysema, or bronchospastic pulmonary disease.
3. In patients with ventricular arrhythmias.
4. In geriatric patients in small doses.
5. When analgesia without sleep is desired.
6. For visceral pain, especially urinary or intestinal.

It is undesirable or poorly effective when:

1. Patients are medicated with antiarrhythmic drugs.
2. Patients have atrial arrhythmias.
3. Patients have hypotensive states.

4. Biliary colic is present.
5. Severe cutaneous pain exists.
6. Patients have anticholinergic effects with large doses.

Effective Pain Relief with Morphine and Meperidine

Plasma Levels for Analgesia

Plasma levels from a given adequate dose of narcotic are effective and above pain threshold for about 2.5 hours. After morphine administration, some analgesia is provided when plasma levels are between 0.05 and 0.1 μg/ml. This is a threshold level for pain relief. Good analgesia is observed at plasma levels of 0.1 to 0.5 μg/ml.

A minimum analgesic blood concentration for meperidine is approximately 0.5 μg/kg. Meperidine analgesia is good at plasma levels of 0.5 to 1.0 μg/ml.[209] To maintain these plasma levels, narcotics need to be administered on a more frequent and flexible schedule of every 2 to 3 hours. Intravenous administration remains the logical method, however; giving smaller fractional doses every hour maintains a steady, effective plasma level.

Route of Administration

Absorption from intramuscular injections of narcotics is usually the single largest cause of variability in blood concentration and, hence, of unpredictable pain relief.

Intramuscular injections at fixed intervals of 4 hours as needed result in highly variable blood concentrations. These concentrations are only above the analgesic threshold for 35% of the time during a 4-hour dose schedule.[210]

Intramuscular injections on a more frequent basis are not well tolerated. The intravenous route may be used through an established intravenous infusion line, which obviates the absorption process. Multiple injections are avoided, and wide swings in plasma concentrations are avoided. Frequent small intravenous doses can be titrated against a readily observable response; a continuous infusion of a dilute solution of narcotic can be used to accomplish the same end steady blood level.

Dosage

Present practice reveals that patients are underdosed by about 30%. A substantial number suffer postoperative pain significantly.[211] Therefore, pain should be treated on "demand" and a dose titrated to an effective end point.[212]

Doses should be based primarily on *lean* body mass and modified by other factors. Consideration should first be given to a *loading dose* to achieve satisfactory pain relief; *morphine* doses of 0.1 to 0.2 mg/kg achieve a satisfactory result. The larger dose is needed for healthy, vigorous subjects under 50 years of age and 70 kg, whereas patients over 65 years of age require less morphine (Fig. 31–17).[50]

The calculated loading dose should be administered fractionally by the intravenous route over a period of 10 minutes until adequate effect is achieved, that is, until pain relief is reported by the patient.

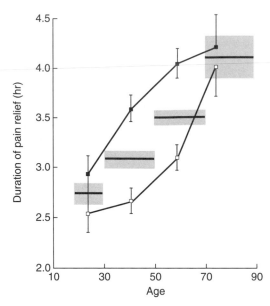

Fig. 31–17. Duration of pain relief in relation to age after 8 mg (lower curve) and 16 mg (upper curve) morphine. The duration of pain relief is the hour after drug that the patient reports the last positive pain relief score. Each point represents mean duration of relief concurrent with the mean ages of four age groups. The vertical bars represent ± SEM. The shaded areas represent comparable data for the combined doses, extending horizontally to define the range of each age group. Redrawn from Kaiko, R. F.: Age and morphine analgesia in cancer patients with postoperative pain. Clin Pharmacol Ther *28*:823, 1980.

Maintenance doses are then provided intravenously to keep the plasma level in the effective range.[213] In healthy adults of 50 to 100 kg lean mass, a dose of 1.0 mg, administered intravenously starting 2 hours after the loading dose and given every hour thereafter, affords continuous relief and maintains an effective plasma level.

One pharmacologic axiom that must guide the physician in controlling pain states is as follows: "The dose of a narcotic analgesic required to relieve ongoing pain is larger than the dose required to prevent pain."[213]

To achieve adequate analgesia with meperidine, the dosage ranges from 1.0 to 1.5 mg/kg. Thus, 80 mg of meperidine equates with 1.0 mg of morphine and a satisfactory, safe intravenous dose schedule can be established. After an effective loading dose, the maintenance dose intravenously ranges between 5.0 and 8.0 mg every hour. A dose of 1.0 to 2.0 mg intravenously every hour for the adult male of 70 kg lean mass maintains an effective plasma level.

Derivatives of Meperidine

Two analogues of meperidine were introduced soon after its widespread clinical use with a view to increase potency and to limit adverse effects: (1) alphaprodine (Nisentil) was prepared by Ziering and Lee in 1947 with a potency two to three times that of the parent; the pharmacology was studied by Gottschalk and associates;[214]

(2) anileridine, a substituted meperidine, was synthetized by Weijlard in 1956 and was studied pharmacologically by Orahovats.[215]

Neither drug has fulfilled some of the early promises of lower adverse effects and higher potency. No significant advantages over meperidine were determined.[215a]

METHADONE (DOLOPHINE)

Chemistry

Continued research for newer analgesics similar to meperidine resulted in the discovery of methadone. This simple compound is a striking analgesic.

It is a synthetic drug chemically designated as a diphenyl heptanone derivative.[216] The chemical name is 6-dimethyl-amino-4-4-diphenylheptanone.

Structure

Methadone contains a dimethyl amino group. Gero has shown that this group could be rearranged to assume a τ-phenyl-N-methylpiperidyl form and thus subscribe to the concept of a common structural moiety for narcotic drugs (Fig. 31–18).[217]

Analgesic activity resides in the levo isomer *l* methadone and is 50 times more potent than the dextro form.

Dosage[218,219]

The oral analgesic dose for adults is 2.5 to 15 mg and is varied with the intensity of pain. The parenteral dose ranges from 2.5 to 10 mg, an average dose being about 0.1 mg/kg body weight. Tablets in doses of 5 and 10 mg are available for oral use; solutions are available for parenteral injection. The potency of 10 mg of methadone is equivalent to 15 mg of morphine.

Administration and Absorption

The drug may be given by all routes. It is well absorbed from the gastrointestinal tract after oral administration. Its efficacy by this route is impressive, and the bioavailability is about 90%, indicating that first-pass destruction by the gut and liver is minimal. Methadone is also readily absorbed from the buccal mucosa.[220]

Subcutaneous injection results in erratic absorption and is accompanied by tissue irritation and pain. It is not recommended.

Intramuscular injection is a desirable route with good absorption and a more rapid onset of action.

Pharmacodynamics[221]

After oral ingestion, the onset of analgesic action occurs in 30 to 60 minutes and coincides with its appearance in plasma. The peak analgesic effect is seen soon after 1 hour, and the duration of action is between 5 and 8 hours.[222]

After parenteral administration, the onset of analgesia is between 10 and 20 minutes. The duration of analgesia, however, remains at about 5 to 8 hours only, despite the prolonged plasma levels for as long as 24 or more hours.

Pharmacokinetics[221]

Binding[215]

Plasma protein binding has been measured as well as the portion bound to the red blood cells; about 30% is associated with the red blood cell mass. The red cell to plasma partition coefficient has been calculated as R/P = 0.32, and the mean blood to plasma ratio is B/P = 0.75. The overall binding reveals that about 88% is bound in the blood, resulting in a free fraction of about 12% in the plasma.

Methadone has great lipoid solubility, and the amount bound is twice that of morphine.[223] The plasma bound drug is released to various tissues and bound to the lipoid fraction,[224] particularly the brain, where the peak concentration is reached in 1 to 2 hours. With repeated doses, accumulation occurs. When medication is discontinued,[223] there is a slow release from the extravascular sites to the circulation, and the drug is then eliminated over 1 to 2 days[224] (Fig. 31–19).

Disposition

After intravenous administration, the plasma methadone concentration declines in a manner fitted by a triexponential equation. The distribution is rapid and extensive to vascular-rich tissues and to receptors, and the volume is calculated as 3.5 to 3.8 L/kg body weight.

Plasma Concentrations[215]

After parenteral injection, methadone is detected in the plasma within 15 minutes and correlates with the onset of analgesia.[225] Peak plasma concentrations are reached in

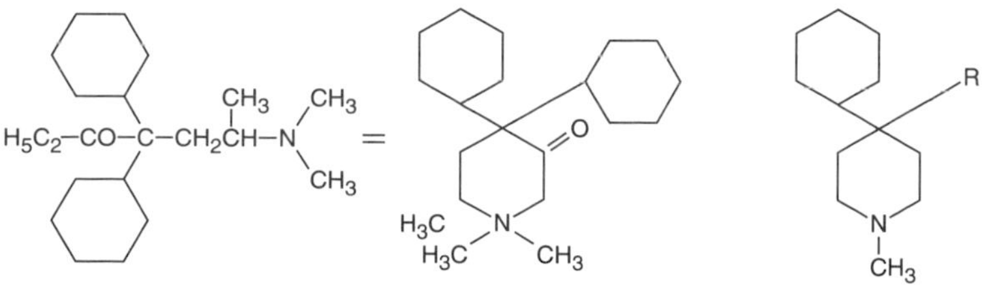

methadone   methadone   γ-phenyl-N-methyl
                                      piperidine moiety

Fig. 31–18. Methadone structural relationships. After Gero in Cutting.

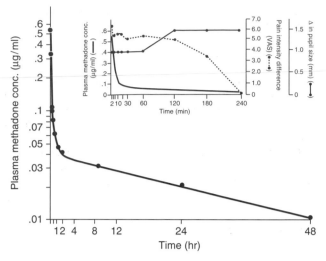

Fig. 31–19. Plasma concentration-time profiles of methadone after a single intravenous dose of 10 mg methadone HCl administered to patient No. 1. The points represent the observed concentrations and the solid line the theoretic line obtained by fitting the data with a triexponential equation. The insert shows measures of pharmacodynamic effect (pain intensity difference [VAS] and changes in pupil size) and the simultaneously determined plasma methadone profile for patient 1 for the 240 minutes after drug administration. Redrawn from Inturrisi, C. E., et al.: Clin Pharmacol Ther 41:392, 1987.

30 to 60 minutes and are accompanied by brain tissue uptake where the peak concentration is reached in less than 2 hours.

The effective analgesic concentration in the plasma is 30 ng/ml.[226] It remains high as the methadone is released from the brain and other tissues. After 6 hours, a slow decline and a slow release from tissues occur, which results in a half-life of 1 to 1½ days or an average of 35 ± 12 hours.

Biotransformation[225]

Extensive degradation of methodone occurs in the liver by N-demethylation and cyclization. The metabolites formed are pyrrolidines and pyrroline.

Excretion[227]

The metabolites are excreted as such by the kidney to the extent of 24% into the urine. Acidification of the urine increases the amount of methadone excreted. Some of the metabolites are also excreted by the liver into bile.

In both instances, the excretion is accompanied by small amounts of unchanged methadone.

The clearance rate is set at $1.4 \pm 0.5 \ ml \cdot min^{-1} \cdot kg^{-1}$ (Table 31–6).

Advantages and Uses

1. Excellent analgesia for chronic pain.
2. Suppression of withdrawal symptoms in physically dependent individuals.
3. Minimal and slow tolerance phenomenon; the drug may be used as a substitute for strong opioids in the weaning process.

Pharmacologic Actions

Central Nervous System

Methadone is primarily a μ agonist. It has many characteristics of morphine and has a greater analgesic activity by about 30%, especially after oral administration. Sedation is minimal.[218] The drug is less prone to cause addiction than morphine[219] and is a useful drug in intractable pain states (cancer).[226] The duration of action is long, between 8 and 12 hours.

Analgesia is more pronounced on a weight-for-weight basis with methadone than with morphine.[222] In a clinical evaluation of pain, relief was obtained in 81% of the cases, which is on a par with morphine.[228] Tolerance develops slowly.[229] Although one sees a relaxing effect in the presence of pain, sedation is minimal, but it becomes marked in some patients with repeated doses, and mental confusion is rare.[228] In obstetrics,[230] the pain relief is inferior to that induced by meperidine, and with the lack of hypnotic action there is little amnesia. Furthermore, the respiratory depressant effect on the fetus is greater than is seen with meperidine.

The pain and muscle spasm of poliomyelitis are significantly relieved by methadone.[228] The pain of renal ureteral or colic is also promptly relieved,[231] and the discomfort of bladder spasm incident to the use of catheters following prostatic and bladder surgery is particularly alleviated.

Parasympathetic System

Among the autonomic actions are increased intestinal tone with constriction of sphincters.[218] Some miosis occurs, which is seen after a single dose, persists for 24

Table 31–6. Pharmacokinetic Data: Methadone

Availability (Oral) (%)	Urinary Excretion (%)	Bound in Plasma (%)	Clearance $(ml \cdot min^{-1} \cdot kg^{-1})$	Vol. Dist. (L/kg)	Half-Life (h)	Effective Concentrations
92 ± 21	24 ± 10*	89 ± 1.4	1.4 ± 0.5*†	3.8 ± 0.6‡	35 ± 12‡	>100 ng/ml§

*Inversely correlated with urine pH.
†Blood-to-plasma ratio = 0.75 ± 0.03.
‡Directly correlated with urine pH.
§Prevention of withdrawal symptoms.
Gilman, A. G., et al.: From Goodman & Gilman's The Pharmacological Basis of Therapeutics, 8th Ed. New York, McGraw-Hill, 1990.

hours, and can be detected for as long as 24 hours after a single dose.

Cardiovascular System

Most cardiovascular effects are not prominent in the recumbent subject. Bradycardia occurs presumably through a parasympathetic action because it does not occur if the vagus nerve is cut. Systolic blood pressure is lowered through peripheral vasodilatation. The electrocardiogram remains unchanged.

Respiratory System

Methadone is a respiratory depressant like morphine.[231] Single doses of 15 mg of methadone decreases the minute volume about 14%. The cough reflex is also significantly depressed, and this effect has been found useful in controlling coughs of bronchiectasis and bronchogenic carcinoma.[231] The respiratory depression can be counteracted to some extent by ephedrine or methedrine.

Miscellaneous Effects

As a preanesthetic medicant,[231] methadone is generally not satisfactory. Apprehension especially is not sufficiently allayed. Some usefulness, however, has been found during regional anesthesia, where the drug has been used to supplement spinal or a block anesthesia that is wearing off.[232,233] Methadone has also been investigated in regard to local anesthetic properties and has been found to possess strong local effects on the rabbit's cornea,[234] although the irritant properties preclude its use as a surface anesthetic. Some side effects include lightheadedness, feelings of weakness, nausea, and vomiting. Generally, these are more frequent than with other narcotics.

PROPOXYPHENE (DARVON)

Chemistry

In the course of synthetizing various substitutes for morphine, a series of four isomers similar to methadone was isolated.[235] Of these, only the α-racemate designated a propoxyphene had analgesic activity, and this property was present only in the dextrorotary isomer. The levopropoxyphene was found to have antitussive activity, however.

The structural formula is similar to that of methodone and is an analogue.

The hydrochloride salt is the basic preparation and has been studied pharmacologically.

Pharmacologic Effects

Central Nervous System Action

Analgesia is produced by binding to the μ-receptors in the CNS. Other CNS actions are similar those of codeine.

Dosage and Potency[236]

Propoxyphene is about half as potent as codeine when taken orally. About 90 to 120 mg is required to equal the analgesic effect of 60 mg of codeine. These doses are about equal to 600 mg of aspirin.[237] A combination of propoxyphene with aspirin provides a more effective medication for mild to moderate pain. The usual oral dose is 65 mg every 4 hours.[237]

Respiratory System

These effects are minimal, and the relative action is about one third that of codeine in producing any depression. Sedatives and hypnotics and alcohol especially exaggerate the depression.[238]

Pharmacokinetics[239]

Absorption

After oral intake of a single dose, progressive uptake from the intestinal tract occurs. Plasma concentrations are detected within 1 hour, reach a peak concentration in 2½ hours, and then slowly decline with a mean half-life of 4 hours.[239] After a 100-mg dose, the peak plasma concentration achieved is 0.05 to 0.1 μg/ml at about 4 hours.[239] With repeated doses, one sees an increase in the plasma concentration and the half-life is extended to 6 to 12 hours. The normetabolite has a longer half-life of over 30 hours.[240,240a] With repeated doses, a steady state of concentration is reached in 48 hours.

Metabolism

Degradation occurs in the liver by N-demethylation. The principal metabolite is norpropoxyphene.

Excretion

Both the parent drug and its metabolite are excreted by the kidney.[241]

Comments and Uses

Propoxyphene is a useful analgesic for mild to moderate pain in patients who have not had a positive response to aspirin. A combination of 35 mg of propoxyphene with 120 mg of aspirin is frequently prescribed. The potential for abuse is about the same as for codeine. The concern about addiction potential with codeine is unrealistic.

BENZMORPHAN DERIVATIVES: OPIOIDS WITH MIXED AGONIST-ANTAGONIST ACTION

In 1954, Lasagna and Beecher[242] noted that the morphine antagonist nalorphine[243] possessed analgesic properties. The analgesia was found to be potent and of the order of two to three times that of morphine. Because the antagonist does not support addiction, it was evident that potent analgesia could be separated from addiction. In addition, Keats and Telford and their associates[244,245] noted that some morphinan derivatives, inactive by laboratory testing, were found to be potent human analgesics. The antagonist also possessed two undesirable side effects, namely, (1) an undesirable sedative effect and (2) psychic effects of a hallucinogenic nature. These findings prompted investigators to prepare and evaluate a series of analgesic antagonists with the benzmorphan nucleus.[246,247]

Modification of the phenanthrene nucleus of morphinans produces the benzmorphan series of compounds. In this modification, the benzene ring containing the alcoholic hydroxyl group is eliminated, leaving only a methyl residue. The heterocyclic nitrogen-containing ring remains (Fig. 31-20), and various substitutions may be made on the nitrogen.

These compounds have three principal characteristics: analgesic activity, opiate antagonism, and minimal addiction liability.

Pentazocine

This derivative is the N-dimethyl-allyl analogue of benzmorphan. It is available as the racemic mixture, and the levo-isomer possesses the analgesic and respiratory depressant properties.

Study of the analgesic action by Telford and associates[245] showed that it was a potent analgesic without addiction liability and without psychomimetic action. Because the drug has low abuse liability, it was not placed under narcotic regulations.[248,249]

This agent is a partial agonist at μ receptors and may have an extensive agonist action at κ receptors. It is a weak antagonist with a potency about $\frac{1}{50}$ that of naloxone.

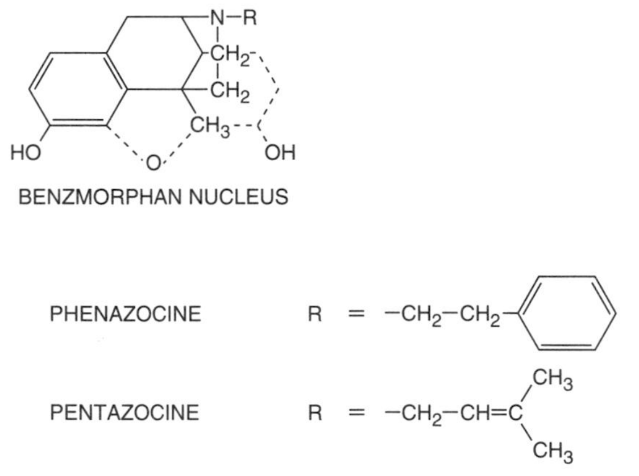

BENZMORPHAN NUCLEUS

PHENAZOCINE   R = $-CH_2-CH_2-$ phenyl

PENTAZOCINE   R = $-CH_2-CH=C$ with CH_3, CH_3

Fig. 31–20. Basic structure of benzmorphan derivates. Eliminated from the morphine nucleus is the third ring containing the alcoholic hydroxyl and the oxygen bridge (dotted part). A methyl group remains.

Pharmacokinetics[250]

Absorption

Absorption readily occurs from the gastrointestinal tract and from parenteral subcutaneous and intramuscular sites. The drug may also be given intravenously. Distribution is rapid to all vascular-rich tissues. The drug passes through the placental barrier but in lesser amounts than meperidine. About 65% is bound to plasma protein.[250]

After oral ingestion of 40 mg of pentazocine, uptake is good from the intestinal tract, and the bioavailability is about 50%, indicating some first-pass loss in the gut and the liver. The onset of analgesia occurs less than 1 hour after oral intake, and a peak plasma concentration is reached between 1 and 3 hours.[251] Plasma levels are still elevated at 5 hours.[252]

After intramuscular injection, the onset of action is less than 15 minutes, coinciding with initial plasma levels. Peak plasma concentrations are achieved between 30 minutes and 1 hour. The half-life is about 4.5 hours.[251] The analgesic and other effects coincide with the plasma levels of pentazocine.[252]

After intravenous administration, the onset of analgesia occurs in 2 to 5 minutes, and peak concentrations are seen in less than 20 minutes.

Biotransformation

Degradation of most of the drug occurs rapidly in the liver by oxidation of the terminal methyl groups and conjugation with glucuronides.

Excretion

The metabolites are excreted by the kidney, and a small portion of intact drug is also excreted in the urine. Approximately 60% of the total drug is elmiminated in 24 hours. The clearance rate is 17 $\pm$ 5 ml $\cdot$ min^{-1} $\cdot$ kg^{-1} (Table 31-7).

Pharmacologic Effects[253,254]

Analgesia

Pain relief scores show *dl*-pentazocine to be a potent analgesic with a relative potency of 0.26. Pain relief is afforded by doses of 20 to 40 mg, and the analgesic potency is one fourth that of morphine; that is, 40 mg, given parenterally, is equivalent to 10 mg of morphine. The *l*-isomer has an analgesic potency of 0.42, which is greater than the racemic mixture or one half that of morphine. In controlled pain studies, however, Moertel[255] found that

Table 31–7. Pharmacokinetic Data: Pentazocine

Availability (Oral) (%)	Urinary Excretion (%)	Bound in Plasma (%)	Clearance (ml·min^{-1}·kg^{-1})	Vol. Dist. (L/kg)	Half-Life (h)	Effective Concentrations
47 ± 15	15 ± 7	65	17 ± 5*	7.1 ± 1.4*	4.6 ± 1.0	—

*CLIF and V$_{area}$/F for intramuscular dose, assuming 70-kg weight.
From Gilman, A. G., et al.: Goodman and Gilman's The Pharmacological Basis of Therapeutics, 8th Ed. New York, McGraw-Hill, 1990.

650 mg of aspirin equaled the activity of 50 mg of oral pentazocine.

After an intramuscular injection of this drug, the onset of action occurs in 15 minutes. Pain relief persists for about 3 hours and then wanes over 4 to 6 hours.

Central Nervous System

Subjective effects similar to those produced by morphine are noted, although some qualitative differences are apparent.[256] The l-isomer produces good relaxation of the patient's psyche, and cognition values are diminished; sedation occurs with both isomers. With large doses of the dl-mixture, however, relaxation is less prominent and anxiety is noted with a 40-mg dose. This response parallels the response to the d-isomer, which at doses of 60 mg, produces anxiety. Lightheaded and dreamy reactions were frequent.

Respiration[257]

The respiratory rate is maximally decreased about 40 minutes after injection, but the tidal volume is elevated. The net effect is a mild decrease in ventilation.

The potency of the dl-mixture is 0.39 relative to morphine in this regard. Controlled studies of pulmonary gas by Bellville and Forrest[257] indicate that the l-isomer is the potent respiratory depressant and that equianalgesic doses produce as much respiratory depression as morphine. Doses of 20 mg administered parenterally were found to be equivalent to 10 mg of morphine, and the relative potency of the l-isomer has been set at 0.76. Little respiratory depressant activity resides in the d-isomer, and if there is any, it is probably less than one tenth the effect of l-pentazocine.

Cardiovascular System[254]

Cardiovascular changes are not significant. Doses of 40 mg produce variable blood pressure changes. A general tendency for the pressure to increase is noted in about one third of the patients, whereas approximately 10% show mild hypotension. The extent of these changes is minimal.

High doses cause a consistent increase in blood pressure and heart rate. Intravenous administration of such doses elevates the mean aortic pressure, left ventricular and diastolic pressure, and mean pulmonary artery pressure. The work of the heart is thereby increased.[172]

Side Effects[250]

Euphoria is not seen. Sedative effects are noted in most patients. Psychomimetic and hallucinogenic effects have not been observed with ordinary doses. Dizziness, headache, nausea, and vomiting do occur but are rare. Impaired judgment and thinking occur.

With doses larger than 60 to 90 mg or repetitive smaller doses, however, psychomimetic effects are seen similar to those seen with nalorphine and probably represent an action at the κ-opioid receptor: dysphoria, racing thoughts, distortion of body image.

Subcutaneous or intramuscular injection of the penta-

zocine lactate solution may result in a peculiar woody sclerosis of the skin and subcutaneous tissues. A fibrous myopathy may also ensue.[258] At the site of injection, flat and nodular sclerosis and ulceration may develop.[256]

Pentazocine can lead to abuse and should be prescribed judiciously.[259,259a] Tolerance does occur but slowly.[49] Because this agent is a weak narcotic antagonist, it may precipitate withdrawal symptoms when administered to patients dependent on opioids.

In patients with severe liver disease, pentazocine may precipitate hepatic coma. Occasionally, grand mal seizures may be triggered. This effect limits its use in ambulatory patients.

Nalbuphine

Nalbuphine[260] belongs to the class of narcotic agonist-antagonists. It is a potent analgesic that, at low doses, is equivalent to morphine in its effect. Apparently, however, a ceiling effect exists at doses greater than 0.45 mg/kg in that no increase in respiratory depression occurs.[261]

Structure-Activity Relations

This drug is basically a phenanthrene derivative. The alcoholic -OH at position 6 of morphine remains and the ring to which it is attached becomes saturated. This is not unlike oxymorphone. Because an -OH group is attached to the fourteenth position, it thus resembles oxymorphone in this particular structuring (Fig. 31–21).

The unique structural feature of nalbuphine is the replacement on the nitrogen methyl group of a cyclic butyl ring. In this structuring, with a relatively large molecule on the piperadine active site, the drug then resembles naloxone. One would thus expect that this drug should have partial antagonist type actions, and this has been clinically confirmed.

Dosage

The doses are similar to morphine and it is, in low doses, equivalent. Thus, it is a potent analgesic. The low doses providing significant analgesia are set at 0.1 to 0.3 mg/kg body weight. This has also been used as the base dose for a nitrous-oxide narcotic balanced anesthesia technique.

At doses greater than 0.45 mg/kg, respiratory depression is no greater than that which appears at low doses.

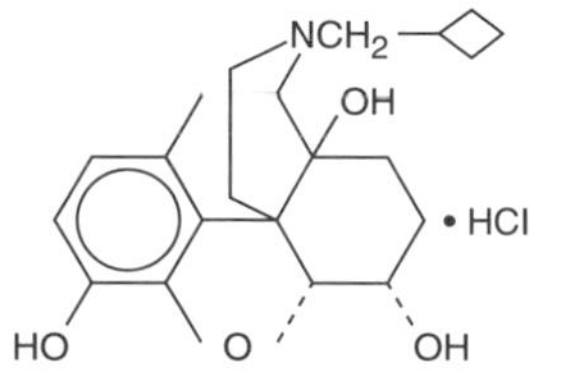

Fig. 31–21. The structure of nalbuphine: (−)-17-(cyclobutyl-methyl)-4,5α-epoxymorphinan-3,6α,14-triol hydrochloride. Its molecular formula is $C_{21}H_{27}NO_4 \cdot HCl$.

Site of Action

The principal site of action is at the μ receptors, and thus it is similar to morphine.

Administration[262]

Nalbuphine may be given by all routes. Oral administration provides only about 20% of the potency of parenteral injection.

Pharmacokinetics[262]

Bioavailability

By the oral route, only 16% is effective.

Disposition[263]

Uptake from parenteral sites is rapid and is similar to that of morphine. Distribution is to parenchymatous tissues initially, and the volume of distribution is set at 3.8 L/kg. The drug is detected in the plasma within 2 minutes, and peak concentration is achieved 8 to 15 minutes after intravenous injection.

Pharmacodynamics

The analgesic effects coincide with the plasma levels. Onset of action is seen in 2 to 3 minutes, and a peak effect occurs in 8 to 15 minutes. The plasma concentration initially decreases rapidly from its peak level, and the half-life is about 2.3 hours.[262] The duration of action is between 3 and 4 hours.

Binding

About 90% of a given dose is bound to plasma protein.

Metabolism

This occurs in the liver and is extensive.

Excretion

The degradation products are excreted by the kidney, and in addition, about 4% of the intact drug appears in the urine (Table 31–8).

Pharmacologic Effects

Respiration[260]

Respiration is depressed in low doses of 0.1 to 0.2 mg/kg of body weight, and the respiratory depression is similar to that of equianalgesic doses of morphine in this range. At doses larger than 0.45 mg/kg, however, one sees no increase in respiratory depression with nalbuphine. Thus, this is categorized as having a ceiling effect. A study of the CO_2 ventilatory response curve shows a shift to the right of 5.0 to 7.0 mm Hg with the low doses recommended for analgesia. With doses of 0.5 mg/kg and up to 1.0 mg/kg, little or insignificant further shift to the right occurs.[260]

Analgesia

The analgesic effect is equivalent to that of morphine; however, a ceiling effect also occurs. With larger doses, greater than 30 mg, no additional depression of respiration is observed, nor is any increase in analgesic effect seen.

Cardiovascular System[264]

This drug does not produce any significant adverse effects on the cardiovascular system. No increase in cardiac work, stroke work, or index occurs.[265] Only a slight decrease in cardiac index has been identified. No increase in pulmonary arterial pressure occurs, and systemic systolic pressure does not show significant change. One sees some increase in systemic vascular resistance; a decrease in heart rate is usual.[261]

Central Nervous System[266]

At ordinary doses of 10 mg in a 70-kg patient, patients have distortion of the body image and nalorphine-like side effects. Sedation, sweating, and headache are occasionally seen. With larger doses, dysphoria and racing thoughts, as well as distortion of the body image, occur.

Tolerance and Addiction

Although this drug was introduced with the hope of limiting the abuse potential, there is a definite degree of euphoria and a certain sense of liking the drug, as expressed by former addicts.

The antagonistic action is approximately *one fourth that of nalorphine* but 10 times that of pentazocine. In patients subject to morphine dependency, the administration of nalbuphine precipitates an abstinence-type syndrome. As higher doses are employed, most subjects consider that the effects are more sedative in nature and similar to those of barbiturates and less similar to the pure opiate agonists.

Table 31–8. Pharmacokinetic Data: Nalbuphine

Availability (Oral) (%)	Urinary Excretion (%)	Bound in Plasma (%)	Clearance $(ml \cdot min^{-1} \cdot kg^{-1})$	Vol. Dist. (L/kg)	Half-Life (h)	Effective Concentrations
16 ± 8 ↑ Aged	4 ± 2 ⟷ Aged	89.4 ± 2.9	22 ± 5 ↑ Child ⟶ Aged	3.8 ± 1.1 ⟷ Aged, Child	2.3 ± 1.2 ↓ Child ⟶ Aged	—

From Gilman, A. G., et al.: Goodman and Gilman's The Pharmacological Basis of Therapeutics, 8th Ed. New York, McGraw-Hill, 1990.

Gastrointestinal Motility[267]

Nalbuphine delays gastric emptying. In a study using paracetamol, which is absorbed from the intestine and is a marker for gastric emptying, nalbuphine delayed emptying 2 to 4 hours, whereas morphine-associated gastric emptying was longer, at 3 to 5 hours. Bowel sounds, however, were heard at 30 to 60 minutes in all instances; hence, this is a poor marker of gastrointestinal progression.

Passing of flatus is a good index of purposeful intestinal motility after anesthesia and surgery. In a control group not receiving medication, or undergoing anesthesia or surgery, but resting in bed after an overnight fast, the time to passing flatus (TPP) was 1 to 2 hours. With diazepam as a premedicant to light general anesthesia and no relaxants, the TPP was about 4 hours. Nalbuphine delayed TPP for 5.5 hours, whereas morphine delayed TPP for 11 to 12 hours. Thus, nalbuphine has a much less depressing effect on bowel activity than morphine.[267]

Therapeutic Uses

Nalbuphine is usually administered parenterally for acute pain. An injectable solution is available for subcutaneous intramuscular or intravenous administration. For intravenous use, several studies have been carried out at dosage levels of 2.0 to 3.0 mg/kg body weight. The drug has been found quite effective and provides stable cardiovascular conditions in patients with coronary or valvular heart disease.[264]

As an agonist-antagonist, nalbuphine has been used to antagonize the ventilatory depression following high-dose fentanyl anesthesia.[268] Although the drug is effective in many patients, the frequency of renarcotization 2 to 3 hours after apparent recovery from ventilatory depression requires continuous monitoring of these patients postoperatively. Because the technique is unpredictable, it is not recommended in view of availability of other antagonists that have some agonist action and retain a degree of analgesia.[269]

Magruder and colleagues[270] demonstrated that nalbuphine is capable of antagonizing the respiratory depression of oxymorphone and hydromorphone. In Julien's study,[260] the significant shift in the CO_2-response curve consequent to the administration of oxymorphone in doses of 1.5 mg can be antagonized, and the CO_2-response curve shifted to the left back to a relatively normal control value with modest doses of nalbuphine.

Side Effects

A study of respiratory effects on resting end-tidal CO_2, the slope of the end-tidal CO_2 when inspiratory effort was occluded, and the slope of the ventilatory V_E/P_{ETCO_2}, demonstrated that morphine significantly depresses all three parameters. With the administration of naloxone, all parameters returned to normal and the analgesic effect was also antagonized. The administration of nalbuphine resulted in further depression of the three respiratory parameters studied, however, but did not alter the pain threshold significantly. From this study, it can be concluded that, at least with morphine in usual therapeutic analgesic doses, nalbuphine does not reverse the respiratory depression, and, indeed, it potentiates the depression.[271] Moreover, with the administration of nalbuphine, the patient may have an immediate onset or increase in pain, as has been reported by Moldenauer and co-workers.[269] In severe respiratory depression, with large doses or morphine and probably other opioids, it appears that naloxone is the antagonist of choice. Additional doses of nalbuphine may alleviate the pain, and the mechanism may be different from the usual analgesic μ-receptor mediation, and the κ-receptor may be the mechanism for this supplemental analgesia.

In ambulatory surgical patients, more adverse effects have been noted with the use of nalbuphine in balanced anesthetic technique. The following have been noted: more psychologic side effects; more nausea and vomiting—about 60% versus 40% with fentanyl; and longer surgical stays.

Buprenorphine

This is a semisynthetic narcotic agonist-antagonist.

Chemical Structure[272]

Buprenorphine is a highly lipophilic agent. The alcoholic -OH on the sixth position of the morphine-phenanthrene nucleus is replaced by a methoxy group, $-OCH_3$. Because the phenanthrene nucleus has a ring that is double bonded and hence is similar to thebaine, buprenorphine may be considered a derivative of thebaine. The nitrogen of the piperidine ring is occupied by a methyl group to which is attached a distinctive cyclopropyl ring.

Potency and Dose[273]

The narcotic potency of this drug in terms of its ability to relieve pain is about 25 to 50 times greater than that of morphine. In adults, the intramuscular dose is about 5.0 μg/kg. The intravenous dose should be slightly less. The dose, therefore, is of the order of 0.4 mg, being equivalent to 10 mg morphine sulphate.

In children, the conventional intravenous dose is about 3.0 μg/kg.

Receptors[274]

The affinity of this drug is for both the μ and the σ receptors and, hence, is nonselective. Some affinity for the κ receptor exists and resembles benzomorphan. It is a partial agonist to the μ receptor. There is a high lipid solubility and a very high receptor affinity, but the overall intrinsic agonist activity is limited.[275]

The κ receptor binding may account for the antagonist action versus a pure μ receptor effect.[274]

Pharmacokinetics

The onset of full effect is slower after intramuscular injection, but once established, the receptor binding is tight, and such binding is resistant to naloxone antagonism. The duration of action is significantly longer than that of morphine sulphate. The plasma half-life is set at 3.5 to 5.0 hours and the overall duration of effective analgesia extends for over 6 hours.

Pharmacologic Effects

All the effects are similar to those of morphine. Some antagonist action exists, however, and in patients who have already received one of the agonist narcotics, the effectiveness of these narcotics will be reduced with the administration of buprenorphine.[273]

Clinical Uses

This drug has been found useful to relieve postoperative pain, especially because of its longer duration of action.[276]

Competitive displacement of fentanyl is produced by the administration of buprenorphine. This is related to the strong lipophilic and dominant displacement capacity over other opiate-type agonists. The drug has been proposed as an antagonist to large-dose fentanyl-type anesthesia. In addition, investigators have suggested that this drug can be useful in the treatment of drug withdrawal effects and in the reversal of acute opioid effects.[277]

Butorphanol

Butorphanol is a morphine congener and belongs to the class of narcotic agonist-antagonists.[278] The predominant action is agonistic, but a portion of its action is antagonistic to opiate analgesics. The actions are similar to those of pentazocine in the pharmacologic profile. A ceiling effect with regard to respiratory depression action probably exists, but then there is also the ceiling effect to analgesia. The drug is not a controlled substance and may have utility in the long-term management of pain.

Structure-Activity Relations

This agent, as noted, is a morphine-type derivative, and the two principal structural changes from the basic morphine nucleus are represented by a replacement of the methyl group on the piperidine nitrogen by a methylbutyl cyclic ring (Fig. 31–22). Position 6 of the morphine nucleus is replaced by a single hydrogen atom, so the attached ring is unsaturated. On the other hand, a single

Molecular weight: 504.09

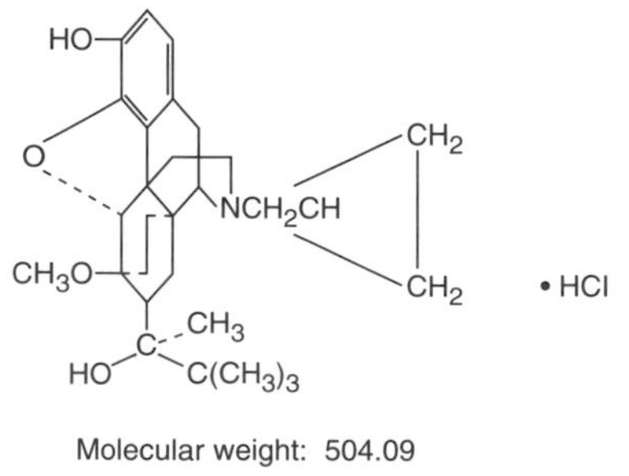

Fig. 31–22. The structure of butorphanol.

-OH group is attached to the fourteenth position. In this sense, it does resemble oxymorphone.

Dosage[279]

The dose of butorphanol is approximately one fifth to one fourth that of morphine. A dose of 2 to 3 mg is approximately equivalent to 10 mg morphine. Abuse of this drug is primarily in the management of acute somatic pain.

Site of Action

The principal site of action of this drug is different from that of morphine. Butorphanol acts primarily as an agonist on κ and σ receptors and on μ receptors as both agonist and antagonist. It is a weak antagonist.

Pharmacologic Effects[278]

Respiration

Respiratory depression approximately equal to that of morphine. Like pentazocine, which acts primarily on κ and σ receptors, as the dose is increased, respiratory depression is less pronounced than it is with morphine and other μ receptor agonists.[278]

A study of the CO_2-response curve following intravenous butorphanol reveals a significant respiratory depression. Using the CO_2 ventilatory response curve, the slopes of the curve for butorphanol, in doses of approximately 10 mg/70 kg body weight, resulted in a depression of 2.42 ± 0.56. This is a significantly greater depression than observed with nalbuphine.[280]

Analgesia

The analgesic effect is similar to that obtained with morphine, as noted previously.

Cardiovascular System

The principal cardiovascular effect is a slight decrease in systemic arterial pressure. Of greater importance, however, is an increase in pulmonary arterial pressure and an increase in the work of the right side of the heart. Cardiac output decreases.

Central Nervous System

Psychomimetic side effects of this drug exist, and they are similar to those of pentazocine. The subjective effects are similar to those of pentazocine or nalorphine. Addiction does develop, but those who have been addicted complain of drowsiness and an inability to actually sleep. Constipation and difficulty in urination are also common. Most previous addicts identify the drug more as a sedative, such as a barbiturate, and are not likely to desire the use of this drug. Acute abstinence may be precipitated in patients who are physiologically dependent on narcotics by the administration of butorphanol. Withdrawal may even be precipitated by a small dose of this drug administered epidurally.[281]

Therapeutic Uses

The drug is available only in parenteral form and is, therefore, of use in acute pain of a somatic type rather than chronic pain problems. It should not be used in patients with myocardial disease. In general, the drug is useful neither in anesthesia practice nor in management of chronic pain.

Epidural Administration[282]

Epidural analgesia can be achieved with butorphanol and has been investigated with the view to diminish the undesirable effects of epidural morphine. The doses studied varied from 1 to 4 mg dissolved in 10 ml saline and so administered epidurally. The 4.0-mg dose provided a rapid onset of analgesia (22 minutes) and a duration of approximately 8 hours. This is compared with morphine, 5.0 mg epidurally, which produced analgesia of a slower onset (51 minutes) and a duration of about 20 hours. The principal side effect with butorphanol is a persistent somnolence, whereas morphine results in pruritus in over two thirds of patients. In a study of ventilatory response to CO_2, definite depression in the slope of the curve occurs of about 20 to 40% with butorphanol, with the greatest depression occurring at about 12 hours after administration; the depression of the CO_2-response curve with morphine varied between 30 and 50%, with the peak depression at 12 hours. Hence, in the use of butorphanol, no increase in safety is seen over morphine, and patients must be carefully monitored after epidural injection. Satisfactory pain relief with butorphanol was found in only 73% of patients, compared with 100% with morphine.[282]

REFERENCES

1. Jaffe, J. H., Martin, W. R.: Narcotic Analgesics and Antagonists. *In* Goodman, L., Gilman, A. G. (eds.). Pharmacological Basis of Therapeutics, 5th Ed. New York, Macmillan, 1975, p. 245.
2. Kirby, G. W.: Biosynthesis of morphine alkaloids. Science *155*:170, 1967.
3. Gulland, J. M., Robinson, R.: Constitution of codeine and thebaine. Mem Proc Manchester Lit Phil Soc *69*:79, 1925.
4. Gates, M., Tschudi, G.: The synthesis of morphine. J Am Chem Soc *74*:1109, 1952.
5. Gates, M.: Analgesic drugs. Sci Am *215*:131, 1966.
6. Gero, A.: The spatial structure of morphine. Science *119*:12, 1954.
7. Lowney, L. I., Schulz, K., Lowery, P. J., Goldstein, A.: Partial purification of an opiate receptor from mouse brain. Science *183*:749, 1974.
8. Pert, C. B., Snyder, S. H.: Opiate receptor: demonstration in nervous tissue. Science *179*: 1011, 1973.
9. Beckett, N., Casey, A. F.: Receptor attachment of morphine to the piperidine group. J Pharm Pharmacol *6*:986, 1954.
10. Snyder, S. H., Matthysse, S. (eds.): Opiate receptor mechanisms. Neurosci Res Prog Bull *13*:1, 1975.
11. Yaksh, T. L., Rudy, T. A.: Analgesia mediated by a direct spinal action of narcotics. Science *192*:1357, 1976.
12. Wang, J. K.: Antinociceptive effect of intrathecally administered serotonin. Anesthesiology *47*:269, 1977.
13. Simanton, R., Snyder, S. H.: Endorphans. Life Sci *18*:781, 1976.
14. Hughes, J., et al.: Peptides with opiate-like activity. Nature *258*:577, 1975.
15. Hughes, J.: Centrally Acting Peptides. New York, MacMillan, 1978.
16. Feinberg, A. P., Creese, I., Snyder, S. H.: The opiate receptor: a model explaining structure, activity, relationships. Proc Natl Acad Sci USA *13*:4215, 1976.
17. Snyder, S. H.: Opiate receptors and internal opiates. Sci Am *236*:44, 1977.
18. Smith, G. D., Griffin, J. F.: Conformation of enkephalin from X-ray refraction recognition and opiate receptor. Science *199*:1214, 1978.
19. Jacquet, Y. F.: Opiate effects after adrenocorticotrophin. Science *201*:1032, 1978.
20. Lord, J. A. H., Waterfield, J., Hughes, H., Kosterlitz, W.: Two types of opiate receptors. Nature *207*:495, 1977.
21. Kostervitz, H. W., Lord, J. A. H., Paterson, S. J., Waterfield, A. A.: Effects of changes in structure of encephalins and of narcotic analgesic drugs on their interactions with μ and δ-receptors Br J Pharmacol *68*:333, 1980.
22. Wei, E., Loh, H.: Physical dependence on opiate-like peptides. Science *193*:1262, 1976.
23. Frederickson, R. C. A., et al.: Metkephamid: a systemically active analogy of methionine enkephalin with potent opioid-receptor activity. Science *211*:603, 1981.
24. Yaksh, T. L.: In vivo studies on spinal opiate receptor systems mediating antinociception. 1. Mu and delta receptor profiles on the primate. J Pharmacol Exp Ther *226*:303, 1983.
25. Goldstein, A.: Opioid peptides (endorphins) in pituitary and brain. Science *193*:1081, 1976.
26. Snyder, S. H.: Receptors, neurotransmitters and drug responses. N Engl J Med *300*:465, 1979.
27. Krieger, D. T., Martin, J. B.: Brain peptides. N Engl J Med *304*:876, 1981.
28. Snyder, S. H.: Brain peptides as neurotransmitters. Science *209*:976, 1980.
29. Willer, J.C., Dehen, H., Cambier, J.: Stress-induced analgesia in humans: endogenous opiates and naloxone reversible depression of pain reflexes. Science *218*:689, 1981.
30. Guillman, R., Vargo, T., Rossier., J.: β-endorphin and adrenocorticotropin are secreted concommitantly by the pituitary gland. Science *197*:1367, 1977.
31. Rossier, J., Pittman, Q., Guillman, R.: Distribution of opioid peptides in the pituitary: a new hypothalamic-pars nervosa enkephalinergic pathway. Fed Proc *39*:2555, 1980.
32. Simantov, R., Snyder, S.: Opiate receptor binding in the pituitary gland. Brain Res *124*:178, 1977.
33. Trouwborst, A., Erdmann, W., Yanagida, H., Corssen, G.: Electrophysiologic evidence for involvement of the pituitary region in opiate analgesia. Anesth Analg *64*:781, 1985.
34. Gilbert, P. E., Martin, W. R.: Multiple opioid receptor systems. J Pharmacol Exp Ther *198*:66, 1976.
35. Martin, W. R.: Pharmacology of opioids. Pharmacol Rev *35*:283, 1984.
36. Iwamoto, E. T., Martin, W. R.: Multiple opioid receptors. Med Res Rev *1*:411, 1981.
37. Cowan, A.: Classification of opioids on the basis of change in seizure threshold in rats. Science *206*:465, 1979.
38. Yaksh, A. L.: Multiple opioid receptor systems in brain and spinal cord. Eur J Anaesthesiol *1*:171, 1984.
39. Fujita, S., Yasuhara, M., Agm, K.: Studies on sites of action of analgesics. Jpn J Pharmacol *3*:27, 1953.
40. Bernheim, F., Bernheim, M. L. C.: Action of drugs on choline esterase of brain. J Pharmacol Exp Ther *57*:427, 1936.

41. Lasagna, L., Beecher, H. K.: The optimal dose of morphine. JAMA 156:230, 1954.

42. Wikler, A.: Opiates and opiate antagonists. Public Health Rep 73:11, 1959.

43. Gravenstein, J., Beecher, H. K.: The effect of preoperative medication with morphine on postoperative analgesia with morphine. J Pharmacol Exp Ther 119:506, 1954.

44. Waters, R. M., Bennett, J. H., Leigh, M. D.: Effects upon human subjects of morphine and scopolamine, alone and combined. J Pharmacol Exp Ther 63:38, 1938.

45. Wangeman, C. R., Hawk, M. H.: The effects of morphine, atropine and scopolamine. Anesthesiology 3:24, 1942.

45a. Collins, V. J. (ed.): Principles of Anesthesiology, 3rd Ed. Philadelphia, Lea & Febiger, 1993.

46. Way, W. L., Costley, E. C., Way, E. L.: Respiratory sensitivity of the newborn infant to meperidine and morphine. Clin Pharmacol Ther 6:454, 1965.

47. Frederickson, R. C.: Diurnal rhythm in response to pain and to action of morphine: hyperalgesic induced by naloxone. Science 198:756, 1977.

48. Belleville, J. W., Forrest, E. M.: Influence of age on pain relief from analgesics. JAMA 217:1035, 1971.

49. Jaffe, J. H., Martin, W. R.: Opioid analgesics and antagonists. In Gilman, A. G., et al. (eds.). Goodman and Gilman's The Pharmacological Basis of Therapeutics, 8th Ed. New York, McGraw-Hill, 1990, p. 485.

49a. Idem. In Goodman, L. S., Gilman, A: The Pharmacological Basis of Therapeutics. Macmillan Publishing Co., 5th Ed., New York, 1975.

50. Hoskins, P. J., et al.: The bioavailability and pharmacokinetics of morphine after intravenous, oral and rectal administration in healthy volunteers Br J Pharmacol 27:499, 1989.

51. Spector, S.: Quantitative determination of morphine sulfate by radioimmune assay. J Pharmacol Exp Ther 178:253, 1971.

52. Stanski, D. R., Greenblatt, D. J., Lowenstein, E.: Kinetics of intravenous and intramuscular morphine. Clin Pharmacol Ther 24:52, 1978.

53. Dahlstrom, B., Tamsen, A., Paalzow, L., Hartvig, P.: Patient-controlled analgesic therapy. Part IV: Pharmacokinetics and analgesic plasma concentrations of morphine. Clin Pharmacol Ther 7:266, 1982.

54. Owen, J. A., et al.: Age-related morphine kinetics. Clin Pharmacol Ther 34:364, 1983.

55. Kaiko, R. F.: Age and morphine analgesia in cancer patients with postoperative pain. Clin Pharmacol Ther 28:823, 1980.

56. Säwe, J., Dahlstrom, B., Paalzow, L., Rane, A.: Morphine kinetics in cancer patients. Clin Pharmacol Ther 30:629, 1981.

57. Spector, S.: Disposition of morphine sulfate in man. Science 174:421, 1972.

58. Stanski, D. R., et al.: Kinetics of high-dose intravenous morphine in cardiac surgery patients. Clin Pharmacol Ther 19:752, 1976.

59. Rapoport, S. I.: Blood-Brain Barrier in Physiology and Medicine. New York, Raven Press, 1976, p. 1.

60. Rapoport, S. I., Ohno, K., Pettigrew, K. D.: Drug entry into the brain. Brain Res 172:354, 1979.

61. Schulman, D. S., Kaufman, J. J., Eisenstein, M. M., Rapoport, S. I.: Blood pH and brain uptake of ^{14}C-morphine. Anesthesiology 61:540, 1984.

62. Kaufman, J. J., Koski, W. S., Benson, D. W., Seno, N. M.: Narcotic and narcotic antagonist pK$_a$'s and partition coefficients and their significance in clinical practice. Drug Alcohol Depend 1:103, 1975/1976.

63. Yeh, S. Y.: Urinary excretion of morphine and its metabolites in morphine-dependent subjects. J Pharmacol Exp Ther 192:201, 1975.

64. Yeh, S. Y., Gorodetzky, C. W., Krebs, H. A.: Isolation and identification of morphine 3- and 6-glucuronides, morphine 3,6-diglucuronide, morphine 3- ethereal sulfate, normorphine, and normorphine 6-glucuronide as morphine metabolites in humans. J Pharm Sci 66:1288, 1977.

65. Shimomura, K., et al.: Analgesic effect of morphine glucuronides. Tohoku J Exp Med 105:45, 1971.

66. Paul, D., Standifer, K. M., Inturrisi, C. E., Pasternak, G. W.: Pharmacological characterization of morphine-6β-glucuronide, a very potent morphine metabolite. J Pharmacol Exp Ther 251:477, 1989.

67. Mazoit, J. X., Sandouk, P., Scherrmann, J.-M., Rocke, A.: Extrahepatic metabolism of morphine occurs in humans. Clin Pharmacol Ther 48:613, 1990.

68. Lynn, A. M., Slattery, J. T.: Morphine pharmacokinetics in early infancy. Anesthesiology 66:136, 1987.

69. Dahlstrom, B., et al.: Morphine kinetics in children. Clin Pharmacol Ther 26:354, 1979.

70. Olsen, G. D., Bennett, W. M., Porter, G. A.: Morphine and phenytoin binding to plasma proteins in renal and hepatic failure. Clin Pharmacol Ther 17:677, 1975.

71. Mazoit, J.-X., Sandouk, P., Zetlaoui, P., Scherrmann, J.-M.: Pharmacokinetics of unchanged morphine in normal and cirrhotic subjects. Anesth Analg 66:293, 1987.

72. Lebrec, D., Bataille, C., Bercoff, E., Valla, D.: Hemodynamic changes in patients with portal venous obstruction. Hepatology 3:550, 1983.

73. Chauvin, M., et al.: Morphine pharmacokinetics in renal failure. Anesthesiology 66:327, 1987.

74. Keats, A. S., Mithoefer, J. C.: The mechanism of increased intracranial pressure induced by morphine. N Engl J Med 252:1110, 1955.

75. Dripps, R. D., Comroe, J. H.: Clinical studies on morphine: I. The immediate effect of morphine administered intravenously and intramuscularly upon the respiration of normal man. Anesthesiology 6:462, 1945.

76. Eckenhoff, J. E., Helrich, M., Hege, J. N.: Effects of narcotics upon respiratory responses to carbon dioxide in man. Surg Forum 15:681, 1954.

77. Dripps, R. D., Dumke, P. H.: Effects of narcotics on the balance between central and chemoreceptor control of respiration. J Pharmacol Exp Ther 77:290, 1943.

78. Hibma, O. V., Jr., Curreri, A. B.: A study of the effect of morphine, atropine and scopolamine on the bronchi. Surg Gynecol Obstet 74:851, 1942.

79. Orkin, L. R., Egge, R. K., Rovenstine, E. A.: Effect of Nisentil, meperidine and morphine on respiration in man. Anesthesiology 16:699, 1955.

80. Arunasalam, K., Davenport, H. T., Painter, S., Jones, J. G.: Ventilatory response to morphine in young and old subjects. Anaesthesia 38:529, 1983.

81. Tenney, S. M., Miller, R. M.: Respiratory response in the aged. J Am Geriatr Soc 3:937, 1955.

82. Daykin, A. P., Bowen, D. J., Saunders, D. A., Norman, J.: Respiratory depression after morphine in the elderly: a comparison with younger subjects. Anaesthesia 41:910, 1986.

83. Eckenhoff, J. E., Helrich, M., Hege, M.: A method for studying respiratory function in awake and anesthetized patients. Anesthesiology 17:66, 1956.

84. Bellville, J. W., Fleischli, G.: The interaction of morphine and nalorphine on respiration. Clin Pharmacol Ther 9:152, 1968.

85. Keats, A. S.: The effect of drugs on respiration in man. Annu Rev Pharmacol 25:41, 1985.

86. Hudson, H. E., Harber, P. I., Smith, T. C.: Respiratory depression from alkalosis and opioid interaction in man. Anesthesiology 40:543, 1974.

87. Bellville, J. W., Howland, W. S., Seed, J. C., Honde, R. W.: The effect of sleep on the respiratory response to carbon dioxide. Anesthesiology 20:628, 1959.

88. Lam, A. M., Clement, J. L., Chung, D. C., Knill, R. L.: Respiratory effects of nitrous oxide during enflurane anesthesia in humans. Anesthesiology 56:298, 1982.

89. Fourcade, H. E., et al.: The ventilatory effects of Forane, a new inhaled anesthetic. Anesthesiology 35:26, 1971.

90. Munson, E. S., et al.: The effects of halothane, fluroxene, and cyclopropane on ventilation: a comparative study in man. Anesthesiology 27:716, 1966.

91. Johnstone, R. E., et al.: Reversal of morphine anesthesia with naloxone. Anesthesiology 41:361, 1974.

92. Gross, J. B., et al.: Time course of ventilatory depression after thiopental and midazolam in normal subjects and in patients with chronic obstructive pulmonary disease. Anesthesiology 58:540, 1983.

93. Bourke, D. L., Rosenberg, M., Allen, P. D.: Physostigmine: effectiveness as an antagonist of respiratory depression and psychomotor effects caused by morphine or diazepam. Anesthesiology 61:523, 1984.

94. Attia, J., et al.: Epidural morphine in children: pharmacokinetics and CO_2 sensitivity. Anesthesiology 65:590, 1986.

95. Twum-Barima, Y., Ahmad, D., Hamilton, J. T., Carruthers, S.G.: Ineffectiveness of beta-adrenergic blockers on ventilatory response to carbon dioxide. Clin Pharmacol Ther 32:289, 1982.

96. Drew, J. D., Dripps, R. D., Comroe, J. H.: Clinical studies on morphine. II. The effect of morphine upon the circulation of man and upon the circulatory and respiratory responses to tilting. Anesthesiology 7:44, 1946.

97. Papper, E. M., Bradley, S. E.: Hemodynamic effects of intravenous morphine and pentothal sodium. J Pharmacol Exp Ther 74:319, 1942.

98. Slocum, H. C.: Problems of overtreatment of surgical patients with depressant drugs. JAMA 156:1573, 1954.

99. Allen, C. R., Echols, R. S., O'Neal, K. C., Slocum, H. C.: Effects of premedication upon the signs of asphyxia during nitrous oxide-oxygen anesthesia. Anesthesiology 10:164, 1949.

100. Ward, A., McGrath, R. L., Weil, J. V.: Effects of morphine on the peripheral vascular response to sympathetic stimulation. Am J Cardiol 29:659, 1972.

101. Flaim, S. F., Zelis, R., Eisle, J. H.: Differential effect of morphine on forearm blood flow.

102. Alderman, E. L.: Analgesics in acute phase of myocardial infarction. JAMA 229:1646, 1974.

103. Strauer, B. E.: Contractile responses to morphine, piritramide, meperidine and fentanyl on isolated ventricular myocardium. Anesthesiology 37:304, 1972.

104. Moyer, J., Pontius, R., Morris, G., Hershberger, R.: Effects of morphine and n-allyl normorphine on cerebral hemodynamics and oxygen metabolism. Circulation 15:379, 1957.

105. Kromer, W.: Endogenous and exogenous opioids in the control of gastrointestinal motility and secretions. Pharmacol Rev 40:121, 1988.

106. Duthie, D. J. R., Nimmo, W. S.: Adverse effects of opioid analgesic drugs. Br J Anaesth 59:61, 1987.

107. Yukioka, H., et al.: Gastric emptying and small bowel transit times in volunteers after intravenous morphine and nalbuphine. Anaesthesia 42:704, 1987.

108. Gaensler, E. A., McGowan, J. A., Henderson, F. F.: A comparative study of the action of Demerol and opium alkaloids in relation to biliary spasm. Surgery 23:211, 1948.

109. Vieira, Z. G., et al.: Double-blind ultrasonographic demonstration of morphine induced spasm of the common bile duct (Abstract 232). Anesthesiology 71(Suppl), 1989.

110. Yaksh, T. L., Noueihed, R.: The physiology and pharmacology of spinal opiates. Annu Rev Pharmacol Toxicol 25:433, 1985.

111. DeBodo, R. E.: The antidiuretic action of morphine and its mechanism. J Pharmacol Exp Ther 82:74, 1944.

112. Mostert, J. W., et al.: Cardiorespiratory effects of anaesthesia with morphine or fentanyl in chronic renal failure and cerebral toxicity after morphine. Br J Anaesth 43:1053, 1971.

113. Don, H. F., Dieppa, R. A., Taylor, P.: Narcotic analgesics in anuric patients. Anesthesiology 42:745, 1975.

114. DeBodo, R. E., Brooks, McC.: The effects of morphine on blood sugar and reflex activity in the spinal cat. J Pharmacol Exp Ther 61:82, 1937.

115. Eisenman, A. J., Isbell, H., Fraser, H., Sloan, J.: Ketosteroid excretion in morphine addiction and withdrawal. Fed Proc 12:200, 1953.

116. McDonald, R. K., et al.: Effect of morphine and nalorphine on plasma hydrocortisone levels in man. J Pharmacol Exp Ther 125:231, 1959.

117. Grossman, A.: Opioids and stress in man. J Endocrinol 119:377, 1988.

118. Gill, G. N.: Endocrine system: the hypothalamic-pituitary system. In West, J. B. (ed.). Best and Taylor's Physiological Basis of Medical Practice, 12th Ed. Baltimore, Williams & Wilkins, 1990.

119. Seevers, M. H., Deneau, H.: Psychopharmacological elements of drug dependence. JAMA 206:1263, 1968.

120. Rojas, E., Tobias, J. M.: Membrane model: "association of inorganic calcium and phospholipid membrane." Acta Biochim Biophys 94:394, 1965.

121. Ross, D. H., Medina, M. A., Cardenas, H. L.: Norphine and ethanol: selective depletion of regional brain calcium. Science 86:63, 1974.

122. Bellville, J. W., Cohen, E. N., Hamilton, J.: The interaction of morphine and d-tubocurarine on respiration and grip strength in man. Clin Pharmacol Ther 5:35, 1964.

123. Lang, D. A., Kimura, K. K., Unna, K. R.: Combination of skeletal muscle relaxing agents with various central nervous system depressants used in anesthesia. Arch Int Pharmacodyn 85:257, 1951.

124. Duke, P. C., Johns, C. H., Pinsky, C., Goertzen, P.: The effect of morphine on human neuromuscular transmission. Can Anaesth Soc J 26:201, 1979.

125. Rumore, M. M., Schlichting, D. A.: Clinical efficacy of antihistamines as analgesics. Pain 25:7, 1986.

126. Moore, J., Dundee, J.: Alteration in response to somatic pain associated with anesthesia. VII. The effect of newer phenothiazine derivatives. Br J Anaesth 33:422, 1961.

127. Forrester, W. H., et al.: Dextro-amphetamine with morphine for treatment of postoperative pain. N Engl J Med 296:712, 1977.

128. Spector, M., Bourke, D. L.: Anesthesia, sleep paralysis and physostigmine: clinical report. Anesthesiology 46:296, 1977.

129. Snir-Mor, I., Weinstock, M., Davidson, J. T., Bahar, M.: Physostigmine anatgonizes morphine induced respiratory depression in human subjects. Anesthesiology 59:6, 1983.

130. Fahmy, N. R.: Hemodynamics, plasma histamine, and catecholamine concentrations during an anaphylactoid reaction to morphine. Anesthesiology 55:329, 1981.

131. Philbin, D. M., et al.: The use of H_1 and H_2 histamine antag-

onists with morphine anesthesia: a double-blind study. Anesthesiology 55:292, 1981.

132. Fahmy, N. R., Sunder, N., Soter, N. A.: Role of histamine in the hemodynamic and plasma catecholamine responses to morphine. Clin Pharmacol Ther 33:615, 1983.

133. Flacke, J. W., et al.: Histamine release by four narcotics: a double-blind study in humans. Anesth Analg 66:723, 1987.

134. Rosow, C. E., Moss, J., Philbin, D. M., Savarese, J. J.: Histamine release during morphine and fentanyl anaesthesia. Anesthesiology 56:93, 1982.

135. Wasserman, S. I.: Mediators of immediate hypersensitivity. J Allergy Clin Immunol 72:101, 1983.

136. Scott, P. V., Fisher, H. B. S.: Pruritis of face following morphine use. Br Med J 284:1015, 1982.

137. Johnson, C. D.: Methods for relief of postoperative pain. Ann R Coll Surg 65:137, 1983.

138. Charway, C. L., Calvey, T. N., Williams, N. E., Murray, G. R.: Postoperative analgesia with duromorph. Br J Anaesth 57:949, 1985.

139. Bradley, J. R.: Comparison of morphine and duromorph for analgesia after abdominal surgery. Anaesth Intensive Care 12:303, 1984.

140. Physicians Desk Reference, 49th Ed. Montvale, NJ, Medical Economics Data, 1995, p. 975.

141. Hanks, G. W., Trueman, T.: Controlled-release morphine tablets are effective in twice-daily dasage in chronic cancer pain. In Wilkes, E., Levy, J. (eds.). Advances in Morphine Therapy. London, Royal Society of Medicine, 1983, p. 103.

142. Aitkenhead, A. R., Pinnock, C. A., Smith, G.: Pharmacokinetics of two preparation of slow-release oral morphine sulfate in volunteers. Anesthesiol Rev (Int) 15:31, 1988.

143. Simpson, K. H., Dearden, M. J., Ellis, F. R., Jack, T. M.: Premedication with slow release morphine (MST) and adjuvants. Br J Anaesth 60:825, 1988.

144. Reidenberg, M. M., et al.: Hydromorphone (Dilaudid) levels and pain control. Clin Pharmacol Ther 44:376, 1988.

145. Brown, C. R., Frorest, W. H., Hayden, J., James, A. T.: Respiratory effects of hydromorphine in man. Clin Pharmacol Ther 14:33, 1973.

146. Schneider, O., Grussner, A.: Synthese von Oxy-morphmanen. Helvet Chim Acta 32:821, 1949.

147. Junkerman, C. L., Heen, R. C., Pohle, H. W.: Clinical experience with a new analgesic agent. Lancet 1:263, 1951.

148. Stoelting, V. K., Theye, R. A., Graf, J. P.: The use of Dromoran hydrobromide for preoperative medication. Anesthesiology 12:225, 1951.

149. Brotman, M., Cullen, S. C.: Intravenous supplementation during nitrous oxide anesthesia. J Pharmacol Exp Ther 4:98, 1950.

150. Inturrisi, C. E., et al.: The pharmacokinetics of heroin in patients with chronic pain. N Engl J Med 310:1213, 1984.

151. Sawynok, J.: The therapeutic use of heroin: a review of the pharmacological Literature. Can J Physiol Pharmacol 64:1, 1986.

152. Kaiko, R. F., et al.: Analgesic and mood effcts of heroin and morphine in cancer patients. N Engl J Med 304:1501, 1981.

153. Lasagna, L., Beecher, H. K.: The analgesic effectiveness of codeine and meperidine. J Pharmacol Exp Ther 112:306, 1954.

154. Bellville, J. W., et al.: The respiratory effects of codeine and morphine in man. Clin Pharmacol Ther 9:435, 1968.

155. Lasha, E. M., et al.: Caffeine as an analgesic adjuvant. JAMA 251:1711, 1984.

156. Beaver, W. T.: Caffeine revisited (Editorial). JAMA 251:1732, 1984.

157. Bellville, J. W., Sneed, J. C.: A comparison of the respiratory depressant effects of dextropoxyphene and codeine in man. Clin Pharmacol Ther 9:42, 1962.

158. Eisleb, O., Schaumann, O.: Dolantin, ein Newartiges Spasmolytikum und Analgetikum. Dtsch Med Wochenschr 65:967, 1939.

159. Batterman, R. C.: Clinical effectiveness and safety of a new synthetic analgesic drug, Demerol. Arch Intern Med 71:345, 1943.

160. Batterman, R. C., Himmelsbach, C. K.: Demerol. JAMA 122:222, 1943.

161. Wolff, H. G., Wolfe, S. G.: Pain. Springfield, IL, Charles C. Thomas, 1948.

162. Yonkerman, F. F.: Pharmacology of Demerol and its analogues. Ann NY Acad Sci 51:59, 1948.

163. Batterman, R. C., Mulholland, J.: Demerol, a substitute for morphine in the treatment of postoperative pain. Arch Surg 46:404, 1943.

164. Rovenstine, E. A., Batterman, R. C.: The utility of Demerol as a substitute for the opiates in preanesthetic medication. Anesthesiology 4:126, 1943.

165. Kepes, E. R.: Effect of Demerol on cerebrospinal fluid pressure. Anesthesiology 13:281, 1952.

166. Eckenhoff, J. E., Oech, S. R.: The effects of narcotics and antagonists upon respiration and circulation in man. Clin Pharmacol Ther 1:483, 1960.

167. Orkin, L. R., Egge, R. R., Rovenstine, E. A.: Effect of Nisentil, meperidine and morphine on respiration in man. Anesthesiology 16:699, 1955.

168. Prescott, S. Rauson, S. G., Thorp, R. H., Wilson, A.: Effect of analgesics on respiratory response to carbon dioxide in man. Lancet 1:340, 1949.

169. Lambertsen, J., Wendel, H., Longhagen, J. B.: The separate and combined respiratory effects of chlorpromazine and meperidine in men controlled at 46 mmHg alveolar p CO_2. J Pharmacol Exp Ther 131:381, 1961.

170. Edwards, D. J., Svensson C. K., Visco, J. P., Lalka, D.: Clinical pharmacokinetics of pethidine. Clin Pharmacokinet 7:421, 1982.

171. McDermott, F. F., Papper, E. M.: Respiratory complications associated with Demerol. NY State J Med 50:1721, 1950.

172. Lee, G., et al.: Comparative effects of morphine, meperidine and pentazocine on the cardiocirculatory dynamics in patients with acute myocardial infarction. Am J Med 60:949, 1976.

173. Abajian, J., Jr., Brazell, E. H., Dente, G. A., Mills, E. L.: Experience with halothane in more than five thousand cases. JAMA 171:535, 1959.

174. Harvey, W., Proctor, F., Leonard, J.: Caution against the use of meperidine hydrochloride in patients with heart disease, particularly auricular flutter. Am Heart J 49:758, 1955.

175. Sugioka, K., Boniface, K. J., Davis, D. A.: The influence of meperidine on myocardial contractility in the intact dog. Anesthesiology 18:623, 1957.

176. Calesnick, B., Smith, N. H., Beutner, R.: Combined action of cardiotonic drugs. J Pharmacol Exp Ther 102:138, 1951.

177. Way, E. L.: Studies on the local anaesthetic properties of isonipecaine. J Pharm Sci 35:44, 194?.

178. Ready, L. B.: Regional anesthesia with intraspinal opioides. In Bonica, J. J. (ed.). The Management of Pain, 2nd Ed., Vol. II. Philadelphia, Lea & Febiger, 1990.

179. Grimmond, T. R., Brownridge, P.: Antimicrobial activity of bupivacaine and pethidine. Anaesth Intensive Care, 14:418, 1986.

180. Levy, J. H., Kochoff, M. A.: Anaphylaxis to meperidine. Anesth Analg 61:301, 1992.

181. Kaiko, R. F., et al.: Central nervous system excitatory effects of meperidine in cancer patients. Ann Neurol 13:180, 1983.

182. Lieberman, A. N., Goldstein, M.: Reversible parkinsonism related to meperidine (Letter). N Engl J Med 312:509, 1985.

183. Kuhnert, B. R., et al.: Meperidine and normeperidine levels following meperidine administration during labor. I. Mother. Am J Obstet Gynecol 133:904, 1979.

184. Kuhnert, B. R., Kuhnert, P. M., Tu, A. L., Lin, D. C. K.: Meperidine and normeperidine levels following meperidine administration during labor. II. Fetus and neonate. Am J Obstet Gynecol 133:909, 1979.

185. Morrison, J. C., et al.: Metabolites of meperidine related to fetal depression. Am J Obstet Gynecol 115:1132, 1973.

186. O'Donoghue, S. E. F.: Distribution of pethidine and chloropromazine in maternal, fetal and neonatal biological fluids. Nature 229:124, 1971.

187. Lieberman, B. A., et al.: The effects of maternally administered pethidine or epidural bupivacaine on the fetus and newborn. Br J Obstet Gynaecol 86:598, 1979.

188. Koch, G., Wendel, H.: The effect of pethidine on the postnatal adjustment of respiration and acid base balance. Acta Obstet Gynecol Scand 47:27, 1968.

189. Scanlon, J. W.: Effects of obstetric anesthesia and analgesia on the newborn: a select, annotated bibliography for the clinician. Clin Obstet Gynecol 24:649, 1979.

190. Hodgkinson, R., Farkhandsa, J. H.: The duration of effect of maternally administered meperidine on neonatal neurobehavior. Anesthesiology 56:51, 1982.

191. Kuhnert, B. R., Linn, P. L., Kennard, M. J., Kuhnert, P. M.: Effects of low doses of meperidine on neonatal behavior. Anesth Analg 64:335, 1985.

192. Burns, J. J., et al.: The physiological disposition and fate of meperidine in man and a method for its estimation in plasma. J Pharmacol Exp Ther 114:289, 1955.

193. Klotz, U., McHorse, T. S., Wilkinson, G. R., Schekner, S.: The effect of cirrhosis on the disposition and elimination of meperidine in man. J Clin Pharm Ther 16:667, 1974.

194. Shambaugh, H. E., Wainer, I. W., Sanstead, J. R., Hemphill, D. M.: The clinical pharmacology of meperidine: comparison of routes of administration. J Clin Pharm Ther 16:245, 1976.

195. Mather, L. E., et al.: Meperidine kinetics in man. J Clin Pharm Ther 17:21, 1975.

196. Koska, A. J., III, et al.: Pharmacokinetics of high-dose meperidine in surgical patients. Anesth Analg 60:8, 1981.

197. Herman, R. J., McAllister, C. B., Branch, R. A., Wilkinson, G.R.: Effects of age on the disposition of meperidine. Clin Pharmacol Exp Ther 37:19, 1985.

198. Verbeeck, R. K., Branch, R. A., Wilkinson, G. R.: Meperidine disposition in man: influence of urinary pH and route of administration. Clin Pharmacol Ther 30:619, 1981.

199. Dundee, J. W., Price, H. L., Dripps, R. D.: Acute tolerance to thiopentone in man. Br J Anaesth 28:344, 1956.

200. Hug, C. C.: Improving analgesic therapy. Anesthesiology 53:441, 1980.

201. Austin, K. L., Stapleton, J. V., Mather, L. E.: Relationship between blood meperidine concentrations and analgesic response: a preliminary report. Anesthesiology 53:460, 1980.

202. Glynn, C. J., Mather, L. E.: Clinical pharmacokinetics applied to patients with intractable pain: studies with pethidine. Pain 13:237, 1982.

203. Mather, L. E., Gourlay, G. K.: Biotransformation of opioids: significance for pain therapy. In Nimmo, W. S., Smith, G. (eds.). Opioid Agonist/Antagonist Drugs in Clinical Practice. Amsterdam, Excerpta Medica, 1984.

204. Inturrisi, C. E., Umans, J. G.: Pethidine and its active metabolite, norpethidine. Clin Anesthesiol 1:123, 1983.

205. Armstrong, P. J., Bersten, A.: Normeperidine toxicity. Anesth Analg 65:536, 1986.

206. Szeto, H. H., et al.: Accumulation of normeperidine, an active metabolite of meperidine, in patients with renal failure or cancer. Ann Intern Med 86:738, 1977.

207. Ausherman, H. W., Nowill, W. K., Stephen, C. R.: Controlled analgesia with continuous drip meperidine. JAMA 160:175, 1956.

208. Randall, H. S., Belton, M. K., Leigh, M. D.: Continuous infusion of Demerol during anesthesia. Can Med Assoc J 67:511, 1952.

209. Austin, K. L., Stapleton J. V., Mather L. E.: Relationship between blood meperidine concentrations and analgesic response: a preliminary report. Anesthesiology 53:460, 1980.

210. Austin, K. L., Stapleton, J. V., Mather, L. E.: Multiple intramuscular injections: a major source of variability in analgesic response to meperidine. Pain 8:46, 1980.

211. Sriwatanakul, K., et al.: Analysis of narcotic analgesic usage in the treatment of postoperative pain. JAMA 250:926, 1983.

212. Hull C. J., Sibbald A., Johnson, M. K.: Demand analgesia for postoperative pain. Br J Anaesth 51:570, 1979.

213. Shimm, D. S., et al.: Medical management of chronic cancer pain. JAMA 241:2408, 1979.

214. Gottschalk, C., Orkin, L. R., Rovenstine, E. A.: Nisentil: preliminary screening study of its clinical applicability. NY J Med 55:90, 1955.

215. Orahovats, P. D., Lehman, E. G., Chapin, E. W.: Anileridine: new potent synthetic analgesic. J Pharmacol Exp Ther 119:26, 1957.

215a.Collins, V. J. (ed.): Principles of Anesthesiology, 2nd Ed. Philadelphia, Lea & Febiger, 1977.

216. Scott, C. C., Chen, K. K.: The action of 1,1-diphenyl-1-(dimethylaminoisopropyl)-butanone-2, a potent analgesic agent. J Pharmacol Exp Ther 87:63, 1946.

217. Gero, A.: The spatial structure of methadone. Science 119:112, 1954.

218. Scott, C. C.: Further observations on the pharmacology of Dolophine. J Pharmacol Exp Ther 91:147, 1947.

219. Isbell, H. Eisenman, A. J., Wikler, A., Frank, K.: Effects of single doses of methadone on human subjects. J Pharmacol Exp Ther 92:83, 1948.

220. Weinberg, D. S., et al.: Sublingual absorption of selected opioid analgesics. Clin Pharmacol Ther 44:335, 1988.

221. Inturrisi, C. E., et al.: Pharmacokinetics and pharmacodynamics of methadone in patients with chronic pain. Clin Pharmacol Ther 41:392, 1989.

222. Kirchhof, A. C., David, N. A.: Clinical experience with methadone. Anesthesiology 9:585, 1948.

223. Olsen, G. D.: Methadone binding to human plasma proteins. Clin Pharmacol Ther 14:338, 1973.

224. Dole, V. P., Kreek, M. J.: Methadone plasma level: sustained by a reservoir of drug in tissue. Proc Natl Acad Sci USA 70:10, 1973.

225. Kreek, M. J.: Methadone in treatment: physiological and pharmacological issues. In Dupont, R. I., Goldstein, A., O'Donnell, J. (eds.). Handbook on Drug Abuse. Washington, D.C., U.S. Government Printing Office, 1979, p. 57.

226. Gourlay, G. K., Cherry, D. A., Cousins, M. J.: A comparative study of the efficacy and pharmacokinetics of oral methadone and morphine in the treatment of severe pain in patients with cancer. Pain 25:297, 1986.

227. Sawe, J.: High dose morphine and methadone in cancer patients: pharmacokinetic considerations of oral treatment. Clin Pharmacokinet 11:87, 1986.

228. Troxil, E. B.: Clinical evaluation of the analgesic methadone. JAMA 136:920, 1948.

229. Isbell, H., et al.: Tolerance and addiction liability of 6-

dimethylamino-4-4-diphenylheptanone-3. JAMA *135:*888, 1947.

230. Prescott, F., Ransom, S. G.: Amidone as an obstetric analgesic. Lancet *1:*501, 1947.

231. Scott, W. W., Livingstone, H. M., Jacoby, J. J., Bromberg, G. R.: Early clinical experience with Dolophine. Anesth Analg *26:*18, 1947.

232. Scott, C. C., Kohlstaedt, K. G., Chen, K. K.: Comparison of the pharmacologic properties of some new analgesic substances. Anesth Analg *26:*12, 1947.

233. Gentling, A. A., Lundy, J. C.: Use of methadone in anesthesia. Proc Staff Meet Mayo Clin *22:*249, 1947.

234. Everett, F. G.: The local anesthetic properties of amidone. Anesthesiology *9:*115, 1948.

235. Braenden, O. J., Eddy, N. B., Halbach, H.: Synthetic substances with morphine-like effect: relationship between chemical structure and analgesic action. Bull World Health Organ *13:*937, 1955.

236. Beaver, W. T.: Mild analgesics: a review of their clinical pharmacology. Part II. Am J Med Sci *251:*576, 1966.

237. Beaver, W. T.: Impact of non-narcotic oral analgesics on pain management. Am J Med *84(Suppl 5A):*3, 1988.

238. Bellville, J. W., Seed, J. C.: A comparison of the respiratory depressant effects of dextropropoxyphene and codeine in man. Clin Pharmacol Ther *9:*428, 1968.

239. Chan, G. L. C., Matzke, G. R.: Effects of renal insufficiency on the pharmacokinetics and pharmacodynamics of opioid analgesics. Drug Intell Clin Pharm *21:*773, 1987.

240. Wolen, R. L., Gruber, C. M., Jr., Kiplinger, G. F., Scholz, N. E.: Concentration of propoxyphene in human plasma following oral, intramuscular, and intravenous administration. Toxicol Appl Pharmacol *19:*480, 1971.

240a. Wolen, R. L., Gruber C. M., Jr., Kiplinger, G. F., Scholz, N. E.: Concentration of propoxyphene in human plasma following repeated oral doses. Toxicol Appl Pharmacol *19:*493, 1971.

241. McMahon, R. E., et al.: The fate of radiocarbon-labelled propoxyphene in rat, dog and humans. Toxicol Appl Pharmacol *19:*427, 1971.

242. Lasagna, L., Beecher, H. K.: Analgesic effectiveness of nalorphine and nalorphine-morphine combination in man. J Pharmacol Exp Ther *112:*356, 1954.

243. Weijlard, J., Erickson, A. F.: N-allylnormorphine. J Am Chem Soc *64:*869, 1942.

244. Keats, A. S., Telford, J.: Nalorphine, potent analgesic in man. J Pharmacol Exp Ther *117:*190, 1956.

245. Telford, J., Papadopoulos, C. N., Keats, A. S.: Studies of analgesic drugs. VII. Morphine antagonists as analgesics. J Pharmacol Exp Ther *133:*106, 1961.

246. May, E. L., Eddy, N. B.: Potent analgesia. J Organ Chem *24:*294, 1959.

247. Harris, L. S., Pierson, A. K.: Some narcotic antagonists in benzomorphan series. J Pharmacol Exp Ther *143:*141, 1964.

248. Houde, R. W., et al.: A method of assaying analgesic effects. Clin Pharmacol Ther *1:*163, 1960.

249. Fraser, H. F., Rosenberg, D. S.: Studies on human addiction liability of 2′,hydroxy-5,-9-dimethyl-2-(3,3-dimethylallyl)-6,7-benzomorphan (win 20,228): weak narcotic antagonist. J Pharmacol Exp Ther *143:*149, 1964.

250. Beckett, A. H., Taylor, J. F., Kourounakis, P.: The absorption, distribution and excretion of pentazocine in man after oral and intravenous administration. J Pharm Pharmacol *22:*123, 1970.

251. Berkowitz, B. A., Asling, J. H., Shnider, S. M., Way, E. L.: Relationship of pentazocine plasma levels to pharmacological activity in man. Clin Pharmacol Ther *10:*320, 1969.

252. Yeh, S. Y., et al.: The pharmacokinetics of pentazocine and tripelennamine. Clin Pharmacol Ther *39:*669, 1986.

253. Cass, L. J., Frederik, W. S., Teodoro, J. V.: Pentazocine as an analgesic. JAMA *188:*112, 1964.

254. Sadove, M., Balagot, R. C., Pecora, F. N.: Pentazocine: a new non-addicting analgesic. JAMA *189:*199, 1964.

255. Moertel, C. G.: Relief of pain by oral medications. JAMA *229:*55, 1974.

256. Bellville, J. W.: Pentazocine vs. morphine. JAMA *189:*332, 1964.

257. Bellville, J. W., Forrest, W. H.: Respiratory and subjective effects of d- and l-pentazocine. Clin Pharmacol Ther *9:*142, 1968.

258. Schiff, B. L., Kern, A. B.: Unusual cutaneous manifestation of pentazocine addiction. JAMA *238:*1542, 1971.

259. Jasinski, D. R.: Effects of short- and long-term administration of pentazocine in man. Clin Pharmacol Ther *11:*385, 1970.

259a. Sadove, M.: Personal communication, 1963.

260. Julien, R. M.: Nalbuphine antagonism of opiate-induced respiratory depression. Anesthesiol Rev *12:*29, 1985.

261. Ramagnoli A., Keats, A. S.: Ceiling effect for respiratory depression by nalbuphine. Clin Pharmacol Ther *27:*478, 1980.

262. Aitkenhead, A. R., Lin, E. S., Achola, K. J.: The pharmacokinetics of oral and intravenous nalbuphine in healthy volunteers. Br J Clin *25:*264, 1988.

263. Jaillon, P., et al.: Pharmacokinetics of nalbuphine in infants, young healthy volunteers, and elderly patients. Clin Pharmacol Ther *46:*226, 1989.

264. Lake, C. L., et al.: Cardiovascular effects of nalbuphine in patients with coronary or valvular heart disease. Anesthesiology *57:*498, 1982.

265. Lee, G., et al.: Hemodynamic effects of morphine and nalbuphine in acute myocardial infarction. Clin Pharmacol Ther *29:*576, 1981.

266. Gomez, Q. J. (ed.): Nalbuphine as a component of surgical anesthesia. *In* Proceedings of a Symposium/VIIIth World Congress of Anaesthesiologists. Manila, Philippines, 1984.

267. Shah, M., Rosen, M., Vickers, M. D.: Effect of premedication with diazepam, morphine or nalbuphine on gastrointestinal motility after surgery. Br J Anaesth *56:* 1235, 1984.

268. Tran, L., et al.: Hemodynamic and endocrine effects of reversal of fentanyl-induced respiratory depression by nalbuphine. Anesthesiology *61:*A476, 1984.

269. Moldenhauer, C. C., et al.: Nalbuphine antagonism of ventilatory depression following high dose fentanyl anesthesia. Anesthesiology *62:*647, 1985.

270. Magruder, M. R., Delaney, R. D., DiFazio, C. A.: Reversal of narcotic-induced respiratory depression with nalbuphine hydrochloride. Anesthesiol Rev *4:*34, 1982.

271. Bailey, P. L., et al.: Failure of nalbuphine to antagonize morphine: a double-blind comparison with naloxone. Anesth Analg *65:*605, 1986.

272. Boas, R. A., Villiger, J. W.: Clinical actions of fentanyl and buprenorphine: the significance of receptor binding. Br J Anaesth *57:*192, 1985.

273. Wallenstein, S. L., Kaiko, R. F., Rogers, A. G., Houde, R. W.: Crossover trials in clinical analgesic assay: studies of buprenorphine and morphine. Pharmacotherapy *6:*228, 1986.

274. Sadee, W., Rosenbaum, J. S., Herz, A.: Buprenorphine: differential interaction with opiate receptor sub-types in vivo. J Pharmacol Exp Ther *223:*157, 1982.

275. Villiger, J. W.: Binding of buprenorphine to opiate receptors: regulation by guanyl nucleotides and metal ions. Neuropharmacology *23:*373, 1984.

276. De Castro, J.: Use of narcotic antagonists in anaesthesia. Br J Clin Pharmacol 7:319S, 1979.

277. Jasinski, D. R.: Opiate withdrawal syndrome: acute and protracted aspects. Ann NY Acad Sci 362:183, 1981.

278. Nagashima, H., et al.: Respiratory and circulatory effects of intravenous butorphanol and morphine. Clin Pharmacol Ther 19:738, 1976.

279. Gilbert, M. S., Hanover, R. M., Moylan, B. S., Caruso, F. S.: Intramuscular butorphanol and meperidine in postoperative pain. Clin Pharmacol Ther 20:359, 1976.

280. Zucker, J. R., Neuenfeldt, T., Freund, P. R.: Respiratory effects of nalbuphine and butorphanol in anesthetized patients. Anesth Analg 66:879, 1987.

281. Weintraub, S. J., Naulty, J. S.: Acute abstinence syndrome after epidural injection of butorphanol. Anesth Analg 64:452, 1985.

282. Abboud, T. K., et al.: Epidural butorphanol or morphine for the relief of post-cesarean section pain: ventilatory responses to carbon dioxide. Anesth Analg 66:887, 1987.

Chapter 32

ANTAGONISTS TO NARCOTICS

KENNETH D. CANDIDO, VINCENT J. COLLINS

Overdosage of narcotic analgesics is a frequent problem. It is characterized by profound respiratory and cardiovascular depression. The principles of treatment are similar to those in other forms of coma, unconsciousness, and depression. One may consider an immediate resuscitative phase, a phase of drug reversal or neutralization, and a delayed or prolonged phase of supportive therapy. In the early phase, the desired aim is to eliminate the offending drug. To achieve this goal, specific antagonists to the narcotic analgesics are available. To understand how these agents exert their pharmacologic effect in vivo, it is important to review the concept of receptor mechanics briefly.

OPIOID RECEPTORS

The discovery of the opioid receptor led to a rapid increase in our understanding of opioid neurophysiology, as well as providing a rationale for the mechanisms of action of both opiate agonists as well as antagonists. In 1967, Goldstein[1] developed an assay technique that indirectly demonstrated the existence of opioid receptors. In 1973, the classic report of Pert and Snyder appeared in which these investigators demonstrated the existence of opioid receptors in brain and other nervous tissues using Goldstein's assay technique.[2] Pert also reasoned that these receptors did not develop in anticipation of the use of exogenous morphine substances, but they exist for the reception of endogenous substances. This bit of serendipity led to the identification in the brain and other nervous tissue of peptides with opiate-like activity and functioning as neurotransmitters.

In 1975, Hughes and associates[3] isolated endogenous pentapeptides with opiate-like activity (leu- and met-enkephalin). By studying the effects of various types of opiates in dogs, Martin and associates[4] proposed three classes of opioid receptors: μ (for morphine sulfate); κ (for ketocyclazocine); and σ (for SKF 10,047, now named N-allylnormetazocine).

By 1977, two additional receptor types had been proposed; δ[5] and ϵ.[6]

Current evidence strongly suggests the existence of three opioid receptor types: mu, δ, and κ. An opioid receptor is one that can also bind with the opiate antagonist naloxone. Further work in opioid receptor typing has been accomplished using a variety of extremely selective opiate antagonists and agonists.

For example, Pasternak and colleagues[7] demonstrated μ_1 and μ_2 receptor subtypes associated with widely divergent activities.

Distribution

Opioid receptors are found throughout the central nervous system (CNS), and also the peripheral nervous system (PNS), and are inhibitory in nature. For example, μ receptors are found in the neocortex, striatum, limbic system, thalamus and substantia gelatinosa of the spinal cord, and also the nucleus tractus solitarii and related nuclei concerned with vagal reflexes. These receptors are located at presynaptic sites and produce presynaptic inhibition[8]:

κ receptors inhibit activity of voltage-dependent calcium channels leading to decreased nerve action potentials.

μ and δ receptors increase activity of potassium channels leading to hyperpolarization of resting membrane potentials.

Both these ion channel actions of opioid receptors decrease the size of the nerve action potential, thus limiting the release of transmitter at the synapse.

Narcotic antagonists bind competitively to the opioid receptors and occupation of the site by an agonist is thus prevented. The competition depends on local concentrations of each agent present at the biophase. Affinity varies with the different drugs for different sites. The binding of naloxone, for example, to μ receptors is much stronger than to κ or δ receptors. This preferential binding is relative, and if high concentrations of the antagonist are present, binding to nonpreferential sites may occur, with the subsequent production of other effects.

ENDOGENOUS PAIN-REGULATING SYSTEMS

At least two endogenous pain-regulating systems are recognized: the descending opioid-serotonergic and the descending adrenergic system.

Opiate application within the periaqueductal gray produces a disinhibition (activation) of the serotonin secretory neurons of the nucleus raphe magnus, which, in turn, activates the opioid interneurons at presynaptic sites of the primary afferents. These opioid interneurons produce presynaptic inhibition of substance P release.

The second source of endogenous analgesia is the descending adrenergic system. When stimulated, the α_2 receptors produce membrane hyperpolarization that inhibits the propagation of second-order afferent nerve action potentials. Therefore, inhibitors of analgesia or antagonists may serve to block either the opioid or adrenergic influences of pain transmission, or both concurrently.

DEVELOPMENT OF OPIOID ANTAGONISTS

In 1915, Pohl[9] of Breslau showed that N-allyl ($-CH_2CH = CH_2$) derivatives of codeine antagonized the depressant effects of morphine. This observation was ignored until 1941, when Weijlard and Erickson reviewed Pohl's findings and substituted the allyl group for the methyl group on the tertiary nitrogen of morphine.[10] This N-allyl derivative or nalorphine proved to be an effective antagonist to the parent morphine.

In the same year, Unna[11] presented the classic description of the pharmacology of N-allyl-morphine and showed it to be a potent antagonist to morphine. Other investigators[12] showed this drug to be a more potent antagonist than the codeine derivative.

Later, Lasagna and Beecher[13] combined the N-allyl-normorphine with morphine and determined that the respiratory depression of morphine could be antagonized. Results were not predictable, but unexpectedly nalorphine proved to be effective in relieving pain. Later, Isbell[13a] demonstrated that nalorphine appeared to have only mild addicting properties in human subjects. For the first time, analgesia to some extent was divorced from the addiction liability. The administration of the allyl derivatives produces hallucinations when given in analgesic doses, however, so their use as agonist agents was severely limited.

Subsequently, other allyl derivatives of opiates were shown to have antagonistic action of the parent compound and also to related narcotic derivatives.[14]

CHEMISTRY OF ANTAGONISTS

Narcotic antagonists are semisynthetic drugs formed from the parent opiate or narcotic compounds by replacement with an allyl group of the radical attached to the nitrogen. Such replacement produces antagonists of varying degrees of activity. Thus, N-allyl-normeperidine does not have significant antagonistic action. The steric configuration is also important because the dextro isomer of levallorphan is inactive.

The allyl group is not specific because substitutions on the N- by other groups such as propyl and isobutyl also produce narcotic antagonists.

AGONISTS AS MINOR ANTAGONISTS

Benzmorphan Antagonists

In 1958, Archer and Harris[15] (Sterling-Winthrop Institute) sought nonaddicting analgesics among morphine antagonists structurally related to benzmorphans (i.e., phenazocine). Further modification of the allyl group produced effective antagonists and potent analgesic drugs.

In 1959, Gates[15a] showed that the cyclopropylmethyl group conferred activity similar to the allyl group when substituted on the nitrogen. Derivatives were prepared with both antagonism to morphine and inherent analgesia. Among the effective derivatives with these structures are cyclazocine (a benzmorphan) and cyclophene (a morphinan). Both are effective antagonists. Cyclazocine is one of the most potent, with an antagonism activity 28 times on a weight basis more effective than nalorphine. Both are also extremely potent analgesics, having 30 to 50 times the activity of morphine.

Minor changes in the structure of an opioid convert the agonist activity to antagonist activity. This activity may be manifest at all receptors or partial. Older congeners such as N-allyl-nor-morphine (nalorphine) or the N-allyl derivative of levorphanol* (Lorfan) are competitive antagonists at the μ receptor but have agonist action at the κ receptor.

Naloxone and naltrexone appear to act as antagonists at all receptors. Nalmefene is a pure μ antagonist with no evident activity at κ or other opioid receptors.

Several nonpeptide antagonists have been designed and synthesized that are selective for a specific opiate receptors. These have not been completely studied as yet in humans.[16]

ANTAGONISTS IN CURRENT USE

Since the 1950s, beginning with naloxone hydrochloride,[17] agents with little or no agonist activity have been available for use as antagonists of opiates for treating respiratory depression and acute overdosage. Agents in clinical use today are also employed in the detection of chronic opiate abuse and in a wide experimental range of conditions and addictions in which endogenous or exogenous opioid receptor agonists are suspected or proved causes.

This chapter emphasizes the uses of naloxone, naltrexone, and nalmefene, as antagonists to the narcotic analgesics. These three antagonists are considered to be "pure antagonists" because they have no intrinsic agonist activity. They are able to occupy μ-, κ-, δ-, and σ type opioid receptors; however, they have a greater preference for μ than for δ or κ receptors.

Naloxone

Naloxone hydrochloride is a semisynthetic opiate antagonist derived from thebaine. Naloxone differs structurally from oxymorphone only in that the methyl group on the nitrogen atom of oxymorphone is replaced by an allyl group (Fig. 32–1).

Naloxone is essentially a pure opiate antagonist. It is devoid of agonist effects, and when it is administered to individuals who have not recently received opiates, naloxone produces little or no pharmacologic effect. In patients who have received large doses of morphine or other narcotic analgesics, naloxone reverses most of the opiate effects. An increase in respiratory rate and minute volume occur. $Paco_2$ returns toward normal, and, if previously depressed, blood pressure returns to normal. Even mild respiratory depression induced by opiates can be antagonized by naloxone. The duration of action of naloxone is generally shorter than that of many opiates, however, resulting in a return of the effects of the opiate as the effects of the antagonist dissipate. Sedation induced

---

*Nalorphine and levallorphan are no longer available in the United States

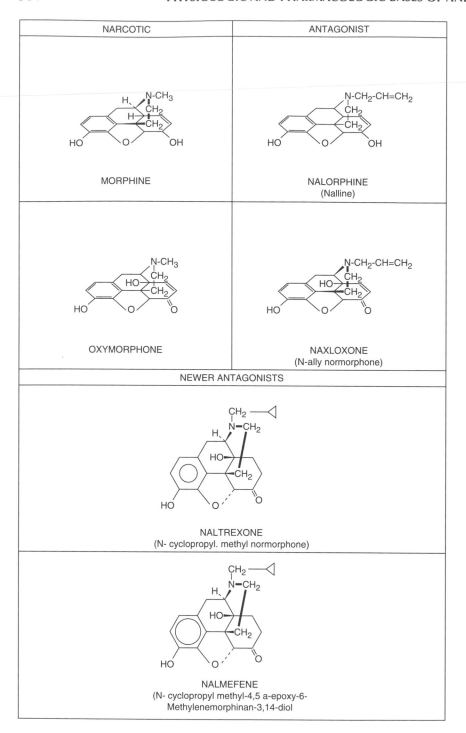

NARCOTIC	ANTAGONIST
MORPHINE	NALORPHINE (Nalline)
OXYMORPHONE	NAXLOXONE (N-ally normorphone)

NEWER ANTAGONISTS

NALTREXONE
(N- cyclopropyl. methyl normorphone)

NALMEFENE
(N- cyclopropyl methyl-4,5 a-epoxy-6-
Methylenemorphinan-3,14-diol

Fig. 32–1. Structural formulas of some opioids and antagonists.

by opiates is also antagonized by naloxone, unless the dose is carefully individualized.

Naloxone is nonaddicting, nor does it produce tolerance when administered over prolonged periods. Although naloxone antagonizes opioid receptors competitively, its greatest effect is on the μ receptor.

Pharmacokinetics

Naloxone is rapidly inactivated after oral administration, and although it may be effective by this route, much larger doses than those required for parenteral use are necessary for complete opiate antagonism. Following in-travenous administration, onset of action is about 1 to 2 minutes. After subcutaneous or intramuscular administration, about 2 to 5 minutes. Duration of action is dose and route dependent and is more prolonged after intramuscular than after intravenous use. Using 0.4 mg/70 kg intravenously, the expected duration of action is on the order of 45 minutes. The drug may also be given by endotracheal tube in emergency situations.

Distribution in Tissues

After parenteral administration, naloxone is rapidly and widely distributed into various tissue compartments including the brain, kidney, spleen, lung, heart, and skeletal muscle. It readily crosses the placenta. In adults, plasma half-life is 60 to 90 minutes, whereas in neonates, it is closer to 3 hours.

Metabolism and Excretion

Metabolism is hepatic, principally by conjugation with glucuronic acid. The major metabolite is naloxone-3-glucuronide. N-dealkylation and reduction also occur to the 6-keto group followed by conjugation. From 25 to 40% of an oral or intravenous dose of the drug is excreted as metabolites in urine in 6 hours, about 50% in 24 hours, and 60 to 70% in 72 hours.

Clinical Uses

Naloxone is used for the treatment of respiratory depression induced by opiate agonists and partial agonist agents, including butorphanol, nalbuphine, pentazocine, and cyclazocine. Postoperatively, the usual initial dose is 0.1 to 0.2 mg intravenously in adults and 0.005 to 0.01 mg intravenously in children, given at 2- to 3-minute intervals until the desired response is obtained. Additional doses may be necessary at 1- to 2-hour intervals, depending on the response of the patient and the dosage and duration of action of the opiate administered. Supplemental intramuscular doses given after the initial intravenous dose may result in a more prolonged duration of antagonist effect. Continuous intravenous infusions, made by diluting naloxone in D_5W or 0.9% normal saline to a concentration of 0.004 mg/ml (4 μg/ml), may alternatively be given in a dose of 0.0037 mg/kg/hour until the agonist effect is ablated.

When the drug is used to reverse opiate-induced asphyxia of the newborn, the usual initial dose is 0.01 mg/kg into the umbilical vein at 2- to 3-minute intervals until the desired effect is attained.

In cases of known or suspected opiate overdosage, the dosage of naloxone for adults is 0.4 to 2.0 mg intravenously, administered at 2- to 3-minute intervals as necessary, or until a total of 10 mg has been administered; if no response is forthcoming after this dose, then other causes of depression or disease must be ruled out.

Other Applications

Naloxone has found a wide variety of potential uses that, not surprisingly, follow the virtual explosion of research into the chemical and neurophysiologic elucidation of opioid receptors and the understanding of their role in various physiologic states.

Experimentally, naloxone has been associated with an increased number and density of μ receptors after long-term administration. The potential to increase the analgesic potency of opiate agonists exists, while avoiding the necessity to increase dosing continuously in chronic pain states.[18-22]

Naloxone has been used in intoxicated patients to reverse alcohol-induced coma, by a mechanism not completely understood. Experimentally, naloxone may have utility in the treatment of chronic ethanol abuse, by attenuating the reinforcing actions of that drug.[23]

Naloxone has also been used in managing some of the systemic manifestations of hypovolemic and septic shock states.[24-28]

In addition, several types of neurologic insults have been variably treated using naloxone. Acute hemiplegia,[29] poststroke pain (thalamic syndrome),[30] acute ischemic stroke,[31,32] and spinal cord traumatic injury[33-36] have all been studied to determine the results, if any, naloxone has in preventing or reversing neurologic deficits. Other types of spinal cord ischemia, that is, thoracic and thoracoabdominal aneurysms, are also being evaluated as clinical situations in which naloxone might prevent neurologic deficits and improve survival.[37]

Some forms of encephalopathy possibly caused by opioid receptor stimulation have been successfully reversed using naloxone in isolated case reports.[38] One report of reversal of schizophrenia-related pathologic behavior offers promise for use of this antagonist in severe forms of organic mental disorders.[39] Likewise, a case of improvement in consciousness in an epileptic patient helps researchers to evaluate the endogenous pentapeptide opiate systems in various forms of illness.[40] Mood and cognition may be linked to the endogenous opioid system.[41]

Some investigators of addictive phenomena such as cigarette smoking and chronic eating disorders have linked the endogenous opioid receptors with the positive-reinforcing aspects of these conditions. Naloxone has been shown experimentally to ameliorate partially cravings for cigarettes, or, in the case of overeating, to blunt some of the physiologic effects of appetite sensation or hunger.[42-45]

Unusual Therapeutic Uses

Preliminary studies detailing the use of naloxone to treat migraine headaches,[46] to use in memory facilitation,[47] to attenuate the pruritis of chronic cholestasis,[48] to reinforce clonidine analgesia,[49] and to treat the chronic constipation of persons habituated to narcotics[50] have been reported.

Although naloxone does not influence breathing in normal conscious humans,[51] it does influence ventilation in several clinical circumstances: chronic obstructive pulmonary disease,[52] ventilatory failure,[53] and depressed ventilation from benzodiazepines.[54-57] The salutary effects are thought to be due to reversal of endogenous opioid action.

Although an area of some controversy, naloxone appears to have some influence on the ventilatory depression caused by some anesthetics. The analgesic effect of nitrous oxide is partially antagonized by naloxone in moderate or large doses.[58] Other studies, however, have shown that naloxone does not influence the anesthetic action of nitrous oxide on reflexes.[59] Prolonged exposure to nitrous oxide has been shown to decrease opioid receptor density in the brain stem of rats.[60] Whereas the minimum alveolar concentrations of potent inhalation anesthetics are unaffected by naloxone, previously it was believed that naloxone could reduce halothane levels. Ventilatory depression due to isoflurane anesthesia is not antagonized by naloxone.[61]

Premature infants are prone to develop recurrent apnea, treatable by naloxone.[62] These infants have high levels of endorphins in the cerebrospinal fluid.[63] Because unacceptably large fluid volumes can result with the use of neonatal naloxone hydrochloride injection (i.e., containing 0.02 mg/ml), especially in small neonates, the American Academy of Pediatrics recommends that use of this preparation be avoided when large doses are needed.[64]

For naloxone administration before delivery, during the second stage of labor this drug is rapidly transferred to the fetus via the placenta.[65] After a single dose of 400 μg, the mean maternal serum concentration has been determined to be 5.8 ng/ml (range 2.0 to 14.0 ng/ml). The highest maternal concentrations were found after 2 minutes. A similar naloxone concentration was noted in the fetus, as evidenced by umbilical-fetal serum concentrations ranging from 0.175 to 7.90 ng/ml, 2 to 4 minutes after intravenous maternal administration. The mean umbilical serum concentration was found to be 3.0 ng/ml. About one-half the infants had serum levels of naloxone of less than 2.5 ng/ml. The intramuscular route of administration has been unpredictable as to serum concentrations, both in the mother as well as in the neonate. The usual circumstance is to administer naloxone to the baby after delivery as detailed in the section: uses of naloxone, examined earlier in this chapter.

Adverse Effects and Contraindications

Naloxone has produced a variety of adverse effects when administered to combat depression produced by opiates. Although a definitive relationship has not been proved, naloxone administration has been associated with hypotension, hypertension, ventricular tachycardia and ventricular fibrillation, and pulmonary edema. These effects have tended to occur most frequently in patients having underlying disorders of the cardiovascular system.[66-71]

Naloxone has also been shown to reverse hypotension due to captopril overdosage[72] and to demonstrate an antiarrhythmic action in animal studies.[73] Several reports demonstrate a positive inotropic action of naloxone, and a possible modification of the cellular responsiveness to catecholamines has been postulated.[74-76]

Naltrexone Hydrochloride

Chemistry

Naltrexone is a synthetic opiate antagonist derived from thebaine.[77] Whereas the methyl group on the nitrogen atom of oxymorphone is replaced by an allyl group to make naloxone, here the methyl group is replaced by a cyclicproplmethyl group (see Fig. 32-1). The result, as per naloxone, is essentially a pure opiate antagonist. The structural modification from naloxone to naltrexone results in the latter's having greater oral bioavailability and also a longer duration of action.

Pharmacology[77]

Naltrexone is approximately two to nine times more potent than naloxone on a weight basis, as regards opiate

antagonist activity. A major metabolite, 6-β-naltrexol also has antagonist actions.

Naltrexone antagonizes most of the subjective and objective effects of opiate agonists and partial agonists. Like naloxone, naltrexone acts competitively at μ, κ, and δ receptors in the CNS, with its highest affinity for the μ receptor. Like naloxone, naltrexone administration is associated with increased plasma concentrations of luteinizing hormone, corticotropin, and cortisol, whereas follicle-stimulating hormone and serum testosterone concentrations do not increase, nor do levels of growth hormone or serum prolactin.

Naltrexone appears to be similar to naloxone as regards utility in clinical situations where blockade of endogenous or exogenous opiates has demonstrable physiologic effects.

Although naltrexone is rapidly and almost completely absorbed from the gastrointestinal tract following oral administration, it does undergo extensive first-pass metabolism in the liver. Following oral administration, only 5 to 20% reaches the systemic circulation unchanged.[78]

Pharmacokinetics[77]

Peak plasma concentrations usually occur within 1 hour following oral administration of a single 100-mg dose with a concentration of 43.6 ng/ml. The primary metabolite, 6-β-naltrexol, usually has peak concentrations 1 to 10 times greater than the parent compound.

Following oral administration, the onset of opiate antagonism is about 15 to 30 minutes. Duration of effect is dose dependent and is longer than with equipotent doses of naloxone.

Naltrexone is widely distributed throughout the body. Following a single 1-mg intravenous dose in healthy adults, the estimated volume of distribution was 1350 L. Following oral use, the volume of distribution averages 16 L/kg after a single 100-mg dose. Protein binding is about 21 to 28%.[79]

Plasma concentrations of naltrexone and 6-β-naltrexol decline in a biphasic manner with T½ of 1 to 3 hours and T½-β 10 to 17 hours, approximately, after oral dosing. Metabolism in the liver is by reduction of the 6-keto group of naltrexone to 6-β-naltrexol (6 to 8% as potent as naltrexone). It is also metabolized by catechol-O-methyl transferase to 2-hydroxy-3-methoxy-6-β-naltrexol and 2-hydroxy-3-methoxynaltrexone. Conjugation with glucuronic acid also occurs.

Naltrexone and its metabolites are excreted principally in the urine.

Uses[80]

Naltrexone is used to antagonize the depressant effects of narcotic analgesics in a manner similar to naloxone.[80]

Additionally, because of its effectiveness orally and its prolonged duration of action, naltrexone is useful as an adjunct in the maintenance of opiate cessation programs in persons previously physically dependent on opiates and who have already been detoxified.

Naltrexone may reduce or eliminate opiate-seeking behavior and may also prevent the conditioned abstinence syndrome that occurs following abrupt cessation of opiate use.

Other Applications

Essentially, naltrexone might be useful in any clinical situation where naloxone has shown effectiveness in blunting the activity of endogenous or exogenous opiates (see the section on naloxone in this chapter).

Precautions and Adverse Effects

Gastrointestinal distress occurs in up to 10% of individuals using this agent chronically. Naltrexone can cause dose-related hepatocellular injury, usually not seen in clinically relevant doses.[78]

Most important, possibly, this agent may precipitate mild to severe signs and symptoms of opiate withdrawal in persons physically dependent on opiates.

To avoid precipitating opiate withdrawal following the administration of naltrexone, some clinicians rely on a naloxone challenge test in patients previously physically dependent on opiates who have been detoxified.

The usual daily oral dose is 50 to 100 mg for maintenance therapy for opiate cessation.

Nalmefene

Nalmefene is a pure narcotic antagonist, structurally similar to naloxone and naltrexone.[81] It contains an exocyclic methylene group, which increases its potency at the opioid receptor level and enhances its oral bioavailability. The structure and chemical name are represented in Figure 32-1.

Like naloxone and naltrexone, nalmefene has a greater preference for μ than δ or κ opioid receptors as demonstrated by IC_{50} (inhibitory concentration of 50%) studies.[82] Intravenous doses of 1.0 to 2.0 mg/70 kg have been demonstrated to be clinically useful for the reversal of narcotic overdosage. Doses as high as 6 to 12 mg/70 kg have been administered with only mild transient side effects, such as lightheadedness. This comparison between the therapeutic doses and doses producing adverse effects is large and represents a wide margin of safety. The usual oral dose is 0.5 to 3.0 mg/kg, which results in a long duration of action.[82] The duration of reversal of fentanyl and morphine-induced respiratory depression is dose dependent.[83] To reverse the depression after general anesthesia with narcotics, the dose is 0.25 to 1.0 μg/kg at two to five minute intervals until the desired effect is achieved.[86]

Pharmacokinetics

Immediately after intravenous injection, nalmefene undergoes an initial rapid distribution in the vascular volume (π phase) with a T½-π of 2 to 6 minutes. This is followed by a slower distribution phase into vascular rich tissues with a T½-α of 1.0 to 2.5 hours. The terminal phase of T½-β has been determined to be about 8 hours. Plasma concentrations decline in a triphasic manner, following a triexponential equation.[84]

Metabolism

The drug is highly extracted by the liver. It shows extensive first-pass metabolism after oral administration. The oral bioavailability is in the range of 40 to 50%, with peak plasma concentrations reached in 1 to 2 hours. One metabolite identified in the plasma and urine is a conjugate subject to β-glucuronidase-sulfatase hydrolysis. Thus, conjugation with glucuronic or sulfuric acid represents a major route of transformation. Only about 5% of nalmefene is excreted unchanged in the urine.

Clinical Uses

Because nalmefene has a longer duration of action than naloxone (T½-β of 8 to 10 hours versus 1 to 2 hours), the possibility of the return of CNS and respiratory depression is reduced in individuals given large doses of narcotic analgesics, for example, during balanced anesthesia techniques. Nalmefene is particularly useful for the same reason in the emergency treatment of narcotic abuse overdosage.

A comparison with naloxone shows that 1.0 mg of naloxone was ineffective after 90 minutes in reversing narcotic-induced respiratory depression.[85] A dose of 2.0 mg/kg of nalmefene was still active after 8 hours for reversal of fentanyl-induced respiratory depression.[83] It is also more effective against meperidine depression or of methadone.[87]

REFERENCES

1. Davis, J.: Endorphins: New Waves in Brain Chemistry. New York, Doubleday, 1984.
2. Pert, C. B., Snyder, S. H.: Opiate receptors: demonstration in nervous tissue. Science *179:*1011, 1973.
3. Hughes, J., et al.: Identification of two related pentapeptides from the brain with potent opiate agonist activity. *258:*577, 1975.
4. Martin, W. R., et al.: The effects of morphine- and morphine-like drugs in the nondependent and morphine dependent chronic spinal dog. J Pharmacol Exp Ther *197:*517, 1976.
5. Kosterlitz, H. W., Paterson, S. J.: Characterization of opioid receptors in nervous tissue. Proc R Soc Lond *210:*113, 1980.
6. Lemnaire, S., Magnan, J., Regoli, D.: Rat vas deferens: a specific bioassay for endogenous opioid peptides. Br J Pharmacol *64:*327, 1978.
7. Pasternak, G. W., Childer, S. R., Snyder, S. H.: Sigma receptors: from molecules to man. J Neurochem *57:*729, 1991.
8. Duggin, A. W., North, R. A.: Electrophysiology of opioids. Pharmacol Rev *35:*219, 1984.
9. Pohl, J.: Uber das N-allylnorcodeine, einen Antagonisten des Morphins. Z Exp Pathol Therap *17:*370, 1915.
10. Weijlard, J., Erickson, A. E.: N-allylnormorphine. J Am Chem Soc *64:*869, 1942.
11. Unna, K.: Antagonistic effects of N-allyl-normorphine upon morphine. J Pharmacol Exp Ther *79:*27, 1943.
12. Hart, E. R., McCawley, E. L.: The pharmacology of N-allylnormorphine as compared with morphine. J Pharmacol Exp Ther *82:*339, 1944.
13. Lasagna, L., Beecher, H. K.: Respiratory and circulatory effects of Nalorphine. J Pharmacol Exp Ther *112:*356, 1954.
14. Wickler, A., Cartier, R. L.: Test for addiction. Fed Proc *11:*402, 1952.

14a. Isbell, H.: Addicting properties of nalorphine. *In* Wickler, H. (ed.). The Addictive States. Baltimore, Williams & Wilkins, 1968.

15. Archer, S., Harris, L. S.: Narcotic antagonists. Prog Drug Res 8:261, 1965.

15a. Gates, M.: Analgesic drugs. Sci Am 215:131, 1966.

16. Portoghese, P. S.: Bivalent ligands and the message-address concept in the design of selective opioid receptor antagonists. Trends Pharmacol Sci 10:230, 1989.

17. Sadove, M. S., Balagot, R. C., Hatano, S., Jobgen, E.A.: Study of a narcotic antagonist -N-allyl-noroxymorphone. JAMA 182:339, 1954.

18. Kosten, T. R., Morgan, C., Kreek, M. J.: Beta endorphin levels during heroin methadone, buprenorphine, and naloxone challenges: preliminary findings. Biol Psychiatry 32:523, 1992.

19. Cantor, A., et al.: Asymptomatic or mildly symptomatic effort-induced myocardial ischemia: plasma beta-endorphin and the effect of naloxone. Isr J Med Sci 26:67, 1990.

20. Levesque, D., Holtzman, S. G.: The potentiating effects of restraint stress and continuous naloxone infusion on the analgesic potency or morphine are additive. Brain Res 617:176, 1993.

21. Alcaraz, C., Vargas, M. L., Fuente, T., Milanes, M. V.: Chronic naloxone treatment induces supersensitivity to a mu but not to a kappa agonist at the hypothalamus-pituitary-adrenocortical axis level. J Pharmacol Exp Ther 266:1602, 1993.

22. Gouarderes, C., et al.: Opioid and substance P receptor adaptations in the rat spinal cord following sub-chronic intrathecal treatment with morphine and naloxone. Neuroscience 54:799, 1993.

23. Hyytia, P., Sinclair, J. D.: Responding for oral ethanol after naloxone treatment by alcohol-preferring AA rats. Alcohol Clin Exp Res 17:631, 1993.

24. Peters, W. P., Johnson, M. W., Friedman, P. A., Mitch, W. E.: Pressor effect of naloxone in septic shock. Lancet 1:1529, 1981.

25. Weissglass, I. S.: The role of endogenous opiates in shock. Adv Shock Res 10:87, 1983.

26. Hackshaw, K. V., Parker, G. A., Roberts, J. W.: Naloxone in septic shock. Crit Care Med 18:47, 1990.

27. Safani, M., et al.: Prospective, controlled, randomized trial of naloxone infusion in early hyperdynamic septic shock. Crit Care Med 17:1004, 1989.

28. Dziki, A. J., Lynch, W. H., Ramsey, C. B., Law, W. R.: Beta-adrenergic-dependent and -independent actions of naloxone on perfusion during endotoxin shock. Circ Shock 39:29, 1993.

29. Hans, P., et al.: Reversal of neurological deficit with naloxone: an additional report. Intensive Care Med 18:362, 1992.

30. Bainton, T., Fox, M., Bowsher, D., Wells, C.: A double-blind trial of naloxone in central post-stroke pain. Pain 48:159, 1992.

31. Federico, F., et al.: A double blind randomized pilot trial of naloxone in the treatment of acute ischemic stroke. Ital J Neurol Sci 12:557, 1991.

32. Olinger, C. P., et al.: High-dose intravenous naloxone for the treatment of acute ischemic stroke. Stroke 21:721, 1990.

33. Bracken, M. B., et al.: Methylprednisolone or naloxone treatment after acute spinal cord injury: 1-year follow-up date. Results of the second National Acute Spinal Cord Injury Study. J Neurosurg 76:23, 1992.

34. Baskin, D. S., et al.: The effect of long-term high-dose naloxone infusion in experimental blunt spinal cord injury. J Spinal Disord 6:38, 1993.

35. Cherian, L., Kuruvilla, A., Abraham, J., Chandy, M.: Evaluation of drug effects on spinal cord injury: an experimental study in monkeys. Indian J Exp Biol 30:509, 1992.

36. Benzel, E. C., Khare, V., Fowler, M. R.: Effects of naloxone and nalmefene in rat spinal cord injury induced by the ventral compression technique. J Spinal Disord 5:75, 1992.

37. Archer, C. W., Wynn, M. M., Archibald, J.: Naloxone and spinal fluid drainage as adjuncts in the surgical treatment of thoracoabdominal and thoracic aneurysms. Surgery 108:755, 1990.

38. Mattana, J., et al.: Naloxone-responsive encephalopathy in end-stage renal disease. Am J Kidney Dis 21:559, 1993.

39. Nishikawa, T., et al.: Nalaxone attenuates drinking behavior in a schizophrenic patient displaying self-induced water intoxication. Clin Neuropharmacol 15:310, 1992.

40. Turner, M., Stewart, M.: Reversal of unconsciousness by use of naloxone in a profoundly mentally handicapped epileptic. J Ment Defic Res 35:81, 1991.

41. Martin-del-Campo, A. F., McMurray, R. G., Besser, G. M., Grossman, A.: Effect of 12 hour infusion of naloxone on mood and cognition in normal male volunteers. Biol Psychiatry 32:344, 1992.

42. Gorelick, D. A., Rose, J., Jarvik, M. E.: Effect of naloxone on cigarette smoking. J Subst Abuse 1:153, 1988-1989.

43. Vettor, R., et al.: Possible involvement of endogenous opioids in beta-cell hyperresponsiveness in human obesity. Int J Obes 13:425, 1989.

44. Yeomans, M. R.: Prior exposure to low or high fat milk enhances naloxone anorexia in rats. Appetite 20:125, 1993.

45. Alavi, F. K., McCann, J. P., Mauromoustakis, A., Sangiah, S.: Feeding behavior and its responsiveness to naloxone differ in lean and obese sheep. Physiol Behav 53:317, 1993.

46. Nicolodi, M., Sicuteri, P.: Chronic naloxone administration, a potential treatment for migraine, enhances morphine-induced miosis. Headache 32:348, 1992.

47. Tomaz, C., Aguiar, M. S., Nogueira, P. J.: Facilitation of memory by peripheral administration of substance P and naloxone using avoidance and habituation learning tasks. Neurosci Biobehav Rev 14:447, 1990.

48. Bergasa, N. V., et al.: A controlled trial of naloxone infusions for the pruritis of chronic cholestasis. Gastroenterology 102:544, 1992.

49. Porchet, H. C., Piletta, P., Dayer, P.: Objective assessment of clonidine analgesia in man and influence of naloxone. Life Sci 46:991, 1990.

50. Culpepper-Morgan, J. A., et al.: Treatment of opioid-induced constipation with oral naloxone: a pilot study. Clin Pharmacol Ther 52:90, 1992.

51. Fleetham, J. A., et al.: Endogenous opiates and chemical control of breathing in humans. Am Rev Respir Dis 121:1045, 1980.

52. Santiago, T. U., Remolina, C., Scoles, V., Edelman, N. H.: Ability of naloxone to restore flow-resistive load compensation in chronic obstructive pulmonary disease. N Engl J Med 304:1190, 1981.

53. Ayres, J., Rees, J., Lee, T., Cochrane, G. M.: Intravenous naloxone in acute respiratory failure. Br Med J 284:927, 1982.

54. Jordan, C., Lehane, J. R., Jones, J. G.: Respiratory depression following diazepam: reversal with high dose naloxone. Anesthesiology 53:293, 1980.

55. Rocha, L., Tatsukawa, K., Chugani, H. T., Engel, J., Jr.: Benzodiazepine receptor binding following chronic treatment with nalaoxone, morphine and met-enkephalin in normal rats. Brain Res 612:247, 1993.

56. Baraban, S. C., Stornetta, R. L., Guyenet, P. G.: Respiratory

control of sympathetic nerve activity during naloxone-precipitated morphine withdrawal in rats. J Pharmacol Exp Ther 265:89, 1993.

57. Johnson, A., Bengtsson, M., Soderlind, K., Lofstrom, B. J.: Influence of intrathecal morphine and naloxone intervention on postoperative ventilatory regulation in elderly patients. Acta Anaesthesiol Scand 36:436, 1992.

58. Yang, J. C., Clark, W. C., Ngai, S. H.: Antagonism of nitrous oxide analgesia by naloxone in man. Anesthesiology 52:414, 1980.

59. Smith, R. A., Wilson, M., Miller, K. W.: Naloxone has no effect on nitrous oxide anesthesia. Anesthesiology 49:6, 1978.

60. Ngai, S. H., Finck, D. A.: Prolonged exposure to nitrous oxide decreases opiate receptor density in rat brain stem. Anesthesiology 57:26, 1982.

61. Drummond, G. B., Brkown, D. T.: Naloxone does not influence breathing during isoflurane anaesthesia. Br J Anaesth 59:444, 1987.

62. Beilin, B., et al.: Naloxone reversal of postoperative apnea in a premature infant. Anesthesiology 63:317, 1985.

63. Orlowsky, J. P.: Endorphins in infants' apnea. N Engl J Med 307:186, 1982.

64. Committee on Drugs: Naloxone dosage and route of administration for infants and children: addendum to emergency drug doses for infants and children. Pediatrics 86:484, 1990.

65. Hibbard, B. M., Rosen, M., Davies, D.: Placental transfer of naloxone. Br J Anaesth 58:45, 1986.

66. Brimacombe, J., Archdeacon, J., Newell, S., Martin, J.: Two cases of naloxone-induced pulmonary edema: the possible use of phentolamine in management. Anaesth Intensive Care 19:578, 1991.

67. Olsen, K. S.: Naloxone administration and laryngospasm followed by pulmonary edema. Intensive Care Med 16:340, 1990.

68. Azar, I., Turndorf, H.: Severe hypertension and multiple atrial premature contractions following naloxone administration. Anesth Analg 58:524, 1979.

69. Michaelis, L. L., Hickey, P. R., Clark, T. A., Dixon, W. M.: Ventricular irritability associated with the use of naloxone hydrochloride. Ann Thorac Surg 18:608, 1974.

70. Andree, R. A.: Sudden death following naloxone administration. Anesth Analg 59:782, 1980.

71. Prough, D. S., Roy, R., Bumgarner, J., Shannon, G.: Acute pulmonary edema in healthy teenagers following conservative doses of intravenous naloxone. Anesthesiology 50:485, 1984.

72. Varon, J., Duncan, S. R.: Naloxone reversal of hypotension due to captopril overdose. Ann Emerg Med 20:1125, 1991.

73. Lin, C. J., Chen, Y. T., Kuo, J. S., Lee, A. Y.: Antiarrhythmic action of naloxone: suppression of picrotoxin-induced cardiac arrhythmias in the rat. Jpn Heart J 33:365, 1992.

74. Gu, H., Barron, B. A., Gaugl, J. F., Caffrey, J. L.: (+) Naloxone potentiates the inotropic effect of epinephrine in the isolated dog heart. Circ Shock 40:206, 1993.

75. Levin, G., Gafni, M., Roz, N., Sarne, Y.: The involvement of sodium ions in the positive inotropic effect of naloxone. Gen Pharmacol 24:423, 1993.

76. Lechner, R. B.: Naloxone potentiates inotropic but not chronotropic effects of isoproterenol in vitro. Circ Shock 39:226, 1993.

77. Gonzalez, J. P., Brogden, R. N.: Naltrexone: a review of its pharmacodynamic and pharmacokinetic properties and therapeutic efficacy in the management of opioid dependence. Drugs 35:192, 1988.

78. Branen, L. S., Capone, T. J., Capone, D. M.: Naltrexone: lack of effect on hepatic enzymes. J Clin Pharmacol 28:64, 1988.

79. Wall, M. E., Brine, D. R., Perez-Reyes, M.: Metabolism and disposition of naltrexone in man after oral and intravenous administration. Drug Metab Dispos Biol Fate Chem 9:369, 1981.

80. Stile, I. L., et al.: The pharmacokinetics of naloxone in the premature newborn. Dev Pharmacol Ther 10:454, 1987.

81. Michel, M. E., Bolger, G., Weisman, B. A.: Binding of a new opiate antagonist nalmefene to rat brain membranes. Pharmacologist 26:201, 1988.

82. Konieczko, K. M., et al.: Antagonism of morphine-induced respiratory depression with nalmefene. Br J Anaesth 61:318, 1988.

83. Gal, T. J., DiFazio, C. A.: Prolonged antagonism of opioid action with intravenous nalmefene in man. Anesthesiology 64:175, 1986.

84. Dixon, R., et al.: Nalmefene: intravenous safety and kinetics of a new opioid antagonist. Clin Pharmacol Ther 39:49, 1986.

85. Aitkenhead, A. R., et al.: Pharmacokinetics of intravenous naloxone in healthy volunteers. Anesthesiology 61:A381, 1984.

86. Glass, P. S. A., Jhavery, R. M., Smith, L. R.: Comparison of potency and duration of action of nalmefene and naloxone. Anesth Analg 78:536, 1994.

87. Kaplan, J. L., Mark, J. A.: Effectiveness and safety of intravenous nalmefene for emergency department patients with suspected narcotic overdosage. Ann Emerg Med 22:87, 1993.

Chapter 33

TRANQUILIZERS AND HALLUCINOGENS IN ANESTHESIA

VERNA L. BAUGHMAN

DEFINITION[1,2]

Agents capable of producing a state of calmness by primary subcortical action have been designated as "tranquilizers." This state of detached serenity without clouding of consciousness has prompted the use of another term to describe these drugs, namely "ataraxics." This is a Greek derivative that means "freedom from confusion" or "peace of mind." Although one may occasionally see reference to this term, the use of the term "tranquilizer" has become entrenched in both the medical and lay vocabulary.

Many agents meeting this definition have been used in medicine, especially psychiatry. Their use in anesthesiology is primarily of historical interest. This chapter reviews the use of tranquilizers in anesthesia and the use of two hallucinogens. The discussion focuses on several drug groups: phenothiazines (promethazine, chlorpromazine), rauwolfia compounds (reserpine), chloral hydrate, hydroxyzine, butyrophenones (droperidol), and the hallucinogens (lysergic acid diethylamide [LSD] and marijuana). The purpose is to describe these drugs briefly and to recount the historical role these agents played in the development of anesthesiology.

PHENOTHIAZINES

During the search for synthetic substitutes for quinidine, several drugs with a phenothiazine nucleus were investigated. The phenothiazines provided the anesthesiologist with a new approach to providing calm without clouding consciousness because this group of drugs acts primarily on the subcortical arousal areas rather than on the cortex. Specifically, these agents depress the alerting pattern of the ascending reticular activating system. In addition, they have inhibiting effects on the hypothalamus, and last, they possess sympatholytic and anticholinergic properties (Table 33–1).

The antipsychotic effects are apparently related to the ability of phenothiazines to block dopamine receptors in the central nervous system (CNS).[3]

Chemistry (Table 33–2)

The phenothiazine nucleus is a three-ring structure; the center ring contains sulfur and nitrogen. Substitutions on the nitrogen and radicals attached to the 2 position produce clinically useful drugs. Potency of action (tranquilization) is achieved in two ways. The first is by insertion of a halogen in the 2 position. Thus, chloride in this position produces chlorpromazine (Thorazine), which is four times as effective as promethazine (Phenergan). The second way of attaining potency is by substituting a piperazine ring for the simple amino group of the side chain at 10. Thus, prochlorperazine (Compazine) is about five times more potent than chlorpromazine.

The prototype drug of this group is phenothiazine. It has been used in animals as a urinary tract antiseptic and as an anthelmintic. Because of significant side effects (anemia, hepatitis, skin reactions), it has never been used in humans. It is still used in veterinary medicine and as an insecticide.

This discussion focuses on two phenothiazines commonly associated with anesthesia: promethazine and chlorpromazine.

Promethazine (Phenergan)

Promethazine is a synthetic phenothiazine. It was initially introduced by Halpern and Ducrot in 1946 in France.[4] Chemically, it is N-(2-dimethylamino-2-methyl) ethyl phenothiazine hydrochloride. As with the other phenothiazine derivatives, the primary site of action is on the ascending reticular formation and the hypothalamus. This drug possesses strong antihistaminic, antianaphylactic, and anticholinergic properties,[4,5] which distin-

Table 33–1. Pharmacodynamic Actions of Phenothiazines

Depression of reticular activating system and hypothalamus: potentiation of other CNS depressants
Depression of medullary chemoreceptor trigger zone for vomiting
Moderate adrenergic blocking action: variable peripheral anticholinergic effects
Central blockade of norepinephrine
Major side reactions including Parkinson syndrome, excitement, dystonias (spastic torticollis), convulsions, hypotension, agranulocytosis, jaundice, and skin rashes

Adapted from Hollister, L. E.: Drugs in emotional disorders. Scientific exhibit, American Medical Association Convention, June 13, 1962.

Table 33–2. Chemical Structure and Pharmacodynamic Properties of Selected Phenothiazines

Drug Name	Formula	Antipsychotic Dose Range		Single Intramuscular Dose* (mg)	Extrapyramidal Effects†	Antiemetic Effects	Sedative Effects†	Hypotensive Effects†
		Usual (mg)	Extreme (mg)					
Aliphatic Group								
Chlorpromazine	$R_1 = $ —CH$_2$—CH$_2$—CH$_2$—N(CH$_3$)$_2$ $R_2 = $ —Cl	300–800	30–2000	25–100	Moderate	Moderate	High	Moderate
Promazine	$R_1 = $ —CH$_2$—CH$_2$—CH$_2$—N(CH$_3$)$_2$ $R_2 = $ —H	500–1000	50–1600	50–200	Moderate	Moderate	Moderate	High
Triflupromazine	$R_1 = $ —CH$_2$—CH$_2$—CH$_2$—N(CH$_3$)$_2$ $R_2 = $ —CF$_3$	100–300	50–400	20–50	High	High	High	Low
Perperazine Group								
Fluphenazine (Prolixin)	$R_1 = $ —CH$_2$—CH$_2$—CH$_2$—N◯N—CH$_2$—CH$_2$OH $R_2 = $ —CF$_3$	2–10	1–20	1.25–2.5	High	High	Moderate	Low
Perphenazine (Trilafon)	$R_1 = $ —CH$_2$—CH$_2$—CH$_2$—N◯N—CH$_2$—CH$_2$OH $R_2 = $ —Cl	16–32	6–64	5–10	High	High	Low	Low
Prochlorperazine (Compazine)	$R_1 = $ —CH$_2$—CH$_2$—CH$_2$—N◯N—CH$_3$ $R_2 = $ —Cl	75–100	15–150	5–10	High	High	Moderate	Low
Trifluoperazine (Stelazine)	$R_1 = $ —CH$_2$—CH$_2$—CH$_2$—N◯N—CH$_3$ $R_2 = $ —CF$_3$	3–15	2–64	1–2	High	High	Moderate	Low
Pipiderine Group								
Thioridazine (Mellaril)	$R_1 = $ —CH$_2$—CH$_2$—◯ N—CH$_3$ $R_2 = $ —SCH$_3$	100–500	30–800	—	Low	Low	Moderate	Moderate

*The lowest effective dose should be used.
†Incidence expected in usual antipsychotic doses.
Modified from Gilman, A. G., et al.: Goodman and Gilman's The Pharmacological Basis of Therapeutics, 8th Ed. New York, McGraw-Hill, 1990.

guish it from the other phenothiazines. Used alone, the phenothiazine derivatives must be administered in relatively large doses to exert any sedative effect; however, when combined with a narcotic or a barbiturate, the desired quieting effects can be achieved using smaller doses of both. Therefore, a common and effective preanesthetic regimen was the intramuscular administration of promethazine (50 mg), meperidine (50 mg), and scopolamine (0.4 mg) 2 hours before surgery. Potentiation of barbiturates was demonstrated by Winter.[6] He determined that the sedative effects of various short-acting barbiturates were prolonged by 40% when given in combination with promethazine. Laborit and Leger[7] described both its use as a sedative and its ability to reduce the amount of anesthesia drugs needed.

Physiologic Effects

Promethazine causes a slight increase in heart rate and fall in systolic pressure; however, these changes are rarely clinically significant. This is in contrast to the cardiovascular effects produced by chlorpromazine. Most patients have a calm recovery from anesthesia if promethazine is part of preoperative medication. If, however, during recovery a patient becomes excited or delirious, promethazine alone will not exert an adequate calming influence. In general, by depressing the alerting mechanism (although it does not posses any true analgesic activity), the drug makes pain more endurable and allows analgesics to be more effective by reducing the extent to which afferent stimuli are perceived. Promethazine's antiemetic property has been demonstrated by many workers.[8] The agent can be administered either prophylactically or therapeutically (20 mg).

Chlorpromazine (Thorazine)

This compound was synthesized in 1950 by Carpentier in France during the search for phenothiazine derivatives similar to promethazine but with a more marked central action.[9]

Metabolism

Chlorpromazine is metabolized in the liver, with less than 1% excreted intact in the urine. Over 30 metabolites have been identified with little or no pharmacologic activity. The principal product is the sulfoxide metabolite. When given orally, less than 24% is absorbed. The level of free plasma chlorpromazine correlates with physiologic effects.

Physiologic Effects

Depression of the reticular activating system results in a cortex that is more susceptible to the action of cortical sedative drugs. Thus, hypnotic and analgesic drugs, and even hypnosuggestion, are more effective in smaller doses in producing a calm patient.[10] Chlorpromazine exerts a quieting effect on excited and anxious subjects. Its action on the hypothalamus results in general autonomic nervous system blockade. Temperature regulation is modified: heat production is diminished while heat loss is enhanced. Thus, body temperature is lowered, and the body tends to take on the environmental temperature.

The hypothalamic depression is also responsible for the improved reaction to stress. Much clinical and experimental evidence indicates that the chlorpromazine-treated patient is better able to respond to "external aggression." Thus, trauma and blood loss are better tolerated.

Medullary center depression is absent. Thus, no significant respiratory changes occur; the cardiac and vasomotor centers are little influenced. The activity of the vagal centers is modified, however. Chlorpromazine prevents drug-induced emesis by directly affecting the medullary chemoreceptor trigger zone (by blocking dopamine receptors). Thus, apomorphine is ineffective.[8]

Cardiovascular System

Clinical studies have indicated that chloropromazine-induced hypotension is not clinically significant.[11] When patients with normal blood pressure were divided into two groups, one treated with standard premedication and the second treated with chlorpromazine, little difference could be noted in the extent of the blood pressure fall. When hypotension follows the administration of chlorpromazine in an otherwise normotensive subject, it is usually due to hypovolemia. Chlorpromazine can produce a small increase in heart rate, probably compensatory to low blood pressure produced by ganglionic blockade and peripheral α-adrenergic blockade. On isolated dog papillary muscle, chlorpromazine depresses the force of contraction in a dose-dependent manner with a decrease in cardiac output. Chlorpromazine also reduces myocardial irritability and protects the heart against epinephrine-induced arrhythmias as well as against rapid administration of calcium chloride.[12] These antiarrhythmic effects are due either to a local anesthetic effect or a quinidine-like action on the myocardium.

Administration of peripherally acting vasopressors, such as phenylephrine or desoxyephedrine, does not produce the elevation of blood pressure one usually expects. In animal experiments, chlorpromazine abolishes or diminishes the pressor effect of epinephrine and norepinephrine. Whether epinephrine reversal also occurs clinically is controversial.[13] Chlorpromazine-treated patients (10 to 15 mg) were given infusions of epinephrine in doses of 0.15 to 0.30 μg/kg of body weight. The only effect was an attenuation of the pressor response. Therefore, it was recommended that peripheral-acting vasopressors be used in larger doses to treat hypotension.

Hypothermic Effects

Chlorpromazine was used by Laborit to provide "artificial hibernation" in combination with surface cooling and to protect patients from the stresses of surgery, trauma and hemorrhage.[7] The term "artificial hibernation" refers to the state of hypothermia achieved by pharmacologic means. The procedure involved blockade of the autonomic nervous system by a combination of promethazine (for its antihistamine effect), chlorpromazine (for ganglionic blockade), and meperidine (to provide some analgesic and cortical sedation). The combination of these drugs has been referred to as the "lytic cocktail." Many anesthesiologists have used chlorpromazine as part of a cooling protocol. Experience indicates that chlorpromazine possesses great utility in facilitating reduction of total body temperature.

Clinical Uses

Chlorpromazine has been used in preanesthetic medication combined with a barbiturate or with a narcotic.[14] The dosage in adults ranges from 12.5 to 50 mg, administered intramuscularly 1 to 2 hours before operation. For children, the dose is 0.25 mg/lb.

The actions of barbiturates, narcotics, and even alcohol are greatly enhanced. Anesthetic agents must be administered in smaller doses to achieve adequate surgical depth. Doses of thiopental sodium are reduced by half to two thirds the usual amount. Postoperatively, the use of chlorpromazine reduces the dose of analgesic drugs. This has the advantage of avoiding respiratory depression and a clouded mental state.

Chlorpromazine is capable of enhancing the effects of succinylcholine by cholinesterase inhibition. A smaller dose of succinylcholine is able to produce adequate relaxation when chlorpromazine is part of the premedication. A consequence of this may be a prolonged recovery period from succinylcholine apnea.[15]

When chlorpromazine is used postoperatively, hiccups[16] and emergence delirium are reduced in number and severity. The antiemetic action is outstanding. Postanesthetic vomiting is reduced in incidence and severity. The effect is believed to be exerted chiefly on the chemoreceptor trigger zone in the medulla.[8] Apparently, chlorpromazine selectively depresses this area and hence is pharmacologically unique.

RAUWOLFIA DRUGS (RESERPINE)

Although reserpine and rauwolfia compounds are not useful for preanesthetic medication, their therapeutic use in general medicine once posed a hazard in anesthesia. Because these drugs are no longer available for use, however, this section presents only a historical perspective.

Because these drugs have a long duration of action (up to 10 days), Coakley and colleagues recommended that they be withheld for 2 weeks before surgery.[17] It was believed that patients could experience significant hypotension and bradycardia during anesthesia if these drugs were not discontinued a significant time before anesthesia. This circulatory depression represented a parasympathetic response that could be enhanced by vagomimetic anesthetics, especially thiopental. Reserpine was used as an orphan drug to treat reflex sympathetic dystrophy, but the results are equivocal.

CHLORAL HYDRATE[18–21]

Chloral hydrate is a sedative and hypnotic. It was first made in 1832 by Liebig. It appears to react with alkali to cause a slow release of chloroform. It is used primarily as a hypnotic to treat insomnia and as a preoperative sedative before surgery or diagnostic procedures (i.e., computed tomography, endoscopy). Sleep latency is decreased, as is the number of awakenings. Rapid eye movement (REM) sleep is rarely suppressed, and rebound is rarely seen after discontinuation. The drug is frequently used in children and elderly patients because it is believed to produce paradoxic excitement less frequently than barbiturates. Chloral hydrate is administered either orally or rectally (dose range of 500 to 1000 mg) approximately 30 to 60 minutes before surgery and lasts 4 to 8 hours. It is usually administered diluted with water or milk because gastric irritation occurs when the drug is taken on an empty stomach. If chloral hydrate is mixed with alcohol, a potent mixture frequently called a "Mickey Finn" or "knock out drops" is created. "Hangover" or malaise may occur, but it is much less severe than that seen with most barbiturates and some benzodiazepines. CNS effects such as lightheadedness, ataxia, and nightmares are occasionally noted. Disorientation and paranoid behavior are rarely seen. Allergic reactions include erythema and urticaria, but they are infrequent. These may be accompanied by eosinophilia and/or leukopenia.[21] A transient enhancement of hypothrombinemia during the administration of oral anticoagulants has been reported. Tolerance occurs within 2 weeks if administered daily. The lethal dose is approximately 10 g, although a dose of 4 g has caused death in some patients, whereas other patients have survived doses as large as 30 g. Treatment consists of respiratory and cardiac supportive measures.

HYDROXYZINE (VISTARIL)

Hydroxyzine is a piperazine derivative of the diphenylmethane tranquilizers. It has been used as an anxiolytic, a preoperative sedative, an antiemetic, and an antihistamine. Its mild anxiolytic and sedative actions are only slightly better than placebo.[22] An oral dose of 25 mg exerts its antianxiety effects for 6 to 12 hours. Forty five to 60% of the drug undergoes oxidative metabolism to a carboxylic acid metabolite (cetrizine), which possesses significant activity at the H_1 histamine receptor but is devoid of CNS effect.[23]

NEUROLEPTIC DRUGS

Neuroleptic drugs act on the subcortical centers of the brain stem and are characterized by the following effects: antiemesis, catalepsies, tremor, barbiturate and opiate potentiation, temperature lowering, and inhibition of sympathetic reflex.[24] Because of their dopaminergic blocking effect, butyrophenones counter the inhibitory effect of dopamine. Unfortunately, approximately 1% of patients have a dysphonic response to these drugs that limits their use as preanesthetic medications.

Haloperidol is a long-acting neurolept agent used primarily as an antipsychotic drug. Droperidol is frequently administered during anesthesia for its antiemetic effect (10 to 20 μg/kg). It also blocks α-adrenergic receptor binding sites, which produce vasodilation and attenuation of the cardiovascular response to sympathomimetic agents.

Neurolept Malignant Syndrome

One of the unusual complications is a hyperpyrexia syndrome entitled the neurolept malignant syndrome (NMS).[25,26] This syndrome was first described in 1968 by DeLay and Deniker. The incidence is estimated to be between 0.5 and 1.0% of all patients exposed to neurolepts. The syndrome affects young men predominantly, but it may be seen at any age and in both sexes. The syndrome develops over 24 to 72 hours or may even occur several days after discontinuing neuroleptic therapy. Characteristics of NMS are hyperthermia, hypertonicity of skeletal muscles, variable level of consciousness, and instability of the autonomic nervous system. The common autonomic dysfunctions include pallor, diaphoresis, fluctuating blood pressure, tachycardia, and cardiac dysrhythmias. The muscular hypertonia is of a "lead pipe" increase in tone. Rigidity and akinesia develop at about the time the temperature evaluation is noted. Laboratory abnormalities include leukocytosis and electrolyte alterations suggesting dehydration. Liver function abnormalities consist of elevated transaminases, lactic dehydrogenase, and alkaline phosphatase. Creatinine kinase is often elevated and may exceed 16,000 IU/L.

A drug's potential for inducing NMS appears to parallel its antidopaminergic potency. Discontinuation of antiparkinsonian agents and the use of dopamine-depleting agents can produce NMS. The predisposing factors include exhaustion, dehydration, and, especially, the use of long-acting depo-neurolepts. Of importance to the anesthesiologist is the differential diagnosis of NMS, which includes the heat stroke associated with phenothiazines (which inhibit sweating), central anticholinergic syndrome, and malignant hyperthermia.

HALLUCINOGENIC DRUGS

Several groups of consciousness-altering drugs were used by anesthesiologists in the past. One such group of drugs produces changes in perception often referred to as hallucinations.[27-29] If a subject can distinguish visions from reality, these drugs are said to produce "illusions." Because of similarities between drug-induced behavior and natural psychosis, these drugs are also called "psychomimetics." Ingestion of these drugs produces many different subjective and objective effects. Subjective effects are reversible and may be classed as somatic, perceptive, and psychic.

Three members of this class of drugs are important: (1) mescaline, derived from the peyote cactus (*Lophophora williamsii*); (2) psilocybin and psilocin,[30] from certain mushrooms (*Psilocybe mexicana* and *Stropharia cubensis*); and (3) d-lysergic acid diethylamine (LSD), derived from the ergot fungus (*Claviceps purpurea*).[31]

Lysergic Acid Diethylamide (Fig. 33–1)

The following discussion focuses on LSD, because it is the only one that was tested clinically as an analgesic and a preanesthetic medication.[30] Chemically, LSD is a semisynthetic derivative obtained by the condensation of d-lysergic acid (an alkaloid extract of the ergot fungus that grows on rye and wheat) with diethylamine.[31] LSD is thought to exert its effect through release of norepinephrine and activation of the sympathetic nervous system. On the other hand, it causes depression of the phosphorylase enzyme system, and it increases binding of serotonin and histamine. Some investigators believe that LSD facili-

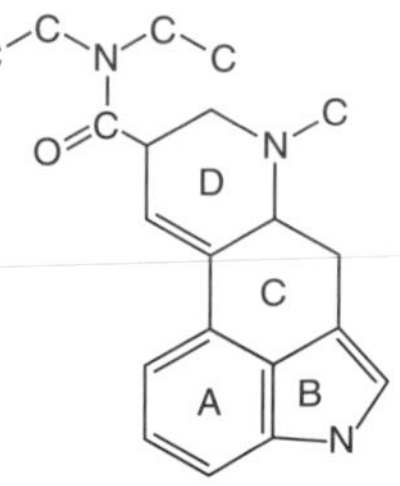

Fig. 33–1. Chemical structure of the lysergic acid diethylamide molecule. Note the four ring structures. One is a five-membered ring with nitrogen and one is a six-membered ring with nitrogen. From Baker, R. W., Chothia, C., Pauling, P.: Molecular structure of LSD. Science *178*:614, 1972.

tates the access of drugs into brain structure otherwise inaccessible.

Physiologic Actions

LSD stimulates the respiratory center, producing tachypnea and hyperventilation, and can partially reverse the respiratory depressant effects of thiopental.[28] Although LSD may block the peripheral vasoconstricting effects of serotonin, norepinephrine, and ephedrine, it acts as a sympathomimetic agent on the cardiovascular system. It accelerates the heart rate and appears to increase cardiac output. It causes localized flushing of the skin and produces fine tremors, elevation of the body temperature, leukocytosis, and perspiration. It expands consciousness, alters the affective behavior of animals and humans, and produces visual distortions. It produces illusions of time and space.

Clinical Uses[32,33]

LSD reduces goal-directed and purposeful activity. Under its influence, a regression to infantile sexuality may occur. Because of its ability to lessen anticipation and anxiety, LSD showed promise as a preanesthetic agent. No adverse affect on circulation, respiration, or anesthetic requirements was noticed with the preanesthetic dosage of 10 µg. The patients showed little apprehension, were preoccupied with miscellaneous sensory input, and had an uneventful postoperative recovery, obviating analgesics postoperatively for approximately 36 hours.

For postoperative analgesia, LSD doses of 20 to 50 µg were used. In a series of 80 preterminal patients, it was demonstrated that LSD was not only a potent analgesic agent, but it also altered the patient's attitude and approach to a desperate situation. In general, panic was converted to serene contemplation for 12 hours to 2 weeks following a single dose of 100 µg.

LSD has been used in psychotherapy; however, the consensus of the literature shows it to have disappointing results, and it has been abandoned as a psychotherapeutic agent. Abnormalities in chromosome structure of leukocytes have been reported, and injections of LSD into mice in early pregnancy cause grossly abnormal embryos in about 60% of offspring.[34]

Marihuana (Tetrahydrocannabinol)

Cannabis is the generic term for the more than 300 compounds obtained from the hemp plant.[29,35,36] Common hemp is a herbaceous annual of a single species (*Cannabis sativa*) with several varieties, including *C. indica* and *C. americana*. Many extracts have been prepared and given special names in different parts of the world. The resinous exudate of the female plant contains most of the potent active ingredients; in the Middle East, this exudate is called "hashish," and in the Far East, it is called "charas." A smaller amount of the active drug is found in the young flowering shoots of the female plant and dried leaves, and this preparation is called "bhang." An exudate from small leaves is called "ganja." In the United States, the term marijuana refers to any part of the plant or extract that induces psychophysiologic changes in man.

Chemistry[37]

The compounds from the hemp plants are known as cannabinoids. Over 400 compounds have been identified from cannabis. Most of the characteristic effects are due to an isomer of tetrahydrocannabinol (THC). Δ-9-THC is the most active compound.

Three other compounds are usually present in the extracts of cannabis. These are nonpsychoactive: cannabinol, cannabidol, and cannabigerol. These appear to be especially toxic and inhibit testosterone production by a direct effect on the Leydig cells and by blockade of the pituitary gonadotropin hormone.

Pharmacodynamics[35]

Following oral ingestion, LSD-like effects occur in 30 to 60 minutes and last 3 to 5 hours. When smoked, marijuana produces its effects in 2 to 3 minutes, and they last only a short time. The average "joint" contains about 10 mg of THC. A cigarette containing 5 mg results in a maximal plasma concentration of 100 ng/ml after 5 minutes. In contrast, ingestion of 20 mg of THC results in effects noted in about 20 to 30 minutes and in a plasma concentration of only 10 ng/ml. Bioavailability from smoking is thus 5 to 10 times greater than after ingestion. As the hydroxymetabolite appears, a secondary, delayed, or additional high is experienced.[35]

Pharmacokinetics[38]

The psychoactive compound THC (Δ-9-THC) is fat soluble (unlike alcohol), and its kinetics are concentration dependent and first order (not dose dependent). After absorption, rapid disappearance from plasma into body tissue compartments occurs.

A single dose of THC has a half-life ($T_{1/2}$) in tissues of 7 days and requires 30 days for complete elimination. After smoking, there is rapid absorption and an initial rise in plasma concentrations to peak levels within 15 minutes. After ingestion, THC is slowly absorbed from the gut and reaches a peak in 1 hour. The α phase accompanies the increasing plasma concentration, and after peak serum concentrations, one sees a rapid disappearance of THC from serum and distribution to tissues and rapid tissue uptake. Within 1 hour, plasma levels fall to one tenth the peak concentration. The $T_{1/2}$-α phase is 30 minutes.[39] Thereafter, one notes a gradual decline in plasma concentration in the β phase, and the $T_{1/2}$-β is about 18 hours. The serum level is further reduced by 50% every 18 hours, referred to as the terminal half-life.

Metabolism[40]

The major metabolic route is hydroxylation to form 11-hydroxy-Δ-9-THC (11-OH-THC), followed by hepatic oxidation to form a carboxylic acid derivative, 9-carboxy-THC. After ingestion, the peak concentration of the 11-OH-THC metabolite occurs in 1 hour and may exceed the plasma peak of the parent drug. The hydroxy metabolite is not easily detected in the plasma after inhaling; however, it is detectable in urine within 1 hour. In the infrequent smoker, the major active components, THC, 11-OH-THC, and 9-carboxy-THC, are detectable in the urine within 1 hour and for as long as 5 days after smoking.[41] In heavy or chronic smokers in whom storage in adipose tissue (THC is strongly lipophilic) occurs, these compounds are detectable in urine for as long as 4 weeks.[42]

Excretion[39]

At the end of 5 days, 50% of the intact drug will have been excreted in the feces, whereas about 15% will have been metabolized and the products excreted in the urine. A glucuronide conjugate is detectable in the urine, but THC itself is not excreted by the kidney. Two thirds of cannabinoid metabolites are excreted via the feces, and the remaining acid metabolites are excreted by the urine.[39] Acid metabolites are detectable in urine by 1 hour after smoking.

The urinary metabolites are principally the acid forms and 9-carboxy-THC. Some 20 other structurally similar acids are recognized. Of the total dose, only about 20% is excreted in the urine as metabolites, whereas most of the intact THC and the rest of the metabolites are excreted in feces.

Pharmacologic Effects

Cardiovascular System[43]

A marked increase in heart rate is seen at the high dose level, but little change occurs at the low doses. A concomitant increase in systolic pressure may be noted even though vasodilatation occurs. Cannabis is believed to be a β-adrenergic agent, and the effects on the heart are prevented by β-adrenergic blockade. After oral administration of 0.6 mg/kg daily for 3 days, changes in the electrocardiograph are noted: ST-segment elevation and decreased amplitude of T waves occur.

Respiratory System[44,45]

Airway resistance falls rapidly after either high or low doses of THC. Specific airway conductance increases 40 to 60%, reaches peak levels in 15 minutes, and lasts for 60 minutes. Because thoracic gas volume (FRC) remains unchanged, these changes are due to relaxation of smooth muscle of tracheobronchial tree. Such a bronchodilator effect is also observed in flow-volume curves. The mean expiratory flow rate at one quarter vital capacity increases 45% or more. In the carbon dioxide response test, the airway changes are largely of greater magnitude and last longer than after therapeutic doses of isoproterenol. Asthma attacks have been effectively treated by THC ingestion. Aerosols of THC have not been satisfactory, however, because the drug is insoluble in water. Long-term smoking (> 30 days) produces alveolar destruction and inflammatory responses that are more pronounced than those seen with tobacco smoking.

Psychic and Mood Effect[38,44]

Most subjective effects depend on the personality of the individual and the circumstances of the drug taking. Altered consciousness includes a dreamy state and/or disconnected ideas. Perception of time, place, and space is distorted, and illusions are created. Mood elevation generally occurs. Large doses produce vivid hallucinations; this may be followed by fear and panic. Basic personality structure is not changed, and it is believed that many of the psychic effects can be suppressed by the user.[46]

Of therapeutic significance is the sedative hypnotic effect. In humans, a "sleepy-high" is produced by Δ-9-THC after oral administration. The electroencephalogram is altered by an increase in stage IV sleep and a decrement in REM sleep. A significant increase in barbiturate sleeping time is induced by THC.[47] Of anesthetic significance is the effect on minimum alveolar concentration (MAC) values:[48,49] one sees a dose-related lowering of MAC 1 hour after intake. Intravenous doses of 0.5 mg/kg of THC decrease halothane MAC by 32%. After larger doses, MAC may remain reduced for 24 hours.

The electroencephalogram in animals may show permanent brain wave changes in the limbic system. Irritative tracings with high-amplitude waves and spikes are found. This forms the basis for the street rule that epileptics should avoid smoking marijuana. A nonpsychoactive cannabinoid—cannabidiol—appears to be an anticonvulsant.

Glaucoma[50,51]

THC eyedrops or oral THC can reduce intraocular tension in normal subjects and can lower ocular hypertension in patients with open-angle glaucoma.

Antiemetic Effect[52,53]

THC is effective in relieving severe nausea and vomiting associated with chemotherapeutic agents. A comparative study showed THC to be superior to phenothiazines (prochlorperazine). The oral antiemetic THC dose is 10 mg/m^2, which produces a blood level of 10 ng/ml. At this level, fewer than 6% of patients continue to experience nausea.

Tolerance[45]

Continued administration for 4 to 6 days results in tolerance. On discontinuance, no early withdrawal symptoms are noted, but after 2 days insomnia and poor appetite are observed. Because the abstinence syndrome seen following morphine withdrawal can be blocked by Δ-THC, THC may be of value in facilitating narcotic detoxification.[54]

Miscellaneous Effects[55]

Blood sugar is slightly elevated, and urinary frequency occurs. Dryness of mouth and throat occur. Nausea and vomiting have been noted, whereas appetite is markedly increased. Conjunctivae are usually inflamed due to dilatation of blood vessels and remain so for 2 to 3 hours. Long-term intensive marijuana use in males alters reproductive physiology by a central hypothalamic (pituitary) mecha-

Table 33–3. Signs and Symptoms of Drug Use

Behavioral signs
  Chronic lying about whereabouts
  Sudden disappearance of money or valuables from home
  Marked dysphoric mood changes that occur without good reason and that cause pain to the family and patient
  Abusive behavior toward self or others
  Frequent outbursts of poorly controlled hostility with lack of insight or remorse for this behavior

Social Signs
  Driving while impaired, auto accidents
  Frequent truancy
  Underachievement over past 6–12 months with definite deterioration of academic performance

Circumstantial evidence
  Drugs or drug paraphernalia in room, clothes, or automobile
  Drug terminology in school notebooks or in school yearbook.
  Definitive change in peer group preference to those peers who lack purpose, are unmotivated, and may be known to use marihuana.

Physical symptoms
  Chronic fatigue and lethargy
  Chronic dry irritating cough, chronic sore throat
  Chronic conjunctivitis (red eyes), otherwise unexplained.

From Schwartz, R. H., Hawks, R. L.,: Laboratory detection of marihuana use. JAMA 254:788, 1985.

nism. Testosterone synthesis is significantly reduced in a dose-related manner. Oligospermia occurs frequently (35%) as a result of inhibition of spermatogenesis, and impotence is occasionally seen. Involution of the prostate and seminal vesicles occurs. In females, heavy marijuana use decreases levels of follicle-stimulating and luteinizing hormones and disrupts the menstrual cycle. Marijuana disrupts placental circulation and function, induces abortion, and produces abnormal behavior in offspring.

Effects on cell metabolism are twofold.[56] First, cell division is impaired. Formation of nucleic acids and proteins is disordered. The cannabinoids dissolve in cell membranes and prevent transport of substrates. DNA and RNA synthesis is impaired. Second, interference with nuclear membrane exchange occurs. Synthesis of chromosomal proteins is reduced.

Signs and Symptoms of Abuse

Behavioral signs and social signs of abuse have been summarized by Schwartz and Hawks.[57] Additional circumstantial evidence and physical symptoms are included in Table 33–3.

Laboratory Detection (Schwartz Principle)

Analytic methods have been described for detection of cannabinoids in body fluids:

1. Mass spectrometry combined with chromatography (accurate, specific, but slow and costly) for blood and urine (carboxy compounds), then layer chromatography for urine.
2. Radioimmunoassay: This is a primary method for blood and urine analysis of cannabinoids.
3. Enzyme immunoassay of drug in urine, for analysis of cannabinoid metabolites. This is the homogenous enzyme immunoassay.
4. Urine testing can reveal the use of marijuana.[40]

REFERENCES

1. Symposium: The pharmacology of psychomimetic and psychotherapeutic drugs. Ann NY Acad Sci 66:471, 1957.
2. National Institutes of Mental Health Bulletin: Psychopharmacologic Agents. Bethesda, MD, Pharmacological Service Center Clearing House for Mental Health Information, 1960.
3. Snyder, S. H., Greenberg D.: Drugs, neurotransmitters and schizophrenia. Science 184:1243, 1974.
4. Halpern, B., Ducrot, R.: Recherches experimentales sur une nouvelle serie chiminique de corps boues de proprietés antihistaminiques puissantes: les dérivés de la thiodiphenylamine. C R Soc Biol 140:361, 1946.
5. Danielopolu, D.: Efficacy of so-called antihistaminic drugs in paraphylastic (anaphylactic) shock does not prove its histaminic origin. Acta Med Scand 130:183, 1948.
6. Winter, C. A.: Potentiating effect of antihistaminic drugs upon sedative action of barbiturates. J Pharmacol Exp Ther 94:7, 1948.
7. Laborit, H., Leger, L.: Utilisation d'un antihistaminique de synthèse en Therapeutique pré, per et post-operatoire. Presse Med 58:492, 1950.
8. Wang, S. C., Chum, H. I: Experimental motion sickness in dogs: functional importance of chemoreceptive-emetic trigger zone. Am J Physiol 178:111, 1954.
9. Courvaisier, S., Fournel, J., Ducrot, R., Kolsky, J.: Dynamiques de chlorhydrate de chloro-3-(dimethylamino-3-propyl)-10-phenothiazine. Arch Intern Pharmacodyn 92:305, 1953.
10. Sadove, M., et al.: Chlorpromazine and narcotics in the management of pain of malignant lesions. JAMA 155:626, 1954.
11. Moyer, J. H., Kent, B., Knight, R., Morris, G.: Hemodynamic and toxicological studies of chlorpromazine. Am J Med Sci 227:283, 1954.
12. Nieschulz, O., Papendiker, K., Hoffman, B.: Pharmacological investigations of 1-methyl piperdye (3)-methyl phenothiazine. Arzneimittelforsch 5:680, 1955.
13. Lear, E., Chiron, A., Pallur, I.: A clinical study of mechanisms of action of chlorpromazine. JAMA 163:30, 1957.
14. Albert, S. N., Spencer, W. A., Finkelstein, M., Coakley, C. S.: The place of chlorpromazine in anesthesia. Curr Res Anesth Analg 35:101, 1956.
15. Kotkin, S.: Preliminary studies on muscle relaxing properties of chlorpromazine. Anesthesiology 17:494, 1958.
16. Friedgood, C. E., Ripstein, C. B.: Chlorpromazine in the treatment of intractable hiccups. JAMA 167:309, 1955.
17. Coakley, C. S., Albert, S., Bohug, J. S.: Anesthesia During rauwolfia therapy. JAMA 161:1143, 1956.
18. Rall, T. W.: Hypnotics and sedatives. In Gilman, A.G. (ed.). Goodman and Gilman's The Pharmacological Basis of Therapeutics, 8th Ed. New York, McGraw-Hill, 1990, p. 364.
19. Kay, D. C., Blackburn, A. B., Buckingham, J. A., Karacan, I.: Human pharmacology of sleep. In Williams, R. I., Karacan, I. (eds.). Pharmacology of Sleep. New York, John Wiley & Sons, 1976, p. 83.
20. Hartman, E.: Long term administration of psychotropic drugs: effects on human sleep. In Williams, R. I., Karacan, I. (eds.). Pharmacology of Sleep. New York, John Wiley & Sons, 1976, p. 211.
21. Christianson, H. B., Perry, H. O.: Reactions to chloral hydrate. Arch Dermatol 74:232, 1956.
22. Mehta, P., et al.: Comparative evaluation of preanesthetic medications. Curr Ther Res 35:715, 1984.
23. Gengo, F. M., et al.: The relative antihistaminic and psychomotor effects of hydroxyzine and cetirizine. Clin Pharmacol Ther 42:265, 1987.
24. Saarne, A.: Experience with haloperidol as a premedicant. Acta Anesth Scand 7:21, 1963.
25. Guze, B. H., Baxter, L. R., Jr.: Neurolept malignant syndrome. N Engl J Med 313:163, 1985.
26. Delay, J., Deniker, P.: Drug-induced extrapyramidal syndromes. In Vinken, P. J., Bruyn, G. W. (eds.). Handbook of Clinical Neurology. Vol. 6. Diseases of the Basal Ganglia. Amsterdam, North-Holland, 1968, p. 248.
27. Silva Sankar, D. V., Broer, H. H., Cates, N.: Effect of administration of lysergic acid diehylamine on serotonin levels in the body. Nature 200:582, 1963.
28. Dobkin, A. B., Harland, J. H.: Drugs which stimulate affective behavior. Anaesthesia 15:48:1960.
29. Barron, F., Jarvik, M.E., Bunnell, S., Jr.: The hallucinogen drugs. Sci Am 210:29, 1964.
30. Wasson, R. G.: The hallucinogen mushroom of Mexico. Trans NY Acad Sci 27:325, 1959.
31. Baker, R. W., Chothia, C., Pauling, P.: Molecular structure of LSD. Science 178:614, 1972.
32. Jacobsen, E.: The clinical pharmacology of the hallucinogens. Clin Pharmacol Ther 4:480, 1963.
33. Kast, E. C., Collins, V. J.: A study of lysergic acid diethylamide as an analgesic agent. Anesth Analg 43:285, 1964.
34. Merbach, R., Rugowski, J. A.: Lysergic acid diethylamide and effect on embryos. Science 157:1325, 1967.

35. Hollister, L. E., Richards, R. K., Gillespie, H. K.: Comparison of tetra-hydro cannibinol and synhexyl in man. Clin Pharmacol Ther 9:783, 1968.

36. Pars, H. G.: The other side of marihuana research (editorial). Anesthesiology 38:519, 1973.

37. Mechoulam, R.: Marihuana chemistry. Science 158:1159, 1970.

38. Nahas, G. G.: Marihuana. JAMA 233:79, 1975.

39. Hunt, C. A., Jones, R. T.: Tolerance and disposition of THC in man. J Pharmacol Exp Ther 215:135, 1980.

40. Wall, M. E., Perez-Reyes, M.: The metabolism of delta-9-tetrahydrocannabinol and related compounds in man. J Clin Pharmacol 21:1785, 1980.

41. McBay, A. J., Dubowski, K. M., Finkle, B. S.: Urine testing for marijuana use. JAMA 249:881, 1983.

42. Dakis, C. A., et al.: Persistence of urinary marijuana levels after supervised abstinence. Am J Psychiatry 139:1196, 1982.

43. Kochar, M. S., Hosko, M. J.: Electrocardiographic effects of marijuana. JAMA 225:25, 1973.

44. Hollister, L. E.: Marijuana in man. Science 722:21, 1971.

45. Tashkin, D. P., Shapiro, B. J., Frank, I. M.: Acute pulmonary physiologic effects of smoked marihuana and oral delta-tetrahydrocannabinol in healthy young men. N Engl J Med 289:336, 1973.

46. Freeman, F.: Effect of marihuana on sleeping states. JAMA 220:1364, 1972.

47. Talbott, J. A., Teague, J. W.: Marihuana psychosis. JAMA 210:299, 1969.

48. Stoelting, R. K., et al.: Effects of delta-9-tetrahydrocannabinol on halothane MAC in dogs. Anesthesiology 38:521, 1973.

49. Vitez, T. S., Way, W. L., Miller, R. D., Eger, E. I., II: Effects of delta-9-tetrahydrocannabinol on cyclopropane MAC in the rat. Anesthesiology 38:525, 1973.

50. Cohen, S.: Marijuana: possible therapeutic use. JAMA 240:1761, 1978.

51. Helper, R. S., Petrus, R. J.: Experiences with the administration of marihuana to glaucoma patients. In Cohen, S., Stillman, R. C. (eds.). The Therapeutic Potential of Marihuana. New York, Plenum Medical Book, 1976, p. 63.

52. Sallan, S. E., Zinberg, N. E., Frei, E., III: Antiemetic effect of delta-9- THC. N Engl J Med 293:795, 1975.

53. Sallan, S. E., et al.: Antiemetics in patients receiving chemotherapy for cancer. N Engl J Med 302:135, 1980.

54. Hine, B.: Morphine-dependent rats: blockade of precipitated abstinence by tetrahydrocannabinol. Science 187:433, 1975.

55. Kolodny, R. C., Masters, W. H., Kolodner, R. M., Toro, G.: Depression of plasma testosterone after chronic marihuana. N Engl J Med 290:872, 1974.

56. Nahas, G. G.: Marihuana chemistry, biochemistry and cellular effects. JAMA 242:2775, 1979.

57. Schwartz, R. H., Hawks, R. L.: Laboratory detection of marijuana use. JAMA 254:788, 1985.

Chapter 34

NONOPIOID ANALGESICS: USE IN THE PERIOPERATIVE PERIOD

HAK Y. WONG

Many drugs possess analgesic activity independent of the opioid receptors. Examples are acetaminophen and nonsteroidal anti-inflammatory drugs (NSAIDs). Less familiar examples include α_2-adrenoceptor agonists and, possibly, metoclopromide.

Traditionally, the nonopioid analgesics (acetaminophen and NSAIDs) have been considered weak analgesics and unsuitable for the severe pain seen in the immediate postoperative period. Concern for opioid side effects such as sedation and respiratory depression and the addictive and abuse potential of opioids, however, have renewed interest in the use of nonopioids in the postoperative period. Recent understanding about pain mechanisms and signal processing also suggests that the nonopioids have an important role in the prevention and relief of postoperative pain.[1,2] One United States federally sponsored panel went as far as stating that NSAIDs should be the first and essential component of all postoperative analgesic therapy, barring contraindications.[3]

NSAIDs have a crucial role in the treatment of rheumatoid disease and have also found use in a variety of painful conditions. The literature on specific pharmacology and on conventional uses of the numerous agents grouped together under the class NSAID is extraordinarily extensive and well beyond the scope of this text. The goal of this chapter is to discuss the rationale and principles of using (selective) NSAIDs on a short-term basis during the perioperative period. The status of the α_2-adrenergic system and metoclopramide is also discussed.

ACUTE PAIN MECHANISMS

Pain after surgical trauma is a complex phenomenon, the culmination of complex interactions of sensory signals produced by the initial injury and incorporating sociologic, cultural, and psychologic influences. Postsurgical pain is therefore highly subjective and personal. Nevertheless, tissue injury that causes pain produces distinct, objective changes in the injured tissue and the nervous system.[4,5] Elucidation of the mechanisms underlying these changes is an ongoing effort. A brief overview of current understanding is important for understanding the role of various analgesic drugs, however.

Somatic Pain

Acute injury produces pain directly by action on the pain receptors (nociceptors) at the site of injury. This direct action produces immediate, intense, but short-lived pain. A series of changes then results in abnormal sensory functions commonly seen after tissue injury: increased response to noxious stimuli (hyperalgesia), reduced pain threshold (allodynia), increase in duration of response to brief stimulation (persistent pain), and a spread of pain and hyperalgesia to uninjured areas. These abnormalities are slower in onset but persist long beyond the duration of the trauma, and in real time they probably embody the postoperative pain felt by most patients who have been unconscious during the surgery. The processes that lead to these altered sensory functions occur both at the injury site and at the spinal cord level.[6]

Peripheral Changes

Sensitization of nociceptors, nerve endings, and pain fibers at the site of injury may be caused by chemical mediators such as potassium ion and adenosine triphosphate (ATP) release by tissue trauma and cell destruction. The peripheral terminals of C-fibers also release a variety of neuropeptides and amino acids such as substance P, serotonin, bradykinin, and histamine, all of which can trigger inflammatory response, can sensitize nociceptors, and cause hyperalgesia. The effects of these substances, especially those of bradykinin are enhanced by prostaglandins PGI_2 and PGE_2, the synthesis of which is stimulated by injury.

Spread of hyperalgesia to areas away from the site of injury is probably mediated by propagation of signals antidromally along peripheral branches of the sensory nerve and release of substance P, which induces vasodilation and further release of algogenic substance and inflammation mediators in the surrounding tissues.

Central Changes

Repetitive afferent activation of $A\delta$ and C fibers leads to altered characteristics in spinal cord dorsal horn neurons.[7] The changes include sensitization (increasing frequency of discharge in response to a stimulus), wind-up (prolonged discharge to a stimulus), expansion of the receptive field, and enhancement of spinal reflexes, especially the flexor reflex. The most probable underlying mechanism is release of excitatory neurotransmitters from the nerve terminals, such as substance P, glutamate, and aspartate, which interact with N-methyl-D-aspartate (NMDA) receptor complex and non-NMDA receptors of dorsal horn neurons.[8] Prostaglandins again play a facilitory role by augmenting the release of neurotransmitters from the nerve terminals.

Other receptor systems known to modulate the activation state of spinal dorsal horn neurons include α_2-adrenergic receptors[9] and opioid receptors. Activation of the sympathetic nervous system also may stimulate synthesis of prostaglandins.

Visceral Pain

The mechanisms underlying visceral pain may include peritoneal inflammation, visceral distention, and exaggerated smooth muscle motility.[10] Adrenergic sympathetic and cholinergic parasympathetic innervations are well-known mediators of smooth muscle motility. Dopaminergic and other peptidinergic systems also play a role.

The prostaglandins are also involved in the genesis of visceral pain. Gastrointestinal motility is increased by PGE. The prostaglandins promote fluid secretion into the gallbladder and contraction of the gallbladder musculature, a mechanism that may be involved in biliary colic and acalculous cholecystitis.[11] In the urinary tract, prostaglandins increase renal blood flow and smooth muscle tone of the pelviureteral system, inhibit the action of antidiuretic hormone, and also increase inflammation at the sites of obstruction, all of which may contribute to the genesis of ureteric colic. The effects of peritoneal irritation is ameliorated by administration of prostaglandin synthesis inhibitors.

The products of arachidonic acid metabolism therefore play significant and complex roles in the genesis and processing of signals that are associated with both somatic and visceral components of postoperative pain.

ARACHIDONIC ACID METABOLISM

A brief overview of the major metabolic pathways of arachidonic acid[12,13] is presented (Fig. 34-1). The precursor and enzymes for prostaglandin synthesis are ubiquitous in the body. Physiologic effects of prostaglandins depend on continual activities of cyclooxygenase pathway because prostaglandins are rapidly catabolized and are not stored in tissues. The cyclooxygenase pathway leads to unstable endoperoxides PGG_2 and PGH_2, and then onto thromboxane A_2 and thromboxane B_2, which are vasoconstrictive and mediate platelet adhesion and aggregation, and PGI_2 (prostacyclin), which mediates vasodilation and platelet deaggregation and blocks leukotriene release. The lipoxygenase pathway leads to formation of leukotrienes and hydroxyeicosatetraenoic acid (HETE), which have bronchoconstrictive, vasoconstrictive, and chemotactic activities. The NSAIDs exert their major effects by inhibiting cyclooxgyenase. The activity of the lipoxygenase pathway may be increased with potential pathophysiologic results.

NONSTEROIDAL ANTI-INFLAMMATORY DRUGS (NSAIDs)

Many compounds have been developed worldwide as NSAIDs, and new agents continue to be developed. Only a fraction of these have withstood the criteria of efficacy and safety, and even fewer are approved for use in the United States (Table 34-1). These agents are a chemically diverse group of drugs, and as the nomenclature indicates, they are primarily anti-inflammatory in action. The designation "nonsteroidal" distinguishes them from steroids, which are also anti-inflammatory and antirheumatic, but are devoid of analgesic effects. Although acetaminophen is not usually considered a NSAID because of its weak inhibitory effect on peripheral cyclooxygenase and negligible anti-inflammatory effect, the mechanism of its analgesic and antipyretic effects is thought to be inhibition of prostaglandin synthesis in the brain. It is therefore included in this section.

Rationale for Use in the Perioperative Period

Role of Cyclooxygenase and Prostaglandin in Pain

Because the products of arachidonic acid metabolism play an important part in inflammation, genesis and processing of pain signals, and facilitation of other algogenic substances, inhibition of cyclooxygenase and reduction of prostaglandins can be expected to interrupt the cascade that leads to exaggerated and prolonged pain. In addition, early use of NSAIDs may prevent sensitization of the nervous system and may decrease the response to subsequent nociceptive signals. By decreasing the inflammatory response, NSAIDs may also modulate the postsurgical stress response, although the benefits and universality of this effect have not been tested.[14]

Value of Multimodal Balanced Analgesia

Single-drug therapy of severe postoperative pain often comes at a cost of excessive side effects. Analgesia is more efficiently attained using a combination of agents that act on different sites along the cascade of pain signals, reducing the dose of each agent required and the accompanying adverse effects.[15,16] In addition, investigators have demonstrated in an animal model that ketorolac has a synergistic action on spinal opioid-mediated analgesia.[17]

Absence of Opioid Effects

Sedation, narcosis, respiratory depression, and intestinal ileus are among the undesirable (sometimes lethal) effects of opioid therapy that are largely absent from the NSAIDs. The absence of addictive and abuse potential also reduces the administrative cost of using these drugs.

General Clinical Pharmacology[18]

With the exception of acetaminophen and nabumetone, all NSAIDs are weakly acidic, with pK_As ranging from 3 to 5. Therefore, in the acid gastric environment,

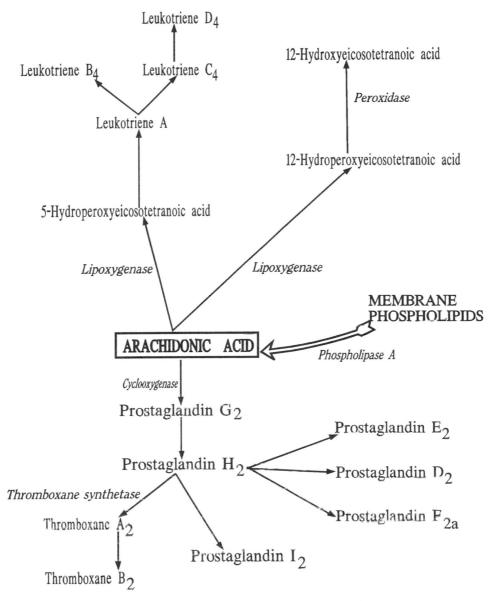

Fig. 34–1. Scheme of arachidonic acid metabolism.

dissociation readily occurs followed by rapid absorption and trapping in gastric mucosal cells. First-pass metabolism in the liver is negligible. With the exception of acetaminophen, all are highly (> 95%) bound to albumin and have small volume of distribution. Hepatic clearance is not flow dependent and low. NSAIDs are extensively metabolized by the liver. Enterohepatic recirculation occurs to a significant degree with sulindac and indomethacin, but is insignificant with nabumetone. Renal elimination of unchanged drug accounts for a small percentage of an administered dose (ketorolac being an exception[19]). In the presence of renal failure, however, metabolites of NSAID accumulate and undergo enterohepatic circulation, which may lead to increased drug level. The elimination half-lives of NSAIDs vary greatly, ranging from short (diclofenac, 1 hour) to intermediate (ketorolac, 5 hours) to long (piroxicam, 50 hours).

Sulindac and nabumetone are prodrugs and represent two exceptions to the general rule. After absorption in the duodenum, nabumetone is rapidly metabolized by the liver to the active metabolite 6-methoxy-2-naphthylacetic acid, which does not undergo enterohepatic circulation and is not eliminated by the kidneys. Sulindac, a sulfoxide, is metabolized to pharmacologically active sulindac sulfide in the liver. Only the prodrug sulindac sulfoxide and the inactive metabolic sulindac sulfone, but not the active sulfide, depend on the kidney for excretion.

Despite the diversity of chemical structures, inhibition of cyclooxygenase appears to be the unifying mechanism for the many clinical and adverse effects of all NSAIDs. Subclasses (or isoenzymes) of cyclooxygenase have been identified,[20] which may permit development of more selective NSAIDs. Some drug and tissue specificities do exist. For example, the effect of acetylated salicylates on

Table 34–1. Chemical Classification of Nonsteroidal Anti-inflammatory Drugs

General Chemical Classes	Specific Chemical Classes		Generic Names	Available in USA	Sample Trade Names
Carboxylic Acids	Salicylic acids and esters				
			Aspirin	Yes	Various
			Diflunsial	Yes	Dolobid
	Acetic acids	Phenylacetic acid	Diclofenac	Yes	Voltaren
			Alcofenac	No	
			Fenclofenac	No	
		Carbo- and heterocyclic acetic acids	Indomethacin	Yes	Indocin
			Sulindac	Yes	Clinoril
			Tolmetin	Yes	Tolectin
			Ketorolac	Yes	Toradol
			Etodolac	Yes	Lodine
	Propionic acid		Ibuprofen	Yes	Motrin, Advil
			Flurbiprofen	Yes	Ansaid
			Naproxen	Yes	Naprosyn
			Ketoprofen	Yes	Orudis
			Fenoprofen	Yes	Nalfon
			Fenbufen	No	
			Tiaprofen	No	
			Pirprofen	No	
			Oxaprozin	Yes	Daypro
	Fenamic acids		Mefanamic	Yes	Ponstel
			Flufenamic	No	
			Meclofenamic	Yes	Meclomen
			Nifumic	No	
Enolic Acids	Pyrazolone		Dipyrone	No	
			Aminopyrone	No	
			Antipyrine	No	
	Pyrazolidines		Phenylbutazone	Yes	Butazolidin
			Feprazone	No	
			Azapropazone	No	
	Oxicams		Piroxicam	Yes	Feldene
			Sudoxicam	No	
			Isoxicam	No	
			Tenoxicam	No	Mobiflex
Nonacidic Phenols			Nabumetone	Yes	Relafen
			Acetaminophen	Yes	Tylenol

platelets is irreversible, whereas that of the other NSAIDs is reversible on elimination of the drugs. Platelet cyclooxygenase is more sensitive than vascular endothelial cyclooxygenase to the effect of salicylates.

Other cell membrane and intracellular processes are affected by NSAIDs (Table 34-2). Most of these have been demonstrated only in vitro, they require a higher drug concentration, and their significance is not defined.

Choice for Perioperative Use

From the drug administration standpoint, options in the perioperative period are limited because the enteral route is often not feasible, either because the patient is unable to take them orally or because the gastrointestinal tract is nonfunctional. Thus, of the many NSAIDs available for treatment of inflammatory conditions, only the few with suitable parenteral formulations, including lysine acetylsalicylate, indomethacin, diclofenac, and ibuprofen have been used in a systematic fashion for perioperative analgesia.

Table 34–2. Cellular and Membrane Processes (Unrelated to Cyclooxygenase) Affected by Nonsteroidal Anti-inflammatory Drugs

Leukotriene synthesis
Superoxide generation
Lysosomal enzyme release
Neutrophil aggregation and adhesion
Lymphocyte function
Rheumatoid factor production
Cartilage and bone metabolism
    Synthesis of proteoglycan
Cell-membrane function
    Enzyme activity
    (NADPH oxidase, phospholipase C)
    Transmembrane anion transport
    Oxidative phosphorylation
    Uptake of arachidonate

In the United States, only indomethacin is available in the injectable form, and that is only approved for use in neonates to induce closure of patent ductus arteriosus. Oral NSAIDs, especially the longer-acting agents (e.g., piroxicam), are gaining popularity. Acetaminophen is widely used (with or without prescription), but for the perioperative period it is often combined in a preparation with an opioid, and few formal studies exist about acetaminophen itself for postoperative pain.

Ketorolac

This addition to the pharmacopeia, ketorolac tromethamine, is one of the most potent NSAIDs. It was developed and marketed in the United States not as an anti-inflammatory drug, but as an analgesic. It is the only injectable NSAID analgesic readily available in the United States and therefore has seen widespread use in the perioperative period since its release.

The pharmacology of ketorolac in general parallels that of the other NSAIDs.[21,22] The oral form is rapidly absorbed by the gastrointestinal tract, with peak blood level attained 20 to 60 minutes after ingestion, and bioavailability of 80 to 100%. After intramuscular injection, peak blood level is attained in 45 to 50 minutes. Ketorolac is highly (< 99%) protein-bound and has a small volume of distribution. The terminal half-life is 4.5 hours in healthy adults, 6.1 hours in elderly patients, 5.4 hours in patients with liver dysfunction, and 9.6 hours in patients with renal dysfunction. The principal metabolic pathway is glucuronic acid conjugation, and urinary excretion of conjugated drug is the major pathway of elimination. Compared with morphine, ketorolac, like the other NSAIDs, has negligible effects on respiration,[23] hemodynamics,[24,25] and the central nervous system.[26] The dosage for intramuscular use includes a loading dose of 30 to 60 mg, followed by 15 to 30 mg every 6 hours. The dosage for oral therapy is 10 mg every 8 hours.

Experience with Use in the Perioperative Period

Many clinical studies on the use of NSAIDs for postoperative analgesia have been conducted, but interpretation and generalizations are difficult because of the nonuniformity of experimental designs, doses of NSAIDs, dosing method (compounded by the delay in onset of analgesia), statistical power, and type of surgical procedures. Consequently, comparison among different NSAIDs is difficult: NSAIDs in oral form are usually used where gastrointestinal function is not interrupted (and in general associated with less severe pain), such as dental surgery, whereas only NSAIDs with parenteral formulations are used during major surgery such as abdominal or thoracic surgery, which are associated with more severe pain and gastrointestinal dysfunction. Direct comparison of different NSAIDs using the same subpopulation of patients is rare.

Mild to Moderate Pain

In general, NSAIDs are efficacious for treatment of mild to moderate pain. Pain after dental procedures,[27-29] superficial procedures (e.g., inguinal hernia repair), and minor gynecologic procedures[30,31] is representative of this category. A variety of oral or parenteral NSAIDs (including salicylate,[32] diclofenac,[33,34] indomethacin, ketorolac,[35,36] ibuprofen,[37,38] piroxicam,[39,40] etodolac,[41] nabumetone,[42] and naproxen[43]) provide effective relief. For these conditions, these drugs are comparable to opioid analgesics, although the onset of analgesia is typically delayed by 15 to 30 minutes.[44] This delay is consistent with the mechanism of analgesia of NSAIDs.

Severe Pain

Ureteric colics are among the most severe nontraumatic pain encountered clinically. Many NSAIDs given parenterally are effective, and are even superior to opioids, in providing pain relief from ureteric colics.[45-48] Ureteric colics are common after extracorporeal shock wave lithotripsy and have been successfully treated by parenteral indomethacin.[49-50]

For patients who have severe pain after major abdominal, thoracic, or orthopedic surgery, the choice of NSAIDs has been limited because only few intramuscular or intravenous preparations are generally available; rectal administration is not always practical or acceptable. NSAIDs that have been most frequently used are indomethacin, diclofenac, and ketorolac.

In the immediate postoperative period when pain is particularly severe, the aforementioned delay in analgesic action is more obvious and problematic. Up to 70% of patients in clinical studies drop out or require supplementation with opioid analgesic.[51] To compensate for the delay in onset of analgesia for postoperative pain, NSAIDs must be administered before or during the operation. The results of clinical studies are mixed, however.[52-55] Beyond this immediate postoperative period, NSAIDs can decrease pain significantly, although the extent of analgesia is more variable than seen in mild to moderate pain, and additional opioid supplements are almost invariably required.[56-58] Several reasons can be hypothesized for this limited potency. First, in contrast to opioids, which interact directly with opioid receptors in a dose-dependent fashion, NSAIDs interfere with pain only indirectly by inhibiting the synthesis of mediators with facilitatory roles in pain signaling. Second, NSAIDs only inhibit cyclooxygenase and prostaglandin synthesis, leaving the lipooxygenase pathway unimpeded, or even accelerated. The products of the lipooxygenase pathway of metabolism can be algogenic and can increase inflammation. Third, not all prostaglandins are algogenic. Some are analgesic and may be decreased by NSAIDs.

Given the delay and relative lack of potency in relieving severe postoperative pain, NSAIDs are unlikely to be used as sole analgesics. They may lower the amount of potent opioids needed and/or potentiate the effect of other analgesic modalities.

Reduction in opioid requirement by about 30% is demonstrated uniformly by a variety of NSAIDs in various doses: diclofenac,[59] ketorolac,[60,61] indomethacin,[62] ibuprofen,[63] naproxen,[64] and tenoxicam.[65]

NSAIDs can be a component of a multimodal or multidrug analgesic strategy that targets several sites along the pain-processing pathway. Several clinical studies using a combination of NSAID and systemic opioids suggest the presence of synergistic effect.[66-69] The NSAIDs can also be an adjuvant to epidural opioid or anesthetic administration, although in the latter case, where effective analgesia is already achieved by the local anesthetic, the addition of NSAID has not improved pain relief.[70,71]

Adverse Effects

Because prostaglandins are ubiquitous in the body and subserve many physiologic functions, inhibition of cyclooxygenase has widespread consequences. Toxic or idiosyncratic reactions independent of cyclooxygenase inhibition are also seen. A partial list of the many adverse effects associated with NSAID therapy is presented in Table 34-3. Knowledge about the adverse effects of NSAIDs is mostly obtained from patients receiving long-term treatment. The spectrum of adverse reactions during short-term use in the perioperative period can be expected to be similar, but the risk is currently undefined.

Renal Function

The prostaglandins are closely involved with maintenance of renal blood flow and glomerular filtration,[72,73] release of renin and aldosterone,[74] sodium and potassium homeostasis,[75] and water metabolism.[76]

Inhibition of prostaglandin synthesis by NSAIDs allows unopposed action of endogenous vasoconstrictors, the consequences of which are more serious when renal perfusion is diminished or when circulating neurohumoral vasoconstrictors are increased. Examples of such circumstances include hypovolemia, congestive heart failure, sodium depletion, cirrhosis with ascites, and general anesthesia. Intrinsic renal diseases lead to diminished local production of vasodilatory prostaglandins, thus increasing the risk of further decrease in prostaglandin due to NSAIDs. Reduced renin and aldosterone secretion, sodium retention, and unopposed action of antidiuretic hormone may lead to hyporeninemic hyperkalemia,[77-79] water retention, and hyponatremia. The effect of loop diuretics is diminished by NSAIDs.[80-82]

Among the NSAIDs, sulindac reportedly has the least deleterious effect on renal function, because its active metabolite, the sulfide, is eliminated directly in the feces and is not eliminated by the kidney. Data on this are conflicting, however, and no NSAID can be considered completely devoid of renal effect. Sulindac has not been studied in the perioperative period.

Concern about the risk of NSAIDs and increased circulating vasoconstrictor has led one major reviewer to recommend that NSAIDs not be used during surgery.[83] Clinical data to date and a recent study[84] appear to support the safety of a variety of NSAIDs in the perioperative period, absent other contraindications and conditions that should evoke caution (Table 34-4).

Cardiovascular System

In addition to the regulation of sodium and water metabolism, prostaglandins also play a complex role in the regulation of vascular beds. By causing renal sodium retention, reduced free water clearance, and enhancement of vascular response to pressor hormone, and by interference with the action of β-adrenergic blocking agents and angiotensin-converting enzyme inhibitors,[85-87] NSAIDs can aggravate systemic hypertension or can interfere with antihypertensive treatment.[88] In most patients, the significance of this cardiovascular effect during a short period of NSAID treatment is probably small.[89]

Coagulation

Inhibition of platelet cyclooxygenase by NSAIDs decreases thromboxane A_2 synthesis and impairs platelet aggregability and hemostasis. Clinically, the bleeding time is

Table 34-3. Potential Adverse Effect of Nonsteroidal Anti-inflammatory Drugs

Area Affected	Adverse Effects
Renal system	↓ Renal blood flow
	↓ Glomerular filtration
	Sodium retention
	Hyperkalemia
	↓ Response to loop diuretic
Gastrointestinal system	Nausea, vomiting
	Dyspepsia
	Gastric mucosal ulceration
	Gastric mucosal bleeding
	Hepatocellular jaundice
Cardiovascular system	↓ Response to β blockade
	Hypertension
	Edema
	Congestive heart failure
Hematologic system	Platelet dysfunction
	Leukopenia
	Thrombocytopenia
	Aplastic anemia
Respiratory system	↑ Bronchial tone
	Asthma
Skin	Pruritus, urticaria
	Stevens-Johnson syndrome
Central nervous system	Confusion
	Headache
	Dizziness

Table 34-4. Contraindications to Nonsteroidal Anti-inflammatory Drugs (NSAID)

Known allergy to aspirin/NSAID
Active erosive gastrointestinal disease
   Peptic ulcer disease
   Inflammatory bowel disease
Concomitant anticoagulation
Intrinsic renal disease and insufficiency
Contracted intravascular volume with high renal vascular tone
   Uncontrolled hypertension
   Severe congestive heart failure
   Cirrhosis with ascites
   Hypovolemia
Asthma and nasal polyps, chronic urticaria

prolonged. Variation among NSAIDs is significant. Acetaminophen has little effect on platelet function. At the other end of spectrum, acetylsalicylate (aspirin) irreversibly acetylates platelet cyclooxygenase,[90,91] and recovery of platelet function depends on the senescence of circulating platelets and replacement by new platelets (a process that takes 10 to 14 days). The other NSAIDs reversibly inhibit cyclooxygenase, and platelet function recovers when the pharmacologic activity of the NSAID has dissipated, about six to seven times its elimination half-life. For example, ketorolac raised bleeding time from 4.9 to 7.8 minutes in one study,[92] and this effect lasted approximately 30 hours (six times the half-life of 5 hours). The effect of piroxicam (half-life 50 hours) lasts 300 hours, or 12 days.

Impairment of platelet function has special significance during the perioperative period because of concern about surgical hemostasis and safety of regional (especially neuraxial) anesthesia. The well-established propensity of NSAIDs to cause gastric erosion further raises the stake of abnormal platelet function. Few studies have specifically addressed the issue of perioperative blood loss, but available data demonstrate no evidence of excessive blood loss in the perioperative period after short-term NSAID treatment.[93-96] NSAIDs are contraindicated where absolute hemostasis is critical, for example, after neurosurgery or when coagulopathy or clinical anticoagulation is present.

The presence of abnormal platelet function tests or coagulation profiles preoperatively precludes the performance of central neuraxial blockade such as continuous epidural anesthesia. The safety of administering NSAIDs subsequent to establishment of a block and the safety of manipulating indwelling catheters in the presence of platelet dysfunction are issues that remain to be resolved.

During long-term NSAID therapy, drug interaction with anticoagulants may lead to hyper- or hypoanticoagulation. Whether this poses a problem during short-term treatment is not clear.[97]

Gastrointestinal Effect

Gastrointestinal adverse effects represent the most frequent complications of NSAID treatment. Dyspepsia is a frequent symptom. Long-term NSAID treatment is associated with de novo gastroduodenal ulceration, as well as exacerbation of peptic ulcer disease and increase in ulcer complication such as perforation and hemorrhage.[98] Advanced age, female gender, alcohol use, and anticoagulation appear to increase the risk of serious complications. Histamine-2 receptor antagonists have not been effective in preventing gastroduodenal complications, whereas misoprostol, a prostaglandin analogue, is effective. Nabumetone is inactive in the stomach and is absorbed only in the small intestine. It might have less effect on the stomach, but the data are not conclusive.

The risk of gastroduodenal ulceration and hemorrhage during a short course of treatment in the perioperative period is unknown. Cumulative uncontrolled data suggest that, in the absence of preexisting peptic ulcer disease, the risk is minimal.[99]

Respiratory System

Products of cyclooxygenase play a role in maintaining bronchodilation by counteracting the bronchoconstrictive effect of leukotriene. Aspirin can provoke asthma in some patients (aspirin-induced asthma). A syndrome of aspirin intolerance, asthma, and nasal polyp has been described as the "aspirin triad."[100] Other NSAIDs can trigger acute asthmatic attack, and cross-sensitivity occurs in patients who have aspirin intolerance or the aspirin triad.[101] The NSAIDs should be used with great caution in patients who have asthma.

Bone Formation

Products of arachidonic acid metabolism may play a role in the early stages of bone formation.[102] NSAIDs can inhibit the synthesis of connective tissue, cartilage, and bone not only by inhibiting cyclooxygenase, but also by acting directly on the synthesis of proteoglycan by chondrocytes.[103] Considerable variation exists among the different NSAIDs.[104] Concerns about wound healing, including healing of bone fractures and prosthesis, have been raised.[105] Currently, no data are available on the effect of short-term perioperative NSAID use.

Special Circumstances

Pregnant and Lactating Women

Prostaglandins play a complex and important role in the maintenance of gestation and the process of parturition. They are also crucial in the regulation of fetal development and fetal circulation. By interfering with prostaglandin synthesis, NSAIDs can have widespread consequences. For example, constriction of ductus arteriosus in utero has been demonstrated after maternal indomethacin administration. During pregnancy, NSAIDs should be considered contraindicated, except when used under specialized protocols to alter the course of pregnancy.

NSAIDs are excreted into human milk to a variable extent, but usually in minimal amounts, up to 2% of a maternal dose.[106] After repeated dosing, the ratio of milk to plasma concentration (M:P ratio) of ketorolac ranged from 0.015 to 0.037, indicating low potential exposure to the breast-fed infant.[107] NSAIDs with shorter half-lives and that form no active metabolites (such as ibuprofen and diclofenac) would be preferred for the lactating patient, however.

Children

Experience with use of NSAIDs in children for acute postoperative pain is limited. Acetaminophen is generally the first drug of choice. No other NSAID has been officially approved in the United States for use in children for acute pain. Ketorolac has been studied as an analgesic and adjuvant in the perioperative period, however.

Some changes in pharmacokinetic parameters are recognized in children. The volume of distribution and plasma clearance for ketorolac are twice as high as adult values, whereas the elimination half-life is unchanged.[108]

Analgesia from ketorolac has the same delay in onset seen in adults.[109] Given intraoperatively, ketorolac 0.9 mg · kg^{-1} is as efficacious as morphine 0.1 mg · kg^{-1} for relief of moderate postoperative pain and is associated with less emesis.[110] Preoperative oral administration of ketorolac is also effective in relief of postmyringotomy pain.[111]

Elderly Patients

In the elderly, changes occur in the pharmacokinetics of NSAIDs that are not predictable based on chemical structure.[112] Significant changes are seen with salicylate,[113] diflunisal, ibuprofen,[114] naproxen,[115] ketoprofen, sulindac, and ketorolac. The clearance of ketorolac is reduced, and plasma half-life is increased by about 25%, from 4.7 to 6.1 hours.[116] No significant changes are seen with prioxicam, tenoxicam, etodolac, diclofenac, or indomethacin.

Pharmacodynamically, serious complications from NSAIDs, such as gastrointestinal bleeding and heart failure, are more common in the elderly.[117,118] Less serious adverse effects of NSAID therapy, such as dizziness and temporary cognitive dysfunction, can assume a significant impact in the elderly.[119] At present, whether short-term treatment with NSAID poses increased risk for the elderly is unclear. The potential risk of alternative analgesia therapy, that is, opioids, must be taken into consideration.

Further Questions

A major attraction of the NSAIDs in the perioperative period is the absence of typical opioid side effects, ranging from potentially lethal effects such as respiratory depression and narcosis to more mundane effects such as nausea and constipation. Substituting an NSAID for an opioid analgesic, or adding an NSAID to an opioid regimen, should reduce the number and severity of side effects that prolong immediate postoperative recovery, increase use of health care facilities, and impinge on the patient's quality of life. Clinical studies have not consistently demonstrated a definitive difference in adverse effects experienced by patients in the immediate postoperative period. This may be secondary to study design and the effect of residual general anesthetic. In one study,[36] nausea and somnolence were less common, and bowel function returned earlier in patients receiving intravenous and oral ketorolac. Subjective assessment of quality of life by these patients was not better, however. Another study found that the discharge time from the postanesthesia recovery room was not shortened by using ketorolac instead of fentanyl.[120] Because many of the newer NSAIDs, and ketorolac in particular, are much more costly than opioid analgesics, further studies and analyses are needed to define the role of these drugs in the current socioeconomic climate.

ADRENERGIC AGONISTS

The role of the descending medullospinal noradrenergic pathway in modulating spinal nociceptive processing appears to be mediated by α_2-adrenergic receptors located on dorsal horn neurons of the spinal cord.[121] These receptors can inhibit the release of nociceptive neurotransmitters such as substance P, adenosine, or tryptamine.[122-124]

A synergistic interaction also exists between α_2 receptors and opioid receptors; α_2-adrenoceptor agonists may therefore have a role in analgesia.

Dexmedetomidine is a superselective α_2 agonist available for clinical trial only in Europe. Clonidine, guanabenz, and guanfacine are relatively selective for α_2-adrenergic receptors, with a ratio of α_1 to α_2 of 1:200.[125]

The role of α_2-adrenoceptor agonist in the perioperative period is beginning to be investigated. Clonidine, administered intraspinally, acts primarily at the spinal cord level to produce analgesia, and parenteral administration of clonidine is much less potent for analgesia.[126] Subarachnoid clonidine has prolonged the duration of spinal bupivacaine[127] and has also attenuated tourniquet pain under tetracaine spinal anesthesia.[128] The efficacy of epidural clonidine has not been consistent in clinical studies available to date,[129-134] probably as a result of varying doses. Mild decrease in blood pressure and sedation are common.

Systemic administration of clonidine produced only weak analgesia.[135] Intravenous dexmedetomidine given intraoperatively appears to have some opioid-sparing effect, but results are not impressive from the analgesic standpoint.[136] The place of α_2-adrenoceptor agonist in postoperative analgesia therefore requires further study and definition.

METOCLOPRAMIDE

Metoclopramide (3-methoxy-5-chloroprocainamide) is chemically related to the antiarrhythmic procainamide, but has no local anesthetic or antiarrhythmic activity. It is rapidly absorbed after oral intake, with a maximum blood level after 2 hours. The plasma half-life is 4 hours, and most of the drug is excreted by the kidney either in unchanged form or as conjugated sulfate or glucuronides. This drug increases gastrointestinal motility through action on postsynaptic cholinergic neurons of the gastrointestinal tract as well as by central mechanisms. It is also an antagonist at central dopamine (D_2) receptors and serotonin (5-HT$_3$) receptors.[137]

Current knowledge of the complex modulating mechanisms of pain signal suggests that metoclopramide, through its action on dopaminergic and tryptaminergic receptors, may have a role in the genesis and process of pain.

Animal studies show that metoclopramide has antinociceptive activity, although the mechanism of antinociception is unclear. Changes in neuronal calcium ion flux may be involved because metoclopromide antinociception appears to be enhanced by calcium channel blockers and inhibited by calcium chloride.[138,139] Increasingly, metoclopramide has been used to treat a variety of neurogenic conditions such as vomiting and migraine headache.

In patients in acute pain, metoclopramide, 20 mg intravenously, was as effective as morphine, 20 mg, plus atropine, 0.5 mg, for ureteric colic.[140] Whether the antismooth muscle spasm activity of metoclopramide played a role in this study is unclear. In a study of patients who underwent hip arthroplasty under subarachnoid anesthesia, metoclopramide, 1 mg · kg^{-1}, followed by an infusion of 1.5 mg · kg^{-1} over 9 hours, appeared to decrease the morphine requirement.[141] A subsequent study by the same group of investigators concluded, however, that a clinically relevant analgesic action could not be demonstrated.[142] The analgesic potential of metoclopramide for the acute postoperative setting is therefore unclear.

REFERENCES

1. Editorials: Postoperative pain relief and non-opioid analgesics. Lancet *337:*524, 1991.
2. Murphy, D. F.: Editorials: NSAIDs and Postoperative Pain. Br Med J *306:*1493, 1993.
3. Acute Pain Management Guideline Panel: Acute Pain Management: Operative or Medical Procedures and Trauma. Clinical Practice Guideline. AHCPR Pub. No. 92-0032. Rockville, MD, Agency for Health Care Policy and Research, Public Health Service, U.S. Department of Health and Human Services, 1992.
4. Cousins, M. J.: Acute pain and the injury response: immediate and prolonged effects. Reg Anesth *14:*162, 1989.
5. Woolf, C. J.: Recent advances in the pathophysiology of acute pain. Br J Anaesth *63:*139, 1989.
6. Raja, S. N., Meyer, R. A., Campbell, J. N.: Peripheral mechanisms of somatic pain. Anesthesiology *68:*571, 1988.
7. Cook, A. J., et al.: Dynamic receptive field plasticity in rat spinal dorsal horn following C-primary afferent input. Nature *325:*151, 1987.
8. Woolf, C. J., Thompson, S. W. N.: The induction and maintenance of central sensitization is dependent on N-methyl-D-aspartic receptor activation; implications for the treatment of post-injury pain hypersensitivity states. Pain *44:*293, 1991.
9. Yaksh, T. L.: Pharmacology of spinal adrenergic systems which modulate spinal nociceptive processing. Pharmacol Biochem Behav *22:*845, 1985.
10. Cervero, F.: Neurophysiology of gastrointestinal pain. Baillieres Clin Gastroenterol *2:*183, 1988.
11. Thornell, E., Jansson, R., Svanvick, J.: Indomethacin intravenously: a new way for effective relief of biliary pain: a double-blind study in man. Surgery *90:*468, 1981.
12. Kuehl, F. A., Jr., Egan, R. W.: Prostaglandins, arachidonic acid, and inflammation. Science *210:*978, 1980.
13. Samuelsson, B., et al.: Prostaglandins and thromboxanes. Annu Rev Biochem *47:*997, 1978.
14. Kehlet, H.: Surgical stress: the role of pain and analgesia. Br J Anaesth *63:*189, 1989.
15. Eng, J., Sabanathan, S.: Post-thoracotomy analgesia. J R Coll Surg Edinb *38:*62, 1993.
16. Code, W.: NSAIDs and balanced analgesia (editorial). Can J Anaesth *40:*401, 1993.
17. Malmberg, A. B., Yaksh, T.: Pharmacology of the spinal action of ketorolac, morphine, ST-91, U50488H, and L-PIA on the formalin test and an isobolographic analysis of the NSAID interaction. Anesthesiology *70:*270, 1993.
18. Day, R. O., Graham, G. G., Williams, K. M.: Pharmacokinetics of nonsteroidal antiinflammatory drugs. Baillieres Clin Rheumatol *2:*363, 1988.
19. Mroszczak, E. J., et al.: Ketorolac tromethamine pharmacokinetics and metabolism after intravenous, intramuscular, and oral administration in humans and animals. Pharmacotherapy *10:*33S, 1990.
20. DeWitt, D. L., Meade, E. A., Smith, W. L.: PGH synthase isoenzyme selectivity: the potential for safer nonsteroidal antiinflammatory drugs. Am J Med *95:*40S, 1993.
21. Mroszczak, E. J., et al.: Ketorolac tromethamine absorption, distribution, metabolism, excretion, and pharmacokinetics in animals and humans. Drug Metab Dispos *15:*618, 1987.
22. Jung, D., Mroszczak, E., Bynum, L.: Pharmacokinetics of ketorolac tromethamine in humans after intravenous, intramuscular and oral administration. Eur J Clin Pharmacol *35:*423, 1988.
23. Bravo, I. J., et al.: The effects on ventilation of ketorolac in comparison with morphine. Eur J Clin Pharmacol *35:*491, 1988.
24. Camu, F., van Overberge, L., Bullingham, R., Lloyd, J.: Hemodynamic effects of two intravenous doses of ketorolac tromethamine compared with morphine. Pharmacotherapy *10:*122S, 1990.
25. Murray, A. W., Brockway, M. S., Kenny, G. N.: Comparison of the cardiorespiratory effects of ketorolac and alfentanil during propofol anaesthesia. Br J Anaesth *63:*601, 1989.
26. MacDonald, F. C., Gough, K. J., Nicoll, R. A., Dow, R. J.: Psychomotor effects of ketorolac in comparison with buprenorphine and diclofenac. Br J Clin Pharmacol *28:*453, 1989.
27. Seymour, R. A., Walton, J. G.: Pain control after third molar surgery. Int J Oral Surg *13:*457, 1984.
28. Winter, L., Jr., Bass, F., Recant, B., Cahaly, J. F.: Analgesic activity of ibuprofen in postoperative oral surgery pain. Oral Surg Oral Med Oral Pathol *45:*159, 1978.
29. Redden, R. J.: Ketorolac tromethamine: an oral/injectable nonsteroidal anti-inflammatory for postoperative pain control. J Oral Maxillofac Surg *50:*1310, 1992.
30. Bloomfield, S. S., Barden, T. P., Mitchell, J.: Comparative efficacy of ibuprofen and aspirin in episiotomy pain. Clin Pharmacol Ther *15:*565, 1974.
31. Huang, K. C., et al.: Effects of meclofenamate and acetaminophen on abdominal pain following tubal occlusion. Am J Obstet Gynecol *155:*624, 1986.
32. Cashman, J. N., Jones, R M, Foster, J. M. G., Adams, A. P.: Comparison of infusions of morphine and lysine acetyl salicylate for the relief of pain after surgery. Br J Anaesth *57:*255, 1985.
33. Fredman, J.: Analgesia for lithotripsy: opioid sparing by diclofenac. J Clin Anesth *5:*141, 1993.
34. McLoughlin, C., McKinney, M. S., Fee, J. P. H., Boules, Z.: Diclofenac for day-care arthroscopy surgery: comparison with a standard opioid therapy. Br J Anaesth *65:*620, 1990.
35. Galasko, C. S. B., Russell, S., Lloyd, J.: Double-blind investigation of multiple oral doses of ketorolac tromethamine compared with dihydrocodeine and placebo. Curr Ther Res *45:*844, 1989.
36. Wong, H. Y., et al.: A randomized, double-blind evaluation of ketorolac tromethamine for postoperative analgesia in ambulatory surgery patients. Anesthesiology *78:*6, 1993.
37. Owen, H., Glavin, R. J., Shaw, N. A.: Ibuprofen in the management of postoperative pain. Br J Anaesth *58:*1371, 1986.
38. Rosenblum, M., et al.: Ibuprofen provides longer lasting analgesia than fentanyl after laparoscopic surgery. Anesth Analg *73:*255, 1991.
39. Sunshine, A., et al.: Analgesic efficacy of piroxicam in the treatment of postoperative pain. Am J Med *84:*16, 1988.
40. Brevik, H., Stenseth, R., Apalseth, K., Spilsberg, A. M.: Piroxicam, acetylsalicylic acid and placebo for postoperative pain. Acta Anaesth Scand *28:*37, 1984.
41. Pena, M.: Etodolac: analgesic effects in musculoskeletal and postoperative pain. Rheumatol Int *10(Suppl):*9, 1990.

42. Movilia, P., et al.: Analgesic activity of nabumetone in postoperative pain. Drugs 40(Suppl 5):71, 1992.

43. Dueholm, S., Forrest, M., Hjortso, E., Lemvigh, E.: Pain relief following herniotomy; a double-blind randomized comparison bnetween naproxen and placebo. Acta Anaesth Scand 33:391, 1989.

44. Rice, A. S. C., et al.: A double-blind study of the speed of onset of analgesia following intramuscular ketorolac tromethamine in comparison to intramuscular morphine and placebo. Anaesthesia 46:541, 1991.

45. Basar, I., et al.: Diclofenac sodium and spasmolytic drugs in the treatment of ureteral colic: a comparative study. Int Urol Nephrol 23:27, 1991.

46. el-Sherif, A. E., Foda, R., Norlen, L. J., Yahia, H.: Treatment of renal colic by prostaglandin synthetase inhibitors and avafortan (analgesic antispasmodic). Br J Urol 66:602, 1990.

47. Vignoni, A., et al.: Diclofenac sodium in ureteral colic: a double-blind comparison trial with placebo. J Int Med Res 11:303, 1983.

48. Sjodin, J. G., Holmlund, D.: Indomethacin by intravenous infusion in ureteral colic: a multicentre study. Scand J Urol Nephrol 16:221, 1982.

49. Ou, Y. C., et al.: Use of indomethacin in the prophylaxis of ureteral colic following extracorporeal shock wave lithotripsy. Scand J Urol Nephrol 26:351, 1992.

50. Cole, R. S., Palfrey, E. L., Smith, S. E., Shuttleworth, K. E.: Indomethacin as prophylaxis against ureteral colic following extracorporeal shock wave lithotripsy (see comments). J Urol 141:9, 1989.

51. Pierce, R. J., Fragen, R. J., Pemberton, D. M.: Intravenous ketorolac tromethamine versus morphine sulfate in the treatment of immediate postoperative pain. Pharmacotherapy 10:111S, 1990.

52. Dundee, J. W., McAteer, E.: Intravenous salicylate for postoperative pain. Lancet 1:154, 1981.

53. Liu, J., et al.: Effects of ketorolac on postoperative analgesia and ventilatory function after laparoscopic cholecystectomy. Anesth Analg 76:1061, 1992.

54. Ding, Y., Fredman, B., White, P.F.: Use of ketorolac and fentanyl during outpatient gynecologic surgery. Anesth Analg 77:205, 1993.

55. Ding, Y., White, P.: Comparative effects of ketorolac, dezocine, and fentanyl as adjuvants during outpatient anesthesia. Anesth Analg 75:566, 1992.

56. Kenny, G. N. C.: Ketorolac tromethamine—a new non-opioid analgesic. Br J Anaesth 65:445, 1990.

57. Powell, H., Smallman, J. M. D., Morgan, M.: Comparison of intramuscular ketorolac and morphine in pain control after laparotomy. Anaesthesia 45:538, 1990.

58. Power, I., Noble, D. W., Douglas, E., Spence, A. A.: Comparison of i.m. ketorolac trometamol and morphine sulphate for pain relief after cholecystectomy. Br J Anaesth 65:448, 1990.

59. Hodsman, N. B. A., et al.: The morphine sparing effects of diclofenac sodium following abdominal surgery. Anaesthesia 42:1005, 1987.

60. Gilles, G. W. A., Kenny, G. N. C., Bullingham, R. E. S., McArdle, C. S.: The morphine sparing effect of ketorolac tromethamine. Anaesthesia 42:727, 1987.

61. Kenny, G. N. C., McArdle, C. S., Aitken, H. H.: Parenteral ketorolac: opiate-sparing effect and lack of cardiorespiratory depression in the perioperative patient. Pharmacotheraphy 10:127S, 1990.

62. Pavy, T., Medley, C., Murphy, D. F.: Effect of indomethacin on pain relief after thoracotomy. Br J Anaesth 65:624, 1990.

63. Owen, H., Glavin, R. J., Shaw, N. A.: Ibuprofen in the management of postoperative pain. Br J Anaesth 58:1371, 1986.

64. Martens, M.: A significant decrease of narcotic drug dosage after orthopaedic surgery: a double-blind study with naproxen. Acta Orthop Belg 48:900, 1982.

65. Merry, A. F., et al.: Prospective, controlled, double-blind study of i.v. tenoxicam for analgesia after thoracotomy. Br J Anaesth 69:92, 1992.

66. Sunshine, A., et al.: Analgesic efficacy of two ibuprofen-codeine combinations for the treatment of postepisiotomy and postoperative pain. Clin Pharmacol Ther 42:374, 1987.

67. McQuay, H. J., et al.: Codeine 20 mg increases pain relief from ibuprofen 400 mg after third molar surgery: a repeat-dosing comparison of ibuprofen and ibuprofen-codeine combination. Pain 37:7, 1989.

68. Beaver, W. T.: Aspirin and acetaminophen as constituents of analgesic combinations. Arch Intern Med 141:293, 1981.

69. Grass, J. A., et al.: Assessment of ketorolac as an adjuvant to fentanyl patient-controlled epidural analgesia after radical retropubic prostatectomy. Anesthesiology 78:642, 1993.

70. Bigler, D., et al.: Effect of piroxicam in addition to continuous thoracic epidural bupivacaine and morphine on postoperative pain and lung function after thoracotomy. Acta Anaesthesiol Scand 36:647, 1992.

71. Mogensen, T., et al.: Systemic piroxicam as an adjunct to combined epidural bupivacaine and morphine for postoperative pain relief: a double-blind study. Anesth Analg 74:366, 1992.

72. Lifschitz, M. D.: Prostaglandins and renal blood flow: in vivo studies. Kidney Int 19:781, 1981.

73. Levenson, D. J., Simmons, C. E., Jr., Brenner, B. M.: Arachidonic acid metabolism, prostaglandins and the kidney. Am J Med 72:354, 1982.

74. Mene, P., Simonson, M. S., Dunn, M. J.: Physiology of the mesangial cell. Physiol Rev 69:1347, 1989.

75. Dunn, M. J., Hood, V. L.: Prostaglandins and the kidney. Am J Physiol 233:F169, 1977.

76. Gross, P. A., Schrier, R. W., Anderson, R. J.: Prostaglandins and water metabolism: a review with emphasis on in vivo studies. Kidney Int 19:839, 1981.

77. Nadler, J. L., Lee, F. O., Hsueh, W., Horton, R.: Evidence of prostaglandin deficiency in the syndrome of hyporeninemic hypoaldosteronism. N Engl J Med 314:1015, 1986.

78. Rotenberg, F. A., Giannini, V. S.: Hyperkalemia associated with ketorolac. Ann Pharmacother 26:778, 1992.

79. Pearce, C. J., Gonzalez, F. M., Wallin, J. D.: Renal failure and hyperkalemia associated with ketorolac tromethamine. Arch Intern Med 153:1000, 1993.

80. Williamson, H. E., Bourland, W. A., Marchand, G. R.: Inhibition of furosemide induced increase in renal blood flow by indomethacin. Proc Soc Exp Biol Med 148:164, 1975.

81. Patak, R. V., et al.: Antagonism of the effects of furosemide by indomethacin in normal and hypertensive man. Prostaglandins 10:649, 1975.

82. Tiggeler, R. G. W. L., Koene, R. A. P., Wijdeveld, P. G. A. B.: Inhibition of furosemide-induced natriuresis by indomethacin in patients with the nephrotic syndrome. Clin Sci Mol Med 52:149, 1977.

83. Clive, D. M., Stoff, J. S.: Renal syndromes associated with nonsteroidal antiinflammatory drugs. N Engl J Med 310:563, 1984.

84. Aitken, H. A., Burns, J. W., McArdle, C. S., Kenny, G. N. C.: Effects of ketorolac tromethamine on renal function. Br J Anaesth 68:481, 1992.

85. Durao, V., Prata, M. M., Goncalves, L. M. P.: Modification of antihypertensive effect of beta-adrenoreceptor-blocking agents by inhibition of endogenous prostaglandin synthesis. Lancet 2:1005, 1977.

86. Wong, D. G., et al.: Effects of non-steroidal antiinflammatory drugs on control of hypertension by beta-blockers and diuretics. Lancet 1:997, 1986.

87. Brown, J., Dollery, C., Valdes, G.: Interaction of nonsteroidal anti-inflammatory drugs with antihypertensive and diuretic agents. Am J Med 81(Suppl 2B):43, 1986.

88. Radack, K., Deck, K.: Do nonsteroidal anti-inflammatory drugs interfere with blood pressure control in hypertensive patients? J Gen Intern Med 2:108, 1987.

89. Camu, F., Van Lersberghe, C., Lauwers, M. H.: Cardiovascular risks and benefits of perioperative nonsteroidal antiinflammatory drug treatment. Drugs 44(Suppl 5):42, 1992.

90. Smith, J. B., Willis, A. L.: Aspirin selectively inhibits prostaglandin production in human platelets. Nature 31:235, 1971.

91. Roth, G. J., Stanford, N., Majerus, P. W.: Acetylation of prostaglandin synthetase by aspirin. Proc Natl Acad Sci USA 72:3073, 1975.

92. Conrad, K. A., Fagan, T. C., Mackie, M. J., Mayshar, P. V.: Effects of ketorolac tromethamine on hemostasis in volunteers. Clin Pharmacol Ther 43:542, 1988.

93. McGlew, I. C., et al.: A comparison of rectal indomethacin with placebo for pain relief following spinal surgery. Anaesth Intensive Care 19:40, 1991.

94. Bricker, S. R. W., Savage, M. E., Hanning, C. D.: Perioperative blood loss and non-steroidal anti-inflammatory drugs: an investigation using diclofenac in patients undergoing transurethral resection of the prostate. Eur J Anaesth 4:429, 1987.

95. Jones, R. M., et al.: Comparison of infusions of morphine and lysine acetyl salicylate for the relief of pain following thoracic surgery. Br J Anaesth 57:259, 1985.

96. Serpell, M. G., Thomson, M. F.: Comparison of piroxicam with placebo in the management of pain after total hip replacement. Br J Anaesth 63:354, 1989.

97. Spowart, K., et al.: Haemostatic effects of ketorolac with and without concomitant heparin in normal volunteers. Thromb Haemost 60:382, 1988.

98. Soll, A. H., Weinstein, W. M., Kurata, J., McCarthy, D.: Nonsteroidal antiinflammatory drugs and peptic ulcer disease. Ann Intern Med 114:307, 1991.

99. Kehlet, H., Dahl, J. B.: Are perioperative nonsteroidal anti-inflammatory drugs ulcerogenic in the short term? Drugs 44(Suppl 5):38, 1992.

100. Snyder, R. D., Siegal, G. L.: An asthma triad. Ann Allergy 25:377, 1967.

101. Szczeklik, A., Gryglewski, R. J.: Asthma and anti-inflammatory drugs: mechanisms and clinical patterns. Drugs 25:533, 1983.

102. Yazdi, M., et al.: Effects of non-steroidal anti-inflammatory drugs on demineralized bone-induced bone formation. J Periodontal Res 27:28, 1992.

103. Herman, J. H., et al.: Cytokine modulation of chondrocyte metabolism: in vivo and in vitro effects of piroxicam. Inflammation 8(Suppl):S125, 1984.

104. Kalbhen, D. A.: The influence of NSAIDs on morphology of articular cartilage. Scand J Rheumatol 77:13, 1988.

105. Hogevold, H. E., Grogaard, B., Reikeras, O.: Effects of short term treatment with corticosteroids and indomethacin on bone healing: a mechanical study of osteotomies in rats. Acta Orthop Scand 63:607, 1992.

106. Knowles, J. A.: Excretion of drugs in milk: a review. J Pediatr 66:1068, 1985.

107. Wischnik, A., et al.: The excretion of ketorolac tromethamine into breast milk after multiple oral dosing. Eur J Clin Pharmacol 36:521, 1989.

108. Olkkola, K. T., Maunuksela, E.L.: The pharmacokinetics of postoperative intravenous ketorolac tromethamine in children. Br J Clin Pharmacol 31:182, 1991.

109. Maunuksela, E. L., Kokki, H., Bullingham, R. E.: Comparison of intravenous ketorolac with morphine for postoperative pain in children. Clin Pharmacol Ther 52:436, 1992.

110. Watcha, M. F., et al.: Comparison of ketorolac and morphine as adjuvants during pediatric surgery. Anesthesiology 76:368, 1992.

111. Watcha, M. F., et al.: Perioperative effects of oral ketorolac and acetaminophen in children undergoing bilateral myringotomy. Can J Anaesth 39:649, 1992.

112. Woodhouse, K. W., Wynne, H.: The pharmacokinetics of non-steroidal antiinflammatory drugs in the elderly. Clin Pharmacokinet 12:111, 1987.

113. Roberts, M. S., et al.: Pharmacokinetics of aspirin and salicylates in elderly subjects and in patients with alcoholic liver disease. Eur J Clin Pharmacol 25:253, 1983.

114. Greenblatt, D. J., et al.: Absorption and disposition of ibuprofen in the elderly. Arthritis Rheum 27:1066, 1984.

115. Upton, R. A., Williams, R. L., Kelly, J., Jones, R. M.: Naproxen pharmacokinetics in the elderly. Br J Clin Pharmacol 18:207, 1984.

116. Jallad, N. S., et al.: Pharmacokinetics of single-dose oral and intramuscular ketorolac tromethamine in the young and elderly. J Clin Pharmacol 30:76, 1990.

117. Griffin, M. R., Ray, W. A., Schaffner, W.: Non-steroidal anti-inflammatory drug use and death from peptic ulcer in elderly persons. Ann Intern Med 109:359, 1988.

118. Van den Ouweland, F. A., Gribnau, F. W., Meyboom, R. H.: Congestive heart failure due to non-steroidal anti-inflammatory drugs in the elderly. Age Ageing 17:8, 1988.

119. Goodwin, J. S., Regan, M.: Cognitive dysfunction associated with naproxen and ibuprofen in the elderly. Arthritis Rheum 25:1013, 1982.

120. Ding, Y., Fredman, B., White, P. F.: Use of ketorolac and fentanyl during outpatient gynecologic surgery. Anesth Analg 77:205, 1993.

121. Fitzgerald, M.: Monoamines and descending control of nociception. Trends Neurosci 9:51, 1986.

122. Kuraishi, Y., et al.: Noradrenergic inhibition of the release of substance P from the primary afferents in the rabbit spinal dorsal horn. Brain Res 359:177, 1985.

123. Sweeney, M. I., White, T. D., Sawynok, J.: Involvement of adenosine in the spinal antinociceptive effects of morphine and noradrenaline. J Pharmacol Exp Ther 243:657, 1987.

124. Duan, J., Sawynok, J.: Enhancement of clonidine-induced analgesia by lesions induced with spinal and intracerebroventricular administration of 5,7-dihydroxytryptamine. Neuropharmacology 26:323, 1987.

125. Maze, M., Tranquilli, W.: Alpha-2 adrenoceptor agonists: defining the role in clinical anesthesia. Anesthesiology 74:581, 1991.

126. Eisenach, J., Detweiler, D., Hood, D.: Hemodynamic and analgesic actions of epidurally administered clonidine. Anesthesiology 78:277, 1993.

127. Racle, J. P., Benkhadra, A., Poy, J. Y.: Prolongation of isobaric bupivacaine spinal anesthesia with epinephrine and clonidine for hip surgery in the elderly. Anesth Analg 66:442, 1987.

128. Bonnet, F., et al.: Prevention of tourniquet pain by spinal isobaric bupivacaine with clonidine. Br J Anaesth 63:93, 1989.

129. Eisenach, J. C., Lysak, S. Z., Viscomi, C. M.: Epidural cloni-dine analgesia following surgery: phase I. Anesthesiology 71:640, 1989.
130. Gordh, T., Jr.: Epidural clonidine for treatment of postoperative pain after thoracotomy: a double-blind placebo-controlled study. Acta Anaesthesiol Scand 32:702, 1988.
131. Bonnet, F., et al.: Postoperative analgesia with extradural clonidine. Br J Anaesth 63:465, 1989.
132. Bonnet, F., et al.: Clonidine-induced analgesia in postoperative patients: epidural versus intramuscular administration. Anesthesiology 72:423, 1990.
133. Mendez, R., Eisensach, J. C., Kashtan, K.: Epidural clonidine analgesia after cesarean section. Anesthesiology 73:848, 1990.
134. Huntoon, M., Eisenach, J. C., Boese, P.: Epidural clonidine after cesarean section: Appropriate dose and effect of prior local anesthetic. Anesthesiology 76:187, 1992.
135. Segal, I. S., et al.: Clinical efficacy of oral-transdermal clonidine combinations during the perioperative period. Anesthesiology 74:220, 1991.
136. Aho, M. S., et al.: Effect of intravenously administered dexmedetomidine on pain after laparoscopic tubal ligation. Anesth Analg 73:112, 1991.
137. Peringer, E., Jenner, P., Marsden, C. D.: Effect of metoclopramide on turnover of brain dopamine, noradrenaline and 5-hydroxytryptamine. J Pharm Pharmacol 27:442, 1975.
138. Ramaswamy, S., Bapna, J. S.: Analgesic effect of metoclopramide and its mechanism. Life Sci 38:1289, 1986.
139. Ramaswamy, S., Lenin Kamatchi, G., Bapna, J. S.: Involvement of calcium in metoclopramide analgesia. IRCS J Med Sci 14:769, 1986.
140. Mueller, T. F., et al.: Metoclopramide (Primperan) in the treatment of ureterolithiasis: a prospective double-blind study of metoclopramide compared with morphatropin on ureteral colic. Urol Int 45:112, 1990.
141. Kandler, D., Lisander, B.: Analgesic action of metoclopramide in prosthetic hip surgery. Acta Anaesthesiol Scand 37:49, 1993.
142. Lisander, B.: Evaluation of the analgesic effect of metoclopramide after opioid-free analgesia. Br J Anaesth 70:631, 1993.

Chapter 35

ANESTHETIC MANAGEMENT OF THE CHEMICALLY DEPENDENT PATIENT

RICHARD McCAMMON, VINCENT J. COLLINS

The problem of substance abuse or chemical dependency in our society may seem remote to an anesthesiologist. Yet, it is with increasing frequency that an anesthesiologist may confront patients for elective surgery with substance abuse histories who may be chronically dependent on a drug(s) or on some type of substitution (i.e., clonidine, methadone) or antagonist (i.e., disulfiram, naltrexone) therapy or currently drug free (i.e., rehabilitated). Similarly, an anesthesiologist may be asked to help resuscitate or anesthetize the traumatized, acutely drug-intoxicated patient. This chapter thus focuses on pertinent medical and anesthetic considerations associated with these problems.

"Prolonged" substance abuse can lead to tolerance, psychologic, and/or physical dependence.[1] Tolerance is a state in which tissues become accustomed to the presence of a drug such that increased quantities of that drug become necessary to produce the effects observed with the original dose. Acquired tolerance often occurs with chronic substance abuse secondary to an increased rate of biotransformation of the drug due to stimulation of microsomal enzymes in the liver by the drug itself (i.e., pharmacokinetic changes). This accelerated rate of breakdown means that less pharmacologically active drug is available to act at receptor sites. Likewise, receptors may become less responsive (i.e., adapt) to the effects of a given blood level of an abused drug (i.e., pharmacodynamic changes). Additionally, substance abusers can develop clinically significant cross-tolerance to many anesthetic drugs or medications administered during the perioperative period. As a result, predicting analgesic or anesthetic requirements can be difficult. Most often, chronic substance abuse results in greater than normal analgesic and anesthetic requirements. In contrast, additive or even synergistic depressant drug interactions among drugs of the same class should be anticipated in the case of acute substance abuse. Finally, an anesthesiologist must appreciate that the level of tolerance is a dynamic, changing phenomenon. In the case of certain classes of drugs (i.e., barbiturates, narcotics), a relatively "normal" response may occur to clinically utilized doses by the peak or soon after completion of the withdrawal syndrome associated with that particular drug. Failure to appreciate this phenomenon can lead to a relative overdose with dramatic adverse consequences.

Physical dependence has developed when the presence of the drug in the body is necessary for normal physiologic function. In the case of certain substances (i.e., narcotics, barbiturates), an altered physiologic state develops in which the continued administration of the drug is necessary to prevent the appearance of a stereotypical syndrome, the withdrawal or abstinence syndrome, characteristic of that particular drug. In general, the withdrawal syndrome consists of a rebound in the physiologic systems modified by the drug itself. Knowing the physiologic impact of the abused substance on specific organ systems thus allows one to predict the manifestations of withdrawal from a given drug. Failure to recognize the withdrawal syndrome not only can confuse the diagnosis of perioperative events, but also may be life-threatening in its own right.

The timing and severity of withdrawal depend on the specific drug abused and the amount, duration, and continuity of abuse as well as the health and personality of the patient. In general, abrupt discontinuation of drugs with short elimination half-lives that are metabolized to inactive compounds results in a brief, intense withdrawal syndrome. Conversely, drugs with longer elimination half-lives and active metabolites are associated with more prolonged, milder withdrawal syndromes. Thus, when confronted with substance-abuse patients, an anesthesiologist must try to find out which drugs have been abused and to know their pharmacokinetic characteristics as well as their impact on organ system physiology.

CHRONIC SUBSTANCE ABUSE

Narcotics

Narcotics are well absorbed from the gastrointestinal tract as well as from subcutaneous and intramuscular injection sites. First-pass hepatic extraction and metabolism primarily account for the less intense effects of a given oral dose of several narcotics such as morphine as compared with their parenteral administration. Narcotics are most commonly abused orally, subcutaneously (i.e., skin popping), or intravenously for their euphorigenic or analgesic effects. Although narcotic and, in particular, heroin abuse seemed to have leveled off or declined in the last decade, a resurgence has occurred in the abuse of narcotics such as fentanyl and several of its analogues.

Certain medical problems can be confronted in the narcotic addict, particularly the intravenous abuser.[2] These problems include cellulitis, superficial skin abscesses and septic thrombophlebitis, tetanus (seen in skin poppers; additives such as quinine used to adulterate heroin lower the redox potential of tissues and promote growth of anaerobes), bacterial or fungal endocarditis, which may be associated with both right- and left-sided valvular lesions as well as both pulmonary (may result in pulmonary hypertension) and systemic septic emboli and infarctions, chronic atelectasis and aspiration pneumonitis, cirrhosis, hepatitis, acquired immunodeficiency syndrome, gastric atony, suppression of adrenal cortical function, varying states of malnutrition, a high incidence of both true and false-positive Venereal Disease Research Laboratory (VDRL) test results, pancytopenia, and rarely, transverse myelitis. Evidence of these medical problems should be sought in every narcotic addict because of the impact of these conditions on the conduct of anesthesia.

Tolerance may develop to some of the effects of narcotics (analgesic, sedative, emetic, euphorigenic, and respiratory depressant), but not to others (miotic, constipating).[1] Fortunately, as tolerance increases, the lethal dose of a narcotic also increases. In general, a high degree of cross-tolerance exists among drugs with morphine-like actions. Tolerance can wane rapidly, however, when patients are withdrawn from narcotics.

Physical dependence also occurs with chronic narcotic abuse, so it is important for the anesthesiologist to recognize the symptoms and signs of narcotic withdrawal. Failure to provide the narcotic addict with his or her "normal" dose of narcotic at frequent enough intervals can result in the development of an abstinence syndrome. Table 35–1 depicts the times of onset, peak intensity, and duration of withdrawal following the abrupt discontinuation of several commonly abused narcotics.[3] In contrast, the narcotic withdrawal syndrome develops a few minutes following parenteral administration of a narcotic antagonist and reaches its peak intensity within 30 minutes.

The narcotic abstinence syndrome predominantly consists of manifestations of adrenergic excess (Table 35–2). Initially, craving for the drug and anxiety develop. Next, yawning, diaphoresis, lacrimation, rhinorrhea, and restless sleep (yen) occur. As these symptoms worsen, mydriasis, piloerection (gooseflesh—origin of the term "cold turkey"), tremors, hot and cold flashes, muscle and bone aches, and anorexia ensue. These are followed by insomnia, hypertension, tachycardia, tachypnea, hyperpyrexia, abdominal cramps, and diarrhea. Muscle spasms and jerking of the legs ("kicking the habit") follow, and cardiovascular collapse has been reported. Seizures are rare, and their occurrence should make one think of other causes. Metabolic alterations of concern to the anesthesiologist that may occur during narcotic withdrawal include dehydration, lactic acidosis, and ketoacidosis.

Although withdrawal from narcotics is rarely life-threatening, it is unpleasant and confuses the diagnosis of perioperative events. Usually, however, regardless of the stage of withdrawal, one can abort the abstinence syndrome by reinstituting the abused narcotic or by substituting methadone. Indeed, it is recommended to give methadone (10 mg) intramuscularly or orally and to repeat doses (5 to 10 mg) every 2 to 6 hours as needed to control and to reverse symptoms.[3] Usually, only 20 to 40 mg of methadone are required in the first 24 hours.

Clonidine has also proved its beneficial role in narcotic withdrawal.[4] Clonidine is thought to act by replacing narcotic-mediated inhibition (absent during withdrawal)

Table 35–1. Time Course of Narcotic Withdrawal in Addicts

	Onset (hours)	Peak Intensity	Duration
Meperidine Dihydromorphine	2–6	8–12 H	4–5 D
Codeine Morphine Heroin	6–18	36–72 H	7–10 D
Methadone	24–48	3–21 D	6–7 WK

Antagonist Syndrome develops within minutes; peak intensity within 30 minutes

Table 35–2. Signs and Symptoms of Opiate Withdrawal

Early	Intermediate	Late
Anxiety	Mydriasis	Hyperpyrexia
Craving drug	Piloerection "goose flesh"	Vomiting
Yawning	Tremors	Diarrhea
Diaphoresis	Hot and cold flashes	Involuntary muscle spasm
Lacrimation	Muscle and bone aches	"Kicking the habit"
Rhinorrhea	Anorexia	Increases in:
"Yen" sleep	Insomnia	Blood sugar
	Restlessness	WBC
	Tachycardia	Cardiovascular collapse
	Hypertension	
	Tachypnea	
	Mild hyperthermia	

—Metabolic alterations: Dehydration, lactic acidosis, ketosis
—Seizures rare: Think of other causes

with α_2 agonist-mediated inhibition of the sympathetic nervous system in the brain. This unfortunately has led to self-administered withdrawal trials by addicts; thus, an anesthesiologist may on rare occasion be confronted with a patient manifesting significant side effects of clonidine. These side effects include dizziness, dysrhythmias, hypotension, congestive heart failure, and marked sedation.

The patient addicted to narcotics or receiving methadone or clonidine should have the narcotic requirements (or substitution therapy) maintained during the perioperative period. These patients should therefore receive a generous preoperative medication that includes their usual narcotic or equivalent dose of methadone.[5,6] No advantage exists in trying to maintain anesthesia with an opiate in a chronic narcotic addict. Doses of narcotics greatly in excess of normal are likely to be required to suppress adrenergic responses to surgical stress. A volatile anesthetic would seem to be a better choice; one must remember, however, that these patients are likely to have underlying liver disease. Similarly, agonist-antagonist analgesics and certainly pure narcotic antagonists should be avoided in these patients because their administration precipitates a withdrawal syndrome.[1,7]

In one large anecdotal series, few perioperative anesthetic problems were noted in narcotic addicts.[5] Fifteen to 20% of patients did, however, exhibit some symptoms or signs of withdrawal in the perioperative period. Likewise, a tendency for perioperative hypotension has been noted, the mechanism of which is unclear. Postulated mechanisms to which narcotic addiction may have been contributory include (1) inadequate intravascular fluid volume secondary to chronic infections and fever or malnutrition, (2) adrenocortical insufficiency,[8] and (3) inadequate levels of narcotics in the central nervous system (CNS), a manifestation of withdrawal.[9] Although the short-term administration of narcotics reduces anesthetic requirements, long-term narcotic usage leads to cross-tolerance to other CNS depressants. In fact, in morphine-addicted dogs, the minimum alveolar concentration (MAC) of halothane increased linearly during the course of addiction.[10] Similarly, rats made tolerant to morphine exhibited a decreased analgesic response to nitrous oxide (Fig. 35-1).[11] A report by one group of investigators, who noted that narcotic addicts needed higher doses of anesthetic agents than nonaddicted adults, lends support to the findings in these animal studies.[8]

These patients seem to have an exaggerated degree of postoperative pain. For reasons that are not entirely clear, satisfactory postoperative analgesia has purportedly been achieved when average doses of meperidine are administered in addition to the patients' usual daily intake of methadone or other narcotics.[12]

An anesthesiologist may also encounter rehabilitated narcotic addicts as well as patients receiving antagonist therapy such as naltrexone. In such patients, it would again seem wise to avoid narcotics and instead to use volatile agents. Postoperatively, serious consideration should be given to the use of transcutaneous electrical nerve stimulation (TENS) or a continuous regional anesthetic technique to provide postoperative pain relief. If narcotics are still required, only the smallest possible

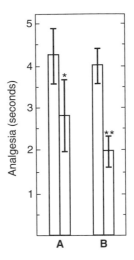

Fig. 35–1. Rats tolerant to morphine are cross-tolerant to nitrous oxide. Long-Evans rats (A, n = 10 per group) or Sprague-Dawley rats (B, n = 35 per group) were made tolerant to morphine as described in Methods. Open bars represent controls, darkened bars, morphine-treated rats. Nitrous oxide (80%) was administered to all animals and analgesia was measured by tail-flick latency. Results are means ± SE. *P < 0.05 compared with nontolerant rats. **P < 0.005 compared with nontolerant rats. Redrawn from Berkowitz, B. A., Finck, A. D., Hynes, M. D., Ngai, S. H.: Anesthesiology *51*:309, 1979.

dose should be employed. Conceivably, epidural or subarachnoid narcotics should be tried in lieu of parenterally administered narcotics.

Finally, regional anesthesia for surgery has a role in some of these patients. One should keep in mind, however, some of the previously noted medical problems such as the tendency to hypotension, the increased incidence of positive serology (hepatitis; viral disorders, including HIV), the occasional case of peripheral neuritis and phlebitis, and the rare occurrence of transverse myelitis.

CNS Depressants: Barbiturates and Benzodiazepines

Various barbiturates, nonbarbiturate sedative-hypnotics (meprobamate, glutethimide, methyprylon, methaqualone, and benzodiazepines are available, differing primarily in their lipid solubilities and elimination half-lives. These general CNS depressant drugs produce similar effects on mood and consciousness presumably by either direct γ-aminobutyric acid (GABA)-like actions or by enhancing the effects of this inhibitory neurotransmitter within the CNS.[1,13] These drugs are most commonly abused orally for their euphorigenic effects, for production of sleep, or to counteract the CNS stimulatory effects of other drugs. Tolerance occurs to most of the actions of this group of drugs, as does cross-tolerance to other general CNS depressants. Unfortunately, although the dosage of barbiturates required to produce sedative or euphorigenic effects increases quickly, the lethal dose does not increase at the same rate or magnitude.[1] Thus, a barbiturate abuser's margin of error decreases as the dose is increased to produce the desired effects.

Table 35–3. Time Course of CNS Depressant Withdrawal

	Onset	Peak Intensity	Duration
Short-acting barbiturates (Pento- and secobarbital) Meprobamate Methaqualone	12–24 H	2–3 D	7–10 D
		Convulsions-Delirium	
Long-acting barbiturates (Phenobarbital) Most benzodiazepines	2–3 D	6–10 D	10 D–WK

Physical dependence occurs with barbiturates as well as with most other sedative-hypnotic drugs. In contrast to narcotics, withdrawal from barbiturates is potentially life-threatening.[13,14] The expected times of onset, peak intensity, and duration of withdrawal for some commonly abused CNS depressants are listed in Table 35–3. Symptoms and signs of barbiturate withdrawal include anxiety, restlessness, tremors, weakness, hyperreflexia, insomnia, nausea and vomiting, tachycardia, diaphoresis, and postural hypotension (Table 35-4). The most serious problem associated with barbiturate withdrawal is the occurrence of grand mal seizures. Likewise, a toxic delirium (disorientation, hallucinations) often develops if the abstinence syndrome is inadequately treated. Hyperpyrexia and cardiovascular collapse have also been reported in severe cases. Many of the manifestations of barbiturate withdrawal, and in particular the seizures, are reportedly difficult to abort once they develop.

Prevention (i.e., maintenance of barbiturates) is thus the mainstay of treatment in the perioperative period. If withdrawal symptoms develop, the most success has been reported with "substitution" therapy with the intermediate-acting barbiturate, pentobarbital, in an initial oral dose range of 200 to 400 mg, with subsequent doses titrated to effect (sedation, slurred speech, ataxia). These doses should be titrated carefully, however, because tolerance has been reported to disappear rapidly (even by the peak of the abstinence syndrome itself) in these patients.[1,15] Phenobarbital and diazepam have also been used successfully to suppress the abstinence syndrome resulting from the withdrawal of barbiturates.

Long-term barbiturate abuse is not associated with major pathophysiologic changes in most organ systems.[2] Exceptions to this general statement include an increased incidence of emotional problems and respiratory disorders that may coexist in these patients and must be dealt with in their total perioperative care. In addition to the many problems previously described with intravenous narcotic abuse, intravenous barbiturate abuse also results in significant sclerosis of the venous system secondary to the high alkalinity of these compounds.

Although few hard data exist concerning the anesthetic management of long-term barbiturate abusers, several practical points are described in the literature. For example, cross-tolerance to the sedative effects of anesthetic drugs is described. Mice tolerant to thiopental awakened at higher tissue levels of barbiturates than control animals.[16] Similarly, anecdotal reports describe the need for increased doses of ultrashort-acting barbiturates for induction of anesthesia and shorter duration of sleep itself in long-term barbiturate abusers.[6,17] Although short-term administration of barbiturates has been shown to decrease anesthetic requirements,[16] to date no reports of increased MAC requirements in long-term barbiturate abusers have been published.[2] Another practical concern is that chronic barbiturate abuse leads to significant induction of the hepatic microsomal enzymes. Several drug interactions of concomitantly administered medications have been well described (warfarin, digitalis, phenytoin, volatile anesthetics), and these must be taken into consideration.

As with barbiturates, tolerance and physical dependence occur with chronic benzodiazepine abuse.[18] Symptoms of withdrawal generally occur later than with barbiturates and are less severe because of the longer elimination half-lives of most benzodiazepines and because many are metabolized to pharmacologically active metabolites (these also have prolonged elimination half-lives). Benzodiazepines do not significantly induce microsomal enzymes. Anesthetic considerations in long-term benzodiazepine abusers are otherwise similar to those described previously in long-term barbiturate abusers.

Table 35–4. Characteristics of Barbiturate Withdrawal Syndrome and General Depressant Withdrawal Syndrome

Early	Late
Anxiety, irritability	1–4 Grand mal convulsions in up to 80% of patients
Tremors, restlessness, weakness	
Nausea, vomiting, anorexia	
Sleep disturbances	Status epilepticus
Hyperreflexia	Toxic delirium
Dizziness, visual distortions	Hallucinosis
Muscle spasms, abd. cramps	Hyperpyrexia
Postural hypotension	Cardiovascular collapse
Tachycardia	
Diaphoresis	

CNS Stimulants: Amphetamines and Cocaine

Some of the currently abused CNS stimulants include amphetamine (Benzedrine), dextroamphetamine (Dexedrine), methamphetamine (Desoxyn), phenmetrazine (Preludin), methylphenidate (Ritalin), diethylpropion (Tepanil), and cocaine. In addition, abuse of newer amphetamine analogues such as 3,4-methylene-dioxymetham-phetamine (MDMA, "Ecstasy") and methylenedioxyethamphetamine (MDEA, "EVE"), has now surfaced as a significant health hazard.[19]

Amphetamines exert their pharmacologic effects either directly or indirectly by stimulating the release of catecholamines from or inhibiting the reuptake of catecholamines into the nerve terminals in the CNS and peripheral sympathetic nerve endings.[2,20] As such, they increase cortical alertness and electrical activity throughout the brain. Such an alerting effect on the CNS results in the decreased need for sleep and food—two of the primary reasons for abuse of these agents. Similarly, amphetamines can produce a feeling of increased ability and well-being. Amphetamines are most commonly abused orally or, in the case of methamphetamine, intravenously. Amphetamines in general are slowly metabolized by hepatic enzymes.

Long-term amphetamine use is associated with tolerance (particularly as regards appetite suppression and euphorigenic and sympathomimetic effects) and psychologic dependence.[1] Although most authorities do not believe that physical dependence occurs, discontinuation of administration after long-term use results in depression, prolonged sleep, lassitude, fatigue, suicidal ideations, and hyperphagia. Neither fatalities nor convulsions have, however, been reported as the result of abrupt amphetamine withdrawal.[2]

Long-term use of amphetamines results in a depletion of body stores of catecholamines. Such depletion may manifest in the form of somnolence or other abnormal sleeping disorders and anxiety or psychotic-like states. Other physiologic abnormalities reported with long-term amphetamine abuse include hypertension, a variety of dysrhythmias, and malnutrition. A rare medical problem associated with amphetamine abuse is that of necrotizing angiitis with microvascular damage to several organ systems.[21] Intravenous amphetamine abuse may be associated with the same problems as noted previously with intravenous narcotic or barbiturate abuse.

Reports in the literature regarding the anesthetic management of chronic amphetamine abusers are sparse. Consideration must of course be given to the potential consequences of the foregoing concomitant medical problems. Unique to anesthesia, Johnston and co-workers found that long-term administration of dextroamphetamine, 5 mg/kg for 7 days, decreased MAC for halothane in dogs by 21 ± 3%.[22] Conceivably, one should similarly anticipate (1) an attenuated response to indirect-acting vasopressors and (2) a prolonged or unexpected duration of somnolence following general anesthesia.

Cocaine became "the recreational drug of choice" in the 1980s.[23] Cocaine is a naturally occurring alkaloid derived from the leaves of the coca plant (*Erythroxylon coca*). Its CNS-stimulant effects may result from direct action of cocaine on dopamine receptors or from release or potentiation of dopamine centrally.[24] Similarly, some of cocaine's pharmacologic effects arise secondary to its ability to prevent uptake of norepinephrine back into postganglionic sympathetic nerve endings.

Cocaine produces a sense of euphoria, well-being, and generalized stimulation. It is most commonly sold as a powder (i.e., as a hydrochloride salt) and is often diluted with other compounds. Although most often snorted, it may also be inhaled, taken orally, or abused intravenously. When snorted intranasally, cocaine limits its own absorption by causing vasoconstriction of the nasal mucous membranes. Plasma drug concentrations peak at 30 to 60 minutes.[23] The hydrochloride preparation is not as suitable for smoking because heat causes it to decompose. Likewise, oral absorption of cocaine is significantly reduced by gastric hydrolysis. Most cocaine is metabolized within 2 hours in the liver to its principal metabolite, benzoylecgonine, which is promptly excreted in the urine. It can also be metabolized by plasma cholinesterases.

Smoking (inhalation) of cocaine "free-base" preparations (rock, crack) is an especially dangerous form of cocaine abuse.[25,26] "Free-base" cocaine is prepared by first mixing the cocaine hydrochloride preparation with an alkaline solution, then adding a solvent such as ether. The mixture separates into two layers; the top layer contains cocaine dissolved in the solvent. The solvent mixture can then be evaporated, leaving relatively pure cocaine crystals. The resulting "free-base" preparations not only are purer but also are not destroyed by moderate heating and are thereby more suitable for smoking. Smoking delivers large quantities of cocaine to the vascular bed of the lung and produces an effect comparable to that of intravenous injection. Higher blood levels are thus achieved and account for the great increase in cocaine-related fatalities reported.[27] Intracranial hemorrhage, both intracerebral and subarachnoid, has been associated with fatalities.[28]

Tolerance can develop to the euphorigenic effects of cocaine, although this is an inconsistent observation. Although psychologic dependence develops with long-term use, physical dependence per se does not occur. Symptoms associated with abstinence after long-term cocaine abuse include prolonged sleep, fatigue, increased hunger, and depression.[27]

Medical problems of consequence associated with long-term cocaine abuse include nasal septal atrophy, nervousness, agitated behavior, paranoid thinking, heightened reflexes, and a parkonsonian-like syndrome. Although no anesthetic interactions have been reported to date in patients chronically abusing cocaine (that is, those not acutely intoxicated), the same considerations as discussed for the chronic amphetamine abuser would seem to be pertinent.

Psychedelics: Lysergic Acid Diethylamide[1,2,29]

Lysergic acid diethylamide (LSD) is an indolealkylamide similar in structure to ergonovine. It is the prototypical drug for a group of drugs that includes psilocybin, psilocin, dimethyltryptamine (DMT), diethyltryptamine (DET), and mescaline. Most often abused for their "mind-expanding" effects, these drugs produce alterations in perception, thought, feeling, and behavior. LSD is relatively easily synthesized as a clear liquid, and when abused, it is usually placed on some material for oral ingestion. Its exact mechanism of action is uncertain, although multiple sites in the CNS seem to be involved.[1] The usual hallucinogenic dose is 20 to 200 μg. Onset of sympathomimetic effects occur about 20 to 40 minutes after oral ingestion of LSD and consists of mydriasis, tachycardia, hypertension, hyperthermia, piloerection, and increased alertness. These physiologic effects last about 6 hours. Psychic effects become evident 1 to 2 hours after ingestion and may last up to 8 to 12 hours.[30] LSD has a relatively short half-life (3 hours) and is essentially totally inactivated in the liver.

Tolerance to the behavioral effects of LSD occurs rapidly, whereas tolerance to the cardiovascular effects is less pronounced. Although a high degree of psychologic dependence occurs, patients have no evidence of physical dependence or withdrawal symptoms when LSD is abruptly discontinued.

No major physiologic derangements associated with long-term LSD abuse have been described in most organ systems. An exception is the immune system, in which long-term LSD abuse may inhibit or disrupt antibody formation. Likewise, LSD has an in vitro anticholinesterase effect.[31] It has thus been suggested that succinylcholine and ester-type local anesthetics be used with caution in such patients, although data to support this contention are scant.[12] Flashbacks are known to occur in about 1 to 2% of LSD users. Anesthesia and surgery have been reported to "precipitate" such responses, the mechanism of which is unclear.[2] In the event of flashback or panic reaction, diazepam is reported to be efficacious. No other interactions with anesthetic drugs have been described.

Cannabis: Marihuana and Hashish

Cannabis is the genus of plants that produce hemp. These plants contain psychoactive compounds known as cannabinoids. Cannabis is primarily abused because it produces feelings of well-being, relaxation, and emotional disinhibition. Marijuana is a general term indicating any part of the hemp plants with psychoactive compounds. Hashish more specifically refers to the resin extracted from the tops of the hemp plant (these contain a higher percentage of active constituents). δ-9-Tetrahydrocannabinol (THC) is the primary psychoactive constituent in cannabis. Its exact mechanism of action in the CNS is unknown, although effects on the hypothalamus and the striate bodies are prominent.[32]

Cannabis is usually abused by smoking the plant, although it may be taken orally and retain its effects. Smoking increases bioavailability 5 to 10 times over that of ingestion. Rarely, boiled marijuana may be abused intravenously. This latter route of abuse has been associated with gastroenteritis, hepatitis, acute renal failure, anemia, and thrombocytopenia. Cannabinoids are primarily metabolized in the liver and eliminated in the feces.

Tolerance to most of the psychoactive effects of THC has been reported. Although physical dependence is not believed to occur, abrupt cessation after long-term use is characterized by mild symptoms including irritability, restlessness, anorexia, insomnia, sweating, nausea, vomiting, and diarrhea.

Long-term cannabis abuse leads to increased tar deposits in the lung, impaired pulmonary defense mechanisms, and decreased pulmonary functions.[33] As such, an increased incidence of sinusitis and bronchitis has been reported, as has an increased incidence of lung cancer. Additionally, long-term abuse may provoke seizures in individuals so predisposed. No major interactions with anesthetic drugs have been reported in the chronic abuser who is not acutely intoxicated at the time of anesthesia.

Cyclohexylamines: Phencyclidine (PCP) and Ketamine

These drugs are still commonly abused for their euphorigenic and mind-expanding properties. Such compounds are easily manufactured in clandestine laboratories and are available in forms that are usually taken orally, smoked, or injected intravenously.[1] Their exact mechanisms of action are unknown although they are believed to interact with several neurotransmitter systems. Phencyclidine is predominantly metabolized by the liver and excreted in the urine. It can also undergo significant enterohepatic circulation.

Tolerance to phencyclidine and related compounds does occur with long-term abuse. Physical dependence per se does not seem to occur. Long-term PCP abuse has not been reported to result in any major organ system derangements or in any interactions with anesthetic drugs.

ACUTE SUBSTANCE ABUSE

Patients acutely intoxicated with various substances often suffer traumatic injuries and thus may present on an emergency basis to the operating room. Likewise, drug ingestions account for a large proportion of the successful or attempted suicides that occur annually in the United States.[34] Similarly, approximately 5 million poisonings occur each year in this country.[35,36]

An anesthesiologist should therefore have a rudimentary understanding of the principles of management in these circumstances. Initially, one should establish the level of consciousness and evaluate and stabilize the patient's respiratory and cardiovascular status. If the level of consciousness is depressed, this should be quickly assessed and recorded, based on the Glasgow coma scale or similar schema.

Concomitantly, attention should be focused on the patient's respiratory and circulatory status, keeping in mind that the principles of management of drug overdose or poisonings are similar irrespective of the drugs taken. If the patient's level of consciousness is reduced or if the gag reflex is absent or diminished, a cuffed endotracheal tube should be placed to protect the lungs from aspiration. Likewise, mechanical ventilation may be necessary if hypoventilation is present.

The extent of cardiovascular monitoring and support is dictated by individual circumstances. The presence of hypotension may reflect direct cardiac depression from the ingested drug, venous pooling, or decreased intravascular fluid volume due to increased capillary permeability. The resulting hypotension may respond to maneuvers as basic as head-down positioning and volume infusion, or it may require the addition of an inotrope or vasopressor.

Body temperature should also be monitored and at times requires aggressive treatment. Hypothermia frequently accompanies unconsciousness due to narcotic or barbiturate overdoses. In contrast, the CNS stimulants and some of the hallucinogens may result in severe life-threatening hyperthermia.

Once supportive care has been instituted and the patient's cardiopulmonary status has stabilized, attention should be turned to a more thorough historical, physical, and laboratory evaluation. One should attempt to obtain as much information as possible from family, associates, and police records regarding the nature and quantity of substances ingested and the time of ingestion. This latter piece of information is important when one remembers that overdoses or poisonings are a dynamic process with ongoing absorption and elimination of the drugs. As such, knowing the time of ingestion affects decisions regarding the efficacy of various modes of therapy that can be employed to decrease absorption or promote elimination of the drugs and the interpretation of blood levels (as with acetaminophen) of various drugs. Nevertheless, the history is often sparse and just as often barely credible. Just as significant, however, and usually more reliable is the patient's past medical history. One must establish the physiologic status of various organ systems and thus their ability to withstand the toxic effects as well as to eliminate the ingested toxins.

Although the physical examination is often nonspecific, clues to the particular type of drug ingested based on certain distinctive clinical findings may be present.[37] Likewise, the toxicology laboratory may be of help in identifying the drugs ingested. Thus, samples of blood, urine, and gastric aspirate should be collected for possible toxicologic analysis. One should be cautioned, however, that results of toxicology studies are usually not immediately available, and different laboratories have a wide range of reliability. Similarly, the significance of a given blood level in a patient varies considerably, depending primarily on that patient's own tolerance level for the particular drugs. Indeed, only with a few drugs, namely, acetaminophen and salicylates, do blood levels have an impact on management.

Moreover, many conditions other than drug overdoses or poisonings result in stupor or coma.[34,37] For example, a host of metabolic derangements can closely mimic drug-induced coma. Thus, laboratory testing should include determinations of electrolytes, blood glucose and ketones, blood urea nitrogen, creatine phosphokinase, liver function tests, and arterial blood gases. The physical examination should also focus on findings that help distinguish between diffuse pathologic processes, such as produced by drug intoxications, endogenous metabolic disturbances, or infections, and focal pathologic processes due to a structural mass lesion such as intracranial hematoma, brain stem infarct, brain abscess, or tumor. In general, unconsciousness due to a diffuse disorder lacks localizing signs (symmetric motor or neurologic findings).

After ensuring adequate ventilatory and cardiovascular support and after completion of a more thorough examination and laboratory evaluation, attention can be focused on measures to prevent any further ongoing absorption of the ingested substance or to promote elimination of the toxins. This is normally accomplished by inducing emesis or performing gastric lavage with the subsequent administration of activated charcoal and cathartics.

For example, approximately 70% of poisonings occur by ingestion. Whether emesis should be induced depends on certain factors including the specific substance ingested (as well as the form in which the drug was dispensed; i.e., liquids are absorbed more rapidly than solids, enteric-coated or timed-release products are absorbed more slowly than standard capsules or tablets), the time elapsed since ingestion (for several drugs induction of emesis is only indicated if the drug was ingested within the previous 2 to 4 hours), the status of gastrointestinal motility (certain drugs, such as narcotics, anticholinergics, and tricyclic antidepressants, and food slow motility and thus absorption), and the level of alertness of the patient. Emesis should not be induced if the patient is not awake or easily arousable with intact protective gag and laryngeal reflexes or if the substance ingested was caustic or corrosive or a petroleum product. Syrup of ipecac is used most commonly to induce emesis because it is safe and generally effective. Forceful emesis generally occurs within 15 to 20 minutes after oral administration of syrup of ipecac.

Gastric lavage is indicated when attempts to induce emesis fail or when the patient's level of consciousness is sufficiently depressed to make aspiration with induced emesis a risk. When the gag reflex is depressed, gastric lavage should not be done until a cuffed endotracheal tube is in place. When lavage is undertaken, as large a bore of tube as feasible should be used to assist in removal of partially dissolved tablets or capsules. Contraindications to lavage include the presence of convulsions and the ingestion of caustic substances or petroleum distillate hydrocarbon products.

Following emesis or lavage, activated charcoal can be given to absorb any drug remaining in the gastrointestinal tract. This compound binds organic compounds and creates a stable complex that does not dissociate. It is not effective for rapidly absorbed compounds such as cyanide, heavy metals, agents ingested in gram quantities (i.e., ethanol), and complex compounds (i.e., petroleum distillates). A cathartic is also often employed to try to speed the rate of transfer of a toxic product through the intestinal tract and thus to limit overall absorption from the small and large bowels. Cathartics may be particularly useful in treating ingestions of drugs that slow peristalsis.

In certain drug overdoses, one may enhance elimination of the drug by forced diuresis and ion trapping. Forced diuresis is accomplished by the parenteral administration of large fluid volumes as well as by the use of osmotic agents and diuretics. This produces an increase in glomerular filtration rate and renal tubular flow that results in an increased filtration of the drug and a decreased reabsorption in the distal tubules. Similarly, ionized diuresis is based on the principle that a drug in its ionized form crosses lipid membranes poorly. Alkalinization of the urine increases the ionized fraction of weak acids (i.e., aspirin or phenobarbital) and decreases their renal tubular absorption. In a similar fashion, urinary excretion of weak bases (i.e., amphetamines or phencyclidine) may be enhanced by acidification of the urine. Little incontrovertible evidence exists of the benefits of forced diuresis and ion trapping, however. Likewise, all these methods carry some risk of fluid overload or iatrogenically induced electrolyte abnormalities (i.e., most commonly hypokalemia).

Utilization of dialysis and hemoperfusion techniques can also prove invaluable in select cases. For example, dialysis may be considered when normal excretory pathways are compromised (i.e., in renal or hepatic failure). Hemoperfusion (i.e., charcoal or resin) is the newest and seemingly more effective method of removing toxins. Adverse effects are minimal (hemolysis, thrombocytopenia), although clinical experience with this technique is still in a preliminary stage.

Last, although the majority of toxic ingestions may be managed by conservative supportive measures, specific and effective antidotes are available for certain toxins. Several specific drug overdoses are now reviewed.

Narcotic Overdose

The manifestations of narcotic overdose most often occur in the CNS and cardiovascular systems.[1,38,39] The CNS manifestations run the gamut from euphoria, dysphoria, drowsiness, and mental clouding to stupor and coma. In the case of some narcotics (meperidine, propoxyphene, pentazocine), convulsions can occur. Respiratory depression initially occurs as a slow ventilatory rate with normal to increased tidal volume. The pupils are usually miotic. As blood levels rise, apnea ensues, and the pupils may dilate because of the hypoxic insult.

The primary cardiovascular manifestations are orthostatic hypotension and syncope due to narcotic-induced peripheral vasodilation of capacitance vessels. Narcotic-induced bradycardia, hypoxemia, and hypercarbia further aggravate hypotensive states. Additionally, in heroin abusers, significant myocardial depression may result from the commonly used adulterant quinine. On occasion, pulmonary edema occurs in patients who take an overdose of narcotics (most often heroin) and has been attributed to an "anaphylactoid" reaction. The cause is poorly understood, but arterial hypoxemia, hypotension, neurogenic mechanisms, and drug-related pulmonary endothelial damage are considerations.[1] Last, gastric atony is a near-universal accompaniment to acute narcotic intoxication. Fatal narcotic overdoses are most frequently an accidental outcome of the dangerous fluctuations in the purity of street products or of the combination of narcotics with other CNS depressants.

Naloxone is a specific narcotic antagonist that should be administered intravenously (0.2 to 0.4 mg every 2 to 5 minutes; 0.01 mg/kg in infants) up to three doses or until ventilatory rate increases to at least 12 breaths/min.[38,39] When naloxone is given, however, it must be titrated to effect to avoid overreversal and subsequent sympathetic nervous system hyperactivity. Moreover, the half-life of naloxone (1 to 2 hours) is shorter than that of most narcotics, and repeated administration or a naloxone infusion may be necessary.[1]

Otherwise, treatment and anesthetic management of acutely narcotic-intoxicated patients presenting for resuscitation and surgery are largely supportive. Supplemental oxygen and airway control are essential. In more severe overdoses or in the presence of narcotic-induced pulmonary edema, controlled mechanical ventilation and positive end-expiratory pressure therapy may be required. Narcotic-induced hypotension most often responds to measures as simple as head-down positioning, intravenous fluid challenges, and, on occasion, anticholinergics or vasoactive drugs. Because of the associated gastric atony, all such patients should be treated with full-stomach precautions. Finally, acute opiate intoxication is associated with decreased anesthetic (MAC) requirements.[10]

CNS Depressants: Barbiturates and Benzodiazepines

CNS depression is the primary pharmacologic effect of barbiturate or benzodiazepine overdose.[1,38,39] In the case of barbiturates, blood levels correlate well with the degree of CNS depression. Such depression may manifest as somnolence, slurred speech, ataxia, and disinhibition (lability of mood, irritability, and combativeness). Higher blood levels result in loss of pharyngeal and deep tendon reflexes and coma. No specific antidote or antagonist exists to reverse this CNS depression, and the use of nonspecific CNS stimulants is to be discouraged in such situations. Barbiturates also cause significant respiratory depression, particularly if taken in large doses or by patients with coexisting lung disease. As with narcotic overdoses, control of the airway and support of ventilation are essential.

Acute overdoses of barbiturates may also be associated with cardiovascular depression due to central vasomotor depression, direct myocardial depression, and an increase in venous capacitance. Barbiturate-induced hypotension usually responds to correction of coexisting hypoxemia or hypercarbia, to head-down positioning, and to volume infusion. Occasionally, vasopressors or inotropes may be required. A predictable additive or even synergistic depression occurs between CNS depressants and anesthetic drugs known to depress the CNS and cardiovascular systems. Hypothermia is a frequent occurrence in CNS depressant overdoses and may necessitate aggressive therapy to warm the patient. Acute renal failure due to hypotension and rhabdomyolysis may also occur.

Forced diuresis and alkalinization of the urine promote elimination of phenobarbital, but these measures are less useful with many of the other CNS depressants. Induced emesis or gastric lavage is indicated if less than 6 hours have elapsed since the time of suspected ingestion. This should be followed by the instillation of activated charcoal and a cathartic.

An acute overdose with benzodiazepines is much less likely to produce fatal respiratory depression as compared with a barbiturate overdose.[18] The combination of benzodiazepines and other CNS depressants such as alcohol have proved lethal, however. In general, supportive measures suffice in the case of benzodiazpine overdoses. Physostigmine is sometimes efficacious in reversing disorientation or hallucinations resulting from benzediazepine overdoses. In the future, specific benzodiazepine antagonists will provide an obvious method of treatment of benzodiazepine overdose.

CNS Stimulants: Amphetamines and Cocaine

Amphetamines in toxic doses cause anxiety, a psychotic state, and progressive CNS irritability manifesting as hyperactivity, hyperreflexia, and occasionally convulsions.[1,38,39] Other physiologic effects include an increase in blood pressure (case reports of subarachnoid hemorrhage), an increase in heart rate, dysrhythmias, a decrease in gastrointestinal motility, mydriasis, diaphoresis, and hyperthermia. Metabolic imbalances such as dehydration, lactic acidosis, and ketosis have also been reported.

In the case of acute oral amphetamine intoxications, emesis and lavage are effective and should be followed by instillation of activated charcoal and a cathartic. Phenothiazines and other major tranquilizers have been reported to antagonize many of the acute CNS effects of amphetamines. Similarly, diazepam is reported to be useful to control amphetamine-induced seizures. Acidification of the urine promotes elimination of amphetamines.

Anesthetic considerations in the patient acutely intoxicated with amphetamines include the admonitions to (1) monitor body temperature and aggressively treat hyperthermia if present; (2) appreciate the well-documented associated increases in anesthetic (MAC) requirements; indeed, in animals, acute intravenous administration of dextroamphetamine produces a dose-related increase in anesthetic requirements for halothane (Fig. 35–2);[22] (3) appreciate the likelihood of coexisting hypovolemia and metabolic derangements; (4) use with caution direct-acting vasopressors and drugs that sensitize the heart to catecholamines; and (5) aggressively treat convulsions (barbiturates, benzodiazepines), hypertension, and dysrhythmias if present.

Many of the manifestations and anesthetic considerations arising from acute cocaine intoxication are similar to those of acute amphetamine intoxication. Because of its rapid metabolism, anesthesiologists are rarely confronted with acutely intoxicated cocaine abusers. Nevertheless, increased anesthetic requirements for halothane following acute intravenous administration of cocaine in dogs are believed to reflect elevated levels of catecholamines in the CNS (Fig. 35–3).[40] This effect was dose related and of relatively short duration (less than 24 hours). Similarly, the arrhythmogenic dose of epinephrine was significantly decreased in dogs given cocaine, 2 mg/kg intravenously, during halothane-nitrous oxide-oxygen anesthesia.[41] In contrast, cocaine (1.5 mg/kg), administered topically in human patients before nasal intubation and after 25 minutes of anesthesia with 0.5% halothane and 60%-40% nitrous oxide-oxygen, caused no apparent increase in heart rate, arterial pressure, or cardiac index, nor did it result in any dysrhythmias.[42]

Marked hyperpyrexia can also follow cocaine intoxication and results from a generalized vasoconstriction, from the increased skeletal muscle activity, and possibly from an effect on CNS centers that regulate temperature. Aggressive treatment of cocaine-induced seizures, with par-

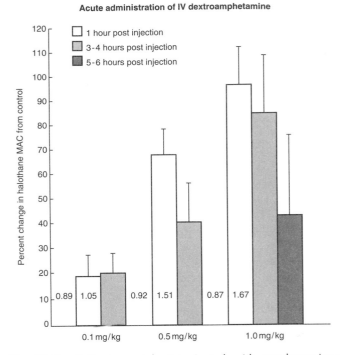

Acute administration of IV dextroamphetamine

☐ 1 hour post injection
▨ 3-4 hours post injection
▨ 5-6 hours post injection

Fig. 35–2. Patients acutely intoxicated with amphetamines have an associated increase in anesthetic requirements (MAC values) for inhalation agents as demonstrated for halothane. The increase in MAC values is related to the doses of amphetamine. Further, with the larger doses, there is a prolongation of the time during which the increase in anesthetic is necessary for the maintenance of anesthesia. Data from Johnson, R. R., et al.: Anesthesiology 36:357, 1972.

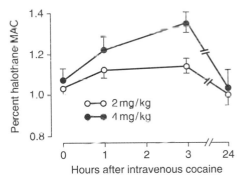

Fig. 35–3. Intravenous injection of cocaine (2 and 4 mg/kg) produces a dose-related increase in dog halothane MAC as measured 1 and 3 hours later. Anesthetic requirements were not different from control measurements 24 hours following cocaine. Data adapted from Stoelting, R. K., Creasser, C. W., Martz, R. C.: Effect of cocaine administration on halothane MAC in dogs. Anesth Analg 54:422, 1975; redrawn from Stoelting, R. K., Dierdorf, S. F. (eds.): Anesthesia and Co-Existing Disease, 2nd Ed. New York, Churchill Livingstone, 1988.

ticular attention focused on the correction of the accompanying acidosis, is of prime importance.[43] Either a barbiturate or diazepam should be effective against seizure activity.

Finally, several recent studies and clinical reports have demonstrated that acute cocaine administration can result in dramatic decreases in coronary artery blood flow.[44] Presumably, such cocaine-induced vasospasm is responsible for the reports of angina and myocardial infarction that have been described in cocaine-intoxicated patients.

Psychedelics: Lysergic Acid Diethylamide

LSD, in addition to its euphorigenic and hallucinogenic properties, causes stimulatory effects on the sympathetic nervous system (via stimulation of the hypothalamus) including mydriasis, piloerection, tremor, hyperreflexia, and increases in temperature, heart rate, and blood pressure. On rare occasions, LSD produces convulsions and respiratory arrest.[1,2] LSD can likewise produce an acute panic reaction characterized by hyperactivity, extreme lability of mood, and illogical reasoning patterns. This syndrome typically lasts 24 to 48 hours. Overt psychosis can also occur in which the patient loses touch with reality.

In humans, no deaths directly attributable to the use of these drugs have been reported. Often, however, these patients suffer traumatic injuries that may go undetected because of the intrinsic analgesic activity of LSD and the inability of the patient to perceive the injury. LSD is reported to prolong the analgesic and ventilatory depressant responses to narcotics; thus, caution in the use of narcotics seems warranted.[45] Diazepam or other sedatives may be needed to control the patient's anxiety. Blood pressure, heart rate and rhythm, and temperature should be monitored, and abnormalities may need to be aggressively treated. Similarly, an exaggerated response to sympathomimetics is predictable. Finally, one should avoid any other CNS delirants because of the already ongoing CNS effects of these drugs.

Cannabis: Marijuana and Hashish

Acute cannabis (THC) intoxication results in signs of increased sympathetic nervous system activity and inhibition of the parasympathetic nervous system. Pharmacologic effects occur within minutes after smoking begins, whereas plasma concentrations reach their peak at 10 to 30 minutes, generally lasting no more than 2 to 3 hours. Oral administration delays onset of effects to 30 to 60 minutes, peak effects to 2 to 3 hours, and duration of effects to 3 to 5 hours.[1] The most consistent cardiovascular changes are an increase in resting heart rate and orthostatic hypotension. Drowsiness is a frequent side effect.

Treatment of acute THC intoxication is primarily supportive. THC significantly prolonged pentobarbital sleeping time in rats[46] and ketamine sleeping time in mice.[47] Similarly, THC can potentiate the respiratory depression of narcotics (Fig. 35–4).[48] Moreover, barbiturates intensify the hallucinations caused by THC.[2] Clinically, however, this admonition only applies to intermediate-acting barbiturates and not to the ultrashort-acting barbiturates used for induction of anesthesia. Finally, two groups of investigators have shown in animal models that the short-term administration of THC can reduce the MAC requirements of inhalation agent[49,50] (Fig. 35–5).

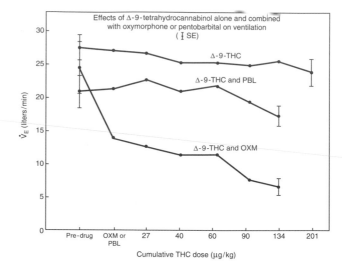

Fig. 35–4. Ventilatory effects of δ-9-tetrahydrocannabinol (THC) alone and preceded by oxymorphone or pentobarbital in three groups of seven to nine subjects. Some subjects did not complete all THC doses. PETCO$_2$ of each subject was held constant at approximately 50 mm Hg. THC-alone data are from a previous study. Redrawn from Johnstone, R. E., Lief, P. L., Kulp, R. A., Smith, T. C.: Anesthesiology 42:674, 1975.

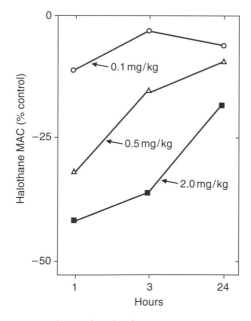

Fig. 35-5. A dose-related decrease in dog anesthetic requirements for halothane (MAC) after intravenous injection of δ-9-tetrahydrocannabinol (THC). Data are plotted as percentage of decrease from control. Changes after THC 0.1 mg/kg were not statistically significant (P > 0.05). MAC was significantly increased (P < 0.05) 1 hour following THC 0.5 mg/kg, and at 1.3 and 24 hours following THC 2.0 mg/kg. From Stoelting, R. K., et al.: Anesthesiology 38:521, 1973.

Cyclohexylamines: Phencyclidine and Ketamine

Acute phencyclidine toxicity is largely dose related. Mild to moderate intoxication causes agitation as well as combativeness and violent behavior. Speech is often slowed and slurred. The patient's eyes are open, but they have a "blank stare." Nystagmus and ataxia are common. Muscle tone is increased, and frank rigidity can occur. Other features include flushing, hypersalivation, facial grimacing, and grunting noises. Additionally, signs of increased CNS activity predominate, including tachycardia, hypertension, diaphoresis, and hyperthermia. More severe intoxication can result in profound CNS and respiratory depression and coma. Muscle rigidity becomes even more pronounced, and seizures may occur. Rhabdomyolysis may likewise result from the muscle spasms and hyperthermia.

The patient should be placed in a calm, quiet environment with minimal external stimuli. No specific antidote exists. Benzodiazepines may be used to control agitation. Supportive care in the form of airway control, support of ventilation, and treatment of seizures and the manifestations of CNS hyperactivity when appropriate is warranted. Forced diuresis and acidification of the urine promote PCP elimination.

Aside from the foregoing medical consideratons associated with acute cyclohexylamine intoxication, unique anesthetic considerations include (1) a well-documented decrease in anesthetic (MAC) requirements[51] and (2) an enhanced response to vasopressors. Similarly, anecdotal reports attest to the difficulty in managing patients acutely intoxicated with PCP or related drugs under regional anesthetic techniques.[2]

MANAGEMENT OF THE ALCOHOL-DEPENDENT PATIENT

Alcoholism is a psychosomatic disease. It exists when the intake of alcohol produces a problem. The problem may be personal (physical health, socioeconomics) or a public health issue. An alcoholic is a human being escaping from intolerable stresses.[52,53]

Incidence

About 6% of American males are problem drinkers, and almost an equal percentage of women are as well; that is, 20 million people are afflicted. Of these, 2 million are chronic inebriates.

Definition

The difficulty with formulating a simple definition is that the criteria for the condition remain indefinite. One general definition of the condition is that of Gordon,[54] which states that alcoholism is the use of alcohol as a beverage, irrespective of time, amount, periodicity, or practice. The World Health Organization Expert Committee defines alcoholism as any form of drinking that goes beyond traditional or customary use. Of practical importance, and leaving aside psychosocial factors, is to consider the use of alcohol in quantitative terms. A biologic gradient can then be recognized, and this serves a useful purpose in understanding pathophysiologic consequences.

Pathogenesis

As a complex disease with multiple characteristics, alcoholism may be considered to develop as follows: life stresses coupled with psychologic factors → personal problems → alcoholic solution → habituation → psychologic dependence → physical dependence → functional disturbances → organic changes → organic deterioration.

Classification[54]

The extent of alcohol use and the corresponding effects provide a biologic gradient of alcoholism from nothing to maximum. The entire population can thus be classified into five groups[54]:

1. Abstainers: a *large fraction* of the population is first distinguished as those who abstain from alcohol.
2. Social or cultural consumers: a *second major part* of the population consists of those who take alcohol customarily in diet or social use, but in limited amounts.
3. *Symptomatic alcoholics* are those who consume alcohol to deal with a current problem but not regularly or systematically.
4. *Addictive alcoholics* represent those with an overpowering psychologic craving and physiologic need for alcohol. Both tolerance and dependence phenomena are present. Withdrawal produces the abstinence syndrome, which leads to increased dosage and further total dependence. This state is produced by consumption of approximately 1 pint of whiskey (80 proof) per day or about 150 g of alcohol over an extended but variable period. This amount is approximately equivalent to 12 to 15 standard cocktails. Usually, if the subject is in otherwise good health, no organic disorder is produced (1 pint of 100 proof provides 190 g of alcohol).
5. *Advanced alcoholics* are those in whom the consumption of alcohol has produced organic or psychic deterioration. Subjects who consume more than 1 pint and up to 1 quart of whiskey, usually an intake of 250 g of alcohol, invariably develop organ disease.

Metabolism of Alcohol[55]

Alcohol is neither selectively excreted nor stored or converted to a storage form in the body. Studies on alcohol labeled with radioactive carbon show that 90% appears as carbon dioxide. Less than 10% of alcohol is eliminated by renal, pulmonary, or cutaneous avenues. After ingestion, blood alcohol rises to a maximum during the absorption phase within 20 minutes. As it is distributed to the tissues, the alcohol disappears essentially in a linear fashion from the blood. Low alcohol concentrations cause a maximal release of the enzyme alcohol dehydrogenase.[56]

Absorption is rapid and occurs throughout the gastrointestinal tract. After ingestion, it quickly passes down the tract and about 80% is absorbed from the small intestine. There is no limit to rate of absorption, which is proportional to its concentration. Concentrations of alcohol of 50% or more have a depressant effect on absorption, "a local narcosis."

Distribution occurs throughout the body and is proportional to the water content of the tissues.[57,58] Thus, blood, which is 90% water, contains a higher level than the rest of the body tissues, which are about 60% water. Actually, blood contains about one and a quarter times as much alcohol per unit as the other body tissues. At equilibrium, most organs have a concentration 70 to 80% of the plasma concentration.

Plasma levels are determined by many variables;[56] however, the following is a quick approximation: ingestion of 1 ml (800 mg) of alcohol/kg body weight/hour will give a maximum blood alcohol concentration of about 100 mg per 100 ml, or 0.1% in 1 hour (equivalent to 5 ounces of whiskey in a man of 70 kg). Each ounce of whiskey (100 proof) raises the blood level of alcohol approximately 20 mg/100 ml or to 0.02%.

Rate of Metabolism[58]

This is essentially slow. The rate of alcohol metabolism has been estimated to vary between 100 and 200 mg/kg body weight/hour. The value of 200 mg is equivalent to 0.25 ml alcohol. Thus, it is expected that the average male of 70 kg can completely metabolize about 1.0 oz whiskey per hour (i.e., 12.5 ml alcohol or 10 g alcohol = 12 oz beer). An average male of 70 kg can metabolize 840 ml whiskey (about a fifth of whiskey) per day, whereas the actual upper limit appears to be one full quart (80 proof = 380 ml alcohol) per day or 240 mg/kg/hour.

Factors Influencing Rate[56,59]

Metabolism is essentially linear. With higher levels, however, carbohydrate metabolism may speed up, and the increased pyruvates may participate in coupled oxidation-reduction reactions with alcohol. The rate is insensitive to overall metabolic needs.

Hyperthyroidism has no effect. Exposure to cold or muscular exercise does not significantly influence the metabolic rate. Reducing body temperature slows all body reactions including alcohol metabolism. The relationship between metabolism and body temperature appears to be the usual one for chemical reactions, namely, a doubling of rate for each 10° rise in temperature.

Proteins effectively increase rate of metabolism, and alanine and glycine are potent amino acids in this respect.

Substances such as insulin, pyruvate, and fructose have been reported to increase the rate of metabolism. This is controversial. All three may stimulate a sluggish or minimal initial rate. The phenomenon of tolerance is simply an adaptation of the CNS to alcohol, not an alteration in metabolism of alcohol.

A diet high in carbohydrate may be considered to increase alcohol utilization, and the combination with insulin is apparently salutary. Moreover, a protein-free diet or fasting reduces the rate of alcohol oxidation.

Pathways[58,59]

Oxidation is the principal mechanism of metabolism (Fig. 35–6), and it occurs in three chief stages:

Stage I

Conversion of alcohol occurs in the liver to acetaldehyde by oxidation by a liver enzyme, alcohol dehydrogenase. This is a zinc enzyme, which requires a nucleotide as a cofactor (dephosphopyridine nucleotide) and the cytochrome chain for complete reaction. Hepatotoxic substances diminish the rate of destruction. During the metabolism of alcohol, one sees a rise in blood pyruvic acid and lactic acid.

Stage II

The second step is the oxidation of acetaldehyde to acetic acid by means of the enzyme acetaldehyde dehydrogenase. This occurs not only in the liver, but in other organs as well. Studies with isotopic alcohol indicate that acetaldehyde is converted to acetyl coenzyme A without the intermediate acetic acid being formed.[55]

Stage III

The final stage is the conversion of acetic acid to carbon dioxide and water. This can occur universally in all tissues and is usually part of the tricarboxylic acid cycle (Krebs). The acetyl group of the coenzyme is also transformed to carbon dioxide and water. Cerebral tissues can transform alcohol to acetaldehyde, to acetyl coenzyme, and presumably to acetic acid.

Pharmacology[56]

Effects on the Central Nervous System

The most important effect of alcohol is on the brain. It evokes a form of narcotic depression that is probably due to interference with synaptic transmission. Actually, investigations have shown that the nerve impulse is inhibited, and this occurs before any decrease in oxygen consumption. Thus, depression of function occurs first and depression of cerebral metabolic rate second.

As a CNS depressant, alcohol is similar to general anesthetic agents. The depression is a descending type, and the pattern of depression corresponds to the stages of anesthesia.[56]

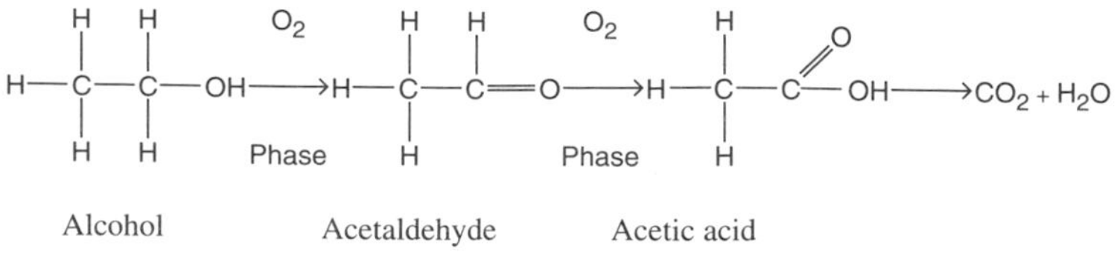

Fig. 35–6. Oxidation of ethyl alcohol.

Stage I

With small doses of alcohol, the higher and complex functions of the cortex such as judgment, self-control, learning, and discrimination are diminished. This releases the lower cerebral centers from higher control and inhibition. A form of excitement may be manifest, as seen in the induction of anesthesia. At the same time, the person becomes less aware of the environment. Perception is lessened. Euphoria, loss of inhibition, less efficient hearing, and impaired vision are present. The reaction of an individual is altered, and the apparent analgesia produced is probably due to a modified appreciation of the pain stimulus so pain is considered unimportant.

The blood level of alcohol necessary for these changes is about 0.05 to 0.1%. At a concentration of 0.05%, the higher cortical areas are blunted. At a concentration of 0.1%, the motor cortical areas are depressed (Table 35-5).

Stage II

In addition to the foregoing, motor incoordination now occurs. Voluntary muscles are affected first. Speech is slurred, and muscular incoordination appears. Staggering gait may appear and, subsequently, generalized motor weakness and paralysis. At the same time, the patient becomes progressively stuporous. The blood alcohol content varies between 0.1 and 0.45%. At a blood level of 0.2%, the entire motor cortical area is depressed, and the midbrain is affected. Emotional behavior is changed. At 0.3%, the more primitive areas, thalamic and others, are affected. During this time, vomiting may occur, and it appears at a blood alcohol level of about 0.12%. This emetic effect is central and occurs whether the alcohol is taken orally or intravenously.[60]

Stage III

Additional doses of alcohol now produce unconsciousness or coma. The person in this condition is often said to be "dead drunk." This occurs at a blood level of 0.50 to 0.6%. Such a level is achieved by the ingestion of 1 pint of whiskey or 200 to 250 ml of alcohol within 1 hour.

Table 35–5. Signs and Symptoms of Alcoholism Correlated with Blood Levels*

Blood Levels	Signs and Symptoms
0.05%	Not under influence
0.05–0.9%	Only corroborative of intoxication considered with signs and symptom; near 0.1% more certain of influence
0.10%–above	Prima facie evidence; subject under influence
	Unfit for driving (driving while intoxicated)
0.25%	*Marked intoxication*, disorientation, stupor
0.40%	*Coma levels*

*Intake Dose: 1 oz 100 proof liquor = 12 oz beer = 4 oz wine = 15 ml absolute alcohol
From Sellers, E. M., Kalant, H.: Alcohol intoxication and withdrawal. N Engl J Med, *294*:757, 1976.

Stage IV

Degrees of depression involving paralysis of medullary centers—the respiratory first, followed by the circulatory centers—are not quickly produced. It does occur at levels of alcohol in the blood of 0.60 to 0.70%. This is fatal. The dose capable of producing unconsciousness is near the fatal dose; that is, the dose necessary to induce an anesthetic state approaches the dose producing death. The margin of safety is small, and hence alcohol is a poor anesthetic.

Effects on Organ Physiology[56]

Gastrointestinal Tract

Concentrations of about 7% alcohol when ingested stimulate gastric secretions and acidity. This effect also occurs after intravenous administration. Concentrations of 15 to 20% inhibit gastric secretion and cause mucosal inflammation. Vomiting is also produced by central action.

Heart and Circulation[61]

At a blood alcohol concentration of about 0.05%, an increase of 5 to 10% in pulse rate, blood pressure, and total blood flow occurs. This effect wanes in 30 minutes. No significant effect on human coronary blood flow has been established; however, in dogs, a marked augmentation of coronary flow occurs after intravenous injection. No significant electrocardiographic responses are to be seen after moderate or nonintoxicating doses.

Skin

Small to moderate doses produce dilatation of skin vessels. Large doses result in impaired circulation. These effects are central.

Liver

Impairment of liver function does occur after drinking moderate to large amounts of alcohol. A drop in liver glycogen can be expected. The relation between chronic alcoholism and cirrhosis is well known.

Kidney

Alcohol has a diuretic effect. It inhibits the production of antidiuretic hormone of the posterior pituitary by action on the supraoptic hypophyseal system. Moderate rises do not produce kidney damage.

Neuromuscular Junction

A blood alcohol level of 0.1% provides a muscle tissue level of about 0.07%. At this concentration, the following neuromuscular effects are produced: a depolarization block; potentiation of functional effects of potassium ion; and antagonism of nondepolarizing relaxants.[62] An increase in blood creatine phosphokinase is found.

Catecholamine Effect

Ethanol causes a dose-dependent rise in plasma norepinephrine. Ordinarily, some norepinephrine is excreted intact (most is removed by neuronal reuptake). The plasma clearance is about 75 ml/kg/min in the urine, but after consumption of 50 g ethanol (five drinks), the plasma clearance is reduced to 50 ml/kg/min. This appears to be the principal reason for the rise of plasma norepinephrine.[63]

Metabolic Effect[59]

Acidosis occurs from alcoholic intoxication. This is both metabolic and respiratory. First is a decrease in the alkali binding power of the blood. Lactic acid increases.

Cardiac Arrhythmias[64]

In the absence of clinical evidence of heart disease and a normal heart size confirmed by x-ray study, chronic alcoholics may experience arrhythmias only when drinking ("holiday heart"). Both atrial tachycardia and ventricular tachycardia are seen. Experimental studies indicate that the presence of alcohol lowers the threshold of the left ventricle to electrical stimulation by 60%.[65]

Cardiac Mechanical Dysfunction

After an episode of drinking and in the absence of a blood alcohol level, the evidence of pump dysfunction is the presence of abnormal systolic time intervals. The PR, QRS, and QT intervals are prolonged. Such delays are fundamental to reentry arrhythmias.[66]

Cardiac contractility is considerably decreased, and ventricular function curves are lowered.[67]

Alcoholic Myopathy[68]

Excessive ingestion of alcohol affects both skeletal and cardiac muscle (Table 35–6).

Skeletal Muscle[68]

Most chronic alcoholics have some abnormality of striated muscle, and half have histologic changes. Weakness and myoglobulinuria are frequent. After 1 month of ethanol ingestion (50 ml of alcohol or five drinks per day), serum creatine phosphokinase activity is increased.

By electron microscopy of skeletal muscle biopsies 1 month after an ethanol ingestion program, significant morphologic changes are noted. Among the findings are intracellular edema, lipid droplets, excessive glycogen, abnormal mitochrondria, and deranged sarcoplasmic reticulum.

Table 35–6. Alcoholic Myopathy

Intracellular edema
Lipid droplet accumulation
Excessive glycogen
Abnormal mitochondria
Deranged sarcoplasmic reticulum

Alcoholic myopathy: diagnosis by alcohol challenge. From Spector, R., Choudury, A., Cancilla, P., Lakin, R.: JAMA 242:1648, 1979.

Alcoholic Cardiomyopathy[69]

Cardiac muscle ultrastructural changes are similar to those in skeletal muscle. Functional derangement also occurs, manifested by an increase in the pressure-rate product after submaximal work indicating loss of efficiency.[70]

Because the electron microscopic changes are similar in both skeletal and cardiac muscle, the following comments pertain to both and correlated functional changes noted.

Sarcolemma

The plasma membrane shows disordered function. Transport of sodium-potassium ions is inhibited. The activity of adenosine triphosphatase (ATPase) is reduced, and the inhibition is dose dependent.

Mitochondria

Ethanol inhibits protein synthesis.

Sarcoplasmic Reticulum

After alcohol ingestion, calcium transport is depressed. Acetaldehyde, a metabolic product, depresses microsomal protein synthesis in the heart. Ethanol inhibits both binding and uptake of calcium by sarcoplasmic reticulum. The role of ethanol in skeletal muscle relaxation is not clear, but ethanol has a negative inotropic effect.

Contractile Proteins

Both ethanol and acetaldehyde inhibit the association of actin and myosin. One also notes a failure of calcium to bind to troponin.

Tolerance and Dependence[71]

The phenomenon of tolerance is related to individual susceptibility and is inherent in the ability of the individual to adapt. The patient becomes practiced in controlling and compensating for overt reactions. During the tolerance phase, larger doses of alcohol are required to produce the same effect. This is only apparent, and careful studies at Yale University show that actual mental and physical impairment are about equal in the habitual drinker and in the inexperienced drinker.

Habituation is a psychologic desire for drink and is acquired. It requires practice. No evidence indicates that in such subjects alcohol is absorbed or detoxified differently. The ability to handle alcohol is probably, again, an adaptive reaction whereby the CNS appears to react to a lesser degree and the individual learns to compensate for deficiencies.

Addiction involves both psychologic and physiologic factors and is evident when alcohol is withdrawn. The reaction may be mild, with craving, anxiety, weakness, perspiration, and tremor. This is often classified as "the shakes." It may be moderate, with anorexia, nausea, vomiting, fever, tachycardia, and bizarre imagery classified as acute hallucinosis. It may progress to convulsions and delerium tremens. The mechanism of addiction is likely to be a cellular adaptation in which alcohol assumes the role of a foodstuff.

Mechanism of Abstinence Syndrome[52]

A cellular electrolyte imbalance appears to be fundamental. A deficiency of intracellular potassium occurs, along with a retention of sodium. The consequence is hyperirritability of the CNS.

Phenytoin uniquely is able to reverse the intracellular sodium-potassium imbalance by enhancing migration outward of sodium and inward passage of potassium. This restores the normal cell polarity and has been successfully used to control the psychomotor and other reactions.

Hypomagnesemia occurs, but this is probably an effect and not a cause. Nevertheless, administration of the magnesium ion often ameliorates the reactions.

Cerebral edema also occurs to some extent as part of the abstinence syndrome, but it is an effect rather than a cause.

When tendon reflexes become depressed, magnesium deficiency, indeed, probably exists and should be treated with the administration of magnesium salts.

General Clinical Considerations

Various significant problems presented by the alcoholic are considered with the goal of understanding the dangers and possible complications in an alcoholic patient who is to be submitted to anesthesia and surgery. Proper evaluation depends on these considerations and subsequently provides a rational basis for preoperative preparation and anesthetic management.

The management of the alcoholic involves both short-term treatment and long-term rehabilitation. The latter is not germane to our review.

Psychologic Problem[71]

Most alcoholics have an unusual amount of anxiety. They attempt to control their tensions and even to escape from some of their conflicts and stresses by drinking. In many instances, the preoperative preparation of an alcoholic patient may involve emergency psychotherapy. The anesthesiologist performs an important service to these patients by observing the following guidelines:

1. Demonstrate a genuine interest in the patient's surgical problem as well as any associated problems brought up by the patient.
2. Cultivate confidence and use generous doses of reassurance.
3. Use tranquilizers generously.
4. Avoid coercion, restriction, or threats; as a group, alcoholics respond poorly to these approaches.

In anesthesia practice, the last recommendation is well taken. Attempts to force an inebriated patient are met by force and violence. Force can be avoided to a large extent and only occasionally is necessary.

Second, any restriction evokes a violent response. Patients should not be "tied." Wrist cuffs and leg straps are greatly resented. "Prepared restraint" is recommended. Adequate personnel are strategically assembled about the surgical table and on the alert to restrain a patient but are not actively doing it. Excitement is even seen with the administration of intravenous barbiturates.

Acute Intoxication

Alcohol is a basal hypnotic. As the intake increases, the blood level increases, and one sees concomitant progressive disturbances of behavior and function. At present, most states have laws designating a blood level of 0.1% as evidence of inebriation (see Table 35–5).

Acute intoxication includes exaggerated attitudes, combative and wild behavior, and uncontrolled and uncoordinated activity, including seizures, depression, and stupor.

Aspiration is a frequent complication of alcoholic depression and stupor. Pneumonia with atelectasis may exist. Careful examination and treatment are essential. These patients have poor gas exchange, and a high FIO_2 is necessary. Many patients have chronic pulmonary disease and a low blood oxygen tension.

Occasionally, one must operate when these complications exist. If a life-saving surgical procedure is indicated in a wild, stuporous person, the following is recommended:

1. Tranquilization: IV diazepam (10 to 15 mg; max, 0.15 mg/kg) or midazolam (0.12 mg/kg) or promethazine (H_1 blocker).
2. Gastric content control: H_1 and H_2 block, IV promethazine and ranitidine; gastric emptying: metoclopramide (5.0 mg IV).
3. Endotracheal intubation: while the patient is awake, if possible.
4. Rapid sequence induction: thiopental 4.0 mg/kg or midazolam 0.25 mg/kg.
5. Immediate relaxation: paralysis: large doses of vecuronium 0.15 mg/kg with priming; alternatively by pretreatment with succinylcholine.
6. Inhalation agents for maintenance: these are controllable and can be eliminated by the assisted ventilation of the anesthesiologist; enflurane is advised; isoflurane is less satisfactory because of the frequency of concomitant alcoholic withdrawal phenomena.

Because the direct effect of alcohol is to induce a state of cellular poisoning and to cause a form of histotoxic hypoxia, oxygenation is most important. The use of high atmospheric concentrations or positive pressure increases the amount of oxygen dissolved and raises oxygen tension.

Coma is not infrequent from excess alcohol. The patient should be handled as a resuscitation problem, and attention should be given to both lifesaving procedures such as airway and ventilation and circulatory assistance and to supportive measures such as parenteral feeding and attention to processes of elimination. Care of the respiratory tract is essential. The patient should be turned frequently to avoid atelectasis. It is rarely necessary to operate on a patient in coma. Delay and preparation are recommended.

Abstinence Syndromes of Chronic Alcoholism[52]

Hangover

Hangover (the shakes) is essentially a water and electrolyte imbalance, with gastrointestinal complaints and vomiting; muscle tremor is present. The key to therapy and preparation of such patients is hydration. Injections of saline-glucose solutions intravenously containing insulin, thiamine, and nicotinamide afford significant improvement. Comparisons of results with each ingredient separately show only minimal benefit. All substances are needed. If the "jitters" is present, the use of mephenesin (Myanesin) has been shown to be an effective single remedy. Tapering doses of alcohol are helpful, but they only prolong or delay recovery. If these measures are employed, one can safely proceed with urgent operations. Generally, it is preferable to wait approximately 3 days or until all hangover symptoms have subsided.

Hallucinosis

Approximately 25% of patients develop tremors, which are usually accompanied by imaginary visual or auditory sensations and referred to as the "horrors." These are exaggerated when the eyes are closed. Nightmares occur, and patients misinterpret reality with respect to time and space. The auditory features are not common and carry a more serious prognosis. The duration is usually about 6 days. This state may progress into paranoia, and occasionally suicide attempts are made.

Seizures and Convulsions

The term for marked muscular activity and convulsions in a nonepileptic alcoholic is "rum fits." In the seizure-free intervals, the electroencephalogram (EEG) is normal. During seizures, however, the EEG shows a grand mal pattern without any focal identification. This is an advanced phase of abstinence.

Delirium Tremens

This is a state of profound confusion, delusions, vivid hallucinations, tremors, agitation, seizures, and intermittent but persistent convulsions. Autonomic sympathetic activity is increased. This usually occurs 1 to 3 days after the last drink, but it may be seen as early as 8 hours after drinking. This form of abstinence occurs in about 5% of patients hospitalized for alcoholic withdrawal. It is attended by a mortality of 10 to 15%.[72,73]

Diagnosis[52]

The clinical features of the abstinence syndrome occur when the alcohol intake falls below maintenance levels. The severity and intensity of the reaction vary with the amount regularly taken and the duration. The reactions range from mild to severe.

Initially, signs are mild and consist of coarse tremors, increased by movement (tremulousness); patients are jumpy and easily startled. Sweating, tachycardia, elevated temperature, exaggerated reflexes, and hypertension are commonly encountered. Time distortion occurs. Symptoms of nausea, anorexia, shakiness, vomiting, and feelings of restlessness are present. At this time, the appearance is one of some anxiety, with a flushed face and injected conjunctivae. Drinkers refer to this as the period of "the shakes" or the "jitters." This type of reaction is frequent in those subjects who consume 15 to 20 ounces of whiskey (8 to 10 ml alcohol) a day for at least 2 weeks. If a greater amount is imbibed, such as 25 to 30 ounces of whiskey, for 1 to 3 months, the reactions become progressively more severe and intense.

In the intermediate phase, the intensity is moderate to severe. Drinkers call this phase the "horrors." All the foregoing features are present and become progressively intense. At the same time, disorientation, mental confusion, delusions, and mild hallucinations occur. Muscle twitching is present, along with spasms, and this phenomenon is called the "rams."

Finally, the patient has the intense phase of withdrawal seen as early as 8 hours after the last drink. One sees a rapid progression through the initial and moderate phases to marked delirium and convulsions.

Withdrawal Phenomena[52]

Management

Steady and excessive alcohol intake results in addiction. This is essentially a manifestation of the late stages of alcoholism. On cessation of alcohol consumption, withdrawal phenomena appear. Three clinical entities are distinguished: acute hallucinosis; the psychosis of the Korsakoff type; and delirium tremens. Because the last is the most severe disturbance and actually incorporates most of the features of the other two entities, a brief discussion of delirium tremens is in order.

Delirium tremens accompanies or follows a long alcoholic bout. Besides the mental panic, extreme anxiety, and high suggestibility, these patients show marked autonomic nervous system activity and bizarre neuromuscular phenomena. The course of the abstinence syndrome is characteristic. In the incipient stage, the patient has tremors and marked apprehension; this is called "the shakes." In the intermediate stage, extensor spasms occur and progress to shaking and clonic muscular activity of the extremities—in the jargon of the alcoholic, this is called "the rams." This is invariably followed by or accompanied by hallucinations and delirium called "the horrors." In uncomplicated cases and in poorly treated cases, the mortality is about 5%.

The mechanism of these acute episodes appears to be a true withdrawal syndrome. During the drinking phase, some cerebral edema may exist, and wetbrain is the term used in describing the appearance of the brain. Dehydration then develops during the abstinence phase.

Treatment

Hydration and the administration of sodium chloride are essential. If dehydration is allowed to persist, the mortality may reach 16%. If polyneuritis is known to have been present, vitamins must be liberally supplied. Otherwise, the mortality may be nearly 100%. Glycogenation of the liver must be promoted and hypoglycemia corrected. In addition, the use of corticosteroids is most effective in shortening the acute process.

Sedation

Classic sedation involves the use of chloral hydrate, 2.0 g initially and 1.0 g every 3 hours, and paraldehyde administered as follows: 16 ml initially and 8 ml every 4 hours. The latter's effect must be carefully observed. Paraldehyde is prone to produce pulmonary capillary hemorrhages and must not be given to excess. The short-acting barbiturates are not well tolerated, except for phenobarbital, sodium amytal, and mephobarbital.

The benzodiazepines are effective in controlling withdrawal phenomena. Diazepam should be administered intravenously. Midazolam may be administered intramuscularly.

Because many of the symptoms resemble those of schizophrenia, the major tranquilizers, such as promethazine, promazine, and chlorpromazine, are effective.

Organic Deterioration

Besides the cerebral deterioration, serious changes in hepatic function are common. Cirrhosis may be of all grades of severity. A severe grade of liver dysfunction with cephalin flocculation of 2+, depressed serum albumin, and elevated serum bilirubin signifies a severe degree of damage. This situation poses its own hazards, and such a patient represents a poor anesthetic and surgical risk.

Some of the consequences of diminished liver function to be appreciated in the alcoholic are as follows:

1. Decreased capacity to detoxify drugs.
2. Deficient clotting ability due to diminished fibrinogen and various accelerator factors.
3. Decreased circulating proteins and, hence, diminished resistance to shock; tendency to ascites.
4. Myocardiopathy; skeletal myopathy.
5. Potential of hepatic coma.
6. Jaundice: bilirubin effect on cardiac mechanism (bradycardia).

In addition to these problems, the presence of significant portal hypertension with or without ascites and the occurrence of upper gastrointestinal hemorrhage are complicating features.

Morbidity and Mortality[73]

The abstinence or withdrawal phenomenon lasts for 3 to 5 days and then begins to subside. In untreated patients and in uncomplicated cases, the mortality is set at about 8% for the severe abstinence syndromes. In patients with other complicating illnesses including surgical conditions, the mortality of delirium tremens is approximately 24%.

Diazepam administration maintains alcohol dependency and enhances the preference or desire of rats to seek alcohol. The use of diazepam may therefore be counterproductive in the diagnosis of alcoholism.

General Considerations

Because the direct effect of alcohol is to induce a state of cellular poisoning and to cause a form of histotoxic hypoxia, oxygenation is most important. The use of high atmospheric concentrations or positive pressure breathing increases the amount of oxygen dissolved in plasma and raises the oxygen tension.[74]

In 1926, Palthe and Ueber demonstrated that animals given fatal doses of alcohol would survive if placed in an oxygen atmosphere.[75] Human subjects could be given large amounts of alcohol without developing signs of intoxication if they breathed oxygen by mask. On the other hand, if delirium existed, intermittent inhalation of oxygen for a period of 20 minutes benefited most patients. The precise mechanism of the cellular hypoxia has been elucidated to some extent. Davis and Robertson[74] have shown that increasing the cerebral oxygen tension can overcome the retarding effect of alcohol on the enzymatic reactions of oxidation.

In acute intoxication, orthodox methods of treatment should be used. The use of stimulants in an attempt to shorten the period of intoxication and perhaps to hasten oxidation of alcohol is unsupported and introduces hazards. One should allow the patient to sleep in mild to moderate intoxication. These episodes are self-limited and are seldom life-threatening.

Endocrine Factor[76]

Although alcoholism develops as a personality problem based on emotional immaturity, nevertheless, definite metabolic factors and organic changes become part of the disease.

The most striking aspect is the biochemical similarity to adrenal insufficiency.[76] This is especially evident in the advanced stages. Endocrinologic investigations reveal definite adrenal and hypophyseal deficiencies. Hypoglycemia is often present, especially in fasting or in the postdrinking stage. Glucose tolerance curves are of the hyperinsulin variety. An abnormal water tolerance also is shown by many alcoholics, and in addition low serum sodium and chloride concentrations are seen. The steroid plasma values are only slightly below normal in most alcoholics, but in patients developing delirium tremens or who show peripheral neuropathy, the serum 17-ketosteroid level is low. Further, ascorbic acid levels are usually low in the alcoholic patient.

In the alcoholic patient, adrenocorticotropic hormone produces an adequate adrenal response. The administration of epinephrine or alcohol, both of which cause adrenal activity through stimulation of the pituitary, however, produces a poor response. The eosinophil response and the release of cortical hormone are poor. Thus, the metabolic defect appears to be principally one of pituitary insufficiency.

Alcohol intake also affects the adrenal medulla. As little

as 2.5 to 3.0 g of alcohol, that is, about 3 to 4 ml taken in 10 minutes, will raise level of blood circulating epinephrine as much as 500%. The norepinephrine levels are also greatly increased.[63]

Drug Interactions

Interactions of drugs with alcohol and in the alcoholic patient occur under three circumstances:
1. Effect of alcohol on drug metabolism[77]
   a. In the presence of blood alcohol, the metabolism of drugs dependent on hepatic enzymes is slowed.
   b. In the absence of blood alcohol, the rate of metabolism of many drugs in the alcoholic is increased.
2. Effect of drugs on alcohol metabolism[78]: in the presence of some drugs, alcohol itself is not readily oxidized, and high plasma levels of alcohol ensue; chlorpromazine inhibits alcohol dehydrogenase, and the blood level of alcohol rises.
3. Action of drugs in the presence of alcohol[79] (Table 35-7)
   a. Additives (barbiturates, sedatives, hypnotics, tranquilizers and benzodiazepines).
   b. Disulfiram (Antabuse) action: intermediate metabolism of alcohol is blocked.
   c. Disulfiram-type action: some drugs have a disulfiram-like action by interfering with hepatic enzyme action; either alcohol levels increase or intermediate metabolites of alcohol accumulate.

Drug Absorption

The effect of oral diazepam is greatly enhanced in the presence of alcohol, and the combination can be lethal. The effect is not only additive, but also the administration of diazepam mixed with alcohol results in higher levels of diazepam than when given with water; that is, the absorption of diazepam is enhanced by alcohol.[77] This effect is unique because increased absorption of other drugs by alcohol is not supported.

Chlorpromazine enhances the absorption of alcohol.[78] After administration of chlorpromazine, the ingestion of alcohol results in much higher blood levels of the alcohol.

Effect of Stimulants

No antidote to alcohol is known. Coffee does not effectively antagonize either the psychologic or the motor impairment due to alcohol. The antagonistic effects of amphetamines and other stimulants are negligible.

Role of Disulfiram (Antabuse)[80,81]

Disulfiram (tetraethylthiuram disulfide; TETD) was introduced by Hald, Jacobsen, and Larsen[81a] as an adjunct in the treatment of alcoholism. This substance interferes with the metabolism of alcohol in the second phase of metabolism. Thus, acetaldehyde is formed at a normal rate, but its further combustion is inhibited and it accumulates. This produces the "acetaldehyde syndrome."

High levels of acetaldehyde produce toxic effects as follows:

Flushing, with marked vasodilatation
Palpitation and tachycardia
Nausea and vomiting
Dyspnea and tachypnea
Occasional fainting, coma, and death

These symptoms and signs occur in a patient receiving disulfiram who ingests alcohol. The reaction occurs at alcohol levels of only 5 to 10 mg/dl, but it is full blown at blood alcohol levels of 50 mg/dl. The unpleasantness of the reaction is considered helpful in discouraging the patient from using alcohol. Ascorbic acid and oxygen therapy reduce the severity of symptoms.

Electrocardiographic changes due to acetaldehyde include flattening of the T wave and depression of the ST segment. Disulfiram administration also appears to reduce oxygen consumption by the liver, as shown by Warberg's experiments.[81a]

In addition to interfering with acetaldehyde combustion, disulfiram inhibits xanthine oxidase. The consequence of this is that sodium thiopental levels are increased and the detoxification is slower. Hence, a given dose produces a more pronounced and prolonged effect.

Workers in the rubber industry (and other industries) where TETD was used as an antioxidant were noted to be hypersensitive to ethanol.

Preanesthetic Preparation

General Supportive Therapy

Environment

Patients should be placed in a pleasant environment in a well-lighted room. Constancy of personnel is desired, and familiar persons and friends should be present and allowed to visit.

Hydration

Most patients are dehydrated and, therefore, need water therapy.

Electrolyte Restoration

Chloride, bicarbonate, and potassium are essential. Calcium and magnesium are usually required. An electrolyte profile is immediately necessary. Magnesium can be given intramuscularly as a 50% magnesium-sulfate solution (1 to 2 g).

Caloric Intake

Parenteral glucose, 10% solution, should provide sufficient calories.

Vitamin Supplements

Included in the parenteral solution should be such vitamins as folic acid, thiamine, and pyridoxine. Glucose should *not* be given without thiamine.

Table 35–7. Some Drug Interactions with Alcohol

Drug	Effect	Probable Mechanism
Disulfiram (Antabuse)	Flushing, diaphoresis, hyperventilation, vomiting, confusion, drowsiness	Inhibition of intermediary metabolism of alcohol
Anticoagulants, oral	Increased anticoagulant effect with acute intoxication	Reduced metabolism
	Decreased anticoagulant effect after chronic alcohol abuse	Enhanced microsomal enzyme activity
Antihistamines	Increased CNS depression	Additive
Antimicrobials		
Chloramphenicol (Chloromycetin; and others)	Minor disulfiram-like reaction	Inhibition of intermediary metabolism of alcohol
Furazolidone (Furoxone)	Minor disulfiram-like reaction	Inhibition of intermediary metabolism of alcohol
Griseofulvin (Fulvicin-U/F; and others)	Minor disulfiram-like reaction	Inhibition of intermediary metabolism of alcohol
Isoniazid (many mfrs.)	Decreased effect after chronic alcohol abuse	Undetermined
Metronidazole (Flagyl)	Minor disulfiram-like reaction	Possible CNS effect
Quinacrine (Atabrine)	Minor disulfiram-like reaction	Inhibition of intermediary metabolism of alcohol
Hypoglycemics		
Chlorpropamide (Diabinese)	Minor disulfiram-like reaction	Inhibition of intermediary metabolism of alcohol
Tolbutamide (Orinase)	Decreased hypoglycemic effect after chronic alcohol abuse	Enhanced microsomal enzyme activity
	Increased hypoglycemic effect with ingestion of alcohol particularly in fasting patients	Suppression of gluconeogenesis
	Minor disulfiram-like reaction	Inhibition of intermediary metabolism of alcohol
Narcotics	Increased CNS depression with acute intoxication	Additive
Salicylates	Gastrointestinal bleeding	Additive
Sedatives and tranquilizers		
Barbiturates	Increased CNS depression with acute intoxication	Additive; reduced metabolism
	Decreased sedative effect after chronic alcohol abuse	Enhanced microsomal enzyme activity; decreased CNS sensitivity
Chloral hydrate (Noctec; and others)	Prolonged hypnotic effect	Mutual potentiation
Chlordiazepoxide (Librium; and others)	Increased CNS depression	Additive
Chlorpromazine (Thorazine; Chlor-PZ)	Increased CNS depression	Additive; inhibition of oxidation of alcohol
Clorazepate (Azene; Tranxene)	Increased CNS depression	Additive
Diazepam (Valium)	Increased CNS depression	Additive; possible increased absorption
Meprobamate (Miltown; and others)	Increased CNS depression with acute intoxication	Additive; reduced metabolism
	Decreased sedative effect after chronic alcohol abuse	Enhanced microsomal enzyme activity
Oxazepam (Serax)	Increased CNS depression	Additive
Phentolamine (Regitine)	Minor disulfiram-like reaction	Inhibition of intermediary metabolism of alcohol
Phenytoin (Dilantin; and others)	Increased anticonvulsant effect with acute intoxication	Reduced metabolism
	Decreased anticonvulsant effect after chronic alcohol abuse	Enhanced microsomal enzyme activity
Other*		

*Many alcoholic beverages contain tyramine, which can cause reactions with MAO inhibitors.
Modified from Abramowicz, M. (ed.): Interactions of alcohol with drugs. Med Lett Drugs Ther *19*:47, 1977.

Nutritional Needs

Protein concentrates are required.

Preanesthetic Management of Acute Alcoholic Complications

Severe complications include seizures, hyperthermia, and vascular collapse. Only seizures are considered at this point.

For tremulousness, twitching and mild seizures, and generalized irritability, small doses of diazepam are recommended. For more prolonged seizures and convulsions, phenobarbital or phenytoin is effective. The half-life of these drugs is only slightly prolonged. The half-life of the short-acting barbiturates, however, is markedly prolonged.

Hyperthermia is considered elsewhere, but hydration, cooling techniques, chlorpromazine, and oxygen are key needs.

Sedative therapy is essential to management of the seizure complex. This should be done without depressing vital functions. For the milder forms of restlessness and agitation, chlordiazepoxide or diazepam in doses of 50 to 100 mg may be given orally every 4 to 6 hours. The half-life of this drug is prolonged for 22 hours. Ordinarily, it is 6 hours.

Phenobarbital and phenytoin are useful for the severe forms of CNS irritability.

Diazepam is most valuable in severe withdrawal syndromes. It is administered intravenously in doses of 5 to 10 mg. The drug should be titrated and administered in fractional portions to a desired response effect. The half-life of diazepam in alcoholism with concomitant liver dysfunction is increased twofold. Although its half-life is prolonged, it is well tolerated, and the presence of liver disease does not increase its toxicity.

Anesthetic Management[82] (Table 35–8)

Evaluation

The alcoholic patient who is presented for surgery represents a special type of risk depending on the considerations reviewed. These situations confront the anesthesiologist: either the management of an acute alcoholic condition during inebriation or withdrawal requiring emergency surgery or the management of chronic alcohol-dependent patient in a nonintoxicated state. The presence of the following peculiar problems must be noted:

1. Emotional attitude.
2. Nutritional defects.
3. Degree of liver damage.
4. State of hydration.
5. Incipient withdrawal phenomena.

Commonly encountered surgical conditions include gastrointestinal hemorrhage, injury, and acute abdomen such as ruptured ulcer, cholecystitis, and appendicitis. Gastrectomy is a more formidable procedure than cholecystectomy or appendectomy. The physical condition or status of the patient plays the major role in determining risk, whereas the surgery is of secondary importance, however. If the alcoholism is of long duration with many of its organic stigmata, the risk is indeed poor. Without evidence of prolonged alcoholism, the risk is good.[73]

Whenever possible, all defects should be corrected. Elective surgery should be postponed, function improved, and psychiatric consultation obtained to enable the patient to develop a proper attitude.

Preanesthetic Medication

The guiding principle is to be cautious about the administration of depressant drugs when the patient is still intoxicated. Synergism occurs between alcohol and the narcotics or barbiturates.

If an acute delirious or hallucinatory reaction exists, some restoration to normality can be accomplished by hydration with glucose-saline and vitamin supplements together with adrenal cortical therapy. Such an infusion is preceded by or accompanied by a generous dose of a tranquilizer such as a benzodiazepine.

The technique of intravenous alcohol administration is based on the concept that many acute symptoms in the alcoholic are the results of abstinence and providing alcohol should curtail these symptoms—"a bit of the tail of the dog that bit you." It has real merit for calming a boisterous, demanding, and belligerent patient who is uncooperative and wants whiskey. The alcohol is administered as a 10 or 20% by volume solution. Blood levels up to 0.1% are sought. The problem of recovery with the complication of emergence delirium remains, however.

In the intervals between acute intoxication, the alcoholic who requires surgery needs generous medication and sedation. Large doses of barbiturates were used in the past, and such doses are usually needed to achieve a desired effect. Thus, some cross-tolerance seems to exist. The narcotics have not been particularly satisfactory, and frequently bizarre behavioral reactions are noted that interfere with preoperative preparations. A calm state can be achieved by the use of phenothiazine derivatives, followed by a generous dose of morphine. Promethazine (or promazine) has been used and is most effective in calming the alcoholic. It is also a good antihistaminic and antiemetic. An anticholinergic agent should be part of the premedication to reduce autonomic reflex excitability and to diminish gastrointestinal motility.

The benzodiazepines have become widely used.[72] They may prevent seizures when used early. Diazepam has been effective in oral doses of 10 to 20 mg 2 to 3 times daily. Shorter-acting agents, such as lorazepam or oxazepam, are a better choice in patients with liver disease.[83]

Central sympathetic blockade with clonidine has become an effective measure to reduce MAC and UD requirements of anesthetic agents.[84]

Dosage Requirements[82]

The long-term use of alcohol in amounts of one-half pint of whiskey per day (8 oz) or even less increases the anesthetic requirement of various drugs.[85] For halothane, the MAC value increases from 0.76 to 1.10%.[86] Fentanyl

Table 35–8. Considerations in Anesthetic Management

Anesthesia in Acute Intoxication

    The alcohol acts as a basal hypnotic
    Anesthetics and CNS depressants are additive to alcohol effect
    Difficulties are minimal
        Overdosage during injection is easy
        Withdrawal symptoms are frequent in a patient; management must be careful;
            use: psychosedative drugs in modest doses

Anesthesia in Chronic Dependent Patient (Sober at time of anesthesia)

    Problems

        Psychic dependency
        Tolerance
        Physical dependency
        Nervous system dysfunction
            Neuritis
            Brain damage
            Psychotic manifestations

        Other system dysfunctions
            Liver
            Renal
            Cardiac
            Psychomotor
            Gastrointestinal varices
            Pulmonary infections

    Choice of Anesthesia (If possible use regional anesthesia; when general anesthesia is
        necessary, the following are characteristic reactions)

        Prolonged stage II: rapid passage through stage III to stage IV
        Tolerance
            To all aliphatic, hypnotic hydrocarbons
            To all fluorinated compounds
            To chloral hydrate barbiturates

Postoperative

    Tranquilization
    Pain relief
    Constant monitoring of arousal

---

supplementation is increased by 30% in the nitrous oxide-oxygen-relaxant technique. Thiopental requirement is increased and may be doubled in poorly prepared or premedicated patients for elective surgery.[87,88]

On the other hand, when alcohol is present in the body, the metabolism of many drugs is slowed, and the effect of this agent on other CNS depressants is one of potentiation. Chlorpromazine inhibits alcohol dehydrogenase, and hence high blood levels of alcohol are attained. One sees a simultaneous increase in the depressant effect of chlorpromazine. The benzodiazepines midazolam or diazepam are generally well tolerated; however, in the acute alcoholic patient, the presence of a blood alcohol level may result in prolonged unconsciousness.

Induction[89]

Intravenous induction with a short-acting barbiturate or with midazolam followed by inhalation of nitrous oxide-oxygen-isoflurane or ethrane, or any other maintenance combination, is a safe technique. Halothane is not recommended because it is accompanied by an appreciable and disturbing number of complications; these include hypotension, myocardial insufficiency, hepatic dysfunction, and more prolonged emergency delirium.

Maintenance Agents

Alcoholics are preferably maintained by an inhalation agent. Enflurane has been found most satisfactory. Ketamine is to be avoided. An unusually high incidence of psychotic reactions is experienced. The incidence of cardiovascular complications and of emergence excitement has been lowest (approximately 15%) when a neurolept-enflurane combination is employed.

Liver function tests do not show a worsening of biochemical activities in alcoholics with mild to moderate liver disease.[90]

Technical Aspects

All other aspects of management are followed as in the nonalcoholic patient. During surgery, much can be accomplished by attention to hydration and steroid therapy. This will ensure a smooth recovery. A patient who has recently eaten—a common situation in patients acutely intoxicated and who have been injured—is handled in the usual fashion, with the aim to prevent aspiration. If cooperation is obtainable, intubation is attempted while the patient is awake. Often, however, the patient must be anesthetized.

A rapid sequence induction with midazolam, followed by a relaxant and intubation with cricoid pressure, has decided merit. It is not a guarantee against aspiration, however. Oxygenation must be excellent throughout. Patients who undergo a bout of hypoxia have a stormy emergence from anesthesia.

Regional anesthesia is ideal for surgery, when feasible, in the intervals between acute bouts of inebriation and when the patient will cooperate.

Recovery

The key to smooth recovery appears to be adequate hydration, as previously described, and steroid therapy. In addition, the continued use of chlorpromazine is essential. If satisfactory results are not obtained with this regimen, we have resorted to intravenous alcohol administration, and this usually controls the situation, albeit temporarily. As soon as the patient is rational and surgically fit, small quantities of oral alcohol may be permitted. Otherwise, these patients are uncooperative.

At the conclusion of surgery, an additional small dose of lorazepam or, to prevent seizures, of chlorpromazine, may be given. It is also advisable to provide adequate pain relief. Postoperative pain should be managed as in any patient after surgery.

Sympathetic blockade with clonidine can be successfully used to relieve withdrawal symptoms, such as tremor, sweating, and tachycardia.[91] Atenolol (a β-adrenergic blocker) also has been useful in treating alcohol withdrawal, and patients receiving this drug usually require less treatment with benzodiazepines.[92] Propranolol produces psychotic reactions.

REFERENCES

1. Jaffe, J. H.: Drug addiction and drug abuse. In Goodman and Gilmans The Pharmacological Basis (Gilman, A., Rall, T. W., Nies, A., Taylor, P. (eds.) New York, MacMillan, 1985, p. 532.
2. Caldwell, T.: Anesthesia for patients with behavioral and environmental disorders. *In* Katz, J., Benumof, J., Kadis, L. B. (eds.). Anesthesia and Uncommon Diseases. Philadelphia, W. B. Saunders, 1981, p. 672.
3. Blachly, P. H.: Management of the opiate abstinence syndrome. Am J Psychiatry 122:742, 1966.
4. Gold, M. S., Pottash, A. C., Sweeney, D. R., Kleber, H. D.: Opiate withdrawal using clonidine: a safe, effective, and rapid nonopiate treatment. JAMA 243:343, 1980.
5. Giuffrida, J. G., Bizzarri, D. V., Saure, A. C., Sharoff, R. L.: Anesthetic management of drug abusers. Anesth Analg 49:273, 1970.
6. Adriani, J., Morton, R. C.: Drug dependence: important considerations from the anesthesiologist's viewpoint. Anesth Analg 47:472, 1968.
7. Weintraub, S. J., Naulty, J. S.: Acute abstinence syndrome after epidural injection of butorphanol. Anesth Analg 64:452, 1985.
8. Eisman, B., Lam, R. C., Rush, B.: Surgery in the narcotics addict. Ann Surg 159:748, 1964.
9. Mark, L. C.: Hypotension during anesthesia in narcotic addicts. NY State J Med 66:2685, 1966.
10. Quasha, A. C., Eger, E. I.: MAC. *In* Miller, R.D. (ed.). Anesthesia. New York, Churchill Livingstone, 1981, p. 257.
11. Berkowitz, B. A., et al.: Tolerance to N20 anesthesia in rats and mice. Anesthesiology 51:309, 1979.
12. McGoldrick, K. E.: Anesthetic implications of drug abuse. Anesthesiol Rev 7:12, 1980.
13. Winchester, J. F.: Barbiturates. *In* Haddad, L. M., Winchester, J. F. (eds.). Poisoning and Drug Overdose. Philadelphia, W. B. Saunders, 1983, p. 413.
14. Wikler, A.: Diagnosis and treatment of drug dependence of the barbiturate type. Am J Psychiatry 125:759, 1968.
15. Eddy, N. B., Hallbach, H., Isbell, H., Seevers, M. H.: Drug dependence: its significance and characteristics. Psychopharmacol Bull 3:96, 1966.
16. Hubbard, T. F., Goldbaum, L. R.: The mechanism of tolerance to thiopental in mice. J Pharmacol 97:488, 1949.
17. Lee, P. K. Y., Cho, M. H., Dobkin, A. B.: Effects of alcoholism, morphinism, and barbiturate resistance on induction and maintenance of general anesthesia. Can Anaesth Soc J 11:366, 1964.
18. Litovitz, T.: Benzodiazepines. *In* Haddad, L. M., Winchester, J. F. (eds.). Poisoning and Drug Overdose. Philadelphia, W.B. Saunders, 1983, p. 475.
19. Dowling, G. P., McDonough, E. T., Bost, R. O.: "Eve" and "Ecstasy." JAMA 257:1615, 1987.
20. Kramer, J. C., Fichman, V. S., Littlefield, D. C.: Amphetamine abuse. JAMA 201:89, 1967.
21. Citron, H. P., et al.: Necrotizing angiitis associated with drug abuse. N Engl J Med 283:1103, 1970.
22. Johnston, R. R., Way, W. L., Miller, R. D.: Alteration of anesthetic requirements by amphetamine. Anesthesiology 36:357, 1972.
23. Haddad, L. M.: Cocaine. *In* Haddad, L. M., Winchester, J. F. (eds.). Poisoning and Drug Overdose. Philadelphia, W.B. Saunders, 1983, p. 443.
24. Caldwell, J., Sever, P. S.: The biochemical pharmacology of abused drugs. Clin Pharmacol Ther 16:625, 1974.
25. Jekel, J. H., et al.: Epidemic free-base cocaine abuse: case study from the Bahamas. Lancet 1:459, 1986.
26. Abramowicz, M. (ed.): Crack. Med Lett Drugs Ther 28:69, 1986.
27. Gay, G. R., et al.: Cocaine in current perspective. Anesth Analg 55:582, 1976.
28. Tuchman, A. J., et al.: Intracranial hemorrhage after cocaine abuse (letters). JAMA 257:1175, 1987.
29. Litovitz, T.: Hallucinogens. *In* Haddad, L. M., Winchester, J. F. (eds.). Poisoning and Drug Overdose. Philadelphia, W. B. Saunders, 455, p. 1983.
30. Freedman, D. X.: The psychopharmacology of hallucinogenic agents. Annu Rev Med 20:409, 1969.
31. Zsigmond, E. K., Foldes, F. F., Foldes, V. M.: The inhibitory effect of psilocybin and related compounds on human cholinesterases. Fed Proc 20:393, 1961.
32. Lieberman, C. M., Lieberman, B. W.: Marijuana: a medical review. N Engl J Med 284:88, 1971.
33. Nahas, G. G.: Current status of marijuana research. JAMA 242:2775, 1979.
34. Nicholson, D. P.: The immediate management of overdose. Med Clin North Am 67:1279, 1983.
35. Robertson, W. O.: Common accidental poisonings. *In* Wyngaarden J. B., Smith, L. H., Jr. (eds.). Cecil Textbook of Medicine. Philadelphia, W. B. Saunders, 1982, p. 2213.
36. McGuigan, M. A., Lovejoy, F. H., Jr.: Poisoning. *In* May, H.

L. (ed.). Emergency Medicine. New York, John Wiley & Sons, 1984, p. 805.

37. Lewis, D. C., Gomolin, I. H.: Drug overdose and withdrawal. *In* May, H. L. (ed.) Emergency Medicine. New York, John Wiley & Sons, 1984, p. 823.

38. Khnatzian, E. J., McKenna, G. J.: Acute toxic and withdrawal reactions associated with drug use and abuse. Ann Intern Med *90:*361, 1979.

39. Millman, R. B.: Drug abuse, dependence, and intoxication. *In* Wyngaarden, J. B., Smith, L. H., Jr. (ed.). Cecil Textbook of Medicine. Philadelphia, W. B. Saunders, 1982, p. 2005.

40. Stoelting, R. K., Creasser, C. W., Martz, R. C.: Effect of cocaine administration of halothane MAC in dogs. Anesth Analg *54:*422, 1975.

41. Koehntop, D. E., Liao, J. C., Van Bergan, F. H.: Effects of pharmacologic alteration of adrenergic mechanisms by cocaine, tropolone, aminophylline, and ketamine on epinephrine-induced arrhythmias during halothane-nitrous oxide anesthesia. Anesthesiology *46:*83, 1977.

42. Barash, P., et al.: Is cocaine a sympathetic stimulant during general anesthesia? JAMA *243:*1437, 1980.

43. Jonsson, S., O'Meara, M., Young, J. B.: Acute cocaine poisoning. Am J Med *75:*1061, 1983.

44. Kossowsky, W. A., Lyon, A. F., Chou, A. Y.: Cocaine and ischemic heart disease. Pract Cardiol *12:*164, 1986.

45. Kast, E. C., Collins, V. J.: Lysergic acid diethylamide. Anesth Analg *43:*285, 1964.

46. Siemons, A. J., Kalant, H., Khanna, J. M.: Effect of cannabis on pentobarbital-induced sleeping time and pentobarbital metabolism in the rat. Biochem Pharmacol *23:*447, 1974.

47. Sofia, R. D., Knoblock, L. C.: The effect of delta-9-tetrahydrocannabinol pretreatment on ketamine, thiopental, or CT-1341-induced loss of righting reflex in mice. Arch Int Pharmacodyn Ther *207:*270, 1974.

48. Johnstone, R. C., Lief, P. L., Kulp, R. A., Smith, T. C.: Combination of delta-9-tetrahydrocannabinol with oxymorphone or pentobarbital. Anesthesiology *42:*674, 1975.

49. Vitez, T. S., Way, W. K., Miller, R. D., Eger, E. I.: Effects of delta-9-tetrahydrocannabinol on cyclopropane MAC in the rat. Anesthesiology *38:*525, 1973.

50. Stoelting, R. K., et al.: Effects of delta-9-tetrahydrocannabinol on halothane MAC in dogs. Anesthesiology *38:*521, 1973.

51. White, P. F., Johnston, R. R., Pudwill, C. R.: Interaction of ketamine and halothane in rats. Anesthesiology *42:*179, 1975.

52. Sellers, E. M., Kalant, H.: Alcohol intoxication and withdrawal. N Engl J Med *294:*757, 1976.

53. Block, M. A.: Alcoholism (editorial). JAMA *163:*550, 1957.

54. Gordon, J. E.: The epidemiology of alcoholism. N Y State J Med *58:*1911, 1958.

55. Westerfeld, W. W., Schulman, M. P.: Metabolism and caloric value of alcohol. JAMA *170:*197, 1959.

56. Harger, R. N.: The pharmacology and toxicology of alcohol. JAMA *167:*2199, 1958.

57. Fazekas, J.: Influences of CP and alcohol on cerebral hemodynamics. Am J Med Sci *230:*128, 1955.

58. Greenberg, L. A.: Alcohol in the body. Sci Am *189:*86, 1953.

59. Himwich, H. E.: The physiology of alcohol. JAMA *163:*545, 1957.

60. Newman, H. W.: Emetic action of ethyl alcohol. AMA Arch Intern Med *94:*417, 1954.

61. Grollman, A.: Influence of alcohol on circulation. Q J Stud Alcohol *3:*5, 1942.

62. Rummel, W., Schmitz, J.: Die Anti-curare wirking des Alkahols. Arch Exp Pathol Pharmakol 222:257, 1954.

63. Eisenhofer, G., Lambie, D. G., Johnson, R. H.: Effects of ethanol on plasma catecholamines and norepinephrine clearance. J Clin Pharm Ther *14:*143, 1983.

64. Regan, T. J.: Of beverages, cigarettes, and cardiac arrhythmias. N Engl J Med *301:*1060, 1979.

65. Greenspan, A. J., Stang, J. M., Lewis, R. P., Schaal, S. F.: Provocation of ventricular tachycardia after consumption of alcohol. N Engl J Med *301:*1049, 1979.

66. Ettinger, P. O., et al.: Arrhythmias and the "holiday heart": alcohol-associated cardiac rhythm disorders. Am Heart J *95:*555, 1978.

67. Bing, R. J., Tillmanns, H.: *In* Lieber, C. S. (ed.). The Effects of Alcohol on the Heart: Metabolic Aspects of Alcoholism. Baltimore, University Park Press, 1977, p. 117.

68. Rubin, E., et al.: Muscle damage produced by chronic alcohol consumption. Am J Pathol *83:*499, 1976.

69. Rubin, E.: Alcoholic myopathy in heart and skeletal muscle. N Engl J Med *301:*28, 1979.

70. Spector, R., Choudry, A., Cancilla, P., Lakin, R.: Alcoholic myopathy: diagnosis by alcohol challenge. JAMA *242:*1648, 1979.

71. Smith, J. A.: Psychiatric treatment of the alcoholic. NY State J Med *58:*3157, 1958.

72. Sellers, E. M.: Diazepam loading: simplified treatment of alcohol withdrawal. Clin Pharmacol Ther *34:*822, 1983.

73. Lewis, A.: The relation between operative risk and the patient's general condition: alcohol, other habits of addiction and psychogenic factors. Bull Soc Int Chir *14:*421, 1955.

74. Davis, C. W., Robertson, H. T.: Oxygen in acute alcoholic intoxication. Q J Stud Alcohol *10:*59, 1959.

75. Palthe, P. M., Ueber, V. W.: Alkoholaerogeftung. Dtsch S F Nerven *92:*791, 1926.

76. Smith, J. J.: The endocrine basis and hormonal therapy of alcoholism. NY State J Med *50:*1704, 1956.

77. Hayes, S. L., et al.: Effects of alcohol on drug absorption. N Engl J Med *296:*186, 1977.

78. Sutherland, V. S., et al.: Effects of drugs on alcohol metabolism. J Appl Physiol *15:*189, 1960.

79. Abramowicz, M. (ed.). Interactions of alcohol with drugs. Med Lett Drugs Ther *19:*47, 1977.

80. Cooper, J., Slocum, N. C., Allen, C. R.: Tetraethyl-thiuram disulfate and the anesthetic agents. Anesthesiology *14:*875, 1951.

81. Fuller, R. K., et al.: Disulfiram treatment of alcoholism: a Veterans Administration Cooperative Study. JAMA *256:*1449, 1986.

81a. Hald, J., Jacobsen, E., Larsen, V.: The Antabuse effect of some compounds related to Antabuse and cyanamide. Acta Pharmacol Toxicol *8:*329, 1952.

82. Orkin, L. R., Chien-Hsu, C.: Addiction, alcoholism and anesthesia. South Med J *70:*1172, 1977.

83. Miller, W. C., Jr., McCurdy, L.: Choice of benzodiazepine in alcoholic patients. Clin Ther *6:*364, 1984.

84. Ghignone, M., Calvillo, O., Quintin, L.: Anesthesia and hypertension: the effect of clonidine on perioperative hemodynamics and isoflurane requirements. Anesthesiology *67:*3, 1987.

85. Han, Y. J.: Why do chronic alcoholics require more anesthesia? Anesthesiology *30:*341, 1969.

86. Barber, R. E.: Anesthetic requirement in alcoholic patients. *In* Abstracts of Scientific Papers: Annual Meeting of the American Society of Anesthesiologists. Park Ridge, IL, American Society of Anesthesiologists, 1978, p. 623.

87. Metabolic fate of thiopental (editorial). JAMA *147:*875, 1958.

88. Mirsky, H., Giarmian, N. J.: Studies on potentiation of pentothal. J Pharmacol Exp Ther *114:*240, 1955.

89. Lee, P. K., Cho, M. H., Dobkin, A. B.: Effects of alcoholism, morphinism, and barbiturate resistance on induction and maintenance of general anesthesia. Can Anaesth Soc J *11:*354, 1964.

90. Zinn, S. E., Fairley, H. B., Glenn, J. D.: Liver function in patients with mild alcoholic hepatitis, after enflurane, nitrous oxide-narcotic, and spinal anesthesia. Anesth Analg *64:*487, 1985.

91. Wilkins, A. J., et al.: Treatment of alcohol withdrawal symptoms. Psychopharmacology *81:*78, 1983.

92. Kraus, M. L., et al.: Effects of beta-adrenergic blockade in the treatment of alcohol withdrawal. N Engl J Med *313:*905, 1985.

Chapter 36

ANTICHOLINERGIC AGENTS IN ANESTHESIA

USHARANI NIMMAGADDA AND VINCENT J. COLLINS

GENERAL MECHANISMS OF ACTION[1]

Acetylcholine exerts both muscarinic and nicotinic actions. At the neuromuscular junction, the receptors are exclusively nicotinic. In the spinal cord and at the autonomic ganglia, the receptors are predominantly nicotinic, whereas at the postganglionic neuroeffector cells, the receptors are muscarinic. Ganglia also contain some muscarinic receptors. Subcortical and cortical regions of the brain contain both muscarinic and nicotinic receptors. The term anticholinergic agents usually refers to those drugs that block the actions of acetylcholine at the muscarinic receptors, whereas those drugs that block the nicotinic actions of acetylcholine are referred to as either ganglionic blocking agents or neuromuscular blocking agents, depending on the site of blockade. The term "muscarinic" comes from the alkaloid muscarine derived from the mushroom *Amanita muscaria*, which has actions similar to acetylcholine on the receptors located at the postganglionic parasympathetic nerves. The muscarinic actions of acetylcholine are shown in Table 36–1.

SUBCLASSES OF MUSCARINIC RECEPTORS

In recent years, many subclasses of muscarinic receptors have been identified in both the central nervous system (CNS) and peripheral organs.[2] Thus far, five human genes that encode structurally distinct muscarinic receptors have been identified by molecular cloning studies.[3] These genes have been found to differ from each other in their ligand-binding properties and in their capacity to produce different functional responses. At this time, considerable confusion exists regarding the nomenclature of these receptors. In general, those receptors that have been pharmacologically defined are called M_1, M_2, and M_3 receptors, whereas those that are identified through molecular cloning are called m_1, m_2, m_3, m_4, and m_5 receptors.[4] M_1, M_2 and M_3 receptors seem to correspond well with m_1, m_2, and m_3 receptors.

LOCATION OF MUSCARINIC RECEPTORS

Most tissues contain several subtypes, but in predominance, M_1 receptors are located in various secretory glands and in ganglia. M_2 receptors are in the myocardium and in the smooth muscle. M_3 receptors are in the secretory glands and in the smooth muscle. The locations of m_4 and m_5 receptors have not been identified at this time. The CNS contains all five subtypes of these receptors.

MEDIATION OF MUSCARINIC RECEPTOR ACTION

The receptor action is mediated by interaction with G proteins. Two different pathways of G protein interaction have been described. One pathway involves m_1, m_3, and m_5 receptors activating a yet-unidentified G protein that stimulates phospholipase C activity. This results in hydrolysis of phosphatidylinositol polyphosphates of the plasma membrane to form inositol polyphosphates. Some of the inositol polyphosphate isomers (chiefly inositol-1,4,5 tris-phosphate) cause release of intracellular calcium (Ca^{2+}) from stores in the endoplasmic reticulum that then causes all the Ca^{2+}-dependent actions such as secretions and contraction of smooth muscle.[5] The second pathway involves the m_2 and m_4 receptors, which react with a group of G proteins (especially G_i proteins) causing several actions. They inhibit adenylate cyclase, activate K^+ channels, and modulate the action of Ca^{2+} channels in certain cell types.[6,7] These actions are predominantly exerted in the myocardium, resulting in the negative inotropic and chronotropic effects of acetylcholine.

Table 36–1. Muscarinic Actions of Acetylcholine

Secretions	
Salivary	↑ ↑
Sweat	↑ ↑ ↑
Respiratory	↑ ↑ ↑
Gastrointestinal	↑ ↑
Heart	
Rate	↓ ↓ ↓
Conduction	↓
Contractility	↓ ↓
Smooth muscle	
Bronchial	↑ ↑
Vascular	
Iris	↑ ↑
Gastrointestinal	
Motility	↑ ↑
Sphincter	↓ ↓
Genitourinary	
Motility	↑ ↑
Sphincter	↓ ↓
Biliary tract	↑ ↑

↑ = slight increase; ↑ ↑ = moderate increase; ↑ ↑ ↑ = large increase; ↓ = slight decrease; ↓ ↓ = moderate decrease; ↓ ↓ ↓ = large decrease.

Anesthesiologists use antimuscarinic drugs during the perioperative period to reduce the undesirable side effects of excessive cholinergic stimulation. The most important objectives are reduction of secretions from salivary glands and from alimentary and respiratory tracts and suppression of untoward cardiovascular effects. Other actions of these drugs include the following: relaxation of smooth muscles of bronchi, trachea, and urinary tract; reduction of secretions of sweat glands; decrease in excessive motility and spasm of the gastrointestinal (GI) tract; and dilatation of the pupil (mydriasis) and paralysis of accommodation (cycloplegia).

CLASSIFICATION OF ANTICHOLINERGIC DRUGS

Anticholinergic drugs can be broadly classified into naturally occurring and synthetic agents. The naturally occurring agents are atropine and scopolamine. The synthetic anticholinergics include both quaternary and nonquaternary compounds. In addition, many other pharmacologic agents possess some anticholinergic activity (Table 36-2).

Naturally Occurring Alkaloids

These are belladonna derivatives and are widely distributed in nature, especially in Solanaceae plants. Atropine (*dl*-hyoscyamine) is mainly found in two plants: *Atropa belladonna*, the deadly night shade, and *Datura stramo-*

nium (known as jimsonweed, Jamestown weed, stinkweed, devil's apple, or thorn apple), which grows wild in wasteland. The shrub *Atropa belladonna* is named after Atropos, the oldest of the Three Fates who cuts the thread of life. The name belladonna derives from the alleged use of this drug by Italian women to dilate their pupils. Scopolamine (hyoscine) is found mainly in the shrub *Hyoscyamus niger* (henbane), which grows wild in the Rocky Mountains and Canada, and it is also found in *Scopolia carniolica*.

Chemistry and Structure-Activity Relationship

Belladonna alkaloids are organic esters formed by a combination of an aromatic acid, tropic acid, and an organic base, either tropine (tropanol) or scopine. Scopine differs from tropine only in having an oxygen bridge between carbons 6 and 7 (Fig. 36-1). The intact ester of tropine or scopine and tropic acid is essential for antimuscarinic activity. The presence of a free OH group in the acid portion of the ester is also important. Atropine is an alkaloid with properties of a base. Chemically, the nitrogen exists in the tertiary form. It has a pKa value of 9.7 and at body pH is largely in the ionized form (protonated);[8] however, the protonated nitrogen is in a rapid dynamic equilibrium with the nonionized tertiary form, which is constantly available to diffuse through blood-membrane boundaries; such as blood-brain and placental barriers.[9] It is racemized during extraction and contains

Table 36-2.   Anticholinergic Drugs in Common Use

Generic Name	Trade Name	Oral Dosage Unit
Belladonna alkaloids		
Atropine sulfate		0.4–0.6 mg
Scopolamine hydrobromide		0.4 mg
Tincture of belladonna		10 drops of 0.03% solution
Belladonna extract		15 mg
Synthetic anticholinergics		
Quaternary ammonium compounds		
Glycopyrrolate	Robinul	1 and 2 mg
Hematropine methylbromide	Mesopin, Novatrin, Malcotran	2.5 and 5.0 mg
Methantheline bromide	Banthine	50 mg
Propantheline bromide	Pro-Banthine	7.5 and 15 mg
Oxyphenonium bromide	Autrenyl	0.5–1.0 mg
Nonquaternary compounds		
Homatropine hydrobromide		(Ophthalmic solution, 2%)
Benztropine mesylate	Cogentin	0.5 1 and 2 mg
Trihexyphenidyl hydrochloride	Artane, Pipanol, Tremin	2 and 5 mg
Other drugs with anticholinergic properties		
Ethanolamine antihistamines		
Dimenhydrinate	Dramamine	50 mg
Diphenhydramine hydrochloride	Benadryl	25 and 50 mg
Piperazine antihistamines		
Cyclizine hydrochloride	Marezine	50 mg
Meclizine hydrochloride	Bonine	25 mg
Phenothiazines		
Promethazine hydrochloride	Phenergan, Remsed	12.5, 25 and 50 mg

Modified from Greenblatt, D. J.: Medical intelligence. Drug therapy: anticholinergics. N Engl J Med *288*:1216, 1973.

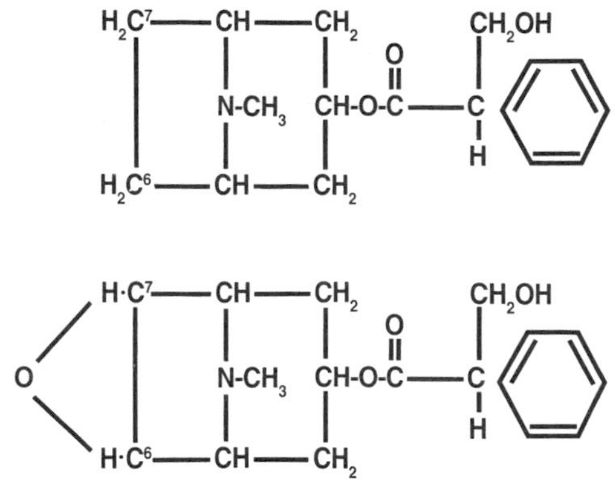

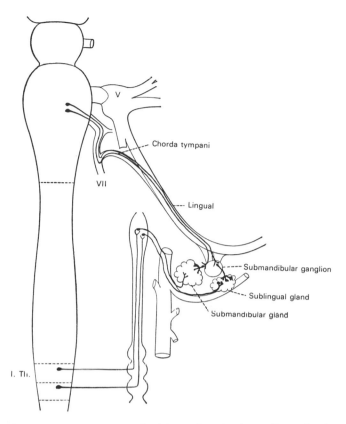

Fig. 36–1. Chemical structure of atropine and scopolamine.

equal parts of *d*- and *l*- hyoscyamine, but the antimuscarinic activity is due to the levo form. Scopolamine is *l*-hyoscine and is more active than *d*-hyoscine.

Atropine

Atropine is the oldest anticholinergic drug and has been used for centuries to treat various ailments. Because it is the prototype for other antimuscarinic drugs, which are sometimes referred to as "atropine-like" drugs, pharmacologic actions of atropine are discussed in detail, and the actions of other drugs that are of interest to anesthesiologists are compared with that of atropine.

Pharmacologic Actions

Secretory Glands

Many types of stimuli provoke salivation. In the mouth, this may be either by taste of a favorable substance or by mere physical stimulation of the receptors for common sensibility. Simple contact with buccal mucosa, grinding of teeth, chewing, or movement of jaws evokes salivation. Salivary secretion is essentially dependent on nervous mechanisms. Because rapid responses are needed, the slow hormonal mechanism of excitation would be inadequate. All the glands have a dual autonomic innervation consisting of both parasympathetic and sympathetic fibers.

The submaxillary and sublingual glands receive their parasympathetic supply from the superior salivatory nucleus. These are located in the upper portion of the medulla in the region of the nucleus of the seventh cranial nerve (facial nerve) (Fig. 36–2). Preganglionic fibers pass from this nucleus in the facial nerve. They course in the facial nerve to the point behind the tympanic cavity where a branch arises called the chorda tympani nerve. After traversing the tympanic cavity, the chorda tympani nerve descends medial to the sphenoid bone and joins the lingual nerve near the cavity of the mouth. In the floor of the mouth, fibers arise from the lingual nerve to synapse with small ganglia. In the case of the sublingual gland, the submaxillary ganglion is located outside the gland where postganglionic cholinergic fibers arise to enter the gland and arborize around secretory cells. In the case of the submaxillary gland, the ganglia are numerous and are situated in the hilum of the gland. From these ganglia, short postganglionic fibers arise to surround se-

Fig. 36–2. Innervation of sublingual and submaxillary glands. From Clemente, C. D.: Gray's Anatomy, 30th Ed. Philadelphia, Lea & Febiger, 1985.

cretory cells. Stimulation of the chorda tympani results in a profuse watery juice; stimulation of vasodilator fibers causes an increase in blood flow.

The sympathetic nerve supply is derived from the upper three thoracic segments of the spinal cord. The preganglionic fibers synapse in the superior cervical ganglia. The postganglionic fibers pass to the plexus about the external carotid artery and the branches extend to the glands. Stimulation causes the production of a thick mucinous saliva of small volume.

Parasympathetic supply to the parotid gland (Fig. 36–3) consists of preganglionic fibers arising in the inferior salivary nucleus situated at the upper end of the medulla near the glossopharyngeal nucleus. The fibers travel in the glossopharyngeal nerve initially, but they separate at the jugular foramen to form the tympanic nerve. This then courses in the small superficial petrosal nerve to the otic ganglion. At this point, the fibers synapse and postganglionic cholinergic fibers arise which are then transmitted by the auriculotemporal branch of the fifth cranial nerve to the gland cells. The sympathetic supply is similar to that of the other glands. Atropine decreases the secretions of not only the three salivary glands, but also the secretions of the mucus glands of the nose, sinuses, mouth, and tracheobronchial tree.

Cardiovascular System

The main action of atropine on the cardiovascular system is on the heart rate. Three distinct phases of heart

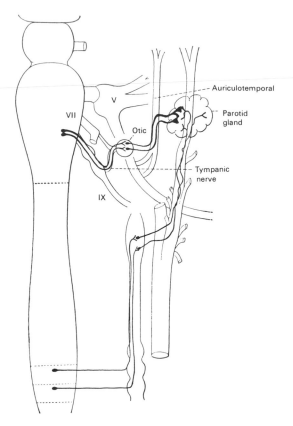

Fig. 36–3. Innervation of parotid gland. From Clemente, C. D.: Gray's Anatomy, 30th Ed. Philadelphia, Lea & Febiger, 1985.

rate change may occur: (1) an initial vagotonic effect; (2) a transient period of vagal imbalance at different levels of the conduction system; and (3) a final period of parasympathetic block. With smaller doses or with slow intravenous injection, the heart rate may initially decrease.[10,11] This initial slowing action of atropine was once thought to be due to direct stimulation of the medullary vagal nuclei, which precedes the blocking action at the vagal nerve terminals on the sinoatrial node.[11] Later, it was found that this paradoxic action of atropine is due to its peripheral cholinomimetic activity and not due to a central action.[12] More recent studies indicate that the decreased heart rate is produced by blockade of excitatory M_1 receptors at the autonomic ganglia.[13]

The predominant effect of atropine is an increase in the heart rate because of blockade of vagal effects on M_2 receptors at the sinoatrial nodal pacemaker. In addition to the increase in heart rate, atropine can cause cardiac arrhythmias. The effects of anticholinergic drugs on heart rate or rhythm may be greater in magnitude in anaesthetized than in conscious adults.[14,15] This greater response is probably due to depression of vagal centers by anesthetic agents.[15] Atrial arrhythmias are seen usually in children when small doses of the drug that slow the heart rate are given. Atrioventricular dissociation is more commonly seen in adults after small or large doses.[16,17] Ventricular extrasystoles are prone to occur, especially in patients with coronary artery disease. The increased heart rate increases myocardial oxygen demand and may in-

crease the degree of ischemia in patients with myocardial infarction.[18,19]

With the increase in the heart rate, the rate-pressure product (RPP) increases, which then stimulates baroreceptors resulting in a reflex decrease in the sympathetic tone and norepinephrine levels. The plasma norepinephrine decreases by 30 to 40% from about 350 to 245 pg/ml.[20] The muscle relaxant pancuronium selectively blocks muscarinic receptors in the heart[21] and has effects similar to those of atropine on RPP and on norepinephrine levels. When pancuronium is administered after atropine premedication (5 to 6 mg/kg), however, no significant changes in heart rate, plasma catecholamine levels, or RPP occur.[22]

Anesthetized patients receiving atropine show heart rate changes that vary with the individual anesthetic agent. Under halothane anesthesia, one sees a greater increase in heart rate in both children[23] and adults[24] when compared with enflurane anesthesia. Narcotic anesthesia produces rises in heart rate similar to those seen with halothane anesthesia. Atropine has been found not to alter the heart rate significantly in patients with either lumbar or cervical epidural anesthesia.[24] A comparison of propofol and enflurane anesthetics has shown that with lower atropine doses (1.8 μg/kg), no difference occurred in heart rate responses, but with higher atropine doses (3.6 μg/kg), propofol anesthesia is associated with reduced heart rate responses more than with enflurane anesthesia.[25]

Atropine can abolish reflex vagal slowing or asystole from many causes such as oculocardiac reflex (OCR) caused by pressure on the eyeballs or pulling on the eye muscles, stimulation of the carotid sinus, or pulling on the peritoneal structures. Intravenous (IV) administration of larger than usual doses is required to accomplish this. Although intramuscular (IM) premedication with atropine reduces the incidence of OCR from 90 to 50%, IV administration is more effective.[26] Atropine is also effective in treating the bradycardia associated with repeated doses of succinylcholine. The degree of tachycardia produced by atropine depends on the degree of preexisting vagal tone. Young healthy adults who have a high resting vagal tone show the greatest increase in heart rate whereas elderly and very young patients show lesser increase. Atropine is an effective first-line drug therapy in patients with heart block, especially if the heart block arises in the atrioventricular node or above (e.g., Mobitz type I). Second- and third-degree heart blocks occurring below the atrioventricular node are generally refractory to atropine, although atropine should also be tried in these patients.

Central Nervous System

Being tertiary amines, both atropine and scopolamine cross the blood-brain barrier. In therapeutic doses, atropine can cause mild excitation as a result of stimulation of the medulla and higher cerebral centers. With larger doses, disorientation, hallucinations, or delirium can occur. Impairment of memory function may be caused by atropine. The effect appears to be on information storage. Associative memory tasks score poorly, whereas retrieval processes appear to be unimpaired.[27] With even larger doses, excitation is followed by medullary depression, resulting in paralysis and coma.

Atropine and some related drugs have antitremor activity and are used for the treatment of parkinsonism and in the management of extrapyramidal symptoms caused by antipsychotic and other drugs. Atropine shifts normal electroencephalogram rhythm to slow activity. The frequency and voltage of the α-rhythm decrease.

Respiratory System

Atropine and some of its congeners were the earliest bronchodilators used in all varieties of airways disease.[28] Over the years, many studies have shown the effectiveness of antimuscarinic drugs in patients with emphysema, chronic bronchitis, and asthma.[29,30] Basic differences exist in the mechanisms of airflow obstruction in patients with asthma and emphysema. Patients with asthma have many causes of airflow obstruction involving smooth muscle contraction and inflammation. Some of the causes can be treated with adrenergic agents and some with anticholinergic agents and most often with a combination of drugs. On the other hand, in emphysema and, to a lesser extent, in chronic bronchitis, airflow obstruction is mainly due to structural changes in and around the airways. Although the structural changes may not be altered, the airway tone mediated by the cholinergic nerves can be abolished effectively by anticholinergic agents.

Inhalation of 1% atropine or IV administration of 0.6 to 1.2 mg of atropine increases airway conductance by 80%. This is accomplished by an increase in anatomic dead space of 17%.[31] Another study[32] comparing the effects of atropine and glycopyrrolate administered intravenously has shown that with atropine, airway resistance (RAW) decreases, and specific airway conductance ($_s$GAW) (which is airway conductance divided by functional residual capacity) increases (Fig. 36–4). The increase in $_s$GAW reaches its maximum of 88 ± 5% above control in about 30 minutes and declines progressively reaching control levels within 3 to 4 hours. One sees an increase in V_{max} 40 (expiratory flow at total lung capacity: 60% of forced vital capacity [FVC], i.e., 40% of FVC above residual volume) and a decrease in lung elastic recoil pressure (Fig. 36–5). Atropine also increases maximum expiratory flow, midexpiratory flow, and forced expiratory volume in 1 second (FEV_1).[33]

Airway hyperresponsiveness seen with viral infections can be blocked by atropine.[34] Two categories of neural abnormalities have been found in airways of patients with viral infections: increased vagal reflex bronchoconstriction and increased response to tachykinins. Both acetylcholine and tachykinins, in addition to causing bronchoconstriction, also stimulate airway submucosal gland secretions and change the quality and character of airway secretions. Normally, the M_3 receptors in the smooth muscle cause contraction of the airway smooth muscle, and the M_2 receptors on vagal nerve endings have a negative feedback activity and inhibit additional release of acetylcholine. The enzyme neuraminidase that is present in the viruses damages the M_2 receptors and eliminates the negative feedback mechanism and causes more release of acetylcholine.[35] A selective anticholinergic agent

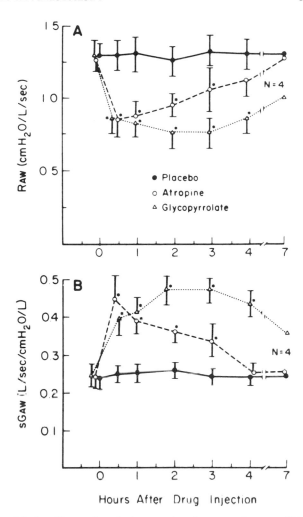

Fig. 36–4. Time-related changes in airway resistance (RAW) (A) and changes in specific airway conductance ($_s$GAW) (B) after placebo, atropine, and glycopyrrolate. From Gal, T. H., Surratt, P. M.: Atropine and glycopyrrolate effects on lung mechanics in normal man. Anesth Analg 60:87, 1981.

that would block only the M_3 receptors but not the M_2 receptors would be ideal to treat the airway symptoms. At this time, no such drugs have been tested in humans. For elective surgical procedures, several weeks of recovery from viral infection should be allowed before the patient undergoes general anesthesia.[36] If general anesthesia has to be administered, atropine-like drugs should be given before the surgical procedure, especially before endotracheal intubation.

Disadvantages of atropine on the respiratory system are its inhibition of ciliary activity, the decrease in mucociliary clearance, and the increase in the viscosity of secretions.[37]

Ocular Effects

Therapeutic doses of atropine administered systemically have only slight ocular effects, in contrast to locally applied atropine, which causes significant dilatation of the pupil and paralysis of accommodation by blocking the responses of the iris and the ciliary muscle of the lens to the cholinergic stimulation. Systemically administered

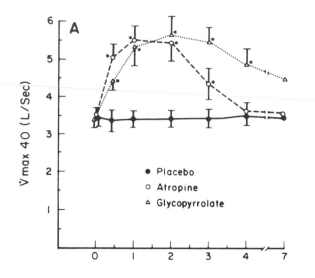

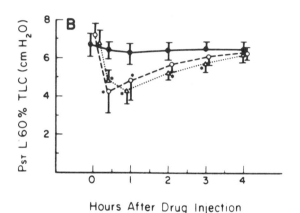

Hours After Drug Injection

Fig. 36–5. Time-related changes in V_{max} 40 (A) and changes in lung elastic recoil pressure (PSTL) at 60% of total lung capacity (TLC) (B) after placebo, atropine, and glycopyrrolate. From Gal, T. H., Surratt, P. M.: Atropine and glycopyrrolate effects on lung mechanics in normal man. Anesth Analg 60:87, 1981.

atropine does not increase intraocular pressure in normal patients. Even in patients with glaucoma, the increase in intraocular pressure with premedicant doses of atropine is insignificant.[38,39] With larger doses, atropine occasionally can cause an increase in intraocular pressure in these patients.

Gastrointestinal System

Atropine decreases the secretions throughout the GI system. In children, 15 to 20 μg/kg of atropine given IM 1 hour before induction of anesthesia increases the gastric pH.[40] In adults, however, traditional preanesthetic doses of atropine have been found not to increase the pH or to decrease the volume of gastric contents.[41] In addition, atropine decreases the lower esophageal sphincter pressure.[42] Thus, atropine is not of much benefit in the prevention of aspiration of gastric contents in adults. It decreases the amplitude and frequency of peristaltic contractions throughout the GI system and is used as an antispasmodic agent.

Urinary System

Atropine decreases the tone and amplitude of contractions of the ureter and bladder and can cause urinary retention. Large doses of atropine dilate the pelves, calyces, ureters, and urinary bladder and improve the visualization of kidneys during urologic examinations.

Biliary Tract

Atropine has only mild antispasmodic action on bile ducts and the gallbladder and thus is not very effective in relieving the spasm of biliary tract during intraoperative cholangiogram. Nitrates and glucagon are probably better agents for this purpose.

Temperature

Atropine decreases sweating by decreasing the activity of sweat glands. Skin becomes dry, and the temperature increases. Increase in temperature is more common in children, and the so-called "atropine fever" has been mistaken for allergic reactions because of the flushing associated with it. The atropine flush is either due to a compensatory reaction to the rise in temperature permitting the radiation of heat or due to a direct cutaneous vasodilatation, especially in the blush area. In addition to the absence of sweating, disturbance of central regulation of temperature may also contribute to the fever.

Dosage

For infants and children, the IM dose is set at 10 μg/kg. It is usual to use 0.1 mg up to 1 year of age. In adolescents, the dose is 0.2 to 0.4 mg; in adults, it is 0.3 to 0.6 mg. Occasionally in adults, for procedures such as bronchography and bronchoscopy, a dose of 0.75 mg may be given. In recent years, IM use of atropine has decreased. Anesthesiologists administer atropine IV before induction of anesthesia or intraoperatively only as needed.

Pharmacokinetics

Metabolism

Plasma concentrations of atropine following IV or IM administration have been determined by radioimmunoassay.[43] After administration of 1.0 mg IV, one sees a rapid decline from 250 ng/ml at 1 minute to 10 ng/ml at 10 minutes. At this time, the amount in the circulation is less than 5% of the administered dose. Plasma concentration then decreases slowly over the following 50 minutes. At 1 hour, the concentration is slightly less than 3 ng/ml (Fig. 36–6). Total clearance rate is 5.9 $\pm$ 1.3 ml/min/kg. Inhibition of salivation after an IV dose is delayed and, although significant at 45 minutes to 1 hour, does not reach its peak effect until 90 minutes. Cardiac accelerating effect corresponds to the plasma levels and is greatest when plasma levels are highest (Table 36–3).

After 1.0 mg IM, rapid absorption occurs with an optimum level at 15 minutes of 2.5 ng/ml and a peak level at 30 minutes of 3.0 ng/ml. At 1 hour, the concentration is only slightly less than 3.0 ng/ml. A slow decline continues, but atropine is still detectable at 4 hours at 1.5 ng/ml

(Fig. 36–7). With IM administration, one sees great individual variation in adults. The vastus lateralis and gluteal muscles have been recommended as injection sites in children; however, in adults and in elderly patients, the deltoid muscle offers more predictable absorption, it is preferred by patients, and it is associated with more rapid absorption (t_{max} 9 to 13 minutes).[44] Furthermore, the plasma concentrations of the racemic atropine (*dl*-hyoscamine) were found to be three times higher than after the active *l*-hyoscamine alone. A further finding is that plasma levels after the racemis atropine did not decline until 2 hours after administration.[45]

Inhalation of atropine sulfate by nebulization from a controlled-delivery device has been used in the management of acute respiratory obstructive disease. This method of atropine administration is variable and unpredictable, however, as are the absorption and serum levels.[46] Intermittent dosage over a period of several hours may lead to high serum levels, even higher than following IV administration.

When radioactive atropine (^{3}H-atropine) is given orally to adults, absorption takes place mainly in the duodenum and jejunum and not in the stomach.[47] Maximal plasma radioactivity is reached in 1 hour. With 2.0 mg of atropine given orally, a maximal serum concentration of about 5.5 ng/ml is reached. The half-life of plasma levels can be placed at 2.5 hours. Clinical effects such as CNS impairment occur at 1 hour, coinciding with the maximal plasma level of the agent. Peripheral antimuscarinic effects occur at 2 to 4 hours after administration, however.[48] Although theoretically the oral dose of atropine should be twice as high as the IM dose to produce equivalent response such as an equal tachycardia, the antisialagogue action, inhibition of sweating, and ocular effects are much less dramatic than following IM injection. In children, oral administration of 0.03 mg/kg results in a maximal serum concentration of 2.0 ng/ml at 2 hours.

Pharmacokinetics of atropine following rectal adminis-

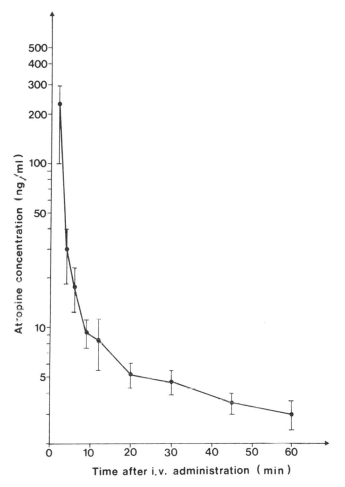

Fig. 36–6. Serum atropine concentration after atropine sulfate, 1 mg IV. From Berghem, L., Bergman, U., Schildt, B., Sörbo, B.: Plasma atropine concentrations determined by radioimmunoassay after single dose IV and IM administration. Br J Anaesth *52:*597, 1980.

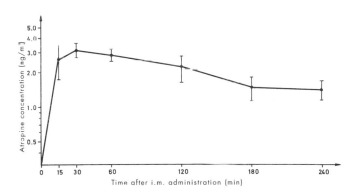

Fig. 36–7. Serum atropine concentration after atropine sulfate, 1 mg IM. From Berghem, L., Bergman, U., Schildt, B., Sörbo, B.: Plasma atropine concentrations determined by radioimmunoassay after single dose IV and IM administration. Br J Anaesth *52:*597, 1980.

Table 36–3. Atropine*: Pharmacokinetic Data

Availability (Oral) (%)	Urinary Excretion (%)	Bound in Plasma (%)	Clearance (ml · min^{-1} · kg^{-1})	Vol. Dist. (Liters/kg)	Half-Life (hours)	Effective Concentrations
50	57 ± 8	14–22 ⟷ Aged	5.9 ± 3.6† ↓ Aged	1.7 ± 0.7†‡ ↑ Child§	4.3 ± 1.7† ↑ Aged, Child	5–10 ng/ml

*Racemic mixture of active S-(−)-hyoscyamine and inactive R-(+)-hyoscyamine.
†Values for active S-(−)-enantiomer.
‡V$_{area}$.
§Less than 2 years of age.

tration have been studied only in children. When the influence of body weight on pharmacokinetics has been observed, it has been found that in smaller children weighing less than 15 kg, the plasma levels are lower and decline faster than in older children weighing more than 15 kg.[49] This may be either due to larger distribution volume[50] or to increased "first-pass" metabolism in the liver.

Excretion

Atropine has a half-life of approximately 4 hours. About half of the administered dose is excreted in the urine unchanged. The other half of the atropine dose is metabolized in the liver.[51] The types of metabolic products differ from those noted in animals (rat and mouse), and neither hydroxylation of the aromatic ring nor glucuronide formation has been demonstrated. No activity is found in expired air, and traces of atropine are found in various secretions including breast milk.

Scopolamine

Pharmacologic Actions

Secretory Glands

At one time, scopolamine was considered to be a more effective antisecretory agent than atropine.[52,53] Some newer studies have shown, however, that when 0.4 mg of scopolamine and 0.6 mg of atropine are compared, the antisialic actions are similar.[54] A significant reduction in salivary flow rate also occurs with transdermal scopolamine.[55]

Cardiovascular System

With low doses of scopolamine, the heart rate slows more than with atropine. With higher doses, the increase in the heart rate is less than with atropine.

Central Nervous System

Scopolamine crosses the blood-brain barrier much more easily than atropine and thus has more CNS effects. In therapeutic doses, scopolamine causes cortical depression resulting in amnesia, drowsiness, and dreamless sleep, with a reduction in rapid eye movement sleep, and thus it can be used for preanesthetic medication and as an adjunct to the anesthetic agents. In elderly patients or in the presence of severe pain, however, scopolamine can sometimes cause excitement, disorientation, and delirium leading to the central anticholinergic syndrome (CAS). It is more potent than atropine on the antitremor activity and thus is more useful in parkinsonism.

An important use of scopolamine is for the control of nausea and vomiting. Oral bioavailability is unpredictable, but absorption through the skin is good. Transdermal scopolamine has been found to be more effective than dimenhydrinate (Dramamine),[56] and meclizine (Antivert)[57] for the protection against nausea and vomiting associated with motion sickness. It is available as 2.5-cm^2 disks containing 1.5 mg of scopolamine, which is programmed to deliver 0.5 mg at a constant rate over 3 days. It should be applied behind the ear at least 4 hours before motion. The exact mechanism of action is not known, but it is probably related to inhibition of vestibular input to CNS. Direct action on the vomiting center within the reticular formation of the brain stem may also play a role. Transdermal scopolamine has been found to be effective in reducing the incidence of postoperative emesis following strabismus surgery in children,[58] after minor surgical procedures under general anesthesia in adults,[59,60] and after major gynecologic surgery performed while the patient is under epidural morphine anesthesia.[61] This form of scopolamine has also been used in the treatment of vertigo.[62] The advantage of transdermal scopolamine over oral or parenteral routes is a decreased incidence of side effects.

Respiratory System

Like atropine, scopolamine decreases airway resistance and increases anatomic dead space. These effects occur even with smaller doses and persist longer than with atropine. A well-controlled study[63] has shown that, following the IM administration of 0.0022, 0.0044 and 0.0066 mg/kg of scopolamine, the greatest decrease in airway resistance was obtained with the intermediate dose. The average decrease is 0.51 cm H_2O/L/sec. The maximum decrease occurs at 40 minutes after the administration, and the effect persists for several hours. The respiratory dead space increases progressively with increasing doses and also lasts longer than with atropine.

Ocular Effects

Unlike atropine, therapeutic doses of scopolamine when given systemically cause definite mydriasis and cycloplegia, so caution should be used in patients with glaucoma because cycloplegia can lead to an increase in intraocular pressure. In general, all mydriatic agents have lesser effect in darkly pigmented eyes than in nonpigmented eyes, and scopolamine is no exception. It causes more mydriasis than atropine in white patients[64] and should probably be avoided in elderly white women, in whom angle-closure glaucoma occurs more frequently than in other groups.

Gastrointestinal System

Like atropine, scopolamine has been widely used as an antispasmodic. A combination of atropine, scopolamine, and phenobarbital (Donnatal) is used frequently for this purpose.

Temperature

In children, scopolamine is more than 60% more effective than atropine in preventing sweating[65] and thus at equal dose levels is more likely to cause a rise in temperature.

Dosage

Because atropine is a mixture of levo and dextro hyoscyamine and scopolamine is only levo-hyoscine, to have equal efficacy, only half the scopolamine should be

Table 36–4. Scopolamine: Pharmacokinetic Data

Availability (Oral) (%)	Urinary Excretion (%)	Bound in Plasma (%)	Clearance ($ml \cdot min^{-1} \cdot kg^{-1}$)	Vol. Dist. (Liters/kg)	Half-Life (hours)	Effective Concentrations
27 ± 12	6 ± 4	—	16 ± 13*	1.4 ± 0.7†	2.9 ± 1.2	40 pg/ml‡

*Assuming 70-kg weight.
†V_{area}.
‡Prevention of motion sickness.
Data from Kanto, J., Klotz, U.: Pharmacokinetic implications for the clinical use of atropine, scopolamine and glycopyrrolate. Acta Anesthesiol Scand 32:69, 1988; and Putcha, L., Cintron, N. M., Tusi, J., Kramer, W. G.: Pharmacokinetics and oral availability of scopolamine. Pharm Res 6:481, 1989.

given; this is usually not the case, however. For small children aged 6 months to 3 years, the dose is 0.1 to 0.15 mg, and for older children, the dose is 6 μg/kg. For adults, the dose is 0.3 to 0.6 mg IM or 8 μg/kg. IV doses should be decreased depending on the age of the patient and the purpose.

Pharmacokinetics

Although scopolamine was used extensively at one time, little is known regarding the pharmacokinetics of the drug.[66,67] IV injection of 0.005 mg/kg produces rapid distribution (half-life ≈ 5 min) in healthy women undergoing cesarean section under general anesthesia.[68] The distribution and elimination have been found to be comparable to those of atropine. The elimination half-life is about 3.0 hours, which is more rapid than atropine. With IM injection, the absorption is faster than with atropine, whereas oral scopolamine has slow absorption similar to that of atropine. Like atropine, scopolamine has a rapid placental transfer, but unlike atropine, it is also transferred into lumbar cerebrospinal fluid (Table 36–4).

Synthetic Anticholinergics

Many synthetic and semisynthetic drugs with anticholinergic activity are available. These include tertiary amines and quaternary ammonium compounds.

Tertiary amines are useful as antispasmodics, as antitremor agents, and in ophthalmology. The antispasmodics include dicyclomine hydrochloride (Bentyl), oxiphencyclamine hydrochloride (Daricon), and others. The antitremor agents are trihexyphenidyl hydrochloride (Artane) and benztropine mesylate (Cogentin). Those that are used in ophthalmology include homatropine hydrobromide (Isopto Homatropine), cyclopentolate hydrochloride (Cyclogyl), and tropicamide (Mydriacyl).

The quaternary ammonium compounds have significant differences in their pharmacologic actions from the natural alkaloids. They are poorly absorbed orally and through the conjunctiva. Their CNS effects are minimal because they do not cross the blood-brain barrier readily. They exert more ganglionic blockade, and in toxic doses they can even produce neuromuscular blockade. The duration of action of many of these drugs is usually longer than that of belladonna alkaloids. This group includes many drugs such as homatropine methylbromide, methantheline bromide (Banthine), propantheline bromide (Pro-Banthine), oxyphenoium (Antrenyl), meth-

scopolamine bromide (Pamine), anisotropine methylbromide (Valpin), and others. In addition, two quaternary ammonium compounds are of interest to anesthesiologists. These are glycopyrrolate and ipratropium bromide.

Glycopyrrolate (Robinul)

The chemistry and pharmacology of glycopyrrolate were described in 1960.[69] Since the 1970s, it has become an important pharmacologic agent in anesthesiology. Chemically, it is 3-hydroxy-1,1-dimethylpyrrolidinium bromide, α cyclo pentylmandelate (Fig. 36–8).

Pharmacologic Actions

Secretory Glands

Several studies comparing the antisialic actions of belladonna alkaloids with glycopyrrolate have found that all of them have similar ability to decrease salivation.[53,54] Glycopyrrolate has the advantage over atropine, however, because it produces less tachycardia, blurred vision, or fever and over scopolamine because it produces less sedation. The duration of antisialic action may last several hours, which may be undesirable.

Cardiovascular System

Glycopyrrolate certainly produces less tachycardia than atropine and thus is preferable in many situations such as during reversal of neuromuscular blockade. It has been found to be equally effective in treating OCR when compared with atropine in children (15 μg/kg atropine and

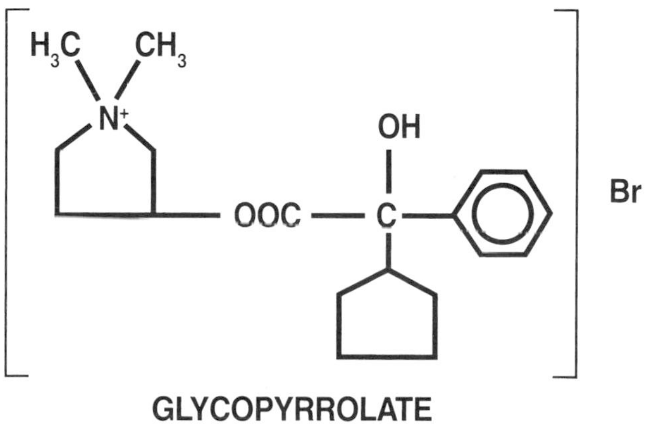

GLYCOPYRROLATE

Fig. 36–8. Chemical structure of glycopyrrolate.

7.5 μg/kg glycopyrrolate), but it produces less tachycardia.[26] During induction of anesthesia, cardiac rate and rhythm following IM administration of these two drugs were compared in adult patients,[70] and glycopyrrolate was found to be associated with a low incidence of arrhythmias. When compared as prophylactic agents in preventing succinylcholine-induced changes in heart rate and rhythm, glycopyrrolate was found to offer similar or greater protection than atropine.[71]

Central Nervous System

The highly polar quaternary ammonium group of glycopyrrolate limits its passage across lipid membranes, such as the blood-brain and placental barriers. Because of this, in therapeutic doses, it does not produce any CNS effects or adversely affect the fetus.[72]

Respiratory System

Like atropine, glycopyrrolate is a bronchodilator, and its effects are much superior to those of atropine[32] (see Figs. 36-4 and 36-5). Glycopyrrolate increases $_sGAW$ 100% above control with both smaller (3.2 μg/kg) and larger (10 μg/kg) doses (Fig. 36-9), but atropine increases $_sGAW$ 100% above control only with larger doses (20 μg/kg) and increases less than 50% with smaller doses (6 to 8 μg/kg) (Fig. 36-9). In addition, the duration of bronchodilation is much longer with glycopyrrolate.

Gastrointestinal System

Glycopyrrolate reduces gastric acidity and volume to a greater degree than atropine but to a much lesser degree than cimetedine or antacids.[41,73,74] In addition, like atropine, it decreases the lower esophageal sphincter pressure[75] and thus is not an effective agent for the prevention of acid aspiration. It is used in the treatment of peptic ulcer disease and other GI disorders, however.

Dosage

For premedication, 0.002 mg/lb IM 30 to 60 minutes should be given before surgery. For intraoperative use, smaller (0.1 mg, increments) IV doses should be given. For reversal of neuromuscular blockade, 0.2 mg with each 1.0 mg of neostigmine or 5.0 mg pyridostigmine is the recommended dose. Because of poor absorption by mouth, it is not used orally.

Pharmacokinetics

The fate of radioactive ^{3}H-glycopyrrolate administered intravenously has been studied.[76] More than 90% of radioactivity disappears from serum in 5 minutes, and almost all is gone in 30 minutes. In the urine, highest radioactivity is seen between 0 and 3 hours, and only insignificant amounts are seen after 6 hours. In the bile, highest activity is seen between 30 and 60 minutes, and small amounts are measurable until 48 hours. In both urine and bile, over 80% corresponds to unchanged glycopyrrolate. The comparative pharmacokinetics of atropine, scopolamine, and glycopyrrolate are shown in Table 36-5.

Ipratropium Bromide (Atrovent)

This agent is a quaternary ammonium congener of atropine. Chemically, it is 8-isopropyl noratropine methobromide. It is freely soluble in water and insoluble in lipids.

Pharmacologic Actions

It is available as a metered-dose inhaler, and its use is only as a bronchodilator. Ipratropium has been found to be superior to other anticholinergic agents not only because of its local effect on the respiratory system, but also because of the lack of side effects. Side effects are lacking because much of the ipratropium when used as an inhaler is swallowed and is not absorbed into the systemic circulation either from the surface of the lung or from the GI tract. Although ipratropium is effective by itself in both chronic obstructive lung disease and asthma, when used in combination with β-adrenergic agents such as salbutamol, the relief of airflow obstruction is superior and longer lasting.[77] For patients with emphysema and chronic bronchitis, combination therapy increases the bronchodilation more than is achieved with β-adrenergic agents alone. For patients with asthma, the combination therapy may only slightly increase the maximal bronchodilation achievable with β-adrenergic agonists alone, but it allows a reduction in the dosage of β-adrenergic agonists without loss of efficacy and prolongs the duration of action (Fig 36-10). In addition, the onset of action of ipratropium is slower, and the β-adrenergic agonists fill in that time because they have a shorter onset of action. Unlike atropine, it has no ad-

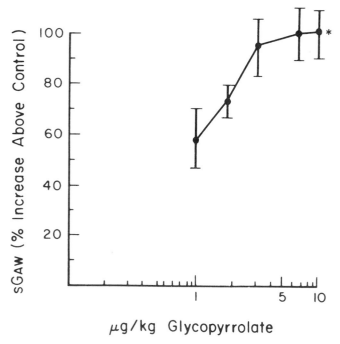

Fig. 36–9. Dose-response curve for bronchodilation after glycopyrrolate. Percentage of increase in $_sGAW$ is plotted as a function of increasing dose on a log scale. From Gal, T. H., Surratt, P. M.: Atropine and glycopyrrolate effects on lung mechanics in normal man. Anesth Analg 60:87, 1981.

Table 36–5. Pharmacokinetics of Anticholinergics in Adults

Agent	Plasma Binding	V^B (L/kg)	T½ (hrs)	CL (ml/min/kg)	Urinary Excretion
Atropine	(1) 14–22%	1.7 ± 0.7	4.3	5.9	57%
Scopolamine	(2) 5%	1.4 ± 0.5	2.9 ± 1.2	16 ± 13	6%
Glycopyrrolate	(3) minimal	3.9 ± 0.15	5 minutes	30	intact 80%

V^B = Volume of distribution; T½ = Elimination half life; CL = Total serum clearance.
Data from references 43, 66, and 76.

verse effects on the function of the ciliated bronchial epithelium.

Dosage

In patients in stable condition, the dosage is 40 to 80 μg (each inhalation provides about 18 μg) four times a day. In patients with severe disease, however, a larger dose of 80 to 120 μg is advised because penetration into the airways is impaired,[78] and these doses of ipratropium are relatively innocuous.[79]

Pharmacokinetics

When the drug is inhaled, blood levels rise slowly, and less than 1% is absorbed into the circulation. About half the 1% is biotransformed, and the metabolites along with the intact agent are excreted in the urine. Most of the inhaled drug is swallowed and is then excreted in the feces.

USES AND COMPARATIVE EFFECTS OF ANTICHOLINERGICS IN ANESTHESIA

The three most important uses of anticholinergic agents in the routine practice of anesthesia are to coun-
teract the muscarinic effects of anticholinesterases that are used to reverse neuromuscular blockade, to decrease salivary secretions, and to prevent or treat reflex vagal bradycardia. Other desirable anticholinergic effects include sedation without causing CNS excitement, decrease in gastric acidity and volume, and bronchodilation in patients with respiratory diseases. Some of the foregoing effects are compared in Tables 36–6 and 36–7.

Anticholinesterase drugs such as edrophonium, neostigmine, and pyridostigmine are used to reverse the actions of neuromuscular blocking agents. Because anticholinesterase agents exert their action by accumulating acetylcholine at the neuromuscular junction, both muscarinic and nicotinic effects are seen with these agents. Only the nicotinic effects are desired, however, and the muscarinic effects have to be blocked. This is the most common use of anticholinergic drugs. Both atropine and glycopyrrolate are useful for this purpose. Atropine has a shorter onset of action than glycopyrrolate, and so atropine is preferable with edrophonium, which has a faster onset of action, and glycopyrrolate is preferred with neostigmine or pyridostigmine, which have a slower onset of action. Usually, if glycopyrrolate is used with edrophonium, an initial bradycardia will occur, and if atropine is used with neostigmine, an initial tachycardia will occur.

Premedication

Routine administration of anticholinergics as premedicants has decreased over the last few years because excessive secretions are not a major concern with newer inhalational anesthetic agents. Patients who are anxious and deprived of fluids have a dry mouth even without the use of anticholinergics,[80] and addition of an anticholiner-

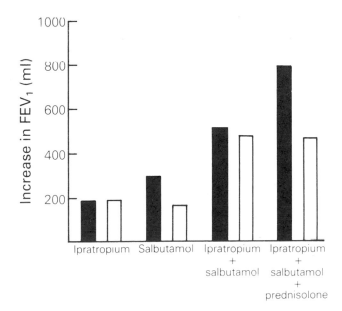

Fig. 36–10. Mean increases in FEV₁ in patients with asthma (solid squares) or chronic obstructive bronchitis (open squares) after 3 days of treatment with ipratropium alone, with salbutamol alone, with the combination and with prednisolone. From Lightbody, et al.: Br J Dis Chest *72*:184, 1978.

Table 36–6. Comparison of Anticholinergic Agents

Effect	Atropine	Scopolamine	Glycopyrrolate
↓ In salivary secretions	+	+ +	+ +
↓ Gastric secretions	+	+	+ +
↑ Heart rate	+ + +	+ +	+
CNS effects	+ +	+ + +	0
Bronchodilation	+	+	+ +
Duration of action (IV)	15–30 min	30–60 min	2–4 h

0 = no effect; + = small effect; + + = moderate effect; + + + = large.

Table 36–7. Comparative Pharmacodynamic Activity of Anticholinergic Agents Used in Preanesthetic Medication, Including Special Preparations

Drug	Dose (mg)	Onset (min)	Duration	Antisecretory	Cardiac Rate Increase (%)	Vagolytic
Levo-hyoscyamine (Bellafoline)	0.5	10	1 h	1	40	1
Scopolamine Methyl Bromide (Pamine)	0.1	15	2 h	1	75	
Scopolamine (*l*-hyoscine)	0.5	15	1½ h	1	25–30	1
Antrenyl (Oxyphenonium)	0.5	10–15	3–4 h	2	40	1
Methantheline Bromide (Banthine)	25.0	5–10	30 min	3	41	3
Diphenmethanil Methyl SO$_4$ (Prantal)	25.0	5–10	15 min	4	—	—
Atropine (mixture *d*- and *l*-hyoscyamine)	0.5	15–20	1 h	5	30	2
Dextro-hyoscyamine	0	0	0	0	0	0

gic drug can make it more uncomfortable to the patient. For intraoral procedures such as tonsillectomy and adenoidectomy and dental rehabilitations and for bronchoscopic procedures, however, anticholinergics can be useful. All three agents produce similar decreases in secretions,[53,54] but because glycopyrrolate is associated with lesser side effects, it has become the most commonly used drug for this purpose.

Management of Intraoperative Bradycardia

The prophylactic use of anticholinergics to reduce intraoperative bradycardia associated with certain procedures or with repeated use of succinylcholine is also becoming uncommon, especially in adults. This decrease may be due to two reasons. First, the use of succinylcholine is decreasing, and second, many anesthesiologists prefer to choose the anticholinergic drug and its dosage when the bradycardia occurs. Both atropine and glycopyrrolate are effective for this purpose, and if an excessive rise in heart rate is not desired, glycopyrrolate would be the drug of choice.

With the availability of antacids, histamine-2 blockers, and metaclopramide, anticholinergics are no longer used to prevent aspiration of gastric contents.

Scopolamine is still given IM as a premedicant drug (along with morphine and diazepam) for its sedative and amnesic actions to patients undergoing cardiac surgery. It should not be given to patients older than 70 years of age, however, because of the concern of CNS effects.

UNDESIRABLE EFFECTS

The undesirable effects are more common with tertiary amines and are related to the dosage. The higher the dosage, the more common the adverse effects. Dry mouth is the first and dry skin is the second most common side effect. Thirst and difficulty in swallowing follow. Increase in temperature and flushing are seen, especially in children. Mydriasis, palpitations, blurring of vision, difficulty in urination, and urinary retention may follow with even larger doses. Nausea, vomiting, drowsiness, restlessness, disorientation, hallucinations, delirium, and coma can result, leading eventually to respiratory and circulatory collapse and death. Dose-related effects of atropine are shown in Table 36–8.

The behavioral changes and other effects that are produced by anticholinergic drugs in the CNS are referred to as central anticholinergic syndrome (CAS). Besides atropine and scopolamine, many other drugs when given in large doses or in combination can cause this syndrome. Some of these agents are listed in Table 36–9.

Therapeutic doses of scopolamine and larger than therapeutic doses of atropine can cause CAS. Most often, CAS is first noticed in the postanesthesia care unit and manifests as agitation, excitement, confusion, and somnolence. Many other symptoms and signs such as ataxia, asynergia, stereotyped movements, hallucinations, and even convulsions can follow. Elderly patients have decreased CNS cholinergic fibers with associated cholinergic dysfunction.[81] In addition, they are also more prone to take various drugs with anticholinergic effects and thus are more prone to CAS. Patients with a history of mental depression who have decreased levels of CNS neurotransmitter substances are also more prone to CAS. In addition, investigators have suggested that early postoperative hypoxemia may contribute to CAS.[82]

Increasing the acetylcholine levels in the brain is necessary to treat CAS. Although drugs such as 4-aminopyridine and galanthamine hydrobromide can increase acetylcholine levels in the CNS, their actions are unpredictable. The acetylcholinesterase inhibitor physostigmine (Antilirium) is a predictable and rapidly acting drug. Unlike neostigmine and pyridostigmine, physostigmine is a tertiary amine and enters the brain rapidly and reverses the CAS. Although it is specific in the treatment of CAS caused by belladonna drugs, it can also reverse the effects of tricyclic antidepressants[83] phenothiazines,[84] antihistamines,[85] and antiparkinsonian drugs[86] that cause CAS, but it also can reverse the effects of certain drugs that have no anticholinergic activity such as diazepam,[87-89] probably by a nonspecific analeptic effect (Table 36–10). It has been shown only transiently to antagonize the somnolence caused by halothane in dogs.[90] The dosage is 0.5 mg increments up to 2 to 3 mg IV, until the response is seen. It acts within 1 to 10 minutes. Side effects are minimal, but transient bradycardia, nausea, intestinal cramps, and increased salivation can occur.

Table 36–8. Effects of Atropine in Relation to Dose

Dose (mg)	Effects
0.5	Slight cardiac slowing; some dryness of mouth; inhibition of sweating
1.0	Definite dryness of mouth; thirst; acceleration of heart, sometimes preceded by slowing; mild at dilatation of pupil
2.0	Rapid heart rate; palpitation; marked dryness of mouth; dilated pupils; some blurring of near vision
5.0	All the foregoing symptoms marked; speech disturbed; difficulty in swallowing; restlessness and fatigue; headache; dry, hot skin; difficulty in micturition; reduced intestinal peristalsis
10.0 and more	Foregoing symptoms more marked; pulse rapid and weak; iris practically obliterated; vision blurred; skin flushed, hot, dry, and scarlet; ataxia, restlessness, and excitement; hallucinations and delirium; coma.

From Gilman, A. G., et al.: Goodman and Gilman's The Pharmacological Basis of Therapeutics, 8th Ed. New York, McGraw-Hill, 1990, p. 158.

Table 36–9. Agents That Can Cause Anticholinergic Syndrome

Belladonna alkaloids
Opioids
Anesthetic agents
Antidepressants
Antipsychotics
Antispasmodics
Antiparkinson agents
Tranquilizers
Hallucinogens
Psychotogenic warfare chemicals

Table 36–10. Use of Physostigmine in Treatment of Central Anticholinergic Syndrome

Used to reverse adverse effects of:

Neuroleptics
  Phenothiazines
  Droperidol
  Diazepam
Belladonna alkaloids
Antiparkinsonian drugs
Antihistamines
  Promethazine
Tricyclic antidepressants

Patients with Down's syndrome are known to be sensitive to atropine. Pupillary dilation is exaggerated in these patients when atropine is instilled in the eye because of the hypoplasia of the peripheral stroma of the iris.[91] With small IV doses, these patients develop bradycardia similar to normal patients, but with larger doses, they develop exaggerated tachycardia. This increased sensitivity to the cardioacceleratory effects of atropine probably results from the genetic imbalance caused by the extra chromosome 21 in Down's syndrome.[92]

For patients with cystic fibrosis, atropine and probably scopolamine should be avoided because they can cause inspissation of secretions, with resultant increase in airway resistance.

NEWER ANTICHOLINERGIC AGENTS

In addition to the quaternary ammonium compound ipratropium, which causes bronchodilation without other anticholinergic actions, many newer drugs that selectively block different muscarinic receptors are being developed. One of these drugs is pirenzepine hydrochloride, which has been extensively used in Europe. It is a tricyclic benzodiazepine that blocks specific M_1 receptors and is used for the treatment of peptic ulcer disease.[93] It selectively suppresses both basal and stimulated acid and pepsin secretion with lesser effects on other muscarinic sites (e.g., salivary secretion). AF-DX 116 is a drug that has great affinity for cardiac (M_2) receptors. It has been found to have cardioselectivity in humans[94] and will be useful for the treatment of bradycardia and atrioventricular block of vagal origin. Methoctramine and himbacine are two other investigational drugs with cardioselectivity,

and hydrosiladifenidol is a drug with selectivity for M_3 receptors in exocrine glands.

REFERENCES

1. Brown, J. H.: Atropine, scopolamine and related anti-muscarinic drugs. In Gilman, A. G., et al. (eds.). Goodman and Gilman's The Pharmacological Basis of Therapeutics, 8th Ed. New York, McGraw-Hill, 1990.
2. Hammer, R., et al.: Pirenzepine distinguishes between different subclasses of muscarinic receptors. Nature 283:90, 1980.
3. Bonner, T. I., Buckley, N. J., Young, A. C., Brann, M. R.: Identification of a family of muscarinic acetylcholine receptor genes. Science 237:527, 1987.
4. Bonner, T. I.: The molecular basis of muscarinic receptor diversity. Trends Neurosci 12:148, 1989.
5. Berridge, M. J.: Inositol lipids and calcium signalling. Proc R Soc Lond (Biol) 234:359, 1988.
6. Brown, A. M., Birnbaumer, L.: Direct G protein gating of ion channels. Am J Physiol 254:H401, 1988.
7. Gilman, A. G.: G proteins: transducers of receptor generated signals. Annu Rev Biochem 56:615, 1987.
8. Zimmerman, J., Feldman, S.: Physical-chemical properties and biologic activity. In Foye, N. O. (ed.). Principles of Medicinal Chemistry. Philadelphia, Lea & Febiger, 1974, p. 8.
9. Meyerhoffer, A.: The molecular structure of some anticholinergic drugs. FOA Rep 6:1, 1972.
10. Chamberlain, D. A., Turner, P., Sneddon, J. M.: Effects of atropine on heart rate in healthy man. Lancet 2:12, 1967.
11. Das, G., Talmers, F. N., Weissler, A. M.: New observations on the effects of atropine on the sinoatrial and atrio ventricular nodes in man. Am J Cardiol 36:281, 1975.
12. Kottmeier, C. A., Gravenstein, J. S.: The parasympathomimetic activity of atropine and atropine methyl bromide. Anesthesiology 29:1125, 1968.

13. Wellstein, A., Pitschner, H. F.: Complex dose response curves of atropine in man explained by different functions of M_1 and M_2 cholinoceptors. Naunyn Schmiedebergs Arch Pharmacol 338:19, 1988.

14. Jones, R. E., Deutsch, S., Turndorf, H.: Effects of atropine on cardiac rhythm in conscious and anesthetized man. Anesthesiology 22:67, 1961.

15. Eger, E. I.: Atropine, scopolamine and related compounds. Anesthesiology 23:365, 1962.

16. Hayes, A. H., Jr., Copelan, H. W., Ketchum, J. S.: Effects of large intramuscular doses of atropine on cardiac rhythm. Clin Pharmacol Ther 12:482, 971.

17. Dauchot, P., Gravenstein, J. S.: Effects of atropine on the electrocardiogram in different age groups. Clin Pharmacol Ther 12:274, 1971.

18. Knoebel, S. B., McHenry, P. L., Phillips, J. F., Widlansky, S.: Atropine induced cardioacceleration and myocardial blood flow in subjects with and without coronary artery disease. Am J Cardiol 33:327, 1974.

19. Tsang, H. S.: Less commonly recognized hazards of atropine as preanesthetic medication. Anesthesiol Rev 4:15, 1977.

20. Roizen, M. F., et al.: Similarity between effects of pancuronium and atropine on plasma norepinephrine levels in man. J Pharmacol Exp Ther 211:419, 1979.

21. Saxena, P. R., Bonka, I. L.: Mechanism of selective cardiac vagolytic action of pancuronium bromide: specific blockade of cardiac muscarinic reception. Eur J Pharmacol 11:332, 1970.

22. Zsigmond, E. K., et al.: The effect of pancuronium bromide on plasma norepinephrine and cortisol concentrations during thiamylal induction. Can Anaesth Soc J 21:147, 1974.

23. Samra, S. K., Cohen, P. J.: Modification of chronotropic response to anticholinergics by halogenated anaesthetics in children. Can Anaesth Soc J 27:540, 1980.

24. Yamaguchi, H., Dohi, S., Sato, S., Naito, H.: Heart rate response to atropine in humans anaesthetized with five different techniques. Can J Anaesth 35:451, 1988.

25. Cross, G., Gaylord, D., Lim, M.: Atropine induced heart rate changes: a comparison between midazolam, fentanyl-propofol-N_2O and midazolam-fentanyl-thiopentone-enflurane-N_2 anaesthesia. Can J Anaesth 37:416, 1990.

26. Mirakhur, R. K., Jones, C. J., Dundee, J. W., Archer, D. B.: IM or IV atropine or glycopyrrolate for the prevention of oculocardiac reflex in children undergoing squint surgery. Br J Anaesth 54:1059, 1982.

27. Whetherell, A.: Some effects of atropine on short-term memory. Br J Clin Pharmacol 10:627, 1980.

28. Gandivia, B.: Historical review of the use of parasympatholytic agents in the treatment of respiratory disorders. Post Grad Med J 51(Suppl 7):13, 1975.

29. Crompton, G. K.: A comparison of responses to bronchodilator drugs in chronic bronchitis and chronic asthma. Thorax 23:46, 1968.

30. Chick, T. W., Jenne, J. W.: Comparative bronchodilator responses to atropine and terbutaline in asthma and chronic bronchitis. Chest 72:719, 1977.

31. Hensley, M. J., O'Cain, C. F., McFadden, E. R., Jr., Ingram, R. H., Jr.: Distribution of bronchodilatation in normal subjects: beta agonist versus atropine. J Appl Physiol 45:778, 1978.

32. Gal, T. H., Surratt, P. M.: Atropine and glycopyrrolate effects on lung mechanics in normal man. Anesth Analg 60:85, 1981.

33. Groto, H., Whitman, R. A., Arakawa, K.: Pulmonary mechanics in man after administration of atropine and neostigmine. Anesthesiology 49:91, 1978.

34. Aquilina, A. T., Hall, W. J., Douglas, R. G., Utell, M. J.: Airway reactivity in subjects with viral upper respiratory infections: the effects of exercise and cold air. Am Rev Respir Dis 122:3, 1980.

35. Fryer, A. D., Jacoby, D. B.: Parainfluenza virus infection damages inhibitory M_2 muscarinic receptors on pulmonary parasympathetic nerves in guinea pig. Br J Pharmacol 102:267, 1991.

36. Jacoby, D. B., Hirshman, C. A.: General anesthesia in patients with viral respiratory infections: an unsound sleep (editorial). Anesthesiology 74:969, 1991.

37. Annis, P., Landa, J., Lichtiger, M.: Effects of atropine on velocity of tracheal mucus in anesthetized patients. Anesthesiology 44:74, 1976.

38. Mehra, K. S., Chandra, P.: The effect on the eye of premedication with atropine. Br J Anaesth 37:133, 1965.

39. Garde, T. F., et al.: Racial mydriatic response to belladonna premedication. Anesth Analg 57:572, 1978.

40. Salem, M. R., et al.: Premedicant drugs and gastric juice pH and volume in pediatric patients. Anesthesiology 44:216, 1976.

41. Stoelting, R. K.: Responses to atropine, glycopyrrolate and riopan of gastric fluid pH and volume in adult patients. Anesthesiology 48:367, 1978.

42. Dow, T. G. B., et al.: The effect of atropine on the lower esophageal sphincter in late pregnancy. Obstet Gynecol 51:426, 1978.

43. Berghem, L., Bergman, U., Schildt, B., Sörbo, B.: Plasma atropine concentrations determined by radioimmunoassay after single dose IV and IM administration. Br J Anaesth 52:597, 1980.

44. Kentala, E., Kaila, T., Iisab, E., Kanto, J.: Intramuscular atropine in healthy volunteers: a pharmacokinetic and pharmacodynamic study. Int J Clin Pharmacol Ther Toxicol 28:399, 1990.

45. Ali Melkkilá, T., Kanto, J., Iisalo, E.: Pharmacokinetics and pharmacodynamics of anticholinergic drugs Acta Anaesthesiol Scand 37:633, 1993.

46. Kradjan, W. A., Smallridge, R. C., Davis, R., Verma, P.: Atropine serum concentrations after multiple inhaled doses of atropine sulfate. Clin Pharmacol Ther 38:12, 1985.

47. Beermann, B., Hellstrom, K., Rosen, A.: The gastrointestinal absorption of atropine in man. Clin Sci 40:95, 1971.

48. Seppala, T., Visakorpi, R.: Psychophysiological measurements after oral atropine in man. Acta Pharmacol Toxicol 52:68, 1983.

49. Bejersten, A., Olsson, G. L., Palmer, L.: The influence of body weight on plasma concentration of atropine after rectal administration. Acta Anaesthesiol Scand 29:782, 1985.

50. Virtanen, R., et al.: Pharmacokinetic studies on atropine with special reference to age. Acta Anaesthesiol Scand 26:297, 1982.

51. Gosselin, R. E., Gabovrel, J. D., Wills, J. H.: The fate of atropine in man. Clin Pharmacol Ther 1:597, 1960.

52. Wyant, G. M., Dobkin, A. B.: Antisialogogue drugs in man: comparison of atropine, scopolamine (l-hyoscine) and l-hyoscyamine (Bellafoline). Anaesthesia 12:203, 1957.

53. Mirakhur, R. K., Dundee, J. W., Connelly, J. D. R.: Studies of drugs given before anesthesia. XVII: Anticholinergic premedicants. Br J Anaesth 51:339, 1979.

54. Sengupta, A., Gupta, P. K., Pandey, K.: Investigation of glycopyrrolate as a premedicant drug. Br J Anaesth 52:513, 1980.

55. Gordon, C., et al.: Effect of transdermal scopolamine on salivation. J Clin Pharmacol 25:407, 1985.

56. Price, N. M., et al.: Transdermal scopolamine in the prevention of motion sickness at sea. Clin Pharmacol Ther 29:414, 1981.

57. Dahl, E., et al.: Transdermal scopolamine, oral meclizine

and placebo in motion sickness. Clin Pharmacol Ther *36*:116, 1984.

58. Horimoto, Y., Tomie, H., Hanzausak, B., Nishida, Y.: Scopolamine patch reduces postoperative emesis in paediatric patients following strabesmus surgery. Can J Anaesth *38*:441, 1991.

59. Tolksdorf, W., Meisel, R., Miller, P., Bender, H. J.: Transdermales Scopolamine (TTS-Scopolamine) zur prophylaxe postoperative äbelkeit und Erbrechen. Anesthetist *34*:656, 1985.

60. Tigerstedt, I., Salmela, L., Aromaa, V.: Double blind comparison of transdermal scopolamine, droperidol and placebo against postoperative nausea and vomiting. Acta Anesthesiol Scand *32*:454, 1988.

61. Loper, K. A., Ready, L. B., Dorman, B. H.: Prophylactic transdermal scopolamine patches reduce nausea in postoperative patients receiving epidural morphine. Anesth Analg *68*:144, 1989.

62. Babin, R. W., Balkany, T. J., Willard, E. F.: Transdermal scopolamine in the treatment of acute vertigo. Ann Otol Rhinol Laryngol *93*:25, 1984.

63. Smith, T. C., DuBois, A. B.: The effects of scopolamine in the airways of man. Anesthesiology *30*:12, 1969.

64. Garde, T. F., et al.: Racial mydriatic response to belladonna premedication. Anesth Analg *57*:572, 1978.

65. Eger, E. I., Kraft, I. D., Keasling, H. H.: Comparison of atropine or scopolamine plus pentobarbital, mepiridine or morphine as pediatric preanesthetic medication. Anesthesiology *22*:962, 1961.

66. Kanto, J., Klotz, U.: Pharmacokinetic implications for the clinical use of atropine, scopolamine and glycopyrrolate. Acta Anesthesiol Scand *32*:69, 1988.

67. Putcha, L., Cintron, N. M., Tusi, J., Kramer, W. G.: Pharmacokinetics and oral availability of scopolamine. Pharmacol Res *6*:481, 1989.

68. Pihlajämaki, K. K., Kanto, J. H., Oksman-Caldentey, K. M.: Pharmacokinetics and clinical effects of scopolamine in cacsarean section patients. Acta Pharmacol Toxicol *59*:259, 1986.

69. Franko, B. V., Lunsford, C. D.: Derivations of 3-pyrrolidinols III. The chemistry, pharmacology and toxicology of some N-substituted-3-pyrrolidyl α-substituted phenylacetates. J Med Pharm Chem *2*:523, 1960.

70. Mirakhur, R. K., Clarke, R. S., Elliott, J., Dundee, J. W.: Atropine and glycopyrronium premedication: a comparison of the effects on cardiac rate and rhythm during induction of anaesthesia. Anaesthesia *33*:906, 1978.

71. Cozanitis, D. A., Dundee, J. W., Khan, M. M.: Comparative study of atropine and glycopyrrolate on suxamethonium induced changes in cardiac rate and rhythm. Br J Anaesth *52*:291, 1980.

72. Proakis, A. G., Harris, G. B.: Comparative penetration of glycopyrrolate and atropine across the blood-brain and placental barriers in anesthetized dogs. Anesthesiology *48*:339, 1978.

73. Manchikanti, L., Roush, J. R.: Effect of preanesthetic glycopyrrolate and cimetidine on gastric fluid pH and volume in outpatients. Anesth Analg *63*:40, 1984.

74. Keating, P. J., Black, J. F., Watson, D. W.: Effects of glycopyrrolate and cimetedine and gastric volume and acidity in patients awaiting surgery. Br J Anesth *50*:1247, 1978.

75. Brok-Utne, J. G., et al.: The effect of glycopyrrolate (Robinul) on the lower esophageal sphincter. Can Anaesth Soc J *25*:144, 1978.

76. Kaltiala, E., et al.: The fate of intravenous [^{3}H]glycopyrrolate in man. J Pharm Pharmacol *26*:352, 1974.

77. Boushey, H. A.: Combination therapy with anticholinergic agents for airflow obstruction. Postgrad Med J *63(Suppl 1)*:69, 1987.

78. Pavia, D., Thomson, H. L., Clarke, S. W., Shannon, H. S.: Effect of lung function and mode of inhalation on penetration of aerosol into the human lung. Thorax *32*:194, 1977.

79. Gross, N. J.: Anticholinergic agents in chronic bronchitis and emphysema. Postgrad Med J *63(Suppl 1)*:29, 1987.

80. Forrest, W. H., Jr., Brown, C. R., Brown, B. W.: Subjective responses to six common preoperative medications. Anesthesiology *47*:241, 1977.

81. Bartus, R. T., Dean, R. L., III, Beer, B., Lippa, A. S.: The cholinergic hypothesis of geriatric memory dysfunction. Science *217*:408, 1982.

82. Berggren, D., et al.: Postoperative confusion after anesthesia in elderly patients with femoral neck fractures. Anesth Analg *66*:497, 1987.

83. Heiser, J. F., Wilbert, D. E.: Reversal of delirium induced by tricyclic antidepressant drugs with physostigmine. Am J Psychiatry *131*:1275, 1974.

84. Bernards, W. (discussion by Katz, R.): Case history #74: reversal of phenothiazine induced coma with physostigmine. Anesth Analg *52*:938, 1973.

85. Lee, J., Turndorf, H., Poppers, P. J.: Physostigmine reversal of antihistamine induced excitement and depression. Anesthesiology *43*:683, 1975.

86. El-Yousef, M. K., Janowsky, D. S., Davis, J. M., Sekerke, H. J.: Reversal of anti-parkinsonian drug toxicity by physostigmine: a controlled study. Am J Psychiatry *130*:141, 1973.

87. Bidwai, A. V., et al.: Reversal of diazepam induced postanesthetic somnolence with physostigmine. Anesthesiology *51*:256, 1979.

88. Larson, G. F., Hurlbert, B. J., Wingard, D. W.: Physostigmine reversal of diazepam induced depression. Anesth Analg *56*:348, 1977.

89. Bidwai, A. V., Cornelius, C. R., Stanley, T. H.: Reversal of Innovar induced postanesthetic somnolence and disorientation with physostigmine. Anesthesiology *44*:249, 1976.

90. Horrigan, R. W.: Physostigmine and anesthetic requirement for halothane in dogs. Anesth Analg *57*:180, 1977.

91. Priest, J. H.: Atropine response of eyes in mongolism. Am J Dis Child *100*:869, 1960.

92. Harris, W. S., Goodman, R. H.: Hyperreactivity to atropine in Down's Syndrome. N Engl J Med *279*:407, 1968.

93. Carmine, A. A., Brogden, R. N.: Pirenzepine: a review of its pharmacodynamic and pharmacokinetic properties and therapeutic efficacy in peptic ulcer disease and other allied diseases. Drugs *30*:85, 1985.

94. Pitschner, H. F., et al.: AF-DX 116 discriminates heart from gland M_2 cholinoceptors in man. Life Sci *45*:493, 1989.

Chapter 37

DIETHYL ETHER AND CHLOROFORM

MARK V. BOSWELL
VINCENT J. COLLINS

Although of only historical interest today, ether and chloroform formed the cornerstones of the early practice of anesthesiology. The introduction of surgical anesthesia is generally attributed to Dr. William T.G. Morton, a medical student and dentist from Boston, who first demonstrated the use of diethyl ether as a surgical anesthetic in 1846. Crawford Long, a physician from Georgia, had used ether since 1842, but had not published his experiences prior to the public demonstration by Morton. Ether was widely used in the United States until it was largely replaced by cyclopropane, which had a better clinical profile but was highly explosive in an oxygen-enriched atmosphere. Chloroform was introduced into clinical practice by the Scottish obstetrician James Simpson, in 1847. Despite its potential for toxic side effects, such as cardiac arrhythmias and hepatotoxicity, chloroform was widely used in Great Britain for nearly 100 years, perhaps because it has a more pleasant odor than ether and is non-flammable. The chemical structures of ether and chloroform are shown in Figure 37–1. For historical purposes, the essential pharmacology of diethyl ether and chloroform is reviewed in the following sections.

DIETHYL ETHER

Essential Pharmacology

Family of Ethers

Ethers may be considered alcohol derivatives in which the H of R-O-[H] is replaced by another R group. They are organic oxides with the following general structure:

$$[R]\text{-}C\text{-}O\text{-}C\text{-}[R]$$

Two generic forms are recognized. When both "R" groups are the same, a simple ether is formed. When the R radicals are of different groups, a mixed ether results. Certain ethers, such as divinyl ether and ethylvinyl ether, were used in clinical practice during the "ether era," because they appeared to offer certain clinical advantages, such as a more rapid induction, more pleasant odor, rapid emergence, or less postoperative nausea and emesis. These agents never came into widespread use, however, and were finally rendered obsolete with the introduction of the nonflammable halogenated ether anesthetics, such as halothane.

History[1,2]

Diethyl ether was first prepared by Valerius Cordus in 1546, who named the compound *oleum vitrioli dulce* or sweet vitriol. The term *spiritus aethereus* was introduced by Frobenius in 1730.[3] He derived the term aethereus from the Greek word aither (aithen) meaning to burn or shine. Many other usages of the word aether have been introduced. Homer described the "clear blue sky" as the aether, and early scientists applied the term to the hypothetic substance filling the void between particles of matter. Today, the word ether almost universally connotes the anesthetic agent.

Physiochemical Factors (Table 37–1)

Ether is a colorless, pungent, volatile liquid. The boiling point of the commercially available anesthetic is 36.2°C. The most common method of preparation is by dehydration of alcohol with sulfuric acid.

Decomposition to acetaldehyde and ether peroxides is favored by air, light, and moisture and is retarded by copper. Concentrations of 1% of these substances may cause respiratory irritation or cardiovascular depression. This is rarely attained. Traces of ketones may also be formed, and small amounts of such sulfur compounds as ethyl mercaptan may be present because of the manufacturing process. Ether is stable and is best preserved with 4% ethyl alcohol in small cans, but large stock cans may be used.[4]

Ether Impurities[5]

The purity of ether has been a subject of extensive investigation. Two sources of impurities exist. Contamina-

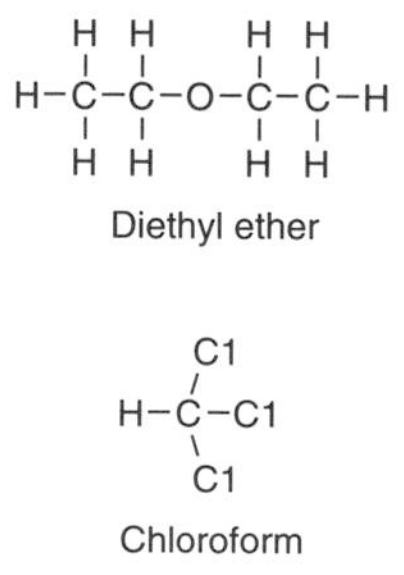

Fig. 37–1. Chemical structures of diethyl ether and chloroform.

Table 37–1. Physiochemical Constants—Diethyl Ether

Appearance	Colorless, clear, volatile liquid
Odor	Pungent characteristic standard
Flammability	Anesthetic range in the flammability range
Air	1.83–48.0%
Oxygen	2.10–82.5%
Molecular weight	74.12
Specific gravity of liquid (at 15°C)	0.719
Specific gravity of vapor (at 25°C)	2.60
Vapor density (at 25°C)	3.12 g
Heat capacity of liquid	0.547 g cal
Latent heat of vaporization (at 20°C)	87.5 g cal
Boiling point (pure ether)	34.6°C
Boiling point anesthetic ether (4% alcohol)	36.2°C
Freezing point	−116.3°C
Vapor pressure at 20°C	460 mm Hg
at 25°C	540 mm Hg

Solubility in water (at 25°C), one part ether in 7 parts water.

Water/gas partition coefficient	13.1	(Eger)
	15.6	(Ronzoni)
Blood/gas partition coefficient	12.1	(Eger)
	15.4	(Ronzoni)
Oil/water solubility 50/15.4	3.2	
Oil/gas	65	(Eger)
	50	(Ronzoni)
Tissue/blood	1.14	(brain)
	1.20	(lung)

Prepared from the following data: Adriani,[8] Steward,[8a] Larson,[10a] and Eger.[10b]

tion by the manufacturing process with thio acids, sulfuric oxides, thioethers, sulfates, and aldehydes may occur. During storage, ether peroxides and acetaldehyde may form slowly if water and air are present. The peroxides are the first to appear and form within 6 months, after which they gradually disappear. Meanwhile, aldehydes are formed. Formation of these impurities is inhibited by heavy metals; therefore, ether containers are usually lined with copper.

After exposure to air and light, the formation of both peroxides and aldehydes is favored. Ether should always be stored in original containers. If one has any question as to the presence of peroxides, the following simple test may be carried out: Shake 1 ml of 10% aqueous solution of potassium iodide (freshly prepared) with 10 ml of ether. The presence of as little as 0.001% peroxide will give the liquid a yellow coloration within 5 minutes.[6] Bourne[5] has shown that aldehydes up to 0.5% produce no significant effect on animals. The same holds true for concentrations of mercaptans up to 1% and peroxides up to 0.5%. Even these concentrations of aldehydes and perox-

ides have a definite injurious effect on cilia of respiratory tract, however.[7]

Preanesthetic Medication

An anticholinergic agent is an essential premedication. It minimizes both salivary and mucous secretions. Scopolamine is more effective in this regard and is preferred in patients under 50 years of age.

Narcotics are by far the most advantageous agents to secure an acquiescent and mentally relaxed patient. Morphine in particular provides a sedated, serene, and easily anesthetized subject. The patient does not need to be in pain for the singular advantages of morphine to be observed; the occurrence of untoward responses is insignificant.[8] Experience and evidence both indicate a definite ease of induction, a reduction in the amount of anesthetic agent, and minimization of the immediate need for postoperative pain relief.

Morphine is preferred because it is vagomimetic and balances the sympathetic effects of ether.

Administration

All inhalation techniques may be used for the administration of ether. The breathing mixture required for induction is 12%, that for maintenance is 3.5 to 4.5%, and that for respiratory arrest is 6.7 to 8.0%. Absorption of ether occurs through the alveolar-capillary membrane and is rapid. The first objective in administration is to attain an adequate alveolar concentration and to establish an equilibrium with the inspired mixture. The agent then passes into the capillary blood according to its partial pressure gradient and solubility in the blood; a second level of equilibrium is thereby established. Blood then circulates to tissues and delivers the agent to set up a third level of equilibrium.

This process was described in 1924, in a classic paper by Haggard.[9] It is simple and concise: "At the commencement of inhalation the ether taken up by the blood is carried in the arterial stream to the capillaries, where it diffuses into the tissues. The venous blood leaves the tissues with a concentration of ether identical with that of the tissues through which the blood has passed and returns to the lungs for a fresh charge. As this continues, the amount of ether, and hence the tension, constantly rises in the tissues. The amount of ether in the venous blood also rises correspondingly and tends to approach that of the arterial. More and more ether is thus carried back to the lungs by the venous blood and a decreasing amount is taken up by the blood from the air in the lungs and by the tissues from the blood. The limit approached is a state of saturation at which the body will contain an amount of ether equal to the weight of the body multiplied by the concentration in the air breathed, and by the coefficient of solubility."

Uptake

Assuming that an anesthetic state is related to the central nervous system concentration of the anesthetic agent, one needs to know the rate and amount of uptake. Using Burkhardt's intravenous ether technique to achieve and

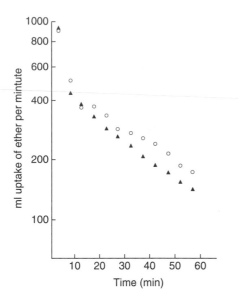

Fig. 37–2. The experimental wane (open circle) is compared with the predicted total uptake (closed triangles) of diethyl ether at an alveolar concentration of 2.3% ether. Redrawn from Eger, E.I., Johnson, E.A., Larson, C.D., Severinghaus, J.W.: The uptake and distribution of intravenous ether. Anesthesiology 23:144, 647, 1962.

maintain a constant arterial level of the agent and a constant anesthetic state as determined by electroencephalogram (EEG), Eger and associates studied the process of uptake[10] (5% ether in saline solution volume per weight).

In this study, the intravenous rate of administration was adjusted to attain an EEG level 4.[11] This represents an arterial concentration of ether of about 100 mg/100 ml of blood or an alveolar concentration of 2.3%. The relationship of EEG and arterial concentration is constant over a period of time. If the EEG is maintained, it is assumed that the arterial concentration is constant. Thus, in the study by Eger and Johnson, because the brain equilibrates rapidly with any inert agent in the blood, the uptake of ether occurred at a constant anesthetic level (Fig. 37–2).

The values of ether uptake were as follows: During the first 5 minutes, about 900 ml of pure vapor per minute (approximately 4 ml liquid ether) entered peripheral tissues. During the second 5 minutes, this value was halved. During the succeeding 5-minute intervals, uptake fell by ever-decreasing amounts, so by the sixtieth minute (1 hour), only 180 ml per minute was required.

Ether is not altered in the body: 90% is eliminated through the lungs, half is eliminated in 5 minutes, most is eliminated in 1 hour, and all is eliminated in an average of 8 hours, but may be as long as 13 hours.

Physiologic Effects (Table 37–2)

Respiratory System

Ether is irritating to the respiratory mucous membranes, stimulates the copious flow of mucus, and may induce coughing and laryngeal spasm. The use of premedications such as atropine or scopalamine is desirable to attenuate the flow of secretions. During the early stages of anesthe-sia, ether causes marked stimulation of respiration. Although tidal volume is decreased, the increase in respiratory rate may result in a higher minute ventilation and a normal or slightly decreased $PaCO_2$. Respiration is generally well maintained until high blood concentrations are reached. Ether, like halothane, is potentially useful with asthmatic patients, because it has a bronchodilating effect.

Central Nervous System

An irregular descending depression occurs. The classic signs of anesthesia are basically those of the effects of ether. On a neural basis, one may conceive of the central effects as one of successive pharmacologic transections of the cerebrospinal axis.

Thus, one sees first a decorticate preparation; with higher concentrations of ether, a thalamic-like picture is evident, followed by a decerebrate and midbrain syndrome.

Investigations of the precise mechanism and site of action of the anesthetic reveal blockade of central synaptic paths. French, Verzeano, and Magoun[14] found depression of the *multisynaptic* paths in the tegmental midbrain reticular formation. Davis and co-workers[15] found that the *oligosynaptic* lemniscal paths were also blocked (in the cat) by ether but at a slower rate, and the action was longer.

EEG tracings during ether anesthesia show a progressive depression of activity. Characteristic patterns were noted for ether and were separated into seven levels by Courtin and associates.[11] The *ether* pattern is discussed under EEG signs of anesthesia[16] (Table 37–3).

Reflexes

Deep tendon reflexes are exaggerated in light anesthesia. Carotid sinus reflex is depressed in humans. It is slightly decreased in light ether anesthesia, but it is profoundly depressed in levels deeper than planes 1 and 2 of the surgical stage. In tilt-tests, the pressoreceptor reflex response is diminished, so a 30° head-up position causes a pronounced fall in blood pressure. Milowsky and Rovenstine have also demonstrated depression of carotid sinus pressoreceptors.[17]

In cats, some increase in sensitivity of pressoreceptor reflexes is evident.

Circulation (Table 37–4)

During induction, the blood pressure increases because of increases in cardiac output and in pulse rate, both results of the release of catecholamines. This effect occurs even when induction is smooth. During maintenance, the blood pressure gradually returns to the preanesthetic level or below, whereas the pulse remains elevated. If the anesthetic time is prolonged beyond an hour, and even in the absence of blood loss, the blood pressure stabilizes at a lower level.

Characteristically, the peripheral circulation tends to become inefficient before either respiratory arrest or cardiac arrest. In turn, respiratory arrest occurs earlier than cardiac arrest in the healthy anesthetized patient. Rob-

Table 37–2. Summary of Actions of Diethyl Ether

Administration	By all techniques Induction time: 10–15 minutes		
		Inhaled Mix (%)	*Blood Level* (%)
	Analgesia	1	
	Unconscious	3	
	Anesthesia	3–5	100–140 mg
	Respiratory arrest	6–8	160 mg
	Induction	10–12	
Fate	Eliminated by lungs 90% Some by skin and urine 50% in 5 minutes; most in 1 hour Complete on average of 8 hours		
Central nervous system	Irregular descending depression Temperature regulating and vomiting centers depressed in 1st plane Tissue oxidation and vasomotor center are depressed		
Respiratory system	Local: irritation; copious sec.; cilia are depressed General: amplitude increased; bronchial muscles relaxed Chemoreceptors: depressed sensitivity		
Cardiovascular system	Heart: output increased 20%; rate increased; arrhythmia during induction; blood pressure elevated Peripheral dilatation especially of face and meninges; peripheral system becomes inefficient before the heart		
Gastrointestinal system	Tone decreased; also motility Secretions decreased All liver functions depressed		
Genitourinary system	Function decreased; anuria		
Miscellaneous	Bleeding time:	Unchanged	
	Clotting time:	Decreased 25%	
	White cells:	Increased: maximum 48 h	
	Red cells:	Increased 15%	
	Cholesterol:	Increased 50–100%	
	Blood glucose:	Increased 100–200%	
	Blood amylase:	Increased 75–100%	
	Acidosis:	Yes—lactate and pyruvate	

Table 37–3. Relation of Electroencephalogram (EEG) Level to Blood Ether Concentrations

EEG Level	Arterial Blood Ether (mg/dl)
I	60
II	80
III	100
IV	110–115
V	120–130
VI	130–140
VII	140–160

Data from Faulconer, A.: Correlation of concentrations of ether in arterial blood with EEg patterns. Anesthesiology *13*:361, 1952.

Table 37–4. Effects of Ether on Circulation and Electrocardiographic (ECG) Patterns

First Changes:

Heart sounds muffled or distant
Pulse in small peripheral arteries lost

Intermediate Changes:

Blood pressure unobtainable
ECG complexes deteriorated

Fatal Changes:

Disappearance of heart sounds
Pulse in large arteries lost
Electrocardiographic acitivity lost

bins[18] has shown that, to produce cardiac arrest in dogs, a blood concentration of ether of about 50% higher (230 to 260 mg/dl) than that needed to produce respiratory arrest (150 to 160 mg/dl) is required.

Maintenance of blood pressure at a normal level during ether anesthesia depends on a continued functioning of the sympathetic nervous system. Ether causes an increased sympathoadrenal activity. Some epinephrine is released and increases in plasma. The catecholamine principally responsible for good circulatory status is norepinephrine, which is greatly increased in the blood.[19] It is liberated from sympathetic nerve endings and possibly from the central nervous system. Patients with nearly normal blood pressure during ether anesthesia have significantly higher levels of circulating norepinephrine, whereas those who develop hypotension have much lower levels. Exhaustion of the amine stores can occur during prolonged or traumatic surgery.

Central venous pressure in healthy persons is only slightly elevated and is generally reduced. This appears to be related to the increased norepinephrine as well as the separate effect of ether in depressing vagal tone,[20] which together increase cardiac output. Some increase in venomotor tone has been reported.[21]

Peripheral resistance tends to be lowered during ether anesthesia. Smooth muscle tone of arteries and arterioles is directly reduced or unchanged. Similarly, the microcirculation shows decreased vasomotion and responsiveness. To some extent, the effect on arteries is minimized by the increased level of norepinephrine.

Myocardial Function[22]

Myocardial function can be best understood by examination of ventricular function curves in which external work (stroke volume) is performed and is related to the initial muscle length before contraction, that is, end-diastolic ventricular pressure (preload) (Fig. 37–3). The slope of the ventricular function curve is an index of the rate of performing ventricular stroke work and, hence, an index of muscle power.

In practice, because afterloads are not controlled, ether exerts a differential effect on right and left ventricles with systemic hypotension and relative pulmonary hypertension. Therefore, one can decrease left-to-right shunts. Evidence exists that raising aortic pressure may increase intrinsic contractility.

Deep ether anesthesia depresses the left ventricular function curve, which indicates that at any given left ventricular end-diastolic pressure, less stroke work is performed. In contrast, no change occurs in the right ventricular function curve. Because aortic impedance has decreased when the function curve was depressed, however, it has been considered that an increased afterload (raised aortic resistance) improves function, and such occurs. When mean aortic pressure is maintained near control values, the capacity of the heart to perform work is not altered.

Examination of the force-velocity curves demonstrates alteration in power under ether anesthesia (Fig. 37–4). If the aortic impedance is kept constant, the mean ejection rate is greater than control values. An actual shift of the curve to the right occurs, indicating increased myocardial contractility and power, a positive inotropic effect.

Arrhythmias

Most arrhythmias are of supraventricular origin. Electrocardiographic (ECG) studies reveal the occurrence of premature ventricular contractions in 20% of patients under ether anesthesia. A descending depression of the conduction mechanism is characteristic, and a displaced pacemaker is seen in 65% with the development of nodal rhythm.

Ether is known to prevent or ameliorate ventricular arrhythmias during cyclopropane anesthesia in humans.[17] It also protects against halothane-induced ventricular arrhythmias.[23] The mechanism of antiarrhythmic effects

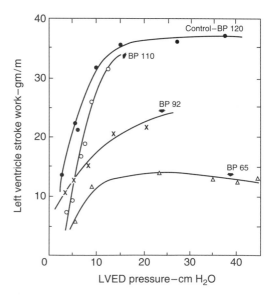

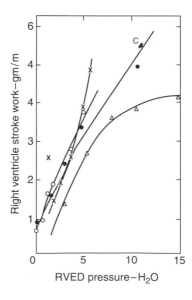

Fig. 37–3. Left and right ventricular function curves obtained before and during deep ether anesthesia at different afterload levels. Left, Left ventricular stroke work is plotted as a function of left ventricular end-diastolic (LVED) pressure. The relationship is obtained during deep ether anesthesia (open triangles), and with intentionally increased mean aortic pressure of 92 mm Hg (X) and 110 mm Hg (open circles). Right, Right ventricular stroke work is plotted against right ventricular end-diastolic (RVED) pressure. Redrawn from Etsten, B., Shimosato, S.: Myocardial contractility: performance of the heart during anesthesia. Clin Anesth 3:56, 1964.

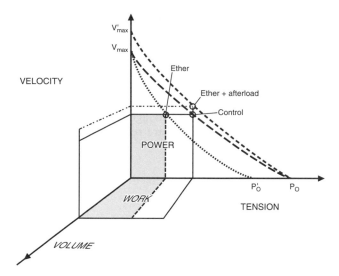

Fig. 37–4. Tension (mean aortic pressure)-velocity (mean ejection rate)-volume (stroke volume) diagram before and during deep ether anesthesia with and without increased afterload. Positive inotropic effect due to the experimentally increased afterload during ether anesthesia is shown by the increase in maximal velocity (V max → V' max). Redrawn from Ftsten, B., Shimosato, S.: Myocardial contractility: performance of the heart during anesthesia. Clin Anesth 3:56, 1964.

may be due to the following: (1) respiratory stimulation by ether whereby the hypercarbia of unassisted cyclopropane anesthesia is minimized (hypercarbia during cyclopropane is one cause of arrhythmias)[24]; (2) blocking of catecholamine action; although ether causes a release of amines, it also appears to interfere with the action of these mediators at the myocardium, and catecholamines may sensitize the heart during cyclopropane and produce ventricular arrhythmias; (3) depression of sympathetic ganglia; the stellate ganglia may be blocked by ether because other sympathetic ganglia are blocked, and local anesthetic block of stellate ganglia or stellectomy prevents the development of arrhythmias where hypercarbia is permitted; (4) depression of the vagus; cyclopropane increases vagal tone and permits vagal escape with appearance of ventricular arrhythmias; ether appears to block the vagus nerve.

Autonomic Nervous System

The salutary effect of ether on cardiovascular function depends on a functioning sympathoadrenal system and represents a safety factor. Ether causes a release of norepinephrine at postganglionic adrenergic fibers. At the same time, some evidence exists that the sympathetic ganglia are depressed.[25] Thus, lowering the pressure in the carotid sinus fails to evoke a good pressor response in dogs. Elevation of pressure causes a relatively great vasodepressor response over that seen in the unanesthetized subject.

Depression of vagal activity occurs during ether anesthesia. This is a separate effect not related to the positive release of sympathetic amines at postganglionic fiber endings. Thus, the infusion of norepinephrine during ether anesthesia does not evoke the typical vagal response of cardiac slowing.

As noted, the sympathetic nervous system is activated by ether. The classic work of Brewster and colleagues[26,27] demonstrated this in a concise manner. After adrenalectomy and total sympathetic blockade in dogs, the administration of ether results in circulatory failure with direct myocardial depression. Fall in cardiac output, a decrease in ventricular stroke work, and an increase in mean auricular pressure occur. Debilitated patients and those with poor cardiocirculatory status should not be anesthetized with ether.

Endocrine Effects

In addition to the adrenal medullary stimulation, the adrenal cortex is also affected. During ether anesthesia, approximately a two-thirds increase in 17-hydroxycorticosteroids occurs.[28] Human thyroid activity is irregularly increased.[29]

Action on Skeletal Muscle

Three actions of ether affect the skeletal muscle. First is depression of the several (motor, premotor, pyramidal, and extrapyramidal) centers that impinge on the motor horn cells. Second is dilatation of skeletal muscle vessels thereby increasing the concentration of ether locally. Third, a direct effect occurs at the motor end plate.

Blockade of the neuromuscular junction was first considered in 1914 by Auer and Meltzer.[30] Subsequently, Gross and Cullen[31] demonstrated the similarity of the peripheral effects of ether on muscle to those of curare. Neostigmine can reverse the ether blockade. Sabawala and Dillon,[32] however, consider that the site of action of ether, Vinethene, and trichloroethylene (also halothane) is at the muscle membrane, rather than at the junction.

Experimentally, Karis and colleagues[33] showed that the neuromuscular junction is the site of the blocking effect of ether. The postjunctional membrane was demonstrated to be the most sensitive synaptic structure.

Extreme Depths

Beyond the depths of tissue saturation producing clinical signs of stage IV of Guedel's chart (approximately 150 mg ether/100 ml of blood),[1] one may continue to administer an excessive dose of ether if ventilation is maintained. The signs and changes are important as evidence of overdose. Pearcy[34] observed the effects of such ether doses on circulation and ECG patterns and has tabulated the changes.

When circulation begins to fail, as evidenced by loss of arterial pulsation, one sees brief reactivation of the silent ECG pattern.[2,35]

Gastrointestinal System

Tone and movements are inhibited by the peripheral action of ether; dilatation tends to occur postanesthetically, and distention occurs in about 16% of cases. The small intestine recovers function first. Nausea and vomiting are seen in about 57% of cases. The spleen may decrease as much as 40% in size.

Liver Effects

Ether is not a direct hepatotoxic agent, and evidence of cytologic damage has not been adduced. Impairment of function does occur, however, and liver profile tests show depression when examined serially under controlled conditions.

In normal human liver, the functional changes are mild in a significant number of cases and may persist for several days postoperatively. In patients with preexisting abnormal liver function, the depression of hepatic function by ether is more intense and frequent, and it persists for a much longer period; the extent of the depression is directly related to the degree of the initial dysfunction.

Bile secretion is decreased, but recovery is seen after 24 hours. Liver glycogen is rapidly depleted to 50% or less in the first hour of ether anesthesia.

Genitourinary System

Urine flow diminishes during ether anesthesia, and oliguria is frequent postoperatively; albuminuria also occurs.

Renal vasoconstriction is produced by ether. This causes a decrease in effective renal plasma flow and in glomerular filtration. An increase in tubular reabsorption and a rise in the filtration fraction also occur. This last effect is due to the enhanced release of the antidiuretic hormone.

Uterine Effects

In light levels of ether anesthesia, uterine physiology is only slightly affected. The agent may be employed for analgesia and for delivery. Equilibrium between the maternal blood levels and the fetal blood concentrations requires about 15 to 20 minutes.

In deeper levels of anesthesia, such as planes 2 or 3 of stage III, uterine tone and the strength of contractions are depressed and the frequency of contractions is decreased. Deep ether anesthesia may be used for version and extraction.

Metabolic Changes

Metabolic acidosis occurs during ether anesthesia. It is chiefly due to elevation of serum lactate, but increases in pyruvate also occur. Elevation of nonesterified fatty acids occurs, and ketones are detectable.

Hyperglycemia is pronounced and is due to glycogenolysis from both liver and muscle glycogen. Glucose intolerance is induced. Both the hyperglycemia and the increase in serum lactate can be abolished by sympathetic blockade and adrenal medullectomy.

Miscellaneous Actions

A small reduction in plasma volume occurs during ether anesthesia. Lymph flow increases. A rise in red cell hematocrit occurs of about 15%. It is pronounced in dogs and is related to splenic contraction. A marked leukocytosis occurs. Most other blood elements show only slight changes. Some decrease in clotting time occurs, indicating enhanced prothrombin effect. Cholesterol and esters are usually unchanged.

Ether Convulsions

No evidence exists that ether is peculiarly capable of producing convulsions. Convulsions can occur during administration of any anesthetic agent. Most commonly, they are seen in children and are related to many factors, as follows.

1. Miscalculation of belladonna drug (overdosage).
2. Dehydration.
3. Elevated temperature.
4. Toxemia, acidosis, alkalosis.
5. Poor elimination of carbon dioxide.
6. The final common denominator: tissue and cellular hypoxia.

Treatment consists of hypothermia, oxygen, fluids, and use of chlorpromazine.

Clinical Use

Contraindications

Known contraindications include the following:

1. Acidosis.
2. Acute respiratory disease.
3. Increased intracranial pressure.
4. Diabetes.
5. Debilitation.

Indications

Known indications include asthma, bronchospastic disease, and coronary artery disease.

Other Aliphatic Ethers

These are no longer used or available. The reader is directed to other texts for a discussion of these agents.[35]

CHLOROFORM

Essential Pharmacology

History[36]

Chloroform was discovered in 1831 and was described by three independent workers: Samuel Guthrie of Sacket Harbor, New York; E. Soubeiran of France; and J. Von Liebig of Germany. The important physical and chemical properties were described by Jean Baptiste Dumas in 1835, who also outlined the formula for the agent and named the compound. The narcotic properties were discovered by Flourens, the French physiologist in 1847, when he showed that the inhalation of chloroform produced a state of insensibility in animals similar to that produced by ether.

Simpson introduced the use of chloroform into clinical practice in 1847. He was dissatisfied with ether because of its disagreeable qualities and searched for a replacement. On the recommendation of D. Waldie, a chemist in Liverpool, Simpson began the use of chloroform analgesia in obstetrics.

Physiochemical Factors[37] (Table 37–5)

Chloroform is a chlorinated hydrocarbon prepared by chlorination of acetone or acetaldehyde. The most common method of preparation is by chlorination of alcohol in alkaline solution. Chloroform is a colorless, clear liquid with a sweet odor. Its boiling point is 61°C. The specific gravity of the vapor is 4.12. It is nonflammable.

It decomposes in presence of heat and light to form aldehydes and formates. Heating causes the formation of phosgene. Stabilization is accomplished commercially by the addition of enough ethyl alcohol to make a 1% solution. This counteracts the formation of phosgene, because the alcohol combines to form ethyl carbonate and ethyl chloride. Chloroform should be stored in tight-stoppered ambered glass bottles, protected from light, heat, and air.

Administration[37]

Administration is by all inhalation techniques. The open system is the one most commonly used. It is a simple and a safe method and is the only one recommended. With current precision vaporizers, experienced anesthesiologists are using either a nonrebreathing system or a closed system. The closed systems are fraught with the danger of overdosage and rapid depression to lethal levels, however. Induction requires a 4.0% inhaled mixture and maintenance a 1.4% mixture. Respiratory arrest occurs if a 2.0% mixture is administered continuously. Oxygen should be administered throughout even with the open mask system.

Open Technique of Administration[38]

This technique is basically similar to the procedure for administering ether. The principles of preparation and use of the open mask are the same, and recommendations are as follows:

1. Administration must be slow and smooth; the drug must be given by drops. Do not alter rate of drip rapidly; do not ever pour; a single breath of a high concentration may be lethal.
2. Use entire vaporizing surface.
3. Keep mask one finger breadth off face; do not enclose mask with a towel; a special mask with an air space between the mask proper and the rim contracting the face has been devised[55] (Fig. 37–5).
4. Administer with oxygen.
5. Approximate dropping rate (Table 37–6).

During the first minute, about 3 to 4 drops are carefully allowed to fall on the mask at different points. Subsequently, the rate is increased by doubling the number of drops for each successive minute to the fourth minute and then continued at this rate or less until surgical anesthesia is attained. Maintenance is attained by a rate of about 8 drops per minute. The mask should be removed when the patient holds his or her breath or stops breathing.

Table 37–5. Physiochemical Properties of Chloroform

Appearance	Colorless, clear, liquid
Odor	Sweet
Flammability	Nonflammable
Molecular weight	119.5
Specific gravity— liquid	1.5 (1.476 at 20°C)
Specific gravity— vapor	4.12
Heat capacity of liquid	0.231 cal/g at 20°C
Latent heat of vaporization	62.8 cal/g at 20°C
Vapor pressure	166 mm Hg at 20°C
Boiling point	61.0°C
Solubility in water	1 ml dissolves in 210 ml water (20°C)
Water/gas solubility	3.8 at 37°C
Blood/gas solubility	10.3
Oil/gas solubility	265
Oil/water solubility (partition)	100

Solubility data from Larson, C. P.

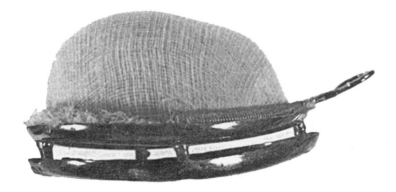

Fig. 37–5. Chloroform mask for open-drop administration developed by Lenehan and Babbage of Buffalo. Note air space provided by use of a second face rim.

Table 37–6. Chloroform Anesthesia: Open Drop Administration

Time	Drops	Concentration Inhaled (%)	Concentration Blood (mg/dl)
First minute	4	0.25	1–4
Second minute	8	0.50	4–8
Third minute	16	1.00	8–12
Fourth minute	32	1.50	12–14
Maintenance	6–12	0.75–1.00	10.0

Table 37–7. Chloroform Anesthesia Blood Concentration

Plane I	8 mg/dl
Plane II	10 mg/dl
Plane III	12 mg/dl
Plane IV	15 mg/dl

From Waters, R. M.: Chloroform: A Study After 100 Years. Madison, WI, University of Wisconsin Press, 1951.

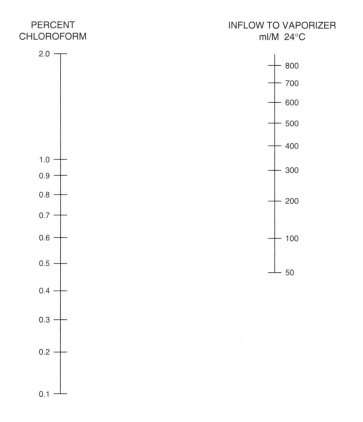
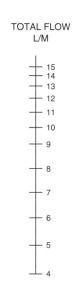

Fig. 37–6. Nomogram for chloroform. Modified from Thomas, D. M.: Nomogram for chloroform. Anesthesiology *20*:378, 1959.

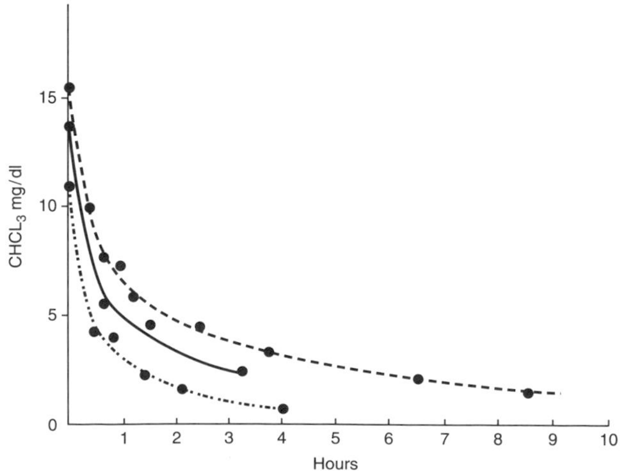

The blood levels[39,40] for clinical planes for surgical anesthesia are tabulated (Table 37-7).

Semiclosed System

This technique provides a measure of controllability. A precision vaporizer is essential, and the Copper Kettle properly calibrated or a modified Fluotec vaporizer called the Chlorotec is quite satisfactory. The latter is temperature compensated. Using the Copper Kettle, a chloroform nomogram has been devised (Fig. 37-6).[41] Such a nomogram relates three variables: (1) oxygen flow into kettle to produce a vapor mixture; (2) the total gas flow; (3) the resultant final concentration.[41] One should always be guided by the clinical condition of the patient, however, and not use a predetermined concentration of agent.

The vapor pressure curve of the agent provides the vapor pressure value for a given temperature. For any given temperature, the carrier gas-vapor mixture is saturated. Chloroform vapor at 20°C is about 20% and at 24°C, the concentration of the vapor is about 24%. Dilution of

Fig. 37–7. Blood levels of chloroform at intervals after cessation of administration. Redrawn from Morris: *In* Waters, R. M.: Chloroform: A Study After 100 Years. Madison, WI, University of Wisconsin Press, 1951.

Table 37–8. Summary of Actions of Chloroform

Administration	By all techniques		
	Induction time:	5–10 min	*Blood Level*
		Inhaled Mix (%)	*(Waters 1951)*
	Analgesia	0.5	
	Unconscious	1.0	
	Anesthesia	1.35–1.65	
	Plane I		5– 8 (7.5)
	Plane II		8–10 (10.4)
	Plane III		10–12 (12.8)
	Plane IV		12–20 (13.5)
	Respiratory arrest	2.0	30–40 mg/dl
	Induction	4.0	
Fate	Eliminated by lungs 70%		
	Most in 30 minutes		
Central nervous system	Same as diethyl ether except carotid sinus is depressed more and the vasomotor center is depressed directly		
Respiratory system	Local: irritation not so great as diethyl ether		
	General: effects same; minute volume decreased; muscles relaxed		
	Chemoreceptors: decreased sensitivity		
Cardiovascular system	Heart: Output decreased 30%		
	A direct muscle depressant		
	Irritability increased; diastolic arrest		
	Rate variable to decreased; blood pressure depressed		
	Peripheral dilatation; heart fails first		
Gastrointestinal system	Tone and motility decreased		
	Secretions decreased		
	More depression of liver function		
	Glycogen depleted; hepatitis prone		
Genitourinary system	Function decreased; anuria		
Miscellaneous	Bleeding time:	Unchanged	
	Clotting time:	Decreased after 30 min	
	White cells:	Increased; normal in 48 min	
	Red cells:	Increased	
	Cholesterol:	Blood lipase increased	
	Blood glucose:	Increased 200%	
	Blood amylase:	Increased	
	Acidosis:	Yes	

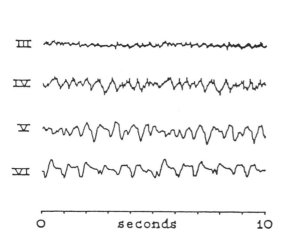

Level - I

II

III

IV

V

VI

0   seconds   10

Fig. 37–8. Levels of chloroform anesthesia in dog. Six characteristic and reproducible levels are noted. Level I, appearance of waves of slow frequency 2 to 3 cps and slightly higher amplitude superimposed on fast-low amplitude background activity; level II, return of low-voltage fast activity; level III, appearance of high-frequency 20 to 30 cps moderate amplitude waves of "β type;" level IV, slow-high voltage "δ waves" appear and gradually dominate the pattern, and one sees a superimposed fast β activity; level V, disappearance of β waves (20 to 30 cps) leaving the slow waves of δ type (100 to 200 mV); θ-type activity (4 to 7 cps) is present; level VI, decreased amplitude of δ waves, with minimal to no θ activity. Modified from Pearcy, W. C., Knott, J. R., Pittinger, C. B., Keasling, H. H.: Electroencephalographic and circulatory effects of chloroform anesthesia in dogs. Anesthesiology *18*:88, 1957.

the vapor mixture is achieved by admitting this mixture into a nitrous oxide-oxygen mixture. A sufficient flow of the latter should be present to cause a dilution of 25 times.

Nonrebreathing System

This technique is also safe in experienced hands. Various inhalers are used, as follows: (1) modified Duke inhaler (which is similar to Trilene Inhaler); (2) Emutril; and (3) Tecota Chloroform Inhaler. Details of the application of the inhalers are outlined by Ngai and co-workers.[42]

Fate and Elimination

Chloroform is not altered in the body. It is eliminated by the lungs, and most of this occurs in 30 minutes. During the first 15 minutes, 30 to 50% is removed (Fig. 37-7).

Physiologic Effects (Table 37–8)

Respiratory System

Locally, this agent is not irritating. Secretions are stimulated at the onset of anesthesia and during recovery but are depressed during anesthesia. The degree of stimulation is not great as compared with ether.

A slight early increase in respiratory rate occurs. Minute volume is decreased, and bronchial muscles are relaxed.

Cardiovascular System

The cardiac rate is variable but usually decreased. The output is decreased about 30%. Chloroform is a direct cardiac muscle depressant, but at the onset of anesthesia, irritability is increased, and fibrillation may occur. In later periods of anesthesia, cardiac arrest in diastole may occur. Various reflexogenic arrhythmias, as demonstrated by Levy.[43]

The peripheral vascular system shows depression with lowered blood pressure and dilatation of vessels. Generally, the heart fails before the circulation.[44]

Central Nervous System

One sees an irregular descending depression of the entire central nervous system. Hence, the drug is a complete anesthetic. The vasomotor center is depressed directly. Depression of respiratory, vomiting, and temperature-regulating centers occurs. Intracranial pressure is raised.

The EEG shows typical changes according to the general pattern (Fig. 37–8).[45]

Gastrointestinal System

Tone and motility are decreased, as are secretions. Liver function is definitely depressed more than with ether, and glycogen is depleted rapidly. Hepatitis is prone to occur with central lobular necrosis. Regeneration is rapid, and fibrosis is rare.

Genitourinary System

Function is depressed, and anuria occurs. Fatty changes may occur in the tubules.

Miscellaneous Actions

Acidosis occurs with an increase in pyruvates and lactates of blood. Blood sugar is increased about 200%. One sees an increase in both white and red cells. Oxygen content is decreased because chloroform inhibits combination of hemoglobin with oxygen. Clotting time is decreased, and capillary permeability is increased. Platelets are unchanged, and bleeding time is normal. Blood lipoids are increased.

Clinical Use

Contraindications

Cardiac Disease

Chloroform produces a direct cellular depression of the cardiac muscle fibers; an increased irritability of the conduction mechanism occurs. Cardiac output is decreased. Sympathomimetic amines, especially epinephrine, must not be administered because they easily induce arrhythmias.

Hepatic Disease

Function of liver is depressed; glycogen stores are depleted. A direct cytotoxic effect may result in central lobular necrosis.

Diabetes

Carbohydrate metabolism is used; blood sugar elevated and glycogen stores are depleted; pyruvate levels are increased.

Acidosis

The carbon dioxide combining power of blood is depressed, indicating depressed buffer mechanism.

Renal Disorders

Urine formation and secretion are suppressed. Oliguria and anuria are prone to occur.

Chronic Diseases

Malnourished, anemic, and debilitated patients are more susceptible to toxic effects of this drug. With anemia, hypoxia occurs, and the liver is especially more vulnerable. Diseases of respiratory tract tend to produce hypoxia and poor gas exchange.

Advantages and Indications

1. Chloroform is the most potent anesthetic agent available; induction is rapid and pleasant.
2. The drug is nonflammable.
3. This agent has low volatility (B.P. 61°C.); this allows use in warm climates (tropics).

4. Minimal equipment is needed.

5. Excellent relaxation occurs, with a quiet abdomen.

6. The drug may be used with air because a low partial pressure produces anesthesia.

7. The agent is stable.

8. Chloroform does not irritate the respiratory tract; secretions are minimal; respiration is not stimulated.

9. This agent is useful for short, simple operations and for obstetric analgesia and anesthesia.

Disadvantages

This drug has a narrow margin of safety, and deep anesthesia can be rapidly attained with small changes in concentration of inhaled mixture. Furthermore, mild degrees of obstruction or hypoxia potentiate the adverse effects of nontoxic doses to the point of toxicity. One sees derangement in function of the liver, the kidney, and the buffer systems of the body. The effect on the myocardium is serious, and arrhythmias are produced both in reflex manner and directly.

REFERENCES

1. Guedel, A. E.: Inhalation Anesthesia. New York, Macmillan, 1951.

2. Dodd, R. B., Bunker, J. P.: Diethyl Ether: Its Effects in the Human Body. Springfield, IL, Charles C Thomas, 1962.

3. Schmidt, K. R., Greene, N. M.: Etymology in terms of interest to the anesthetist. Anesth Analg 39:167, 1960.

4. Gold, H.: The use of bulk ether in anesthesia. JAMA 120:44, 1942.

5. Bourne, W.: Pure ether and impurities: a review. Anesthesiology 7:599, 1946.

6. Thomas, G. J.: Do you know? Newslett ASA 20:33, 1956.

7. Mendenhall, W.: Pharmacological effects of impurities of ethers. Anesth Analg 12:264, 1933.

8. Adriani, J.: The Chemistry and Physics of Anesthesia. 2nd Ed. Charles C. Thomas, Springfield, IL 1962.

8a. Steward, A., Allott, P. B., Cowles, A. L. and Mapleson: Solubility coefficients for inhaled anaesthetics for water, oil and biological media. Br J Anaesth 45:282, 1973.

9. Haggard, H. W.: The absorption, fate and elimination of diethyl ether. J Biol Chem 59:737, 1924.

10. Eger, E. I., Johnson, E. A., Larson, C. D., Severinghaus, J. W.: The uptake and distribution of intravenous ether. Anesthesiology 23:144, 647, 1962.

10a. Larson, C. P. Jr., Eger, E. I. (II), Severinghaas, J. W., Ostwald solubility coefficients for anesthetic gases in various fluids and tissues. Anesthesiology 23:868, 1962.

10b. Eger, E. I. (II): Anesthetic Uptake and Action. Williams and Wilkins, Baltimore, 1974.

11. Courtin, R. F., Rickford, R. G., Faulconer, A., Jr.: The classification and significance of electro-encephalographic patterns produced by nitrous-oxide-ether anesthesia. Proc Staff Meet Mayo Clin 25:197, 1950.

12. Waters, R. M.: Fundamentals of Anesthesia. Chicago, American Medical Association, 1942.

13. Thomas, G. J.: Fundamentals of Anesthesia. Philadelphia, W. B. Saunders, 1954.

14. French, J. D., Verzeano, M., Magoun, H. W.: A neural basis of the anesthetic state. AMA Arch Neurol Psychiatry 69:519, 1953.

15. Davis, H. S., Dillon, W. H., Collins, W. F., Randt, C. T.: The effect of anesthetic agent on evoked central nervous system responses. Anesthesiology 19:441, 1958.

16. Faulconer, A.: Correlation of concentrations of ether in arterial blood with EEG patterns. Anesthesiology 13:361, 1952.

17. Milowsky, J., Rovenstine, E. A.: The use of ether to abolish arrhythmias during cyclopropane anesthesia. Anesth Analg 21:353, 1942.

18. Robbins, E. H.: Ether anesthesia. J Pharmacol Exp Ther 85:192, 1945.

19. Price, H. L., et al.: Sympatho-adrenal responses to general anesthesia in man and their relation to hemodynamics. Anesthesiology 20:563, 1959.

20. Gordh, T.: Postural circulatory and respiratory changes during ether and intravenous anesthesia. Acta Chir Scand 92(Suppl 102), 1945.

21. Bartelstone, H. J.: Vasomotor activity and venous return. Fed Proc 18:8, 1959.

22. Etsten, B., Shimosato, S.: Myocardial contractility: performance of the heart during anesthesia. Clin Anesth 3:56, 1964.

23. Dobkin, A. B., Harland, J. H., Fedoruk, S.: Comparison of the cardiovascular and respiratory effects of halothane and the halothane-diethyl ether azeotrope in dogs. Anesthesiology 21:13, 1960.

24. Lurie, A. A., et al.: Cyclopropane anesthesia. I. Cardiac rate and rhythm during steady levels of cyclopropane anesthesia at normal and elevated end-expiratory carbon dioxide tensions. Anesthesiology 19:457, 1958.

25. Normann, N., Lofstrom, B.: Interaction of d-tubocurarine, ether, cyclopropane and thiopental on ganglionic transmission. J Pharmacol Exp Ther 114:231, 1955.

26. Brewster, W. R., Isaacs, J. P., Waino-Andersen, T.: Depressant effects of ether on myocardium of the dog and its modification by reflex release of epinephrine and norepinephrine. Am J Physiol 175:399, 1953.

27. Brewster, W. R., Bunker, J. P., Beecher, H. K.: Metabolic effects of anesthesia. VI. Mechanism of metabolic acidosis and hyperglycemia during ether anesthesia in the dog. Am J Physiol 171:37, 1952.

28. Hammond, W. G., et al.: Studies in surgical endocrinology anesthetic agents as stimuli to changes in corticosteroids. Ann Surg 148:199, 1958.

29. Goldenberg, I. S., Hayes, M. A., Greene, N. M.: Endocrine responses during operative procedures. Ann Surg 150:196, 1959.

30. Auer, J., Meltzer, S. J.: The effect of ether inhalation upon skeletal motor mechanism. J Pharmacol Exp Ther 5:521, 1914.

31. Gross, E. G., Cullen, S. C.: Effect of anesthetic agents on muscular contraction. J Pharmacol Exp Ther 78:358, 1943.

32. Sabawala, P. B., Dillon, J. B.: The positive inotropic action of cyclopropane on human intercostal muscle in vitro and its modification by d-tubocurarine. Anesthesiology 19:473, 1958.

33. Karis, J. H., Gissen, A. J., Natsuk, W. L.: Mode of action of diethyl ether in blocking neuromuscular transmission. Anesthesiology 27:42, 1966.

34. Pearcy, W. C.: Circulatory and electroencephalographic effects of extreme ether anesthesia in dogs. Anesthesiology 23:605, 1962.

35. Collins, V. J.: Principles of Anesthesiology, 2nd Ed. Philadelphia, Lea & Febiger, 1976.

36. Keys, T. E.: History of Surgical Anesthesia. New York, Schumanns, 1945.

37. Waters, R. M.: Chloroform: A Study After 100 Years. Madison, WI, University of Wisconsin Press, 1951.

38. Lenahan, R. M., Babbage, E. D.: A review of chloroform anesthesia in obstetrics. NY State J Med *50:*1717, 1950.

39. Pittinger, C., et al.: Observations on the kinetics of transfer of xenon and chloroform between blood and brain in the dog. Anesthesiology *17:*4, 1956.

40. Morris, L., Frederickson, E., Orth, S.: Differences in concentration of chloroform in blood of man and dog during anesthesia. J Pharmacol Exp Ther *101:*6, 1951.

41. Thomas, D. M.: Nomogram for chloroform. Anesthesiology *20:*378, 1959.

42. Ngai, S. H., Green, H. D., Knox, J. R., Slocum, H. C.: Evaluation of inhalers for trichloroethylene, chloroform and fluothane. Anesthesiology *19:*488, 1958.

43. Levy, A. G.: Heart irregularities resulting from the inhalation of low percentages of chloroform vapor and their relationship to ventricular fibrillation. Heart *3:*99, 1911.

44. Troch, E. E.: Study on chloroform, Adrenalin, and cyclopropane Adrenalin induced cardioventricular fibrillation. Arch Int Pharmacodyn *94:*175, 1953.

45. Pearcy, W. C., Knott, J. R., Pittinger, C. B., Keasling, H. H.: Electroencephalographic and circulatory effects of chloroform anesthesia in dogs. Anesthesiology *18:*88, 1957.

Chapter 38

HALOTHANE

MARK V. BOSWELL
VINCENT J. COLLINS

ALIPHATIC FLUORINATED ANESTHETICS

Fluorine Chemistry

Fluorine, the most chemically active of the halogens, was isolated by Moissan in 1886. The free element is a pale yellow gas slightly heavier than air with an extremely pungent odor. Fluorine has properties distinct from the other halogens. For example, it is considerably more electronegative and forms a stronger bond with carbon than do the other halogens. A single fluorine atom on a compound results in an easily hydrolyzable chemical, whereas difluoro and trifluoro compounds are extremely stable. Properties of the halogens are listed in Table 38-1.

Generally, the element can replace hydrogen in a hydrocarbon series, producing a fluorinated series called fluorocarbons, which are commonly used as refrigerants and solvent-propellants for aerosols (e.g., Freon-12, dichlorodifluoromethane). Concerns about fluorocarbon-induced damage to the Earth's ozone layer, however, have resulted in phased elimination of these compounds, except in certain instances, such as for medical uses.

Development of Fluorinated Hydrocarbons

Pioneering work on fluorinated hydrocarbons began with studies in 1940 to 1950 by B.H. Robbins. Subsequent investigations were related to specific agents, such as studies by Krantz at Maryland and Sadove at Illinois on fluroxene (trifluoroethyl vinyl ether, the first fluorinated anesthetic introduced into clinical use) in 1953, by Raventos and Suckling of England on halothane in 1956 and by Fabian, of halopropane, in 1959 (Fig. 38-1). All these anesthetics have become obsolete, because of various adverse clinical effects such as a propensity to cause cardiac arrhythmias, except halothane.

ESSENTIAL PHARMACOLOGY OF HALOTHANE

With the use of electrocautery in surgery, the need for a potent nonflammable inhalation anesthetic was evident, and investigations were directed toward halogenated hydrocarbons. Suckling[1] screened several nonexplosive fluorinated compounds and synthesized 2-bromo-2-chloro-1,1,1-trifluoroethane ($CF_3CHBrCl$) in 1951. This compound called halothane was investigated pharmacologically by Raventos[2] in animals and released for clinical use shortly thereafter, in 1956.

Physicochemical Properties (Table 38-2)

Halothane is a clear, colorless liquid with a molecular weight of 197.4 and a relatively sweet pleasant odor similar to that of trichloroethylene. Synthesis of the compound is accomplished by halogenation of ethane. At room temperature, the drug is relatively stable if kept in a light resistant amber bottle. To enhance stability, thymol (0.01% weight) is added as a preservative. Otherwise, slow decomposition may occur, with formation of hydrochloric acid and phosgene. In addition, spontaneous decomposition may occur in closed-circle breathing systems on exposure to soda lime, with generation of trace amounts of potentially toxic compounds. Halothane also chemically attacks rubber in breathing circuits and causes softening and swelling. At clinically useful concentrations, halothane in 70% nitrous oxide and 30% oxygen is not flammable; the minimal flammable concentration is 4.75%, and combustion requires optimum conditions (i.e., no water vapor) and a spark generated by 60 mA of current.[3] In all proportions, it is not explosive.

Administration

Because halothane is a volatile liquid, it has to be vaporized for use as an anesthetic. For safe administration, accurate methods of vaporization are mandatory, although theoretically the drug may be given by all inhalation techniques. Modern vaporizers, such as the Fluotec Mark II (Fraser Harlake, Orchard Park, NY), the Ohmeda Tec 4 (Ohio Medical Products, Madison, WI), and the Drager Vapor 19.1, provide accurate anesthetic output concentrations within the temperature range of 20 to 35°C over a useful range of flow rates (2 to 10 L/min).

Table 38–1. Some Properties of the Halogens

Halogen	van der Waals' Radius (Å)	Electronegativity	Bond Energy (kcal/mol) To Carbon	Bond Energy (kcal/mol) To Hydrogen
F	1.35	4.0	107	147.5
Cl	1.80	3.0	66.5	102.7
Br	1.95	2.8	54.0	87.3
I	2.15	2.4	45.5	71.4

From Goldman, P.: Properties of halogens. Science *164*:1173, 1969.

CHART OF THE FLUORINATED HYDROCARBON
ANESTHETICS

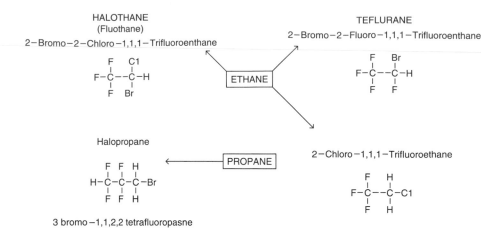

Fig. 38–1. Structural formulas of aliphatic fluorinated hydrocarbon anesthetics.

Table 38–2. Physiochemical Characteristics of Halothane

Appearance	Colorless, clear
Odor	Sweet, pleasant
Flammability	Non-flammable
Molecular weight	197.4
Specific gravity—liquid (g/ml)	1.86 at 20°C.
Heat capacity of liquid (25°C)	0.42 cal/g
Vapor pressure	243 mmHg at 20°C; 290 mmHg at 25°C
Boiling point (at 760 mmHg)	50.2°C.
Solubility in water	0.345 g dissolves in 100 ml at 23°C
Solubility in blood	1.160 g dissolves in 100 ml at 37°C
Partition coefficients:	
Water/gas (at 37°C)	0.63
Blood/gas (at 37°C)	2.3
Brain/blood (at 37°C)	2.9
Oil/gas (at 37°C)	224
Oil/water (at 23°C)	330

From Steward, A., Allott, P. R., Mapelson, W. W. Solubility coefficients for inhaled anaesthetics for water, oil and biological fluids Br: J Anaesth *45*:282, 1973. Wyeth-Ayerst Laboratories, Philadelphia, 1995.

Preanesthetic Medications

Halothane can safely be used with anticholinergic agents, barbiturates, opioids, and muscle relaxants. For mask induction, an intravenous dose of atropine or other anticholinergic is recommended, to counteract the bradycardic effect of halothane, which may permit deeper levels of anesthesia. Because halothane, unlike ether, does not stimulate copious airway secretions, the antisialagogue action of atropine is not as important as in the days of ether anesthesia. Meperidine has also been suggested as an appropriate premedicant, because of its vagolytic effect, but if atropine has been given, the vagotonic effects of morphine or other opioids are minimized. Premedica-

tion with a barbiturate or benzodiazepine may also be useful for preoperative sedation or anxiolysis.

Potency

Halothane is the most potent inhalation anesthetic currently in use. Minimum alveolar concentration (MAC) values for halothane vary with age[4,5] (Table 38-3). In neonates, MAC expressed as percentage of inspired gas, is 0.87, which is about 25% lower than for infants. MAC progressively falls with increasing age thereafter; the often-quoted value of 0.76 applies to patients about 42 years of age (range 31 to 55 years).

Induction

A vapor concentration of 2.0 to 3.5% is often used for induction, to achieve anesthetic blood concentrations (overpressure) rapidly, whereas maintenance is readily accomplished with concentrations of 0.5 to 1.5%. These concentrations may be reduced when halothane is used in conjunction with nitrous oxide or larger doses of opioid (e.g., fentanyl, 2 to 3 μg/kg). Induction is rapid, and the vapor is nonirritating. A short period of excitement

Table 38–3. Age and Halothane

Age	Minimum Alveolar Concentration (% Inspired Gas)
Neonates	0.87
1–6 mo	1.20
0.5–2.5 y	0.97
2.5–6 y	0.91
7–11 y	0.87
12–18 y	0.92
19–30 y	0.84
31–55 y	0.76
70–96 y	0.64

Data from Gregory, G. A., Eger, E. I., II, Munson, E. S.: The relationship between age and halothane requirements in man. Anesthesiology *30*:489, 1969; and Lerman, J., Robinson, S., Willis, M. M., Gregory, G. A.: Anesthetic requirements for halothane in young children 0–1 months and 1–6 months of age. Anesthesiology *59*:421, 1983.

with mask induction lasts about 1 minute or less. Generally, coughing, vomiting, and laryngospasm are not seen, because pharyngeal and laryngeal reflexes are obtunded early and the masseter muscle is quickly relaxed. At sufficient anesthetic depth (which may require approximately 10 minutes to achieve using mask induction), intubation is possible without the aid of muscle relaxants, while maintaining spontaneous respirations. The potency of halothane permits the use of high concentrations of nitrous oxide, which can speed induction by the second gas effect. Although newer volatile agents are more commonly used, halothane remains an excellent anesthetic for mask induction, particularly for infants and children without intravenous lines. Halothane may also be used effectively in the unusual case in which an adult requires mask induction, although concerns about hepatic toxicity have markedly reduced the general use of this agent with adult patients.

Maintenance

Anesthesia is maintained by a continuation of the induction procedure; however, the concentration of halothane required is less. For patients not requiring deep anesthesia (minimal surgical stimulation), anesthesia is readily maintained with inspired concentrations of 0.5 to 1.0% in nitrous oxide. The depth of anesthesia can be altered with three or four respirations. Assisted ventilation or complete ventilatory control is easily attained. Indeed, care must be exercised, because increasing depth often occurs. Muscle relaxation by halothane is only moderate, and relaxant agents are needed to provide adequate surgical relaxation.

Absorption and Elimination

Absorption from the lung is rapid. In normal individuals, the arterial partial pressure of halothane is approximated by the alveolar partial pressure. The actual arterial concentration is a function of the blood/gas solubility coefficient, which is 2.3 for halothane. The partial pressure of halothane in vessel-rich tissues reaches equilibrium with the partial pressure of inspired halothane in approximately 12 minutes ($T_{1/2}$ of 3 minutes), with muscle tissue in about 360 minutes ($T_{1/2}$ of about 90 minutes) and with fat tissue in about 130 hours ($T_{1/2}$ of 32 hours).[6,7] Partition coefficients of halothane for various tissues are shown in Table 38–4.

Halothane is eliminated from the body mainly by the lungs, at a rate similar to that of uptake. Because fat and muscle (except during long anesthesia) do not reach

Table 38–4. Partition Coefficients for Halothane at 37°C

Blood/Gas	Brain/Blood	Muscle/Blood	Fat/Blood
2.3	2.9	3.5	60

Data from Eger, E. I., II (ed.): MAC, Anesthetic Uptake and Action. Baltimore, Williams & Wilkins, 1974.

equilibrium with blood by the completion of anesthetic administration, however, the rate of fall of alveolar halothane partial pressure may be faster than the rate of rise on induction. This occurs because tissues that have not equilibrated with blood will continue to remove halothane from blood, accelerating the fall of blood and alveolar anesthetic partial pressures. One minute after discontinuing halothane (following 1 hour of anesthesia), the concentration of expired halothane drops to about half the value seen immediately before stopping the agent. At 10 minutes, the expired concentration falls to 25%, but at 1 hour it is still about 10% of the anesthetic level (Fig. 38–2).[8] The fall of alveolar halothane is delayed with longer anesthetic times, because of higher tissue concentrations of halothane. This effect is more pronounced for halothane than nitrous oxide, whose lower blood and tissue solubilities allow for a rapid fall in alveolar partial pressure at the cessation of anesthesia. Hyperventilation at the end of anesthetic administration enhances the elimination of the inhalation anesthetics.

Biotransformation

Degradation of halothane in humans was established in 1964 by Van Dyke and colleagues.[9] The primary site of metabolism is the liver. Between 20 and 45% of absorbed halothane is metabolized,[10,11] with an average of approximately 20% on first exposure; after a second exposure, about 30% is formed, and greater amounts are formed after repeated exposures. Of the metabolites, approximately 18% are organic fluoride compounds, 12 to 25% is trifluoroacetic acid, and about 1% is inorganic fluoride.[10,12–14] Essentially all the bromide is released from the halothane molecule during metabolism; serum concentrations of bromide far exceed those of fluoride.

Halothane is metabolized by oxidative pathways involving the mixed function oxidases (cytochrome P-450 mono-oxygenases) in hepatocyte smooth endoplasmic reticulum, which require NADPH as the electron donor and molecular oxygen. The predominant reactions are hydroxylation and dehalogenation, which produce nonvolatile metabolites of halothane that are excreted in the urine. Two halogens on the terminal carbon provide optimal conditions for oxidative dehalogenation, whereas the trifluoro moiety is relatively resistant to oxidative enzymatic attack.

Oxidative urinary metabolites of halothane include the following: (1) trifluoroacetic acid (TFA), the major metabolite, comprising about 12% to 25% of total metabolic products[10,14]; (2) free bromide[15]; and (3) free chloride.[10]

Only trace amounts of fluoride are produced by oxidative metabolism, because, as noted previously, the trifluoro carbon is relatively resistant to oxidation. Most of the free fluoride (about 1% of total metabolites) is released by an alternate, reductive metabolic process that is not oxygen dependent. Reductive metabolism of halothane appears to involve cytochrome P-450, with generation of a reactive free radical intermediate. Halothane is the only volatile anesthetic known to undergo reductive metabolism.

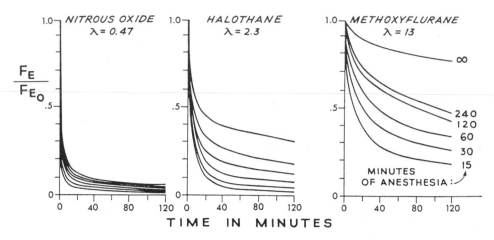

Fig. 38–2. Decrease in anesthetic partial pressures after cessation of anesthetic administration is dependent on blood solubility of the agent and duration of the preceding anesthetic. Nitrous oxide, with a blood/gas solubility coefficient of 0.47, has a much quicker alveolar washout than halothane, which has a blood/gas solubility coefficient of 2.3. In contrast, the fall in alveolar partial pressure of methoxyflurane, with a blood/gas solubility of 13, is markedly delayed. Longer anesthetic times also slow the fall of anesthetic partial pressures, although the effect is minimal with nitrous oxide. From Stoelting, R. K., Eger, E. I.: The effects of ventilation and anesthetic solubility on recovery from anesthesia: an in vivo analog analysis before and after equilibration. Anesthesiology 30:290, 1969.

In addition to free fluoride and bromide, certain reductive metabolites of halothane are produced, which are excreted by the lungs.

Reductive volatile metabolites of halothane include the following:

1. Carbon dioxide, comprising about 1% of total metabolites,[9] formed during complete dehalogenation of halothane.
2. 2-Chloro-1,1,1-trifluoroethane CF_3-CH_2Cl (CTF), 0.35 ppm, produced in a semiclosed circuit with 1% halothane (10,000 ppm) for 1 hour.[16]
3. 2-Chloro-1,1-difluoroethylene CF_2=CHCl (CDF), 0.14 ppm, generated in a semiclosed circuit with 1% halothane for 1 hour.[16]
4. 2-Bromo-2-chloro-1,1-difluoroethylene CF_2=CbrCl (BCDF), 4 to 5 ppm, formed in closed circuits on exposure to soda lime.[16]

Some of the foregoing oxidative and reductive metabolites undergo conjugation and are excreted in the urine. Conjugated urinary metabolites of halothane include the following:

1. An ethanolamine derivative, N-trifluoroacetyl-ethanolamide[17]; the reactive intermediate is the trifluoroacetyl moiety (TFA, from oxidative metabolism), capable of covalent binding to lipid constituents of hepatocyte cell membranes.
2. A cysteine conjugate, N-acetyl-S-(2-bromo-2-chloro-1,1-difluoroethyl) cysteine, formed by conjugation with bromochloro-difluorethylene (BCDF, a reductive metabolite of halothane) and glutathione.[16,17]

The trifluoroacetyl residue, an oxidative metabolite of halothane, may covalently bind to liver proteins. Conjugation to liver proteins may generate haptens, capable of provoking an immunologic response.[18] Free radical inter-mediates generated during reductive metabolism can attack hepatocyte proteins and membrane phospholipids, producing a biochemical or metabolic insult that may result in cell injury or necrosis.[19] (See the section of this chapter on hepatic pathophysiology and Figures 38-12 and 38-13).

Biotransformation in Children

Hepatic dysfunction or injury is rare in children. This may be related to differences in metabolism or to greater levels of endogenous protective agents, such as free radical scavengers. A study of the extent of reductive metabolites of halothane in children shows that the volatile metabolites, CTF and CDF, are quickly formed and exhaled within 10 minutes of anesthetic exposure, although the levels reached are slightly lower than in adults.[20] The metabolites reach a stable plateau within 10 to 15 minutes, in contrast to adults, in whom metabolites gradually rise to a plateau by 60 minutes.[21] In children, one sees little evidence of increased biotransformation or of enzyme induction with repeated halothane administration at short intervals (10 to 30 exposures),[22] although this has been observed in adults with repeated exposure to halothane.[14,23] Levels of CTF in expired air are not significantly different between the first and last exposures. Peak serum bromide levels range from 1.0 to 3.5 mmol/L, below the toxic range. Because metabolites are readily formed in children, it is suggested that either the hepatocytes are resistant to chemical attack or children have more effective protective mechanisms such as more free radical scavengers.

Bromide Metabolite

In 1964, Stier and associates[15] demonstrated that significant amounts of bromide are released from halothane during anesthetic administration to humans. Bromide re-

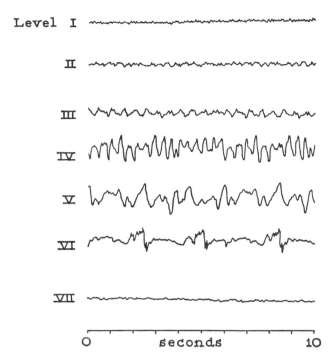

Fig. 38–3. Electroencephalographic levels of halothane anesthesia in humans. Level I = Induction; awake pattern changes to fast low voltage waves (15 to 20 cps and 10 to 25 μV); level II = corresponds to stage II; slow waves with low voltage appear (3 to 6 cps and 20 μV) superimposed on the fast, low voltage activity; level III = stage III; slow waves of 4 cps and amplitude of 50 to 100 μV and disappearance of fast activity; level IV = no fast activity; slow waves of 2 to 3 cps and 100 to 200 μV; level V = slow waves of 1 cps and amplitude of 100 to 200 cps; appearance of smaller faster waves; level VI = burst suppression; level VII = no cortical activity. From Gain, F. A., Paletz, S. G.: An attempt to correlate the clinical signs of Fluothane anaesthesia with the electroencephalographic levels. Can Anaesth Soc J 4:289, 1957.

covered in the urine on the first postoperative day was in the range of 0.1 to 0.6 mmol/L, as the free ion. On the fifth to seventh postoperative day, peaks of from 0.4 to 1.0 mmol/L were detected in urine. These levels occurred after only 1 to 2 hours of light halothane anesthesia (1.0 to 1.4 MAC). Subsequently, more sensitive analytic techniques have substantiated significant biotransformation of halothane, with release of bromide. Markedly elevated levels of bromide (normally undetectable in serum), in the range of 4.5 mmol/L, have been measured in human serum following halothane anesthesia.[24,25] Of the bromide that is released from halothane, 95% is the inorganic ion that is excreted entirely in the urine.

Elevated serum bromide levels may account for prolonged sedative effects in adults after administration of halothane. Bromism, a syndrome characterized initially by headache, lethargy, and dizziness and, in more severe cases, by mental confusion, tremors, ataxia, slurred speech, and dermatitis can result from high serum levels of bromide. Serum levels associated with an early toxic response are in the range of 5 to 10 mmol/L, and a full-blown syndrome is noted when serum levels reach 20 mmol/L.[26]

Anesthesiologists exposed daily to trace amounts of halothane may have elevated bromide levels. After 1 week of exposure to an ambient level of 20 ppm for 3 to 4 hours per day, mean serum bromide levels were 0.1 mmol/L, and at the end of the second week they were 0.2 mmol/L, although peak concentrations reached 0.6 mmol/L.[26] The serum half-life of bromide is approximately 10 days in healthy men. The half-life in chronically exposed individuals is longer, however, with a mean of 15 days. The clinical significance of bromide accumulation in occupationally exposed persons is unclear.

PHYSIOLOGIC EFFECTS OF HALOTHANE

General Body Metabolism

Whole-body oxygen consumption has been studied in dogs, in which halothane has been found to cause a dose-dependent decrease in Vo₂. Concentrations of halothane from 0.2 to 1.5% decrease Vo_2 approximately 27 to 59%.[27] In humans, halothane reduces oxygen consumption (normal 250 ml/min) at 1 MAC by about 30% and at 2 MAC by about 40%.[28] The overall changes in body metabolism are related to the summated effects of reduction in Vo_2 for various organs. Contributions of individual organs to the total decrease expressed as percentages are: myocardial, 47%; skeletal muscle, 23%; splanchnic, 9%; and renal, 5%.

Generally, a pattern of reduction in oxygen consumption with different organs is observed and is probably common to most anesthetic agents. Any general reduction in metabolism is a reflection of the different contributions made by reduction in Vo_2 in individual organ systems. Metabolic changes in the most active organs make the greatest contributions, and reduction in myocardial Vo_2 is the major component decreasing whole-body Vo_2. Such changes can be reproduced by measures that reduce arterial pressure and cardiac output, such as vagal stimulation.

Central Nervous System

A smooth descending depression of the nervous system is achieved with increasing concentrations between 0.5 and 3.0% of halothane. The depth of anesthesia varies to some extent at a given concentration among individuals. Electroencephalographic changes caused by halothane were described by Gain and Paletz,[29] as shown in Figure 38-3. Seven patterns were noted, with good surgical conditions occurring at level III. In clinical practice, changes in pupil size are similar to those caused by other agents and can serve as a guide to depth of anesthesia; however, changes in depth of anesthesia are reflected best by changes in respiratory and cardiovascular parameters.

Halothane is a cerebral vasodilator, producing a significant increase in cerebral blood flow (CBF) and cerebral blood volume at usual anesthetic concentrations, which can increase intracranial pressure (ICP) in the presence of intracranial disorders. Among the inhalation anesthetics in common use, halothane has the most effect on ICP (halothane > enflurane > isoflurane)[30,31] (Fig. 38-4).

Murphy and colleagues[32] found that halothane at 1 MAC increased CBF nearly threefold over baseline, and at

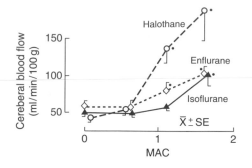

Fig. 38–4. Cerebral blood flow in normal individuals during normocapnic controlled ventilation. Redrawn from Eger, E. I.: Isoflurane (Forane): A Compendium and Reference. Madison, WI, Ohio Medical Products, 1981; and Eger, E. I.: Isoflurane: a review. Anesthesiology 55:559, 1981.

1.6 MAC, it increased CBF about 3.5 times. In comparison, enflurane increased CBF about 1.5 and 2.0-fold, respectively, and isoflurane increased CBF 1.2 and 2.0-fold. In a more recent study,[33] using radioactive xenon to measure regional CBF in patients with intracranial masses, halothane and enflurane in 70% nitrous oxide at 1.5 MAC equivalents both increased CBF (0.58% halothane increased CBF by 2.7-fold and 1.14% enflurane by 1.3-fold), whereas 1.0% isoflurane in 70% nitrous oxide had no effect on CBF. The increase in CBF observed with halothane appears to be time dependent and may return to normal after several hours of anesthesia.[34] Moreover, this effect on CBF is attenuated or abolished unless systemic blood pressure is maintained. The dependence of CBF on systemic blood pressure during halothane anesthesia indicates a loss of CBF autoregulation, which normally maintains CBF at about 50 ml/min/100 g despite wide fluctuations in blood pressure. At high halothane concentrations, autoregulation is abolished.[35] Whether halothane-induced alteration of CBF is a passive phenomenon resulting from metabolic effects on brain or a direct effect on cerebral vasculature is unclear. Halothane and the other inhalation anesthetics cause a dose-dependent inhibition of cerebral metabolic rate (CMRo_2), however, while paradoxically increasing CBF (which is normally tightly coupled to CMRo_2),[36] an effect that appears to be unique to the inhalation agents. In contrast, reactivity of cerebral vessels to carbon dioxide is not markedly changed by inhalation anesthetics in normal brain, and increases in CBF associated with inhalation agents can be blunted or abolished by hyperventilation-induced hypocapnia. The reduction in CBF by hypocapnia appears to be more pronounced with isoflurane than halothane.[37] The clinical significance of retained carbon dioxide reactivity in pathologic states during anesthesia is unpredictable, however.

Respiration

With deepening halothane anesthesia, the respiratory centers become progressively depressed. Respirations become shallow and rapid, with decreased minute volume. Generally, respiratory depression is continuous and gradual, until well into third-plane anesthesia, when apnea may abruptly occur, coincident with complete intercostal and diaphragmatic paralysis. The ease with which control of respiration can be achieved with halothane is striking, however. Bronchial secretions (compared with ether) are markedly absent, bronchomotor tone is reduced, and bronchospasm that may occur with manipulation of the airway in lighter planes of anesthesia is relieved.

Mechanisms of Respiratory Depression

Halothane produces a dose-related depression of respiration, with increased respiratory rate and decreased tidal volume. Minute volume is decreased because tachypnea does not compensate for the reduced tidal volume. Tachypnea caused by inhalation agents has been attributed to sensitization of pulmonary stretch receptors,[38] although a central bulbopontine mechanism is more likely. As halothane concentration increases, the phasic output of phrenic motoneuron activity progressively decreases. According to the theory of bulbopontine rhythmicity,[39] timing of the respiratory cycle is controlled by inspiratory center activity in the dorsal medulla and a reciprocal, inhibitory "off-switch" mechanism in the pons, which terminates inspiration. Shortening of either inspiratory or expiratory time may lead to increased respiratory frequency, however. In the cat, Nishino and Honda[40] demonstrated that halothane shortens expiratory time while lengthening inspiratory time, in which the off-switch mechanism in the pons (the pneumotaxic center) is inhibited, leading to prolongation of inspiration (apneusis) but rapid expiration. Evidence also exists for suprapontine influences. The cortex is thought to be inhibitory, whereas the diencephalon is facilitative to the pontomedullary centers[41]; thus, removal of cortical influences by halothane may also cause tachypnea.

Effects on Mechanics of Respiratory Muscles

Halothane causes a profound depression of intercostal muscle activity, with a relative sparing of diaphragmatic function, although the diaphragm is displaced cranially.[42] The tonic activity of inspiratory muscles is reduced,[43,44] functional residual capacity is decreased,[45] and inspiratory mean gas flow and occlusion pressure are reduced. In spontaneously breathing patients, halothane causes atelectasis in dependent lung regions, and it is impressive that atelectasis develops promptly with the induction of anesthesia. Full paralysis with muscle relaxants enhances the degree of atelectasis. Tokics and colleagues[46] proposed that anesthetic-induced atelectasis in dependent lung regions results from compression of lung resulting from loss of diaphragmatic muscle tone and not from resorption of pulmonary gas. Awake subjects have been able voluntarily to relax their diaphragms and produce a reduction in lung volume in dependent regions.[47]

Ventilatory Response to Carbon Dioxide

The ventilatory response to carbon dioxide is mediated by central and peripheral chemoreceptors. The central chemoreceptors, however, located in the ventral medulla, are most important in the minute to minute control of ventilation. Denervation of the carotid bodies by carotid endarterectomy causes only a minor decrease in sensitivity to carbon dioxide.

All volatile anesthetics depress the ventilatory response to carbon dioxide, which most likely results from a direct inhibitory effect on the medulla. Of the volatile anesthetics, halothane produces the least depression, followed by isoflurane and then enflurane. In spontaneously breathing anesthetized patients, in the absence of surgical stimulation, $PaCO_2$ rises in a dose-dependent manner[31] (Fig. 38-5). At 1 MAC, halothane and isoflurane increase $PaCO_2$ to about 45 mm Hg, and enflurane increases $PaCO_2$ to approximately 60 mm Hg. At 1.5 MAC, the effect is more pronounced, with halothane increasing $PaCO_2$ to approximately 50 mm Hg, isoflurane to about 60 mm Hg, and enflurane to more than 70 mm Hg.

Surgical stimulation increases minute ventilation by about 40%, owing to increased tidal volume and respiratory rate, but $PaCO_2$ only decreases about 10%. This paradoxic response may result from increased metabolic production of carbon dioxide caused by activation of the sympathetic nervous system, which counteracts the effect of increased ventilation on $PaCO_2$.[31,48]

Effects on Hypoxic Ventilatory Drive

In humans, the peripheral chemoreceptors in the carotid bodies are responsible for the increase in ventilation seen with hypoxemia, and complete denervation of the carotid bodies abolishes hypoxic ventilatory drive. Indeed, hypoxemia has no effect on the central chemoreceptors, and in the absence of peripheral chemoreceptors, severe hypoxemia depresses respiration by inhibiting the respiratory centers in the pons and medulla. The peripheral chemoreceptors are extremely sensitive to halothane and the other inhalation anesthetics (including nitrous oxide). Extremely low concentrations of halothane (e.g., 0.1 MAC) reduce the ventilatory response to hypoxemia by 50 to 70%, and 1 MAC abolishes the hypoxic drive[49]; in contrast, 0.1 MAC of halothane does not have a significant effect on the ventilatory response to carbon dioxide.

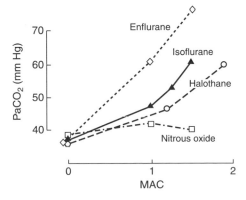

Fig. 38-5. Dose-response effect of volatile anesthetics on $PaCO_2$ in spontaneously breathing subjects in the absence of surgical stimulation. Redrawn from Eger, E. I. Isoflurane (Forane): A Compendium and Reference. Madison, WI, Ohio Medical Products, 1981; and Eger, E. I.: Isoflurane: a review. Anesthesiology 55:559, 1981.

Inhibition of peripheral chemoreceptors by low concentrations of inhalation anesthetics increases the risk of postoperative hypoxemia. After cessation of anesthesia, blood levels of anesthetic persist for some time. Moreover, elimination is delayed with the more soluble agents, such as halothane, and with prolonged anesthetic times. Therefore, blood levels sufficient to inhibit hypoxic ventilatory drive should be expected in the immediate postoperative period.

Cardiac Arrhythmias

Generally, halothane does not change heart rate, although bradycardia may sometimes occur, from reduction in sympathetic tone and vagal dominance. Direct slowing of the sinoatrial node may also occur, resulting from reduction in the rate of phase 4 depolarization and elevation of the threshold for generation of the action potential.[50] Sinoatrial node depression may allow ectopic discharges to occur, which are more likely during rapid induction and deep anesthesia. Manipulation of the airway can accentuate vagal tone, during which time sinus bradycardia, first-degree atrioventricular block and nodal rhythms may occur, but these are usually benign. With increasing levels of anesthesia, His-Purkinje conduction times are prolonged, an effect that contrasts with enflurane. In addition, the atrial refractory period, the functional refractory period of the atrioventricular node and atrioventricular nodal conduction times are prolonged with halothane. Thus, reentrant supraventricular tachyarrhythmias may occur.[51] Halothane anesthesia also increases the incidence of ventricular arrhythmias, an effect enhanced by hypercarbia and endogenous and exogenous catecholamines.

Sensitization to Epinephrine

The propensity for epinephrine to cause arrhythmias with halothane, particularly ventricular premature beats, has been known for years. Katz and colleagues[52] identified certain factors influencing their incidence and severity. Adults are susceptible to these arrhythmias, whereas children can tolerate larger doses of epinephrine. The site of injection is also important. Infiltration of epinephrine into tissues that are highly vascular, especially the nasopharynx, mouth, and face, results in rapid absorption and higher levels of epinephrine, increasing the risk of arrhythmias. The chance of intravascular injection in these tissues is also increased. Baseline heart rate and blood pressure are additional factors to consider.[53] When either is elevated, as in anxiety states or hypertension, arrhythmias with halothane are more likely, and epinephrine further increases their incidence. Likewise, the fasting state, which is associated with increased levels of plasma fatty acids, has been demonstrated experimentally by Miletich and colleagues[54] to render the heart more sensitive to epinephrine and to increase the incidence of arrhythmias during halothane anesthesia. Indeed, the administration of lipid infusions lowers the threshold for epinephrine-induced arrhythmias with halothane. Other factors that have been implicated include prostaglandins[55] and certain drugs including muscle relaxants,[56] local anesthetics[57] (although low doses of lidocaine appear to be protective[58]), and thiopental sodium.[59] The proarrhythmic effect of thiopental with halothane and epinephrine is seen with low doses; when larger doses of thiopental are used (i.e., full induction doses), the incidence of arrhythmias is diminished.

Epinephrine Doses Producing Arrhythmias

In adults during halothane anesthesia (1.25 MAC), the mean effective dose (ED_{50}) for the production of ventricular premature beats (three or more considered a positive response) with epinephrine is 2.1 μg/kg.[58] This compares with an ED_{50} of 6.7 μg/kg for isoflurane and 10.9 μg/kg for enflurane. The dose-response curve for enflurane is nearly horizontal, however, and the actual dose is probably difficult to predict. Of further concern is evidence that the simultaneous administration of nitrous oxide increases the arrhythmic potential of epinephrine.[60]

Children have a decreased likelihood of developing epinephrine-produced ventricular arrhythmias. Karl and associates[61] observed that doses up to 10 μg/kg were not arrhythmogenic in the presence of halothane.

Mechanism of Halothane-Epinephrine Arrhythmias

Extensive studies of cardiac arrhythmias by halothane and catecholamines have been carried out, and the conclusion is that the mechanism of halothane sensitization does not materially differ from that of cyclopropane-induced arrhythmias. The site of origin of the abnormal beats and the typical bigeminal rhythm are probably in the basal portion of the intraventricular septum, near the right ventricular surface.[62] The mechanism of the arrhythmia is one of reentry rather than increased automaticity. The arrhythmia is sensitive to changes in blood pressure and heart rate and can be converted to sinus rhythm by vagal stimulation, whether or not the atrial rate is controlled.[62] In view of the relationship of halothane arrhythmias with catecholamines, clinical and experimental studies have demonstrated that a myocardial α_1-adrenergic mechanism is involved. Prazosin, a selective α_1-adrenergic antagonist, raises the threshold for epinephrine-induced arrhythmias with halothane,[63] as does droperidol.[64] Indeed, selective α_1 blockade is more effective than selective β_1 blockade, such as with metoprolol.

Recommendations

1. When epinephrine is to be used in surgical practice for hemostasis in head and neck surgery, and in perineal and vaginal surgery, halothane should not be administered.
2. Although halothane is contraindicated in adults when epinephrine hemostasis is needed, some degree of safety may exist in the use of dilute solutions of epinephrine with children.
3. Regardless of the anesthetic agent used, or if epinephrine is to be used in children during halothane anesthesia, solutions of epinephrine stronger than 1:200,000 (5 μg/ml) should not be used; a dilution of 1:200,000 is prepared by mixing 0.5 mg of epinephrine in 100 ml of saline.

Cardiac Output

Halothane reduces cardiac output in a dose-related manner because of a fall in stroke volume.[28] Generally, halothane does not change heart rate, although the bradycardia sometimes seen may result from direct depression of sinoatrial node activity. In humans, 1 MAC halothane reduces cardiac output by about 25%. Price and co-workers[65] showed that the initial reduction of cardiac output returns toward normal with time, except in the presence of β blockade.

Myocardial Function

Halothane reduces myocardial contractility. Analyses of ventricular function and force-velocity curves during halothane anesthesia show a progressive depression of stroke work. One sees a negative inotropic effect without any inherent compensation as occurs with ether or cyclopropane. Left and right ventricular function curves show that both ventricles produce less stroke work at any end-diastolic pressure[66] (Fig. 38–6). The slopes of the curves decrease in proportion to increasing halothane concentration. If mean aortic pressure is raised to control values, no change in stroke velocity or ventricular stroke work occurs, and the volume of blood ejected remains the same. Tension-velocity curves during halothane anesthesia demonstrate a negative inotropic effect (Fig. 38–7).

Inotropic Effect of Calcium

The negative inotropic effect of halothane (1.2 MAC) can be partially antagonized by the administration of calcium chloride[67]: 10% calcium chloride at a dose of 7 mg/kg produces an approximate 10% increase in cardiac index. Left ventricular stroke and work index are also mildly increased, whereas small decreases in heart rate,

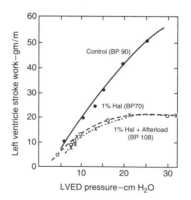
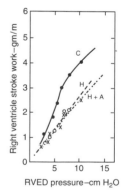

Fig. 38–6. Left and right ventricular function curves obtained before and during halothane anesthesia at different afterload levels, showing that there was no improvement of stroke work in either ventricle when mean aortic pressure was increased (from decreased value during halothane anesthesia) to the control value. LVEDP = left ventricular end-diastolic pressure; RVEDP = right ventricular end-diastolic pressure. Redrawn from Etsten, B. E., Shimosato, S.: Myocardial contractility: performance of the heart during anesthesia. Clin Anesth *3*:56, 1964.

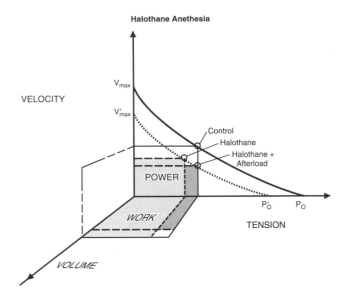

Fig. 38–7. Tension-velocity-volume diagram before and during halothane anesthesia at different afterload levels. Halothane anesthesia resulted in a shift of the tension-velocity curve to the left, indicating negative inotropic effect. Shaded areas demonstrate that experimentally increased afterload during halothane anesthesia did not increase power and work of the heart. Redrawn from Etsten, B. E., Shimosato, S.: Myocardial contractility: performance of the heart during anesthesia. Clin Anesth 3:56, 1964.

total peripheral vascular resistance, and preejection time period are noted.

Circulation

Halothane reduces mean arterial blood pressure from 25 to 50%, in a dose-related fashion, from about 1 to 2 MAC.[28] Fall in systolic pressure is greater than the fall in diastolic pressure. This hypotensive effect is due chiefly to a reduction in cardiac output, because halothane does not significantly change total systemic vascular resistance.[28] Halothane does appear to have direct vasoactive effects on specific vascular beds, however. For example, prominent cutaneous venodilation is characteristic with halothane (and the other volatile anesthetics), which makes it easier to insert intravenous lines in the anesthetized than the awake patient. In experimental studies using canine and primate models, Vatner and Smith[68] showed that halothane causes vasodilation in the renal and iliac circulations and vasoconstriction in the mesenteric circulation, effects not altered by adrenergic blockade. Moreover, in addition to direct effects on the vasculature, indirect effects mediated by changes in resting sympathetic tone may also occur, and the relative clinical importance of each is difficult to assess.

In infants, halothane anesthesia is associated with depression of systolic blood pressure, mean arterial pressure, and heart rate.[69] Infants have a low ventricular compliance, and cardiac output is largely rate dependent. Therefore, it is necessary to maintain blood pressure, which can be accomplished by keeping the heart rate at a sufficiently high level with atropine. Depres-

sion is also less likely if halothane concentrations are kept under 1.0%.

Renal Function

A depression of renal function comparable to that produced by other anesthetic agents occurs during halothane anesthesia and is generally attributed to reductions in cardiac output and blood pressure. Studies describing specific effects on renal function are contradictory, however. Clearance studies in humans indicate that 1% halothane decreases renal blood flow by about 50% and glomerular filtration rate by about 65%.[70] In contrast, animal studies by Vatner and Smith[68] indicate that 1 to 2% halothane does not alter renal blood flow, despite a 50% reduction in renal vascular resistance. This observation is consistent with other experimental studies[71] indicating that autoregulation of renal blood flow is maintained during halothane anesthesia. In the clinical setting, the sympathetic nervous system probably plays a role in the variable responses, because excessive sympathetic activity can markedly reduce urine output. Overall, during halothane anesthesia, the net effect is a decrease in urine production, which can be reversed by intraoperative administration of saline or mannitol.

Little or no direct effect on renal tubular transport is noted.[72] The presence of casts, albumin, cells, or other evidence of renal toxicity has not been reported. An immediate postoperative diuresis is sometimes seen, however, and may lead to electrolyte depletion.

The Liver

Halothane, as a halogenated hydrocarbon, has the potential for causing liver injury. Early clinical studies indicated, however, that the extent of hepatic dysfunction after halothane was comparable to that seen with other inhalation anesthetics then in use.[73] Mild elevations in serum alanine aminotransferase (ALT; serum glutamate pyruvate transaminase [SGPT]) occurred in 12.5% of patients, similar to the incidence following anesthesia with cyclopropane,[74] an inhalation agent not associated with direct hepatotoxic effects. The incidence of postoperative jaundice was about 4 per 1000 halothane anesthetics, again similar to that seen with other inhalation agents.[75] In addition, liver dysfunction could be demonstrated in halothane-anesthetized patients when associated hypotension was present; typical abnormalities included elevated serum bromsulphthalein (cleared by the liver and excreted in bile after conjugation) and serum bilirubin.[76]

Based on widespread clinical experience, halothane was considered to be a safe anesthetic. Shortly after its introduction into clinical use, however, several reports, especially by Burnap and colleagues,[77] Bunker and Blumenfeld,[78] and Brody and Sweet,[79] implicated halothane in a severe, potentially fatal form of postoperative hepatitis, associated with fulminant hepatic necrosis. Subsequently, the United States National Halothane Study[80] retrospectively reviewed approximately 255,000 halothane anesthetic administrations and found it to be a remarkably safe anesthetic, with a better safety record than the other agents then in use. Nonetheless, the study identified 7 cases of unexplained massive hepatic necrosis (e.g., other causes, such as shock, sepsis, or preexisting liver disease, were excluded) in the patients who received halothane, with an incidence of 1 per 36,400 anesthetic administrations. The overall incidence of massive hepatic necrosis (from all causes) was 1 per 10,000 halothane anesthetic administrations, which was less than the incidence with cyclopropane (1.7 per 10,000 anesthetic administrations). Only 1 case of unexplained massive hepatic necrosis occurred in over 147,000 cyclopropane anesthetic administrations, however. Therefore, halothane did appear to be associated with a rare, often fatal hepatitis not attributable to other causes, although the incidence was actually less than the often-quoted rate of 1 per 10,000 anesthetic administrations. The topic of halothane-associated hepatitis is reviewed in the section of this chapter on hepatic pathophysiology.

Splanchnic Blood Flow

Halothane, 1.5 MAC, reduces splanchnic blood flow by 25 to 30%, which appears to be a passive phenomenon due to reduction in cardiac output.[81] During spontaneous ventilation, splanchnic vascular resistance is unchanged, and as systemic blood pressure falls, splanchnic perfusion pressure is reduced, thereby accounting for the observed decrease in blood flow. This is in contrast with elderly patients during light halothane anesthesia, in whom splanchnic blood flow decreases approximately 30%, despite a reduction in splanchnic vascular resistance of about 20%.[82] In contrast, during controlled ventilation, splanchnic vascular resistance may increase, which can further reduce splanchnic blood flow.[81] The increase in splanchnic vascular resistance was shown to be due to hypocapnia from hyperventilation, an effect that could be attenuated by adding carbon dioxide to the inspired mixture.

In general, halothane anesthesia does not appear to cause visceral hypoxia. Although splanchnic arteriovenous oxygen differences are increased with halothane, indicating a greater uptake of oxygen, elevated splanchnic lactate levels are not observed.[83] The clinical relevance of these alterations in splanchnic blood flow is speculative, and other variables such as trauma, surgical manipulation of the viscera, hypovolemia, and preexisting liver disease may be more important.

Gastrointestinal Tract

At anesthetic levels, halothane depresses gastrointestinal tone and depresses motility of stomach, jejunum, and colon. On discontinuance of halothane, activity promptly returns. Halothane also blocks contractions produced by neostigmine or methacholine.[84]

Neuromuscular Junction

Early studies by Gissen and co-workers[85] with amphibian nerve-muscle preparations demonstrated that 1.5% halothane blocked muscle twitch by nerve stimulation, but higher concentrations, in the range of 4%, were required to block axonal conduction or direct stimulation of muscle. Therefore, the neuromuscular junction was shown to be more sensitive to inhibition than nerve or muscle. Later studies[86] indicate that two mechanisms are involved: (1) depression of the twitch response to nerve stimulation (indirect simulation) by interference with depolarization of the motor end plate by acetylcholine (stabilization of the postsynaptic membrane); and (2) depression of the twitch response to direct stimulation by a postjunctional mechanism, which may involve inhibition of excitation-contraction coupling or interference with the contractile mechanism. The indirect response is clearly more sensitive to inhibition by volatile anesthetics than the direct response. End plate depolarization must be depressed by at least 50% before the indirect twitch begins to fail, however. At 1 MAC, most anesthetics produce only 20 to 40% depression, which clinically is not detectable. Inhibition of the direct response occurs only at much higher concentrations. For halothane, concentrations in the range of 8 to 10 MAC are required to depress the direct twitch response by 50%. Therefore, observed relaxant effects of halothane probably reflect depression of the central nervous system with reduction in resting tone of skeletal muscle.[86,87]

Clinically, effects of halothane on the neuromuscular junction are manifested by a reduced requirement for nondepolarizing blockers. Halothane, at 0.5 to 1.0%, reduces the ED_{50} of d-tubocurarine by 40 to 60%, compared with nitrous oxide without the volatile anesthetic.[88] Potentiation of pancuronium and vecuronium blockade is similar to that seen with d-tubocurarine.

Halothane also enhances neuromuscular blockade by succinylcholine, a depolarizing agent. The effect is small, however, only about 20%.[89,90]

Skeletal Muscle

With light anesthesia, surgical relaxation is fair to moderate and may be adequate for lower abdominal surgery. It is not satisfactory for upper abdominal surgery, however, and adequate relaxation can be secured only at the cost of marked hypotension and cardiac arrhythmias, so administration of a muscle relaxant is necessary.

Halothane Contracture Test

As noted previously, halothane does not produce significant direct relaxation of skeletal muscle at usual clinical concentrations. At high concentrations, in the range of 4%, however, halothane does cause direct relaxation of normal skeletal muscle, evident by suppression of the direct twitch response. Paradoxically, skeletal muscle biopsies from patients who are susceptible to malignant hyperthermia often develop a contracture with direct electrical stimulation in the presence of halothane. This abnormal response appears to result from an increased sensitivity of the calcium release mechanism to halothane. With repeated electrical stimulation in the presence of halothane, enhanced calcium release results in a sustained contracture of the test muscle strip. Under precisely defined conditions, the force developed by the abnormal contracture is reproducible and can be quantified. This is the basis for the halothane contracture test, one of the tests used to diagnose susceptibility to malignant hyperthermia. A second method, the caffeine contracture test, is used to complement the results of the halothane contracture test. Caffeine enhances the twitch response in normal and abnormal skeletal muscle by increasing calciumpermeability of the sarcoplasmic reticulum. Again, with precise techniques, the difference between normal and abnormal responses can be quantified. An additional test employs both halothane and caffeine in the protocol, in which the concentration of caffeine in the Krebs-Ringer solution bathing the muscle specimen is incrementally increased during simultaneous exposure to halothane, and the resulting force of contracture is measured. As with all laboratory tests, validation of results requires standardization of techniques and appropriate controls.

For diagnostic purposes, most laboratories use specimens of fresh muscle obtained from the vastus lateralis. To increase the diagnostic value of these protocols, the North American Malignant Hyperthermia Group has developed a set of general guidelines to be used in interpreting the results of the muscle tests.[91] These are reproduced in Table 38–5.

The halothane contracture test may have the greatest specificity, but the least sensitivity, and the standard appears to be the joint halothane-caffeine assay.[92] Currently, both the halothane-only and the caffeine-only contracture tests are considered mandatory, whereas the combined test is optional. A positive clinical diagnosis of susceptibility to malignant hyperthermia is made if one viable muscle strip demonstrates an abnormal contracture response after exposure to either 3% halothane alone, caffeine alone, or for those laboratories performing the test, the combined halothane-caffeine assay.[91]

The indications for biopsy appear controversial, because some physicians suggest that the management of patients suspected of having malignant hyperthermia will not be altered. On the other hand, negative contracture tests indicate that a patient may be safely exposed to triggering agents. Moreover, indiscriminate labeling of patients as susceptible to malignant hyperthermia is avoided.[92] The North American Malignant Hyperthermia Group recommends that all patients with a clinical history of unequivocal malignant hyperthermia have a biopsy performed. In addition, all patients who have had

a clinical episode consistent with this disorder, and one or both parents of a proband, should be tested.[91]

Reflexes

Halothane depresses the patellar monosynaptic reflex arc by central synaptic inhibition. Halothane also causes a progressive inhibition in the firing rate of dorsal horn neurons in response to skin stimulation. Neuronal activity in response to pain and light touch is often abolished within 5 to 45 minutes, but fairly high concentrations of halothane are required (2 to 3%).[93] The area of skin evoking a dorsal horn response to stimulation is also progressively diminished, indicating reduction in size of the receptive field. Of clinical importance, these findings indicate that usual anesthetic concentrations of halothane do not prevent afferent sensory input to the spinal cord.

Ganglionic Blockade

Halothane can weaken ganglionic transmission and can potentiate the effects of ganglionic blockers, such as hexamethonium. Synaptic transmission in the stellate ganglion is markedly depressed by halothane at concentrations of 0.75 to 1.5%,[94] and in conjunction with cardiac depression and central sympathetic inhibition, it probably contributes to the arterial hypotension seen with halothane. Sympathetic blockade may also contribute to the cutaneous venodilation seen with halothane, although the anesthetic has direct relaxant effects on vascular smooth muscle if it is injected intra-arterially.[68] Salivary and mucous secretions may also be suppressed. Similarly, halothane enhances blockade by d-tubocurarine, which has ganglionic as well as neuromuscular junction effects.

The Uterus

Relaxation of uterine muscle occurs in both the pregnant and nonpregnant women. The degree is directly related to the depth of anesthesia: 1% halothane causes depression of uterine tone and reduced frequency and amplitude of contractions, which can be counteracted with pitocin; however, 2% halothane results in complete uterine relaxation, which cannot be antagonized by pitocin. A direct effect on uterine smooth muscle appears to be one mechanism causing relaxation, but stimulation of β-adrenergic receptors may also contribute.[95] On this basis, halothane has been used to provide uterine relaxation for inversions, breech

Table 38–5. Criteria for Abnormal Contracture Response in the Diagnosis of Malignant Hyperthermia Susceptibility*

Positive halothane contracture test: A positive response is considered to be a contraction > 0.2–0.7 g, after exposure to 3% halothane for 10 min; exact value shall be determined by each testing laboratory after evaluation of at least 30 normal muscle biopsies.

Positive caffeine contracture test: A positive response is defined as (1) development of ≥ 0.2 g tension at 2 mmol/L caffeine, or (2) concentration of caffeine required to produce a net increase in tension (above baseline) of 1 g is < 4 mmol/L, or (3) percentage of maximal tension is > 7% above baseline at 2 mM caffeine.

Positive halothane-caffeine contracture test: A positive response is defined as the development of a 1-g contracture after exposure to a concentration of 1 mmol/L or less caffeine in the presence of 1% halothane.

*These are suggested values and must be modified by each laboratory.
Adapted from Larach, M. G.: Standardization of the caffeine halothane muscle contracture test. Anesth Analg 69:511, 1989.

birth, and extraction of retained placenta; the last is still a recognized indication for halothane. Halothane readily crosses the placental barrier.

Endocrine Effects

Halothane anesthesia causes inhibition of insulin release.[96] A variable change in blood glucose occurs in normal subjects, but in most instances, a mild hyperglycemic response (about 20 mg/dl) persists for the duration of anesthesia.[97] Mild progressive hypoglycemia may develop during prolonged anesthesia, however.

The actions of insulin and glucagon are reduced, and glucose utilization is impeded.[98] Wide variations in free fatty acids are observed. Preoperative elevations of free fatty acids are often encountered related to apprehension and do not correlate with fasting. Preoperative levels are markedly reduced after 30 minutes of anesthesia, however, followed by a progressive rise to approximately normal levels. Insignificant changes in pyruvate occur, but one sees a mild increase in serum lactate that progressively increases in subjects anesthetized for more than 3 hours, without surgery.[97] With the associated stresses related to surgery, elevations of pyruvate and more marked increases in lactate occur.[99]

Elevations in cortisol are associated with halothane anesthesia, and they most likely reflect the stresses related to surgery. In contrast, blood levels of testosterone, an anabolic steroid, are reduced slightly during anesthesia (12%) and show a progressive fall in the postanesthetic period, reaching a 50% reduction on the first postoperative day.[100] Low values persist for a week. The clinical significance of this effect, also seen following ether and thiopental administration, is unclear. Hormonal changes associated with anesthesia and surgery reflect the catabolic state characteristic of the postoperative period, however.

Recovery from Anesthesia

Recovery is rapid and is generally free from excitement. Protective reflexes return in a matter of minutes, and nausea and vomiting are infrequent. Transient shivering is seen in about 5% of patients. Consciousness and orientation return in 5 to 20 minutes; however, cognitive activity may be impaired for several days after halothane anesthesia. Features noted include memory difficulties, reduced ability to concentrate, and impairment of psychomotor tasks.[101] This effect appears to be specific for halothane, because these cognitive changes are not seen after enflurane anesthesia. Bromide, released during the metabolism of halothane, is the probable culprit.[24,25]

HEPATIC PATHOPHYSIOLOGY AND HALOTHANE HEPATITIS

Mechanisms of Liver Injury

The phenomenon of halothane hepatitis is confounded by the many factors associated with anesthesia and surgery that can cause liver injury. Indeed, conditions and drugs with the potential for causing liver damage are multiple. Individually and in combination, these can contribute to the production of jaundice, to liver dysfunction, to hepatic failure, and to death in the postoperative period. The liver has an enormous functional reserve, so extensive damage may be incurred before clinical manifestations of injury become evident. Etiologic factors include trauma, hepatitis viruses, and drugs and hepatotoxins.

Trauma

Hepatic damage may be sustained as a result of direct or indirect trauma. During operations on the liver or contiguous structures, direct injury to the biliary tract or hepatic blood vessels may occur, such as with retraction of the liver or viscera.

Indirect injury is more subtle, but probably fairly common, and can result from the following: traction reflexes impairing liver blood flow by vasoconstriction; blood loss and shock, which markedly decrease hepatic blood flow; and excessive use of vasopressors. The typical hepatic lesion is centrilobular necrosis, which emphasizes the key role of reduced blood flow and hypoxia in the pathogenesis of indirect injury. The morphologic changes are generally reversible and do not result in fibrosis.

Viral Hepatitis

Numerous viruses may infect the liver, including cytomegalovirus, rubella, adenoviruses, and enteroviruses. The term viral hepatitis usually refers to liver infections caused by a small group of hepatotropic viruses that includes hepatitis A, hepatitis B, and non-A, non-B hepatitis virus, however. The morphologic changes in acute viral hepatitis are similar regardless of the infective agent. The characteristic lesion is lobular disarray with spotty or focal hepatocyte necrosis, distributed randomly throughout the lobule, although injury is often more pronounced around the central vein.[102] An inflammatory exudate is evident in the portal areas and is dominated by lymphocytes and histiocytes. Cholestasis and bile duct changes may also occur, but they can be absent in anicteric hepatitis. Regeneration proceeds concurrently with necrosis, and the lesions usually heal without fibrosis.

Acute hepatitis may progress into a chronic necrotizing and fibrosing disease known as chronic active hepatitis.[102] The characteristic morphologic picture is confluent hepatic necrosis, also known as bridging hepatic necrosis. In addition to the spotty and random injury of viral hepatitis, bridges of necrosis exist between liver lobules and triads. This syndrome carries a significant mortality from liver failure, whereas survivors may develop cirrhosis.

The least common result of acute viral infection is a fulminant hepatitis that results in submassive to massive hepatic necrosis. Although this entity occurs in less than 5% of cases, viral hepatitis accounts for the majority of cases of acute hepatic failure.[103] Lobular or multilobular necrosis is referred to as submassive necrosis, whereas widespread and extensive destruction of the hepatic parenchyma is called massive necrosis. Fatal cases may run a protracted course lasting up to 3 months or a fulminant course, rapidly progressing to coma and death in 2 to 3 weeks. The pathogenesis of fulminant viral hepatitis appears to be an overwhelming immune response to infected hepatocytes, because little evidence indicates that hepatitis viruses are directly cytopathic.[103] One sees confluent necrosis of hepatocytes, involving the entire lobule, although necrosis is more extensive centrally, sometimes sparing portal areas. Early on, minimal inflammatory infiltrate is present, but during later stages, a mononuclear infiltrate develops in portal areas. In those who survive, disorganized nodular regeneration eventually occurs, with little or no scarring. On morphologic grounds, massive hepatic necrosis of viral origin cannot be distinguished from that resulting from drugs or halothane.

The incidence of viral hepatitis is obviously much higher than that of halothane hepatitis, and therefore, from a clinical standpoint, viral hepatitis is of considerably more importance. Indeed, the postoperative mortality rate of patients with viral hepatitis undergoing anesthesia is high and ranges from 9 to 100%, regardless of the inhalation anesthetic used.[104]

Hepatotoxic Drugs

Drug-induced liver injury is a common medical problem that should be considered in the differential diagnosis of any patient presenting with liver disease. Although drug reactions account for a minority of clinical cases of jaundice, drug toxicity may be involved in up to a quarter of patients with fulminant hepatic necrosis.[102,105]

Drugs may be categorized as predictable (intrinsic) or unpredictable (idiosyncratic) hepatotoxins, depending on the frequency with which they produce liver injury (Klatskin's principles)[106]:

Drugs causing predictable liver injury share several important characteristics[106]: (1) hepatic injury occurs in all individuals if the drug is given in sufficient dosage; (2) the extent of damage is dose-dependent; (3) similar lesions can be readily produced in experimental animals; (4) the morphology of the lesions is characteristic; and (5) the latent period between exposure and manifestation of injury is predictable and brief.

Cell injury inflicted by intrinsic toxins may involve several mechanisms. For example, direct physicochemical destruction of cell membranes can occur, such as with lipid peroxidation. This is the mechanism involved in carbon tetrachloride (CCl_4) toxicity. Carbon tetrachloride is metabolized by cytochrome P-450 to the highly reactive trichloromethyl free radical CCl_3, which can abstract hydrogen ions from cell membrane polyenoic fatty acids, causing lipid peroxidation. The process is self-sustaining and rapidly produces cell necrosis.

A different mechanism is responsible for the toxicity of chloroform ($CHCl_3$). Although small amounts of the trichloromethyl radical may be generated during metabolism (again by cytochrome P-450), the extent of lipid peroxidation is much less than that seen with carbon tetrachloride.[107] Little $CHCl_3$ is observed to covalently bind to cellular constituents.[108] Hepatic toxicity of chloroform most likely results from oxidation of the C-H bond of $CHCl_3$ to trichloromethanol (Cl_3COH), an unstable intermediate.[108] Trichloromethanol undergoes spontaneous dehydrochlorination, yielding the toxic compound phosgene ($COCl_2$), which covalently binds to tissue macromolecules, causing cellular injury.

Acetaminophen is another example of a drug with a potentially toxic metabolite. A small proportion of acetaminophen undergoes N-hydroxylation by cytochrome P-450, yielding the highly reactive intermediate, N-acetylbenzoquinoneimine.[109] When taken in overdose, sufficient product may accumulate to deplete hepatic glutathione, which usually scavenges the metabolite. Covalent binding to liver macromolecules can result in potentially fatal hepatic necrosis.

The majority of drug-induced reactions causing liver injury are unpredictable or idiosyncratic, however.[103] Classically, idiosyncratic drug toxicity has been thought to involve an immunologic mechanism, because the incidence of hepatotoxicity is unpredictable, and extrahepatic manifestations of hypersensitivity, such as rash, fever, arthralgias, leukocytosis, and eosinophilia, occur in about 25% of cases.[110] According to this theory, injury results from an immunologic response directed at altered cellular constituents. More recent evidence suggests, however, that liver injury with some of these drugs may be consequent to direct toxicity of metabolites; that is, the metabolites may be intrinsic toxins. Susceptibility is mediated by the propensity to form metabolites, which may differ widely among individuals. Therefore, the term hypersensitivity should be reserved for reactions exhibiting clinical or morphologic features of drug allergy.

The hepatic response associated with idiosyncratic toxicity is unpredictable in that[106]: (1) lesions develop in only a small number of exposed individuals; (2) no proportionality to dose exists; (3) animal models are difficult to produce; (4) lesions are inconsistent and may show focal necrosis, cholestasis, or changes reminiscent of viral hepatitis; and (5) a variable interval exists between exposure to the drug and appearance of hepatitis; patients may take these drugs for long periods of time before manifestations of hepatic injury appear.

Morphologic Forms of Toxic Injury

Drugs that cause predictable hepatic injury (intrinsic toxins) produce direct or indirect cytologic damage, characterized by cell necrosis and fatty change (steatosis).[111] The end result is parenchymal damage. Necrosis is typically zonal, limited to parts of the hepatic lobule, and may be centrilobular, midzonal, or portal.[111] The particular zonal site of injury may reflect the location in the lobule where enzymes that metabolize the particular drug are concentrated. For example, chloroform typically causes centrilobular necrosis; the mixed-function oxidases that metabolize chloroform are concentrated in the central part of the lobule.

In contrast, cell necrosis associated with idiosyncratic reactions is usually diffuse, which denotes a panlobular, rather than zonal, distribution. The degree of necrosis may range from mild to severe. Massive necrosis, which indicates destruction of entire lobules, may be an extreme form of diffuse necrosis.[111]

Cholestatic hepatitis is a more common form of injury associated with idiosyncratic reactions and is characterized by centrilobular cholestasis and a portal inflammatory infiltrate consisting of lymphocytes, neutrophils, and eosinophils.[103] Generally, little or no necrosis is present. Clinical and laboratory findings are those of obstructive jaundice. Examples of drugs causing cholestatic hepatitis are chlorpromazine and erythromycin estolate.

The most serious type of idiosyncratic drug reaction resembles viral hepatitis, with diffuse, spotty necrosis. Severe cases are typified by bridging necrosis, and occasionally massive necrosis, and have a high mortality.[103] Drugs producing this type of injury include isoniazid and halothane.

Clinical Features and Epidemiology of Halothane Hepatitis

Shortly after the introduction of halothane into clinical practice, reports appeared, implicating the anesthetic as a cause of a severe form of hepatitis.[77-79] Subsequently, the National Halothane Study demonstrated a low incidence of severe hepatitis, apparently specific for halothane (after excluding other causes), in the range of 1 in 36,000 halothane administrations.[80] Later studies showed that severe hepatic injury following halothane was more common, from 1 in 6000 to 1 in 20,000 administrations.[112,113]

Currently, little doubt exists that halothane exposure can result in a severe form of hepatitis. The rarity of severe halothane-associated hepatitis in humans, the difficulty in producing similar lesions in animal models except under certain experimental conditions (e.g., hypoxia), and the delayed appearance of hepatic injury, however, suggest that halothane is not a direct hepatotoxin, but probably a sensitizing agent involving reactive metabolites. A genetic predisposition leading to an idiosyncratic immunologic reaction has been suggested. This conclusion is strengthened by the finding that prior exposure to halothane increases the incidence and severity of liver injury. Some of the morphologic patterns of injury, discussed later, indicate that a direct toxic mechanism may also be involved, however.

The pathogenesis of halothane hepatotoxicity is further complicated by the fact that mild elevations in transaminases may occur in up to 20% of patients following halothane anesthesia,[114-116] particularly after repeat administrations. This effect may not be specific for halothane, however. Cousins and co-workers[117] prospectively evaluated 24 patients undergoing abdominal surgery randomly assigned to receive halothane, enflurane, or meperidine as a supplement to nitrous oxide anesthesia. Transaminase levels were elevated about threefold above control levels, and bilirubin levels were approximately 1.5 times control levels, following both halothane and enflurane anesthesia. In 3 patients, liver biopsies showed several foci of necrosis and neutrophilic infiltrates near central veins; 2 patients had received halothane and 1 enflurane. Clearance of antipyrine, a

drug metabolized by hepatic mixed-function oxidases, was delayed only with halothane, however. Meperidine had no effect on any of the parameters. Therefore, the clinical picture of halothane hepatitis is far from clear. From an epidemiologic viewpoint, however, two types of hepatic injury may be associated with halothane.[19] The common mild form is basically asymptomatic and of little clinical consequence (and not necessarily specific for halothane). The second type of reaction is the rare, often fatal form of hepatitis that physicians usually associate with halothane.

Clinical Characteristics

Common clinical manifestations of halothane hepatitis include fever, moderate leukocytosis, and eosinophilia, occurring during the first week.[118] Jaundice develops about 10 days after exposure, and earlier after multiple exposures. Nausea and vomiting may precede the occurrence of jaundice. Hepatomegaly is usually mild, but the liver is often tender. Hepatic enzymes are moderately to markedly elevated. The pathologic changes in fatal cases are similar to the massive hepatic necrosis seen with severe viral hepatitis. The fatality rate is unknown, but probably approaches 50%[112]; the diagnosis is basically one of exclusion, often made at autopsy.

Incrimination of halothane rests on several considerations. One assumes that the patient did not have severe hypotension during the surgical procedure, the course was not complicated by administration of blood products, and other potentially hepatotoxic drugs were not given. These complicating factors are often present and make the diagnosis difficult. Certain clinical characteristics appear to typify halothane hepatitis, however, as described in the following paragraphs.

Multiple Exposures

One of the most important factors appears to be a history of previous exposure. Halothane hepatitis occurs much more frequently in patients who have received the anesthetic on one or more occasions; of those who develop hepatitis, approximately 80% have had a previous exposure.[112,114-119] The process may occur in individuals not previously exposed, however.

Fever

Patients who develop halothane hepatitis have a secondary febrile episode, characteristically seen between the fourth and seventh postoperative day.[118] This is in addition to the low-grade temperature elevation often seen postoperatively in patients on the first and second days, which usually subsides by the third day. The onset is denoted by rigors, chills, and a high fever of 102°F (39°C) or more, in the majority of patients. Fever of this magnitude is rarely seen in viral hepatitis. If the patient has had multiple halothane administrations, the secondary fever tends to occur earlier; that is, the time of appearance of halothane hepatitis is shortened by prior exposure—a feature suggesting a hypersensitivity reaction.

The Latent Period

This is shorter than in viral hepatitis. Infectious hepatitis (hepatitis A virus) has an incubation period of 2 to 6 weeks, and that of serum hepatitis (hepatitis B virus) is 4 to 24 weeks. Patients who develop halothane hepatitis do so usually within the first 15 days. In the individual patient, however, the short latency period typical of halothane hepatitis is not particularly helpful in making the diagnosis, because the patient may be harboring a subclinical viral infection at the time of surgery, which becomes clinically evident in the postoperative period. Therefore, to implicate halothane, a viral cause must be excluded.

Laboratory Data

In halothane hepatitis, laboratory studies reflect the severity of hepatic damage.[118,120] Serum transaminases may be above 2000 IU. Leukocytosis is characteristic, with counts greater than 10,000; eosinophilia may occur in about a quarter of patients. This contrasts with viral hepatitis, wherein leukopenia without eosinophilia is observed. In addition, patients in whom fulminant hepatic failure develops may have circulating antibodies that react with a specific halothane-hepatocyte membrane determinant.[121] Marked prolongation of the prothrombin time is the most important adverse prognostic sign; loss of synthetic liver function indicates extensive hepatic injury.[111]

Epidemiology

A variety of factors may contribute or may simply represent "other causes" of hepatitis. Fasting, malnutrition, and hypoxia may increase the susceptibility to halothane-induced liver injury.[122] Hypoxia per se may induce liver injury, however, unrelated to the production of reductive metabolites of halothane.[123,124] Therefore, liver injuries due to hypoxia from hypoventilation, shock, passive congestion, liver retraction, and compression of liver blood supply by packs and retractors are confounding factors that frequently can not be excluded. No evidence indicates that preexisting acute (other than viral hepatitis) or chronic liver disease, including cirrhosis, is exacerbated by halothane or any of the other inhalation agents.[104]

Physical characteristics appear to play a role.

Age

Patients older than 40 years appear more vulnerable. Hepatitis from other causes is also more common in older people, however. Conversely, children seem relatively resistant.

Gender

Females develop halothane-associated hepatitis more often than males in a ratio of 60:40.[125]

Obesity

The residence of halothane in the body is prolonged in obese patients because of the high lipid solubility of halothane, which increases the duration of exposure and presumably the risk. A study by Walton and colleagues[126] found that 38% of patients with unexplained hepatitis following halothane anesthesia were obese. In addition, enhanced biotransformation of halothane occurs in obese subjects, as demonstrated by increased levels of serum fluoride and bromide, compared with nonobese controls.[127] This may be related to decreased hepatic and respiratory reserves in obese patients, which increase the propensity for reductive metabolism. Again, this implicates hypoxia and reduced hepatic blood flow in the pathogenesis of halothane hepatitis.

Some studies suggest that a genetic susceptibility to halothane-induced hepatotoxicity may exist. Cascorbi and colleagues[128] showed that the rate of metabolism is similar in identical twins but different in fraternal twins. HLA typing has demonstrated a genetic susceptibility to halothane hepatitis,[129] which has also been reported in Hispanic first-degree relatives.[125] In addition, a constitutional susceptibility factor has been proposed on the basis of an in vitro lymphocyte cytotoxicity test.[130] Lymphocytes from patients presumed to have halothane hepatitis showed an eightfold increase in cytotoxicity from metabolites of phenytoin. Family members of these patients also had cytotoxic responses, whereas healthy controls and patients with other forms of liver disease had a normal response.

Morphologic Features of Halothane Hepatitis

The accumulation of case reports since the first association of halothane with hepatic injury has led to a near consensus regarding the reality of the clinical syndrome, but it has left many unanswered questions, including the role of the surgical procedure and the precise morphologic characteristics of the hepatic injury. The large number of cases available for review at the Armed Forces Institute of Pathology provided Benjamin and colleagues[131] with the opportunity to perform a detailed study of biopsy and autopsy samples and to correlate the findings with clinical histories. Cases were excluded from analysis if the interval between exposure to halothane and onset of symptoms was greater than 15 days, blood products were given within 2 months preceding surgery, HBsAg was detected in blood samples, patients had been exposed to other potentially hepatotoxic drugs, or hypotension occurred before the onset of liver injury.

After exclusion of unsuitable cases, 77 cases remained for analysis. There were 34 nonfatal and 43 fatal cases. Overall, the ratio of females to males was approximately 60:40, and the mean age was about 50 years. Obesity was noted in 46% of cases, and 60% of the nonfatal and 84% of the fatal cases were in patients who had been exposed to halothane. One child was included in the study (a fatal case).

The clinical histories indicated a causal relationship between previous exposure to halothane and the incidence of halothane hepatitis. A new finding of this study was that the severity of injury was also related to the number of exposures, especially when repeated within 3 months. The average interval between the last exposure to halothane and the onset of symptoms was about 5 days, with a range of 1 to 13 days. Aminotransferase levels (aspartate aminotransferase [AST] and ALT), although moderately to markedly elevated, were generally lower than 1000 IU in the survivors and higher than 2000 IU in the fatalities. Total bilirubin levels ranged from about 10 mg/dl in the nonfatal cases to 25 mg/dl in the fatal cases. The type of surgical procedure was unrelated to the severity of liver injury; the frequency of severe hepatic injury was similar whether minor (nonabdominal) surgery or major surgery had been performed.

Samples of liver were obtained by biopsy from the nonfatal cases and by autopsy from the fatal cases. The opportunity to examine tissue from nonfatal cases, as well as from severe, fatal cases, allowed a spectrum of histologic patterns of injury to emerge. Pathologic changes ranged from panlobular spotty necrosis, resembling viral hepatitis, through submassive confluent zonal necrosis to massive necrosis.

Spotty Necrosis (Fig. 38–8)

Biopsies (from nonfatal cases) revealed spotty necrosis alone in about one third of cases. The characteristic finding was panlobular involvement, with multiple foci of hepatocellular injury, variable degrees of fat accumulation, and inflammation consisting predominately of lymphocytes, eosinophils, and plasma cells.

Submassive (Confluent) Necrosis (Fig. 38–9)

A more severe hepatic injury was evident in about two thirds of the biopsy and autopsy cases. In the nonfatal cases, confluent necrosis was preferentially localized to centrilobular areas in the majority of cases, but it involved periportal areas preferentially in one third. In the fatal cases, confluent necrosis always preferentially involved the centrilobular areas. In both cases, hepatocellular degeneration, focal necrosis, and inflammation were scattered throughout the surviving parts of the acini. Mild to moderate fat accumulation was noted in half the cases, and canalicular and intracellular cholestasis was prominent in the majority of cases. Early fibrosis was evident in about a third of cases. The inflammatory response in nonfatal cases was characterized by a striking predominance of eosinophils and neutrophils (Fig. 38-10). In fatal cases, lymphocytes predominated, and although neutrophils were common, eosinophils were usually less conspicuous.

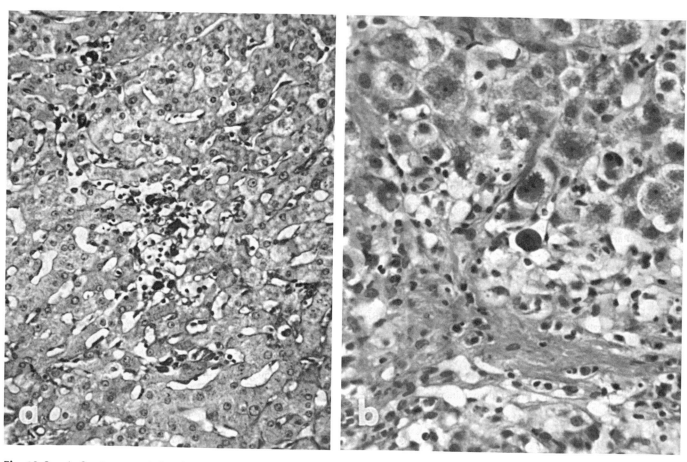

Fig. 38–8.   A. Spotty necrosis in a liver biopsy from a patient who developed elevated serum aminotransferase levels 3 days following halothane anesthesia. The biopsy shows focal hepatocellular necrosis and an inflammatory infiltrate, predominately lymphocytic (160×). B. Spotty necrosis with ballooning and acidophilic degeneration of hepatocytes and a mixed inflammatory infiltrate (250×). From Benjamin, S. B., et al.: The morphologic spectrum of halothane-induced hepatic injury: analysis of 77 cases. Hepatology 5:1163, 1985 and the Armed Forces Institute of Pathology.

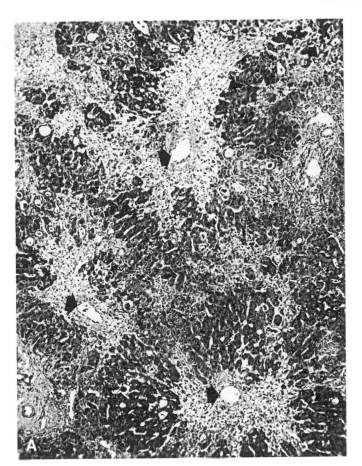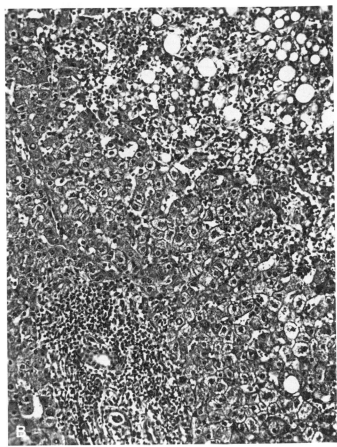

Fig. 38–9. A. Biopsy specimen from a patient with multiple exposures to halothane over a 4-week period, demonstrating submassive centrilobular necrosis. Arrows indicate central veins (60×). B. Submassive centrilobular necrosis with hepatocellular fat accumulation limited to the area of necrosis (160×). From Benjamin, S. B., et al.: The morphologic spectrum of halothane-induced hepatic injury: analysis of 77 cases. Hepatology 5:1163, 1985 and the Armed Forces Institute of Pathology.

Massive Necrosis (Fatal Cases) (Fig. 38–11)

Livers from one third of the fatal cases had all or nearly all the hepatocytes destroyed. Necrosis involved all parts of the acini. Lymphocytes predominated, with a variable admixture of neutrophils and eosinophils.

Previous reports described anecdotal observations from cases with a fatal outcome. The study by Benjamin and colleagues[131] demonstrates that halothane can produce diverse patterns of injury, ranging from focal necrosis to complete hepatocyte destruction. Moreover, it demonstrates the relationship of prior halothane exposure to both the incidence and severity of the injury. Indeed, prior exposure seemed more important than the extensiveness of the surgical procedure; severe hepatic injury was seen even after minor surgery, in which trauma to the liver, altered hepatic blood flow, or inadequate oxygenation most probably did not occur.

The precise pathologic mechanisms involved remain obscure. More than one mechanism is likely involved in the severe form of halothane-induced injury, however. The patterns of injury observed by Benjamin and colleagues[131] show both direct cytotoxic effects and the characteristics of a hypersensitivity reaction. The histologic picture of zonal centrilobular necrosis with varying amounts of fat accumulation is evident in the more severe cases (fatal and nonfatal) and is reminiscent of lesions caused by intrinsic toxins, such as chloroform. On the other hand, diffuse, spotty necrosis and infiltrates of eosinophils were common findings in the less severe cases (nonfatal), both of which are features of idiosyncratic drug toxicity, suggesting an immunologic mechanism. The high incidence of previous halothane exposures in fatal and nonfatal cases would appear to support an immunologic mechanism in both.

Halothane Hepatitis in Children

Halothane is a widely used and safe inhalation agent in children. Liver injury has been reported in children under 2 years of age following halothane administration, however. The risk of hepatitis is extremely low, probably less than 1 per 100,000 halothane administrations.[132,133] Usually, patients have a history of multiple exposures within a relatively short time. For example, Whitburn and Sumner[134] reported the occurrence of hepatitis in an 11-month-old infant after 7 exposures. The infant had postoperative pyrexia and developed jaundice, and studies demonstrated specific antibodies against the surface of halothane-altered rabbit hepatocytes. Kenna and col-

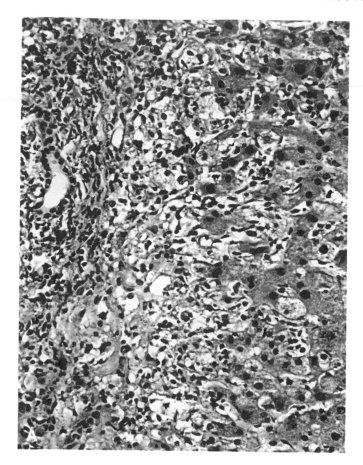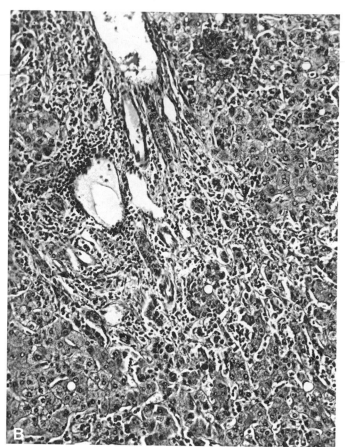

Fig. 38–10. A. Submassive confluent necrosis of zone 1. The portal area (left side of photograph) is surrounded by a zone of hepatocellular necrosis and dropout with a mixed cellular infiltrate of eosinophils, neutrophil, plasma cells, and lymphocytes (× 250, Armed Forces Institute of Pathology negative 83-7860). B. Submassive necrosis of zone 1 with periportal inflammatory infiltrates simulating piecemeal necrosis (×250, Armed Forces Institute of Pathology negative 83-8046). From Benjamin, S. B., et al.: The morphologic spectrum of halothane-induced hepatic injury: analysis of 77 cases. Hepatology 5:1163, 1985 and the Armed Forces Institute of Pathology.

leagues[135] reported 7 children with halothane hepatitis, confirmed by serologic tests for antibodies. Detection of antibodies specific for halothane using an enzyme-linked immunosorbent assay may be useful in establishing the diagnosis in children.[136]

As in adults, mild degrees of hepatitic dysfunction, without jaundice, may occur, but at a substantially lower frequency than in adults. In a prospective study of liver function in children having two halothane anesthetic administrations within 28 days, minor elevations of AST occurred in 11%, ALT was elevated in 5%, and alkaline phosphatase and τ-glutamyl transferase (GGT) were elevated in 3% of children.[137] This supports the view that mild postoperative liver dysfunction is relatively common in children, but it is of little clinical significance. As in adults, mild elevations of liver enzymes following halothane anesthesia and the severe form of hepatitis associated with fulminant hepatic failure appear to be two separate, unrelated entities.

Metabolites of Halothane and Liver Injury

Theories explaining the pathogenesis of halothane-induced liver injury must account for both types of hepatitis seen after halothane exposure: the relatively common, mild form causing a slight elevation of hepatic enzymes, and the rare, severe form of hepatitis physicians usually associate with halothane.[19] Metabolites of halothane play key roles in the pathogenesis of both types of injury. (See also the section of this chapter on biotransformation.)

Mild Liver Dysfunction with Low Mortality (Fig. 38–12)

Under hypoxic conditions, halothane is reduced to reactive metabolites, such as the 2-chloro-1,1,1-trifluorethane free radical, which can react with hepatocyte macromolecules and membrane lipids.[16,138,139] Associated stresses, such as fasting, pretreatment with enzyme-inducing drugs, and hypoxia markedly enhance the formation of reductive metabolites and may increase the incidence or severity of hepatic injury.[122] Therefore, the mild form of hepatic injury associated with halothane exposure may involve direct cytotoxic effects of reductive metabolites of halothane. The end result appears to be a metabolic or biochemical derangement, which is usually of little clinical significance.

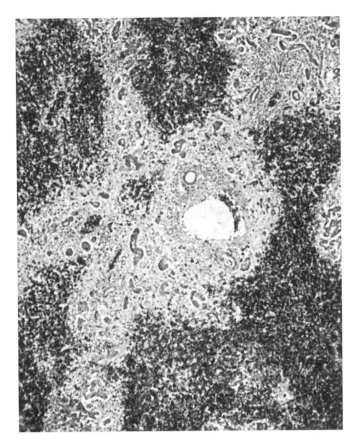

Fig. 38–11. Massive hepatic necrosis with dropout of all hepatocytes and extravasation of blood in areas of collapse (60×). From Benjamin, S. B., et al.: The morphologic spectrum of halothane-induced hepatic injury: analysis of 77 cases. Hepatology 5:1163, 1985 and the Armed Forces Institute of Pathology.

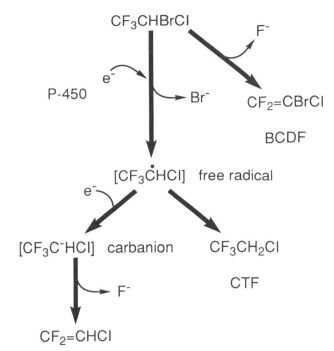

Fig. 38–12. Reductive metabolism of halothane. Hypoxic conditions favor reductive metabolism of halothane. One or two electron reduction, mediated by cytochrome P-450, may occur. Molecular oxygen is not required and inhibits the enzymatic process. The direct precursor of 2-chloro-1,1,1-trifluoroethane (CTF) appears to be the chlorotrifluorothane free radical, which may react with hepatocyte proteins and membrane lipids, causing cellular injury. Additional metabolites include 2-chloro-1,1-difluoroethylene (CDF), also generated from the free radical with a carbanion intermediate, and 2-bromo-2-chloro-1,1-difluoroethylene (BCDF), which was first detected in closed-circle breathing systems in the presence of soda lime. Modified from Ahr, H.J., King, L.J., Nastainczyk, W., Ullrich, V.: The mechanism of reductive dehalogenation of halothane by liver cytochrome P450. Biochem Pharmacol 31:383, 1982.

Severe Hepatitis with High Mortality (Fig. 38–13)[140]

Serum antibodies to the trifluoroacetyl moiety, an oxidative metabolite of halothane, have been identified in patients with hepatic failure after halothane anesthesia.[18,141,142] Immunofluorescence demonstrates granular deposits of immunoglobulin on surface membranes of hepatocytes, which are specific for halothane.[121] No such antibodies have been found on liver cells exposed to the other anesthetics, nor have been found in patients with toxic or viral liver injuries. More recently, a neoantigen recognized by antibodies from the sera of patients with halothane hepatitis has been isolated from microsomal fractions of halothane-treated rats.[143] The altered cellular component appears to be a trifluoroacetylated endoplasmic reticulum carboxylesterase. These studies provide fairly strong circumstantial evidence that an immunologic mechanism plays a role in the pathogenesis of halothane hepatitis. In this scenario, metabolites covalently bind to cell proteins and act as haptens, invoking an immunologic response that causes progressive and often fatal hepatotoxicity. Finally, centrilobular necrosis is a typical pathologic alteration seen in severe cases of halothane hepatitis. This type of lesion is characteristic of classic hepatotoxic agents, such as chloroform. Therefore, a direct cytotoxic effect of oxidative metabolites of halothane may also be involved in the pathogenesis of halothane hepatitis.

Synopsis: The Pathogenesis of Halothane Hepatitis

Two types of hepatic injury appear to occur following halothane anesthesia. The rather common, mild form of hepatitis appears to result from a direct cytotoxic mechanism, involving reductive metabolites of halothane, and is accentuated by liver hypoxia, such as can occur with hypovolemia and surgical stress. Fortunately, this form of halothane-associated hepatitis is usually of little or no clinical significance.

On the other hand, the more severe form of hepatitis, which physicians usually associate with the term "halothane hepatitis," is fortunately rare, but often fatal. The pathologic features of severe cases are indistinguishable from those seen in fulminant viral hepatitis. In less severe cases, pathologic alterations include spotty, panlobular necrosis and a prominent leukocytic infiltrate,

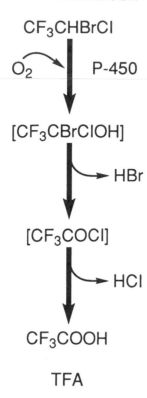

TFA

Fig. 38–13. Oxidative metabolism of halothane. In the presence of molecular oxygen, halothane is metabolized to trifluoroacetic acid (TFA). Several reactive intermediates are generated in the process that can acylate liver proteins. It is suggested that these TFA-altered proteins can act as haptens, capable of inducing an immunologic response. Modified from Sipes, I. G., et al.: Comparison of the biotransformation and hepatotoxicity of halothane and deuterated halothane. J Pharmacol Exp Ther *214:*716, 1980.

typically consisting of lymphocytes and eosinophils. Thus, the histologic picture is consistent with an immunologic mechanism of injury. Liver injury with viral hepatitis is also probably immunologically mediated, because hepatitis viruses do not appear to be directly cytopathic. The most compelling evidence for an immunologic mechanism in halothane hepatitis is the association of prior exposure to halothane, however, which increases the incidence and severity of hepatic injury. Moreover, the clinical presentation is often suggestive of a hypersensitivity reaction, with fever, arthralgias, and eosinophilia. The identification of antibodies from patients with fulminant halothane hepatitis, specific for halothane-modified determinants on hepatocytes, provides additional evidence for an immunologic mechanism. The identification of covalently bound trifluoroacetic acid moieties, which may act as haptens capable of invoking an immunologic response, suggests that oxidative metabolism of halothane plays a key role in the pathogenesis of severe halothane hepatitis. The precise immunologic mechanisms that result in cell injury are unclear at present, however; both cell-mediated and humoral mechanisms may be involved.[144,145] The possibility also exists that the immunologic response represents an epiphenomenon, with antigenic responses occurring secondarily to cell injury. Indeed, a direct cytotoxic mechanism may also be involved; centrilobular necrosis with steatosis, a typical form of injury caused by direct hepatotoxins is another frequent pathologic feature of halothane hepatitis. Both immunologic and direct cytotoxic mechanisms appear to be involved. At present, the precise pathogenesis of halothane hepatitis remains unclear. Better animal models will eventually clarify the picture.[144]

Finally, the newer volatile agents, such as enflurane, have been associated with postoperative hepatitis. Although the incidence of hepatitis associated with enflurane is extremely rare, in the range of 1 in 800,000 anesthetic administrations, potential hepatotoxicity cannot be excluded.[146,147] Again, a hypersensitivity reaction may occur, involving the covalent binding of oxidative metabolites to liver microsomal proteins.[148] Fortunately, available evidence indicates that isoflurane is unlikely to cause postoperative hepatitis.[149] Additional clinical experience will be required to evaluate the newest of the volatile agents, desflurane and sevoflurane.

RECOMMENDATIONS FOR USE OF HALOTHANE

Halothane has largely been replaced by other anesthetics in the United States, because of concerns about toxicity. It is still widely used with pediatric patients, however, because it is less irritating to the upper airways and allows smooth and "atraumatic" inhalation inductions. Indeed, halothane is still widely used in other countries for patients of all ages. Based on the available evidence, certain recommendations can be made regarding the use of halothane:

1. Do not administer halothane if a patient had experienced an undiagnosed hepatic reaction following a previous exposure to the agent; a more conservative approach would be to avoid halothane in all patients previously exposed.
2. Halothane should probably be avoided in obese patients.
3. Although no evidence indicates that halothane increases the risk of liver damage in patients with preexisting liver disease (except viral hepatitis), postoperative hepatic dysfunction will undoubtedly raise the issue of halothane hepatitis; because other anesthetics are readily available, halothane should not be used in these patients.
4. Halothane still appears to be a safe anesthetic for pediatric patients; however, prudence dictates using another anesthetic when a patient had experienced an undiagnosed hepatic reaction following a previous halothane exposure.

REFERENCES

1. Suckling, C. W.: Some chemical and physical factors in the development of Fluothane. Br J Anaesth *29:*466, 1957.
2. Raventos, J.: The action of Fluothane: a new volatile anaesthetic. Br J Pharmacol *11:*394, 1956.
3. Leonard, P. F.: The lower limits of flammability of halothane, enflurane, and isoflurane. Anesth Analg *54:*238, 1975.

4. Gregory, G. A., Eger, E. I., II, Munson, E. S.: The relationship between age and halothane requirements in man. Anesthesiology 30:489, 1969.

5. Lerman, J., Robinson, S., Willis, M. M., Gregory, G. A.: Anesthetic requirement for halothane in young children 0–1 months and 1–6 months of age. Anesthesiology 59:421, 1983.

6. Robson, J. G., Gillies, D. M., Cullen, W. G., Griffith, H. R.: Fluothane (halothane) in closed circuit anesthesia. Anesthesiology 20:251, 1959.

7. Eger, E. I., II (ed.): MAC, Anesthetic Uptake and Action. Baltimore, Williams & Wilkins, 1974.

8. Stoelting, R. K., Eger, E. I.: The effects of ventilation and anesthetic solubility on recovery from anesthesia: an in vivo analog analysis before and after equilibration. Anesthesiology 30:290, 1969.

9. Van Dyke, R. A., Chenowith, M. B., Larsen, E. R.: Synthesis and metabolism of halothane $1-^{14}C$. Nature 204:471, 1964.

10. Rehder, K., et al.: Halothane biotransformation in man: a quantitative study. Anesthesiology 28:711, 1967.

11. Carpenter, R. L., et al.: The extent of metabolism of inhaled anesthetics in humans. Anesthesiology 65:201, 1986.

12. Saki, T., Tabaori, M.: Biodegradation of halothane, enflurane, and methoxyflurane. Br J Anaesth 50:785, 1978.

13. Stier, A.: Trifluoroacetic acid as metabolite of halothane. Biochem Pharmacol 13:1544, 1964.

14. Cascorbi, H. F., Blake, D. A., Helrich, M.: Differences in biotransformation of halothane in man. Anesthesiology 32:119, 1970.

15. Stier, A., et al.: Urinary excretion of bromide in halothane anesthesia. Anesth Analg 43:723, 1964.

16. Sharp, J. H., Trudell, J. R., Cohen, E. N.: Volatile metabolites and decomposition products of halothane in man. Anesthesiology 50:2, 1979.

17. Cohen, E. N., Trudell, J. R., Edmunds, H. N., Watson, E.: Urinary metabolites of halothane in man. Anesthesiology 43:392, 1975.

18. Callis, A. H., et al.: Evidence for the role of the immune system in the pathogenesis of halothane hepatitis. In Roth, S. H., Miller, K. W. (eds.): Molecular and Cellular Mechanisms of Anesthesia. New York, Plenum Publishing, 1986.

19. Brown, B. R., Jr.: Hepatotoxicity of inhalation anesthetics. In Anesthesia in Hepatic and Biliary Tract Disease. Philadelphia, F.A. Davis, 1988, p. 93.

20. Plummer, J. L., Van Der Walt, J. H., Cousins, M. J.: Reductive metabolism of halothane in children. Anaesth Intensive Care 12:293, 1984.

21. Gourlay, G. K., Adams, J. F., Cousins, M. J., Sharp, J. H.: Time-course of formation of volatile reductive metabolites of halothane in humans and in an animal model. Br J Anaesth 52:331, 1980.

22. Plummer, J. L., Steven, I. M., Cousins, M. J.: Metabolism of halothane in children having repeated halothane anaesthetics. Anaesth Intensive Care 15:136, 1987.

23. Nimmo, W. S., Thompson, P. G., Prescott, L. F.: Microsomal enzyme induction after halothane anaesthesia. Br J Clin Pharmacol 12:433, 1981.

24. Johnstone, R. E., et al.: Increased serum bromide concentration after halothane anesthesia in man. Anesthesiology 42:598, 1975.

25. Tinker, J. H., Gandolfi, A. J., Van Dyke, R. A.: Elevation of plasma bromide levels in patients following halothane anesthesia: time correlation with total halothane dosage. Anesthesiology 44:194, 1976.

26. Duvaldestin, P., et al.: Halothane biotransformation in anesthetists. Anesthesiology 51:41, 1979.

27. Theye, R. A.: The contributions of individual organ systems to the decrease in whole-body VO_2 with halothane. Anesthesiology 37:367, 1972.

28. Eger, E. I., et al.: Cardiovascular effects of halothane in man. Anesthesiology 32:396, 1970.

29. Gain, E. A., Paletz, S. G.: An attempt to correlate the clinical signs of Fluothane anaesthesia with the electroencephalographic levels. Can Anaesth Soc J 4:289, 1957.

30. Adams, R. W., et al.: Isoflurane and cerebrospinal fluid pressure in neurosurgical patients. Anesthesiology 54:97, 1981.

31. Eger, E. I.: Isoflurane: a review. Anesthesiology 55:559, 1981.

32. Murphy, F. L., Kennell, E. M., Johnstone, R. E.: The effects of enflurane, isoflurane and halothane on cerebral blood flow and metabolism in man. Anesthesiology 42:A61, 1974.

33. Eintei, C., Leszniewski, W., Carlsson, C.: Local application of ^{133}xenon for measurement of regional cerebral blood flow (rCBF) during halothane, enflurane, and isoflurane anesthesia in humans. Anesthesiology 63:391, 1985.

34. Albrecht, R. F., Miletich, D. J., Madala, L. R.: Normalization of cerebral blood flow during prolonged halothane anesthesia. Anesthesiology 58:26, 1983.

35. Miletich, D. J., et al.: Absence of autoregulation of cerebral blood flow during halothane and enflurane anesthesia. Anesth Analg 55:100, 1976.

36. Smith, A. L., Wollman, H.: Cerebral blood flow and metabolism: effects of anesthetic drugs and techniques. Anesthesiology 36:378, 1972.

37. Scheller, M. S., Todd, M. M., Drummond, J. C.: Isoflurane, halothane, and regional cerebral blood flow at various levels of $PaCO_2$ in rabbits. Anesthesiology 64:598, 1986.

38. Dundee, J. W., Dripps, R. D.: Effects of diethylether, trichloroethylene, and trifluoroethylvinyl ether on respiration. Anesthesiology 18:282, 1957.

39. Euler, C. Von: The functional organization of the respiratory phase-switching mechanisms. Fed Proc 36:2375, 1977.

40. Nishino, T., Honda, Y.: Changes in the respiratory pattern induced by halothane in the cat. Br J Anaesth 52:1191, 1980.

41. Tenney, S. M., Ou, L. C.: Ventilatory response of decorticate and decerebrate cats to hypoxia and CO_2. Respir Physiol 29:81, 1977.

42. Froese, A. B., Bryan, A. C.: Effects of anesthesia and paralysis on diaphragmatic mechanics in man. Anesthesiology 41:242, 1974.

43. Muller, N., et al.: Diaphragmatic muscle tone. J Appl Physiol 47:279, 1979.

44. Tusiewicz, K., Bryan, A. C., Froese, A. B.: Contributions of changing rib cage-diaphragm interactions to the ventilatory depression of halothane anesthesia. Anesthesiology 47:327, 1977.

45. Hickey, R. F., et al.: Effects of halothane anesthesia on functional residual capacity and alveolar-arterial oxygen tension difference. Anesthesiology 38:20, 1973.

46. Tokics, L., et al.: Computerized tomography of the chest and gas exchange measurements during ketamine anaesthesia. Acta Anaesthesiol Scand 31:684, 1987.

47. Roussos, C. S., Fukuchi, Y., Macklem, P. T., Engel, L. A.: Influence of diaphragmatic contraction on ventilation distribution in horizontal man. J Appl Physiol 40:417, 1976.

48. France, C. J., et al.: Ventilatory effects of isoflurane (Forane) or halothane when combined with morphine, nitrous oxide and surgery. Br J Anaesth 46:117, 1974.

49. Knill, R. L., Gelb, A. W.: Ventilatory responses to hypoxia

and hypercapnia during halothane sedation and anesthesia in man. Anesthesiology 49:244, 1978.

50. Reynolds, A. K., Chiz, J. F., Pasquet, A. F.: Halothane and methoxyflurane: a comparison of their effects on cardiac pacemaker fibers. Anesthesiology 33:602, 1970.

51. Atlee, J. L., Rusy, B. F.: Atrioventricular conduction times and atrioventricular nodal conductivity during enflurane anesthesia in dogs. Anesthesiology 47:498, 1977.

52. Katz, R. L., Matteo, R. S., Papper, E. M.: The injection of epinephrine during anesthesia with halogenated hydrocarbons and cyclopropane in man: 2. Halothane. Anesthesiology 23:597, 1962.

53. Zink, J., Sasyniuk, B., Dresel, P. E.: Halothane-epinephrine induced cardiac arrhythmias and the role of heart rate. Anesthesiology 43:548, 1975.

54. Miletich, D. J., Albrecht, R. F., Seals, C.: Responses to fasting and lipid infusion of epinephrine-induced arrhythmias during halothane anesthesia. Anesthesiology 48:245, 1978.

55. Pace, N. L., Ohmura, A., Wong, K. C.: Epinephrine induced arrhythmias: effect of exogenous prostaglandins and prostaglandin synthesis inhibition during halothane-O_2 anesthesia in the dog. Anesth Analg 58:401, 1979.

56. Schick, L. M., Chapin, J. C., Munson, E. S., Kushins, L. G.: Pancuronium, d-tubocurarine, and epinephrine-induced arrhythmias during halothane anesthesia in dogs. Anesthesiology 52:207, 1980.

57. Chapin, J. C., Kushins, L. G., Munson, E. S., Schick, L. M.: Lidocaine, bupivicaine, etidocaine, and epinephrine-induced arrhythmias during halothane anesthesia in dogs. Anesthesiology 52:23, 1980.

58. Johnston, R. R., Eger, E. I., Wilson, C.: A comparative interaction of epinephrine with enflurane, isoflurane and halothane in man. Anesth Analg 55:709, 1976.

59. Atlee, J. L., Malinson, C. F.: Thiopental potentiation of epinephrine sensitization with halothane. Anesthesiology 53:S133, 1980.

60. Liu, W. S., Wong, K. C., Port, J. D., Andriano, K. P.: Epinephrine-induced arrhythmias during halothane anesthesia with the addition of nitrous oxide, nitrogen or helium in dogs. Anesth Analg 61:414, 1982.

61. Karl, H. W., Swedlow, D. B., Lee, K. W., Downs, J. J.: Epinephrine-halothane interactions in children. Anesthesiology 58:142, 1983.

62. Smith, E. R., Dresel, P. E.: Site of origin of halothane-epinephrine arrhythmia determined by direct and echocardiographic recordings. Anesthesiology 57:98, 1982.

63. Maze, M., Hayward, E., Jr., Gaba, D. M.: Alpha$_1$-adrenergic blockade raises epinephrine-arrhythmia threshold in halothane-anesthetized dogs in a dose-dependent fashion. Anesthesiology 63:611, 1985.

64. Bertolo, L., Novakovic, L., Penna, M.: Anti-arrhythmic effects of droperidol. Anesthesiology 37:529, 1972.

65. Price, H. L., Skovshrd, P., Panca, A. L., Cooperman, L. H.: Evidence for B-receptor activation produced by halothane in man. Anesthesiology 32:329, 1970.

66. Etsten, B. E., Shimosato, S.: Myocardial contractility: performance of the heart during anesthesia. Clin Anesth 3:56, 1964.

67. Denlinger, J. K., Kaplan, J. A., Lecky, J. H., Wollman, H.: Cardiovascular responses to calcium administered intravenously to man during halothane anesthesia. Anesthesiology 42:390, 1975.

68. Vatner, S. F., Smith, N. T.: Effects of halothane on left ventricular function and distribution of regional blood flow in dogs and primates. Circ Res 34:155, 1974.

69. Friesen, R. H., Lichtor, J. L.: Cardiovascular depression during halothane anesthesia in infants: a study of three induction techniques. Anesth Analg 61:42, 1982.

70. Mazze, R. I., Schwartz, F. D., Slocum, H. C., Barry, K. G.: Renal function during anesthesia and surgery. I. The effects of halothane anesthesia. Anesthesiology 24:279, 1963.

71. Bastron, R. D., Perkins, F. M., Pyne, J. L.: Autoregulation of renal blood flow during halothane anesthesia. Anesthesiology 46:142, 1977.

72. Miller, T. R., Stoelting, R. K., Rhamy, R. K.: A comparison of effects on renal tubular function of halothane-oxygen vs. halothane-nitrous oxide-oxygen. Anesth Analg 45:41, 1966.

73. Little, D. M., Barbour, C. M., Given, J. B.: Effects of Fluothane, cyclopropane and ether anesthesia on liver function. Surg Gynecol Obstet 107:712, 1958.

74. Collins, W. F., Fabian, L. W.: Transaminase studies following anesthesia. South Med J 57:555, 1964.

75. Henderson, J. C., Gordon, R. A.: The incidence of postoperative jaundice with special reference to halothane. Can Anaesth Soc J 11:453, 1964.

76. Morris, W. L., Feldman, S. A.: Influence of hypercarbia and hypotension upon liver damage following halothane anaesthesia. Anaesthesia 18:32, 1963.

77. Burnap, T. K., Galla, S. J., Vandam, L. D.: Anesthetic, circulatory and respiratory effects of Fluothane. Anesthesiology 19:307, 1958.

78. Bunker, J. P., Blumenfeld, C. M.: Liver necrosis after halothane anesthesia. Cause or coincidence? N Engl J Med 268:531, 1963.

79. Brody, G. L., Sweet, R. B.: Halothane anesthesia as a possible cause of massive hepatic necrosis. Anesthesiology 24:29, 1963.

80. Summary of the National Halothane Study. JAMA 197:775, 1966.

81. Epstein, R. M., et al.: Splanchnic circulation during halothane anesthesia and hypercapnia in normal man. Anesthesiology 27:654, 1966.

82. Tokics, L., Brismar, B., Hedenstierna, G.: Splanchnic blood flow during halothane-relaxant anaesthesia in elderly patients. Acta Anaesthesiol Scand 30:556, 1986.

83. Price, H. L., et al.: Can general anesthetics produce splanchnic visceral hypoxia by reducing regional blood flow? Anesthesiology 27:24, 1966.

84. Marshall, F. N., Pittinger, C. B., Long, J.: Effects of halothane on GI motility. Anesthesiology 22:363, 1961.

85. Gissen, A. J., Karis, J. H., Natsuk, W. L.: Effect of halothane on neuromuscular transmission. JAMA 197:110, 1966.

86. Waud, B. E., Waud, D. R.: Effects of volatile anesthetics on directly and indirectly stimulated skeletal muscle. Anesthesiology 50:103, 1979.

87. Waud, B. E., Waud, D. R.: The effects of diethyl ether, enflurane and isoflurane at the neuromuscular junction. Anesthesiology 42:275, 1975.

88. Stanski, D. R., Ham, J., Miller, R. D., Sheiner, L. B.: Pharmacokinetics and pharmacodynamics of d-tubocurarine during nitrous oxide-narcotic and halothane anesthesia in man. Anesthesiology 51:235, 1979.

89. Smith, C. E., Donati, F., Bevan, D. R.: Potency of succinylcholine at the diaphragm and at the adductor pollicis muscle. Anesth Analg 67:625, 1988.

90. Smith, C. E., Donati, F., Bevan, D. R.: Dose-response curves for succinylcholine: single *versus* cumulative techniques. Anesthesiology 69:338, 1988.

91. Larach, M. G.: Standardization of the caffeine halothane muscle contracture test. Anesth Analg 69:511, 1989.

92. Larach, M. G.: Should we use muscle biopsy to diagnose malignant hyperthermia susceptibility? (Editorial.) Anesthesiology 79:1, 1993.

93. de Jong, R. H., Robles, R., Moikawa, K. T.: Actions of halothane and nitrous oxide on dorsal horn neurons. Anesthesiology *31*:205, 1969.

94. Bosnjak, Z. J., et al.: The effects of halothane on sympathetic ganglionic transmission. Anesthesiology *57*:473, 1982.

95. Klide, A. M., Penna, M., Aurade, D. M.: Stimulation of adrenergic beta-receptors by halothane and its antagonism. Anesth Analg *48*:58, 1969.

96. Merin, R. G., Samuelson, P. N., Schalch, D. S.: Major inhalation anesthetics and carbohydrate metabolism. Anesth Analg *50*:625, 1971.

97. Hall, G. M., et al.: Substrate mobilization during surgery. Anaesthesia *33*:924, 1978.

98. Galla, S. J., Wilson, E. P.: Hexose metabolism during halothane anesthesia in dogs. Anesthesiology *25*:96, 1964.

99. Lowenstein, E., Clark, J. D., Villareal, Y.: Excess lactate production during halothane anesthesia in man. JAMA *190*:110, 1964.

100. Oyama, T., Aoki, N., Kudo, T.: Effect of halothane anesthesia and surgery on plasma testosterone levels in man. Anesth Analg *51*:130, 1972.

101. Storms, L. H., Stark, A. M., Calverley, R. K., Smith, N. T.: Psychologic functioning after halothane or enflurane anesthesia. Anesth Analg *59*:245, 1980.

102. Koff, R. S., Galambos, J. T.: Viral hepatitis. *In* Schiff, L., Schiff, E. R. (eds.). Diseases of the Liver, 6th Ed. Philadelphia, J.B. Lippincott, 1987, p. 457.

103. O'Brien, M. J., Gottlieb, L.: The liver and biliary tract. *In* Robbins, S. R., Cotran, R. S. (eds.). Pathologic Basis of Disease, 2nd Ed. Philadelphia, W.B. Saunders, 1979, p. 1009.

104. Brown, B. R., Jr.: Hepatitis. *In* Anesthesia in Hepatic and Biliary Tract Disease. Philadelphia, F.A. Davis, 1988, p. 183.

105. Trey, C., et al.: Fulminant hepatic failure: presumable contribution of halothane. N Engl J Med *279*:798, 1968.

106. Klatskin, G.: Toxic and drug-induced hepatitis. *In* Schiff, L. (ed.). Diseases of the Liver, 4th Ed. Philadelphia, J.B. Lippincott, 1975, p. 604.

107. Sagai, M., Tappel, A. L.: Lipid peroxidation induced by some halomethanes as measured by *in vivo* pentane production in the rat. Toxicol Appl Pharmacol *49*:283, 1979.

108. Pohl, L. R., Martin, J. L., George, J. W.: Mechanism of metabolic activation of chloroform by rat liver microsomes. Biochem Pharmacol *29*:3271, 1980.

109. Insel, P. A.: Analgesic-antipyretics and antiinflammatory agents: drugs employed in the treatment of rheumatoid arthritis and gout. *In* Gilman, A. G. (ed.). The Pharmacologic Basis of Therapeutics, 8th Ed. New York, McGraw-Hill, 1990, p. 657.

110. Dienstag, J. L., Wands, J. R., Koff, R. S.: Acute hepatitis. *In* Braunwald, E., et al (eds.). Harrison's Principles of Internal Medicine, 11th Ed. New York, McGraw-Hill, 1987, p. 1325.

111. Zimmerman, H. J., Maddrey, W. C.: Toxic and drug-induced hepatitis. *In* Schiff, L., Schiff, E. R. (eds.). Diseases of the Liver, 6th Ed. Philadelphia, J.B. Lippincott, 1987, p. 591.

112. Inman, W. H. W., Mushin, W. W.: Jaundice after repeated exposure to halothane: a further analysis of reports to the Committee on Safety in Medicine. Br Med J *2*:1455, 1978.

113. Bottinger, L. E., Dalen, E., Hallen, B.: Halothane-induced liver damage: an analysis of the material reported to the Swedish Adverse Drug Reaction Committee 1966–1973. Acta Anaesthesiol Scand *20*:40, 1976.

114. Trowell, J., Peto, R., Crampton-Smith, A.: Controlled trial of repeated halothane anaesthetics in patients with carcinoma of the uterine cervix treated with radium. Lancet *1*:821, 1975.

115. Wright, R., et al.: Controlled prospective study of the effect on liver function of multiple exposures to halothane. Lancet *1*:817, 1975.

116. Klatskin, G., Kimbert, D. V.: Recurrent hepatitis attributable to halothane sensitization in an anesthetist. N Engl J Med *280*:515, 1969.

117. Cousins, M. J., et al.: A randomized prospective controlled study of the metabolism and hepatotoxicity of halothane in humans. Anesth Analg *66*:299, 1987.

118. Moult, P. J. A., Sherlock, S.: Halothane-related hepatitis: a clinical study of twenty six cases. Q J Med *44*:99, 1975.

119. Fee, J. P. H., et al.: A prospective study of liver enzyme and other changes following repeat administration of halothane and enflurane. Br J Anaesth *51*:1133, 1979.

120. Carney, F. M. I., Van Dyke, R. A.: Halothane hepatitis: a critical review. Anesth Analg *51*:135, 1972.

121. Vergani, D., et al.: Antibodies to the surface of halothane-altered rabbit hepatocytes in patients with severe halothane-associated hepatitis. N Engl J Med *303*:66, 1980.

122. Van Dyke, R. A.: Hepatic centrilobular necrosis in rats after exposure to halothane, enflurane, or isoflurane. Anesth Analg *61*:812, 1982.

123. Shingu, K., Eger, E. I., Johnson, B. H.: Hypoxia per se can produce hepatic damage without death in rats. Anesth Analg *61*:820, 1982.

124. Shingu, K., Eger, E. I., Johnson, B. H.: Hypoxia may be more important than reductive metabolism in halothane-induced hepatic injury. Anesth Analg *61*:824, 1982.

125. Hoft, R. H., Bunker, J. P., Goodman, H. I., Gregory, P.B.: Halothane hepatitis in three pairs of closely related women. N Engl J Med *304*:1023, 1981.

126. Walton, B., et al.: Unexplained hepatitis following halothane. Br Med J *1*:1171, 1976.

127. Bentley, J. B., Vaughan, R. W., Gandolfi, A. J., Cork, R. C.: Halothane biotransformation in obese and nonobese patients. Anesthesiology *57*:94, 1982.

128. Cascorbi, H. F., Vessell, E. S., Blake, D. A., Helrich, M.: Halothane biotransformation in man. Ann NY Acad Sci *179*:244, 1971.

129. Otsuka, S., et al.: HLA antigens in patients with unexplained hepatitis following halothane anesthesia. Acta Anaesthesiol Scand *29*:497, 1985.

130. Farrell, G., Prendergast, D., Murray, M.: Halothane hepatitis: detection of a constitutional susceptibility factor. N Engl J Med *313*:1310, 1985.

131. Benjamin, S. B., et al.: The morphologic spectrum of halothane-induced hepatic injury: analysis of 77 cases. Hepatology *5*:1163, 1985.

132. Wark, H. J.: Postoperative jaundice in children: the influence of halothane. Anaesthesia *38*:372, 1983.

133. Warner, L. O., Beach, T. P., Garvin, J. P., Warner, E. J.: Halothane and children: the first quarter century. Anesth Analg *63*:838, 1984.

134. Whitburn, R. H., Sumner, E.: Halothane hepatitis in an 11-month old child. Anaesthesia *41*:611, 1986.

135. Kenna, J. G., et al.: Halothane hepatitis in children. Br Med J *294*:1209, 1987.

136. Hals, J., Dodgson, M. S., Skulberg, A., Kenna, J. G.: Halothane-associated liver damage and renal failure in a young child. Acta Anaesthesiol Scand *30*:651, 1986.

137. Wark, H., O'Halloran, M., Overton, J.: Prospective study of liver function in children following multiple halothane anaesthetic at short intervals. Br J Anaesth *58*:1224, 1986.

138. Gandolfi, A. J., White, R. D., Sipes, I. G., Pohl, L. R.: Bioactivation and covalent binding of halothane *in vitro:* studies with [3H]- and [14C]halothane. J Pharmacol Exp Ther *214:*721, 1980.

139. Ahr, H. J., King, L. J., Nastainczyk, W., Ullrich, V.: The mechanism of reductive dehalogenation of halothane by liver cytochrome P450. Biochem Pharmacol *31:*383, 1982.

140. Sipes, I. G., et al.: Comparison of the biotransformation and hepatotoxicity of halothane and deuterated halothane. J Pharmacol Exp Ther *214:*716, 1980.

141. Hubbard, A. K., Gandolfi, A. J., Brown, B. R., Jr.: Immunological basis of anesthetic-induced hepatotoxicity (editorial). Anesthesiology *69:*814, 1988.

142. Kenna, J. G., Satoh, H., Christ, D. D., Pohl, L. R.: Metabolic basis for a drug hypersensitivity: antibodies in sera from patients with halothane hepatitis recognize liver neoantigens that contain the trifluoracetyl group derived from halothane. J Pharmacol Exp Ther *245:*1103, 1988.

143. Satoh, H., et al.: Human antiendoplasmic reticulum antibodies in sera of patients with halothane-induced hepatitis are directed against a trifluoroacetylated carboxylesterase. Proc Natl Acad Sci USA *86:*322, 1989.

144. Clark, J. B., Lind, R. C., Gandolfi, A. J.: Mechanism of anesthetic hepatotoxicity. Adv Anesth *10:*219, 1993.

145. Ray, D. C., Drummond, G. B.: Halothane hepatitis. Br J Anaesth *67:*84, 1991.

146. Brown, B. R., Jr., Gandolfi, A. J.: Adverse effects of volatile anaesthetics. Br J Anaesth *59:*14, 1987.

147. Elliot, R. H., Strunin, L.: Hepatotoxicity of volatile anaesthetics. Br J Anaesth *70:*339, 1993.

148. Christ, D. D., Satoh, H., Kenna, J. G., Pohl, L. R.: Potential metabolic basis for enflurane hepatitis and the apparent cross-sensitization between enflurane and halothane. Drug Metab Dispos *16:*135, 1988.

149. Stoelting, R. K., Blitt, C. D., Cohen, P. J., Merin, R. G.: Hepatic dysfunction after isoflurane anesthesia. Anesth Analg *66:*147, 1987.

Chapter 39

FLUORINATED ETHER ANESTHETICS

MARK V. BOSWELL
VINCENT J. COLLINS

In the search for nonflammable volatile anesthetics, halogenation is considered essential. Halogenation also affects other properties of anesthetics, however, including stability, potency, and toxicity.[1] Iodinated and brominated compounds tend to be unstable and are subject to degradation, with potentially toxic products. Bromination and chlorination tend to increase the potency of anesthetics, whereas totally fluorinated compounds are devoid of anesthetic activity. Halogenated alkanes are arrhythmogenic, and bilaterally halogenated diethyl ethers tend to cause convulsions and apneustic respirations. Partially fluorinated methyl ethyl ethers (most also containing a chlorine atom) have proved suitable, however, and several have been introduced into clinical practice (Fig. 39-1). They are chemically stable, possess sufficient potency, have minimal toxicity, and are generally devoid of central nervous system (CNS) excitatory effects.

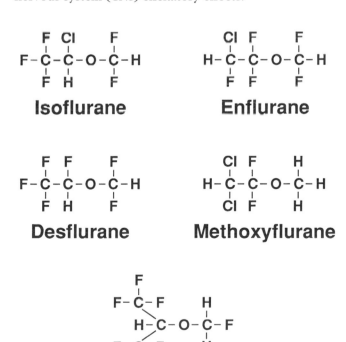

Fig. 39–1. Structures of fluorinated ether anesthetics.

ISOFLURANE

Essential Pharmacology

Isoflurane is currently the most widely used volatile anesthetic in North America, partly because of its excellent safety profile, but also because of the perceived shortcomings of the other volatile agents. Halothane and enflurane remain useful anesthetics and have not been rendered obsolete. Indeed, halothane remains the best agent for inhalation induction available today, although concerns about hepatic toxicity generally limit its use to pediatric patients, at least in the United States. Enflurane also has suitable anesthetic properties, and it is safe and inexpensive. As the various physicochemical and clinical properties of isoflurane are discussed in the following sections, frequent comparisons are made with the other volatile agents.

Properties

Isoflurane (Forane) is a volatile methyl ethyl ether (1-chloro-2,2,2-trifluoroethyl difluoromethyl ether), synthesized by Terrell and colleagues in 1965 (compound 469) and introduced into clinical practice in 1981. Its discovery followed that of its isomer, enflurane, which was easier to synthesize. Physicochemical properties of isoflurane are shown in Table 39-1. Isoflurane is a clear, colorless liquid with a pungent odor. The vapor pressure is similar to that of halothane, but unlike halothane,

Table 39–1. Physicochemical Properties of Isoflurane

Chemical name: 1-chloro-2,2,2-trifluoroethyl difluoromethyl ether	
Structure	$CF_3CHCl\text{-}O\text{-}CHF_2$
Molecular weight	184.5
Specific gravity (25°C)	1.496
Boiling point	48.5°C
Vapor pressure (mm Hg at 20°C)	238
Vapor/liquid (ml at 25°C)	198
Partition coefficients (37°C)	
Oil/gas	90.8
Blood/gas	1.4
Water/gas	0.61
Flammability	None
Chemical stabilizer	None

Ohmeda Pharmaceuticals Division

687

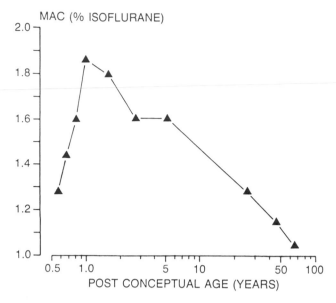

Fig. 39–2. The MAC of isoflurane as related to all ages. Values for post-conceptual age were obtained by adding 40 weeks to the mean post-natal age for each age group. From LeDez, K. M., Lerman, J.: The minimum alveolar concentration (MAC) of isoflurane in preterm neonates. Anesthesiology 67:301, 1987.

it can be irritating to the airway if high concentrations are used initially during mask induction. Isoflurane is nonflammable at concentrations less than 7% (in 70% nitrous oxide and 30% oxygen),[2] it is stable in soda lime, it does not attack metals, and it is not affected by light.

Potency

Isoflurane is an inhalation anesthetic of intermediate potency. The minimum alveolar concentration (MAC) of isoflurane varies with age, as depicted in Figure 39–2[3] and Table 39–2.[4] Although the MAC for 1-year-old patients is about 1.9, the agent is considerably more potent in younger and older patients. The MAC of isoflurane for patients 30 to 55 years old is 1.15. As with the other volatile agents, anesthetic effects of nitrous oxide are generally additive with isoflurane; 70% nitrous oxide reduces its MAC by about 60% for all age groups. The MAC of isoflurane does not appear to be significantly affected by gender, although pregnancy may reduce MAC by 40%.[5]

Table 39–2. Minimum Alveolar Concentrations of Isoflurane

	Age (years)	MAC
Isoflurane	20–30	1.28
	30–55	1.15
	55+	1.05
Isoflurane (with 70% nitrous oxide)	20–30	0.56
	30–55	0.50
	55+	0.37

From Stevens, W. C., et al.: Minimum alveolar concentrations (MAC) of isoflurane with and without nitrous oxide in patients of various ages. Anesthesiology 42:197, 1975.

Administration

Inhalation of isoflurane by mask in adult patients is an acceptable method of delivery. The single "vital capacity breath" technique with 5% isoflurane (4.5 MAC) produces unconsciousness in about 40 seconds, in patients premedicated with 5 μg/kg of fentanyl.[6] In comparison, 3.5% halothane (4.5 MAC) induces unconsciousness in about 90 seconds; these characteristics are consistent with the blood/gas solubilities of the two anesthetics. Isoflurane is pungent, however, and a slow induction is recommended to lessen the irritating effects of the vapor, to avoid breath-holding and coughing. Indeed, respiratory complications can be pronounced in infants. Friesen and Lichtor[7] demonstrated that inhalation induction with isoflurane, using inspired concentrations up to 3.5% (a value that is roughly equivalent to 3.0% halothane—the MAC of halothane in infants is 1.2[8]), is associated with an unacceptably high frequency of laryngospasm and coughing, often severe. Moreover, in infants, inhalation induction with isoflurane causes significant decreases in heart rate, systolic blood pressure, and mean arterial pressure.[7] Premedication with atropine minimizes the bradycardia, but it does not prevent the decrease in blood pressure, which is significantly more pronounced than with halothane and atropine. In infants at least, use of halothane for inhalation induction is clearly preferable to isoflurane.

As with the other volatile agents, the technique of overpressure can be used to hasten induction, but as noted previously, the pungency of isoflurane limits the rate at which its concentration can be increased. In practice, a short-acting barbiturate is usually administered to facilitate the process. Concomitant use of nitrous oxide can also help to circumvent the problem, by achieving a similar MAC equivalent of total anesthetic at a lower inspired concentration.

Absorption and Elimination

Partition coefficients of isoflurane are shown in Table 39–3.[9,10] The rise in the alveolar concentration of isoflurane occurs more rapidly than that of halothane, and slightly faster than enflurane, because the blood/gas parti-

Table 39–3. Partition Coefficients of Volatile Anesthetics

	Blood/Gas	Brain/ Blood	Muscle/ Blood	Fat/ Blood
Isoflurane	1.4	2.6	4.0	45
Enflurane	1.9	1.4	1.7	36
Halothane	2.3	2.9	3.5	60

More recent determinations of tissue/blood partition coefficients by Lerman et al.[10] for isoflurane and three other volatile anesthetics (enflurane, halothane, and methoxyflurane) are approximately 30% lower than those of earlier studies, which they attributed to their efforts to prevent loss of intracellular water (volatile anesthetics are poorly soluble in water). Compare with more recent solubility data in Table 39–9. From Eger, E. I., II: Anesthetic Uptake and Action. Baltimore, Williams & Wilkins, 1974.

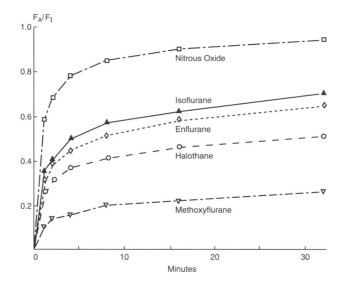

Fig. 39–3. Alveolar (uptake) concentration curves for inhaled anesthetics. From Eger, E. I., II: Isoflurane: a review. Anesthesiology 55:559, 1981.

tion coefficient of isoflurane is only 1.4 (which is less than any of the other volatile agents except desflurane and sevoflurane). Within 5 to 10 minutes of induction, the alveolar concentration of isoflurane is approximately 50% of the inspired concentration, and by 30 minutes it is about 70% of the inspired concentration (Fig. 39-3).[11,12]

Despite its low blood/gas partition coefficient, the tissue solubilities of isoflurane more closely resemble those of halothane than those of isoflurane's isomer, enflurane. Therefore, a considerable amount of isoflurane is taken up by tissues during the course of an anesthetic administration, requiring an alveolar concentration in the range of 2% to maintain a blood partial pressure 30% above MAC.[11] At 1.3 MAC, the calculated blood concentration of isoflurane (in mg/dl), based on a blood/gas solubility coefficient of 1.4 and a blood partial pressure of 1.5% (1.15 × 1.3 MAC) is approximately 15 mg/dl. Again, adding nitrous oxide to the inhaled mixture reduces the isoflurane requirement, and with 70% nitrous oxide, inspired concentrations in the range of 1.3% maintain an alveolar partial pressure about 30% above MAC.[11]

As noted previously, except for a lower blood/gas solubility compared with halothane, the tissue solubilities of isoflurane and halothane are similar. As a result, the elimination curves of both agents are nearly identical (see Fig. 39-7).[12] The lower brain/blood solubility of isoflurane results in a faster emergence than with halothane, however. Patients anesthetized with isoflurane for less than 1 hour open their eyes on command about 7 minutes after discontinuation of anesthesia.[11] Even after prolonged anesthesia, in the range of 5 to 6 hours, emergence is relatively rapid, occurring on average in about 11 minutes. In a more recent study by Frink and co-workers,[13] response to command occurred in about 18 minutes following 2.5 MAC-hours of anesthesia. In addition, cognitive function returns more quickly than with halothane.[14]

Biotransformation

Isoflurane is an extremely stable chemical compound. Its stability is primarily related to halogenation of the carbon on each side of the ether bond with fluorine and chlorine and the complete fluorination of the terminal ethyl carbon. Metabolism of isoflurane in humans is less than that any of the halogenated agents in current use, except desflurane.

Some oxidative metabolism does occur, to the extent of about 0.2%, but this is considered clinically insignificant. Oxidation occurs at the α ethyl carbon-hydrogen bond, with release of the chloride ion and generation of difluoromethanol and trifluoroacetic acid. The difluoromethanol residue undergoes further metabolism, with release of two free fluoride ions, whereas trifluoroacetic acid is resistant to further degradation and is the major metabolite in humans. A peak serum fluoride concentration of 4.4 μmol/L is reached after 4.9 MAC hours of anesthesia,[15] which is less than one tenth the serum concentration seen after enflurane anesthesia. In obese subjects, metabolism is slightly increased, and the free fluoride ion concentration peaks at about 6.5 μmol/L after 2 hours of anesthesia.[16] Reductive metabolism and generation of free radicals do not occur.

Physiologic Effects

Central Nervous System

A progressive obtundation of consciousness and sensory perception occurs with increasing concentrations of isoflurane. A stage of anesthesia denoted by absence of somatic responses, but some sympathetic activation, is produced. The sequence follows that of the usual signs of anesthesia, especially as seen with diethyl ether. In the postanesthesia period, decreased mental acuity may persist for 2 to 3 hours, which may be an important consideration in ambulatory surgery.

Isoflurane does not produce CNS excitation. Burst suppression occurs at 1.5 MAC, and the electroencephalogram (EEG) becomes isoelectric at 2.0 MAC.[17,18] Among the volatile anesthetics, the ability to produce an isoelectric EEG at clinically relevant concentrations appears to be unique to isoflurane.

Cerebral Metabolism and Blood Flow

Isoflurane causes a dose-related reduction in cerebral metabolic rate ($CMRo_2$), which correlates with a decrease in cortical electrical activity. At 2 MAC, isoflurane produces an isoelectric EEG, with a maximal reduction in $CMRo_2$ of about 50%, to 1.5 ml/min/100 g.[18] The reduction in $CMRo_2$ with isoflurane is more than twice that seen with enflurane or halothane. Higher concentrations of isoflurane do not produce a further reduction in $CMRo_2$, but the cerebral energy state remains normal; that is, cellular integrity is preserved.[19]

In studies by Newburg and Michenfelder,[20] the investigators suggested that isoflurane may provide some protection for the brain from the effects of global hypoxemia or ischemia. During isoflurane anesthesia, cerebral energy stores of adenosine triphosphate (ATP) and phosphocreatine and the cerebral energy charge are sustained. In addition, cerebral lactate concentrations are considerably lower than seen during halothane anesthesia. Indeed, the effect of isoflurane on cerebral metabolism is identical to that seen with barbiturates.[21,22]

Average values for cerebral metabolism and cerebral blood flow (CBF), during stable isoflurane administration at less than 1 MAC, are 2.0 ± 0.6 ml/100 g/min (CMRo$_2$; the normal human awake value is approximately 3.5 ml/100 g/min) and 49 ± 14 ml/100 g/min (CBF; normal is 45 to 50 ml/100 g/min), with a mean arterial blood pressure (MAP) of 78 mm Hg.[23] Thus, concentrations of isoflurane below 1.0 MAC reduce CMRo$_2$, but have an insignificant effect on CBF. On the other hand, higher concentrations increase CBF, which is doubled at 1.5 MAC.[11] Autoregulation of CBF appears relatively intact during isoflurane anesthesia. In contrast, enflurane and, particularly, halothane disrupt autoregulation,[24] which means that CBF is dependent on systemic blood pressure.

CMRo$_2$ and CBF have been determined for isoflurane in patients undergoing craniotomy for small supratentorial tumors.[25] One hour after induction of anesthesia with an inspired isoflurane concentration of 0.75%, CMRo$_2$ averaged 2.1 ± 0.2 ml/100 g/min and CBF averaged 31 ± 3 ml/100 g/min. When isoflurane was increased to 1.5% (1.3 MAC), CBF did not change, but CMRo$_2$ was significantly reduced from 2.4 ml to 1.9 ml/100 g/min, which confirms the experimental studies.

Anesthetic-induced increases in CBF are of concern in patients with space-occupying lesions, because of the associated risk of increasing intracranial pressure. Because carbon dioxide reactivity is maintained (or possibly enhanced with isoflurane), however, hyperventilation can blunt or prevent increases in CBF that would otherwise occur. This effect is more pronounced with isoflurane than with enflurane or halothane. As a result, hyperventilation appears to prevent increases in intracranial pressure (ICP). Adams and colleagues[26] evaluated the effect of 1% inspired isoflurane on cerebrospinal fluid (CSF) pressure (measured with a lumbar needle) in 20 neurosurgical patients undergoing craniotomy for supratentorial tumors or hematoma. In 15 patients, Paco$_2$ was maintained between 25 to 30 mm Hg with hyperventilation, which was begun simultaneously with administration of isoflurane. The other 5 patients were hyperventilated during administration of isoflurane, but they were kept normocapnic with inspired carbon dioxide. The study demonstrated that hypocapnia prevents the rise in CSF pressure that would otherwise accompany isoflurane administration. Moreover, CSF pressures were reduced to below baseline values. This salutary effect can be achieved with hyperventilation begun with introduction of isoflurane, and unlike the situation with halothane, hypocapnia need not be established before administering the anesthetic. Cerebral perfusion pressure (CPP) was reduced in both groups of patients to a similar degree, because arterial blood pressure decreased more in the hypocapnic patients. This raises the important point that in the presence of increased ICP, maintaining an adequate CPP depends on maintaining a sufficient MAP.

In patients undergoing clipping of cerebral aneurysms, effects on metabolism and blood flow have been measured during induced hypotension.[18] Deliberate hypotension was produced with isoflurane at a mean inspired concentration of 2.3% (2 MAC), and cerebral metabolism and blood flow were measured when the MAP was reduced to about 50 mm Hg. Under these conditions, the CMRo$_2$ decreased to 1.5 ± 0.5 ml/100 g/min, but the global CBF of about 45 ml/100 g/min was close to normal, maintaining an adequate oxygen supply-demand balance. An isoelectric EEG occurred at 2 MAC, corresponding to a maximal reduction in CMRo$_2$.[18] Again, the low CMRo$_2$ confirms the potent metabolic depressant effects of isoflurane noted in animals.

In patients undergoing carotid endarterectomy, one may see a reduction in regional CBF (rCBF) in the distribution of the middle cerebral artery. Critical rCBF has been defined as the flow below which EEG signs of ischemia occur.[23] During normocapnic isoflurane anesthesia, rCBF less than 10 ml/100 g/min produces EEG changes indicative of ischemia.[27] This contrasts with normocapnic halothane anesthesia, in which the critical rCBF is 18 to 20 ml/100 g/min.[23,28] This suggests that isoflurane maintains cellular integrity at a lower CBF than halothane, providing a margin of safety during carotid endarterectomy.

Respiration

Isoflurane is a potent respiratory depressant, as are the other inhalation agents. With increasing depth of anesthesia, minute ventilation decreases and the ventilatory response to carbon dioxide is diminished. In spontaneously breathing subjects, the Paco$_2$ concomitantly rises. In anesthetized patients breathing 1.3% isoflurane (approximately 1 MAC), the Paco$_2$ averages 50 mm Hg, compared with 40 mm Hg in the awake subject.[29] When ventilation is assisted, thereby reducing the Paco$_2$, the apneic threshold is about 46 mm Hg. The magnitude in reduction of Paco$_2$ that is required to produce apnea is not different from that of the other volatile agents, however.[30]

Comparing isoflurane with the other volatile anesthetics reveals few differences in overall respiratory depressant effects. In spontaneously breathing subjects anesthetized with approximately equal MAC multiples of the various agents, minimal differences in minute ventilation are observed. Differences in respiratory rate and tidal volume do occur, however. For example, tidal volume is greater with isoflurane than with halothane. On the other hand, the respiratory rate increases more with halothane than with isoflurane. Nonetheless, the result is that the Paco$_2$ increases more in the spontaneously breathing subject anesthetized with halothane than with isoflurane.[31]

Heart

Isoflurane does not depress human myocardial contractility at light levels of anesthesia, when the sympathetic nervous system is intact. No significant changes in cardiac output, ballistocardiogram I-J wave amplitude, ejection time, or mean rate of ventricular ejection occur. With deeper levels of anesthesia, a decrease in stroke volume occurs, but this is offset by an increase in heart rate. Even at 2 MAC, the cardiac output remains about 90% of control.[11] During spontaneous ventilation with an elevated Pa_{CO_2}, one sees a further increase in heart rate and an accompanying rise in cardiac output. Little predisposition to arrhythmias exists, and the dose of epinephrine required to produce premature ventricular contractions is at least 7 μg/kg, which is probably the same as in the awake state.[32] Earlier work by Johnston and co-workers[33] had determined that the median effective dose (ED_{50}) during isoflurane anesthesia is 6.7 μg/kg. Thiopental lowers the arrhythmogenic dose of epinephrine for both isoflurane and halothane.[34,35]

Coronary Circulation

Isoflurane is a potent coronary vasodilator with direct effects on coronary resistance vessels.[36] Experimental studies indicate that the vasodilatory effect is limited to the small coronary vessels, with little or no effect on the epicardial conductance arteries.[37] The dose-dependent decrease in coronary vascular resistance probably occurs at the level of the myocardial arterioles, which are the major determinants of coronary vascular resistance.

Isoflurane is similar to dipyridamole, adenosine, and papaverine in producing arteriolar dilation. In contrast, nitrates and calcium channel blockers have predominant effects on the epicardial arteries. Thus, isoflurane may divert flow away from compromised regions by vasodilating small vessels in well-perfused regions. This effect is similar to that seen in patients with coronary artery disease, in whom dipyridamole may produce angina or ischemic changes on the electrocardiogram (ECG).[38,39]

Coronary "Steal" Phenomenon

As noted previously, in the presence of borderline regional myocardial perfusion, ischemia may occur as a result of small vessel dilation.[36,38-41] Moreover, 1 MAC isoflurane decreases coronary perfusion pressure by about 35%, because of systemic vasodilation and decreased myocardial contractility, which may further compromise blood flow to poorly perfused regions of myocardium. Deleterious effects may be partially offset by a reduction in myocardial contractility, however, which is associated with a decrease in myocardial oxygen consumption of about one third. The capacity to produce "coronary steal" or maldistribution of blood flow as well as hypotension may pose a risk to the patient with coronary artery disease.[42] One study using a chronically instrumented canine model of coronary artery disease (left anterior descending occlusion and left circumflex stenosis) did not demonstrate a "steal" phenomenon with isoflurane, whereas adenosine markedly decreased coronary collateral blood flow.[43]

Experimental Myocardial Effects

Depression of myocardial contractility occurs with higher concentrations of isoflurane. Left ventricular performance and oxygen consumption are decreased in a dose-dependent manner.[11] Experimentally, isoflurane depresses contractility of isolated cat papillary muscles.[44] In the dog, right and left ventricular function are affected differently, but in a dose-dependent manner.[45] At lower isoflurane concentrations, one tends to see an increase in right ventricular preload with unchanged pulmonary vascular resistance and a decrease in left ventricular afterload. At a mean aortic pressure of 70 mm Hg, right ventricular dimensions are unchanged, whereas left ventricular dimensions decrease. At higher isoflurane concentrations and lower mean aortic pressures, right ventricular dimensions increase, whereas left ventricular dimensions do not decrease further. In general, left ventricular function is better preserved, a characteristic that appears to be due to a decrease in afterload.

Circulation

Isoflurane is a potent systemic vasodilator that reduces systemic vascular resistance by 50% at about 2 MAC.[46] Decreases in systemic vascular resistance are associated with a fall in blood pressure, on the order of 25 to 50% at 1 to 2 MAC, which occurs despite a normal cardiac output. This contrasts with halothane, with which hypotension is primarily a result of decreased cardiac output. Significant effects on pulmonary vascular resistance have not been observed. Large increases in muscle and skin blood flow occur, however, consequent to the fall in systemic vascular resistance. Noxious stimulation maintains blood pressure during light anesthesia, as does adding nitrous oxide. In addition to reducing the concentration of isoflurane required, nitrous oxide appears to maintain systemic vascular resistance by increasing sympathetic tone.

Kidney

Isoflurane and the other volatile agents in use today produce similar reductions in renal blood flow, glomerular filtration, and urine output.[15] Renal autoregulation remains intact. The effects are attributed to decreases in blood pressure and cardiac output and do not reflect toxic effects on the kidney. Indeed, the release of fluoride from metabolism of isoflurane is too small to result in nephrotoxicity.

Liver

Isoflurane has not been implicated in postanesthetic hepatitis.[47] A slight elevation in postoperative serum liver enzymes may occur, however, but the magnitude is similar to that seen after nitrous oxide-narcotic anesthesia.[11]

Neuromuscular Effects

Adequate muscle relaxation accompanies surgical levels of anesthesia. In anesthetized patients, tetanus is not maintained with nerve stimulation, although twitch amplitude is preserved. The action of d-tubocurarine is markedly potentiated by isoflurane, and doses needed to produce relaxation are one third those needed with halothane.[48] The effect of succinylcholine is also increased and is attributed to increased muscle blood flow and enhanced delivery of the drug.

Table 39–4. Physicochemical Properties of Enflurane

Chemical name: 2-chloro-1,1,2-trifluoroethyl difluoromethyl ether

Structure	CHF_2-O-CF_2CHFCl
Molecular weight	184.5
Specific gravity (25°C)	1.517
Boiling point	56.5°C
Vapor pressure (mm Hg at 20°C)	175
Vapor/liquid (ml at 25°C)	201
Partition coefficients (37°C)	
Oil/gas	98.5
Blood/gas	1.91
Water/gas	0.78
Flammability	None
Chemical stabilizer	None

ENFLURANE

Essential Pharmacology

Properties

Synthesized by Speers and colleagues in 1963, enflurane (Ethrane) was the 347th compound produced in their search for an improved, nonexplosive volatile anesthetic. Krantz and his colleagues at the University of Maryland tested enflurane and found it to be a potent anesthetic, and subsequent studies demonstrated that it was safe and had a satisfactory clinical profile. Enflurane was introduced into clinical practice in 1972.

Enflurane is a volatile methyl ethyl ether (2-chloro-1,1,2-trifluoroethyl difluoromethyl ether). The anesthetic is a clear, colorless liquid with a pleasant odor, and it causes minimal irritation to the airway, thereby making it a suitable agent for inhalation induction. Physicochemical properties are shown in Table 39-4. Enflurane is nonflammable at concentrations below 5.8% (in 70% nitrous oxide and 30% oxygen),[2] is stable in the presence of soda lime, does not react with metals, and is not affected by light.

Potency

The MAC of enflurane decreases with the patient's age, as shown in Table 39-5,[49] with the highest value in infants (2.4) and the lowest in elderly subjects (1.4). For adults about 40 years of age, the MAC of enflurane in oxygen is 1.7. Adding 50% nitrous oxide decreases the apparent MAC of enflurane by about 50% to 0.9, and 70% ni-

Table 39–5. Minimum Alveolar Concentrations of Enflurane

Infants	6 mo	2.4
Children	3–6 y	2.0
Adults	25 y	1.8
	40 y	1.7
	80 y	1.4

Percentage of inspired concentration in oxygen. From Gion, H., Saidman, L. J.: The minimum alveolar concentration of enflurane in man. Anesthesiology 35:361, 1971.

trous oxide by about 70% to 0.5. Thus, the anesthetic effects of the two agents are additive.[50]

Administration

Induction of anesthesia may be accomplished quickly with an intravenous agent, such as thiopental, or more slowly by inhalation, gradually increasing the inspired concentration of enflurane to about 4.0%. With a mask induction technique, surgical anesthesia is attained in 7 to 10 minutes. Indeed, enflurane is a suitable anesthetic for inhalation induction and compares favorably with halothane.[51]

Absorption and Elimination

A commonly quoted blood/gas partition coefficient for enflurane is 1.9 (37°C), but variations in solubility occur, related to patient weight and blood hemoglobin concentration. A body mass index (BMI) above 30 is associated with a slightly lower blood/gas solubility of 1.8 compared with an average value of 2.0 in the nonobese individual. Hemoglobin concentration appears to have a greater effect; with a hemoglobin of 8.0 g/dl, the blood/gas coefficient is 1.2; at 12.0 g/dl, it is 1.8; and at 15.0 g/dl, it is 2.2.[52]

Partition coefficients of enflurane are shown in Table 39-6. The average blood/gas solubility coefficient of enflurane of 1.9 suggests that induction with enflurane should be slower than with isoflurane. Tissue solubilities of enflurane are about half those of isoflurane, however, and consequently, uptake by tissues is slower and thereby tends to compensate for enflurane's higher blood solubility. The net effect is that the rate of rise of alveolar enflurane is only slightly less than that of isoflurane (see Fig. 39-3). Within 10 minutes of induction, the alveolar concentration of enflurane is about 50% of the inspired concentration, and by 30 minutes it is approximately 60% of the inspired concentration.

Equilibration of the vessel-rich group of tissues is essentially complete after the first 10 minutes. During the next 30 minutes, enflurane uptake by tissues gradually declines, and lower concentrations, in the range of 3.0 to 3.5%, maintain an alveolar concentration approximately 30% above MAC. At 1.3 MAC, the calculated blood concentration of enflurane (in mg/dl), based on a blood/gas solubility coefficient of 1.9 and a blood partial pressure of 2.2% (1.7% × 1.3 MAC) is approximately 30 mg/dl. With 70% nitrous oxide, an alveolar concentration about 1.3 times MAC can be maintained with an inspired enflurane concentration of about 1.5%.

The time of awakening after discontinuing enflurane varies according to the length of the anesthetic. For procedures lasting less than 30 minutes, the average time to

Table 39–6. Partition Coefficients of Enflurane

Blood/Gas	Brain/Blood	Muscle/Blood	Fat/Blood
1.9	1.4	1.7	36

Adapted from Eger, E. I., II: Anesthetic Uptake and Action. Baltimore, Williams & Wilkins, 1974.

recovery is about 4 minutes, compared with about 10 minutes for halothane. Thus, recovery following short anesthetic administrations is more rapid with enflurane than with halothane, and enflurane is suitable for ambulatory surgery.[53,54] For longer procedures, however, time to recovery with enflurane is about twice as long as it is with isoflurane, although for anesthesia lasting about an hour, awakening occurs in less than 15 minutes in the majority of patients.

Biotransformation

From 2[55] to 8%[56] of absorbed enflurane is metabolized, and the products are excreted in the urine as nonvolatile fluorinated compounds and free fluoride. The major metabolite is difluormethoxydifluoroacetic acid, which results from hydroxylation and dehalogenation of the β carbon of the ethyl group.[57] The half-life ($T_{1/2}$) for inorganic fluoride excretion is 1.5 days, and 3.7 days for organic fluoride. Elimination of unaltered enflurane in exhaled air is triexponential, with a $T_{1/2}$ of 17.8 minutes, 3.2 hours, and 36.2 hours.[55]

Serum Fluoride Levels

In usual clinical practive, inorganic serum fluoride levels rarely reach 50 μmol/L, which is considered the threshold for subclinical toxicity.[58] Following 2 MAC hours of enflurane anesthesia, the average serum fluoride level is less than 20 μmol/L.[59,60] Higher fluoride levels are seen in obese patients, with peak levels about 30 μmol/L, because of increases in metabolism of the anesthetic, a phenomenon also observed with isoflurane.[61] Of the free fluoride produced, about half is rapidly deposited in bone and half is excreted in the urine.[62] Subsequently, fluoride is gradually leached from bone and excreted as fluoride by the kidney.

Renal fluoride excretion is enhanced with increasing urinary pH, which decreases tubular reabsorption of fluoride.[60] Conversely, acidic conditions enhance reabsorption, probably because of diffusion of nonionic hydrogen fluoride into the interstitium. As long as creatinine clearance exceeds 16 ml/min, fluoride excretion is normal. Although high fluoride levels generally do not occur in most patients with poor renal function, fluoride nephrotoxicity may be seen,[63] suggesting that enflurane be avoided in these patients. Similarly, enflurane should be avoided in patients with tuberculosis who are being treated with isoniazid. In a study by Rice and Talcott[64] of patients treated with isoniazid and given enflurane, some patients showed enhanced defluourination of enflurane and were prone to develop high blood levels of fluoride, far exceeding the threshold for clinical toxicity.

Physiologic Effects

Central Nervous System

A progressive descending depression of the CNS ensues with increasing blood levels of enflurane, in the range of 15 to 20 mg/dl.[65-67] Signs of motor area irritability appear in 2% of patients,[67] however, manifested by twitching movements of the jaw, neck, or extremities,

which seem to be related to deep anesthesia and hypocarbia. Seizure activity is generally self-limited and does not persist when anesthesia is lightened and normal ventilation is resumed, although lower concentrations of enflurane (below 2.0%) may be associated with EEG activation or seizures in patients taking tricyclic antidepressants, such as amitriptyline.[68] Despite a propensity for producing seizures at high concentrations, however, usual clinical concentrations of enflurane (without hypocarbia) do not appear to increase the risk of seizures in patients with epilepsy.[69]

Electroencephalography

Increasing depth of anesthesia is characterized by the appearance of high-voltage spikes, with subsequent development of spike waves and burst suppression (Fig. 39-4).[70] Spike voltage is between 150 and 200 μV, interspersed with an 8- to 10-Hz pattern. The EEG spike activity increases with increasing inspired enflurane concentrations up to 3% and is aggravated by hypocarbia or alkalosis.[70] In patients with hypercarbia, however, cerebral irritability appears to be reduced. During deep enflurane anesthesia, with inspired concentrations above 3.0%, most patients show bilateral symmetric spike-dome formations and posterior δ activity. Small doses of thiopental may provoke δ changes, but larger doses (5.0 mg/kg) diminish δ activity. The addition of nitrous oxide does not alter the predominant EEG patterns. Diazepam can provoke seizure activity with enflurane that may persist for several days.[71] Enflurane has also been used as a diagnostic tool to activate epileptogenic foci.[72]

In animal studies, EEG seizure activity is noted with inhaled enflurane concentrations between 3 and 4%, but below and above this range, the agent has anticonvulsant effects. At light levels of anesthesia, enflurane has significant anticonvulsive action, and it is difficult to induce convulsions by injection of penicillin and penicillin G benzathine (Bicillin).[72]

Cerebral Blood Flow and Metabolism

Compared to halothane, enflurane only modestly increases CBF. Nonetheless, the potential effect on ICP may be of concern in the presence of intracranial lesions. At 1 MAC, enflurane increases CBF about 50%, which is considerably less than with halothane, which increases CBF about 2.5-fold. In contrast, isoflurane at 1 MAC has a negligible effect on CBF. At 1.5 MAC, however, both enflurane and isoflurane increase CBF about twofold, and halothane increases CBF at least threefold.[11] Although the rise in CBF with enflurane can be attenuated by hyperventilation, (which indicates that carbon dioxide reactivity is maintained), hypocarbia may increase the likelihood of seizure activity at deeper levels of anesthesia.

During enflurane-induced seizures with "moderately deep" anesthesia (2.5 to 3.0% enflurane) in humans, jugular venous oxygen tension increases.[65,73] Although $CMRO_2$ may increase by 50% during seizures, a concomitant increase in CBF appears to maintain adequate oxygenation.

Enflurane also produces CNS depressive effects, as do the other volatile agents; 1 to 2 MAC enflurane decreases

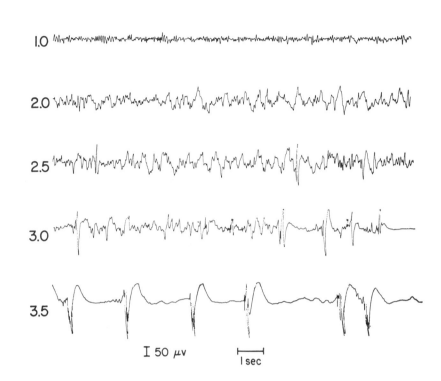

EEG with Ēthrane-Oxygen Anesthesia
Pa_{CO_2} — 35–39 mm Hg

Inspired Ēthrane Concentration (%)

awake

1.0

2.0

2.5

3.0

3.5

$\bar{\text{I}}$ 50 μv

I sec

Fig. 39–4. Electroencephalogram.

CMR_{O_2} 10 to 15% in human studies[74] and about 30% in canine studies.[21] Furthermore, some evidence indicates that enflurane also has anticonvulsive effects in humans.[69,75]

Effects of enflurane on CSF secretion are unique.[76] Initially, one sees an increase in CSF production of about 50%, which may increase ICP in the presence of reduced intracranial compliance. Thereafter, a gradual decline in secretion occurs, of about 7% per hour.

In patients with cerebral tumors, 2% enflurane has little effect on ICP, although CPP is decreased.[77] At lower anesthetic concentrations, ICP is reduced without significant change in CPP. Thus, monitoring MAP and maintaining an adequate perfusion pressure may be essential in the presence of cerebral tumors.[77] Enflurane does appear to provide some protection against ischemia, however; the critical CBF with enflurane is about 15 ml/100 g/min.[78]

Respiration

Ventilatory depression with enflurane parallels anesthetic depth. The moderate changes in ventilatory parameters during light anesthesia with 1.5 to 2% enflurane in 50% nitrous oxide may be an improvement over the tachypnea and shallow tidal volume observed with halothane, however. Nonetheless, enflurane sufficiently depresses respiration so assisted or controlled ventilation is required.

During spontaneous ventilation in unpremedicated patients with higher concentrations of enflurane (in oxygen), ventilation is profoundly depressed. This is evident by a marked rise in Pa_{CO_2} to more than 70 mm Hg at an alveolar concentration of approximately 1.5 MAC.[11] In contrast, the rise in Pa_{CO_2} is considerably less with halothane and isoflurane (about 55 to 60 mm Hg) at 1.5 MAC, and it is negligible with nitrous oxide. All the inhalation anesthetics depress the ventilatory response to inhaled carbon dioxide to a similar degree, however, which is abolished at approximately 2 MAC.[11] In addition, all the anesthetics decrease the ventilatory response to hypoxia, which is markedly depressed at 0.1 MAC and eliminated at 1 MAC.[79]

Bronchomotor Tone

Shortly after induction, only a slight change in airway conductance is evident with enflurane, but at 15 minutes, airway resistance is decreased by 56%.[80] This compares favorably with halothane.

Heart

Depression of myocardial contractility occurs with enflurane,[81,82] as with the other inhalation anesthetic agents. The primary effect on contractility is to decrease the force of contraction; a less prominent effect is to shorten the duration of the active state.[83] The following parameters are depressed: velocity of shortening dl/dt; net shortening; peak developed tension and maximal velocity of isotonic contraction; power and work. The result is a decrease in cardiac output of about 30%, which is similar in magnitude to that seen with halothane and is attributable mainly to a decrease in stroke volume.[11] With isoflurane, an increase in heart rate may compensate for the fall in stroke volume, maintaining a normal cardiac output.

In patients with hypercarbia (a $Paco_2$ of 60 mm Hg), however, a marked increase in cardiac index (5.0 L/min/m^2),[84] is probably attributable to the direct effects of carbon dioxide. Similar cardiovascular effects are seen in awake subjects with hypercarbia, including increased cardiac output, stroke work, MAP, and right heart filling pressures, together with a decreased peripheral vascular resistance (carbon dioxide is a direct vasodilator). In addition, increased circulating catecholamines and enhanced sympathetic nervous activity have been demonstrated in awake subjects, consequent to increased $Paco_2$, which indicates that these responses are unimpaired by enflurane.

Cardiac Rate and Rhythm

Enflurane has a positive chronotropic action in humans, increasing heart rate about 33%.[85,86] As noted previously, however, it is insufficient to offset decreases in stroke volume. This is likely a direct effect, but a vagolytic action may also occur. Thus, the effect of atropine on heart rate may be attenuated.

Cardiac rhythm is remarkably stable.[87,88] Arrhythmias, which are generally infrequent, include premature ventricular contractions, bradycardia, nodal rhythms and premature atrial contractions. Increasing concentrations of enflurane from 1 to 2 MAC prolong atrioventricular node conduction time, which is rate-dependent, and increasing heart rate enhance the effect (in contrast to halothane). The atrial effective refractory period is also prolonged; however, the His-Purkinje system and ventricular conduction times are not altered.[89] Arrhythmias tend to be of short duration and disappear with increased ventilation or correction of hypotension.[90]

Enflurane does not sensitize the myocardium to catecholamines to the same degree as halothane (the ED$_{50}$ for ventricular arrhythmias with halothane is 2.1 μg/kg), and larger amounts of epinephrine may be used with enflurane (the ED$_{50}$ is 10.9 μg/kg).[33] Although this value is also higher than that for isoflurane (at least 7 μg/kg), the dose-response curve with enflurane is relatively flat, and some patients experience arrhythmias with considerably lower doses of epinephrine.

Coronary Circulation

Enflurane in oxygen decreases coronary vascular resistance about 20%, whereas myocardial oxygen consumption decreases an average of 40%. With the addition of nitrous oxide, one sees a further decrease in coronary vascular resistance of approximately 30%. In patients with ischemic heart disease, the potential exists for maldistribution of blood flow when enflurane is administered in oxygen, but apparently this is abolished by the simultaneous administration of nitrous oxide. Enflurane is a coronary vasodilator, and the addition of nitrous oxide augments the effect.[91]

Circulation

Enflurane at 1 to 1.5 MAC reduces arterial blood pressure by about 35 to 40%,[92] an effect that is more pronounced than with halothane, but similar to that with isoflurane. Central sympathetic depression does not appear to be an important cause of hypotension with enflurane.[93] Because enflurane decreases systemic vascular resistance only 20 to 25%, arterial hypotension is due in part to a fall in cardiac output.[92] In contrast, isoflurane decreases blood pressure by reducing systemic vascular resistance, and cardiac output remains essentially unchanged. Blood pressure generally returns toward normal with surgical manipulation, although systolic hypotension of more than 30 mm Hg may persist in about 10% of patients anesthetized with enflurane.

Capillary and venular flow is little changed, although precapillary sphincters and capillaries show a decreased response to norepinephrine. This suggests improved flow in the microcirculation with a possible protective effect from tissue ischemia.[94]

Sympathetic Nervous System

Adrenal medullary catecholamine secretion and release, from spontaneous sympathetic nervous system activation or from splanchnic nerve stimulation, is inhibited by enflurane. The decrease is due to a direct effect on chromaffin cells of the adrenal gland and from reduced secretion of ganglionic acetylcholine. In addition, CNS suprasegmental activation of sympathetics is inhibited,[95] with depression of "pressor" mechanisms in the hypothalamus and medulla. Baroreceptor reflexes are maintained, however.[93]

Kidney

Enflurane decreases renal blood flow, glomerular filtration rate, and urine output, as do the other volatile agents in use today, because of reductions in blood pressure and cardiac output. After prolonged enflurane anesthesia, elevated fluoride levels occasionally may be associated with reductions in renal concentrating ability.[58] Fluoride released during metabolism of enflurane is usually below the level associated with nephrotoxic effects (see the preceding section about serum fluoride levels), however.

Liver

During routine enflurane anesthesia, significant impairment of liver function does not occur. Liver function tests (bilirubin, alkaline phosphatase, thymol turbidity, alanine aminotransferase [ALT], and cephalin flocculation), performed preoperatively and 5 days postoperatively are within normal limits, except for sulfobromophthalein sodium (Bromsulphalein; BSP), which is slightly elevated. With prolonged anesthesia, volunteers given 9.6 MAC hours of enflurane do not have increased BSP retention, but may have a transient increase in ALT.[96] Repeated enflurane exposure does not increase BSP retention or alter enzyme levels.[97]

Hepatic Toxicity

Enflurane hepatotoxicity is extremely rare, with an incidence of less than 1 in 800,000 exposures,[98,99] if it occurs at all. Most case reports of hepatitis following enflurane exposure are poorly documented or can be attributed to other causes. Eger and colleagues[100] studied this issue in detail. Of 88 patients who were reported to have some evidence of hepatic injury following enflurane anesthesia, 15 cases were "possibly" related to enflurane exposure. A causal relationship could not be established, however, in view of the presence of other risk factors for hepatic dysfunction and injury. For example, a major cause of postoperative liver injury is non-A, non-B hepatitis (hepatitis C), from subclinical infection present at the time of surgery or acquired from blood transfusions. Indeed, the incidence of non-A, non-B hepatitis in the general population is relatively high, in the range of 3%,[101] which far exceeds the incidence of any reported enflurane associated hepatic injury.

If enflurane is a hepatotoxin, it is one of the least toxic agents used in anesthesia, especially when compared with halothane. An immune-mediated mechanism for hepatic injury with enflurane has been suggested, however. Christ and colleagues[102] demonstrated that the major product of enflurane metabolism, the difluoromethoxydifluoroacetyl moiety, may form adducts by covalently binding to rat liver proteins, which are recognized by antibodies from sera of patients with halothane hepatitis. This suggests a possible hypersensitivity mechanism, such as has been postulated for halothane hepatitis. In any case, a specific histologic picture has not been described, and as noted by Eger and colleagues,[100] "if severe injury is caused by enflurane, it is an extremely rare event."

Neuromuscular Effects

Enflurane depresses the indirect twitch response at 1.5 to 2.5 MAC in isolated nerve-muscle preparations, a finding indicating that enflurane has a more potent effect at the neuromuscular junction than either halothane or isoflurane.[103] Clinical concentrations of enflurane inhibit transmission at the neuromuscular junction,[104] and adequate surgical muscle relaxation can be obtained at inspired concentrations in the range of 3 to 3.5%.

Muscle relaxants allow a reduction in enflurane concentration, which avoids the hypotension that would otherwise result. Enflurane potentiates the effects of nondepolarizing muscle relaxants, an action that likely occurs at the motor end plate. Potentiation of nondepolarizing agents is similar to that seen with isoflurane, and it is more pronounced than with halothane. As with the other volatile agents, depression of the direct twitch response occurs only at concentrations well above those used clinically.

DESFLURANE

Essential Pharmacology

Properties

Desflurane (Suprane) is a volatile methyl ethyl ether (1,2,2,2-tetrafluoroethyl difluoromethyl ether), introduced into clinical practice in 1992. Desflurane differs from isoflurane only in the substitution of fluorine for chlorine on the α ethyl carbon. The agent was the 653rd compound in a series of over 700 synthesized by Terrel and colleagues. Physicochemical properties of desflurane are shown in Table 39–7.[105] The agent is a clear, colorless liquid (below 22.8°C) with a pungent odor. The vapor is irritating to the airway, particularly at high concentrations, and when used as an inhalation induction agent, it may cause coughing and laryngospasm.

Desflurane is nonflammable over the range of clinical concentrations, in oxygen and nitrous oxide, and is an extremely stable compound. The only known degradation reaction results from direct contact with soda lime, producing trace levels of fluoform (CHF_3), also a breakdown product of isoflurane. Desflurane does not react with light under normal conditions, or with metals, such as stainless steel, brass, copper, or aluminum.

The extremely low solubility of desflurane in blood and tissues is the major physicochemical characteristic that sets it apart from the other volatile anesthetics and probably was the major impetus for its introduction into clinical practice. Indeed, a volatile agent that provides all aspects of general anesthesia and has the low blood and tissue solubilities of nitrous oxide would be exceedingly useful. Induction and emergence would be rapid, with few or no lingering effects on respiration and mentation. Intraoperative titration to effect would also be rapid, and the depth of anesthesia could be deepened quickly, without concern for prolonging the recovery time at the conclusion of surgery. The need for an induction agent, such as thiopental, would be reduced, because the low solubility of the anesthetic would allow unconsciousness to be produced in just a few breaths. This would have the added benefit of further speeding recovery, by avoiding the use of sedating intravenous agents that usually have relatively long elimination half-lives and prolonged ef-

Table 39–7. Physicochemical Properties of Desflurane

Chemical name: 1,2,2,2-tetrafluoroethyl difluoromethyl ether	
Structure	$CF_3CHF-O-CHF_2$
Molecular weight	168.04
Specific gravity (15°C)	1.467
Boiling point	22.8°C
Vapor pressure (mm Hg at 20°C)	669
Vapor/liquid (ml at 15°C)	206
Partition coefficients (37°C)	
Oil/gas	18.7
Blood/gas	0.42
Saline/gas	0.22
Flammability	None
Chemical stabilizer	None

Partition coefficients from Eger, E. I., II: Partition coefficients of I-653 in human blood, saline, and olive oil. Anesth Analg 66:971, 1987.

fects. These goals appear to be only partially met by desflurane. Unfortunately, several adverse effects of desflurane have been identified, including a high incidence of coughing and laryngospasm during induction and cardiovascular stimulation due to apparent sympathetic activation, which will certainly limit use of the agent. Considerably more experience with desflurane will be needed to determine the role of this anesthetic in clinical practice.

Potency

Desflurane is considerably less potent than any of the currently used volatile anesthetics. The low potency of desflurane reflects its low oil/gas solubility coefficient (18.7 at 37°C). Replacement of chlorine with fluorine at the α ethyl carbon produces a smaller, less lipid soluble molecule. Comparing the oil/gas solubility of desflurane with isoflurane (90.8) suggests that desflurane should be about one fifth as potent as isoflurane, which is close to experimentally derived values. Currently accepted values for the MAC of desflurane are shown in Figure 39–5[106] and Table 39–8.[107] As is true with the other volatile agents, the MAC of desflurane varies with age. For subjects 31 to 65 years of age, the MAC is 6.0%, about five

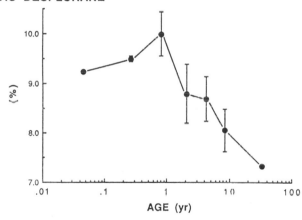

MAC DESFLURANE

Fig. 39–5. The MAC of desflurane in neonates, infants, and children. From Taylor, R. H., Lerman, J.: Minimum alveolar concentration of desflurane and hemodynamic responses in neonates, infants, and children. Anesthesiology 75:975, 1991.

Table 39–8. Minimum Alveolar Concentrations of Desflurane

	Age (years)	MAC
Desflurane	18–30	7.2
	31–65	6.0
Desflurane (with	18–30	4.0
60% nitrous oxide)	31–65	2.8

From Rampil, I. J., et al.: Clinical characteristics of desflurane in surgical patients: minimum alveolar concentration. Anesthesiology 74:429, 1991.

times greater than the MAC of isoflurane. This relationship holds across the various age groups. As with the other volatile agents, the MAC of desflurane is highest for infants 1 year of age (about 10%), which again is approximately five times higher than that of isoflurane for this age group (about 1.9%). The addition of 60% nitrous oxide reduces the MAC of desflurane by about 50%,[107] an effect that is similar in magnitude to that seen with the other volatile agents.

The MAC-awake (defined as the MAC of an inhalation anesthetic at which awakening occurs) of desflurane in volunteers has been reported to be 2.4%.[108] Although the MAC of desflurane in this study was 4.6%, approximately 35% less than subsequent determinations,[107] the ratio of MAC-awake and the lower value for MAC is 0.5, which is identical to the MAC-awake/MAC for halothane.[109] This means that the dose-response curve for desflurane is relatively steep (as it is with the other volatile agents), and patients lose consciousness at alveolar concentrations that are about 50% of MAC.

Administration

Desflurane, because of its high vapor pressure (669 mm Hg at 20°C; room temperature is near its boiling point, 23.5°C) requires a new type of vaporizer. The Tec 6 vaporizer, produced by Ohmeda (Ohio Medical Products, Madison, WI), is electrically heated and calibrated to deliver saturated desflurane vapor into an internally pressurized system. The anesthetic is then metered into the gas flow administered to the patient.

The low blood/gas solubility of desflurane results in rapid induction of anesthesia. Indeed, with inhalation induction, loss of the eyelash reflex occurs in about 2 minutes. Concomitant use of nitrous oxide speeds the process by 25%.[110] This compares with an induction time with propofol of about 1.5 minutes.[110]

As noted previously, inhalation induction is associated with a high incidence of troublesome and potentially severe respiratory complications. The cause appears to be related to the pungency and presumably irritant properties of the drug. Inhalation induction is associated with coughing, breathholding, apnea, and secretions requiring suctioning in about 25% of adult patients. Laryngospasm is also common, occurring in 4 to 12% of adults.[107,110] Use of nitrous oxide does not appreciably alter the incidence of respiratory complications.[107,110] All these problems are more common in infants and children, with moderate to severe laryngospasm occurring in 49% and moderate to severe coughing occurring in 58% of pediatric patients.[111] The use of premedication does not appear to alter the incidence of respiratory complications. Clearly, desflurane will not replace any of the currently used volatile agents for induction, and for safety reasons, an intravenous drug will be required to facilitate the process.

The deleterious respiratory effects may be predictable, based on similar effects noted with isoflurane. Because desflurane is markedly less potent than isoflurane, however, much higher concentrations must be used to induce anesthesia, a finding that may explain the higher incidence of respiratory problems with desflurane.

Table 39–9. Partition Coefficients of Desflurane and Other Inhalation Anesthetics

	Blood/Gas	Brain/Blood	Muscle/Blood	Fat/Blood
Desflurane	0.42	1.3	2.0	27
Isoflurane	1.46	1.6	2.9	45
Halothane	2.54	1.9	3.4	51
Sevoflurane	0.68	1.7	3.1	48
N_2O	0.47	1.1	1.2	2.3

Solubilities of desflurane and other volatile anesthetics in blood and tissues are shown. The solubilities of desflurane are lower than any of the volatile agents currently in use. The values for the other agents are generally lower than previously reported by other groups, however. The specific reasons for the differences are not known. Please compare with coefficients shown in Table 39–3. The solubility coefficients for nitrous oxide are included here for comparison with the volatile agents. Except for the lower blood/gas solubility of desflurane, nitrous oxide is less soluble in all tissues than any of the volatile agents. From Eger, E. I., II: Desflurane animal and human pharmacology: aspects of kinetics, safety, and MAC. Anesth Analg 75:53, 1992.

Absorption and Elimination

Partition coefficients of desflurane are shown in Table 39-9. For comparative purposes, recently determined coefficients for other anesthetics are included. The rise in the alveolar concentration of desflurane occurs more rapidly than any of the anesthetics in current use, except nitrous oxide. As determined in volunteers breathing 2.0% desflurane, the alveolar concentration of desflurane is 80% of the inspired concentration within 5 minutes, 83% of the inspired concentration at 10 minutes, and 90% at 30 minutes.[112] Alveolar concentration curves for the various anesthetics are depicted in Figure 39-6.[113] Although desflurane has a lower blood solubility than nitrous oxide, the alveolar concentration of nitrous oxide rises more rapidly than that of desflurane. The faster rise in alveolar nitrous oxide has been attributed to the concentration effect.[114] During recovery, the decline in the alveolar concentration of desflurane is more rapid than that in any of the other volatile agents.[112] Elimination curves for the various anesthetics, expressed as alveolar concentration ratios, which are defined as the quotient of the end-tidal concentration (FA) and the alveolar concentration immediately before discontinuing the anesthetic (FAO), are shown in Figures 39-7 and 39-8.[113] After 30 minutes of anesthesia, the FA of desflurane falls to 12% of FAO within 5 minutes of terminating the anesthetic. Ten minutes after discontinuing desflurane, the FA is about 10% of FAO, a value close to that for nitrous oxide,[108] and 30 minutes following termination of anesthesia, FA is about 3% of FAO.[114] Similar values are obtained after 1.5 hours of exposure to desflurane.[108]

Time to awakening is rapid. Following inhalation induction and 1.5 hours of anesthesia with 0.5 to 1 MAC of desflurane, volunteers responded to command in less than 4 minutes after discontinuing desflurane, with an average of 2.7 minutes.[108] In patients undergoing surgery, after induction with thiopental and maintenance with approximately 1 MAC of desflurane for 45 to 50 minutes, emergence was also rapid, with awakening in about 9

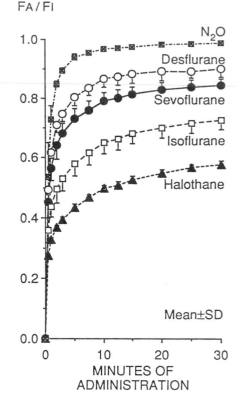

FA / FI

Fig. 39–6. The pharmacokinetics of inhalation anesthetics during administration, expressed as the ratio of alveolar concentration (FA) to inspired concentration (FI). From Yasuda, N., et al.: Comparison of kinetics of sevoflurane and isoflurane in humans. Anesth Analg 72:316, 1991.

minutes after discontinuing the anesthetic.[115] The slightly longer time to emergence compared with the volunteers may have been due to thiopental induction. Patients anesthetized for 2 to 3 hours with 0.65 MAC desflurane awoke within 9 minutes, and after 1.25 MAC desflurane (approximately 3 MAC-hours), they awoke within 16 minutes.[116] In contrast, emergence times for isoflurane were approximately twice as long, about 16 and 30 minutes, respectively. Cognitive function also returns more quickly with desflurane than with isoflurane, although psychomotor ability and discharge times may not be significantly different from those seen after isoflurane anesthesia.[117]

Biotransformation

Substitution of chlorine with fluorine predictably results in a more stable chemical compound than isoflurane, which is reflected in the decreased spontaneous breakdown of desflurane on exposure to soda lime and heat.[118] Similarly, desflurane resists biodegradation. Fluoride levels in serum and urine were not elevated following up to 7 MAC hours of desflurane anesthesia.[119] Serum and urine trifluoroacetic acid levels were mildly elevated for about a week postoperatively, however; a peak level of 0.4 μmol/L was detected at 24 hours, which is about 1000-fold lower than levels measured after halothane anesthesia,[120] and at least 10-fold less than levels following exposure to isoflurane.[119] Although desflurane does undergo some degradation in vivo, compared with the other volatile agents (including isoflurane), metabolism is trivial.

Physiologic Effects

Central Nervous System

EEG effects of desflurane parallel those of isoflurane. Rampil and colleagues[121] evaluated the effects of desflurane on the EEG in 12 volunteers exposed to concentrations up to 2.08 MAC. Increasing concentrations of desflurane produced increasing cortical depression, with progressive slowing in electrical activity. At 0.8 MAC, activity was predominately α, θ, and δ. At 1.2 MAC, activity shifted to predominately θ and δ, and burst suppression was evident in most subjects. Higher concentrations of desflurane produced more pronounced burst suppression, without a further slowing in frequency. Electrical silence was not produced at the desflurane levels used in this study, although a burst suppression ratio of about 80% was obtained at 2.08 MAC. Exchange of 3% desflurane (approximately 0.45 MAC) for 60% nitrous oxide decreased burst suppression when present and increased EEG frequencies. Hyperventilation and repetitive auditory stimuli did not produce EEG evidence of seizure activity. In a canine model, cerebral metabolic rate for oxygen ($CMRo_2$) decreased in a dose-dependent manner with desflurane, to about 2.5 ml/min/100g at 2.0 MAC, an effect similar to that seen with isoflurane.[122] Similarly, in this canine model, desflurane increased CBF in a dose-dependent manner. At 1.5 MAC, CBF was about 1.3-fold above baseline, and at 2.0 MAC, it was increased about 1.5-fold.[123]

As with isoflurane, the cerebral vasculature appears to remain responsive to carbon dioxide with desflurane, and hyperventilation appears to decrease CBF. In human patients undergoing surgery for removal of supratentorial masses, in the presence of mild to moderate hypocarbia, the effects of desflurane are similar to those of isoflurane.[124] At 1.0 to 1.2 MAC desflurane or isoflurane, CBF was approximately 20 ml/min/100 g at a $PaCO_2$ of 25 mm Hg, which increased to about 35 ml/min/100 g at a $PaCO_2$ of 35 mm Hg.

The effect of desflurane on CSF pressure was examined by Muzzi and colleagues,[125] who measured lumbar CSF pressures in patients with supratentorial masses, anesthetized with 1 MAC desflurane or isoflurane. In the presence of hypocarbia, desflurane increased lumbar CSF pressure to 18 mm Hg, from a baseline of 11 mm Hg. In contrast, isoflurane had no effect on CSF pressures. During the course of the study, MAP was kept within 20% of patients' preoperative values. At present, the effects of desflurane on ICP in the presence of decreased intracranial compliance remain unclear.

Respiration

In unpremedicated volunteers, desflurane causes a dose-dependent reduction in tidal volume that is partially compensated by an increase in respiratory rate. The increase in respiratory rate is not sufficient to prevent a reduction in minute ventilation, however. As a result, $PaCO_2$ progressively rises with increasing desflurane concentrations. At 1 MAC, the $PaCO_2$ is about 55 mm Hg, and at 1.7 MAC, it is about 85 mm Hg.[126] At the higher concentration, minute ventilation is reduced to about half of normal, and the degree of respiratory depression is similar to that seen with enflurane.

Despite the low blood and tissue solubilities of desflurane, which indicate that the agent should be useful for inhalation induction, the respiratory irritant properties of desflurane will probably prevent its widespread use for this purpose. The common respiratory complications seen with desflurane are discussed in the section of this chapter on administration.

Cardiovascular System

The effects of desflurane on cardiovascular function have been studied by Weiskopf and colleagues.[127] Volunteers received desflurane at three different concentrations (approximately 0.8, 1.2, and 1.7 MAC), and ventilation was controlled to maintain normocarbia. Desflurane caused a progressive reduction in systemic vascular resistance, MAP, and stroke volume and an increase in preload, heart rate, and pulmonary artery pressure. Unlike isoflurane, desflurane did not increase muscle blood flow. Despite changes in the various parameters noted previously, cardiac index remained in the normal range, suggesting that desflurane is less of a cardiac depressant than the other volatile agents. Indeed, stroke volume index does appear to be better maintained with desflurane than with isoflurane, and it is much better preserved than with halothane.[127] At deeper levels of anesthesia, the increase in heart rate may also partially offset the cardiac depressant effects that would otherwise be evident. Prolonged anesthesia with desflurane (longer than 90 minutes) may be associated with less cardiac depression. In the studies by Weiskopf and colleagues,[127] evidence of mild sympathetic stimulation was noted, with mean heart rates elevated compared with the first 90 minutes of anesthesia. Addition of 60% nitrous oxide and reduction of desflurane concentrations by approximately 50% (yielding MAC equivalents of 0.9, 1.3, and 1.7) also appear to cause less cardiovascular depression than the use of desflurane alone.[128]

Despite a propensity for causing tachycardia, desflurane does not appear to sensitize the myocardium to catecholamines. The incidence of epinephrine-induced arrhythmias with desflurane is the same as with isoflurane.[32]

Sympathetic Activation

The studies with volunteers described previously demonstrated signs of sympathetic activation by desflurane, such as elevation in heart rates, although the specific role of sympathetic activation in the observed cardiovascular parameters was not evaluated. Subsequent work suggests that sympathetic activation may have important implications in patients with hypertension or cardiac disease. To evaluate the role of sympathetic activation in the observed cardiovascular effects of desflurane specifically, Ebert and Muzi[129] measured sympathetic nerve activity (peroneal nerve) in normotensive, healthy volunteers receiving desflurane or isoflurane under carefully controlled conditions. The study demonstrated consistent and pronounced sympathetic activation with desflurane, which was most evident during transition periods from a lower to higher concentration of desflurane (1.0 to 1.5 MAC). Sympathetic activation resulted in transient but pronounced tachycardia and hypertension. Minimal activation was noted at less than 1.0 MAC desflurane. In contrast, sympathetic activation did not occur with isoflurane at any concentration. Indeed, increasing concentrations of isoflurane caused a decline in sympathetic activity and blood pressure, although heart rates remained mildly elevated. Also of importance was the observation that thiopental, administered for induction, did not block the sympathetic response that occurred with desflurane.

An added finding by Ebert and Muzi[129] was that desflurane, like isoflurane, decreased vascular resistance and increased muscle blood flow, findings that contrast with the observations of Weiskopf and co-workers.[127]

The hemodynamic consequences of sympathetic activation by desflurane are of concern in patients with cardiovascular disease. Helman and colleagues[130] observed a significant increase in the incidence of ischemia with desflurane in patients undergoing cardiac surgery, as assessed by ECG and echocardiography. Induction with desflurane (inhalation by mask) was associated with significant increases in heart rate and systemic and pulmonary blood pressures. The incidence of prebypass tachycardia and hypotension was also higher than in the sufentanil control group. In contrast, no evidence of cardiac ischemia was seen during induction or prebypass in patients given sufentanil rather than desflurane. During maintenance anesthesia with desflurane, the risk of myocardial ischemia did not appear to be increased when hemodynamic parameters were tightly controlled.[130]

Desflurane does not cause a "cardiac steal" phenomenon in a chronically instrumented canine model of cardiovascular disease (total occlusion of the left anterior descending artery and stenosis of the left circumflex arteries).[131]

The currently available product literature for desflurane (Suprane) reflects a concern about potential hemodynamic and ischemic changes in patients with coronary artery disease and suggests that desflurane not be used for induction or as the sole anesthetic agent in such patients. Moreover, desflurane may only partially block the cardiovascular responses to noxious stimulation. Yasuda and co-workers[132] observed that desflurane (up to 1.7 MAC) did not abolish cardiovascular responses to supramaximal electrical stimulation of the ulnar nerve. Thus, the effects of surgical stimulation appear to accentuate the sympathetic activation caused by desflurane.

Kidney and Liver

Fluoride levels following desflurane anesthesia are normal, and toxic effects on the kidney appear unlikely. Renal blood flow is not appreciably altered by up to 2.0 MAC of desflurane (or isoflurane), as measured in chroni-

cally instrumented dogs.[133] Because desflurane decreases both MAP and renal vascular resistance in this model, renal blood flow is maintained.

In the chronically instrumented dog, hepatic vascular resistance is unchanged during desflurane anesthesia.[133] Although hepatic arterial blood flow is maintained, portal flow is slightly decreased. Consequently, total hepatic blood flow is reduced by desflurane. In contrast, isoflurane decreases hepatic vascular resistance, an effect that may explain why isoflurane does not alter total hepatic blood flow in this model.

Neuromuscular Effects

The effects of desflurane on the neuromuscular junction are similar to those of isoflurane. At 1.5 MAC, desflurane depresses twitch amplitude (indirect) and train-of-four ratio (TOF) by about 20%. Although lower concentrations of desflurane (0.5 to 1.5 MAC) do not affect twitch or TOF, tetanic fade of at least 10% is observed.[134] The effects of desflurane on succinylcholine and pancuronium requirements are similar to those seen with isoflurane.[134] Compared with nitrous oxide-opioid anesthesia, desflurane reduces the ED_{95} of succinylcholine by about 30%, and it lowers the ED_{95} of atracurium and pancuronium by approximately 50%.[135]

SEVOFLURANE

Essential Pharmacology

Properties

Sevoflurane is a fluorinated isopropyl methyl ether recently approved for clinical use in the United States. The chemical name of sevoflurane is 1,1,1,3,3,3-hexafluoro-2-propyl fluoromethyl ether (or, alternatively, fluoromethyl-2,2,2-trifluoro-1-[trifluoromethyl] ethyl ether). The anesthetic was first described by Wallin and Napoli of Travenol Laboratories, in 1971.[136] The low blood/gas solubility and pleasant odor of sevoflurane provide for rapid inhalation induction and recovery.

In Japan, sevoflurane has become the leading inhalation anesthetic agent used in clinical practice.[137] Concerns about possible toxicity of breakdown products, including compounds formed on exposure to soda lime and fluoride released during biotransformation in the body, however, delayed release of sevoflurane into clinical practice in the United States. Were toxic side effects not an issue, sevoflurane would replace halothane, and most likely isoflurane, in routine clinical anesthetic practice in the United States.

Physicochemical properties of sevoflurane are shown in Table 39–10.[138] Sevoflurane is nonflammable at concentrations below 12% in oxygen and is stable in the presence of light and oxygen.[139] The agent is less soluble in rubber and plastic than any other volatile agent, except desflurane.

Potency

The MAC of sevoflurane in oxygen in humans has been reported to be 1.7[140] and 2.05.[141] When administered in 64% nitrous oxide-oxygen, the MAC of sevoflurane is

Table 39–10. Physicochemical Properties of
Sevoflurane

Chemical name: 1,1,1,3,3,3-hexafluoro-2-propyl fluoromethyl
  ether

Structure	$(CF_3)_2CH\text{-}OCH_2F$
Molecular weight	200.0
Specific gravity (20°C)	1.505
Boiling point	58.5°C
Vapor pressure (mm Hg at 20°C)	160
Vapor/liquid (ml at 20°C)	181
Partition coefficients (37°C)	
Oil/gas	53.4
Blood/gas	0.68
Water/gas	0.36
Flammability	None

Blood/gas solubility from Malviya, S., Lerman, J.: The blood/gas solubilities of sevoflurane, isoflurane, halothane, and serum constituents concentrations in neonates and adults. Anesthesiology 72:793, 1990.

0.66%,[140] which is a reduction of 61%, indicating that the anesthetic effects of nitrous oxide are additive with sevoflurane. The MAC-awake of sevoflurane is approximately 0.6%. The MAC-awake/MAC is about 0.3, as determined by a slow alveolar washout technique, which is close to that of isoflurane.[142]

Administration

The low blood/gas solubility of sevoflurane produces a rapid anesthetic induction by inhalation. Equally important, however, is sevoflurane's lack of pungency, which provides a smooth inhalation induction, without airway irritability or increased secretions. Sevoflurane is probably the least irritating to the respiratory tract of any of the currently used volatile anesthetics.[143]

Absorption and Elimination

Partition coefficients for sevoflurane are shown in Table 39–9, and the alveolar concentration curve during administration of anesthesia is shown in Figure 39–6. Because of a slightly greater blood/gas solubility than desflurane, the rise in alveolar concentration of sevoflurane is slower than that of desflurane, but it is considerably faster than isoflurane.[113] Tissue solubilities of sevoflurane and isoflurane are similar, however, and multicompartment analysis demonstrates that elimination of both anesthetics from tissues occurs at about the same rate.[113]

Despite the lower blood/gas solubility of desflurane, in clinical practice, anesthesia can be achieved more rapidly with sevoflurane, which does not produce the respiratory irritation seen with desflurane. Indeed, unconsciousness can be achieved within five breaths with 2% sevoflurane.[144]

Alveolar elimination curves of sevoflurane and desflurane are shown in Figures 39–7 and 39–8.[113] For comparison, curves for nitrous oxide, halothane, and isoflurane are also depicted. Alveolar washout curves of sevoflurane and desflurane are similar, at least during the first 2 hours following anesthesia, and emergence compares favorably with that after desflurane administration. In healthy pa-

tients following 2 to 3 MAC-hours of anesthesia, emergence time is about 7.5 minutes with sevoflurane,[13] 16 minutes with desflurane,[116] and 18 to 30 minutes with isoflurane.[13,116] Thereafter, elimination curves of the two agents diverge slowly, with sevoflurane lagging. This is more apparent after several days, reflecting the higher muscle and fat solubilities of sevoflurane.[113] In contrast, the alveolar washout of isoflurane is similar to that of halothane.

Biotransformation

Sevoflurane undergoes spontaneous, temperature-dependent decomposition in contact with carbon dioxide absorbents (soda lime and baralyme). At 80°C, sevoflurane rapidly decomposes at a rate of 92% per hour. This compares with a rate of 16% per hour for halothane, 13% per hour for isoflurane, and 0.4% per hour for desflurane.[118] In addition to methanol, at least five products are produced, several of which are toxic to laboratory animals at sufficient dosage.[145,146] At temperatures likely to occur in the absorber canister during anesthesia (less than about 50°C), however, only one or two products are detectable. Morio and co-workers[145] detected two products, designated compound A [$CF_2{=}C(CF_3)OCH_2F$] and compound B [$CH_3OCF_2CH(CF_3)OCH_2F$], after 8 hours of exposure to soda lime at 54°C or less. The peak concentration of compound A was less than 80 ppm. The lethal concentration of compound A in rats was found to be about 1100 ppm

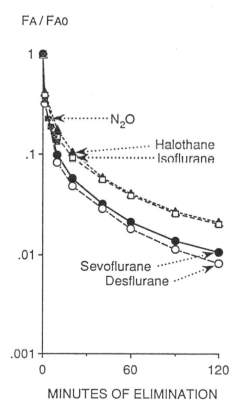

Fig. 39–7. Elimination of inhaled anesthetics, expressed as the ratio of alveolar concentration (FA) to inspired concentration (FI). From Yasuda, N., et al.: Comparison of kinetics of sevoflurane and isoflurane in humans. Anesth Analg 72:316, 1991.

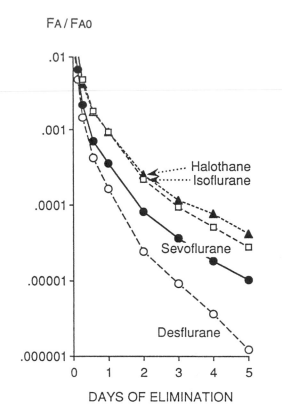

Fig. 39–8. The terminal elimination of volatile anesthetics. From Yasuda, N., et al.: Comparison of kinetics of sevoflurane and isoflurane in humans. Anesth Analg 72:316, 1991.

for a 1-hour exposure, and about 400 ppm for an exposure of 3 hours. Animals died from 30 minutes to 9 days after exposure. Acute deaths were associated with lung congestion, and animals dying later succumbed to acute tubular necrosis. Long-term exposure to low levels (> 120 ppm) caused no adverse effects except weight loss. Mutations were not induced in the Ames test. Mutagenesis is an important consideration, because compound A is a vinyl derivative that could react with nucleic acids. Compound B was not toxic and did not induce mutagenesis.

Using a low-flow anesthetic technique of more than 3 hours' duration with surgical patients, Frink and colleagues[146] quantified the degradation products of sevoflurane in soda lime and baralyme. In their study, only compound A was detectable, and the average concentration was less than 20 ppm, although one patient was exposed to a peak concentration of 61 ppm. No toxic effects were evident in any of the patients.

The clinical significance of degradation products remains unclear. In a toxicity study using a rat model, sevoflurane was no more toxic than isoflurane, and both were less toxic than halothane.[147] Moreover, halothane undergoes degradation in soda lime, to bromochlorodifluoroethylene (BCDE), reaching approximately 5 ppm in low-flow circuits.[148] The lethal concentration of the halothane breakdown product is 250 ppm in rats. The toxic potential of BCDE and compound A appears to be

about the same, and clinically, toxicity of BCDE has never been an issue.[149] In any case, this unfortunate characteristic of sevoflurane is still a matter of considerable controversy, and it will likely delay approval of the anesthetic in the United States.

Sevoflurane also undergoes biotransformation to about the same extent as enflurane (about 3%). The principal products are inorganic fluoride and hexafluoroisopropanol (organic fluoride).[144] The organic fluoride compound is rapidly conjugated to inert byproducts, a property that probably precludes covalent bonding to hepatic proteins,[143] a proposed mechanism for halothane hepatitis.

Peak plasma inorganic fluoride concentrations in nonobese patients after 1.4 MAC-hours of sevoflurane were 28 μmol/L, 1 hour after discontinuing anesthesia,[150] similar to the value obtained by Holaday and Smith[144] during initial human studies with sevoflurane. Similar plasma fluoride levels were obtained with obese patients, indicating that obese patients are at no greater risk for potential fluoride nephrotoxicity than nonobese individuals, after a short exposure to sevoflurane. Low blood solubility and rapid elimination may reduce the rate of fluoride production. After longer anesthetic administrations, however, obesity may be associated with fluoride levels near the threshold for renal toxicity. After 3.5 hours of anesthesia with sevoflurane, fluoride levels in obese patients were significantly higher than in nonobese controls. Peak serum fluoride was 52 μmol/L in obese patients, and levels exceeded 50 μmol/L for about 2 hours.[151] Animal studies indicate that sevoflurane may have less nephrotoxic potential than enflurane, however, even when animals were exposed to 10 MAC-hours of sevoflurane and enzyme inducers, which enhance hepatic metabolism of the anesthetic.[152] At present, it appears that sevoflurane may have about the same or slightly less potential for causing nephrotoxicity as enflurane, at least in nonobese patients and for anesthetic administrations of moderate duration.

Physiologic Effects

Central Nervous System

Unconsciousness may occur after five breaths with approximately 2% sevoflurane.[144] The EEG effects are similar to those of other potent inhaled agents. With increasing concentrations, one sees an increase in voltage and a decrease in frequency.[153] Higher concentrations produce burst suppression.

In rats, CBF increases by about 35% at 1.0 MAC.[154,155] In a study comparing the effects of sevoflurane, enflurane, and halothane on ICP, CPP, and MAP in hypocarbic dogs, enflurane and halothane caused small increases in ICP at 0.5 to 1.5 MAC, but no changes were seen with sevoflurane.[156] All three agents caused significant decreases in MAP and CPP, however. In the rabbit, the effects of sevoflurane on CBF, CMR_{O_2}, ICP, and the EEG are similar to those of isoflurane.[157]

In patients with cerebrovascular disease who were anesthetized with 1.5% sevoflurane (0.9 MAC in 33% nitrous oxide and 33% argon, used to determine CBF and CMR_{O_2}), CBF was 28 ml/100 g/min and CMR_{O_2} was 1.31

ml/100 g/min, at a Paco$_2$ of 40 mm Hg and a MAP of 90 mm Hg.[158] Reactivity of CBF to changes in Paco$_2$ was maintained, and autoregulation of CBF in response to changes in MAP was intact. These preliminary data suggest that sevoflurane should be suitable for neuroanesthesia.

Respiration

Sevoflurane at 1.4 MAC decreases tidal volume by about 60%, and respiratory rate approximately doubles.[159] Because the increased rate does not compensate for a decrease in tidal volume, minute ventilation falls by about 25% and Paco$_2$ rises to about 55 mm Hg. In comparison, respiratory rate increases more with halothane at 1.4 MAC, which tends to maintain a normal minute ventilation. At concentrations less than 1.4 MAC, however, sevoflurane appears to produce about the same amount of respiratory depression as halothane. Similar results were obtained by Kochi and colleagues,[160] except that the duration of inspiration and expiration were longer with sevoflurane than with halothane, suggesting slightly different effects of the two agents on the medullary respiratory center.

Cardiovascular System

In the chronically instrumented dog, cardiovascular hemodynamics with sevoflurane are similar to those seen with isoflurane.[161] At 1.2 and 2.0 MAC, sevoflurane produced an increase in heart rate of about 60%, a reduction in systemic vascular resistance of about 20%, and dose-related decreases in arterial blood pressure of 20 to 40% and stroke volume of 30 to 50%. Cardiac output was decreased only at 2.0 MAC, by about 20%. Coronary blood flow increased about 30%. Except for a slightly greater increase in heart rate with sevoflurane, hemodynamic changes were almost identical to those seen with isoflurane.

In a dose-response study in rats, hemodynamic variables were maintained similar to awake values at up to 1.5 MAC sevoflurane, except for a modest reduction in MAP of 12%.[154,155] Coronary blood flow was not altered. Similar results were obtained by Conzen and colleagues.[162]

In healthy patients, 1 MAC sevoflurane or isoflurane produces similar systolic and diastolic blood pressures, although heart rate following incision is faster with isoflurane than with sevoflurane (about 100 bpm versus 90 bpm, respectively).[13] In humans, sevoflurane appears to have fewer cardiac depressant effects than enflurane.[163]

The arrhythmogenic threshold of epinephrine with sevoflurane is midway between that of isoflurane and that of enflurane.[164] As with halothane and isoflurane, thiopental administration lowers the arrhythmogenic threshold of epinephrine with sevoflurane.[34,35]

Renal and Liver

Fluoride toxicity is a potential complication of sevoflurane anesthesia. The risk is probably about the same as with enflurane, at least in nonobese patients given anesthetic administrations of moderate duration.[150] At 1 MAC, renal blood flow did not change in rats, as determined by a microsphere technique.[154,155]

Patients submitted to prolonged sevoflurane anesthesia for orthopedic surgery have been tested for their urine concentrating ability. With the vasopressin test, the urinary osmolality averaged 700 to 800 mOsmol/kg. The concentrating ability was not impaired, and no evidence of subclinical nephrotoxicity was noted.[155a]

In the rat model, total hepatic blood flow was unchanged, although hepatic arterial flow increased by about 60% at 1.5 MAC.[154,155] In chronically instrumented dogs, sevoflurane at less than 2 MAC preserves hepatic arterial blood flow and oxygen delivery.[165] Effects on the hepatic circulation are similar to those seen with isoflurane.[166]

The principal metabolite of sevoflurane, hexafluoroisopropanol, is rapidly conjugated to inert compounds. Because of the rapid elimination, covalent bonding to liver macromolecules is unlikely.[143]

Neuromuscular Effects

Significant muscle relaxation occurs at moderate depths of anesthesia.[140] Following inhalation induction, laryngoscopy and endotracheal intubation can be accomplished without the aid of muscle relaxants.

METHOXYFLURANE

Essential Pharmacology

Methoxyflurane (Penthrane) is manufactured by Abbott Laboratories and is still available in the United States, although concerns about nephrotoxicity have eliminated its use as an anesthetic. It is still used as an analgesic, however, delivered by self-administration with an inhaler device, such as the Cyprane (Fluotec 4 vaporizer, Cyprane, England, distributed by Fraser Harlake, Orchard Park, NY) inhaler. More than 500 hospitals per year still purchase methoxyflurane for use as an inhaled analgesic, largely for obstetric use. The agent is also used by some hospice institutions, particularly for patients with AIDS. Methoxyflurane is especially attractive as an analgesic for terminally ill patients, because it can be administered without intravenous access to patients who are unable to take oral medications.

Toxicity associated with the use of methoxyflurane as an analgesic appears to be minimal, and adverse drug reactions have not been reported concerning its use as an analgesic. The United States Food and Drug Administration has required extensive labeling restrictions for methoxyflurane, however, restrictions that describe in detail the potential toxic side effects of the drug.

Methoxyflurane was synthesized by Larsen in 1958. Clinical development of the drug was due to the efforts of Van Poznak.[167]

Properties

Methoxyflurane (2-dichloro-1-difluoroethyl methyl ether) is a clear, colorless liquid with a fruity odor. Physicochemical properties are shown in Table 39–11. It is stable in soda lime but may undergo oxidation when exposed to air or light. Therefore, butylated hydroxy-

Table 39–11. Physicochemical Properties of Methoxyflurane

Chemical name: 2-dichloro-1-difluoroethyl methyl ether	
Structure	$CHCl_2CF_2$-O-CH_3
Molecular weight	165.0
Specific gravity (25°C)	1.411
Boiling point	104.6°C
Vapor pressure (mm Hg 20°C)	25 mmHg
Vapor/liquid (ml at 20°C)	204 ml
Partition coefficients (37°C)	
Oil/gas	825
Blood/gas	13.0
Water/gas	4.5
Flammability	Insignificant
Chemical stabilizer	Yes

toluene (0.01%) is added as an antioxidant, and the agent is stored in a light-resistant bottle. Methoxyflurane reacts with metals such as aluminum and brass, but usually, no deleterious effects of the liquid or vapor are noted on the stainless steel parts of the anesthesia machine. It is considered good practice to empty the vaporizer daily (the agent can be returned to its container), however. Polyethylene and polypropylene plastics are not affected, although polyvinyl plastics and pure gum rubber extract methoxyflurane.

The vapor concentration of methoxyflurane at room temperature is limited to about 3.5%, because of its low vapor pressure. This concentration is not readily achieved in practice, however, because of the cooling effect of vaporization. The vapor pressure and boiling point of methoxyflurane are similar to those of water, although the compound vaporizes 12 times as rapidly as water. Methoxyflurane does not burn at concentrations below 5% in oxygen, and it is not explosive at ordinary room temperatures.

Uptake by Rubber and Other Losses[168]

Uptake of methoxyflurane by rubber components of a breathing system influences the final concentration inspired by the patient. The partition coefficient of methoxyflurane in conductive rubber is about 650, which is one of the highest of all anesthetics. In closed-system anesthesia, losses to rubber may account for 50% of the delivered agent during the first 10 minutes, and it may take over an hour for equilibration to occur.

Absorption of methoxyflurane by soda lime is also rapid. Although moist soda lime is quickly saturated and the amount absorbed is relatively small, about 14 ml of vapor per 100 g of soda lime, dry soda lime may trap 100 ml of vapor per 100 g of absorbent. Thus, in the "jumbo" canister, as much as 1400 ml vapor (7 ml of liquid) may be absorbed. This process can delay induction inordinately.

The problem is partially overcome by employing baralyme, which has intrinsic water of crystallization. Water can, of course, be added to a soda lime canister to increase the moisture content of the lime; about 100 to 200 ml moisturizes each 1000 g of dry lime.

During recovery, the release of methoxyflurane by the machine components can provide sufficient agent to inspired air to maintain a state of unconsciousness. Recovery is thereby delayed.

Potency

Methoxyflurane is the most potent anesthetic agent available, with a MAC of 0.16% in oxygen. The administration of 60% nitrous oxide reduces the MAC of methoxyflurane by 56%.[169]

Administration

Demand flow methods of administration of methoxyflurane employ inhaler vaporizers such as the Cyprane inhaler and the Duke inhaler, which provide *analgesic* concentrations of the drug. As noted previously, methoxyflurane was commonly employed in obstetrics for self-administration, and this is still an approved use of the drug. Using the Duke inhaler with the setting "full on" and a respiratory minute volume of 8 L/min, a vapor concentration of 0.8% methoxyflurane is provided. In practice, intermittent inhalation of vapor concentrations in the range of 0.3 to 0.8% is recommended, and appropriate monitoring of the patient is necessary. Methoxyflurane is dispensed in 15-ml bottles, specifically for use with the inhaler devices. The usual dosage is limited to a single 15-ml charge of liquid methoxyflurane, and total dosage and time of exposure should conform to the limits determined for the agent when it is used as an anesthetic.

Although now largely of historical interest, techniques of administration of methoxyflurane for use as an anesthetic are worth reviewing. Semi-closed or partial rebreathing systems are satisfactory methods of administration. The agent may be used alone for induction. Because of its low vapor pressure and high blood solubility, however, 10 to 15 minutes may be required to attain surgical anesthesia. For these reasons, other anesthetics or supplements are needed to obtain rapid induction. In the days when methoxyflurane was widely used, the following methods were employed to hasten induction:

1. Nitrous-oxide-oxygen-methoxyflurane sequence.
2. Intravenous thiopental followed by methoxyflurane in oxygen or nitrous-oxide-oxygen mixture.
3. Induction with cyclopropane and then switch-over to nitrous-oxide-oxygen-methoxyflurane mixture.

A vapor concentration of 2.0 to 4.0% is needed to establish a blood concentration sufficient for surgical levels of anesthesia; that is, to quickly establish an alveolar concentration of about 0.2% in 2 to 4 minutes (Fig. 39–9).[170] These initial concentrations are best attained by introducing the methoxyflurane vapor into the breathing mixture by small increments of 0.5% as tolerated, to the desired induction concentration. When surgical anesthesia is established, the concentration of methoxyflurane is reduced and adjusted according to the patient's needs.

Absorption and Elimination

Partition coefficients for methoxyflurane are shown in Table 39–12. Methoxyflurane is extremely soluble in blood. The blood/gas solubility coefficient is 13.0, which

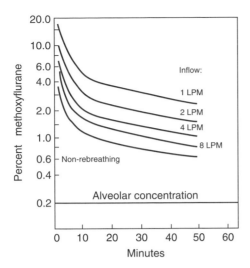

Fig. 39–9. Inflowing methoxyflurane concentration required to maintain the alveolar concentration at 0.2% at various flow rates.

Table 39–12. Partition Coefficients of Methoxyflurane

Blood/Gas	Brain/Blood	Muscle/Blood	Fat/Blood
13.0	2.0	1.3	49

From Eger, E. I., II: Anesthetic Uptake and Action. Baltimore. Williams & Wilkins, 1974.

is higher than any other anesthetic agent, including diethyl ether (which has a blood/gas coefficient of 12). Despite its low vapor pressure and the low concentration gradients achieved at anesthetic doses, a large fraction of the inspired methoxyflurane is removed by the blood. Because of its high blood solubility, however, the rate of rise in *alveolar* concentration of methoxyflurane is the slowest of all of the anesthetics (see Fig. 39–3).

The uptake of methoxyflurane in tissues is related to regional blood flow and tissue solubilities. Tissue/blood solubilities of methoxyflurane are slightly less than those of halothane. Because of the high blood solubility of methoxyflurane, however, absolute uptake of methoxyflurane by tissues is high, despite the low inspired concentrations used. The venous plasma concentration during light anesthesia (1 MAC) is about 15 mg/dl, which is similar to that for halothane, although methoxyflurane is 14 times more potent than halothane. As a result of tissue uptake, arterial concentrations of methoxyflurane are higher than venous concentrations during induction and early maintenance.[171]

Elimination of methoxyflurane occurs through the lungs, although a large fraction is metabolized and the products are excreted by the kidneys. An insignificant amount of unchanged drug is excreted in the urine. After discontinuing the anesthetic, pulmonary elimination is enhanced by promoting ventilation with oxygen or nitrous oxide-oxygen mixtures to wash out the agent. If pulmonary elimination is begun 15 to 30 minutes before the end of surgery, most patients regain their protective

reflexes by completion of the operation. Response to verbal stimuli may be delayed for 1 to 2 hours, however, depending on the duration of anesthesia and the technique. The odor of methoxyflurane may persist on the breath for many hours. Some investigators have claimed that the prolonged recovery reduces the need for postoperative analgesics.

Biotransformation

Methoxyflurane undergoes rapid and extensive metabolism, and 50 to 75% of absorbed methoxyflurane is metabolized in humans.[56,172] Among the metabolites identified are dichloroacetic acid and methoxydifluoroacetic acid. The final products are inorganic fluoride and oxalic acid. High serum and urinary inorganic fluoride levels and high urinary oxalic acid concentrations occur in *all* patients receiving methoxyflurane.[173]

Two principal P-450-dependent metabolic pathways have been proposed. First is initial ortho-demethylation, with cleavage of the methylether group. This results in defluorination, producing dichloroacetic acid. Second is initial dechlorination, and subsequent defluorination and hydrolysis to form oxalic acid.

After 3 to 4 hours of anesthesia, the uptake of methoxyflurane is largely by the fat compartment. This provides a postoperative pool of drug available for continued biotransformation and the production of organic and inorganic fluoride metabolites. Blood levels of methoxyflurane remain high during the postanesthesia period, and fluoride is greatly elevated on the first postoperative day.

Principal factors in the development of high blood fluoride are the dose of methoxyflurane and the duration of exposure. The anesthetic dose should be reported in MAC hours, that is, by multiplying the alveolar anesthetic concentration converted to MAC by the duration of anesthesia in hours. Studies have demonstrated that the total methoxyflurane dose should not exceed 2.0 to 2.5 MAC hours, if nephrotoxicity is to be avoided.

Phenobarbital induction enhances the rate of metabolism of methoxyflurane. In addition, a greater fraction of methoxyflurane is metabolized when the agent is administered in subanesthetic doses and during the recovery period when lower blood concentrations prevail. Indeed, metabolism of methoxyflurane accelerates the rate of decline of alveolar partial pressure.[56]

Physiologic Effects

Central Nervous System

A generalized and progressive descending depression of the CNS occurs. Based on the obtundation of the various reflexes, one can estimate the depth of anesthesia. Ocular changes of the classic sequence (Guedel) are not reliable as an index of anesthetic depth, however. This is consistent with the general observation that the ocular signs are variable even with the other agents such as ether and cyclopropane. With methoxyflurane, the pupils change little; slight dilatation of pupils may occur in stages I and II. During maintenance in stage III, the pupils remain constricted unless extreme doses are administered. When patients lose consciousness, their pupils become centered and fixed.

Electroencephalography

As soon as analgesia and light anesthesia are achieved, the EEG pattern is one of decreased voltage and an increased frequency of 16 to 20 cps.[174] During early surgical anesthesia, amplitude increases. Further deepening of anesthesia produces a spindle pattern with slight slowing of frequency to 14 to 16 cps. This is followed by a mixed pattern of slow waves (3 to 4 cps) of 50 to 75 μV superimposed on the basic pattern of fast frequency and low voltage. Deepening anesthesia further results in burst suppression.

Respiration

Methoxyflurane is only slightly irritating to the respiratory mucous membranes at concentrations up to 1.5%. During induction, the respiratory rate is slightly increased, whereas the tidal volume is full and regular, even in second-stage anesthesia. When surgical anesthetic levels are reached, respiratory minute volume is mildly reduced. At 2 MAC tidal volume is decreased by 50% and the respiratory rate increased by about 30%, however. Thus, minute ventilation is reduced by about the same degree as with halothane.[175] During spontaneous ventilation with methoxyflurane, the $Paco_2$ at 2 MAC is about 55 mm Hg.

Cardiovascular System

Some slowing of the heart rate may occur, especially in deeper planes of anesthesia. Generally, rate and rhythm are stable. Blood pressure and cardiac output are mildly reduced, on the order of 25%. Pulmonary vascular resistance does not change. At 1 MAC, contractility is reduced about 20%.[83]

Kidney

During methoxyflurane anesthesia, decreased urine output is common, although urine osmolarity and serum osmolarity usually do not change significantly.[177] After anesthesia, however, some patients may have increased production of dilute urine, and in some cases, a striking rise in blood urea nitrogen (BUN) and serum creatinine and hypernatremia can occur.[178,179] In addition, patients who receive tetracycline are at higher risk of developing renal failure.[180]

Renal failure following methoxyflurane anesthesia was first reported by Crandell in 1966.[181,182] In typical cases, surgery was longer than 2 hours in duration, often involving complicated bowel procedures. A serum fluoride level of 50 μmol/L is considered the threshold for subclinical toxicity, and serum fluoride levels above 80 μmol/L are associated with tubular injury. Contributing factors include preexisting renal disease, diabetes, drug interactions, enzyme inducers, other nephrotoxic drugs such as antibiotics (tetracycline, gentamicin, kanamycin), weaker nephrotoxins such as cephaloridine when combined with furosemide, and aortorenal surgery.

Methoxyflurane nephropathy is dose-related and appears to be caused by oxalic acid and fluoride.[183-185] The early phase of polyuria may be caused by fluoride, which inhibits sodium transport in the loop of Henle.[186,187] Permanent renal failure is attributed to the combined effects of oxalic acid and fluoride.[186,188]

In biopsy specimens, large numbers of oxalic acid crystals are noted in renal tubules and interstitium.[183,189] Tubular dilation and widening of the interstitium occur, but obvious tubular necrosis is absent, and glomeruli are intact. Similar morphologic changes can be produced by administration of large doses of oxalic acid to rats.[188] Oliguria and permanent renal damage appear to result from obstruction of tubules by oxalate crystals.

Liver

Retention of BSP occurs in the postoperative period and is maximal on the third to fifth day. The degree of retention is related to the duration of anesthesia. After operations over 4 hours in length, one may see 30 to 35% BSP retention by the fifth postoperative day.

Muscle Relaxation

A striking effect of methoxyflurane is the degree of skeletal muscle relaxation produced, even with light surgical anesthesia. Ngai and Hanks[190] suggested that this represents an effect on spinal cord reflexes.

Uterus

The strength of uterine contractions is not altered, and the rate and rhythm remain essentially unchanged. Hence, the agent is useful for analgesia in the first stage of labor, often self-administered by the patient. Methoxyflurane is still marketed for this purpose.

Placental Transfer

Methoxyflurane is rapidly transferred across the placenta. During labor analgesia, maternal arterial concentrations range from 2 to 9 mg/dl. Umbilical venous concentrations are between 50 and 70% of maternal concentrations, whereas umbilical arterial concentrations stabilize at 1.0 to 2.0 mg/dl. Thus, considerable amounts of methoxyflurane are taken up by fetal tissues.[191] Adverse effects on the fetus have not been demonstrated, however.

Disadvantages and Contraindications

Certain problems with methoxyflurane were recognized during the time when the agent was widely used as an anesthetic, including the slow rate of induction and prolonged recovery periods required. The most worrisome characteristic of methoxyflurane was its propensity to cause renal dysfunction, and in some cases renal failure, however. Therefore, preexisting renal disease, diabetes, and concomitant use of potentially nephrotoxic drugs were contraindications to the use of methoxyflurane. The following precautions should be observed with methoxyflurane: (1) limit the duration of high dose exposure; (2) use a maintenance concentration of inhaled agent of 0.2 to 0.4% after the first hour; (3) limit the total duration of anesthesia to 4 hours (no more than 2 to 2.5 MAC hours); (4) use accurate, calibrated flowmeters; and (5) do not use this agent in patients with renal disease or in patients undergoing urinary tract surgery.

Methoxyflurane is still occasionally used in the United States as an analgesic, mostly for obstetric use, and for this purpose it appears to be a safe drug. The low concentrations achieved and the intermittent nature of the exposure probably reduce the potential for toxicity. In addition, methoxyflurane is currently used by some hospice programs as an analgesic for terminally ill patients. The ability to administer a potent analgesic without the need for intravenous access, particularly in patients who are unable to take oral medications, makes methoxyflurane an attractive alternative to more traditional analgesics.

REFERENCES

1. Halsey, M. J.: A reassessment of the molecular structure-functional relationship of the inhaled general anaesthetics. Br J Anaesth 56:9S, 1984.
2. Leonard, P. F.: The lower limits of flammability of halothane, enflurane and isoflurane. Anesth Analg 54:238, 1975.
3. LeDez, K. M., Lerman, J.: The minimum alveolar concentration (MAC) of isoflurane in preterm neonates. Anesthesiology 67:301, 1987.
4. Stevens, W. C., et al.: Minimum alveolar concentrations (MAC) of isoflurane with and without nitrous oxide in patients of various ages. Anesthesiology 42:197, 1975.
5. Palahniuk, R. J., Shnider, S. M., Eger, E. I., II: Pregnancy decreases the requirement for inhaled anesthetic agents. Anesthesiology 41:82, 1974.
6. Loper, K., et al.: Comparison of halothane and isoflurane for rapid anesthetic induction. Anesth Analg 66:766, 1987.
7. Friesen, R. H., Lichtor, J. L.: Cardiovascular effects of inhalation induction with isoflurane in infants. Anesth Analg 62:411, 1983.
8. Lerman, J., et al.: Anesthetic requirements for halothane in young children 0-1 month and 1-6 months of age. Anesthesiology 59:421, 1983.
9. Eger, E. I., II: Anesthetic Uptake and Action. Baltimore, Williams & Wilkins, 1974.
10. Lerman, J., et al.: Effect of age on the solubility of volatile anesthetics in human tissues. Anesthesiology 65:307, 1986.
11. Eger, E. I., II: Isoflurane: a review. Anesthesiology 55:559, 1981.
12. Yasuda, N., et al.: Comparison of kinetics of sevoflurane and isoflurane in humans. Anesth Analg 72:316, 1991.
13. Frink, E. J., et al.: Clinical comparison of sevoflurane and isoflurane in healthy patients. Anesth Analg 74:241, 1992.
14. Davison, L. A., et al.: Psychological effects of halothane and isoflurane anesthesia. Anesthesiology 43:313, 1975.
15. Mazze, R. I., Cousins, M. J., Barr, G. A.: Renal effects and metabolism of isoflurane in man. Anesthesiology 40:536, 1974.
16. Strube, P. J., Hulands, G. H., Halsey, M. J.: Serum fluoride levels in morbidly obese patients: enflurane compared with isoflurane anaesthesia. Anaesthesia 42:685, 1987.
17. Eger, E. I., II, Stevens, W. C., Cromwell, T. H.: The electroencephalogram in man anesthetized with Forane. Anesthesiology 35:504, 1971.
18. Newman, B., Gelb, A. W., Lam, A. M.: The effect of isoflurane-induced hypotension on cerebral blood flow and cerebral metabolic rate for oxygen in humans. Anesthesiology 64:307, 1986.
19. Newberg, L. A., Milde, J. H., Michenfelder, J. D.: The cerebral metabolic effects of isoflurane at and above concentrations that suppress cortical electrical activity. Anesthesiology 59:23, 1983.
20. Newberg, L. A., Michenfelder, J. D.: Cerebral protection by isoflurane during hypoxemia or ischemia. Anesthesiology 59:29, 1983.
21. Stullken, E. H., Jr., Milde, J. H., Michenfelder, J. D., Tinker, J.H.: The nonlinear responses of cerebral metabolism to low concentrations of halothane, enflurane, and thiopental. Anesthesiology 46:28, 1977.
22. Cucchiara, R. F., Theye, R. A., Michenfelder, J. D.: The effects of isoflurane on canine cerebral metabolism and blood flow. Anesthesiology 40:571, 1974.
23. Sundt, T. M., Jr., et al.: Correlation of cerebral blood flow and electroencephalographic changes during carotid endarterectomy with results of surgery and hemodynamics of cerebral ischemia. Mayo Clin Proc 56:533, 1981.
24. Miletich, D. J., et al.: Absence of autoregulation of cerebral blood flow during halothane and enflurane anesthesia. Anesth Analg 55:100, 1976.
25. Madsen, J. B., Cold, G. E., Hansen, E. S., Bardrum, B.: The effect of isoflurane on cerebral blood flow and metabolism in humans during craniotomy for small supratentorial cerebral tumors. Anesthesiology 66:332, 1987.
26. Adams, R. W., et al.: Isoflurane and cerebrospinal fluid pressure in neurosurgical patients. Anesthesiology 54:97, 1981.
27. Messick, J. M., Jr., et al.: Correlation of regional cerebral blood flow (rCBF) with EEG changes during isoflurane anesthesia for carotid endarterectomy: critical rCBF. Anesthesiology 66:433, 1987.
28. Sharbrough, F. W., Messick, J. M., Jr., Sundt, T. M.: Correlation of continuous electroencephalograms with cerebral blood flow measurements during carotid endarterectomy. Stroke 4:674, 1973.
29. Eger, E. I., II, et al.: Surgical stimulation antagonizes the respiratory depression produced by Forane. Anesthesiology 36:544, 1972.
30. Hickey, R. F., et al.: The effects of ether, halothane and Forane on apneic thresholds in man. Anesthesiology 35:32, 1971.
31. Alagesan, K., Nunn, J. F., Feeley, T. W., Heneghan, C. P. H.: Comparison of the respiratory depressant effects of halothane and isoflurane in routine surgery. Br J Anaesth 59:1070, 1987.
32. Moore, M. A., et al.: Arrhythmogenic doses of epinephrine are similar during desflurane or isoflurane anesthesia in humans. Anesthesiology 79:943, 1993.
33. Johnston, R. R., Eger, E. I., II, Wilson, C. L.: A comparative interaction of epinephrine with enflurane, isoflurane and halothane in man. Anesth Analg 55:709, 1976.
34. Atlee, J. L., Malkinson, C. E.: Potentiation by thiopental of halothane-epinephrine-induced arrhythmias in dogs. Anesthesiology 57:285, 1982.
35. Atlee, J. L., Robert, F. L.: Thiopental and epinephrine-induced dysrhythmias in dogs anesthetized with enflurane or isoflurane. Anesth Analg 65:437, 1986.
36. Reiz, S., et al.: Isoflurane: a powerful coronary vasodilator in patients with coronary artery disease. Anesthesiology 59:91, 1983.
37. Sill, J. C., et al.: Effects of isoflurane on coronary arteries and coronary arterioles in the intact dog. Anesthesiology 66:273, 1987.
38. Brown, B. G., et al.: Intravenous dipyridamole combined with isometric handgrip for near maximal acute increase in coronary flow in patients with coronary artery disease. Am J Cardiol 48:1077, 1981.

39. Brown, B. G., Bolson, E. L., Dodge, H. T.: Dynamic mechanisms in human coronary stenosis. Circulation 70:917, 1984.

40. Priebe, H. J., Foex, P.: Isoflurane causes regional myocardial dysfunction in dogs with critical coronary artery stenosis. Anesthesiology 66:280, 1987.

41. Buffington, C. W., et al.: Isoflurane induces coronary steal in a canine model of chronic coronary occlusion. Anesthesiology 66:280, 1987.

42. Becker, L. C.: Is isoflurane dangerous for the patient with coronary artery disease? (Editorial.) Anesthesiology 66:259, 1987.

43. Hartman, J. C., Kampine, J. P., Schmeling, W. T., Warltier, D. C.: Alterations in collateral blood flow produced by isoflurane in a chronically instrumented canine model of multivessel coronary artery disease. Anesthesiology 74:120, 1991.

44. Kemmotsu, O., Hashimoto, Y., Shimosato, S.: Inotropic effects of isoflurane on mechanisms of contraction in isolated papillary muscles from normal and failing hearts. Anesthesiology 39:470, 1973.

45. Priebe, H. J.: Differential effects of isoflurane on right and left ventricular performances, and on coronary, systemic, and pulmonary hemodynamics in the dog. Anesthesiology 66:262, 1987.

46. Stevens, W. C., et al.: The cardiovascular effects of a new inhalation anesthetic, Forane, in human volunteers at constant arterial carbon dioxide tension. Anesthesiology 35:8, 1971.

47. Stoelting, R. K., Blitt, C. D., Cohen, P. J., Merin, R. G.: Hepatic dysfunction after isoflurane anesthesia. Anesth Analg 66:147, 1987.

48. Miller, R. D., et al.: Comparative neuromuscular effects of Forane and halothane alone and in combination with d-tubocurarine in man. Anesthesiology 35:38, 1971.

49. Gion, H., Saidman, L. J.: The minimum alveolar concentration of enflurane in man. Anesthesiology 35:361, 1971.

50. Torri, G., Damia, G., Fabiani, M. L.: Effect of nitrous oxide on the anesthetic requirement of enflurane. Br J Anaesth 46:468, 1974.

51. Helrich, M., Cascorbi, H. F.: Crossover study of Ethrane and halothane in volunteers. Anesthesiology 31:370, 1969.

52. Borel, J. D., Bentley, J. B., Vaughan, R. W., Gandolfi, A. F.: Enflurane blood-gas solubility: influence of weight and hemoglobin. Anesth Analg 61:1006, 1982.

53. Padfield, A.: Recovery comparison between enflurane and halothane techniques. Anaesthesia 35:508, 1980.

54. Storms, L. H., et al.: Psychologic functioning after halothane or enflurane anesthesia. Anesth Analg 59:245, 1980.

55. Chase, R. E., et al.: The biotransformation of Ethrane in man. Anesthesiology 35:262, 1971.

56. Carpenter, R. L., et al.: The extent of metabolism of inhaled anesthetics in humans. Anesthesiology 65:201, 1986.

57. Burke, T. R. J., Branchflower, R. V., Lees, D. E., Pohl, L. R.: Mechanisms of defluorination of enflurane: identification of an organic metabolite in rat and man. Drug Metab Dispos Biol Fate Chem 9:19, 1981.

58. Cousins, M. J., Greenstein, L. R., Hitt, B. A., Mazze, R. I.: Metabolism and renal effects of enflurane in man. Anesthesiology 44:44, 1976.

59. Maduska, A. L.: Serum inorganic fluoride levels in patients receiving enflurane anesthesia. Anesth Analg 53:351, 1974.

60. Jarnberg, P. O., et al.: Renal fluoride excretion during and after enflurane anaesthesia: dependency on urinary pH. Acta Anaesthesiol Scand 24:129, 1980.

61. Strube, P. J., Hulands, G. H., Halsey, M. J.: Serum fluoride levels in morbidly obese patients: enflurane compared with isoflurane anaesthesia. Anaesthesia 42:685, 1987.

62. Sargent, E. T.: Metabolism of fluorides in man. Arch Indust Health 24:318, 1960.

63. Carter, R., Heerdt, M., Acchiarb, G.: Fluoride kinetics after enflurane anesthesia in healthy patients and in patients with poor renal function. Clin Pharmacol Ther 20:565, 1976.

64. Rice, S. A., Talcott, R. E.: Effects of isoniazide treatment on selected hepatic mixed function oxidases. Drug Metab Dispos Biol Fate Chem 7:260, 1979.

65. Wollman, H., Smith, A. L., Hoffman, J. C.: Cerebral blood flow and oxygen consumption in man during electroencephalographic seizure patterns induced by anesthesia with Ethrane. Fed Proc 28:356, 1969.

66. Hoscik, E. C., Clark, D. L., Adam, N., Rosner, B. S.: Neurophysiological effects of different anesthetics in conscious man. J Appl Physiol 31:892, 1971.

67. Bart, A. J., Homi, J., Linde, H. W.: Changes in power spectra of electroencephalograms during anesthesia with Ethrane, fluroxene and methoxyflurane. Anesth Analg 50:53, 1971.

68. Sprague, D. H., Wolf, S.: Enflurane seizures in patients taking amitriptyline. Anesth Analg 61:67, 1982.

69. Opitz, A., Oberwetter, D.: Enflurane of halothane anaesthesia for patients with cerebral convulsive disorders? Acta Anaesthesiol Scand Suppl 71:43, 1979.

70. Neigh, J. L., Garman, J. K., Harp, J. R.: The electroencephalographic pattern during anesthesia with Ethrane. Anesthesiology 35:482, 1971.

71. Castro, A. D., Smith, R. E., Neigh, J. L.: The effects of IV diazepam on enflurane-induced CNS excitation. In Abstracts of the Annual Meeting of the American Society of Anesthesiologists. New Orleans, American Society of Anesthesiologists, 1977, p. 272.

72. Oshima, E., Urabe, N., Shingu, K., Mori, K.: Anticonvulsant actions of enflurane on epilepsy models in cats. Anesthesiology 63:29, 1985.

73. Rolly, G., Van Aken, J.: Influence of enflurane on cerebral blood flow in man. Acta Anaesthesiol Scand Suppl 71:59, 1979.

74. Sakabe, T., et al.: Cerebral circulation and metabolism during enflurane anesthesia in humans. Anesthesiology 59:532, 1983.

75. Gallagher, T. J., Galindo, A., Richey, E. T.: Inhibition of seizure activity during enflurane anesthesia. Anesth Analg 57:130, 1978.

76. Artru, A. A., Nugent, M., Michenfelder, J. D.: Enflurane causes a prolonged and reversible increase in the rate of CSF production. Anesthesiology 57:255, 1982.

77. Moss, E., Dearden, N. M., McDowell, D. G.: Effects of 2% enflurane on intracranial pressure and on cerebral perfusion pressure. Br J Anaesth 55:1083, 1983.

78. Michenfelder, J. D., Sundt, T. M., Fode, N., Sharbrough, F. W.: Isoflurane when compared to enflurane and halothane decreases the frequency of cerebral ischemia during carotid endarterectomy. Anesthesiology 67:336, 1987.

79. Knill, R. L., Clement, J. L.: Variable effects of anaesthetics on the ventilatory response to hypoxemia in man. Can Anaesth Soc J 29:93, 1982.

80. Lehane, J. R., Jordan, C., Jones, J. G.: Influence of halothane and enflurane on respiratory airflow resistance and specific conductance in man. Br J Anaesth 52:773, 1980.

81. Etsten, B. E., Sugai, N., Iwatsuki, N., Shimosato, S.: Effect

of Ethrane on cardiac muscle mechanics. Anesthesiology *30:*513, 1969.

82. Jwatsuk, N., Shimosato, S., Etsten, B. E.: The effects of changes in time interval of stimulation on mechanics of isolated heart muscle and its response to Ethrane. Anesthesiology *32:*11, 1970.

83. Brown, B. R. Jr., Crout, J. R.: A comparative study of the effects of five general anesthetics on myocardial contractility. Anesthesiology *34:*236, 1971.

84. Marshall, B. E., et al.: Some pulmonary and cardiovascular effects of enflurane (Ethrane) anesthesia with varying Paco$_2$ in man. Br J Anaesth *43:*996, 1971.

85. Levesque, P. R., Nanagas, V., Shanks, C., Shimosato, S.: Circulatory effects of enflurane in normocapnic human volunteers. Can Anaesth Soc J *21:*580, 1974.

86. Christensen, V., Sorensen, M. B., Klauber, P. V., Skovsted, P.: Haemodynamic effects of enflurane in patients with valvular heart disease. Acta Anaesthesiol Scand Suppl *67:*34, 1978.

87. Doblin, A. B., et al.: Clinical and laboratory evaluation of a new inhalation agent: compound 347. Anesthesiology *29:*275, 1968.

88. Botty, C., Brown, B., Stanley, V., Stephen, C. R.: Clinical experiences with compound 347, a halogenated anesthetic agent. Anesth Analg *47:*499, 1968.

89. Atlee, J. L., Rusy, B. F.: Atrioventricular conduction times and atrioventricular nodal conductivity during enflurane anesthesia in dogs. Anesthesiology *47:*498, 1977.

90. Lebowitz, M. H., Blitt, C. D., Dillon, J. B.: Clinical investigation of compound 347. Anesth Analg *49:*1, 1970.

91. Reiz, S., Rydvall, A., Haggmark, S.: Coronary haemodynamic effects of surgery during enflurane-nitrous oxide anaesthesia in patients with ischemic heart disease. Acta Anaesthesiol Scand *29:*106, 1985.

92. Calverley, R. K., et al.: Cardiovascular effects of enflurane anesthesia during controlled ventilation in man. Anesth Analg *57:*619, 1978.

93. Skovsted, P., Price, H. L.: The effects of Ethrane on arterial pressure, preganglionic sympathetic activity, and barostatic reflexes. Anesthesiology *36:*257, 1972.

94. Novelli, G. P.: Effects of enflurane and halothane on the microcirculation. Acta Anaesth Scand Suppl *71:*59, 1979.

95. Gothert, M., Wendt, J.: Inhibition of adrenal medullary catecholamine secretion. I. Investigations in vivo. Anesthesiology *46:*400, 1977.

96. Eger, E. I., II, Calverley, R. K., Smith, N. T.: Changes in blood chemistry following prolonged enflurane anesthesia. Anesth Analg *55:*547, 1976.

97. Fee, J. P. H., et al.: A prospective study of liver enzymes and other changes following repeat administration of halothane and enflurane. Br J Anaesth *51:*1133, 1979.

98. Brown, B. R., Jr., Gandolfi, A. J.: Adverse effects of volatile anaesthetics. Br J Anaesth *59:*14, 1987.

99. Elliot, R. H., Strunin, L.: Hepatotoxicity of volatile anaesthetics. Br J Anaesth *70:*339, 1993.

100. Eger, E. I., II, et al.: Is enflurane hepatotoxic? Anesth Analg *65:*21, 1986.

101. Stevens, C. E., et al.: Hepatitis B virus antibody in blood donors and the occurrence of non-A, non-B hepatitis in transfusion recipients. Ann Intern Med *101:*733, 1984.

102. Christ, D. D., et al.: Enflurane metabolism produces covalently bound liver adducts recognized by antibodies from patients with halothane hepatitis. Anesthesiology *69:*833, 1988.

103. Waud, B. E., Waud, D. R.: Effects of volatile anesthetics on directly and indirectly stimulated skeletal muscle. Anesthesiology *53:*103, 1979.

104. Lebowitz, M. H., Blitt, C. D., Walts, L. F.: Depression of twitch response to stimulation of the ulnar nerve during Ethrane anesthesia in man. Anesthesiology *33:*52, 1970.

105. Eger, E. I., II: Partition coefficients of I-653 in human blood, saline, and olive oil. Anesth Analg *66:*971, 1987.

106. Rampil, I. J., et al.: Clinical characteristics of desflurane in surgical patients: minimum alveolar concentration. Anesthesiology *74:*429, 1991.

107. Taylor, R. H., Lerman, J.: Minimum alveolar concentration of desflurane and hemodynamic responses in neonates, infants, and children. Anesthesiology *75:*975, 1991.

108. Jones, R. M., et al.: Kinetics and potency of desflurane (I-653) in volunteers. Anesth Analg *70:*3, 1990.

109. Stoelting, R. K., Longnecker, D. E., Eger, E. I., II: Mimimum alveolar concentrations in man on awakening from methyoxyflurane, halothane, ether and fluroxene anesthesia: MAC awake. Anesthesiology *33:*5, 1970.

110. Hemelrijck, J. V., Smith, I., White, P. F.: Use of desflurane for outpatient anesthesia: a comparison with propofol and nitrous oxide. Anesthesiology *75:*197, 1991.

111. Zwass, M. S., et al.: Induction and maintenance characteristics of anesthesia with desflurane and nitrous oxide in infants and children. Anesthesiology *76:*373, 1992.

112. Yasuda, N., et al.: Kinetics of desflurane, isoflurane, and halothane in humans. Anesthesiology *74:*489, 1991.

113. Yasuda, N., et al.: Comparison of kinetics of sevoflurane and isoflurane in humans. Anesth Analg *72:*316, 1991.

114. Eger, E. I., II: Desflurane animal and human pharmacology: aspects of kinetics, safety, and MAC. Anesth Analg *75:*S3, 1992.

115. Fletcher, J. E., et al.: Psychomotor performance after desflurane anesthesia: a comparison with isoflurane. Anesth Analg *73:*260, 1991.

116. Smiley, R. M., et al.: Desflurane and isoflurane in surgical patients: comparison of emergence time. Anesthesiology *74:*425, 1991.

117. Ghouri, A. F., Bodner, M., White, P. F.: Recovery profile after desflurane-nitrous oxide versus isoflurane-nitrous oxide in outpatients. Anesthesiology *74:*419, 1991.

118. Eger, E. I., II: Stability of I-653 in soda lime. Anesth Analg *66:*983, 1987.

119. Sutton, T. S., et al.: Fluoride metabolites after prolonged exposure of volunteers and patients to desflurane. Anesth Analg *73:*180, 1991.

120. Bentley, J. B., Vaughan, R. W., Gandolfi, A. J., Cork, R. C.: Halothane biotransformation in obese and nonobese patients. Anesthesiology *57:*94, 1982.

121. Rampil, I. J., et al.: The electro-encephalographic effects of desflurane in humans. Anesthesiology *74:*434, 1991.

122. Lutz, L. J., Milde, J. H., Milde, L. N.: The cerebral functional, metabolic, and hemodynamic effects of desflurane in dogs. Anesthesiology *73:*125, 1990.

123. Lutz, L. J., Milde, J. H., Milde, L. N.: The response of the canine cerebral circulation to hyperventilation during anesthesia with desflurane. Anesthesiology *74:*504, 1991.

124. Ornstein, E., Young, W. L., Fleischer, L. H., Ostapkovich, N.: Desflurane and isoflurane have similar effects on cerebral blood flow in patients with intracranial mass lesions. Anesthesiology *79:*498, 1993.

125. Muzzi, D. A., et al.: The effect of desflurane and isoflurane on cerebrospinal fluid pressure in humans with supratentorial mass lesions. Anesthesiology *76:*720, 1992.

126. Lockhart, S. H., et al.: Depression of ventilation by desflurane in humans. Anesthesiology *74:*484, 1991.

127. Weiskopf, R. B., et al.: Cardiovascular actions of desflurane in normocarbic volunteers. Anesth Analg *73:*143, 1991.

128. Cahalan, M. K., et al.: Hemodynamic effects of desflu-

rane/nitrous oxide anesthesia in volunteers. Anesth Analg 73:157, 1991.

129. Ebert, T. J., Muzi, M.: Sympathetic hyperactivity during desflurane anesthesia in healthy volunteers: a comparison with isoflurane. Anesthesiology 79:444, 1993.

130. Helman, J. D., et al.: The risk of myocardial ischemia in patients receiving desflurane versus sufentanil anesthesia for coronary artery bypass graft surgery. Anesthesiology 77:47, 1992.

131. Hartman, J. C., et al.: Influence of desflurane on regional distribution of coronary blood flow in a chronically instrumented canine model of multivessel coronary artery obstruction. Anesth Analg 72:289, 1991.

132. Yasuda, N., et al.: Does desflurane modify circulatory responses to stimulation in humans? Anesth Analg 73:175, 1991.

133. Merin, R. G., et al.: Comparison of the effects of isoflurane and desflurane on cardiovascular dynamics and regional blood flow in the chronically instrumented dog. Anesthesiology 74:568, 1991.

134. Caldwell, J. E., et al.: The neuromuscular effects of desflurane, alone and combined with pancuronium or succinylcholine in humans. Anesthesiology 74:412, 1991.

135. Effect of Desflurane on Doses of Muscle Relaxants. Madison, WI, Ohmeda Pharmaceutical Products Division, 1992.

136. Wallin, R. F., Regan, B. M., Napoli, M. D., Stern, I. J.: Sevoflurane: a new inhalational anesthetic agent. Anesth Analg 54:758, 1975.

137. Morio, M., Fujii, K., Satoh, N.: The safety of sevoflurane in humans: I. (letter) Anesthesiology 79:200, 1993.

138. Malviya, S., Lerman, J.: The blood/gas solubilities of sevoflurane, isoflurane, halothane, and serum constituents concentrations in neonates and adults. Anesthesiology 72:793, 1990.

139. Terrell, R. C.: Physical and chemical properties of anaesthetic agents. Br J Anaesth 56:3S, 1984.

140. Katoh, T., Ikeda, K.: The minimum alveolar concentration (MAC) of sevoflurane in humans. Anesthesiology 66:301, 1987.

141. Scheller, M. S., Saidman, L. J., Partridge, B. L.: MAC of sevoflurane in humans and the New Zealand white rabbit. Can J Anaesth 35:153, 1988.

142. Katoh, T., Suguro, Y., Kimura, T., Ikeda, K.: Cerebral awakening concentration of sevoflurane and isoflurane predicted during slow and fast alveolar washout. Anesth Analg 77:1012, 1993.

143. Brown, B. R. Jr., Frink, E. J.: Whatever happened to sevoflurane? (Editorial.) Can J Anaesth 39:207, 1992.

144. Holaday, D. A., Smith, F. R.: Clinical characteristics and biotransformation of sevoflurane in healthy human volunteers. Anesthesiology 54:100, 1981.

145. Morio, M., et al.: Reaction of sevoflurane and its degradation products with soda lime. Anesthesiology 77:1155, 1992.

146. Frink, E. J., et al.: Quantification of the degradation products of sevoflurane in two CO_2 absorbents during low-flow anesthesia in surgical patients. Anesthesiology 77:1064, 1992.

147. Strum, D. P., et al.: Toxicity of sevoflurane in rats. Anesth Analg 66:769, 1987.

148. Sharp, J. H., Trudel, J. R., Cohen, E. N.: Volatile metabolites and decomposition products of halothane in man. Anesthesiology 50:2, 1979.

149. Brown, B. R., Jr., Frink, E. J.: The safety of sevoflurane in humans: II. (Editorial.) Anesthesiology 79:201, 1993.

150. Frink, E. J., et al.: Plasm inorganic fluoride levels with

sevoflurane anesthesia in morbidly obese and nonobese patients. Anesth Analg 76:1333, 1993.

151. Higuchi, H., et al.: Serum inorganic fluoride levels in mildly obese patients during and after sevoflurane anesthesia. Anesth Analg 77:1018, 1993.

152. Malan, T. P., et al.: Renal function after sevoflurane or enflurane anesthesia in the Fischer 344 rat. Anesth Analg 77:817, 1993.

153. Avramov, M. N., et al.: Effects of different speeds of induction with sevoflurane on the EEG in man. J Anaesth 1:1, 1987.

154. Crawford, M. W., Lerman, J., Saldivia, V., Carmichael, F.J.: Hemodynamic and organ blood flow responses to halothane and sevoflurane anesthesia during spontaneous ventilation. Anesth Analg 75:1000, 1992.

155. Crawford, M. W., Lerman, J., Pilato, M., Orrego, H.: Haemodynamic and organ blood flow responses to sevoflurane during spontaneous ventilation in the rat: a dose-response study. Can J Anaesth 39:270, 1992.

155a. Higuchi, H.: Urinary concentrating ability after prolonged servoflurane anesthesia. Br J Anaesth 73:239, 1994.

156. Takahashi, H., Murata, K., Ikeda, K.: Sevoflurane does not increase intracranial pressure in hyperventilated dogs. Br J Anaesth 71:551, 1993.

157. Scheller, M. S., Tateishi, A., Drummond, J. C., Zornow, M. H.: The effects of sevoflurane on cerebral blood flow, cerebral metabolic rate for oxygen, intracranial pressure, and the electroencephalogram are similar to those of isoflurane in the rabbit. Anesthesiology 68:548, 1988.

158. Kitaguchi, K., et al.: Effects of sevoflurane on cerebral circulation and metabolism in patients with ischemic cerebrovascular disease. Anesthesiology 79:704, 1993.

159. Doi, M., Ikeda, K.: Respiratory effects of sevoflurane. Anesth Analg 66:241, 1987.

160. Kochi, T., et al.: Breathing pattern and occlusion pressure waveform in humans anesthetized with halothane or sevoflurane. Anesth Analg 73:327, 1991.

161. Bernard, J. M., et al.: Effects of sevoflurane and isoflurane on cardiac and coronary dynamics in chronically instrumented dogs. Anesthesiology 72:659, 1990.

162. Conzen, P. F., et al.: Systemic and regional hemodynamics of isoflurane and sevoflurane in rats. Anesth Analg 74:79, 1992.

163. Kikura, M., Ikeda, K.: Comparison of effects of sevoflurane/nitrous oxide and enflurane/nitrous oxide on myocardial contractility in humans. Load-independent and noninvasive assessment with transesophageal echocardiography. Anesthesiology 79:235, 1993.

164. Hayashi, Y., et al.: Arrhythmogenic threshold of epinephrine during sevoflurane, enflurane, and isoflurane anesthesia in dogs (letter). Anesthesiology 69:145, 1988.

165. Frink, E. J., et al.: The effects of sevoflurane, halothane, enflurane, and isoflurane on hepatic blood flow and oxygenation in chronically intrumented greyhound dogs. Anesthesiology 76:85, 1992.

166. Bernard, J. M., et al.: Effects of sevoflurane and isoflurane on hepatic circulation in the chronically instrumented dog. Anesthesiology 77:541, 1992.

167. Van Poznak, A.: Clinical administration of methyoxyflurane. Clin Anesth 1:105, 1962.

168. Eger, E. I., II, Brandstater, B.: Solubility of methoxyflurane in rubber. Anesthesiology 24:679, 1963.

169. Stoelting, R. K.: Effect of nitrous oxide on mimumum alveolar concentration of methoxyflurane needed for anesthesia. Anesthesiology 34:353, 1971.

170. Eger, E. I., II: Uptake of methoxyflurane in man at constant

alveolar and at constant inspired concentration. Anesthesiology 25:284, 1964.

171. Chenoweth, M. B., Robertson, D. N., Erley, D. S., Golhke, R.: Blood and tissue levels of ether, chloroform, halothane and methoxyflurane in dogs. Anesthesiology 23:101, 1962.

172. Sakai, T., Takaori, M.: Biodegradation of halothane, enflurane, and methoxyflurane. Br J Anaesth 50:785, 1978.

173. Holaday, D. A., Rudofsky, S., Treuhalf, P. S.: The metabolic degradation of methoxyflurane in man. Anesthesiology 33:579, 1970.

174. Campbell, M. W., Hvolboll, A. P., Brechner, V. L.: Penthrane: a clinical evaluation of 50 cases. Anesth Analg 41:134, 1962.

175. Larson, C. P., et al.: The effects of diethyl ether and methoxyflurane on ventilation. Anesthesiology 30:174, 1969.

176. Dobkin, A. B., Fedoruk, S.: Comparison of the cardiovascular, respiratory and metabolic effects of methoxyflurane and halothane in dogs. Anesthesiology 22:355, 1961.

177. Austin, L. M., Villandy, P. J.: Methoxyflurane and renal function. Anesthesiology 28:637, 1967.

178. Pezzi, P. J., Frobese, A. S., Greenberg, S. R.: Methoxyflurane and renal toxicity. Lancet 1:823, 1966.

179. Mazze, R. I., Shue, G. L., Jackson, S. H.: Renal dysfunction associated with methoxyflurane anesthesia: a randomized prospective clinical evaluation. JAMA 216:278, 1971.

180. Kuzucu, E. Y.: Methoxyflurane, tetracycline and renal failure. JAMA 211:1162, 1970.

181. Crandell, W. B., Pappas, S. G., Macdonald, A.: Nephrotoxicity associated with methoxyflurane anesthesia. Anesthesiology 27:591, 1966.

182. Crandell, W. B.: Nephropathy associated with methoxyflurane anesthesia. JAMA 205:798, 1968.

183. Frascino, J. A., Vanamee, P., Rosen, P. P.: Renal oxalosis and azotemia after methoxyflurane anesthesia. N Engl J Med 283:676, 1970.

184. Hollenberg, N. K., et al.: Irreversible acute oliguric renal failure: a complication of methoxyflurane anesthesia. N Engl J Med 286:877, 1972.

185. Hook, J. B.: Fluoride and methoxyflurane nephropathy. Anesthesiology 35:238, 1971.

186. Cousins, M. J., Mazze, R. I.: Methoxyflurane nephrotoxicity: a study of dose response in man. JAMA 225:1611, 1973.

187. Whitford, G. M., Taves, D. R.: Fluoride-induced diuresis: renal tissue solute concentrations, functional, hemodynamic and histological correlates in the rat. Anesthesiology 39:416, 1973.

188. Cousins, M. J., et al.: The etiology of methoxyflurane nephrotoxicity. J Pharmacol Exp Ther 190:530, 1974.

189. Panner, B. J., Freeman, R. B., Roth-Mayo, L. A., Markowitch, W.: Toxicity following methoxyflurane anesthesia. I. Clinical and pathological observations in two fatal cases. JAMA 214:86, 1970.

190. Ngai, S. H., Hanks, E. C.: Effect of methoxyflurane on electromyogram, neuromuscular transmission and spinal reflex. Anesthesiology 23:158, 1962.

191. Siker, E. S., Wolfson, B., Dubnansky, J., Fitting, G. M. J.: Placental transfer of methoxyflurane. Br J Anaesth 40:588, 1968.

Chapter 40

PHARMACOLOGY OF INORGANIC GAS ANESTHETICS

MARK V. BOSWELL
VINCENT J. COLLINS

NITROUS OXIDE

Essential Pharmacology

Soon after the discovery of nitrous oxide (dinitrogen monoxide, N_2O) by Joseph Priestley in 1772, Sir Humphry Davy recognized that it was capable of relieving physical pain and suggested that it be used to alleviate the pain of surgical procedures.[1] Not until December 1844, however, was the gas used for this purpose. At that time, an itinerant chemist lecturer, Gardner Quincy Colton, visited Hartford, Connecticut, and put on a public demonstration of nitrous oxide or laughing gas. Among those attending was Horace Wells, a dentist. In the course of the demonstration, a man who had just inhaled nitrous oxide ran into a bench and lacerated his leg, but apparently felt no pain. Wells thereupon asked Colton to give him nitrous oxide on the following day, for the extraction of one of his own teeth. Colton consented, and the result was successful, Wells stating that the operation was painless.[2]

Later, Wells put on a demonstration at Massachusetts General Hospital. For technical reasons it failed, however, and Wells was ridiculed. Not until 1868, when Edmund Andrews, a surgeon in Chicago, introduced oxygen with nitrous oxide was it again seen as useful. Methods of storage and administration were worked out by Andrews, who found that nitrous oxide could be stored as a liquid under pressure and delivered as a gas for anesthesia. At about the same time, Paul Bert of Paris demonstrated that hyperbaric administration (2 atm) was also effective, which provided both sufficient anesthetic and adequate oxygen.[3] Because of its clinical characteristics, nitrous oxide remains widely used today.

Physicochemical Properties[4] (Table 40–1)

Nitrous oxide is a colorless, inert gas with a slightly sweet taste and odor. The density of the gas is 1.5 times that of air. Ordinarily, nitrous oxide is stored as a liquid and gas in pressurized cylinders. Its critical temperature is 36.5°C (97.7°F), however, and so when environmental temperatures exceed this temperature, at any pressure it is entirely a gas.

Nitrous oxide is prepared from ammonium nitrate crystals at high temperature. The crystals are first heated at 190°C until liquified and then further heated to 240°C, whereupon nitrous oxide and other gaseous compounds are released. Conditions are carefully controlled to prevent detonation of the ammonium nitrate and scrubbers are used to remove contaminants and water vapor.

The chief impurities generated during synthesis are (1) nitrogen, which dilutes the anesthetic, (2) nitric oxide, which can combine with hemoglobin to produce hypoxia or to form nitric acid in tissues and cause pulmonary edema, and (3) nitrogen dioxide and higher oxides, which may cause damage to machine valves. Some ammonia is also formed, along with water vapor. Most of these contaminants are removed during the purification process.

Contamination with water vapor originally presented a problem. On release of compressed nitrous oxide, a temperature drop occurs across the reducing valve attached to the cylinder, and internal condensation of water with freezing of the valve occurred. Currently, the water content is less than 0.0015% (3 mg/20 L), which eliminates the problem. On warm, humid days, however, frost may appear on the cylinder valve and shoulder.

Nitrous oxide produced for medical purposes is at least 99.0% pure and must conform to the standards of the United States Pharmacopeia.[5] Each batch of nitrous oxide is tested for purity, and after transfer to cylinders for distribution, additional samples from each lot of gas are

Table 40–1. Physicochemical Properties of Nitrous Oxide

Formula	N_2O; $N{=}N{=}O \geqq$ $N{\equiv}N{-}O$
Molecular weight	44.01
Density of gas (0°C and 1 atm)	1.96 g/L
(37°C and 1 atm)	1.73 g/L
Specific gravity (air = 1.0)	1.5
Flammability	Supports combustion
Boiling point	−88.44°C
Critical pressure	71.7 atmospheres
Critical temperature	36.4°C (97.7°F)
Solubility coefficients	
Oil/gas	1.4
Blood/gas	0.47
Water/gas	0.44
Heart/blood	1.0
Brain/blood	1.1
Lung/blood	1.0
Muscle/blood	1.2

From Adriani.[4]

again tested for purity. For anesthetic use, nitrous oxide is stored in blue cylinders, compressed to 750 psi (51 atm) at 20°C. Under these conditions, a full tank contains mostly liquid nitrous oxide, although a small amount of compressed gas is present on top of the liquid; the E cylinder contains 1500 L of gas (1 atm) in liquified and compressed form. As gas is removed from the cylinder, the remaining liquid vaporizes, replacing the removed gas. Because the density of the compressed gas is about one fourth that of the liquid, as all the liquid is exhausted, approximately one fourth of the original contents of the cylinder will remain. At this point, the pressure in the cylinder falls as the remaining gas is removed.

Nitrous oxide does not react with soda lime, other anesthetic drugs, or metal parts of equipment. It does impregnate and diffuse through rubber, however.[6] Solubility of nitrous oxide in water is limited, and bubbling the gas through water does not change its pH. Unlike some of the oxides of nitrogen, nitrous oxide has minimal toxicity. It has a long shelf-life and remains stable at room temperature.

Nitrous oxide does not burn or explode, but it is a mild oxidizing agent. Structurally, it is a linear molecule, with the two nitrogen atoms bonded to each other and the oxygen bonded to one of the nitrogen atoms (see Table 40-1). Pauling proposed that the molecule exists in two forms called resonating hybrids.[7] By giving up its oxygen, nitrous oxide supports combustion.

Principles of Administration

Nitrous oxide is the least potent of the currently used anesthetics, with a minimum alveolar concentration (MAC) of 104.[8] Nonetheless, certain characteristics make it an attractive anesthetic, including low blood and tissue solubilities, analgesic effects at subanesthetic concentrations, few clinically significant cardiovascular effects, and minimal toxicity. In addition, nitrous oxide is nonirritating to the airway and is well tolerated during mask induction.

Because of its low solubility, uptake by the blood and tissues is slow compared with the volatile agents; nitrous oxide causes a rapid rise in alveolar, blood, and brain partial pressures on induction. In a similar manner, washout and, therefore, emergence are rapid. Moreover, compared with the volatile agents, nitrous oxide is used at high inspired concentrations, a method that partially overcomes its lack of potency.

Except under hyperbaric conditions, however, concentrations of nitrous oxide higher than 80% cannot be used, or hypoxia will result. Thus, in usual clinical practice, "subanesthetic" concentrations are administered. Despite this limitation, nitrous oxide can be used to advantage, because the anesthetic effects of nitrous oxide and the volatile agents are generally additive. Indeed, adding nitrous oxide can substantially reduce the amount of volatile agent that would otherwise be required. For example, 70% nitrous oxide (0.67 MAC) reduces the concentration of halothane required to achieve 1 MAC of total anesthetic to about 0.25% (the MAC of halothane is 0.77). Moreover, because of a rapid rise in alveolar concentration, surgical anesthesia is achieved more rapidly than with the volatile agent alone. Administration of nitrous oxide also results in a more rapid rise in the alveolar concentration of the volatile agent, because of the second gas effect.[9] For the foregoing reasons, on termination of anesthesia, emergence is also faster.

The MAC-awake of nitrous oxide is approximately 65%.[10] Above this concentration, patients may be rendered unconscious or amnestic to the surgical procedure,[11] although the depth of anesthesia with unsupplemented nitrous oxide is insufficient to blunt more than a mild surgical stimulus. As noted previously, however, its anesthetic, analgesic, and amnestic properties are useful when combined with other agents.

Adjunctive Drugs

Many drugs are available to support and complement the effects of nitrous oxide. By this means, its usefulness is enhanced. The selection of the adjunct should be guided by the effect desired. During monitored anesthetic care, analgesia is an important objective when painful stimulation is expected. The analgesia provided by 50% nitrous oxide is approximately equal to that provided by 10 mg of morphine.

Sedation and anxiolysis become the important objectives when a patient is unduly nervous or anxious or is responding without correlation to painful stimulation. Unwanted effects, however, such as excitement, confusion, exhilaration, laughing, or inability to cooperate may be encountered when concentrations of nitrous oxide of 50% or higher are used in unanesthetized patients. Therefore, an anxiolytic drug such as a benzodiazepine, or a hypnotic agent such as a barbiturate, may be useful to complement the sedative and analgesic effects of nitrous oxide.

Absorption, Fate, and Elimination

Rate of Absorption

Total uptake of nitrous oxide by the body in humans was first studied by Severinghaus[12] (Fig. 40-1). During the first minute, nitrous oxide is rapidly absorbed, at about 1000 ml/min. By 5 minutes, the rate falls to around 600 ml/min, and at 10 minutes, it is about 350 ml/min. At 50 minutes, the rate of absorption is still about 100 ml/min, but thereafter it slowly declines and eventually approaches zero. Note that during the first 30 minutes of anesthesia with nitrous oxide, 10 to 12 L of gas is absorbed by blood and tissues. During a 2-hour anesthetic administration, about 30 L is absorbed.

The rate at which the alveolar concentration approaches the inspired concentration is illustrated in Figure 40-2.[13] Three main factors determine the alveolar concentration of an anesthetic: (1) the inspired concentration of the gas; (2) alveolar ventilation; and (3) uptake by the circulation, as governed by blood solubility and cardiac output.[14,15] Because blood solubility of nitrous oxide is low, changes in cardiac output do not greatly influence the alveolar content. Therefore, the alveolar concentration of nitrous oxide largely depends on inspired

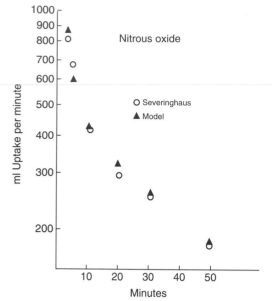

Fig. 40–1. A comparison of experimental uptake for nitrous oxide (open circles) with that predicted (filled triangles). Experimental uptake in this and the remaining figures is corrected to uptake per 70 kg, except for the study of ether at a constant inspired concentration, for which no weight figures are available. Average alveolar ventilation is 3 L/min with a concentration of 75% nitrous oxide. Redrawn from Severinghaus, J. W.: Rate of uptake of nitrous oxide in man. J Clin Invest *33*:1183, 1954.

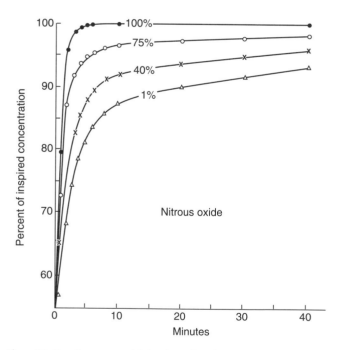

Fig. 40–2. Rate at which the alveolar concentration approaches the inspired concentrations. The curves apply to a 70-kg man with an alveolar ventilation of approximately 4 L/min. Cardiac output is 6 L/min with normal distribution. Redrawn from Eger, E. I., II: Applications of a mathematical model of gas uptake. *In* Papper, E. M., Kitz, R. J. (eds.). Uptake and Distribution of Anesthetic Agents. New York, McGraw-Hill, 1963.

concentration and on ventilation. For a patient breathing 75% nitrous oxide with an alveolar ventilation of 4 L/min, the alveolar concentration reaches approximately 95% of the inspired concentration (71%) within 4 to 5 minutes.

Distribution

Nitrous oxide is distributed to all tissues. The concentration in a particular tissue is a function of the perfusion per unit volume of the tissue, the time of exposure, and the solubility of the agent in the specific tissue.

Four tissue compartments are recognized, each with a different rate of uptake (Fig. 40–3):

1. Highly perfused tissues (75% of cardiac output for the vessel-rich group) such as brain, kidney, heart, and liver absorb the greatest portion of nitrous oxide during the first 10 minutes. Because the total mass of this type of tissue is small (approximately 10%), saturation is quickly attained.
2. At the same time, other tissues take up some drug, but early on this is a relatively small fraction of the total. As the vessel-rich tissues become saturated, the uptake by these tissues becomes more evident. Thus, muscle uptake soon predominates. It is delayed because of a smaller perfusion rate of only 18% of cardiac output, but the total amount eventually absorbed (because this tissue compartment represents 50% of body mass) is great. Uptake continues over a period of 30 minutes at a rate 200 to 300 ml/min. At 45 minutes, the rate falls to 100 ml/min, and by 90 minutes, it is 25 ml/min. Some nitrous

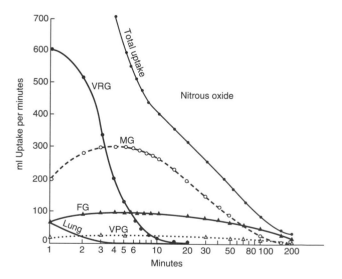

Fig. 40–3. Calculated uptake of nitrous oxide in a 70-kg man by various groups of tissues. VRG (vessel-rich group) refers to the highly perfused tissues such as brain, heart, kidney, and hepatoportal system. MG refers to muscle and skin, FG refers to fat, and VPG (vessel-poor group) refers to bone, cartilage, ligament, and tendon. Inspired concentration is 75%, and alveolar ventilation is 4 L/min. Redrawn from Eger, E. I., II: Applications of a mathematical model of gas uptake. *In* Papper, E. M., Kitz, R. J. (eds.). Uptake and Distribution of Anesthetic Agents. New York, McGraw-Hill, 1963.

oxide continues to be absorbed slowly for as long as 3 to 5 hours.

3. Fat tissue (approximately 5% of cardiac output and 20% of body mass) takes up nitrous oxide at a much slower, but steady rate, of 50 to 100 ml/min for the first 100 minutes. Thereafter, absorption continues at a declining rate for as long as 18 to 30 hours. The total amount absorbed is small in most patients, however.

4. Tissues with the least perfusion rates (vessel-poor group; less than 1% of cardiac output and 20% of body mass) are the last to be saturated. The rate of uptake is below 25 ml/min, and the total capacity is small.

In addition to saturation of various tissue groups, constant loss of nitrous oxide occurs through the skin and through the rubber components of the anesthesia circle.

Elimination

Nitrous oxide is almost entirely eliminated through the lungs, although as noted previously, some excretion occurs through the skin. After saturation (skin belongs to the vessel-rich group), cutaneous loss of 5 to 10 ml/min occurs.[16] This may be compared with the loss of nitrogen through the skin of about 0.3 ml/min. Small amounts of nitrous oxide also appear in sweat, urine, and intestinal gas.

The pattern of pulmonary elimination is generally the reverse of the alveolar uptake curve.[17,18] Elimination is slower than uptake, however, because induction can be accelerated by the technique of overpressure, but the inspired concentration of the anesthetic cannot be made less than zero. Nonetheless, the alveolar concentration of nitrous oxide falls to about 5% of that seen immediately before cessation of anesthetic administration within about 5 to 10 minutes. Because of continued elimination from tissue stores, detectable levels of nitrous oxide may be present in exhaled gas for 1 to 2 hours, depending on the duration of the anesthetic.

Diffusion Hypoxia

The rapid elimination of nitrous oxide from the body following cessation of anesthesia can lead to a complication referred to as diffusion hypoxia.[19] During the first 5 to 10 minutes of recovery, between 500 and 800 ml/min of nitrous oxide enters the alveoli from the capillary circulation, which dilutes and displaces alveolar oxygen. To prevent diffusion hypoxia, 100% oxygen should be administered for the first 5 to 10 minutes of recovery.

A second phenomenon that may occur is dilution of alveolar carbon dioxide by nitrous oxide. Low concentrations of carbon dioxide may inhibit respiratory drive, resulting in depression of ventilation, further exacerbating hypoxia. Moreover, blood levels of the volatile agents sufficient to inhibit hypoxic ventilatory drive persist for approximately 30 minutes following cessation of administration, again necessitating vigilance during the recovery period.

Biotransformation

Although most of absorbed nitrous oxide is eventually exhaled, it does undergo limited biotransformation. Some nitrous oxide may be metabolized to nitric oxide or to nitrate ions;[20] this can occur in the intestine.[21] Other gaseous products possibly are formed, such as nitric oxide, nitrogen dioxide and ammonia, or water-soluble nonvolatile ions (NO^-_3, NO^-_2, NH^+_4) possibly may be formed; however, evidence with radiolabeled $^{15}N_2O$ indicates that nitrogen is the only significant derivative.

Exposure of nitrous oxide to x-rays has been shown to produce nitric oxide and nitrogen dioxide.[22] Long exposure increases the amount of both products in the presence of abundant oxygen. A potential interaction may result when used in the presence of x-rays during procedures such as angiography, pulmonary fluoroscopy, bronchoscopy, or cardiac catheterization. The clinical significance is probably limited, however.

Physiologic Actions

Central Nervous System

At an inspired concentration of 25%, nitrous oxide causes mild sedation, although excitement may occur at higher concentrations. With increasing concentrations, all modalities of sensation are affected, as evidenced by decreased activity of the special senses such as acuity of sight, hearing, taste, and smell, followed by decreased responsiveness to somatic sensations such as touch, temperature, pressure, and pain. The decreased sense of smell makes the agent suitable for induction and administration of other more irritating agents.

Most studies indicate that 70% nitrous oxide alone has only a small influence on the cerebral metabolic rate of oxygen ($CMRO_2$) in humans. A variable effect has been reported, from no significant change to a 25% reduction. Nitrous oxide is a cerebral vasodilator, however; a 50% alveolar concentration doubles cerebral blood flow. Barbiturates, benzodiazepines, etomidate, and propofol can blunt this effect. Despite this limitation, nitrous oxide continues to be widely used for neurosurgical procedures.

Electroencephalographic Pattern

Faulconer and colleagues[23] noted changes in the electroencephalogram (EEG) during nitrous oxide anesthesia, without hypoxia, in humans. With unsupplemented nitrous oxide anesthesia, however, EEG changes are minimal. During induction, the waking pattern shows a reduction in amplitude and an increase in frequency. During unconsciousness, the waking frequency of the α type (8 to 10 Hz) is replaced by slow waves of 2 to 4 Hz (δ rhythm), with an increased amplitude. Deeper anesthesia shows a further increase of amplitude. Burst-suppression patterns are not observed. Deeper anesthesia can only be achieved with hyperbaric administration, hypoxic mixtures, or supplementation with other agents (Fig. 40-4).[24]

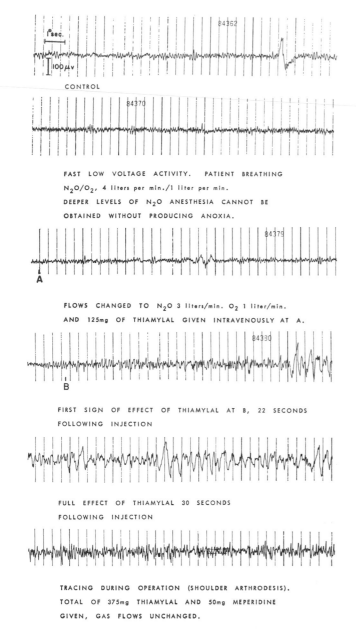

CONTROL

FAST LOW VOLTAGE ACTIVITY. PATIENT BREATHING
N₂O/O₂, 4 liters per min./1 liter per min.
DEEPER LEVELS OF N₂O ANESTHESIA CANNOT BE
OBTAINED WITHOUT PRODUCING ANOXIA.

FLOWS CHANGED TO N₂O 3 liters/min. O₂ 1 liter/min.
AND 125mg OF THIAMYLAL GIVEN INTRAVENOUSLY AT A.

FIRST SIGN OF EFFECT OF THIAMYLAL AT B, 22 SECONDS
FOLLOWING INJECTION

FULL EFFECT OF THIAMYLAL 30 SECONDS
FOLLOWING INJECTION

TRACING DURING OPERATION (SHOULDER ARTHRODESIS).
TOTAL OF 375mg THIAMYLAL AND 50mg MEPERIDINE
GIVEN, GAS FLOWS UNCHANGED.

Fig. 40–4. Electroencephalographic pattern during nitrous oxide anesthesia supplemented by intravenous thiobarbiturate (thiamylal). Courtesy of Dr. V. L. Brechner and Eden Division of Epsco Corporation, Westwood, MA.

Anesthesia and Analgesia

Nitrous oxide produces analgesia in a dose-dependent manner; 50% nitrous oxide is approximately equivalent to 10 mg of morphine.[25-27] Evidence indicates that nitrous oxide has agonist effects at opioid receptors or activates the endogenous opioid system.[28] Indeed, tolerance to subanesthetic nitrous oxide has been shown to occur with morphine administration (although the converse is not true). A 50:50 nitrous oxide-oxygen mixture alleviates opiate withdrawal symptoms.[29,30] In addition, naloxone has been demonstrated to antagonize nitrous oxide anal-

gesia in humans.[28] The state of nitrous oxide anesthesia is unaffected by naloxone, however.[31] Thus, investigators have proposed that a distinction be made between the mechanism of analgesia with subanesthetic concentrations of nitrous oxide and the analgesic and anesthetic effects of the other inhaled agents.[32]

Receptors

In 1981, Gillman and Lichtigfeld[26] proposed that analgesic effects of low-dose nitrous oxide are due to action at opioid receptors. This is supported by the observation that nitrous oxide interferes with binding of (^{3}H)naloxone.[33] In contrast, anesthetic action correlates with lipid solubility, which implies a hydrophobic site of anesthetic action shared by the other inhaled agents. In any case, nitrous oxide anesthesia does not increase the concentration of opioid peptides in cerebrospinal fluid of human subjects.[34,35]

Effect on Noxious Stimuli

Certain noxious stimuli are obtunded by nitrous oxide: cutaneous pain stimuli are tolerated; ischemic pain is reduced; and evoked potentials to painful tooth pulp stimulation are depressed. Analgesic or anesthetic mechanisms (or both) may be involved.

The blink response, a brain stem reflex elicited by a stimulus applied to the cornea or conjunctiva, is depressed by nitrous oxide. The reflex can be produced by an electrical stimulus applied to the supraorbital nerve, and efferent activity can be measured by the electromyographic response of the orbicularis oculi muscle. Low concentrations of nitrous oxide (33%) produce an 80% depression of this response, which is not reversed by naloxone.[31] This suggests a depressant effect on nociceptive input to the central nervous system (CNS) or inhibition of central synaptic transmission, and it appears to be an anesthetic rather than an analgesic effect.

Subcortical centers are variously affected by nitrous oxide. Thalamic centers appear to be depressed, consistent with its anesthetic action. Although nitrous oxide does not alter temperature regulation by the hypothalamus,[36] it does produce sympathetic activation, which may have cardiovascular effects. Nystagmus is seen, and cerebellar function is altered; ataxia and uncoordinated movements occur.

Medullary centers do not show depression. Eckenhoff and Helrich[37] demonstrated that minute ventilation is actually increased. If a supplemental drug is used, however, a greater depression of respiration occurs than would be anticipated by the adjunct alone. Although the respiratory centers are not depressed by nitrous oxide, sensitivity of the larynx is decreased and the cough reflex is suppressed.

The vomiting center is unpredictably affected. At present, little evidence suggests that nitrous oxide increases the incidence of postoperative nausea.[38] When postoperative nausea and emesis are encountered after nitrous oxide administration, however, consideration should be given to the possibility of increased middle ear pressure, which may cause vestibular stimulation (vestibular activation also occurs with opioids), bowel distention, or coexisting hypoxia.

Reflexes

Deep tendon reflexes are not affected.

Cardiovascular System

Nitrous oxide has only minimal effects on heart rate and cardiac output, and a mild increase in cardiac output may reflect increased sympathetic activity. No significant changes in the electrocardiogram occur. The sensitivity of the carotid sinus does not change in humans.[39]

Direct myocardial effects of nitrous oxide have been compared with those of nitrogen.[40] Both gases depress peak isometric tension and maximum rates of rise of tension. A fall in cardiac output on the order of 12% is seen with 50:50 nitrous oxide-oxygen and with 50:50 nitrogen-oxygen; this effect may result from the increased oxygen concentration.[41] Decreases in cardiac output and slight rises in systemic vascular resistance occur with oxygen enriched air mixtures and with hyperbaric oxygenation.[42] Paired electrical stimulation reverses the negative inotropic action of both nitrous oxide and nitrogen, and the relative potentiation of contractility with electrical stimulation is the same for nitrogen, oxygen, and nitrous oxide. This finding suggests that nitrous oxide has minimal direct myocardial depressant effects.[40]

In the absence of hypoxia and hypercarbia, nitrous oxide administered to healthy subjects has minimal effects on blood pressure, venous pressure, or peripheral resistance. The addition of nitrous oxide to steady-state oxygen-halothane anesthesia produces signs of sympathetic activation, however. This includes increased mean arterial and right atrial pressure, systemic vascular resistance, and central blood volume. Forearm blood flow and venous compliance decrease.[43] Although cutaneous vasoconstriction may occur with nitrous oxide alone, the vasodilation seen with halothane is enhanced. Addition of nitrous oxide can antagonize the cardiovascular depressant effects of morphine.[44]

As noted previously, studies with human subjects indicate that nitrous oxide mildly stimulates the sympathetic nervous system in healthy volunteers, but the effect is transient.[45] During the first hour of exposure to 60% nitrous oxide, the mean arterial pressure is mildly elevated. Heart rate and stroke volume are slightly increased, but they return to preanesthetic levels during the second hour. More prolonged inhalation of nitrous oxide results in an increased $PaCO_2$ and a progressive, mild decrease in arterial pH. The early stimulation of the cardiovascular system by nitrous oxide possibly may be related to CNS excitation, secondary to incomplete anesthesia or an increase in $PaCO_2$, rather than direct stimulation of the hypothalamus.

In patients with coronary artery disease, administration of a mixture of 50% nitrous oxide and 50% oxygen, after premedication with diazepam, produces a decrease in the determinants of myocardial oxygen demand. Although left ventricular systolic pressure, left ventricular end-diastolic volume, a measure of preload, and left ventricular end-diastolic pressure are not changed,[46,47] the maximum rate of rise of ventricular pressure declines slightly. The pressure-rate product and left ventricular minute work index decrease.

In patients with coronary artery disease undergoing coronary bypass surgery during anesthesia with intravenous morphine, however, administration of 50% nitrous oxide may result in cardiovascular effects.[48] Mean arterial pressure, cardiac index, stroke index, and left ventricular stroke work index decrease, whereas pulmonary artery pressure, left ventricular end-diastolic pressure, and pulmonary vascular resistance increase. Therefore, nitrous oxide can reduce left ventricular performance and can increase pulmonary artery pressure, suggesting the need for extra care in patients with pulmonary hypertension. On discontinuing nitrous oxide, one sees a prompt return of all parameters to normal.

Respiratory System

Respiration is only minimally affected. An increase in depth may occur with unsupplemented nitrous oxide administration. No change in bronchomotor tone occurs, but the patient may have a decrease in chest wall compliance. Exhalation, which is ordinarily passive, becomes active, as demonstrated myographically.[49] Sensitivity of the larynx and trachea to manipulation is reduced, and the occurrence of laryngospasm is minimized. Secretions are not stimulated; indeed, mucociliary clearance may be depressed. The ventilatory response to carbon dioxide is not affected.

Because nitrous oxide is rapidly eliminated at the conclusion of anesthesia, alveolar dilution of oxygen may occur, producing hypoxia. As with other inhaled anesthetics, hypoxic respiratory drive is markedly inhibited by nitrous oxide. In addition, if mild bronchiolar obstruction exists at the end of surgery, alveolar nitrous oxide may be rapidly absorbed, producing atelectasis. For these reasons, ventilation with 100% oxygen for at least 5 to 10 minutes is indicated at the conclusion of the anesthetic administration.

Effect on Oxyhemoglobin Dissociation Curve

Nitrous oxide at 70% causes a small but significant shift of the oxygen half-saturation pressure (P_{50}) to the right. In the study by Kambam and Holaday,[50] the shift was from 26.8 to 28.4 mm Hg and was found to be rapidly inducible and reversible.

Hazard of Hypoxia

Nitrous oxide is a weak anesthetic and must be given in high percentages to be effective. At least 20%, and preferably 30% oxygen, should be provided in the inspired mixture. Intention to do this is usual, but accomplishment is not always guaranteed. Only when high flows of gases are used does the calculated percentage meet the recommendation. Thus, 8 L of nitrous oxide and 2 L of oxygen flowing into a reservoir such as a rebreathing bag furnish a mixture close to 80%/20%. At lower flow rates, the actual mixtures may have a lower percentage of oxygen than the calculated value. Special care is required for patients with sickle cell disease, and avoiding nitrous oxide in these patients may be advisable. In all patients, the risk of hypoxia with nitrous oxide is real, and the use of this agent to its full potential requires skill and careful monitoring of inspired oxygen concentrations with a properly calibrated oxygen sensor.

Gastrointestinal System[51]

Gastrointestinal motility and tone are not affected. Some distention may occur as a result of swallowing air or a gas mixture, or as a result of the transfer of nitrous oxide to the intestinal lumen. Salivary and gastrointestinal secretions are unaffected. Liver and pancreatic functions are not altered, except in the presence of hypoxia or hypercarbia. When these two conditions occur during nitrous oxide anesthesia, however, they do not provoke the marked changes that may be seen with the volatile anesthetics.

Despite bowel distention associated the nitrous oxide anesthesia, one sees a subtle effect on gastrointestinal motility compared with the effect of surgery, and abdominal surgery in particular.[52] No significant delay of the return of bowel function has been observed.[53]

Genitourinary System

No changes in kidney function, bladder activity, or urine formation have been observed. Postoperative urine retention is usually due to the decreased sense of urgency for urination. Other factors include the excessive administration of fluids and the effect of other drugs.

Reproductive System

Uterine tone and contractility are not appreciably altered by this agent during pregnancy and labor.[54] Transmission across the human placenta is rapid. The equilibration between mother and fetus is not as fast as saturation in other vessel-rich organs because of nonhomogeneity of blood in intervillous spaces and the uptake of anesthetic by placental tissue, however. After 10 to 14 minutes, the fetal-maternal concentration ratio is about 0.8.[55]

Experimental studies in rats show that prolonged exposure to nitrous oxide has toxic effects on testicular structure and function; 20% nitrous oxide produces injury of seminiferous tubules in some animals after 2 days and in all animals by 14 days.[56] The injury is confined to spermatogenic cells with reduction in mature spermatozoa. Recovery of spermatogenesis occurs on return to room air after 3 days.

Skeletal Muscle

Skeletal muscle relaxation is not produced by unsupplemented nitrous oxide. Indeed, slight increases in flexor muscle tone and then in extensor muscle tone are seen during induction. Muscles show good contractility and respond to direct stimulation or to motor nerve stimulation.

Animal Toxicity

In ordinary anesthetic use, nitrous oxide in the absence of hypoxia exhibits no untoward effect or toxicity. Administration for longer than 12 hours can be associated with significant toxic effects, however.

Benigno[57] demonstrated that nitrous oxide has some bacteriostatic activity. At high pressures (28 to 50 atm) and when all oxygen is excluded, coliform bacterial growth is inhibited. Inhibition of oxygen consumption of various brain hemogenates occurs, and certain enzyme systems, such as the hydrogen transport system involving cytochrome *b* and the flavoproteins, appear to be blocked.[58] Mammalian cells grown in culture show a block of cell division when exposed to nitrous oxide under pressure. A metaphase block of mitosis is induced, but it is reversible and results in a synchronization of cell division.[59]

Human Toxicity

Hematologic Effects

Nitrous oxide has been used for prolonged postoperative analgesia and as an anticonvulsant in tetanus. A classic report by Lassen and co-workers in 1956[60] on the prolonged use of nitrous oxide for the control of the signs and symptoms of tetanus demonstrated hematologic effects. Patients developed leukopenia and, in some instances, megaloblastic anemia. Subsequently, Lassen reported on the remission of chronic myeloid leukemia following the administration of nitrous oxide over prolonged periods.[61]

Further studies by Eastwood and associates in 1963[62] showed the beneficial effects of nitrous oxide in patients with leukemia. In these studies, granulocytopenia, thrombocytopenia, and bone marrow depression were recognized. These hematologic effects occurred after 3 to 4 days of 50% nitrous oxide oxygen inhalation. By the third day, leukocyte counts dropped abruptly to 2000 to 4000 cells/mm^3. Thrombocytopenia was frequent, but it was usually delayed as long as 12 days. After discontinuing treatment, remission commenced in 3 to 4 days and continued indefinitely.

In patients without myeloproliferative disorders, prolonged administration of nitrous oxide may also cause bone marrow depression, with megaloblastic changes resembling those seen in pernicious anemia.[63-65] Short-term administration of nitrous oxide decreases human polymorphonuclear leucocyte chemotaxis,[66] an effect not seen with halothane.

Nitrous oxide has been found to undergo a conventional chemical reaction in vivo. In this reaction, the cobalt ion of vitamin B_{12} is oxidized, resulting in inactivation of this co-factor essential in folate related pathways.[67] The resulting hematologic defect is considered to be related to methionine depletion consequent to reduced activity of methionine synthetase, which requires active vitamin B_{12}. With the lack of methionine, megaloblastic anemia and leukopenia follow, and bone marrow changes resemble those of pernicious anemia.

Some anticancer drugs, such as methotrexate, are potentiated by the inactivation of cobalamine. Hence, greater bone marrow depression may occur with administration of nitrous oxide. The reversal of high-dose methotrexate therapy by leucovorin may be attenuated.[68] Nitrous oxide should be avoided in children and others subjected to this type of therapy.

Seriously ill patients and those suffering from massive hemorrhage may have preexisting bone marrow changes. Administration of nitrous oxide in such patients may have further deleterious effects. Amos and co-workers[69] reported a high mortality in patients with preexisting megaloblastic changes who received nitrous oxide.

To detect indirectly the occurrence of impaired methionine synthetase activity and inactivation of vitamin B_{12} associated with megaloblastic changes, a deoxyuridine-suppressant test (dU test) can be carried out using marrow cells incubated with deoxyuridine, which assesses the capacity to methylate deoxyuridine to thymidine.

In these circumstances, the administration of folinic acid at the time of surgery and postoperatively for 3 to 5 days may restore hematopoiesis to a normoblastic state.[70] Folate requirements are more than doubled in the third trimester of pregnancy, and folinic acid should be administered before anesthesia when nitrous oxide is used in pregnant patients.

Effects on the Fetus

Embryonic toxicity was studied by Fink and colleagues[71] in pregnant animals (rats) exposed to 70% nitrous oxide and 20% oxygen for 24 hours. The embryonic and teratogenic effects include an appreciable incidence of embryonic death, an increase in female offspring (female-to-male ratio, 2:1), and defects in vertebral and rib ossification.

In the first and second trimesters of human pregnancy, nitrous oxide may be potentially hazardous to the fetus. This is more likely during the first trimester, particularly during the initial 8 weeks of embryogenesis. A retrospective study by Aldridge and Tunstall,[72] however, who evaluated fetal outcome after short-duration anesthesia with nitrous oxide during the first and second trimesters, did not demonstrate adverse effects. Moreover, an earlier study by Brodsky and co-workers[73] did not show an increased in the incidence of congenital abnormalities following nitrous oxide anesthesia in early pregnancy, although a higher incidence of spontaneous abortion was noted, thought to be related to the stress of surgery.

Effects on Pregnancy

Despite the experimental work on the proposition that nitrous oxide should not be administered to women in the first or second trimester of pregnancy because of an increased risk of spontaneous abortion, this has not been supported by clinical studies. Crawford and Lewis[74] compared the abortion rate and the incidence of low-birth-weight babies in a series of cervical cerclage and other operations during pregnancy, conducted with the patient under general anesthesia, as compared with a series conducted with the patient under regional anesthesia. The incidence of spontaneous abortion was identical in the two series. Hence, whether nitrous oxide increases the risk of first-trimester spontaneous abortion is uncertain.

Neurologic Dysfunction

As noted previously, clinical reports indicate that megaloblastic anemia may occur following the use of nitrous oxide for anesthesia. In patients with vitamin B_{12} deficiency, exposure to nitrous oxide may exacerbate the clinical syndrome of myeloneuropathy known as subacute combined degeneration of the spinal cord.[75] Myeloneuropathy has also been reported in subjects abusing nitrous oxide.[76]

Regular exposure of professionals (dentists and anesthetists) to nitrous oxide is associated with an increased frequency of complaints suggesting peripheral polyneuropathy. Reports include tingling, numbness, and muscle weakness. In heavily exposed individuals, the incidence is increased about fourfold.[77] This is especially so for persons who abuse nitrous oxide.[76]

Safe Levels in the Operating Room

In the United States, the National Institute for Occupational Safety and Health (NIOSH) has recommended that nitrous oxide levels in the operating room not exceed 25 ppm (on a time-weighted average).[78] Trace levels of halogenated anesthetics should not exceed 0.5 ppm, when used with nitrous oxide; without nitrous oxide, levels should not exceed 2.0 ppm.

Transfer to Body Air Cavities

During nitrous oxide anesthesia, a significant transfer of the gas into closed air spaces of the body occurs. Nitrogen is the predominant gas filling these spaces, and because its blood solubility is low (0.013) compared with that of nitrous oxide (0.47), the rate of transfer of nitrous oxide into air spaces is some 35 times faster than the rate of washout of nitrogen. Consequently, nitrous oxide accumulates in air-filled cavities. The result is either an increase in *volume* of compliant spaces or an increase in *pressure* in noncompliant spaces (Table 40–2). At equilibrium, the rate of molecular exchange is proportional to the ratio of the coefficients of blood solubilities. The magnitude of the change depends on the partial pressure of the gases in the alveoli, and at equilibrium the concentrations must approach the concentration in the alveoli.

Several theoretic considerations apply to transfer of nitrous oxide into closed air spaces: (1) nitrogen does not readily leave enclosed spaces; (2) the blood solubility of the gas in question must be significantly greater than that of nitrogen to enter the nitrogen-filled space rapidly; and (3) the concentration of the gas must be high. In practice,

Table 40–2. Air-Containing Body Spaces

COMPLIANT SPACES
Gastrointestinal tract
Pneumoperitoneum
Pneumothorax
Air emboli
Endotracheal tubes
Air-filled balloon catheters
NONCOMPLIANT SPACES
Middle ear
Paranasal sinuses
Cerebral ventricles
Eyeball

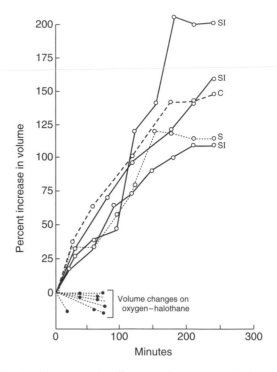

Fig. 40–5. These graphs illustrate the increase in bowel gas volume produced by nitrous oxide administration (large open circles). All parts of the bowel (C = colon, dashed line; SI = small intestine, solid line; and stomach, dotted line) show a similar change with time. Note that no volume increase occurs during halothane administered in oxygen (small filled circles). Redrawn from Eger, E. I., II, and Saidman, L. J.: Hazards of nitrous oxide anesthesia in bowel obstruction and pneumothorax. Anesthesiology 26:61, 1965.

a limit to the expansion or pressure increase actually observed exists, because impedance to blood flow occurs in the given space as volume or pressure rises and thereby prevents further transfer of gas.

Gastrointestinal Tract

Bowel gas is a mixture of swallowed air and of gases such as hydrogen and methane from decomposition of food by intestinal bacteria. Because any oxygen in the swallowed air is rapidly absorbed, the principal residual gas is nitrogen.

Actual volume changes have been determined experimentally.[79] After 2 hours of exposure to 70 to 80% nitrous oxide, volume increased about 1.5-fold, and at 4 hours, it increased about 2.5-fold (Fig. 40–5). An approximate geometric relationship exists between the concentration of nitrous oxide in alveoli and the increase in bowel volume. The change in volume occurs slowly, and for short procedures is probably not clinically significant, although administration of nitrous oxide in the presence of intestinal obstruction may be deleterious. Similarly, nitrous oxide is probably best avoided in patients with diaphragmatic hernia, in those with omphalocele, and in anxious patients exhibiting aerophagia.

Pneumoperitoneum

This condition is occasionally encountered in the management of abdominal hernias and in diagnostic laparoscopy. The administration of nitrous oxide in concentrations greater than 50% increases the intra-abdominal gas volume and may result in tamponade of the abdominal vessels; decreased venous return and cardiocirculatory depression can occur.

Pneumothorax

Changes in intrapleural gas volume produced by nitrous oxide administration in the presence of pneumothorax are rapid. The inspiration of 75% nitrous oxide doubles the pneumothorax volume in 10 minutes and triples the volume in 45 minutes[79] (Fig. 40–6). Profound effects on ventilation and circulation may ensue, with possible respiratory failure and circulatory collapse. A closed pneumothorax represents an absolute contraindication to nitrous oxide administration.

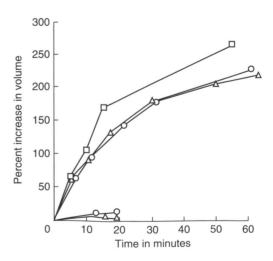

Fig. 40–6. Intrapleural gas volume increases rapidly in the presence of 75% inspired nitrous oxide plus halothane in oxygen (open circles, squares, and triangles) but shows little change when only halothane in oxygen is respired (triangle and circles). Redrawn from Eger, E. I., II, and Saidman, L. J.: Hazards of nitrous oxide anesthesia in bowel obstruction and pneumothorax. Anesthesiology 26:61, 1965.

In cystic lung disease, administration of nitrous oxide increases pressure in bullae, and rupture of the bullae or compression of adjacent alveoli may occur. A pneumothorax may result from rupture of surface bullae, whereas rupture into blood vessels lining a cyst wall can produce an air embolism.

Venous Air Embolism

Because nitrous oxide in the blood is in direct contact with the "cavity" surface of bubbles, an air embolus rapidly increases in size and may cause profound circulatory effects. Therefore, when an air embolus is suspected, nitrous oxide should be immediately discontinued.

Endotracheal Tube Cuffs

Diffusion of nitrous oxide into endotracheal tube cuffs readily occurs, increasing cuff volume and pressure. The rate of change is proportional to the concentration of nitrous oxide administered to the patient[80,81] (Fig. 40-7). Studies by Konchigeri and Lee[82] demonstrated that the changes in volume and pressure can be prevented by using a sample of the inspired gas mixture to inflate the endotracheal cuff. This simple procedure can prevent ischemic damage to tracheal mucosa. The alternative to this simple procedure is the frequent adjustment of cuff pressure during the course of prolonged anesthesia. Other air-filled balloon type catheters, such as pulmonary artery catheters, are also subject to increased volume and pressure during the administration of nitrous oxide.[83]

Noncompliant Gas Spaces

Middle Ear and Paranasal Sinuses

In upper respiratory infections and disease states, air passageways to the noncompliant spaces in the middle ear and paranasal sinuses are blocked, resulting in disruption of the normal equilibrating mechanisms. When a patient breathes nitrous oxide, significant amounts of the anesthetic enter the middle ear and raise the pressure. The rate of pressure rise is proportional to the alveolar concentration of the gas and is relatively rapid. In 10 to 30 minutes, ear pressure may rise to 20 to 30 cm H_2O[84,85] (Fig. 40-8). If the eustachian tube is not open, barotrauma may result. Nitrous oxide may continue to enter the middle ear for as long as 20 minutes after discontinuing the anesthetic.

Conversely, with anesthesia lasting more than 3 hours, sufficient nitrogen may be displaced from these cavities that, on discontinuing anesthesia, rapid reabsorption of nitrous oxide will occur, with a lowering of middle ear pressure. Congestion and middle ear hemorrhage or implosion of the eardrum can result. Instances of pain, vertigo, nausea, and temporary hearing loss have occurred. Similar changes on breathing nitrous oxide occur in the paranasal sinuses, with comparable difficulties.

Nitrous oxide should be avoided during anesthesia for middle ear surgery or surgery on the eardrum (except for tympanostomy tubes), to minimize the risk of injury. Nitrous oxide should also be avoided in patients with an ab-

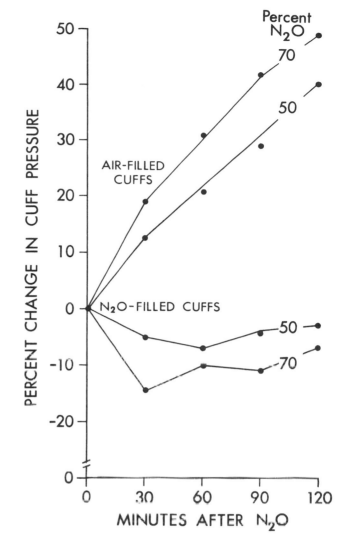

Fig. 40–7. Percentage of change in endotracheal cuff pressure before and after exposure to 50 and 70% nitrous oxide. Note that pressure change is proportional to nitrous oxide concentration and cuffs filled with nitrous oxide show no increase in pressure. Drawn from the data of Konchigeri and Lee, 1979, in Munson, E. S.: Nitrous oxide and body air spaces. Middle East J Anaesth 7:193, 1983.

normality of the eustachian apparatus or with an upper respiratory infection.

Pneumoencephalography

Although largely of historical interest since the advent of the computed tomography scanner, administration of nitrous oxide following pneumoencephalography results in transfer of the anesthetic into the air-filled cerebral ventricles. Because the ventricular system is a closed, relatively rigid space, the cisternal cerebrospinal fluid pressure can rise within 5 minutes to 90 mm Hg.[86] Resorption of instilled air may require 48 to 72 hours.

Philippart[87] demonstrated that the rise of pressure and the magnitude of the rise is greatest in the upright and

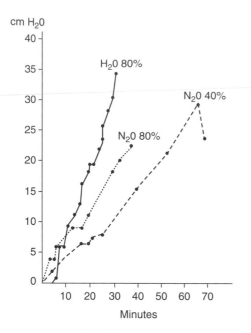

Fig. 40–8. Nitrous oxide inhalation increases middle ear pressure in man. The rate of increase is directly related to the inspired nitrous oxide concentration. From Thomsen, K. A., Terkildsen, K., Arnfred, I.: Middle ear pressure variations during anesthesia. Arch Otolaryngol *82*:609, 1965.

prone positions. In these positions, the air is in close contact with the choroid plexus and, hence, the transfer of nitrous oxide from the blood is enhanced. If the supine position is used, the pressure rise is blunted, because air rises to the anterior portion of the ventricular system away from the choroid plexus. Nevertheless, nitrous oxide should not be employed within several days of pneumoencephalography. This caution may also apply following neurosurgical procedures, when air has entered the cerebral ventricles or cranium.

Ophthalmologic Procedures

In the vitrectomy procedure, the eye may be filled with a mixture of sulfur hexafluoride and air, to prevent retinal detachment. Nitrous oxide rapidly diffuses into the intraocular gas mixture and can increase the intraocular pressure by up to 200%, which can impair the retinal circulation. Nitrous oxide should not be used during these operations.[88]

Tolerance and Dependence

Several studies indicate that tolerance to the anesthetic action of nitrous oxide can develop with time. Long-term exposure to subanesthetic concentrations of nitrous oxide increases tolerance to nitrous oxide and other anesthetics.[89] Tolerance to nitrous oxide has also been demonstrated during short exposures, which is maximal within 10 minutes.[90]

Concomitant development of dependence or neuroadaptation with withdrawal symptoms on abrupt discontinuation has been demonstrated for many drugs that depress the CNS. Drugs of the sedative-hypnotic class are especially likely to result in neuroadaptation. In addition, convulsions may occur during abrupt discontinuation of such drugs. Offending agents include barbiturates, benzodiazepines, ethanol, meprobamate, opioids, and anticonvulsants. Such phenomena can occur with the gaseous anesthetics, particularly nitrous oxide. Convulsions have been produced in animals after exposure to nitrous oxide for 15 minutes, followed by abrupt withdrawal.[91] The duration of this effect is about 90 minutes, and thereafter convulsions are not elicitable.

Tolerance to the analgesic effects of nitrous oxide has also been demonstrated. One mechanism suggested for nitrous oxide analgesia involves the endogenous opioid system.[92] As noted previously, nitrous oxide analgesia is in part related to the activity of enkephalins, and inhibition of enkephalinase appears to prevent the development of tolerance to nitrous oxide.[93]

Contraindications

Nitrous oxide is remarkably safe when hypoxia is avoided, and its excellent clinical characteristics make it a widely used anesthetic. Indeed, few clinically significant deleterious effects occur, and hence few contraindications to its use exist. Nevertheless, certain situations preclude the use of nitrous oxide. In patients with pulmonary hypertension, nitrous oxide may cause a significant increase in pulmonary vascular resistance, compromising cardiac function. Prolonged exposure to nitrous oxide may result in megaloblastic changes and associated hematologic effects. In addition, prolonged exposure and abuse of nitrous oxide can be associated with neurologic toxicity. Teratogenic effects have been demonstrated in rodents, but the clinical relevance to humans is still an area of active investigation. Clinical studies to date suggest that nitrous oxide is generally a safe anesthetic during pregnancy, however. Finally, appropriate consideration should be given to accumulation of nitrous oxide in closed air cavities, particularly when the risk of pneumothorax or air embolism exists, during operations on the ear and eye, and in patients with upper respiratory infections.

XENON

Essential Pharmacology

Xenon, the rarest and heaviest of the noble gases, was discovered by Ramsey and Travers in 1898, in the residue after evaporation of liquid air. Anesthetic properties were first described by Cullen and Gross based on the solubility characteristics of xenon and its similarity to ethylene.[94]

Physical Properties

Xenon is an inert, monoatomic element and does not form stable compounds with other elements. It does form various crystalline hydrates, however.

Preparation of the gas in pure form is achieved by fractional distillation of liquid air. It is a colorless, odorless,

Table 40–3. Physicochemical Properties of Xenon

Molecular weight	131.3
Boiling point	$-108.1°C$
Density (STP)	5.4 g/L (air = 1.3 g/L) [96]
Solubilities (37°C)	
Water/gas	0.085
Blood/gas	0.14
Oil/gas	1.9

tasteless, and nonirritating gas, present in air in the proportion of 1 part in 20 million parts of air (Table 40–3).

Administration

Xenon may be administered by the semiclosed or closed system. The former is used for induction to denitrogenate the patient. Thereafter, a closed carbon dioxide absorption system is used because of the expense of xenon.

Fate and Elimination[95]

Xenon is unchanged in the body and is eliminated by the lungs. It is distributed to all tissues, as determined using radioactive xenon.

Potency[96,97]

The MAC of xenon is 71, which is similar to that of ethylene.

Physiologic Actions

Central Nervous System[98,99]

Clinical signs are those of a descending depression of the CNS. The EEG shows patterns of burst suppression at anesthetic levels. The frequency is slowed, and a δ rhythm of 6 cps appears.

Respiratory System

Ventilation is not depressed. Irritation is not evident, and salivary secretions and tracheobronchial mucus formation are not stimulated. Laryngeal spasm does not occur.

Cardiovascular System[98]

A mild slowing of cardiac rate occurs, blood pressure remains unchanged, and arrhythmias are not produced.

Relaxation

In general, skeletal muscle relaxation sufficient for abdominal surgery does not occur. The jaw muscles relax so pharyngeal airways may be inserted, however. Abnormal neuromuscular activity is not seen.

Hepatorenal Effects

No demonstrable adverse effects have been noted.

Metabolic Effects

No changes of significance are demonstrable.

Use

Because of its high cost, the use of xenon as an anesthetic remains a curiosity. Closed-circle systems can be used to minimize loss of the anesthetic, however, and they may eventually be cost effective.[100,101] Indeed, if cost were not an issue, xenon would probably be an attractive anesthetic, because its water/gas solubility is considerably less than that of nitrous oxide.[102] Also of interest are other potential medical uses of xenon, such as as a contrast agent for radiologic procedures. Because of its density, it can be used to visual bronchi with computed tomography, and it may also be useful as a contrast agent with magnetic resonance imaging techniques.

REFERENCES

1. Keys, T. E.: The History of Surgical Anesthesia. New York, Schumanns, 1945.
2. Erving, H. W.: The discoverer of anesthesia: Dr. Horace Wells of Hartford. Yale J Biol Med 5:521, 1933.
3. Heironimus, T. W.: History of nitrous oxide. Clin Anesth 1:1, 1964.
4. Adriani J. The Chemistry and Physics of Anesthesia, 2nd Ed. Springfield, IL, Charles C Thomas, 1972.
5. United States Pharmacopeia: The National Formulary, 20th Rev. Washington, D.C., United States Pharmacopeial Convention, 1980.
6. Wineland, A. J., Waters, R. M.: The diffusibility of anesthetic gases through rubber. Anesth Analg 8:322, 1929.
7. Pauling, L.: College Chemistry. San Francisco, W.H. Freeman, 1957.
8. Hornbein, T. F., et al.: The minimum alveolar concentration of nitrous oxide in man. Anesth Analg 61:553, 1982.
9. Epstein, et al.: In Collins, V. J. (ed.). Principles of Anesthesiology, 3rd Ed. Philadelphia, Lea & Febiger, 1993.
10. Stoelting, R. K.: MAC awake. Anesthesiology 33:5, 1970.
11. Frumin, M. J.: Clinical use of a physiological respirator producing nitrous oxide amnesia-analgesia. Anesthesiology 18:290, 1957.
12. Severinghaus, J. W.: Rate of uptake of nitrous oxide in man. J Clin Invest 33:1183, 1954.
13. Eger, E. I., II: Applications of a mathematical model of gas uptake. In Papper, E. M., Kitz, R. J. (eds.). Uptake and Distribution of Anesthetic Agents. New York, McGraw-Hill, 1963.
14. Eger, E. I., II: Factors affecting the rapidity of alteration of nitrous oxide concentration in a circle system. Anesthesiology 21:238, 1960.
15. Eger, E. I., II: Effect of inspired anesthetic concentration on the rate of rise of alveolar concentration. Anesthesiology 24:153, 1963.
16. Orcutt, F. S., Waters, R. M.: The diffusion of nitrous oxide, ethylene and carbon dioxide through human skin during anesthesia, including a new method for estimating nitrous oxide in low concentrations. Anesth Analg 12:45, 1933.
17. Frumin, M. J., Salanitre, E., Rackow, H.: Excretion of nitrous oxide in anesthetized man. J Appl Physiol 16:720, 1961.
18. Salanitre, E., et al.: Uptake and excretion of subanesthetic concentrations of nitrous oxide in man. Anesthesiology 23:814, 1962.

19. Fink, B. R.: Diffusion anoxia. Anesthesiology 16:511, 1955.
20. Matsubara, T., Mori, T.: Studies on denitrification. IX: Nitrous oxide, its production and reduction of nitrogen. J Biochem 64:871, 1968.
21. Hong, K., et al.: Metabolism of nitrous oxide by human and rat intestinal contents. Anesthesiology 52:16, 1980.
22. Yanagida, H., Nakajima, M.: Exposure of nitrous oxide to x-rays. Anaesthesia 33:1169, 1981.
23. Faulconer, A., Pender, J. W., Bickford, R. G.: The influence of partial pressure of nitrous oxide on the depth of anesthesia and the electroencephalogram in man. Anesthesiology 10:601, 1949.
24. Brechner, V. L., Dornette, W. H. L.: Electroencephalographic pattern during nitrous oxide-trifluoroethyl-vinyl ether anesthesia. Anesthesiology 18:321, 1957.
25. Gillman, M. A., Lichtigfeld, F. J.: A Comparison of the effects of morphine sulphate and nitrous oxide analgesia on chronic pain states in man. J Neurosurg Sci 49:41, 1981.
26. Gillman, M. A., Lichtigfeld, F. J.: The similarity of the action of nitrous oxide and morphine. Pain 10:110, 1981.
27. Gillman, M. A., Lichtigfeld, F. J.: Nitrous oxide acts directly at the Mu opioid receptor. Anesthesiology 62:375, 1985.
28. Yang, J. C., Clark, W. C., Ngai, S. H.: Antagonism of nitrous oxide analgesia by naloxone in man. Anesthesiology 52:414, 1980.
29. Koblin, D. D., Deady, J. E., Dong, D. E., Eger, E. I., II: Mice tolerant to nitrous oxide are also tolerant to alcohol. J Pharmacol Exp Ther 213:309, 1980.
30. Koblin, D. D., et al.: Mice tolerant to nitrous oxide are not tolerant to barbiturates. Anesth Analg 60:138, 1981.
31. Smith, R. A., Wilson, M., Miller, K. W.: Naloxone has no effect on nitrous oxide anesthesia. Anesthesiology 49:6, 1978.
32. Gillman, M. A., Footeman, D. S.: The need for a clearer distinction between anesthesia and analgesia in relation to the opiate system. Anesthesiology 54:524, 1981.
33. Daras, C., Cantrill, R. C., Gillman, M. A.: (^{3}H) Naloxone displacement: evidence for nitrous oxide as opioid receptor agonist. Eur J Pharmacol 89:177, 1983.
34. Way, W. L., et al.: Anesthesia does not increase opioid peptides in cerebrospinal fluid of humans. Anesthesiology 60:45, 1984.
35. Morris, B., Livingston, A.: Effects of nitrous oxide exposure on met-enkephalin levels in discrete areas of rat brain. Neurosci Lett 45:11, 1984.
36. Eastwood, D. W.: Clinical Use of Nitrous Oxide. Philadelphia, F.A. Davis, 1964.
37. Eckenhoff, J. E., Helrich, M.: The effects of narcotics, thiopental and nitrous oxide upon respiration and the respiratory response to hypercapnia. Anesthesiology 19:340, 1948.
38. Watcha, M. F., White, P. F.: Postoperative nausea and vomiting: its etiology, treatment, and prevention. Anesthesiology 77:162, 1992.
39. Price, H. L.: General anesthesia and circulatory homeostasis. Physiol Rev 40:187, 1960.
40. Goldberg, A. H., Sohn, Y. Z., Phear, W. P. C.: Direct myocardial effects of nitrous oxide. Anesthesiology 37:373, 1972.
41. Thornton, J. A., Fleming, J. S., Goldberg, A. D., Gaird, D.: Cardiovascular effects of 50% nitrous oxide and 50% oxygen mixture. Anesthesiology 28:484, 1973.
42. Eggers, G. W. N., Jr., et al.: Hemodynamic responses to oxygen breathing in man. J Appl Physiol 17:75, 1962.
43. Smith, N. T.: The cardiovascular and sympathetic numeric responses to the addition of nitrous oxide to halothane in man. Anesthesiology 32:410, 1970.
44. Stoelting, R. K., Gibbs, P. S.: Hemodynamic effects of morphine and morphine-nitrous oxide in valvular heart disease and coronary artery disease. Anesthesiology 38:45, 1973.
45. Kawanura, R., et al.: Cardiovascular responses to nitrous oxide exposure for two hours in man. Anesth Analg 59:93, 1980.
46. Wynne, J., et al.: Hemodynamic effects of nitrous oxide administered during cardiac catheterization. JAMA 243:1440, 1980.
47. Eisele, J. H., Smith, N. T.: Cardiovascular effects of 40% nitrous oxide in man. Anesth Analg 51:956, 1972.
48. Lappas, D. G., et al.: Left ventricular performance and pulmonary circulation following addition of nitrous oxide to morphine during coronary artery surgery. Anesthesiology 43:61, 1975.
49. Freud, F. G., Roos, A.: Abdominal muscle activity during general anesthesia (abstract). Fed Proc 22:363, 1963.
50. Kambam, J. R., Holaday, D. A.: Effect of nitrous oxide on the oxyhemoglobin dissociation curve and PO_2 measurements. Anesthesiology 66:208, 1987.
51. Miller, G. H.: The effects of general anesthesia on the muscular activity of the gastrointestinal tract. Anesth Analg 5:226, 1926.
52. Cundy, R. I., Aldrete, A., Thomas, T. J.: Intestinal distention produced by nitrous oxide or ethylene inhalation. Surg Gynecol Obstet 129:108, 1969.
53. Giuffre, M., Gross, J. B.: Effects of nitrous oxide on postoperative bowel motility. Anesthesiology 65:699, 1986.
54. Vasicaka, A., Kretschmer, H.: Conduction and inhalation anesthesia on uterine contractions: experimental study of the influence of anesthesia on the entra-amniotic pressure. Am J Obstet Gynecol 82:600, 1961.
55. Marx, G. F., Joshi, C. W., Orkin, L. R.: Placental transmission of nitrous oxide. Anesthesiology 32:429, 1970.
56. Kripe, B. J., et al.: Testicular reaction to prolonged exposure to nitrous oxide. Anesthesiology 44:104, 1976.
57. Benigno, P.: Toxicity and antibacterial action of nitrous oxide. Boll Soc Ital Biol Sper 16:127, 1941.
58. Hosein, E. A., Stachiewicz, E., Bourne, W., Denstedt, O. F.: Influence of nitrous oxide on metabolic activity of brain tissue. Anesthesiology 16:708, 1955.
59. Rao, P. N.: Mitotic synchrony in mammalian cells treated with nitrous oxide at high pressure. Science 160:774, 1968.
60. Lassen, H. C. A., Henriksen, E., Neukirch, F., Kristensen, H.S.: Treatment of tetanus: severe bone marrow depression after prolonged nitrous oxide anaesthesia. Lancet 1:527, 1956.
61. Lassen, H. C. A.: Remission in chronic myeloid leukemia following prolonged nitrous oxide anaesthesia. Dan Med Bull 6:252, 1959.
62. Eastwood, D. W., Green, C. D., Lambdin, M. A., Gardner, R.: Effect of nitrous oxide on the white-cell count in leukemia. N Engl J Med 268:297, 1963.
63. Amess, J. A. L., et al.: Megaloblastic haemopoiesis in patients receiving nitrous oxide. Lancet 2:339, 1978.
64. Kripke, B. J., et al.: Hematologic reaction to prolonged exposure to nitrous oxide. Anesthesiology 47:342, 1977.
65. Nunn, J. F., Sturrock, J. E., Howell, A.: Effect of inhalation anaesthetics on division of bone-marrow cells in vitro. Br J Anaesth 48:75, 1976.
66. Hill, G. E., et al.: Nitrous oxide and neutrophil chemotaxis in man. Br J Anaesth 50:555, 1978.
67. Nunn, J. F., Chanarin, I.: Nitrous oxide inactivates methionine synthetase. In Eger, E. I., II (ed.). Nitrous Oxide. London, Edward Arnold, 1985.
68. Ueland, P. M., Refsumtt, H., Wesenberg, F.: Methotrexate

therapy and nitrous oxide anesthesia. N Engl J Med *314:*1514, 1986.

69. Amos, R. J., Amess, J. A. L., Hinds, C. J., Mollin, D. L.: Incidence and pathogenesis of acute megaloblastic bone marrow changes in patients receiving intensive care. Lancet *2:*835, 1982.

70. Amos, R. J., Amess, J. A. L., Nancekievill, D. G., Rees, G. M.: Prevention of nitrous oxide-induced megaloblastic changes in bone marrow using folinic acid. Br J Anaesth *56:*103, 1984.

71. Fink, B. R., Shepard, T. H., Blandau, R. J.: Teratogenic activity of nitrous oxide in the rat. Nature *214:*146, 1967.

72. Aldridge, L. M., Tunstall, M. E.: Nitrous oxide and the fetus. Br J Anaesth *58:*1348, 1986.

73. Brodsky, J. B., et al.: Surgery during pregnancy and fetal outcome. Am J Obstet Gynecol *138:*1165, 1980.

74. Crawford, J. A., Lewis, M.: Nitrous oxide in early human pregnancy. Anaesthesia *41:*900, 1986.

75. Schilling, R. F.: Is nitrous oxide a dangerous anesthetic for vitamin B_{12} deficient subjects? JAMA *255:*1605, 1986.

76. Blanco, G., Peters, H. A.: Myeloneuropathy and macrocytosis associated with nitrous oxide abuse. Arch Neurol *40:*416, 1983.

77. Brodsky, J. B., Cohen, E. N., Brown, B. W., Jr.: Exposure to nitrous oxide and neurologic disease among dental professionals. Anesth Analg *60:*297, 1981.

78. Occupational exposure to waste anesthetic gases and vapors. DHEW (NIOSH) Pub 77:140. Cincinnati, Center for Disease Control, National Institute for Occupational Safety and Health, 1977.

79. Eger, E. I., II, Saidman, L. J.: Hazards of nitrous oxide anesthesia in bowel obstruction and pneumothorax. Anesthesiology *26:*61, 1965.

80. Munson, E. S., Stevens, D. S., Redfern, R. E.: Endotracheal tube obstruction by nitrous oxide. Anesthesiology *52:*275, 1980.

81. Munson, E. S.: Nitrous oxide and body air spaces. Middle East J Anaesth *7:*193, 1983.

82. Konchigeri, H. N., Lee, Y. E.: Preventive measures against nitrous oxide induced volume and pressure changes of endotracheal tube cuffs. Middle East J Anaesth *5:*369, 1979.

83. Kaplan, R., Abramowitz, M. D., Epstein, B. S.: Nitrous oxide and air-filled balloon-tipped catheters. Anesthesiology *55:*71, 1981.

84. Thomsen, K. A., Terkildsen, K., Arnfred, I.: Middle ear pressure variations during anesthesia. Arch Otolaryngol *82:*609, 1965.

85. Matz, G. J., Rattenborg, C. G., Holaday, D. A.: Effects of nitrous oxide on middle ear pressure. Anesthesiology *28:*948, 1967.

86. Saidman, L. J., Eger, E. I., II: Change in cerebrospinal fluid pressure during pneumoencephalography under nitrous oxide anesthesia. Anesthesiology *26:*67, 1965.

87. Philippart, C.: Contrast gas analysis with air myelography and ventriculography during nitrous oxide anaesthesia. Anaesthesist *18:*367, 1969.

88. Mirakhur, R. K.: Anaesthetic management of vitrectomy. Ann R Coll Surg Engl *67:*34, 1985.

89. Smith, R. A., Winter, P. M., Smith, M., Eger, E. I., II: Tolerance to and dependence on inhalational anesthetics. Anesthesiology *50:*505, 1979.

90. Smith, R. A., Winter, P. M., Smith, M., Eger, E. I., II: Rapidly developing tolerance to acute exposures to anesthetic agents. Anesthesiology *50:*496, 1979.

91. Smith, R. A., Winter, P. M., Smith, M., Eger, E. I., II: Convulsions in mice after anesthesia. Anesthesiology *50:*501, 1979.

92. Berkowitz, B. A., Finck, A. D., Ngai, S. H.: Nitrous oxide analgesia: reversal by naloxone and development of tolerance. J Pharmacol Exp Ther *203:*539, 1977.

93. Rupreht, J., et al.: Enkephalinase inhibition prevented tolerance to nitrous oxide analgesia in rats. Acta Anesthesiol Scand *28:*617, 1984.

94. Cullen, S. C., Gross, E. G.: Anesthetic properties of xenon and krypton. Science *113:*580, 1951.

95. Pittinger, C. B., et al.: Xenon concentrations in brain and other body tissues. J Pharmacol Exp Ther *70:*110, 1954.

96. Pittinger, C. B.: New drugs. Anesth Analg *36:*36, 1957.

97. Cullen, S. C., Eger, E. I., II, Cullen, B. F., Gregory, P.: Observations on the anesthetic effect of the combination of xenon and halothane. Anesthesiology *31:*305, 1969.

98. Pittinger, C. B., et al.: Electroencephalographic and other observations in monkeys during xenon anesthesia at elevated pressures. Anesthesiology *16:*551, 1955.

99. Morris, L. E., Knott, J. R., Pittinger, C. B.: Electroencephalographic changes in human surgical patients during xenon anesthesia. Anesthesiology *16:*312, 1955.

100. Lachmann, B., et al.: Safety and efficacy of xenon in routine use as an inhalation anaesthetic. Lancet *335:*1413, 1990.

101. Boomsma, F., et al.: Haemodynamic and neurohumoral effects of xenon anaesthesia: a comparison with nitrous oxide. Anaesthesia *45:*273, 1990.

102. Steward, A., Allott, P. R., Cowles, A. L., Mapleson, W. W.: Solubility coefficients for inhaled anaesthetics for water, oil and biological media. Br J Anaesth *45:*282, 1973.

Chapter 41

ELIMINATION OF INHALATION ANESTHETICS

DUNCAN A. HOLADAY

Four pathways are currently recognized for the clearance of the volatile inhalation anesthetics. These are as follows:

1. Pulmonary excretion: This is the major route of elimination of the more chemically stable, parent drugs and for volatile metabolites.
2. Renal excretion: The major route of removal of most water-soluble drug metabolites.
3. Biotransformation: Almost all the volatile, organic anesthetics are subject to enzymatic degradation to a degree that is inversely proportional to the drug's chemical stability. The metabolic products are almost always more water soluble and are eliminated by renal or pulmonary excretion.
4. Long-term tissue binding: Fluoride ion (F^-) is rapidly cleared from the plasma approximately equally by binding strongly to apatite crystal of bone and renal excretion.

Volatile anesthetics are excreted to a negligible extent through skin and are lost to an indeterminate extent from open, surgical fields.

PULMONARY EXCRETION

The recovery from anesthesia depends on the reduction of the partial pressure of the anesthetic in the brain. The latter reflects the anesthetic partial pressure in the alveolar gas with a brief lag resulting from circulatory transport time. Thus, pulmonary clearance is important to the initial phase of awakening because the alveolar gas can be exchanged almost completely in 2 minutes.[1] The next phase of pulmonary excretion depends on the solubility of the anesthetic.[2] As alveolar gas tension falls, a pressure gradient is created between the air space and the pulmonary circulation. Rate of diffusion of anesthetic from blood to air space depends on the amount of drug in the blood, which is a function of its solubility. The more soluble the drug, the more it slows recovery by maintaining its partial pressure in the alveolar gas. In this manner, pulmonary excretion resembles uptake. Recovery is usually slower than induction, however, because of the use during induction of anesthesia of "over pressure," inhaled concentrations higher than those required to maintain anesthesia. During recovery, the partial pressure in the blood is a mixture of those coming from the various tissue compartments. It is lower following anesthesia of short duration than after anesthesia of longer duration because the venous contributions from muscle and fatty compartments reflect less complete approaches to equilibrium.

Mass Balance Method

A precise measurement of how much of an inhalation anesthetic has undergone metabolic breakdown can be obtained by carefully determining the difference between the amount of drug absorbed during exposure and the amount exhaled following exposure.[3-5] Carpenter and associates exposed a group of patients to an approximately equipotent mixture of four anesthetics—isoflurane, enflurane, halothane, and methoxyflurane—and compared the amounts of each drug exhaled to the amounts absorbed. Because the amount of isoflurane exhaled equaled 93% of the uptake, and because less than 0.2% of isoflurane has been recovered as urinary metabolites,[6] it was assumed, as a first approximation, that no appreciable amount of isoflurane underwent metabolism. The amount of isoflurane recovered was normalized to 100%, and a similar correction was applied to the recoveries of the other drugs. Thus, investigators estimated that enflurane is metabolized to the extent of 8%, halothane 46%, and methoxyflurane 75%.[4]

RENAL EXCRETION

The inhalation anesthetics undergo essentially no clearance through the kidney because of their high lipid solubility. The renal tubular epithelium is highly lipophilic and readmits to the tubular capillary blood all lipophilic substances lost into the glomerular urine. Metabolites of lipophilic drugs are water soluble, however, and are readily eliminated by renal excretion. In fact, the discovery that all volatile organic anesthetics undergo some degree of biotransformation was made by identifying metabolites of isotopically labeled anesthetics in the urine of exposed laboratory animals.[7]

DRUG METABOLISM

All the inhalation anesthetics in use at the time of this printing are metabolized to some extent. All except nitrous oxide are subject to attack by the mixed function oxidase system of the endoplasmic reticulum (or enzyme

P-450 system).[8] The endoplasmic reticulum is a tubule or canal system extending from nucleus to plasma membrane, consisting of a lipoprotein membrane, rich in enzymes, that is distributed throughout all organs and tissues of the body, but principally in the liver and to lesser extent in the kidney, lung, and brain. When isolated by homogenization of the tissue and staged centrifugation, the endoplasmic reticulum is broken into many small, spherical liposomes, called microsomes, in which are contained the mixed function oxidase system and other enzymes.

The effect of drug metabolism is to increase the water solubility of drugs, that is, to form more polar substances and thereby enhance their renal elimination.[9] Without this mechanism, the body would have no way to rid itself of highly lipid-soluble, nonvolatile xenobiotics. The metabolites may be less active or more active and may exhibit more or less toxicity than the parent compounds.

Pathways

Two phases of metabolism are apparent,[9] as discussed in the following paragraphs.

Phase I

Phase I reactions result in biochemical degradations. The *mixed function oxidase system* is one of several enzyme systems in the body capable of degrading endogenous compounds and xenobiotics. It is responsible for the metabolism of most drugs, including all of the organic, inhalation anesthetics. It includes reduced nicotinamide adenine dinucleotide phosphate (NADPH), cytochrome P-450 reductase, cytochrome P-450 (one of several cytochrome enzymes), and molecular oxygen. The reaction involves the transfer of an electron from NADPH by cytochrome P-450 reductase to cytochrome P-450. The reduced cytochrome, in turn, transfers the electron to molecular oxygen, activating one atom of oxygen and producing a molecule of water with the second atom of oxygen. The reduced cytochrome P-450 combines the active oxygen to a susceptible drug, forming an hydroxylated intermediate that can proceed to an O-dealkylation (ether cleavage) or a dehalogenation, in the case of the volatile anesthetics. Other oxidation reactions include aliphatic and aromatic hydroxylations, N-dealkylation, sulfoxidation, desulfuration, epoxidation (of fatty acids), and N-oxidation. In the absence of sufficient dissolved oxygen, cytochrome P-450 transfers an electron from NADPH to a certain few drugs that can accept an electron, resulting in reduction. Halothane is the only volatile anesthetic susceptible to reduction.

Other pathways include *hydrolysis,* which involves the splitting of a compound containing an ester or amide linkage by addition of water. This reaction applies to local anesthetics and certain other injectable drugs and occurs in the cytosol or extracellular fluids. It affects none of the inhalation anesthetics.

Nitrous oxide is not metabolized by the microsomal enzymes. Hong and co-workers[10] demonstrated, however, that *intestinal bacteria* are able to reduce it to nitrogen to a minute extent. These investigators warn that other carcinogenic and teratogenic nitroso compounds and free radical intermediates may also be formed. Never in the course of the many millions of administrations of nitrous oxide to human patients, on the other hand, has overt evidence of such a reaction been identified.

Phase II

Phase II reactions are *conjugations,* or molecular additions.[8] The enzymes on which phase II reactions depend are specific to certain chemical groups, rather than to drug or molecular species. These groups are NH_2, SH, OH, and COOH. The effect of the conjugation is to increase the polarity and water solubility and, hence, renal excretion of a metabolite. Additions include the formation of glucuronides catalyzed by glucuronyl transferase, methylations in which S-adenosylmethionine serves as a methyl donor, acetylations dependent on coenzyme A (for coenzyme of acetylation), and mercapturic acids that result from conjugation with glutathione.

Factors Influencing Rate

The extent of metabolic change and the rate of metabolism are related to factors dependent on characteristics of the drug and on other factors that influence enzyme activity.

Drug-Dependent Factors

The *chemical reactivity* of the compound is of primary importance. The more stable the molecular structure, the less the breakdown. Replacement of protons that are susceptible to enzymatic attack with deuterium reduces the oxidation of a drug because the deuterium carbon (D-C) bond has a significantly higher bond energy than the H-C bond.[11,12]

The *solubilities* of the drug, that is, the lipophilic and hydrophilic natures of the drug are important factors. Anesthetic agents with low lipid solubilities are metabolized less and hence are less likely to cause toxicity as a result of undergoing enzymatic activation to a free radical or other highly reactive intermediate metabolite.[9]

The *concentration* and duration of stay of the drug in the body also must be considered. The longer a drug is present in the plasma, the greater is its exposure to hepatic enzymes. Trace amounts of more soluble anesthetics may be released from lipid stores for days or weeks.[13]

Factors Affecting Enzyme Activity

The activity of an enzyme is a function of the rate of its production and the rate of removal. Both processes depend on protein synthesis.[8] The turnover rate of the P-450 isozymes vary from slow to rapid. When something perturbs either production or removal rate, the rate at which a new equilibrium activity is reached is determined by the turnover rate.

Enzyme induction is a process by which the amount and activity of an enzyme can be increased. Prior exposure to certain drugs, or to other substances, increases the activity of the enzyme by increasing the amount of the enzyme in the liver as a result of increasing rate of formation of the enzyme.[14]

Substances that are known to increase the activity of the P-450 isozymes that metabolize the volatile anesthetics include the barbiturates, isoniazid, phenytoin, the polychlorbiphenyls, the steroid hormones, and a host of other drugs, including certain of the anesthetics, themselves, such as halothane and methoxyflurane.[15,16]

Enzyme inhibition can diminish metabolism by several mechanisms. The enzyme may be occupied by a competitively binding substance, or it may be destroyed by another drug such as carbon tetrachloride or chloroform, on which the enzyme acts. The production of the enzyme may be reduced, or its rate of removal may be increased, or another element in the mixed function oxidase system may be blocked, such as the activation of molecular oxygen.[17] Substances that are known to inhibit enzyme activity include SKF 525A, an inhibitor of drug oxidations,[18] disulfiram, a substance that interferes with the oxidation of acetaldehyde by reducing the activity of aldehyde dehydrogenase, and antimetabolites such as puromycin and actinomycin, which block protein synthesis.[14]

Other factors[9] include *age,* which exerts important influence on drug metabolism. The fetus and newborn are essentially devoid of conjugating, mixed function oxidases and other microsomal drug-metabolizing enzymes. These appear gradually and at rates characteristic of each enzyme. Doses of barbiturates that are readily tolerated by adult animals may produce prolonged sleeping times or death in juveniles. Senility is also accompanied by decreased tolerance to many drugs, presumably as a result of decline in hepatic function and rates of protein synthesis.

Gender makes a considerable difference to drug metabolism in experimental animals. Males metabolize greater amounts of the inhalation anesthetics than females.[9,19] *Obesity* tends to enhance drug metabolism. Two factors contribute: (1) increased storage of fat soluble drugs in adipose tissues support continued slow leakage of drug over long periods of time for increased exposure to liver enzymes; and (2) fatty infiltration of the liver occurs in 75% of people who are 50% or more overweight and is associated with significantly higher plasma concentrations of halothane and methoxyflurane metabolites.

Starvation causes a reduction of drug metabolism as a result of depressed liver function. Obstructive jaundice, liver tumors, and alloxan diabetes have similar effects, as do conditions interfering with protein synthesis.[8]

METABOLISM OF THE INHALATION ANESTHETICS

Twenty or 30 compounds, mostly hydrocarbons or ethers, have been proposed, entered into clinical trials, or incorporated into routine clinical practice for a time. All but 4 of these compounds have been discarded because of flammability, toxicity, or arrhythmogenicity.[20] Only those that remain in use at this time and those that show promise for future acceptance are discussed here.

Halothane

The first of the halogenated drugs to receive wide acceptance because of its lack of flammability and rapid and pleasant induction, halothane has become the most investigated drug with respect to its biotransformation because of its rare association with severe hepatic necrosis. It is subject to both oxidation and reduction by the mixed function oxidase system. In experimental animals, the extent of each depends on the concentration of oxygen to which the animal is exposed.[21]

Oxidation proceeds in steps, one of which produces trifluoroacetylchloride, a reactive, hydrolyzable compound known to bind covalently to proteins.[22] The final product of oxidation is trifluoroacetate, a nontoxic, highly polar, readily excreted substance. The other products of oxidative metabolism are chloride (Cl^-) and bromide (Br^-). Mass balance studies indicate that humans metabolizes up to 46% of absorbed halothane.[4]

Halothane is the only anesthetic among those discussed here that is subject to *reductive metabolism.* The requirements are NADPH, cytochrome P-450, and reduced oxygen partial pressure.[23] Prior treatment with phenobarbital enhances the reaction in experimental animals. Following uneventful halothane anesthesia, normal persons, not subjected to a hypoxic atmosphere, exhale for a brief period a certain, minimal amount of the volatile products of reductive metabolism;[24] this finding suggests the possible presence of some areas within the liver that are hypoxic under normal circumstances.

Reductive metabolism proceeds by several pathways[23] (Fig. 41–1). The products include at least two reactive intermediates: an electron is transferred to halothane from a reduced cytochrome P-450, Br^- is lost, creating a free radical; or a second electron is acquired, creating a carbanion. Both activated forms can react with a nearby protein, lipid, or water to acquire a proton and form the volatile metabolite, 2-chloro-1,1,1-trifluoroethane, or lose F^- to form a second volatile metabolite, 2-chloro-1,1-difluoroethylene.

Methoxyflurane

The most-lipid soluble of the inhalation anesthetics and, associated with this, the most extensively metabolized of currently marketed drugs, methoxyflurane has fallen into disuse except as a self-administered analgesic for second-stage obstetric labor because of fear of renal toxicity associated with fluoride release (Fig. 41–2).

Methoxyflurane is subject to enzymatic attack at two sites, dehalogenation of the β carbon and cleavage of the ether linkage.[13] The metabolic products of the former are Cl^- and methoxydifluoroacetic acid, which is excreted in the urine or can decompose to oxalate, formaldehyde, and F^-. The formaldehyde joins the one carbon pool and ultimately is excreted as carbon dioxide. The products of ether cleavage are formaldehyde, F^-, and dichloroacetic acid, which apparently is rapidly metabolized further to Cl^- and oxalate.[13,25] Clinical mass balance studies indicate that as much as 85% of absorbed methoxyflurane is metabolized.[4,6]

Enflurane

Because one of its metabolites is F^-, enflurane has been suspected of being nephrotoxic.[26] It is, however, resistant to metabolism; on average, only 1.8% of absorbed en-

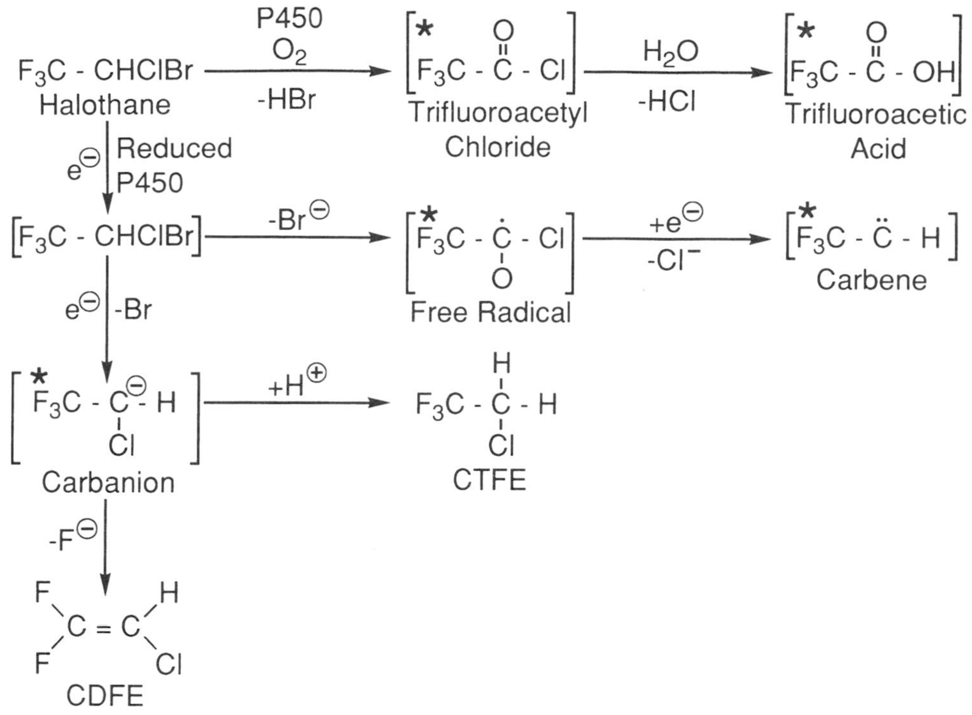

$F_3C - CHClBr$ (Halothane) $\xrightarrow[\text{-HBr}]{\text{P450 } O_2}$ $[\overset{*}{F_3C} - \overset{O}{\overset{\|}{C}} - Cl]$ (Trifluoroacetyl Chloride) $\xrightarrow[\text{-HCl}]{H_2O}$ $[\overset{*}{F_3C} - \overset{O}{\overset{\|}{C}} - OH]$ (Trifluoroacetic Acid)

Halothane $\xrightarrow[]{e^{\ominus} \text{ Reduced P450}}$ $[F_3C - CHClBr]$ $\xrightarrow{-Br^{\ominus}}$ $[\overset{*}{F_3C} - \overset{\cdot}{\underset{O}{C}} - Cl]$ (Free Radical) $\xrightarrow[\text{-Cl}^-]{+e^{\ominus}}$ $[\overset{*}{F_3C} - \overset{\cdot\cdot}{C} - H]$ (Carbene)

$[F_3C - CHClBr] \xrightarrow[\text{-Br}]{e^{\ominus}}$ $[\overset{*}{F_3C} - \overset{\ominus}{\underset{Cl}{C}} - H]$ (Carbanion) $\xrightarrow{+H^{\oplus}}$ $F_3C - \underset{Cl}{\overset{H}{C}} - H$ (CTFE)

Carbanion $\xrightarrow{-F^{\ominus}}$ $\underset{F}{\overset{F}{C}} = \underset{Cl}{\overset{H}{C}}$ (CDFE)

Fig. 41–1. Proposed metabolic pathways of halothane. Bracketed forms are transients; the asterisks indicate highly reactive compounds that may covalently bind to, or react with, cellular macromolecules, providing a basis for halothane hypersensitivity or for an acute toxic reaction. Oxidation requires cytochrome P-450 and activated oxygen. Reduction depends on transfer of electrons from reduced P-450. CTFE and CDFE stand for chlorotrifluoroethane and chlorodifluoroethylene, respectively, the volatile reductive metabolites that occur in exhaled air briefly following halothane anesthesia. Data from Sipes, I. G., et al.: Comparison of the biotransformation and hepatotoxicity of halothane and deuterated halothane. J Pharmacol Exp Ther *214:*716, 1980; and Sharp, J. H., Trudell, J. R., Cohen, E. N.: Volatile metabolites and decomposition products of halothane in man. Anesthesiology *50:*2, 1979.

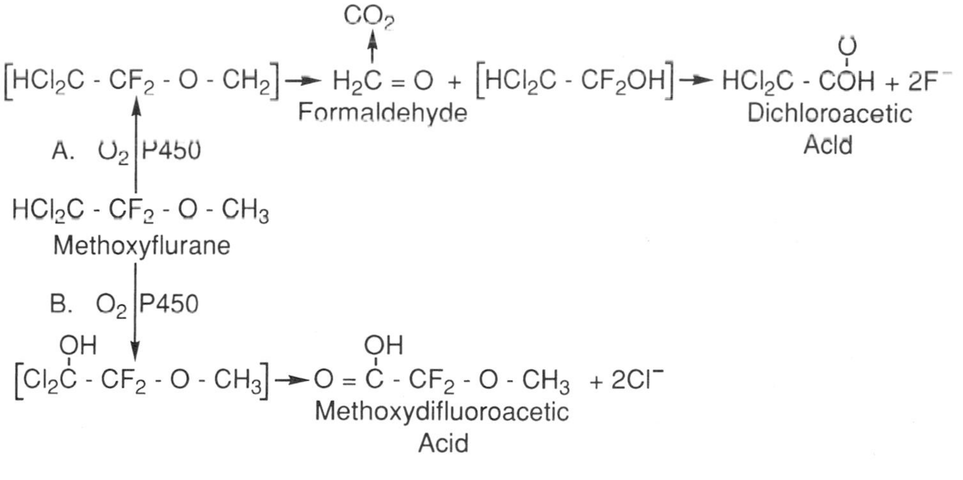

$[HCl_2C - CF_2 - O - CH_2] \rightarrow H_2C = O$ (Formaldehyde) $+ [HCl_2C - CF_2OH] \rightarrow HCl_2C - \overset{O}{\overset{\|}{C}}OH + 2F^-$ (Dichloroacetic Acid)

A. $O_2 \mid$ P450

$HCl_2C - CF_2 - O - CH_3$ (Methoxyflurane)

B. $O_2 \mid$ P450

$[Cl_2\overset{OH}{\overset{|}{C}} - CF_2 - O - CH_3] \rightarrow O = \overset{OH}{\overset{|}{C}} - CF_2 - O - CH_3 + 2Cl^-$ (Methoxydifluoroacetic Acid)

Fig. 41–2. Proposed pathways of metabolism of methoxyflurane. Methoxyflurane has two sites of attack by the mixed function oxidase system: A, on a proton of the methoxy group; and B, on the β carbon of the ethyl group. Pathway B is preferred by a ratio of about 4:1. From Holaday, D. A., Rudofsky, S., Treuhaft, P. S.: The metabolic degradation of methoxyflurane in man. Anesthesiology *33:*579, 1970.

flurane is excreted as urinary metabolites,[27] and mass balance studies support that a maximum of 15% is metabolized.[4] Metabolism of enflurane is not induced by phenobarbital or phenytoin,[26] but it is induced by pretreatment with isoniazid.[28,29]

The principal metabolites of enflurane are difluoromethoxy-difluoroacetic acid, Cl^-, and F^-, as a consequence of oxidative dehalogenation of the β carbon.[30] In the rat, a small fraction, 9%, of enflurane tagged with ^{14}C in the methoxy moiety undergoes ether cleavage, liberating $^{14}CO_2$ and four atoms of F^{-31} (Fig. 41–3).

Isoflurane

Isoflurane is the most resistant to enzymatic attack of the marketed anesthetics. Less than 0.2% of absorbed drug is excreted in human urine.[5] Identified metabolites are F^- and trifluoroacetic acid.[32,33] (Fig. 41–4).

Experimental Drugs

Sevoflurane is an experimental drug submitted for licensure for clinical use in Japan. It is characterized by low water, blood, and lipid solubilities;[34] its distribution

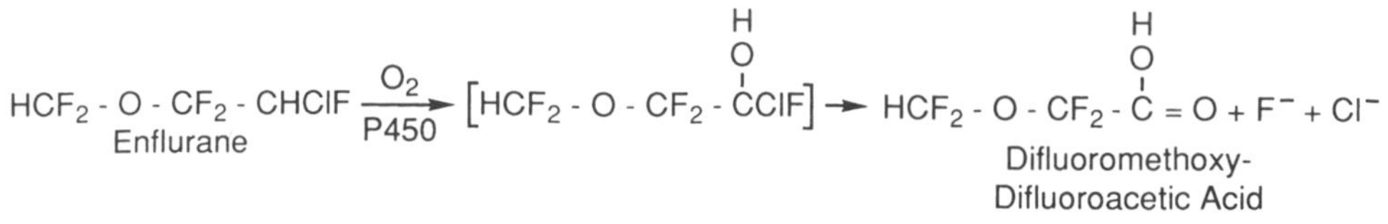

$$HCF_2 - O - CF_2 - CHClF \xrightarrow[P450]{O_2} \left[HCF_2 - O - CF_2 - \overset{\overset{\displaystyle H}{\overset{|}{\overset{\displaystyle O}{|}}}}{C}ClF\right] \rightarrow HCF_2 - O - CF_2 - \overset{\overset{\displaystyle H}{\overset{|}{\overset{\displaystyle O}{|}}}}{C} = O + F^- + Cl^-$$

Enflurane

Difluoromethoxy-
Difluoroacetic Acid

Fig. 41–3.   The major metabolites of enflurane are fluoride ion and difluoromethoxydifluoroacetic acid. Organic and inorganic fluoride are released into the urine at a ratio of 4:1.[27] Less than 10% of the amount of enflurane metabolized results from cleavage of the ether linkage.[31]

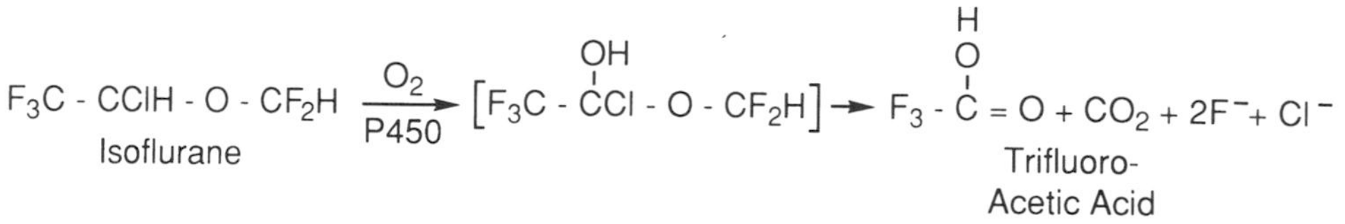

$$F_3C - CClH - O - CF_2H \xrightarrow[P450]{O_2} \left[F_3C - \overset{\overset{\displaystyle OH}{|}}{C}Cl - O - CF_2H\right] \rightarrow F_3 - \overset{\overset{\displaystyle H}{\overset{|}{\overset{\displaystyle O}{|}}}}{C} = O + CO_2 + 2F^- + Cl^-$$

Isoflurane

Trifluoro-
Acetic Acid

Fig. 41–4.   Isoflurane is resistant to metabolism. The proton on the α carbon of the ethyl group is the likely site of attack to release F⁻ and trifluoroacetic acid. From Davidkova, T. I., et al.: Biotransformation of isoflurane: urinary and serum fluoride ion and organic fluorine. Anesthesiology 69:218, 1988.

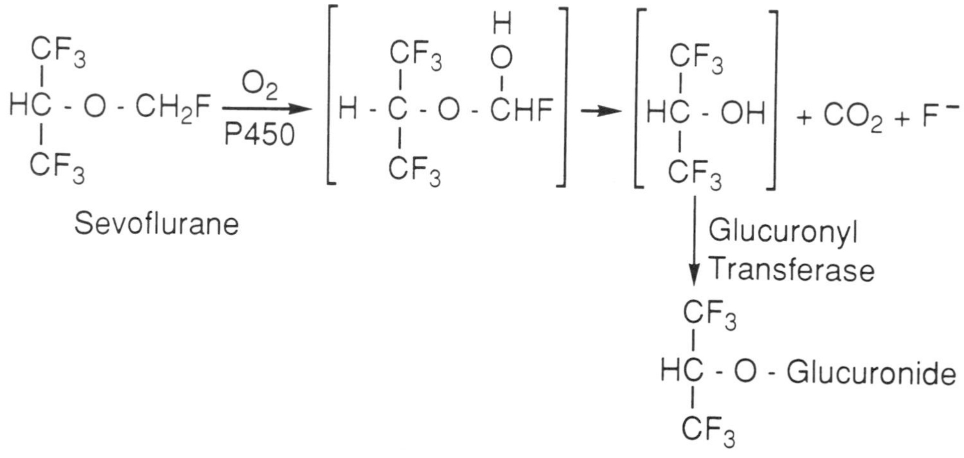

$$\underset{\text{Sevoflurane}}{\overset{\overset{\displaystyle CF_3}{|}}{\underset{\underset{\displaystyle CF_3}{|}}{HC}} - O - CH_2F} \xrightarrow[P450]{O_2} \left[\overset{\overset{\displaystyle CF_3}{|}}{\underset{\underset{\displaystyle CF_3}{|}}{H - C}} - O - \overset{\overset{\displaystyle H}{\overset{|}{\overset{\displaystyle O}{|}}}}{C}HF\right] \rightarrow \left[\overset{\overset{\displaystyle CF_3}{|}}{\underset{\underset{\displaystyle CF_3}{|}}{HC} - OH}\right] + CO_2 + F^-$$

Glucuronyl
Transferase

$$\overset{\overset{\displaystyle CF_3}{|}}{\underset{\underset{\displaystyle CF_3}{|}}{HC} - O - Glucuronide}$$

Fig. 41–5. Sevoflurane metabolism includes both phase I and phase II biotransformations. The ether linkage undergoes oxidative cleavage, following which the trifluoroethyl moiety is conjugated with glucuronic acid. The F⁻ released by hydrolysis of the methoxyl group, and the glucuronide are rapidly excreted in the urine. From Martis, L., et al.: Biotransformation of servoflurane in dogs and rats. Anesth Analg 60:186, 1981.

coefficients are: water/gas, 0.36; blood/gas, 0.60; and olive oil/gas, 53.4.[35] Because of its low solubilities, induction of and recovery from anesthesia are rapid, and exposure to hepatic microsomal enzymes is limited.[36] Sevoflurane is the fluoromethyl ether of bistrifluoromethylisopropanol (Fig. 41–5). The ether linkage is broken following hydroxylation of the methyl group, releasing a fluoride ion from the methyl group and a fluorine containing glucuronide. Treatment of the glucuronide with glucuronidase yields hexafluoroisopropanol.[36,37] Humans metabolize sevoflurane to about the same extent as enflurane. Serum fluoride concentrations peak at 14 to 22 μm during and for approximately 1 hour after anesthesia and fall rapidly during the next 24 hours.[36,38,39] Deuteration reduces significantly the metabolism of sevoflurane in the rat.[40] Sevoflurane is subject to alkaline degradation in soda lime.[41] No renal or hepatic toxicity has been reported following sevoflurane anesthesia.

Desflurane (I-653) is an isomer of isoflurane; it contains six fluorine atoms and no chlorine. It has a vapor pressure of 700 mm Hg at 22° to 23°C. Its solubility in bi-ologic fluids is lower than that of any other inhalation anesthetic; its saline, blood, and lipid partition coefficients are 0.225, 0.42, and 19, respectively.[42] In the rat pretreated with phenobarbital, F⁻ rose slightly immediately following exposure to I-653.[43] Urinary F⁻ concentrations were not different from those of unexposed rats, but organic fluorine rose significantly following ethanol pretreatment, and to a lesser extent following pretreatment with phenobarbital or no pretreatment.

DRUG METABOLISM AND TOXICITY

This subject, the toxicity of inhalation anesthetics, has many interesting aspects: history, incidence, epidemiology, actions of the general anesthetics on hepatic mitochondrial functions in hyperthyroidism, and roles of age, gender, obesity, immunology, genetics, and ethnic background. All are important to the complete understanding of each manifestation of toxicity and for development of safe practices of clinical anesthesia. In this brief account of elimination of the inhalation anesthetics, discussion is limited to the role of drug metabolism and its principal determinants in producing toxic reactions.

Drug metabolism results in more polar, and hence more readily excreted, compounds, but not necessarily more inert substances.[8] The more frequent result of drug metabolism is to detoxify, that is, to render xenobiotics inert and nontoxic. This is achieved not only by converting lipid-soluble substances into water-soluble derivatives that can be excreted, but by conjugation, which increases further water solubility. Thus, most end products are in low concentration and are nontoxic. Metabolism can also produce undesirable products, however, and high concentrations of some metabolites can be toxic.

Two mechanisms can result in a toxic reaction. The first is easily monitored and readily understood, namely, the production of an *intrinsically poisonous substance,* such as trifluoroethanol from oxidation of fluroxene by most species of laboratory animals, but not by humans.[44] Exposure of a rat, cat, or dog to anesthetic concentrations of fluroxene for as little as 1 hour can result in death.[45]

The second mechanism involves the formation of an *unstable intermediate,* which, because of its high reactivity, can bind covalently to an intracellular constituent. Most reactive intermediates react with water or other dispensable cellular constituent and become benign, excretable metabolites, such as trifluoroacetate. Some intermediates can bind to vital macromolecules, however, including proteins and phospholipids, can destroy cytochrome P-450, and can cause hepatic necrosis.[9] The liver failure that follows exposure to carbon tetrachloride and chloroform proceeds by this mechanism.

Halothane Hepatitis

The elucidation of the mechanism underlying the rare massive hepatic necrosis that has tainted the otherwise favorable reputation of halothane has followed a twisted and rambling course from the first indecisive attempt to establish its existence.[46] The search for a reason has touched on an immunologic explanation, ties to drug metabolism—first oxidative, then reductive, oxidative, genetic, and finally, most of these together. In the course of the search, much has been learned about the interactions of the inhalation anesthetics with vertebrate biochemical and immunologic systems.[47]

Early recognition of covalent binding of halothane metabolites to liver in induced mice by radioautography[48] suggested that a metabolite of halothane might be acting as a haptene, in conjunction with a cellular component, to produce the hypersensitivity reaction associated with fulminant halothane hepatitis. Attempts to generate an antigen using trifluoroacetate resulted in only weak antigenic activity.[49] When Uehleke and associates[50] demonstrated that anaerobic conditions altered the character of the metabolites and, more significantly, increased the amount of covalent binding, attempts were made to define an animal model of fulminant halothane hepatitis. Employing phenobarbital pretreatment, mild hypoxia (14% oxygen), and 1% halothane, McLain and associates[51] were able to cause reproducible hepatic necrosis in the rat, and Cousins and associates[52] were able to produce a similar condition in the guinea pig without enzyme induction or a hypoxic atmosphere. These experiments have established that exposure to halothane, particularly prolonged or repeated exposures, or exposure during reduced liver blood flow or other condition resulting in liver hypoxia during exposure, can produce mild, temporary hepatitis, sufficient to classify halothane as a weak hepatotoxin. These reactions do not explain the pathogenesis of fulminant hepatic necrosis.

Hoft and co-workers[53] provided confirmation of the genetic factor predicted to be required to explain the rarity of occurrence.[54] Vergani and associates[55] first employed a leukocyte migration test to demonstrate that 8 of 12 patients who had suffered severe hepatitis following halothane anesthesia had become sensitized to halothane. These investigators confirmed the presence of an IgG antibody that was sensitive to an antigen associated with hepatocytes of rabbits that had been exposed to halothane by direct lymphocyte and indirect cytotoxic assays and by indirect immunofluorescence staining.[56,57] They further established that the sensitivity was augmented by exposing the rabbits to an oxygen-rich rather than hypoxic atmosphere during exposure to halothane.[58] Finally, Satoh,[59] Kenna, and their associates[60] demonstrated that the trifluoroacetyl halide of halothane reacts directly with constituents of the plasma membrane or with other cellular components, and antibodies in sera of patients with a history of halothane hepatitis recognize only a neoantigen that contains both the trifluoroacetyl group and structural features of the carrier protein.

Fluoride Nephrotoxicity

Although suspected previously, the nephrotoxicity of methoxyflurane was established when 5 of 12 surgical patients subjected to methoxyflurane-oxygen anesthesia lasting 2.75 to 5.5 hours in a prospective study developed hypernatremia, serum hyperosmolality, and weight loss postoperatively as a result of polyuria unresponsive to vasopressin (antidiuretic hormone). Ten control patients anesthetized with halothane showed none of these changes.[61] A subsequent study based on dose, measured as the product of inspired concentration and hours of exposure (minimum alveolar concentration [MAC] hours), revealed that serum F^-, sodium, and urea nitrogen concentrations and serum osmolality increased proportionally to the dose of methoxyflurane, but bore no relation or an inverse relation to the dose of halothane.[62] No nephrotoxicity was observed when methoxyflurane doses remained at 2 MAC hours or less and peak serum concentrations of F^- remained below 40 μmol/L. Subclinical nephrotoxicity occurred at doses of 2.5 to 3 MAC hours (serum F^- = 50 to 80 μmol/L); mild clinical toxicity was seen after 5 MAC hours (90 to 120 μmol/L); and clinical toxicity with thirst and polyuria occurred at doses over 7 MAC hours (80 to 175 μmol/L).

The mode of fluoride injury to the renal concentrating mechanism is interference with the generation of the medullary interstitial hyperosmolality that permits passive diffusion of water from the collecting ducts when these membranes are rendered permeable to water by antidiuretic hormone. This mechanism depends on an energy-consuming Cl^- pump in the ascending limb of Henle's loop, which is fueled by adenosine triphosphate.[63] This corroborates the finding of high concentrations of F^- and low sodium in the inner medulla of the kidneys of rats infused with amounts of F^- similar to those released from methoxyflurane.[64]

Enflurane, isoflurane, and halothane release F^- following anesthesia. Isoflurane and halothane carry no threat of nephrotoxicity because they release so little F^-, isoflurane because it is so resistant to biotransformation,[6] and halothane because F^- is released only during reductive metabolism, and this is limited.[65] Enflurane metabolism is also limited,[27] but not to the extent of the foregoing. Enflurane metabolism is induced significantly in patients receiving isoniazid on a long-term basis,[29] however, and it is augmented in the obese.[66] Healthy volunteers who were anesthetized for 9.6 MAC hours exhibited a brief but significant reduction in renal concentrating ability following exposure.[67] Although no report of renal failure following enflurane anesthesia has been published, except in one patient who was receiving isoniazid,[26] caution should be exercised when administering enflurane to the obese and to patients receiving hydrazide-containing drugs.

REFERENCES

1. Eger, E. I., II: Anesthetic Uptake and Action. Baltimore, Williams & Wilkins, 1974.
2. Eger, E. I., II: Respiratory factors in uptake and distribution of volatile anaesthetic agents. Br J Anaesth 36:155, 1964.
3. Holaday, D. A., Fiserova-Bergerova, V.: Fate of fluorinated metabolites of anesthetics in man. Drug Metab Rev 9:61, 1979.
4. Carpenter, R. L., et al.: The extent of metabolism of inhaled anesthetics in humans. Anesthesiology 65:201, 1986.
5. Fiserova-Bergerova, V., Holaday, D. A.: Uptake and clearance of inhalation anesthetics in man. Drug Metab Rev 9:43, 1979.
6. Holaday, D. A., Fiserova-Bergerova, V., Latto, I. P., Zumbiel, M.A.: Resistance of isoflurane to biotransformation in man. Anesthesiology 43:325, 1975.
7. Van Dyke, R. A., Chenoweth, M. B., Van Posnak, A.: Metabolism of volatile anesthetics: I. Conversion *in vivo* of several anesthetics to $^{14}CO_2$ and chloride. Biochem Pharmacol 13:1239, 1964.
8. Goldstein, A., Aronow, L., Kalman, S. M.: Principles of Drug Action: The Basis of Drug Action. New York, Harper & Row, 1968, p. 206.
9. Van Dyke, R. A.: Toxic metabolites from biotransformation: major organ damage. Int Anesthesiol Clin 19:39, 1981.
10. Hong, K., Trudell, J. R., O'Neil, J. R., Cohen, E. N.: Metabolism of nitrous oxide by human and rat intestinal contents. Anesthesiology 52:16, 1980.
11. McCarty, L. P., Malek, R. S., Larsen, E. R.: The effects of deuteration on the metabolism of halogenated anesthetics in the rat. Anesthesiology 51:106, 1979.
12. Sipes, I. G., et al.: Comparison of the biotransformation and hepatotoxicity of halothane and deuterated halothane. J Pharmacol Exp Ther 214:716, 1980.
13. Holaday, D. A., Rudofsky, S., Treuhaft, P. S.: The metabolic degradation of methoxyflurane in man. Anesthesiology 33:579, 1970.
14. Goldstein, A. A., Aranow, L., Kalman, S. M.: Principles of Drug Action: The Basis of Drug Action. New York, Harper & Row, 1968, p. 280.
15. Brown, B. R., Jr., Sipes, G. I.: Commentary: biotransformation and hepatotoxicity of halothane. Biochem Pharmacol 26:2091, 1977.
16. Berman, M. L., Bochantin, B. S.: Nonspecific stimulation of drug metabolism in rats by methoxyflurane. Anesthesiology 32:500, 1970.
17. Fiserova-Bergerova, V.: Inhibitory effect of isoflurane upon oxidative metabolism of halothane. Anesth Analg 63:399, 1984.
18. Kato, R., Chiesara, E., Vasanelli, P.: Further studies on the stimulation and inhibition of microsomal drug-metabolizing enzymes of rat liver by various compounds. Biochem Pharmacol 13:69, 1964.
19. Plummer, J. L., Hall, P., Jenner, M. A., Cousins, M. J.: Sex differences in halothane metabolism and hepatotoxicity in a rat model. Anesth Analg 64:563, 1985.
20. Terrell, R.: Physical and chemical properties of anaesthetic agents. Br J Anaesth 56:3S, 1984.
21. Lind, R. C., et al.: Oxygen requirements for reductive defluorination of halothane by rat hepatic microsomes. Anesth Analg 65:835, 1986.
22. Hall, P., Cousins, M. J., Plummer, J. L., Lunan, C. A.: Pathogenic mechanisms for halothane hepatotoxicity in animals and man. *In* Roth, S. H., Miller, K. W. (eds.). Molecular and Cellular Mechanisms of Anesthetics. New York, Plenum, 1986.
23. Ahr, H. J., King, L. J., Nastainczyk, W., Ullrich, V.: The mechanism of reductive dehalogenation of halothane by liver cytochrome P450. Biochem Pharmacol 31:383, 1982.
24. Sharp, J. H., Trudell, J. R., Cohen, E. N.: Volatile metabolites and decomposition products of halothane in man. Anesthesiology 50:2, 1979.
25. Yoshimura, N., Holaday, D. A., Fiserova-Bergerova, V.: Metabolism of methoxyflurane in man. Anesthesiology 44:372, 1976.
26. Dooley, J. R., Mazze, R. I., Rice, S. A., Borel, J. D.: Is enflurane defluorination inducible in man? Anesthesiology 50:213, 1979.
27. Chase, R. E., et al.: The biotransformation of Ethrane in man. Anesthesiology 35:262, 1971.
28. Rice, S. A., Sbordone, L., Mazze, R. I.: Metabolism by rat hepatic microsomes of fluorinated ether anesthetics following isoniazid administration. Anesthesiology 53:489, 1980.
29. Mazze, R. I., Woodruff, R. E., Heerdt, M. E.: Isoniazid-induced enflurane defluorination in humans. Anesthesiology 57:5, 1982.
30. Burke, T. R., Branchflower, R. V., Lees, D. E., Pohl, L. R.: Mechanism of defluorination of enflurane: identification of an organic metabolite in rat and man. Drug Metab Dispos Biol Fate Chem 9:19, 1981.
31. Holaday, D. A., Oda, M., Smith, F.: Is the ether linkage of enflurane subject to cleavage? *In* Abstracts of Scientific Papers, 1978 Annual Meeting of the American Society of Anesthesiologists. Chicago, American Society of Anesthesiologists, 1978, p. 231.
32. Hitt, B. A., et al.: Metabolism of isoflurane in Fischer 344 rats and man. Anesthesiology 40:62, 1974.
33. Davidkova, T. I., et al.: Biotransformation of isoflurane: urinary and serum fluoride ion and organic fluorine. Anesthesiology 69:218, 1988.
34. Wallin, R. F., Regan, B. M., Napoli, M. D., Stern, I. J.: Sevoflurane: a new inhalation anesthetic agent. Anesth Analg 54:758, 1975.
35. Strum, D. P., Eger, E. I., II: Partition coefficients for sevoflu-

rane in human blood, saline, and olive oil. Anesth Analg 66:654, 1987.

36. Holaday, D. A., Smith, F. R.: Clinical characteristics and biotransformation of sevoflurane in healthy human volunteers. Anesthesiology 54:100, 1981.

37. Fujii, K., et al.: Ionchromatographical analysis of a glucuronide as a sevoflurane metabolite. Hiroshima J Anesth 23:3, 1987.

38. Fujii, K., et al.: Pharmacokinetic study on excretion of sevoflurane. Hiroshima J Med Sci 36:89, 1987.

39. Davidkova, T. I., et al.: Urinary excretion of inorganic and organic fluoride after inhalation of sevoflurane. Hiroshima J Med Sci 99:99, 1987.

40. Holaday, D. A., England, R.: Deuteration reduced significantly the biotransformation of sevoflurane (abstract). Anesthesiology 57:A246, 1982.

41. Hanaki, C., Fujii, K., Morio, M., Tashima, T.: Decomposition of sevoflurane in sodalime. Hiroshima J Med Sci 36:61, 1987.

42. Eger, E. I., II: Partition coefficients of I-653 in human blood, saline and olive oil. Anesth Analg 66:971, 1987.

43. Koblin, D. D., et al.: I-653 resists degradation in rats. Anesth Analg 67:534, 1988.

44. Gion, H., et al.: Biotransformation of fluroxene in man. Anesthesiology 40:553, 1974.

45. Johnstone, R. R., et al.: The toxicity of fluroxene in animals and man. Anesthesiology 38:313, 1973

46. National Halothane Study: Summary of the National Halothane Study: possible association between halothane anesthesia and postoperative hepatic necrosis. JAMA 197:775, 1966.

47. Stock, J. G. L., Strunin, L.: Unexplained hepatitis following halothane. Anesthesiology 63:424, 1985.

48. Cohen, E. N., Hood, N.: Application of low temperature autoradiography to studies of uptake and metabolism of volatile anesthetics in the mouse: III. Halothane. Anesthesiology 31:553, 1969.

49. Mathieu, A., et al.: Correlation between specific immunity to a metabolite of halothane and hepatic lesions after multiple exposures. Anesth Analg 54:332, 1975.

50. Uehleke, H., Hellmer, K. H., Tabarelli-Poplawfski, S.: Metabolic activation of halothane and its covalent binding to liver endoplasmic proteins in vitro. Naunyn Schmiedebergs Arch Pharmacol 279:39, 1973.

51. McLain, G. E., Sipes, I. G., Brown, B. R., Jr.: An animal model of halothane hepatotoxicity: roles of enzyme induction and hypoxia. Anesthesiology 51:321, 1979.

52. Cousins, M. J., et al.: Hepatotoxicity and halothane metabolism in an animal model with application for human toxicity. Anaesth Intensive Care 7:9, 1979.

53. Hoft, R. H., Bunker, J. P., Goodman, H. I., Gregory, P. B.: Halothane hepatitis in three pairs of closely related women. N Engl J Med 304:1023, 1981.

54. Sherlock, S.: Halothane and the liver: occurrence of halothane hepatitis—a genetic factor. Proc R Soc Med 57:305, 1964.

55. Vergani, D., et al.: Sensitization to halothane-altered liver components in severe hepatic necrosis after halothane anaesthesia. Lancet 2:801, 1978.

56. Vergani, D., et al.: Antibodies to the surface of halothane-altered rabbit hepatocytes in patients with severe halothane-associated hepatitis. N Engl J Med 303:66, 1980.

57. Neuberger, J., Gimson, A. E. S., Davis, M., Williams, R.: Specific serological markers in the diagnosis of fulminant hepatic failure associated with halothane anaesthesia. Br J Anaesth 55:15, 1983.

58. Neuberger, J., et al.: Oxidative metabolism of halothane in the production of altered hepatocyte membrane antigens in acute halothane-induced hepatic necrosis. Gut 22:669, 1981.

59. Satoh, H., et al.: Immunological studies on the mechanism of halothane-induced hepatotoxicity: immunohistochemical evidence of trifluoroacetylated hepatocytes. J Pharmacol Exp Ther 233:857, 1985.

60. Kenna, J. G., Satoh, H., Christ, D. D., Pohl, L. R.: Metabolic basis for a drug hypersensitivity: antibodies in sera from patients with halothane-hepatitis recognize liver neoantigens that contain the trifluoroacetyl group derived from halothane. J Pharmacol Exp Ther 245:1103, 1988.

61. Mazze, R. I., Shue, G. L., Jackson, S. H.: Renal dysfunction associated with methoxyflurane anesthesia. JAMA 216:278, 1971.

62. Cousins, J. M., Mazze, R. I.: Methoxyflurane nephrotoxicity: a study of dose response in man. JAMA 225:1611, 1973.

63. Roman, R. J., Carter, J. R., North, W. C., Lauker, M. L.: Renal tubular site of action of fluoride in Fischer 344 rats. Anesthesiology 46:260, 1977.

64. Whitford, G. M., Taves, D. R.: Fluoride-induced diuresis: renal-tissue solute concentrations, functional, hemodynamic, and histologic correlates in the rat. Anesthesiology 39:416, 1973.

65. Cousins, M. J., et al.: A randomized prospective study of the metabolism and hepatotoxicity of halothane in humans. Anesth Analg 66:299, 1987

66. Miller, M. S., Gandolfi, A. J., Vaughan, R. W., Bentley, J. B.: Disposition of enflurane in obese patients. J Pharmacol Exp Ther 215:292, 1980.

67. Mazze, R. I., Calverley, R. K., Smith, N. T.: Inorganic fluoride nephrotoxicity: prolonged enflurane and halothane anesthesia in volunteers. Anesthesiology 46:265, 1977.

Suggested Readings

Cohen, E. N., VanDyke, R. A.: Metabolism of Volatile Anesthetics. Reading, MA, Addison-Wesley, 1977.

Chapter 42

VASOACTIVE AND INOTROPIC AGENTS

JAMES A. DINARDO

In clinical practice, vasoactive and inotropic agents are used alone or in combination to alter blood pressure. Blood pressure is the product of cardiac output and systemic vascular resistance. Cardiac output, in turn, is the product of heart rate and stroke volume. In simple terms, systemic vascular resistance can be considered to constitute ventricular afterload. This is a gross simplification, and more detailed discussion is offered elsewhere.[1] Preload is the ventricular end-diastolic volume. With afterload, heart rate and contractility constant increases in preload will increase stroke volume and therefore cardiac output. Contractility is defined as the state of cardiac performance independent of preload and afterload. Increases in contractility decrease end-systolic volume. With afterload, heart rate and preload constant increases in contractility increase stroke volume and cardiac output.

The ability of the ventricle to maintain stroke volume in the face of increased afterload by increasing preload is defined as preload reserve.[2] Preload reserve is exhausted when the sacromeres are stretched to their maximum diastolic length. When this occurs, one sees no further augmentation of the velocity of shortening by increasing diastolic fiber length, and the ventricle behaves as if preload is fixed. For a given level of contractility, once preload reserve is exhausted, additional increases in afterload are accompanied by parallel decreases in stroke volume. This is defined as a state of afterload mismatch.[2] Therefore, afterload mismatch is the inability of the ventricle at a given level of contractility to maintain stroke volume in the face of an increased wall stress.

Vasoactive agents alter vascular smooth muscle tone. Venoconstrictors reduce venous capacitance, and because 60 to 80% of the blood volume is on the venous side of the circulation, venoconstriction can augment preload significantly. Constriction of arterioles increases systemic vascular resistance and afterload. Postive inotropic agents increase contractility, whereas negative inotropes depress contractility.

This chapter reviews the major classes of drugs used by anesthesiologists to alter and control blood pressure.

ADRENERGIC AGONISTS

Interaction of endogenous catecholamines, synthetic catecholamines, and sympathomimetics with the myocardium and vascular smooth muscle occurs by means of adreneric receptors. Adrenergic receptors have been extensively classified since Ahlquist postulated the existence of α and β receptors in 1948.[3] We now know that subsets of both α (α_1 and α_2)[4] and β (β_1 and β_2)[5] adrenoceptors exist. In addition are peripheral adrenoceptors specific for dopamine. Two subsets of these dopaminergic (DA) receptors are recognized: DA_1 and DA_2.[6] Genetic cloning techniques are being used to identify an ever increasing number of α_1, α_2, β_1, β_2, DA_1, and DA_2 subtypes.

Adrenoceptors have both presynaptic and postsynaptic locations in the sympathetic nervous system. Adrenoceptor synaptic site, anatomic location, and action are summarized in Table 42–1. Stimulation of presynaptic α_2 receptors inhibits postsynaptic release of norepinephrine. This effect is offset by stimulation of presynaptic β_2 receptors, which enhance postsynaptic norepinephrine release. Postsynaptic α_2 and β_2 receptors are more responsive to hormonal epinephrine than to the neurotransmitter norepinephrine. This finding has led to the suggestion that these receptors are extrasynaptic and noninnervated.[7] α_1 Adrenoceptors are widely distributed in the periphery and are largely responsible for peripheral (arterial and venous) vasoconstriction. The distribution and role of peripheral α_2 adrenoceptors are less clear.

Approximately 80% of the β receptors located in the myocardium are of the β_1 subset, whereas the remaining 20% are of the β_2 subset.[8,9] In congestive heart failure, selective down-regulation of β_1 receptors occurs such that β_2 adrenoceptors account for as much as 40% of the total myocardial β adrenoceptor population.[8–10] Thus, one sees a progressive dependence on β_2 agonism to enhance contractility in the failing heart. In addition, α_1 adrenoceptors play a greater role in producing positive inotropy in the setting of β_1 down-regulation.

DA_1 receptors are postsynaptic and are preferentially distributed in the renal and mesenteric vasculature. Postsynpatic DA_1 receptors are also distributed on renal tubules and juxtaglomerular cells. DA_2 receptors are primarily presynaptic; stimulation inhibits norepinephrine release similar to that seen with presynaptic α_2 stimulation.

Receptor stimulation is the first in a series of steps that initiate a cellular response to adrenergic agonism. The structure of the β adrenergic receptor and the intracellular response to β-adrenergic agonism is well characterized. The β-adrenergic receptor complex consists of a receptor site for specific hormones coupled to a stimulatory G protein that binds guanosine triphosphate and

Table 42–1. Adrenoceptors: Synaptic and Anatomic Sites and Actions

Receptor	Synaptic Site	Anatomic Site	Action
α_1	Postsynaptic	Peripheral vascular smooth muscle	Constriction
		Renal vascular smooth muscle	Constriction
		Coronary arteries: epicardial	Constriction
		Myocardium	Positive inotropism
		Renal tubules	Antidiuresis
α_2	Presynaptic	Peripheral vascular smooth muscle release	Inhibits norepinephrine (NE)
		Central nervous system (CNS)	Secondary vasodilation
			Inhibition of CNS activity
			Sedation
			Decrease MAC
	Postsynaptic	Coronary arteries: endocardial	Constriction
		CNS	Inhibition of insulin release
			Decrease bowel motility
			Inhibition of antidiuretic hormone
			Analgesia
		Renal tubule	Promotes Na^{++} and H_2O excretion
β_1	Postsynaptic	Myocardium	Positive inotropism and chronotropism
		Sinoatrial (SA) node	
		Ventricular conduction	
		Kidney	Renin release
β_2	Presynaptic	Myocardium	Accelerates NE release; opposite action to presynaptic α_2 agonism
		SA node ventricular	
		Conduction vessels	Constriction
	Postsynaptic	Myocardium	Positive inotropism and chronotropism
		Vascular smooth muscle	Relaxation
		Bronchial smooth muscle	Relaxation
		Renal vessels	Relaxation
DA_1	Postsynaptic	Blood vessels (renal, mesentery, coronary)	Vasodilation
		Renal tubules	Natriuresis
			Diuresis
		Juxtaglomerular cells	Renin release
		Sympathetic ganglia	Minor inhibition
DA_2	Presynaptic	Postganglionic sympathetic nerves	Inhibit NE release
			Secondary vasodilation
	Postsynaptic	Renal and mesenteric vasculature	?Vasoconstriction

stimulates the enzyme adenyl cyclase (AC).[11] AC catalyzes the conversion of adenosine triphosphate to cyclic adenosine monophosphate (cAMP). Sutherland is credited with identifying cAMP as the second messenger.[12] As such, increased concentrations of cAMP initiate a cascade of phosphorylation reactions in the cell that leads to a cell-specific response such as positive inotropy or chronotropy. In cardiac muscle, phosphorylation of a cAMP-dependent protein kinase is necessary to open the inner calcium gate on the myocyte. Thus, calcium is the final mediator of effects and is referred to as the third messenger.

Recent evidence supports the existence of second messengers for both α_1 and α_2 receptors. α_1 Receptors are coupled to regulatory G proteins that bind guanosine triphosphate and regulate the interaction of the receptor site with the enzyme phospholipase C (PLC). PLC catalyzes the formation of the second messengers inositol 1,4,5-triphosphate (IP_3) and diacyl glycerol (DAG). Both produce increased intracellular calcium IP_3 by releasing calcium from intracellular stores and DAG by initiating opening of calcium channels to allow an influx of extracellular calcium.[13] α_2 Receptors are coupled to an inhibitory G protein that binds guanosine triphosphate and inhibits AC. As a result, reduced levels of cAMP serve as a second messenger.

ENDOGENOUS CATECHOLAMINES

The sympathetic nervous system is distributed to all areas of the peripheral circulation. Blood vessels in the skin and splanchnic bed are extensively innervated, whereas vessels in heart, brain, and muscle are less extensively innervated. Activity of the sympathetic nervous system on the myocardium and peripheral vasculature is mediated by the endogenous catecholamines norepinephrine and epinephrine. Stimulation of the postganglionic fibers that terminate in the myocardium and vascular smooth muscle cause release of norepinephrine. In addition, stimulation of postganglionic fibers that terminate in the adrenal medulla cause release of large quantities of epinephrine and some norepinephrine into the circulation, where they act as hormones.

Dopamine is a neurotransmitter in the central nervous system; few, if any, peripheral dopaminergic neurons are known. Dopamine that reaches the peripheral circulation presumably comes from the central nervous system (CNS).

The chemical structures of both endogenous and exogenous catecholamines are depicted in Figure 42-1.

Epinephrine

Epinephrine possesses β_1-, β_2-, and α_1-adrenergic activities. At doses of 0.01 to 0.03 μg/kg/min, epinephrine has a potent positive inotropic effect mediated through β_1 stimulation with little effect on vasomotor tone resulting from the balance of β_2 and α_1 stimulation. As the dose increases above 0.03 μg/kg/min, progressively more α_1 activity occurs, with resultant mixed positive inotropic and vasoconstrictive effects. Doses above 0.03 μg/kg/min also cause progressive decreases in renal blood flow because of renal vasoconstriction.[14] Above 0.1 μg/kg/min, epinephrine is primarily a vasoconstrictor. Epinephrine's vasoconstrictive effects also reduce venous capacitance. Although coronary blood flow is maintained at high doses, epinephrine may not be favorable to myocardial energetics because, in addition to increasing contractility, it increases systolic blood pressure, increases left ventricular end-diastolic volume and pressure, and reduces diastolic blood pressure while increasing heart rate. Epinephrine is a potent chronotrope and is also dysrhythmogenic.

Epinephrine has been demonstrated to increase cardiac index more reliably during termination of cardiopulmonary bypass than either dopamine or dobutamine.[15] For this reason, epinephrine, at 0.015 to 0.04 μg/kg/min, has been described as the agent of choice to terminate cardiopulmonary bypass.[16] The potent intopic and balanced peripheral vascular effects allow prompt, reliable termination of cardiopulmonary bypass while avoiding the ventricular distention and systemic hypotension that

compromise subendocardial perfusion. Critics point out that the potent inotropic effects of epinephrine may not be necessary in every instance, and thus epinephrine's potentially deleterious effects on myocardial energetics and renal blood flow can be avoided.

Norepinephrine

Norepinephrine possesses β_1- and α_1-adrenergic activity. The α_1 effects of norepinephrine are mainfest at low doses (0.01 to 0.02 μg/kg/min), producing vasoconstriction that predominates as the dose increases. Contractility increases as a result of β_1 agonism, but usually no increase occurs in cardiac output because any potential reduction in end-systolic volume is offset by the increased afterload. Norepinephrine reduces renal blood flow, elevates both systolic and diastolic blood pressure, reduces venous capacitance, and generally causes a reflex decrease in heart rate. Although coronary blood flow is maintained, norepinephrine may not be favorable to myocardial energetics because, in addition to increasing contractility, it increases systolic and diastolic blood pressure and left ventricular end-diastolic volume and pressure.

Dopamine

Dopamine possesses β_1- and α_1-adrenergic and DA$_1$ and DA$_2$ activities. Some of the α_1 activity is due to release of endogenous norepinephrine. At doses of 2 to 3 μg/kg/min, the DA$_1$ activity is maximal and results in preferential dilation of renal, mesenteric, and coronary vasculature. Stimulation of presynaptic DA$_2$ inhibits norepinephrine release, which enhances vasodilation. β_1-Induced enhanced inotropy is seen at doses between 2 and 5 μg/kg/min, resulting in increased cardiac output and renal blood flow. Beginning at doses of 5 μg/kg/min, dopamine's α_1-adrenergic activity increases because of release of norepinephrine. This results in increased peripheral resistance, pulmonary vascular resistance, and pulmonary capillary wedge pressure with little concomitant increase in cardiac output.[17] This combination of increased ventricular wall radius and afterload may cause detrimental increases in myocardial oxygen consumption. At doses above 10 μg/kg/min, release of norepinephrine

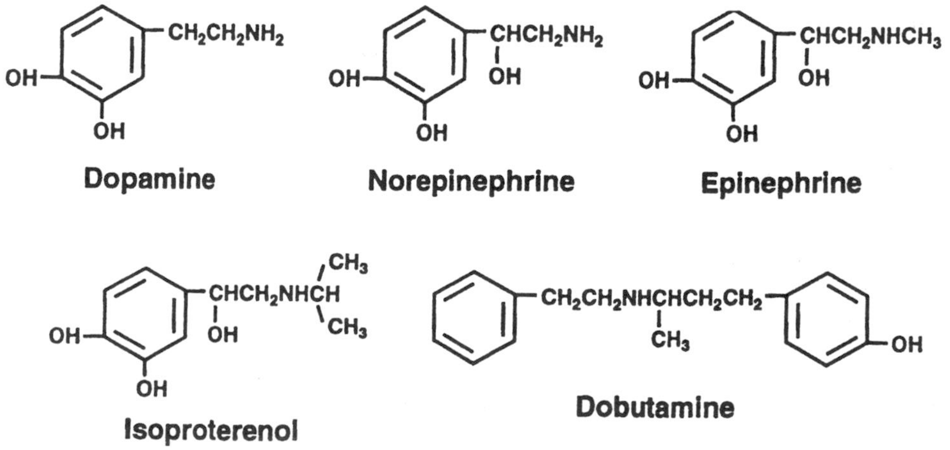

Fig. 42–1. Chemical structures of endogenous (dopamine, norepinephrine, epinephrine) and exogenous (isoproterenol, dobutamine) catecholamines.

is such that dopamine is hemodynamically similar to norepinephrine. This intense α_1 activity reverses the renal vasodilation seen at lower doses. Dopamine's chronotrophic and dysrhythmic effects increase as the dose increases.

SYNTHETIC CATECHOLAMINES (EXOGENOUS)

Isoproterenol

Isoproterenol is a pure β_1- and β_2-adrenergic agonist. Isoproterenol at standard doses (0.01 to 0.05 µg/kg/min) enhances contractility and reduces peripheral resistance. The increase in cardiac output that should accompany the increased contractility and reduced afterload is attenuated by reductions in preload. Preload is reduced as the result of venodilation and tachycardia.

Isoproterenol can produce unfavorable myocardial energetics by reducing diastolic blood pressure in the face of increased contractility and heart rate. Finally, isoproterenol is the most dysrhythmogenic of the catecholamines.

Dobutamine

Dobutamine possesses β_1-, β_2-, and α_1-adrenergic activities. The predominant effect is enhanced inotropy through β_1 stimulation. The β_2 and α_1 activities are balanced such that mild vasodilation occurs at the commonly used doses of 5 to 20 µg/kg/min. Dobutamine decreases pulmonary vascular resistance,[18] blunts hypoxia pulmonary vasoconstriction,[19] and increases coronary blood flow.[20] Dobutamine may actually reduce myocardial oxygen consumption in the failing heart because, although it increases contractility, it reduces left ventricular radius and end-diastolic pressure while increasing arterial pressure and maintaining heart rate.[21] Dobutamine appears to have less of a chronotrophic effect than dopamine.[22]

SYMPATHOMIMETICS (NONCATECHOLAMINES) (FIG. 42–2)[14]

These agents by definition do not contain the catecholamine moiety but have many of the same properties as catecholamines. The largest clinically useful class of sympathomimetics are the phenylisopropylamines.

Ephedrine

Ephedrine has both direct and indirect β_1-, β_2-, and α_1-adrenergic effects. The indirect effect is secondary to release of norepinephrine from nerve terminals. As a result of this mixed activity, the drug produces a β_1 effect and weaker β_2 and α_1 effects. Ephedrine can be considered a less potent epinephrine. The α_1 effect is such that more constriction of venous capacitance than of arterial resistance vessels occurs.

Typical adult doses of 5 to 10 mg as a bolus produce an increase in blood pressure by increasing preload, contractility, and heart rate, with a lesser increase in peripheral resistance. Heart rate increases from β_1 agonist may be attenuated by baroreceptor reflexes secondary to increases in blood pressure. The onset of action of a single ephedrine dose is within 1 minute, whereas the duration of action is 10 to 15 minutes.

Ephedrine is the agent of choice for treatment of hypotension in the obstetric patient because of its lack of uterine artery vasoconstrictive effects. As a result, uterine blood flow varies directly with blood pressure.

Phenylephrine

Phenylephrine is a pure α_1-adrenergic agent. It binds α_2 receptors only at extremely high concentrations. Some β-adrenergic activity occurs at concentrations 10 times those seen clinically. Phenylephrine at clinically relevant doses is a pure vasoconstrictor. It has equal vasoconstrictive activity on arterial resistance and venous capacitance vessels. Thus, typical doses of 40 to 100 µg as a bolus produce increases in both preload and afterload. Blood pressure elevation may produce a reflex bradycardia. The onset of action a single phenylephrine dose is within 1 minute, whereas the duration of action is 5 to 10 minutes.

Methoxamine

Methoxamine, like phenylephrine, is a pure α_1-adrenergic agent. In contrast to phenylephrine, it has little effect

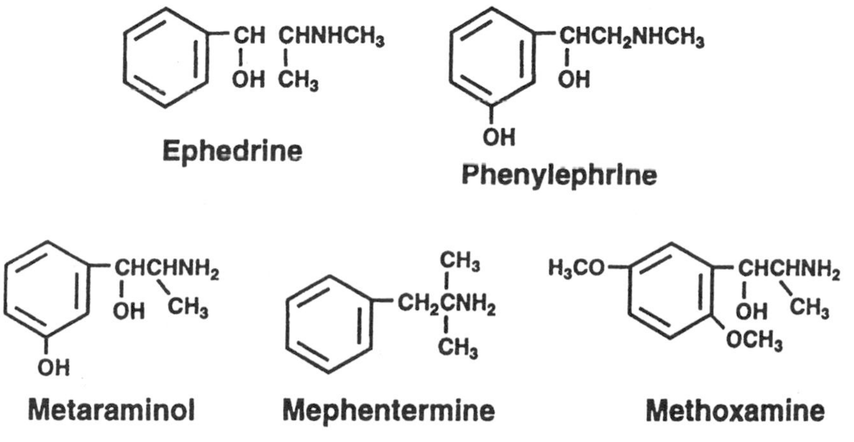

Fig. 42–2. Chemical structures of sympathomimetics.

on venous capacitance vessels. Thus, a typical bolus dose of 5 to 10 mg produces an increase in afterload with subsequent blood pressure elevation. Blood pressure elevation may produce a reflex bradycardia. The onset of action of a single methoxamine dose is within 1 minute, whereas the duration of action is 60 to 90 minutes.

Vasopressin (Pitressin)

Posterior pituitary hormones are formed in the hypothalamic nuclei. Packets of the material migrate as granules down axons to the posterior lobe of the pituitary where they are stored. The mechanism of release is not established, but it is likely neurogenic.

Oxytocin is an octapeptide containing isoleucine and leucine, whereas the pressor principle is an octapeptide containing phenylalanine-arginine. The latter, known as vasopressin, is also the antidiuretic hormone, which increases reabsorption of water in distal tubules of the kidney. It is a direct smooth muscle stimulant of blood vessels including coronary and perhaps cerebral vessels. Altering the structure of oxytocin can completely change its type of activity. Thus, 4-leucine-oxytocine is a diuretic natriuretic, antivasopressin polypeptide.[23]

The duration of effect is about 3 hours. Its clinical use is limited to treatment of diabetes insipidus and to increasing intestinal motility in paralytic ileus.

Angiotensin

A hypertensive agent formed in ischemic kidneys was recognized as early as 1928. Page and co-workers in 1958 isolated and synthetized the substance named angiotensin.[24] Several intermediate analogues were also identified, and each of the angiotensins is a polypeptide. Steps in the formation of the most active material are as follows:

ANGIOTENSINOGEN   →   ANGIOTENSIN I   →   ANGIOTENSIN II
(Renin substrate from   (Decapeptide)   (Octapeptide)
 kidney or blood)

The mechanism by which the process is activated is a reduction of blood pressure, which stimulates baroreceptors in the kidneys to release renin from juxtaglomerular cells.

The end product, angiotensin II, acts predominantly on the circulation. A powerful pressor response results from constriction of renal and splanchnic arteriolar beds. Little or no action on veins is seen, and no change in heart rate or cardiac output occurs.

Phenylpressin

A specific polypeptide containing eight amino acids is known as phenylpressin or PLV$_2$. The letters stand for (2) phenylalanine (8) lysine vasopressin. It differs from the antidiuretic hormone of the posterior pituitary in that lysine is substituted for arginine of the antidiuretic hormone.

Selective microcirculatory effects have been demonstrated. A greater degree of reactivity is exhibited on the venular side, with a diminishing gradient to the arteriolar

Table 42–2. Comparison of Norepinephrine, Angiotensin, and the Octapeptide PLV-2 in Regard to Effects on Peripheral Circulation

Microcirculatory Effects of Selected Pressor Drugs	
Drugs	Effects
Norepinephrine	
Arterioles	Intense constriction
Capillary inflow	Reduced
Epinephrine reactivity	Increased
Vasomotion	Depressed
Venules	Predisposed to stasis
Microcirculation	Ultimately damaged
Capillaries	Ischemic
Angiotensin	
Arterioles	Less intense constriction
Capillary inflow	Improved
Epinephrine reactivity	Decreased
Vasomotion	Depressed
Venules	Predisposed to atony and stasis
Microcirculation	Ultimately damaged
Capillaries	Stasis
PLV-2	
Arterioles	Less intense constriction
Capillary inflow	Improved
Epinephrine reactivity	Decreased
Vasomotion	Sustained
Venules	Normal tone
Microcirculation	Virtually no damage
Capillaries	Normal flow

After Hershey and Altura-Scientific Exhibit Third Postgraduate Seminar on Anesthesiology, Miami, 1966.

side. In contrast, norepinephrine and epinephrine show a pronounced effect on the arteriolar site and a diminishing gradient toward the venules. Clinical investigations of the use of this drug in management of hypotension and in shock are currently underway (Table 42-2).

PHOSPHODIESTERASE INHIBITORS

This group of agents acts not by interaction with the adrenergic receptor, but also by directly influencing the intracellular concentration of cAMP. Normally, three phosphodiesterase enzymes (PDE I, PDE II, and PDE III) are responsible for hydrolyzing cyclic nucleotides including cAMP. PDE III is specific for converting 3'5'-cAMP to the less active 5'-cAMP. This activity attenuates the effect of β agonism by reducing the quanity of the second messenger.

Phosphodiesterase inhibitors inhibit these enzymes and increase the concentration of cAMP and other cyclic nucleotides. Thus, they are capable of eliciting cellular responses identical to those obtained with β agonism even in the presence of β antagonism. In addition, these agents may produce synergistic adrenergic activity when combined with β agonists. In cardiac tissue (β_1 receptors), PDE III inhibition leads to an increase in intracellular calcium and increased contractility, whereas in vascular tissue (β_2 receptors), it leads to a decrease in intracellular calcium and vasodilation.

Amrinone

Amrinone is a specific inhibitor of PDE III. As a result, amrinone produces mild positive inotropy and strong vasodilation, effects similar to β_1 and β_2 agonism. This inodilator is useful when afterload mismatch exists in conjunction with depressed systolic function. Amrinone increases cardiac index, reduces left ventricular end-diastolic pressure and volume, reduces systolic blood pressure, and has little effect on heart rate. Like dobutamine, in the failing heart this increase in cardiac index may be associated with a decrease in myocardial oxygen consumption because of the concomitant reduction in wall stress.[25]

In addition, amrinone, in combination with traditional β agonists, has been shown to be additive or synergistic in improving left ventricular function.[26,27] Amrinone is usually administered as a bolus (0.75 to 1.5 mg/kg over 5 minutes) followed by an infusion at 2 to 10 μg/kg/min. Intense vasodilation may follow the bolus. Enoximone is also a PDE III inhibitor that, in early clinical trials, appears to have a hemodynamic profile similar to that of amrinone.

EDRF/NO

An endogenous vasodilator known as endothelium-derived relaxing factor (EDRF) has been described. This substance, derived from endothelium, is labile, diffusible, and capable of inducing vasodilation in response to many substances that increase intracellular calcium.[28-30] In fact, an increase in intracellular calcium stimulates production of EDRF/NO from L-arginine. EDRF is nitric oxide (NO) or an NO-containing moiety.[31,32] Once formed, EDRF/NO diffuses from endothelium to vascular smooth muscle, where it binds to and activates guanylate cyclase to produce cyclic guanosine monophosphate (cGMP). cGMP acts as a second messenger to catalyze reactions that lead to a reduction of vascular smooth muscle calcium by reduced calcium influx, increased calcium efflux, and reduced release of intracellular calcium.[33] This, in turn, produces relaxation of vascular smooth muscle and vasodilation. EDRF/NO is involved in modulation of basal vascular smooth muscle tone as well. This modulation capacity is lost in vessels where entholethium is removed or damaged.

DIRECT-ACTING VASODILATORS

Nitrovasodilators such as nitroglycerin and sodium nitroprusside are not dependent on vascular endothelium to exert their vasodilatory effects. These agents interact directly with vascular smooth muscle to form S-nitrosothiol intermediates.[33] Subsequent interaction of an NO moiety with guanylate cyclase produces the second messenger cGMP, which catalyzes reactions that lead to a reduction of calcium and to relaxation in vascular smooth muscle.

All direct-acting vasodilators produce reflex increases in heart rate and contractility. Thus, they are commonly used in conjunction with β-adrenergic antagonists, as discussed later in this chapter.

Sodium Nitroprusside

Sodium nitroprusside is a widely used, intravenous vasodilator with a short half-life. Infusions start at 0.5 μg/kg/min and are titrated upward for control of blood pressure. Nitroprusside dilates primarily precapillary arterioles, resulting in an decrease in systemic vascular resistance and a reduction in afterload. Some increase in venous capacitance occurs as well, producing preload reduction. Because sodium nitroprusside is a potent arteriolar dilator, it can induce a coronary steal in the presence of the appropriate anatomy.[34] In addition, it also induces a reflex increase in heart rate and contractility. Nitroprusside dilates cerebral resistance and capacitance vessels and thereby increases intracranical pressure in patients with reduced intracranial compliance.[35]

Chemically, nitroprusside is structurally an unusual agent[36] (Fig. 42-3). It consists of a ferrous core bristling with five formidable cyanides (CN^-) and an ominous nitrosol (NO^+) group. Each CN group possesses a negative charge, whereas the iron possesses two, and the NO group one positive charge. The NO moiety is the effective group. It may act like nitrites or nitrates, but it is 30 to 1000 times more potent; and unlike these agents, nitroprusside does not induce tolerance. It is dissimilar in other modes as well.

Biodegradation of nitroprusside is initiated by a very rapid transfer of electrons from intracellular ferrous oxyhemoglobin Fe^{2+} to the nitroprusside forming an unstable cyanoferrate radical of nitroprusside and yielding the ferric form, Fe^{2+} methemoglobin.[37]

A major nonenzymatic chemical reaction also occurs by an interaction of nitroprusside with sulfhydryl groups (SH) bound in the membranes of the red blood cells and in the membranes of vascular walls with the formation of cyanogen (HCN).[38,39] Both the cyanoferrate and the cyanogen liberate free CN^- ions. Normally, one of the CN ions interacts with methemoglobin to form cyanomethemoglobin.

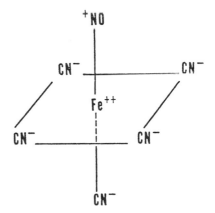

Fig. 42-3. Schematic representation of the iron coordination complex of nitroprusside. The overall complex has a net negative charge and must be associated with cations such as the two sodiums in sodium nitroprusside. Reprinted with permission from Palmer, R. F., Lasseter K. C.: Drug therapy: sodium nitroprusside. N Engl J Med *294*:1403, 1976. See Collins, V. J. Principles of Anesthesiology, Third Ed. Philadelphia, Lea & Febiger, 1070–1082, 1993.

1. $Fe(CN_5) NO + SH$ groups (RBC) $\xrightarrow{\text{Blood}}$ HCN (cyanogen) $\rightarrow H^+ + CN^-$

2. CN^- + thiosulfate (from cysteine) $\xrightarrow[\text{Rhodanese}]{\text{Hepatic}}$ SCN (thiocyanate)

Fig. 42–4. Biotransformation of nitroprusside.

The four remaining molecules of CN are converted by the liver-kidney enzyme rhodanase in conjunction with hydroxyocobalamin (B_{12}) and thiosulfate to thiocyanate,[37] which is renally excreted (Fig. 42–4). High plasma levels of thiocyanate produce CNS toxicity; these high levels are more common in patients with poor renal function. Quanities of CN excessive enough to overwhelm the rhodanase-thiosulfate system result in CN binding to cytochrome oxidase. This binding interferes with the final stages of electron transport and prevents tissue oxygen utilization.

Cyanide toxicity is due to a cellular poisoning by the excess cyanide that binds tightly to the Fe^{3+} of cytochrome oxidase.[38] This results in a metabolic acidosis in the face of high mixed venous oxygen saturations because of the inability of tissues to utilize oxygen. Signs of inpending CN toxicity are tachyphylaxis, muscle twitching, labored respirations, rigidity, and convulsions. Doses greater than 10 $\mu g/kg/min$ are needed for response, and an immediate resistance to the hypotensive effect of the drug ensues. Treatment consists of discontinuing the infusion and giving 150 mg/kg of thiosulfate over 10 to 15 minutes. Some clinicians recommend the use of sodium nitrite, 5 mg/kg over 5 minutes, to convert hemoglobin to methemoglobin because methemoglobin has a greater affinity for CN than cytochrome oxidase. Methemoglobin does not carry oxygen, however, and that this limitation may add an anemic hypoxia to the existing cytotoxic hypoxia.

Nitroglycerin

Systematically, nitroglycerin has it greatest dilating capacity on the venous beds resulting in preload reduction. Arterial dilation (large arteries more than smaller arteries and arterioles) occurs only at higher doses.[40] Despite their predominant effects on venous capacitance when used in appropriate doses, nitroglycerin and nitroprusside have been shown to be equally effective in the treatment of hypertension.[41,42] With comparable reductions in systolic blood pressure, nitroglycerin causes less reduction in diastolic blood pressure than does nitroprusside.[42] Therefore, coronary perfusion pressure may be better preserved with nitroglycerin than with nitroprusside.

Furthermore, nitroglycerin dilates large epicardial vessels, collateral vessels, and stenotic coronary lesions. Because it does not dilate coronary arterioles, it is not implicated in producing the coronary steal phenomenon. For these reasons, nitroglycerin may be the preferred agent for treatment of hypertension associated with myocardial ischemia. For treatment of hypertension, nitroglycerin is started at 0.5 $\mu g/kg/min$ and is titrated upward.

Toxicity of nitroglycerin is limited to production of small quantities of methemoglobin. This is the result of a nitrite metabolite that oxides hemoglobin. Methemoglobin levels average 1.5% in patients receiving long-term intravenous nitroglycerin therapy.[43] These levels are well below the 20% considered clinically important.

Hydralazine[44]

Hydralazine produces direct smooth muscle relaxation with a subsequent reduction in systemic vascular resistance and afterload. It also causes a reflex increase in heart rate and contractility. Hydralazine is administered in incremental intravenous doses of 2.5 to 5 mg. Onset time is delayed (10 to 15 minutes), and duration of action is 2 to 4 hours.

Hydralazine-induced hypotension, in combination with a reflex tachycardia, can seriously compromise subendocardial perfusion.[44] This situation is particularly dangerous in patients with concentric hypertrophy from long-standing hypertension. Thus, if hydralazine is chosen, it may be necessary to administer a β_1 antagonist as well. Propranolol is commonly used in combination with hydralazine.

ADRENERGIC ANTAGONISTS

β-Adrenergic antagonists have a basic structure similar to that of β agonists. β_1-Selective (cardioselective) antagonists have been developed to avoid the problems associated with β_2 blockade in patients with reactive airway disease and diabetes mellitus. These agents are selective for β_1 receptors and are not specific. At higher doses, all β_1-selective agents possess some β_2-antagonist activity.

The manner in which β antagonists reduce blood pressure is not well understood. Long-term administration produces a reduction in cardiac output, but this does not appear to be a major antihypertensive mechanism.[45] Inhibition of renin release with a subsequent reduction in aldosterone may also play a role.[46] Prejunction β_1 blockade inhibits release of norepinephrine from postjunction neurons, this effect may play a role as well. On a short-term basis, β antagonists are rarely used alone to decrease blood pressure. In fact, they are more commonly used to counteract reflex increases in heart rate and contractility, which accompany the use of vasodilators.

Many α-adrenergic antagonists are available,[47-49] but few are clinically relevant. α_1-Receptor blockade produces vasodilation because tonic α_1 stimulation contributes substantially to resting vascular tone.

The following is a review of the commonly used α, β, and combined α-β antagonists.

Propranolol[46]

Propranolol is a nonselective β antagonist with an elimination half-life of 4 hours. A usual intravenous dose is 0.5 to 5 mg.

Atenolol

Atenolol is a β_1-selective antagonist with an elimination half-life of 6 hours. A usual intravenous dose is 5 to 10 mg.

Metoprolol

Metoprolol is a β_1-selective antagonist with an elimination half-life of 3.5 hours. A usual intravenous dose is 5 to 15 mg.

Esmolol[49]

Esmolol is an ultrashort-acting β antagonist. Esmolol has an elimination half-life of 9 minutes because of metabolism by red cell esterases and is relatively β_1 selective.[49] Esmolol is started with a bolus of 0.5 mg/kg given over several minutes, followed by an infusion of 50 μg/kg and titrated up to 300 μg/kg as necessary. Esmolol is useful in patients with poor ventricular function or broncospastic disease because if it is not tolerated therapy can be quickly terminated.

Phentolamine

Phentolamine is an α_1 and α_2 antagonist that is rarely used clinically. Doses of 2 to 5 mg are given to control blood pressure. A reflex increase in heart rate uniformly occurs.

Labetalol[50]

Labetalol has α_1- and nonselective β-antagonist activity. This drug also has some intrinsic β_2-agonist activity that promotes vasodilation.[50] When given intravenously, labetalol has β-antagonist activity that is seven times that of its α_1-antagonist activity. Labetalol reduces systemic vascular resistance and prevents reflex increases in heart rate and contractility. The net result is a reduction in systemic vascular resistance with little or no change in cardiac output.

Labetalol is given as an intravenous bolus of 0.1 to 0.25 mg/kg over 1 to 2 minutes. The drug is metabolized by the liver and has an elimination half-life of 5.5 hours. Infusion doses start at 0.02 mg/kg/min. Caution must be used in patients with compromised systolic function because large doses of labetalol may induce afterload mismatch resulting from the unbalanced α and β effects.

CALCIUM CHANNEL ANTAGONISTS[51]

Calcium is a universal messenger in myocytes and vascular smooth muscle cells. Two basic types of calcium channels exist: voltage-dependent channels and receptor-operated channels.[51] Voltage-dependent channels require a change in transmembrane potential to open. Three types of voltage-dependent calcium channels are recognized: T (transient), L (long-lasting), and N (neuronal). T and L channels are located in cardiac tissue and vascular smooth muscle. T channels are activated at low voltage, may have some role in cardiac tissue depolarization (phase 0), and are not blocked by calcium antagonists.[52] L

channels are the slow calcium channels. They are responsible for phase 2 of the action potential of cardiac cells, for automaticity (phase 0) in the sinoatrial and atrioventricular nodes, and for allowing calcium influx into vascular smooth muscle. These are the channels blocked by calcium antagonists.

Receptor-operated channels require the binding of an agonist (such as α and β agonists) to recruit voltage-dependent calcium channels (L channels) or to open calcium channels directly by a second messenger.

Drugs from three different classes constitute the calcium antagonists in current use today. Verapamil is a phenylalkylamine, nifedipine and nicardipine are dihydropyridines, and diltiazem is a benthothiazepine. These structural differences help to account for their diverse hemodynamic effects. Verapamil and diltiazem produce frequency-dependent block, whereas nifedipine and nicardipine produce slow channel block at rest. Frequency-dependent block is more likely to affect cells with repetitive activity such as the sinoatrial and atrioventricular nodes.

To simplify comparison of these agents, one must consider inotropy, chronotropy, dromotropy, and vasodilation. As a rule, the calcium antagonists have little effect on venous capacitance vessels. This is true even of those agents that are potent arterial vasodilators. Finally, reflex cardiovascular responses accompany the use of these agents. As a result, the effects of a calcium antagonist in isolated tissue and in the intact organism can differ.

Nifedipine

Nifedipine is a potent arterial vasodilator. This intense vasodilation elicits a reflex increase in heart rate and contractility such that the inherent negative inotropic, chronotropic, and dromotropic activity of the drug is not seen clinically. This makes nifedipine a good antihypertensive agent. Nifedipine can be given sublingually (5 to 10 mg) or intravenously (5 to 15 μg/kg) to treat hypertension.

Nicardipine

Nicardipine is similar to nifedipine, but with a longer half-life (8 to 9 hours) and selectivity for the coronary and cerebrovascular vascular beds. Nicardipine can be titrated intravenously to control blood pressure because it reduces systemic vascular resistance with little reflex increase in heart rate. Intravenously, it has an immediate onset, with a 10- to 15-minute duration of action. A loading dose of 0.15 to 0.2 mg/kg may be given over 15 minutes, followed by an infusion of 0.05 mg/kg/hour.

Verapamil

Verapamil is less of a vasodilator than nifedipine and less of a negative inotrope. Clinically, however, verapamil depresses systolic function to a greater degree than nifedipine because of the lack of reflex sympathetic stimulation. Verapamil's negative chronotropic and dromotropic activity depresses the rate of sinus node discharge, slows conduction velocity, and prolongs the atrioventricular nodal refractory interval. This makes verapamil a good agent for treatment of supraventricular tachycardia. Verapamil can be given intravenously in doses of 50 to 100 μg/kg.

Diltiazem

Diltiazem's hemodynamic profile can be considered to lie between that of nifedipine and that of verapamil. Like verapamil, diltiazem depresses the rate of sinus node discharge, slows conduction velocity, and prolongs the atrioventricular nodal refractory interval. It is less of a negative inotrope than verapamil and is a poor peripheral vasodilator, although it is an excellent coronary vasodilator. Diltiazem can be given intravenously in doses of 50 to 100 μg/kg.

ANGIOTENSIN-CONVERTING ENZYME INHIBITORS (ACE INHIBITORS)

Two ACE inhibitors are in current use, namely, captopril and enalapril. These are taken orally for control of hypertension and inhibit the formation of the active angiotensin II (see Chapter 23 for details).

REFERENCES

1. DiNardo, J. A.: Interpreting cardiac catheterization data. *In* DiNardo, J. A., Schwartz, M. S. (eds.): Anesthesia for Cardiac Surgery. East Norwalk, CT, Appleton and Lange, 1990, p. 17.
2. Ross, J.: Cardiac function and myocardial contractility: a perspective. J Am Coll Cardiol *1*:52, 1983.
3. Ahlquist, R. P.: A study of adrenotropic receptors. Am J Physiol *153*:586, 1948.
4. Hoffman, B. B., Lefkowitz, R. J.: Alpha-adrenergic receptor subtypes. N Eng J Med *302*:1390, 1980.
5. Lands, A. M., et al.: Differentiation of receptor systems activated by sympathomimetic amines. Nature *214*:597, 1967.
6. Kebabian, J. W., Calne, D. B.: Multiple receptors for dopamine. Nature *277*:93, 1979.
7. Reid, J. L., Hamilton, C. A., Hannah, J. A. M.: Peripheral alpha$_1$ and alpha$_2$ adrenoreceptors mechanisms in blood pressure control. Chest *83(Suppl)*:302, 1983.
8. Brodde, O. E., et al.: Regional distribution of beta-adrenoreceptors in the human heart: coexistence of function beta$_1$ and beta$_2$ adrenergic in both atria and ventricles in severe congestive cardiomyopathy. J Cardiovasc Pharmacol *8*:1235, 1986.
9. Bristow, R. M., et al.: Beta$_1$ and beta$_2$ adrenergic receptor subpopulations in non-failing and failing human ventricular myocardium: coupling of both receptor subtypes to muscle contraction and selective beta$_1$ receptor down-regulation in heart failure. Circ Res *59*:297, 1986.
10. Port, J. D., et al.: Differences in ventricular myocardial beta receptor expression in ischemic versus idiopathic dilated cardiomyopathy. Circulation *80(Suppl IV)*:8, 1989.
11. Kobilka, B.: Molecular and cellular biology of adrenergic receptors. Trends Cardiovasc Med *5*:198, 1992.
12. Sutherland, E. W., Robison, G. A.: The role of cyclic 3' 5' AMP in response to catecholamines and other hormones. Pharmacol Rev *18*:145, 1966.
13. Fleming, J. W., Wisler, P. L., Watanabe, A. M.: Signal transduction by G proteins in cardiac tissue. Circulation *85*:425, 1991.
14. Weiner, N.: Norepinephrine, epinephrine, and the sympathomimetic amines. *In* Gilman, A. G., Goodman, L. S., Gilman, A. (eds.): The Pharmacological Basis of Theraputics, 6th Ed. New York, Macmillan, 1980, p. 146.
15. Steen, P. A., et al.: Efficacy of dopamine, dobutamine, and epinephrine during emergence from cardiopulmonary bypass in man. Circulation *57*:378, 1978.
16. Tinker, J. H.: Pro: Strong inotropes (ie, epinephrine) should be drugs of first choice during emergence from cardiopulmonary bypass. J Thorac Cardiovasc Anesth *1*:256, 1987.
17. Leier, C. V., et al.: Comparative systemic and regional hemodynamic effects of dopamine and dobutamine in patients with cardiomyopathic heart failure. Circulation *58*:466, 1978.
18. Makabali, C., Weil, M. H., Henning, R. J.: Dobutamine and other sympathomimetic drugs for the treatment of low cardiac output failure. Semin Anesth *1*:62, 1982.
19. Furman, W. R., Summer, W. R., Kennedy, T. P., Sylvester, J. T.: Comparison of the effects of dobutamine, dopamine and isoproteronol on hypoxic pulmonary vasoconstriction in the pig. Crit Care Med *10*:371, 1982.
20. Fowler, M. B., Alderman, E. L., Oesterle, S. N.: Dobutamine and dopaminew after cardiac surgery: greater augmentation of myocardial blood flow with dobutamine. Circulation *70(Suppl 1)*:105, 1985.
21. Amin, D. K., Shah, P. K., Shellock, F. G.: Comparative hemodynamic effects of intravenous dobutamine and MDL-17,043, a new cardioactive drug in severe congestive heart failure. Am Heart J *109*:91, 1985.
22. Benoti, J. R., McCue, J. E., Alpert, J. S.: Comparative vasoactive therapy for heart failure. Am J Cardiol *56*:19B, 1985.
23. Chen, W. Y.: 4-Leucine-oxytocin: natriuretic, diuretic and antivasopressin polypeptide. Science *161*:280, 1968.
24. Page, I. H.: Isolation of angiotensin and serotonin. Physiol Rev *38*:277, 1958.
25. Baim, D. S.: Effects of amrinone on myocardial energetics in severe congestive heart failure. Am J Cardiol *56*:16B, 1985.
26. Gage, J., et al.: Additive effects of dobutamine and amrinone on myocardial contractility and ventricular performance in patients with severe congestive heart failure. Circulation *74(Suppl II)*:II-367, 1986.
27. Goenen, M., Pedemonte, O., Baele, P., Col, J.: Amrinone in the management of low cardiac output after open heart surgery. Am J Cardiol *56*:33B, 1985.
28. Smith, N. A., et al.: Clinical pharmacology of intravenous enoximone: pharmacodynamics and pharmacokinetics in patients with heart failure. Am Heart J *122*:755, 1991.
29. Johns, R. A.: EDRF/nitric oxide: the endogenous nitrovasodilator and a new cellular messenger. Anesthesiology *75*:927, 1991.
30. Moncada, S., Palmer, R. M. J., Higgs, E. A.: Nitric oxide: physiology, pathophysiology and pharmacology. Pharmacol Rev *43*:109, 1991.
31. Palmer, R. M. J., Ferrige, A. G., Monacada, S. A.: Nitric oxide release accounts for the biological activity of endothelium-derived relaxing factor. Nature *327*:524, 1987.
32. Johns, R. A.: Endothelium-derived relaxing factor: basic review and clinical implications. J Cardiothorac Vasc Anesth *5*:69, 1991.
33. Ignarro, L. J., et al.: Mechanism of vascular smooth muscle relaxation by organic nitrates, nitrites, nitroprusside and nitric oxide: evidence for the involvement of S-nitrosothiols as active intermediates. J Pharmacol Exp Ther *218*:739, 1981.
34. Mann, T., et al.: Effect of nitroprusside on regional myocardial blood flow in coronary artery disease: results in 25 pa-

tients and comparison with nitroglycerin. Circulation *57:*732,1978.

35. Cottrell, J. E., Patel, K. P., Ranshohoff, J. R.: Intracranial pressure changes induced by sodium nitroprusside in patients with intracranial mass lesions. J Neurosurg *48:*329, 1978.

36. Palmer, R. F., Lasseter, K. C.: Drug therapy: sodium nitroprusside. N Engl J Med *294:*1403, 1976.

37. Norris, J. C., Hume, A. S.: In vivo release of cyanide from sodium nitroprusside. Br J Anaesth *59:*236, 1987.

38. Ivankovich, A. D., Militch, D. J., Tinker, J. H.: Sodium nitroprusside: metabolism and other considerations. Int Anesthesiol Clin *16:*1, 1978.

39. Tinker, J. H., Mitchenfelder, J. D.: Sodium nitroprusside: pharmacology, toxicity and therapeutics. Anesthesiology *45:*340, 1976.

40. Abrams, J.: Nitroglycerin and long-acting nitrates. N Engl J Med *302:*1234:1980.

41. Flaherty, J. T., et al.: Comparison of intravenous nitroglycerin and sodium nitroprusside for treatment of acute hypertension developing after coronary artery bypass surgery. Circulation *65:*1072, 1982.

42. Kaplan, J. A., Jones, E. L.: Vasodilator therapy during coronary artery surgery: comparison of nitroglycerin and nitroprusside. J Thorac Cardiovasc Surg *77:*301, 1977.

43. Kaplan, K. J., et al.: Association of methemoglobinemia and intravenous nitroglycerin therapy. Am J Cardiol *55:*181, 1985.

44. Brent, B. N., et al.: Contrasting acute effects of vasodilators (nitroglycerin, nitroprusside, and hydralazine) on right ventricular performance. Am J Cardiol *51:*1682, 1983.

45. Tarazi, R. C., Dustan, H. P.: Beta-adrenergic blockade in hypertension: practical and theoretical implications of long term hemodynamic variation. Am J Cardiol *29:*633, 1972.

46. Morgan, T. O., et al.: Beta-adrenergic receptor blocking agents, hypertension and plasma renin. Br J Clin Pharmacol *2:*159, 1975.

47. Hoffman, B. B., Lefkowitz, R. J.: Alpha-adrenergic receptor subtypes. N Engl J Med *302:*1990, 1980.

48. Flacke, J. W.: Alpha 2 antagonists in cardiovascular anesthesia. J Cardiothorac Vasc Anesth *6:*344, 1992.

49. Newsome, L. R., Roth, J. V., Hug, C. C., Nagle, D.: Esmolol attenuates hemodynamic responses during fentanyl-pancuronium anesthesia for aortocoronary bypass surgery. Anesth Analg *65:*451, 1986.

50. Dage, R. C., Hsieh, C. P.: Direct vasodilation by labetalol in anesthetized dogs. Br J Pharmacol *70:*287, 1980.

51. Braunwald, E.: Mechanisms of action of calcium channel blocking agents. N Engl J Med *307:*1618, 1982.

52. Hess, P., et al: Calcium channel types in cardiac myocytes: modulation by dihydropyridines and beta adrenergic stimulation. J Cardiovasc Pharmacol *8(suppl 9):*S11, 1986.

Chapter 43

ANESTHETIC IMPLICATIONS OF MATERNAL PHYSIOLOGIC CHANGES DURING PREGNANCY

HAROLD J. HEYMAN

Most of the maternal physiologic changes occurring during pregnancy that are important to anesthesiologists are caused by changes in blood levels of estrogen and progesterone.

BLOOD VOLUME CHANGES

The total blood volume increases 35 to 40% during pregnancy.[1,2] The plasma volume component begins to rise early in the first trimester, and because it increases to a greater volume than does the red cell mass, the phenomenon has been referred to as the "physiologic anemia of pregnancy."[3,4] This entity is not a true anemia, of course, and represents a relative hemodilution. If the maternal hemoglobin concentration falls below 11 g/dl, however, this will represent a true anemic state.[5] The rise in plasma volume has been attributed to sodium and water retention.[6] This rise in blood volume and the autotransfusion caused by uterine emptying allow the parturient to tolerate the blood loss at delivery and cesarean section.[2]

AORTOCAVAL COMPRESSION

With the assumption of the supine position by the pregnant woman, both the inferior vena cava and the abdominal aorta above the origin of the uterine artery are compressed by the gravid uterus. This process is referred to as aortocaval compression. The aortic component begins by week 19 of gestation[7] and the caval component by week 28. With vena caval compression, most individuals do not develop symptomatic hypotension because of compensatory physiologic mechanisms—vasoconstriction, increased heart rate, and increased myocardial contractility. About 10 to 15% of pregnant women at term develop symptomatic hypotension in the supine position, however, and therefore they try to avoid this position.[8,9] When regional anesthesia is administered, compensatory vasoconstriction for supine vena caval obstruction is eliminated below the upper level of sympathetic blockade and can result in significant reduction in maternal blood pressure and cardiac output. Left or right uterine displacement or assumption of the lateral decubitus position compensates for the aortocaval obstruction. Even without sympathetic blockade from regional anesthesia, and with a normal brachial blood pressure in the supine position, the fetus can be adversely affected[10] from the de- creased uterine blood flow due to abdominal aortic obstruction, hence the importance of avoidance of the supine position in the parturient.

CARDIOVASCULAR CHANGES (FIG. 43–1)

Cardiac output changes result from increases in stroke volume and heart rate. By term pregnancy, cardiac output has risen by 30 to 50% over the nonpregnant state.[11,12] Measurements have demonstrated a rise in stroke volume of about 30% and a rise in heart rate of 10 to 15%. Systolic blood and diastolic blood pressures show a slight decrease in pregnancy,[13] whereas the central venous pressure does not change. The systemic vascular resistance decreases maximally by the second trimester.[14] Left ventricular stroke work increases. Maximal periods of cardiovascular stress in the pregnant woman may occur because of increases in cardiac output at 28 to 32 weeks of gestation, during labor and delivery, and at 12 to 24 hours post partum.[15] These periods of cardiac stress may be of significance in the management of the parturient with heart disease.

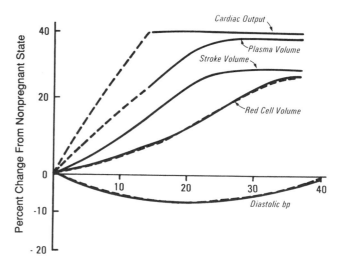

Fig. 43–1. Changes in cardiovascular hemodynamics throughout the course of gestation. From West, J. B.(ed.): Best & Taylor's Physiological Basis of Medical Practice, 12th Ed. Baltimore, Williams & Wilkins, 1993, p. 893.

Stress During Labor

During the first stage of labor, heart rate, cardiac output, blood pressure, and central venous pressure increase significantly with each contraction. These changes result from catecholamine release secondary to the stimuli of labor pain and from autotransfusion of 200 to 400 ml of blood with each uterine contraction.[16] The physiologic work of "pushing" during the second stage of labor increases the cardiac output. In the immediate postdelivery period, the acute blood loss associated with delivery or cesarian section, decreased aortocaval compression, and rapid hormonal changes often results in a postdelivery tachycardia and a rise in cardiac output. The absence of an increased pulmonary capillary wedge pressure (PCWP) or central venous pressure in the presence of a marked increase in blood volume reflects the decrease in systemic vascular resistance and pulmonary vascular resistance.[17]

The colloid osmotic pressure (COP) decreases 14% during pregnancy, but the increased COP-PCWP gradient indicates a greater tendency to develop pulmonary edema than in the nonpregnant state. These periods of cardiac stress may precipitate congestive heart failure in the parturient with significant mitral stenosis, mitral regurgitation, aortic insufficiency, coronary artery disease, or cardiomyopathy.

Epidural analgesia may be of benefit in these situations by effecting a reduction in the cardiac preload and heart rate.[18,19] In parturients with cardiac lesions such as aortic stenosis, pulmonary hypertension, or Eisenmenger's syndrome, however, the usual local anesthetic-based epidural technique may be harmful because of vasodilation and reduction in cardiac preload; such patients need invasive monitoring and an epidural technique that combines a low dose of a local anesthetic with an opioid.[20,21] The physical examination of the parturient may reveal the following: displacement of the cardiac point of maximal impulse (PMI) to the left; the presence of a functional systolic murmur; appearance of the heart to be large and displaced in a cephalad direction in a chest radiograph; and left axis deviation evident on the electrocardiogram (ECG).

RESPIRATORY CHANGES (FIG. 43–2)

Several important changes occur in respiratory physiology. Although the diaphragm is pushed in a cephalad direction during the course of pregnancy, the total lung capacity remains essentially the same. The inspiratory capacity, which consists of the inspiratory reserve volume and the tidal volume, increases in size throughout pregnancy. These changes are due to conformational changes in the bony architecture of the chest by progestational influences.[22,23]

The functional residual capacity, which consists of the expiratory reserve volume and the residual volume, is reduced 15 to 20% by term.[24] In the supine position, the closing volume of the lung is above the functional residual capacity, which causes airway closure and an increased alveolar-to-arterial oxygen gradient during normal tidal ventilation. Moreover, in the supine position, the de-

creased blood flow to the lungs occurring as a result of vena caval compression may increase the ventilation-perfusion (V/Q) mismatch. The basal metabolic rate increases 10 to 20% during pregnancy. Because of the changes in functional residual capacity and metabolic rate, parturients may rapidly become hypoxemic with the onset of apnea.

The major respiratory change is a 70% increase in alveolar ventilation during pregnancy.[25] This is partially due to an increase in the respiratory rate, but it is mostly from the increase in tidal volume. No change in respiratory dead space is noted. No change occurs in lung compliance itself, although total pulmonary compliance decreases because of changes in the elasticity of the chest wall. Because of the increase in alveolar ventilation, the arterial P_{O_2} increases 5 to 10 mm Hg, to a value of about 106 mm Hg in the healthy parturient breathing room air.[26] Therefore, an arterial blood gas determination obtained with the parturient breathing 50% oxygen, for example, who has an arterial P_{O_2} of 110 mm Hg, probably has significant pulmonary shunt. The arterial P_{CO_2} decreases to 32 mm Hg. Therefore, the subject at term pregnancy who is not in labor is chronically hyperventilating and has a compensated respiratory alkalosis.

During general anesthesia administered to the parturient, the end-tidal carbon dioxide should be kept at about 30 mm Hg to keep within this physiologic parameter.[27] If the parturient develops acute hyperventilation during labor and delivery as a result of the experience of painful contractions, an acute, uncompensated maternal respiratory alkalosis may develop. If this maternal respiratory alkalosis is prolonged, it may cause maternal metabolic acidosis due to decreased maternal cardiac output secondary to an increase in mean intrathoracic pressure. Fetal acido-

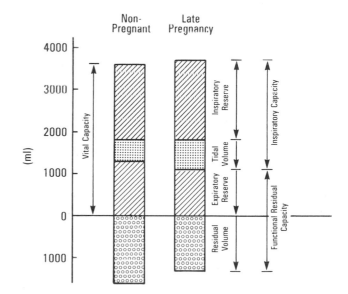

Fig. 43–2. Comparison of lung volumes in the nonpregnant and late-pregnant female. Adapted from Hytten, F., et al.: Clinical Physiology and Obstetrics. Oxford, Blackwell Scientific Publications, 1980, In West, J. B. (ed.): Best & Taylor's Physiological Basis of Medical Practice, 12th Ed. Baltimore, Williams & Wilkins, 1993.

sis may result from the transplacental passage of maternal fixed acids,[28] as well as from reduced uterine blood flow, secondary to reduced maternal cardiac output. Normally, the maternal oxyhemoglobin dissociation curve shifts to the right (higher P_{50} value, which is an expression of the affinity of oxygen for hemoglobin; this value represents the oxygen tension at which hemoglobin is 50% saturated and is about 25 mm Hg under normal conditions), facilitating the unloading of oxygen transplacentally to the fetus. A maternal left shift of the P_{50}, occurring as a result of hyperventilation in labor, can decrease oxygen unloading to the fetus and can contribute to the development of fetal acidosis. These maternal and fetal respiratory changes occurring as a result of maternal hyperventilation during labor can be prevented and treated by the proper use of epidural analgesia.

Upper airway edema occurs in pregnancy. This is caused by progesterone-induced submucous venous engorgement.[23] This edema involves the nose, mouth, nasopharynx, and larynx. This edema can increase in preeclampsia. Trauma or manipulation may increase the edema, or it may cause bleeding, making mask ventilation difficult and obscuring visibility during laryngoscopy. Epistaxis may occur easily, from the use of nasal airways, endotracheal tubes, and suction catheters. The laryngeal edema suggests the use of smaller than usual size endotracheal tubes for endotracheal intubation. A 7.0-mm (ID) should be the largest endotracheal tube size used. For most patients, a 6.5-mm tube size suffices, and in certain preeclamptic patients, and some adolescents, a 6.0- or 5.5-mm tube is appropriate.

Effect of Pregnancy on Anesthetic MAC Values

The minimal alveolar concentration (MAC) of the inhalation anesthetic agents is decreased by 25 to 40%.[29] The sedative effect of progesterone may contribute to this effect. There may also be an increase in endogenous opiates (β endorphins) present at the opiate receptors. Local anesthetic agents are also more potent during pregnancy. The elevated maternal cardiac output increases the maternal uptake of inhalation agents; however, the rise in alveolar ventilation is greater than that of the cardiac output, so induction of anesthesia is faster in pregnancy than in the nonpregnant state. The reduced MAC of the inhalation agents also facilitates the rate of induction. These factors place the parturient at risk for rapid and unexpected induction of general anesthesia during inhalation of normally subanesthetic concentrations of volatile agents or nitrous oxide.

GASTROINTESTINAL CHANGES

The following gastrointestinal changes occur during pregnancy: by the end of the first trimester, the lower esophageal sphincter relaxes, leading to a loss of barrier pressure (the difference between the intraesophageal and intragastric pressure) and functional incompetence of the gastroesophageal pinchcock mechanism; cephalad gastric displacement during pregnancy also decreases the oblique angle at the gastroesophageal junction, decreas-

ing the competence of the lower esophageal sphincter; placental gastrin production increases maternal gastric acid output; the enlarging uterine fundus may partially cause gastric outlet obstruction; and gastric emptying is delayed with the onset of labor.

Roberts and Shirley[30] estimated from animal studies that, in humans, gastric aspiration of 25 ml of gastric juice with a pH of 2.5 or less would be sufficient to cause acid damage to the maternal lung. In animal studies, acid can cause greater damage to pregnant than to nonpregnant lungs. Because aspiration of gastric contents is still a leading cause of maternal death during the administration of general anesthesia,[31] nonparticulate antacids have been given to the parturient before anesthetic induction in an effort to neutralize gastric contents rapidly.

HEPATIC CHANGES

Hepatic changes during pregnancy include elevation of serum glutamate oxaloacetate transaminase, lactate dehydrogenase, alkaline phosphatase, and cholesterol levels. The total protein level and the albumin/globulin ratio decrease. Plasma cholinesterase activity decreases during pregnancy and reaches its lowest level about 24 hours after delivery.[32] Prolonged paralysis rarely occurs after clinically appropriate doses of succinylcholine, despite the decrease in enzyme activity. In the presence of homozygous atypical plasma cholinesterase, the duration of succinylcholine action would be obviously prolonged. Although the rate of metabolism of the local anesthetic, chloroprocaine, is also prolonged in presence of enzyme,[33] the plasma half-life has been measured at 100 seconds instead of the usual 40 seconds.

COAGULATION CHANGES

Blood coagulation changes are mainly those related to the hypercoagulable state of pregnancy. All coagulation factors show increased activity, except for factors XI and XIII.[34] Fibrinolytic activity decreases in the third trimester. The hypercoagulable state confers some protective effect against postpartum bleeding, but it also increases the risk of postpartum deep vein thrombosis and pulmonary embolism. The risk of thrombotic events is doubled if a cesarean section is performed.

RENAL CHANGES (FIG. 43–3)

Renal changes in pregnancy include a rise in the glomerular filtration rate of 30 to 50% and an increase in the renal plasma flow of 30 to 50%. These changes begin during the first trimester. The serum creatinine decreases to 0.5 mg/dl, and the blood urea nitrogen decreases to 9 mg/dl. Any elevation of serum creatinine above 0.8 mg/dl or of blood urea nitrogen greater than 13 mg/dl is considered abnormal. Maternal progesterone secretion causes dilatation of the ureters, pelves, and calyces, leading to state of physiologic hydronephrosis and hydroureter. This can predispose the parturient to the development of bacteriuria and pyelonephritis. Glycosuria occurs during pregnancy because of greater quantities of glucose traversing the glomerulus per unit of time.[35]

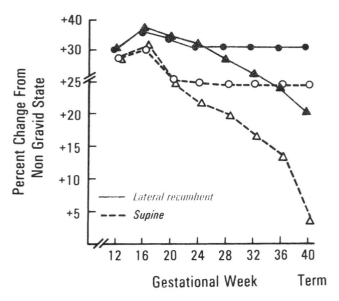

Fig. 43–3. Gestational changes in glomerular filtration rate measured in the supine and lateral recumbent positions. Adapted from Lindheimer, M. D., Katz, A. I.: Kidney Function and Disease in Pregnancy. Philadelphia, Lea & Febiger, 1977, p. 20, In West, J. B.(ed.): Best & Taylor's Physiological Basis of Medical Practice, 12th Ed. Baltimore, Williams & Wilkins, 1993.

UTEROPLACENTAL CHANGES

Uterine blood flow comprises about 10% of maternal cardiac output at term, 700 ml/min;[36] 80% of uterine blood flow perfuses the placenta and is not autoregulated. Therefore, uterine blood flow can drop in response to a decrease in maternal blood pressure. The uterine vascular bed is almost maximally vasodilated;[37] it is, however, capable of marked vasoconstriction. The uterine blood flow is equal to the uterine arterial pressure minus the uterine venous pressure, divided by the uterine vascular resistance. Any condition that causes a drop in uterine arterial pressure, a rise in uterine venous pressure, or a rise in uterine vascular resistance therefore causes a decrease in uterine blood flow.[37]

Aortocaval compression by the gravid uterus in the supine position can drop the uterine arterial pressure, increase the venous pressure, and increase the vascular resistance. Preeclampsia can decrease the uterine arterial pressure and can increase the uterine vascular resistance.

Factors that can decrease the uterine blood flow include the following[37]: uterine contractions; uterine hypertonus; maternal hypertension; and peripheral vasoconstriction. α Adrenergic agonists such as methoxamine or norepinephrine can decrease uterine blood flow. Ephedrine, a mixed α and β agonist, tends to protect the uterine blood flow. Phenylephrine has been shown to produce no adverse fetal effects when used as a vasopressor agent to treat spinal hypotension in humans,[38,39] even in those subjects with placental insufficiency. It appears to be an effective alternative to the use of ephedrine in that clinical situation and may be valuable in situations in which hypotension secondary to sympathetic blockade develops in parturients with idiopathic hypertrophic

subaortic stenosis, aortic stenosis, or Eisenmenger's syndrome. Placental blood flow using Doppler velocimetry was not measured in these parturients, however. Uteroplacental insufficiency occurring as a result of pregnancy-induced hypertension, diabetes, and postmaturity can decrease uterine blood flow.[37] In the absence of maternal hypotension, sympathetic blockade resulting from an epidural anesthetic can improve intervillous blood flow, including in parturients with preeclampsia. In experimental hypertension in the pregnant sheep model, nitroglycerin and hydralazine, but not sodium nitroprusside, can lower maternal blood pressure without decreasing uterine blood flow.[40,41] Toxic levels of local anesthetic agent can constrict uterine arteries.[42] No known agents directly increase uterine blood flow. Experimentally, in the pregnant sheep, magnesium diverts more blood to the uterus. In vitro, nitric oxide can cause uterine vasodilation.[43]

Effect of Anesthetic Agents on Uterine Contractility

Volatile inhalation agents can decrease uterine contractility when they are administered at end-tidal concentrations of greater than two thirds MAC. Nitrous oxide has little effect on uterine contractility. Opioids can slightly increase or decrease uterine contractility. Ketamine increases contractility, as does paracervical block. Local anesthetic toxicity can cause uterine hypertonus and fetal distress. Uterine artery vasoconstriction and uterine hypertonus may be responsible for severe fetal bradycardia reported after paracervical block.[44] Lumbar epidural blockade can either increase, decrease, or have no effect on uterine contractility and the length of the first stage of labor, depending on the upper sensory level achieved, the concentration of local anesthetic agent, the use of epinephrine, and the presence of dystocia. α Adrenergic stimulation, as with agents such as norepinephrine, methoxamine, and metaraminol, can cause an increase in uterine contractility.

OXYTOCIN

Drugs Specifically Affecting Uterine Motility

Oxytocic agents are used in obstetrics to increase uterine contractility. They may be used to "induce" labor in the pregnant patient or to augment uterine contractility following delivery. Oxytocin, a synthetic hormone, was originally extracted from the posterior lobe of the pituitary gland. These pituitary extracts were contaminated with vasopressin, could cause maternal hypertension, and are no longer available. The synthetic compound does not cause a directly acting vasoconstrictive or hypertensive response. The sensitivity of the uterus to this agent is maximal at the end of pregnancy, during labor, and immediately post partum. The onset of uterine action in response to intravenous injection occurs almost immediately and lasts about 1 hour.

Systemic Reactions To Oxytocin

Systemic reactions include anaphylactoid reactions, arrhythmias, and nausea and vomiting. Oxytocin is a direct-acting vasodilator. With rapid intravenous injection of 0.1

U/kg, one may see hypotension, decreased systemic vascular resistance, decreased mean arterial pressure, and a compensatory reflex tachycardia and increase in cardiac output. These cardiovascular effects are dose related and last 2 to 5 minutes. When this agent is administered as a dilute intravenous solution, rather than as an intravenous bolus injection, these cardiovascular reactions do not occur.

Oxytocin has been shown to have intrinsic antidiuretic activity, usually attributed to the structural similarity of the compound to vasopressin. This activity results in increased renal resorption of water and can result in hyponatremia, oliguria, and water intoxication leading to seizures, coma, and maternal death.[45] Parturients receiving large doses or prolonged infusions of oxytocin combined with large volumes of electrolyte-free intravenous fluids should be observed for symptoms of an acute hyponatremic state such as drowsiness, listlessness, headaches, nausea, and abdominal pain. The serum sodium and osmolality are low in this state, and the fetus-neonate may also experience a hyponatremic overhydration.

Prostaglandins

Prostaglandin E and F compounds are used in obstetrics as stimulants of uterine muscle contraction. The majority of their actions on the myometrium appear to be controlled by changes in intracellular calcium flux, mediated through alterations of either cyclic adenosine monophosphate (cAMP) or guanosine monophosphate. Prostaglandin use in pregnancy includes the "ripening" of the cervix as part of the induction of labor and in the control of postpartum hemorrhage secondary to uterine atony. The latter action of the F series is of usual concern to the anesthesiologist.

In the United States, the compound of the F class agent used for control of postpartum hemorrhage is carboprost tromethamine (15-methyl $PGF_2\alpha$). This compound stimulates both uterine contraction and cervical dilatation, although the effect on myometrial contractility predominates. Because of its effect on smooth muscle stimulation, nausea, vomiting, and diarrhea are common. This agent also stimulates bronchial smooth muscle, leading to bronchoconstriction.[46] Marked maternal oxygen desaturation because of significant ventilation/perfusion mismatch may occur after intramyometrial injections. Hemodynamic alterations associated with $PGF_2\alpha$ compounds include an increase in blood pressure, heart rate, cardiac output, pulmonary vascular resistance, pulmonary capillary wedge pressure, and pulmonary edema.[47,48] Elevation of the patient's temperature has also occurred.

TOCOLYTIC AGENTS

β-Mimetic Agents

β-Adrenergic agents stimulate the postulated β-adrenergic receptors of the uterus, causing uterine relaxation. This property makes this class of agents useful in the treatment of preterm labor and, occasionally, of value in the management of uterine hypertonus or acute fetal distress accompanying labor contractions. The β-adrenergic agents are the most important tocolytic agents in use; ritodrine and terbutaline are the usual choices, although ritodrine is the only agent specifically approved by the United States Food and Drug Administration for this purpose.

Mechanism of Action

Stimulation of the β_1-adrenergic receptor at the myometrial cell activates intracellular cyclic AMP and causes sequestration of intracellular calcium, thus blocking the contractile interaction of actin and myosin, and resulting in cellular relaxation.[49] β_2-Adrenergic receptors are found mainly in the smooth muscle of the blood vessels, bronchioles, and the uterus. Although the β_2 agonists utilized as tocolytic agents are selected for their predominantly β_2-adrenergic receptor activity, they have side effects related to their action on both β_2- and β_1-adrenergic receptors.

Side Reactions

β_1 Receptors are located in the myocardium and produce tachycardia and increased inotropy when stimulated. The most frequent and serious maternal complications from the use of β_2-adrenergic agents, therefore, are cardiovascular and may present the anesthesiologist caring for these patients with some serious challenges, such as hypotension, tachycardia, arrhythmias, chest pain, ST-segment changes, and T-wave inversion.[50,51] Most of these changes are dose related and usually diminish with cessation of therapy.

Pulmonary edema has been reported in approximately 5% of patients receiving β-mimetic agents.[52-54] The risk of developing this complication is increased in the presence of twin gestation, prolonged exposure to the drug, and fluid overload. The pathophysiologic features of pulmonary edema have not clearly established either cardiogenic or noncardiogenic causes. Neither invasive nor noninvasive studies have been able to document cardiac failure in pregnant patients with previously normal hearts. No reports of invasive monitoring have taken measurements as a baseline, however, before the start of β-mimetic therapy, then followed with serial measurements in patients who did and did not develop edema. Possible noncardiogenic causes of pulmonary edema include increased capillary hydrostatic pressure secondary to fluid overload and increased pulmonary capillary permeability. Hypoxia may seem to be excessive, relative to the amount of pulmonary edema present, and may be due to the inhibition of hypoxic pulmonary vasoconstriction by this group of agents.

The metabolic alterations related to β-mimetic agents include hyperglycemia and hypokalemia. The stimulation of glucagon release from the pancreas by these agents, with resultant glycogenolysis, is responsible for this action. As serum glucose and secondarily released insulin levels rise, potassium is driven intracellularly. Total serum potassium stores are not depleted, however. Although some investigators have recommended that serum glucose and potassium levels be monitored, intravenous administration of insulin or potassium is usually not recommended.

Magnesium Sulfate

Magnesium sulfate therapy inhibits uterine contractions by causing a decrease in myometrial muscle contractility. Although the mechanism of action is not completely understood, in vitro studies appear to show that magnesium competes with calcium in the muscle cytoplasm, lowering free levels of free calcium and thereby inhibiting the coupling of the actin-myosin unit.[55] This property makes magnesium useful in the treatment of preterm labor. It is also used as an anticonvulsant in patients with preeclampsia. An advantage of magnesium over the β-mimetic agents clinically is a decreased number of side effects, as long as serum levels are kept below the toxic range.

Indications for Use[56,57]

Indications for use of magnesium sulfate are as follows:

1. Pregnancy-induced hypertension (selective patients).
2. Prevention of eclampsia.
3. Management of eclamptic convulsions.

Administration and Dosage[56]

The usual recommended method of administration is the intravenous route, which is less painful than intramuscular injection. A loading dose of 10 mg is first given, followed by maintenance doses of 5 mg every 4 hours for preeclampsia. For severe preeclampsia, or for treatment of seizures, the recommended intravenous loading dose is 14 mg.

Phenytoin has been used for the management of eclampsia. It is about one third as effective as magnesium, however, which is the superior agent and the first choice in the prevention of eclampsia and in the control of seizures.[57]

Toxicity of Magnesium

Signs of magnesium toxicity become evident above serum levels of 9 mg/dl. The earliest signs of toxicity consist of a prolongation of the PR interval and a widened QRS complex on the ECG trace.[58] With progressively toxic levels, decreased deep tendon reflexes occur, followed by central nervous system, respiratory, and myocardial depression. Because magnesium sulfate excretion depends on renal function, it should be used with caution in patients with kidney disease. Because of the possibility of acute respiratory depression, magnesium should not be used in patients with myasthenia gravis.

Side effects are more commonly observed during the initial intravenous loading dose and include hypotension, flushing, headache, nystagmus, blurred vision, chest pain, nausea, drowsiness, and subjective sensation of heat.[59]

Magnesium sulfate therapy has also been associated with about a 1% incidence of pulmonary edema,[59] which may be associated with other risk factors, such as twin gestation and intravenous fluid overload. Placental transfer of the agent is possible, and cases of neonatal hypotonia have been reported following intravenous maternal infusion lasting over 24 hours. Preterm neonates may show hypotonia after magnesium infusions to the mother.

Calcium gluconate or chloride should be available to treat maternal or neonatal toxicity. Other management of toxicity includes discontinuation of the infusion, documentation of serum levels, and supportive therapy.

The major anesthetic consideration in patients receiving magnesium sulfate therapy is the increased sensitivity to both depolarizing and nondepolarizing agents. The dosage of nondepolarizing agents should be regulated by the twitch response to the nerve stimulator.

Prostaglandin Synthetase Inhibitors

Prostaglandins are hormone-like substances that are important stimulators of uterine contraction in humans. This class of compounds inhibits the formation of cyclooxygenase, an enzyme utilized in the synthesis of prostaglandins. This property makes these compounds potentially useful in the treatment of preterm labor. Indomethacin is the most frequently used compound of this class, because, unlike aspirin, it has only a transient effect on platelet function. Indomethacin is an effective tocolytic agent and has no cardiovascular side effects. Concern has existed that maternal administration of indomethacin may cause in utero closure of the ductus arteriosus. Diverse neonatal effects are unlikely to occur, however, if indomethacin is used for only 24 to 48 hours, is given to patients of less than 34 weeks' gestation, and is discontinued before delivery.[60]

Calcium Channel Blocking Agents

Nifedipine is a calcium channel blocking agent that is a smooth muscle relaxant useful in the treatment of hypertension and coronary artery disease. This class of agents prevents the increase of intramyometrial cytoplasmic calcium necessary for actin-myosin coupling and thereby has shown some promise for use as a tocolytic agent. These agents have been generally considered potentially safer than the β-mimetic agents because of less severe side effects.[61,62] Maternal headache, constipation, and nausea have been reported, as well as decreased uterine blood flow and fetal acidosis in laboratory animals.

Nitroglycerin

Nitroglycerin is a smooth muscle dilator that is used most often in clinical medicine for purposes of cardiac preload reduction in patients with coronary artery disease and myocardial failure. Intravenous nitroglycerin has been utilized to produce acute uterine relaxation for the performance of certain emergency obstetric maneuvers.[63-65] These include the following: removal of retained placenta; extraction of a trapped aftercoming head in breech delivery; and management of acute uterine inversion. This agent shows some promise of becoming an alternative to general endotracheal anesthesia, with its associated risks of delay, airway management difficulties, aspiration risk, and systemic hypotension due to the use of deep inhalation agents. Maternal blood pressure must be continually monitored because of nitroglycerin's vasodilatory action. Nitroglycerin may be used with regional anesthesia, general anesthesia, or intravenous sedation.

REFERENCES

1. Pritchard, J. A.: Changes in the blood volume during pregnancy and delivery. Anesthesiology 26:193, 1965.
2. Ueland K.: Maternal cardiovascular dynamics. VII. Intrapartum blood volume changes. Am J Obstet Gynecol 126:671, 1976.
3. Assali, N. S., and Brinkman, C. R., III: Disorders of maternal circulatory and respiratory adjustments. In Assali, N. S., Brinkman, C. R., III (eds.). Pathophysiology of Gestation: Maternal Disorders, Vol. 1. New York, Academic American, 1972.
4. Hytten, F. E., Paintin, D. B.: The Physiology of Human Pregnancy. Philadelphia, F.A. Davis, 1964.
5. Cheek, T. G., Gutsche, B. B.: Maternal physiologic alterations during pregnancy. In Shnider, S.M., Levinson, G. L. (eds.). Anesthesia for Obstetrics, 3rd Ed. Baltimore, Williams & Wilkins, 1993.
6. Laidlaw, J. C., Ruse, J. L., Gomall, A. G.: The influence of estrogen and progesterone on aldosterone excretion. J Clin Endocrinol Metab 22:161, 1962.
7. McClennan, C. E.: Antecubital and femoral venous pressure in normal and toxemic pregnancy. Am J Obstet Gynecol 45:568, 1943.
8. Lees, M. M., Scott, D. B., Kerr, M. G., Taylor, S. H.: The circulatory effects of recumbent postural change in late pregnancy. Clin Sci 32:453, 1967.
9. Holmes F.: Incidence of the supine hypotensive syndrome in late pregnancy: a clinical study in 500 subjects. J Obstet Gynaecol Br Comm 67:254, 1960.
10. Marx, G. F.: Aortocaval compression: Incidence and prevention. Bull NY Acad Med 50:443, 1974.
11. Robson, S. C., Hunter, S., Moore, M., Dunlop, W.: Hemodynamic changes during the puerperium: a Doppler and M-mode echocardiographic study. Br J Obstet Gynaecol 94:1028, 1987.
12. Robson, S. C., Hunter, S., Boys, R. J., Dunlop, W: Serial study of factors influencing changes in cardiac output during human pregnancy. Am J Physiol 256:H1060, 1989.
13. MacGillivray, I., Rose, G. A., Rowe, B.: Blood pressure survey in pregnancy. Clin Sci 37:395, 1969.
14. Clark, S. L., et al.: Central hemodynamic assessment of normal term pregnancy. Am J Obstet Gynecol 161:1439, 1989.
15. Ueland, K., Hansen, J. M.: Maternal cardiovascular dynamics. III. Labor and delivery under local and caudal analgesia. Am J Obstet Gynecol 103:8, 1969.
16. Robson, S. C., Dunlop, W., Boys, R. J., Hunter S.: Cardiac output during labour. Br Med J 295:1169, 1987.
17. Clark, S. L., et al.: Central hemodynamic assessment of normal term pregnancy. Am J Obstet Gynecol 169:1439, 1989.
18. Clark, S. L., et al.: Labor and delivery in the presence of mitral stenosis: central hemodynamic observations. Am J Obstet Gynecol 152:984, 1985.
19. Hemmings, G. T., et al.: Invasive monitoring and anaesthetic management of a parturient with mitral stenosis. Can J Anaesth 34:182, 1987.
20. Choi, H. J., Chiu, L., Hurd, J. M., Tremper, K. K.: Epidural anesthesia for a woman with severe aortic stenosis undergoing a cesarean section. Anesthesiol Rev 19:61, 1992.
21. Brian, J. E., et al.: Aortic stenosis, cesarean delivery, and epidural anesthesia. J Clin Anesth 5:1504, 1993.
22. Pernoll, M. L., et al.: Ventilation during rest and exercise in pregnancy and post partum. Respir Physiol 25:295, 1975.
23. Leontic, E. A.: Respiratory disease in pregnancy. Med Clin North Am 61:111, 1977.
24. Knuttgen, H. G., Emerson, K., Jr.: Physiological response to pregnancy at rest and during exercise. J Appl Physiol 36:549, 1974.
25. Prouse, C. M., Gaensler, E. A.: Respiratory acid-base changes during pregnancy. Anesthesiology 26:381, 1965.
26. Templeton, A., Kelman, G. R.: Maternal blood gases (PAO_2-PaO_2), physiological shunt and VD/VT in normal pregnancy. Br J Anaesth 48:1001, 1976.
27. Shnider, S. M., Levinson, G. L.: Anesthesia for obstetrics. In Shnider, S. M., Levinson, G. L. (eds.). Anesthesia for Obstetrics, 3rd Ed. Baltimore, Williams & Wilkins, 1993.
28. Levinson, G. L., Shnider, S. M., de Lorimier, A. A., Steffenson, J. L.: Effects of maternal hyperventilation on uterine blood flow, fetal oxygenation, and acid-base status. Anesthesiology 40:340, 1974.
29. Palahniuk, R. J., Shnider, S. M., Eger, E. I., II: Pregnancy deceases the requirement for inhaled anesthetic agents. Anesthesiology 41:82, 1974.
30. Roberts, R. B., and Shirley, M. A.: Reducing the risk of acid aspiration during cesarean section. Anesth Analg 53:859, 1974.
31. Chadwick, H. S., et al.: A comparison of obstetric and nonobstetric anesthesia malpractice claims. Anesthesiology 74:242, 1991.
32. Shnider, S. M.: Serum cholinesterase activity during pregnancy, labor, and puerperium. Anesthesiology 26:335, 1965.
33. Kuhnert, B. R., Philipson, E. H., Pimental, R., Kuhnert, P. M.: A prolonged chloroprocaine epidural block in a postpartum patient with abnormal pseudocholinesterase. Anesthesiology 56:477, 1982.
34. Hellgren, M., Blöuback, M.: Studies on blood coagulation and fibrinolysis in pregnancy, during delivery, and in the puerperium. I. Normal conditions. Gynecol Obstet Invest 12:141, 1981.
35. Davison, J. M., Hytten, F. E.: The effect of pregnancy on the renal handling of glucose. Br J Obstet Gynecol 82:374, 1975.
36. Wehrenberg, W. B., et al.: Vascular dynamics of the reproductive tract in the female rhesus monkey: relative contributions of ovarian and uterine arteries. Biol Reprod 17:148, 1977.
37. Assali, N. S., Brinkman, C. R., III: The uterine circulation and its control. In Longo, L. D., Bartels, H. (eds.). Respiratory Gas Exchange and Blood Flow in the Placenta. Washington, D.C., U.S. Department of Health, Education, and Welfare, 1972.
38. Ramanathan, S., Grant, V. J.: Vasopressor therapy for hypotension due to epidural anesthesia for cesarean section. Acta Anaesthesiol Scand 32:559, 1988.
39. Moran, D. H., et al.: Phenylephrine in the prevention of hypotension following spinal anesthesia for cesarean section. J Clin Anesth 3:301, 1991.
40. Craft, J. B., Jr., Co, E. G., Yonekura, M. L., Gilman, R. M.: Nitroglycerin therapy for phenylephrine-induced hypertension in pregnant ewes. Anesth Analg 69:494, 1980.
41. Ring, G., et al.: Comparison of nitroprusside and hydrolazine in hypertensive pregnant ewes. Obstet Gynecol 50:598, 1977.

42. Greiss, F. C., Jr., Still, A. G., Anderson, S. G.: Effects of local anesthetic agents on the uterine vasculatures and myometrium. Am J Obstet Gynecol 124:889, 1976.

43. Magness, R. R., Rosenfeld, C. R., Carr, B. R.: Protein kinase C in uterine and systemic arteries during ovarian cycle and pregnancy. Am J Physiol Endocrinol Metab 260:E464, 1991.

44. Asling, J. H., et al.: Paracervical block in obstetrics. II. Etiology of fetal bradycardia following paracervical block anesthesia. Am J Obstet Gynecol 107:626, 1970.

45. Hughes, S. A., Partridge, B. L.: Oxytocics, tocolytics, and prostaglandins. Anesthesiol Clin North Am 8:27, 1990.

46. Smith, A. P.: The effect of intravenous infusion of graded doses of prostaglandins F_2 alpha and E_2 on lung resistance in patients undergoing termination of pregnancy. Clin Sci 44:17, 1973.

47. Secher, N. J., et al.: Effect of prostaglandin E_2 and F_2 alpha on the systemic and pulmonary circulation in pregnant anesthetized women. Acta Obstet Gynecol Scand 61:213, 1982.

48. Cates, W., Jordaan, H. V. F.: Sudden collapse and death of women obtaining abortions induced with prostaglandin F_2 alpha. Am J Obstet Gynecol 133:398, 1979.

49. Huddleton, J. F.: Preterm labor. Clin Obstet Gynecol 25:123, 1982.

50. Nuwayhid, B. A., et al.: Hemodynamic effects of isoxuprine and terbulaline in pregnant and nonpregnant sheep. Am J Obstet Gynecol 137:25, 1980.

51. Hosenpud, J. D., Morton, M. J., O'Grady, J. P.: Cardiac stimulation during ritodrine hydrochloride tocolytic therapy. Obstet Gynecol 62:52, 1983.

52. Benedetti, T. J.: Maternal complications of parenteral β-sympathomimetic therapy for premature labor. Am J Obstet Gynecol 145:1, 1983.

53. Wheeler, A. S., Patel, K. F., Spain, J.: Pulmonary edema during beta$_2$ tocolytic therapy. Anesth Analg 60:695, 1981.

54. Pisari, R. J., Rosenow, E. C.: Pulmonary edema associated with tocolytic therapy. Ann Intern Med 110:714, 1989.

55. Iseri, L. T., French, J. H.: Magnesium: nature's physiologic calcium blocker. Am Heart J 108:188, 1984.

56. Luca, M. J., Leveno, K. J., Cunningham, F. G.: Comparison of magnesium sulfate with phenytoin for prevention of eclampsia. N Engl J Med 333:201, 1995.

57. Eclampsia Trial Collaborative Group: Which anti-convulsant drug for women with eclampsia? Evidence from the Collaborative Eclampsia Trial. Lancet 345:1455, 1995.

58. Gutsche, B. B., Cheek, T. G.: Anesthetic considerations in pre-eclampsia-eclampsia. In Shnider, S. M., Levinson, G. L. (eds.). Anesthesia for Obstetrics, 3rd Ed. Baltimore, Williams & Wilkins, 1993.

59. Elliot, J. P.: Magnesium sulfate as a tocolytic agent. Am J Obstet Gynecol 147:277, 1983.

60. Niebyl, J. R., Witter, F. R.: Neonatal outcome after indomethacin treatment for preterm labor. Am J Obstet Gynecol 155:747, 1986.

61. Ferguson, J. E., et al.: Cardiovascular and metabolic effects associated with nifedipine and ritodrine tocolysis. Am J Obstet Gynecol 161:788, 1989.

62. Bucero, L. A., Leikin, E., Kirshenbaum, N., Tejani, N.: Comparison of nifedipine and ritodrine for the treatment of preterm labor. Am J Perinatol 8:365, 1991.

63. DeSimone, C. A., Norris, M. C., Leighton, B. L.: Intravenous nitroglycerin aids manual extraction of a retained placenta (letter). Anesthesiology 73:787, 1990.

64. Mayer, D. C., Weeks, S. K.: Antepartum uterine relaxation with nitroglycerin at caesarean delivery. Can J Anaesth 39:166, 1992.

65. Ley, S. J., Scheller, J., Jones, B. R., Slotnick, N.: Intrauterine pressure during administration of nitroglycerin for extraction of retained placenta. Anesthesiol Rev 20:95, 1993.

Chapter 44

PHYSIOLOGY OF THE NORMAL PEDIATRIC PATIENT

TERRANCE A. YEMEN

Fundamental to providing anesthesia to infants and children is an understanding of their developmental physiology. Some anesthesiologists commonly refer to children as small adults. This is true, in part, for children of school age, but certainly not for infants. This chapter addresses the developmental physiology of infants, with emphasis on the first few months of life. This is appropriate; developmental differences in physiology between a newborn and a 1-year-old infant are greater than those changes that occur over the next 12 to 14 years. A functional knowledge of the physiology of infants in the first 6 months of life is the cornerstone of pediatric anesthesia.

NEUROBIOLOGY OF THE NEONATE

A discussion of the neurobiology of neonates addresses two key questions: (1) do children feel pain? and (2) are neonates and premature infants capable of mounting a stress response to surgery? Significant information has been gained over the past decade that reveals premature and, in particular, full-term neonates have a neurologic system considerably more advanced than previously thought.

Neuroanatomy

To answer the first question, we must consider recent discoveries regarding the neuroanatomy of neonates. Neuropathways for pain extending from sensory receptors in the skin to areas in the cerebral cortex have been demonstrated in newborn infants.[1-3] In fact, the density of nociceptive nerve endings in the skin of newborn infants is similar to, or greater than, that in adult skin. Cutaneous sensory receptors appear in the perioral area of the human fetus by the seventh week of gestation. The development of synapses between sensory fibers and interneurons in the dorsal horn of the spinal cord occurs in the sixth week of gestation.[4,5] Subsequently, sensory receptors spread throughout the face, palm of the hands, and soles of the feet by the eleventh week and include the proximal aspects of the arms and legs by the fifteenth week of gestation. Complete spread to all cutaneous and mucous tissues occurs by the twentieth week.[6]

Studies have also shown that a variety of cell types appear in the dorsal horn complete with laminary arrangement, synaptic interconnections, and neurotransmitter vesicles before weeks 13 and 14 of gestation. The development of these structures is actually complete by the thirtieth week.[7]

Myelinization of Nerve Tracts

A lack of myelination in newborn infants was previously proposed to promote the concept that infants are incapable of pain perception.[8] This concept is inaccurate. In adults, nociceptive impulses are carried through unmyelinated and thinly myelinated fibers. The presence or absence of myelination is primarily related to the speed of conduction velocity. The most recent neuroanatomic data of infants show that nociceptive nerve tracts in the spinal cord and central nervous system have, in fact, undergone complete myelination by the third trimester.[9]

Pathways for Pain Transmission

Pathways responsible for the transmission of pain are complete between the brain stem and the thalamus by 30 weeks' gestation, and thalamocortical pain fibers of the internal capsule and corona radiata are myelinated by 37 weeks' gestation.[7,9] The fetal neocortex begins development at 8 weeks' gestation, and by 20 weeks' gestation, each cortex has a complement of 109 neurons. Dendritic arborization of corticoneurons is complete and established by 20 to 24 weeks' gestation. Encephalography has been used to demonstrate functional maturity of the cerebral cortex in the neonatal age group. Intermittent bursts have been shown in both cerebral hemispheres by 20 weeks' gestation and are sustained by 22 weeks' gestation. Using this criterion, by 30 weeks' gestation, the distinction between wakefulness and sleep can be well defined. Quick sleep, active sleep, and wakefulness have been shown to occur in utero, beginning at approximately 8 weeks' gestation. On the basis of this current information, one can reasonably believe that newborns have both the anatomic and functional capacity required for the perception of painful stimuli and, quite possibly, its memory.

Effect of Pain on Brain Metabolism

Finally, in addressing the functional capacity of the premature and newborn to perceive pain, in vivo measurements of metabolic activity of the neonatal brain are available. They show that regions associated with pain perception, such as the cortex, thalamus, and mindbrain, have the maximum metabolic activity and capability necessary for the interpretation of pain.[9]

Stress Response

To answer the second question, whether infants can mount a stress response to surgery, we must consider certain investigations examining neonatal endocrine and metabolic capabilities. Several elaborate experiments done by Anand and colleagues have addressed this question by examining the same markers for surgical stress as in adults.[9-11] Their data suggest that newborn infants can indeed mount a substantial endocrine and metabolic response, highlighted by hyperglycemia and hyperlactatemia, with associated release of catecholamines and the inhibition of insulin secretion.

Some specific differences differentiate preterm from term infants regarding the stress response.[9,10] Glucose levels increase equally in both, although a trend exists toward greater postoperative hyperglycemia in premature infants. Preterm neonates also develop a significant degree of hyperlactatemia during surgery. This may be due to a deficiency in key hepatic enzymes, but that remains to be proved. Insulin levels increase postoperatively in term neonates, but they do not change substantially in preterm neonates. This may represent a decreased responsiveness of cells in the premature pancreas. It may also explain the tendency of preterm neonates to maintain higher blood glucose levels than term neonates. This is especially true during the postoperative phase of the stress response to surgery.

Effect of Anesthetics

Studies have also been conducted to examine the relationship between the stress response and the choice of anaesthesia in infants. In a study by Anand and Hickey, neonates receiving high doses of sufentanil for intraoperative anesthesia were compared with infants assigned to receive halothane and morphine.[11] These investigators found that, in neonates undergoing cardiac surgery, the physiologic responses to stress were attenuated by high dose sufentanil and by the postoperative analgesia afforded by it, as compared with the halothane-morphine control group. In addition, these investigators suggested that moderation of the neuroendocrine response is related to morbidity and mortality, which may be reduced by the choice of such anesthesia. Although a discussion of the full implications of such studies is beyond the scope of this chapter, these findings give us pause to reconsider the choice of anesthesia we administer to critically ill infants.

To appreciate the effect of narcotic analgesics on neonates, we must consider the development of opioid receptors in the neuroaxis. Little is still known about the development of opioid receptors in humans, but it is believed to occur within the fetus.[12] Endogenous opiates have been detected in the human fetal dorsal horn at 12 to 14 weeks of gestation and have been shown to be released late in pregnancy when fetal distress is present.[13,14]

Traditional anesthesic literature includes the statement that neonates and infants are more sensitive to narcotics than their older counterparts. Much of this information stemmed from experiments done in the 1960s that found the median lethal dose of morphine to be lower in newborn rats as compared with adult rats.[15] Further studies showed that similar doses of morphine, on a milligram-per-kilogram basis, resulted in similar plasma concentrations in newborn and adult rats but dissimilar brain tissue levels, with higher levels appearing in the newborns.[16] Other studies suggested that infants sedated with intramuscular morphine had a greater ventilatory depression than nonsedated infants. As a result, some researchers have concluded that infant sensitivity to narcotics, such as morphine, is related to its water solubility, reduced protein binding, and incomplete development of the neonatal blood-brain barrier. These factors would explain the higher concentration of morphine in the brain tissue of the newborn infant as compared with that of the adult.

Opiate Receptors in Neonates

Research has shown that opiate receptor binding sites in rats undergo developmental changes regarding the receptor types present.[17] Receptor ontogen may well be a factor responsible for the respiratory depression and analgesic effects of opiates used in newborns. These studies have shown that low- and high-affinity opiate receptors are present in rats. Low-affinity receptors are associated with respiratory depression, and high-affinity receptors are associated with analgesia. Low-affinity receptors are present in large numbers at birth, and the number of receptors appears to be constant from 1 to 18 days of life. High-affinity receptors are scarce at birth, however, and do not reach a significant proportion until 15 to 18 days of life. The large number of low-affinity receptors offers an explanation of the respiratory depression and lack of analgesic attained with opiods in the newborn rat. The pharmacodynamic changes that occur as the animal matures may be closely related to the maturation of opiate receptors.

Pharmacokinetics of Opiates in Neonates

What about the pharmacokinetics of opiates in neonates? In general, most studies have shown age-related changes in pharmacokinetics.[18,19] These changes are particularly notable with the use of synthetic narcotics. The volume of distribution is larger, clearance is slower, and the elimination half-life is prolonged in both full-term and preterm newborns.

The aforementioned studies suggest that narcotics be used with great caution in neonates. This is true, but we must put these concerns in proper perspective. Robinson and Gregory originally demonstrated that fentanyl could be used as a safe and effective anesthetic agent for premature infants undergoing ligation of a patent ductus arteriosus.[20] Anand and Hickey suggested that the use of analgesics, in particular synthetic narcotics, may decrease morbidity and mortality.[11] Narcotics are valuable anesthetic agents with unique characteristics in the neonate. The safe use of opioids must take into consideration both the pharmacokinetics and the pharmacodynamics of these drugs in neonates.

NEUROMUSCULAR PHYSIOLOGY

Neonates have been shown to have a myasthenic response to repetitive or tetanic stimulation.[21,22] This means that the contraction was not sustained at 100%, but in fact the fourth twitch was decreased to 95% of the first. In preterm infants, the ratio of the fourth to first twitch is reduced to 83%. Post-tetanic exhaustion is seen after higher-frequency tetanic stimulation. In nonanesthetized neonates, the frequency sweep electromyogram shows a markedly decreased response at higher frequencies compared with that seen in older infants and adults. All these responses change to the pattern seen in adults within the first 2 months of life. Generally, the differences between neonatal and adult responses to tetanic stimulation are interpreted as indicating a decreased reserve for neuromuscular transmission in the preterm and full-term neonate.

In the past, infants have been reported to have an increased sensitivity to the effects of neuromuscular blocking agents. When determining neonatal sensitivity to a neuromuscular blocking agent, however, one must consider whether the drug administered was indexed to body weight or to body surface area.[23] Most neuromuscular blocking agents are distributed in the extracellular fluid, primarily the circulating blood volume, and this extracellular fluid is directly related to the body surface area. Therefore, dosage requirements for neuromuscular blocking agents must be correlated with the surface area of the subject, rather than with body weight.

In one study, the sensitivity of the infant to neuromuscular blockade, in this case tubocurare, was examined.[24] This investigation determined that the steady-state plasma concentration associated with a 50% neuromuscular blockade was lower in infants in the first few months of life, as compared with older children. When the volume of distribution, which is larger in infants than in older children, is taken into consideration, and the appropriate calculation is made, little difference was seen between the infants and the older children.

Most pharmacokinetic data demonstrate similar clearance values for infants and older children.[25-27] A larger volume of distribution subsequently results in a longer elimination half-life in infants, however. As a result, infants generally need fewer and/or smaller supplemental doses to maintain the same degree of neuromuscular blockade compared with older children.

CARDIOVASCULAR PHYSIOLOGY

Neonatal Circulation and Transitional Changes

Shortly after birth, the neonatal circulation is in transition, between that present in the fetus (Fig. 44–1) and that found in normal infants.[28] This persists until the foramen ovale and the ductus venosus and ductus arteriosus close. Systemic vascular resistance increases because of the loss of placenta, and pulmonary blood flow increases 450% as pulmonary vascular resistance decreases with lung expansion. As arterial oxygenation increases, the pulmonary vascular smooth muscle relaxes, resulting in dilation of the pulmonary arteries. Leukotrienes and prostaglandins are also involved in this complex picture,

much of which is mediated by nitric oxide. Right ventricular and pulmonary artery pressures decrease significantly during the first 24 hours of life. The pulmonary arterial wall thickness of infants is comparable to that of adults by 4 months of age.

Although the right and left ventricles are similar in thickness at birth, left ventricular wall thickness increases rapidly during the first few weeks of life secondary to an increased work load.[29] The increase in left ventricular mass occurs by hyperplasia rather than as a result of hypertrophy. Functional closure of the ductus arteriosus occurs first, by constriction of the medial muscle layers of the vasculature, within the first 3 to 4 days of life. This structure undergoes permanent anatomic closure, by fibrosis, within 3 weeks of life. Physiologic closure of the foramen ovale occurs shortly after birth. Shunting through this foramen may occur, in a few individuals, for the first year of life. The physiologic ability of the ductus arteriosus to close is not related to gestational age.[30] Failure of the ductus to close is almost invariably the result of pulmonary hypertension.

Persistence of Fetal Circulation

Failure to achieve these complex and rapid changes in vascular resistance and ductal closure is common in many conditions. When this occurs, it is called persistent fetal or transitional circulation and is commonly life-threatening.

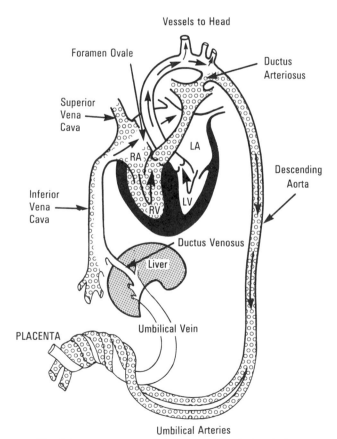

Fig. 44–1. Diagram of the normal fetal circulation.

Persistence of the transitional circulation beyond the first day of life may occur in both full-term and premature infants, especially in children with a respiratory distress syndrome, such as with a diaphragmatic hernia or meconium aspiration, or in those with congenital heart disease. Transient right-to-left shunting may occur in normal infants during coughing or straining and is inconsequential. In addition, acute or chronic hypoxia occurring either pre- or postnatally may affect the normal reduction of pulmonary resistance that occurs with the onset of respiration at birth. The development of the pulmonary vasculature can also be affected, and the response to hypoxia can be altered.[29,30]

Comparison of Infant and Adult Cardiac Physiology

The major differences between the heart of the infant and that of the adult are heart rate, contractility, compliance, afterload mismatch susceptibility, ventricular interdependence, and the response to catecholamines (Table 44-1). Cardiac output in the neonate is largely said to be rate dependent, with heart rates below 90 to 100 beats per minute associated with hypotension and inadequate tissue perfusion. Increases in cardiac output are primarily achieved by increasing the heart rate rather than stroke volume. In patients with a patent ductus arteriosus, however, an increase in preload and a decrease in afterload can result in significant increases in stroke volume. During the first 6 weeks of life, cardiac output increases markedly and continues to do so at a lesser rate until about 2 years of age.

Character of Myocardial Cells in Infants

The immature myocytes of the infant myocardium shorten less rapidly than those of the adult.[30] Reduced myocardial contractility in newborns is due in part to lower cytosolic calcium concentrations. Maturation in the structure and organization of myofilaments, membrane systems controlling cytosolic calcium concentration, and contractile proteins controlling the sensitivity of myofilaments to calcium produce the gradual increase in contractility found in adults.

Table 44–1. Comparison of Cardiovascular Variables

	Neonate	Infant	5 Years of Age	Adult
Weight (kg)	3	6–10	18	70
Oxygen consumption (ml·kg^{-1}·min^{-1})	6	5	6	3
Systolic arterial blood pressure (mmHg)	65	90–95	95	120
Heart rate (beats·min^{-1})	130	120	90	80
Blood volume (ml·kg^{-1})	85	80	75	65
Hemoglobin (g·dl^{-1})	17	11–12	13	14

From Stoelting, R. K., Miller, R. D.: Basics of Anesthesia, 3rd Ed. New York, Churchill Livingstone, 1994.

Ventricular Performance

The immature ventricles of the infant are less compliant than those of an adult. The physiologic consequence is that increases in preload do not produce the increase in stroke volume expected in the adult. In the infant, Starling's law relating stroke volume to end-diastolic pressure shows a short, steep ascending limb with a plateau occurring at 5 to 7 mm Hg.

Effect of Vasoactive Agents on Myocardial Action

Responses to exogenous catecholamines are reduced in the neonate, probably because of reduced receptor responsiveness and incomplete development of myocardial sympathetic receptors. Infusions of pressor drugs, especially dopamine and dobutamine, need to be increased significantly from those used in older children and adults.

Myocardial Metabolism in the Neonate

Changes in myocardial metabolism occur within hours of birth. Mitochondrial and enzymatic activity increases and is directly related to gluconeogenic activity. The neonatal myocardium converts completely to fatty acid oxidation by 1 to 2 years.

Effect of Anesthetic Agents

A discussion of cardiovascular physiology in neonates would be incomplete without mentioning the effects of inhalational agents on that physiology. First, the MAC of all neonates is not the same. In studies done 10 to 20 years ago, neonates and infants 1 to 6 months of age were considered a homogeneous group. More recent studies, however, have determined that the MAC of halothane is 25% less in neonates than it is in infants 1 to 6 months of age.[31] The same is true of isoflurane, with a 17% reduction of MAC demonstrated in neonates as compared with older infants.[32] The MAC values of inhalational anesthetics in preterm infants have also been studied.[33] The MAC of isoflurane in preterm neonates less than 32 weeks' gestational age is 10% less than it is in neonates 32 to 37 weeks of age. The results of these studies demonstrate that MAC values are lowest in severely premature infants and increase to the peak values for MAC determined for infants 6 months of age.

The cause of age-dependent decreases in MAC is unclear. Previously, the anesthetic literature suggested that preterm infants are more susceptible to myocardial depression than are full-term infants; however, more recent literature suggests that, when MAC is controlled for gestational age, circulatory depression is similar, comparing preterm and older infants.[32,34]

Some work has suggested that halothane and isoflurane are equipotent myocardial depressants in neonates and infants.[34] At 1 MAC concentrations of halothane and isoflurane, cardiac outputs decreased to 74% of controls from awake levels in both groups. At 1.5 MAC, a 35% decrease from awake values was seen. The only difference between these two agents on the cardiovascular system appears to be related to heart rate changes, with significant decreases in heart rate occurring with halothane but not with isoflurane.

Intravenous atropine increases the heart rate and cardiac output when either halothane or isoflurane is used, but stroke volume and ejection refraction remain unchanged from measurements before atropine administration.[34,35] This finding suggests that all increases in cardiac output are related to changes in heart rate, and the myocardial depression of halothane and isoflurane is unchanged. In addition, the use of atropine in children less than 6 months of age does not result in a significant increase in systolic blood pressure.

Finally, anesthesiologists must appreciate that neonates are more susceptible than adults to baroreceptor depression by volatile agents.[36] The normal increase in heart rate that occurs when systemic blood pressure decreases is abolished.

RESPIRATORY PHYSIOLOGY

The first inspiration after birth generates negative intrapleural pressures equivalent to −70 to −80 cm of water. This pressure change is essential to overcome the surface tension of the newborn lung. Gas exchanged in the lung is facilitated by removal of fluids from the airways and alveoli (Table 44–2). This is accomplished by oral drainage and increased pulmonary lymphatic flow in the first few hours after birth. The presence of surfactant is essential to create a low surface tension at the gas/liquid interface on the alveolar walls, which allows the alveoli to stay inflated, even at end-expiration. The absence of surfactant in severely premature infants is the cause of neonatal respiratory syndrome.[37] Fortunately, commercial preparations of surfactant are now available to prevent and treat this disorder.

Respiratory Control in the Neonate

Respiratory control is not well developed in the neonate. Immaturity of respiratory control predisposes the neonate to respiratory complications.[38] During the

Table 44–2. Comparison of Pulmonary Variables

	Neonate	Infant	5 Years of Age	Adult
Weight (kg)	3	6–10	18	70
Breathing frequency (breaths·min⁻¹)	35	24–30	20	15
Tidal volume (ml·kg⁻¹)	6	6	6	6
Vital capacity (ml·kg⁻¹)	35			70
Alveolar ventilation (ml·kg⁻¹·min⁻¹)	130			60
Carbon dioxide production (ml·kg⁻¹·min⁻¹)	6			3
Functional residual capacity (ml·kg⁻¹)	25	25	35	40

From Stoelting, R. K., Miller, R. D.: Basics of Anesthesia, 3rd Ed. New York, Churchill Livingstone, 1994.

first 3 weeks of life, the response of the infant to hypoxia is paradoxic. Hypoxia produces an increase in ventilation initially, followed rapidly by respiratory depression. In addition, hypoxia depresses the neonate's response to carbon dioxide.

Respiratory Mechanics

The neonatal rib cage is at a disadvantage with its high compliance and circular configuration, versus the elliptic shape present in adults (Table 44–3). In addition, the horizontal angle of diaphragmatic insertion, as compared with the oblique insertion in the adult, causes distortion of the rib cage and inefficient diaphragmatic contraction.

Muscle Fibers and Muscle Tone

In the full-term infant, only 25% of the diaphragmatic and intercostal fibers are type 1, or "fatigue-resistant fibers."[39] In the preterm infant, only 10% are type "1" fibers. This low number of type 1 fibers predisposes the respiratory muscles to fatigue. Maturation and presence of type "1" fibers in both the diaphram and intercostal muscles is complete by 6 to 8 months of age.

In infants, continuous tone of the inspiratory muscles of the thorax is important. The immature neonatal thoracic cage lacks the intrinsic rigidity to oppose the elastic recoil of the lung. One could presuppose therefore that loss of muscle tone during anesthesia, in infants, would result in a reduction of functional residual capacity (FRC) and airway to closure. This, in fact, seems to be the case.[38] FRC is markedly reduced in infants receiving general anesthesia compared with their older counterparts.

Role of Fetal Hemoglobin in the Neonate

Fetal hemoglobin, which helps to facilitate oxygen transport in utero, presents a slight problem for the neonate as they adapt to extrauterine life.[37] Fetal hemoglobin causes a shift in the hemoglobin oxygen disassociation curve to the left. Increased oxygen uptake and higher oxygen saturations at the lower partial pressures of oxygen are present in the placenta and fetus. After birth, oxygen unloading to tissues may be less efficient. Generally speaking, compensatory mechanisms such as a higher hemoglobin level, greater blood volume, and increased cardiac output help to compensate and allow adequate oxygen delivery as oxygen demands increase in the newborn. Clinically, however, a sick newborn may require a higher hemoglobin level than older infants to maintain an adequate oxygen delivery. Fetal hemoglobin is gradually replaced by hemoglobin A. By the third month of life, hemoglobin F levels are inconsequential.

METABOLIC DIFFERENCES

Significant metabolic differences exist among neonates, infants, and adults with respect to the pharmacokinetics of local anesthetics. Local amide anesthetics are metabolized in the liver and bound to plasma proteins. Neonates and infants less than 3 months of age have immature metabolic pathways and significantly decreased liver blood flow.[40,41] Together, these factors have a significant effect on the clearance and elimination of local anesthet-

Table 44–3.   Structural Differences in Respiratory System of Pediatric Patients

	Anatomic Characteristic	Importance
All pediatric patients	Narrow larynx and trachea	Increased susceptibility to upper airway obstruction from mucosal edema, granulation tissue, and so on
	Short tracheal length	Position of endotracheal tube critical to prevent accidental dislodgment or endobronchial intubation
	Smaller terminal airways and alveoli	Increased tendency to small airway obstruction and alveolar collapse
Infants	Greater dependence on diaphragm for respiratory work	Significant respiratory impairment from interference with movement of diaphragm (phrenic nerve palsy, abdominal distention)
Newborns	Greater elasticity of chest wall	Tendency to retraction of thoracic cage with inspiration; inefficient ventilatory effort
	Increased thickness of muscular layer of wall of pulmonary arterioles; smaller lumina	Increased pulmonary vascular resistance
Premature infants	Immature central control of respiration	Periodic breathing; apneic episodes
	Surfactant deficiency	Increased surface tension and tendency to atelectasis; respiratory distress syndrome

Data from Motoyama, E. K., Cook, C. D.: Respiratory Physiology. In Smith RM (eds.): Anesthesia for Infants and Children, 4th Ed. St. Louis, C. V. Mosby, 1980, p. 38; Doershuk, C. F. et al.: Pulmonary physiology of the young child. In Scarpelli, E., Auld, P. (eds.). Pulmonary Physiology of the Fetus, Newborn, and Child. Philadelphia, Lea & Febiger, 1975, p. 174; and Polgar G., Weng, T. R.: Functional development of the respiratory system. Am Rev Respir Dis *120*:625, 1979.

ics. Proteins that usually bind in these drugs, particularly albumin and α_1-acid glycoprotein, are significantly reduced in preterm and term infants.[42] With a decrease in the metabolism and protein binding of amide local anesthetics, greater levels of unbound drug can be expected. This increase in unbound drug is offset, at least in part, by the greater volume of distribution of local anesthetics in infants.

Ester local anesthetics are generally metabolized by plasma cholinesterase. Infants less than 6 months old have reduced enzyme levels.[40,41] The elimination of local ester anesthetics can therefore be expected to be prolonged. The data to support this conclusion, however, do not exist.

No evidence currently suggests that developmental differences exist between neonates and adults regarding the myocardial depressant effects of local anesthetics. Nor do conclusive data indicate that children are more prone to central nervous system toxicity, as compared with adults. One might speculate that the immature conduction system of the child's myocardium may alter sensitivity to amide local anesthetics, but this remains to be shown.

Children with cyanotic congenital heart disease may be particularly vulnerable to local anesthetic toxicity.[43] Lung tissue is normally responsible for the clearance of a significant fraction of circulating lignocaine. Children with right-to-left shunts have a significant decrease in clearance of local amide anesthetics. Additionally, α_1-glycoprotein is reduced in children with congenital heart disease.

TEMPERATURE REGULATION

Temperature regulation is an important physiologic function in the neonate. Immediately after delivery, the infant is exposed to a cooler and drier environment than that in utero and begins to lose heat by evaporation, convection, conduction, and radiation. Neonates have limited compensatory mechanisms that allow them to maintain temperature during a narrow temperature range once they are exposed to the cold. Nonshivering thermogenesis is the main compensatory mechanism by which infants respond to cold-induced stress.[44] Norepinephrine is released and thereby activates triglyceride and fatty acid metabolism of brown fat present in newborns. Hypothermia affects oxygen consumption in the newborn infant, and therefore one should keep the neonate in a thermally neutral environment. Prematurity, hypoglycemia, and general anesthesia all inhibit the neonatal metabolic response to hypothermia.

Prolonged hypothermia in neonates can cause cardiopulmonary decompensation and can result in tissue acidosis. In addition, hypothermia eliminates the hyperventilation that occurs as a normal response to hypoxia. Hypoventilation or apnea is a common finding in the hypothermic premature infant.

Finally, the large ratio of body surface to body weight of the infant, combined with the lack of subcutaneous fat and the inability to shiver, makes the neonate at particular risk of hypothermia.

RENAL PHYSIOLOGY OF THE NEONATE

The discussion of developmental renal physiology requires two considerations: (1) a discussion of the anatomy of fluid spaces in the infant; (2) the physiology of the neonatal kidney. In the neonate, as in the adult, total body water is divided into two compartments, intracellular and extracellular. The extracellular fluid is divided into two unequal compartments, plasma volume and interstitial fluid.

Total Body Water

Total body water is related to age and changes accordingly.[45] In full-term infants, 70 to 80% of body weight is total body water. Approximately 40% of the body weight is extracellular fluid at birth. Total body water decreases to 60% of body weight at 1 year of age, and extracellular fluid decreases to 20 to 25% of body weight. Intracellular fluid remains at 40% of body weight.

At birth, renal function of both preterm and full-term infants is immature as compared with the adult kidney.[46,47] The immaturity of renal function is directly related to gestational age; the greater the prematurity, the more the kidney is immature, both structurally and functionally.

Glomerular Filtration

Glomerular filtration rates (GFR) are lower in neonates than in adults. On the basis of surface area, the GFR of term neonates is 30% of adults. It reaches the adult level by 1 year of age. The neonatal kidney initially has a high vascular resistance and a resultant low renal blood flow. The low GFR is presumably the result of this reduced perfusion and a low filtration coefficient. The increase in GFR that occurs during the first few days of life is greater in term than in premature infants. The rapid increase in GFR at birth is related to the hemodynamic changes that occur in the first few days of life, with structural maturation less important.

Tubular Capacity

The tubular capacity for active transport is also poorly developed in the neonatal kidney. Reabsorption of sodium occurs along the entire nephron. Relative to the distal segment of the nephron is a lower reabsorption capacity of sodium in the proximal tubule and loop of Henle. Premature infants demonstrate this immature renal physiology by an inability to conserve sodium effectively during hyponatremia.

Production of Hormones

Neonates can produce aldosterone, cortisol, and antidiuretic hormone and have enhanced renin-angiotensin activity, but the distal tubule has a limited response to aldosterone. Tubular immaturity, therefore, accounts for much of the salt wasting that occurs in premature infants. Reabsorption of glucose, phosphates, and amino acids is also decreased, as is the threshold for bicarbonate reabsorption.

In the neonate, large amounts of solute free water are difficult to manage.[46,47] In the full-term infant, the response to a pure water load approximates the adult capacity by 1 month of age. Additionally, the neonate is, relative to an adult, incapable of concentrating the urine, with the urine commonly found to contain 700 to 800 mOsm/L, versus the adult value of 1200 to 1400 mOsm/L.[48] The reason for this phenomenon appears to be the reduced medullary solute gradient in the newborn.

Immaturity in the neonatal kidney (limited ability to concentrate urine and to conserve sodium adequately) requires paying greater attention to fluid and electrolyte management.

FLUID MANAGEMENT

In healthy neonates undergoing surgery, preoperative hydration is important. In the past, neonates have commonly remained NPO (nothing by mouth) for prolonged periods. Traditionally, infants were "NPO after midnight." Our views have changed substantially in the past decade.[49] In fact, the necessity for such an order is questionable even in children and adults. Studies in the past few years have demonstrated that clear fluids can be given safely up to 2 to 4 hours before the induction of anesthesia, without increasing the risk of aspiration.[49,50] Hence, neonates are rarely required to remain NPO for clear fluids for longer than 2 hours before induction. Solids take much longer to be evacuated from the stomach, and therefore, NPO for solids 6 to 8 hours before anesthesia is still appropriate. In addition, some medications, particularly narcotic analgesics, may slow gastric emptying. These factors should be taken into account when ordering NPO times.

In general, although it may be annoying for the parents of neonates to have their children NPO for solids for 4 to 6 hours, such a precaution is reasonable and does not have detrimental effects. Maintaining children NPO for clear fluids, however, does result in discomfort, causes dehydration preoperatively, and may increase the likelihood of difficult intravenous access and hypotension during induction of anesthesia.

Maintenance Fluid Requirements

Maintenance fluids are required to fulfill five basic requirements: (1) evaporation from the skin; (2) excretion of waste products by the kidney; (3) water in the stool; (4) water losses from the respiratory tract; (5) water needed for growth. Maintenance fluid requirements vary and depend on the caloric requirements and metabolic rate of the infant. The volume of water needed is generally equated with the estimated energy expenditure in calories. Thus, without unusual loss or gain, water requirement is 100 ml/100 calories.[45]

Changes in the metabolic rate alter fluid requirements. Fever and hypermetabolic states increase fluid requirements. Fever increases caloric consumption by 12% per degree centigrade rise in body temperature. A decrease in metabolic rate, secondary to hypothermia, decreases fluid requirements by a similar fraction. Ambient humidity affects evaporative water losses, with high humidity decreasing the losses and vice versa.

For infants, preoperative maintenance fluids can be described as follows:

4 ml/kg	for the first 10 kg body weight
2 ml/kg	for the second 10 kg body weight
1 ml/kg	for every kg of body weight over 20 kg

Electrolytes must also be supplied in the daily maintenance fluids. The usual daily requirements for sodium are 3 to 4 mEq/kg. For potassium, 2.5 to 3 mEq/kg is appropriate, and for chloride it is 3 to 4 mEq/kg. Potassium is not routinely needed for intraoperative maintenance fluids, and a maintenance solution of 0.25% normal saline is appropriate, for short-term use.

Intraoperative Fluid Management

The intraoperative fluid management of the child must take in to account the length of time the child has been fasting, preoperative fluid losses, maintenance fluid requirements, third-space losses that occur as a consequence of the surgery, and finally fluids that are required to replace blood loss.

Typically, isotonic fluid losses occur with trauma, burns, peritonitis, bleeding, and losses from the upper gastrointestinal tract. All these losses are high in sodium and, for the purpose of discussion, can be considered as a loss of extracellular fluid. Therefore, these types of losses should be replaced by a balanced salt solution.

Hypotonic fluid losses occur with sweating and diarrhea. Generally, the replacement of fluid for these losses requires a hypotonic solution between 0.25 and 0.5% normal saline. For practical purposes, balanced salt solutions are often used to replace these hypotonic losses, because the neonatal kidney handles excesses of sodium better than it compensates for the losses of sodium not appropriately replaced.

Although NPO guidelines have changed over the last few years, some children are invariably kept NPO for a longer period of time. From a practical point of view, those losses do not need to be replaced based on values calculated by taking the number of NPO hours and multiplying by the hourly maintenance fluid rate. Rather, one should replace deficits based on whether or not the child has had normal fluid requirements during the NPO period. For those with normal fluid requirements during the NPO period, one can simply administer 15 ml/kg of fluid on establishment of intravenous access. For children who have had a fever or gastrointestinal losses, one should administer 25 ml/kg of fluid during the immediate induction period. Ringer's lactate is a resonable choice for this purpose. Ringer's lactate is chosen over normal saline because Ringer's lactate contains less chloride than does normal saline. The high chloride content of normal saline results in hyperchloremic acidosis in children.

Following replacement of NPO losses, calculate maintenance fluid needs for the child during the surgery as previously discussed.[45] Fluids for maintenance can be either a balanced salt solution or a hypotonic solution of 0.25 to 0.5% normal saline.

Third-Space Fluid Requirements

Third-space fluid losses must also be calculated for the infant during surgery. These losses are divided into three categories: mild trauma, moderate trauma, and severe trauma. Mild trauma requires an additional 2 ml/kg/hour of balanced salt solution added to maintenance fluids. For moderate trauma, an additional 4 ml/kg/hour of balanced salt solution is needed. Finally, for severe trauma, 6 to 8 ml/kg/hour of additional balanced salt solution is required, although occasionally 10 to 12 ml/kg/hour is needed. For discussion purposes, an inguinal hernia re-

pair is considered minimal trauma, a thoracotomy is moderate trauma, and severe trauma is represented by repair of an omphalocele or the presence of necrotizing entercolitis.

Replacement of Blood Losses

Replacement of blood losses require three considerations.

Role of Volume Lost

This first consideration deals with the amount of fluid necessary to replace a given quantity of blood loss. When blood loss is replaced with colloid solutions, such as 5% albumin, hetastarch, or blood itself, 1 ml of fluid for each milliliter of blood loss is appropriate. If balanced salt solution is used, 3 ml of crystalloid must be given for every milliliter of blood lost.

Role of Normal Blood Volume in Children

This second consideration in replacing blood loss relates to the blood volume of children at any given age. In general, the younger the neonate, the greater the blood volume. For simplicity, the blood volume of children can be divided into three categories: (1) for severely premature, low-birth-weight infants, blood volumes can be considered to be between 100 and 110 ml/kg; (2) for premature infants between 34 and 38 weeks' gestation, blood volumes can be considered to be 90 to 100 ml/kg; (3) for children 36 to 40 weeks' gestation, blood volumes can be considered 90 ml/kg.

Role of Hematocrit Values

The third consideration is in regard to acceptable hematocrits. Normal hematocrit values vary with the age of the child. Premature infants have a mean hematocrit of approximately 45% and newborns 55%. The hematocrit value decreases rapidly, and at 3 months of age it is 35%. The lowest hematocrit value acceptable in these children is arbitrary. General guidelines include the following: premature infants' hematocrits may fall to between 30 and 35%, 30% for newborns, and 25% for infants in the first 3 months of life. The decrease in hemoglobin F may allow older infants to tolerate lower hematocrit levels. Obviously, hematocrit levels must be adjusted to take into account the underlying medical condition, particularly cardiac and respiratory problems. Most important, one *should not* use the acceptable blood loss and hematocrit values calculated for adults and apply them to neonates.

Postoperative Fluid Needs

The switch to hypotonic fluids, in the immediate postoperative period, can lead to acute dilutional hyponatremia.[45] The high antidiuretic hormone levels in the immediate postoperative period, combined with ongoing third-space losses in the first 2 to 24 hours after surgery, can result in a reduction in free water clearance unless appropriate replacement of salt needs occurs. Vomiting often complicates the postoperative picture, aggravating fluid losses high in sodium. When hypotonic solutions are used to replace these fluid losses, the sodium intake may be inadequate to meet the needs of the body. Five percent dextrose in water (D5W) should never be used in children, especially after surgery.

Acute symptomatic hyponatremia is a medical emergency that is fortunately rare.[51] It does require immediate therapy. The drug of choice is probably sodium bicarbonate, which is a 6% sodium solution. The dose of this solution is usually 2 ml/kg given rapidly over 1 to 2 minutes. Each 2 ml/kg of sodium bicarbonate raises serum sodium levels by 6 mEq/L.

Glucose Requirements

Recent studies have resulted in a complete reevaluation of glucose usage in routine operative fluids for neonates.[51,52] In the past, the neonate was presumed to be at special risk of developing hypoglycemia in the operative period. Glucose solutions were therefore recommended for all infants. To appreciate the risk of hypoglycemia, however, the condition must first be defined. Glucose levels are age related. Normally, premature infants have a glucose level of approximately 30 to 40 mg/dl. Older infants have levels of approximately 40 to 50 mg/dl. These levels are obviously lower than values accepted in older children and adults.

Studies determining glucose levels in children fasting between 6 and 18 hours did not demonstrate any child with symptomatic hypoglycemia.[51-53] Using age-dependent neonatal definitions of hypoglycemia, none of the patients had hypoglycemia on the basis of their serum glucose concentrations. From these studies, one may conclude that glucose is not routinely needed.

Are certain high-risk patients in danger of hypoglycemia? The most frequent children at risk are those who are receiving glucose-containing solutions, especially hyperalimentation. These patients should have glucose infusions continued in the operative period, preferably in the form of continuous hyperalimentation. Other patients at risk include the infants of diabetic mothers in the immediate delivery period and neonates who are small for gestational age.

To decide whether infants should receive routine glucose infusions intraoperatively, one must consider whether the use of glucose will be harmful or beneficial.[54] The use of glucose is potentially harmful. Besides the well-known risks of hypergylcemia is the risk of hypoxia in infants, during our anesthetic management. This consideration relates to the concept that the administration of glucose solutions results in an increase of glucose levels in the brain, so, with hypoxia and ischemia, anaerobic metabolism produces large quantities of lactic acid. Lactic acid may lower the pH of brain cells and may increase the potential for neurologic damage. Neurologic deficits have been associated with the administration of glucose.[55,56]

Because the risk of hypoglycemia in infants is less than previously thought, we should use glucose as a drug, just like any other. Glucose should be administered to neonates only when necessary and not as routine practice. The administration of glucose, particularly in those infants undergoing long procedures, should be based on serum glucose levels. These same children should have serum glucose levels monitored if a nonglucose-containing solution is used, avoiding rare occurrences of hypoglycemia. Only by monitoring serum levels of glucose can appropriate decisions be made. Infusions of glucose as small as 1% are often more than adequate to maintain normal serum glucose levels in infants at risk of hypoglycemia.

REFERENCES

1. Okado, N.: Onset of synapse formation in the human spinal cord. J Comp Neurol 201:211, 1981.
2. Pernow, B.: Substance P. Pharmacol Rev 35:85, 1983.
3. Charney, Y., et al.: Distribution of substance P-like immunoreactivity in the spinal cord and dorsal root ganglia of the human foetus and infant. Neuroscience 10:41, 1983.
4. Humphrey, T.: Some correlations between the appearance of human fetal reflexes and the development of the nervous system. Prog Brain Res 4:93, 1964.
5. Marin-Padilla, M.: Structural organization of the human cerebral cortex prior to the appearance of the cortical plate. Anat Embryol 165:21, 1983.
6. Rakic, P., Goldman-Rakic, P. S.: Development and modifiability of the cerebral cortex. Early developmental effects: cell lineages, acquisition of neuronal positions, and areal and laminar development. Neurosci Res Prog Bull 20:433, 1982.
7. Gilles, F. J., Shankle, W., Dooling, E. C.: Myelinated tracts: growth patterns. In Gilles, F. H., Leviton, A., Dooling, E. C. (eds.). The Developing Human Brain: Growth and Epidemiologic Neuropathology. Boston, John Wright, 1983, p. 117.
8. Jansco, G., Kiraly, E., Jansco-Garbor, A.: Pharmacologically induced selective denervation of chemosensitive primary sensory neurons. Nature 270:741, 1977.
9. Anand, K. J. S., Hickey, P. R.: Pain and its effects in the human neonate and fetus. N Engl J Med 317:1321, 1987.
10. Anand, K. J. S., et al.: Can the human neonate mount an endocrine and metabolic response to surgery? J Pediatr Surg 20:41, 1985.
11. Anand, K. J. S., Hickey, P. R.: Halothane-morphine compared with high-dose sufentanil for anesthesia and postoperative analgesia in neonatal cardiac surgery. N Engl J Med 326:1, 1992.
12. Fitzgerald, M., McIntosh, N.: pain and analgesia in the newborn. Arch Dis Child 64:441, 1989.
13. Charney, Y., et al.: Distribution of enkephalin in human fetus and infant spinal cord: an immunofluorescence study. J Comp Neurol 223:415, 1984.
14. Gautray, J. P., et al.: Presence of immunoassayable B-endorphin in human amniotic fluid: elevation in cases of fetal distress. Am J Obstet Gynecol 129:211, 1977.
15. Way, W. L., Costley, E. C., Way, E. L.: Respiratory sensitivity of newborn infants to meperidine and morphine. Clin Pharmacol Ther 6:454, 1965.
16. Loren, G., et al.: Postoperative morphine infusion in newborn infants: assessment of disposition characteristics and safety. J Pediatr 107:963, 1985.
17. Zhang, A. Z., Pasternak, G. W.: Ontogeny of opioid pharmacology and receptors: high and low affinity site differences. Eur J Pharmacol 73:29, 1981.
18. Koehntop, D. E., et al.: Pharacokinetics of fentanyl in neonates. Anesth Analg 65:227, 1986.
19. Yaster, M.: The dose response of fentanyl in neonatal anesthesia. Anesthesiology 66:433, 1987.
20. Robinson, S., Gregory, G. A.: Fentanyl air oxygen anesthesia for ligation of patent ductus arteriosis in preterm infants. Anesth Analg 60:331, 1981.

21. Goudsouzian, N. G.: Maturation of neuromuscular transmission of the infant. Br J Anaesth 52:205, 1980.

22. Goudsouzian, N. G., Standaert, F. G.: The infant and the myoneural junction. Anesth Analg 65:1208, 1986.

23. Goudsouzian, N. G., Shorten, G.: Myoneural blocking agents in infants: a review. Paediatr Anaesth 2:3, 1992.

24. Fisher, D. M., et al.: Pharmacokinetics and pharmacodynamics of d-tubocurarine in infants, children and adults. Anesthesiology 57:203, 1982.

25. Fisher, D. M., Castagnoli, K., Miller, R. D.: Vecuronium kinetics and dynamics in anesthetized infants and children. Clin Pharmacol Ther 37:402, 1985.

26. Meretoja, O. A., Luosto, T.: Dose-response characteristics of pancuronium in neonates, infants and children. Anaesth Intensive Care 18:455, 1990.

27. Matteo, R. S., et al.: Distribution, elimination, and action of d-tubocurarine in neonates, infants, children and adults, Anesth Analg 63:799, 1984.

28. Lake, C. L.: Cardiovascular diseases. In Berry, F. A., Steward, D.J. (eds.). Pediatrics for the Anesthesiologist. New York, Churchill Livingstone, 1993, p. 25.

29. Lake, C. L.: Cardiovascular embryology, growth, and development. In Lake, C. L. (ed.). Pediatric Cardiac Anesthesia, 2nd Ed. Norwalk, CT, Appleton & Lange, 1993, p. 21.

30. Reller, M. D., Rice, M. J., McDonald, R. W.: Review of studies evaluating ductal patency in the premature infant. J Pediatr 122:S59, 1993.

31. Lerman, J., Robinson, S., Willis, M. M., Gergory, G. A.: Anesthetic requirements for halothane in young children 0-1 month and 1-6 months of age. Anesthesiology 59:421, 1983.

32. Lerman, J.: Pharmacology of inhalational anaesthetics in infants and children. Paediatr Anaesth 2:191, 1992.

33. LeDez, K. M., Lerman, J.: The minimum alveolar concentration (MAC) of isoflurane in pertern infants. Anesthesiology 67:301, 1987.

34. Friesen, R. H., Lichtor, J. L.: Cardiovascular depression during halothane anesthesia in infants: a study of three induction techniques. Anesth Analg 61:42, 1982.

35. Murray, D. J., et al.: Hemodynamic effects of atropine during halothane and isoforane anaesthesia in infants and small children. Can J Anaesth 36:295, 1989.

36. Gregory, G. A.: The baroresponses of preterm infants during halothane anesthesia. Can Anaesth Soc J 29:105, 1981.

37. Wensley, D., Seear, M.: Respiratory disease. In Berry, F. A., Steward, D. J. (eds.). Pediatrics for the Anesthesiologist. New York, Churchill Livingstone, 1993, p. 1.

38. Davis, G. M., Bureau, M. A.: Pulmonary and chest wall mechanics in the control of ventilation in the newborn. Clin Perinatol 14:551, 1987.

39. Keens, T. G., Bryan, A. C., Levison, H., Zanuzzo, C. D.: Developmental pattern of muscle fiber types in human ventilatory muscles. J Appl Physiol 144:909, 1978.

40. Yaster, M., Maxwell, L. G.: Pediatric regional anesthesia. Anesthesiology 70:324, 1989.

41. Dalens, B.: Regional anesthesia in children. Anesth Analg 68:654, 1989.

42. Lerman, J., et al.: Effects of age on the serum concentration of alpha 1-acid glycoprotein and the binding of lidocaine in pediatric patients. Clin Pharmacol Ther 47:219, 1989.

43. Burrows, F. A., Lerman, J., Ledez, K. M., Strong, H. A.: Pharmacokinetics of lidocaine in children with congenital heart disease. Can J Anaesth 38:196, 1991.

44. Jessen, K.: An assessment of human regulatory nonshivering thermogenesis. Acta Anaesthesiol Scand 24:138, 1980.

45. Berry, F. A.: Practical aspects of fluid and electrolyte therapy. In Berry, F. A. (ed): Anesthetic Management of Difficult and Routine Pediatric Patients, 2nd Ed. New York, Churchill Livingstone, 1990, p. 89.

46. Al-Dahhan, J., et al.: Sodium homeostasis in term and preterm neonates: effect of salt supplementation. Arch Dis Child 59:945, 1984.

47. Spitzer, A.: The role of the kidney in sodium homeostasis during maturation. Kidney Int 21:539, 1982.

48. Costarino, A. T., Baumgart, S.: Controversies in fluid and electrolyte therapy for the premature infant. Clin Perinatol 15:863, 1988.

49. Cote, C. J.: NPO after midnight for children: a reappraisal. Anesthesiology 72:589, 1990.

50. Schreiner, M. S., Triebwasser, A., Keon, T. P.: Ingestion of liquids compared with preoperative fasting in pediatric out patients. Anesthesiology 72:593, 1990.

51. Welborn, L. G., et al.: Perioperative blood glucose concentration in pediatric outpatients. Anesthesiology 65:543, 1986.

52. Sarnaik, A. P., et al.: Management of hyponatremic seizures in children with hypertonic saline: a safe and effective strategy. Crit Care Med 19:758, 1991.

53. Doze, V. A., White, P. F.: Effects of fluid therapy on serum glucose levels in fasted outpatients. Anesthesiology 66:223, 1987.

54. Steward, D. J., DaSilva, C. A., Flegel, T.: Elevated blood glucose levels may increase the danger of neurological deficit following profoundly hypothermic cardiac arrest. Anesthesiology 68:653, 1988.

55. Michaus, L. J., et al.: Elevated initial blood glucose levels and poor outcome following severe brain injuries in children. J Trauma 31:1356, 1991.

56. Glauser, T. A., et al.: Acquired neuropathologic lesions associated with the hypoplastic left heart syndrome. Pediatrics 85:991, 1990.

Chapter 45

SELECTED ACUTE AND CHRONIC DISEASES

VINCENT J. COLLINS, RAGHUBAR P. BADOLA

CONTENTS

BULLOUS DISORDERS (EPIDERMOLYSIS BULLOSA)

These disorders are a heterogenous group of both heritable and acquired lesions, primarily of the skin, produced by trivial trauma. The more appropriate term for these diseases is mechanobullous disorders, which stresses the relation between mechanical trauma and blister formation.[1]

These disorders are unified under the pathologic concept of impaired skin adherence. The disruption within the skin may occur between epidermal cells, forming intradermal bullae, or below the epidermis. Epidermal cells are held together by dense circular attachment bodies; the epidermis and dermis are attached to each other by a basal lamina, with anchoring fibers of glycose amines. Disorders of either of these two sites may result in bulla formation.

Two classes of bullous disorders of the skin are recognized, namely, acquired and genetic. The acquired forms represent a large group and include toxic epidermal necrolysis with separation of the basal layer, staphylococcal scalded skin syndrome with separation of the granular layer, and pemphigus vulgaris with separation at the subepidermal site.

Epidermolysis bullosa was originally described by von Hebra and was designated as pemphigus.[2] In recent years, many syndromes have been identified, and at least 14 have been classified by Briggaman.[1] The genetic or inherited forms are of 2 types, according to dominant or recessive inheritance. These are subdivided into the dominant simple generalized type, the dominant dystrophic type, and the recessive dystrophic type.[3] A further division recognizes whether the disorder is characterized by scarring or nonscarring consequences.

In all situations, bulla formation occurs as a result of skin trauma. In this sense, these dystrophic disorders are designated mechanobullous disorders. Friction, pressure, or any shearing force causes disruption of the skin. Separation occurs at the subepidermal layer, causing a split between the epidermis and the dermis, with extravasation of fluid. Perpendicular trauma does not seem to produce any damage resulting in the formation of bullae. The trauma need only be minor and may even arise spontaneously, however.

Dominant simple generalized epidermolysis bullosa has an autosomal dominant inheritance, and the incidence is approximately 1 per 50,000 live births. This form is nonscarring.

Dominant dystrophic epidermolysis bullosa and recessive epidermolysis bullosa dystrophica are scarring disorders. The recessive genetic form is rare, with an incidence of 1 per 300,000 live births.

CONSIDERATIONS

The most important objective in patient care is to avoid damaging epithelial surfaces. Minimal contact with skin is to be sought. Particularly vulnerable areas are the skin surface and the oropharyngeal mucous membrane lid, where stratified squamous epithelium is found. From experience with endotracheal intubation, the tracheobronchial membranes consisting of pseudostratified ciliated columnar epithelium are not affected by the presence of the endotracheal tube; however, caution in the use of inflated cuffs is recommended. Kelly stated that a search of the literature did not reveal a single report of laryngeal bullous formation.[4]

ANESTHETIC MANAGEMENT

A preoperative visit is necessary for the following reasons:

1. To review the associated medical problems of maldevelopment, malnourishment, anemia, cachexia, amyloidosis, and impairment of renal function.
2. To determine drug intake, such as phenytoin and/or steroids often used for treatment.
3. To reassure the patient that the best of care will be provided, and to calm the patient.
4. To ensure a regimen in which preanesthetic medication is minimal; an oral tranquilizer of the benzodiazepine type is warranted.

Choice of Anesthesia

Either general anesthesia[5] or regional anesthesia[6] can be safely administered if certain precautions are taken, as discussed later in this section.

Monitoring

Blood pressure recording by sphygmomanometry may be chosen, but frictional or shearing force must be avoided. This goal is accomplished by careful wrapping of the arm with soft moist cotton padding (Webrol), over which the blood pressure cuff is smoothly wrapped without creases.[7] Alternatively, a percutaneous intra-arterial catheter may be inserted into a peripheral artery for direct measurement.

Electrocardiographic (ECG) monitoring should be done, provided the electrode pads are lightly applied without the encircling adhesive and are allowed to remain attached by means of the electrode gel.

Antisepsis

For antisepsis at intravenous or intra-arterial sites, cotton alcohol sponges may be placed over the site for puncture and allowed to remain for several minutes. One should not rub the area or use ordinary gauze sponges. For regional anesthesia, an alternative to cotton alcohol sponges is the use of a povidone-iodine spray. Securing of an intravascular catheter is accomplished by soft cotton padding, and the catheter is wrapped with cotton gauze (Webrol).

Administration of Oxygen and Inhalational Agents

For supplemental breathing oxygen or administration of an inhalation anesthetic, a face mask is necessary. The mask should be cushioned from direct contact with the skin of the face by patting a dermal steroid cream on the patient's face, especially about the mouth, cheeks, and chin. Soft cotton padding should then be applied to the patient's face and over the chin. The mask should be gently applied and held without force and without movement.

Airway[5]

A patent airway must be maintained at all times. Positioning of the patient's head in the sniffing posture, with the head slightly extended, is often sufficient. Oropharyngeal or nasopharyngeal airways must be avoided; bullae of the pharynx can be produced.

Endotracheal Intubation

If this procedure is necessary, the following are recommended[5]:

1. Intravenous induction is accomplished with ketamine.[8]
2. Profound muscle relaxation is induced. Our best experience is with vecuronium. These patients have dystrophic muscle masses, and the dose need not be greater than warranted by the general physical condition. Succinylcholine has been used, but a hyperkalemic response is likely.[9,10]
3. Laryngoscopy is best accomplished by using the Macintosh curved blade. This instrument is passed over the tongue (not subject to bullous formation) and lifts the tongue forward exposing the glottis, and it does not touch the posterior part of the epiglottis (subject to bullous formation).
4. Introduction of a well-lubricated endotracheal tube should be gentle, and contact with the pharynx should be avoided as much as possible. Scarring of the oral cavity occurs in up to 50% of patients.[5]
5. Cuffs are inflated only if absolutely necessary, and the intracuff pressure is kept to a minimum.
6. The endotracheal tube is secured. The tube should remain in the midline and should not exert a lateral force on the corner of the mouth. Soft cotton tape, such as used to secure tracheostomy tubes, may be wrapped about the endotracheal tube and held by adhesive to the tube or stitched to the tube and then taken laterally and tied behind the patient's neck.
7. Extubation must be equally as careful as intubation; catheter suction of the pharynx should be avoided.

Choice of General Anesthetic Agents

Intravenous anesthesia is probably the most satisfactory approach to management of general anesthesia, because it avoids problems related to masks and airways. This presumes that adequate spontaneous respiration is maintained. Sedative doses of benzodiazepines—diazepam or midazolam—have been used, in conjunction with local peripheral nerve blocks.

Many surgical procedures require full surgical stage III anesthesia and complete pain relief, however, and the experienced anesthesiologist may accomplish this goal and may maintain the patient's spontaneous respiration with the potent volatile agents plus nitrous oxide (oxygen as a carrier).

Intravenous ketamine has many desirable characteristics.[8,10] Experience in several institutions has shown it to be highly successful and safe. It produces unconsciousness, provides excellent analgesia, and maintains competence of the airway and laryngeal reflexes. Cardiovascular stability, even in the presence of shock states, is maintained.

The problem of postoperative behavioral difficulties can be avoided by pretreatment with a dose of 1 to 2 mg diazepam or midazolam. If necessary, rapid induction followed by administration of a muscle relaxant allows quick and easy intubation without ever applying a face mask.

Regional Anesthesia

Regional anesthesia is in many circumstances the technique of choice.[7,11] With certain precautions, it is both safe and more satisfactory than general anesthesia and has fewer complications. Spinal,[7] epidural,[7] and plexus block[6] have all been administered.

The essential consideration for any anesthesia and the special management techniques in the bullous disorders are previously outlined. These include preoperative reassurance and explanation, monitoring of blood pressure and ECG, establishment of intravenous lines by proper antisepsis and security without adhesive tape, and procedures for oxygen therapy.

Spinal or Epidural Anesthesia[7,11]

Considerations include the following:

1. Gentle and careful positioning are essential, allowing patient to do most of the moving.
2. Cleaning and antisepsis of back with 70% alcohol cotton sponges are indicated, followed by application of a povidone-iodine spray, with no rubbing or scrubbing.
3. Do not press to identify the intervertebral space. Most patients are thin and poorly nourished, so the vertebral column and spines are readily visible.
4. A small hypodermic needle size (26 to 28 gauge) should be used and directed perpendicular to the skin and 1.0% lidocaine injected subcutaneously.
5. Insertion of spinal or epidural needle proceeds according to ordinary technique.
6. When a continuous catheter technique is employed, the catheter can be secured by application of collodion at the insertion site. The catheter may then be brought up a few centimeters along the back, fastened to the skin with 4-0 silk stitches (this can be omitted). The entire area should be covered with soft cotton padding and the catheter should be brought to the side or along the back to the patient's head and covered by cotton wadding.

Brachial Plexus Block[6]

The axillary approach with secondary block of the musculocutaneous and thoracobrachialis nerves has been successfully used and found safe.

Comment

Sedation or supplemental anesthesia for regional techniques can be achieved by the use of ketamine 1 to 2 mg intravenously.

REFERENCES

1. Briggaman, R. A.: Hereditary epidermolysis bullosa with special emphasis on newly recognized syndromes and complications. Dermatol Clin 1:263, 1983.
2. Von Hebra, F.: Phemphigus. Vienna, Arzlicher Bericht des K. K. Allgemeinen Krankenhauses, 1870, p. 362.
3. Tomlinson, A. A.: Recessive dystrophic epidermolysis bullosa. Anaesthesia 38:485, 1983.
4. Kelly, A. J.: Epidermolysis bullosa dystrophica: anesthetic management. Anesthesiology 35:659, 1971.
5. James, I., Wark, H.: Airway management during anesthesia in patients with epidermolysis bullosa dystrophica. Anesthesiology 56:323, 1982.
6. Kelly, R. E., et al.: Brachial plexus anesthesia in eight patients with recessive dystrophic epidermolysis bullosa. Anesth Analg 66:1318, 1987.
7. Broster, T., Placek, R., Eggers, G. W. N.: Epidermolysis bullosa: anesthetic management for cesarean section. Anesth Analg 66:341, 1987.
8. LoVerme, S. R., Oropollo, A. T.: Ketamine anesthesia in dermolytic bullosous dermatosis (epidermolysis bullosa). Anesth Analg 56:398, 1972.
9. Hamann, R. A., Cohen, P. J.: Anesthetic management of a patient with epidermolysis bullosa dystrophica. Anesthesiology 34:389, 1971.
10. Lee, C., Nagel, E. L.: Anesthetic management of a patient with recessive epidermolysis bullosa dystrophica. Anesthesiology 43:122, 1975.
11. Spielman, F. J., Mann, E. S.: Subarachnoid and epidural anaesthesia for patients with epidermolysis bullosa. Can Anaesth Soc J 31:549, 1984.

CROUP

Croup is a common cause of acute upper airway obstruction in infants and children. It is properly defined as acute laryngotracheobronchitis. The incidence is approximately 3 cases per 100 children below the age of 6 years. About 1.3% of affected children are hospitalized. The need for hospitilization is determined by the criteria of a croup score of 7 or more based on clinical signs.[1]

ETIOLOGY

Viruses are the causative agent in most cases of croup. The parainfluenza virus is most frequently found and is accompanied by high titers of specific IgE for the virus as well as histamine in nasal secretions. Bacterial membraneous tracheitis and epiglottitis should be ruled out.[2]

PATHOLOGY

The basic pathologic feature is an inflammatory process of the vocal cords, the subglottis, trachea and bronchi, with varying degrees of edema.

DIAGNOSIS OF SEVERITY: THE CROUP SCORE

To evaluate the clinical state of a patient objectively, a croup score was devised by Westley and associates[3] and modified by Downes and Godinez.[4] Five symptoms and signs are assessed:

1. The cardinal sign is the respiratory stridor or crow, which may occur on inspiration initially but may progress and be present on both inspiration and expiration. It is present at rest but is more pronounced when the patient is agitated.
2. On coughing or crying, the child may respond with a coarse cry or a barking cough.
3. Chest movements may begin with suprasternal *retractions* accompanied by some nasal flaring; this may progress to include intercostal and subcostal retractions.
4. Inspiratory breath sounds on auscultation are likely to be harsh, with wheezing and rhonchi; an attempt at inspiration may be accompanied by delayed air entry into the lungs.
5. Cyanosis while breathing air at rest but especially on agitation may be seen; if this condition is present while the patient is breathing 40% oxygen, it is ominous.

Each sign is scored as follows: not present (0); present (1); or advanced (2). A score of 4 or more requires therapy. If the score is over 7 despite initial treatment, hospitalization is indicated.[4-6]

Respiratory and heart rates should be recorded as part of the examination. These parameters increase with the severity of the disease. At croup scores of 4, the respiratory rate may be 40 to 50 breaths per minute and the heart rate 140 to 170 beats per minute in 2-year-old children.

RADIOLOGIC EXAMINATION

On lateral neck projections, one sees blurring of the tracheal air shadow consistent with edema of the subglottic region. On an anteroposterior projection, one sees narrowing of the subglottic air shadow, designated the "church steeple sign."[5]

TREATMENT[6]

Although in the majority of children croup is a self-limited illness, it is not predictable, and treatment at an early stage reduces the severity of symptoms, diminishes the progression to obstruction and hospitalization, and prevents the occurrence of epiglottitis.

Initial and Early Treatment of Mild-To-Moderate Croup (Croup Score of 4 or More)

1. Glucocorticoids are firmly established as therapy for croup and should be given early when inspiratory stridor is persistent. Intramuscular dexamethasone, in doses of 0.3 mg/kg, is effective in reducing the inflammation. Nebulized budesonide provides prompt and important clinical improvement and avoids the discomfort of intramuscular injection.[7] Budesonide is a synthetic glucocorticoid with relatively strong topical anti-inflammatory effects and low systemic activity.[8] The drug begins to act in about 1 hour, with significant improvement seen within 2 to 4 hours and a prolonged effect in controlling symptoms.
2. Racemic epinephrine delivered by nebulizer is a major effective component for treatment of croup.[9-15] The mechanism of action is through the α-adrenergic effect producing mucosal vasoconstriction and decreasing the edema of the subglottic region and the glottis.[10] Improvement is evident within 10 minutes and reaches an optimum effect by 30 minutes, with a significant reduction in the croup score. A single treatment provides clinical improvement for about 2 hours. Repeated doses can be administered until relief is attained.[11] Ordinarily, a 2.25% solution of the racemic form is administered in a 1.8% dilution. Because the effective component of the racemic epinephrine is the levo-rotory form, a 1% aqueous solution of L-epinephrine is equally effective.[12]
3. The use of humidified air in tents[16] has been a routine treatment for children with croup. Little evidence indicates any beneficial effect on the glottic and subglottic edema,[17] however, as demonstrated by controlled studies.

ROLE OF ANTIBIOTICS

Because viruses are the causative agents, little justification to use antibiotics exists. If bacterial membranous tracheitis and epiglottitis is present, however, then antibiotics are needed. For patients hospitalized with severe croup due to influenza A virus and persistent, uncontrolled symptoms, amantadine, an antiviral agent, maybe used.[16]

MANAGEMENT OF SEVERE CROUP

When a patient has increasing inspiratory airway obstruction and a croup score above 7, hospitalization is required.[6,18] If one sees a rising $Paco_2$ blood gas analysis and hypoxemia is developing despite high inspired oxygen concentrations, then translaryngeal intubation with an orotracheal or nasotracheal tube OR a transtracheal airway is needed.[19] A smaller tube of diameter 0.5 mm less than that predicted for the child's age should be used. This procedure should be planned for the short term, and extubation should be considered by 24 to 48 hours. Although tracheosteomy is often recommended in patients requiring intubation of longer duration, this procedure has not been necessary, and the complication rate of sub-glottic stenosis and vocal cord has not been found to be greater than after tracheostomy.[19,20]

REFERENCES

1. Denny, F. W., et al.: Croup: an 11-year study in a pediatric practice. Pediatrics 71:871, 1983.
2. Welliver, R. C., et al.: Role of parainfluenza virus-specific IgE in pathogenesis of croup and wheezing subsequent to infection. J Pediatr 101:889, 1982.
3. Westley, C. R., Cotton, E. K., Brooks, J. G.: Nebulized racemic epinephrine by IPPB for the treatment of croup: a double-blind study. Am J Dis Child 132:484, 1978.
4. Downes, J. J., Godinez, R. I.: Acute upper airway obstruction in the child. American Society of Anesthesiologists Refresher Courses in Anesthesiology, Vol. 8. Philadelphia, J. B. Lippincott, 1980, p. 29.
5. Mills, J. L., et al.: The usefulness of lateral neck roentgenograms in laryngotracheobronchitis. Am J Dis Child 133:1140, 1979.
6. Diaz, J. R.: Croup and epiglottitis in children: the anesthesiologist as a diagnostician. Anesth Analg 64:621, 1985.
7. Klassen, T. P., et al.: Nebulized budesonide for children with mild-to-moderate croup. N Engl J Med 331:285, 1994.
8. Johansson, S. A., et al.: Topical and systemic glucocorticoid potencies of budesonide and beclomethasone in man. Eur J Clin Pharmacol 22:523, 1982.
9. Singer O. P., Wilson, W. J.: Laryngotracheobronchitis: two years' experience with racemic epinephrine. Can Med Assoc J 115:132, 1976.
10. Skolnik, N. S.: Treatment of croup: a critical review. Am J Dis Child 143:1045, 1989.
11. Fogel, J. M., Berg, U., Gerber, M. A., Sherter, C. B.: Racemic epinephrine in the treatment of croup: nebulization alone versus nebulization with intermittent positive pressure breathing. J Pediatr 101:1028, 1982.
12. Ellis, E. F., Taylor, J. C., Jr., Lefkowitz, A.: Use of levo-rotary epinephrine (letter). Pediatrics 53:291, 1971.
13. Super, D. M., et al.: A prospective randomized double-blind study to evaluate the effect of dexamethasone in acute laryngotracheitis. J Pediatr 115:323, 1989.
14. Kuusela, A. L., Vesikari, T.: A randomized double-blind, placebo-controlled trial of dexamethasone and racemic epinephrine in the treatment of croup. Acta Paediatr Scand 77:99, 1988.
15. Super, D. M., et al.: A prospective randomized double-blind study to evaluate the effect of dexamethasone in acute laryngotracheitis. J Pediatr 115:323, 1989.
16. Landau, L. I., Geelhoed, G.C.: Aerosolized steroids for croup (editorial). N Engl J Med 331:322, 1994.
17. Bourchier, D., Dawson, K. P., Fergusson, D. M.: Humidification in vital croup: a controlled trial. Aust Paediatr J 20:289, 1984.
18. Diaz, J. H.: Further modifications of the Miller blade for difficult pediatric laryngoscopy. Anesthesiology 60:612, 1984.
19. Schuller, D. E., Birck, H. G.: The safety of intubation in croup and epiglottitis: an eight-year follow-up. Laryngoscope 85:33, 1975.
20. Tos, M.: Nasotracheal intubation instead of tracheotomy in acute epiglottitis in children. Acta Otolaryngol 75:382, 1973.

SUPRAGLOTTITIS (EPIGLOTTITIS)

Epiglottitis is an acute fulminant inflammatory disease of supraglottic structures and is more appropriately designated a supraglottitis.

PATHOLOGY

The inflammation is of the *supraglottic structures.*[1] including the epiglottis, arytenoids, supraglottic folds, and the uvula[2] and the posterior tongue. It occurs as a life-threatening disease in children and must be differentiated from croup.[1] Acute supraglottitis (epiglottitis) also occurs in adults and is a serious disease producing fatal airway obstruction in healthy persons.[3]

Sporadic descriptions of the disease first appeared in the latter part of the eigtheenth century. A classic patient was George Washington.[4] During the early part of the twentieth century, this condition was recognized as a distinct disease entity,[5] resulting from an acute infection localized to the epiglottis.[6]

ETIOLOGY

The usual cause of this disorder in children is *Haemophilus influenzae* type B.[7-9] Blood cultures have revealed bacteremia in 96%. Rarely, other bacterial agents have been reported to cause the disease, namely, *Staphylococcus aureus* and phenolytic streptococcus.

Other viruses have been demonstrated to cause the disease, namely, parainfluenzae myxoviruses (30%), respiratory synctial virus 6%, and adenovirus type 5 (4%).[10]

Blood cultures have been positive for *Haemophilus influenzae* type b in a high percentage of children (more than 90%) with epiglottitis.[11] This is more reliable than pharyngeal-epiglottitic cultures for diagnosis.[12]

Transmission of the virus in supraglottitis has been well documented as a person-to-person contact spread. This is in contrast to transmission in croup, which is by inhalation of the airborne virus.[13]

In adult patients hospitalized with the diagnosis of epiglottitis, however, a careful study of the multiple sites of the supraglottic inflamed tissues revealed that the epiglottis was often not the most involved area of the inflammatory process.[14,15]

Second, *Haemophilus influenzae* could not be demonstrated in any of the tissues or in blood, and few patients developed respiratory complications. This non-*Haemophilus influenzae* adult type of supraglottitis (usually described as epiglottitis) usually follows a less pernicious course.[15] In another clinical study of patients with supraglottitis, pharyngeal and blood cultures revealed *Haemophilus influenzae* in 32%, and bacteremia was demonstrated in 23% of the blood cultures.[3]

INCIDENCE

In children, supraglottitis is an uncommon bacterial infection that usually occurs in the 2- to 7-year age group. Males are at a slightly greater risk than females.[16] This disorder is less common in those under 2 years of age. The incidence is estimated at 10 cases per 100,000 children.

The incidence is greater than in adults, however, in whom this infection is rare; it occurs overall in about 1 in 100,000 population, with lower rates in those between 15 and 30 years and over the age of 70 years. The rate is about equal in men and women.[3]

SIGNS AND SYMPTOMS[17,18]

This airway disease develops rapidly in older preadolescent children (2 to 7 years of age) and more rarely in adults (age 20 to 50 years) without preceding coryza. The patient has an abrupt onset of fever, severe sore throat, and marked irritability with intermittent lethargy. Pathognomonic signs are the "four Ds": dysphagia (painful swallowing), dysphonia, drooling and marked respiratory distress with delayed expiration, and diminished breath sounds.[14] Coughing is weak.

The tripod posture is characteristic and unique. This posture is an attempt at airway protection, by sitting with chin thrust forward, slight cervical flexion, and slight forward flexion at the waist. Retractions of the chest at the suprasternal and supraclavicular sights are noted. This posture should be maintained when an enriched oxygen atmosphere of 40% or more is provided. Nevertheless, cyanosis is common.

LABORATORY

Marked leukocytosis is usual, with WBC counts between 15,000 and 25,000, with a relative lymphocytosis usually greater than 30% characteristic of viral disease.[14]

RADIOLOGIC EXAMINATION

Soft tissue radiographs may be useful if they can be expeditiously obtained without interfering with the physical examination or care of the patient and without interfering with the natural protective sitting posture of the patient. Characteristic of lateral neck films is the thickening of supraglottic tissues. A rounded thickening of the epiglottic shadow gives a configuration of a rounded "thumb."[19] The radiograph shows obliteration of the valleculae and pyriform sinuses.

DIAGNOSIS

The "historical findings" and the postural tripod sign are usually sufficient to make a diagnosis, but lateral neck radiographs are an excellent diagnostic tool and have confirmatory value.[11] One may also confirm the diagnosis by early indirect pharyngoscopy, followed by indirect laryngoscopy for epiglottic visualization. If both these procedures are easily accomplished, direct laryngoscopy in the operating room can be done. This examination is quick and more reliable than neck radiography.[20]

TREATMENT

The immediate objective is to provide an airway and to supply an oxygen-enriched breathing mixture into the lungs. Nasotracheal or orotracheal intubation of conscious or anesthetized patients can be accomplished under careful direct laryngoscopy.[21]

For awake intubation, topical anesthetization of the nasal or oropharyngeal structures can be accomplished with 4% cocaine, preceded by mask preoxygenation for 5 minutes with 100% oxygen. The child should be kept in the seated posture. Direct laryngoscopy is recommended. Diaz[22] recommends the use of the Miller blade, modified with an open C-flange and a side-arm insufflation port attached.

In adults, tracheostomy is often performed, but oral nasotracheal intubation is equally effective and is a short-term treatment, whereas a tracheostomy requires more care and postoperative management.[3] Nasotracheal intubation in the operating room is as effective as tracheostomy and has a lower rate of complications.[23-25]

MORBIDITY AND MORTALITY

In children, the mortality, when management consists of observation and medical treatment alone without early airway intervention, is about 6%. The use of early airway intervention by prophylactic short-term nasotracheal intubation has dropped the mortality to 0.9%.[26]

Adults have a significantly higher mortality of over 8% related to management by observation and medical therapy followed by tracheostomy, usually under emergency circumstances. Since 1975, emphasis has been placed on early airway prophylactic intervention by the use of orotracheal or nasotracheal intubation.[23-26] By 1980, the feasibility and success of endotracheal management instead of tracheostomy in adults had demonstrated that this was the method of choice. Mortality in adults has dropped to about 1%, similar to that seen in children.[3]

REFERENCES

1. Benjamin, B., O'Reilly, B.: Acute epiglottitis in infants and children. Ann Otol Rhinol Laryngol 85:565, 1976.
2. Rapkin, R. H.: Simultaneous uvulitis and epiglottitis. JAMA 243:1848, 1980.
3. MayoSmith, M. F., Hirsch, P. J., Wodzinski, S. F., Schiffman, F. J.: Acute epiglottitis in adults: an eight-year experience in the state of Rhode Island. N Engl J Med 314:1133, 1986.
4. Lewis, F. O.: Washington's last illness (quinsy). Ann Med Hist 4:245, 1932.
5. Theisen, C. F.: Angina epiglottidea anterior: report of three cases. Albany Med Annu 21:395, 1900.
6. Key, S. N.: Angina epiglottidea anterior: report of a case caused by the bacillus influenzae. JAMA 67:116, 1916.
7. Sinclair, S. E.: H. influenzae type b, in acute laryngitis with bacteremia. JAMA 117:170, 1941.
8. Jones, H., Camps, F.: Acute epiglottitis: supraglottitis. Practitioner 178:223, 1957.
9. Lewis, J. K., Galvis, A. G., Michaels, R. H.: Occurrence of haemophilus epiglottitis. Am J Dis Child 132:424, 1978.
10. Chanock, R. M.: In Debre, R., Celers, J. (eds.). Clinical Virology. Philadelphia, W. B. Saunders, 1979, p. 551.
11. Vernon, D.D., Sarnaik, A. P.: Acute epiglottitis in children: a conservative approach to diagnosis and management. Crit Care Med 14:23, 1986.
12. Hansman, D.: Ampicillin-insensitive Haemophilus influenzae type b causing acute epiglottitis. Lancet 1:1354, 1979.
13. Ginsburg, C.: Epiglottitis, meningitis, and arthritis due to Haemophilus influenzae type b presenting almost simultaneously in sibling. J Pediatr 87:492, 1975.

14. Diaz, J. H.: Group and epiglottitis in children: the anesthesiologist as a diagnostician. Anaesth Analg 64:621, 1985.
15. Shapiro, J. O., Eavey, R. D., Baker, A. S.: Adult supraglottitis: a prospective analysis. JAMA 259:563, 1988.
16. Molteni, R. A.: Epiglottitis. Incidence of extraepiglottic infection: report of 72 cases and review of the literature. Pediatrics 58:526, 1976.
17. Jones, H. M. Acute epiglottitis: a personal study over 20 years. Proc R Soc Med 63:706, 1970.
18. Jones, H. M.: Acute epiglottitis. Practitioner 215:732, 1975.
19. Podgore, J. K., Bass, J. W.: The "thumb sign" and "little finger" sign in acute epiglottitis. J Pediatr 88:154, 1976.
20. Edelson, P. J.: Radiographic examination in epiglottitis. J Pediatr 81:1036, 1972.
21. Diaz, J. H., Lockhart, C. H.: Early diagnosis and airway management of acute epiglottitis in children. South Med J 75:399, 1982.
22. Diaz, J. H.: Further modifications of the Miller blade for difficult pediatric laryngoscopy. Anesthesiology 60:612, 1984.
23. Schuller, D. E., Birck, H. G.: The safety of intubation in croup and epiglottitis: an eight-year follow-up. Laryngoscope 85:33, 1975.
24. Tos, M.: Nasotracheal intubation instead of tracheotomy in acute epiglottitis in children. Acta Otolaryngol 75:382, 1973.
25. Oh, T. H., Motoyama, E. K.: Comparison of nasotracheal intubation and tracheostomy in management of acute epiglottitis. Anesthesiology 46:214, 1977.
26. Cantrell, R. W., Bell, R. A., Morioka, W. T.: Acute epiglottitis: intubation versus tracheostomy. Laryngoscope 88:994, 1978.
27. Bishop, M. J.: Epiglottitis in the adult. Anesthesiology 55:701, 1981.
28. Ward, C. F., Benumof, J. L., Shapiro, H. M.: Management of adult acute epiglottitis by tracheal intubation. Chest 71:93, 1977.
29. From, L. J., Manlee, J.: Adult epiglottitis in a community hospital. Wis Med J 82:21, 1983.

CYSTIC FIBROSIS (MUCOVISCIDOSIS)

Cystic fibrosis (CF) is the most common serious genetic disorder of the white population. The disease is defined as a dysfunction of all exocrine glands, including mucous glands and is *inherited* as an autosomal recessive disorder.[1,2]

INCIDENCE[3]

The disease occurs in approximately 1 per 2000 live births (1 per 1600 to 1 per 2500 live births). This represents the homozygous form and requires that both parents contain the genetic defect.[4] The prognosis has been poor until recently and, at the present time, about one third of these patients reach adulthood. With antibiotic therapy and tracheobronchial clearing techniques, the survival averages approximately 25 years in females and 30 years in males.[5] Hence, the disease is not exclusive to a pediatric population. The mean age at death is approximately 19 years. The heterozygous form, that is, the carrier state, is asymptomatic and occurs in approximately 4% of the population.

MECHANISM[2]

A generalized dysfunction of the exocrine glands, including the mucous glands, is accompanied by an increased protein and mucopolysaccharide synthesis. The biochemical basis of these abnormal physiochemical processes is incompletely known.

Traditionally a disease of exocrine glands proper, especially of the submucosal glands bordering the airways, of sweat glands, and of the pancreas, the disorder may not be of the exocrine gland cells themselves but of specialized epithelial cells that comprise, in part, the exocrine glands. Inability of chloride to cross into or out of these cells appears to be the defect in airway glands[6] and sweat glands.[7] Ordinarily, during sweating, sodium is reabsorbed, accompanied by chloride from the sweat, and water is largely excreted. When chloride ion is not reabsorbed, the sodium is retained in the secretions. This accounts for the high sodium content in the secretion of the dysfunctioning glands—the hallmark of the disorder. The defect is in the chloride ion transfer.[7]

Prenatal diagnosis of CF may develop with the measurement of an enzyme, α-phosphatase, in amniotic fluid. A deficiency of this enzyme predicts the development of CF in infants.[6]

Associated with the glandular dysfunction is a significant autonomic dysfunction with abnormally increased adrenergic and cholinergic sensitivity.[8]

PATHOPHYSIOLOGY

CF is a multisystem disease, whose hallmark is abnormal secretion of all exocrine and mucous glands,[9] particularly excessive tracheobronchial secretions and a deficiency of pancreatic enzymes. Patients have poor fat utilization, and the pancreas may develop obstruction of its ducts. Carbohydrates are easily used, and protein is well tolerated. Persistent bronchial infection leads to irreversible changes in airways.

CLINICAL SIGNS

The secretions of all glands are thick and viscid because of a complex of glycoprotein and calcium. An accumulation of mucopolysaccharides in cytoplasm of glands is noted.[9]

These patients are prone to superimposed pulmonary and upper respiratory infection.[10] Sinusitis is usual, with excessive secretion and pneumatization. Nasal polyps are frequently found, leading to nasal obstruction and wide-mouth breathing. Pulmonary problems dominate the clinical picture. The patient is subject to various chronic diseases, and cough is a dominant presenting symptom. Bronchopneumonia is frequent and obstructive emphysema, as well as an acute adult respiratory distress syndrome, may occur. Hemoptysis is common.

Gastrointestinal symptoms are also frequent.[11] A meconium ileus is often present soon after birth, followed by a malabsorption syndrome and pancreatic insufficiency. The pancreatic insufficiency is often manifested by abdominal distention, foul-smelling stools, and steatorrhea.

Biliary disease is present in about one third of the patients. Portal hypertension and gastrointestinal bleeding are frequent complications.

Of diagnostic interest is the occurrence of abnormally composed sweat. One notes increased electrolytes in the sweat, and usually the sodium level exceeds 60 mEq/L.[12]

When the malabsorption syndrome dominates the picture, one must differentiate CF from celiac disease.[11]

DIAGNOSIS[2]

Four criteria (the tetrad) establish a correct diagnosis: (1) the presence of chronic lung disease and acute pulmonary dysfunction; (2) the absence of pancreatic enzymes in duodenal drainage; (3) increased electrolytes in sweat; and (4) a family history of this disorder.

ABNORMAL AUTONOMIC NERVOUS SYSTEM RESPONSES[8] (Table 45–1)

Autonomic dysfunction is denoted by increased adrenergic and cholinergic activity. Simultaneously, one notes diminished sensitivity of the β-adrenergic autonomic mechanisms. These abnormalities of function are outlined as follows: (1) diminished sensitivity of β-adrenergic mechanisms; (2) enhanced α-adrenergic response; and (3) enhanced cholinergic responsiveness. Although the parents of a child with CF may be asymptomatic, nevertheless, these heterozygotes also have altered sensitivity of the autonomic nervous system. In both the homozygous and heterozygous conditions, a defect apparently exists at the receptor levels of the autonomic nervous system.

THERAPY

The most important aspect of therapy is pulmonary physiotherapy to minimize the obstructive and hypoxic component due to the thick viscid tracheobronchial secretions: postural drainage, liquefaction of secretion by

Table 45–1. Abnormal Autonomic Nervous System Response

Diminished sensitivity of β-adrenergic mechanisms
    More isoproterenal needed for response
    Similar in mild allergic asthma
Enhanced α-adrenergic response
    Phenylephrine response greater than usual; small doses dilate pupil readily
    Response to darkness (mydriasis) less than usual; diminished α-mediator release
Enhanced cholinergic responsiveness
    Increased sensitivity to carbachol; pupils constrict readily
    Increased response to inhalants; a form of atopy (asthmalike) present
    Hypertrophy, hyperplasia, and hypersecretion of mucus glands
    Production of abnormal secretions by the parotid gland
    Parents' (heterozygotes) altered sensitivity of the autonomic nervous system

---

means of mist nebulizers,[13] deep breathing exercises, and chest percussion. Prophylactic antimicrobial drugs are indicated to minimize a superimposed bacterial infection. An ampicillin dose schedule of 4 days each week is usual.

Diet restriction is important. Medium-chain triglycerides are advised. The administration of pancreatic extracts is also effective in the management of the gastrointestinal signs.

ANESTHETIC CONSIDERATIONS[10,14–16]

1. Response to β-acting drugs:
   Agonist action is diminished.
   Diminished cardiac response to isoproterenol is seen.
   Diminished bronchodilator effect is noted.
   Increased dose is needed for chronotropic effect.
   β-blockers, both selective and nonselective, show an enhanced effect.
2. Response to α-acting agents:
   Exaggerated response to agonists is seen.
   Vasopressors should be diminished.
   Enflurane is recommended because of its effect in blocking chromaffin cells and norepinephrine release.
3. Increased response to cholinergic drugs[8]:
   Thiopental is prone to produce laryngospasm.
   Increased secretions are seen.
   Anticholinergic drugs are needed in larger doses— 60 to 80 μg/kg atropine; glycopyrrolate 30 to 40 μg/kg.
4. Relaxants:
   Because of the increased cholinergic response,[8] succinylcholine's effect is enhanced, and lower doses should be employed. Bradycardia and arrhythmias are frequent. Indeed, this drug should be avoided.[15] Pancuronium is without undesirable cholinomimetic effects, but it should be given in lower doses of 25 to 50 μg/kg. Vecuronium for short surgical procedures is the coice. Atracurium is an alternative relaxant. D-tubocurarine is required in larger doses for neuromuscular block, but its cholinomimetic and histamine releasing effects militate against its use.
5. Choice of anesthesia:
   Regional anesthesia is desirable whenever feasible. Inhalation general anesthesia with the volatile ethers enflurane and isoflurane is recommended. Halothane is tolerated in young children under 5 years of age, but it should be avoided in older children or when chronic hypoxemia is present.
   The breathing mixture should be humidified and warmed.
6. Effect of general anesthesia[16]:
   Regardless of the anesthetic agent used to produce general anesthesia, one sees significant deterioration of the principal parameters of lung function: forced vital capacity; forced expiratory volume at 1.0 second; peak expiratory flow rate; and forced expiratory flow between 25 and 75% of vital capacity.[10]

Evidence indicates increased airway resistance not related to bronchospasm. Such changes have been reported after brief minor surgical procedures performed in these patients. Nasal polypectomy for example, is one of the common procedures performed in these patients. One must be extremely vigilant in managing the most minor procedures.[16]

MORBIDITY AND MORTALITY FROM ANESTHESIA[10]

In 1964, Salanitre reported the perioperative morbidity as being approximately 27%.[15] Doershuk reported a 4% mortality from anesthesia.[17] In 1985, Lamberty and Rubin reported a complication rate of approximately 9% without any anesthetic deaths.[14] These low morbidity and mortality rates are consonant with the present aggressive therapeutic regimens and the longer lifespans of these patients.

REFERENCES

1. Nelson, W. E.: Textbook of Pediatrics, 11th Ed. Philadelphia, W. B. Saunders, 1979, p. 1988.
2. Nussbaum, E.: Pediatric Respiratory Disorders: Clinical Approaches. Orlando, FL, Grune and Stratton, 1984.
3. National Cystic Fibrosis Research Foundation: Cystic Fibrosis: Most Serious Lung Problem in Children. New York, 1979, p. 1.
4. Sing, C. F., Risser, D. R., Horvatt, W. F., Erickson, R. P.: Phenotypic heterogeneity in cystic fibrosis. Am J Med Genet 13:179, 1982.
5. Wilmott, R. W., Tyson, S. L., Dinwiddie, R., Matthew, D. J.: Survival rates in cystic fibrosis. Arch Dis Child 58:835, 1983.
6. Arehart-Treichal, J.: Ninth International Cystic Fibrosis Congress, Brighton, England: reports summarized. JAMA 252:2519, 1984.
7. Quinton, P. M., Bijman, J.: Higher bioelectric potentials due to decreased chloride absorption in the sweat glands of patients with cystic fibrosis. N Engl J Med 308:1185, 1983.
8. Davis, P. B., Shelhamer, J. R., Kaliner, M.: Abnormal adrenergic and cholinergic sensitivity in cystic fibrosis. N Engl J Med 302:1453, 1980.
9. Boat, T. F., Dearborn, D. G.: Etiology and pathogenesis. In Taussig, L. M. (ed.). Cystic Fibrosis. New York, Thieme-Stratton, 1984, p. 25.
10. Robinson, D. A., Branthwaite, M. A.: Pleural surgery in patients with cystic fibrosis. Anaesthesia 39:655, 1984.
11. Park, R. W., Grand, R. J.: Gastrointestinal manifestations of cystic fibrosis: a review. Gastroenterology 81:1143, 1981.
12. Davis P. B., Del Rio, S., Muntz, J. A., Dieckman, L.: Sweat chloride concentration in adults with pulmonary disease. Am Rev Respir Dis 138:34, 1983.
13. Boucher, R. C., et al.: Acute toxicity of intravenous and aerosolized amiloride in the dog cystic fibrosis. Cystic Fibrosis Soc Abstract 23:83, 1992.
14. Lamberty, J. M., Rubin, B. K.: The management of anaesthesia for patients with cystic fibrosis. Anaesthesia 40:448, 1985.
15. Salanitre, E., Klonymus, D., Rackow, H.: Anesthetic experience in children with cystic fibrosis of the pancreas. Anesthesiology 25:801, 1964.
16. Price, J. F.: The need to avoid general anesthesia in cystic fibrosis. J R Soc Med 79(Suppl 12):10, 1986.
17. Doershuk, C. F., Reyes, A. L., Regan, A. G., Matthews, L. W.: Anesthesia and surgery on cystic fibrosis. Anesth Analg 51:413, 1972.

CARCINOID TUMORS AND CARCINOID SYNDROME

CARCINOID TUMORS

Carcinoid tumors were first observed in 1888, by Lubarsch,[1] who referred to them as "little carcinomas." Oberndorfer named them carcinoid (Karzinoide—resembling carcinoma).[2] The slow growth and homogeneous appearance of the tumor cells led early investigators to underestimate the malignant potential of these lesions. Although these tumors are rare, with an incidence of 1.3 cases per 100,000 of the general population,[3] they are of particular significance in the gastrointestinal tract because they are the most common tumors of the appendix and small intestine.

Pathophysiology

Carcinoid tumor is a neoplasm of the neuroendocrine cells. Kultschitsky, in 1897, recognized the neuroendocrine cells as a population of cells with dense neurosecretory granules in the cytoplasm distinct from other mucosal epithelium in the gastrointestinal tract; these cells have since been named Kultschitsky cells,[4] although they were first described by Heidenhain in 1870.[5] In 1906, Ciaccio proposed their endocrine nature, and because they closely resembled chromaffin cells in the adrenal medulla, they were called enterochromaffin cells.[6] In 1910, researchers suggested that carcinoid tumors originated from these chromaffin cells.[7]

Masson, in 1930, demonstrated that carcinoid tumor cells had an affinity for silver salt similar to the Kultschitsky cells and proposed that carcinoid tumors originated from these neuroendocrine cells and called them argentaffinomas.[8]

Biochemistry and Origin of Tumor Cells

Pearse, in 1968, recognized that these neuroendocrine cells have similar ultrastructure and cytochemical characteristics and have the ability to synthesize amines and polypeptides by the process of amine precursor uptake and decarboxylation (APUD), a process essential for the production of monoamine neurotransmitters such as serotonin, dopamine, and histamine. The amines or peptides thus synthesized are stored in secretory granules in the cytoplasm[9] and are liberated by exocytosis. Pearse also postulated that all the APUD cells were of a common neuroectodermal origin derived from the embryonic neural crest.[10]

Newer evidence indicates that some APUD cell types, particularly the gastropancreatic neuroendocrine cells, are not of neural crest origin but are derived from endoderm.[11,12] Therefore, two related systems exist, one derived from the primitive endoderm, the diffuse endodermal endocrine system, and the other derived from the neural crest, the diffuse neuroendocrine system.[13] The possibility, however, remains of a common ectoblastic neuronal precursor cell.[14]

These neuroendocrine cells of the gastrointestinal tract secrete peptides and amines and have a physiologic function in regulating and modulating normal control of carbohydrate metabolism digestion of proteins and fats and in adjusting pH appropriate for assimilation of nutrients. This physiologic control is achieved on the neighboring cells by means of paracrine activity through aminergic and peptidergic neurotransmitters and by humoral endocrine function.[15]

Tumors arising from the APUD cells are labeled apudomas. The APUD cells, although closely related in terms of their biosynthetic mechanisms, histochemical, and ultrastructural features, demonstrate clear-cut differences in morphologic factors and endocrine activity. As many as 19 gastroenteropancreatic neuroendocrine cells have been identified, and as many as 40 of their humoral products have been discovered[16] (Table 45–2). Tumors arising from these cells may produce the expected hormone (entopic) in large quantities, or (ectopic) substances not expected from those tissues, or the tumor may be nonfunctioning despite the histologic appearance of endocrine cells.[15] Tumors that produce ectopic hormones tend to be more malignant.

Immunocytochemical methods have demonstrated many more enteroendocrine cells than are visible by current silver methods, and these methods also indicate their main secretion of these cells. Cells are customarily classified now according to their hormone content, which is demonstrated by immunohistochemical staining using antibody to each hormone type, and such classification techniques have effectively replaced empiric silver methods for demonstrating such cells.[17]

Diagnosis

Diagnostic tests that demonstrate excess serotonin production are as follows: (1) urinary 5-hydroxyindoleacetic acid (5-HIAA) levels higher than 50 mg per 24 hours (normal range less than 10 mg per 24 hours); (2) elevated plasma 5-hydroxytryptamine (5-HT) levels; (3) elevated platelet 5-HT levels;[18] (4) elevated liver functions values cases of liver metastasis.

Table 45–2. Some Amines and Peptides that May Be Produced by Carcinoid Tumors

Kinin peptides	Prostaglandins
Histamine	Neuropeptide K
Catecholamines	Somatostatin
Insulin	Substance P
Glucagon	Kallikrein
Calcitonin	5-Hydroxytryptophan
Bombesin	Endorphins
5-Hydroxytryptamine	Adrenocorticotrophin
Enkephalins	Bradykinins
Vasopressin	Tachykinins
Gastrin	

Provocation Tests

Provocation tests to liberate 5-HT and other tumor products can be dangerous. Microgram doses of epinephrine, small doses of pentagastrin, and alcohol have been used.

Localization Studies

In addition to the use of conventional methods to locate the primary and metastatic sites (computed tomographic [CT] scan, upper gastrointestinal tract study, barium enema, endoscopy, ultrasonography, chest radiograph, bronchoscopy, liver scan, and echocardiography), the use of somatostatin analogue scintigraphy with indium-111-labeled octreotide allowed the localization of more tumor sites than with other imaging techniques. Apart from its use for tumor localization, octreotide scintigraphy, in consequence of its ability to demonstrate receptor positive tumors, can be used to select those patients with carcinoid syndrome who are likely to respond favorably to octreotide therapy.[19]

Distribution[15]

About 85% of carcinoid tumors occur in the gastrointestinal tract, 10% in the lungs as bronchial carcinoid, and the remaining 5% in other organs such as the larynx, thymus, thyroid (c cells), kidney, ovary, prostate, and skin (melanocytes). Three fourths of abdominal carcinoid are from the midgut. The most frequent locations are: appendix, 46%; small intestine, 28%; rectum, 16%. These tumors appear as firm submucous nodules with a characteristic bright yellow color. The incidence of gastric carcinoid may increase in patients with pernicious anemia, achlorhydria, and Hashimoto's thyroiditis.[15] Gastrointestinal carcinoids frequently cause abdominal pain, gastrointestinal bleeding, and intussusception causing intestinal obstruction. The tumor may spread to the mesentery causing mesenteric fibrosis, intestinal kinking, intestinal obstruction, and vascular compromise to the bowels, or symptoms may be from tumor-secreted hormones.

Histology and Metastatic Potential

By histologic appearance, one cannot determine whether the carcinoid tumor is benign or malignant. The presence of metastasis or spread to adjacent tissues is the true indicator of malignancy. If the tumor is confined to the submucosa, then no metastasis is present. If the muscularis propria is invaded, then metastasis is about 8%. If the spread is beyond the serosa, then metastasis is 70%.[20]

The risk of metastasis seems to be related to the size of the primary tumor. If the tumor is less than 1 cm in diameter, the chances of metastasis are less than 2%. Between 1 and 2 cm, the risk is 50%, and above 2 cm, the incidence of metastasis rises to 80 to 90%.[21]

The site of origin is closely related to the malignant potential of the tumor. Only 2% of appendicular carcinoids metastasize; the incidence of metastasis for ilial carcinoids is 35%, and it is 60% for colonic carcinoids. The malignant potential of carcinoid tumors is also related to the nuclear DNA content.[22] The tumor's ability to arise in several sites (multicentricity) is found in 30% of patients with ilial carcinoids.[15] Along with carcinoid tumor of the small intestines, a second tumor of different histologic character can be present in 30% of cases.[21]

Bronchial Carcinoid

Bronchial carcinoids represent 1.5% of all lung tumors. They are locally invasive and capable of metastasis. Most patients are younger than 40 years, and the incidence is equal in both sexes. No relationship with smoking exists.

Bronchial carcinoids are neoplasms of the neuroendocrine cells in the bronchial mucosa. The cells contain dense neurosecretory granules in their cytoplasm and secrete hormonally active amines and peptides. The neurosecretory granules, when analyzed by immunochemistry, are found to contain serotonin, nonspecific enolase, bombesin, calcitonin, or other peptides. Intraluminal growth can cause persistent cough, hemoptysis, secondary infection, atelectasis, and bronchiectasis.

CARCINOID SYNDROME

Etiology

Carcinoid syndrome is a collection of signs and symptoms that manifest when large amounts of biologic amines and or peptides liberated by the carcinoid tumor are released into the systemic circulation. Only 7% of patients with carcinoid tumors develop the syndrome.[28] The signs and symptoms of the carcinoid syndrome are related to two distinct major neurohormonal peptide systems, namely, the serotoninergic and the kininergic.

Serotonin Dysfunction: Clinical Features (Table 45–3)

Serotonin (5-HT) has been implicated in the pathophysiology of the carcinoid syndrome since 1952 when it was isolated from the enterochromaffin cells,[23] and later in 1953, it was the first biologic amine isolated in an autopsy specimen from a carcinoid tumor.[24] (The synthesis, metabolism, and excretion of 5-HT are explained in Figure 45–1).

Increased synthesis and metabolism of serotonin remains an important diagnostic feature of carcinoid syndrome, although immunohistochemical techniques have demonstrated the ability of carcinoid tumor to secrete a variety of hormonal mediators. Midget tumors show the larger plasma concentration of serotonin; foregut tumors show a moderate increase, whereas hindgut tumors rarely show any increase.[25]

Table 45–3. Clinical Features of Serotoninergic Dysfunctions

Somnolence: central serotonin mechanism (Jouvet)
Hyperkinetic: cardiovascular response
Hyperpnea: hyperactivity of carotid chemoreceptors
Hyperglycemia: increased glycogenolysis
Hypermetabolism: increased protein catabolism; hypoproteinemia

Serotonin is synthesized in the enterochromaffin cells of the gastrointestinal tract and the serotonergic neurons of the central nervous system (CNS). The substrate for serotonin is tryptophan and the uptake is about 10% of the dietary content. In the presence of carcinoid tumors, about 60% or more of the dietary content is taken up by the cellular granules. Normally, 10 to 25 mg of serotonin is formed each day and is released into the circulation. Ninety percent of serotonin is present in the enterochromaffin cells, whereas 10% is present in the serotoninergic neurons and platelets; the latter store serotonin but do not manufacture it. Human mast cells do not contain serotonin. Little 5-HT can cross the blood-brain barrier, and plasma levels of 5-HT may be attributed to release by enterochromaffin cells. Serotonin not taken up by platelets is subjected to enzymatic degradation in the liver, lung, and blood. The lung is an important degradation site for 5-HT, and 30 to 90% of an administered dose of 5-HT is taken up by the pulmonary epithelium. The final product excreted in the urine is 5-hydroxyindoleacetic acid (5-HIAA). In malignant carcinoid syndrome, large amounts of 5-HIAA are excreted, and its quantitative estimation is used as a diagnostic and prognostic test of the syndrome.[26] Reliability of this test increases if foods high in tryptophan are excluded from patients' diets before the test. These substances include bananas, plantain, pineapple, walnuts, plums, and pecans, as well as acetaminophen. Conversely, falsely low values may be obtained if aspirin or levodopa is ingested.[27] Normal values of 5-HIAA in urine range from 1.5 to 10 mg per 24 hours.

The presence of tumors of enterochromaffin cells should be suspected if excretion of 5-HIAA exceeds 15 mg in 24 hours. If the urinary 5-HIAA exceeds 150 mg in 24 hours, survival is less than 1 year.[28] Large amounts of 5-HT produced by carcinoid tumors may cause nutritional disorder. Dietary tryptophan, an essential amino acid and a precursor of 5-HT synthesis, is 99% converted to nicotinic acid and protein in healthy individuals; 1% is used for 5-HT production. In patients with carcinoid tumors, 60% of tryptophan may be consumed for 5-HT production.[29]

As a result, tryptophan available for the production of protein and nicotinic acid becomes limited, resulting in hypoproteinemia and pellagra.

Exceptional patients may present with full-blown carcinoid syndrome with generalized metastasis, even without increased urinary 5-HIAA excretion.[30]

Serotonin has positive myocardial chronotropic and inotropic effects mediated by 5-HT receptors, and coupled with vasoconstriction, these effects lead to hypertension. At higher concentrations, 5-HT releases norepinephrine from the nerve endings.[31] Serotonin also amplifies the activity of other vasocontrictors (angiotensin II, prostaglandin F_2 [PGF_2]).

Ketanserin, a 5-H_2 receptor antagonist, can block these vasoconstrictive actions. Diarrhea, abdominal cramps, nausea, and vomiting have been attributed to serotonin.

Slow awakening from anesthesia in patients with carcinoid syndrome has been noted, and although 5-HT crosses the blood-brain barrier poorly, 5-HT may be responsible, released during surgical manipulation of the

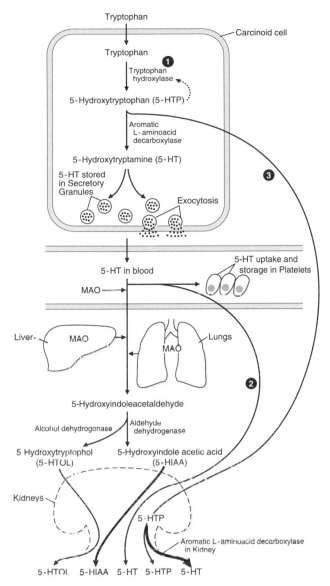

Fig. 45–1. Synthesis, secretion and metabolism of serotonin (5-HT). 1. The activity of tryptophan hydroxylase is rate limiting. 2. 5-Hydroxyindoleacetyldehyde is also reduced by alcohol dehydrogenase to 5-Hydroxytryptophol (5-H TOL); all three enzymes (i.e., monoamine oxidase, aldehydedehydrogenase, and alcohol dehydrogenase) are present in liver and in various tissues that contain 5-HT including the brain; 5-HIAA is the principal metabolite normally excreted, and 5-HTOL is excreted in much smaller amounts, but ingestion of ethyl alcohol greatly increases excretion of 5-HTOL (reduction pathway) and correspondingly reduces the 5-HIAA (oxidative pathway) excretion in urine. 3. Many gastric carcinoid tumors lack the enzyme aromatic L-amino acid decarboxylase, and conversion to 5-HT is impaired. Blood levels of 5-HTP rises. Renal cells contain aromatic L-amino acid decarboxylase and convert 5-HTP to 5-HT. Urine in these patients shows high levels of 5-HT.

tumor.[32] Serotoeninergic cells in the nuclei of raphe can induce sleep.[27]

Kinins and the Role of Lysosomes

Kinin levels may rise acutely in carcinoid patients. These substances may contribute to flushing, bronchospasm, and hypotension during a carcinoid crisis.[29]

Kinins are small polypeptides lysed by proteolytic enzymes from α_2 globulins in the plasma or tissue fluids. Kallikrein, an enzyme present in lysosomes of carcinoid cells, blood, and body tissue, is stored in inactive form. Kallikrein stored in the lysosomes may be liberated by anoxia, mechanical trauma, pH variation, alcohol intoxication, catecholamines, and tissue inflammation[33] (Fig. 45–2).

Bradykinin, kallidin (lysylbradykinin), and methionyl-lysyl-bradykinin are three kinins found in mammals, and each contains bradykinin in its structure. These kinins can be converted to bradykinin by various enzymes.

Kinins are 10 times more potent than histamine in producing vasodilation of the arterial bed. Kinins release endothelium-derived relaxing factors (EDRF, nitric oxide) or vasodilator prostaglandins (PGE_2 and PGI_2) to achieve arterial smooth muscle dilatation. Kinins cause venous contraction by direct stimulation of venous smooth muscle and by release of venoconstrictor prostaglandins (PGF_{2a}).

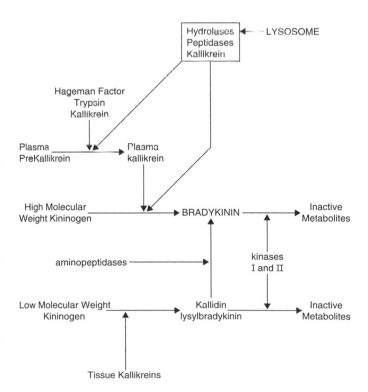

Fig. 45–2. Possible role of lysosome peptidases (kallikrein) in activating kinin cascade in carcinoid syndrome. Schema showing the storage of enzymes in the lysosome. These are in inactive form. When liberated, they act in a cascade manner on various precursors to form active kinins.

Table 45–4. Clinical Features of Bradykininergic Dysfunctions

Vasodilitation
  Cutaneous: flushing
  Peptide-induced
Vasoderpression
  Visceral
Shock
  Microcirculatory failure
  Changes in permeability
Bronchospastic
  Kallikrein: bradykinin
  No response to antihistamines or to antiserotonin

Kininergic Dysfunction: Clinical Features (Table 45–4)

When kinins are injected systemically, a rapid drop in blood pressure results from their arteriolar dilation. Simultaneously, venous constriction causes a rise in pressure and flow in the capillary bed. One also sees contraction of capillary endothelial cells with widening of intercellular junctions, and as a result, intravascular fluid escapes, causing edema. Kinins are potent pain-producing mediators. Two types of kinin receptors are known: B_1 and B_2. (B stands for bradykinin, not for β adrenoreceptors). Most actions of kinins are mediated by B_2 receptors.[34]

Inhibitors of Kallikreins and Kinins

Steroids stabilize lysosomal membrane and diminish the release of proteolytic and hydrolytic enzymes. The predominant mechanism of steroid action is believed to be the inhibition of kallikrein-induced proteolytic cascade. Steroids may inhibit kinin formation and may counteract bradykinin-induced capillary leak. Large doses are required if given prophylactically. Aprotinin (Trasylol), like steroids, inhibits the kallikrein cascade by blocking proteinase activity of kallikrein. Several kinin antagonists have been described.[34] The most selective and potent B_1 (bradykinin receptor) antagonists are des Arg^9 (Leu^8) bradykinin, and des Arg^{10} (Leu^9) kallidin. An example of a B_1 and B_2 (bradykinin receptor) blocker is a nonselective bradykinin antagonist D-Arg (4-hydroxy-Pro^3-D-Phe^7) bradykinin. Most of the biologic effects of bradykinin are blocked by this latter analogue, which has a short half-life. A therapeutic effect has been obtained in the suppression of pain from burns and in treatment of allergic asthma and cold symptoms of rhinovirus. Usefulness of the kinin antagonists in the management of carcinoid syndrome awaits evaluation.

Antagonists of histamine receptors H_1 and H_2 receptors have been used with some success in alleviating flushing associated with carcinoid syndrome. H_1 antagonists alone are ineffective.

Leukocyte interferon had some success in relieving symptoms of flushing, diarrhea, and asthma, and serum levels of polypeptides and of urinary 5-HIAA may decrease. Octreotide is probably the most promising addition to the list of kinin inhibitors.

Carcinoid Heart Disease

Etiology

5-HT was implicated in the origin of carcinoid heart disease in the past, but which of the bioactive products secreted by the carcinoid tumor induces the syndrome of cardiac disease is unclear. Although serotonin is accorded greatest importance, a rough correlation exists among the plasma levels of the tumor-derived tachykinins, neuropeptide K, and substance P, and urinary excretion of the serotonin metabolite 5-HIAA, and the severity of the heart disease.[33] Carcinoid heart disease occurs in more than one third of all patients with carcinoid syndrome. It is seen most frequently in patients with metastatic ileal carcinoid tumors and with tumors in various locations outside the gastrointestinal tract, including the lungs and ovary. Tumor products are released to the systemic circulation. As noted, long-term exposure of the endocardium to bioactive products in the right side of the heart leads to the development of heart lesions. Measurement of plasma atrial natriuretic peptide (ANP) concentration levels has been found useful as a guide in determining the severity of cardiac decompensation and clinical improvement in patients with carcinoid heart disease.[35]

Pathology

Carcinoid heart disease is usually confined to the right heart and consists of the development of plaques of fibrous tissue that are superficial and are separated from the endocardium by a membrane. The tricuspid valve is most commonly involved, with a deformity of the cusp resulting in tricuspid regurgitation. Plaques on the pulmonary valve cause stenosis.[29] Left-sided heart disease can occur in patients with carcinoid tumor of the lung or in patients with coexisting left-to-right shunt. Mitral and aortic valves are frequently involved.

Right-sided heart failure with peripheral edema, hepatomegaly or hepatosplenomegaly, and ascites are the predominant findings. Echocardiographic findings are most helpful in preoperative evaluation.

Pathogenesis

Fewer than 10% of patients with carcinoid tumor exhibit symptoms.[15] Only 4 to 5% of carcinoid tumors produce vasoactive substances in quantities large enough to produce the debilitating clinical syndrome.[36,37] The mediators released by the carcinoid of the gastrointestinal tract are carried to the liver by the portal venous system, where they are normally inactivated by the liver enzymes, and the patient remains symptom free for a long time because these tumors grow slowly. Carcinoid syndrome manifests when an excess amount of mediator is released by the tumor overwhelms the liver enzymes, resulting in an escape into the systemic circulation causing the carcinoid syndrome. It occurs mostly when in the presence of liver metastasis; the vasoactive peptides from the metastasis can enter the suprahepatic venous blood without having been exposed to the destructive action of the liver enzymes. It is also achieved when metastasis is to other sites draining directly into the systemic circulation such as a parietal peritoneal implant or retroperitoneal spread and tumors arising from ovaries, testes, and bronchi releasing their active hormones into the systemic circulation and producing clinical manifestations before metastatic disease occurs.

Two thirds of all carcinoid syndromes occur from tumors from the mid-gut, and 9% of all carcinoid from the ilium produce carcinoid syndrome.[15]

Symptoms and their Causes

Not all patients with carcinoid syndrome suffer from all its manifestations. Episodic or permanent cutaneous flushing of the head and torso is the most common feature (95% of patients), followed by abdominal pain and cramping (50% of patients), right-sided cardiac valvular lesions (50% of patients), and wheezing (6%).[28] Other changes include telangiectasis and pellagra dermatosis.[15]

Serotonin alone cannot account for all the symptoms of the syndrome. In fact, the mediator or mediators responsible for flushing is not known.[38,39]

Exogenous infusions of serotonin and substance P in combination failed to reproduce the symptoms.[40] Serotonin and bradykinin are thought responsible for the majority of features seen in the carcinoid syndrome, and the other peptides secreted modulate the effects of these major mediators and give rise to many of the symptoms seen in the syndrome.[41]

Carcinoid cells secrete many more amines and peptides in addition to serotonin and are capable of secreting more than one hormone simultaneously producing a particular clinical syndrome. They can change the hormone secreted at any time to produce a different picture. Metastasis may produce different hormones from that of the primary site, and different metastases can produce different hormones.[42] Whether these products are expressions of genetic programs into the endocrine cells or are "ectopic hormones" resulting from neoplastic alterations of genetic programs is not clear.

Anesthetic Implications of Carcinoid Tumors

Excision of the primary tumor is usually not curative in patients exhibiting carcinoid syndrome because fewer than 90% of patients have extensive metastases, but removal of the primary tumor may be required because of obstruction of bowels, bronchi, or blood vessels. Curative surgery is possible in rare cases of isolated ovarian tumor or tumors with resectable lymph nodes or single liver metastasis. More often, symptomatic relief is obtained by debulking surgery before hepatic arterial embolization. Such operative techniques include dissection of the central mesenteric lymph nodes, intestinal resection, cholecystectomy, and division of collateral vessels to the liver.

The rationale behind hepatic arterial embolization is that secondary hepatic tumors depend largely on hepatic arterial blood, whereas normal liver can survive purely on the portal venous blood supply. Therefore, one can selectively destroy the tumor within the liver by obliterating the hepatic arterial flow.[43] Open heart surgery may be required in patients with carcinoid heart disease for correction of incompetent tricuspid valves.

Anesthetic management has a potential for life-threatening complications by the release of tumor products into the general circulation. Every effort therefore is made to prevent the release of tumor hormones during anesthesia and surgery and to prepare to treat the consequences as they arise.

Factors Precipitating Symptoms

The provocation of carcinoid symptoms and crisis (i.e., flushing, tachycardia, hypo- or hypertension) has been associated with a variety of stimuli, as discussed in the following paragraphs.

Physiologic Factors

Eating (in patients with gastric carcinoids), defecating (in patients with rectal carcinoids), or excitement or exertion (mediated by the release of catecholamines) may induce a carcinoid crisis.

Chemical/Hormonal Factors

Catecholamines and sympathomimetic amines, especially β stimulants, release tumor products in carcinoid syndrome, and their use should be avoided in treating hypotension during carcinoid crisis (e.g., epinephrine, norepinephrine, dopamine). Other amines and chemicals capable of releasing tumor products include histamine, ethanol, and pentagastrin.

Medical Preparation and Treatment of Carcinoid Crisis

Asymptomatic patients (i.e., without carcinoid crisis) do not present problems in their management. Several drugs have been useful in the treatment of carcinoid crisis, as described in the following paragraphs.

Somatostatin

This agent named for its activity as a growth-hormone release-inhibiting hormone. It is a naturally produced hormone with a short half-life but may be given by a dilute intravenous infusion. It is a 14-amino acid peptide with cyclic configuration, isolated from sheep hypothalamus in 1973. Functions attributed to somatostatin include its effects as a neurohumoral regulator, neurotransmitter, and endocrine and paracrine hormone.[43] It is found throughout the CNS and also in the gastrointestinal tract and pancreas. In the human gut, the hormone is confined to the mucosal layer, where it is localized in endocrine cells termed D cells.

Somatostatin inhibits secretion in both endocrine and exocrine glands. In the pituitary, growth hormone and thyrotropic and lactotropic hormones are suppressed. In the pancreas, secretion of insulin and glucagon are inhibited. Gastrointestinal motility is reduced, and secretions are suppressed, including gastrin, gastric acid, secretin, cholecystokinin, digestive enzymes, and bicarbonates. Prolonged use of somatostatin can cause dyspepsia, hypochlorhydria, cholelithiasis, and watery diarrhea. In the kidneys, renal plasma flow is reduced, glomerular filtration is decreased, and urinary output is reduced. Blood flow to the liver, spleen, and gastric mucosa is reduced, as is saliva production.[44]

Somatostatin exerts these effects by binding to specific receptors on the surface of target cells. These ligand receptors interact with G proteins that mediate certain intracellular events, including inhibition of adenyl cyclase activity and suppression of the accumulation of cyclic adenosine monophosphate (AMP).[45] Intracellular calcium available to support secretion is decreased. The half-life of somatostatin is extremely short (T½ = 3 minutes)[46] and limits its clinical usefulness. Because somatostatin receptors in different tissues are pharmacologically heterogeneous, somatostatin agonists with greater selectivity are under investigation.

Octreotide Acetate (Sandostatin)

This is an octapeptide analogue of somatostatin and hence is a semisynthetic agent. It has a long duration of action with a mean plasma half-life of 100 minutes (100 μg subcutaneously). Octreotide has been described as "endocrine cyanide" because of its ability to prevent regulatory peptide release from the gastropancreatic system[47] and therefore is the basis of its use in the carcinoid syndrome.

Its use reduces both symptoms and biochemical indicators of tumor activity. It also reduces release of 5-HT from the carcinoid tumor and the excretion of 5-HIAA in urine.[48]

Pentagastrin-provoked release of 5-HT is markedly reduced, and the basal level of 5-HT is reduced in patients with initial high levels. Like somatostatin, somatostatin analogues may block an intracellular mechanism common for activation of monoamine and tachykinin receptors on both tumor cells and normal cells.

Somatostatin receptors have been identified in both in vivo and in vitro preparations of carcinoid tumors.[49] Octreotide bends to these receptors and has peripheral effects such as stabilizing arterial blood pressure despite high levels of circulating 5-HT and other peptides and amines. Octreotide also inhibits the release of tumor products. The severe hypotension encountered during a carcinoid crisis is best controlled by octreotide. Conventional vasopressors such as ephedrine, phenylephrine, and epinephrine are usually ineffective and may aggravate the crisis by causing further release of the biologic amines from carcinoid tumors. In a large series, diarrhea was abolished or significantly reduced in 83% of patients, and flushing improved in 100%. Bronchospasm improved in all patients, and airway resistance decreased. The blood 5-HT level was changed insignificantly, and urinary 5-HIAA was decreased marginally in 75% of cases.

Octreotide has been used successfully in the treatment of carcinoid crisis[50] and for the prevention and treatment of intractable hypotension during anesthesia in these cases.[41] In one case report, carcinoid-induced life-threatening bronchospasm was successfully treated with intravenous bolus administration of 200 μg octreotide. Within 15 seconds, bronchospasm had decreased and ventilation

was confirmed by chest motion. Hypoxia and cardiovascular symptoms were resolved within the next 3 minutes.[51]

Octreotide is effectively used in the long-term management of patients with carcinoid tumor with metastasis.[47] Octreotide is administered subcutaneously or intravenously. The subcutaneous dose is 50 to 500 μg every 8 hours.

Intravenously, octreotide can be administered 100 μg/ml in normal saline, and peak plasma concentration is achieved in 4 minutes, with a plasma half-life of 72 to 113 minutes.[52] Adverse side effects are uncommon. Complaints of pain on injection and gastrointestinal symptoms may be seen. Octreotide inhibits insulin secretion in response to hyperglycemia, which is mild because glucagon is also inhibited. Its use in obese patients or in noninsulin-dependent diabetics, in combination with high-dose corticosteroids, may complicate blood sugar management.

Ketanserin

This 5-HT$_2$ receptor antagonist blocks 5-HT-induced vasoconstriction, bronchoconstriction, platelet aggregation, and hypertension. Prophylactic use of kentanserin is a useful adjunct to octreotide in patients with carcinoid syndrome who are undergoing surgery for hepatic arterial embolization. Other 5-HT receptor-blocking agents include methysergide, cyproheptadine, methotrimeprazine, and droperidol.

Special Problems in Carcinoid Syndrome

Carcinoid syndrome can develop in the perioperative period with life-threatening complications, including hypotension, bronchospasm, and hypertension.

Hypotension may be caused by release of bradykinins, histamine, and tachykinins. It is aggravated by accompanying dehydration and hypovolemia secondary to 5-HT-induced diarrhea. A hypotensive episode may stimulate the release of tumor products by reflex adrenergic mechanism, worsening the crisis. Right-sided cardiac disease also may predispose to hypotension.

In the presence of carcinoid heart disease, cardiovascular variables are monitored by pulmonary arterial catheterization. Drugs used to treat hypotension include octreotide, methoxamine, and angiotensin II.

One case report emphasized the need for precautions in patients with carcinoid syndrome undergoing even minor procedures. Immediately following a fine-needle biopsy of a carcinoid liver metastasis, the patient developed severe flushing, nausea, and faintness, followed by seizure activity, profound hypotension, and cardiopulmonary arrest refractory to resuscitation. Massive release of vasoactive substances into the systemic circulation, caused by manipulation of the tumor at biopsy and aggravated by resuscitative efforts, was considered causative. Intravenous cannulae should be in place before any studies are done, and octreotide should be available. Catecholamine administration and compression of the tumor metastasis in the liver can only aggravate symptoms during resuscitation.

Bronchospasm can occur at any time with or without a prior history of pulmonary disease. It is often associated with hypotension and flushing. Adrenergic agonists (epinephrine or β_2 stimulants) and phosphodiesterase inhibitors such as aminophylline may aggravate the crisis by reflex release of catecholamines that liberate tumor products. Prophylactic use of steroids in large doses (30 mg/kg hydrocortisone hemisuccinate) has been found beneficial. Intraoperative bronchospasm treatment includes steroids, diphenhydramine, halothane, and ketamine, but none are as effective as octreotide.

Hypertension is attributed to 5-HT release, and the 5-HT_2 receptor antagonist ketanserin is effective in achieving hemodynamic stability even when the plasma serotonin level is elevated.

Preanesthetic management of patients with carcinoid heart disease includes the use of diuretics and digitalis. Valvular surgery may be required in patients who are unresponsive to medical therapy. These persons are managed like other patients with heart disease with an additional risk of perioperative carcinoid crisis.

ANESTHETIC MANAGEMENT

Preoperative Preparation

The goals of anesthetic management are to avoid the triggering stimuli that may precipitate carcinoid crisis.

Mechanical stimuli: (1) Mechanical palpation of the tumor through abdominal wall or inadvertent pressure on the tumor during surgical preparation; (2) surgical manipulation of the tumor intraoperatively

Physiologic states as triggers: Hypotension, hypercarbia, hypoxemia, and hypothermia all increase sympathetic activity and may precipitate crisis by releasing tumor products.

Pharmacologic triggering agents: These include agents that release histamine, such as morphine,

and curare. Sympathomimetic agents include β- and α-adrenergic stimulants, vasopressors, and bronchodilators in common use. Indirectly acting vasopressors such as ephedrine and phosphodiasterase inhibitors, the release catecholamines, are not indicated.

Alternate anesthetic methods and agents that do not trigger the release of tumor products should be used. Hypotension is best treated by adequate preoperative hydration with central venous pressure and urine output measurements. Severe hypotension during the crisis is best treated with intravenous boluses of octreotide, angiotensin II, and directly acting methoxamine. Hypertension is treated with octreotide to inhibit release of vasoactive tumor products and vasodilators.

Depending on the severity of the condition, the patient should be managed in an intensive care unit for 2 to 6 days before surgery. Tests should include blood analysis for electrolytes, renal and hepatic function tests, complete cell count, and assessment of gastrointestinal hormones. Arterial and central venous catheters are placed to measure central venous pressure to ensure adequate hydration and volume expansion and for monitoring and frequent sampling for measurement of 5 HT. Twenty-four hour urine is collected for 5-HIAA determination.

Good communication among anesthesiologist, surgeon, internist, and endocrinologist is important, to determine which mediators are responsible for the symptoms and the response of the patient to various therapies.

Medications are continued up to the day of surgery. Before the availability of octreotide in 1988, several agents were used in the preoperative period to prevent the effects of circulating peptides (Table 45–5). In a large series involving anesthetic management of all 21 patients with carcinoid syndrome,[41] octreotide seemed to replace most drugs used to control the untoward symptoms of carcinoid syndrome and prepare the patient for surgery. Treatment is commenced with octreotide at least 24 hours before

Table 45–5. Specific Agents Used in the Prevention of Endocrine Effects in Carcinoid Syndrome

Endocrine Mediator	Inhibitor of Synthesis	Preventor of Release	Receptor Antagonist
Serotonin	Parachlorophenylalanine α-Methyldopa	Phenoxybenzamine Octreotide Somatostatin*	Ketanserin Pizotifen Methysergide Octreotide Droperidol Cyproheptadine Methotrimeprazine
Bradykinin	Aprotinin ϵ-aminocaproic acid	Octreotide Steroids Somatostatin*	Octreotide Somatostatin*
Histamine	—	—	Cimetidine Ranitidine Cyproheptadine Chlorpheniramine

*Natural hormone

surgery and is continued as part of premedication. Patients should be asymptomatic after treatment with octreotide.

Octreotide treatment is started at 50 to 500 μg 8 hourly or at 50 to 500 μg subcutaneously 1 hour before operation in emergency. Further intravenous bolus doses of 10 to 20 μg are injected during surgery as needed.[40]

Anxiety may precipitate crisis,[1] and adequate sedation with an oral benzodiazapine is preferred. Narcotics may depress respiration, thereby causing hypoxemia. Morphine is avoided because it may release histamine. Patients should continue taking their medications up to the morning of operation. These medications include steroids, H_1 and H_2 receptor blockers, especially in histamine-releasing tumors, $5-HT_2$ receptor blockers ketanserin, droperidol and octreotide, and medications to treat cardiac and associated conditions.

Anesthetic Procedure

A smooth anesthetic technique is as important as the choice of agents used. During anesthesia, drugs that release histamine should be avoided. These include morphine, d-tubocurarine, thiopental,[53] and atracurium. Succinylcholine may increase intra-abdominal pressure during fasciculation and may release peptides from the liver.[54] It also has a potential for histamine release. Midazolam and etomidate are suitable agents for induction of anesthesia because of their cardiovascular stability and lack of histamine-releasing properties. Pressure responses to laryngoscopy and intubation can be avoided by preliminary orolaryngeal topical anesthesia with a potent agent such as 1½% tetracaine (no cocaine). Pressure response to intubation with etomidate can be effectively controlled by fentanyl. Vecuronium, a nondepolarizing muscle relaxant, is the drug of choice to provide surgical relaxation and to allow controlled ventilation. It does not liberate histamine while pulse rate and cardiovascular stability is maintained, and the drug's effects are easily reversed.

For maintenance of anesthesia, the inhalation agent isoflurane or enflurane (which blocks chromaffin cells) with supplements of boluses of fentanyl can meet the requirement of providing surgical anesthesia and an early postoperative recovery. This is important because high levels of 5-HT in blood have been associated with prolongation of sleep.[55]

Most patients with the carcinoid syndrome have metastases, and complete surgical cure is not possible. Octreotide treatment is therefore continued in the postoperative period and should be available by the patient's bedside for intravenous administration to treat episodes of sudden hypotension in this period. These episodes of hypotension have been reported within 1 hour postoperatively or even on the second or third postoperative day.

Pain relief can be obtained by patient-controlled analgesia (PCA) using fentanyl. Morphine is to be avoided because it releases histamine. Extradural analgesia has also been found to provide excellent pain relief. If liver disease is present, clotting studies should be done before an extradural catheter is inserted. A weak concentration of bupivacaine (0.1% or less) is used to avoid sympathetic blockade and to preserve motor activity. It is supplemented with fentanyl, 2 to 5 μg/ml, in the PCA solution.

REFERENCES

1. Lubarsch, O.: Uber den primaren Krebs des lieum nebst: Bemerkungen uberdas gleichzeitige Vorkommen Von Krebs und Tuberkulose. Virchows Arch A 3:280, 1888.
2. Oberndorfer, S.: Karzinoide Tumoren des Dunndarms. Frankf Z Pathol 1:426, 1907.
3. Watson, R. G. P., et al.: The frequency of gastrointestinal endocrine tumors in a well-defined population, Northern Ireland 1970–1985. Q J Med 267:647, 1989.
4. Kultschitsky, N.: Zinf frage uber den bau des Darmkanals. Arch Microsk Anat 49:7, 1897.
5. Heidenhain, R.: Untersuchungen Uber den bau der Labdrusen. Arch Mikrosk Anat 6:368, 1870.
6. Ciaccio, C.: Sur une nouvelle espèce cellulaire dans les glandes de Lieberkuhn. C R Seances Soc Biol 60:76, 1906.
7. Hebschmann, P.: Sur le carcinome primitif de l'appendice vermiculaire. Rev Med Suiss Romande 30:317, 1910.
8. Masson, P.: Significance of muscular "struma" of argentaffin tumors (carcinoids). Am J Pathol 6:499, 1930.
9. Pearse, A.: Common cytochemical and ultrastructure characteristics of cells producing polypeptide hormones (the APUD series), and their relevance to thyroid and ultimobrachial C cells and calcitonin. Proc R Soc Lond (Biol) 170:71, 1968.
10. Pearse, A. G. E.: The cytochemistry and ultrastructure of polypeptide hormone producing cells of the APUD series and the embryologic, physiologic and pathologic implications of the concept. J Histochem Cytochem 17:303, 1969.
11. Sidhu, G. S.: The endodermal origin of digestive and respiratory tract APUD cells. Am J Pathol 96:5, 1979.
12. Andrew, A., Kramer, B., Rawdon, B. B.: Gut and pancreatic amine precursor uptake and decarboxylation cells are not neural crest derivatives. Gastroenterology 84:429, 1983.
13. Dawson, I. M. P.: Diffuse endocrine and neuroendocrine cell tumors. In Anthony, P. P., MacSween, R. N. (eds.). Recent Advances in Histopathology. Vol. 12. Edinburgh, Churchill Livingstone, 1984.
14. Pearse, A. G. E.: Genesis of the neuroendocrine system. In Friesen, S. R., Thompson, N. W. (eds.). Surgical Endocrinology. Philadelphia, J.B. Lippincott, 1990, p. 15.
15. Delcore, R., Friesen, S.: Gastrointestinal neuroendocrine tumors (review). J Am Coll Surg 178:187, 1994.
16. Hrejs, A. J.: Gastrointestinal endocrine tumors. Am J Med 82:1, 1987.
17. Stevens, A., Lowe, J.: Histology. London, Gower Medical Publishing, 1992, p. 266.
18. Wall, R. T., III: Anesthetic management of pheochromocytoma, insulinoma and carcinoid syndrome. In Barash, P. G. (ed.). ASA Refresher Courses in Anesthesiology. Vol. 21. Philadelphia, J. B. Lippincott, 1993, p. 142.
19. Kwekkeboom, D. J., et al.: Somatostatin analog scintigraphy in carcinoid tumors. Eur J Nucl Med 20:283, 1993.
20. Zeitels, J., et al.: Carcinoid tumors: a 37 year experience. Arch Surg 117:732, 1982.
21. Moertel, C. G., et al.: Life history of carcinoid tumor of the small intestines. Cancer 14:901, 1961.
22. Falkner, S., et al.: Pattern of DNA distribution and neurohormone immunoreactivity in tumor cells: tools for the histopathological assessment of gastrointestinal carcinoids. Digestion 35:144, 1986.
23. Erspamer, V., Asero, B.: Identification of enteramine, the specific hormone of the enterochromaffin cell system, as 5-hydroxytryptamine. Nature 169:800, 1952.
24. Lembeck, F.: 5-Hydroxytryptamine in a carcinoid tumor. Nature 172:910, 1953.

25. Norheim, I., et al.: Malignant carcinoid tumors. Ann Surg 206:115, 1987.
26. Godwin, D. J.: Carcinoid tumors: an analysis of 2,837 cases. Cancer 36:560, 1975.
27. Jouvet, M.: Biologic amines and the state of sleep. Science 163:32, 1969.
28. Moertel, C. G.: Treatment of the carcinoid tumor and the malignant carcinoid syndrome. J Clin Oncol 1:727, 1983.
29. Grahame Smith, D. F.: The carcinoid syndrome. Am J Cardiol 21:376, 1968.
30. Lundin, L., et al.: Carcinoid heart disease: relationship of circulating vasoactive substances to ultrasound-detectable cardiac abnormalities. Circulation 77:264, 1988.
31. Houston, D. S., Vanhaulte, D. M.: Serotonin and vascular system: role in health and disease and implications for therapy. Drugs 31:149, 1986.
32. Mason, R. A., Stean, P. A.: Anaesthesia for a patient with carcinoid syndrome. Anaesthesia 31:243, 1976.
33. Dery, R.: Theoretical and clinical considerations in anesthesia for secreting carcinoid tumors. Can Anaesth Soc J 18:245, 1971.
34. Burch, R. M., Farmer, S. G., Steranka, L. R.: Bradykinin receptor antagonists. Med Res Rev 10:143, 1990.
35. Lunding, L., et al.: Plasma atrial natriuretic peptide in carcinoid heart disease. Am J Cardiol 63:969, 1989.
36. Ureles, A.: Diagnosis and treatment of malignant carcinoid syndrome. JAMA 229:1346, 1974.
37. Weidner, F. A., Zitler, F. M. II.: Carcinoid tumors of the gastrointestinal tract. JAMA 245:1153, 1981.
38. Lucas, K. G., Feldman, J. M.: Flushing in the carcinoid syndrome and plasm kallikrein. Cancer 58:2290, 1986.
39. Oates, J. A.: The carcinoid syndrome (editorial). N Engl J Med 315:702, 1986.
40. Zinner, M. G., Yeo, C. J., Jaffe, B. M.: The effects of carcinoid levels of serotonin and substance P on hemodynamics. Ann Surg 199:197, 1984.
41. Veall, G. R. Q., Peacock, J. E., Bax, N. D. S.: Review of anesthetic management of 21 patients undergoing laperotomy for carcinoid syndrome. Br J Anaesth 72:335, 1994.
42. Vink, A., Moattari, A.: Use of somatostatin analog in management of carcinoid syndrome. Dig Dis Sci 34:14S, 1989.
43. Brazeau, P., et al.: Somatostatin: isolation, characterization, distribution, and blood determination. Metabolism 27(Suppl 1):1133, 1978.
44. Lucey, M. R., Yamada, T.: Biochemistry and physiology of gastrointestinal somatostatin. Dig Dis Sci 34:5S, 1989.
45. Park, J., Chiba, I., Yamada, I.: Mechanisms of direct inhibition of canine gastric parietal cells by somatostatin. J Biol Chem 262:4190, 1987.
46. Sheppard, M., et al.: Metabolic clearance and plasma half disappearance time of exogenous somatostatin in man. J Clin Endocrinol Metab 48:50, 1979.
47. Bloom, S. R., Polak, J. M.: Somatostatin. Br Med J 295:288, 1987.
48. Lawrence, J. P., et al.: Effect of somatostatin on 5-hydroxytryptamine release from a carcinoid tumor. Surgery 108:1131, 1990.
49. Reubi, J. C., et al.: In vitro and in vivo detection of somatostatin receptors in human malignant tissues. Acta Oncol 30:463, 1991.
50. Marsh, H. M., Martin, K., Kvols, L. K.: Carcinoid crisis during anesthesia: successful treatment with a somatostatin analogue. Anesthesiology 66:89, 1987.
51. Quinlivan, J. K., Roberts, W. A.: Intraoperative octreotide for refractory carcinoid-induced bronchospasm. Anesth Analg 78:400, 1994.
52. Dollery, C.: Therapeutic Drugs. Vol. 2. London, Churchill Livingstone, 1991, p. 1.
53. Clarke, R. S. J., et al.: Adverse reactions to intravenous anesthetics. Br J Anaesth 47:575, 1975.
54. Parris, W. C. V., et al.: Pretreatment with somastatin in the anesthetic management of a patient with carcinoid syndrome. Can J Anaesth 35:413, 1988.
55. Mason, R. A., Steane, P. A.: Anaesthesia for a patient with carcinoid syndrome. Anaesthesia 31:243, 1976.

DEMYELINATING DISEASES (MULTIPLE SCLEROSIS)

These acquired diseases include the encephalitides and other infections. Presumably, such infections result in diffuse sclerosis, disseminated myelitis, and disseminated sclerosis (multiple sclerosis [MS]). Of these conditions, the most common is disseminated sclerosis, and half a million Americans have this disease. The incidence is approximately 60 to 70 patients per 100,000 population in the United States.

PATHOLOGY[1]

The neuropathologic changes occur principally in the white matter of the brain and spinal cord, at multiple sites and in a random fashion. The peripheral nervous system is virtually intact. One sees a loss of myelin and an ingrowth of oligodendroglia into the myelin sheath of axons. These changes are accompanied by an increase in oxydative enzyme in the myelin sheath. The oligodendroglial cell membrane produces myelin in the CNS, whereas the Schwann cell produces myelin in the peripheral nervous system. Thus, in the CNS, myelin covering the axons is lost.

Sclerotic plaques in multiple brain areas appear, and edema of the neurons and conduction block occurs. Accompanying the progress of the disease is an increased level of immunoglobulin G (IgG) in the cerebrospinal fluid.[2]

DIAGNOSIS

The diagnosis is made on clinical grounds.[3] No laboratory tests are specific. In suspected patients, the "hot bath" test may confirm the diagnosis.[4] Immersing a subject in a hot bath at 41°C and then elevating the temperature of the bath to 43°C for 10 minutes increases body temperature. In patients with MS, preexisting signs are worsened, and in 60% of patients, new neurologic signs may develop.[4]

A second confirmatory study in patients presumed to have MS is done during an attack. This concerns the examination of cerebrospinal fluid. In such patients who indeed do have MS, one sees a significant elevation of IgG.[5]

CLINICAL COURSE

The onset of this disease is usually in the second or third decade of life, is usually rapid, and can be one of two types. One type of onset is denoted by the development of visual disorders and weakness of the eye muscles. The second type of onset is the development of generalized motor weakness, along with numbness and paresthesias. Bladder control is lost.

Classically, the course is accompanied by exacerbations and plateauing of symptoms, with some remissions in certain patients.[6] Usually, a remission does occur after an acute attack. Serious exacerbations may occur every 2 to 3 years. The relapse rate is approximately 0.44 per patient per year. The aforementioned tests of Malhotra and Goren indicate that heat elevations of the body cause an exacerbation of the condition.

EPIDEMIOLOGIC FACTORS[7,8]

The incidence of this disease is low in latitudes near the equator. The disease occurs in a characteristic geographic distribution. The incidence is higher as one moves away from the equator. Thus, one sees a high prevalence in the northern temperate zones (higher in Seattle than in Los Angeles) and in southern temperate zones (higher in southern Australia than in New Zealand).[7]

Latitude also affects the course of the disease. Thus, when the disease occurs in a low-risk area, it tends to be more disabling and shows a malignant course.[8]

ETIOLOGY

A familial or host factor is evident in that a 12- to 15-fold increase of the disease occurs among first-degree relatives of patients with MS. Several viruses can cause CNS demyelination. A high incidence of MS occurs in persons with certain tissue types; that is, those with the human leukocyte antigen (HLA)-DW2[9] have a 4- to 5-fold increased risk, and those with HLA-B7 have only a 2- to 3-fold greater risk.

Several studies suggest a genetic susceptibility. MS has been associated with specific genotypes: those coded for in the HLA of chromosome 6 and the IgG allotypes coded on chromosome 14.[10]

Several viruses can cause CNS demyelination in animals and, in turn, the prediction of an overall disease similar to MS.[11]

Nonspecific viruses may break down myelin and may induce antibodies against the myelin protein. Once the host's immune system is sensitized to myelin, the immune system continues to destroy it.[12] Under certain stress conditions, the process is augmented, and clinical exacerbations occur. Thus, an autoimmune hypothesis linked to a viral infection has gained significant support.[14]

Genetic factors, in combination with biochemical factors and a prior viral infection, whichever may set in motion an antibody response to myelin, once initiated, continue in the absence of the virus. In the ensuing inflammatory process, infiltrating lymphocytes (predominantly T cells) and macrophages lead to degradation of the myelin sheath.

NERVE CONDUCTION[1]

Nerve impulses are conducted down a nerve fiber from one node of Ranvier to the next. When the internodal portion becomes demyelinated, the current is leaked (shunted), and the excitation of successive nodes is blunted. When several contiguous segments are demyelinated, conduction fails. Contributing to conduction failure are other factors, including changes in extracellular fluid composition, disturbances of the sodium (Na)/potassium (K) channels, and temperature changes. Circulating agents that block synaptic transmission also alter conduction. One consequence is the appearance of more sodium channels in the demyelinated axon membrane, which attempts to restore impulse propagation as a natural means. This is inadequate, however, and some remyelination is impaired.

Under normal conditions, the development of myelination depends on the integrity of the Na/K channels: Na channels in nodes, K channels in internodes. Disturbances of these channels lead to both demyelination and poor remyelination.

FACTORS OF PROGNOSIS[13]

Several host and environmental factors are associated with a benign or malignant course. A *benign* course is more likely when the onset is at an early age (averaging 29 to 30 years) and symptoms are sensory, such as numbness and unusual feelings in arms, hands, or legs. Visual and speech difficulties are among the initial symptoms. Double vision, some loss of vision, and "electric" or shooting sensations also occur. A *malignant* course is associated with a later onset, with a mean age of 35 years. Motor disability and coordination symptoms occur early. Adverse responses to heat exposure are common, and improvement is reported on cold exposure.

Some amelioration and limitation of exacerbations have been obtained by daily injection of a synthetic polymer of amino acids simulating myelin basic protein.[15] At least this regimen has been beneficial in limiting the number (by over half) and the intensity of the exacerbations.[16]

CLASSIFICATION OF DISABILITY

Patients can be classified on the basis of disability into three categories: (1) walking without aids (benign); (2) walking with aids; (3) restricted to a wheelchair or bed and unable to perform essential self-care activities (malignant).

Onset of the disease after 40 years of age has a graver prognosis, and the progress of the disease is more rapid.

DIAGNOSTIC TESTS[3]

Relevant testing includes the following:

1. Complete conduction block with elevation of body temperature.[4,17]
2. Central evoked potentials: These include visual brain stem auditory and somatosensory responses, which reveal slowing of conduction in CNS pathways before significant clinical symptoms.
3. CT brain scanning has demonstrated large demyelination plaques and can detect ventricular dilatation and cerebral atrophy.

PREOPERATIVE PREPARATION

The following measures are necessary in patients with MS:

1. Control of spasticity by diazepam or midazolam.
2. Myotonia syndrome not seen with nondepolarizing agents (EMG is normal).
3. Minimizing of psychologic and physical stresses.

GENERAL ANESTHESIA

Despite abnormalities of blood-brain transfer (perivascular block), the response to general anesthetic agents is customary. The rate of new symptoms appears to be less than expected after anesthesia, and such symptoms may be related to pyrexia. Some reports suggest new symptoms on awakening after thiopental administration.

TEMPERATURE MONITORING

Patients with MS require the following measures:

1. Prevention of shivering.
2. Use of adrenocorticotropic hormone (ACTH).
3. Use of antibiotics prophylactically to prevent postoperative infections and pyrexia.

REFERENCES

1. Waxman, S. G.: Membranes, myelin, and the pathophysiology of multiple sclerosis. N Engl J Med 306:1529, 1982.
2. Link, H.: Some aspects of immune reactions of the brain. In Rose, F. C. (ed.). Clinical Neuroimmunology. Oxford, Blackwell Scientific Publications, 1979, p. 12.
3. Gilman, S.: Diagnosis of multiple sclerosis (editorial). JAMA 246:1122, 1981.
4. Malhotra, A. S., Goren, H.: The hot bath test in the diagnosis of multiple sclerosis. JAMA 246:1113, 1981.
5. Link, H.: Immunoglobin G and low molecular weight proteins in human cerebrospinal fluid: chemical and immunological characterization with special reference to multiple sclerosis. Acta Neurol Scand Suppl 43:1, 1967.
6. Bamford, C., et al.: Anesthesia in multiple sclerosis. Can J Neurol Sci 5:41, 1978.
7. Kurtzke, J. F.: Geography in multiple sclerosis. J Neurol 215:1, 1977.
8. Detels, R., et al.: Factors associated with a rapid course of multiple sclerosis. Arch Neurol 39:337, 1982.
9. Aronson, S. M., et al. (eds.): Therapeutic Claims in Multiple Sclerosis. New York, International Federation of Multiple Sclerosis Societies, 1982.
10. McDonald, W. I.: Multiple sclerosis: epidemiology and HCL association. Ann NY Acad Sci 436:109, 1984.
11. Lublin, F.: Experimental allergic encephalomyelitis in heterotrophic brain transplants. Ann Neurol 18:128, 1985.
12. Lublin, F.: Demyelinative lesions demonstrated by MRI in Vogt-Koyanagi-Harava syndrome. J Neurol 35(Suppl), 1985.
13. Clark, V. A., et al.: Factors associated with a malignant or benign course of multiple sclerosis. JAMA 248:856, 1982.
14. Waksman, B. H., Reynolds, W. E.: Multiple sclerosis as a disease of immune regulation. Proc Soc Exp Biol Med 175:282, 1984.
15. Weiner, H. L.: Cop 1 therapy for multiple sclerosis. N Engl J Med 314:442, 1987.
16. Bornstein, B. B., et al.: A pilot trial of Cop 1 in exacerbating-remitting multiple sclerosis. N Engl J Med 314:408, 1987.
17. Berger, J., Ontell, R.: Intrathecal morphine in conjunction with combined special and general anesthesia in a patient with multiple sclerosis. Anesthesiology 66:400, 1987.

DISORDERS OF THE UPPER AND LOWER MOTOR NEURON (AMYOTROPHIC LATERAL SCLEROSIS)

Progressive degeneration of the upper and lower motor neuron cells and of the corticospinal tracts characterizes amyotrophic lateral sclerosis (ALS). Bulbar motor nuclei are also involved.

COMMON SIGNS AND SYMPTOMS

Muscular weakness and atrophy occur early, but they may be preceded by muscle cramps, which are common. The onset of muscle disturbance is random and occurs in an asymmetric pattern. Muscle fasciculations are visible, and spasticity occurs. Involvement of the corticospinal tracts is accompanied by hyperactive deep tendon reflexes and extensor plantar responses (Babinski sign).

CLASSIFICATION (TABLE 45–6)[1]

This classification is based on the site of onset of neuronal degeneration and the related signs and symptoms. In typical ALS, the common motor neuron disturbance initially shows evidence of anterior spinal cord horn cell dysfunction, but this is soon followed by strong evidence of concomitant motor cortex and corticospinal nerve tract dysfunction.[2]

When the anterior horn cell degeneration outpaces corticospinal involvement, it may be considered an adult variant and is termed progressive muscular atrophy (PMA). The lower motor neuron dysfunction predominates. Progression is usually more benign and is slower. Muscle weakness and wasting usually begin in the hands and progresses to the arms, shoulders, and legs, but eventually it becomes *generalized*, with cortical neuronal involvement. Fasciculations are often the earliest sign of the disease. Onset occurs at any age, and survival for 25 or more years is possible.

Table 45–6. Degenerative Motor Neuron Diseases

Amyotrophic lateral sclerosis (ALS)
  Progressive muscular atrophy
  Primary lateral sclerosis
  Pseudobulbar palsy
Inherited motor neuron diseases
  Autosomal recessive spinal muscular atrophy
    Type I: Werdnig-Hoffmann, acute
    Type II: Werdnig-Hoffmann, chronic
    Type III: Kugelberg-Welander
    Type IV: Adult onset
  Familial ALS
  Familial ALS with dementia or Parkinson's disease (Guam)
Acquired
  Acute: poliomyelitis, coxsackie, other enteroviruses
  Chronic: ALS in parkinsonism, Shy-Drager syndrome, Creutzfeldt-Jakob disease, Guillain-Barré syndrome

Modified from Tandan, R., Bradley, W. A.: Amyotrophic lateral sclerosis. Part I: clinical features, pathology and ethical issues in management. Ann Neurol 18:271, 1985.

An autosomal dominant pattern of inheritance is present in about 10% of these patients, and the onset of PMA in the genetically linked disorder generally occurs at a younger age, that is, the late teens.

When anterior horn cell involvement is the singular or only pattern of involvement, this rare variant is designated primary lateral sclerosis (PLS). The limbs are principally affected, showing signs of stiffness and distal motor weakness.

PROGRESSIVE BULBAR PALSY

This variant affects striated muscles innervated by the cranial nerves.[3] Corticobulbar tracts are predominantly involved, namely, the ninth, tenth, and twelfth cranial nerves. Early symptoms are often related to defects in speech, and talking becomes difficult (dysarthria). Chewing and swallowing are abnormally affected, and dysphagia presents an increased risk of regurgitation and pulmonary aspiration. The prognosis is poor, and death within 1 to 3 years is common and is related to respiratory complications.

With this CNS dysfunction, patients may have disturbances in control of emotional responses that induce facial muscular spasms and labile or inappropriate emotions. This phenomenon has been designated pseudobulbar palsy. Less than 1% of all patients have dysfunction restricted to the medullary areas.[3]

DIAGNOSIS

Principal diagnostic features are those of the common signs and symptoms of progressive and generalized motor involvement. The onset is usually during middle age, with a peak incidence at 40 to 50 years. This onset occurs without involvement of the sensory system; voluntary eye movements by extraocular muscles are unimpaired. Regulatory mechanisms for the control and coordination of movements of intact muscles remain (i.e., cerebellar mechanisms are intact).

The intellect remains intact. The sympathetic and parasympathetic nervous systems are spared, and hence bladder and bowel control remains.

Electromyography is a useful laboratory test. Fibrillations, positive waves, and fasciculations are observed along the large motor nerves. Conduction velocities remain normal until late in the disease process, however.

COURSE OF THE DISEASE AND PROGNOSIS

ALS is a progressive and fatal neurodegenerative disease.[3] It affects the motor muscular system. The progression is relentless, without periods of improvement. Respiratory function is impaired, and death is usually related to failure of respiratory mechanics or pulmonary infection.

A rare patient may survive for 30 years from onset of the disease; 50% die within 3 years of onset; 20% live for 5 years; and 10% live for 10 years.[4]

Evidence for an autoimmune disorder has been presented for ALS by Appel and colleagues,[5] but further studies are needed.

TREATMENT

No specific treatment exists. Physical therapy helps to maintain some muscle function. Rehabilitative measures with mechanical aids may overcome some of the disabilities. Respiratory support may be indicated, but, in the long term, it raises ethical questions.

Thyrotropin-releasing hormone infusions have been observed to improve motor function for short periods of time.

Drugs that modulate the *glutaminergic* system have been proposed as treatment.[6] Some studies[7,8] have demonstrated that a benzothiazole agent, riluzole, was found to modulate glutaminergic transmission. A controlled clinical trial with this agent slowed the progression of ALS and appeared to improve survival in patients with disease of bulbar onset.[9]

ANESTHETIC CONSIDERATIONS

A few points are in order. Because the sensory system is intact, peripheral nerve block regional anesthesia for minor surgical procedures has been successful. Epidural or spinal anesthesia has not been reported or recommended. General anesthesia can be used. Succinylcholine is definitely contraindicated, whereas nondepolarizing muscle blocking agents may not be needed. Most inhalation agents, such as isoflurane and enflurane, have been tolerated.

REFERENCES

1. Tandan, R., Bradley, W. A.: Amyotrophic lateral sclerosis. Part I: Clinical features, pathology and ethical issues in management. Ann Neurol *18:*271, 1985.
2. Plaitakis, A., et al.: Pilot trial of branched chain amino acids in amyotrophic lateral sclerosis. Lancet *1:*1015, 1988.
3. Morris, F., et al.: Anset, natural history and outcome in idiopathic adult motor neuron disease. J Neurol Sci *118:*48, 1993.
4. Nealon, N. M.: Disorders of peripheral nervous system. *In* Merck Manual, 16 Ed. Rahway, NJ, Merck Research Laboratories, 1992.
5. Appel, S. H., Smith, R. G., Englehardt, J. I., Stefani, E.: Evidence for auto immunity in amyotrophic lateral sclerosis. J Neurol Sci *118:*109, 1993.
6. Lipton, S. A., Rosenberg, P. A.: Excitatory amino acids as a final common pathway for neurologic disorders. N Engl J Med *330:*613, 1994.
7. Plaitakis, A., Caroscio, J. T.: Altered glutaminergic mechanism and selective motor neuron degeneration in amyotrophic lateral sclerosis: possible role of glycine. Adv Neurol *56:*319, 1991.
8. Bensimon, G., Lacomblez, L., Meninger, V., ALS/Riluzole Study Group: A controlled trial of riluzole in amyotrophic lateral sclerosis. N Engl J Med *330:*585, 1994.
9. Rowland, L. P.: Riluzole for the treatment of amyotrophic lateral sclerosis: too soon to tell (editorial) N Engl J Med *330:*636, 1994.

DOWN SYNDROME (TRISOMY 21)

GENETIC ORIGIN

About 95% of patients with Down syndrome[1] have an extra chromosome 21 coming from the nuclei of the fa-ther. This anomaly is one of the most common chromosomal abnormalities in humans, with an overall incidence of 1 in 600 to 800 live births. Marked variability exists, depending on maternal age in the child-bearing years. For women under 40 years, the incidence is 1 in 2000 live births; for those over 40 years, the incidence rises to 1 in 80 live births.[2] These older mothers, however, have only 7 to 8% of the children born.

Possible causes of the anomaly include radiation exposure, diabetes, malnutrition, thyroid dysfunction, and viral diseases.[3]

CHROMOSOMAL TRANSLOCATION

A familial form of Down syndrome exists in which the usual 46 chromosome number is present, but the patient is a phenotype of the congenital form. In this familial form, the extra chromosome is translocated and is attached to other chromosomes, namely, chromosomes 13, 14, 15, 22. The most common attachment is to chromosome 14 (21:14); the next most frequent attachment is to chromosome 22 (21:22). These forms represent about 5% of patients with Down syndrome.[3,4]

PATHOGENESIS

Because the chromosomal abnormality affects every cell in the patient with Down syndrome, all organs and systems are affected, and the clinical manifestations are extensive.[4]

SYMPTOMS AND SIGNS

The infant with Down syndrome tends to be placid and rarely cries, but shows muscular hypotonicity. The classic physical features include a small head and facial stigmata of a small nose with a flat bridge, upward slanting of the palpebral fissures, and strabismus. A small mouth with macroglossia is a distinct characteristic. The neck is short and broad, and nuchal edema is noted. Extremities are short, hands and feet are small, and a single line crease across the palm is noted in many patients (the simian crease).

Mental retardation is common and is mild to moderate in most instances. Growth is retarded. Adults are usually obese and of short stature. Muscular strength is also poor in most patients; ligamentous laxity is present, and atlantoaxial instability is usually seen.[5,6]

Associated problems include the presence of congenital heart disease, which is responsible for the high mortality in childhood. A compromised immune system is the cause of frequent infections, such as disorders of the upper airway and especially infection of the lower respiratory tract. Anomalies of the gastrointestinal tract require early surgery. Sleep apnea is frequent.[7] Myelomeningocele is common, and the incidence of leukemia is increased. Thyroid abnormalities are likely in adults.

SURVIVAL AND MORTALITY

At present, 76% of patients with Down syndrome survive beyond the tenth year of life.[8] Most surgery is performed during childhood and is for the correction of congenital defects. Up to 50% of such surgery is for correction of cardiac defects. Otolaryngeal ophthalmologic and orthopedic procedures account for most of the other surgical procedures.[9]

Life expectancy is decreased by heart disease and acute leukemia. Patients without a major heart defect survive to adulthood, but the aging process seems accelerated, and death occurs in the fourth or fifth decade. The microscopic findings in the brain of those afflicted with Down syndrome are typical of those in Alzheimer's disease, and a connection between genes on chromosome 21 and Alzheimer's disease is under investigation.

ANESTHETIC CONSIDERATIONS[9,10]

Preanesthetic assessment is the cornerstone of identification of systemic disorders and the correction of functional disturbance. It also enables one to identify likely technical problems in anesthetic management. One important feature of institutionalized children with Down syndrome is the high incidence of low-grade asymptomatic hepatitis and of hepatitis B antigen seropositivity.[11] This warns the anesthetist to avoid halothane or other direct or indirect (facultative) hepatotoxins.

Sympathetic activity (both central and peripheral) is reduced. Reduced levels of norepinephrine and dopamine are related to abnormalities of catecholamine metabolism, including reduced levels of dopamine β-hydroxylase.[12] Blood pressure is usually lower than in normal or other mentally handicapped children.[13] Plasma levels of epinephrine are usually normal, although urinary excretion is decreased.

Premedication

Because of the decreased sympathetic activity, patients should receive atropine in small doses. This drug should, preferably, be given intravenously at the time of induction of anesthesia. The cardiac acceleratory effect is usually normal.[14]

Sedatives and tranquilizers may be given, but responses may be erratic. Midazolam or ketamine may be administered intramuscularly, especially in the obstreperous or frightened child. Intramuscular ketamine has been especially effective in the experience with anesthesia and minor surgical procedures at St. Mary of Providence School for handicapped children in Chicago.[15] The presence of a family member in whom the child has confidence and with whom the child has rapport is often desirable.

Choice of Anesthesia

Usually, in the younger patient, general anesthesia is preferred. In older children (15 to 20 years) and in the adult afflicted with Down syndrome, some local and regional anesthetic techniques are readily accepted and are successful. Dental procedures and other minor operations can be readily performed using local anesthesia or block techniques such as intraoral maxillary and alveolar blocks.

For *general anesthesia,* induction by intravenous or intramuscular injection of midazolam (or other benzodiazepines) or ketamine provides a smooth course to be followed by an inhalation agent (as previously noted, halothane is not recommended). Most other inhalation agents are acceptable; however, the maximal concentrations should be reduced.[16]

Oral administration of midazolam is particularly effective for producing sleep in infants and children and in those with Down syndrome.[17] The drug is prepared by dissolving the aqueous parenteral preparation (5 mg/ml) in an equal volume of a chocolate-cherry syrup or an equal volume of simple syrup (NF) flavored with oil of peppermint as follows:

To 15 ml of the aqueous parenteral preparation (total 75 mg) add 14.5 ml of the simple syrup (NF) mixed with 0.5 ml of oil of peppermint.

This mixing provides a final concentration of 2.5 mg/ml. This solution is stable at room temperature for up to 14 days.[18]

The usual dose for children 1 to 6 years of age (8 to 25 kg) is 0.5 mg/kg of body weight. This amounts to about 4 ml of the solution (1 teaspoonful) for those 1 to 2 years of age; at 6 years of age, the volume dose is about 1 to 2 teaspoonsful.

Absorption is relatively rapid, and onset of sedation is seen in 10 to 15 minutes.[19] The bioavibility is about 50% because of extensive first-pass metabolism in the liver.

A chloral hydrate syrup may also be used for sedation and is available as an oral preparation in units of 500 mg/10 ml. Chloral hydrate is particularly useful to provide a mild sleep without interfering with normal or abnormal brain waves. It provides mild sleep for electroencephalography (EEG). The dose for children who have some degree of mental retardation is 5 to 10 ml (250 to 500 mg). For older children and adults, the dose is 10 to 20 ml, or about 1 g.

Muscle relaxants of the nondepolarizing type may not be needed because of the muscle hypotonicity. A short-acting nondepolarizing muscle relaxant such as mivicurium may be useful, however. Succinylcholine may be used for endotracheal intubation if atropine has been provided.

Monitoring includes ECG, pulse oximetry, and capnography, as well as temperature and blood pressure recording.

REFERENCES

1. Down, J. L.: Observations on an ethnic classification of idiots. Clin Lect Rep Lond Hosp *25*, 1866.
2. Merck Manual, 16th Ed. Rahway, NJ, Merck Research Laboratories, 1992, p. 2299.
3. Patterson, D.: The causes of Down syndrome. Sci Am *257:*52, 1987.
4. Lejeune, M.J., Gauthier, M., Turpin, M. R.: Les chromosomes humains en culture de tissues. C R Seances Acad Sci *248:*602, 1959.
5. Williams, J. P., et al.: Atlantoaxial subluxation and trisomy 21. Anesthesiology *67:*253, 1987.
6. Pueschel, S. M., Scala, F. H.: Atlantoaxial instability in individuals with Down syndrome. Pediatrics *80:*555, 1987.
7. Southall, D. P., et al.: Upper airway obstruction with hypox-
8. Baird, P. A., Sadornick, A. D.: Causes of death to age 30 in Down syndrome. Am J Hum Genet *43:*239, 1988.
9. Kobel, M., Creighton, R. E., Steward, D. J.: Anesthetic considerations in Down syndrome: experience with 100 patients and a review of the literature. Can Anesth Soc J *29:*593, 1982.
10. Sofair, D.: The patient with trisomy 21: preanesthetic assessment. Anesthiol News *Sept:*13, 1989.
11. Skinhoj, P., et al.: Hepatitis and hepatitis-associated antigen HAA in Down syndrome. J Ment Defic Res *15:*236, 1971.
12. Coleman, M., et al.: Serum dopamine beta hydroxylase levels in Down syndrome. Clin Genet *1:*312, 1974.
13. Richards, B. W., Enver, F.: Blood pressure in Down syndrome. J Ment Defic Res *23:*123, 1979.
14. Wark, H. J., Overton, J. H., Marian, P.: The safety of atropine pre-medication in children with Down syndrome. Anesthesia *38:*871, 1983.
15. Collins, V. J.: Anesthesia for Down's children and other mentally handicapped children at St. Mary of Providence School for Handicapped Children (Chicago, IL) 1963–1980. Personal Reports, 1985.
16. Eger, E. I. (ed.): MAC: Anesthetic Uptake and Action. Baltimore, Williams & Wilkins, 1974, p. 1.
17. McMillan, C. O., et al.: Pre-medication of children with oral midazolam. Can J Anaesth *39:*545, 1992.
18. Gregory, D. F., Koestner, J. A., Tobias, J. D.: Stability of midazolam prepared for oral administration. South Med J *89:*771, 1993.
19. Levin, M. F., et al.: Oral midazolam pre-medication in children: the minimum time interval for separation from parents. Can J Anaesth *40:*726, 1993.

EPILEPSY

Basic Management Considerations

Epilepsy means seizure; it is a syndrome characterized by recurring attacks of (1) of impaired consciousness or (2) of involuntary muscle movements. The latter, with clonic and tonic generalized muscular contractions or convulsions with loss of consciousness, may not always occur. Sudden loss of consciousness may occur without muscle activity. This is *petit mal*, to distinguish the occurrence from the major convulsive attack or *grand mal*.

A stupor follows, and the patient tends to perform automatic acts. Seizures may be due to a lesion localized in some part of the cortex and is called focal epilepsy or jacksonian epilepsy.[1] When no gross organic lesion can be identified, this condition is called idiopathic epilepsy, and it represents a problem in anesthetic management.

Certain pathogenic factors are associated with the seizures and are considered responsible.[2] A disturbance in *water balance* is encountered. Water retention and increased volume of cerebrospinal fluid occur increase intracranial pressure. Hypotonic solutions precipitate attacks, whereas hypertonic solutions and those effective in reducing cerebral edema decrease the tendency to convulsions. Cerebral edema from any cause and especially *hypoxia* precipitates convulsions. On the other hand, metabolic acidosis or ketosis decreases the number and severity of attacks, whereas alkalosis has an undesirable effect. This finding raises questions as to how vigorous ventilation should be during anesthesia. Certainly, a patient should not be hyperventilated.

Acute hypoxia causes pial constriction and provokes an attack. Procedures that cause cerebral vascular constriction similarly induce seizures. Physiologic changes in the brain that may influence seizures have been summarized by Lennox and Cobb.[3]

Penfield observed the brains of conscious epileptics and noted that constriction of pial arteries and diminution of pulsation invariably accompany an epileptic seizure.[4-6]

A commonly used classification of epilepsy is as follows[4-6]:

1. Grand mal or classic seizure.
2. Petit mal triad (pyknoepilepsy; myoclonic jerks; akinetic seizures); onset in childhood.
3. Psychomotor epilepsy (adults).

Each class has a characteristic clinical picture and a typical EEG pattern.[7] These types of seizure also respond to certain classes of antiepileptic drugs. The term "petit mal" is restricted to seizures characterized by brief lapses of consciousness with absence of any but minimal muscular movement. The onset is in childhood, and a seizure is readily precipitated by hyperventilation; the accompanying EEG shows a 3-per-second spike-wave activity. This must be distinguished from psychomotor seizures of adults.

Preparation[8]

Drug therapy must be continued, and the patient's condition must be under control. Because the drugs used occupy a cardinal position in preventing seizures, the different classes of antiepileptic agents and their field of usefulness should be recognized (Table 45-7). Thus, the barbituric acid derivatives, especially phenobarbital, are keystones in controlling grand mal seizures. If a drug used is not available as a parenteral preparation (primidone),

Table 45-7. Drugs Used in Management of Epilepsy

Drug	Clinical condition

Barbituric acid derivatives
  Phenobarbital, 3–5 mg/kg d
  Mephobarbital
  Primidone
	Grand mal in infants and children; also in adults

Phenytoin (Dilantin)	Grand mal and psychomotor epilepsy in older children and adults

Succinimide derivatives
  Ethosuximide
  Methsuximide
  Trimethadione
	Petit mal triad

Straight chain compounds Phencacemide	Psychomotor attacks
Diazepam (5–30 mg children and adults; 1–2 mg for infants) Phenobarbital (50–500 mg IV)	Status epilepticus

then it is recommended that one of the standard agents be prescribed. A ketogenic diet and water restriction are desirable.

Choice of Anesthesia

Drugs should be chosen with the objective of avoiding seizures. Hypoxia and heat retention alkalosis are most undesirable. Preanesthetic sedation should be fairly generous. It should include the regular anticonvulsant drug administered 1 to 2 hours before induction. In addition, a barbiturate such as phenobarbital or amobarbital sodium is recommended as part of the preanesthetic medication. Patients so medicated are less susceptible to anesthetic convulsions. The short-acting barbiturates, except amobarbital, cause an increased cerebrovascular constriction and preferably are not used for night sedation or for preanesthetic medication. Morphine is tolerated well and, because it reduces oxygen requirements, is useful. Scopolamine is preferred to atropine because of its cortical sedative effect. Stimulant drugs and centrally acting vasopressors such as ephedrine methedrine are not recommended.

Local anesthetic agents cause more reactions than general anesthetic agents. Therefore, infiltration anesthesia for other than minor surgical procedures requiring small amounts of the local anesthetic solution is contraindicated. Spinal anesthesia, but not epidural, is satisfactory because the dose of local agent usually used is small.

Epileptic patients are best managed with general anesthesia, and preliminary basal narcosis is often desirable. Excitement must be avoided. Intravenous thiopental or methohexital for induction and for basal narcosis are indicated. They can be followed by nitrous oxide and oxygen (at least 30% oxygen). The total dosage of an intravenous barbiturate for induction must be carefully estimated by incremental dose-response observations. Larger than usual doses may be required because barbiturates are well tolerated in treated epileptics because of the intense enzyme induction action of phenobarbital on the liver.

Ether use in patients without hypoxia or hypercarbia has been recommended as an anesthetic and has been used to control status attacks.[9] By creating a mild metabolic acidosis, ether limits the development of epileptic convulsions. The so-called ether convulsions are mostly due to associated hyperpyrexia and hypoxia; however, ether is the only agent shown to produce spike-wave activity in EEG. This phenomenon is especially precipitated when ether is combined with hyperthermia.[2]

Vinyl ether is contraindicated, because it is associated commonly with the production of abnormal motor movements. Cyclopropane tends to conserve heat and requires a closed system. As a consequence, the temperature tends to rise, and this is undesirable in epileptics. This agent is no longer available.

Isoflurane does not produce excitation of the CNS. Spike-wave formations are not produced, and epileptiform tracings are not seen. Enflurane, on the other hand, produces high-voltage spikes, and spike-wave formations occur with increasing depth of anesthesia. About 2% of patients show motor cortex irritability without sequelae.[10]

Muscle relaxants are not contraindicated; however, our preference is the blocking group of agents. The depolarizing agents not only enhance muscular activity but exert a mild central cholinergic effect. A good airway and excellent oxygenation are necessities. Hyperventilation from excess control of respiration may produce alkalosis and should be avoided, however. At the same time carbon dioxide excess must be avoided. In young epileptics, mild hyperthermia should be studiously avoided because it precipitates a seizure. In severe cases, monitoring with EEG is desirable.

REFERENCES

1. Jackson, J. H.: On the anatomical, physiological and pathological investigation of the epilepsies. West Riding Lunatic Asylum Med Rep 3:315, 1873.
2. Jackson, J. H.: Selected Writings of John Hughlings Jackson. Vol. 1. On Epilepsy and Epileptiform Convulsions. J. Taylor (ed.). London, Hodder and Stoughton, 1931.
3. Lennox, N. G., Cobb., S.: Convulsive disorders. Medicine 7:105, 1928.
4. Penfield, W.: Epilepsy, neurophysiology, and some brain mechanisms related to consciousness. In Jasper, H. H., et al. (ed.). Basic Mechanisms of the Epilepsies. Boston, Little, Brown, 1969.
5. Penfield, W.: Epileptic automatism and the centrencephalic integrating system. Res Nerv Ment Disord Proc 30:513, 1952.
6. Penfield, W.: The Excitable Cortex in Conscious Man: The Fifth Sherrington Lecture. Springfield, IL, Charles C Thomas, 1958.
7. Commission on Classification and Terminology of the International League Against Epilepsy. Epilepsia 26:268, 1985.
8. Rall, T. W., Schleifer, L.S.: Drugs effective in the therapy of the epilepsies. Summarized in Gilman, A.G., et al. (eds.). Goddman and Gilman's The Pharmacological Basis of Therapeutics, 8th Ed. New York, McGraw-Hill, 1990.
9. Owens, G., Dawson, R. E., Scott, H. W., Jr.: Clinical and experimental experiences with ether convulsions. Surg Gynecol Obstet 105:681, 1957.
10. Bart, A. J., Homi, J., Linde, H.: Changes in power spectra of electroencephalograms during anesthesia with Ethrane. Anesth Analg 50:53, 1971.

GLAUCOMA

DEFINITION

Glaucoma is defined by the presence of three main features: (1) an increase in ocular pressure; (2) development of increased cupping with pallor of optic disc; and (3) loss of visual field.[1]

Normal intraocular pressure ranges from 10 to 22 mm Hg. It is about 12 to 15 mm Hg higher than intracranial pressure. Ocular hypertension is defined as ocular pressures between 21 and 30 mm Hg without loss of vision. Pressures greater than 21 mm Hg increase markedly with age; at 45 years, 5% of the population have ocular hypertension; at 55 years, 10%; and at 75 years of age, 15%. About 3.5% of persons with ocular hypertension develop visual field loss within 5 years. A higher percentage of patients with pressures greater than 30 mm Hg develop visual field loss and open-angle glaucoma. The prevalance

in the population at large of abnormal readings is about 5%, whereas the prevalence of abnormal readings with visual loss is about 0.7% at age 65 and 1.3% at 75 years of age.

The essential basis of chronically elevated intraocular pressure is an obstruction to outflow of aqueous humor.

FORMATION OF AQUEOUS HUMOR[2]

Aqueous humor is formed from plasma by the ciliary body (supplied by choroidal vessels) at a rate of about 2.0 μl per minute, and the humor is completely replaced every 2 hours. It enters the posterior chamber and passes through the pupil into the anterior chamber. From this chamber, the fluid leaves the eye at the angle between the iris and cornea through a trabecular meshwork (of Fontana) into Schlemm's canal and thence is absorbed into episcleral veins. These veins empty into superior and inferior ophthalmic veins.

Two thirds of the aqueous humor is secreted by an active enzymatic process (carbonic anhydrase and cytochrome oxidase systems) and enters the posterior chamber; one third filters through the anterior surface of the iris into the anterior chamber.

The volume of the anterior chamber is about 0.25 ml, and that of the posterior chamber is about 0.06 ml.[1]

CLASSIFICATION OF GLAUCOMA[1]

Primary and secondary groups are recognized based on the type of obstruction (Table 45–8). The most common form of glaucoma is primary open- or wide-angle glaucoma, representing about 80% of patients. In this condition, the obstruction exists on a microscopic level in the fine connective tissue meshwork through which the fluid in the anterior chamber drains into the canal of Schlemm.

Primary angle-closure (narrow-angle) glaucoma, which is the less common form, representing about 15 to 20%, of patients is due to forward displacement of the iris. This condition may be related to a higher posterior chamber pressure than anterior chamber or to overproduction of aqueous humor. The patient usually has a shallow anterior chamber, and the iris encroaches on the absorption meshwork at the angle. Commonly, obstruction of the pupillary opening by the lens also occurs, and the outflow of aqueous from posterior chamber to the anterior chamber is impeded.

Table 45–8. Classification of the Glaucomas

Primary glaucoma
  Open-angle glaucoma
  Angle-closure glaucoma: acute, intermittent or subacute, or chronic
  Congenital or developmental glaucoma
Secondary glaucoma
  Uveitis, trauma, intraocular tumor, corticosteroid-induced disease

From Schwartz, B.: Concepts in ophthalmology. N Engl J Med 299:183, 1978.

Congenital or developmental glaucomas are rare, whereas secondary glaucomas are due to a variety of causes corrected by other means.

THERAPY

Open-angle (wide-angle) glaucoma is primarily treated by medications that lower intraocular pressure to a safe level. The basic drugs are miotics. *Three drug types* are employed:[3] (1) topical cholinomimetics—topical pilocarpine (0.5 to 4.0%), a naturally ocurring alkaloid, or carbachol (1.5%), a synthetic cholinergic stimulant; (2) topical anticholinesterases,[4] such as physostigmine (0.02 to 1.0%); demecarium bromide, a bis compound with longer duration than simple anticholinesterase; and echothiophate iodide (0.03 to 0.25%), a long-lasting and widely used organic phosphate and anticholinesterase derivative; (3) and inhibitors of aqueous humor formation.[5] This last category includes systemic carbonic anhydrase inhibitors, such as acetazolamide, which drug inhibits the formation of carbonic acid from CO_2 and diminishes the subsequent formation of bicarbonate.[6] Because aqueous humor has a high content of bicarbonate, the production of aqueous humor is greatly decreased by this drug. Another means by which to inhibit the formation of aqueous humor is to block β adrenoreceptors, for example, with timolol eyedrops (0.25 to 0.5%), one drop twice a day;[7] this drug is a nonspecific β blocker, and its duration of action is 7 to 12 hours.[6]

δ-Tetrahydrocannabinal (THC), the active principle of marihuana, has been found to lower ocular hypertension in patients with wide-angle glaucoma.[8] Administration of a solution of THC by eyedrops or by a dose of 5 to 10 mg orally is effective.[9] Intravenous urea (1.0 g) may be needed in acute narrow-angle glaucoma.

Sympathomimetic agents[10] (epinephrine, 1.0%) paradoxically reduce intraocular pressure by increasing outflow (in open-angle chronic glaucoma) and by vasoconstriction of chorioidal vessels, thereby decreasing the rate of secretion. These agents must not be used in closed-angle glaucoma.

Formation of aqueous humor may depend on β-adrenergic receptors, and studies demonstrate that β-adrenergic blocking drugs (timolol) are effective topically in reducing formation of aqueous humor.[7]

In open-angle glaucoma, drugs may not always be effective, and disease may progress. When changes in the optic disc appear, the visual field narrows, and ocular pressure remains high, surgery is needed.[3] The procedure consists of creating a drain route from the anterior chamber into the subconjunctival or intrascleral space.

Angle-closure glaucoma and congenital glaucoma are treated best by operation. A small opening in the iris is created, permitting easy flow from posterior chamber into anterior chamber. This procedure decreases pressure in posterior chamber and allows the iris to fall away from absorption trabeculae.

DRUG INTERACTIONS[6]

Corticosteroids administered both topically and systemically can raise ocular pressure, can produce optic disc change, and can cause visual field loss.

Anticholinergic agents,[11,12] such as belladonna derivatives, drugs used in gastrointestinal disorders, and agents used in parkinsonism, may greatly elevate intraocular pressure in patients predisposed to angle-closure (narrow-angle) glaucoma. This condition is the less prevalent form of glaucoma, however.

Other drugs that elevate intraocular pressure in angle-closure glaucoma include tranquilizers and nitrites.[11] Precipitation of narrow-angle glaucoma by tricyclic drugs may occur. Depolarizing muscle relaxants, such as succinylcholine, also elevate intraocular pressure significantly in angle-closure glaucoma. These drugs have not been found to elevate intraocular pressure in *open-angle type* glaucoma.[6]

COMPLICATIONS OF DRUGS USED IN THERAPY

Most of the adverse responses to the principal drugs used in glaucoma are exaggerated parasympathomimetic effects due to systemic absorption.[6] These include the following:

1. Sinus bradycardia.
2. Occasional cardiac arrest.[13]
3. Vasodepression followed by hypertension; both depressor and pressor responses are blocked by atropine.
4. Bronchospasm.
5. Sweating and salivation.
6. Increased gastric secretion with low pH.
7. Arousal effects.
8. Hallucinogenesis.

That the topical instillation of miotic drugs has systemic consequences should be appreciated.

A 1% pilocarpine solution has 10 mg/ml. Thus, 2 drops in the eye may result in 1.5 to 2.0 mg of the agent being absorbed.[14] Similarly, 2 drops of an 0.5% physostigmine solution may quickly introduce 0.5 to 1.0 mg of this agent into the circulation.

Anticholinesterases used as eyedrops are absorbed systemically and repress both erythrocyte and *plasma cholinesterase*. Depolarizing (succinylcholine) muscle relaxants administered to patients receiving this therapy may be prolonged in action and may produce concomitant prolonged respiratory depression.

Echothiophate, marketed as Phospholine, is a potent organophosphorous compound.[13,15] It is useful in chronic simple wide-angle glaucoma and is a potent miotic. One to two drops of 0.25% solution may be administered topically one to two times a day. As with the other topical agents instilled into the eye, this drug is readily absorbed, and after a few weeks of therapy, pseudocholinesterase activity may be reduced by 60 to 80%.[16] The combination of this compound with the esterase is virtually irreversible. Recovery of levels depends on synthesis of the enzyme. In the absence of inhibitors, this process requires 7 to 14 days. If therapy is discontinued, the excretion of the inhibitor requires 2 to 3 weeks. Thus, a significant reduction of enzyme continues for 4 to 6 weeks. After 1 week of therapy, plasma enzyme levels are 50% of normal. After 2 weeks of therapy, plasma enzyme levels are reduced to 30% of normal, and by 1 month, levels are less than 10% of normal. Thereafter, one sees a slow decline for a year to levels of 5%. Red blood cell activity is reduced to below 50% by 6 weeks of therapy. Because this drug taken daily is cumulative, other systemic adverse reactions of anticholinesterase action may be manifested.

β Blockers[17,18] and, specifically, timolol,[7] as an eyedrop solution are frequently used in glaucoma and decreases humor formation. These agents have minimal effects on vision and do not cause conjunctivitis, although they do have systemic effects at cardiac and pulmonary receptors.[19] Sinus bradycardia and reduction in cardiac output may be seen; cardiac arrest and bronchospasm have been reported.[13] Sensitivity to insulin occurs from systemic nonspecific β blockers, and glycogenolysis in muscle is decreased. Hence, hypoglycemia may ensue. A central effect may produce respiratory depression and apnea in infants.[20,21]

Newer β blockers, betaxolol and levobunolol, appear to be more selective in blocking β_1 receptors at concentrations below those required to block β_2 receptors in the bronchi.

ANESTHETICS: EFFECT ON INTRAOCULAR PRESSURE

Most inhalation anesthetic agents decrease intraocular pressure.[22] The decrease is nonspecific for these agents, but Magora and Collins indicated that the decrease is proportional to the depth of anesthesia, and the pressure reaches a common value or "floor" for all agents during deep anesthesia (EEG level III).[23] The following inhalation agents have been studied and confirm this general principle:

- Diethylether and cyclopropane[22]
- Chloroform and trichlorethylene[23]
- Carbon dioxide[24]
- Halothane[25,26]
- Methoxyflurane[27]
- Enflurane[26,28,29]

A "floor" level of intraocular pressure is often produced without regard to dosage or anesthetic depth. Enflurane appears to have this effect and produces a 40% decrease in intraocular pressure in light anesthesia with little or no further decline.[29]

Most of the following intravenous agents also lower intraocular pressure:

- Thiopental[22] (reduces intraocular pressure by 30%)
- Hydroxydione[23]
- Fentanyl (neuroleptanesthesia)[27,30]
- Diazepam[31]
- Etomidate[32] (reduces intraocular pressure by 50%)

With neurolept narcotics, one sees little or no change in light levels, but a uniform drop to a stable level at EEG level II or III.

Ketamine, the one exception of the commonly used intravenous agents, produces either a slight increase[33] or no significant change.[34]

MUSCLE RELAXANT DRUGS

With d-tubocurarine,[35] a significant fall occurs due probably to paralysis of extraocular striated muscles and intraocular ciliary muscles. However, d-tubocurarine decreases the coefficient of facility of outflow. Pretreatment with d-tubocurarine before succinylcholine fails to inhibit succinylcholine-induced elevations of intraocular pressure.[36]

Pancuronium produces no change or transient decreases in intraocular pressure.[37] The reduction amounts to about 20% in unanesthetized patients and about 30% after induction with thiopental-oxygen-nitrous oxide. The reduction remains for 3 to 8 minutes and continues lower, even after intubation.

The depolarizing muscle relaxants and, specifically, succinylcholine, produce a marked increase in intraocular pressure, approximately doubling the pressure and lasting 10 minutes or more.[38] This effect is due principally to the contraction of the extraocular striated muscles. Pretreatment with an antidepolarizing agent (d-tubocurarine) does not significantly alter the rise, nor does a large dose of thiopental immediately preceding the succinylcholine.[39]

MECHANISMS OF ANESTHETIC ACTION ON INTRAOCULAR PRESSURE

The usual decreases in intraocular pressure noted for most anesthetic agents may be related to several mechanisms:

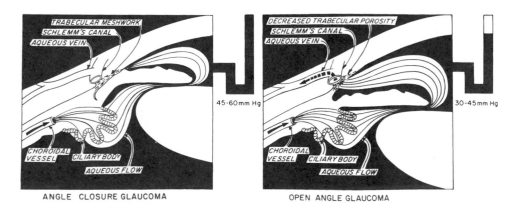

ANGLE CLOSURE GLAUCOMA

OPEN ANGLE GLAUCOMA

Fig. 45–3. Mechanism of the rise of intraocular pressure in angle-closure glaucoma (A) and in open-angle glaucoma due to trabecular obstruction preventing access to the canal of Schlemm (B). From Schwartz, B.: Concepts in ophthalmology. N Engl J Med 299:182, 1978.

- Depression of central control at ocular centers in hypothalamus, diencephalon and, midbrain[40]
- An increased coefficient in facility of outflow of aqueous humor by general anesthetics[22]
- Paralysis of extraocular striated muscles
- Paralysis of intraocular smooth muscles

REFERENCES

1. Schwartz, B.: Current concepts in ophthalmology: the glaucomas. N Engl J Med 299:182, 1978.
2. Adler, F. H.: Physiology of the Eye, 5th Ed. St. Louis, C. V. Mosby, 1970.
3. Hoskins, H. D., Jr., Kass, M.: Diagnosis and Therapy of the Glaucomas, 6th Ed. St. Louis, C. V. Mosby, 1989, p. 406.
4. Taylor, P.: Anticholinesterase agents. In Gilman, A.G., et al. (eds.). Goodman and Gilman's The Pharmacological Basis of Therapeutics, 8th Ed. New York, McGraw-Hill, 1990.
5. Maren, T. H.: Carbonic anhydrase: chemistry, physiology and inhibition. Physiol Rev 47:595, 1967.
6. Grant, W. M.: Systemic drugs and adverse influence on ocular pressure. In Leopold, I. H. (ed.). Symposium on Ocular Therapy. Vol. 3. St. Louis, C. V. Mosby, 1968, p. 57.
7. Boger, W. P.: Comparison of timolol and pilocarpine in glaucoma. Am J Ophthalmol 86:8, 1978.
8. Hepler, R. S., Frank, I. M.: Marihuana smoking and intraocular pressure. JAMA 217:1392, 1971.
9. Cohen, S.: Marihuana: possible therapeutic use. JAMA 240:1761, 1978.
10. Potter, D. E.: Adrenergic pharmacology of aqueous humor dynamics. Pharmacol Rev 33:133, 1981.
11. Spence, A. A.: Symposium on anaesthesia and the eye. Br J Anaesth 52:641, 1980.
12. McGoldrick, K.: Current concepts in anesthesia for ophthalmic surgery. Anesthesiol Rev 7:7, 1980.
13. Hiscox, P. E. A., McCulloch, C.: Cardiac arrest occurring in a patient on echothiophate iodide therapy. Am J Ophthalmol 60:425, 1965.
14. Epstein, E., Kaufman, I.: Systemic pilocarpine toxicity from over-dosage. Am J Ophthalmol 59:109, 1965.
15. Ellis, P. P., Esterdahl, M.: Echothiophate iodide therapy in children. Arch Ophthalmol 77:598, 1967.
16. De Roetth, W., et al.: Effect of phospholine on blood cholinesterase levels of normal and glaucoma subjects. Am J Ophthalmol 59:586, 1965.
17. Samuels, S. I., Maze, M.: Beta-receptor blockade following the use of eye drops. Anesthesiology 52:369, 1980.
18. Phillips, C. I., Howitt, G., Rowlands, D. J.: Propranolol as ocular hypotensive agent. Br J Ophthalmol 51:222, 1967.
19. Britman, N. A.: Cardiac effects of topical timolol. N Engl J Med 300:566, 1979.
20. Bailey, P. L.: Timolol postoperative apnea in neonates and young infants. Anesthesiology 61:622, 1984.
21. Two new beta-blockers for glaucoma. Med Lett 28:45, 1986.
22. Kornbleuth, W., et al.: Influence of general anesthesia on intraocular pressure in man. Arch Ophthalmol 61:84, 1959.
23. Magora, F., Collins, V.: The influence of anesthetic agents on intraocular pressure. Arch Ophthalmol 66:806, 1965.
24. Duncalf, D., Weitzner, S. W.: The influence of ventilation and hypercapnea on intraocular pressure during anesthesia. Anesth Analg 42:232, 1963.
25. Esposito, A. C.: The role of general anesthesia (halothane) in cataract surgery. South Med J 58:922, 1965.
26. Runciman, J. C., et al.: Intraocular pressure changes during halothane and enflurane anesthesia. Br J Anaesth 50:371, 1978.
27. Ivankovic, A. D., Lowe, J. H.: Influence of methoxyflurane and neurolept anesthesia on intraocular pressure in man. Anesth Analg 48:933, 1969.
28. Presbitero, J. V., et al.: Intraocular pressure during enflurane and neurolept anesthesia in adult patients undergoing ophthalmic surgery. Anesth Analg 59:50, 1980.
29. Zindel, G., Meistelman, C., Gandy, J. H.: Effects of increasing enflurane concentration on IOP. Br J Anaesth 59:440, 1987.
30. Feneck, R. O., Durkin, M. A.: A comparison between the effects of fentanyl, droperidol and halothane in intraocular pressure. Anaesthesia 42:266, 1987.
31. Cunningham, A. J., Albert, O., Cameron, J., Watson, A. G.: The effect of intravenous diazepam on rise of intraocular pressure following succinylcholine. Can Anaesth Soc J 28:581, 1981.
32. Calla, S., Gupta, A., Sen, N.: Comparison of effect of etomidate with thiopental. Br J Anaesth 59:437, 1987.
33. Corssen, G., Hay, J. E.: A new parenteral anesthetic CL-581: its effect on intraocular pressure. J Pediatr Ophthalmol 3:20, 1967.
34. Peuler, M., Glass, D. D., Arens, J. F.: Ketamine and intraocular pressure. Anesthesiology 43:575, 1975.
35. Al-Abrak, M. H., Samuel, J. R.: Effects of general anaesthesia on the intraocular pressure in man: comparison of tubocurarine and pancuronium with nitrous oxide and oxygen. Br J Ophthalmol 58:806, 1974.
36. Myers, E. F., et al.: Failure of non-depolarizing neuromuscular blockers to inhibit succinylcholine-induced increases in intraocular pressure. Anesthesiology 48:149, 1978.
37. Smith, R. B., Leano, N.: Intraocular pressure following pancuronium. Can Anaesth Soc J 20:742, 1974.
38. Lincoff, H. A.: The effect of succinylcholine on intraocular pressure. Am J Ophthalmol 40:501, 1955.
39. Cook, J. H.: The effect of succinylcholine on intraocular pressure. Anaesthesia 36:359, 1981.
40. Schmerl, E., Steinberg, B.: The role of the diencephalon in regulating ocular tension. Am J Ophthalmol 31:155, 1948.

IRON BALANCE AND HEMOCHROMATOSIS

IRON CONTENT OF THE BODY[1-9]

To maintain basic iron content and balance, the human body needs to replenish the daily losses. Iron is found in the body primarily in the hemoglobin of the red blood cells and in the myoglobin of muscle cells.[1] In a 70-kg man, about 2.5 g is located in the hemoglobin; 1 g of hemoglobin contains 3.4 mg of iron. Specifically, the four atoms of iron per molecule amount to 1.1 mg of iron per milliliter of red blood cells or the loss of 2.0 ml of whole blood; muscle myoglobin contains about 150 mg of iron, and traces of iron of about 15 mg are found in iron-dependent heme and nonheme tissue enzymes.[2] A small amount of iron, about 3.0 mg, is also found in plasma bound to transferrin being transported to the erythroid cells. A serum ferritin level less than 12 μg/L is diagnostic of iron deficiency.[3]

An excess of iron above that required for essential functions and amounting to 1.0 g is stored in the reticuloendothelial system and in the parenchymal cells of the liver bound to the protein ferritin.[4] This protein exists as individual molecules or in an aggregated form. The aggregated form represents the storage iron and is referred to as *hemosiderin*. The stored iron is about one third of the total body iron.

EXCRETION OF IRON

Normally, physiologic losses of iron are minimal and represent a remarkable ability of the body to conserve body iron. Only about 0.6 to 2.0 mg of iron is lost per day, or an average of 1.0 mg per day in adult men.[5] The turnover of total body iron is thus only about 10% per year.

About two thirds of the iron loss is through the gastrointestinal tract, as follows: as extravasated red blood cells; iron in the bilirubin (about 200 mg) derived from the breakdown of 6.0 g of hemoglobin by phagocytosis in the parenchymal cells of the liver; iron in the exfoliated intestinal mucosal cells containing iron bound to ferritin in a transitional stage or in storage. Another third of the iron is lost in the urine; trace amounts are lost in desquamated skin.

Apoferritin, a glycoprotein in the mucosal cells of the small intestine, has two binding sites for ferric iron.[4] Similarly, the plasma protein transferrin has two binding sites for ferric iron.

Additional losses occur in the female during menstruation, and this amounts to about 2.0 to 3.0 mg per day. Because the blood volume lost during the menstrual period is averaged at 45 ml,[8] the total iron lost during this period is about 22 mg. The loss of 2.0 ml of blood results in the loss of 1.0 mg or iron. Normally, 100 ml of blood contains approximately 50 mg of iron; the donation of 500 ml of blood results in the loss of 250 mg of iron.

IRON REQUIREMENTS[6]

About 20 mg of iron is required daily to form new hemoglobin for incorporation into the erythroid cells. This iron is furnished mostly by the recycling of heme. A smaller amount is needed to replenish the iron lost from the total amount in storage or reserve. This is accomplished by absorption of dietary iron.

RECYCLING OF IRON[7]

Part of the conservation of body iron is through the recycling of the heme iron following the destruction of senescent red blood cells. Normally, the red cells circulate for about 120 days before being catabolized by mononuclear phagocytes in the reticular endothelial system and in the hepatocytes. These mononuclear phagocytes are also located in the spleen and bone marrow and recognize senescent cells, engulf them, and proceed with their destruction intracellularly. The heme is dissociated from the globin chain and is oxidized, causing opening of the porphyrin ring with the release of iron. The iron is then carried by the protein transferrin to normoblasts in the bone marrow to be incorporated into new hemoglobin. About 6 g of hemoglobin is broken down in this manner each day. About 10% of the daily breakdown of red blood cells occurs intravascularly.

ABSORPTION

Only enough iron is absorbed daily from the diet to balance the iron loss of about 1.0 to 2.0 mg per day. The average for men is 1.0 mg (13 μg/kg per day), and it is 1.4 mg for menstruating women (21 μg/kg per day).

The bioavailability of iron in the food is of great importance. After partial digestion of food in the stomach and acidification of the contents, the iron is made available to the intestinal mucosa, mostly the duodenum or the upper intestine (where low pH and bile acids promote solubilization) as inorganic or heme-iron. Heme-iron is derived from meats, egg yolks, and fruits and represents 30% of the iron absorbed, although it constitutes only about 6% of the dietary iron.[8]

The amount of iron absorbed into the plasma or to be stored in absorptive mucosal cells depends on the iron content of the diet, but also to a large extent on an intrinsic mucosal regulatory mechanism.[4] In iron deficiency states, however, the most iron that can be absorbed is 3 to 4 mg of dietary iron per day.[9]

HEMOCHROMATOSIS: RECKLINGHAUSEN-APPLEBAUM DISEASE

Definition[10]

Hemochromatosis is an iron storage disease that results in cellular damage and fibrosis in many tissues and in multiple organs. Storage of iron in the body in the form of ferritin aggregates (hemosiderin) initially occurs in the mononuclear phagocytes of the reticuloendothelial system (hemosiderosis) and in the hepatocytes.

Major overload that results in the deposition of ferritin throughout the body, and in many organs so impaired, it is designated hemochromatosis. Such deposition then leads to organ failure and usually occurs when the total body iron exceeds 15 g.

Etiology

The disease can be inherited, and this form is the most common, designated primary hemosiderosis. It affects 3 to 8 of every 1000 persons and results from an autosomal recessive trait linked to the histocompatibility locus on chromosome 6p (the short arm).

Secondary hemochromatosis is an acquired form related to disorders that promote iron overload. Two principal causes are blood transfusions and increased dietary absorption. The disorder may result from long-term transfusion therapy (or massive transfusion) when a patient has received 60 to 100 units. Each unit of packed red blood cells contains 200 mg of iron. Accumulation of 10 g of iron generally correlates with the onset of clinical symptoms. Hemochromatosis also results from increased dietary absorption from excess ferric or ferrous salts or from an inherited intestinal failure of regulation of absorption.[10]

Signs and Symptoms[11]

Hemochromatosis is rare before middle age. The appearance of clinical symptoms is usually correlated with the accumulation of 10 g of iron. The typical manifestations are a triad of cirrhosis of the liver, diabetes mellitus (overt in 50 to 60% of patients), and bronze pigmentation of the skin.

Hepatic involvement leads to fibrosis or cirrhosis with esophageal varices, ascites, encephalopathy, and jaundice. Splenomegaly, platelet sequestration, and thrombocytopenia occur and are related to altered synthetic function of the liver. Hepatomas frequently occur in patients with long-standing siderosis.

Cardiac involvement is common.[12] Cardiomyopathy due to accumulation of over 50 g of iron is manifested by cardiomegaly, arrhythmias, atrioventriclar node dysfunction, and congestive heart failure.

In patients with endocrine involvement, adrenal gland infiltration leads to primary hyperaldosteronism. Thyroid gland accumulation of iron may result in hypothyroidism, and this occurs in about 10% of patients.

Pituitary failure is common and may be the cause of the frequently noted testicular atrophy and loss of libido.

Pathophysiology[12]

Presumably, all the symptoms and signs are due to the parenchymal iron deposition. The diabetes appears to be related to the destruction of the β cells in the pancreas and to problems secondary to hepatic gluconeogenesis; however, these patients have an increased familial incidence of diabetes.

Laboratory Studies

The serum iron and the percentage of saturation of transferrin are elevated early in the disease process. The serum iron is greater than 200 μg/dl, and the transferrin saturation is usually over 70%. The serum ferritin is usually 2000 ng/ml, and the red blood cell ferritin is 400 attogram per red blood cell. Liver biopsy demonstrates hepatic siderosis and cirrhosis and confirms the diagnosis. Family members should be screened by HLA typing and serum iron studies.

Treatment[13]

Phlebotomy and chelation therapy are the methods for removing excess iron from the body, and these treatments do improve survival. Phlebotomy should be initiated before advanced liver disease develops. Venisection should be done ideally twice a week for 6 months or more. Removal of 500 ml of blood removes about 250 mg of iron. This process should be continued until serum iron levels are normal and then every 3 to 4 months to maintain the serum levels below 150 μg/dl. The hemoglobin level may be maintained at 10 g/dl.

If anemia develops during venisection therapy, then chelation therapy should be instituted with deferoxamine. A daily dose of 20 to 40 mg/kg has a slow infusion either subcutaneously or intravenously over night by pump. Newer oral iron-chelating agents are now available.

Focal Hemosiderosis

This disorder occurs chiefly in the lungs and kidneys. Pulmonary hemosiderosis is due to recurrent hemorrhage into the lungs as an idiopathic entity and in mitral stenosis. The iron sequestration in the lungs may be severe and

may produce an iron deficiency anemia. Renal hemosiderosis is due to intravascular hemolysis from trauma and fragmentation of red blood cells. Such fragmentation can also occur in association with prosthetic valves and is seen in paroxysmal nocturnal hemoglobinuria. In these situations, free hemoglobin is filtered at the glomerulus and iron deposition occurs. No damage to the renal parenchyma occurs, but a severe hemosiderinuria may result in an iron deficiency. The treatment of these conditions is supportive, and the anemia responds to oral iron therapy.

Anesthetic Considerations[14]

Preanesthetic evaluation rests on the appraisal of the degree of organ impairment. *Hepatic involvement* may cause encephalopathy producing disorientation and somnolence that should be recognized and managed preoperatively. Ascites can compromise ventilatory function by reducing functional residual capacity. A distended abdomen may require a rapid sequence induction. The coagulation status should be evaluated, and measures should be taken to correct deficiencies.

Blood glucose levels should be monitored and abnormalities rectified to prevent complications of diabetic ketoacidosis or hyperosmolar coma. Fluid administration with Ringer's lactate solution may cause a metabolic acidosis because these patients may not be able to metabolize the lactate to bicarbonate.

Cardiac status review may reveal the presence of arrhythmias because the conduction system is often impaired.[12] When evidence of congestive heart failure exists, appropriate therapy is indicated, and caution must be exercised in the administration of fluids.

REFERENCES

1. Hillman, R. S.: Hematopoietic agents: iron and iron salts. *In* Gilman, A. G., et al. (eds.). Goodman and Gilman's The Pharmacological Basis of Therapeutics, 8th Ed. New York, McGraw-Hill, 1990.
2. Sigel, H.: Metal Ions in Biological Systems. Vol. 7. Iron in Model and Natural Compounds. New York, Marcel Dekker, 1977, p. 1.
3. Cook, J. D.: Clinical evaluation of iron deficiency. Semin Hematol 19:6, 1982.
4. Huebers, H. A., Finch, C. A.: The physiology of transferrin and transferrin receptors. Physiol Rev 67:520.
5. Green, R., et al.: Body iron excretion in man. A collaborative study. Am J Med 45:336, 1968.
6. Cook, J. D., Skikne, B. S., Lynch, S. R., Reusser, M. D.: Estimates of iron sufficiency in the U.S. population. Blood 68:726, 1986.
7. Hillman, R. S., Finch, C. A.: Red Cell Manual, 5th Ed. Philadelphia, F. A. Davis, 1985.
8. Hallberg, L.: Bioavailability of dietary iron in man. Annu Rev Nutr 1:123, 1981.
9. Bothwell, T. H., Charlton, R. W., Cook, J. D., Finch, C. A.: Iron Metabolism in Man. Oxford, Blackwell Scientific Publications, 1979.
10. Milder, M. S., et al.: Idiopathic hemochromatosis. Medicine 59:34, 1980.
11. Cazzola, M., et al.: Natural history of idiopathic refractory sideroblastic anemia. JAMA 257:2814, 1988.

12. James, T. N.: Pathology of the cardiac conduction system in hemochromatosis. N Engl J Med *271:*92, 1964.
13. Modell, B.: Advances in the use of iron-chelating agents for the treatment of iron overload. Prog Hematol *11:*267, 1979.
14. Levine, J. M.: Hemochromatosis: anesthetic implications. Anesthesiol Rev *21:*121, 1994.

LUPUS ERYTHEMATOSUS

SYSTEMIC LUPUS ERYTHEMATOSUS

Definitions[1,2]

Systemic lupus erythematosus is a multisystemic chronic inflammatory disorder characterized by changes in blood vessels and connective tissue and accompanied by autoantibody production. The antibodies are produced against the host antigens, and the inflammatory response causes tissue injury to various organs and systems of the host.

Origin of Terms[3]

The term "lupus" was used in the thirteenth century to describe skin conditions with erythema of the malar region of the face and the nose that produced a pattern resembling a wolf. Later, the pattern was described as resembling a butterfly.[4]

Incidence

This disorder is most frequently found in young women.[5] In the third and fourth decades of life, the incidence is in a ratio of 10 women to 1 man. Systemic lupus erythematosus also is seen in children and is more prevalent in dark-skinned people. The disease occurs in 1 of every 1000 persons. In a healthy population, under ordinary hygienic conditions, however, the risk of occurrence is less, at about 1 in 7000 persons.

Etiology

The cardinal feature of this disease is an immune-mediated tissue injury.[6] The major components of the immune system are three: (1) cellular elements (lymphocytes, plasma cells, macrophages); (2) humoral products of cells (immunoglobulins); and (3) complement. Ordinarily, these three components interact to rid the body of foreign substances and pathogenic organisms. If the immune response is directed toward discrete body tissue antigens, however, then autoantibodies are produced that induce inflammatory responses and destruction of different tissues and organs.

The precise inciting cause is unknown. Two mechanisms have been implicated. Trauma to mast cells is proposed as a mechanism causing the release of edema-producing substances that invade cells and lead to fibrin formation[3] and a classic inflammatory response.

A second mechanism suggests that the disorder is due to an autoimmune response. The sera of most patients contain antinuclear antibodies (ANA), which bind to diverse nucleic acid antigens, such as DNA or RNA. These antibodies are produced against host antigens, inducing the inflammatory response that leads to tissue injury.[6]

Another group of antibodies, known as antilipid antibodies, is responsible for the anticoagulant activity in lupus and for the anticardiac activity. These antibodies are of the IgG or IgM class and are found in 10 to 34% of patients with systemic lupus erythematosus.[7]

A genetic factor appears to play a role. The increased incidence in women may be related to X-chromosome determinant. Autoimmune disorders are also seen in relatives.

The formation of the autoantibodies may be induced by a virus, and viral antibody titers are known to be elevated in these patients.[8]

Pathology[9]

The histopathologic features are those of connective tissue, and the mechanism is uncertain. Blood vessels and the connective tissues of many organs are damaged, however.

Clinical Features[10]

Presenting symptoms and signs depend on the acuteness of the disease process and the systemic distribution. Usually, the patient complains of fever, which may develop abruptly or insidiously over several months. This is accompanied by an erythematous skin rash, as previously noted, in the face, appearing in the "butterfly pattern." Maculopapular lesions may be observed in areas of the skin exposed to the sun, such as the fingers, neck, upper chest, and elbows. These lesions may become bulbous and infected. Photosensitivity occurs in 40% of patients. Oral and nasal mucosal ulcerations may also occur and are seen in 50% of these patients.

Besides the characteristic rashes, an acute polyarthritis with significant pain is a common presenting manifestation. The joint pain is present in most patients and is the most frequent complaint, affecting the joints of the fingers, wrists, knees, and ankles. Major joints are not commonly afflicted.

Kidney damage[11] is common and may become evident at any time. The cardiovascular,[12] respiratory,[14] and nervous systems[15] are all affected. (See the discussion in this section on treatment.)

The following symptoms and signs are common:

- Recurrent pleurisy with or without effusion
- Pericarditis with or without myocarditis
- Pulmonary hypertension
- Generalized adenopathy
- Splenomegaly in 10% of patients (histologically, the spleen show periarterial fibrosis—"onion skin lesion")
- CNS involvement including organic brain syndrome

The American College of Rheumatology has classified criteria of systemic lupus erythematosus and has proposed that four of these criteria are required for the designation of this disease (Table 45-9).[2]

Table 45–9. Criteria for Classification of Systemic Lupus Erythematosus

Malar rash
Discoid rash
Photosensitivity
Oral ulcers
Arthritis
Serositis
  Pleuritis
  Pericarditis
Renal disorders
  Proteinuria
  Casts
Neurologic disorders
  Seizures
  Psychosis
Hematologic disorders
  Hemolytic anemias
  Leukopenia and lymphopenia
  Thrombocytopenia purpura
Immunologic disorders
  Type III immune complex disease
  Antilipid antibodies
  Lupus anticoagulant of the IgG or IgM class (in 10–34% of patients)
Antinuclear antibodies

Laboratory Findings

Leukopenia and serum hypoalbuminemia together with hyperglobulinemia are usually present. Anti-DNA antibodies in serum are characteristic and are found in 90% of patients. As the disease progresses, complement levels decrease.

A screening test for ANAs is the fluorescent test. It is positive in this disease, and a high titer is found in over 90% of the patients. The screening procedure should be followed by a more specific test for anti-DNA antibodies.

Diagnosis

The diagnosis requires evidence of disease in more than one organ system (usually four) together with serologic evidence of a disordered immune system, particularly antibodies to components of the cell nucleus.[10]

Treatment

Treatment varies with the severity of the disease, which may be either a mild process or a life-threatening disease.

Mild disease[16] is denoted by low fever, arthritis, pleurisy, headache, and rash. Such patients may require only symptomatic management. Arthralgia is usually controlled with nonsteroidal anti-inflammatory drugs. Aspirin is effective in relieving pain and is useful in counteracting any thrombolic tendency due to anticardiolipin antibodies. Antimalarial drugs are effective when skin and joint manifestations are prominent.

Severe disease is denoted by hemolytic anemia, thrombocytopenia, purpura, massive pleural and pericardial involvement, renal damage, and acute vasculitis of the extremities or of the gastrointestinal tract. The cardiovascular system is involved in over half these patients, and this involvement is manifested by myocarditis.[12] The respiratory system is involved in over 70% of the patients by pleural effusions; a friction rub represents pleurisy, is accompanied by pain, and may be one of the early symptoms. Noninfectious pulmonary infiltrates may be seen in radiographs.

Renal system involvement is commonly takes the form of glomerulitis and glomerulonephritis. This involvement usually occurs in at least 50% of patients within 2 years of onset.[13]

Neuropsychiatric changes occur in 50% of patients.[15] Fear and anxiety referable to the chronicity of the illness render the patient irritable, confused, and often psychotic. Peripheral neuropathies are frequently observed.[15]

Immediate corticosteroid (prednisone) therapy combined with immunosuppressive agents is recommended in acute systemic lupus erythematosus, especially when lupus nephritis appears. Immunosuppression is accomplished by azathioprine, 2.5 mg/kg per day, or cyclophosphamide, 2.5 mg/kg per day.[16]

Anesthetic Considerations

One must recognize two elements: (1) the multisystemic nature of the disease and the severity of organ involvement; and (2) the effect of the drugs used in treatment on the anesthetic regimen.

A systematic approach in evaluating the patient enables one to identify the organs damaged and permits one to select anesthetic agents appropriately. Intraoperative monitoring should be tailored to the disease, and the principles applied to that disease in other circumstances should be utilized.

Special attention should be directed to the pregnant patient.[18] The occurrence of pregnancy-induced hypertension is of particular concern, and spontaneous abortion occurs. The hypertension should be managed as in other patients. Similarly, patients with a history of coronary artery disease should be managed as other such patients.

Conditions in the Patient Selected for Anesthetic Comment

1. Ulcers on oral and nasal mucous membranes, especially on the central part of the hard palate near junction with soft palate, the buccal and gum mucosa, and the anterior nasal septum are common. Difficulties in inserting airways or laryngoscopes may be encountered, and mask fits are traumatic or poor.

2. Mobility of the temporomandibular joint may be impaired.[19] Laryngeal cartilages may be affected and may cause narrowing of the glottis. The arytenoid cartilage is often immobilized, and abduction of the vocal cords is reduced. The use of smaller endotracheal tubes may be indicated.

3. The lupus anticoagulant may have significant effects on the coagulation screen, and clotting times should be assessed preoperatively. The patient may have a prolonged partial thromboplastin time and, rarely, a

prolonged prothrombin time. This is not corrected by plasma.[20] These patients are at increased risk of thromboembolic complications, however.[7,21] Antibodies to coagulation proteins, particularly factor VIII and prothrombin, predispose the patient to hemorrhage.[22]

4. Peripheral neuropathies or fixed neurologic deficits may contraindicate regional anesthesia. Because psychologic features may be prominent, such as great anxiety and confusion, this situation may also preclude spinal-epidural and other regional anesthetic techniques.[15]

Medication Concerns

1. Long-term corticosteroid medication warrants perioperative steroid coverage. Prednisone seems to be the preferred agent.
2. Aspirin intake for rheumatic pain should be assessed and consideration given to discontinuing its preoperative use.[21,23]
3. Antimalarial drugs are used when joint and skin manifestations are prominent (hydroxychloroquine, 200 mg/day preferred). These drugs may cause diplopia but has low retinal toxicity.
4. Immunosuppressive agents as indicated in lupus nephritis should be followed by complete blood counts.
5. Some drugs, such as hydralazine, procainamide, and β blockers, produce positive ANA tests and occasionally a lupus-like syndrome in these patients. If such a drug is withdrawn, the adverse features disappear.[2]
6. Hypersensitivity rashes are produced by sulfonamides, sulfamethoxazole (with trimethoprim), penicillin, and other similar drugs.
7. When renal involvement is evident, drugs that are metabolized or cleared by the kidney should be avoided. Included are curare and enflurane.[24]

DISCOID LUPUS ERYTHEMATOSUS (CUTANEOUS LUPUS ERYTHEMATOSUS)

This chronic and recurrent disorder primarily affects the skin. It is characterized by circumscribed macules and papules displaying erythema, follicular plugging, scaling of the skin, telangiectasia, and atrophy.[2]

Symptoms and Signs

The disease is more common in females than in males, and it appears most often in women in their thirties, but the age range is wider than in systemic lupus erythematosus. The cause is unknown.

The active lesions are first presented as erythematous, round, scaling papules about 5 to 10 mm in diameter. Plugging of the skin follicles is usual. Appearance of the lesions is most often on the malar region, the bridge of the nose, the scalp, and the external auditory canals. They may be generalized over the trunk and extensor surfaces of the extremities. Mucous membranes are commonly involved, with blistering of the lips. Untreated lesions extend peripherally, and the center atrophies. Scars

form and are noncontractile. Mild systemic features include arthralgia and chronic synovitis. Eventually, 10% develop mild systemic disease.

Treatment

Exposure to sunlight must be minimized. A sunscreen preparation is advised. Small lesions may be involuted by applying topical corticosteroid ointments or creams three or four times daily (triamcinolone acetonide 0.1% or 0.5%; fluocinolone 0.025 or 0.2%). Betamethasone dipropionate 0.05% is most effective. In resistant cases, antimalarial agents, such as hydroxychloroquine, 200 mg per day, are useful.

REFERENCES

1. Dubois, E. L.: Lupus Erythematosus. Los Angeles, University of Southern California Press, 1978
2. Hughes, G. R.: Systemic lupus erythematosus (SLE). *In* Berbow, R. (ed.). Merck Manual of Diagnosis and Therapy. Rahway, NJ, Merck Research Laboratories, 1992, p. 1317.
3. Schur, P. H.: Systemic lupus erythematosus. *In* Syngaarden, J., Smith, L. H., Jr. (eds.). Cecil Textbook of Medicine. Philadelphia, W. B. Saunders, 1982, p. 1852.
4. Hebra, F., Kaposi, M.: On Diseases of the Skin, Including the Exanthemata. Vol. 4. (Fagge, H., Smith, P., Tay, W., trans. and eds.) London, New Sydenham Society, 1874.
5. Nicholas, N. S.: Rheumatic diseases in pregnancy. Br J Hosp Med *39:*50, 1988.
6. Hartley, J. B., Gaither, K. K.: Autoantibodies. Rheum Dis Clin North Am *14:*43, 1988.
7. Love, P. E., Santoro, S.A.: Antiphospholipid antibodies: anticardiolipin and the lupus anti-coagulant in systemic lupus erythematosus (SLE) and non-SLE disorders. Ann Intern Med *112:*682, 1990.
8. Tan, E. M.: Autoantibodies to nuclear antigens: their immunobiology and medicine. Adv Immunol *33:*167, 1982.
9. Klemperer, P., Pollack, A. D., Baehr, G.: Pathology of disseminated lupus erythematosus. Arch Pathol *32:*569, 1941.
10. Pisetsky, D. S.: Systemic lupus erythematosus. Med Clin North Am *70:*337, 1986.
11. Smith, M. F.: Skin and connective tissue disorders. *In* Katz, J., Steward, D. (eds.). Anesthesia and Uncommon Pediatric Diseases. Philadelphia, W. B. Saunders, 1987, p. 406.
12. Bulkley, B. H., Roberts, W. C.: The heart in systemic lupus erythematosis and the changes induced in it by corticosteroid therapy. Am J Med *58:*243, 1975.
13. Balow, J. E., et al.: Effective treatment of the evolution of renal abnormalities in lupus nephritis. N Engl J Med *311:*491, 1984.
14. Divertie, M. B.: Lung involvement in the connective tissue disorders. Med Clin North Am *48:*1015, 1964.
15. Feinglass, E. J., et al.: Neuropsychiatric manifestations of systemic lupus erythematosus: diagnosis, clinical spectrum and relationship to other features of the disease. Medicine *55:*323, 1976.
16. Muller, S. B.: Systemic lupus erythematosus. *In* Hurst, J. W. (ed.). Medicine for the Practicing Physician, 2nd Ed. Boston, Butterworth, 1988, p. 228.
17. Carette, S.: Cardiopulmonary manifestations of systemic lupus erythematosus. Rheum Dis Clin North Am *14:*135, 1988.
18. Davies, S. R.: Systemic lupus erythematosus and the obstetrical patient: implications for the anaesthetist. Can J Anaesth *38:*790, 1991.

19. Sourander, L. B., Pulkkinen, K.: Simultaneous occurrence of ankylosis of the cricoarytenoid joints with dyspnea and LE syndrome in rheumatoid arthritis. Acta Rheumatol Scand 8:255, 1962.
20. Espinoza, L. R., Hartman, R. C.: Significance of the lupus anticoagulant. Am J Hematol 22:331, 1986.
21. Malinow, A. M., et al.: Lupus anticoagulant. Anaesthesia 42:1291, 1987.
22. Triplett, D. A., Brandt, J. T.: Lupus anticoagulants: misnomer, paradox, riddle, epiphenomenon. Hematol Pathol 2:121, 1988.
23. Hindman, B. J., Koka, B. V.: Usefulness of the post-aspirin bleeding time. Anesthesiology 64:368, 1986.
24. Cousins, M. J., Mazzi, R. I.: Methoxyflurane nephrotoxicity. JAMA 225:1611, 1973.

MASTOCYTOSIS

Mastocytosis is an abnormal proliferation and accumulation of mast cells commonly in the skin, but not limited to this area, and is likely to involve multiple organs and sites selectively, such as the bone marrow, lymph nodes, liver, and gastrointestinal tract.[1] The dermal proliferation is manifested by macules, papules, or nodules with vesicle and bulla formation, particularly in infants and children.

Manifestations are related to the release of stored mediators from the mast cells. These are largely vasodepressor products, including heparin and prostaglandin D, as well as serotonin, hyaluronic acid, and histamine.

PATHOLOGY

Three principle forms are recognized.

1. Solitary mastocytomas of the skin
2. Urticaria Pigmentosa including telangiectasia macularis
3. Systemic mastocytosis involving organs: bone, liver, spleen and G-I tract.

Variants include diffuse cutaneous mastocytosis and isolated dermal infiltrates.

SYMPTOMS

Symptoms are protean. Episodic flushing, tachycardia, hypotension, abdominal pain, headache, and cardiovascular collapse are representative. Provocative and aggravating conditions include such stress situations as emotional upset, cold, physical exertion, anxiety, and trauma. Certain foods, such as beans, have also been implicated. Urine assay for prostaglandin D metabolites and histamine, usually elevated, is confirmatory. Treatment is generally symptomatic and includes antihistaminics, both H_1 and H_2 blockers, antimetabolites, steroids, and adrenocorticotropic hormone (ACTH). Ephedrine is an effective vasopressor agent, as are β_2 adrenergic stimulants. Chlorpheniramine, 25 mg, is frequently used to avoid or to attenuate a response.

ANESTHETIC CONSIDERATIONS[2,3]

Anesthetic considerations (Table 45–10) include careful preoperative evaluation, especially with intradermal

Table 45–10. Anesthetic Guidelines

1. Suspect the diagnosis: symptoms of unexplained episodes of pruritus, urticaria, flushing, dizziness.
2. Perform preoperative studies
   a) Skin biopsy: 10 mast cells/HPF is indicative
   b) Bone marrow biopsy: presence of mast cells
   c) Elevated serum and urine histamine
   d) Elevated urine levels of 5-hydroxy-indole acetic acid
   e) Elevated prostaglandin D_2 usually confirmatory
3. Determine sensitivity by intradermal skin injections of drugs to be used for anesthesia: e. g. butorphanol; glycopyrollate; pancuronium or vecuronium; IV induction agent: ketamine; propofol
4. Determine need for perioperative corticosteroid coverage
5. Position patient carefully to avoid skin friction
6. Determine use of prophylactic preoperative H_1 and H_2 blocking drugs
7. Choose drugs used in anesthesia
   Avoid:
   a) histamine releasing agents
   b) morphine and related congeners
   c) relaxants metocurine, curare, atracurium
   d) thiopental and pancuronium are suspect
8. Choose anesthetics and techniques
   Recommended: inhalational anesthetics
   Regional anesthesia: nerve blocks and epidural anesthesia have been successfully used (Scott)
   Use amide–type local anesthetic agent
9. Minimize rubbing the skin
10. Avoid fluctuations in temperature
11. Determine premedication; butorphanol has been successful
12. Manage airway as indicated
    Oral mucosa may be involved but not with bullae
    Note: Intravenous epinephrine solution should be readily available

Modified from Partridge. B. L., Skin and Bone Disorders, in Katz, J. Benumof, J. Kadis, L. B., eds. *Anesthesia and Uncommon Diseases,* W. B. Saunders, Third Edition, Philadelphia, 1990 p. 678-680.

testing of drugs intended to be used during the anesthetic state. Regional anesthesia with the amide local anesthetics has been recommended as safe, but lidocaine or bupivacaine should be skin tested. Analgesia with butorphanol, 0.5 mg, has been used without untoward effect and avoids the use of morphine and analogues. General anesthesia with ketamine induction and maintenance with nitrous oxide oxygen is recommended. Safe muscle relaxants include, first, vecuronium, and alternatively, pancuronium and atracurium.

REFERENCES

1. Kovenblat, P. E., et al.: Systemic mastocytosis. Arch Intern Med 144:2249, 1984.
2. Parris, W. C. V., Smith, B. E.: Management of mastocytosis in pregnancy. Anesthesiol Rev 13:17, 1986.
3. Katz, J., Benumof, J., Kaolis, L.: Mastocytosis. In Anesthesia and Uncommon Diseases. Philadelphia, W. B. Saunders, 1990, p. 678.
4. Scott, H. W., Parris, W. C. V., Sandidge, P. C., Oates, J. A., Roberts, L. J.: Hazards in operative management of patients with systemic mastocytosis. Ann Surg 197:507-513, 1983.

MIXED MULTIPLE ENDOCRINE NEOPLASTIC SYNDROMES (APUDOMAS)

DEFINITION[1]

Multiple endocrine neoplastic (MEN) syndromes are a group of genetically distinct familial diseases denoted by adenomatous hyperplasia and malignant tumor formation in several endocrine glands. Three distinct syndromes have been identified. Each is inherited as an autosomal dominant trait with a great penetrance, variable expressivity, and extensive pleiotropism. Although the syndromes are considered distinct, overlap is significant.

PATHOGENESIS[2]

These endocrine neoplasias are also called APUD-omas because they participate in the formation and secretion of amine hormones. This term, APUD, is an acronym for tumor cells of the Amine Precursor Uptake and Distribution system. Tumors of this system arise from two proposed cell lines derived embryologically from a common progenitor cell of the neural crest (Fig. 45–4).

- One cell line is of neuroentodermal origin and gives rise to carcinoid tumors of the gastrointestinal tract and lung, pituitary tumors, parathyroid tumors, and pancreatic islet tumors.[3]
- The second cell line is of ectodermal origin and gives rise to neurofibromas, medullary carcinoma of the thyroid gland, and pheochromocytomas.

CLASSIFICATION OF MULTIPLE ENDOCRINE NEOPLASIAS

The three syndromes are considered (Table 45–11).[1]

MEN I (Type I) Wermer's Syndrome

Parathyroid hyperplasia, or tumor, is the most common neoplasia of the MEN I syndrome and occurs in 90% of these patients. Asymptomatic hypercalcemia is the most common manifestation; about 25% of patients have symptoms of nephrolithiasis or nephrocalcinosis. Solitary adenomas are usually not seen.

Tumors of the islet cells of the pancreas occur in 80% of affected patients and are of two types:[4] about 40% are of the β cell and secrete insulin, causing fasting hypoglycemia; about 60% are of non-β cells and secrete excessive amounts of gastrin, causing hypersecretion of gastric juice and associated with complicated peptic ulceration (Zollinger-Ellison syndrome).[5] Investigation of patients presenting with Zollinger-Ellison syndrome reveals other tumors of the MEN complex in 20 to 30% of affected patients.

Some patients with non-β cell tumors have hypersecretion of glucagon and the ectopic secretion of ACTH and growth hormone-releasing hormone with appearance of acromegaly (Cushing's syndrome).[6]

Pituitary tumors are found in 65% of patients with MEN I; 25% of these patients show hypersecretion of growth hormone and present with acromegaly. These patients may have an associated enlarged tongue and epiglottis. Airway problems may be encountered. An equal number of these tumors secrete prolactin, and in these prolactinomas, a defect in dopaminergic regulation is probable. About 3% of the tumors secrete ACTH, producing Cushing's disease.[7]

MEN II Type II (Sipple's Syndrome) (IIa)

This syndrome is characterized by medullary carcinoma of the thyroid gland, pheochromocytoma, and hyperparathyroidism.[8] A chromosomal abnormality has been shown to be located on chromosome 10 by linkage studies. The disorder is inherited as a mendelian autosomal dominant trait. In several kindreds, a chromosomal deletion has also been noted on the short arm of chromosome 20.

Medullary carcinoma (MCT) of the thyroid occurs in over 90% of all patients with the MEN II syndrome.[9] The tumor is denoted by extensive biosynthetic activity, including the production of serotonin, histamines, ACTH, prostaglandins, and calcitonin. Elevated calcitonin levels are present in all patients with MCT.[10]

Pheochromocytoma is an integral part of this syndrome and occurs in over 75% of patients with MEN II.[11] The syndrome begins with adrenal medullary hyperplasia, it is multicentric, and it is usually bilateral (75%).

The tumor usually produces epinephrine. This feature may be the only abnormality early in the disease and is evident by hypertensive episodes that are paroxysmal and not sustained. The hyperplasic cells and the tumors are benign.

The diagnostic hallmark of a pheochromocytoma is the hypertension and the associated triad of diaphoresis, tachycardia, and headaches.[1] Less than 0.1% of all patients who are hypertensive have a pheochromocytoma. Up to 50% of patients who have an unrecognized tumor die in the perioperative period, however. Diagnosis is established by measurement of free catecholamines and specifically epinephrine levels in a 24-hour urine specimen. In the common sporadic forms of pheochromocytoma, norepinephrine is the predominant catecholamine secreted.

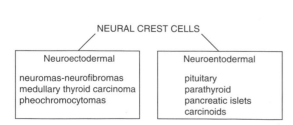

APUDOMAS: An acronym for amine precursor uptake and decarboxylation tumors

PATHOGENESIS: (Ellison and Neville)
Neoplasma of cell lines of neural crest cells

APUD System — Neoplasia
1) neuroectodermal
2) neuroentodermal

NEURAL CREST CELLS

Neuroectodermal	Neuroentodermal
neuromas-neurofibromas medullary thyroid carcinoma pheochromocytomas	pituitary parathyroid pancreatic islets carcinoids

Fig. 45–4. Mixed multiple endocrine neoplasia syndromes.

Table 45–11. Classification Mixed Multiple Endocrine Neoplastic Syndromes Apudomas (Acronym: Amine Precursor Uptake and Distribution)

MEN I (Wermer's syndrome; multiple endocrine adenomatosis)
  Inherited autosomal dominant
  Neuroentodermal neural crest cell origin
    1. Parathyroid (neoplasia): most common tumor of this syndrome (90%), either adenoma or hyperplasia
    2. Pancreatic (diffuse hyperplasia of islets or tumor): 80% of affected patients
       May produce gastrin non-β cell tumors (gastrointestinal ulcer)
       May produce insulin or glucagon-islet cell tumors in 40%
    3. Pituitary (neoplasia) prolactinoma (defect in dopaminergic regulation)
    4. Occasional pheochromocytoma
  Variants
    Thyroid
    Adrenal cortex
    Carcinoid: frequent
    Lipomas
    Brown fat tumors
  Gastric Polyps
    Schwannomas
    Thymomas
  G-tumors (non-β cell)
MEN II (MEN IIa; Sipple 1961)
  Autosomal dominant
  Genetic disorder of chromosome 10
  Neuroectodermal neural crest cell origin
    1. Pheochromocytoma: integral part, 76%; usually bilateral; rarely extra-adrenal or malignant
    2. Thyroid: medullary carcinoma (asymptomatic), 100% of patients
    3. Hyperparathyroidism (hyperplasia), 60% of patients
    4. Neurofibromatosis, 5% of patients
MEN III (MEN IIb)
    1. Pheochromocytoma (usually bilateral), 50% of patients
    2. Thyroid: medullary carcinoma, 100% of patients
    3. Mucosal neuromas: lips, tongue, eyelids
    4. Corneal neuromas (Marfan appearance)
    5. Parathyroid disorders: rare (Das Gupta)
Zollinger-Ellison Syndrome (MEN I)
    Jejunal ulcer
    Gastric hypersecretion
    Islet tumor (G-cells)
    Secretion 10 mEq/h
    Gastrinoma (Wolfe)
Probably a separate endocrine tumor entity

Modified from Albert;[2] Ellison;[3] Cagel[14] and Landsberg.[1]

About 25% of patients within the MEN II kindred have clinical evidence of *hyperparathyroidism* with hypercalcemia, nephrolithiasis, or renal dysfunction, hypophosphatemia, and increased parathormone levels. Another 25% of patients without biochemical evidence of these abnormalities have parathyroid hyperplasia.

MEN Type III Syndrome (IIb)

This type III syndrome is also designated multiple endocrine adenomatosis (MEA III).[12] The hallmark is the presence of multiple mucosal neuromas, which are found in 100% of patients, and a marfanoid habitus. Medullary carcinoma of the thyroid gland is present in over 90% of patients in this category, whereas 60% of these patients manifest pheochromocytoma signs.

A specific genetic marker for MEN III has not been determined; however, the kindred of MEN III patients have a deletion of the short arm of chromosome 20, as in MEN II kindreds.

Gastrointestinal abnormalities are common, consisting of altered motility and occasionally megacolon. This condition is considered to be related to a diffuse intestinal ganglioneuromatosis. Skeletal abnormalities of the spine and of the chest (pes cavus) and talipes equinovarus are common. The complete syndrome is seen in only 50% of the patients.

This syndrome is usually not diagnosed until the presence of medullary carcinoma of the thyroid or pheochromocytoma is recognized in later life. Early diagnosis of medullary carcinoma is important. If pheochromocytoma is present, it should be surgically excised first, followed by total thyroidectomy.

CLINICAL FEATURES

These features depend on the type of endocrine tumors presented. Onset of symptoms may appear as early as the first decade of life or as late as the second decade. Management is directed specifically to the symptoms of each functionally active tumor as determined. Surgical removal of tumors is generally necessary.

ANESTHETIC CONSIDERATIONS

1. Thorough assessment of the cardinal features of each syndrome is mandatory.
2. Prior medical control of the abnormal functions requires the input of an endocrinologist.
3. Anatomic abnormalities are evident from a careful physical examination that have a bearing on the airway and anesthetic techniques.
4. Induction of anesthesia should be accomplished by slow intravenous administration of midazolam or thiopental.
5. Most inhalation anesthetic agents are acceptable. Preferred agents are enflurane and isoflurane. Enflurane is of particular value in patients with pheochromocytoma because it blocks the output of chromoffin cells.[13]
6. Because many of the surgical procedures are prolonged and require careful monitoring, one should avoid halothane except in young children.
7. Muscle relaxation with current nondepolarizing relaxants is recommended. Succinylcholine is not recommended.
8. In the syndromes with both pheochromocytoma and carcinoma of the thyroid gland, the pheochromocytoma should be excised first.

REFERENCES

1. Landsberg, L., Daly, P.: Multiple endocrine neoplasms: MEN Syndromes. *In* Berkow, R. (ed.). Merck Manual of Diagnosis and Therapy. Rahway, NJ, Merck Research Laboratories, 1992, p. 1100.
2. Albert, W. M., McMeekin, J. O., George, J. M.: Mixed multiple endocrine neoplasia syndromes. JAMA *244:*1236, 1980.
3. Ellison, M. L., Neville, A. M.: Neoplasia and ectopic hormone production. *In* Raven, R. W. (ed.). Modern Trends in Oncology. London, Butterworth, 1973, p. 163.
4. Schimke, R. N.: Multiple endocrine adenomatosis syndromes. Adv Intern Med *21:*249, 1976.
5. Cameron, D., Spiro, H. M., Landsberg, L.: Zollinger-Ellison syndrome with multiple endocrine adenomatosis type II. N Engl J Med *299:*152, 1978.
6. Hermus, A. R., et al.: Transition from pituitary-dependent to adrenal-dependent Cushing's syndrome. N Engl J Med *318:*966, 1988.
7. Findling, J. W.: The Cushing syndromes, an enlarging clinical spectrum. N Engl J Med *321:*1677, 1989.
8. Keiser, H. R.: Sipple's syndrome: medullary thyroid carcinoma, pheochromocytoma and parathyroid disease. Ann Intern Med *78:*561, 1973.
9. Wells, W. A., Jr., Norton, J. A.: Medullary carcinoma of the thyroid and multiple endocrine neoplasia-II syndrome. *In* Fiesen, S. R., Boliknger, R. E. (eds.). Surgical Endocrinology: Clinical Syndromes. Philadelphia, J. B. Lippincott, 1978, p. 287.
10. Tashjian, A. H., Jr.: Immunoassay of human calcitonin: clinical measurement relations to serum calcium and to patients with medullary carcinoma. N Engl J Med *283:*890, 1970.
11. Bravo, E. L., Gifford, R. W.: Pheochromocytoma: diagnosis localization and management. N Engl J Med *311:*1298, 1984.
12. Khairi, M. R. A., et al.: Mucosal neuroma, pheochromocytoma and medullary thyroid carcinoma: multiple endocrine neoplasia type III. Medicine *54:*89, 1975.
13. Gothert, M., Wendt, J.: Inhibition of adrenal medullary catecholamine secretion. Anesthesiology *46:*400, 1977.
14. Cagel, R. F.: Multiple Endocrine Neoplasia. *In* Williams Textbook of Endocrinology. 8th Ed. pp. 1537–1553. Philadelphia: W. B. Saunders Co. 1992.

MULTIPLE MYELOMA

This disease is the malignant neoplastic form of plasma cell dyscrasias. Multiple myeloma is characterized by abnormal proliferation of one clone of plasma cells in the bone marrow, with bone tumor formation and overproduction of monoclonal immunoglobulins.[1] Polypeptide units of protein of the Bence Jones type are also produced. These are the light chain elements of the globulin fraction. Ordinarily, plasma cells are engaged in immunoglobulin synthesis, and electrophoretic examination of the serum shows an M-component spike. Patients have a significant proteinemia, but some of the immunoglobulins produced in the malignant melanoma condition are abnormal in that they have limited antibody activity and a poor response to antigen challenge.[2]

CLINICAL FEATURES

This disease is a malignant process of unknown origin and with an onset at over 40 years of age. The incidence is approximately 3 per 100,000 population. Men are affected approximately twice as often as women. Exposure to radiation may be a factor in the development of proliferation of the plasma cells. The disease is progressive and ultimately fatal.

PATHOLOGIC FEATURES

Expanding plasma cell tumors are found in the marrow of almost any bone, but most frequently in the pelvis, ribs, and skull, including the mandible. The expanding tumors produce diffuse osteoporosis, as well as lytic lesions. The latter may be related to a humoral factor secreted by the plasma cells. The consequences of this osteoporosis and lysis are hypercalcemia, anemia, and pancytopenia.

Plasma cell infiltrates may be seen in any organ. The kidney is particularly susceptible, with renal tubular cell atrophy and cast formation seen in the renal tubules. Interstitial renal deposits are followed by fibrosis and renal insufficiency or failure. Amyloidosis occurs in about 10% of patients, especially in the presence of Bence Jones-type protein (light chain peptide) production with extensive proteinuria. Of the immunoglobulins, IgG is present in the serum in 50% of patients, and IgA is noted in 20%. About half these patients have Bence Jones protein, whereas amyloidosis occurs in about 10% of the patients.

SYMPTOMS AND SIGNS

Pain is perhaps the earliest symptom, resulting from bone involvement, periosteal distention, and pressure on adjacent nerves.[3]

Pathologic fractures of long bones, sternum, ribs, clavicle, and vertebrae are common. Radicular pain is secondary to vertebral osteoporosis and collapse. The pain is also related to the pressure of the plasma cell tumors on nerves.

NEUROPATHY

Neurologic signs of paresthesis and changes in position sense are frequent.

The anemia that accompanies this disorder results in significant weakness.[4]

Renal insufficiency and failure are common causes of death. Decreasing urine output is a consequence of dehydration, and precipitation of protein occurs in the renal tubules.

Vomiting is a common feature, as well as other gastrointestinal disturbances.

Because of the poor immune response to infections, various types of skin and oral infections recur, and pneumonia is frequent.[5]

LABORATORY FINDINGS

Proteinuria is characteristic, with as much as 20 to 30 g protein excreted per day. Despite the hyperproteinemia and the high τ-globulin fraction, a poor response exists to antigenic insults.

Hypercalcemia and hypercalciuria occur and result in a secondary form of hyperparathyroidism with generalized weakness, apathy, and sluggish gastrointestinal motility.[6] Constipation is a frequent concomitant condition. ECG changes are frequent, and arrhythmias leading up to ventricular fibrillation are noted, especially when the calcium levels exceed 14 mg/dl. This disorder is also associated with cardiovascular collapse. Calcium may affect the anesthetic considerations.

ANESTHETIC CONSIDERATIONS

Osteoporosis

Osteoporosis may be generalized.[3] Gentle care in the movement and positioning of patients must be exercised to prevent pathologic fractures.

Airway Management

With the frequency of plasma cell tumors in the cervical and occipital region, extension of the neck may be hazardous and painful. One should determine the range of motion acceptable to the patient while the patient is awake and without pain. Any involvement of the mandible, as demonstrated by radiographs, or pain or painful movement at the temple or mandibular joint, is a warning sign. Even a pharyngeal airway, when inserted against resistance, may cause fracture of the mandible.

Medications for Pain

These patients are usually receiving high doses of analgesics and opioids. Hydromorphone is a useful drug in older patients, inasmuch as the agent has little or no sedative action, but effective analgesia; 1 mg is equivalent to 8 mg of morphine. Doses of 1.0 to 2.0 mg every 3 to 4 hours are not uncommon. This type of baseline analgesia is frequently prescribed. Superimposed on this basic analgesic regimen may be additional doses of meperidine or alphaprodine. One must be aware that tolerance readily develops.

Therapeutic Medications

Prednisone is used in patients with hypercalcemia as a means for immunosuppression, as are anticancer drugs of the alkylating type, such as cyclophosphamide, melphalan (nitrogen mustard), and cisplatin. Cyclophosphamide lowers plasma cholinesterase and should be considered in the selection of muscle relaxants. Thrombocytopenia and a chronic pneumonitis may exist.

Radiation therapy is often employed, and so fibrosis of the mandible, mouth, and neck may be present.

Neuropathy

The neurologic signs that are often present,[3] particularly when the disease has invaded the vertebral column with pressure on nerve roots and cord compression, are a valid reason for avoiding subarachnoid spinal anesthesia or epidural anesthesia. Moreover, infiltration of peripheral nerves and a demyelinating-type syndrome may be seen.

Anemia

Normocytic, normochromic anemia is common. The patient may have a concomitant bleeding diathesis, and both leukopenia and thrombocytopenia may exist. Erythropoietin has been useful in treating the anemia.[4]

Associated with weight loss is generalized debility, and this becomes pronounced as the disorder progresses.

Renal Insufficiency

Renal failure is a common cause of death. A decrease of urine output occurs as a consequence of both dehydration and precipitation of protein in renal tubules. One must prevent the oliguria by adequate hydration and thereby minimize the precipitation of protein in the renal tubules.

Muscle Relaxants

The antidepolarizing agents are well tolerated. Hypercalcemia does affect the release of acetylcholine.[6] Cyclophosphamide decreases plasma cholinesterase, however, and lower doses of succinylcholine should be used. Calcium levels can be reduced with corticosteroids or by infusion of potassium-containing solutions.

Cardiac Considerations

As previously noted, arrhythmias and cardiovascular collapse are not infrequent, related in large measure to the high levels of plasma calcium. Calcium levels can be lowered with corticosteroid treatment and infusions of potassium-containing solutions.

POSTOPERATIVE COURSE

1. Respiratory insufficiency due to muscle weakness and pulmonary changes necessitates respiratory support.
2. Atelectasis and pneumonia are frequent, and prophylactic measures are warranted.[5]
3. Hydration must be continued vigorously in the postoperative period. For pain relief, it must be continued at a high level to prevent renal failure and nephrolithiasis, to reduce the concentration of calcium, and to prevent hyperviscosity.
4. Pain relief must be pursued vigorously, as in the preoperative period.
5. Measures to prevent cooling must be taken because cryoglobulin precipitation may otherwise occur.

REFERENCES

1. Harvey, A. M., et al.: The Principles and Practice of Medicine, 20th Ed. New York, Appleton-Century-Crofts, 1980.
2. Griffiths, L. L., Brews, V. A. L.: The electrophoretic pattern in multiple myelomatosis. J Clin Pathol 6:187, 1953.
3. Rousseau, J. J., et al.: Osteosclerotic myeloma with polyneuropathy and ectopic secretion of calcitonin. Eur J Cancer 14:133, 1978.
4. Ludwig, H., et al.: Erythropoietin treatment of anemia associated with multiple myeloma. N Engl J Med 322:1693, 1990.
5. Zimmerman, H. H., Hall, W. H.: Recurrent pneumonia in multiple myeloma and some observations on immunological response. Arch Intern Med 103:173, 1959.
6. Hutter, O. R., Kostial, K.: Effect of magnesium and calcium ions on the release of acetylcholine. J Physiol 124:234, 1954.

NEUROFIBROMATOSIS (VON RECKLINGHAUSEN'S DISEASE)

Neurofibromatoses are genetic disorders that primarily affect cell growth of neural tissues. Two distinct forms are recognized, but variant forms may exist. The names used in the past to describe these forms were found to be inaccurate and incomplete. The National Institute of Health Consensus Development Conference on Neurofibromatosis in 1987[1] adopted a numbered classification for these disorders.

The most common type of neurofibromatosis is Von Recklinghausen's neurofibromatosis, previously called peripheral neurofibromatosis but now named neurofibromatosis-1, or NF-1. Bilateral acoustic neuromatosis, previously known as central neurofibromatosis, is now named neurofibromatosis-2 or NF-2. Because NF-1 and NF-2 have both peripheral and central manifestations, these terms should be discarded for classification as misleading.

Table 45–12 lists the diagnostic criteria for the two types of neurofibromatosis as outlined at the consensus conference.

Table 45–12. Diagnostic Criteria for the Neurofibromatoses

Neurofibromatosis 1 (diagnosed when 2 or more of the following are present.)
    Six or more café au lait macules whose greatest diameter is >5 mm in prepubertal patients and >15 mm in postpubertal patients
    Two or more neurofibromas of any type, or one plexiform neurofibroma
    Freckling in the axillary or inguinal region
    Optic glioma
    Two or more Lisch nodules (iris hamartomas)
    A distinctive osseous lesion (e.g., sphenoid dysplasia or thinning of long bone cortex), with or without pseudarthrosis
    A parent, sibling, or child with neurofibromatosis 1 according to the above criteria
Neurofibromatosis 2 (diagnosed when 1 of the following is present)
    Bilateral eighth-nerve masses seen with appropriate imaging techniques (CT or MRI)
    A parent, sibling, or child with neurofibromatosis 2 and either unilateral eighth-nerve mass or any two of the following: neurofibroma, meningioma, glioma, schwannoma, or juvenile posterior subcapsular lenticular opacity

From Martuza, R. L., Eldredge, R.: Neurofibromatosis 2. N. Engl J Med 318:684, 1988.

NEUROFIBROMATOSIS-1 (NF-1)

Patients with NF-1 may have Schwann cell tumors on any nerve in the body, but bilateral acoustic neuromas are virtually nonexistent in this group of patients.[2]

Other forms of neurofibromatosis occur but are not classified:

- Segmental neurofibromatosis is characterized by having café au lait spots and cutaneous neurofibromas limited to a circumscribed body segment. Intrathoracic or intra-abdominal neurofibromas may be present. The ipsilateral extremity may also be involved. This condition represents a somatic postzygotic mutation.
- Multiple café au lait spots present without freckling, neurofibromas, Lisch nodules, or visceral manifestations.
- Intracranial, or spinal, meningiomas appear in the second or third decade in the same family.

Pathophysiology

Taking into account the cellular components of the characteristic lesions of neurofibromatosis, such as, café au lait spots, neurofibromas, and various tumors of the CNS, neural crest is the most likely embryologic origin in broad general terms,[3] and particularly the neuroectodermal line.

The property of APUD, sometimes used to identify cells of neural crest origin, is inadequate, because not all neural crest derivatives have this property and some that are not neural crest derivatives may have it.[4,5]

Clinical Features of Neurofibromatosis-1

Genetic Basis

Von Recklinghausen's disease is a relatively common inherited disorder of the human nervous system. Von Recklinghausen in 1882 described the entity.[6] This syndrome is transmitted as an autosomal dominant mutation without any racial, ethnic, or national restrictions. NF-1 mutation has been localized to the long arm of chromosome 17.[7] Both sexes are affected equally, and penetrance is virtually 100%, so any offspring born has a 50% chance of developing the tumors.[8] NF-1 is a progressive disorder affecting 1 in 350,000 of the population. A nerve growth factor with functional activity may be involved in NF-1. The gene for this factor has been identified.[9]

Diagnostic Elements

The diagnostic triad of NF-1 is as follows: (1) multiple café au lait spots; (2) multiple neurofibromas; and (3) Lisch nodules (pigmented iris hamartomas). One sees an increase with age in the number and size of the hyperpigmented skin lesions and of the tumors in all sites, especially the skin and in the number of Lisch nodules. Except for these defining features, which usually occur more than once in all patients, no other feature is constant or even found in as many as 50% of the patients, and the presence of one feature does not correlate with the severity or presence of any other feature.

Pigmentary Skin Changes

Three types of pigmentary skin changes are seen in classic neurofibromatosis:

1. Café au lait spots are found in over 99% of all patients with NF-1. Six or more of these spots larger than 1.5 cm diameter in adults are one of the diagnostic features of NF-1.[10] These spots vary in size from 1 to 2 mm to 15 cm and appear from the age of 1 year and continue to grow in the first decade. They grow randomly over the body and present no threat to health.
2. Freckling consists of areas of hyperpigmentation up to 2 to 3 m in diameter, occurring frequently in the axilla and groin, in opposing surfaces of skin folds resulting from obesity, and in the inframammary region.
3. Hyperpigmented patches are darker than café au lait spots, and the borders of these patches correspond with an underlying plexiform neurofibroma. If one of these patches extends to the midline in the back, it often indicates that the tumor underneath involves the spinal cord.[11]

Neurofibromas

These lesions occur mostly on skin as nodular, sessile, or pedunculated tumors or may involve deeper peripheral nerves or nerve roots. Viscera and blood vessels may have neurofibromas from the autonomic nerves innervating them. The skin neurofibromas usually do not appear until after puberty.[12]

Plexiform neurofibromas may grow in deeper subcutaneous tissues in a diffuse manner interdigitating with the surrounding tissue (and underlying bone) and producing deformity, which is sometimes grotesque. This has been exemplified in the elephant man, John Merrick.[13-15]

Histopathology

Neurofibromas are benign and comprise various combinations of neurons, Schwann cells, fibroblasts, vascular elements, mast cells, and pigment cells. Puberty and pregnancy cause an increase in the number and size of the neurofibromas.[16]

Neurofibromas may undergo a malignant change into a neurofibrosarcoma. Alteration of p 53, locus on the short arm of chromosome 17, is found to be critical in the progression of a neurofibroma to a neurofibrosarcoma.[17] In this respect, tumors subjected to repeated trauma and friction should be excised.

If neurofibromas in infancy and childhood compress the cervical or mediastinal area, they may be life-threatening because of possible involvement of the airway and vascular or neurologic functions.[8] Timely surgery is recommended to remove cutaneous neurofibromas that are disfiguring or functionally compromising. Early recognition of surgically correctable complications and early surgical intervention minimize serious complications. Some plexiform neurofibromas in mediastinum may be inoperable.

Lisch Nodules

Lisch nodules are the most common clinical feature of NF-1 in adults. They are melanocytic hamartomas that appear as well-defined, dome shaped elevations projecting from the surface of the iris and are clear to yellow or brown. Although these nodules were first described by Waardenburg in 1918,[18] not until 1937 did Lisch[19] report their distinctive association with Von Recklinghausen's disease NF-1.[20] These lesions increase in number with age. In a large series of patients with NF-1,[21] only 5% of the children less than 3 years old had Lisch nodules. Among children aged 3 to 4 years, the prevalence was 42%, and it was 55% among children 5 to 6 years old. All adults 21 years of age or older had Lisch nodules (95%). These nodules often appear before neurofibromas in children. They are not found as a rule in patients with NF-2.[8] Symptoms are not produced by Lisch nodules, but they allow one to discriminate between types of neurofibromatosis and between persons who bear a mutation at the NF-1 locus on the long arm of chromosome 17 and those who do not.[20]

Other Clinical Features

Initial evaluation with history and physical examination should give particular attention to the following possible manifestations of NF-1.[8]

Macrocephaly may be absolute or relative and is postnatal in onset. It is not secondary to hydrocephalus or brain tumor. Half of all cases of congenital pseudoarthrosis are due to neurofibromatosis. The most common site is the tibia, followed by the radius. Tibial bowing should be treated by bracing to prevent fracture and subsequent pseudarthrosis. This feature is more common in males.

Kyphoscoliosis occurs in 2% of patients and involves the lower cervical and upper thoracic spine. The patient has acute anterior angulation and "S" shaped rotatory scoliosis. This condition develops between the ages of 5 and 15. Early fitting with braces, and, if the condition progresses, aggressive surgical intervention in the form of spinal fusion may prevent progression and may thus avoid cardiopulmonary and neurologic complications. Short stature is common and bears no correlation with other features of neurofibromatosis.

Association with malignancy has been reported.[22] In addition to malignant degeneration of a neurofibroma, certain malignant diseases such as Wilms's tumor, rhabdomyosarcoma, and several types of leukemia are more common in patients with neurofibromatosis than in the general population.

Pheochromocytoma occurs in less than 1% of the patients. Some patients have several neurofibromatoses (especially cervical) that secrete excessive amounts of norepinephrine and have catecholamines and their metabolites in the urine.

Optic pathway gliomas occur in 15% of patients with NF-1. Early detection through screening of asymptomatic patients with neuroimaging and visual evoked-response studies may prevent dysfunction.

Hypertension may be coincidental or secondary to pheochromocytoma or secondary to extramural or intramural involvement of the renal artery.

Miscellaneous complaints have been reported.[8] *Headache* is common in patients with neurofibromatosis. It may be secondary to brain tumors, but most frequently the cause is unknown. *Constipation* occurs in 10% of patients and requires life-long attention.[23] It is due to disorganization of Auerbach's plexus and tunica muscularis in the colon. *Pruritus* occurs in the skin overlying the cutaneous neurofibromas or following blunt trauma to the skin. Itching is aggravated by heat and diminished by bath or shower. Antihistamines partially relieve the itching. Mast cells and histamine are probably responsible for the itching. *Seizures* are frequently seen, both major and minor, as complications of neurofibromatosis. *Endocrine disorders* in addition to pheochromocytoma include medullary thyroid carcinoma (C cell) and sometimes hyperparathyroidism.

Pregnancy and NF-1[24]

Fertility does not seem to be impaired, but these patients experience a higher than expected rate of first-trimester spontaneous abortion (20.7%), stillbirths (8.7%), intrauterine growth retardation (13.0%), and a higher rate of cesarean section (26.0%) than the general population. Patients with NF-1 constitute a high-risk group in danger of developing life-threatening complications. With proper antenatal care, however, most patients can be delivered of their infants safely if pregnancy continues beyond the first trimester. Each child born to an affected person has a 50% chance of having NF-1.

Psychologic considerations are important in these patients. Cosmetic disfigurement, functional compromise, and fear of untimely death from cancer and other complications affect the patient's emotional, psychologic, and social well-being. Family members suffer equally. Frank discussions should aim at decreasing adverse concern and should provide a realistic approach for future management.

All patients with neurofibromatosis should undergo baseline evaluation to confirm diagnosis, to identify complications, and to monitor progression. Evaluation should include the following[8]:

- Intelligence quotient and psychologic testing
- EEG, audiography
- Slit-lamp ocular examination
- Radiography of the skeleton with special attention to skull, spine, internal auditory canals
- CT scan of cranium with and without dye contrast to include orbit and optic chiasma
- Visual evoked-response studies
- 24-hour urine testing for measurement of the levels of epinephrine, norepinephrine, and their metabolites

Other tests should be guided by findings on clinical evaluation.

Clinical Course and Prognosis

Progression is a common feature in all patients with neurofibromatosis. Growth of tumors in neurofibromatosis seem to be influenced by hormones. Investigators have suggested that sex hormones, acting directly or through nerve growth factor, influence the appearance of tumors and their growth in both forms of neurofibromatoses.[9] In NF-1, café au lait spots may be present from birth, but neurofibromas usually do not appear until puberty.[12] Acostic neuromas usually become symptomatic during or soon after puberty.[2] During pregnancy, tumors of the skin and spine may appear and enlarge in NF-1,[10] and one usually notes the onset or exaggeration of symptoms during pregnancy in NF-2.[24]

Life span is usually normal unless malignant diseases or other complications develop. No cure for the neurofibromatosis exists, and treatment consists of amelioration of symptoms and surgery.

NEUROFIBROMATOSIS-2

In 1917, Cushing[25] designated the formation of bilateral acoustic neuroma as a form of neurofibromatosis because of the similarity of this disorder to Von Recklinghausen's disease in certain aspects. Family studies of bilateral acoustic neuromas showed consistency with which bilateral acoustic neuromas developed in those affected and indicated that a single mutant gene was responsible for the disorder. The genetic abnormality and clinical expressions of patients with bilateral acoustic neurofibromas are distinct from those of Von Recklinghausen's neurofibromatosis.

Genetic Basis

The inherited gene for NF-2 is on the long arm of chromosome 22,[26,27] and it is inherited also in an autosomal dominant pattern. A glial growth factor may be involved in the abnormal proliferation of Schwann cells in acoustic neuromas.[28]

Clinical Features

The hallmark of diagnosis of NF-2 is bilateral acoustic neuromas in various members of the family tree. NF-2 should be suspected under the following circumstances[29]:

- The parent, sibling, or a child has NF-2; a person under 30 years of age has symptoms of unilateral acoustic neuroma.
- A child has a meningeal or Schwann cell tumor.
- An adolescent or adult has no history of NF-1, but has a few café au lait spots and a few neurofibromas on the skin, but has no Lisch nodules.
- A person has multiple CNS tumors not attributable to another disorder.

These patients require a careful examination for skin tumors and plexiform tumors and an eye examination for lenticular opacity and for Lisch nodules (which should be absent). Neurologic assessment should be made of cranial nerves, balance, and coordination. Tests should include audiogram with brain stem auditory-evoked response (BAER) study. If the abnormal BAER of impaired hearing suggests acoustic neuroma, then magnetic resonance imaging (MRI) of the head should be performed to search for acoustic neuromas and other brain tumors. MRI provides more detailed imaging than CT of the characteristic central nervous system lesions of neurofibromatosis. MRI, especially with gadolinium enhancement, provides superior soft tissue contrast without ionizing radiation and may be the method of choice for following certain patients and screening family members.[30]

If auditory-evoked response and MRI are negative, then no further tests are necessary.

Signs and Symptoms

The symptoms of bilateral acoustic neurofibromatosis usually begin in the teens or early twenties, but patients may become symptomatic in the first decade or as late as the seventh decade of life. One must differentiate between NF-2 and sporadic unilateral acoustic neuroma. The solitary acoustic neuroma tends to develop late in life, is not inherited, and is much easier to manage.

The first symptom of NF-2 is loss of hearing, generally unilateral, and the patient first notices it when using a telephone. The patient may give a history of intermittent ringing or roaring in one or both ears and some unsteadiness in walking at night on uneven ground.

Other symptoms may include facial weakness, headache, seizures, or a change in vision. Café au lait spots may be present, although less commonly than in NF-1. The patient may have a few neurofibromas on the skin and visible or palpable masses under the skin that would indicate plexiform neurofibroma on deeper nerves. Motor, or sensory, changes suggest spinal cord tumor.

Presenile lens opacities, or subcapsular cataract, may be found in about 50% of patients, and these opacities precede the onset of symptoms of acoustic neuroma.[31]

Histopathology[29]

Tumors of the CNS are common in NF-2. The bilateral acoustic neuromas are Schwann cell tumors that arise from the vestibular nerves and hence are vestibular schwannomas. Other tumors of meningial and glial origin may be present in the same patient.

Schwann cell tumors are the most common and may develop on any of the cranial nerves or spinal roots, particularly those involving sensation; the dorsal horns of the spinal cord may be involved with these tumors.[32,33] Removal of the tumors of the acoustic nerve at the early stages without damage to the cochlear nerve may be possible.

Progress of tumor growth is unpredictable. One or both acoustic neuromas may progress rapidly leading to deafness ataxia, headache, visual disturbances, paralysis, and death due to brain stem compression. Alternatively, one may see little growth for many years, and the patient may not have significant limitations.

The growth of individual tumors is best followed by CT and MRI.

Prognosis

Prognosis is unpredictable. The major risks to the patient are the loss of hearing and vestibular function. Underwater activities and climbing are to be avoided. The risk of developing intracranial or intraspinal neoplasms is increased.

Counseling should discuss the possibility of hearing loss, and future education and career should be planned accordingly.

To preserve hearing and to avoid damage to the auditory nerve, it is much better to operate when the tumor is small. During surgery for eighth nerve tumors, auditory and facial nerve monitoring should be used to minimize injury to the nerves.

ANESTHETIC CONSIDERATIONS

Anesthesia for patients with neurofibromatosis is usually uneventful, but careful preanesthetic evaluation is essential before general or regional anesthesia is planned. The following problems need special consideration:

- Unrecognized pheochromocytoma may be lethal.[34] The incidence of pheochromocytoma among patients with neurofibromatosis has been reported to be as high as 13%.[35]
- Renal hypertension caused by compression of renal arteries by neurofibromas may activate the renin-angiotensin system.[36]
- Skin lesions offer a problem in starting arterial or intravenous lines for fluid administration or monitoring.

- Pulmonary function may be compromised by fibrosis of the lung or by cystic disease.
- Truncal obesity is frequent.
- Hypoglycemia may be related to intraperitoneal fibromas affecting the pancreas.
- Medullary thyroid (C cell) carcinoma is occasionally found and may induce secondary hyperparathyroidism. Other endocrine dysfunctions are not a feature of either type.
- Airway patency may be compromised. Tumors causing airway problems during induction of anesthesia include pharyngeal, intraoral, laryngeal, and intratracheal.[37-39] Tumors in the cervical mediastinum may distort the normal anatomy by moving or compressing the larynx, trachea, or bronchi.
- Kyphyscoliosis may influence positioning of patient during operation, and, if advanced, may cause cardiorespiratory and neurologic compromise. Neurofibroma impinging on the dorsal nerve roots may present with radiating pain or pressure on the spinal cord, with neurologic damage. Autonomic nerves may also be involved.
- Headache is a common feature in patients with neurofibromatosis and may indicate increased intracranial pressure and intracranial tumors. They may be primary neurofibromas or associated tumors such as astrocytomas or meningiomas.
- Cranial nerve involvement may impair the swallowing or gag reflex. When spinal or epidural anesthesia is considered, possible future development of neurofibroma involving the spinal cord and its implications should be recognized.
- Seizure incidence is 20 times higher in patients with neurofibromatosis than in the general population.
- Prolonged responses to nondepolarizing muscle relaxants have been reported using d-tubocurarine[40] and pancuronium,[41] and myasthenic responses have been reported with the use of d-tubocurarine.[42] Resistance to succinylcholine has been reported by Baraka, who noticed no fasciculations or significant neuromuscular block when succinylcholine was administered.[42] Yamashita and co-workers noted an increased sensitivity to succinylcholine.[43]

Undue sensitivity to muscle relaxants should suggest the possibility of a malignant neuropathy or a myasthenic syndrome.

Monitoring of neuromuscular block with the administration of the muscle relaxant in incremental doses is recommended. Anesthetic management should be tailored to the pathologic process uncovered preoperatively.

REFERENCES

1. National Institutes of Health Consensus Development Conference on Neurofibromatosis: Conference statement. Arch Neurol 45:575, 1988.
2. Eldridge, R.: Central neurofibromatosis with bilateral acoustic neuroma. Adv Neurol 29:57, 1981.
3. Bolande, R. P.: Neurofibromatosis: the quintessential neurocristopathy: pathogenic concepts and relations. Adv Neurol 29:67, 1981.
4. Pearse, A. G. E., Polak, J. M.: Endocrine tumors of neural crest origin: neurolymphomas apudomas and the APUD concept. Med Biol 52:3, 1974.
5. Andrew, A.: APUD cells, apudomas and the neural crest. S Afr Med J 50:890, 1976.
6. Von Recklinghausen, F.: Ueber die Multiplen Fibroma der Haut und ihre 7. Beziehung zu den multiplen Neuromen. Berlin, A. Hirschwald, 1882.
7. Barker, D., et al.: Gene for Von Recklinghausen neurofibromatosis is in the pericentromeric region of chromosome 17. Science 236:1100, 1987.
8. Riccardi, Vincent M.: Von Recklinghausen, F: Neurofibromatosis N Engl J Med 305:1617, 1981.
9. Ulrich, A., et al.: Human B-nerve growth factor gene Nature 303:821, 1983.
10. Crowe, F. W., Schull, W. J., Neel, J. V.: A Clinical Pathological and Genetic Study of Multiple Neurofibromatosis. Springfield, IL, Charles C Thomas, 1956.
11. Riccardi, V. M.: Cutaneous manifestations of neurofibromatosis: cellular interaction, pigmentation and mast cells. Birth Defects 17:129, 1981.
12. Braesfield, R. D., Gas Gupta, T. K.: Von Recklinghausen's disease: a clinicopathological study. Ann Surg 175:86, 1972.
13. Lott, I. T., Richardson, E. P.: Neuropathological findings and the biology of neurofibromatosis. Adv Neurol 29:23, 1981.
14. Montagu, A.; The Elephant Man: A Study in Human Dignity, 2nd Ed. New York, E.P. Dutton, 1979.
15. Howell, M., Ford, P.: The True History of the Elephant Man. London, Allison and Busby, 1980.
16. Jarvis, G. J., Crompton, A. C.: Neurofibromatosis and pregnancy. Br J Obstet Gynaecol 85:844, 1978.
17. Menon, A. G., et al.: Chromosome 17p deletions and P53 gene mutations associated with the formation of malignant neurofibromatosis in Von Recklinghausen neurofibromatosis. Proc Natl Acad Sci USA 87:5435, 1990.
18. Waardenburg, P. J.: Heterochrome en melanosis. Ned Tijdschr Geneeskd 2:1453, 1918.
19. Lisch, K.: Ueber Beteiligung der Augen, insbesondere das Vorkommen Von irisknotchen bei der Neurofibromastose (Reckenhausen). Z Augenheilkd 93:137, 1937.
20. Riccardi, V. M.: Neurofibromatosis: past, present and future (editorial). N Engl J Med 324:1283, 1991.
21. Lubs M.-L. E., et al.: Lisch nodules in neurofibromatosis type 1. N Engl J Med 324:1264, 1991.
22. Hope, D. G., Mulvihill, J. J.: Malignancy in neurofibromatosis Adv Neurol 29:33, 1981.
23. Monzer, J.: Abnormal responses in Von Recklinghausen's disease Br J Anaesth 42:183, 1970.
24. Weissman, A., et al.: Neurofibromatosis and pregnancy: an update. J Reprod Med 38:890, 1993.
25. Cushing, H.: Tumors of the Nervus Acusticus. Philadelphia, W.B. Saunders, 1917.
26. Rouleau, C. A., et al.: Genetic linkage of bilateral acoustic neurofibromatosis to a DNA marker on chromosome 22. Nature 329:246, 1987.
27. Seizinger, B. R., Martuza, R. L., Gusella, F.: Loss of genes on chromosome 22 in tumorigenis of human acoustic neuroma. Nature 322:644, 1986.
28. Brockes, J. P., Breakefield, X. O., Martuza, R. L.: Glial growth factor-like activity in Schwann cell tumors. Ann Neurol 20:317, 1986.
29. Martuza, R. L., Eldridge, R.: Neurofibromatosis-2 (bilateral acoustic neurofibromatosis). N Engl J Med 318:684, 1988.
30. Truhan, A. P.: Magnetic resonance imaging: its role in the neuroradiologic evaluation of neurofibromatosis, tuberous sclerosis and Sturge-Weber syndrome. Arch Dermatol 129:219, 1993.

31. Pearson-Webb, M. A., Kaiser-Kupfer, M. I., Eldridge, R.: Eye findings in bilateral acoustic (central) neurofibromatosis: association with pre-senile lens opacities and cataracts but absence of Lisch nodules. N Engl J Med *315*:1553, 1986.

32. Rubenstein, L. J.: Tumors of the Central Nervous System. Washington, D.C., Armed Forces Institute of Pathology, 1972.

33. Rubenstein, A. E., Mytilineau, C., Yahr, M. D., Revoltella, R.P.: Neurological aspects of neurofibromatosis. Adv Neurol *29*:11, 1981.

34. Knoonce, C. H., Pollock, B. E., Glassy, F. J.: Bilateral pheochromocytoma associated with neurofibromatosis: death following aortography. Am Heart J *44*:901, 1952.

35. Chapman, R. C., Kemp, V. E., Taliaferro, L.: Pheochromocytoma associated with multiple neurofibromatosis and intracranial hemangioma. Am J Med *26*:883, 1959.

36. Allen, T. N. K., Davies, E. R.: Neurofibromatosis of the renal artery. Br J Radiol *43*:906, 1970.

37. Fisher, M.: Anaesthetic difficulties in neurofibromatosis. Anaesthesia *30*:648, 1975.

38. Crozier, W.: Upper airway obstruction in neurofibromatosis. Anaesthesia *42*:1209, 1987.

39. Morris, H. D., Patterson, W. J.: Neurofibromatosis of the laryngopharynx. Can J Otolaryngol *211*:17, 1973.

40. Manser, J.: Abnormal responses in Von Recklinghausen's disease. Br J Anaesth *42*:183, 1970.

41. Magbagbeola, J. A. O.: Abnormal responses to muscle relaxants in a patient with Von Recklinghausen's disease (multiple neurofibromatosis). Br J Anaesth *42*:710, 1970.

42. Baraka, A.: Myasthenic response to muscle relaxants in Von Recklinghausen's disease. Br J Anaesth *46*:701, 1974.

43. Yamashita, M.: Anesthetic considerations in Von Recklinghausen's disease: abnormal responses to neuromuscular relaxants. Anaesthetist *26*:317, 1977.

OBESITY

Of all the problems encountered in patients coming to surgery, obesity is one of the most frequent. A weight 20% over the predicted is abnormal and a health hazard, whereas double the desired weight is pathologic.[1] The present table of desirable weight is related to habitus or body frame (Tables 45-13 and 45-14).[2,3] Some 20% of the population, in the age group over 20 years, is overweight. One of every 10 males is 30% or more overweight, and one of every 10 females is 40 to 50% overweight (Table 45-15). At any given age, the mortality rate is 30 to 60% over the predicted rate.[4] In the age group from 25 to 35 years, the mortality for obese persons is 12-fold greater than nonobese persons; for ages 36 to 45 years, the mortality in obese persons is 6-fold greater; in the age group from 46 to 55 years, the mortality of obese persons is 3-fold greater than in nonobese persons.[1,5] Such an omnipresent problem must be given serious attention by all physicians.

PATHOPHYSIOLOGY

Obesity is a disease.[6,7] Two types appear to exist[8]: one is *regulatory,* in which food addiction exists beyond body needs, and the other is *metabolic,* in which disturbed metabolism favors deposition of fat. Factors in the development of obesity are varied. These may either alter caloric intake or change energy expenditure. Obesity may

Table 45–13. Desirable Weights for Men

Height (Ft.–In.)	Small Frame	Medium Frame	Large Frame
5–2	128–134	131–141	138–150
5–3	130–136	133–143	140–153
5–4	132–138	135–145	142–156
5–5	134–140	137–148	144–160
5–6	136–142	139–151	146–164
5–7	138–145	142–154	149–168
5–8	140–148	145–157	152–172
5–9	142–151	148–160	155–176
5–10	144–154	151–163	158–180
5–11	146–157	154–166	161–184
6–0	149–160	157–170	164–188
6–1	152–164	160–174	168–192
6–2	155–168	164–178	172–197
6–3	158–172	167–182	176–202
6–4	162–176	171–187	181–207

From Entmacher, P. S.: New Weight Standards for Men and Women. Statistic Bulletins. New York, Metropolitan Life Insurance Company, 1983.

Table 45–14. Desirable Weights for Women

Height (Ft.–In.)	Small Frame	Medium Frame	Large Frame
4–10	102–111	109–121	118–131
4–11	103–113	111–123	120–134
5–0	104–115	113–126	122–137
5–1	106–118	115–129	125–140
5–2	108–121	118–132	128–143
5–3	111–124	121–135	131–147
5–4	114–127	124–138	134–151
5–5	117–130	127–141	137–155
5–6	120–133	130–144	140–159
5–7	123–136	133–147	143–163
5–8	126–139	136–150	146–167
5–9	129–142	139–153	149–170
5–10	132–145	142–156	152–173
5–11	135–148	145–159	155–176
6–0	138–151	148–162	158–179

From Entmacher, P. S.: New Weight Standards for Men and Women. Statistic Bulletin. New York, Metropolitan Life Insurance Company, 1983.

Table 45–15. Obesity Population

General incidence
  Men: 15% } 20 to 75 years of age: 20% overweight
  Women: 25%
Severe obesity
  Men: 5%: 30% + overweight
  Women: 7%: 50% + overweight
Morbid obesity
  Twice average desirable weight
  0.25% of population or 600,000 persons

be the sequela of illness, of a chance inherent gene, or of a multitude of stimuli that derange hypothalamic appetite or satiety control, metabolic paths, and enzymatic processes.[9]

With respect to caloric intake, this is increased because of involvement of the CNS by such processes as organic disease, trauma, or a "functional state," as in habit patterns. Furthermore, low-calorie diets do not appear to curb the basic disease process in severe obesity, and an imposed starvation program may further damage the health of a patient.

Major Etiologic Factors

Constitutional Factors

Heredity may play a role.[10] The trait has been demonstrated in animals and is carried as a dominant gene.[11,12] Obesity tends to be familial. Overweight children become overweight adults 90% of the time. One fourth of adult-onset diabetics were overweight children. Environmental factors appear to play a more dominant role in some instances, however.

Psychologic attributes of those 50% or more overweight are significant. Severely obese patients have low self-esteem, are self-conscious, and feel helpless. They are subject to depression and dislike being disturbed. Hostility is frequent.

Hypothalamic Factors[13]

Overeating may be due either to hyperphagia or to interference with the satiety mechanism. Two diencephalic-hypothalamic centers are involved in the control or appetite: the feeding center and the satiety center. The sensor of the hypothalamic controller is considered to be glucoreceptors in the hypothalamus that respond to the amount of glucose available in the blood perfusing the area.

The feeding center is located in the lateral area and is a constantly activated mechanism.[14] Destruction or injury results in cessation of feeding and loss of appetite. Normally, this center is inhibited by the satiety center located in the ventromedial area. Injury of this area releases the appetite and feeding centers from any inhibition; an uncontrolled appetite follows, accompanied by constant eating, and the result is pathologic obesity.

Metabolic Factors[15]

High-carbohydrate diets increase insulin demands. Glucose intolerance is a common association of obesity, and relative insulin resistance exists. Obese, nondiabetic persons respond to glucose with an excess of insulin in their plasma.[16] Large adipose cells are less sensitive to insulin. These cells are insulin dependent for entrance of glucose into the cell, and, in obesity, the requirement is greater. Decreased membrane and receptor binding may not be the principal defect, however, and intracellular metabolic processes may instead be compromised.

Degree of Physical Activity

This factor bears a close relation to weight gain and loss. Exercise decreases insulin requirements and enhances the entrance of glucose into muscle cells.

Endocrine Factors

Many of the following factors are interrelated: hypothyroidism; prolonged use of insulin; Cushing's syndrome; and adipose-genital disturbances. These factors are common accompaniments of obesity.

CNS Factors

Emotional distress, prefrontal lobotomy, and encephalitis are associated with the development of obesity.

Stress[17]

Under this category is included severe physical injury, infections, shock, emotional upset, and drug stress. The sudden development of obesity following severe infections such as tuberculosis, meningitis, and scarlet fever has been reported.

Evidence indicates that the obese person has a significant reduction in the number of sodium-potassium pump units of about 22%, as compared with nonobese persons. This adenosine triphosphatase (ATPase) pump mechanism uses considerable energy estimated at 20 to 50% of total cellular thermogeneses and metabolism to maintain proper sodium and potassium levels.[18]

These complex factors may be involved primarily or secondarily. Any of the basic mechanisms of weight control, namely, the hypothalamic or metabolic, may be triggered or altered by toxic agents, stress (pregnancy or surgery), infections, and endocrine derangements.

Body Fat[17,19]

The normal fat content of a healthy person is about 5 to 10% of body weight. White fat tissue in the adult has an appreciable blood supply and is active metabolically. Fat tissue has a low specific gravity. Active individuals have a high body specific gravity, and sedentary subjects have a low body specific gravity. This circumstance exists even when heights and weights are the same in the two occupation groups. Thus, various weight tables may be misleading. Furthermore, the aging process is a factor. The bodies of older people contain, in general, about 21% fat, whereas young healthy people have less than 10% body fat.

Brown fat is a specialized form of fat tissue that plays a role in thermogenesis. The cells are rich in mitochondria and lamellated cristae with a high cytochrome oxidase level. The brown fat tissue is highly innervated and richly vascular. It represents 27% of fat in infants, but it is replaced by white fat with age. It is rich in all hibernating species of animals. Exposure to heat causes atrophy. In animals, 50% of warming energy is derived from this fat.

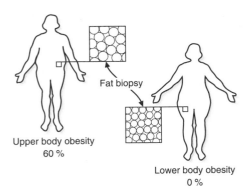

Upper body obesity
60 %

Lower body obesity
0 %

Fig. 45–5. Prevalence of diabetes and relation to fat cell size. Redrawn from JAMA Med News *247:*731, 1982; after Kissebah, A.: J Clin Endocrinol Metab *54:*254, 1982.

Histophysiology[15]

Normal adipose cells number about 30 billion in a person of normal body weight. Each cell has a fat content of 0.25 mg/cell.[20] On a histologic basis, one may define two types of cellular obesity,[21] namely, hypercellular obesity and hypertrophic obesity. In the hypercellular type, the obesity is of the lower body, whereas in the hypertrophic type, the obesity is of the upper body in which the regular fat cells are engorged (Fig. 45-5).

In morbid obesity (100% overweight, or more), the fat content is 50 to 80% of body weight. The excess fat is present in two forms:

1. As increased storage in the normal numbers of fat cells. These cells have a fat content of 0.7 to 1.0 mg/cell.
2. In the increased number of adipose cells, where a fourfold increase from 30 to 120 billion cells may occur.[20]

ESTIMATION OF OVERWEIGHT[11,22]

Determination of overweight should reflect the degree of fatness. The commonly used derivative of weight to height is a relative weight index and compares the weight-height of the subject to a *standard weight* for persons of that height and sex. The standard weights are based on data from insurance populations and provide tables of "desirable weight."

Other indexes avoid reference to standards and use a simple ratio of weight to height (W/H). This ratio underestimates the amount of fat.

The Ponderal index, introduced by Levy in 1887, is also a relationship between weight and height, but it uses a power function of weight to height

$$\sqrt[3]{\frac{W}{H}}$$

This calculation overestimates the degree of fatness and obesity.

The body mass index (BMI), originally called Quetelet's rule (the body weight of an adult should be as many kilograms as the body length is in centimeters), is an anthropometric measurement. It also relates weight to a power function of height as W/H^2 to minimize the influence of height on weight in any correlation to true fatness. The BMI is one of the best indicators of obesity.[7,22] It is determined as a ratio of weight in kilograms to height in meters squared, or kg/m^2 (Table 45-16). An index of 30 represents the cutoff point (Table 45-17), and values above this number are associated with increased mortality.[1]

Brocas' index enables one to estimate the ideal weight in kilograms, but it does not take into account body build. The height in centimeters minus 100 equals the ideal weight of a person.

Lean body mass can be determined accurately by measuring body potassium. In this technique, radioactive potassium-40 (^{40}K) is employed, and total body radiation is counted. Total body potassium is proportional to lean body mass less bone, fat, and water. This is an accurate, but complex, method useful for investigations.

Clinical Estimation of Overweight[23]

A practical and predictable determination of the percentage of fat and an estimation of overweight can be made at the bedside by measurement of skin fat folds.

A skinfold caliper (Lange) is employed. Two sites for measurement may be used:

1. The triceps: an area midway between the shoulder and the elbow on the posterior aspect of the upper arm. This underestimates the percentage of fat.
2. The scapula: a point overlying the inferior (angle) aspect the scapula.

Table 45–16. Body Mass Index

$\dfrac{\text{Weight in Kilograms}}{\text{Height in Meters}^2} = \text{BMI}$	
20–25	Normal
25–30	20% overweight
31–35	Moderate
36*–40	Severe
40–50	Pathologic (double desired weight)
50+	Morbid

*Desirable weight according to current Metropolitan Life Insurance Company tables.
From Entmacher, P. S.: New Weight Standards for Men and Women. Statistic Bulletins. New York, Metropolitan Life Insurance Company, 1983.

Table 45–17. Classification of Obesity

	Degree	Body Fat (%)
Not overweight	Nonobese	<10
5–10% overweight	Mild	16
10–20% overweight	Moderate	20
20–40% overweight	Severe	27
50–100% overweight	Pathologic	62
100%+ overweight	Morbid	75–80

Table 45–18. Scapular Skinfold Test

Skin Fold (mm)	Fat (%)	Overweight (%)
4–5	9–10	Normal lean
10	16	10
15	21	15
20	27	20
25	33	25
40	50	40
50	62	50

From Crook, G. H.: Evaluation of skin-fold measurements and weight chart to measure body fat. JAMA 198:39, 1966.

The skin and subcutaneous tissues are lifted by pinching between the examiner's thumb and forefinger while the caliper is used to measure the thickness of the fold; with experience, the pinched fold may be approximated without the caliper.

Skinfold measurement, percentage of fat, and percentage of overweight are summarized in Table 45–18. Correlation with height-weight table standards is closest with scapular measurements. Accuracy is within 10% of the true fat value. Moreover, correlation with the "potassium technique" shows that a skinfold measurement gives a dependable measurement of fat.

The scapular fold measurement is reliable[23]: a thickness of 5 mm represents less than 10% fat body content of a normal weight. A skinfold thickness of 10 mm corresponds to a fat percentage of 16% (10% overweight); 15 mm corresponds to 21% fat; 20 mm corresponds to 27% fat (20% overweight); and 25 mm corresponds to 33% fat (25% overweight).

BODY FAT DISTRIBUTION: AN INDEX OF MORBIDITY[24] (BY CIRCUMFERENCE OF WAIST-TO-HIP RATIO)

The ratio of waist circumference to hip circumference (W/H ratio) in centimeters has been found to be a better marker than BMI as a risk factor of morbity and mortality in older women (age over 55 years). Measurements are made by a tape measure: the waist circumference is determined at 1 inch (2.5 cm) above the umbilicus, and the hip measurement at the level of the maximal protuberance. These anthropometric measures have been found reliable and valid.

The mean W/H ratio was found to be 0.84 (± 0.09) with a relative risk of 1.0. Mortality rates have been found positively associated with W/H ratio in a monotonic fashion. Waist circumference alone or hip circumference were less strongly associated with mortality. The association of waist circumference shows a J-shaped death rate per 1000 person years, however, whereas the hip circumference alone was found to be U-shaped as regards mortality. For each 0.15-unit increase in W/H ratio (e.g., a 15-cm increase in waist measurement in a woman with a 100-cm (40-inch) hip measurement), the relative risk of death is associated with a 60% increase in the risk of death.[24]

ASSOCIATED DISEASES AND PROBLEMS[7,25]

Obesity is a disease. In addition, it imposes a physical burden on the victim and predisposes to other diseases. It has been aptly stated the "corpulency is not only a disease itself, but the harbinger of others."[7] Among the diseases associated with obesity, the following are significant:

1. *Cardiovascular disorders:* Arteriosclerosis and arterial hypertension are common. Hypertension is 3 times more frequent in obese subjects. In the Framingham Heart Disease Study,[26] hypertension occurred 10 times more frequently in persons 20% overweight than in the normal-weight population. Hypercholesterolemia is usual. Advanced atherosclerosis and particularly coronary and renal involvement are twice as frequent in obese persons as in the general population.[27] Angina pectoris and coronary insufficiency are common, whereas ischemic heart disease occurs twice as often in the obese person.

    Cerebrovascular disease and accidents are three times as frequent in obese subjects[28] as in normal-weight persons. Weight reduction is accompanied by reductions of blood pressure. Accompanying the weight loss is a fall in plasma renin activity and aldosterone levels.[25]

    As a result of increased pulmonary resistance, patients develop pulmonary hypertension and cor pulmonale. The pulmonic second sound is accentuated. Cardiac output is elevated and increases linearly with weight. A 100-kg increase above ideal weight doubles resting cardiac output. This change is expected because of the general body demands. Pulmonary artery pressure is elevated; the pulmonary capillary wedge pressure and the left ventricular end-diastolic pressure are elevated, reflecting left atrial and ventricular stress. Cardiomegaly is demonstrable in obese persons whether they are hypertensive or not.[29]

    A relationship between BMI and left ventricular hypertrophy has been shown to be remarkably strong. Left ventricular mass (normalized for height) was shown to increase by 10.2 g/m² in men and by 9.3 g/m² in women for every 4.0 kg/m² in BMI. This relationship was observed across the full range of obesity. Significant increased left ventricular wall thickness was present and appears to increase with increasing BMI.

    The ECG commonly shows the following: prolonged QT interval; reduced QRS voltage. First- and second-degree heart block are frequent.[28]
2. *Renal disturbances:* Aluminumuria is frequent.
3. *Fat storage:* Abnormal sites of fat storage can be observed. Infiltration of the heart and of the pancreas is seen. An excessive accumulation of fat occurs in the liver. Adipose tissue cysts are a notable abnormality.
4. *Diabetes mellitus:* An elevated blood sugar and impaired glucose tolerance exist in the obese person

whether overt insulin-dependent diabetes exists or not.[30] Diabetes tends to occur in obese persons, however, and 20% of overweight persons develop diabetes; that is, the frequency of diabetes in the obese adult is 3 to 4 times the rate in comparable nonobese adults. Conversely, of patients with adult-onset diabetes, 85% are overweight. In the Pima Indians, glucose intolerance is widely prevalent, and diabetes is common.[31]

Many studies indicate the importance of an intact functioning pancreas in maintaining normal weight. Involvement of the pancreas in obesity with fatty infiltration has been noted and demonstrated experimentally. The action of insulin is reduced.[32]

5. *Endocrine disturbance*[33]: Endocrine abnormalities may not only facilitate the development of obesity, but also seem to be a constant feature. The obesity of Cushing's syndrome is well known; prolonged use of cortisone is recognized as a cause of obesity. Adrenalectomy is often followed by obesity. Abnormalities of 17-ketosteroid excretion have been reported in certain forms of juvenile adiposity. Thus, the presence of obesity should alert one to the possible existence of adrenal dysfunction. Gonadal dysfunction is also a commonly associated problem. The thyroid, the pituitary, and the hypothalamus are all interrelated in an abnormal manner.

6. *Hepatic damage*[34]: Abnormal liver function values are frequent. An enlarged liver occurs in 25% of those 50% overweight. Fatty infiltration occurs. Hepatocellular damage seems to be proportional to the duration of the obesity.[35] Liver enzymes serum glutamic-oxaloacetic transaminase (SGOT) and serum glutamic-pyruvic transaminase (SGPT) are moderately elevated. The liver is under long-term stress, and agents handled by or affecting the liver should not be used. High lipoid-soluble agents tend to be retained in the body. Thus, large amounts of halogenated volatile anesthetic agents become available for biotransformation, and a greater percentage of the halogenated agent is biotransformed. Serum ionic fluoride concentrations increase more rapidly, and peak concentrations are higher and occur sooner than in nonobese patients. Studies of halothane reveal small, but significant, increases in serum fluoride (10.4 mmol/L mean) in the obese patient.[36]

7. *Blood coagulation*[7]: Although significant defects in blood clotting or coagulation are not pronounced, thrombophlebitis and thromboembolism have a much higher incidence in the obese. This may, in part, be mechanical and positional. It also emphasizes the need for early ambulation and minimal sedation in the obese patient.

8. *Blood volume:* When blood volume is estimated on the basis of standard values (72 ml/kg), then obese subjects are hypovolemic. If the volume is calculated on the basis of lean mass and of circulatory capacity of fat tissue, however, the correct blood volume will be more closely approximated. The volume can be estimated by using the standard value of 65 ml/kg. Schwartz[37] has suggested that the ideal weight, plus one third of the difference between obese and ideal weight, will serve this purpose. If volume is actually reduced, it should be restored. The hematocrit is usually in normal range, but with advancing hypoxemia, polycythemia occurs.

9. *Respiratory dysfunction*[38,39]: Mechanical interference with ventilation is obvious in the obese. These patients are respiratory cripples and have poor or borderline respiratory reserves. Bronchitis and emphysema are frequent. A specific diminished pulmonary compliance is not associated with pulmonary diseases as commonly known, but it is related to intrinsic structural changes in the periphery of the lung. Respiratory complications are decidedly more frequent in the obese surgical patient.[40]

10. *Gastric fluids*[41]: The volume and pH of gastric juice in obese patients are significantly altered. The gastric volume at the time of induction was found to be more than 25 ml in over 85% of patients, whereas the pH of the gastric juice was below 2.5. These values are associated with increased regurgitation and an increased risk of aspiration pulmonitis, because parenchymal damage from aspiration of liquid gastric contents increases with acidity, and damage increases as the pH falls below 2.5 (Fig. 45-6).

Respiratory System

The effects of obesity on the mechanics of breathing are of great significance and are discussed in greater detail.

The ventilatory mechanical system is impaired by obesity in three ways[42,43]:

1. A fixed thoracic cage. The intrapleural pressure is generally elevated. An attempt at compensation is noted in the hypertrophy of the intercostal muscles. The efficiency of the respiratory muscles is diminished by the great demands on their work. Compliance is reduced, and elastic resistance is greatly increased.

2. An elevated diaphragm. This is related to the abdominal visceral contents and the increased intra-abdominal pressure. The diaphragm is restricted in its movements by the abdominal wall weight and the abdominal cavity contents, so a shallow bellows mechanism exists. Nonelastic resistance is sharply increased. Obese individuals have an increased incidence of hiatus hernia.

3. Parenchymal changes. Such changes lead to loss of compliance and compression of airways. Flow resistance is increased.[43]

Changes in Respiratory Function

Functional impairment of the respiratory pump progressively increases with overweight and is correlated with the following defects (Fig. 45-7 and Table 45-19):

1. Total lung capacity is decreased.
2. Expiratory reserve volume (ERV) decreases 70% or more.

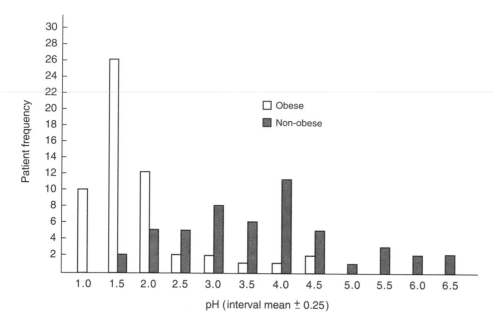

Fig. 45–6. Obesity causes increased gastric aspiration. Obese individuals manifest a composition of gastric juice that differs from their nonobese counterparts. In one study, the median and mode pH for obese patients were 1.3. The median pH for nonobese patients was 3.7, and the mode was 4.0. Because parenchymal damage from aspiration of liquid gastric contents increases with acidity, damage can increase to a maximum as the aspirate decreases below pH 2.5. Redrawn from Vaughan, R.W., et al.: Volume and pH of gastric juice in obese patients. Anesthesiology 43:686, 1975.

OBESITY: POSITION EFFECTS

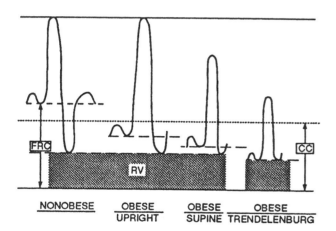

Fig. 45–7. In obesity, decreased chest wall compliance results in functional residual capacity (FRC) decreasing at the expense of expiratory reserve volume (RV). Closing capacity (CC) stays normal. From Vaughan, R.W.: Anesthesiol News, 1987..

Table 45–19. Functional Impairment

Total lung capacity ↓ ↓
Expiratory reserve volume 70% decreased
Residual volume ↓
Functional residual capacity 60% decreased (Dempsey); early airway closure
Vital capacity: moderate ↓
Maximum ventilatory volume ↓ ↓
Dead space/tidal volume ratio ↑
Diffusion capacity: decreased alveolar surface
Alveolar-arterial oxygen tension difference ↑ shunt
Ventilation/perfusion pressure (Barrera): PaO_2 60–70 mm Hg; 60% saturation
Total basal metabolic rate
High minute ventilation (minute volume)

3. Residual volume (RV) is decreased, but this is not as significant as changes in ERV.
4. Functional residual capacity (FRC) is reduced 60% or less.[44] This reduction is due primarily to a reduced ERV. Premature airway closure occurs, especially in dependent portions of the lung. This may lead to the closing capacity's being greater than FRC.
5. Vital capacity may only be moderately reduced.
6. Maximum voluntary ventilation (MVV) value is reduced, as is maximum breathing capacity (MBC).
7. Tidal volume is reduced, and shallow-breathing at a reduced lung volume is usual. This is a partial but inefficient attempt to reduce work of breathing. The ratio of dead space to tidal volume (DS/TV) is increased from a normal value DS/TV = 0.3 to values of 0.4 and higher. One sees an absolute decrease in each, but the decrease in TV is greater.
8. Diffusion capacity is reduced. Alveolar surface is decreased because of compression from a generalized restriction to chest-lung movement, and, second, because of intrapulmonary parenchymal compression.
9. The A-aDO_2 is increased. Varying degrees of shunt are found. An absolute intrapulmonary shunt occurs throughout the respiratory cycle.
10. Ventilation perfusion ratios are low.[45] Perfusion is normal, or even increased, but a maldistribution of ventilation exists, with diminished alveolar ventilation. First, low PaO_2 values result, on the order of 60 to 70 mm Hg (8 to 10 kPa), in the supine position compared with the sitting position in the obese patient.[46] Although one sees some decrease in PaO_2 values in the supine position in nonobese persons, a greatly exaggerated decrease occurs in obese persons. With advancing age, PaO_2 values decline in the nonobese when in the supine position. Thus, a semirecumbent position is preferable for the surgi-

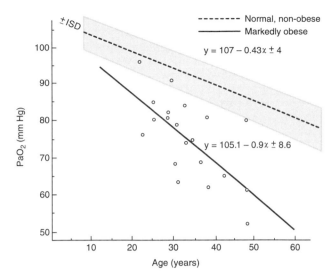

Fig. 45–8. Age, supine position, and rate of decline in PaO₂. The expected resting arterial oxygenation is reduced in markedly obese patients in the supine position (awake, breathing room air), but in contrast to the seated position, the supine PaO₂ drops much more sharply in obese patients as they age than it does in nonobese patients. Redrawn from Vaughan, R.W., et al.: Postoperative hypoxemia in obese patients. Ann Surg *180*:877, 1974.

cal patient (Fig. 45–8). Second, arterial oxygen saturation is reduced to 60%.

11. A total higher body oxygen consumption and a higher CO₂ production occurs than in normal subjects. In obese subjects, this change is due to increase in body mass.[44,47,48]

12. The obese patient has a relatively high minute ventilation, to keep the PaO₂ in the normal range.

Physiologic Effects On Changing Position from Sitting To Supine [49]

Paul and colleagues have measured the physiologic changes occurring in otherwise normal markedly obese patients when they are shifted from the sitting to the supine position while awake and unsedated (Table 45–20).[49] Evidence from these calculations indicates a

Table 45–20. Physiologic Effects Seen Upon Changing From Sitting to Supine Position

17.9% increase in arteriovenous oxygen difference
11% increase in oxygen consumption
17.7% increase in venous admixture
No significant change in alveolar-arterial oxygen tension difference
No significant change in respiratory rate
35.5% increase in cardiac output
35.8% increase in cardiac index
31% increase in mean pulmonary artery
44% increase in pulmonary artery wedge pressure
21.5% decrease in peripheral resistance
6% decrease in heart rate
No significant change in mean arterial pressure

sudden increase in cardiac work and oxygen requirements. One also sees a great increase in the work of breathing. Blood volume is suddenly diverted into the central circulation, adding an extra preload to the cardiac work. Congestive heart failure, arrhythmias, and even sudden death may be induced.

Work of Breathing (Fig. 45–9)

The obese subject must work harder to breath and to supply the oxygen needs of the body. The ventilatory apparatus, because of anatomic changes, is mechanically impeded in its performance; that is, obesity imposes a burden on breathing like "strapping" the chest wall. The energy expended by the obese is related to the following:

1. Greater elastic resistance (decreased compliance). Total compliance C_T is reduced.[42] A pronounced reduction in lung compliance C_L (parenchymal changes) occurs and the chest wall becomes non-compliant C_c.[47]
2. Greater nonelastic resistance (simple chest wall-diaphragm weight).[50]
3. Greater air flow resistance,[42] in part because of narrowed major airways parenchymal compression.

The work of breathing is best analyzed by the amount of oxygen needed for the purpose of breathing; specifically, the amount of oxygen required by the respiratory mechanical apparatus to move 1 L of air (based on the volume in liters ventilated per minute [MV]) is known as the "oxygen cost" of breathing (Fig. 45–9). This increases greatly and progressively with the degree of obesity. In

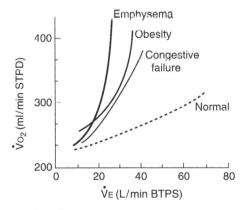

Fig. 45–9. The change in oxygen consumption associated with increases in ventilation in normal subjects and in patients with respiratory insufficiency. In emphysema, oxygen consumption increases 4 to 10 times normal values and may represent 25% of the total body consumption. Obesity increases oxygen consumption by 2 to 4 times normal; this compares with a twofold or more increase in oxygen consumption in congestive heart failure. Ordinarily, the oxygen cost of breathing is about 1% of the total consumption at rest. This is increased up to 10% with activity, and with strenuous work it is about 15% of the total body consumption. Redrawn from Cherniak, R.M.: Respiratory effects of obesity. Can Med Assoc J *80*:613, 1969.

mild to moderate obesity (20% overweight—29% fat), the cost may be doubled or quadrupled.[38]

In obesity, the increase in oxygen cost is greater than the work done; that is, cost is 4 to 12 times the mechanical work done. Converted to absolute amounts, the oxygen needed in the moderately obese person is 4.0 ml of oxygen per liter of air moved. This is compared with an average of 1.0 ml O_2/L of air moved and a range of 0.3 to 1.8 ml/L for the nonobese person at rest. In terms of percentage, the increase is from a normal of 1 to 3% of the total oxygen consumption by the body to 12 to 16% in the moderately obese individual.

In eucapnic obese persons, the oxygen cost may only be 30% above normal, but when hypercapnia exists, the cost may be 3 to 4 times greater than normal.

HYPOVENTILATION SYNDROME[47] (Fig. 45–10)

The increased work of breathing, produced by marked obesity of 50% overweight or more, sets in motion a vicious cycle called the obesity-hypoventilation syndrome. The conditions of respiratory dysfunction set the stage.

Hypoxia is common, and Pao$_2$ values of 50 to 60 mm Hg are observed.[51] Simultaneously, some CO_2 retention exists. In pathologic obesity (over 50%), the CO_2 retention is marked and produces somnolence. Under metabolic stress, oxygen desaturation is aggravated, and CO_2 retention is more pronounced.

Ventilation and gas exchange are impaired, but the ensuing hypoventilation is unrelated to the usual primary obstructive or restrictive lung diseases. Oxygen saturation may be reduced to 70%, and CO_2 tension increased to 75 mm Hg. Such changes can produce cyanosis, on one hand, and somnolence, on the other. The somnolence appears to be due to hypoxemia and is aggravated by CO_2 narcosis. In addition, the sensitivity of the respiratory center is lost.

These disorders are usually reversed when weight is reduced.

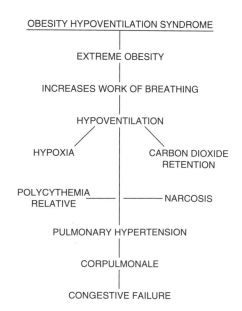

Fig. 45–10. Obesity hypoventilation syndrome.

The somnolence of marked obesity is often accompanied by sleep apnea.[52] This condition is not exclusive to the obese person, and it can occur in persons of normal weight. It is related to arterial oxygen desaturation to below 80% and appears to be a male characteristic. Because of the sex difference, progesterone has been used to prevent abnormal breathing and has been reported effective in both pickwickian somnolence and altitude sickness.[53,54]

Pickwickian Syndrome (Extreme Obesity)

At the extreme end of the scale of obesity is the so-called pickwickian syndrome.[55] The features were classically described by Charles Dickens in 1837. Characteristics (as seen in Mr. Wardel's boy Joe of *The Pickwick Papers*) are epitomized by a classic triad.[56]

Primary characteristics are as follows:

1. Marked obesity.
2. Episodic somnolence.
3. Arterial desaturation with cyanosis (hypoventilation).

Secondary features include the following:

1. Twitching of facial and extremity muscles.
2. Periodic respiration with bouts of apnea.
3. Increase in the red cell mass per meter of surface area and development of secondary polycythemia.
4. Right ventricular hypertension, with an accentuated second pulmonic sound.
5. Possible right ventricular failure.
6. Peripheral edema.

The primary defect is hypoventilation unrelated to obstructive or restrictive disease.

Supine Death Syndrome

A severely obese patient who is already hypoxic and hypercarbic and assumes a supine position has a greater than normal risk of death. Cardiorespiratory collapse is sudden and is rarely reversible.[57]

ANESTHETIC MANAGEMENT

Evaluation of obesity and its associated diseases leads to a recognition of the anesthetic problems.[58,59]

Anatomic Problems

Large facial features, including short neck and enlarged tongue, make airway maintenance difficult. Mask fits are difficult. Second, the size of the subject often poses a problem in accommodation to the standard operating table and in transportation. Landmarks are difficult to identify, and regional procedures are not easily accomplished. Surgical exposure is always a problem. The problem is not a matter of muscle relations as much as it is a mechanical problem of retraction and packing. Veins for intravenous infusion are obscure. The dorsum of the hand is the best site. Venipuncture is difficult.

Sphygmomanometry has many pitfalls; large-diameter cuffs 20 to 25 cm wide should be used. Endoscopy is frequently difficult (note awake intubation). Positioning is difficult.

Physiologic Problems[60]

The major physiologic problem is that of ventilation. Obesity interferes with diaphragmatic movement and also limits chest expansion.[47] Emphysema impairs alveolar gas mixing. Only moderate blood loss readily causes hypertension. Blood volume should be corrected before surgery. Carbohydrate balance is easily upset. Regulation of caloric intake, of hydration, and of insulin needs before operation must be carefully done to avoid ketosis. About 5% of obese individuals show endocrine disturbances exclusive of diabetes. These conditions should be regulated. Hypertension should be under medical control, and the use of antihypertensive drugs should be noted.

Temperature[61] may be subnormal from low metabolism. A tendency to elevated temperatures exists, however, because of poor heat loss in a warm environment. On exposure to cold, the metabolic rate may increase, and hyperthermia may develop.

With regard to *ventilation,* the airway should be established early. Awake intubation is often indicated when any concern or difficulty in airway management is expected. This should be considered in patients 50% or more overweight. Assisted ventilation to oxygenate and eliminate CO_2 before induction is highly desirable.

Pharmacologic Problems[62,63]

Fat tissue represents a storehouse for many agents. All volatile agents and many nonvolatile substances, such as the barbiturates, are included. Volatile agents, however, may be eliminated more readily by good ventilation. In contrast, highly lipoid nonvolatile agents are slowly released from fat depots and need to be metabolized or cleared, and their action is prolonged.

Uptake and Distribution[36,53]

Despite high solubility in fat of halogenated drugs, adipose tissue has poor blood supply and has minimal influence during induction of anesthesia. Any increased induction time is related to airway or ventilation. Maintenance of anesthesia may require a slightly higher inspiratory concentration to compensate for continuous fat tissue uptake. Washout or pulmonary denitrogenation and preoxygenation must begin earlier.

Halothane has an intermediate blood gas coefficient of solubility of 2.3 and a moderate diffusion velocity. At the beginning, the partial pressure of the vapor in the blood is slightly below the alveolar. At equilibrium between blood and alveolar gas, one notes twice the percentage in blood as in gas phase. Equilibrium is moderately rapid compared with ether. Tissues, especially fat, become saturated in time.

Enflurane has a lower blood/gas coefficient of solubility of 1.9, and diffusion velocity is slower than that of halothane. Equilibrium between concentration in alveoli and blood is faster, and the percentage in blood and gas is more rapidly equilibrated.

Finally, nitrous oxide, with low diffusion velocity, but a great concentration effect and a low blood/gas coefficient of solubility (0.47), results in an alveolar gas percentage more than twice that in the blood.

Thiopental is relatively contraindicated in obesity if larger than sleep doses are used. Brodie has shown that this agent is concentrated in the fat deposits and is released slowly.[64] In addition, it is actually metabolized slowly, about 15% per hour, and this leads to prolonged drowsiness postoperatively, an undesirable feature that is pronounced in the obese patient.

Preanesthetic Preparation

The following recommendations stem from the foregoing considerations:

1. Determine blood volume and hemoglobin. Correct hypovolemia and anemia before surgery.
2. Estimate needs for cardiac support; ECG monitoring is essential. Peaked P waves are commonly observed in obese patients.
3. Control diabetes and any ketosis.
4. Clear the patient's respiratory tract.
5. Perform blood gas studies.
6. Obtain a liver profile.
7. Ensure psychologic preparation. Many patients are embarrassed about their weight and have fears and tensions. They need much reassurance.

Choice of Anesthesia

This choice is determined by individualization of each case. Difficulties can be anticipated for either regional or general anesthesia.

Regional Anesthesia

Regional anesthesia presents disadvantages in identification of landmarks. Needles must be longer. Doses of local anesthetic agents generally are lower and should be based on lean body mass.

For operations of the lower abdomen and extremities, spinal or epidural anesthesia is not only feasible, but also is least disturbing to physiology. These regional procedures avoid CNS depression and provide better postoperative respiration, cough, and early ambulation.

Spinal levels are usually higher than ordinarily anticipated, so care in positioning and the use of lower doses are important. For epidural anesthesia, doses of local agents required for a given level should be reduced 30 to 40%.[65] Increased intra-abdominal pressure in the obese patient tends to shift blood from the caval system to the vertebral plexus system, increasing its vascularity and thus reducing the epidural space.

Spinal anesthesia can best be accomplished with the patient in the sitting position. While the patient is sitting, the midline of the back can be identified by a line from the seventh cervical spine, which remains prominent, to the gluteal folds. An assistant may draw pendulous skin folds laterally. If one inserts the regular 3.5-inch spinal needle for moderately obese subjects (and the 5-inch needle for pathologically or morbidly obese subjects) carefully in the midline at a point 6 to 8 inches above the gluteal crease, it will reach the dura and can enter the subarachnoid space in most instances if the needle is advanced to the hub. Dosage should be reduced by about one third. High spinal anesthesia to sensory levels above T6 is not recommended.

General Anesthesia

When general anesthesia is necessary, the following principles are pertinent:

1. Strict maintenance of airway (morbid obesity: consider awake intubation).
2. Adequate tidal volume intra- and postoperatively.
3. Optimum oxygenation.
4. Use of inhalation agents.
5. Adequate relaxation where needed.
6. Complete reversal of muscle relaxant.
7. Pain control.
8. Physiologic positioning.

Consideration of Agents

Ether, halothane, and most agents with a high blood/gas coefficient of solubility, as well as thiopental, are not desirable. Thiopental, which is distributed in body tissues and is retained for 10 to 15 hours,[64] should be used only to produce unconsciousness. Enflurane and isoflurane have a lower blood/gas solubility and are more rapidly eliminated. Agents that are quickly eliminated have been used with great success, such as the gases. These include cyclopropane, ethylene, and nitrous oxide.

An ideal agent for the obese patient is lacking. Some clinicians have suggested that intravenous (fixed) agents are preferred to inhalation agents.[62] The argument is that the highly lipoid-soluble inhalation agents are taken up and stored for prolonged periods, and recovery is prolonged compared with narcotic (fentanyl) techniques. A careful study by Vaughan and colleagues does not support this contention.[60] The time from last suture to opening of the patient's eyes was less with intravenous narcotic-nitrous oxide technique compared with enflurane or with isoflurane inhalation technique. Extubation and total recovery room time were similar for the intravenous and inhalation agents, however. Hence, no disadvantage in regard to recovery is seen using these volatile agents in obese patients. Indeed, hyperventilation toward the end of the surgical procedure markedly reduces body stores of volatile agents, and the eye-opening to command response is just as rapid.

Nitrous oxide is an excellent agent. It needs supplementation, and this can be accomplished with intravenous drip of meperidine or fentanyl, which provides analgesia.

Muscle relaxants are well tolerated. Antidepolarizing derivatives are preferred, because they are better handled in the presence of possible liver disturbance and can be antagonized.

Occult abnormal liver histopathologic features have been documented in over 80% of severely obese subjects despite normal liver function tests. At least one of four types of hepatic histologic abnormalities are observed: lobular hepatitis, fibrosis, portal hepatitis, or steatosis.[66]

Vecuronium depends on hepatic clearance, and 40% is excreted unchanged in the bile within 24 hours. Thus, this relaxant has a longer recovery time: to go from 5 to 25% recovery of twitch response requires 15 minutes, versus 7 minutes in nonobese subjects; and for recovery, from 25 to 75% recovery, the time is 33 minutes, versus 13 minutes in the nonobese.[67] This prolonged duration of action of vecuronium is likely related to impaired hepatic clearance or to an overdose. On the other hand, atracurium shows no difference in recovery when given to obese or nonobese patients.[67]

Mivacurium depends on metabolism by plasma cholinesterase, and its fate is similar to that of succinylcholine. Mivacurium is a suitable agent in the obese patient.[68]

Technical Management

1. *Adequate patent airway:* An endotracheal tube is generally indicated on the basis of obesity itself. During induction of general anesthesia, either by inhalation or by the intravenous route, obstruction may occur before surgical anesthesia is achieved, and insertion of an oral airway may be impractical. A topical spray should be used before induction thereby to permit insertion of a pharyngeal airway in the conscious state or in light planes of anesthesia.

   Markedly obese patients (those double their ideal weight) should be managed by first improving ventilation. An endotracheal tube can be inserted under topical or local anesthesia while the patient is awake. The patient may then have ventilation assisted and oxygenation improved. This can be accomplished before either intravenous or general anesthesia induction. An endotracheal tube is indicated on the basis of obesity itself. During induction of general anesthesia, either by inhalation or by the intravenous route, obstruction may occur before surgical anesthesia is achieved and insertion of oral airway is practical.

2. *Oxygenation:* Inspired oxygen concentrations of 50% are recommended in obese patients for intra-abdominal surgery; 40% inspired oxygen ($Fi_{O_2} = 0.4$) does not regularly produce adequate arterial oxygen tension.[60]

3. *Compensation for respiration:* To counteract the mechanical interference to ventilation of body weight and any deranged pulmonary gas exchange, during positive pressure breathing, avoidance of high positive end-expiratory pressure (PEEP) is desired. Salem and associates have demonstrated that discontinuing PEEP during intraoperative intermittent positive-pressure ventilation increases Pa_{O_2}. PEEP appears only to overinflate nondependent

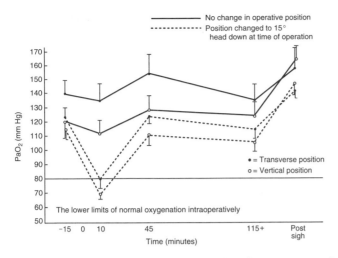

Fig. 45-11. Head down. The relationship between arterial oxygen tension at $F_{IO_2} = 0.4$ and changes in operative position resulted in a statistically significant (p ± 0.001) reduction to a mean Pa_{O_2} of 73 mm Hg; 75% of these patients demonstrated Pa_{O_2} values of less than 80 mm Hg when $F_{IO_2} = 0.4$. The vertical lines extended from the open and closed circles indicate the standard error of the mean. Redrawn from Vaughan, R.W., Wise, L.: Intraoperative arterial oxygenation in obese patients. Ann Surg, 184:35, 1976.

areas of the lung and causes greater mismatching of dependent underinflated portions.[69]

4. *Avoidance of head-down and prone positions:* A change from supine to 15° head-down position reduces Pa_{O_2} from 80 to 85 mm Hg to 70 to 75 mm Hg at inspired oxygen of 40% (Fig. 45-11).[46,70,71]

5. *Surgical packing:* Packing in the upper abdomen results in a consistent fall in Pa_{O_2} to less than 65 mm Hg without any other positional or ventilatory changes. Surgical incisions alter oxygenation, especially during the postoperative period. The midline incision is associated with a significantly lower Pa_{O_2} than transverse incisions.[72]

6. *Avoidance of hypotension.*

Postoperative Problems[71]

Obese patients have significantly greater morbidity than do persons of normal weight. Respiratory insufficiency continues into this period (Fig. 45-12). An airway and assisted ventilation are necessary. In many situations, the endotracheal tube should be left in place, and assisted or controlled ventilation should be provided. Oxygen supplementation is desirable, but the patient's respiratory performance must be monitored. Some hypoxia may be present for days 1 through 5. The semirecumbent position provides an improved Pa_{O_2} of 10 to 15 mm Hg. Early ambulation is needed (Fig. 45-13).[73]

In one study of women over 200 lb, or 40% overweight, the respiratory complication rate was doubled.

Thrombosis and embolism are more frequent. The obese patient has an increased fibrinogen level and diminished fibrinolytic activity.

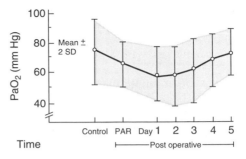

Fig. 45-12. The fall in Pa_{O_2} postoperatively. The solid line represents the mean Pa_{O_2} for 20 markedly obese patients. Some of these patients, on postoperative days 1 and 2, had Pa_{O_2} values that caused a significant reduction in arterial oxygen content. Redrawn from Vaughan, R.W., et al.: Postoperative hypoxemia in obese patients. Ann Surg 180:877, 1974.

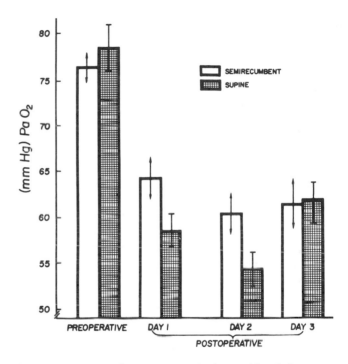

Fig. 45-13. For 2 days postoperatively, position is important. This graph shows the effect of semirecumbent and supine positions on Pa_{O_2} preoperatively and postoperatively for days 1 through 3 in 22 markedly obese female subjects. Preoperatively, position does not have a significant effect on the Pa_{O_2}, but for 48 hours postoperatively, position does have a significant effect. From day 3 on, effects are not significant. From Vaughan, R.W., Wise, L.: Postoperative arterial blood gas measurements in obese patients: effect of position on gas exchange. Ann Surg 182:705, 1975.

Criteria for Gastric Restrictive Surgery[70]

Two surgical procedures have been advocated for the treatment of morbid obesity, namely, gastric bypass (gastric plication with gastrojejunostomy) and gastroplasty. In a 1984 report by the Diagnostic and Therapeutic Technology Assessment,[74] gastric exclusion procedures were considered as effective as intestinal bypass, and safer.

Gastric bypass is attended by a higher risk and more complications than gastroplasty, with a perioperative mortality between 2 and 4%. Gastroplasty appears to have an acceptable risk with a perioperative mortality of 1 to 3%.

A consensus on minimum criteria was reported. Patients should not be accepted unless they are at least 100 lb over standard weight, but most surgical groups require 175 lb over standard weight, or double ideal weight. Criteria are as follows:

- An age limitation of 20 to 55 years.
- Lack of response to medical management or behavioral modification for at least 3 years.
- Abstinence for 3 years for patients with a history of alcoholism.
- No serious diseases, such as pulmonary, cardiovascular, or metabolic disorders.

REFERENCES

1. Van Itallie, T. B.: Health implications of overweight and obesity in the United States. Ann Intern Med *103*:983, 1985.
2. Entmacher, P. S.: New weight standards for men and women. *In* Statistics Bulletin of the Metropolitan Life Insurance Company. New York, 1983.
3. Build Study: Chicago, Chicago Society of Actuaries and Association of Life Insurance Medical Directors of America, 1980.
4. Manson, J., et al.: Body weight and longevity: a reassessment. JAMA *257*:353, 1987.
5. Van Itallie, T. B., Kral, J. G.: The dilemma of morbid obesity. JAMA *246*:999, 1981.
6. National Institutes of Health Consensus Development Conference Statement: Health implications of obesity. Ann Intern Med *103*:1073, 1985.
7. Mann, G. V.: The influence of obesity on health. (First of two parts.) N Engl J Med *291*:178, 1974.
8. Hartcroft, W. S.: The pathology of obesity. Bull NY Acad Med *36*:313, 1960.
9. Mayer, J.: Genetic, traumatic and environmental factors in the etiology of obesity. Physiol Rev *33*:472, 1953.
10. Stunkard, A. M., Harris, J. R., Pedersen, N. L., McClearn, G. E.: The body mass index of twins who have been reared apart. N Engl J Med *322*:1483, 1980.
11. Danforth, C. H.: Hereditary adeposity on mice. J Hered *18*:153, 1927.
12. Anand, B. K., Brobeck, J. R.: Hypothalamic control of food intake in rats and cats. Yale J Biol Med *24*:123, 1951.
13. Mayer, J.: Hunger and hypothalamus. Clin Res Proc *5*:123, 1957.
14. Miller, N. F., Bailey, C. J., Stevenson, J. A. F.: Decreased hunger but increased food intake resulting from hypothalamic lesions. Science *112*:256, 1950.
15. Kissebah, A. H., et al.: Relation of body fat distribution to metabolic complications of obesity. J Clin Endocrinol Metab *54*:254, 1982.
16. Pettitt, D. J., Lisse, J. R., Knowler, W. C.: Mortality as a function of obesity and diabetes mellitus. Am J Epidemiol *115*:359, 1982.
17. Peterson, H. R., et al.: Body fat and activity of the autonomic nervous system. N Engl J Med *318*:1077, 1988.
18. Deluise M., Blackburn, G. L., Flien, J. S.: Reduced activity of the red cell sodium-potassium pump in human obesity. N Engl J Med *303*:1017, 1980.
19. Kissebah, A. H., Peiris, A. N.: Biology and regional body fat distribution relationship to non-insulin-dependent diabetes. Diabetes Metab Rev *5*:83, 1989.
20. Hirsch, J.: Adipose tissue cellularity in human obesity. Clin Endocrinol Metab *5*:299, 1976.
21. Krotkiewski, M.: Adipose tissue cellularity. Int J Obes *1*:398, 1977.
22. Keys, A., et al.: Indices of relative weight and obesity. J Chronic Dis *25*:329, 1972.
23. Crook, G. H., et al.: Evaluation of skin-fold measurements and weight chart to measure body fat. JAMA *198*:39, 1966.
24. Folsom, A. R., et al.: Body fat distribution and 5-year risk of death in older women. JAMA *269*:483, 1993.
25. Tuck, M. L., et al.: The effect of weight reduction on blood pressure plasma renin activity and plasma aldosterone levels in obese patients. N Engl J Med *304*:930, 1981.
26. Dawber, T. R.: The Framingham Study. Cambridge, MA, Harvard University Press, 1980.
27. Terry, B. E.: Morbid obesity and circulation. Med Concepts Cardiovasc Dis *32*:799, 1963.
28. Terry, B. E.: Morbid obesity: cardiac evaluation and function. Gastroenterol Clin *16*:215, 1987.
29. Lauer, M. S., Anderson, K. M., Kannel, W. B., Levy D.: The impact of obesity on left ventricular mass on geometry: the Framingham Heart Study. JAMA *266*:231, 1991.
30. Harris, M. I., Hadden, W. C., Knowler, W. C., Bennett, P. H.: Prevalence of diabetes and impaired glucose tolerance and plasma glucose levels in U.S. population aged 20–74 years. Diabetes *36*:523, 1987.
31. Saad, M. F., Knowler, W. C., Pettit, D. J.: The natural history of impaired glucose tolerance in the Pima Indians. N Engl J Med *319*:1500, 1988.
32. Bogardus, C., et al.: Relationship between degree of obesity and in vivo insulin action in man. Am J Physiol *248*:E286, 1985.
33. Jung, P.: Endocrinological aspects of obesity. Clin Endocrinol Metab *13*:597, 1984.
34. Rosenthal, P., Biava, C., Spencer, H., Zimmerman, H. J.: Liver morphology and function tests in obesity and starvation. Am J Digest Dis *12*:198, 1967.
35. Zelman, S.: Hepatocellular damage and obesity. Arch Intern Med *90*:141, 1957.
36. Young, S. R., et al.: Anesthetic biotransformation and renal function in obese patients. Anesthesiology *42*:451, 1975.
37. Schwartz, H.: The problem of obesity in anesthesia. NY State J Med *55*:3257, 1955.
38. Kaufman, B. J., Ferguson, M. H., Cherniak, R. M.: Hypoventilation in obesity. J Clin Invest *38*:500, 1959.
39. Hackney, J. D., et al.: Studies of extreme obesity and hypoventilation. Arch Intern Med *51*:541, 1959.
40. Bates, D. V., Macklem, P. T., Christie, R. V.: Respiratory Function in Disease. Philadelphia, W.B. Saunders, 1972, pp. 100, 353.
41. Vaughan, R. W., Bauer, S., Wise, L.: Volume and pH of gastric juice in obese patients. Anesthesiology *43*:686, 1975.
42. Sharp, J. T., Henry, J. P., Sweany, S. K.: The total work of breathing in normal and obese men. J Clin Invest *43*:728, 1964.
43. Sharp, J. T., et al.: Effects of mass loading the respiratory system in man. J Appl Physiol *19*:959, 1964.
44. Dempsey, J. A., Redden, W., Rankin, J., Balke, B.: Alveolar-arterial gas exchange during muscular work in obesity. J Appl Physiol *21*:1807, 1966.
45. Barrera, F., Reidenberg, M. M., Winters, W. L., Hungspreugs, S.: Ventilation perfusion relationship in the obese patient. J Appl Physiol *26*:420, 1969.
46. Vaughan, R. W., Wise, L.: Postoperative hypoxemia in obese patients. Ann Surg *180*:877, 1974.
47. Cherniak, R., Cherniak, L., Naimark, A.: Respiration in

Health and Disease, 2nd Ed. Philadelphia, W. B. Saunders, 1972.

48. Rochester, D. F., Enson, Y.: Current concepts in the pathogenesis of obesity-hypoventilation syndrome: mechanical and circulatory factors. Am J Med 57:402, 1974.

49. Paul, D. R., Hoyt, J. L., Boutros, A. R.: Cardiovascular and respiratory changes in response to changes in posture in the very obese. Anesthesiology 45:73, 1976.

50. Cherniak, R. M.: Respiratory effects of obesity. Can Med Assoc J 80:613, 1969.

51. Anderson, J., Rasmussen, P. J., Eriksen, J.: Pulmonary function in obese patients scheduled for jejuno-ileostomy. Acta Anaesth Scand 21:346, 1977.

52. Block, A. J., Boysen, P. G., Wynne, J. W., Hunt, L. A.: Sleep apnea, hypopnea and oxygen desaturation in normal subject. N Engl J Med 300:513, 1979.

53. Lyons, H. A., Huang, C. T.: Therapeutic use of progesterone in alveolar hypoventilation associated with obesity. Am J Med 44:8831, 1968.

54. Sutton, F. D., Jr., et al.: Progesterone for outpatient treatment of Pickwickian syndrome. Ann Intern Med 83:476, 1975.

55. Burwell, C. S., Robin, E. D., Whaley, R. D., Bickelman, A. G.: Extreme obesity associated with alveolar hypoventilation: a Pickwickian syndrome. Am J Med 21:811, 1956.

56. Edelist, G.: Extreme obesity. Anesthesiology 29:846, 1968.

57. Tscuda, K., et al.: Pancuronium bromide requirement during anesthesia for the morbidly obese. Anesthesiology 48:458, 1978.

58. Vaughan, R. W.: In Brawn, B. R. (ed.). Anesthesia and the Obese Patient. Philadelphia, F. A. Davis, 1982.

59. Vaughan, R. W., Vaughan, S.: Anesthetic management of patients with massive obesity. In Nunn, J. F., Utting, J. E., Brown, B. R., Jr. (eds.). General Anesthesia, 5th Ed. London, Butterworth, 1989.

60. Vaughan, R. W., Wise, L: Intraoperative arterial oxygenation in obese patients. Ann Surg 184:35, 1976.

61. Jung, R. T., et al.: Reduced thermogeneses in obesity. Nature 279:322, 1979.

62. Fisher, A., Waterhouse, T. D., Adams, A.D.: Obesity: its relation to anesthesia. Anaesthesia 39:633, 1975.

63. Cork, R. C., Vaughan, R. W., Bentley, J. B.: General anesthesia for morbidly obese patients: an examination of postoperative outcomes. Anesthesiology 54:310, 1981.

64. Brodie, B. R., Bernstein, E., Mark, L. C.: The role of body fat in limiting the duration of action of thiopental. J Pharmacol Exp Ther 105:421, 1952.

65. Hodgkinson, R., Husain, F. J.: Obesity and gravity and the spread of epidural anesthetics. Anesth Analg 60:421, 1980.

66. Galambos, J. T., Wells, J. T.: Relationship between 505 paired liver tests and biopsies in 242 obese patients. Gastroenterology 74:1191, 1978.

67. Weinstein, J. A., et al.: Pharmacodynamics of vecuronium and atrocurium in the obese surgical patient. Anesth Analg 67:1149, 1988.

68. Savarese, J. J., et al.: The clinical neuromuscular pharmacology of mivacurium chloride. Anesthesiology 68:723, 1988.

69. Salem, M. R., et al.: Does PEEP improve intra-operative arterial oxygenation in grossly obese patients? Anesthesiology 48:280, 1975.

70. Vaughan, R. W., Wise, L.: Choice of abdominal operative incision in the obese patient: a study using blood gas measurements. Ann Surg 181:829, 1975.

71. Vaughan, R. W., Wise, L.: Postoperative arterial blood gas measurements in those obese patients: effect of position on gas exchange. Ann Surg 182:705, 1975.

72. Vaughan, R. W., Engelhardt, R. C., Wise, L.: Postoperative alveolar-arterial oxygen tension differences: its relation to the operative incidion in obese patients. Anesth Analg 54:433, 1975.

73. Alpers, D.: Surgical therapy for obesity. N Engl J Med 308:1026, 1983.

74. DATTA: Diagnostic and Therapeutic Technology Assessment: gastric restrictive surgery for morbid obesity. JAMA 251:3011, 1984.

PHENYLKETONURIA

DEFINITION[1]

Phenylketonuria (PKU) is an inborn error of metabolism of the amino acid phenylalanine. The disorder is characterized by the virtual absence of the enzyme hydroxylase and the elevation of plasma phenylalanine first identified in 1934 by J. Folling.[2,3]

GENETIC BASIS[1]

PKU is due to a genetically determined defect in the production of the enzyme hydroxylase and is transmitted in an autosomal recessive pattern. The genetic defect is located on chromosome 12.

INCIDENCE

The incidence in the United States of the classic homozygous type is about 1 in 16,000 live births. The incidence of variants wherein a deficiency (not the absence) exists is about 1 in 100,000.

BIOCHEMISTRY[3]

Phenylalanine is an essential amino acid obtained by ingestion of the substance in various foodstuffs and absorbed into the blood. It is an important amino acid and is a precursor of tyrosine produced by hydroxylation of the phenylalanine at the pars position of the phenyl unit. Tyrosine is utilized in the production of proteins and of hormones, that is, catecholamines, thyroid hormone, melanin, and other biogenic amines, including dopamine. The key to the production of tyrosine is the presence of the enzyme hydroxylase. The oxidative conversion of phenylalanine to tyrosine is an irreversible reaction that occurs only in the liver, kidney, and pancreas. The liver normally is the only place where measurable amounts of hydroxylase are found. Excess phenylalanine normally is partially excreted in the urine, but it is significantly metabolized after being transaminated to three major products: phenylacetic acid, phenyllactic acid, and phenylpyruvic acid, which are all excreted in the urine.

CLINICAL FEATURES

Symptoms of PKU are usually absent in the newborn, and laboratory screening tests are necessary for its diagnosis. The infant may be lethargic and may feed poorly. Untreated children usually show some degree of retarded development and slow response to environmental stimuli ordinarily expected in the growing infant and child. Skin is often a light color, as are hair and eyes, as a result of poor pigmentation. Progressive loss of hair occurs. Occasionally, rash is seen similar to infantile eczema.

Abnormal neurologic signs are manifest in over three fourths of these children. These include hyperreflexia, muscular hypertonicity, and hyperactivity. Seizures are common in older children. Abnormal EEGs are observed in over 75% of untreated children, whereas most treated older children have normal ECGs. Psychomotor development is delayed.

Many children exude an unpleasant "mousy" body odor from the phenylacetic acid in the urine and sweat.

ETIOLOGY

If the enzyme hydroxylase is absent or impaired, phenylalanine accumulates in excessive amounts in the blood, producing phenylalaninemia. Levels in excess of 15 to 20 mg/dl during the neonatal period and the first 6 years of life are associated with the development of mental retardation.

With the abnormal plasma levels of phenylalanine is a significant increase in the renal elimination of intact phenylalanine in the urine. Similarly, metabolism of phenylalanine is greatly increased, and the phenylacid metabolites are greatly increased in the urine over normal. The phenylpyruvic acid also contains a ($-C-C-C-$) carbonyl group and hence is a ketone.

LABORATORY STUDIES

Detection of a high plasma level of phenylalanine and of a normal or low plasma tyrosine level in the newborn is diagnostic. A plasma level of 15 to 20 mg/dl or more has been proposed as a cutoff point for classic PKU. Levels below this may be found in variants or when the hydroxylase is inactive or faulty.

Prenatal diagnosis is possible.[4] DNA isolated from cultured amniotic cells or chorionic villus cells is analyzed by restriction length fragment polymorphism, and this is compared with the DNA of the parents.

PATHOGENESIS

The major pathologic process is found in the brain. Both structure and function are disturbed by the elevated phenylalanine, but the precise mechanism is not clear. Fetal hydroxylase activity is present by the seventh week of gestation.

At birth, all nervous system structures are present. Growth and development of these structures, and particularly the brain, occur during the first 6 months of life. Therefore, the majority of growth occurs as a result of additions in protein, DNA, and lipid content of the existing cells. Maturation and further growth then proceed for at least 6 to 8 years. During this time, myelinization is the principal process and is not complete until well after the eighth year.

In PKU, however, with the excessive levels of phenylalanine,[5] diffuse and focal demyelinization[6] of nerve axons occurs. How the phenylalanine impairs myelinization is not understood. The process of myelinization, however, involves stepwise elaboration of complex lipids and their lamination in lipoprotein layers around nerves. The excess phenylalanine does present an abnormal mix of amino acids, and myelin construction is arrested, as are growth and differentiation of the brain. Intellectual and emotional growth is retarded.

VARIANTS

In some hyperphenylalaninemias, a simple reduction of the phenylalanine hydroxylase activity occurs, in contrast to the classic PKU or type I form. A reduction of activity to 1.5 to 35% of normal designates types II and III. Defects of other enzymes, which are cofactors, designates types IV and V (Table 45-21).

Table 45-21.　Hyperphenylalaninemias: Phenylketonuria (PKU) and Its Variants

Type	Disorder	Enzymatic Disorder	Blood Phenylalanine Concentration	Urine Metabolites
I	Phenylketonuria	Absent phenylalanine hydroxylase	>20 mg/dl on regular diet	Increased phenylalanine metabolites
II	Persistent hyperphenylalaninemia	Decreased phenylalanine hydroxylase	Similar to PKU in early infancy 4–20 mg/dl on regular diet in later years	Normal or transiently increased phenylalanine metabolites
III	Transient hyperphenylalaninemia	Maturational decrease (delay) phenylalanine hydroxylase	Similar to PKU in early infancy Gradual decrease to normal levels with growth	Normal or transiently increased phenylalanine metabolites
IV	Dihydropteridine reductase deficiency	Insufficient or absent dihydropteridine reductase	May be similar to type I	Unpredictable and dependent on other factors
V	Abnormal dihydropteridine function	Synthesis of dihydrobiopterin	≥20 mg/dl	Abnormal biopterin

From Kaufman, S.: Phenylketonison and its variants. Adv Hum Genet *13*:217, 1983.

TREATMENT

Restriction of dietary phenylalanine in early infancy has virtually eliminated PKU as a cause of mental retardation. Special diets without phenylalanine are available. Casein hydroxylates (treated to remove phenylalanine) or mixtures of amino acids constitute the protein portion of a diet. Lofenalac is widely used as a complete food product in place of milk. The phenylalanine requirement is met by supplements to maintain a normal plasma level of 4 to 10 mg/dl.

Evidence indicates that the restricted diets should be continued through 8 years of life to attain satisfactory intellectual achievement levels (scores). The greatest deficiencies were observed when the children were out of diet control before the age of 6 years. The diets were found to be out of control when the blood phenylalanine level exceeded 15 mg/dl.[7]

ANESTHETIC CONSIDERATIONS

These patients are sensitive to opiates and CNS depressants. Phenothiazines and neuroleptic drugs should be avoided. Because seizure phenomena are prone to develop, anticonvulsant treatment should be considered. For premedication, midazolam has proved effective and is also useful for intravenous induction.[8] Glycopyrrolate should be the choice for anticholinergic action. Halothane nitrous-oxide inhalation anesthesia for infants and small children is recommended. For older children, isoflurane is preferred.

Because hypoglycemia is easily provoked, an intravenous glucose solution should be employed. Care of the skin is important, because these patients bruise easily.

REFERENCES

1. Kaufman, S.: Phenylketonuria and its variants. Adv Hum Genet 13:217, 1983.
2. Guttler, F.: Phenylketonuria: 50 years since Folling's discovery and still expanding our clinical and bio-chemical knowledge. Acta Paediatr Scand 73:705, 1984.
3. Knox, W.: Phenylketonuria. In Stanbury, J., Wyngaarden, J., Fredrickson, D. (eds.). The Metabolic Basis of Inherited Disease. New York, McGraw-Hill, 1972, p. 265.
4. Woo, S.: Prenatal diagnosis and carrier detection of classical phenylketonuria by gene analysis. Pediatrics 74:412, 1984.
5. Tourian, A., Sidbury, J.: Phenylketonuria and hyperphenylalaninemia. In Stanbury, J., et al. (eds.). The Metabolic Basis of Inherited Disease, 5th Ed. New York, McGraw-Hill, 1983, p. 270.
6. Jawad, S., et al.: A pharmacodynamic evaluation of midazolam as an antileptic compound. J Neurol Neurosurg Psychiatry 49:1050, 1986.
7. Jackson, S. H.: Inborn errors of amino acid metabolism: phenylketonuria and other hyperphenylalaninemias. In Katz, J., Benumof, J. L., Kadis, L. B. (eds.). Anesthesia and Uncommon Diseases, 3rd Ed. Philadelphia, W. B. Saunders, 1990, p. 34.
8. Holtzman, N., et al.: Effect of age at loss of dietary control on intellectual performance and behavior of children with phenylketonuria. N Engl J Med 314:593, 1986.

PHEOCHROMOCYTOMA

INCIDENCE

The term pheochromocytoma is applied to any tumor producing catecholamines and causing typical clinical features of the disease.[1] These are rare tumors of abnormally secreting gland chromaffin tissue producing excessive epinephrine and/or norepinephrine. The hormones provide for pathophysiology of the pheochromocytoma. Patients with elevated blood pressure and pheochromocytoma account for about 0.1% of all patients diagnosed as hypertensive. The tumor occurs in childhood and adolescence (about 30%) and peaks in the third to fifth decade.

PATHOLOGY[1]

Pheochromocytomas are tumors of chromaffin tissue of ectodermal origin.[2] About 95% are abdominal. About 90% are adrenal, of which 10% are bilateral.[3] About 10% are extra-adrenal, often located along the sympathetic chain of the lumbar region and outflow in the region of Zuckerkandl's body at the bifurcation of the aorta. A rare origin is from a sympathetic ganglion or the wall of the urinary bladder.[4,5] About 1.0% of pheochromocytomas occur outside the abdomen, above the thorax. Though 90% are benign and do not metastasize, they are malignant in the sense of causing abnormal physiologic actions that can incapacitate or can cause death. Death is usually due to congestive heart failure, myocardial infarction, or intracerebral hemorrhage. Of all pheochromocytomas, 10% are actually malignant in the oncologic sense.

The average tumor weighs about 100 g, but variation occurs, from 1 g to 1000 g.

CLINICAL FEATURES[6]

Elevation of blood pressure, either continuous or paroxysmal, is the principal manifestation of this tumor. It must be distinguished from other causes of hypertension, because the hypertension can be cured. Characteristic symptoms represent the following triad: (1) headache with severe pounding, often episodic; (2) heart palpitations (often with a tachycardia or arrhythmias; (3) sweating and pallor attacks. When these symptoms accompany hypertension, they are diagnostic with a 90% specificity. When all three are absent, it is unlikely that pheochromocytoma is present to the extent of 99.9% assurance. The severity of symptoms correlates with the level of blood pressure elevation.

In about half of patients with pheochromocytoma, the hypertension and symptoms occur in paroxysms, with normotensive, asymptomatic intervals. Thus, two clinical types are manifested:

1. Paroxysmal hypertensive type: Hypertension and the triad occur at unexpected intervals and are relatively common. One sees a frequent association of anxiety, tremor, and nausea, usually related to an abundant epinephrine-secreting-type tumor.
2. Sustained hypertensive type: Often confused with

Table 45–22. Conditions Associated with the Three Types of Multiple Endocrine Neoplasia

Condition	MEN I	MEN II	MEN III
Parathyroid adenomas	≥90%	25%	Rare
Pancreatic islet cell tumors	80%	—	—
Pituitary adenomas	65%	—	—
Medullary carcinoma of the thyroid	—	>90%	>90%
Pheochromocytomas	—	50%	60%
Mucosal neuromas/ marfanoid habitus	—	—	≈100%

Landsberg, L., Daly, P.: Multiple endocrine neoplasia (MEN) syndromes. Section 89. In Merck Manual of Diagnosis and Therapy. Rahway, NJ, Merck Research Laboratories, 1992.

Table 45–23. Plasma Levels of Catecholamines (Catecholamine Levels in Arterial Blood)

	Mean	Range
Epinephrine	50 pg/ml (5.0 ng/dl) (0.27 nmol)	20–120 pg/ml
Norepinephrine	250 pg/ml (25 ng/dl) (1.7 nmol)	120–500 pg/ml (12–50 ng/dl)

*Norepinephrine in venous blood from adrenal 40 ng/dl (400 pg/ml): epinephrine: 1.0 nmol = 180 ng/L; norepinephrine: 1.0 nmol = 170 ng/L.

essential hypertension, but with superimposed attacks of severe hypertension. These patients are often thin, under 40 years of age, with features of hypermetabolism (BMR elevated in 20%). Norepinephrine secretion appears to be predominant.

Patients with pheochromocytoma may have a malignant-type hypertension without symptoms. Others are nonresponsive to ordinary antihypertensive therapy and may even have a paradoxic hypertensive response. Unmasking of a tumor is seen during induction of anesthesia, and a hypertensive crisis unresponse to standard intravenous antihypertensive therapy at this time warrants cancellation. The use of antidepressant drugs, such as imipramine, may induce a hypertensive crisis. Both these situations should alert the anesthesiologist to a potentially lethal condition. Sudden persistent hypertension occurring during parturition in the absence of any evidence of toxemia should suggest pheochromocytoma.

ASSOCIATED ENDOCRINE TUMORS[7] (Table 45–22)

Coexistence of pheochromocytoma with other tumors of endocrine origin has been designated as mixed multiple endocrine neoplasia syndromes (MEN).[8] These syndromes are denoted by a common origin of the tumors, from neuroectodermal and neuroentodermal embryologic structures, with subsequent abnormality of amine precursor uptake and distribution (APUDomas).[9] These syndromes are usually familial. Most often, pheochromocytoma is seen in association with medullary carcinoma of the thyroid. This is MEN type II or Sipple syndrome. When found in addition to mucosal and corneal neuromas, it is designated as MEN type III syndrome (see Table 45–10).[8] Hence, other hormonal disturbances may exist and should be evaluated.

DIAGNOSTIC TESTS

Biochemical Testing

A definitive diagnosis and confirmation of the presence of pheochromocytoma depends on tests demonstrating excess catecholamine secretion or on tests for the metabolic products of catecholamines.[10] Serum levels must be tested for catecholamines, or excess metabolic products must be demonstrated in the urine.

Serum Assays[1]

Serum catecholamine levels elevated above the range of normal variation are the ultimate test.[11] The range of normal values is summarized in Table 45–23. For the test, conditions should be standardized: The patient should be in a fasting state; as soon as patient is supine, venous cannulation and a slow infusion to keep cannula patent should be started. Blood sampling is done after the patient has had a 30-minute rest in the supine position. In Bravo and Gifford's study,[1] the 95% confidence limit was found to be 950 pg/ml (5.62 nmol/L) of norepinephrine plus epinephrine. Patients with higher values, over 2000 pg/ml, had pheochromocytomas. Elevations above normal may also be found in patients with neuroblastomas. A rare patient with essential hypertension may have a level above the limit.

Additional assay of the individual's epinephrine and norepinephrine levels may be carried out to identify the predominant catecholamine.

If epinephrine is the only catecholamine abnormally elevated, the tumor is likely located in the adrenal medulla or the organ of Zuckerkandl.[3]

Urinary Assays

These tests are easy to perform. Usually, a 24-hour urine specimen is collected.[10] Obtaining a 24-hour specimen is difficult, however, especially in children, and an overnight specimen or a 4-hour specimen may suffice. The parent catecholamines, the intermediate metabolic metanephrines, and the final metabolite VMA are all assayed (Table 45–24). Of these, metanephrine values are the most reliable index of excess catecholamine production. The urinary 3-hydroxy-4-methoxy mandelic acid (misnamed "VMA") is associated with a high percentage of false-negative results (Fig. 45–14 and Table 45–25).[1,11]

Pharmacologic Testing

These tests are obsolete or play a secondary role. Pharmacologic tests may be used in the unusual situation in

Table 45–24. Excretion of Catecholamines and Metabolites: Daily Urine Values*

Free epinephrine	25–50 μg
Free norepinephrine	100–200 μg
Methoxamines	
Metanephrine (adrenal source)	100–200 μg
Normetanephrine (adrenergic nerve; deaminated in nerve by monoamine oxidase)	100–300 μg/d
"VMA" (3-methoxy-4-hydroxyl mandelic acid)	2–6 mg
MOPEG (3-methoxy-4-hydroxyl phenylethylene glycol)	1.2–1.8 mg

*Dopamine metabolite: homovanillic acid (variable small amounts).
From Weiner, N. Palmer, P.: *In* Gilman, A.G., et al. (eds.). *In* Goodman and Gilman's The Pharmacological Basis of Therapeutics, 7th ed. New York, Macmillan, 1985.

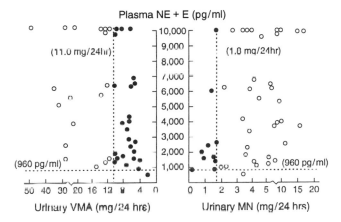

Fig. 45–14. Comparison of simultaneously measured indexes of catecholamine production in 43 patients with surgically confirmed pheochromocytoma. The horizontal broken lines represent the 96% upper confidence limits (i.e., 960 pg/ml) of plasma catecholamine values in 70 subjects with essential hypertension. The broken vertical lines represent the 96% upper confidence limits of values for urinary vanillylmandelic acid (VMA) (i.e., 11 mg/24 hours) and urinary metanephrines (MN) (i.e., 18 mg/24 hours) in 30 subjects with essential hypertension. NE+E denotes norepinephrine plus epinephrine. Solid symbols denote false-negative tests. All determinations were made in hospitalized patients. To convert MN and VMA values to micromoles per liter, multiply by 5.265 and 5.046, respectively; to convert NE+E values to nanomoles per liter, convert to micrograms per liter and multiply by 5.911. Redrawn from Bravo, E.L., Gifford, R.W., Jr.: N Engl J Med *311*:1298, 1984.

which biochemical values are equivocal, even after repeat examination. These tests were classic before catecholamine analysis was available. Two types are recognized: the provocative and the suppressive.[1,6]

Provocative Tests

These tests produce an elevation of blood pressure or symptoms:

Table 45–25. Sensitivity and Specificity of Various Tests of Pheochromocytoma*

Test	Referent Values	Sensitivity	Specificity
Plasma NE + E (after clonidine)	>500 pg/ml‡	0.97 (31/32)	0.99 (69/70)
Plasma NE + E	>950 pg/ml†	0.94 (60/64)	0.97 (68/70)
Urinary MN	>1.8 mg/24 hr†	0.79 (34/43)	0.93 (28/30)
Urinary VMA	>11 mg/24 hr†	0.42 (18/43)	1.00 (30/30)

*NE + E denotes norepinephrine plus epinephrine, MN is metanephrine, and VMA is vanillylmandelic acid. Numbers of patients are shown in parentheses. To convert values for MN and VMA to micromoles per liter, multiply by 5.265 and 5.046, respectively; to covert NE + E values to nanomoles per liter, convert to micrograms per liter and multiply by 5.911.
†Upper 95% confidence limits of basal values in 70 patients with essential hypertension.
‡Upper 95% confidence limits of basal values in 47 normotensive controls.
Data from Bravo, E.L., Gifford, R.W., Jr.: Pheochromocytoma: diagnosis, localization and management. N Engl J Med *311*:1298, 1984.

1. Cold pressor test.
2. Histamine or tyramine: A dose of 25 to 50 μg administered subcutaneously in 0.5 ml normal saline should be followed in a half-minute with a drop in blood pressure, followed by a rise to a level higher than the patient's usual pressure. This was and is used only in patients with blood pressures usually lower than 170/110 mm Hg. Adrenolytic drugs must be immediately available for intravenous use.
3. Glucagon test[12]: To be used after determining responses to cold pressor test. An intravenous bolus dose of 1.0 to 2.0 mg is administered. An increase in pressure of at least 20/15 mm Hg should occur. More important, the patient should have a marked increase of at least threefold (or 2000 pg/ml) in plasma catecholamines.

Suppression Tests

These tests are designed to reduce blood pressure in a hypertensive patient for differential diagnoses and are carried out in a standard manner.

1. Phentolamine (Regitine): A benazoline derivative, which causes dilatation of peripheral arterioles by blockade of α pressoreceptors. An intravenous bolus dose of 5.0 mg is administered. A sharp fall in pressure of 35 mm Hg systolic and 25 mm Hg diastolic in 2 minutes is diagnostic. No effect is seen in essential hypertension.
2. Clonidine suppression: This test should be carefully used according to the technique outlined by Bravo.[13] Clonidine acts by inhibiting central sympathetic outflow. It also has potent vagotonic action and can cause bradycardia. Suppression tests should not be carried out on patients who are taking anti-

hypertensive drugs. β-adrenergic blocking agents should be withheld for 48 hours.

LOCALIZATION OF TUMOR[1]

1. CT scanning is the preferred procedure initially. Tumors larger than 1.0 cm are usually located with precision.[7]
2. Selective arteriography may be necessary.
3. Selective localization may be accomplished by studies using radioactive iodine-131 (^{131}I) metaiodobenzyl guanadine, which is taken up by chromaffin tissue.

ANESTHETIC PRINCIPLES[14]

1. These patients are at significant risk and must be programmed carefully.
2. If the disorder is unsuspected, the risk and mortality are great, with sudden pulmonary edema or irreversible shock.
3. The perioperative objective is stress-free care.

ANESTHETIC CONSIDERATIONS AND RECOMMENDATIONS

Preoperative Preparation[14,15]

1. Appropriate blood volume therapy:
   Re-expand a contracted volume.
   Perform autologous blood replacement during surgery; collect blood 1 to 2 days preoperatively.
   Replace blood collected with substitutes.
   Treat anemia with frozen packed cells.
2. α-Adrenergic blockade (partial block recommended):
   Administer phenoxybenzamine (Dibenzyline), 10 to 20 mg orally three times daily for 4 days.
   Administer prazosin, 2 to 5 mg twice daily for 4 days.
   Note: Do not complete the α-block regimen if extra-adrenal tumors are suspected of coexisting. In high-risk patients, a partial block is desired. When the tumor is removed, an abrupt fall in blood pressure should occur; if not, another tumor is likely present.
3. β Blockade (only after α blockade):
   Administer propranolol, 30 to 40 mg orally 3 to 4 days (for hypertension, 80 mg two to three times per day).
   Administer metoprolol (Lopressor), 0.05 mg/kg.
4. α-Metyrosine blocks hydroxylase:
   It limits synthesis of DOPA precursor.
   The dose is 250 mg four times daily, increased as needed.
   The maximum dose is 1 to 4 g per day.

Premedication

Heavy premedication is desirable, as follows:

1. Barbiturate.
2. Neuroleptic agent: droperidol, which prevents epinephrine arrhythmias.
3. Narcotic: nalbuphine or meperidine; histamine release is limited.
4. Antihistaminics.

5. Anticholinergic agents:
   Atropine: undesirable; CNS stimulation, tachycardia; potentiation of pressor activity of norepinephrine.
   Scopolamine.
   Glycopyrrolate (preferred).

Choice of Anesthesia

General anesthesia provides the best conditions for management of the surgery and control of stress reactions. Some experience with continuous high spinal anesthesia combined with lighter general anesthesia appears to decrease "stress reactions."

Induction: Intravenous Agents

Thiopental, midazolam, droperidol, and fentanyl are recommended.

Inhalation Agents

1. Trichlorethylene, ether, cyclopropane: These agents release catecholamines.
2. Methoxyflurane: The arrhythmia threshold is low, and the drug causes renal damage.
3. Halothane: This drug causes cardiac muscle depression, sensitizes the myocardium, and induces arrhythmias.
4. Enflurane: This drug blocks chromaffin cells,[16] the stable cardiovascular system,[17] and does not sensitize the myocardium.[18]

Muscle Relaxants

1. Succinylcholine: This drug stimulates sympathetic ganglion and increases arterial pressure; muscular fasciculation occurs, and potassium is released; it is relatively contraindicated.
2. Gallamine: This agent causes tachycardia, increases catecholamine release, has cardiac vagolytic action, and is contraindicated.
3. Tubocurarine: This drug promotes the release of histamine and is contraindicated.
4. Pancuronium: This agent causes histamine release, has no ganglion blocking effect, produces cardiovascular stimulation that may be undesirable, and has no effect on plasma free catecholamine.
5. Atracurium: This drug promotes some histamine release.
6. Vecuronium: This is the preferred relaxant, causes no histamine release, promotes cardiovascular stability, is of ideal duration, and is easily reversed.

Monitoring

1. Before induction of anesthesia:
   ECG.
   Direct arterial measurement of blood pressure.
   Sphygmomanometry.
   Chest stethoscope.
2. After induction and intubation:
   Rectal temperature.
   Central venous pressure.
   Pulmonary capillary wedge pressure (Swan-Ganz).

Urine output.
Esophageal stethoscope.
Arterial blood gas determinations.
Measurement of blood loss.

PROBLEMS DURING SURGERY

1. Hypertensive crises: Causes include inadequate depth of anesthesia, excessive handling of the patient generally, and manipulation of time. Treatment is as follows:
   - Hydralazine: 10 to 20 mg IV; repeat as needed.
   - Phentolamine: 1 to 5 mg IV bolus or 100 mg/L drip (α_1 and β_2 block).
   - Sodium nitroprusside: infusion of an 0.01% solution.
   - Nitroglycerin: infusion of 0.01% solution (25 mg in 250 ml).

2. Heart rhythm abnormalities: These abnormalities are usually related to excess catecholamines:
   - Lidocaine: 1.0 mg/kg (ventricular arrhythmia).
   - Propranolol: 0.02 mg/kg increments to 0.2 mg/kg (average 0.035 mg/kg) (tachyarrhythmia; not in elderly patients with congestive heart failure).
   - Metoprolol: 0.05 mg/kg (average dose 2 to 5 mg); this agent does not block the vasodilatory effect of epinephrine and has no β_2 blockade.

3. Heart block: This should be managed with a pacemaker.

4. Hypotension: This problem usually occurs after tumor removal and is resolved by positioning of the anesthetized patient, transfusion of blood (autologous where possible) and plasma, and volume substitutes.

5. Hyperglycemia: This complication is related to glycogenolysis and inhibition of insulin secretion and to glucose intolerance.

6. Hypertrophy of myocardium and susceptibility to heart failure.

7. Adverse response to histamine-releasing drugs.

8. Hypocorticism: This is related to adrenal insufficiency postoperatively.

REFERENCES

1. Bravo, E. L., Gifford, R. W., Jr.: Pheochromocytoma: diagnosis, localization and management. N Engl J Med 311:1298, 1984.
2. Ellison, M. L., Neville, A. M.: Neoplasia and ectopic hormone production. In Raven, R. W. (ed.). Modern Trends in Oncology. London, Butterworth, 1973, p. 163.
3. Engelman, K.: Pheochromocytoma. Clin Endocrinol Metab 6:769, 1977.
4. Van Buskirk, K.: Pheochromocytoma of the bladder. JAMA 196:203, 1966.
5. Higgins, P.: Pheochromocytoma of the urinary bladder. Br Med J 2:274, 1966.
6. Gifford, R. W., Jr., et al.: Clinical features, diagnosis, and treatment of pheochromocytoma: a review of 76 cases. Mayo Clin Proc 39:281, 1964.
7. Thomas, J. L., Bernardino, M. E.: Pheochromocytoma in multiple endocrine adenamatosis: efficacy of computed tomography. JAMA 245:1467, 1981.
8. Alberts, W. M., McMeekin, J. O., George, J. M.: Mixed multiple endocrine neoplasia syndromes. JAMA 244:1236, 1980.
9. Marks, A.: Extra-adrenal pheochromocytoma and medullary thyroid carcinoma with pheochromocytoma. Arch Intern Med 134:1106, 1974.
10. Kaplan, N. M., et al.: Single-voided urine, metanephrine assays in screening for pheochromocytoma. Arch Intern Med 137:190, 1977.
11. Bravo, E. L., Tarazi, R. C., Gifford, R. W., Jr., Stewart, B. H.: Circulating and urinary catecholamines in pheochromocytoma. N Engl J Med 301:682, 1979.
12. Sebel, E.: Responses to glucagon in hypertensive patients with and without pheochromocytoma. Am J Med Sci 267:337, 1974.
13. Bravo, E. L., et al.: Clonidine-suppression test: a useful aid in the diagnosis of pheochromocytoma. N Engl J Med 305:623, 1981.
14. Roisen, M. F., Schreider, B. D., Hassan, S. K.: Anesthesia for patients with pheochromocytoma. Anesthesiol Clin North Am 5:269, 1987.
15. Kumar, S. M., Zsigmond, E. K.: Anesthetic management of pheochromocytoma. Anesthesiol Rev 5:14, 1978.
16. Gothert, M.: Inhibition of adrenal medullary catecholamine secretions. Anesthesiology 46:400, 1977.
17. Skorsted, P., Price, H.: Effects of ethrane on arterial pressure, preganglionic sympathetic activity and barostatic reflexes. Anesthesiology 36:257, 1972.
18. Reddy, K. D., Naraghi, M., Adriani, J.: Enflurane anesthesia for pheochromocytoma. Anesthesiol Rev 3:18, 1976.

SUGGESTED READINGS

Apgar, V., Papper, E. M.: Anesthetic management of patients with pheochromocytoma. Arch Surg 62:634, 1951.
Brunjes, S., Johns, V. J., Jr., Crane, M. G.: Pheochromocytoma: postoperative shock and blood volume. N Engl J Med 262:393, 1960.
Goldenberg, M., Snyder, C. H., Aranow, H.: New test for hypertension due to circulating epinephrine. JAMA 135:971, 1947.
Kvale, W. F., Priestley, J. T., Roth, G.: Pheochromocytoma: clinical aspects and surgical results. AMA Arch Surg 68:769, 1954.
Manager, W. M., et al.: Chemical quantization of epinephrine and norepinephrine in patients with pheochromocytoma. Circulation 10:641, 1954.
Price, H. L., et al.: Cyclopropane anesthesia. II: Epinephrine and norepinephrine in initiation of ventricular arrhythmias by CO_2 inhalation. Anesthesiology 19:619, 1958.
Schull, L. B., Bailey, J. C.: Anesthesia for patients having pheochromocytoma. Anesth Analg 39:400, 1960.
Von Euler, U. S., Floding, I.: Diagnosis of pheochromocytoma. Scand J Clin Lab Invest 8:288, 1956.

SCLERODERMA[1]

In this rheumatic disease, the skin and multiple viscera are affected by inflammation, vascular sclerosis, and fibrosis. No known cause or therapy is known; glucocorticoids are not effective. The prognosis is poor, and morbidity and mortality are related to the visceral involvement and not the skin involvement. The kidneys, heart, and lungs are the organs principally affected. Myocardial function is disordered by sclerosis of the smaller coronary vessels and fibrosis about the conduction system. Pulmonary fibrosis develops as the disease progresses, causing pulmonary hypertension and edema. Pulmonary function may only be mildly disturbed. Sclerosis of the renal vessels may result in acute renal failure. This is usually accompanied by systemic malignant hypertension.

Involvement of the gastrointestinal tract is characterized mainly by incompetence of the lower esophageal sphincter mechanisms. This involvement permits regurgitation and the ever-present risk of aspiration pneumonia.

Musculoskeletal abnormalities include flexion contractures and necrosis of the humeral head.

Skin sclerosis results in easy scar formation and Raynaud's phenomenon. Hardening of the facial skin may limit the opening of the mouth and may compromise control of the airway, as well as limit laryngoscopy. Venipuncture is difficult.

ANESTHETIC CONSIDERATIONS[2,3]

1. Intravenous access is limited by skin involvement.
2. Hypertension should be treated; patients respond poorly to vasodilation therapy.
3. Because of the ease of regurgitation, rapid-sequence anesthesia is recommended.
4. Spread of spinal agents is unpredictable.
5. Airway management may be difficult.
6. Corneal ulcers and conjunctivitis occur; the patient's eyes must be protected.
7. Sepsis and thrombocytopenia are common.
8. Renal failure is always a possibility.
9. Positioning must be careful.
10. A warm operating room environment is desirable to minimize Raynaud's phenomenon.

REFERENCES

1. Siegel, R. C.: Scleroderma. Med Clin North Am *61:*283, 1977.
2. Eisele, J. H., Reitan, J. A.: Scleroderma, Raynaud's phenomenon, and local anesthetics. Anesthesiology *34:*386, 1971.
3. Younker, D., Harrison, B.: Scleroderma and pregnancy: anaesthetic considerations. Br J Anaesth *57:*1136, 1985.

SKELETAL DEFORMITIES

Structural deformities encountered in patients, especially in children, include lordosis, kyphosis, scoliosis, kyphoscoliosis, and pectus excavatum, as well as pectus carinatum. Of these, scoliosis, kyphoscoliosis, and funnel chest cause sufficient intrathoracic changes to impair pulmonary and cardiac function.[1]

Scoliosis is defined as a lateral curvature of the spine.[2] Two main types are recognized: (1) nonstructural scoliosis, which is nonprogressive, and examination of which shows normal mobility of the spine; a shortened lower extremity causes a tilt of the lumbar spine with a convexity to the side of the short limb; and (2) structural scoliosis, which is characterized by a lateral curvature to one or another side of the vertebral column, accompanied by a rotation of the vertebra toward the convex side of the curve; some 80% of the lateral curvature is thoracic and to the right; this produces a bulging of the right chest wall.

Kyphosis is an increased posterior angulation of the spine (or a decreased anterior angulation). Lordosis is an increased anterior angulation of the spine or a decreased posterior angulation. An angulation of 40° or more is abnormal.

TERMINOLOGY (SCOLIOSIS RESEARCH SOCIETY)[1,2]

The term *structural curve* refers to the most significant deformity. Older terms were *major* or *primary* and are not necessarily accurate. The secondary curve is properly designated the *compensatory curve*.

The *end vertebrae* of a curve are designated as those vertebrae that tilt maximally into the concavity of the curve.

MEASUREMENTS AND SEVERITY

The severity of a curvature is determined as the angle of the convexity (the outward bulge). Cobb's method of measurement is used (Fig 45–15).[3]

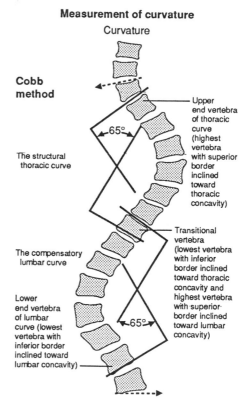

Measurement of curvature

Curvature

Cobb method

The structural thoracic curve

65°

Upper end vertebra of thoracic curve (highest vertebra with superior border inclined toward thoracic concavity)

Transitional vertebra (lowest vertebra with inferior border inclined toward thoracic concavity and highest vertebra with superior border inclined toward lumbar concavity)

The compensatory lumbar curve

Lower end vertebra of lumbar curve (lowest vertebra with inferior border inclined toward lumbar concavity)

65°

Fig. 45–15. Schematic view of idiopathic scoliosis for measurement. The end vertebrae of a curve are those that maximally tilt into the concavity of the curvature. In this schematic, the structural curve is right thoracic. For this curve, the upper or proximal thoracic end vertebra is the fifth thoracic, and the distal end vertebra is the first lumbar. Cobb's method of measuring the bulge is followed: A line is drawn parallel to the superior cortical plate of the proximal end vertebra (T5) and to the inferior cortical plate of the distal end vertebra (L1). A perpendicular is erected to these two lines, and the angle of intersection of the perpendiculars is the angle of the outward curve—the bulge. For the structural curve, there is a compensatory curve in this example, namely, the lumbar curve bulging in the opposite direction. Modified from Netter, F., Goldstein, L.A., Waugh, T.R.: Clin Orthop *93:*10, 1972.

The severity of a curve may be classified into one of seven groups:

- Group I: Less than 20°
- Group II: 20 to 30°
- Group III: 31 to 50°
- Group IV: 51 to 75°
- Group V: 76 to 100°
- Group VI: 101 to 125°
- Group VII: Over 125°

The degree of rotation is preferably determined by the Pedicle method of Moe[4] and is classified into five grades (Fig 45–16).

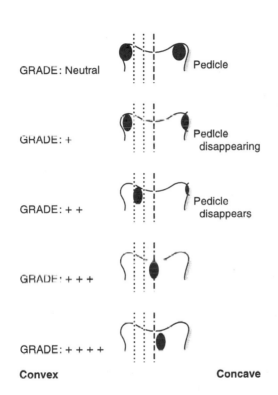

Pedicle method of determining vertebral rotation

	Pedicle	
	Convex	**Concave**
GRADE: Neutral	No asymmetry.	No asymmetry. No rotation.
GRADE: +	Migrates within first segment.	Pedicle disappearing overlaps edge of vertebra.
GRADE: + +	Migrates to second segment. Early distortion.	Pedicle almost disappears. Early distortion.
GRADE: + + +	Migrates to middle segment.	Pedicle not visible.
GRADE: + + + +	Migrates past midline to concave side of vertebral body.	Pedicle not visible.

Fig. 45–16. The grading of the degree of vertebral rotation as determined by the pedicle method. Redrawn from Nash, C.L., Moe, J.H. (eds.): A study of vertebral rotation. J Bone Joint Surg *51A*:223, 1969.

CURVE PATTERNS[5]

These patterns are designated according to the level of the apex of the curvature. Five patterns of curvature are defined in idiopathic scoliosis: (1) lumbar; (2) thoracolumbar; (3) thoracic; (4) cervicothoracic; and (5) double structural or combined.

INCIDENCE

From clinical examinations and roentgenographic surveys of school children, an overall incidence of 1.8 in 1000 has been determined. The occurrence in girls is set at about 3.9 in 1000, and it is 0.3 in 1000 in boys.[6]

CLASSIFICATION OF SCOLIOSIS (TABLE 45–26)

This classification is based on the origin of the structural change. In making a diagnosis, disease and mechanical factors should be identified.[7] A survey of the patient's family is needed. A search for underlying congenital abnormalities is required. A review of infectious diseases, such as poliomyelitis, and of rheumatoid diseases and skeletomuscular disorders is important.[7,8]

The most common type of scoliosis is idiopathic and is usually diagnosed by exclusion.[9] It represents about 85% of patients with scoliosis. Three periods of onset are recognized, each corresponding to peak periods of growth.[2] The thoracic and lumbar areas are involved. The infantile type is usually in males and is characterized as resolving or progressive. The convexity is to the left. The progres-

Table 45–26. Etiologic Classifications of Structural Types (Terminology: Committee on Scoliosis Research Society)

Idiopathic scoliosis (three groups according to age; 85% of scoliosis deformities)
   Infantile (under 4 years)
   Juvenile
   Adolescent
Congenital spine deformity (Failure to develop or abnormal segmentation defects; lordosis)
Neuromuscular scoliosis
   Neuropathic (poliomyelitis; cerebral palsy)
   Myopathic (dystrophies; amyotonia)
Associated with neurofibromatosis
Mesenchymal disorders
   Rheumatoid arthritis
   Marfan's syndrome
   Morquio's syndrome
Traumatic scoliosis
   Vertebral fractures
   Extravertebral trauma: thoracoplasty
   Burns
Scoliosis secondary to irritative phenomena
   Spinal cord tumors
   Osteomas
   Radiculitis
Other types
   Nutritional deficiency (vitamin D deficiency)
   Endocrine disorders
   Infectious tuberculosis

From Goldstein, L. A., Waugh, T. R.: Clinical Orthopaedics and Related Research *93*:10–22, 1973.

sive type is associated with a true kyphosis; it is severe, and the mean angle is about 130°.

The adolescent type occurs between 10 years of age and skeletal maturity. It is the most common and is usually seen in females. It is rapidly progressive and involves 7 to 10 vertebrae. The angle of curvature is severe and ranges from 70 to 130°. A high familial incidence is present, with a dominant inheritance pattern.[6]

MORTALITY

Generally, the greater the primary curve, the poorer the prognosis. Most deaths in patients with idiopathic scoliosis occur before age 45 years, from respiratory or cardiac failure (Fig. 45–17), which account for 60% of the deaths. Mortality of patients with untreated scoliosis who die of other causes is twice that of the general population, and the average age at death is 46 years.

ORTHOPEDIC DESCRIPTION[2]

The deformity of scoliosis is denoted by two structural changes: (1) lateral curvature of the spine; and (2) rotation of the vertebrae, accompanied by deformation of the rib cage. Clinically, 80% of cases of scoliosis present a right-sided deformity. The structural curve (primary) of the spine is convex toward the right and produces a bulging of the right chest wall. In the area of the major curve, the vertebrae and spinous processes rotate toward the convexity of the curve; the disks and bodies become wedge-shaped. Because of the rotation, the ribs on the convex side are pulled back, producing a prominent posterior angle. This appears to be a hump, but is not a typi-

cal kyphosis. On the concave side, the posterior angle of the ribs is flattened, but anteriorly the ribs are prominent. On the concave side, the pedicles and laminae are thin and short and, in addition, the vertebral canal is narrow. The compensatory curve (secondary) bends sharply to the left in the lower thoracic and lumbar region. This causes a compression of the left intrathoracic viscera.

In funnel chest (pectus excavatum),[9] the inward position of the sternum causes displacement of the mediastinum either to the right or to the left, more often to the right. Torsion on the great vessels, rotation of spine, and other mechanical influences impose a burden on both cardiac and pulmonary function. This condition may compound a scoliosis deformity.

SYMPTOMS[10,11]

These patients have symptoms of dyspnea, palpitation, and cough. The angulation of the spine tends to increase up to the age of 10 years, and the distress progresses. Fainting attacks are common. Tachycardia is usual, and the diastolic pressure is elevated. Enlargement of the heart, chiefly the right ventricle, occurs, and peripheral edema or congestion occurs. The right atrium is dilated, and the ECG shows a P wave larger than 2.5 mm in the later stages.

These patients are both pulmonary and cardiac cripples.[11] Ventilation is poor, and pulmonary infection is prone to occur. Congestive heart failure is frequent. The common cause of death is pulmonary-cardiac failure.[12] It is often sudden. Costal respiration is limited, and breathing is accomplished largely by diaphragmatic movement.

FUNCTIONAL DERANGEMENTS

The structural changes impose mechanical restriction on thoracic viscera, which are displaced or compressed. One sees impaired pulmonary and cardiac function; pulmonary insufficiency and cardiac failure are usual complications.[10] The compensatory curve displaces the heart upward.[13]

Pulmonary hypertension is a progressive problem. The increasing pulmonary resistance is due first to a decreased number of vascular units per unit of lung volume, from impaired growth and development, and second to compression of the alveoli, so they approach a residual volume.[14]

Respiratory function is impaired, and a restrictive pattern is observed,[15] accompanied by decreased compliance. The lungs have a diminished volume, mechanically limited. Lung volumes and compliance are inversely related to the angle of the curvature. The greatest reduction is in the vital capacity, which is reduced between 25 and 75%, with an average reduction of only 60% of the predicted. Total lung capacity shows a decrease and averages 70% of predicted, whereas the FRC is 80% of predicted. Most of the reduction in ventilatory capacity is due to a reduced inspiratory capacity. Tidal air in advanced cases may also be diminished with tachypnea.

Alveolar hypoventilation and maldistribution of blood flow are present.[15] These conditions lead to hypoxemia

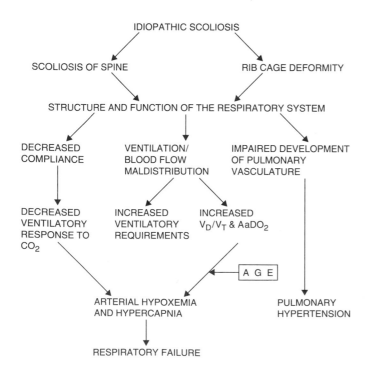

Fig. 45–17. The factors in idiopathic scoliosis that contribute to respiratory function abnormalities and failure. From Kafer, E. R.: Anesthesiology 52:339, 1980.

Table 45–27. Preoperative Evaluation

Hemoglobin, hematocrit, urinalysis, prothrombin time, partial thromboplastin time
Anteroposterior and lateral chest radiographs
Anteroposterior and lateral 36-inch spine films for measurement of the curve
Etiology and degree of the curve
Pulmonary function test: vital capacity, timed vital capacity, functional residual capacity, peak expiratory flow rate
Pulmonary lung scan (both perfusion and ventilation) if necessary
Electrocardiogram; vector electrocardiogram where indicated
Myelogram in patients with myelodysplasia or for other indications

From Dahm, L. S., Dickson, J. U., Harrison, G. H.: Preoperative evaluation, perioperative and anesthetic management in the patient with scoliosis. Anesthesiol Rev 9:13, 1982.

(the common blood gas abnormality). The Pao_2 is reduced, whereas a normal Pao_2 is usual, except in late stages. Patients with a thoracic deformity of less than 50° usually do not have extensive abnormal pulmonary function values.

PREANESTHETIC EVALUATION AND PREPARATION[11,16] (Table 45–27)

Careful attention to the respiratory tract is essential.[11] Infections, including colds, must be absent. Secretions must be removed, and postural drainage is recommended. The patient should be tested in the proposed operative position and observed for physiologic changes or evidence of discomfort. Any position restricting ventilation may induce hypoxia and may produce sudden hypotension and death, and all abnormal positions should be avoided. Usually, the lateral position is best tolerated, with the left side dependent in most instances (right-sided convexity). The kneeling position is often assumed.

Pulmonary function studies should be done. Breathing exercises, including an explanation of their importance, as well as training with positive pressure and respirator devices, are desirable.[7] The conditioning of the accessory muscles of respiration by appropriate exercise enables a patient to increase ventilatory capacity.

As part of patient preparation, if the patient is in a cast, windows should be cut into the body cast over the precordium and over the neck anteriorly. These enable the surgical team to institute such measures as cardiac resuscitation and tracheostomy in an emergency.

GROUPING OF PATIENTS

According to the extent of changes in vital capacity and based on other findings in an extensive preoperative evaluation, Dahm and associates have divided scoliotic patients into four groups[16] (Table 45–28).[8] These groups correlate with the American Society of Anesthesiologists (ASA) physical status classification.

PREANESTHETIC MEDICATION

Patients should arrive in the operating room calm and sleepy but arousable. The opiates in modest doses are tolerated in these patients; morphine often produces an unpredictable response and is considered contraindicated because of its respiratory depression action and, equally important, its bronchoconstrictor action. Meperidine is well tolerated. The barbiturates as a whole are poorly tolerated, with the exception of phenobarbital and amobarbital sodium. The phenothiazine derivatives, promethazine in particular, provide good tranquilization without untoward effects in doses of 12 to 25 mg. Short-acting benzodiazepines, such as triazolam and temazepam, are effective.

Table 45–28. Preoperative Findings: Situations I–IV

Situation	Vital Capacity (% predicted norm)	Expiratory Peak Flow	Hemoglobin/ hematocrit	Electrocardiographic Findings	Arterial Blood Gases
I	70 or greater	Normal for height	Normal	Normal	Normal
II	50–70	Approximately one standard deviation below normal	Slightly elevated*	Normal	Normal
III	30–50	Two standard deviations below mean	16 g or higher*	(Vector) Right ventricular preponderance	Pao_2 greater than 75 mm Hg
IV	10–30	Below second standard deviation below mean	17–18 g*	(Vector) Cor pulmonale	Pao_2 less than 75 mm Hg†

*Because many of the patients seen are adolescent girls, the slight elevation in hemoglobin and hematocrit may be masked; in situation III and IV patients, even a moderate elevation is significant.

†On increased inspired oxygen concentration, the Pao_2 may still be less than 75 mm Hg; in more severe cases, the Pao_2 may be even lower than the $Paco_2$.

From Dahm, L. S., Dickson, J. U., Harrison, G. H.: Preoperative evaluation, perioperative and anesthetic management in the patient with scoliosis. Anesthesiol Rev 9:13, 1982.

CHOICE OF ANESTHESIA[11]

The patient's anatomic abnormalities and associated neuromuscular disease, with any predetermined impairment in cardiovascular and respiratory status, are prime determinants. The type of procedure and the operative position, then, must be considered. Corrective orthopedic procedures present special problems. Nonorthopedic procedures present postoperative problems.

General anesthesia with inhalation agents is recommended for most procedures. These agents have built-in safety and are retrievable. By artificial ventilation, the agents can be removed and postoperative depression can be avoided.

Regional anesthesia may be used safely for carefully selected surgical procedures. Epidural and low spinal anesthesia regimens are suitable for lower extremity operations. Brachial plexus blocks are useful for upper extremity surgery. Regional anesthesia should be selected for short procedures, for noncavity operations, and when position is not a compounding factor. If the severity of the scoliosis curve is greater than 50°, general anesthesia is indicated.

Management by General Anesthesia[16]

General anesthesia is preferred in infants, children, and adolescents. It is also preferred for adults when the severity of the scoliosis has compromised cardiopulmonary function. Induction is usually accomplished with thiopental. When hypersensitivity and allergic conditions exist, midazolam may be used. Ketamine provides an excellent agent for infants and young children and can be given intramuscularly.

After unconsciousness is produced by the induction agents, the anesthetic state is established with an inhalation agent. Halothane is suitable for infants and younger children. During puberty and thereafter, an enflurane-nitrous oxide-oxygen combination is employed.

Intubation is accomplished with pancuronium or vecuronium. Succinyl-choline is avoided. When an unusual position is required, especially the prone position, or when the patient prefers a semilateral (left-side down) posture, a nonkinking spinal wire endotracheal tube is selected.

When lung-chest compliance permits, a ventilator is used. In patients with severe degrees of scoliosis, however, manual ventilation is more effective.

A nasogastric tube should be placed initially and the stomach emptied. As part of preanesthetic medication, the gastric acidity may be lowered by histamine blockers and antacids.

Controlled hypotension is employed in corrective surgery of the spine.

MONITORING

Standard techniques include sphygmomanometry and ECG. For extensive surgery, an arterial line and a central venous pressure monitor are employed. In the severe scoliotics (curvature over 75°), some judgment should be made regarding a Swan-Ganz catheter. This is more likely when the cardiac function is impaired. Blood gases should be determined frequently during the operative procedure.

INTRAOPERATIVE PROBLEMS[16]

The major problems encountered are seen in patients with respiratory insufficiency and cardiovascular impairment. Mild to moderate hypoxemia is frequent and, if accompanied by hypercarbia, represents borderline respiratory failure.

Several potential problems should be considered[11]:

1. Of patients developing malignant hyperthermia, 7% of those reported have scoliosis.[17] A significant number of patients with structural abnormalities have an elevated creatinine phosphokinase level.
2. Sustained muscular contracture is more frequent in these patients following succinylcholine administration, especially without pancuronium pretreatment.[18]
3. Potassium values are often elevated.
4. Myoglobulinemia and cryoglobulinemia are frequent.

POSTOPERATIVE CARE[16,19]

All patients must be carefully monitored, whether following nonorthopedic surgery or following corrective orthopedic surgery.[20]

In mild to moderate scoliosis, the patient may be extubated in the operating room. If a body cast is applied, extubation should be delayed. Humidified oxygen should be administered at a concentration of 30 to 40% by a T-piece, either by endotracheal tube or by mask.

For patients with severe scoliosis, ventilatory assistance should be provided for at least the first 24 hours. Volume-controlled ventilation (e.g., MA-1)[7] is recommended. Blood gases are regularly determined.

Before extubation, a good precaution is to administer dexamethasone, 4 mg IV.[16] This drug minimizes laryngeal edema. Because these patients are prone to pulmonary infection, prophylactic antibiotic therapy is begun intraoperatively or immediately postoperatively. One should be aware of those antibiotics that affect neuromuscular function.

REFERENCES

1. Harrington, P. R.: Aetiology of scoliosis. Clin Orthop 126:17, 1977.
2. Goldstein, L. A., Waugh, T. R.: Classification and terminology of scoliosis. Clin Orthop 93:10, 1973.
3. Cobb, J. R.: Outline for the Study of Scoliosis. Instructional Course Lectures, American Academy of Orthopaedic Surgeons. Vol. 5. Ann Arbor, MI, J. W. Edwards, 1948, p. 261.
4. Moe, J. H.: A critical analysis of methods of fusion for scoliosis: an evaluation in 266 patients. J Bone Joint Surg 40A:529, 1958.
5. Moe, J. H., Kettleson, D. M.: Idiopathic scoliosis: analysis of curve patterns and preliminary results of Milwaukee brace treatment—169 patients. J Bone Joint Surg 52A:1509, 1970.
6. Wynne-Davies, R.: Familial (idiopathic) scoliosis. J Bone Joint Surg 50B:24, 1968.
7. Beck, G., Graham, G., Barach, A.: Respiration and cough ef-

fect of physical methods on the mechanics of breathing in poliomyelitis. Ann Intern Med *43*, 1955.

8. Joos, T. H., Talner, N. S., Wilson, J. L., Arbor, A.: Risk of surgery in poliomyelitis patients dependent on respirators. JAMA *161*:935, 1956.

9. Lester, C. W.: The surgical treatment of funnel chest. Ann Surg *123*:1003, 1946.

10. Cugell, D. W., Gantt, M. E.: Thoracic deformity and cardiopulmonary disease; kyphoscoliosis, rhematoid spondylitis, pectus excavatum, fibrothorax. *In* Clinical Cardiopulmonary Physiology. New York, Grune & Stratton, 1980, p. 670.

11. Kafer, E. R.: Respiratory and cardiovascular functions in scoliosis and the principles of anesthetic management: review. Anesthesiology *52*:339, 1980.

12. Chapman, E. M., Dill, D. B., Graybiel, A. N.: Decrease in functional capacity resulting from deformities of the chest: pulmo-cardiac failure. Medicine *18*:167, 1939.

13. Holmes, J. H., Waill, D. R.: Incomplete heart block produced by changes in posture. Am Heart J *30*:291, 1945.

14. Fishman, A., Bergofsky, E., Turino, G.: Circulation and respiration in kyphoscoliosis. Circulation *14*:935, 1956.

15. Fishman, A. P., Goldring, R. M., Turino, G. M.: General alevolar hypoventilation: a syndrome of respiratory and cardiac failure in patients with normal lungs. Q J Med *35*:261, 1966.

16. Dahm, L. S., Dickson, J. U., Harrison, G. H.: Preop evaluation, perioperative and anesthetic management in the patient with scoliosis. Anesthesiol Rev *9*:13, 1982.

17. Britt, B. A., Kalow, W.: Malignant hyperthermia: a statistical review. Can Anaesth Soc J *17*:293, 1970.

18. Britt, B. A.: Malignant hyperthermia: a pharmacogenetic disease of skeletal and cardiac muscle. N Engl J Med *74*:1140, 1974.

19. Makley, T. J., et al.: Pulmonary function in paralytic and non paralytic scoliosis before and after treatment. J Bone Joint Surg *50A*:1379, 1968.

20. Smith, T. K., Stallone, R. J., Yee, J. M.: The thoracic surgeon and anterior spinal surgery. J Thorac Cardiovasc Surg *77*:925, 1979.

MONITORING SPINAL CORD INTEGRITY

In the correction of scoliosis, certain procedures carry an increased risk of neurologic injury. Predisposing conditions associated with scoliosis correction have been enumerated (Table 45–29).[1]

The orthopedic procedures predisposing to neurologic injury during scoliosis correction are also tabulated (Table 45–30). Patients with mild to moderate scoliosis

Table 45–29. Conditions Predisposing to Neurologic Injury During Scoliosis Correction

Kyphosis
Severe scoliosis (>50° curve)
Congenital scoliosis
Scoliosis associated with neurologic deficits
Scoliosis associated with neurologic deficits acquired during skeletal traction

From MacEwen, G. D., Bunnell, W. P., Sriram, K.: Acute neurological complications in the treatment of scoliosis: a report of the Scoliosis Research Society. J. Bone Joint Surg *57A*:404, 1975.

Table 45–30. Orthopedic Procedures Predisposing to Neurologic Injury During Scoliosis Correction[a]

Preoperative skeletal traction
Spinal osteotomy
Use of Harrington instrumentation to gain correction in congenital scoliosis
Use of Harrington instrumentation to gain further correction after skeletal traction

From MacEwen, G. D., Bunnell, W. P., Sriram, K.: Acute neurological complications in the treatment of scoliosis: a report of the Scoliosis Research Society. J. Bone Joint Surg *57A*:404, 1975.

frequently have accompanied syringomyelia. Spinal fusion, spinal distraction techniques, and Harrington rod instrumentation carry a greater risk of neurologic damage in such patients. To determine whether the surgical procedure has incurred neurologic damage, two techniques are currently employed to monitor spinal cord integrity. These are (1) wake-up techniques and (2) recording of somatosensory evoked potentials (SSEPs).[2,3]

APPLICATION OF WAKE-UP TECHNIQUE

The wake-up technique was introduced in 1973 and has been developed in subsequent years.[4] This consists of discontinuing anesthesia after rodding or other procedures have been completed. The patient is allowed to awaken, and two tests are carried out: (1) response to pinpoint testing of extremities and noting the usual rapid withdrawal-type reflex in the intact patient; and (2) a response to a command to move feet and observation of appropriate movement.

Contraindications or hazards consist of the following: the severely retarded patient, infants and young children, and patients with preexisting paraplegia. This last group needs preoperative assessment of the areas of activity and determination of any decrease in such areas.

Hazards of the technique in spinal fusion for scoliosis correction consist of the following:

• On emergence, the complaint of pain
• Emotional stress and trauma of awaking during surgery
• Postoperative recall and sleep disorders
• Coughing on endotracheal tube, with endotracheal tube dislocation
• Air embolism through exposed epidural veins
• Rod dislocation or fracture with coughing

The successful wake-up technique indicates that there is significant integration and preservation of dorsal column and motor tract functions. Wake-up end points are not seriously affected by the anesthetic agents, by hypotensive anesthesia, or by electrical interference.

Despite the present techniques of monitoring, occasional patients have an increase in their neurologic impairment, and delayed paraplegia has been reported. Similarly, despite proper monitoring, the occurrence of tetraplegia has been reported.[5]

The two commonly used techniques of testing for neurologic responses or deficits have not been compared. Al-

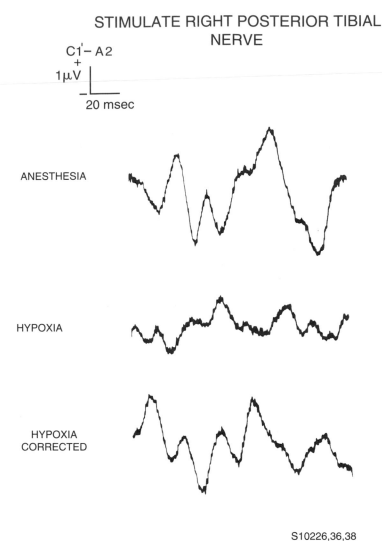

STIMULATE RIGHT POSTERIOR TIBIAL NERVE

C1'– A2
+
1µV
–
20 msec

ANESTHESIA

HYPOXIA

HYPOXIA CORRECTED

S10226,36,38

Fig. 45–18. Somatosensory cortical-evoked potentials (SCEPs) recorded during surgery. Unretouched wave forms show some motion artifact, which could have been removed by additional filtering, but filter settings that smooth wave forms hinder recording of early SCEP components. This amount of artifact does not interfere with monitoring. From Grundy, B.L., International Anesthesia Research Society: Anesth Analg *60:*437, 1981.

though false-negative responses have not been reported with the "wake-up" test, false-positive test results have occurred with SSEP. Both techniques should be employed to corroborate the patient's neurologic status.

SOMATOSENSORY EVOKED POTENTIAL (SSEP)

This technique was introduced by Engler and associates in 1978,[2] and it has become available as a routine in selected situations.

The technique consists of the application of electrodes preoperatively to the lower extremities, usually over the sight of the posterior tibial nerves (Fig. 45–18), as well as to the scalp overlying the corresponding sensorimotor cortex (C_z-F_z); The parameters of the technique are summarized in Table 45–31.[6] Short latency procedures are firmer than those of intermediate latency, and they therefore appear to be less affected by anesthetic and physiopharmacologic factors.[7]

Because SSEPs are sensitive to changes in blood supply and to hypotension and hypoxia,[8] this technique is an important tool for recognizing such changes. This useful-

Table 45–31. Stimulus and Recording Parameters: Somatosensory Cortical Evoked Potentials

Stimulation
  Site: Right posterior tibial nerve at ankle, carthode proximal
  Constant current: 19.9 amp
  Duration: 250 µsec
  Rate: 0.9/sec
Recording
  Site: primary somatosensory area to opposite ear; C1'–A2; international ten twenty system (9); C1', 2 cm behind C1; patient reference electrode, right popliteal fossa
  Filters: 1–1500 Hz
  Sensitivity: ±50 µV full scale
  Sweep time: 262 msec
  Sampling rate for analog to digital conversion: 3906 Hz
  Repetitions per average: 128

*Electrodes for stimulation and recording were 10-mm gold discs, applied with collodion and filled with conductive gel. All impedances were less than 3000 ohm.

From Grundy, B. L., et al: Intraoperative hypoxia detected by evoked potential monitoring. Anesth Analg *60:*437, 1981.

ness has been shown by Grundy and associates.[6] When SSEPs are observed during spinal manipulation, rapid reversal or cessation of the surgical procedure is known to prevent spinal cord damage.[7] The administration of high concentrations of oxygen and the reversal of hypotension have also been found to restore potentials toward normal limits.[9]

REFERENCES

1. MacEwen, G. D., Bunnell, W. P., Sriram, K.: Acute neurological complications in the treatment of scoliosis: a report of the Scoliosis Research Society. J Bone Joint Surg 574:404, 1975.
2. Engler, G. L., et al.: Somatosensory evoked potentials during Harrington instrumentation for scoliosis. J Bone Joint Surg 60A:528, 1978.
3. Spielholz, N. I., Benjamin, M. V., Engler, G. L., Ransohoff, J.: Somatosensory evoked potentials during decompression and stabilization of the spine. Spine 4:500, 1979.
4. Vauzelle, C., Stagnara, P., Jouvinoux, P.: Functional monitoring of spinal cord activity during spinal cord surgery. Clin Orthop 93:173, 1973.
5. Diaz, J. H., Lockhart, C. H.: Postoperative quadriplegia after spinal fusion for scoliosis with intraoperative awakening. Anesth Analg 66:1039, 1987.
6. Grundy, B. L., et al.: Intraoperative hypoxia detected by evoked potential monitoring. Anesth Analg 60:437, 1981.
7. Clark, D. L., Rosner, B. S.: Neurophysiologic effects of general anesthetics. I. Electroencephalogram and sensory evoked responses in man. Anesthesiology 38:564, 1973.
8. Gillian, L. A.: Vascular supply of the spinal cord: clinical significance. In Chou, S. N., Seljeskoy, E. L. (eds.). Spinal Deformities and Neurological Dysfunction. New York, Raven Press, 1978, p. 11.
9. Grundy, B. L., Nash, C. L., Brown, R. H.: Arterial pressure manipulation alters spinal cord function during correction of scoliosis. Anesthesiology 54:249, 1981.

KLIPPEL-FEIL SYNDROME

This syndrome was originally described in 1912 and is characterized by congenital abnormalities of the bony vertebral spine. Deformities consist of fusion of various vertebrae and can be classified into three principal types[1]:

Type I. Fusion of the bodies of cervical vertebrae at two sites, namely, C2 and C3 or C5 and C6. This is the more common occurrence. This is often combined with *atlanto-occipital fusion.*
Type II. Massive fusion of the bodies of many cervical vertebrae combined with fusion of upper thoracic vertebrae may be seen.
Type III. Both cervical vertebral fusion and lower thoracic or lumbar vertebral fusion may occur. Spina bifida may be seen in this type.

GENETIC ASPECT

The syndrome is inherited as an autosomal dominant disorder or as a recessive disorder with variable penetrance and expressivity. Females are affected more often than males.[2]

ASSOCIATED DISORDERS

Type I deformity is often associated with additional skeletal abnormalities,[3] as follows: maxillomandibular deformities; cleft palate; significant khyphoscoliosis and upward displacement of the scapulae (Sprengel's deformity). Skull asymmetry and flattening of the occipital bone are seen.

Congenital cardiac defects are frequent, with an incidence of about 8%.[3] Ventricular septal anomalies are the commonest, but other lesions may be seen.

CLINICAL FEATURES[3,4]

The limited range of neck motion is the dominant manifestation of this skeletal abnormality. It is usually painless and asymptomatic. A low occipital hairline may represent a relation to the flattening of the occipital bone. This platybasia (maldeveloped base of the skull) may permit invagination of the occiput or of the upper cervical spine into the posterior fossa that may manifest itself later in adolescence or adult life. Compression of the medulla and cervical spinal cord can lead to increased intracranial pressure, headache, and vomiting.

Neurologic manifestations are secondary to the compression of the cervical spinal cord or to stretch of the lower cranial nerves. If the cerebellar tonsils descend into the cervical spinal canal, the symptoms of the Arnold-Chiari malformation may be seen.[4]

ARNOLD-CHIARI MALFORMATION[4,5]

The Arnold-Chiari malformation is represented as a group of congenital hindbrain anomalies caused by a downward displacement of the lower pons and medulla. The symptoms of type II Arnold-Chiari malformation appear in infancy and are associated with myelomeningocele and progressive hydrocephalus. The respiratory symptoms are common and include inspiratory stridor (tenth nerve palsy) episodic apnea, depressed gag reflex, nystagmus, and spastic upper extremity weakness.

In type I Arnold-Chiari malformation, which is evident in adulthood, the most common symptoms are pain in the neck shoulders or arms and atrophy of the hand and upper extremity. Headache, nystagmus, vertigo, and ataxia are common. Bulbar symptoms develop, with fasciculations and atrophy of the tongue.

Type III Arnold-Chiari malformation is the second most frequent malformation and involves caudal displacement of the cerebellum and brain stem into a cervical meningocele.

In the usual Klippel-Feil syndrome, syncopal episodes may occur during sudden rotary motion of the head or movement of the neck, causing compression of the basilar artery.

ANESTHETIC CONSIDERATIONS[6,7]

In the preanesthetic evaluation, skeletal deformities should be described in detail, and any neurologic defects identified. Cervical-vertebral conditions should be especially carefully assessed, with a thorough examination of the oropharynx and notation of the extent to which the mouth can be opened. An airway score should be noted for laryngoscopic and airway procedures.

The patient with an upper cervical deformity should be treated as if a neck fracture existed. Movement of the head should be limited, and the neck should be maintained in the neutral axis. If general anesthesia is chosen, these aspects determine whether an awake intubation is necessary or whether laryngoscopy with intubation can be accomplished without difficulty in the sleeping patient. Muscle relaxation should be obtained with nondepolarizing relaxant whether or not neurologic defects are present.

In type I and type II Klippel-Feil syndrome, regional anesthesia can be successfully achieved for many surgical procedures. Even spinal or epidural anesthesia can be used if no lower spinal vertebral abnormalities exist and no neurologic deficiencies are present.[7]

REFERENCES

1. Klippel, M., Feil, A.: Anomalies de la colonne vertebrate par absence des vertebraes cervicales: cage thoracique remontant jusqu'à la base du crane. Bull Mem Soc Anat (Paris) 87:185, 1912.
2. Gunderson, C. H.: The Klippel-Feil syndrome: genetic and clinical evaluation of cervical fusion. Medicine 46:491, 1967.
3. Helmi, C.: Craniofacial and extra cranial malformations in the Klippel-Feil syndrome. Cleft Palate J 17:65, 1980.
4. McLeod, M. E., Creighton, R. E.: Anesthesia for pediatric neurological and neuromuscular diseases. J Child Neurol 1:189, 1986.
5. Bell, W. O., Charney, E. B., Bruce, D. A.: Symptomatic Arnold-Chiari malformation: review of experience with 22 cases. J Neurosurg 66:812, 1987.
6. Naguib, M. G., Heram, F., Wahab, A.: Anesthetic considerations in Klippel-Feil syndrome. Can Anaesth Soc J 33:66, 1986.
7. Ramanathan, J., Maduske A. L.: Epidural anesthesia in Klippel-Feil syndrome. Anesthesiol Rev 9:41, 1982.

VON HIPPEL-LINDAU DISEASE

This rare autosomal dominant disease has a variable expression.[1] The disease is classified as a phakomatosis affecting the CNS. This term implies a congenital dermatologic lesion, from the word *phakos*, from the Greek meaning birthmark (mole or freckle).[2] This disease complex is considered to be a group of congenital neuroectodermal disorders describing dysplasias and some neoplasias originating from the embryonic ectoderm of the skin, eyes, and nervous system.

PATHOLOGY

The characteristic lesion of this hereditary disorder is a capillary hemangioblastoma. It was clearly described by von Hippel in 1895 as an ocular angiomatosis, occurring in 60 to 70% of patients with the complex.[3] Single and

Table 45–32. Incidence of Specific Lesions Associated with von Hippel-Lindau Disease*

Lesion	Incidence (%)	Reference
Ocular Hemangioblastomas/ angiomas	60	Wing et al.[7]
CNS angioblastomas (intracranial)	40	Lamell et al.[1]
Cerebellar hemangioblastomas	2	Hardwig and Robertson[2]
Renal cell cysts and/or adenocarcinomas	30	Neumann[5]
Cystic lesions of the pancreas or islet cells	1	Cornish et al.[12]
Pheochromocytoma	15	Mulshine et al.[12]
Erythrocythesia	5–10	Brody and Rodriguez[10]

*The presence of anocular lesion and that of a CNS angioblastoma represents classic von Hippel-Lindau Disease.

multiple hemangioblastomas were also described in the CNS with an incidence of 30 to 50%. The CNS lesions in combination with the optic lesions define von Hippel-Lindau disease. An intracranial hemangioblastoma with cystic lesions of the pancreas or kidney is designated Lindau's syndrome.[4] In the von Hippel-Lindau disease, the commonest site of the CNS tumors is the cerebellum, but these tumors also occur in the medulla and in the spinal cord. The cerebellar tumor is the commonest cause of death.[2] About 75% of the lesions are cystic, and 25% are solid.[5]

Renal cell carcinoma occurs in about 25% of patients, whereas renal cysts may be found in 50% of von Hippel-Lindau patients. Angiomas and adenomas of the liver and kidney are rather common (Table 45–32).

HISTOLOGY

Most lesions are cystic. Fine vascular networks of endothelial channels compose the tissue, and the tumor is usually devoid of neurons or glial cells. Cystic lesions have a lower mortality of about 25% than the solid tumors, with a mortality of 50%.

GENETIC BASIS

Many studies have demonstrated an autosoma dominant inheritance with almost complete penetrance.[1] Heterozygotes are usually not affected until adulthood. The inheritance of the disease phenotype has been shown to be associated with an abnormal chromosome 3p.[6] The gene is specifically related to the human oncogene that maps to chromosome 3p[25].

CLINICAL CONSIDERATIONS

Basic symptoms include headache, visual disturbances, and incoordination of muscles, especially on the affected side, with cerebellar tumors and ataxia. Nausea and vomiting are common, and changes in the patient's mental state are seen. These are usually evident in the third or fourth decade of life. Vertigo and nystagmus are common, and a broad-based gait may develop.

Ophthalmologic problems are seen in over 60% of patients[7]; these are usually related to retinal angiomatosis and retinal angioblastoma as seen in two thirds of the patients. These are yellow to red lesions surrounded by a tortuous network of arterial vessels. The patient complains of decreased visual acuity and eventual blindness. Glaucoma and retinal detachment are frequent.

When a diagnosis of von Hippel-Lindau disease is determined, a variety of other lesions should be investigated, especially the association with pheochromocytoma. Failure to eliminate this tumor may be the cause of high mortality in the perioperative period.

With the establishment of von Hippel-Lindau disease in a patient, other family members should be screened. The patient should also have more detailed studies besides the standard physical examination and history. Studies should include CT and MRI scans of the CNS and the abdomen and a thorough ophthalmologic examination. Urine should be tested for evidence of pheochromocytoma.

ANESTHETIC CONSIDERATIONS[8]

Because therapy for these patients is essentially surgical, the anesthetic assessment is of considerable importance. The effects of surgical positioning, especially for infratentorial procedures, should be discussed, and complications should be avoided. For example, the sitting position has been associated with frequent cardiovascular changes, and therefore many surgeons have utilized careful prone positions.

Eye care includes careful patching and padding as well as prior eye lubricants. Pressure on the eyes should be minimized.

Drugs aggravating glaucoma such as atropine should be avoided, and those that increase intraocular pressure such as succinylcholine should not be used. Retinal angiomatosis occurs as indicated previously in about 65% of patients with von Hippel-Lindau disease.[7]

Spinal lesions resulting from hemangioblastomas are usually intramedullary 63% of the time; they are extramedullary but intradural 25% of the time and extradural 11% of the time.[9]

Polycythemia due to erythrocythemia from presumed stimulation by increased erythropoietin is often present and represents a risk factor for thrombosis and an additional cardiac load.[10]

REFERENCES

1. Lamiell, J. M., Salazar, F. G., Hsia, Y. E.: von Hippel-Lindau disease affecting 43 members of a single kindred. Medicine 68:1, 1989.
2. Hardwig, P., Robertson, D. M.: von Hippel-Lindau disease: a familial often lethal, multisystem phakomatosis. Ophthalmology 91:263, 1984.
3. Collins, E. T.: Intraocular growths. Trans Ophthalmol Soc UK 14:141, 1894.
4. Lindau, A.: Zur Frage der Angiomatosis retinae und ihrer Hirnkomplikationen Acta Ophthamol (Copenh) 4:193, 1927.
5. Neumann, H. P. H.: Basic criteria for clinical diagnosis and genetic counselling in von Hipple-Lindau syndrome. Vasa 16:220, 1987.
6. Seizinger, B. R., et al.: von Hipple-Lindau disease maps to the region of chromosome 3 associated with renal cell carcinoma. Nature 332:268, 1988.
7. Wing, G. L., et al.: von Hippel-Lindau disease: angiomatosis of the retina and central nervous system. Ophthalmology 88:1311, 1981.
8. Pudimat, P. A.: The patient with von Hippel-Lindau disease: the preanesthetic assessment. Anesthesiol News 17:10, 1991.
9. Yasargil, M. G., et al.: The neruosurgical removal of intramedullary spinal hemangioblastomas: report of twelve cases and a review of the literature. Surg Neurol 6:141, 1976.
10. Brody, J. I., Rodriguez, F.: Cerebellar hemangioblastoma and polycythemia (erythrocythemia). Am J Med 242:579, 1961.
11. Cornish, D., et al.: Metastatic islet cell tumor in von Hippel-Lindau disease. Am J Med 77:147, 1984.
12. Mulshine, J. L., et al.: Clinical significance of the association of the von Hippel-Lindau disease with pheochromocytoma and pancreatic apudoma. Am J Med Sci 288:212, 1984.

MUCOPOLYSACCHARIDOSIS

This group of genetic disorders (Table 45–33) is characterized by increased urinary saccharide excretion and variable clinical manifestations.[1] The genetic defect is probably inherited in an autosomal recessive fashion, with the exception of Hunter's syndrome, which is X linked. The overall incidence of all 7 types of mucopolysaccharidosis (MPS) is approximately 1 in 100,000 births.[2]

PATHOLOGY AND BIOCHEMICAL BASIS

The pathology of these disorders is an abnormality of connective tissues. The basic defect is an enzymatic deficiency of specific lysosomal hydroxylases, such as α-L-iduronidase and iduronate-2-sulfatase. These are responsible for the degradation of dermatan sulfate and heparitin sulfate. Accumulations of these sulfates of chondroitin and of dermatan sulfate and their polymers are then deposited in most organs and tissues. Development of bone and cartilage is abnormal.

HURLER'S SYNDROME

The prototype of these disorders is considered to be Hurler's syndrome, MPS type I, first described in 1919 by Gertrude Hurler.[3]

This syndrome is manifested usually in the first 2 years of life. Clouding of the cornea may be seen soon after birth. Many structural abnormalities occur, denoted by a gargoyle-like facies with a marked increase in the interorbital distance (hypertelorism) and a depressed bridge of the nose. Defective ossification of the cranial bones occurs with large fontanels; one sees dysostosis and the absence of clavicles. A dwarf stature with many skeletal changes is common; the neck and trunk are short;

Table 45–33.   Genetic Mucopolysaccharidoses

MPS Type	Enzymatic Defect	Gene Locus	Glycosaminoglycan	Clinical Diagnosis	Distinguishing Clinical Features
I	α-L-iduronidase	4p16.3	DS,HS	Hurler syndrome	Diagnosis before age 2 years, early corneal clouding and kyphoscoliosis, mental retardation, death before age 10 years
				Hurler-Scheie syndrome	Intermediate age of diagnosis, mild to severe skeletal involvement, corneal clouding, early death
				Scheie syndrome	Late corneal clouding, normal intellect, virtually normal longevity
II	Iduronate 2-sulfatase	Xq27.3	DS,HS	Hunter syndrome, severe	Diagnosis before age 4 years, absence of corneal clouding and kyphoscoliosis, mental retardation, death before age 15 years
				Hunter syndrome, mild	Absence of corneal clouding and kyphoscoliosis, moderate skeletal and respiratory involvement, survival into adulthood with little or no intellectual impairment
IIIA	Heparan N-sulfatase (Sulfamidase)	—	HS	Sanfilippo syndrome, type A	Diagnosis after age 2 years, minimal physical abnormalities, progressive dementia
IIIB	α-N-acetylglucosa-minidase	—	HS	Sanfilippo syndrome, type B	Same as for type A
IIIC	Acetyl-CoA: α-glucosaminide N-acetyltransferase	—	HS	Sanfilippo syndrome type C	Same as for type A
IIID	N-acetylglucosamine 6-sulfatase	12q14	HS	Sanfilippo syndrome, type D	Same as for type A
IVA	Galactose 6-sulfatase	—	KS	Morquio syndrome, type A	Variable extreme-to-mild short stature, corneal clouding, thin tooth enamel, progressive spinal cord damage, survival into adulthood
IVB	β-galactosidase	3p21-cen	KS	Morquio syndrome, type B	Variable extreme-to-mild short stature, corneal clouding, progressive cervical spinalcord damage
VI	N-acetylgalactosamine 4-sulfatase	5q11-q13	DS	Maroteaux-Lamy syndrome	Variable extreme-to-mild short stature, frequent kyphoscoliosis, corneal clouding, cardiopulmonary failure, normal intellect, variable survival
VII	β-glucuronidase	7q11.2-q22	DS,HS,CS	Sly syndrome, neonatal	Hydrops fetalis, lethal in newborn
				Sly syndrome, infantile	Mental retardation, moderate skeletal involvement
				Sly syndrome, juvenile	Mild mental retardation

DS = dermatan sulphate; *HS* = heparan sulfate; *KS* = keratan sulfate; *CS* = chondroitin sulfate.

From Whitley, C. B. The mucopolysaccharidoses. *In* Beighton, P. (ed.). McKusick's Heritable Disorders of Connective Tissue, 5th ed. C.V. Mosby, St Louis, 1993.

kyphoscoliosis with a pronounced hump is evident. Hands are short and broad with stubby fingers.

Major defects include deafness and severe mental retardation. Cardiovascular defects and pulmonary hypertension are marked. Hepatosplenomegaly is significant. The abdominal wall is lax because of poor development of connective tissue. Death occurs before the age of 10 years, from respiratory or cardiac failure.

HUNTER'S SYNDROME

Hunter's syndrome (MPS type II) clinically resembles Hurler's syndrome,[4] but the signs and symptoms are less severe, and the disorder is denoted by the absence of corneal clouding or kyphoscoliosis. It is transmitted by an X-linked recessive trait. Deafness occurs and is progressive. Joints are stiff, including the temporomandibular joint. The larynx is often displaced anteriorly and cephalad. In the severe form of the disorder, death usually occurs before the age of 15 years.

A mild form occurs, with moderate skeletal and respiratory involvement. The dwarfism and gargoyle facies are less prominent. These patients may live to adulthood. Mental impairment is often limited. In the upper Hudson River Valley of New York State, two or more interrelated families of Dutch origin live. Members of these families are usually followed medically at the Albany Medical Center. They exhibit mild dwarfism, but they are adults (40 to 50 years of age), and they have minimal mental impairment.

ANESTHETIC CONSIDERATIONS

The upper airway is markedly compromised[5-7]; airway obstruction readily occurs from anatomic factors and may be enhanced by infiltration of lymphoid tissue. Abnormalities of tracheobronchial cartilages are present, and an extremely short neck causes the head to appear to rest on the thorax. Pulmonary infection is common and must be treated vigorously.

REFERENCES

1. Whitley, C. B. Mucopolysaccharidosis. *In* Beighton, P. (ed.). McKusick's Heritable Disorders of Connective Tissues, 5th Ed. St. Louis ,C. V. Mosby, 1993, p. 367.
2. Lowry, R. B., Renwick, D. H. T.: The relative frequency of Hurler and Hunter syndromes. N Engl J Med *284:*221, 1971.
3. Hurler, G.: Uber einen Typ multipler Abartungen, vorwiegend am Skelettsystem. Z Kinderheilkd *24:*220, 1919.
4. Hunter, C. A.: A rare disease in two brothers: evaluation of scapula, limitation of movement of joints and other abnormalities. Proc R Soc Med *10:*104, 1917.
5. Verma, R., Bonta, S.: Anesthesia for a child with Hurler's syndrome. Anesthesiol Rev *11:*40, 1984.
6. Kreidstein, A., et al.: Delayed awakening from general anesthesia in a patient with Hunter's syndrome. Can J Anaesth *41:*423, 1994.
7. Krovetz, L. J., Lorinez, A. E., Schiebler, G. L.: Cardiovascular manifestations of Hurler's syndrome: hemodynamic and other observations. Circulation *31:*132, 1965.

Chapter 46

RESUSCITATION, COMA RECOVERY SCORES, AND DYING

VINCENT J. COLLINS

RESPIRATORY INSUFFICIENCY

Diseases of any system of the body and specifically diseases of the pulmonary system may progressively diminish ventilatory reserve. Varying degrees of inability to perform the work of respiration are recognized as respiratory insufficiency and may lead to respiratory failure. Such a critical state portends death and must be corrected (Table 46-1).[1]

Definition[2]

A state of acute respiratory failure (ARF) has been best defined as follows:

> A state in which Pao_2 is below the predicted range for the patient's age at the prevailing barometric pressure (in absence of intracardiac right-left shunt) and/or a $Paco_2$ above 50 torr (not due to respiratory compensation for metabolic alkalemia).[2]

Pathophysiology

Primary ventilatory failure is due to derangement in one or all of the nervous, muscular, and skeletal systems (Fig. 46-1). This may lead to secondary morphologic

Table 46–1. Clinical Classification of Respiratory Failure

I. *Acute respiratory failure with previously normal lungs*
  A. Without initial pulmonary pathology
    (Failure of the "respiratory pump")
    Examples: myasthenia, botulism muscle paralysis, drug overdose
  B. With pulmonary pathology
    (Failure of the "gas-exchanger")
    Examples: severe pneumonia, post-traumatic pulmonary insufficiency
II. *Acute failure superimposed on chronic lung disease*
  A. Without preexisting CO_2 retention
    Example: bronchopneumonia in chronic pulmonary fibrosis
  B. With chronic CO_2 retention
    Example: bronchopneumonia in chronic obstructive pulmonary disease

---

From Dripps, R. D. Eckenoff, J. A., Vandam, L.: Introduction to Anesthesia, 7th Ed. Philadelphia, W.B. Saunders, 1988.

changes in the pulmonary system, and such insufficiency and failure can occur in the absence of preexisting lung disease. Several clinical syndromes have been designated to describe this type of ventilatory insufficiency such as "wet lung," "shock lung," and "stiff lung." All represent a nonspecific response to injury. These syndromes are now collectively classified as adult respiratory distress syndromes (ARDS). Two mechanisms have been invoked to explain the development of ARDS: one is interference with the production of surfactant material due to *mechanical* interference with perfusion to type II alveolar cells;[3,4] second is the release of vasoactive substances from injured tissue or brain,[5] which cause vasoconstriction and diminished perfusion of the region of type II alveolar cells and subsequent decrease in the production of surfactant.

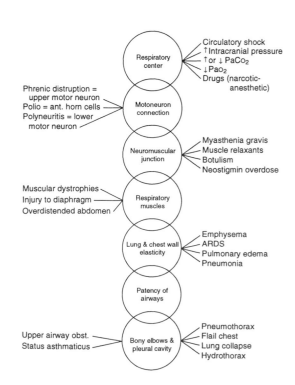

Fig. 46–1. The interconnected anatomic and physiologic links necessary for maintenance of normal alveolar ventilation and some diseases affecting them that can cause acute respiratory failure.

Ventilatory failure may also be secondary to acute and chronic pulmonary disease. Included are such conditions as chronic obstructive lung diseases, restrictive-type lung disease, asthma, pneumonia, pulmonary embolism, and pulmonary edema.

In either instance, primary ventilatory failure or pulmonary disease, two pathophysiologic conditions are present:

1. Abnormal patterns of pulmonary gas distribution and airway closure with air trapping.
2. Increases in pulmonary extravascular fluid with vascular congestion, transudation, and interstitial edema.

Consequences of these abnormalities are a decreased functional residual capacity (FRC), decreased pulmonary compliance, and mismatching of ventilation and perfusion.

Diagnosis[2]

Ventilatory insufficiency or failure is primarily determined by the abnormal values of oxygenation and of CO_2 elimination. Other parameters that indicate impairment of the mechanics of breathing are also abnormal.

A survey of physiologic criteria indicative of ventilatory failure and the need for ventilatory support in the adult is listed in Table 46-2.

Table 46-2. Physiologic Criteria of Respiratory Failure in Adults

Datum	Normal Range	Trachael Intubation and Ventilation Indicated
Mechanics:		
Respiratory rate	12–20	>35
Vital capacity (ml/kg of body weight*)	65–75	<15
FEV₁ (ml/kg of body weight†)	50–60	<10
Inspiratory force (cm H_2O)	75–100	<25
Oxygenation:		
PaO_2 (mm Hg)	100–75 (air)	<70 (on mask O_2)
$P(A-aDO_2)^{1.0}$ (mm Hg‡)	25–65	>450
Ventilation:		
$PaCO_2$ (mm Hg)	35–45	>55§
VD/VT	0.25–0.40	>0.60

*The trend of values is of utmost importance. The numeric guidelines should obviously not be adopted to the exclusion of clinical judgment. For example, a vital capacity below 15 ml/kg may prove sufficient provided the patient can still cough "effectively," if hypoxemia is prevented, and if hypercapnia is not progressive.

†"Ideal" weight is used if weight appears grossly abnormal.

‡After 10 min of 100% oxygen.

§Except in patients with chronic hypercapnia.

From Pontoppidan, H., Geffin, B., Lowenstein, E.: Acute respiratory failure in adult. N Engl J Med 287:749, 1972.

Table 46-3. Criteria of Respiratory Failure in Infants and Children with Acute Pulmonary Disease

Clinical Criteria	Physiologic Criteria
1. Decreased or absent inspiratory breath sounds.	1. $PaCO_2 \geqslant 75$ mm Hg
2. Severe inspiratory retractions and use of accessory muscles.	2. $PaO_2 \leqslant 100$ mm Hg in 100% O_2
3. Cyanosis in 40% ambient oxygen.	3. VDP/VT ratio $\geqslant 0.75$
4. Depressed level of consciousness and response to pain.	
5. Poor skeletal-muscle tone.	
6. Respiratory Rate Infants f > 80 Children f > 40	

From Downes, J.: Mechanical ventilation in management of status asthmaticus in children. In Science and Practice in Anesthesia. Philadelphia, J. B. Lippincott, 1965.

For infants and children, the criteria for respiratory failure (RDS type) are similar to those in the adult.[6] These are summarized in Table 46-3. Infant respiratory distress syndrome is related both to morphologic immaturity of the newborn lung and to deficient synthesis and production of surfactant material.

Neonatal Respiratory Distress[7]

Neonatal respiratory distress can occur after any delivery, but it should be anticipated in high-risk infants. This group includes the following: infants born prematurely; infants born after a difficult labor; infants delivered by cesarean section; and infants of diabetic mothers. This disorder occurs in 50 to 60% of premature infants, and its complications accounted for about 10,000 neonatal deaths per year in 1980. Females are particularly at risk.[8]

Common causes of respiratory distress are as follows: (1) wet lung disease; (2) meconium aspiration syndrome; (3) pneumonia; (4) hyaline membrane disease, classically termed respiratory distress syndrome associated with immaturity of the lungs; (5) pneumothorax; (6) pneumoperitoneum; (7) pneumomediastinum; (8) maternal diabetes (sixfold increase in hyaline membrane disease); (9) erythroblastosis fetalis; (10) congenital heart disease; and (11) surgical conditions. The differential diagnosis has been briefly reviewed by Miller and colleagues, and the reader is referred to this article.[7]

Neonatal Respiratory Distress Syndrome

This syndrome is classically the hyaline membrane disease of the premature infant, the baby born by cesarean section, and the infant of a diabetic mother. The early roentgenogram of the chest shows granular densities throughout both lungs giving the "ground glass" appearance. Hypoaeration of the periphery is evident while the air-filled bronchi and the bronchioles are distended, giving an "air-bronchogram." The clinical picture is that of impaired ventilation—PaO_2 is decreased and $PaCO_2$ is elevated; both metabolic and respiratory acidosis are present. Spontaneous respiration is rapid, and labored and thoracic retraction is observed.

Therapeutic measures can be considered in two parts: the immediate control of the respiratory insufficiency and the more definitive care to improve the pulmonary ventilatory capacity and to enhance maturation of the lung.

Control of Respiratory Insufficiency

Admission to a respiratory intensive care unit or neonatal care unit is necessary. For the neonate, special environmental conditions must be satisfied: nutrition, waterload and humidity, climate and temperature. Airway and ventilatory support are cornerstones of management.

Improvement in Ventilatory Capability

In respiratory distress of prematurity, the need to aid the development and maturation of the lung is evident. Two approaches are available.

Time to Mature

Supportive and maintenance ventilatory therapy must be continued after the resuscitative phase. This may extend over several weeks or months.

Efficacy of Corticosteroids[8]

A collaborative study by a division of the United States National Institutes of Health (NIH) has confirmed the results of a large clinical study performed in New Zealand. Administration of dexamethasone (20 mg in 4 doses) before delivery to mothers at risk of having premature infants showed a reduction of RDS from 18 to 4% in female infants; male infants still had an incidence of 14%.

Thyroid Hormones[9]

Administration of thyroxine speeds maturity of the immature lung. Thyroid hormone preparations also augment the synthesis and storage of lung surfactant.

Naloxone[10]

Endogenous opiates appear to depress the ventilatory responses to chemical stimuli early in the neonatal period. On this basis, naloxone has been used to reverse the depression related to fetal asphyxia.

Etiology

The various causes of respiratory insufficiency may be classified as follows:

1. Increased work requirements.
2. Increased physiologic shunting (venous admixture).
3. Increased physiologic dead space (dead space effect).
4. Decreased oxygen transport.

Increased Effort of Breathing

The work of breathing may be expressed in mechanical terms as pressure times volume ($W = \int P dV$) or in terms of metabolic requirements as reflected in the oxygen con-

sumed by muscles of respiration. The work done by normal humans at rest amounts to an average of 0.5 kg/m per minute (0.3 to 0.7 kg/m per minute) or 0.05 kg/m/L.[11] The oxygen required amounts to 2 to 3% of the total body oxygen consumption.[12] Primarily, the energy is expended for inspiratory activity.[13] Whole body oxygen consumption ($\dot{V}O_2$) at rest varies between 130 and 185 ml O_2/m body surface per minute.

The work is performed to overcome (1) elastic resistance of the lungs and chest wall, (2) airway resistance, and (3) nonelastic resistance, as discussed in Chapter 1 and as listed:

Increased airway resistance
  Diseases: elastic at alveoli (trapping)
  Bronchoconstriction at muscle
  Secretions at lumen
  Edema at mucosa
  Obstruction at lumen tumors
Increased elastic resistance
  (Decreased static compliances: no air moving)
  Air space collapse: quiet breathing
  Alveolar surface tension
  Fibrosis
  Atelectasis
  Pneumonia
  Pulmonary congestion
  Edema alveolar
Nonelastic resistance
  Body weight: obesity
  Fractured ribs
  Pleural fluids
  Crushed chest

In ARF, not only is the work of respiration increased, but also expiration becomes active. When compliance is reduced, the work performed may be up 33%.[14]

Postoperative patients are particularly susceptible to ARF. They may have respiratory muscle fatigue or paralysis, shock, hypoperfusion, and discoordinate muscle activity; obesity emphysema, cardiovascular disease, and debility compromise good ventilation and recovery. Patients susceptible to ARF should have ventilatory support as an extension of the intraoperative anesthetic management. Ventilation can reduce whole-body oxygen consumption $\dot{V}O_2$ postoperatively by as much as 7%.

Increased Dead Space[15]

Generally, disorders of physiologic dead space and specifically of alveolar dead space cause impairment in oxygen uptake and elimination of CO_2 and of respiratory reserve. When dead space is increased, ventilation is wasted. Ventilation in excess of perfusion represents a mismatching and inefficiency and is a frequent cause of respiratory failure. The more common specific causes are listed:

1. Deficient capillary perfusion of alveoli.
2. Nonperfusion of alveoli by pulmonary embolus and continued ventilation of these alveoli.
3. Hemorrhage: redistribution of blood away from pulmonary circulation.

4. Elevation of airway pressure impeding pulmonary capillary flow.
5. Large anatomic shunts.
6. Large tidal volumes (TV).

The measurement of the ratio between the increase in dead space and the TV has been a valuable guide in assessing respiratory failure, indicating the increased ventilation requirement above normal to obtain proper gas exchange.

In certain types of respiratory insufficiency, the ratio of dead space ventilation to toal ventilation (VD/VT ratio) can be misleading in assessing the ventilation requirements in the following situations: (1) in respiratory failure secondary to chronic obstructive lung disease, such as emphysema, the VD/VT ratio is unaffected by even large changes in TV; (2) in respiratory failure characterized by hyperventilation, such as in post-traumatic respiratory insufficiency, increasing the TV results in an increase in the VD/VT ratio; a high VD/VT ratio in such a patient may not imply an increase in ventilation requirements but instead may represent a low cardiovascular reserve.

Increased Physiologic Shunting[7,15]

Conditions that cause an abnormality of the ventilation-perfusion ratio so that blood is not exposed to ventilated alveoli result in venous admixture and a diminution of respiratory reserve. When blood bypasses the alveolar capillary system entirely, the condition is designated a constant or anatomic shunt.

In contrast, when blood does perfuse the alveolar capillary system but is exposed to nonventilated or poorly ventilated alveoli, a variable or capillary shunt is produced. The commonest cause is partial or complete atelectasis.

Clinical Factors

Gas Distribution

At a resting lung volume, alveoli in dependent parts of the lung are smaller than in superior segments. The physical forces accounting for this phenomenon are a uniform air pressure in the alveoli opposed by an increasing vertical gradient of pleural pressure. In the upright posture, this pleural pressure gradient is about 0.3 cm H_2O per centimeter from above downward. Thus, the net distending pressure is minimized in lower segments. On inspiration, however, gas preferentially enters dependent alveoli because distending pressure is maximized at lower segments and the small alveoli expand more per unit pressure differential than larger already inflated superior alveoli.

Abnormal Airway Closure[16]

This situation causes abnormal distribution of pulmonary gas. Early airway closure on exhalation results in gas trapping. Such gas can be absorbed, especially if the fraction of inspired oxygen (FIo2) is high, and atelectasis may ensue.[17] This is likely when closing volume exceeds the FRC and especially when closing volume exceeds FRC + normal TV.[18] Similarly, with early airway closure, the alveolar-arterial oxygen tension (P(A-a)o2) difference is high, and Pao2 diminished. In addition, besides airway

Table 46–4. Nonpulmonary and Pulmonary Causes of Abnormal Airway Closure

Nonpulmonary and pulmonary causes of abnormal airway closure
1. Age: At 65 years of age, closing volume begins to exceed FRC
2. Breathing a low lung volumes; if oxygen alone is the gas, atelectasis may occur rapidly
3. Reduced FRC from supine position; head-down position; general anesthesia; postoperative pain and restricted respiratory movements[18]
4. Obesity
5. Abdominal distention
6. Suctioning: tracheobronchial tube
7. Vigorous exhalatory efforts
8. Loss of sighing mechanism: drugs; paralysis; pain
9. High oxygen concentrations[17]

Pulmonary causes of early airway closure (includes closure of terminal air spaces)
1. Increased surface tension
2. Interstitial edema
3. Bronchial mucosal inflammation or edema
4. Constriction of smooth muscle

closure, the neck of the alveolar sacs or alveolar ducts may close even earlier than the conduits.

Causes of abnormal airway closure may be pulmonary or nonpulmonary (Table 46–4).[15,16]

Edema of Lung[19]

Accumulation of water in lung tissue is an invariable pathophysiologic feature of respiratory failure. A common pathophysiologic response to several clinical conditions is noted. The progression shows fluid appearing first in the interstitial space around large blood vessels and airways; then the fluid appears in the alveolar wall, and it finally appears in the alveolar spaces. The pulmonary capillary endothelium is more permeable to aqueous fluids than is the alveolar epithelium. Time may elapse before the interstitial fluid traverses the alveolar wall and enters the air space. This resistance of the alveolar wall to permeation affords relative protection against the development of alveolar fluid. Only when fluid appears in the alveolar space does one see significant interference with gas exchange. The interstitial edema may contribute to early airway closure, however.

Conditions in which extravascular water accumulates in the lung in significant quantities include shock, trauma, sepsis, mitral stenosis, cor pulmonale, fluid overload, damage to the pulmonary capillary endothelium or alveolar epithelium by drugs or inhalants (alloxan and oxygen in excess of 0.5 FIo2), and the syndrome of prolonged pulmonary ventilation with a positive water balance.

GUIDE TO MANAGEMENT OF PATIENTS REQUIRING MECHANICAL VENTILATION

I. Airway care
1. Sterile tracheal aspiration every hour and as needed.
2. Nasopharyngeal aspiration every hour and as needed.

3. Mobilization of secretions by higher humidity of breathing air and/or ultrasonic nebulizer.
4. Culture of tracheal aspirate *every other day.*

II. Chest physical therapy
1. Bilateral chest percussion, cupping, chest vibration every 3 to 6 hours (depending on disease).
2. Deep breathing by following sequence:
   a. Manual hyperinflation by self-inflating bag system.
   b. Holding at peak inflation for 3 seconds.
   c. Sudden release.
   d. Suction of secretions.
   e. Repetition.
3. Checking of breath sounds bilaterally before and after chest physical therapy and after tracheal aspiration.
4. Positioning: Turning of patient every 2 hours; the recommended sequence is as follows:
   a. Turning of patient side-back-side every 2 hours.
   b. One side: head up 1 hour; head down 1 hour.
   c. Supine: head up 1 hour; head down 1 hour.
   d. Other side: head up 1 hour; head down 1 hour.
   e. Repetition: patient left longer in any given position when abundant secretions are obtained.
5. Artificial coughing and sighing techniques.

III. Oxygen
1. Inspired oxygen (F_{IO_2}) adjusted to maintain Pa_{O_2} at levels between 70 and 100 mm Hg.
2. Specification of oxygen and air flows to ventilator (in L/min) on order sheet.
3. Checking of F_{IO_2} with oxygen analyzer every hour until stable, then every 4 hours.
4. Humidity (75 to 90% relative humidity desired): checking of water level of unit every 4 hours.

IV. Ventilator
For long term ventilation, the volume preset unit is the choice. TVs of at least 10 ml/kg are required. In the conscious patient, TVs less than 10 ml/kg are not well tolerated, and TVs of at least 15 ml/kg are used. Orders should indicate the settings for volume, frequency per minute, pressure, and flow rate, as follows:
1. Type of ventilator.
2. Mode of support (control or assist).
3. Expired TV.
4. Inspiratory-expiratory (I/E) ratio.
5. Flow rate if required by ventilator.
6. Dead space volume to be allowed.

V. Monitoring
1. Continuous electrocardiographic (ECG) oscilloscope monitoring.
2. Alarm system, varying with type of ventilator; not a substitute for constant nursing and medical attendance for oxygen or for ventilator performance (warning of disconnection).
3. Arterial pressure: if circulatory complications are likely, direct arterial pressure monitoring with an intra-arterial catheter and strain gauge is indicated; the same intra-arterial line can be used for frequent blood sampling; otherwise, arterial pressures can be checked every 30 to 50 minutes by sphygmomanometry.

4. Central venous pressure (CVP) monitoring with either a water manometer or a strain gauge.
5. Continuous rectal temperature monitoring for 24 hours or longer; esophageal temperature always to be monitored when hypothermia is used.

VI. Arterial blood studies and acid-base balance
1. Arterial pH, P_{CO_2}, base-excess, P_{O_2}, and hematocrit determined within 1 hour after patient is placed on mechanical ventilator.
2. Studies repeated at 4- to 12-hour intervals as indicated for subsequent 48 hours, and then as often as necessary.
3. Studies repeated within 2 to 4 hours after discontinuing mechanical ventilation.
4. Correction of acid-base balance.
5. Daily determination of pulmonary shunt and dead space.

VII. Intravenous fluids
1. Correction of water and electrolyte imbalances, anemia, and plasma deficits.
2. Cutdown or indwelling plastic cannula for intravenous fluids.
3. Accurate intake/output records; determination of humidity water factor and ultrasonic nebulizer water load to patient; continuous collection of urine included.
4. Recording of daily body weight.

VIII. Narcotic sedation and neuromuscular blockade
1. For sedation euphoria, amnesia, antianxiety, decreased respiratory center sensitivity and analgesic, use of a sedative narcotic. (The drug should have minimal cardiovascular effects and be reversible. Morphine is the agent of choice. This agent is suitable for aiding in synchronization of patient's respiration with ventilator mechanics.)
2. Neuromuscular blockade, used as a last resort to synchronize patient breathing with ventilator. The initial dose of curare is usually 0.3 to 0.6 mg/kg; that of pancuronium is 0.08 to 0.1 mg/kg. Subsequent doses vary from 25 to 75% of initial dose.

IX. Body temperature control
1. Placement of patients on a temperature-controlled mattress pad covered by 4 layers of sheets used for stabilization of temperature (see Chapter 19).
2. Temperature kept at normal levels unless hypothermia is used.

X. Progress notes
1. Progress note written by the critical care team physician at least twice a day for all patients receiving mechanical ventilation.
2. Note written after any significant procedure, such as intravenous cutdown, change in type of mechanical ventilator, or change in antibiotic therapy, by the appropriate physician. NOTE: All care should be the responsibility of the respiratory care physician (critical care) or intensivist. A team approach is mandated. General policies and procedures (including admission) for intensive care should be provided in a unit manual.

Ventilation Lung Syndrome[19]

Prolonged artificial respiration frequently produces a syndrome of positive water balance and radiographic evidence of pulmonary edema. A water intake of 38 ml/kg per day is usual, and although it is within acceptable clinical limits, this may be a relative excess in respiratory failure. Retention of water was shown by Holaday to occur when patients were placed on positive pressure ventilation.[20] A role for antidiuretic hormone has been suggested. Further, the addition of positive end-expiratory pressure (PEEP) to intermittent positive pressure ventilation (IPPV) enhances antidiuretic hormone (ADH) secretion threefold.

Treatment consists of the following:

1. Limiting water intake to 20 to 25 ml/kg per 24 hours. This should include water obtained from humidifiers.
2. Diuretic drugs.
3. An upright or semirecumbent posture.
4. Frequent position changes.
5. Oxygen therapy for hypoxemia and proper ventilatory pattern.
6. Total ventilatory care.

CARDIORESPIRATORY ARREST AND RESUSCITATION*

One of the commonest health and hospital emergencies is cardiopulmonary arrest with interruption of the oxygenation system. Restoration of this system and the establishment of a tissue supply of oxygen are immediate goals.

Causes of cardiopulmonary arrest include ischemic heart disease, and more than half a million deaths occur per year in the United States. Other victims die as a result of such accidental causes as drowning, electrocution, suffocation, drug intoxication, or automobile accidents. A large proportion of these patients could be saved by prompt and proper resuscitation care both in the community and in the hospital by an organized and effective system. In the operating room and in monitored situations, cardiac arrest is precipitated by many factors (Table 46–5). An organized plan of management has resulted in a high survival rate.[21]

Definitions[22,23]

Basic life support is the emergency first aid procedure that consists of the recognition of airway obstruction, respiratory arrest and cardiac arrest, and the proper application of cardiopulmonary resuscitation (CPR). CPR consists of opening and maintaining a patent airway, providing artificial ventilation by means of rescue breathing, and providing artificial circulation by means of external cardiac compression. CPR can be accomplished in the field as well as in the hospital setting. It can be continued by use of specialized equipment and techniques of advanced life support.

---

*This section is an edited version of the "Standards for CPR." Courtesy of Dr. A.R. Gordon, Chairman of CPR Committee, National Academy of Sciences and American Heart Association; JAMA 227(Suppl):834, 1974; and Paraskos, A.: Recommendations of 1992 national conference. JAMA 268:2178, 1992.

Table 46–5. Precipitating Factors in Sudden Cardiac Collapse

I. Factors initiating neurovascular reflexes
  A. Efferent vagal stimulation, especially from cervical and thoracic region
  B. Vasovagal reflexes
  C. Any afferent stimulus with a vagal efferent pathway
    1. Pain skin
    2. Anal dilatation
    3. Pharyngotracheal
    4. Periosteum
    5. Visceral traction
    6. Others
II. Chemical factors and anesthesia
  A. Hypoxia
  B. Hypercarbia
  C. Asphyxia
  D. Epinephrine
  E. Nonanesthetic drugs
  F. Anesthetic agents and overdoses
  G. Errors in technique
III. Physical and physiologic factors
  A. Anomalies: diaphragmatic hernia; congenital cardiac defects
  B. Cardiac tamponade
  C. Torsion, pressure, or retraction of heart or adjacent structures
  D. Surgical position: abnormal or sudden changes
  E. Preoperative hypovolemia
  F. Hyperthermia
  G. Miscellaneous
IV. Surgical factors
  A. Site of surgery; vulnerability during intrathoracic, intra-abdominal and intracranial.
  B. Nature and duration: major and prolonged
  C. Blood loss
V. Factors during anesthesia
  A. Cardiovascular
    1. Hypotension severe (not controlled)
    2. Air embolism
    3. Myocardial infarction
    4. Dysrhythmias
  B. Respiratory factors
    1. Airway obstruction, secretions, laryngospasm
    2. Aspiration
    3. Failure to intubate: difficult intubation, esophageal intubation, accidental extubation
    4. Carbon dioxide retention
    5. Postextubation, airway obstruction, ARI or ARF, premature extubation
    6. Pneumothorax

Collins, V. J.: Principles of Anesthesiology, p. 1323, 2nd Ed. Lea & Febiger Philadelphia, 1976. Modified from Martin, S. J.: Considerations of the etiology and treatment of sudden cardiac collapse. Anesth Analg 39:23, 1960.

Advanced life support is basic life support plus use of adjunctive equipment, intravenous fluid lifeline (infusion), drug administration, defibrillation, stabilization of the victim by cardiac monitoring, control of arrhythmias, and postresuscitation care.

Indications

Indications for resuscitation are as follows:[24-26]

1. Respiratory arrest.
2. Cardiac arrest, which can result from cardiovascular collapse (electromechanical dissociation), ventricular fibrillation, or ventricular standstill (asystole).

In collapsed or unconscious persons, the adequacy or absence of breathing and circulation must be determined immediately. If breathing alone is inadequate or absent, rescue breathing may be all that is necessary. If circulation is also absent, artificial circulation must be started in combination with rescue breathing. The methods of recognizing adequacy or absence of breathing or circulation and the recommended techniques for performing artificial ventilation and artificial circulation are presented.

Essentials of Cardiopulmonary Resuscitation[27,28]

Basic life support is an emergency first aid procedure. A maximum sense of urgency is required. Optimally, only seconds should intervene between recognizing the need and starting treatment. Treatment includes the ABCD steps of CPR (Fig. 46–2).

These steps always should be started as quickly as possible. They are performed in the order shown, except in special circumstances such as in monitored patients or in witnessed cardiac arrests. When cardiac arrest occurs in the monitored patient and trained personnel and defibrillators are available immediately, a precordial thump or advanced life support procedures should be instituted without delay. In a witnessed cardiac arrest, the ABCD sequence should include use of a precordial thump.

Respiratory inadequacy may result from an obstruction of the airway or from respiratory failure. An obstructed airway is sometimes difficult to recognize until the airway is opened. A partially obstructed airway is recognized by labored breathing or excessive respiratory efforts, often involving accessory muscles of respiration, and by soft tissue retractions of the intercostal, supraclavicular, and suprasternal spaces. Respiratory failure is characterized by minimal or absent respiratory effort, failure of the chest or upper abdomen, and inability to detect air movement through the nose or mouth.

Opening of the airway and restoring of breathing are basic steps of artificial ventilation. The steps can be performed quickly under almost any circumstance and without adjunctive equipment or help from another person. They constitute emergency first aid for airway obstruction and respiratory inadequacy or arrest. One must not delay first aid to obtain or apply adjunctive devices and special equipment! No adjuncts are required for effective rescue breathing.

Establishment of Airway (Fig. 46–3)

The initial and most important procedure for successful resuscitation is immediate opening of the airway. The procedure is as follows:

1. Tilting of the patient's head backwards as far as possible. This maneuver opens up the pharynx and is effective in most cases.
2. Chin lift. Pulling the patient's chin forward improves the passageway by further advancing the patient's tongue forward away from pharynx.
3. Jaw-thrust. Additional opening of the air passageway may be achieved by forward displacement of the patient's jaw at the angle of the mandible.
4. In the clinical setting or when trained personnel are present, an oropharyngeal airway or the "S" shaped airway (Resuscitube of Safar[27]) can be inserted.[28] In a hospital program with an anesthesia service, an endotracheal tube may eventually be introduced in the advanced life support procedure.[27]

Often the maneuvers to establish a clear airway result in the patient's breathing. When establishment of airway does not result in the victim's resuming spontaneous breathing, the rescuer must move to the victim's side and provide artificial ventilation.

Artificial Ventilation

1. Mouth-to-mouth ventilation (rescue breathing) is initiated (Fig. 46–4).[21,29-34]

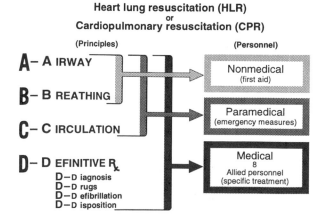

Heart lung resuscitation (HLR)
or
Cardiopulmonary resuscitation (CPR)

(Principles)   (Personnel)

A– **A** IRWAY

B– **B** REATHING

C– **C** IRCULATION

D– **D** EFINITIVE R_x

D–D iagnosis
D–D rugs
D–D efibrillation
D–D isposition

Nonmedical
(first aid)

Paramedical
(emergency measures)

Medical
8
Allied personnel
(specific treatment)

Fig. 46–2. The ABCD steps of resuscitation and the types of personnel who should be trained to perform them.

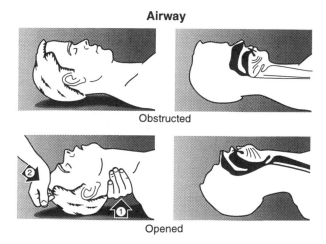

Airway

Obstructed

Opened

Fig. 46–3. Recommended head-tilt method for relieving upper airway obstruction by the tongue. 1, Lift neck. 2, Extend head. (Do *not* lift neck if neck injury is suspected, as in diving accidents.)

2. Mouth-to-nose ventilation is recommended when it is difficult to open the victim's mouth, when it is impossible to ventilate through the victim's mouth, when the victim's mouth is seriously injured, and when it is difficult to achieve a tight seal around the victim's mouth.

3. Direct mouth-to-stoma artificial ventilation should be used for persons who have had a laryngectomy. It is often necessary to seal the patient's nose and mouth.

4. A self-inflating bag and mask unit is used.

For infants and small children, the rescuer covers the mouth and nose of the child with his or her mouth and blows with puffs or small breaths to inflate the child's lungs once every 3 seconds. The neck of an infant is so pliable that forceful backward tilting of the head may ob-

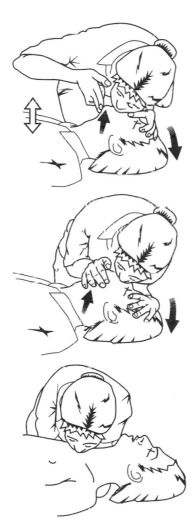

Fig. 46–4. Illustrates the technique of rescue breathing. The airway is provided by the head-tilt/chin-lift maneuver (a maneuver often referred to as the Heiberg-Esmarch maneuver, but this term is inaccurate and obsolete),[29] followed by mouth-to-mouth insufflation (upper sketch); mouth-to-nose insufflation (middle sketch); and mouth-to-stoma or to an artificial airway (pharyngeal, or Safar J airway) (lower sketch). This technique is based largely on the studies and the movies on rescue breathing by Elam and colleagues.[29–35]

struct breathing passages. Therefore, the tilt position should not be exaggerated.

In accident victims, one must use caution to avoid extension of the neck when the possibility of neck fracture exists. If a fracture is suspected, a modification of the jaw thrust maneuver should be used to open the airway. In this variation, the rescuer places his or her hands on either side of the victim's head so the head is maintained in a fixed, neutral position without being extended. The rescuer's index fingers should then be used to displace the patient's mandible forward without tilting the head backward or turning it to either side.

Complications

Artificial ventilation frequently causes distention of the stomach. This complication occurs most often in children, but it is not uncommon in adults. Marked distention of the stomach may be dangerous because it promotes regurgitation, and it reduces lung volume by elevating the diaphragm. In the unconscious victim, distention can be reduced without adjuncts by exerting moderate pressure with one hand over the victim's epigastrium between the umbilicus and the rib cage. To prevent aspiration of gastric contents during this maneuver, the victim's head and shoulders should be turned to one side.

Esophageal Obturator

Smock proposed in 1975[36] that adequate ventilation could be carried out if the esophagus was occluded, and if high-flow oxygen would then be forced by default through the oropharynx into the trachea and lungs. For this purpose, the esophageal obturator airway was developed. In addition, a variation of the esophageal obturator airway, namely, the esophageal gastric tube airway, was recommended by many as an alternative to endotracheal intubation.

Support for these types of airways was meager, and indeed most investigators have not only expressed concern about the original studies, but have subsequently evaluated these airways in an appropriate clinical setting. As a result of the studies by Meislin[37] and by Auerbach and Geehr,[38] it is clear that ventilation by means of the obturator type of airway, forcing air or oxygen, preferentially, into the lungs, is relatively ineffective. Indeed, measured against a simple oropharyngeal airway and proper head positioning, and, of course, the standard of artificial airways, namely, the endotracheal tube, the esophageal techniques are of little merit.

This type of procedure should not be used in prehospital management of the airway. Auerbach and Geehr[38] have indicated that victims of cardiac arrest treated with this class of airway have both inadequate volume ventilation and oxygenation. Further, in the hospital practice, simple measures should be employed in emergency rooms, followed by the expertise of those well trained and adept in providing an endotracheal airway. Training programs have been instituted for paramedics to perform safe laryngoscopy and endotracheal intubation. In the meantime, the esophageal-type obturator and its modification should be discontinued.[39]

Foreign Body Obstruction

The rescuer should not look for foreign bodies in the upper airway unless their presence is known or is strongly suspected. The first effort to ventilate the lungs determines whether an airway obstruction is present. If the first attempts to ventilate are unsuccessful despite proper opening of the airway and provision of an airtight seal around the mouth, an attempt should be made immediately to clear the patient's airway with the rescuer's fingers.

Where skilled advanced life support personnel and equipment are available, direct laryngoscopy may permit the foreign body to be removed.

If the rescuer is unable to dislodge the foreign body, or if it is impacted below the epiglottis, the victim should be rolled onto the side toward the rescuer, who then delivers sharp blows with the heel of the hand between the victim's shoulder blades.

A small child with airway obstruction should be quickly picked up and inverted over the arm of the rescuer while blows are delivered between the child's shoulder blades.

If all these maneuvers fail, emergency cricotracheal† puncture and insertion of a 6-mm tube have been recommended for adults. This procedure requires appropriate instruments and training, however, and must be regarded as an advanced life support technique.

Newborn Resuscitation[40]

Important features of resuscitation in a newborn are the establishment of an airway and the proper technique for ventilation. To this end, appropriate face masks should be employed. An evaluation of the commonly used neonatal face masks has been carried out for their efficiency in terms of degree of leakage and ease of cleaning. Among the face masks used and tested include the ambu neonatal mask, and the Rendell-Baker, Bennet, Laerdal, and Ohio masks.[41] Results show that the triangular molded rubber mask (Rendell-Baker) leaks most and that the circular silicone rubber mask (Laerdal) leaks the least. Leakage was considered to be the most important part of the efficiency of a mask. If leakage is high, the pressure reaching the alveolar system is insufficient to exceed the opening pressures in the lungs. An opening pressure for the newborn infant has been set at approximately 30 cm H_2O to aerate nonexpanded lungs. The evaluation also determined that the Rendell-Baker mask is the most difficult to use, and only on half the babies that were tested did this mask allow an adequate opening pressure. The construction of the mask is also important, and masks constructed of one piece are preferable to all others. This includes the Laerdal and Ohio masks. The ease of cleaning is significantly greater with the Laerdal mask. It can be autoclaved or boiled. The problem of dead space is still a feature that needs further study.

Criteria of Effective Ventilation

Adequate ventilation is ensured on every breath in the following situations:

1. If the patient's chest rises and falls.
2. If the rescuer feels in his or her own airway the resistance and compliance of the victim's lungs as they expand.
3. If the rescuer hears and feels air escape from the patient's lungs during exhalation. The initial ventilatory maneuver should be four quick, full, breaths without allowing time for full lung deflation between breaths.

ARTIFICIAL CIRCULATION: EXTERNAL CARDIAC COMPRESSION

When sudden, unexpected cardiac arrest occurs, all the ABCs of basic life support are required in rapid succession. This includes both artificial ventilation and artificial circulation (external cardiac compression).[7]

Diagnosis

Cardiac arrest is recognized by pulselessness in large arteries in an unconscious victim who has a deathlike appearance and absent breathing. The status of the carotid pulse should be checked as quickly as possible when cardiac arrest is suspected. In an unwitnessed cardiac arrest, however, the rescuer must first open the airway and quickly ventilate the lungs. The rescuer then feels for the carotid pulse in the groove between the patient's larynx and neck muscle.

In hospital situations, palpation of the femoral artery is an acceptable option instead of palpation of the carotid artery. In infants and small children, the rescuer's hand should be placed gently over the precordium to feel the apical beat.

Rationale

The thoracic cage is flexible and the sternum can be easily depressed. Pressure applied on the sternum reduces the anteroposterior axis of the thoracic cavity. Two mechanical effects occur. First, a generalized increase in intrathoracic-intrapleural pressure occurs.[42] This elevation of pressure is transmitted to all vascular structures in the chest including the pericardium and the heart cavities. Blood contained in these structures is pressed forward into the general circulation. Indeed, the elevation of intrapleural pressure is quickly transmitted to the intrathoracic vasculature and, in turn, is transmitted to the extravascular arteries as demonstrated in the cardiac catheterization laboratory.[43] Furthermore, little retrograde flow occurs out of the right side of the heart because of venous valves at the thoracic inlet.[44] The pericardium also prevents lateral expansion of the heart, and the heart valves maintain unidirectional flow. Second, the pressure applied to sternum also imposes a more direct squeezing force on the heart by compressing it between the sternum and the vertebral column. The efficacy of this maneuver under the best of circumstances of exter-

---

†Cricotracheal membrane puncture is recommended. It is more effective than cricothyroid membrane puncture, and injury to the subglottic region does not occur, nor does hemorrhage from the anterior thyroid artery (see Clemente, C. D.: Gray's Anatomy, 30th Ed. Philadelphia, Lea & Febiger, 1985).

nal "cardiac compression" has been questioned.[45] Moreover, cardiac compression can be induced by coughs.[46]

On release of external pressure, the anteroposterior axis of the thoracic cavity returns to normal, allowing the flow of blood into large veins of the chest and into auricular chambers.

Artificial ventilation is always required and is maintained when external cardiac compression is used.

Effective external cardiac compression requires sufficient pressure to depress an adult's lower sternum a minimum of 1½ to 2 inches.

Procedure

For external cardiac compression to be effective, the victim must be on a firm surface and in a horizontal position. The rescuer is positioned close to the victim's side and proceeds as follows:

1. The rescuer feels the tip of the patient's xiphoid and places the long axis of the heel of one hand parallel to and over the long axis of the lower third to half of the sternum (Fig. 46-5). The rescuer should not place the hand over the patient's xiphoid onto the abdomen.
2. The rescuer places the other hand on top of the first (one may interlock the fingers).
3. The rescuer brings his or her shoulders directly over the victim's chest, keeps his or her arms straight, and exerts pressure almost vertically downward to depress the lower sternum a minimum of 1½ to 2 inches toward the spine. The compressions must be regular, rhythmic, smooth, and uninterrupted (Fig. 46-6).
4. Relaxation must immediately follow compression

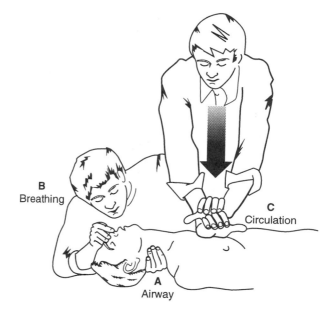

Fig. 46-6. Two-rescuer cardiopulmonary resuscitation cycle: chest compressions at the rate of 80 to 100 per minute, with no pause for ventilation; and 10 lung inflations per minute, after each 8 compressions and delivered over 2 seconds by *slow* inspiratory flow rate. (Redrawn from Paraskos, J. A.: Guidelines for cardiopulmonary resuscitation and emergency cardiac care. JAMA 268:2178, 1992.)

and must be of equal duration. The heel of the rescuer's hand should not be removed from the patient's chest during relaxation, but pressure on the sternum should be completely released so the sternum returns to its normal resting position between compressions. This procedure permits full reexpansion of the lungs and filling of the vascular tree in the chest.

5. The compression rate should be 80 to 100 per minute and need not be interrupted for ventilation. This rate produces a systolic blood pressure of about 80 mm Hg. If the victim's trachea has been intubated, lung inflation is easier, and compression rates of 80 to 100 per minute can be used because breaths can be either interposed or superimposed following endotracheal intubation.
6. When only one rescuer is present, he or she must perform both artificial circulation and artificial ventilation using a 15:2 ratio. This consists of two quick lung inflations after each 15 chest compressions (Fig. 46-7).

Optimization of Compression

Vascular pressures can be optimized by the following:

1. Using the recommended compression force: depressing the sternum 1½ to 2 inches.[47]
2. Prolonging compression duration; the compressing thrust should be at least 50% of the thrust-release cycle.[48]
3. Maintaining a chest compression rate of 80 to 100 per minute for the normal adult.[49,50]

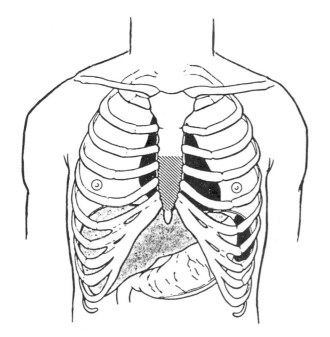

Fig. 46-5. Anatomic relationships of the sternum important for correct performance of external cardiac compression (shaded area).

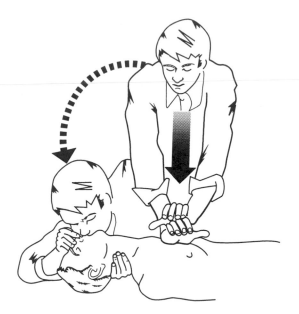

Fig. 46–7. One-rescuer cardiopulmonary resuscitation: 15 chest compressions at the rate of 80 per minute; a pause for ventilation; and 2 quick lung inflations. (Redrawn from Paraskos, J. A.: Guidelines for cardiopulmonary resuscitation and emergency cardiac care. JAMA *268*:2178, 1992.)

4. In emergency basic life support with two rescuers, compression should not be interrupted for ventilation.

Chest Compression in Infants and Children

For small children, only the heel of one hand is used, and, for infants, only the tips of the index and middle fingers are used. The ventricles of infants and small children lie higher in the chest, and the external pressure should be exerted over the midsternum. The danger of lacerating the liver is greater in children because of the pliability of the chest and the higher position of the liver under the lower sternum and xiphoid. Infants require ½- to ¾-inch compression of sternum; young children require ¾ to 1½ inches. The compression rate should be 100 per minute, with breaths delivered as quickly as possible after each 5 compressions.

Alternative External Method of Chest Compression

In certain situations, the standard arm-hand method for external chest compression is ineffective. This is frequent when the rescuer is of small stature, a woman, a child or teenager, or a weak or fatigued individual. A leg-heel (standing) method applied to the lower half of the sternum is offered as an alternative. Pilot studies and tests show that the method is effective. Caution is advised.[51]

Effectiveness

The reaction of the patient's pupils should be checked periodically during CPR, because it provides the best indication that oxygenated blood is being delivered to the victim's brain. Pupils that constrict when exposed to light indicate adequate oxygenation and blood flow to the

brain. If the pupils remain widely dilated and do not react to light, serious dysfunction is present and brain damage is imminent or has occurred. Dilated but reactive pupils are a less ominous sign. Normal pupillary reactions may be altered in the aged and frequently are altered in any individual who has received various drugs.

The carotid pulse should be palpated periodically during CPR to check the effectiveness of external cardiac compression or the return of a spontaneous effective heartbeat.

Precordial Thump

The precordial thump as a basic maneuver has been used following the detection of pulselessness in adults in these cases[52]:

1. Witnessed cardiac arrest (basic life support).
2. Monitored patient (advanced life support).
3. Pacing known atrioventricular block (advanced life support).

The precordial thump is not recommended for use on children.

In cases where the primary cause of cardiac arrest is not hypoxia, a single precordial thump may be effective in restarting cardiac action and may reverse certain dysrhythmias if the maneuver is performed within the first minute after cardiopulmonary arrest.[53]

The precordial thump may be effective in restoring a heartbeat in cases of ventricular asystole due to block and in reversing ventricular tachycardia or ventricular fibrillation of recent onset.

Hazards are also associated with the precordial thumps. In patients with an anoxic heart that is still beating, the low-voltage stimulus may induce ventricular fibrillation. In addition, rescuers who do not restrict themselves to the recommended single blow may delay effective CPR.

In delivering the precordial thump, these rules should be followed[54]:

1. Deliver a sharp, quick single blow over the midportion of the patient's sternum 8 to 12 inches over the chest, hitting with the bottom, fleshy portion of the fist.
2. Deliver the thump within the first minute after cardiac arrest.
3. If no immediate response occurs, begin basic life support at once.

Precautions

Enumerated here are important points to remember in performing external cardiac compression and artificial ventilation[47,50]:

1. *CPR should not be interrupted for more than 5 seconds,* except that endotracheal intubation usually cannot be accomplished in 5 seconds. It is an advanced life support measure and should be performed only by those well practiced in the technique.

2. *The rescuer should not move the patient* until the patient has been stabilized and is ready for transportation or until arrangements have been made for uninterrupted CPR during movement.

3. *The rescuer must never compress the patient's xiphoid process at the tip of the sternum.* (Laceration of the liver can occur.)

4. Between compressions, the heel of the hand must completely release its pressure but should remain in contact with the chest wall over the lower one half of the sternum.

5. The rescuer's fingers should not rest on the victim's ribs during compression.

6. Compressions should be smooth, regular, and uninterrupted (50% of the cycle should be compression, and 50% should be relaxation). Quick jabs increase the possibility of injury and produce only quick jets of flow; they do not enhance stroke volume or provide a mean steady flow and pressure.[48]

7. The rescuer should not maintain continuous pressure on the patient's abdomen.

8. The shoulders of the rescuer should be directly over the victim's sternum. The elbows should be straight. Pressure is applied vertically downward on the lower sternum.

9. The lower sternum of an adult victim must be depressed 1½ to 2 inches by external cardiac compression.

10. Although complications may result from improperly performed external cardiac compression and precordial thumps, even properly performed external cardiac compression may cause rib fractures in some patients. Other complications that may occur with properly performed CPR include fracture of the sternum, costochondral separation, pneumothorax, hemothorax, lung contusions, lacerations of the liver, and fat emboli. These complications can be minimized by careful attention to details of performance; however, during cardiac arrest, effective CPR is required even if it results in complications, because the alternative to effective CPR is death.

SPECIAL RESUSCITATION SITUATIONS[35,55]

Drowning

Basic life support resuscitation procedures should be performed as quickly as possible on a victim of drowning. A few special considerations exist:

1. When attempting to rescue a drowning victim, the rescuer should get to the victim as quickly as possible.

2. External cardiac compression should never be attempted in water because it is impossible to perform it there effectively.

3. Mouth-to-mouth or mouth-to-nose ventilation may be performed in the water.

4. As soon as the rescuer can stand in shallow water, he or she should begin artificial ventilation.

5. In cases of suspected neck injury, as in a *diving* accident, the victim must be floated onto a back support before being removed from the water. If artificial respiration is required, the routine head tilt or jaw thrust maneuvers should not be used.

6. When removed from the water, the victim should have standard artificial ventilation or CPR performed.

7. Drowning victims swallow large volumes of water, and their stomachs usually become distended. This distention impairs ventilation and circulation and should be alleviated as soon as possible by appropriate posture and drainage of fluids from the oropharynx or removal of debris by *finger sweep.* The Heimlich Maneuver should not be used because the danger of pulmonary aspiration of swallowed water and vomitus is real,[56] and its use delays the institution of ventilation by rescue breathing. Actually, only a modest amount of water is inhaled in victims of near drowning and amounts to less than 20 ml/kg body weight because laryngospasm is evoked.[57] Only 10% of victims usually aspirate. When freshwater is aspirated, it is rapidly absorbed into the circulation, and up to 2 L may be absorbed in an average adult in a few minutes.[58] In seawater drowning, the aspiration of hypertonic salt water (3.5% saline) draws fluid from the circulation into lung tissue and produces pulmonary edema. The ensuing obstruction is not in the airways but in the alveoli. Immediate mouth-to-mouth breathing and positive pressure ventilation are the key to successful resuscitation.[58]

8. Every submersion victim, even one who requires only minimal resuscitation, should be transferred to a medical facility for follow-up care.

Electric Shock[59]

Electric shock may induce a variety of phenomena ranging from a benign tingling sensation to lethal cardiac arrest. The outcome depends largely on the amplitude and duration of contact with the current. Other than burns of varying severity and injuries due to falls, possible emergencies include the following[60]:

1. Tetany of the musculature of breathing, which is usually confined to the duration of the shock but may produce secondary cardiac arrest if the tetanizing shock is of a prolonged duration.

2. Prolonged paralysis of respiration, which may result from a massive convulsive phenomenon and may last for minutes after the shock current has terminated.

3. Ventricular fibrillation or other serious cardiac arrhythmias (such as runs of premature ventricular contractions or ventricular tachycardia that may progress to ventricular fibrillation) produced by low-voltage currents (110 to 220 V) sustained for several seconds.

The prognosis for victims of electric shocks is not predictable easily because the amplitude and duration of the charge usually are not known. Failure of either respiration or circulation is likely to result.[61]

After separating a victim from an energized object, the rescuer should determine the victim's cardiopulmonary status immediately. If spontaneous respiration or circulation is absent, the technique of CPR should be initiated.

When electric shock occurs on a public utility pole, a precordial thump should be delivered and mouth-to-mouth ventilation should be started at once. The victim must then be lowered to the ground as quickly as possible. CPR is only effective when performed on a victim who is in the horizontal position.

Lightning Strike

Lightning acts as a massive direct current countershock depolarizing the entire myocardium instantaneously but often followed by resumption of normal rhythm.[62] Death occurs in about 30% of cases and is usually due to cardiac arrest[63]; this may be either asystole or ventricular fibrillation. About 50% of survivors may sustain morbid injuries.

Respiratory arrest due to thoracic skeletal muscle spasm and to suppression of the respiratory center also occurs simultaneously and lasts longer than the cardiac arrest. Hence rescue breathing should be started at once and the program of basic life support, the ABC sequence followed by advanced cardiac life support, should be instituted. Recovery is excellent if cardiac arrest does not occur.

Smoke Inhalation[64]

Pulmonary insufficiency as a result of inhalation of smoke, especially if the air is hot, is the major cause of death among fire victims. The death rate is approximately 50% of fire-related deaths. Three types of respiratory abnormalities are encountered: (1) carbon monoxide poisoning; (2) thermal injury from the heat inspired smoky air; and (3) chemical injury from products of combustion.

Carbon Monoxide Poisoning

The immediate life-threatening problem is the development of tissue hypoxia due to the combination of carbon monoxide with hemoglobin.[65]

Thermal (Heat) Injury

The inhalation of hot air and smoke heated to a temperature of 150°C or higher usually results in burns to the face, oropharynx, and upper airway. Injury to the airway below the vocal cords is less likely. Superheated air is rapidly cooled before reaching the lower respiratory tract because of the tremendous heat-exchange efficiency of the oropharynx and nasopharynx. An exception to this rule is the inhalation of hot steam, which has a heat capacity at least 4000 times that of warm air. Hence, hot steam is capable of burning the distal airways and even the major bronchioles.

Flame exposure that produces facial burns and singes the nasal fibrillae is associated with temperatures sufficiently high to produce mucosal damage, and this injury may result in an obstruction of the upper airway. The injury may be present soon after the burn, but the major physiologic changes may not be seen for several hours.

Edema with hoarseness of the voice and obstruction of the airways may be delayed.

If the victim has extensive bodily burn, in addition to the burns of the face and upper respiratory tract, then the injury to the airways is magnified and is in direct proportion to the size and depth of the skin burn. Edema is also enhanced because of the release of vasoactive substances from thermally injured tissues.

Functional tests, such as spirometry or fiberoptic bronchoscopy, usually do not provide adequate information that would predict the severity of later airway compromise, because edema especially is progressive during the first 18 to 24 hours.

The patient must be closely monitored for any obstruction. The patient should be preferably positioned with the head elevated at about 30°. Hypovolemia should be corrected, and the capability of endotracheal intubation should be assessed. If any distortion exists because of the burn of the upper airway, endotracheal intubation should be carried out as soon as possible. Tracheostomy through burned tissues is generally not done, because of an increase in the risk of infection.

Chemical Injury

Chemical injury of the air passages is more serious than that produced by heat alone. Toxic gases are contained in smoke, as well as particulate carbon. Among the chemicals are aldehydes and organic acids, which irritate and destroy the mucosa of both upper and lower airways. Ordinarily, breath holding and laryngospasm, as a result of irritation, protect against excessive exposure in the conscious patient. In the unconscious patient, however, this protection is lost. In addition, water-soluble gases are found in smoke, especially from the burning of plastics or rubber. Among these agents are ammonia, sulfur dioxide, and chlorine, which react with water in the mucous membranes and produce strong acids and alkalis. Polyvinyl chloride, a common plastic, decomposes into hydrogen chloride when this plastic is heated. Very small concentrations of hydrogen chloride are extremely injurious and are usually carried through the lower airway, producing both bronchiolitis and alveolitis. Phosgene is also liberated from burning plastic and results in the production of hydrochloric acid.

Many gases are lipid soluble, such as nitrogen oxides and various aldehydes liberated from wood and cotton. These substances alter the cellular membrane lipid fraction. Fatal pulmonary edema and ciliary damage are frequent. Hydrogen cyanide is also a product of burning polyurethane and other paddings of upholstery. The cyanide that is released binds with cellular cytochrome oxidase. Besides injury to the respiratory system and the airways, pulmonary vascular changes also occur soon after the inhalation of smoke. Pulmonary vascular constriction, which usually leads to decreased cardiac output and shunting, results in increased dead space ventilation and hypoxemia.

Management

Treatment of smoke inhalation abnormalities must be aggressively pursued. The mortality rate from inhalation injury alone ranges from 5 to 10%. The addition of a cutaneous burn accentuates lung injury and the mortality rate may increase fourfold or more. Among the features of respiratory care are the following: (1) provision of an excellent airway; (2) provision of humidified inspired air; (3) provision of continuous positive airway pressure; (4) administration of intravenous and aerosolized bronchodilators; and (5) administration of chest physical therapy therapy. The corticosteroids have not been found to be effective, and evidence exists that the mortality rate of patients with a combined inhalation injury and cutaneous burn is increased.

Choking Syndrome[66]

Food choking is the sixth leading cause of accidental death. It is often called "café coronary." Choking should be recognized easily: The victim usually cannot speak or breathe, becomes pale, then deeply cyanotic, and collapses. Death may occur within 4 to 5 minutes. The onset, signs, and symptoms are distinct from those of the myocardial infarction. The inability to speak or to breathe and the victim's evident panic are distinctive. Frequently, a victim reaches up and grabs his or her throat. Indeed, this action is recommended as a signal, and the public should be made aware of this particular action and its meaning.

All types of food particles have become embedded either in the posterior pharynx or in the supraglottic region or have become caught within the glottic chink itself.

Usually, food choking occurs during inspiration, which causes a bolus of food to be sucked against the laryngeal orifice. Therefore, the lungs are usually expanded, and a significant movable air volume is contained in the lungs represented by the expiratory reserve volume plus the tidal inspiration. A forcible expiration with a significant air volume can be developed.

Heimlich Maneuver

Pressing one fist into the epigastrium elevates the choking victim's diaphragm. Sudden elevation of the diaphragm compresses the lung within the thoracic cavity, increasing air pressure and causing an increase in pressure in the trachea sufficient to eject the food bolus. This action is likened to an increase in pressure in a bottle of champagne forcing the cork to be popped.

Two procedures are available, depending on the position of the victim. One has to do with a victim who is standing or still sitting and the second with a victim who is supine. The following procedures are verbatim from these proposed by Heimlich.[66]

Rescuer Standing

The rescuer stands behind the victim and wraps his or her arms around the victim's waist. The rescuer grasps his or her own fist with the other hand and places the thumb side of the fist against the victim's abdomen slightly above the navel and below the rib cage. The rescuer presses his or her own fist into the victim's abdomen with a *quick upward thrust*. This maneuver is repeated several times if necessary.

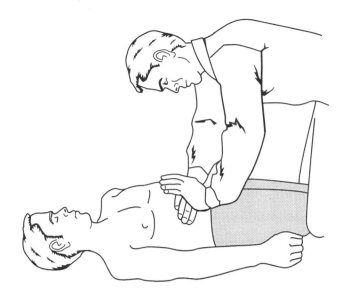

Fig. 46–8. With the victim lying face up, the rescuer presses into the victim's abdomen with an upward thrust. (Redrawn from Heimlich, H. J. JAMA *234*:398, 1975.)

When the victim is sitting, the rescuer stands behind the victim's chair and performs the maneuver in the same manner.

Rescuer Kneeling

A variation of the maneuver can be performed when the victim has collapsed or when the rescuer is unable to lift the victim (Fig. 46–8). The victim is lying on his or her back. Facing the victim, the rescuer kneels astride the victim's hips. With one hand on top of the other, the rescuer places the heel of his or her bottom hand on the victim's abdomen slightly above the navel and below the rib cage. The rescuer presses into the victim's abdomen with a *quick upward thrust*. This maneuver is repeated several times if necessary.

Should the victim vomit, the rescuer should quickly place him or her on the side and wipe out the victim's mouth to prevent aspiration.

Traditional methods of removing objects from the supraglottic region are usually unsuccessful. Moreover, this maneuver has had some measure of success in drowning victims, in which situations water is actually ejected from the tracheal-bronchial tree and the pharynx.

Closed Versus Open Chest Massage[67]

Several controlled studies have compared the effectiveness of closed and open cardiac massage in maintaining circulation and tissue oxygenation. All parameters related to flows and pressures showed higher values with open chest massage, but oxygen saturation of arterial blood was consistently higher with closed chest massage.[68] To assume that the opening of the chest is concurrent with an impairment of ventilation and perfusion of the lungs is logical; thus, availability of oxygen to the circulating blood is reduced. Because in emergency cardiorespiratory resuscitation physicians are are most concerned with restoring oxygenation of the tissues, the near-normal oxy-

Table 46–6.　Open Versus Closed Cardiac Resuscitation

Parameter	Control	Fibril-lation	Closed	Open
Carotid flow (60/min)	248	0	75	86
Carotid flow per stroke	13.4	0	1.27	1.37
Femoral flow (60/min)	138	0	27	49
Central venous pressure	1.5	12.0	7.0	8.6
Blood pressure		20/?	70/35	94/50
Oxygen saturation:				
Arterial	93%	91%	90%	77%
Venous	69%	56%	31%	32%

Data from Pappelbaum, S., et al.: Open versus closed cardiac resuscitation. JAMA *193:*659, 1965.

gen saturation obtained with closed chest massage outweighs by far the advantages of slightly higher flow rates of pressures obtained with open massage (Table 46–6). In the operating room setting, however, open chest massage is superior to closed chest compression.[69] See later in this chapter for other situations and conditions.

ADVANCED LIFE SUPPORT

Advanced life support consists of the following elements (Table 46–7):

1. Initial basic life support.
2. Use of adjunctive equipment and special techniques, such as endotracheal intubation and open chest internal cardiac compression.
3. Cardiac monitoring for dysrhythmia recognition and control.
4. Defibrillation capability.
5. Establishment and maintenance of an intravenous infusion lifeline.
6. Definitive therapy, including drug administration to correct acidosis and to aid in establishing and maintaining an effective cardiac rhythm and circulation.
7. Stabilization of the patient's condition.

Internal Cardiac Compression

Internal cardiac compression is indicated in certain conditions in which external cardiac compression may be ineffective. These circumstances include penetrating wounds of the heart and other internal thoracic injuries, cardiac tamponade, tension pneumothorax with mediastinal displacement, chest or spinal deformities, and severe emphysema causing barrel-type chest. If one suspects or can determine that any of these conditions is present, or if closed chest cardiac compression does not appear to establish sufficiently effective artificial circulation, open chest internal cardiac compression may be performed in conjunction with artificial ventilation.

Open chest cardiac compression should only be performed by a physician with the necessary skill, equipment, and facilities. In this procedure, a thoracotomy is performed through the left fifth intercostal space, and the pericardial sac is opened to allow direct manual cardiac compression.

Patients with crushed chest or flail chest may require only effective artificial ventilation.

If a tension pneumothorax is suspected in an emergency situation, a large-bore needle may be inserted on the side of the pneumothorax through the second intercostal space 2 inches from the midline. If the diagnosis is confirmed, this procedure should be replaced with a chest tube and valve or an underwater seal drainage as soon as possible.

In one experimental study of cerebral preservation during CPR, the open chest technique was found to be superior to the closed chest method. The neurologic deficit scores were not significantly different from control values.[70]

Cardiac Monitoring

ECG monitoring should be established immediately on all patients who have symptoms of suspected heart attack or patients who suddenly collapse.

Most sudden deaths following acute myocardial infarction are due to dysrhythmias. When initial emergency is a cardiac arrest, CPR steps and techniques of basic life support should be initiated. As quickly as possible thereafter, ECG electrodes should be applied. If the patient has a relatively regular ECG rhythm, pulse and blood pressure should be checked immediately to determine whether electromechanical dissociation is present.

Defibrillation[71]

Defibrillation produces a simultaneous depolarization of all muscle fascicles of the heart, after which a spontaneous beat may resume if the myocardium is oxygenated and is not acidotic. Direct current defibrillator shocks should be delivered as soon as possible when the heart is known to be in ventricular fibrillation. Countershocks also are indicated on an emergency basis in the presence of ventricular tachycardia without a peripheral pulse.

The standard electrode position should be used: one electrode just to the right of the upper sternum below the clavicle and the other electrode just to the left of the cardiac apex or left nipple.

A single defibrillator shock does not produce serious functional damage to the myocardium; it should not be withheld in the unconscious, pulseless adult patient when a direct current defibrillator is available even though the patient is unmonitored. Unmonitored defibrillation is not recommended for children.

In instances of apparent cardiac arrest secondary to hypoxemia, such as drug overdose, CPR for a period of 2 minutes is recommended, with reevaluation before the delivery of an unmonitored defibrillator shock.

The output delivered into a 50- to 100-ohm load should range from 200 to at least 250 watt-seconds, preferably 300 watt-seconds for the conventional sine waveform. The average adult transthoracic human impedance is about 70 to 80 ohms.[72,73] In emergency situations, the

Table 46–7. Advanced Cardiac Life Support: Definitive Therapy in Cardiac Resuscitation

DEFINITIVE ℞
- DIAGNOSIS
- DRUGS
- DEFIBRILLATION

DIAGNOSIS (CARDIAC ARREST)

TYPE	HEARTBEAT	ECG	SIGNS
1. Cardiac standstill	Absent	Flat	1. Breathing absent
2. Ventricular fibrillation	Uncoordinated	Erratic	2. Pulse absent
3. Cardiovascular collapse	Rhythmic Ineffective	May be near normal	3. Pupils dilated

Always continue heart-lung resuscitation without interruption during DIAGNOSIS

DRUGS (administer via venous cutdown)
Epinephrine—0.5 to 1.0 ml. (1:1000) ⎫
   Improves blood pressure ⎪
   Improves cardiac tone ⎬ REPEAT
Sodium bicarbonate—3.75 g in 50 ml ⎪ q̄ 10 MIN.
   Combats acidosis ⎪ p.r.n.
   Improves cerebral flow ⎭

Calcium gluconate 10 ml of 10% solution
   Increases myocardial tone
   Increases cardiac output
Vasopressors—As indicated after heartbeat restored
Quinidine or procaine amide—100 mg as needed
   As indicated to decrease myocardial irritability

Always continue heart-lung resuscitation without interruption during ADMINISTRATION OF DRUGS

DEFIBRILLATION
Use external shocks, as needed, with 30 pounds pressure on electrodes over saline pads on standard position, as shown
AC: 440 to 880 volts
DC: 100 to 200 watt-seconds
Repeat shocks, as needed
Repeat drugs, as needed
Always continue heart-lung resuscitation without interruption between DEFIBRILLATIONS

Courtesy of A.S. Gordon, Chairman of Committee on CPR Standards. JAMA *227(suppl)*:834, 1974.

customary procedure has been to deliver a maximum shock up to 360 joules (J; watt-seconds) for patients with ventricular fibrillation. The damage resulting from defibrillator shocks is directly proportional to the energy used, and maximal settings, when not required, may further impair an already damaged myocardium. This can be accomplished by defibrillating up to three times if needed at levels of 200 J, 200 to 300 J, and up to 360 J.

Energy Levels

Conventional effective devices for defibrillation can store up to 400 J of energy and can deliver 300 J or less of energy. In a prospective survey of the energy levels needed for various patients' weights, 1.8 J/kg body weight delivered to the chest wall terminated 98% of episodes of ventricular fibrillation.[74] For patients weighing 91 to 225 kg, the average effective direct current shock was 190 J on the first shock in most patients. Sub-

sequent shocks at the same energy level were even more effective; this effect is explained by the reduced impedence to flow of current through the skin and chest after the first shock.[72] These determinations contrast with retrospective studies of heavy patients that predicted that 3.7 J of energy/kg body weight would be needed to defibrillate.[75] Thus, devices that have a capacity of more than 400 J are unnecessary.

Clinical variables that determine successful defibrillation are the following[76]:

1. Corrected acidemia.
2. Corrected hypoxia.
3. Ventricular fibrillation; if less than 2 minutes' duration, defibrillation can be accomplished at low energies of 70 to 90 J; nonagonal ventricular defibrillation is more readily achieved than agonal defibrillation.

An undesirable consequent of defibrillation is related to the development of resistant tachyarrhythmias. As shocks increase in energy from 100 to 400 J, the frequency of arrhythmias increases from 3 to 65%.

In addition to resistant arrhythmias, passing excessive electric currents through the heart may cause direct damage. Burns of the heart have been reported as well as burns of the chest skeletal muscle.[77]

Studies at two energy levels of 175 and 320 J have been carried out to determine effectiveness and safety. After one or two shocks, a reversion to an organized rhythm usually occurs at either level. Survival is related to the rhythm noted after the first shock. Persistent fibrillation usually occurs in about 70% of patients. Repeated shocks at the high energy level cause a higher incidence of atrioventricular block and other adverse rhythms. In general, initial defibrillatory shocks at 175 J are safe and are as effective as shocks at twice that energy level.[78]

Intravenous Therapy

Providing an intravenous route for the intermittent or continuous rapid administration of drugs and fluids that may be required to reestablish or support a stable cardiac rhythm and adequate circulation is essential. This route must be established as early as possible and must be a routine part of advanced life support.

A large peripheral vein or a central vein is recommended. Intracardiac injections are *not* recommended.

Cardiac Arrest Prognosis

The success of resuscitation is affected by the location of the cardiac arrest and the environment in which the care is provided (Table 46–8).[79,80]

Drugs and Definitive Therapy

Oxygen and Ventilation

Tracheal intubation by trained personnel and the early administration of high concentrations of oxygen are of major importance in reducing hypoxemia during the cardiorespiratory emergency. Although the dangers of hypoxemia are easily demonstrated experimentally and clin-

Table 46–8. Cardiac Arrest Prognosis

Cardiac Arrest	Survival (Discharged Alive) (%)
In hospital emergency room	9
In hospital wards	13
In community, with immediate resuscitation	16
In Community, outside hospital no doctor or paramedics	4
Ventricular fibrillation outside hospital	10
Asystole outside hospital	1
Ventricular fibrillation inside hospital (Seattle)	30

From Warnberg, M., Thomassen, A.: Prognosis after cardiac arrest occurring outside intensive care and coronary care units. Acta Anaesthesiol Scand 23:69, 1979.

ically, no evidence indicates that lung damage occurs with high concentrations of oxygen if it is used for less than 24 hours.

Essential Drug Therapy

Drugs usually are administered intravenously to ensure their delivery into the cardiovascular system as artificial circulation is provided. Intracardiac injections are sometimes used, but this route is usually limited to epinephrine early during the cardiac arrest and before an intravenous infusion has become available.

Sodium Bicarbonate

The administration of sodium bicarbonate in the management of cardiac arrest does not improve outcome. In the first 5 to 10 minutes of CPR after cardiac arrest, one sees a paradox of significant mixed venous respiratory acidosis, with high Pv^-co_2 and normal arterial pH.[81,82] Bicarbonate appears only to increase Pv^-co_2 and tissue Pco_2 further.[83] Therefore, ensuring effective alveolar ventilation is the key to maintaining acid-base balance early after cardiac arrest and during CPR. Base buffers that do not generate CO_2 loads, such as sodium carbonate or tromethamine, may be appropriate.

Other disadvantages of sodium bicarbonate include the following[84]:

1. The oxygen-hemoglobin association curve is shifted to the right, inhibiting the tissue release of oxygen.
2. Hyperosmolality and hypernatremia are induced.
3. The excess CO_2 diffusing into cells depresses both cerebral and myocardial function.
4. An extracellular alkalosis is induced.
5. Catecholamines may be inactivated.

In conclusion, neither the ability to defibrillate nor the survival rate is improved.

Epinephrine

Epinephrine increases myocardial contractility, elevates perfusion pressure, lowers defibrillation threshold, and, in some instances, restores myocardial contractility in electromechanical dissociation. Of great importance is increased myocardial and cerebral blood flow.[85] These effects are related to the α-adrenergic stimulating properties of epinephrine. The β-adrenergic effects are at best undesirable because of increased myocardial work and reduced subendocardial perfusion.[86]

The recommended dose in the management of cardiac arrest is 1.0 mg administered intravenously in a dilute solution of 1/10,000. (This solution is prepared by adding 10 mg of epinephrine to 100 ml of isotonic saline or Ringer's lactate solution.) Thus, 1.0 mg is contained in 10 ml and is repeated every 3 to 5 minutes. Each dose is followed by a 20 ml flush of isotonic saline solution.[87]

Some experimental work has demonstrated that an optimal cardiac response may be obtained with higher doses ranging from 0.045 to 0.20 mg/kg.[88] In clinical studies, however, although a more rapid return of spontaneous circulation was observed, no improvement occurred in survival rates or in neurologic outcomes.[89,90]

An alternative dosage schedule involves a dilute solution. This solution is prepared by adding 1.0 mg of epinephrine to 200 ml of isotonic saline of Ringer's lactate solution. This solution provides a 1/200,000 dilution, so it is 5.0 μg/ml. The initial rate of administration for adults is 1.0 μg/kg for the first minute, increasing rapidly to 4.0 μg/min or until an effect is observed.[91] For infants and children, an infusion rate is based on a dose of 0.1 μg/kg per minute, increasing up to a maximum of 1.5 μg/kg per minute or until an effect is observed.[92]

Dextrose Solutions

Intravenous fluids containing dextrose during resuscitation worsen the outcome when they are used during experimental cardiac arrest. Dogs receiving a dextrose 5% Ringer's lactate solution showed greater neurologic deficits, including convulsive activity and a significantly increased mortality after 8 minutes of cardiac arrest. Hyperglycemia combined with cerebral ischemia worsens the neurologic outcome in patients with cardiac arrest. If brain glucose is increased, one sees an increase in lactic acid and an increase in brain pH. This situation aggravates neuronal injury. In primates, modest increases in blood glucose in a range of 120 to 220 mg/dl during cerebral ischemia, as occurs in cardiac arrest, resulted in a linear increase in the magnitude of neurologic injury.

Special Drug Therapy

Atropine Sulfate

Atropine sulfate reduces vagal tone, enhances atrioventricular condition, and accelerates the cardiac rate in case of sinus bradycardia. This agent is most useful in preventing cardiac arrest in patients with profound sinus bradycardia secondary to myocardial infarction, particularly when hypotension is present.

Atropine sulfate is indicated for the treatment of sinus bradycardia in patients with a pulse of less than 60 beats per minute when accompanied by premature ventricular contractions or systolic blood pressure of less than 90 mm Hg. This drug is also indicated for high-degree atrioventricular block accompanied by bradycardia. It is of no value in ventricular ectopic bradycardia in the absence of atrial activity. The recommended dose is 0.5 mg administered intravenously as a bolus, and it is repeated at 5-minute intervals until a pulse rate greater than 60 is achieved. The total dose of atropine sulfate should not exceed 2 mg, except in cases of third-degree atrioventricular block, in which larger doses may be required.

Lidocaine

Lidocaine raises the fibrillation threshold and exerts its antidysrhythmic effect by increasing the electrical stimulation threshold of the ventricle during diastole. This drug is particularly effective in depressing irritability in which successful defibrillation repeatedly reverts to ventricular fibrillation. This agent also is particularly effective in the control of multifocal premature ventricular beats and episodes of ventricular tachycardia. Fifty to 100 mg should be administered slowly as a bolus intravenously and may be repeated if necessary. It may be followed by a continuous infusion of 1 to 3 mg per minute, usually not exceeding 4 mg/min.

Calcium Chloride

Calcium chloride increases myocardial contractility, prolongs systole, and enhances ventricular excitability. Sinus impulse formation can be suppressed, and sudden death following a rapid intravenous injection of calcium chloride has been described, particularly in fully digitalized patients. Calcium chloride is useful in profound cardiovascular collapse (electromechanical dissociation). It may be useful in restoring an electrical rhythm in patients with asystole and may enhance electrical defibrillation.

The usual recommended dose of calcium chloride is 2.5 to 5 ml of a 10% solution (3.4 to 6.8 mEq Ca^{++}). Calcium gluconate provides less ionizable calcium per unit volume. If it is used, the dose should be 10 ml of a 10% solution (4.8 mEq).

Supplemental Drug Therapy

Vasoactive Drugs (Levarterenol, Metaraminol)

The choice of a vasoconstrictor or a positive inotropic agent remains controversial in the treatment of cardiac arrest and the immediate postresuscitation period. During cardiac compression and the postresuscitation period, however, blood pressure must be supported when low blood pressure and inadequate cerebral and renal perfusion give evidence of shock.

In peripheral vascular collapse, manifested clinically by hypotension and the absence of significant peripheral vasoconstriction, intravenous levarterenol bitartrate (norepinephrine bitartrate; Levophed) in high concentrations of 16 μg/ml or metaraminol bitartrate (Aramine) in concentrations of 0.4 mg/ml of dextrose in water should be titrated intravenously.

Isoproterenol

For patients with profound bradycardia demonstrated to be the result of complete heart block, isoproterenol hydrochloride (Isuprel) is the drug of choice for immediate treatment. It should be infused in amounts of 2 to 20 μg per minute (1 to 10 ml of a solution of 1 mg in 500 ml of 5% glucose in water) and adjusted to increase heart rate to approximately 60 beats per minute. It is useful also for profound sinus bradycardia refractory to atropine.

Propranolol

This agent is useful in patients with repetitive ventricular tachycardia or repetitive ventricular fibrillation in whom maintenance of a rhythmic heart beat cannot be achieved with lidocaine. The usual dose of propranolol is 1 mg intravenously. This may be repeated to a total of 3 mg under careful monitoring. Caution is required in patients with chronic obstructive pulmonary disease and cardiac failure.

Corticosteroids

Present evidence favors the use of pharmacologic doses of synthetic corticosteroids (5 mg/kg of methylprednisolone sodium succinate or 1 mg/kg of dexamethasone phosphate) for prompt treatment of cardiogenic shock or shock lung occurring as complications of cardiac arrest. When cerebral edema is suspected following cardiac arrest, methylprednisolone sodium succinate in doses of 60 to 100 mg every 6 hours may be beneficial. When pulmonary complications, such as postaspiration pneumonitis, are present, dexamethasone phosphate may be used in doses of 4 to 8 mg every 6 hours. In both cerebral anoxic edema and aspiration pneumonitis, corticosteroids may be administered, but this use is empiric.

Postcardiac Arrest Drug Treatment

In addition to corticosteroids, potent diuretic agents, hypothermia and controlled hyperventilation may be useful for the prevention or attenuation of cerebral edema that may follow successful resuscitation. Potent diuretic agents (furosemide and ethacrynic acid) in doses of 40 to 200 mg may help to promote diuresis. Hyperosmolality may be aggravated by these agents.

Protection of Brain

In conditions of global ischemia, as occurs after cardiac or respiratory arrest and successful CPR, the brain needs protection to ameliorate or to prevent progressive functional deterioration and structural disintegration with cell necrosis. These conditions represent global ischemia. Evidence accumulated between 1976 and 1984 indicate that barbiturates may protect the brain, may reduce the edema, may reduce intracranial pressure, and may reduce size of infarctions.[93,94] At the very least, cells at a marginal level of survival have a reduction in their metabolic oxygen requirement.[95] One study of patients by Ruano and colleagues[96] showed some initial improvement in morbidity and mortality, but little long-term advantage.

Laboratory and human trials have not confirmed the foregoing concepts. A multinational study of patients of the effect of barbiturates on the neurologic outcome after cardiac arrest did not reveal improvement over patients not given barbiturates.[97] Indeed, any accompanying hypotensive effect adversely affected outcome.[98] At the end of 1 year, the mortality in patients treated with thiopental and those not so treated (all other therapy being identical in both groups) was about 80%. The conclusion was that the use of barbiturate coma "to preserve brain function after cardiac arrest or stroke has no clinical bases and should be abandoned."[99]

Other causes of acute cerebral injury have not benefited by the barbiturates: (1) local ischemia (strokes); (2) head trauma; (3) global ischemia (anoxia); and (4) direct cell toxic effects of metabolic and infectious processes.

In severe head injury, when the patient is comatose for 6 hours or more and is unable to speak, to open eyes, or to obey commands, the mortality rate is between 40 and 50%. With rapid diagnosis, however, evacuation of intracranial hematomas, artificial ventilation, control of intracranial pressure (mannitol), and intensive monitoring,

mortality may be reduced, but not morbidity. In these patients, intravenous pentobarbital had no protective effect against an increase in intracranial pressure. Outcome at the end of 1 year is essentially the same in barbiturate- and nonbarbiturate-treated patients.

The hypothesis that the failure of high intracranial pressure to respond to barbiturates portends a poor prognosis has not been substantiated. Some patients do show fair to moderate recovery, despite failure to respond to barbiturate treatment of intracranial pressure.[100]

Incomplete Ischemia

In aneurysmal surgery, carotid endarterectomy, and cerebral bypass procedures, the administration of thiopental in doses of 10 mg/kg to achieve a plasma level of 5.0 μg/ml or 20 mg/kg to establish a plasma level of 8.0 to 9.0 μg/ml affords cellular protection. This drug should be given before clamping is performed. Doses should be gauged by electrocerebral function monitor to an electroencephalographic (EEG) level of 10 to 40 seconds and burst suppression.[101]

In certain clinical cardiopulmonary bypass procedures,[102] the administration of thiopental improves the neuropsychiatric outcome. Nussmeier found that a large dose was needed, of about 40.0 mg/kg, and that the EEG should be maintained near total suppression, but not absent. This result is considered to be the first valid demonstration of barbiturate-induced brain protection in human patients.[103]

Experimentally, in global brain ischemia, isoflurane provides some protection. Two conditions appear to be necessary, namely, suppression of the cortical EEG *without* abolition of cortical electrical activity and large doses achieved at 3% isoflurane concentration. Dogs exposed to isoflurane have cerebral energy stores of adenosine triphosphate and phosphocreatine and energy charge sustained at high levels with less accumulation of cerebral lactate.[104]

Deliberate hypotension induced with isoflurane (mean concentration 2.3 $\pm$ 1.0%) in patients undergoing craniotomy for repair of cerebral aneurysms favorably influences the global cerebral oxygen supply-demand balance. Mean cerebral blood flow remained at normal range (49 $\pm$ 15 ml $\cdot$ 100 g^{-1} $\cdot$ min^{-1}) during and after hypotension (mean arterial pressure reduced from 78 $\pm$ 5 to 51 $\pm$ 7 mm Hg). The CMR_{O_2} was reduced from 2.0 $\pm$ 0.6 ml $\cdot$ 100 g^{-1} $\cdot$ min^{-1} to 1.5 $\pm$ 0.5 ml $\cdot$ 100 g^{-1} $\cdot$ min^{-1} during hypotension. This reduction in oxygen demand is significant. The CMR_{O_2} returned to normal after return to normotension.[105]

Calcium Entry Blockade[106]

Studies of primates indicate that at least one calcium-entry blocker, namely, nimodipine, improves outcome when given after complete cerebral ischemia.[107]

CONTINUATION OR TERMINATION OF LIFE SUPPORT

The decision to terminate resuscitative efforts is medical and depends on an assessment by a physician of the cerebral status of the patient. The best criteria of adequate cerebral circulation are the reaction of the pupils, the level of consciousness, movement, and spontaneous respiration.

Beecher was the first to clearly define irreversible coma.[108] Deep unconsciousness, absence of spontaneous respiration, and pupils that are fixed and dilated for 15 to 30 minutes usually are indicative of cerebral death, and further resuscitative efforts are generally futile.[109] Cardiac death is likely in the continuing absence of ventricular ECG activity after 10 minutes or more of adequate cardiopulmonary support including appropriate drug therapy. In children, or in unusual circumstances, such as when the cardiac arrest is associated with hypothermia, resuscitative efforts should be continued for longer periods because recovery has been seen after prolonged unconsciousness.

Life support measures should be continued until one has evidence of recovery or sufficient evidence to pronounce the victim dead.

Postanesthetic Recovery Score[110]

A simple method of evaluation of postanesthetic patients applicable to all situations, regardless of the anesthetic and adjuvant agents administered, has been proposed by Aldrete and McDonald. It is a means of evaluating recovery.[111] The score is based on the observation of five signs. A score of 0, 1, or 2 is given to each sign, depending on whether it is present or absent. A score of 10 indicates a recovered patient in the best possible condition (Table 46-9). Scoring is performed at least every 5 minutes initially and then at longer intervals.

Resuscitation of the Newborn (Apgar Score)[112]

In 1949, Virginia Apgar devoted herself to the anesthetic management of obstetric labor and delivery and developed a system and organization of full-time physicians for this purpose. The problems of the newborn infant received her attention, and, at this time, modernization of techniques of resuscitation were needed. No standard of evaluation of the newborn's transition from intrauterine to extrauterine life existed. The idea of a score was instigated by a question from a medical student of how to evaluate the newborn. Apgar responded by saying, "That's easy! You do it this way," and proceeded to write

down five essential points on a cafeteria table card (Table 46-10). The score was published in 1953 and again in 1958.[112,113]

The score enabled all personnel to observe the newborn in a standard way. It provides the following: (1) a guide to the need for appropriate resuscitation techniques from the simplest to the complex; (2) repeated at 5 minutes, it serves to show the effectiveness of the resuscitation; the highest incidence of neonatal and later complication occurs in infants with the lowest scores; (3) it is a predictor of neonatal survival and of neurologic development[114]; and (4) it provides a basis for comparison of labor interventions and techniques of labor and of anesthesia.

With a standard index of the physical condition of the newborn, the influence of labor and delivery interventions has been assessed.[115] Duncan Holaday and Stanley James introduced new methods of measuring blood gases, the adequacy of oxygenation, acid-base balance, and blood levels of anesthetic agents. The influence of the anesthetic techniques of regional and general anesthesia was readily demonstrated in obstetrics.[115] Umbilical artery cannulation and catheter insertion into the umbilical vein and right atrium were introduced as essential technology. With this background was born the specialty of modern neonatology, and a program for teaching visiting physicians was developed.

This score has become a universal standard. In its simplicity, it is informative and practical. It has served to improve obstetric care and to separate the causes of newborns' problems between those with a prenatal factor from those due to labor trauma.[116] For example, the problem of cerebral palsy is clearly related to risk factors preceding labor[116] and is not directly to the management factors at delivery.[117]

Use of Score as a Guide to Newborn Resuscitation (Table 46-11)

At birth, the newborn is provided standard care including suction of the nose, mouth, and pharynx, placement in a warm environment (radiant-heated bassinet), and provided mild foot and skin stimulation. Within 1 minute, the child is scored; however, resuscitation measures are not to be delayed if the degree of depression is evident.

Table 46-9. Postanesthetic Recovery Score

Assessment	AMD	15M	30M	1 HR	1HR 30M	2 HR
ACTIVITY Purposeful-2 Random-1 None-0						
RESPIRATION Regular Good Depth-2 Limited-1 APNEA or Assist-0						
CONSCIOUSNESS Alert Awake-2 Arousable-1 Nonresponsive-0						
COLOR Pink-2 Pale, Dusky-1 Cyanotic-0						
CIRCULATION BP = 20%-2 ± 2-50%-1 ± 50%-0						
TOTAL						

From Aldrete, J. A., Kronlik, D.: A postanesthetic recovery score. Anesth Analg 49:924, 1970.

Table 46–10. Apgar Score

Sign	0	1	2
1. Heart rate	Absent	Slow	Over 100
2. Respiratory effort	Absent	Slow Irregular	Good Crying
3. Muscle tone	Limp	Some flexion of extremities	Active motion
4. Reflex responses to tangential slap on foot	No response	Grimace	Vigorous cry
5. Color	Blue Pale	Body pink Extremities blue	Completely pink

Note: Score obtained 60 seconds after delivery of infant with evaluation of each objective sign. 10 is characteristic of an infant in the best possible condition. Repeat in 5 minutes. Highest incidence of neonatal and later complications occur in infants with lowest scores.

Table 46–11. Apgar Score: A Guide To Newborn Resuscitation

Apgar Score	Treatment
>8	Suction pharynx Place in a warm environment
5–7	External stimulation Oxygen by mask Mechanical ventilation by mask if no response
3–6	Initial mechanical ventilation by mask Intubation of the trachea if spontaneous ventilation does not occur promptly Analysis of arterial blood gases from a doubly clamped segment of the umbilical cord
<2	Intubation of the trachea and mechanical ventilation of the lungs with oxygen External cardiac compressions if heart rate <60 beats·min^{-1}

Most newborns have a score of 8 to 10, which implies minimal or no depression.

A score of 5 to 7 indicates mild to moderate depression, and these infants respond to external stimulation by tapping the soles of the feet or by further gentle skin surface rubbing and providing oxygen by a face mask.

A score of 3 to 5 represents moderate depression and may warrent initial mechanical ventilation by face mask and oxygen. If spontaneous ventilation does not occur promptly, intubation of the trachea with an appropriate endotracheal tube should be accomplished, and positive pressure at positive airway pressures no higher than 25 cm H_2O is pursued at a rate of 30 to 60 breaths per minute. An end-expiratory positive pressure at 1 to 3 mm Hg may be instituted to maintain an expanded lung.

A score of less than 3 (between 0 and 3) implies severe depression, and vigorous resuscitation should be pursued according to the ABCDs of cardiopulmonary care. If the heart rate is below 60 beats per minute, external cardiac compression is instituted; epinephrine, 5.0 μg/kg, is indicated when the newborn is severely bradycardic and hypotensive.

Contraindications to Resuscitation

CPR is not indicated in certain situations, such as in patients with terminal, irreversible illness in whom death is not unexpected or in whom prolonged cardiac arrest dictates the futility of resuscitation efforts. Resuscitation in these circumstances may represent a positive violation of an individual's right to die with dignity. When CPR is considered contraindicated for hospital patients, it is appropriate to indicate this in the patient's progress notes. It also is appropriate to indicate this on the physicians' order sheet for the benefit of nurses and other personnel who may be called on to initiate or participate in CPR.

Selection of Critically Ill Patients for Treatment

According to the medical factors, a decision must be made about the optimum treatment of critically ill patients.[118] A triage concept is applied, and patients are classified. The following is a classification according to a Massachusetts General Hospital (Boston) protocol and with modifications according to Meisel and Grenvik[119]:

Class A: Total care, a maximal therapeutic effort without time limitation. Effort may be with reservations namely a daily assessment of effect.
Class B: Selective limitation of therapeutic effort; the total effort is made with reservations and daily assessment of effect.
Class C: No extraordinary therapeutic efforts; one should provide comfort and minimal care and apply rational therapeutics and should withdraw ineffective therapeutics.
Class D: No therapy; no CPR.

Orders Not to Resuscitate[120]

Numerous medical, ethical, socioeconomic, family, administrative, and legal factors must be considered. In the final analysis, the medical factors are critical.

Medical judgment forms the basis for decision. This is the responsibility of the primary physician and his or her consultants.[121] The patient must have an *irreversible, irreparable* illness or condition. One must determine that no therapeutic measures would be effective in reversing the disease process.[122] The condition must be beyond repair. The prognosis of imminent death, that is, in less than 2 weeks, is essential.

Minimum ethical and legal considerations are as follows: (1) consent must be given by a conscious, competent patient; the patient may indeed have already requested that no therapeutic measures be employed—only care, and the patient has a right to decline treatment; and

(2) when a patient is unconscious or incompetent, consultation with another physician is necessary and agreement reached on the medical factors; then the responsible next of kin must be consulted, informed of the situation, and requested to give consent.

A decision to resuscitate or not must be weighed heavily in favor of preserving an integrated life.[123] When the decision must be made in an emergency and in a newly unconscious patient who has an undiagnosed condition, the presumption must be made in favor of life.

MEDICAL ETHICAL PRINCIPLES OF CARDIOPULMONARY RESUSCITATION

The fundamental principle guiding one in performing resuscitation measures is that *"the patient must be salvable."*[124] Indications to perform or not to perform resuscitation both medically and ethically are limited, specifically with regard to CPR and advanced life support.[125]

CPR is clearly a medical therapy.[126] The need has emerged to obtain consent based on a patient's advance directive or the designation of surrogate with power of attorney to provide or to withhold complex treatment. As with all other therapies, however, the physician must decide about the benefit of a given therapy. It is therefore more appropriate and accurate to write an order stating *CPR Not Indicated* when the patient is not salvable and when the effort at resuscitation would be futile[127-130] (Table 46–12).

CURRENT ANALYSIS OF THE PHYSIOLOGY OF CARDIOPULMONARY RESUSCITATION[131]

The present standard for CPR, updated in 1992 by the National Conference on Cardiopulmonary Resuscitation and Emergency Care, has changed little since CPR was introduced in 1960. The present approach to CPR is moderately successful in resuscitating patients with initial ventricular fibrillation, with a 24 to 43% hospital discharge survival rate. These rates depend on rapid initiation of CPR (4 minutes) and initiation of advanced life support in 8 minutes. The results after cardiac arrest in patients with asystole, electrical mechanical dissociation, or refractory

Table 46–12. Clinical Situations Where CPR is Unlikely to Prolong Life

Advanced, progressive, ultimately lethal illness
  Bedfast metastatic cancer
  Child's class C cirrhosis
  HIV infection (patient has had ≥2 episodes of *Pneumocystis carinii* pneumonia)
  Dementia requiring long-term care
Acute, near-fatal illness without evidence of improvement after ICU admission
  Coma (traumatic or nontraumatic) lasting >48 hr
  Multiple organ system failure with no improvement after 3 consecutive days in ICU
  Unsuccessful out-of-hospital CPR

From Murphy, D.J., Finucane, T.E.: New do-not-resuscitate policies. Ann Intern Med 153:1641, 1993.

ventricular fibrillation are less than desirable, with a hospital discharge survival rate of less than 16%.

Closed Chest Methods

To analyze the technique of closed chest cardiac massage, attention has been focused on two areas: (1) the mechanics of producing blood flow; and (2) the coronary perfusion pressure during massage.[132]

Several researchers have speculated that the forward blood flow during closed chest CPR may be secondary to a generalized increase in intrathoracic pressure, rather than to true cardiac compression.[132,133] Accordingly, techniques that combine simultaneous ventilation compression of the thorax and abdominal binding have been used in animal experiments. Although cardiac blood flow and aortic systolic pressure did increase, these techniques did not necessarily improve survival. The survival rate was actually associated with aortic diastolic pressure and coronary perfusion.

Because these techniques elevate all pressures in the thorax to approximately equal levels, the coronary perfusion (aortic minus right atrial diastolic pressure) is not high, and the heart does not have an adequate blood supply during chest compression.

The importance of the coronary perfusion pressure has been documented in the dog model, when a higher survival rate was obtained even after 30 minutes of ventricular fibrillation, when the aortic diastolic pressure was maintained above 30 mm Hg.[134] Other studies have shown that the mean aortic-right atrial pressure difference and the diastolic arterial-venous pressure difference are directly correlated with coronary blood flow and the ability to resuscitate dogs undergoing CPR.

Open Chest Massage

Various reports of successful open chest massage after failure with closed chest massage have been published. The few experimental studies comparing the two techniques show that, although open chest massage improves cardiac output, it does not seem to increase arterial pressures, the end result being far from conclusive.[67]

In conclusion, new alternative techniques of CPR with interposed abdominal compressions corresponding with each chest relaxation, the use of pneumatic antishock garments,[135] and high-frequency, high-momentum chest compression are under investigation.[136] These techniques aim to take advantage of the thoracic pump and to improve the mechanism of forward blood flow.

The roles of open chest massage, abdominal bleeding, optimal rate, duration of chest compression, and timing of ventilation are all being reevaluated in the effort to improve the survival of patients in cardiac arrest.

New areas of investigation on drugs that improve the coronary perfusion pressure, such as the continuous intravenous drip of large doses of epinephrine and calcium channel blockers, are also being researched in the attempt to sustain survival after the success of the initial resuscitation.

Finally, the area of resuscitation has broadened its view to the point that investigators and clinicians are starting to act in terms of brain resuscitation by combining drugs and maneuvers to increase brain blood flow and to prevent neurologic deterioration: cardiopulmonary cerebral resuscitation.

CONSIDERATIONS IN COMA, RECOVERY, AND DYING

Definition of Death

A medical definition of death stems from the *nature* of human life. Fundamentally, life is the integration of the biologic functions of nine principal organ systems.[137]

Death is the cessation of these life functions and the destruction of the organ systems. Two forms of death are recognized:

Clinical death is based on the cessation of integrated life functions and the integrity of the organ systems. *Biologic death* refers to the cessation of the simple life processes of organs and a dissolution of cellular activity.

The Nature of Dying[138]

Dying is a progressive process. Each part of the body or each organ system deteriorates progressively at different rates. Each organ has a vulnerability index to stress and a revival time. Thus, the brain has a high degree of vulnerability to lack of oxygen or nutrition. It is more sensitive in this regard than the next most vulnerable organ, namely, the heart. The time during which the brain may recover if restoration of circulation is achieved is approximately 4 minutes.[139] This is a period of relative vulnerability and deterioration. Recovery is probable, but after 4 minutes it becomes improbable, and after 8 minutes it is usually impossible. The heart can withstand loss of circulation for more than 8 minutes, but thereafter, revival of the heart becomes improbable, if not impossible. The revival period to which we refer therefore depends on several factors: (1) time; (2) temperature; (3) perfusion; (4) oxygen tension; and (5) total circulation. (A reduction in total cardiac output to 12% is critical for the brain.)

The Dying Process

Three phases of deterioration leading to absolute clinical death can be recognized. These phases are modified from Kramer[140] and are designated as (1) disordered function (disequilibration), (2) disintegration, and (3) deanimation.

In the first phase, disordered function, each organ system or part of the body functionally deteriorates, insofar as it is integrated with and coordinates with other organ systems of the body. This phase may be considered a period of early clinical death. It is reversible, and complete recovery is possible if direct injury with destruction of the tissue has not occurred at the level of the brain or heart.

The second phase, intrinsic disintegration, represents deterioration of an organ itself with regard to its capacity to respond. In a sense, this is the loss of intrinsic regulation and leaves only an automatic, vegetative, or intrinsic cellular autoregulation. This is a critical period, and revival, indeed, complete reanimation of the entire person,

is not possible. This is a period of intermediate clinical death.

The third phase, deanimation, is actually one of structural and tissue disintegration. It is the period of progressive deanimation in which structural damage begins and has been referred to as annihilation, as evidenced by the isoelectric EEG.[141] During this time, one sees a progressive loss of autoregulation. Some injuries or causative factors, however, may be directly and immediately destructive of cellular integrity. This situation is not reversible. Complete reanimation is not possible. A semblance of life may be attained artificially from 24 to 72 hours, but this existence is vegetative. Human life or, indeed, an organized life is not possible. Some organs may be kept alive at the cellular or biologic level, however, if the resuscitation techniques are applied effectively and before complete loss of autoregulation occurs. Individual organs may be alive at the simple tissue level, but the sum of all these does not result in an integrated whole.

Diagnosis of Death[138]

The recognition of death is one of diagnosis. The decision that no likelihood of recovery exists must be established on customary medical and scientific observations and tests.

No single clinical factor, such as arrest of respiration, stoppage of cardiac action, or cessation of nervous system activity, and no single test, can be considered sufficient by itself to establish a diagnosis of death. The decision to abandon efforts to revive the patient must depend on many signs and observations. The diagnosis is initially presumptive, but with current techniques the decision can be made conclusive.

Establishing Clinical Death

The first task is to establish the fact of death. This fact then enables one to identify the time when resuscitation procedures should be abandoned. At this point, biologic death is imminent, even though the individual life processes of many organs may be present. The diagnosis of clinical death should be in writing on the patient's chart. Thereafter, extraordinary measures of resuscitation may be withdrawn or abandoned.[142]

One should not consider any other factor but the patient's medical status in arriving at this decision. When the virtues of discontinuing life-sustaining measures are questioned, the physician should inform the family about the diagnosis and its pros and cons.[143]

Brain Death[144]

The subsequent discussion relates to the establishment of irreversible coma or brain death, and all the following factors must coexist when considering the diagnosis of brain death.[145]

   I. Coma: the patient must be deeply comatose
     1. Coma is not due to depressant drugs.
     2. Primary hypothermia is excluded.
     3. Metabolic and endocrine causes are excluded.
   II. Ventilator maintenance

1. Spontaneous respiration is absent or inadequate.
2. No neuromuscular blocking agents are involved (stretch reflexes may be present or nerve stimulation may elicit a response).
3. Respiratory center-depressant drugs must be excluded.

III. Condition of coma due to a recognizable nonremedial structural brain damage (disorder should be diagnosed that leads to brain death)

1. Global ischemia (arrested circulation from raised intracranial pressure or pulmonocardiac arrest).
2. Cardiac arrest.
3. Direct Tissue damage (trauma).
4. Massive focal ischemia (stroke).
5. Massive uncontrollable infectious process (meningitis) or metabolic failure (liver; cancer).
6. Cancer, neurologic or metastatic.

Apnea Test[146]

One of the criteria used to determine cessation of brain stem function is persistent absence of spontaneous respiration and, therefore, absence of the brain stem function. The neurologic inability to drive respiration can be tested by the patient's response to endogenous CO_2. Persistent apnea is proof of irreversible brain stem neurologic destruction of respiratory centers.

A standardized protocol has been developed to provide proof of irreversible apnea. The test is performed on comatose patients who lack reflexes and in whom reversible causes of coma are excluded. The EEG should show electrocerebral silence, and the patient should be supported by a mechanical respirator.

The procedure is as follows:

1. The ventilator is set to deliver 100% oxygen for at least 30 minutes.
2. The volume should be adjusted so overventilation and hypocarbia are avoided; that is, a $Paco_2$ of 36 to 40 mm Hg is the base line; a pH of 7.4 is desired.
3. The ventilator is disconnected, and a flow of 6 L/min of oxygen is delivered to the endotracheal tube by a T-piece.
4. The ventilator is disconnected, and oxygen insufflation is continued for 10 minutes.
5. If spontaneous repetitive respiratory efforts are made or if cardiovascular instability develops, the patient is immediately reconnected to the ventilator.
6. If no spontaneous respiratory efforts occur and the $Paco_2$ reaches 60 mm Hg by arterial blood gas study, the patient is considered neurologically apneic, with irreversibly damaged brain stem and loss of function.

Hemodynamic Responses[147]

In the diagnosis of brain death, one considers not only cortical and subcortical death and irreversible function, but also brain stem dysfunction and irreversibility. If an extracorporeal artificial supporting system and artificial ventilation are instituted to maintain the integrity of organs other than the brain, functional viability is presumed in such organs as the heart, the liver, and the kidney. Moreover, the peripheral autonomic nervous system, including the adrenal gland, is still functional. Hemodynamic responses in such brain-dead patients who undergo surgical procedures for organ retrieval have been demonstrated and are often dramatic. Heart rate, blood pressure—both systolic and diastolic—increase at the time of incision. Such pressure response is in part explained by a form of peripheral "mass reflex." This phenomenon is similar to the hypersensitivity of the autonomic nervous system in tetraplegic patients.[148]

The presence of peripheral reflex-type responses and perhaps some residual lower medullary function does not negate the diagnosis of brain death, which, according to current criteria, identifies a degree of loss of function of brain stem neurons and represents irreversible damage with no possible return to independent existence. The responsiveness of the peripheral cardiovascular system has been tested[149] by the administration of, first, atropine and, second, epinephrine to patients who have satisfied most of the criteria of irreversibility of brain function. When such tests are carried out, one sees a cardiac response with an increase in heart rate to atropine, and when epinephrine is administered in small doses, not only does cardiac rate increase, but one also sees a pressor effect. All types of reflex responses are not necessarily obtunded at the same time, but certain vulnerable responses essential to continuing life are indeed irreversibly damaged in the severely comatose, nonresponsive patient. In experimental practice, a single organ isolated from the body and perfused is capable of responding to a variety of stimuli.

Prediction of Risk of Dying

Glasgow Coma Scale[150]

This scale assesses the neurologic impairment of cortical function (Table 46-13). The signs evaluated include eye opening, verbal response, and motor responses, both spontaneous and to commands, and these signs are rated on a scale of 1 to 6. A total score of 20 represents a return to full consciousness.[151] This scale does not provide information about lower brain stem function, such as somatic and autonomic reflexes, respiratory patterns, cardiovascular responses, and evoked motor responses to reflex and pain stimulation. The scale does not correlate with mortality from head injury. It does not provide a complete neurologic assessment.

Apache III

Risk prediction of mortality for critically ill hospitalized adults admitted to intensive care units has been developed under the acronym APACHE (Score) meaning Acute Physiology, Age, Chronic Health Evaluation. The original scores were designated APACHE I and II, and they have been refined by Knaus and colleagues into the APACHE III Prognostic System.[152] Data collected from representative intensive care unit admissions in tertiary-care hospitals have been used to determine the relative value of

Table 46–13. Consciousness (modified Glasgow Coma Scale)

	Response	No.
Eye opening	None	1
	To pain	2
	To speech	3
	Spontaneous	4
Best motor response	None	1
	Extending	2
	Flexing	3
	Withdrawing	4
	Localizing	5
	Obeying commands	6
Best verbal response	None	1
	Incomprehensible	2
	Inappropriate	3
	Confused	4
	Oriented	5
Orientation	No response	1
	Total disorientation	2
	Orientation in space only	3
	Orientation in time only	4
	Excellent orientation in both	5
Total		20

variables in contributing to outcome. The assessment of the likelihood of patients' surviving to hospital discharge is then based on the following predictive variables: major medical or surgical disease categories; acute physiologic abnormalities: preexisting functional limitations; major comorbidities; chronologic age; and type and location of treatment before admission to the intensive care unit (i.e., treatment in other hospitals, by paramedics, or in the emergency room).

In this scoring system, the primary reason for admission to intensive care units is based on a comprehensive list of 212 disease categories. Each category classifies the patient according to medical or surgical status and major organ system. Assignment to one of the major categories is determined by the data in the medical record indicating the disease process most directly responsible for the patient's admission. Assignment is completed within 24 hours of admission to the intensive care unit.

Severity of the disease process is judged by abnormalities of the vital signs and laboratory data. Measurements of 17 physiologic variables are made and are assigned a point value. The physiologic variables selected are those of importance in providing diagnostic information. The patient's prior health status including chronologic age and the presence of preexisting disease is given a point score. APACHE scores range from 0 to 299. At any given time, a 5-point increase in the score is associated with a statistical increase in the relative risk of hospital death.

For predicting hospital mortality, an equation has been developed. For each disease classification, a coefficient of diagnostic and prognostic importance has been determined, and it affects outcome. This is combined with the components of the APACHE III score of physiology, age, and chronic health into an APACHE III *predictive equa-*

tion. This equation has provided a risk estimate of mortality for individual patients in intensive care units.

The reader is referred to the Knaus report for details of scoring and for the calculation of the predictive equation.[152]

Prognosis of Hypoxic Coma

Coma or a state of unconsciousness describes one dimension of a severe hypoxic-ischemic brain dysfunction. The ability to predict the outcome of global ischemia of the brain becomes important in terms of decision making in overall care. The application of a multivariate analysis of the neurologic signs of a comatose patient enables one to estimate, to some extent, the prognosis in a given set of circumstances.[153]

Specific evidence of brain stem dysfunction or of multifocal damage represents a grave prognosis.

Of patients lacking pupillary light reflexes on initial examination and during the first day, none ever became independent, and only 4% regained consciousness in Levy's analysis. Further, no patient who lacked a corneal reflex on the first day ever regained consciousness.

At 1 day, each of the following signs represented at least a 50% chance of the patient's regaining independence and leaving the hospital: confused or inappropriate speech, orienting spontaneous eye movements, normal oculocephalic or oculovestibular response, and obedience to verbal commands.

With regard to coma following cardiac arrest, if the coma lasts 3 days, full recovery should not be expected.

For a working analysis based on neurologic examination, one can categorize patients as semiconscious, vegetative, or comatose.[154] Basically, these categories correspond to the stages of anesthesia and the neurologic signs and reflexes clinically used to determine the depth of anesthesia coma. The semiconscious subject corresponds to stage I of anesthesia. The vegetative state is basically stage II of anesthesia coma, and the comatose category is stage III of surgical anesthesia.

Operational criteria of the levels of brain function assessed by Levy are as follows[153]:

Comatose patients: no eye opening, no comprehensible words and no obedience to command, no oculovestibular response, and no motor withdrawal response

Vegetative patients (comparable to stage II of the neurologic signs of anesthesia): spontaneous eye opening to noise or to pain, no comprehensible words and no obedience to commands

Semiconscious or stage I patients: comprehensible words or obedience to command.

Over one third of patients classified as vegetative at 1 day could be considered likely to remain vegetative on the basis of absent or posturing motor responses.

The overall outcome revealed the following: of comatose-vegetative patients who failed to open their eyes spontaneously or on command on the first day, 51% died; of all patients assessed, 20% became vegetative. Only 13% of all patients regained independence.

Table 46–14. The Viability Score for Differentiation Between Clinical and Biologic Death and For Evaluation of Recovery Potential

Function	2 Normal	1 Abnormal	0 Absent
1. Cerebral	Normal	Depressed	Absent
A. EEG	α	Spikes	Isoelectric (flat)
B. Stimulus			
Light, temperature		Evoked response	No evoked response
2. Reflexive	Present	Diminished	Absent
A. Eyes	Constricted pupils	Pupillary response	Dilated
B. Laryngeal	Pharyngeal reflex	Laryngeal-carinal	
C. Tendon reflexes		Evoked response	No evoked response
D. Neuromuscular			
3. Respiratory	Normal	Abnormal	Absent
	Spontaneous	Assisted	Controlled
A. Doxapram test	Adequate	Evoked response	No evoked response
4. Circulatory	Normal	Depressed	Absent
	Pulse	No pulse	
	Pressure	No pressure	
A. Vasopressor test		Artificial support	
Atropine; epinephrine		Evoked response	No evoked response
5. Cardiac	Normal	Ineffective	Absent
A. Action	Heart sounds	Assisted	
B. ECG	Normal	Abnormal	Isoelectric (flat or fibrillating)
C. Pacemaker	Not needed	Evoked response	No evoked response

From Collins, V. J.: Considerations in prolonging life: a dying and recovery score. IL State J Med, *148*:43, 1975; and Collins, V. J.: AMA Convention Medicine and Religion Covocation, San Francisco, June 1968.

The Dying Score[149]

To assist the physician in determining the end point of life (clinical and biologic), the concept of a multiparameter score to determine death is proposed. To a degree, this score parallels the Apgar score, or viability score for newborn babies (Table 46–14).

Five critical physiologic functions have been selected for appraisal; these are cerebral (consciousness), sensory, motor, reflex, and autonomic activity. Their presence, their potential, or their absence is noted by an arbitrary scoring system of 2, 1, and 0. These functions are all of critical and vital importance; however, they are not all of equal importance but are interdependent for spontaneous life. To some degree, an increasing order of dependence exists. The irrevocable absence of one of these functions or the inability of an organ system to perform spontaneously precludes the ability of the others to perform efficiently.

In application, an initial score is obtained as soon as artificial resuscitation procedures have been instituted and the requirements of emergency care have been satisfied. Serial determinations of a score should then be made every 15 minutes over a period of 1 to 6 hours. Such an action plan shows a trend and has predictive value. A score of 5 or more represents potential life. A score of under 5 represents impending or presumptive death. A persistent score of 0 is conclusive death. Further, an increasing score over a period of 1 to 2 hours indicates effective therapy and probable recovery, whereas a decreasing score over a period of 2 hours indicates failing therapy and clinical deterioration. The clinical observations are supported by laboratory, pharmacologic, and monitoring tests of function and responsiveness.

Cerebral Function

In the absence of consciousness, one assumes depression or loss of cortical function. Initially, this loss may be reversible. During this reversible period, sensory stimulation should be tried to evoke responses. At first, the responses are somatic, but later, if deterioration continues, only the visceral or neurovegetative type of responses will be evoked, and one may define a state of irreversible coma.

Muscular movements may be observed, and if they are noted to be purposeful, coordinated, and spontaneous, a score of 2 is assigned. When such movements are altered, incoordinate, and without purpose, and when they are only observed when induced by strong stimulation (pain reflexes), a score of 1 is assigned. When such movements are absent and cannot be evoked by strong stimulation, a score of 0 is assigned.

The EEG may show progressive deterioration.[139] When spike bursts alternate with periods of suppression, depression of cortical function is evident. This pattern represents a score of 1. When complete silence and an isoelectric potential are observed and when one sees a loss of evoked potentials, a score of 0 is assigned.

The method of EEG study primarily reveals changes in cortical function. This method does not necessarily reflect the capacity of the organism to be revived, nor does it reflect the existence of cellular life throughout the cerebral axis. The actual patterns of electrical activity should be assessed when amplification is maximal. Rather than a flat pattern, one should speak of an isoelectric pattern. These cortical patterns may be easily silenced by many stresses: drugs, shock, and trauma. An isoelectric pattern without evoked responses over 2 to 6 hours is highly suggestive of cortical death and cerebral disorganization. This pattern is not conclusive, however, and it must be assessed concurrently with the other clinical signs and responses of other organs.

Reflex Excitability

This function is evaluated by the observation of several conditions and responses. Pupullary size is significant: constricted pupils are evidence of good central nervous system control at the diencephalic level, and a score of 2 is warranted; dilated pupils indicate a loss of such control. Testing of the dilated pupil by a light stimulus and evoking some constriction indicate the capacity to recover and dictate a score of 1. Many other sensitive reflexes may be stimulated in sequence. One can progress from the eyelid reflex to the pupillary light reflex to the pharyngeal, laryngeal, and carinal reflexes. Stimulating the larynx, trachea, or carina usually evokes a modified cough or "buck." In deep coma, no response occurs, and a score of 0 is indicated.

Respiration

The presence of spontaneous and adequate respiratory efforts dictates a score of 2. When breathing becomes abnormal and requires assistance, a score of 1 is assigned. If spontaneous respiration is absent, but the administration of a respirogenic drug (e.g., doxapram) evokes a spontaneous respiratory effort, a score of 1 is also assigned. When respiration is absent, complete artificial control is required, and the drug challenge to the respiratory center and to the pulmonary apparatus does not evoke a response, a score of 0 is indicated.

Circulation

The presence of the circulation can be determined by detection of a peripheral pulse, estimation of blood pressure, and observation of the capillary refill phenomenon in the skin or nail bed. A more sophisticated method of assessment of circulatory function is the observation of retinal vessels by ophthalmoscopy. The presence of a measurable blood pressure, of a palpable pulse, and of good capillary refill suggests a score of 2.

The absence of an estimable blood pressure and the absence of a peripheral pulse with no capillary refill, but the presence of a detectable large artery pulsation, indicate a score of 1. The score can be further verified by evoking a pressure response with a peripheral-acting vasopressor or by observing movement of blood in the eye grounds.

When no pulsation is detected in large arteries and when no evoked response to a vasopressor occurs, a score of 0 is justified.

Cardiac Action

For a score of 2, a spontaneous palpable cardiac impulse over the chest wall should be present and a peripheral pulse detected. Auscultation should reveal a regular heartbeat, with the ECG of normal configuration.

When the heartbeat is not detected by precordial palpation and when weak, ineffective contractions exist, as evidenced by abnormal heart sounds coupled with an incoordinate bizarre pattern in the ECG, a score of 1 is assigned. Cardiac resuscitation measures are needed, and cardiac assistance is indicated. A pharmacologic stimulus to the heart, such as the injection of isoproterenol or epinephrine, should evoke a response if the patient has functional capability. A transvenous cardiac pacemaker may be used at this critical time.

The absence of any spontaneous cardiac activity and the absence of ECG electrical activity demand artificial circulation by cardiac compression ("massage"). Failure of the patient to respond to pharmacologic stimulus or failure of the electrical pacemaker to produce an effective cardiac contraction indicates a 0 cardiac score.

Secondary Considerations

Other factors than the medical and scientific operate in our complex, pluralistic society. Economic, social, familial, emotional, legal, and religious aspects are recognized. The physician must remain aloof from these influences, however, and must pursue the art of medicine to the best of his or her ability. If the logic of the physician and the science of medicine operate clearly and without encumbrance, a proper decision will probably be reached with regard to the patient's condition, and the best interests of all will be served. Whatever reasonable and rational course of action is best for the patient will inevitably coincide with the best interests of the family if care is humane and personalized.

Legal Aspects[155]

Perhaps the most lucid exposition of the subject of prolonging life and of the legal aspects of any medical decision regarding death is that of Professor George P. Fletcher of the University of Washington.[156] He states:

> The responsibility for the patient's expectations lies with the medical profession as a whole.
> The medical profession (not the legal profession) confronts the challenge of developing humane and sensitive customary standards for guiding decisions to prolong the lives of terminal patients.
> They should have a clear standard for deciding when to render aid or not to the dying patient.

Religious Aspect[157]

Major religious leaders have clearly indicated that it is the doctor's responsibility to establish conclusively that death does, in fact, exist. I should only quote from Pope Pius XII in this regard. In answer to the question "When does death occur?" proposed at the International Congress of Anesthesiologists in Rome, November 24, 1957, Pope Pius XII stated:

> Human life continues for as long as its vital functions, distinguished from the simple life (biologic) of the organs, manifest themselves spontaneously without the help of artificial processes.
>
> The task of determining the exact instant of death is that of the physician.

With regard to discontinuing ineffective extraordinary therapy, Pope Pius XII further stated:

> Since this form of treatment (reanimation of comatose patients) goes beyond ordinary methods, one cannot maintain that it would be obligatory to continue indefinitely.

Summary of Responsibility[156]

In the area of prolonging life and of determining death, the responsibility is clearly medical. Three primary determinants exist regarding the limits of medical responsibility. First is the physician-patient contract, which involves a surrendering of certain features both physical and psychologic of the natural rights of privacy of the individual to the doctor. This contract is founded in the virtue of trust and faith. Second is the ethical guidance of the physician's professional code of conduct. It is founded in the virtue of charity. Third is the science and art of the physician as exemplified in the wise application of knowledge. This is founded in the intellectual virtue of hope.

The concept of "multiparameter scoring" provides an end point defining irreversible clinical death at a time when biologic organ death has not occurred. As the technology of prolonging life and the science of organ transplantation have progressed, the need for such an end point has become increasingly apparent.

At least three objectives may be realized by a multiparameter scoring system:

1. The physician can decide when efforts at resuscitation are no longer successful and should be abandoned. This will allow the patient to die peacefully and not in pieces.
2. The score permits the anesthesiologists and the intensive care physician to quantitate the stages of recovery from coma.
3. A precise system, based on sound medical and scientific principles, protects any potential organ donor from even the possibility of precipitous removal of organs. Death can be pronounced without the shadow of doubt before artificial and extraordinary supports are discontinued and any organ is removed for purposes of transplantation.

ADVANCE MEDICAL DIRECTIVES

The use of life-sustaining medical measures usually concerns patients who anticipate the time when they no longer may be competent to participate in decision-making about their medical care.[158] Treatment decisions are complex and are influenced by moral and ethical considerations, as reported by the President's Commission in 1983.[159] To provide a means for people to extend their interests and desires, Congress passed the Patient Self Determination Act (PL 101-508, Section 4206 and 4751) in 1990.[160] This act became effective on December 1, 1991.

The essence of this act is that it requires hospitals and health care professionals to provide information concerning *advance medical directives,* and that on hospitalization, such directives are documented in the hospital record whether they have been signed or not. The law does not require a person to complete such a document; however, physicians and health care professionals are urged to have their patients prepare such a directive.[161] Indeed, a survey of a population sample in the Boston area reveals that 70 to 93% of patients would refuse life-sustaining treatments if they were faced with coma, a vegetative state, or a terminal illness. Thus, most people, while they are still competent, want to formally specify what medical interventions they would choose or refuse if they were unable to make medical care decisions in the future.[162]

Two common types of *advance directives* are completed in advance of hospitalization, as a statement regarding how patients wish medical decisions to be made[163,164]: a "living will" and a "durable power of attorney for health care."

Living Wills

A living will states in general terms a person's *preferred* medical care choices for when he or she is unable to make such choices. The living will takes effect while the individual is still living; it can be modified at any time. Many states have living will forms. The document constitutes clear evidence of a patient's wishes and should state treatment preferences. It should also direct the physicians who are providing care in a terminal illness.

Concerns about living wills have been raised.[165] The living will should be simple and should express wishes and treatment preferences in general terms. To cover all medical situations is impossible, and such an attempt may actually hinder the physician in providing indicated care of an obligatory nature. Conversely, choosing to want certain complex treatments may be medically undesirable and futile.[166] Therefore, patients should seek counsel from their physician in preparing a living will directive.[167]

Durable Power of Attorney for Health Care

This document names another person (husband/wife; daughter/son; relative; friend) as the surrogate "agent" or "proxy" to make medical decisions for an individual if he or she becomes unable to do so.[164] This "agent" should base decisions on previously established preferences of the patient. If these choices are not known, the medical care decisions should be based on the best interests of the patient. A personal physician or other health care provider involved in the patient's care cannot be named as a surrogate.

People choosing the durable power of attorney can include any instructions about any treatment they would prefer to have or prefer to avoid. Discussion with a physician should ensure that the specific directions are informed. These instructions should be kept up to date by frequent discussion with the individual's physician. This type of document is the preferred advance directive regarding life-sustaining treatment.[165]

ETHICAL CONSIDERATIONS IN THERAPY FOR THE COMATOSE AND DYING PATIENT

Primary Determinants[168]

The basic obligation of the physician is to ensure the patient's existence as a whole human being with a meaningful life. In confronting the problem of death or of life, the physician is challenged by the need for differential diagnoses.

For any course of action, at least three determinants exist. These are (1) contractual (patient-physician relationship), (2) ethical, and (3) scientific.

Physician-Patient Contract

The crux of medical practice is, of course, the physician-patient relationship. This is a contract with an implicit and explicit relationship. In the physician-patient relationship, medical care is implied. The duties of the physician are correlative to those of the patient. The patient expects the services of the physician to be for the patient's benefit and therefore permits an invasion of physical and mental privacy. Incumbent on every physician is the obligation to exert individual judgment, self-discipline, and a conscientious attitude in decisions made regarding another special human being—the patient. The physician must respect the patient's rights.

A "natural right" of humankind is the right of privacy. "It is the claim of an individual to determine for himself when, how, and to what extent information about himself is communicated to others."[169] This right is never absolute, because society has certain claims, and above all, many believe that the only absolute authority over our minds or bodies must remain supernatural.

One might also state that the right to maintain the privacy of one's personality is part of the right of self-preservation. This is the right that is shared and even surrendered by a patient consulting a physician. A patient who visits a physician is reasonably seeking advice and help. Consent for therapy is implied. In the interrelationship, the physician informs the patient of the state of health and the option to maintain health. The physician's duty is to educate the patient as to the patient's condition. This education has popularly been designated informed consent, but it is better termed "educated consent."

Some forms of therapy are implicit. Other more serious complex therapies, such as surgery and anesthesia, may be explicit in a written consent form.

Throughout the physician's practice, a moral understanding and sensibility to the health problems of the individual must be exercised.

The contractual relationship is and must be one governed by the moral virtue of faith and the doctrine of trust.

Ethical Guides[170]

Because an implicit contract exists between a physician and a patient, we must assess the ethical principles guiding the physician in fulfilling this contract. Every contract has *obligations*. Elements that operate in this personal contract include the *faith* of the patient in the doctor, and the doctor's competence, dependability, and expertise; the *hope* of the patient to be relieved of the illness and the hope of the physician that these efforts will be fruitful; and *love* of patient and physician as neighbors in society. Hippocrates stated this in the Physician's Oath:

> I will follow that method of treatment which, according to my ability and judgement, I consider for the benefit of my patient; and abstain from whatever is deleterious and wrong. I will give no medicine deadly to anyone, even if asked, nor suggest any such counsel.

Another way of stating the duties of a physician to a patient is that it should be according to the Golden Rule,[171] the Universal Rule found in all religions but stated in various ways. This rule is a most pertinent guide to human and medical conduct.[172] The words of Christ appear in Luke (6:31):

> As you wish that men would do to you, do so to them.

It is also revealed in the Talmud (Shabbat 31a):

> What is hateful to you, do not to your fellow man. That is the Law; all else is commentary.

Medical ethics are part of general ethics. These are rules of conduct established between men and women dealing with the human rights and with what is good and beneficial. They are exemplified in the duties and in the habits of doing good deeds. Ethics are principles founded in the moral virtue of love (charity).

The fulfillment of our humanitarian duties requires a reverence for human life, a respect for the sanctity of the body, and a recognition of the right to human dignity.

Scientific Determinant[168]

Based on medical facts and good judgment, the physician does those things in any situation that benefits the patient. The physician must do those things that predictably result in improvement of the patient. The techniques of reanimation are proven, sound, and legitimate. They can and do prolong life, *but* it must be determined that the nature of the resultant life is not mere biologic existence of several organs, but totally integrated functional existence at a human rational level.

To continue an act or a procedure of therapy that produces no improvement does not achieve or have the potential to achieve "full human life" and is demonstrably ineffective in its objectives and is imprudent, illogical, and irrational. This is the essence of medical practice.

A physician and the medical team who bring together all the knowledge and skill related to sustaining life processes and treating patients with disease do so rationally. The effectiveness of the physician's therapeutic skill must be constantly assessed. In artificially maintaining life or in arresting a disease process, the physician buys time. The physician provides by assistance time for the patient's natural recovery processes to act, to allow natural restoration of functional organization, and to return the individual to a spontaneous, full personal life.

If, after some time, all measures are obviously not effective and are not reversing the dying process, then the measures are failing. Deterioration may be observed. To persist may produce the appearance of life, but it is most often technical or mechanical life. The final decision will then be made in the face of a late phase or a second end point, namely, that of biologic life. The physician has an obligation to cease efforts early when they are determined to be ineffective in the total reanimation process. The patient should then be allowed to die. The patient has this right and should not be cheated of a peaceful death in the face of a physician powerless to restore consciousness.

A vegetating patient, hopeless and irresponsive and showing no spontaneous activity, should be allowed to die peacefully. Physicians should make the dying process dignified.

The scientific determinant is founded in the moral principle of hope. Science is one of the intellectual virtues denoted by understanding, knowledge, and wisdom. The patient hopes that the physician will apply these virtues and expects the physician to show prudence and respect in the selection of a course of action. To a large extent in modern medical practice, the scientific determinant must also be tempered by distributive justice.

Courses of Action in Treatment[168]

In the unconscious or hopelessly ill patient requiring resuscitation, *three* courses of action are possible:

1. *Active treatment:* prolonged dying versus reanimation.
2. *Active intervention to end life:* euthanasia.
3. *Passive management:* shortening the dying process by withholding or withdrawing extraordinary measures of life support.

The generic duty of a physician is a commitment to save lives[170] to preserve life, to cure disease, to care for the sick, and to tend the dying. The *means* by which various therapies and procedures have been used have been classified on ethical and moral grounds into *ordinary and extraordinary*. The relativity of theses classes is on a continuum determined by the nature of the illness, and the distinction is necessary in the practice of medicine.

Ordinary and Extraordinary Means of Treatment[173]

Ordinary measures of patient care are recognized as elements of essential care. They represent obligatory, proven, and justified therapies and procedures that the patient can obtain and put to his or her own use. They further represent measures that the patient can reasonably undergo with only minimal or moderate danger and maximal effectiveness. Such measures are also not an impossible or excessive burden. Ordinary means of preserving life are thus all medicines, treatments, and operations that offer a reasonable hope of benefit.

Extraordinary measures, on the other hand, are complicated methods. They are impossible for the patient to use or apply alone, and they present a costly and difficult burden. In addition, they represent a high level of danger, and the results expected are not predictable; that is, the effectiveness is minimal or moderate, whereas the dangers are maximal.

Extraordinary measures sustain life artificially at the level it is found. One hopes that, at this point, no organic deterioration exists. The measures in resuscitation may then arrest the lethal process. The aim is to gain time in order for natural restorative processes to operate.

Concept of Therapeutic Rationalism

The fundamental principle of therapeutic rationalism is founded in the dictate that only appropriate and effective therapy as indicated by the nature of the disease should be given. Providing appropriate and medically effective measures within a rational treatment regimen, relieving pain and suffering, and avoiding unnecessary or ineffective measures are part of the everyday practice of medicine. Thus, within the care of the critically ill or injured patient, the corollary to the principle of therapeutic rationalism permits withholding inappropriate or ineffective drugs and procedures or withdrawing medical support that is not beneficial.

A converse theorem should be identified. This concept holds that one should persist with all forms of treatment even if a hopeless prognosis exists. This is a philosophy of vitalism. To continue extraordinary and unusual therapy at all costs means that life is viewed as the absolute good and death as the absolute evil. This is an unacceptable concept in the rational practice of medicine.

Persistence in the use of measures lacking benefit or failing to improve a patient's condition is not only irrational, but indeed is immoral if the concept of therapeutic rationalism forms a conceptual basis for determining the course of action.

Euthanasia

Euthanasia is a term derived from the Greek *eu* (good) and *thantos* (death). It is defined as the act or practice of ending the life of an individual suffering from a terminal illness by means that are lethal such as the injection of an overdose of a drug or the inhalation of a noxious agent (such as carbon monoxide). Euthanasia has been argued as necessary when pain is intractable and suffering intolerable. One term often expressed is "active euthanasia," but this term is redundant because, by definition, euthansia is clearly a positive act. It is used to contrast with an additional inappropiate term, passive euthanasia, which is a complete contradiction.

Advances in pain management and in concepts of emotional and supportive care of patients suffering from a terminal illness invalidate the arguments for euthanasia. Newer effective analgesics and techniques of blocking pain pathways make it possible to control all types of pain. Support by family and friends and a caring physician are clearly needed for the dying patients and most effectively control the emotional aspects of suffering. Patients must not die alone. The fear of desertion provokes great anxiety and aggravated pain. Depression is a common accompaniment of suffering and should be treated by antidepressants. A variety of techniques have been outlined to provide creature comforts. Although dying at home in a familiar environment is ideal, it is not always possible, and for the care of patients with terminal illness the hospice program has been developed.

Euthanasia can be characterized as an act that relieves suffering by destroying the sufferer. The only valid ethical argument for euthanasia rests in the goal of relieving suffering. Although historically, when a person is a direct instrument of death, the law has related this to intention—even a noble motive such as sparing a patient from physical or mental agony does not absolve the act.

When a life is ended by active intercession, harm is caused to the individual, even though this harm may apparently have a good reason. Such an act is nontherapeutic and is abandonment of the patient-physician contract. As such, it is misguided mercy, and the act of killing must be considered the proximate cause of death.

From the legal standpoint, from moral codes, and from the guidelines of ethical practice, the general principle is applied that no one is permitted to actively kill—regardless of intent.

Aspects of Resuscitation or Prolongation of Life[168]

Many of the concepts previously discussed may be applied to a humanistic approach to resuscitation. A physician has a moral responsibility to know when such efforts will be fruitful and when they will not provide any benefit in the total restorative plan for the patient. Criteria may be established as a guide to the physician in decision making, but the fundamental scientific question that must be answered on moral grounds is whether any procedure instituted will be or has a reasonable chance of being beneficial and restorative.

A more complicated question is that of prolonging life. In saving a life, in preventing death, and in prolonging life, three questions must be asked: Is the condition irreversible and the end result inevitable? Is the life artificially sustained one of mere organic existence (vegetative)? Is death inevitable, or can it be diagnosed medically now? In responding to these questions, the distinction between letting a patient die and euthanasia must be retained. The first is mercy dying (not passive euthanasia), the second is mercy killing (murder). These are different moral realities. The intent of the first is to do no harm. The intent of the second is a recognized harm. When one permits death by not continuing therapy, the harm is done by a disease process. This is passive management based on reason and the judgment to shorten the act of dying. It is defended by the concept of therapeutic rationalism wherein treatment is discontinued when the efforts to maintain sound life are manifestly ineffective and futile.[174]

REFERENCES

1. Dripps, R. D., Eckenoff, J. A., Vandam, L.: Introduction to Anesthesia, 7th Ed. Philadelphia, W. B. Saunders, 1988.
2. Pontoppidan, H., Geffin, B., Lowenstein, E.: Acute respiratory failure in adult. N Engl J Med 287:702, 743, 799, 1972.
3. Clements, J. A.: Pulmonary surfactant. Am Rev Respir Dis 101:984, 1970.
4. Scarpelli, E. M.: The Surfactant System of the Lung. Philadelphia, Lea & Febiger, 1968.
5. Moss, G.: Shock, cerebral hypoxia and pulmonary vascular control. Bull NY Acad Med 49:689, 1973.
6. Downes, J.: Mechanical ventilation in management of status asthmaticus in children. In Eckenhoff, J. (ed.). Science and Practice in Anesthesia. Philadelphia, J.B. Lippincott, 1965.
7. Miller, L. K., Calenoff, L., Boehm, J. J., Riedy, J.: Respiratory distress in the newborn. JAMA 243:1176, 1980.
8. Gordon, R. S., NIH Report: Dexamethasone and the incidence of neonatal respiratory distress syndrome. JAMA 246:18, 1981.
9. Redding, R. A., Douglas, W. H., Stein, M.: Thyroid hormone influence upon lung surfactant. Science 175:994, 1972.
10. Chernick, V., Craig, R.: Naloxone reverses neonatal depression caused by fetal asphyxia. Science 216:1252, 1982.
11. Christie, R. V.: The mechanical work of breathing. Proc R Soc Med 46:38, 1953.
12. Otis, A. B.: The work of breathing. Physiol Rev 34:449, 1954.
13. Otis, A. B.: The work of breathing. In Handbook of Physiology. Section 3: Respiration, Vol. I. Bethesda, MD, American Physiological Society, 1961.
14. Peters, R. M.: Energy cost of breathing: physiologic review. Ann Thorac Surg 7:51, 1969.
15. Bendixen, H. H., et al.: Respiratory Care. St. Louis, C. V. Mosby, 1965.
16. Don, H. F., et al.: The measurement of gas trapped in the lungs at functional residual capacity and the effects of posture. Anesthesiology 35:582, 1971.
17. Don, H. F., et al.: The effect of anesthesia and 100 per cent oxygen on the functional residual capacity of the lungs. Anesthesiology 32:521, 1970.
18. Craig, D. B., et al.: "Closing volume" and its relationship to gas exchange in seated and supine positions. J Appl Physiol 31:717, 1971.
19. Pontoppidan, H., et al.: Ventilation and oxygen requirements during prolonged artificial ventilation in patients with respiratory failure. N Engl J Med 273:401, 1965.
20. Salem M. R., Ginsberg, D., Holaday, D. A.: The effect of continuous positive and negative pressure breathing on urine formation. Fed Proc 23:362, 1964.
21. Jude, J. R., Elam, J. O.: Fundamentals of Cardiopulmonary Resuscitation. Philadelphia, F.A. Davis, 1965.
22. Gordon, C. S.: Chairman Committee on CPR Standards. JAMA 227(Suppl):834, 1974.

23. Paraskos, J. A.: Guidelines for cardiopulmonary resuscitation and emergency cardiac care. JAMA *268*:2178, 1992.

24. Stahlgren, L. H., Angelchic, J.: Cardiac arrest: evaluation of cardiac massage in treatment of seventy patients, with emphasis on cardiac arrest occurring outside the operating room. JAMA *174*:226, 1960.

25. Collins, V. J.: Fatalities in anesthesia and surgery. JAMA *172*:549, 1960.

26. Collins, V. J.: Iatrogenic cardiac arrest. NY State J Med *61*:3107, 1961.

27. Safar, P. (ed.): Respiratory Therapy. Philadelphia, F. A. Davis, 1965.

28. Vieira, Z., Collins, V. J.: Emergency cardiorespiratory resuscitation. Postgrad Med *41*:418, 1967.

29. Elam, J. O., Ruben, H. M., Greene, D. G., Schneider, M. A.: Head-tilt method of oral resuscitation. JAMA *127*:812, 1960.

30. Elam, J. O., Brown, E. S., Elder, J. D., Jr.: Artificial respiration by mouth-to-mouth methods. N Engl Med J *250*:749, 1954.

31. Safar, P., Escarraga, L. A., Elam, J. O.: A comparison of the mouth-to-mouth and mouth-to-airway methods of artificial respiration with the chest pressure-arm lift methods. N Engl J Med *258*:671, 1958.

32. Elam, J. O., Ruben, H. M., Greene, D. G., Schneider, M. A.: Rescue Breathing: Improved Techniques of Expired Air Resuscitation (First Movie, 1957), 2nd Ed. Albany, NY, New York State Department of Health, 1961.

33. Ruben, H. M., Elam, J. O., Ruben, A. M., Greene, D. G.: Investigation of upper airway problems in resuscitation. I. Studies of pharyngeal x-rays and performance by laymen. Anesthesiology *22*:271, 1961.

34. Elam, J. O., Ruben, A. M., Greene, D. G., Bittner, T. J.: Mouth-to-nose resuscitation during convulsive seizures. JAMA *176*:565, 1961.

35. National Conference on CPR and ECG (Paraskos, J. A., Chairman): Guidelines for Cardiopulmonary Resuscitation and Emergency Cardiac Care. Part IV. Special Resuscitations Situations. JAMA *268*:2242, 1992.

36. Smock, S. N.: Esophageal obturator airway: preferred CPR technique. J Am Coll Emerg Physicians *4*:232, 1975.

37. Meislin, H. W.: The esophageal obturator airway: a study of respiratory effectiveness. Ann Emerg Med *9*:54, 1980.

38. Auerbach, P. S., Geehr, E. C.: Inadequate oxygenation and ventilation using the esophageal gastric tube airway in the prehospital setting. JAMA *250*:3067, 1983.

39. Bryson, T. K., Benumof, J. L., Ward, C. F.: The esophageal obturator airway: a clinical comparison to ventilation with a mask and oropharyngeal airway. Chest *74*:537, 1978.

40. Palme, C., et al.: An evaluation of the efficiency of face masks in the resuscitation of newborn infants. Lancet *1*:207, 1985.

41. Dorsch, J. A., Dorsch, S. E.: Understanding Anesthesia Equipment, 2nd Ed. Baltimore, Williams & Wilkins, 1984, p. 198.

42. Rudikoff, M. T., et al.: Mechanisms of blood flow during cardiopulmonary resuscitation. Circulation *61*:345, 1980.

43. Chandra, N., et al.: Augmentation of carotid flow during CPR by ventilation at high airway pressure simultaneous with chest compression. Am J Cardiol *48*:1053, 1981.

44. Weisfeldt, M. L., Chandra, N., Tsitlik, J.: Increased intrathoracic pressure not direct heart compression: causes the rises in intra-thoracic vascular pressures during CPR in dogs and pigs. Crit Care Med *9*:377, 1981.

45. Rogers, M. C.: CPR: some old beliefs are no longer valid. ASA Refresher Course No. 226. Annual Convention American Society of Anesthesiologists, New Orleans, October 14, 1989.

46. Criley, J. M., Blaufuss, A. H., Kissel, G. L.: Cough-induced cardiac compression: self-administered form of cardiopulmonary resuscitation. JAMA *236*:1246, 1976.

47. Paradis, N. A., et al.: Simultaneous aortic, jugular bulb, and right atrial pressures during cardiopulmonary resuscitation in humans: insights into mechanisms. Circulation *80*:361, 1989.

48. Taylor, G. J., et al.: Importance of prolonged compression during cardiopulmonary resuscitation in man. N Engl J Med *296*:1515, 1977.

49. Maier, G. W., et al.: The physiology of external cardiac massage: high-impulse cardiopulmonary resuscitation. Circulation *70*:86, 1984.

50. Halperin, H. R., et al.: Determinants of blood flow to vital organs during cardiopulmonary resuscitation in dogs. Circulation *73*:539, 1986.

51. Bilfield, L. H., Regula, G. A.: A new technique for external heart compression. JAMA *239*:2418, 1978.

52. Pennington, J. E., Taylor, J., Lown, B.: Chest thump for reverting ventricular tachycardia. N Engl J Med *283*:1192, 1970.

53. Caldwell, G., et al.: Simple mechanical methods for cardioversion: defence of the precordial thump and cough version. Br Med J *291*:627, 1985.

54. Miller, J., et al.: The precordial thump. Ann Emerg Med *13*:791, 1984.

55. Ornato, J. P.: Special resuscitation situations: near drowning, traumatic injury, electric shock and hypothermia. Circulation *74(Suppl IV)*:23, 1986.

56. Modell, J. H.: Is the Heimlich maneuver appropriate as the first treatment for drowning? Emerg Med Serv *10*:63, 1981.

57. Modell, J. H.: Electrolyte changes in human drowning victims Anesthesiology *30*:414, 1969.

58. Reuben, A., Reuben H.: Artificial respiration: flow of water from the lung and the stomach. Lancet *1*:780, 1962.

59. Kobernick, M.: Electrical injuries: pathophysiology and emergency management. Ann Emerg Med *11*:633, 1982.

60. Browne, B. J., Gaasch, W. R.: Electrical injuries and lightning. Emerg Med Clin North Am *10*:211, 1992.

61. Cooper, M. A.: Electrical and lightning injuries. Emerg Med Clin North Am *2*:489, 1984.

62. Duclos, P. J., Sanderson, L. M.: An epidemiological description of lightning-related deaths in the United States. Int J Epidemiol *19*:673, 1990.

63. Cooper, M. A.: Lightning injuries: prognostic signs for death. Ann Emerg Med *9*:134, 1980.

64. Cahalane, M., Demling, R. H.: Early respiratory abnormalities from smoke inhalation. JAMA *251*:771, 1984.

65. Collins, V. J.: Hyperbaric oxygenation. *In* Principles of Anesthesiology. Philadelphia, Lea & Febiger, 1993.

66. Heimlich, H. J.: A life-saving maneuver to prevent food choking. JAMA *234*:398, 1975.

67. Del Guercio, L. R., et al.: Comparison of blood flow during external and internal cardiac massage in man. Circulation *31*:1, 1965.

68. Pappelbaum, S., et al.: Open versus closed chest cardiac massage. JAMA *193*:659, 1965.

69. Sanders, A. B., et al.: Improved resuscitation from cardiac arrest with open-chest massage. Ann Emerg Med *13*:672, 1984.

70. Bircher, N., Safar, P.: Cerebral preservation during cardiopulmonary resuscitation. Crit Care Med *13*:185, 1985.

71. Kouwenhoven, W. B., Jude, J. R., Knickerbocker, G. G.: Closed Chest cardiac massage. JAMA *173*:1064, 1960.

72. Kerber, R. E., et al.: Energy, current, and success defibrillation and cardioversion: clinical studies using an automated impedance-based method of energy adjustment. Circulation 77:1038, 1988.

73. Sirna, S. J., Ferguson, D. W., Charbonnier, F., Kerber, R. E.: Factors affecting transthoracic impedance during electrical cardioversion. Am J Cardiol 62:1048, 1988.

74. Lown, B., et al.: The energy for ventricular defibrillation. N Engl J Med 298:1252, 1978.

75. Tacker, W. A., Jr., et al.: Energy dosage for human trans chest electrical ventricular defibrillation. N Engl J Med 290:214, 1974.

76. Gascho, J. A., et al.: Energy levels and patient weight in ventricular defibrillation JAMA 242:1380, 1979.

77. Lown, B.: Electrical reversion of cardiac arrhythmias. Br Heart J 29:469, 1967.

78. Weaver, W. D., Cobb, L. A., Copass, M. K., Hallstrom, A. P.: Ventricular defibrillation: a comparative trial using 175-joule and 320-joule shocks. N Engl J Med 307:1107, 1982.

79. Warnberg, M., Thomassen, A.: Prognosis after cardiac arrest occurring outside intensive care and coronary care units. Acta Anaesthesiol Scand 23:69, 1979.

80. Cobb, L. A., Werner, J. A., Trobaugh, G. B.: Sudden cardiac death: a decades experience in out-of hospital resuscitation. Concepts Cardiovasc Dis 49:31, 1980.

81. Weil, M. H., et al.: Difference in acid-base state between venous and arterial blood during cardiopulmonary resuscitation. N Engl J Med 315:153, 1986.

82. Grundler, W., Weil, M. H., Masonobu, Y., Michaels, S.: The paradox of venous acidosis and arterial alkalosis during CPR (abstract). Chest 86:282, 1984.

83. Relman, A. S.: 'Blood gases': Arterial or venous (editorial)? N Engl J Med 315:188, 1986.

84. Standards and guidelines for cardiopulmonary resuscitation and emergency cardiac care. JAMA 255:2942, 1986.

85. Michael, J. R., et al.: Mechanisms by which epinephrine augments cerebral and myocardial perfusion during cardiopulmonary resuscitation in dogs. Circulation 69:822, 1984.

86. Ditchey, R. V., Lindenfeld, J.: Failure of epinephrine to improve the balance between myocardial oxygen supply and demand during closed-chest resuscitation in dogs. Circulation 78:382, 1988.

87. Paradis, N. A., et al.: Coronary perfusion pressure and the return of spontaneous circulation in human cardiopulmonary resuscitation. JAMA 263:1106, 1990.

88. Stiell, I. G., et al.: High-dose epinephrine in adult cardiac arrest. N Engl J Med 327:1045, 1992.

89. Brown, C. G., et al.: A comparison of standard-dose and high-dose epinephrine in cardiac arrest outside the hospital. N Engl J Med 327:1051, 1992.

90. Foine, R. O., Kajaste, S., Kaste, M.: Neuropsychological sequelae of cardiac arrest. JAMA 269:237, 1993.

91. White, R. D.: Cardiovascular pharmacology: part 1. In McIntyre, K. M., Lewis, A. J. (eds.). Textbook of Advanced Cardiac Life Support. Dallas, American Heart Association, 1981, p. VIII-4.

92. Chameides, L., et al.: Resuscitation of infants and children. In McIntyre, K. M., Lewis, A. J. (eds.). Textbook of Advanced Cardiac Life Support. Dallas, American Heart Association, 1981, p. XVII-11.

93. Safar, P., et al.: Resuscitation after global brain ischemic-anoxia Crit Care Med 6:215, 1978.

94. Ping, F. C., Jenkins, L. C.: Protection of the brain from hypoxia: a review. Can Anaesth Soc J 25:468, 1978.

95. Brevik, H., et al.: Clinical feasibility trials of barbiturate therapy after cardiac arrest. Crit Care Med 6:288, 1978.

96. Ruano, M., et al.: Barbiturate therapy of postanoxic encephalopathy. Crit Care Med 9:249, 1981.

97. Abramson, N. S., et al.: Results of a randomized clinical trial of brain resuscitation with thiopental (abstract). Anesthesiology 59:A101, 1983.

98. Abramson, N. S., Safar, P.: Randomized clinical study of thiopental loading in comatose survivors of cardiac arrest. N Engl J Med 314:397, 1986.

99. Yatsu, F. M.: Cardiopulmonary-cerebral resuscitation (editorial). N Engl J Med 314:440, 1986.

100. Marshall, L. F., Smith, R. W., Shapiro, H. M.: The outcome with aggressive treatment in severe head injuries. Part II: Acute and chronic barbiturate administration in the management of head injury. J Neurosurg 50:25, 1979.

101. Searle, J., Collins, C. A.: A brain-death protocol. Lancet 1:287, 1980.

102. Nussmeier, N., Arlund, C., Slogoff, S.: Neuropsychiatric complications after cardiopulmonary bypass: cerebral protection by a barbiturate. Anesthesiology 64:165, 1986.

103. Michenfelder, J.: A valid demonstration of barbiturate induced brain protection in man—at last. Anesthesiology 64:140, 1986.

104. Newberg, L. A., Michenfelder, J.: Cerebral protection by isoflurane during hypoxemia or ischemia. Anesthesiology 59:29, 1983.

105. Newman, B., Gelb, A. W., Lam, A. M.: The effect of isoflurane-induced hypotension on cerebral blood flow and cerebral metabolic rate for oxygen in humans. Anesthesiology 64:307, 1986.

106. Shapiro, H.: Post-cardiac arrest therapy: calcium blockade and brain resuscitation. Anesthesiology 62:384, 1985.

107. Steen, P., et al.: Nimodipine improves outcome when given after complete cerebral ischemia in primates. Anesthesiology 62:406, 1985.

108. Beecher, H. K.: A definition of irreversible coma. JAMA 205:337, 1968.

109. Schneiderman, L. J., Jecker, N. S., Jonsen, A. R.: Medical futility: its meaning and ethical implications. Ann Intern Med 112:949, 1990.

110. Aldrete, J. A., Kroulik, D.: A post-anesthetic recovery score. Anesth Analg 49:924, 1970.

111. Aldrete, J. A., McDonald, J. S.: The post-anesthetic recovery score as a method of evaluation of anesthesia performance. In Symposium Workshop, Proceedings of Demography and Epidemiology. Washington, D.C., December 2, 1977.

112. Apgar, V.: Proposal for a new method of evaluation of the newborn infant. Curr Res Anesth 32:260, 1953.

113. Apgar, V., et al.: Evaluation of the newborn infant: second report. JAMA 168:1985, 1958.

114. Drage, J. S., Kennedy, C., Schwartz, B. K.: The Apgar score as an index of neonatal mortality. Obstet Gynecol 24:222, 1964.

115. Apgar, V., Holaday, D. A., James, L. S.: Comparison of regional and general anesthesia in obstetrics. JAMA 165:2155, 1957.

116. Apgar, V., Beck, J.: Is My Baby All Right? New York, Trident Press, 1972.

117. Nelson, K. B., Ellenberg, J. H.: Antecedents of cerebral palsy. Multivariate analyses of risk. N Engl J Med 315:81, 1986.

118. Clinical Care Committee of the Massachusetts General Hospital, Pontoppidan, H.: Optimum care for hopelessly ill patients. N Engl J Med 295:362, 1976.

119. Meisel, A., Grenvik, A.: Hospital guidelines for deciding about life-sustaining treatment dealing with health limbo. Phys Care Med *14:*239, 1986.

120. Rabkin, M. T., Gillerman, G., Rice, N. R.: Orders not to resuscitate. N Engl J Med *295:*364, 1976.

121. Collins, V. J.: Ethical considerations in therapy for the comatose and dying patient. J Crit Care *8:*1084, 1979.

122. Council on Ethical and Judicial Affairs, American Medical Association: Guidelines for the appropriate use of do-not-resuscitate orders. JAMA *265:*1868, 1991.

123. Fox, M.: The decision to perform cardiopulmonary resuscitation (editorial). N Engl J Med *309:*607, 1983.

124. Jude, J. R., Elam, J. O.: Fundamentals of Cardiopulmonary Resuscitation. Philadelphia, F. A. Davis, 1965.

125. Collins, V. J.: Limits of medical responsibility in prolonging life: guides to decisions. JAMA *206:*389, 1968.

126. Waisel, D. B., Truog, R. D.: The "CPR-Not-Indicated" Order: Futility Revisited. Lackland AFB, TX, Air Force Press, 1994.

127. Truog, R. D.: Withholding and withdrawing life-sustaining therapy. Am Soc Anesth Newslett *58:*21, 1994.

128. Waisel, D., Truog, R.: CPR not indicated order: futility revisited. Ann Intern Med *122:*304, 1995.

129. Murphy, D. J., Finucane, T. E.: New do-not-resuscitate policies. Arch Intern Med *153:*1641, 1993.

130. Orentlicher, D.: Advance medical directives: from the Office of the General Counsel. JAMA *263:*2365, 1991.

131. Sanders, A. B., Meislin, H. W., Ewy, G. A.: The physiology of cardiopulmonary resuscitation: an update. JAMA *252:*3283, 1984.

132. Rudikoff, M. T., et al.: Mechanisms of blood flow during cardiopulmonary circulation. Circulation *61:*345, 1980.

133. Weisfeldt, M. I., et al.: New attempts to improve blood flow during CPR. *In* Schluger, J., Lyon, A. F. (eds.). CPR and Emergency Cardiac Care: Looking to the Future. New York, E. M. Books, 1980.

134. Sanders, A. B., Ewy, G. A., Taft, T.: The importance of aortic diastolic blood pressure during cardiopulmonary resuscitation (abstract). J Am Coll Cardiol *1:*609, 1983.

135. Mahoney, B. D., Mirlek, M. J.: Efficacy of pneumatic trousers in refractory prehospital cardiopulmonary arrest. Ann Emerg Med *12:*8, 1983.

136. Newton, J. R., et al.: Quantitative comparison of several methods of external cardiac massage (abstract). J Am Coll Cardiol *3:*596, 1984.

137. Angrist, A.: Certified cause of death: analysis and recommendations. JAMA *166:*2148, 1958.

138. Collins, V. J.: Considerations in defining death. Linacre Q *38:*94, 1971; Middle East J Anaesth *3:*217, 1972.

139. Sugar, O., Gerald, R. W.: Anoxia and brain potentials. J Neurophysiol *1:*558, 1938.

140. Kramer, W.: Extensive necrosis of the brain: development during reanimation. *In* Proceedings of the Fifth International Congress of Neuropathology. New York, Excerpta Medica, 1966, p. 33.

141. Kimura, J., Gerber, H. W., McCormick, W. F.: The isoelectric encephalogram: significant in establishing death in patients maintained on mechanical respirators. Arch Intern Med *121:*551, 1968.

142. Collins, V. J.: Concepts and ethics in defining death and a scoring system. J IL State Soc Med *38:*94, 1975.

143. Moss, A. H.: Informing the patient about cardiopulmonary resuscitation: when the risks outweigh the benefits. J Gen Intern Med *4:*349, 1989.

144. Plum, F., Posner, J. B.: The Diagnosis of Stupor and Coma, 3rd Ed. Philadelphia, F. A. Davis, 1980, p. 313.

145. Council on Scientific Affairs and Council on Ethical and Judicial Affairs, American Medical Association: Persistent vegetative state and the decision to withdraw or withhold life support. JAMA *263:*426, 1990.

146. Belsh, J. M., Blatt, R., Schiffman, P. L.: Apnea testing in brain death. Arch Intern Med *146:*2385, 1986.

147. Wetzel, R. C., Setzer, N., Stiff, J. L., Rogers, M. C.: Hemodynamic responses in brain dead organ donor patients. Anesth Analg *64:*125, 1985.

148. Ciliberti, B. J., Goldfern, J., Rovenstine, E. A.: Hypertension during spinal anesthesia in patients with spinal cord injuries. Anesthesiology *15:*273, 1954.

149. Collins, V. J.: Considerations in prolonging life: a dying and recovery score. IL Med J *147:*543, 1975.

150. Teasdale, G., Jennett, B.: Assessment of coma and impaired consciousness: a practical scale. Lancet *2:*81, 1974.

151. Jennett, B., et al.: Severe head injuries in three countries. J Neurol Neurosurg Psychiatry *49:*291, 1977.

152. Knaus, W. A., et al.: The APACHE III prognostic system: risk prediction of hospital mortality for critically ill hospitalized adults. Clinical investigations in critical care. Chest *100:*1619, 1991.

153. Levy, D. E., et al.: Predicting outcome from hypoxic-ischemic coma. JAMA *253:*1420, 1985.

154. American Academy of Neurology: Position of the American Academy of Neurology on certain aspects of the care and management of the persistent vegetative state. Neurology *39:*125, 1989.

155. Curran, W. F.: Legal and medical death: Kansas takes the first step. N Engl J Med *284:*260, 1971.

156. Fletcher, G. P.: Legal aspects of the decision not to prolong life. JAMA *203:*65, 1968.

157. Pope Pius XII: The prolongation of life: allocution to the International Congress of Anesthesiologists, Rome, November 24, 1957. Am Q Papal Documents *4:*393, 1958.

158. Emanuel, E. J.: A review of the ethical and legal aspects of terminating medical care. Am J Med *84:*291, 1988.

159. President's Commission for the Study of Ethical Problems in Medicine and Biomedical and Behavioral Research: Deciding to Forego Life-Sustaining Treatment. Washington, D.C., U.S. Government Printing Office, 1983.

160. Omnibus Reconciliation Act 1990. Title IV. Section 4206. Congressional Record, October 26, No. 12638, 1990.

161. Emanuel, L. L., et al.: Advance directives for medical care: a case for greater use. N Engl J Med *324:*889, 1991.

162. Emanuel, L. L., Emanuel, E. J.: The medical directive: a new comprehensive advance care document. JAMA *261:*3288, 1989.

163. Orentlicher, D.: Advance medical directives: from the Office of the General Counsel. JAMA *263:*2365, 1991.

164. Annas, G. J.: The health care proxy and the living will. N Engl J Med *324:*1210, 1991.

165. Wolf, S. M., et al.: Sources of concern about the Patient Self-determination Act. N Engl J Med *325:*1666, 1991.

166. Schneiderman, L. J., Jecker, N. S., Jonsen, A. R.: Medical futility: its meaning and ethical implications. Ann Intern Med *112:*949, 1990.

167. Schneiderman, L. J., Arras, J. D.: Counseling patients to counsel physicians on future care in the event of patient incompetence. Ann Intern Med *102:*693, 1985.

168. Collins, V. J.: Ethical considerations in therapy for the comatose and dying patient. Heart Lung J Crit Care *8:*1084, 1979.

169. Westin, A. F.: Privacy and Freedom. New York, Atheneum, 1968.
170. Ramsey, P.: The Patient as a Person. New Haven, CT, Yale University Press, 1970.
171. DeBakey, M. D.: Medical research and the golden rule. JAMA 203:574, 1968.
172. Beecher, H. K.: Research and the Individual: Human Studies. Boston, Little, Brown, 1970, p. 187.
173. Kelley G.: Medico-Moral Problems. St. Louis, Catholic Hospital Association, 1958.
174. Pope Pius XII: Acta Apostolica Sedis 49: 1033. *In* The Pope Speaks. Vatican City, Vatican Press, 1957.